REHABILITATION MEDICINE

REHABILITATION MEDICINE
Principles and Practice

Edited by
Joel A. DeLisa, M.D., M.S.

Professor and Chairman,
Department of Rehabilitation Medicine
University of Medicine and Dentistry of New Jersey–
 New Jersey Medical School
Newark, New Jersey
Medical Director and Chief Medical Officer,
Kessler Institute for Rehabilitation
West Orange, New Jersey

Section Editors

Donald M. Currie, M.D.
Associate Professor,
Department of Physical Medicine and Rehabilitation
University of Texas Health Science Center at San Antonio
Staff Physician,
Rehabilitation Medicine Service
Audie L. Murphy Memorial Veterans Administration Hospital
San Antonio, Texas

Bruce M. Gans, M.D.
Professor and Chairman,
Department of Rehabilitation Medicine
Tufts University School of Medicine
Physiatrist-in-Chief,
Rehabilitation Institute
New England Medical Center
Boston, Massachusetts

Paul F. Gatens, Jr., M.D.
Clinical Assistant Professor,
Department of Physical Medicine
Ohio State University
Director of Inpatient Rehabilitation,
Mount Carmel Hospital
Columbus, Ohio

James A. Leonard, Jr., M.D.
Clinical Assistant Professor and Associate Chairman,
Department of Physical Medicine and Rehabilitation
Medical Director, Division of Orthotics and Prosthetics
University of Michigan Medical Center
Ann Arbor, Michigan

Malcolm C. McPhee, M.D.
Associate Professor,
Department of Physical Medicine and Rehabilitation
Mayo Medical School
Rochester, Minnesota
Consultant, Department of Physical Medicine and Rehabilitation
Mayo Clinic Scottsdale
Scottsdale, Arizona

J.B. Lippincott *Philadelphia*
London Mexico City New York
St. Louis São Paulo Sydney

With 104 contributors

Dedicated to

- *Our patients, who challenge us to continually strive to improve their health, function, and quality of life*

- *Our teachers, who challenged us to develop a scientific approach to problem solving and instilled in us the need for continuous learning*

- *Our students, who challenge and stimulate us to keep at the cutting edge. They are our hope for the future.*

Manuscript Editor: Jody A. DeMatteo
Indexer: Betty Herr Hallinger
Design Coordinator: Michelle Gerdes
Production Manager: Carol A. Florence
Production Assistant: Kathryn Rule
Compositor: Circle Graphics
Printer/Binder: Murray Printing

3   5   6   4

Library of Congress Cataloging-in-Publication Data

Rehabilitation medicine.

Includes index.
1. Medicine, Physical. I. DeLisa, Joel A.
[DNLM: 1. Rehabilitation. WB 320 R3458]
RM700.R42 1988   615.8′2   88–6854
ISBN 0–397–50764–X

The authors and publisher have exerted every effort to ensure that drug selection and dosage set forth in this text are in accord with current recommendations and practice at the time of publication. However, in view of ongoing research, changes in government regulations, and the constant flow of information relating to drug therapy and drug reactions, the reader is urged to check the package insert for each drug for any change in indications and dosage and for added warnings and precautions. This is particularly important when the recommended agent is a new or infrequently employed drug.

Contributors

Paul Bach-y-Rita, M.D.
Professor and Chairman,
Department of Rehabilitation Medicine
University of Wisconsin Medical School
Chairman, Department of Rehabilitation Medicine
University of Wisconsin Hospital and Clinics
Madison, Wisconsin

Richard D. Ball, M.D., Ph.D.
Attending Physician in Physical Medicine
    and Rehabilitation
Munson Medical Center
Traverse City, Michigan

Richard Balliet, Ph.D.
Associate Professor,
University of Wisconsin Medical School
Department of Rehabilitation Medicine
Neuromuscular Training Clinic
Madison, Wisconsin

Karin J. Barnes, M.S., OTR
Assistant Professor of Occupational Therapy
Assistant Professor of Physical Medicine and Rehabilitation
University of Texas Health Science Center at San Antonio
Assistant Professor of Life Sciences
University of Texas at San Antonio
San Antonio, Texas

David M. Barrett, M.D.
Professor of Urology,
Mayo Medical School
Consultant, Department of Urology
Mayo Clinic and Mayo Foundation
Rochester, Minnesota

Jeffrey R. Basford, M.D., Ph.D.
Assistant Professor,
Department of Physical Medicine
Mayo Medical School
Consulting Physician, St. Mary's Hospital
Rochester Methodist Hospital
Rochester, Minnesota

Kathleen R. Bell, M.D.
Instructor, Department of Rehabilitation Medicine
University of Washington
Assistant Chief, Rehabilitation Medical Service
Seattle Veterans Administration Medical Center
Seattle, Washington

Susan Biener-Bergman, M.D.
Assistant Professor of Rehabilitation Medicine
Boston University School of Medicine
Boston, Massachusetts

Michael G. Boyeson, Ph.D.
Assistant Professor,
Department of Rehabilitation Medicine
University of Wisconsin Medical School
Madison, Wisconsin

H. L. Brammel, M.D.
Associate Clinical Professor of Medicine
University of Colorado Health Sciences Center
Medical Director,
HEALTHSOUTH Rehabilitation Center of Denver
Denver, Colorado
Cardiology Consultant,
Adolph Coors Company
Golden, Colorado

Catherine W. Britell, M.D.
Assistant Professor,
Department of Rehabilitation Medicine
University of Washington
Acting Chief, Spinal Cord Injury Service
Seattle Veterans Administration Medical Center
Seattle, Washington

Beth A. Burkhard, M.S., CCC-SLP
Speech-Language Pathologist,
Department of Rehabilitation Medicine
Thomas Jefferson University Hospital
Philadelphia, Pennsylvania

Jack S. Burks, M.D.
Associate Professor,
Department of Neurology
University of Colorado Health Sciences Center
Center for Neurological Diseases/Rocky Mountain
 Multiple Sclerosis Center
Denver, Colorado

Charles H. Chesnut, III, M.D.
Professor, Medicine and Radiology
Director, Osteoporosis Research Center
University of Washington School of Medicine
Seattle, Washington

Charles H. Christiansen, Ed.D., OTR, FAOTA
Professor and Chairman,
Department of Occupational Therapy
Professor, Department of Physical Medicine and Rehabilitation
University of Texas Health Science Center at San Antonio
Professor of Life Sciences,
University of Texas at San Antonio
San Antonio, Texas

Gary S. Clark, M.D.
Clinical Associate Professor of Rehabilitation Medicine,
University of Rochester School of Medicine and Denistry
Medical Director,
Neurorehab Associates, Inc.
Rochester, New York

Nancy D. Cobble, M.D.
Assistant Professor,
Department of Rehabilitation Medicine
University of Colorado Health Sciences Center
Center for Neurological Diseases/Rocky Mountain
 Multiple Sclerosis Center
Denver, Colorado

Jeffrey L. Cole, M.D.
Clinical Assistant Professor,
Department of Rehabilitation Medicine
Albert Einstein College of Medicine
Bronx, New York
Chief, Neuromuscular Electrodiagnostic Services
Department of Rehabilitation Medicine
St. Luke's/Roosevelt Hospital Center
New York, New York

Donald M. Currie, M.D.
Associate Professor,
Department of Physical Medicine and Rehabilitation
University of Texas Health Sciences Center at San Antonio
Staff Physician,
Rehabilitation Medicine Service
Audie L. Murphy Memorial Veterans Administration Hospital
San Antonio, Texas

Deborah J. Davis, M.A., OTR, CRC
Director of Vocational Rehabilitation
Special Tree Ltd.
Romulus, Michigan

Norman Decker, M.D.
Clinical Associate Professor,
Department of Psychiatry
Baylor College of Medicine
Houston, Texas

Joel A. DeLisa, M.D., M.S.
Professor and Chairman,
Department of Rehabilitation Medicine
University of Medicine and Dentistry of New Jersey–
 New Jersey Medical School
Newark, New Jersey
Medical Director and Chief Medical Officer,
Kessler Institute for Rehabilitation
West Orange, New Jersey

Robert R. Dodaro, Ph.D., CCC/SP
Director, Speech Pathology Service
The Methodist Hospital
Baylor College of Medicine
Houston, Texas

William H. Donovan, M.D.
Professor, Departments of Rehabilitation and
 Physical Medicine
Baylor College of Medicine
Houston, Texas

Stanley Ducharme, Ph.D.
Director, Rehabilitation Psychology
Associate Professor of Rehabilitation Medicine
Boston University School of Medicine
Boston, Massachusetts

Daniel Dumitru, M.D.
Assistant Professor,
Department of Physical Medicine and Rehabilitation
The University of Texas Health Science Center
 at San Antonio
Medical Director,
Department of Physical Medicine and Rehabilitation
Brady/Green Community Health Center
San Antonio, Texas

Rolland P. Erickson, M.D.
Assistant Professor,
Department of Physical Medicine and Rehabilitation
Mayo Medical School
Consultant, Department of Physical Medicine
 and Rehabilitation
Mayo Clinic and Mayo Foundation
Rochester, Minnesota

Louisa Fertitta, M.S.
Assistant Professor of Obstetrics and Gynecology
Tufts University School of Medicine
Boston, Massachusetts

Steven V. Fisher, M.D.
Assistant Professor,
Department of Physical Medicine and Rehabilitation
University of Minnesota Hospitals
Acting Chairman,
Department of Physical Medicine and Rehabilitation
St. Paul-Ramsey Medical Center
St. Paul, Minnesota

Christopher S. Formal, M.D.
Assistant Professor of Rehabilitation Medicine,
Thomas Jefferson University School of Medicine
Staff Physiatrist,
Magee Rehabilitation Hospital
Philadelphia, Pennsylvania

Leonard Forrest, M.D.
Spinal Cord Injury Program
Thomas Jefferson University Hospital
Philadelphia, Pennsylvania

Donna L. Frankel, M.D., R.D.
Clinical Assistant Professor,
Department of Rehabilitation Medicine
University of Washington
School of Medicine
Seattle, Washington

Maureen Freda, OTR/L, B.S.O.T.
Director of Occupational Therapy Department,
Magee Rehabilitation Hospital
Philadelphia, Pennsylvania

William D. Frey, Ph.D.
President and Senior Research Associate,
Disability Research Systems Inc.
East Lansing, Michigan

Bruce M. Gans, M.D.
Professor and Chairman,
Department of Rehabilitation Medicine
Tufts University School of Medicine
Physiatrist-in-Chief,
Rehabilitation Institute
New England Medical Center
Boston, Massachusetts

Susan L. Garber, M.A., OTR
Assistant Professor,
Department of Rehabilitation
Baylor College of Medicine
Houston, Texas

Susan J. Garrison, M.D.
Assistant Professor,
Departments of Physical Medicine and Rehabilitation
Baylor College of Medicine
Houston, Texas

Steve R. Geiringer, M.D.
Assistant Professor,
Department of Physical Medicine and Rehabilitation
University of Michigan
Director, Outpatient Clinics
Physical Medicine and Rehabilitation
University of Michigan Hospitals
Ann Arbor, Michigan

Lynn H. Gerber, M.D.
Associate Professor of Medicine,
George Washington University
Washington, D.C.
Chief, Department of Rehabilitation Medicine
National Institute of Health
Bethesda, Maryland

Arthur M. Gershkoff, M.D.
Clinical Assistant Professor,
Department of Rehabilitation Medicine
Thomas Jefferson University
Attending Physician,
Magee Rehabilitation Hospital
Philadelphia, Pennsylvania

Kathleen Gill, Ph.D.
Assistant Attending Psychologist,
McLean Hospital/Harvard Medical School
Clinical Psychologist,
Braintree Hospital
Cambridge, Massachusetts

Gary Goldberg, M.D., FRCP(C)
Assistant Professor,
Departments of Physiology and Rehabilitation Medicine
Temple University School of Medicine
Director, Electrodiagnostic Center
Moss Rehabilitation Hospital
Philadelphia, Pennsylvania

Martin Grabois, M.D.
Professor and Chairman,
Department of Physical Medicine
Baylor College of Medicine
Houston, Texas

Michael E. Groher, Ph.D.
Assistant Chief, Audiology and Speech Pathology Service
New York Veterans Administration Medical Center
Adjunct Faculty, Adelphi University
Professional Associate,
Department of Rehabilitation Medicine
The New York Hospital
New York, New York

Eugen M. Halar, M.D.
Professor, Department of Medicine and Rehabilitation
University of Washington, Seattle
Chief, Rehabilitation Medical Service
Veterans Administration Medical Hospital
Seattle, Washington

Margaret C. Hammond, M.D.
Associate Professor,
Department of Rehabilitation Medicine
University of Washington
Staff Physiatrist,
Seattle Veterans Administration Medical Center
Seattle, Washington

Steven M. Hamilton, M.D.
Resident,
Department of Plastic Surgery
Baylor College of Medicine
Houston, Texas

Toni Jo Hanson, M.D.
Instructor,
Department of Physical Medicine and Rehabilitation
Mayo Medical School
Consultant, Mayo Clinic
Mayo Medical Center
Rochester, Minnesota

Phala A. Helm, M.D.
Professor and Chairman
Department of Physical Medicine and Rehabilitation
The University of Texas Southwestern Medical Center
  at Dallas
Dallas, Texas

Jeanne E. Hicks, M.D.
Deputy Chief, Department of Rehabilitation Medicine
Clinical Center
Department of Health and Human Services
National Institute of Health
Bethesda, Maryland

Nicholas S. Hill, M.D.
Assistant Professor,
New England Medical Center Hospitals
Assistant Professor, Pulmonary Medicine
Tufts University School of Medicine
Boston, Massachusetts

Judith F. Hirschwald, M.S.W., A.C.S.W.
Director of Social Services,
Magee Rehabilitation Hospital
Philadelphia, Pennsylvania

David Hirsh, M.D.
Assistant Professor,
Physical Medicine and Rehabilitation
Baylor College of Medicine
Houston, Texas

R. L. Joynt, M.D.
Clinical Assistant Professor,
Department of Physical Medicine & Rehabilitation
Wayne State University Medical School
Detroit, Michigan
Medical Director, Department of Physical Medicine
Hurley Hospital
Flint, Michigan

Cynthia B. Kincaid, M.S., P.T.
Assistant Professor, Physical Therapy Program
University of Michigan—Flint
Ann Arbor, Michigan

Ron M. Koppenhoefer, M.D.
Director of Rehabilitation Medicine,
Good Samaritan Hospital
Cincinnati, Ohio

George H. Kraft, M.D.
Professor,
Department of Rehabilitation Medicine
School of Medicine
University of Washington
Seattle, Washington

Thomas A. Krouskop, Ph.D.
Professor, Departments of Rehabilitation
    and Physical Medicine
Baylor College of Medicine
Houston, Texas

Jo-Anne C. Lazarus, Ph.D.
Research Associate,
University of Wisconsin Medical School
Department of Rehabilitation Medicine
Neuromuscular Retraining Clinic and Research Unit
University of Wisconsin Hospitals and Clinics
Madison, Wisconsin

James A. Leonard, Jr., M.D.
Clinical Assistant Professor and Associate Chairman,
Department of Physicial Medicine and Rehabilitation
Medical Director, Division of Orthotics and Prosthetics
University of Michigan Medical Center
Ann Arbor, Michigan

James S. Lieberman, M.D.
Professor and Chairman,
Department of Physical Medicine and Rehabilitation
University of California—Davis Medical Center
Sacramento, California

James W. Little, M.D., Ph.D.
Assistant Professor,
Department of Rehabilitation Medicine
University of Washington
Staff Physician,
Spinal Cord Injury Service
Seattle Veterans Administration Medical Center
Seattle, Washington

Rebecca A. Marburger, M.Eng., OTR
Clinical Instructor,
Department of Occupational Therapy
University of Texas Health Science Center at San Antonio
    and Children's Habilitation Center/Freedom Center
San Antonio, Texas

Gordon M. Martin, M.D., M.S., FACP, FAAPMR
Executive Director,
American Board of Physical Medicine and Rehabilitation
Emeritus Professor,
Physical Medicine and Rehabilitation
Mayo Medical School and Mayo Graduate School of Medicine
Emeritus Consultant and Chairman,
Department of Physical Medicine and Rehabilitation
Mayo Clinic
Rochester, Minnesota

Samuel R. McFarland, M.S.M.E.
Director, Rehabilitation Engineering
National Rehabilitation Hospital
Washington, D.C.

Malcolm C. McPhee, M.D.
Associate Professor,
Department of Physical Medicine and Rehabilitation
Mayo Medical School
Rochester, Minnesota
Consultant, Department of Physical Medicine
    and Rehabilitation
Mayo Clinic Scottsdale
Scottsdale, Arizona

Robert H. Meier, III, M.D.
Associate Professor and Chairman,
Department of Rehabilitation Medicine
University of Colorado Health Science Center
Denver, Colorado

Geno Merli, M.D.
Clinical Associate Professor,
Departments of Medicine and Rehabilitation Medicine
Thomas Jefferson University
Philadelphia, Pennsylvania

John L. Merritt, M.D., FACP
Associate Professor,
Department of Physical Medicine and Rehabilitation
Mayo Medical School
Consultant,
Mayo Clinic and Medical Center
Rochester, Minnesota

Gail D. Miller, B.S., P.T.
Adjunct Clinical Instructor,
Program in Physical Therapy
Hahnemann University
Director, Physical Therapy
Magee Rehabilitation Hospital
Philadelphia, Pennsylvania

Robert M. Miller, Ph.D.
Clinical Assistant Professor,
Departments of Rehabilitation Medicine,
    Otolaryngology/Head and Neck Surgery, and
    Speech and Hearing Sciences
Chief, Audiology and Speech Pathology Service
Seattle Veterans Administration Medical Center
University of Washington
Seattle, Washington

Patrick K. Murray, M.D.
Assistant Professor of Medicine (Rehabilitation),
Case Western Reserve University School of Medicine
Director, Department of Physical
    Medicine and Rehabilitation
Cleveland Metropolitan General/Highland View Hospital
Cleveland, Ohio

Theodore A. Myers, M.D.
Resident,
Department of Rehabilitation Medicine
University of Wisconsin Hospital and Clinics
Madison, Wisconsin

Anthony J. O'Callaghan, M.B.A.
Manager, Physical Medicine and Rehabilitation
The Methodist Hospital
Baylor College of Medicine
Houston, Texas

Patricia K. Olson, R.P.T.
Staff Physical Therapist,
Department of Physical Medicine and Rehabilitation
Mayo Clinic and Mayo Foundation
Rochester, Minnesota

Joachim L. Opitz, M.D.
Associate Professor of Physical Medicine and Rehabilitation,
Mayo Medical School
Consultant, Department of Physical Medicine
    and Rehabilitation
Mayo Clinic and Mayo Foundation
Rochester, Minnesota

Liina Paasuke, M.A., CRC
Counselor, Michigan Rehabilitation Services
Department of Physical Medicine and Rehabilitation
University Hospital
Ann Arbor, Michigan

Alfred P. Pavot, M.D.
Chairman, Department of Rehabilitation Medicine
Greater Southeast Community Hospital
Clinical Associate Professor in Physical Medicine
    and Rehabilitation
Georgetown University
Washington, D.C.

Parminder S. Phull, M.D.
Assistant Professor,
Department of Rehabilitation Medicine
Tufts University School of Medicine
Assistant Physiatrist,
Rehabilitation Institute
New England Medical Center
Boston, Massachusetts

Kristjan T. Ragnarsson, M.D.
Professor and Chairman,
Department of Rehabilitation Medicine
Mount Sinai Medical Center
One Gustave L. Levy Place
New York, New York

Somayaji Ramamurthy, M.D.
Professor,
Department of Anesthesia
The University of Texas Health Science Center at San Antonio
Attending Physician,
Medical Center Hospital
San Antonio, Texas

James J. Rechtien, D.O., Ph.D.
Associate Professor, Departments of Biomechanics
    and Physical Medicine and Rehabilitation
Michigan State University School of Osteopathic Medicine
East Lansing, Michigan

Thomas S. Rees, Ph.D.
Assistant Professor,
Department of Otolaryngology/Head and Neck Surgery
University of Washington
Seattle, Washington

Gladys P. Rodriguez, M.S.
Research, Assistant Professor
Department of Rehabilitation
Baylor College of Medicine
Houston, Texas

Daniel E. Rohe, Ph.D.
Assistant Professor of Psychology,
Mayo Medical School
Consultant, Section of Psychology
Mayo Clinic and Mayo Foundation
Rochester, Minnesota

Loren A. Rolak, M.D.
Assistant Professor,
Department of Neurology
Baylor College of Medicine
Houston, Texas

Robert D. Rondinelli, M.D.
Assistant Professor, Rehabilitation Medicine
University of Colorado Health Sciences Center
Medical Director, Rehabilitation Unit
Rose Medical Center
Chief, Rehabilitation Medicine Services
Veterans Administration Medical Center
Denver, Colorado

Mitchell Rosenthal, Ph.D.
Assistant Professor of Psychology and Rehabilitation Medicine,
Rush Medical College
Chicago, Illinois
Director of Psychological Medicine,
Marianjoy Rehabilitation Center
Wheaton, Illinois

Jeffrey A. Saal, M.D.
Team Physician, Santa Clara University
Consultant Team Physician, San Francisco Forty-Niners
    Professional Football Team
Associate Clinical Professor,
Department of Physical Medicine and Rehabilitation
University of California, Irvine
Founder, Sports, Orthopedic and Rehabilitation Medicine
    Association (S.O.A.R.)
Portola Valley, California

Lawrence S. Schoenfeld, Ph.D.
Professor,
Departments of Psychiatry and Anesthesiology
University of Texas Health Science Center at San Antonio
San Antonio, Texas

Ann H. Schutt, M.D.
Associate Professor of Physical Medicine and Rehabilitation
Mayo Medical School
Consultant, Department of Physical Medicine
    and Rehabilitation
Mayo Clinic and Mayo Foundation
Rochester, Minnesota

Richard K. Schwartz, M.S., OTR
Associate Professor of Occupational Therapy,
Associate Professor of Physical Medicine and Rehabilitation,
University of Texas Health Science Center at San Antonio
Associate Professor of Life Sciences,
University of Texas at San Antonio
San Antonio, Texas

Steven G. Scott, D.O.
Assistant Professor of Physical Medicine and Rehabilitation,
Mayo Medical School
Consultant, Department of Physical Medicine
    and Rehabilitation
Mayo Clinic and Mayo Foundation
Rochester, Minnesota

Neil I. Spielholz, Ph.D.
Research Associate Professor,
Department of Rehabilitation Medicine
Rusk Institute of Rehabilitation Medicine
New York University Medical Center
New York, New York

William E. Staas, Jr., M.D.
Professor of Rehabilitation Medicine
Jefferson Medical College
Thomas Jefferson University
President and Medical Director
Magee Rehabilitation Hospital
Philadelphia, Pennsylvania

Samuel Stal, M.D.
Associate Professor
Department of Plastic Surgery
Baylor College of Medicine
Houston, Texas

Robert G. Taylor, M.D.
Professor and Vice Chairman,
Department of Physical Medicine and Rehabilitation
University of California—Davis Medical Center
Sacramento, California

Gudni Thorsteinsson, M.D.
Assistant Professor of Physical Medicine and Rehabilitation,
Mayo Medical School
Chairman and Consultant, Department of Physical Medicine
    and Rehabilitation
Mayo Clinic and Mayo Foundation
Rochester, Minnesota

Nicolas E. Walsh, M.D.
Associate Professor,
Department of Physical Medicine and Rehabilitation
University of Texas Health Science Center at San Antonio
San Antonio, Texas

Carolyn Wangaard, R.N., C.A.N.P.
Center for Neurological Diseases/Rocky Mountain
    Multiple Sclerosis Center
University of Colorado Health Sciences Center
Denver, Colorado

Robert J. Weber, M.D.
Associate Professor and Chair,
Department of Physical Medicine and Rehabilitation
Wright State University
Dayton, Ohio

John Whyte, M.D., Ph.D.
Assistant Professor,
Department of Rehabilitation Medicine
Tufts University School of Medicine
Assistant Physiatrist,
New England Medical Center
Director of Research and Associate Director
    of Rehabilitation Medicine,
Greenery Rehabilitation and Skilled Nursing Center
Boston, Massachusetts

Kathryn M. Yorkston, Ph.D.
Associate Professor,
Department of Rehabilitation Medicine
University of Washington
Director, Speech Pathology Services
Seattle, Washington

R. Eugene Zierler, M.D.
Assistant Professor,
Department of Surgery
University of Washington
Seattle, Washington

Preface

Rehabilitation medicine is a unique medical specialty that seems to know no boundaries of age or disease entity. It focuses, rather, upon function and interaction of individuals with their environment and society. The editors and authors of this text have attempted to create a book that provides both breadth and depth of coverage to the full scope of topics that are relevant in the field.

Our goal has been to provide a comprehensive and multidisciplinary coverage of both basic principles and practical techniques of patient management. We believe that this text will be appropriate for physiatrists and other physicians interested in rehabilitation medicine as well as for a broad range of allied health professionals who work with physically impaired people. Medical students particularly should appreciate the blend of scientific detail with practical strategies for patient management.

The book is organized into four parts: Principles of Evaluation, Diagnostic and Management Methods, Major Rehabilitation Problems, and Rehabilitation of Specific Disorders. In Part 1, Chapter 1 covers the basic structure of rehabilitation service delivery models and a history of the specialty. Chapters 2 through 9 provide in-depth coverage of the components of evaluation that form the basis for comprehensive rehabilitation care.

Part 2, Diagnostic and Management Methods, contains ten chapters that include electrodiagnosis (peripheral and central), therapeutic exercise, modalities, prosthetics and orthotics, functional electrical stimulation, and rehabilitation engineering. In addition, a detailed discussion of the neurophysiologic basis of motor control is included.

Part 3 contains nine chapters dealing with major rehabilitation problems and two special age groups: children and elderly. Detailed discussions about spasticity, bowel and bladder disorders, pressure ulcers, contractures, movement disorders, nutrition, and sexual dysfunction will be found there.

Part 4 contains sixteen chapters dealing with the rehabilitation of patients with specific conditions. Each chapter follows the general format of disease definition, epidemiology, etiology, functional impairments, natural history, complications, and management strategies.

The editors wish to express their appreciation to each of the authors who have contributed to the textbook. Their hard work and dedication have made this an exciting and productive effort. We hope that this text will contribute to the training of rehabilitation health care professionals so that the care they provide to disabled people will be of the highest quality, contributing to improvement in their health, function, and quality of life.

Joel A. DeLisa, M.D.
Donald M. Currie, M.D.
Bruce M. Gans, M.D.
Paul F. Gatens, Jr., M.D.
James A. Leonard, Jr., M.D.
Malcolm C. McPhee, M.D.

Contents

REHABILITATION MEDICINE

Part 1

Principles of Evaluation

Rehabilitation Medicine: Past, Present, and Future

Joel A. DeLisa

Gordon M. Martin

Donald M. Currie

Rehabilitation is defined as the development of a person to the fullest physical, psychological, social, vocational, avocational, and educational potential consistent with his or her physiological or anatomical impairment and environmental limitations. Realistic goals are determined by the person and those concerned with the patient's care. Thus, one is working to obtain optimal function despite residual disability, even if the impairment is caused by a pathological process that cannot be reversed even with the best of modern medical treatment.

Rehabilitation is a concept that should permeate the entire health care system. It should be comprehensive and should include prevention; early recognition; outpatient, inpatient, and extended care programs. Anticipated patient outcomes of such a comprehensive and integrated rehabilitation program should include increased independence, shortened length of stays, and an improved quality of life.

PATIENT CARE TEAMS

Since rehabilitation is a holistic and comprehensive approach to medical care, the combined expertise of an interdisciplinary team is necessary. The team approach is critical to solve the complex problems. A *health care team* is defined as a group of health care professionals from different disciplines who share common values and work toward common objectives.[17] Halstead surveyed the literature from 1950 to 1975 on team care in chronic illness and found three major broad categories that he described as "bases." The "opinion base" reflects statements of belief and faith in the team approach to chronic illness. The "descriptive base" contains details and personal testimony of programs using team concepts. The "study base" includes serious research efforts to investigate the effectiveness of team care in various settings. Significantly, Halstead found only ten studies in the research category. He concluded that coordinated team care appears to be more effective than fragmented care for patients with long-term illness.[17]

Organization

There are many ways of organizing a team and many differences exist with respect to integration, collaboration, hierarchical organization, and individual responsibilities. Some teams are organized by body systems and others by practice specialty, concepts of delivery of care, and focus of delivery of care. The classic hierarchical model of bureaucratic pyramids of medical and administrative staff with only vertical communication between supervisor and subordinate does not adapt to the communication style used by rehabilitation teams. Matrix organization superimposes a project orientation on the classic organization structure.[12] Because the matrix organization allows for lateral as well as vertical communication it is much better suited for organization of rehabilitation teams.[35] The project orientation of matrix organization meshes well with the problem orientation of medical rehabilitation. Also, matrix organization easily accommodates the concept of diagnostically oriented specialty teams within the broad team.

Rehabilitation teams can use either a multidisciplinary or an interdisciplinary approach.[39] The multidisciplinary approach refers to specially oriented efforts that represent the sum of each discipline, providing its own unique activity. The efforts are discipline oriented; to operate in a multidisciplinary setting one needs only to know the skill of one's own discipline. The interdisciplinary team uses an approach toward a common goal by professionals from different disciplines. However, these people not only require the skills of their discipline but also must be able to contribute to a group effort on behalf of the patient. The program is synergistic, producing more than each discipline could accomplish individually. After team members evaluate patients according to their clinical specialty, they join in a team conference to communicate, collaborate, and consolidate knowledge from which plans are made, actions determined, future decisions reached, and the accomplishment of the goals evaluated. The key to an effective team is establishing and maintaining intrateam communication. The interdisciplinary team concept provides a means for patient diagnosis, goal setting, problem solving, and treatment in a coordinated, nonfragmented, cost-effective manner by specialists representing several disciplines that will produce a positive rehabilitation outcome that would not be possible without this structure. Rothberg states that it is a compromise between the benefits of specialization and the need for continuity and comprehensiveness of care.[44]

Team Development and Dynamics

Although the team concept appears to be straightforward, the development and maintenance of an effective team require a commitment of time and effort from all of its members. The "healthy" team is efficient in reaching its goals and creates an exciting and stimulating work environment for its members. McGregor developed one of the first descriptions of an effective work team, summarized as 11 characteristics (Table 1-1).[9]

Table 1-1
McGregor's Characteristics of an Effective Work Team

1. The "atmosphere" tends to be informal, comfortable, and relaxed. There are no obvious tensions. It is a working atmosphere in which people are involved and interested. There are no signs of boredom.

2. There is a lot of discussion in which virtually everyone participates, but it remains pertinent to the task of the group. If the discussion gets off the subject, someone will bring it back in short order.

3. The task or the objective of the group is well understood and accepted by the members. There will have been free discussion of the objective at some point, until it was formulated in such a way that the members of the group could commit themselves to it.

4. The members listen to each other! The discussion does not have the quality of jumping from one idea to another unrelated one. Every idea is given a hearing. People do not appear to be afraid of being foolish by putting forth a creative thought even if it seems fairly extreme.

5. There is disagreement. The group is comfortable with this and shows no signs of having to avoid conflict or to keep everything on a plane of sweetness and light. Disagreements are not suppressed or overridden by premature group action. The reasons are carefully examined, and the group seeks to resolve them rather than to dominate the dissenter.

   On the other hand, there is no "tyranny of the minority." Members who disagree do not appear to be trying to dominate the group or to express hostility. Their disagreement is an expression of a genuine difference of opinion, and they expect a hearing in order that a solution may be found.

   Sometimes there are basic disagreements that cannot be resolved. The group finds it possible to live with them, accepting them but not permitting them to block its efforts. Under some conditions, action will be deferred to permit further study of an issue between the members. On other occasions, when the disagreement cannot be resolved and action is necessary, it will be taken but with open caution and recognition that the action may be subject to later reconsideration.

6. Most decisions are reached by a kind of consensus in which it is clear that everybody is in general agreement and willing to go along. However, there is little tendency for members who oppose the action to keep their opposition private and thus let an apparent consensus mask real disagreement. Formal voting is at a minimum; the group does not accept a simple majority as a proper basis for action.

7. Criticism is frequent, frank, and relatively comfortable. There is little evidence of personal attack, either openly or in a hidden fashion. The criticism has a constructive flavor in that it is oriented toward removing an obstacle that faces the group and prevents it from getting the job done.

8. Team members are free in expressing their feelings as well as their ideas both on the problem and on the group's operation. There is little pussyfooting, there are few "hidden agendas." Everybody appears to know quite well how everybody else feels about any matter under discussion.

9. When action is taken, clear assignments are made and accepted.

10. The chairman of the group does not dominate it, nor on the contrary, does the group defer unduly to him or her. In fact, as one observes the activity, it is clear that the leadership shifts from time to time, depending on the circumstances. Different members, because of their knowledge or experience, are in a position at various times to act as "resources" for the group. The members use them in this fashion and they occupy leadership roles while they are thus being used. There is little evidence of a struggle for power as the group operates. The issue is not who controls but how to get the job done.

11. The group is self-conscious about its own operations. Frequently, it will stop to examine how well it is doing or what may be interfering with its operation. The problem may be a matter of procedure, or it may be a member whose behavior is interfering with the accomplishment of the group's objectives. Whatever it is, it gets open discussion until a solution is found.

(Modified from McGregor D: The Human Side of Enterprise, pp 232–235. New York, McGraw-Hill, 1960)

In rehabilitation, the focus of the team is the well-being of the patient. This establishes a common goal for the team that all of its members share.[9] When a team exhibits McGregor's characteristics, it has a built-in feedback mechanism with which it constantly reassesses itself and maintains its effectiveness. When a team is not functioning well, healthy team function can be developed or restored through a process known as team building.[9] Team building requires commitments of time and energy, but the rewards of improved patient outcomes and satisfaction of the team members are worth the effort.

Team building is discussed briefly below in the section on communication and in more detail in several references.[9, 14, 46] A newly formed team or a team with several new members faces several major tasks that must be accomplished if the team is to function effectively.[9, 14] The members must build a working relationship and establish a facilitative emotional climate. They must work out methods for setting goals, solving problems, making decisions, ensuring follow-through on task assignments, developing collaboration of effort, establishing lines of open communication, and ensuring an appropriate support system that will let people feel accepted yet allow open discussion and disagreement. In a newly formed team it is advisable to designate specific meetings to share personal expectations and develop the working policies of the team.

Conflict and Disagreement

Conflict is a normal and necessary part of team development.[46] How it is handled determines its effect on team objectives and on the group process. It is important that the team create an atmosphere that encourages the expression of disagreement. In this setting, members can disagree without making personal accusations or faulting another's personality. Conflict is then used as a vehicle for growth.

When conflict repeatedly occurs with no resolution, action must be taken to restore the team's effective functioning. An appropriate setting for conflict resolution is a team building session, which is discussed in the section on communication.

Complacency

Another factor that may be just as detrimental to the team's effectiveness is complacency.[9] A complacent team may be recognized by one or more of the following characteristics: the same members seem to be doing the same things the same way year after year despite changes in the field; products prescribed are predictable; new members transfer out of the team because of the lack of challenge; there is a fear of or resistance to risk taking; and the rewards go to the members with average performance. These characteristics are especially detrimental to the rehabilitation team when the external conditions that define the team's direction are always changing. Despite similar diagnoses, each patient presents a unique picture; thus, treatment goals and procedures will differ. The treatment techniques used in health fields change in response to research findings. Therefore, creativity and problem solving are very important to the functioning of a rehabilitation team. Steiner has identified some of the characteristics of a creative team as follows: it includes unusual types of people, has open channels of communication, encourages contacts with outside sources, experiments with new ideas, and is not run as a "tight ship"; its members have fun; rewards go to people with ideas; and there is a risk-taking ethos.[9]

Leadership

A team is usually led by the physician in charge. Although other physicians interested in rehabilitation may lead the team, the physiatrist has special skills in the evaluation of neuromuscular, musculoskeletal, and cognitive systems. The physiatrist also has been trained in cardiopulmonary and exercise fitness and in treatment of the functional deficits caused by a variety of illnesses. As the leader of a patient care team, the physician has broad responsibilities in that he or she is the pilot of the combined medical treatment and rehabilitation programs. The physician has the primary responsibility for medical and rehabilitative evaluation and treatment and also for coordinating and integrating a complex care program. Managerial skills, such as the ability to motivate and direct the team, and the willingness to acknowledge and appropriately defer to the opinions of team members are desirable and necessary.

The team leader must have the skills to supervise the treatment goals and the medical status of the patient's rehabilitation. Irrespective of who is the team leader, certain leadership qualities are necessary. The qualities of leadership according to Lundberg are noted in Table 1-2.[36]

The traditional model in which the physician assumes an authoritarian role and other team members "obey" may function effectively in some medical settings but not on the rehabilitation team.[46] In this setting every team member should be encouraged to develop leadership to perform the tasks necessary for meeting the patient goals. On a successful interdisciplinary team there is an administrative leader or coordinator, but *leadership* is passed around from one member to another during team meet-

ings. There is coordination, cooperation, and open communication among team members who know each other's skills and are willing to share the responsibility for the team's action. Patients are perceived as co-managers of their rehabilitation and must accept more and more responsibility as the rehabilitation process goes on.

Managing a Team Meeting

A rehabilitation team's success depends on effective team meetings. A good meeting is productive, stimulating, and goal oriented. It involves creativity, problem solving, and interaction. The team leader, the physiatrist, has the responsibility for conducting a meeting to meet these standards.

The organization of a team meeting can facilitate an effective team process. Perhaps the simplest and most popular structure for team meetings is for a member of each discipline to give a progress report sequentially for each patient. This structure can work well, probably because each member tends to concentrate his or her effort on one problem or on a related set of problems.

Another approach is the problem-oriented agenda. The problem list for each patient is the outline for discussion at the meeting. As each problem is discussed, any team member addresses his or her role in managing the problem. For example, when discussing a patient's ischial ulcer, the physician may review a physiologically sound overview of the strategy being applied to allow healing and prevent recurrence, the plastic surgeon may discuss surgical consideration, the nurse may describe the effects of the topical dressings, the dietitian may mention the implications of dietary proteins and nutritional support of optimal wound healing, the occupational therapist may describe how the patient's daily activities have been adapted to avoid ischial pressure, and the physical therapist may note the effects of hydrotherapy and the patient's ability and dependability in weight-shifting maneuvers. It is easier to keep the meeting goal oriented because the problem-oriented agenda inherently defines the objectives for the meeting. However, this model probably requires more skill of the team manager to keep meetings efficient.

Regardless of which model is used, it is the team manager's responsibility to keep the group focused on the task. This involves facilitating discussion, ensuring that ideas are understood, negotiating compromises, and clarifying responsibilities.[2] It is advisable to keep minutes clarifying responsibilities during the meeting and to distribute these to team members as a form of documentation and cross-checking. An action summary of the meeting to supplement or replace traditional narrative minutes clearly identifies all assignments and summarizes deadlines agreed to at the team meeting (Fig. 1-1).

Communication

"Communication is the passing of information and understanding from sender to receiver."[35] An effective communicator must have certain attributes. He or she must be able to accept differences in perspectives of others; function independently; negotiate roles with other team members; form new values, attitudes, and perceptions; tolerate constant review and challenge of ideas; take risks; possess personal identity and integrity; and accept the team philosophy of care.[14] The maintenance of effective communication requires constant application of all these qualities from all team members because the group process is dynamic.

The physical setting is important for facilitating communication within a team meeting. A specific meeting time must be designated and team members must be committed to this time.

Table 1-2
Some Qualities of a Leader

- Knows where he or she is going
- Knows how to get there
- Has courage and persistence
- Can be believed
- Can be trusted not to "sell out" a cause for personal advantage
- Makes the mission seem important, exciting, and possible to accomplish
- Makes each person's role in the mission seem important
- Makes each member feel capable of performing his or her role

(Lundberg LB: What is leadership. J Nurs Admin 12:32–33, 1982)

Decision	Who is to do it	Date of completion	Date to report progress
Train to do safe independent car transfers with a sliding board	Jane Hoover, P.T. Patient's mother is to bring her car in for use in the training sessions.	May 23	May 27 (next scheduled team meeting)

Figure 1-1.   Example of action summary.

The meeting room's size, lighting, and temperature may help or hinder effective group process. The seating should allow for face to face communication among all members. This criterion is typically met by sitting at a round table or in a circle. Having adequate physical space and time can prevent communication barriers. Another consideration for facilitating communication is the identification and resolution of barriers to communication.

Poor team dynamics can interfere with the achievement of treatment goals. Given and Simmons have identified communication barriers.[14] These include autonomy; individual member's personal characteristics that may contribute to personality conflicts; role ambiguity and incongruent expectations; differing perceptions of authority, power, and status differentials; varying educational preparation of the patient care team members; and hidden agendas. These barriers stem from interpersonal, inter-professional, and practice issues and are not intrinsic defects of the team concept.

Lack of communication can be detrimental to the rehabilitation of the patients as well as uncomfortable for the team members. Time must be designated to maintain effective team process and overcome communication barriers. When a team is functioning suboptimally owing to conflict, complacency, or poor communication, the problem can be resolved by the process of team building.[9]

Dyer cites three prerequisites for conflict negotiation: (1) all parties must agree to come together and work on the problems; (2) members must agree that there are problems that need to be solved and that solving them is everyone's responsibility; and (3) members accept the position that the end result is that the team will communicate better, thus enhancing the rehabilitation process.[9] With these prerequisites met, the team may now list the conflicts or barriers to communication in need of resolution. It is important that concrete suggestion be made for the resolution of these problems and that the team agree on the solutions. This creates a problem-solving session rather than a detrimental process in which the members attempt to determine fault or place blame. Once solutions are agreed on, each member has the responsibility to follow through according to his or her role.

Sometimes an outside consultant can be extremely helpful.[9] There are some symptoms of poor team function that are more easily discerned by outsiders than by team participants.[9] Other symptoms are more easily seen by members, but an outside consultant can help the members identify and interpret these symptoms. The outside consultant can guide the team away from interpretations of problems that are not likely to lead to resolution, such as erroneously labeling incomplete or inadequate conflict resolution as an inevitable "personality conflict."[9] He or she can lead the team toward constructive ways to solve its problems, such as the use of the "expectation theory," which states that negative reactions can be predicted whenever the behavior of one person violates the expectations of another. A vicious cycle of escalating conflict can result when the negative reaction itself violates the expectations of the first person. However, because this theory focuses on behavior rather than "personality," it allows a greater possibility for resolution of conflict. If the parties involved, or even if only one of the parties can identify the behaviors that violate expectation, then these behaviors can be changed, or agreements can be reached, so that team members can reward each other's behaviors rather than negatively reinforce each other.[9] The outside consultant can help the team learn ways to sustain healthy communication by developing its own internal mechanisms for problem identification and diagnosis, planning remediation, implementing changes, and evaluating its own results in a healthy feedback loop. The beneficiaries of healthy communication on the rehabilitation team are the patients and the team members.

In order to make rehabilitation teams more effective and interdisciplinary Rothberg[44] believes we must

- Teach the various members how to work together and give them sufficient practice time in team work.
- Ensure that all members learn, understand, and respect the knowledge and skills of others.
- Develop clear definitions of the roles and behaviors expected of team participants and lessen ambiguities regarding expectations of others.
- Encourage utilization of the full potential of each member.
- Direct attention to initiation and maintenance of communication and to the breaking down of those barriers to interdisciplinary communications that are amenable to change; we should be aware that not all barriers can be razed.
- Attend to the maintenance of the teams—in the same way that organizations need to engage in activities that strengthen their cohesion and offer satisfaction to their personnel.
- Acknowledge that leadership should shift as necessary in terms of the patient's paramount needs.
- Ensure that the person in the leadership role respects the other members, as evidenced by consultation, listening, and involving them in planning.
- Develop an internal system for demonstrating the accountability of each team member to the group and to the institution in which the team practices.
- Develop a process to acknowledge conflict as it arises and to deal with it in a manner that strengthens the group and its members.

Team Size and Membership

The following members are usually present on each rehabilitation team. Overlap does occur among the various team members with respect to their areas of expertise and training.

The Occupational Therapist

The occupational therapist can provide many services to rehabilitation patients. These may include the following:

1. Evaluate and train the patient in self-care activities, such as dressing, eating, bathing, and personal hygiene to maximize independence. Use orthoses or adaptive equipment when necessary.
2. Provide training in home management skills, using simpler methods to minimize fatigue and conserve energy.
3. Explore vocational skills and avocational interests. Work with the vocational counselor when a change in employment is anticipated.
4. Aid in maintaining and improving joint range of motion (ROM), muscle strength, endurance, and coordination.
5. Evaluate and train the patient in weak areas to compensate for sensory and perceptual deficits.
6. Evaluate the home and suggest modifications to provide a barrier-free environment.
7. Assess driving habits and retrain when necessary, with the assistance of appropriate devices if required.
8. Educate the patient's family by demonstrating techniques designed to maintain patient independence and to minimize overprotection.
9. Train in the functional use of an upper extremity prosthesis.
10. Evaluate and train patients in the use of environmental control systems.
11. Train patients and/or significant others in the maintenance of equipment.
12. Evaluate and manage dysphagia.

The Physical Therapist

The physical therapist assists the patient in functional restoration. Tasks may include the following:

1. Provide joint range of motion (ROM) and exercises to maintain and increase ROM.
2. Perform muscle strength evaluation and quantification.
3. Evaluate sitting and standing balance, transfers, and ambulation, including wheelchair and bipedal. Progressive gait training with or without ambulatory aids may be offered and includes rough ground, ramps, and stairs.
4. Offer exercises to increase strength, endurance, and coordination for either specific muscle groups or the entire body.
5. Offer various physical therapy modalities, such as both superficial and deep heat and cold, as well as hydrotherapy techniques, electrical stimulation, traction, and massage.
6. Aid in home evaluations to make the environment barrier free and accessible.
7. Assess the patient's wheelchair needs, including maintenance, and assist with individualized wheelchair prescriptions.
8. Assess the patient's wheelchair cushion needs.

The Recreation Therapist

The recreation therapist uses recreational activities for purposive intervention in some physical, social, and/or emotional behavior to bring about a desired change in that behavior and promote the growth and development of the patient.

The therapeutic recreation process includes the following:

1. Assessing, in detail, the patient's interests, resources, level of participation, social capability, cognitive functioning, physical limitations and/or abilities, perceived barriers, emotional functioning, and level of resource awareness.
2. Educating patients in leisure activities, concentrating on the needs of the patient, with topics such as specialized equip-

ment, training, adapted sports, increasing awareness of leisure time and alternatives to prior life-styles, acquiring new leisure skills, self-initiation at leisure pursuits, developing and/or increasing social skills, and much more.
3. Actively participating in patient rehabilitation by using recreational activities to
   - Increase attention span, concentration, and/or maintenance of physical strength, social skills, and motivation
   - Assist in adjustment to disability
   - Assist in the family's adjustment to disability
   - Decrease atypical behaviors
   - Increase independence
   - Reinforce other therapies
   - Provide community integration
   - Further evaluate functioning level
4. Providing recreation activities that are nonstructured and more suited to the patient's wants than needs in order to facilitate participation in previously acquired leisure interests, a form of self-expression, a healthy outlet for frustrations, maintenance of health, and a nonthreatening atmosphere for patient-staff interaction and/or patient social interaction.
5. Developing program plans specifically suited to the patient's needs that include the preceding.
6. Integrating the patient into the community by a safe, nonthreatening, and graduated program of recreational outings into the community.
7. Assisting the patient in exploring resources for postdischarge activities such as support groups.

The Prosthetist-Orthotist

The prosthetist-orthotist is responsible for the design, fabrication, and fitting of the orthosis (brace) and prosthesis (artificial limb). The prosthetist-orthotist makes certain that the device functions and fits properly and that the patient adjusts well to its presence. Patient and family instruction in the care of the prosthesis and follow-up maintenance and repair should be stressed.

The Rehabilitation Nurse

Rehabilitation nursing evaluates the health status of the patient and helps determine short- and long-term goals. The nurse provides information on the physical, social, and behavioral sciences and shows an attitude of awareness toward the disabled.

Rehabilitation nursing therapy is similar to nursing in other settings. However, the functions of the rehabilitation nurse emphasize certain priorities related to promoting maximal function. The nurse must be constantly vigilant for any small skills and environmental modifications that make the difference between dependence and independence. Nursing therapy is responsible, among other things, for assessing the following:

1. Hygienic factors
2. Environmental factors such as heat and noise, control of personal property, sanitation, infection control, and safety
3. The use of adaptive equipment needed by patients to communicate, eat, move, eliminate, dress, and ambulate
4. The need for specific preventive measures to minimize the effects of inactivity
5. The need for specific measures to promote optimal independence
6. The patient's progress in integrating the various therapies into their daily activities
7. Medication management

The Speech Pathologist

The speech pathologist helps the patient and significant others in the area of communication and swallowing. This can involve the following:

1. Evaluation and treatment of neurological communication problems
2. Vocal re-education
3. Preoperative counseling prior to laryngectomy, glossectomy, and other procedures that will potentially influence communication abilities
4. Alaryngeal speech training (esophageal speech or use of a prosthetic larynx)
5. Retraining speech in patients with intraoral defects (*i.e.,* glossectomy, palatectomy)
6. Evaluation of swallowing function and management of dysphagia
7. Patient and family education regarding communication and swallowing problems
8. Evaluating and training the patient in the use of nonvocal communication devices
9. Cognitive retraining

The Psychologist

The psychologist helps the patient and significant others to psychologically prepare for full participation in rehabilitation. This can involve a number of activities:

1. Testing involving
   - Personality, style (manipulative, dependent, dogmatic)
   - Ways of dealing with stress
   - Problem-solving skills
   - Psychological status (neurosis, psychosis)
2. Incorporation of the test results into the care plan
3. Counseling in
   - Adjustment to body changes
   - Development of problem-solving skills
   - Secondary problems caused by the disease and its disability
   - Adjustment to changes in sexual functioning and viable alternatives
   - Death and dying
4. Testing of intelligence, memory, and perceptual functioning

The Social Worker

The social worker interacts with the patient, family, and rehabilitation team and can assist in the following ways:

1. Evaluating the patient's total living situation, including lifestyle, family, finances, and community resources, and assessing the impact of the disease or disability on these areas
2. Maintaining a continuing relationship with the patient and family
3. Discussing arrangements and concerns about finances
4. Helping the family develop the skills needed to actively participate in treatment procedures in the home
5. Providing assistance in locating alternative living situations

The Vocational Counselor

Some major areas of responsibility for vocational counselors with respect to rehabilitation of the patient include

1. Evaluating vocational interests, aptitudes, and skills
2. Counseling patients who must shift to alternate occupations

3. Organizing activities, individual or group, to improve job-related behaviors (*i.e.,* job interview skills, work skills, employer–employee relationship behaviors)
4. Acting as a liaison between agencies that provide training or job placement services and the patient
5. Providing counseling education and support to potential employers of these patients

Allied health care professionals from several other disciplines may be brought onto the team depending on the patient's needs. The following professionals are well known: psychiatrist, enterostomal therapist, maxillofacial prosthetist, podiatrist, dentist, audiologist, dietitian, and chaplain. Although their roles with rehabilitation patients possess some special features, their areas of responsibility are familiar enough to not need clarification here. Other professionals are less well known and not as readily available but can provide important services to selected patients. Some of these are listed below and in Appendix 1-1.

The Child Life Specialist

The child life specialist acts as the advocate for a child who requires health care. Child life specialists work in hospitals, most commonly with inpatients but sometimes also in ambulatory care settings. The philosophy of child life programs is to minimize, as much as possible, the interruption and disruption of normal life experiences caused by hospitalization or illness, and even to make hospitalization a positive growth experience for a child and the family. Some of the specialist's activities include the following:

1. Using play and homelike activities to foster continued development
2. Encouraging and facilitating continuation of school and family relationships during hospitalization and illness
3. Providing developmentally appropriate explanations of health care procedures to children, sometimes using props such as dolls or puppets

Child life specialists work closely with other allied health care team members, but the child life program should be autonomous and equal in status with other departments and have separate facilities. Child life specialists have bachelor's degree academic preparation in fields as varied as nursing, psychology, social work, special education, and occupational therapy.

The Corrective Therapist

The American Corrective Therapy Association defines corrective therapy as "the applied science of medically prescribed therapeutic exercise, education, and adapted physical activities to improve the quality of life and health of adults and children, by developing physical fitness, increasing functional mobility and independence, and improving psycho-social behavior." The corrective therapist seeks a coach–player relationship in which he or she helps the patient reach the goal of becoming an independent, self-sustaining person. The potential overlaps among corrective therapy, physical therapy, occupational therapy, and recreational therapy need to be resolved in each setting. As compared with physical therapists, with whom there is probably the most potential overlap, corrective therapists put more emphasis on geriatric care, extended care, reconditioning and fitness, and psychiatric care. A large percentage of corrective therapists practice in veterans hospitals. Corrective therapists can provide the following:

1. Gross motor and remedial exercise programs
2. Adapted driver education
3. Home maintenance programs for fitness for physically handicapped children
4. Fitness as a means of stress management for psychiatric patients
5. Gait training and fitness programs for amputees
6. Fitness-promoting therapeutic recreation programs for acute, chronic, and convalescent patients

The Horticultural Therapist

The raising of flowers, vegetables, and other plants is thought to have therapeutic value in building or rebuilding personal confidence and self-esteem. There is a tangible, visible difference that results from the work done in raising plants. Horticultural therapists offer the following services:

1. Working with a variety of patients, including those with mental retardation and psychiatric diagnoses as well as physically disabled and hospitalized children and adults, to promote independence, motor skills, and psychological well-being
2. Helping prepare selected patients for vocations involving work with plants, gardening, and groundskeeping

The Music Therapist

The music therapist works with patients with a broad variety of diagnoses and therapeutic goals. The interventions may involve musical performance with instruments, voice, or body movements; listening to music; or attending musical events. Possible goals and treatments include the following:

1. Helping children with cerebral palsy or other paralytic conditions, or adults with paralysis, to improve coordination and develop gross and fine motor skills through playing selected instruments or exercising to music
2. Relaxation, sedation, or control of pain or anxiety for therapeutic procedures or control of acute or chronic pain
3. Improving speech through articulation training or melodic intonation therapy
4. Preparing selected patients for music-related careers (*e.g.,* visually impaired piano tuners)
5. Improving socialization skills, self-confidence, and self-esteem through group music activities
6. Improving quality of life for patients in palliative or hospice care

The Dance Therapist

The dance therapist, sometimes called a movement therapist, focuses on rhythmic body movement as a medium of physical and psychological change. Dance therapy is practiced more often with mental health patients than with physically disabled patients. A master's degree level of training is required by the American Dance Therapy Association in order to award the credentials Dance Therapist Registered (D.T.R.). Dance therapists can use rhythmic movements and music to help patients in the following ways:

1. Improve gross motor control
2. Relieve and improve awareness of tension and stress, and awareness and expression of other emotions, especially when verbal expression is limited
3. Improve body image and awareness
4. Classify and describe body movements

TREATMENT STRATEGIES IN CHRONIC DISEASE

The history and physical examination techniques that, when applied to patients with chronic disease, permit the identification of disability problems are described in Chapter 2. In chronic disease, or chronic disability secondary to severe trauma such as spinal cord injury, the pathological process usually is irreversible. Hence, removal of these disability problems depends on a set of techniques that are directed not at the pathological condition but at achieving maximum independence despite the disorder. These techniques and principles are applicable to the rehabilitation of patients with specific disease states or organ system dysfunctions that will appear throughout this textbook.

There are six classes of treatment strategies to help mitigate disability. A few examples for each strategy are given to help appreciate this approach to disability.

PREVENTION OR CORRECTION OF ADDITIONAL DISABILITY

- Medications to prevent congestive heart failure in patients with cardiac disease
- Good glucose control in diabetes with the hope of delaying retinopathy and nephropathy
- Regular foot care in peripheral vascular disease to avoid skin lesions and decrease the risk of amputation
- High caloric nutritional supplements in specific patients with swallowing impairment to prevent malnutrition
- Passive joint ROM exercises to avoid contractures in paretic limbs
- Adequate bladder hygiene for patients with indwelling catheters to avoid bladder calculi formation, ureter reflux, and/or pyelonephritis
- Muscle stretching exercises to correct contractures in spastic limb muscles
- Periodic pressure relief over anesthetic bony surfaces to avoid pressure ulcers
- Time-contingent medication schedule to prevent drug addiction, especially in managing patients with chronic pain
- Patient education and training in tracheostomy care to prevent formation of mucus plugs and tracheal obstruction

ENHANCEMENT OF SYSTEMS UNAFFECTED BY THE PATHOLOGICAL CONDITION

- Training laryngectomees to trap air in the esophagus and release it through the esophageal-pharyngeal junction for voice production
- Progressive resistive exercises to the nonparalyzed side of a stroke patient or to upper extremities of paraplegic patients to aid in transfers
- Use of visual feedback for hand function in patients with a sensory deficit
- Speech–reading training for patients with severe hearing loss and following cochlear implantation for the patient with total deafness
- Ear–echo training for travel for patients with total deafness
- Development of overarticulation to enhance speech intelligibility for the laryngectomee using an electrolarynx

ENHANCEMENT OF FUNCTIONAL CAPACITY OF AFFECTED SYSTEMS

- Hearing aids to partially compensate for hearing loss
- Graded exercise programs for patients who have recently had a myocardial infarction

- Progressive resistive exercises to weakened muscles to enhance their strength
- Training dysarthric speakers to reduce their speaking rates for improved intelligibility
- Use of visual written cues (prosthetic memory) in brain-damaged patients to assist memory function
- Serial pumping of lymphedema to improve cosmesis and use of extremity

USE OF ADAPTIVE EQUIPMENT TO PROMOTE FUNCTION

- Use of electrolarynx for voice production following laryngectomy
- Use of canes, crutches, and/or orthoses to achieve ambulation
- Use of augmentative communication devices for patients with unintelligible dysarthric speech
- Wheelchair training when walking is not possible
- Use of equipment to extend hand function needs in dressing (*i.e.,* long shoe horns, stocking pullers, button hooks)
- Use of hand controls for the automobile of paraplegic patients
- Shoe modifications to promote standing balance
- Prostheses for amputees to achieve walking or upper extremity function
- Use of "closed caption" television systems for the hearing-impaired patient
- Voice activation to direct a computerized robot or animal assistant to perform duties for patients with severe disabilities

MODIFICATION OF SOCIAL AND VOCATIONAL ENVIRONMENT

- Moving to a one-level home for patients who are unable to climb stairs
- Widening bathroom doorways to allow wheelchair to pass
- Adding rails on stairs to promote stair climbing
- Providing assistance in home for physical dependency needs
- Shifting employment to sedentary activities for patients with reduced ambulation skills
- Redesigning work areas for patients now wheelchair confined
- Modifying diet for certain swallowing problems
- Training family members to not reinforce sick behavior but to reinforce well behavior

PSYCHOLOGICAL TECHNIQUES TO ENHANCE PATIENT PERFORMANCE AND PATIENT EDUCATION

- Using repetition in training self-care in patients with memory problems
- Teaching new skills by verbal instruction for patients with memory problems
- Teaching new skills by demonstration (pantomime) for patients with language deficits
- Developing skill in task performance by operant methods (behavior therapy)
- Group therapy for patients with similar disabilities

HISTORICAL PERSPECTIVES OF PHYSICAL MEDICINE AND REHABILITATION

Background and Early Stages

The history of the beginnings and the evolution of the medical specialty of physical medicine and rehabilitation has proven fascinating to a number of historically oriented physicians and writers.[48] The roots of physical medicine have been traced back as far as the ancients, who were aware of the beneficial effects of various physical agents. Heliotherapy and hydrotherapy were recognized and were operational at the time of the Roman Empire and perhaps even earlier. In the 18th and 19th centuries, applications of galvanic and faradic currents were prescribed as valuable therapeutic methods. About 1890, high-frequency currents from spark-gap diathermy machines were introduced by d'Arsonval in France for both medical and surgical treatment.[31] If this important milestone were singled out as a logical beginning point for the history of the specialty of physical medicine and rehabilitation, we would now be thinking in terms of a century of evolution, growth, and development.

During and after World War I, diathermy, electrical stimulation, heat, massage, and exercise were increasingly used as therapeutic tools in the United States.[7, 27, 32, 40] Army medical hospitals made extensive use of physical therapy and occupational therapy. Colonel Harry Mock of the Army Medical Corps referred to the importance of these services in the "rehabilitation" of wounded and other disabled people in World War I.[40] Dr. John Coulter, an Army Medical Corps physician, promoted physical therapy and rehabilitation before he later became involved in establishing this discipline at Northwestern University.[7] World War I uses of physical therapy were followed by more extensive, updated, and sophisticated uses of physical and rehabilitation medicine in military medicine in World War II.[47]

A medical specialty evolves when a small group of physicians recognize that a special body of knowledge, along with certain procedural skills, should be nurtured and developed so that its benefits can be made available to patients whose needs in that special area are not being adequately met.

A detailed, well-documented account of many highlights in the long and complex history of the specialty of physical medicine and rehabilitation appears as the first chapter in Dr. Frank Krusen's pioneering textbook *Physical Medicine* published in 1941.[31] This classic reference is still recognized as an outstanding source book. Other authors have reviewed various aspects of the evolution of the specialty, particularly reporting on the several physician-oriented organizations that have played significant roles in the development and evolution of the specialty. Dr. Krusen, in 1969, reviewed 40 years of history of interest areas and activities related to the specialty since the decade of the 1920s.[30]

Special reference must be made to Dr. Paul Nelson's notable in-depth study of the origins and evolution of the principal publication of the specialty in the *Archives of Physical Medicine and Rehabilitation*. Nelson's 1969 article, recognizing and honoring 50 years of publication of the *Archives,* includes extensive historical data and pictures of the physicians of the decade from 1915 to 1925 who were pioneers in the medical uses of x-ray and electrotherapeutics.[41] Nelson's article is a unique data source regarding the organizations whose activities, interests, and publications served the new specialty effectively. In a 1973 article, Nelson reviewed the early interrelationships of electrotherapeutics and radiology.[42] In addition to the *Archives,* another significant periodical is the *American Journal of Physical Medicine,* which has a distinguished editorial board and was edited by Dr. H. D. Bouman from 1952 through 1987. In 1988, the journal was renamed the *American Journal of Physical Medicine and Rehabilitation* and is sponsored by the Association of Academic Physiatrists, with Dr. E. W. Johnson as editor.

The historical development of the various methods and devices that are in current use in physical medicine and rehabilitation will be discussed in the chapters pertaining to these topics. The main thrust here will be the important organizations that have evolved to represent this specialty, along with some special clinical areas, that, although now superseded, were milestones in the development of the specialty.

American Congress of Rehabilitation Medicine

The complexities of the evolving specialty can best be appreciated and understood by an overview of several important organizations and their areas of major interests, functions, expertise, and performance in relation to physical and rehabilitation medicine. Nelson stated that among the early organizations related to the specialty was the American Electrotherapeutic Association, founded in 1890.[42] It consisted of physicians with varied interests who banded together for the study and promotion of electrotherapeutic measures. It included physicians who were particularly involved with irradiation; ear, nose, and throat medicine; general surgery; neurology; and general medicine. In 1929, this organization merged with the Western Association of Physical Therapy. It was a regional association of physicians interested in physical therapy, and its leaders and organizers were primarily midwestern, based in Omaha and Des Moines. Another parent organization began in 1923 as the American College of Radiology and Physiotherapy. The name of this organization was changed in 1925 to the American Congress of Physical Therapy, and 10 years of its progress were reviewed by Hollander in 1935.[20]

In 1933, the American Physical Therapy Association, an organization of physicians interested in physical treatment, and the American Congress of Physical Therapy merged. The new organization continued to use the term "congress" while undergoing several other name changes: in 1945, it became known as the American Congress of Physical Medicine; in 1952, the American Congress of Physical Medicine and Rehabilitation; and, in 1966, the American Congress of Rehabilitation Medicine. Through the years, membership in the Congress has been open to any physician with an interest in physical medicine or rehabilitation. In addition to physiatrists, it has included family practitioners, internists, orthopedists, neurologists, surgeons, and dermatologists. Since 1975, membership in the American Congress of Rehabilitation Medicine has been extended to include nonphysicians with advanced degrees in allied health or basic science fields pertinent to rehabilitation. Represented are psychologists, speech–language pathologists, physical therapists, occupational therapists, social workers, vocational rehabilitation specialists, rehabilitation nurses, and others. Those concerned with rehabilitation of the hard of hearing and the visually impaired may also be included.

The membership of the American Congress of Rehabilitation Medicine reached 3,200 in 1987, with 2,260 physicians and 940 nonphysicians. The annual meetings of the Congress are held jointly and concurrently with those of the American Academy of Physical Medicine and Rehabilitation. The administrative officers of the Congress and the Academy have included Dr. Walter Zeiter of Cleveland, Dr. Glenn Gullickson, Jr., of Minneapolis, and Creston Herald and Ike Mayeda of Chicago, the last-named being the current executive director.

The Congress portion of the annual scientific program of the Academy–Congress meeting provides opportunity for nonphysician professionals in rehabilitation medicine to present papers or poster exhibits on research aspects pertinent to their involvement and interests. Five of the past ten presidents of the American Congress of Rehabilitation Medicine have been nonphysicians (Table 1-3), all highly qualified in selected areas of rehabilitation and respected authorities in rehabilitation as well as in their areas of expertise. The expanding of the membership to its current broad scope has strengthened the Congress and broadened its base as a recognized specialty organization.

In addition to scientific involvement, this organization and the Academy are deeply concerned with many aspects of the changing pictures in the economics, organization, and delivery of health care at federal, state, and local levels. The Congress and Academy have for 13 years been represented by a Washington,

Table 1-3
Past Presidents, American Congress of Rehabilitation Medicine

*Samuel B. Childs, 1923–24, Denver
*Curran Pope, 1924–25, Louisville
*John S. Coulter, 1925–26, Chicago
*Disraeli Kobak, 1926–27, Chicago
*James C. Elsom, 1927–28, Madison, WI
*Frank Walke, 1928–29, Shreveport, LA
*Normal T. Titus, 1929–30, New York

*Roy W. Fouts, 1930–31, Omaha
*Frank H. Ewerhardt, 1931–32, St. Louis
*Gustav Kolischer, 1932–33, Chicago
*Albert F. Tyler, 1933–34, Omaha
*William J. Clark, 1934–35, Philadelphia
*John S. Hibben, 1935–36, Los Angeles
*William Bierman, 1936–37, New York
*Frederick L. Wahrer, 1937–38, Marshaltown, IA
*Frank H. Krusen, 1938–39, Rochester, MN
*William H. Schmidt, 1939–40, Philadelphia

*Nathan H. Polmer, 1940–41, New Orleans
*Abraham R. Hollender, 1941–42, Chicago
*Fred B. Moor, 1942–43, Loma Linda, CA
*Kristian G. Hansson, 1943–44, New York
Miland E. Knapp, 1944–45, Minneapolis
Miland E. Knapp, 1945–46, Minneapolis
*Walter S. McClellan, 1946–47, Saratoga Springs, FL
H. Worley Kendell, 1947–48, Chicago
*O. Leonard Huddleston, 1948–49, Denver
*Earl C. Elkins, 1949–50, Rochester, MN

*Arthur L. Watkins, 1950–51, Boston
*Robert L. Bennett, 1952–52, Warm Springs, GA
*Walter M. Solomon, 1952–53, Cleveland
*William B. Snow, 1953–54, New York
*William D. Paul, 1954–55, Iowa City, IA
Gordon M. Martin, 1955–56, Rochester, MN
A.B.C. Knudson, 1956–57, Washington, DC
Donald L. Rose, 1957–58, Kansas City, KS
*Arthur C. Jones, 1958–59, Portland, OR
Frederic J. Kottke, 1959–60, Minneapolis

*Donald A Covalt, 1960–61, New York
Donald J. Erickson, 1961–62, Rochester, MN
Jerome S. Tobis, 1962–63, New York
*Charles D. Shields, 1963–64, Washington, DC
William J. Erdman, II, 1964–65, Philadelphia
*Lewis A. Leavitt, 1965–66, Houston
Edward W. Lowmann, 1966–67, New York
*Sidney Licht, 1967–68, New Haven, CT
William A. Spencer, 1968–69, Houston
Jerome W. Gersten, 1969–70, Denver

Herman J. Flax, 1970–71, Puerto Rico
Leonard D. Policoff, 1971–72, Princeton, NJ
James W. Rae, 1972–73, Ann Arbor, MI
Rene Cailliet, 1973–74, Los Angeles
John W. Goldschmidt, 1974–75, Chicago
Henry B. Betts, 1975–76, Chicago
John E. Affeldt, 1976–77, Chicago
June S. Rothberg 1977–78, Garden City, NY
Thomas P. Anderson, 1978–79, Minneapolis
Wilbert E. Fordyce, 1979–80, Seattle

Marcus J. Fuhrer, 1980–81, Houston
Victor Cummings, 1981–82, New York
Sam C. Colachis, Jr., 1982–83, Phoenix
Alfred J. Szumski, 1983–84, Richmond, VA
Glenn Gullickson, Jr., 1984–85, Minneapolis
Don A. Olson, 1985–86, Chicago
Dorothea D. Glass, 1986–87, Miami
John L. Melvin, 1987–88, Milwaukee

*Deceased.

D.C. legal counsel, Richard E. Verville, who informs both organizations regarding pending and proposed legislation that might affect either recipients or providers of health care and rehabilitation services.

A list of the past presidents of the American Congress (see Table 1-3) indicates the wide geographical base of the top leadership of the organization since early in this century. Each of these leaders and his or her organizational associates have contributed significantly to the evolution and growth of the specialty.

Registry of Physical Therapists and the American Physiotherapy Association

Dr. John Coulter reported that in 1919 Dr. Paul Magnuson established a physical therapy department at Wesley Memorial Hospital at Northwestern University and developed a teaching course for physical therapy technicians in 1927.[7] Dr. Harry Mock developed a program at St. Luke Hospital, Chicago, when he returned from World War I. In 1926, he became the first chairman of the Council on Physical Therapy of the American Medical Association (AMA). In 1944, the AMA trustees changed the name to the Council of Physical Medicine.

The American Registry of Physical Therapists was organized under the auspices of the American Congress of Physical Medicine and the Council on Physical Therapy of the AMA in 1935 to approve training schools and establish educational standards and to provide certification of registered therapists. Physical therapy schools date back to training programs established at Walter Reed Army Hospital during World War I. The American Physiotherapy Association (APTA) started in 1921–22. By 1947, its membership had increased to 4,000 and by 1986 to 37,000. In 1934, the APTA asked the Council on Medical Education and Hospitals of the AMA to assist with the certification of approved training schools. In December 1971, the APTA withdrew from its functionally cooperative status with the AMA and the American Congress of Rehabilitation Medicine and assumed responsibility for approving training programs and for certifying therapists, at first in cooperation with the Council on Allied Health Education Accreditation and, more recently, under the auspices of the Council on Postsecondary Accreditation.

Section Council on Physical Medicine and Rehabilitation of the American Medical Association

The AMA Section Council on Physical Medicine provides specialty representation at the AMA. Beginning in the early 1940s, the Section Council sponsored scientific sessions and exhibits at the annual conventions each June until these were discontinued in the late 1970s. The Section Council maintained active liaison with other specialty section councils regarding topics of mutual concern. The section councils of the various specialties also have representation in the AMA House of Delegates. Currently, Section Council members participate in the AMA nominations for directorships on the American Board of Physical Medicine and Rehabilitation. Beginning in the 1930s as the Council on Physical Therapy, and extending to 1950, the Section Council was involved with the evaluation, testing, and approval of diagnostic and physical therapy devices.

The American Academy of Physical Medicine and Rehabilitation

The American Academy of Physical Medicine and Rehabilitation had its official origin in 1938. Since 1947, Academy membership comprised Board-certified physiatrists, and a current membership status as "Fellow of the American Academy of Physical Medicine and Rehabilitation" is available only to certified diplomates of the American Board of Physical Medicine and Rehabilitation. Its roots and precursor organizations were researched by Dr. G. K. Stillwell and described in the 1982 Zeiter lecture.[49] Some of these earlier organizations had also overlapped with physician groups that could be considered allied to those of the pre–American Congress era. The first president of the Academy of Physical Medicine and Rehabilitation was Dr. John Coulter of Northwestern University, Chicago (Table 1-4). The organization at first consisted primarily of physicians practicing almost full time in physical medicine.

One of the primary aims of the group in the early 1940s was to support the founding and development of a certifying board for the new specialty of physical medicine. This emerging organization (the Academy) provided financial support for a committee that was to be involved in the preliminary planning for a specialty board of physical medicine and rehabilitation. The Academy thus became the primary sponsoring organization of the specialty board, which was established in 1947. When the first diplomates were certified, it was the decision of the Academy that for membership in the Academy an applicant would have to be a board-certified diplomate in physical medicine. At a later date, the Academy decided that fully qualified members of the Academy would be known as Fellows of the American Academy of Physical Medicine and Rehabilitation. Although the growth of the Academy was relatively slow during the early years, membership has increased appreciably during the past 10 years. As of 1987, the Academy has 1,600 fellows and 700 associate and junior members.

The Academy, in collaboration with the American Congress of Rehabilitation Medicine, is involved in the sponsorship, management, and production of the *Archives of Physical Medicine and Rehabilitation*. It co-sponsors the annual joint scientific meetings of the Academy and the Congress. The Academy has a board of governors made up of nine members, including the current officers, the past president, and three members at large. The executive director is currently based at the Chicago office of the Academy and serves in the same capacity for the American Congress of Rehabilitation Medicine. The list of presidents of the Academy (see Table 1-4) reflects the wide geographical distribution of these officers and also the quality and dedication of the leaders of this organization during the past 48 years.

The American Board of Physical Medicine and Rehabilitation

The American Board of Physical Medicine and Rehabilitation was founded in 1947 and celebrated its 40th anniversary in 1987. In 1936, Dr. Louis Wilson, then president of the Advisory Board of Medical Specialties, suggested the need for a certifying board in the special field of physical medicine. In the late 1930s and the early 1940s, plans for the establishment of an accrediting board were developed. Much of the groundwork was laid by Drs. Frank Krusen, John Coulter, and Walter Zeiter. It was believed to be essential to develop a plan of organization of a board of physical medicine that was acceptable to the Advisory Council of Medical Specialties. It was also considered to be necessary to seek the support of other, already established, boards on behalf of the new board when the proposal was presented to the Advisory Board. After considerable exchange of views with the existing boards, and not a little controversy, especially regarding the use of the term *rehabilitation* in the title, the American Board of Physical Medicine was approved by the Advisory Board for Medical Specialties in January 1947. It was authorized to begin

Table 1-4

Past Presidents, American Academy of Physical Medicine and Rehabilitation

*John S. Coulter, 1938–39, Chicago
*F. W. Ewerhardt, 1939–40, St. Louis

*William Bierman, 1940–41, New York
*Frank H. Krusen, 1942–42, Rochester, MN
*K. G. Hansson, 1942–43, New York
*William H. Schmidt, 1943–44, Philadelphia
*Fred B. Moor, 1944–45, Los Angeles
*Fred B. Moor, 1945–46, Los Angeles
*William D. Paul, 1946–47, Iowa City, IA

*Earl C. Elkins, 1947–48, Rochester, MN
Arthur E. White, 1948–49, Washington, DC
Charles O. Molander, 1949–50, Chicago

Miland E. Knapp, 1950–51, Minneapolis
*Frances Baker, 1951–52, San Francisco
*Walter S. McClellan, 1952–53, Saratoga Springs, FL
Donald L. Rose, 1953–54, Kansas City, KS
Harold Dinken, 1954–55, Denver
*Ben L. Boynton, 1955–56, Chicago
*Murray B. Ferderber, 1956–57, Pittsburgh
*George D. Wilson, 1957–58, Asheville, NC
Louis B. Newman, 1958–59, Chicago
Clarence W. Dail, 1959–60, Los Angeles

*Ray Piaskoski, 1960–61, Milwaukee
Robert W. Boyle, 1961–62, Milwaukee
Max K. Newman, 1962–63, Detroit
*Morton Hoberman, 1963–64, New York
*Herman L. Rudolph, 1964–65, Reading, PA
A.B.C. Knudson, 1965–66, Washington, DC
*Michael M. Dacso, 1966–67, New York
Robert C. Darling, 1967–68, New York
G. Keith Stillwell, 1968–69, Rochester, MN
Herman J. Bearzy, 1969–70, Dayton, OH

Glenn Gullickson, Jr., 1970–71, Minneapolis
*Arthur S. Abramson, 1971–72, New York
Justus F. Lehmann, 1972–73, Seattle
Leonard F. Bender, 1973–74, Ann Arbor, MI
Eugene Moskowitz, 1974–75, New York
Carl V. Granger, 1975–76, Boston
Ernest W. Johnson, 1976–77, Columbus, OH
Joseph Goodgold, 1977–78, New York
Frederic J. Kottke, 1978–79, Minneapolis
Joseph C. Honet, 1979–80, Detroit

William M. Fowler, Jr., 1980–81, Los Angeles
John F. Ditunno, Jr., 1981–82, Philadelphia
Murray M. Freed, 1982–83, Boston
Arthur E. Grant, 1983–84, San Antonio, TX
George H. Kraft, 1984–85, Seattle
Myron M. LaBan, 1985–86, Detroit
Richard S. Materson, 1986–87, Houston
Joachim L. Opitz, 1987–88, Rochester, MN

*Deceased.

certification procedures under the advisory capacity of the American Board of Medicine, the American Board of Orthopedics, and the American Board of Radiology.

The 11 original members of the American Board of Physical Medicine were Dr. Kristian Hansson of New York, Dr. Richard Kovacs of New York, and Dr. Walter Zeiter of Cleveland, from the American Society of Physical Medicine (now the American Academy of Physical Medicine and Rehabilitation); Dr. John Coulter of Chicago, Dr. Frank Krusen of Rochester, Minnesota, and Dr. Arthur Watkins of Boston, from the American Medical Association; Dr. Leonard Huddleston of Los Angeles, Dr. Benjamin Strickland, Jr., of Washington, D.C., and Dr. William Schmidt of Philadelphia, from the American Congress of Physical Medicine (now the American Congress of Rehabilitation Medicine); and Dr. Robert Bennett of Warm Springs, Georgia, and Dr. Frank Ewerhardt of St. Louis, from the Section of Physical Medicine of the Southern Medical Association. The Board was incorporated in Illinois on February 27, 1947. The first meeting was held in Atlantic City on June 6, 1947. The officers of the Board elected at this meeting were Dr. Krusen, chairman, Dr. Strickland, vice chairman, and Dr. Bennett, secretary–treasurer.

The American Board of Physical Medicine was organized under the auspices of the Advisory Board for Medical Specialties as an affiliated board functioning under the direction of the Committee on Standards and Examinations of the Advisory Board for Medical Specialties and under the auspices of the boards of medicine, orthopedics, and radiology. After 2 years, it became an independent board with full representation on the Advisory Board for Medical Specialties, and it was approved by the Council on Medical Education and Hospitals (now known as the Council on Medical Education) of the AMA.

The first certifying examinations of the American Board of Physical Medicine were held in Minneapolis in August 1947. At the first certification session, 91 diplomates were certified. About half of these were certified on the basis of peer recognition of full-time practice in the field. This was the only time such "grandfathering" was used as a basis for certification by this Board. It is interesting to note that a large number of those considered eligible to be "grandfathered in" responded to a request of the Board to take the written examinations in order to help the Board and the Examinations Committee establish baseline pass–fail performance standards.

In June 1949, the American Board of Physical Medicine became the American Board of Physical Medicine and Rehabilitation with the approval of the Advisory Board for Medical Specialties (now known as the American Board of Medical Specialties).

The gradual growth of the total number of diplomates certified by the Board from 1947 through 1985 is shown in Figure 1-2; the number certified annually ranged from 17 to 71 up through 1976. Beginning in 1977, the number certified each year increased significantly, having since then ranged from 101 to 168 annually. As of 1987, the total number certified as diplomates is 2,748. Each year since 1947 the Board has given a two-part written and oral examination to candidates who have satisfactorily completed a residency program approved by the Residency Review Committee in Physical Medicine and Rehabilitation and accredited by the Accreditation Council on Graduate Medical Education.

Prior to 1980, candidates applying for admissibility to the certification process could use an option of submitting documented evidence of 2 years of full-time clinical practice in physical medicine and rehabilitation as an alternative for 1 year of satisfactorily completed accredited residency training in the specialty. This option was terminated in July 1981.

The Board has given oral examinations (part II of the certification examinations) annually since 1947 to candidates who present evidence of a minimum of 1 full year of broadly based clinical practice in physical and rehabilitation medicine following satisfactory completion of the residency training program, or an acceptable fifth year of advanced residency involvement or other suitable alternative. Before 1977, the clinical practice requirement had been for 2 years. Essentially the same format for the oral examinations has been used since the founding of the Board. Each candidate has three 45-minute oral examinations with three separate examiners. Before 1965, all oral examinations were given by members of the Board. However, as the number of candidates increased, it became necessary to invite selected certified diplomates to assist the Board members as guest oral examiners. Since 1965, 200 guest oral examiners have assisted the Board in the evaluation process. The format for the oral examinations is specified, and a training manual and a training session are provided by the Board for the oral examiners so that there is a unified, structured format with minimal duplication of subject matter. Principles of scoring and grading candidates are carefully structured and standardized. The format has worked well for many years, and studies have shown that new examiners tend to grade comparably with the experienced examiners and Board members. At variance with procedures used in some specialty Board oral examinations, specific questions and answers are not prescribed by the Board's examination committee.

During the past 10 years, the Board has conducted an annual survey of all the residency training programs in order to obtain current statistical data on numbers of trainees in the various years of the residency plus some demographic aspects of residents in training. These data are shared with the residency training program directors and have proved to be a valuable source of information relating to person-power studies in the speciality.

The progressive growth in the number of residents in training, along with the residency positions available in all accredited training programs, is shown in Figure 1-3. The total number of training programs has remained between 65 and 70 during the past 10 years. Each year two or three programs lose accreditation, or withdraw, while two or three new programs receive provisional approval by the accrediting authority of the Residency Review Committee.

Some demographic aspects of residents in training in recent years in relation to foreign and American medical graduates are shown in Figure 1-4. Changes in percentages of male and female residents are indicated in Figure 1-5.

The 24 specialty boards that are members of the American Board of Medical Specialties provide quality assurance services to the public and medical profession. All of these specialty boards are autonomous, nonprofit corporations maintaining functional liaisons with the AMA and the specialty organizations in their field. Specifically, the purpose of the American Board of Physical Medicine and Rehabilitation is to standardize qualifications for specialists in the field and to certify as specialists the

Figure 1-2. Progressive growth of the number of diplomates in physical medicine and rehabilitation from 1947 through 1985. Total certificates awarded annually ranged from 17 to 166 for a total of 2,378 diplomates, 1,146 certified since 1977.

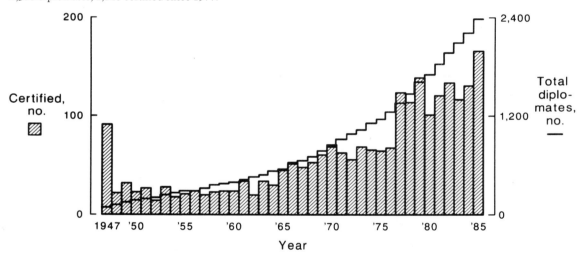

Figure 1-3. The number of training programs in physical medicine and rehabilitation since 1945 increased to 73 in 1960 and remained fairly constant, between 62 and 68, since 1970. Total residency positions reached 819 in 1985.

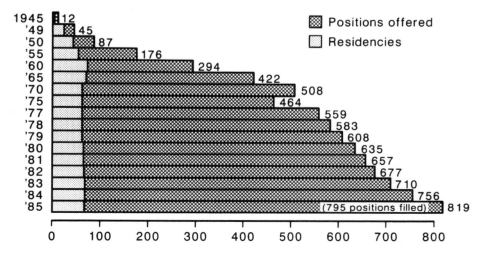

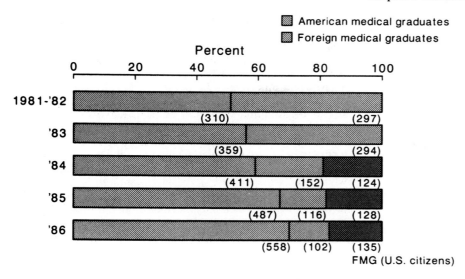

Figure 1-4. Demographics of residents in physical medicine and rehabilitation indicate increasing numbers and percentages of American medical graduates since 1981. Decreases in foreign medical graduates enrolled are indicated.

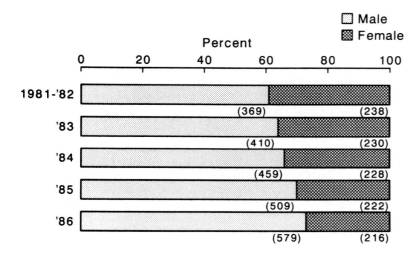

Figure 1-5. Demographics of male and female residents in physical medicine and rehabilitation, 1981 to 1986, indicate an increasing percentage of males, from 61% to 73%, and an essentially constant number of females.

physicians who have voluntarily appeared before it for recognition and certification according to its requirements. Thus, the Board provides assurance to the public and the medical profession that certified physicians possess particular qualifications in their specialty. Qualified applicants for the examinations in 1987 numbered 313 for part I (written) and 316 for part II (oral).

The history of the Board was reviewed by Koepke in the Zeiter lecture of 1971.[24] Its further history, including presentation of statistical studies and analysis related to Board certification, was reviewed by Martin, Gullickson, and Gerken in 1980.[38] The Board comprises 11 directors, and the majority of these have been intimately involved with programs for the training of residents in physical medicine and rehabilitation. New Board directors are elected from lists of five nominees submitted by the American Academy of Physical Medicine and Rehabilitation, the AMA, and the Association of Academic Physiatrists. Members usually serve one or two 6-year terms, and broad geographical representation is considered desirable. The directors of the Board and the oral examiners serve without remuneration. The Board's activities in graduate medical education and certification are coordinated and integrated with the activities of the Residency Review Committee, the Accreditation Council on Graduate Medical Education, the residency training programs, and the American Board of Medical Specialties. The original 1947 incorporation of the American Board of Physical Medicine and Reha-

bilitation in Illinois was dissolved in 1981, and it was then incorporated in 1981 as an autonomous nonprofit corporation in the State of Minnesota.

The current and past Directors of the American Board of Physical Medicine and Rehabilitation are listed in Table 1-5.

Residency Review Committee for Physical Medicine and Rehabilitation

Organizational plans for the establishment of a residency review committee in physical medicine and rehabilitation were undertaken in 1953 following a letter of communication from Dr. Edward Leveroos for the Council on Medical Education of the AMA to the American Board of Physical Medicine and Rehabilitation. Before this time, residencies were granted approval for training by the Council of Medical Education of the AMA. A prototype for the function of the specialty Board as a co-sponsor of a Residency Review Committee had existed for several years in internal medicine. By 1953, there were ten other functioning residency review committees, whose method for the evaluation and approval of residency programs was proving to be effective and efficient. It was proposed that the Residency Review Committee include three representatives of the American Board of Physical Medicine and Rehabilitation and three representatives of the

Table 1-5
Directors and Past Directors, American Board of Physical Medicine and Rehabilitation

Directors (1987)

B. Stanley Cohen, M.D., chairman	Phala A. Helm, M.D.
Murray M. Freed, M.D., vice chairman	Catherine N. Hinterbuchner, M.D.
Robert P. Christopher, M.D.	Malcolm C. McPhee, M.D.
Victor Cummings, M.D.	John L. Melvin, M.D.
Barbara deLateur, M.D.	John W. B. Redford, M.D.
Arthur E. Grant, M.D.	Donald H. See, M.D.
Gordon M. Martin, M.D., executive director	

Past Directors

*Arthur S. Abramson, M.D., 1957–68	H. Worley Kendell, M.D., 1956–65
*Robert L. Bennett, M.D., 1947–63	A. B. C. Knudson, M.D., 1949–66
*Joseph G. Benton, M.D., 1965–76	George H. Koepke, M.D., 1965–76
*Wiliam Bierman, M.D., 1950–56	Frederic J. Kottke, M.D., 1955–69
*John S. Coulter, M.D., 1947–49	*Richard I. Kovacs, M.D., 1947–50
*Donald A. Covalt, M.D., 1951–62	Edward M. Krusen, M.D., 1965–76
John F. Ditunno, Jr., M.D., 1972–84	*Frank H. Krusen, M.D., 1947–49
Alfred Ebel, M.D., 1966–78	Justus F. Lehmann, M.D., 1961–72
*Earl C. Elkins, M.D., 1949–77	*Edward W. Lowman, M.D., 1962–72
*Frank H. Ewerhardt, M.D., 1947–48	Leonard D. Policoff, M.D., 1970–80
Jerome W. Gersten, M.D., 1966–77	Arthur A. Rodriquez, M.D., 1972–80
Edward E. Gordon, M.D., 1968–70	Donald L. Rose, M.D., 1956–67
Glenn Gullickson, Jr., M.D., 1947–48	*William H. Schmidt, M.D., 1947–64
*Kristian G. Hansson, M.D., 1947–60	*Walter M. Solomon, M.D., 1951–54
*Thomas F. Hines, M.D., 1959–64	Benjamin A. Strickland, Jr., M.D., 1947–50
Thomas H. Hohmann, M.D., 1969–74	*Arthur L. Watkins, M.D., 1947–58
*O. Leonard Huddleston, M.D., 1947–60	Walter J. Zeiter, M.D., 1947–55

*Deceased.

Council, two of whom were to be physiatrists. It was stated that the chairman of the committee was to be a Board representative, whereas the secretary was to be a member of the Council. All expenses for the administration and meetings of the committee were to be covered by the Council on Education of the AMA.

The first official meeting of the Residency Review Committee was held in 1954 and included, representing the Board, Drs. Robert L. Bennett, Earl C. Elkins, and Walter M. Solomon; representatives of the Council were Drs. Harold Dinken, Donald L. Rose, and Edward Leveroos. Dr. Elkins was elected the first chairman and Dr. Leveroos the first secretary. The members were, and continue to be, elected or appointed for a 3-year term and are eligible to serve two terms. Original appointments were made on a staggered basis.

The Residency Review Committee meets for one full day twice a year to consider applications for accreditation of new residency programs and applications for renewal of accreditation. Residency survey reports prepared by AMA site visitors are reviewed and discussed. Site visitors are trained as experienced analysts and reporters and sent out by the AMA office to review one or several residency programs at an institution. The members of the Committee are not eligible to serve as specialty site visitors. The site visitors have current information, which is submitted to them by the program directors, plus a protocol and format to be completed for transmission to the Residency Review Committee. The Committee is generally the body that decides when use of a specialist site visitor is indicated. In some instances, additional information or clarification is requested. The Residency Review Committee decides on one of several options regarding the status of a residency program. A new program that appears to have potential for success is given provisional approval for 3 years. Full approval is usually granted after 3 years of effective performance under provisional status, and accreditation is generally renewed after surveys made at 3- to 5-year intervals. Probationary status for a program may be in order when significant questions arise regarding faculty, didactic programs, or clinical teaching and experience. Before a decision is made to give a probationary rating or to withdraw approval, the representatives of the program and the supporting institution have the opportunity to respond to concerns and criticisms by the Residency Review Committee.

The actions of the Residency Review Committee are subject to final approval by the Accreditation Council on Graduate Medical Education, one of its parent bodies. If members of a residency training program, and the sponsoring institution, are dissatisfied with a ruling or action of the Residency Review Committee, they can appeal at the Committee and, if advisable, the Council level.

Usually, 15 to 20 programs are fully or partially considered at a meeting of the Residency Review Committee. The specialty board works closely with the Committee and maintains an up-to-date listing of the accredited programs, the names of the program directors, the names of physiatrists responsible for the residents in training, and details of the training program. Additionally, information is provided by the Board office, from program or institutional staff, from the residents themselves, or by the record of performance of the residents in the certification process. The Executive Secretary of the Residency Review Committee is currently on the staff of the Accreditation Council on Graduate Medical Education and the AMA and provides information on the activities of the Committee to the Council on Education of the AMA, which annually produces the *Directory of Residency Training Programs* (Green Book).

Another important function of the Residency Review Committee is to prepare a statement and detailed description of the special requirements for a residency training program in physical medicine and rehabilitation, which is published annually by the AMA in the *Directory of Residency Training Programs*. The "Special Requirements" section directly follows the section on "General Essentials of a Residency Training Program." These special and general essentials undergo almost constant revision, and occasionally a general rewriting is required. The *Directory* includes a complete listing of all currently accredited residency training programs. The Residency Review Committee welcomes suggestions regarding possible modifications in training program requirements and procedures that might lead to more effective residency training.

The current and past members of the Residency Review Committee in Physical Medicine and Rehabilitation are listed in Table 1-6.

Table 1-6
Past Members of the Residency Review Committee for Physical Medicine and Rehabilitation

Time Period: 1954–82	Current Members 1983–86
Victor Cummings, M.D.*	*American Board of Physical Medicine and Rehabilitation*
Richard S. Materson, M.D.	
Edward M. Krusen, M.D.	John L. Melvin, M.D., chairman
John F. Ditunno, Jr., M.D.	B. Stanley Cohen, M.D.
Gordon M. Martin, M.D.*	Catherine N. Hinterbuchner, M.D.
Glenn Gullickson, Jr., M.D.*	Gordon M. Martin, M.D., ex-officio
Jerome Tobis, M.D.	
Earl C. Elkins, M.D.*	*Council of Medical Education of AMA*
Arthur E. Grant, M.D.	Wiliam J. Erdman II, M.D.,
George H. Koepke, M.D.*	vice-chairman
Oscar Selke, M.D.	Joseph C. Honet, M.D.
Murray M. Freed, M.D.	Roger Pesch, M.D.
Nancy Kester, M.D.	Paul O'Connor, Ph.D., staff
Ernest W. Johnson, M.D.	
Alfred Ebel, M.D.*	
Donald A. Covalt, M.D.	
Leonard D. Policoff, M.D.	
Robert L. Bennett, M.D.*	
Frederic J. Kottke, M.D.*	
Walter J. Zeiter, M.D.	
Arthur L. Watkins, M.D.*	
James W. Rae, M.D.	
Thomas F. Hines, M.D.*	
Edward W. Lowman, M.D.*	
A. B. C. Knudson, M.D.*	
Harold Dinken, M.D.	
Edward Leveroos, M.D.	
Donald L. Rose, M.D.	
Walter M. Solomon, M.D.*	

*Representative of the American Board of Physical Medicine and Rehabilitation.

The American Board of Medical Specialties

The concept of a specialty board in medicine was first proposed in 1908 at the meeting of the American Academy of Ophthalmology and Otolaryngology. The first board to be formed was the American Board for Ophthalmic Examinations, which was incorporated in 1917; the name was changed in 1933 to the American Board of Ophthalmology.[1] The second specialty board was the American Board of Otolaryngology, founded and incorporated in 1924. The third and fourth boards, the American Board of Obstetrics and Gynecology and the American Board of Dermatology and Syphilology, were established in 1930 and 1932. In 1933, a conference was attended by representatives of the four specialty boards, plus the American Hospital Association, the Association of American Medical Colleges, the Federation of State Medical Boards, the AMA Council on Education and Hospitals, and the National Board of Medical Examiners. This group proposed and created the Advisory Board for Medical Specialties, which was organized in 1933 with Dr. Louis Wilson as the first president.

Since 1934, official recognition of specialty boards in medicine has been under the jurisdiction of the Adisory Board for Medical Specialties and later its successor, the American Board of Medical Specialties (ABMS) and the AMA Council on Medical Education.[1] This mechanism was formalized through the establishment of a Liaison Committee for Specialty Boards and the publication of the "Essentials of Approval of Examining Boards in Medical Specialties." This document has undergone several revisions but remains the standard for recognition of new specialty boards. By 1948, eighteen specialty boards had received approval and recognition. Between 1949 and 1969, no new boards were approved by the ABMS and the Liaison Committee for Specialty Boards. Between 1969 and 1979, five specialty boards were approved: Allergy and Immunology, Emergency Medicine, Family Practice, Nuclear Medicine, and Thoracic Surgery. This brought the total to 23 specialty boards.

The ABMS has continued to grow and to expand its interests and concerns, and it provides a forum for representation of all specialty boards. At semiannual sessions, the ABMS considers policies regarding certification procedures and requirements of various boards, length of residency training, and standards for residency programs.

An extensive program involving publications based on several conferences sponsored by the ABMS on examination procedures, educational concepts, and teaching method is functioning effectively. A continuing project of the ABMS is the publication of directories of certified specialists in each specialty.

One division of the ABMS is concerned with research on education in specialty fields, examination procedures for certification, and in-service resident evaluation procedures and their potential role in certification processes. Through annual surveys, the ABMS maintains data regarding residency training and certification in all of the accredited specialties. The American Board of Physical Medicine and Rehabilitation, an active member of the ABMS, has two official delegates and two alternates to provide active participation and voting representation at the annual and semiannual meetings.

The ABMS celebrated its 50th anniversary in 1983.[1] In addition to its own organizational activities, it maintains official functional liaison with the Council for Medical Affairs, the Accreditation Council for Graduate Medical Education, the Accreditation Council for Continuing Medical Education, the National Resident Matching Program, the National Board of Medical Examiners, the Educational Commission for Foreign Medical Graduates, and the Liaison Committee for Specialty Boards.

The Association of Academic Physiatrists

The Association of Academic Physiatrists (AAP) was founded in 1967 in response to a letter from Dr. Ernest Johnson to about 20 academically affiliated physiatrists.[22] Its purpose is to stimulate interest in and share expertise related to undergraduate and graduate academic physiatry. An organization with a strong academic orientation and involvement of its members was needed to gain representation in the Council of Academic Societies. The AAP was selected to be a member of the Association of American Medical Colleges (AAMC) in 1970. It has experienced gradual growth to a membership of 425 in 1986. It has achieved recognition both within the specialty and in several areas of academic medicine. Annual meetings of the AAP have been scheduled to coincide with the meeting of the AAMC with the aim of increasing the visibility of the specialty of physical medicine and rehabilitation as a significant segment of the medical academic community.

The AAP has sponsored workshops and sessions for improving curriculum planning and teaching skills, particularly for physiatrists involved with educational endeavors at all levels. The AAP provides a forum for the American Board of Physical Medicine and Rehabilitation and its residency training program directors and faculties. It encourages increased faculty and resident involvement in high-quality basic and clinical research in both academic-based and other departments of physical medicine and rehabilitation.

The AAP provides advisory services for matching academic positions with potential candidates. It is also one of the nominating organizations for candidates for selection as directors of the American Board of Physical Medicine and Rehabilitation.

The AAP publishes a quarterly newsletter with information of interest to those involved in medical school and graduate medical education and for residents with potential for academic career involvement. It also provides curricular and other academic consultation to medical schools requesting such assistance. In addition, the AAP works with the American Medical Student Association in providing career information.

A listing of AAP presidents serves to reflect the quality and prestige of the leadership this organization has enjoyed:

William J. Erdman, II, M.D.
Henry B. Betts, M.D.
Ray Piaskoski, M.D.
Murray M. Freed, M.D.
Nadene Coyne, M.D.
Joseph Goodgold, M.D.
John F. Ditunno, Jr., M.D.
Justus Lehmann, M.D.
Ernest W. Johnson, M.D.
George H. Kraft, M.D.
Paul Corcoran, M.D.
Martin Grabois, M.D.
John Melvin, M.D.
Paul Kaplan, M.D.

The International Rehabilitation Medicine Association

Since 1940, several international organizations have been formed with various goals and related in various ways to specialty areas pertaining to rehabilitation. Probably the most active international organization, and the one with the widest membership in the 1980s is the International Rehabilitation Medicine Association (IRMA). IRMA was founded by Dr. Sidney Licht in 1969. Dr. Licht, editor of the 11-volume *Physical Medicine Library* and a Connecticut-based physiatrist, had for many years been a world traveler and had established many professional and personal contacts with physicians interested in physical and rehabilitation medicine. Almost single-handedly, he developed the basic plans for the organization, its aims, and its meeting schedules.

IRMA is a society of physicians from all specialties of medicine and surgery who are interested in promoting the art and science of medicine and in the improvement of health through an understanding and utilization of rehabilitation medicine. IRMA's objectives are based on the recognition that at least 300 million people of all ages require rehabilitation services in the treatment of their disabilities. This is perceived as being the most serious public health problem confronting every nation of the world at the present time. The goal of IRMA is to educate and encourage government and society to recognize the reality of this need and to provide rehabilitation medicine services for this vast number of chronically diseased and disabled people, including the aged, and to promote medical research in this area.

IRMA offers its members the opportunity to broaden their professional competence through the formation of and participation in activities of scientific sections geared to medical and surgical specialties and to other areas of interest, including education and research. IRMA sponsors a "world congress" every

4 years. The IRMA I meeting was held in Italy in 1970, IRMA II in Mexico City in 1974, IRMA III in Basel, Switzerland, in 1978, IRMA IV in Puerto Rico in 1982, and IRMA V in Manila in 1986. The IRMA VI meeting is scheduled for 1990 in Madrid. The official journal of IRMA, titled *International Rehabilitation Medicine,* is published four times a year.

This organization maintains liaison with the International Federation for Physical Medicine and Rehabilitation, the Medical Commission of Rehabilitation International, and the World Health Organization. IRMA is governed by an executive committee comprising officers and eight members elected by the general assembly at the business meeting of the World Congress. The presidents of this organization since its founding have included Drs. C. Wynn Perry (Great Britain), Silvano Boccardi (Italy), Luis Ibarra (Mexico), Wilhelm Zinn (Switzerland), Herman Flax (Puerto Rico), and Tyrone Reyes (Philippines). The IRMA Honorary Secretary is Dr. Martin Grabois, Department of Physical Medicine, Baylor College of Medicine, Houston, Texas.

The Baruch Committee on Physical Medicine and Rehabilitation

In the early 1940s, Bernard Baruch, a renowned financier, philanthropist, and personal advisor to the presidents of the United States from World War I until his death in 1965, became vitally interested in the developing new specialty of Physical Medicine and Rehabilitation. His interest was initiated by admiration for his father, Dr. Simon Baruch, who had been a physician involved with care of Civil War soldiers and later a physician practicing in New York City. He had been particularly interested in physical activities and in hydrotherapy in the rehabilitation and return of soldiers to active duty. Dr. Simon Baruch had written the textbook *An Epitome of Hydrotherapy,* published in 1920 and republished in 1950 under Bernard Baruch's auspices in honor of his father.[3] As a memorial to his father, he wished to provide significant support to the development of physical medicine as a specialty area because of what it had meant to the elder Baruch. He approached Dr. Frank Krusen at the Mayo Clinic, in 1942, who assembled and organized a committee of physiatrists and noted consultants from several other specialties and from the basic sciences of physiology and physics.[28, 29] This committee, under the chairmanship of Dr. Ray Lyman Wilbur, and its consultants included about 40 enthusiastic and capable scientists who (1) proposed and initiated opportunities and encouragement for training of residents in physical medicine, (2) established model training and research centers, and (3) encouraged and supported pertinent research projects in specialized institutions, including the Massachusetts Institute of Technology and several other university centers.

The Baruch Committee was extremely active for 4 years, during which time its basic aims were achieved, and its influence has continued within the specialty. Approximately 50 physicians received sponsorship and aid with their residency training from the Baruch Committee. The principal research and development centers that were established with some original funding and other support from the Baruch Committee were Columbia University College of Physicians and Surgeons, to establish a model center for basic research and teaching of physical medicine, the University of Minnesota Medical School, Harvard Medical School, the University of Southern California, the Medical College of Virginia, and New York University College of Medicine. The Massachusetts Institute of Technology was given a grant to establish a center on biophysics, electronics, and instrumentation as related to medicine. Some Baruch Committee–supported residents had opportunity for research experience at this center.

In the post–World War II era, there was rapidly increasing interest and development in rehabilitation concepts and services, which had evolved significantly in military medicine. Dr. Howard Rusk was a prime developer and promoter in this area after his involvement in the Air Force medical services.[45] His enthusiasm, coupled with his organizational, promotional, and communication abilities, rapidly raised the level of interest of many physicians, hospitals, and medical centers in providing effective medical rehabilitation services and training programs for physicians and other essential rehabilitation personnel.

Dr. Rusk developed the outstanding New York University rehabilitation center, which became the largest residency training program, a position it held for many years. His writing for the *New York Times,* as an associate editor, was an important public relations resource regarding physical and rehabilitation medicine. Dr. Rusk is recognized for his efforts in involving many foreign countries and their physicians in rehabilitation medicine. Through the World Rehabilitation Fund, trainees were aided in obtaining training in the United States. In addition, educational and service programs have been organized and implemented in many parts of the world.

The Baruch Committee and the Special Exhibit Committee on Physical Medicine of the AMA sponsored and arranged for extensive state of the art scientific exhibits for the AMA conventions and interim meetings in 1948 and 1949. These were described by Krusen and co-workers.[31]

The Role of Specific Disorders in the Development of Rehabilitation Medicine

Poliomyelitis

In the 1940s there was a revolution in the management of patients with both acute and chronic poliomyelitis. Before the use of new concepts promulgated by the Australian nurse Sister Elizabeth Kenny, patients who had paralytic poliomyelitis were treated for many weeks and months with plaster-shell supports of the extremities and trunk muscles weakened by the anterior horn cell involvement of poliomyelitis. These long periods of supportive bed rest and splinting were generally followed by efforts at reestablishing ambulation, often including extensive bracing, crutches, walkers, and wheelchairs.

Sister Kenny, through her observation of the clinical course and management of poliomyelitis patients in Australia and England, had evolved concepts of the pathophysiology that were not compatible with the pathologists' descriptions of anterior horn cell inflammation and destruction as the basic lesion. A new term, *mental alienation,* was used instead of *paralysis,* and daily treatment with hot packs for pain and spasm followed by passive and retraining exercises was prescribed. Sister Kenny and her co-workers used precise, standardized manual muscle testing and grading procedures done at frequent intervals. A Sister Kenny Institute for treatment of poliomyelitis was established in Minneapolis with a number of affiliated satellite centers, some in conjunction with support from the National Foundation for Infantile Paralysis.

Dr. Miland Knapp, a pioneer physiatrist in Minneapolis, who, with his associates, worked with Sister Kenny for several years in the management of these patients, modified and refined some of her original concepts of disease and its manifestations. At the same time, he acknowledged the important contributions Sister Kenny had made to the subject of poliomyelitis:[23]

(1) She has emphasized muscle shortening as a cause of deformity, and has pointed out that this shortening is not secondary to anterior horn cell damage, but is a positive entity which requires positive treatment in the early stages if future deformity is to be minimized.

(2) She has systematized a technique of muscle re-education which really deserves the name "re-education" and which is based upon sound physiologic principles and logical reasoning.

(3) She has emphasized a positive approach to the treatment, emphasizing stress upon those things which can be treated with some hope of success such as muscle shortening, reversible paralyses and incoordination, and relatively ignoring those things for which no treatment is successful, namely, anterior horn cell degeneration with motor denervation.[23]

As Sister Kenny's methods and observations gained the support of physicians at the University of Minnesota and elsewhere, the importance of the new specialty of physical medicine in providing a new style of treatment for poliomyelitis rapidly evolved. Dr. Robert L. Bennett, long-time medical director and physiatrist at the Georgia Warm Springs Foundation, pointed out the importance of the evolution of a sound basis for the practice of physical medicine.[4]

Polio, more than any other disease, was the workshop and the showcase for demonstration of the physical aspects of medical care. The pathology of polio was never very difficult to understand . . .

Even though confined almost entirely to lower motor neurons, polio is never monotonous in its manifestations. Each patient seen is a neuromuscular puzzle with patterns of weakness and paralysis of endless variety. If the puzzle is not solved—and solved quickly—musculoskeletal complications result which create new and intriguing puzzles for us to solve. Probably from no other disease have we learned so much about the pathogenesis of musculoskeletal deformities and their functional significance.

The severe impairment not infrequently caused by polio has had great influence on the development of the concept of realistic functional goals for these patients . . .

. . . Highly refined methods of muscle evaluation and care were developed which we believe keep impairment within the bounds of irreversible pathology. Such evaluation and the subsequent formulation of the prescription for care required a knowledge of functional anatomy and muscle retraining. It was through our experience with polio that this knowledge became one of the cornerstones of physical medicine.

There is no reason to believe that manual muscle testing was devised entirely for evaluation of the patient with poliomyelitis, but certainly the systems of manual muscle testing now used to determine and record voluntary muscle strength were developed and refined from the demands of caring for such patients.

Muscle re-education was, and of course still is, a natural follow-through of thorough muscle testing. It seems unnecessary to state that exercise of weakened muscles without accurate knowledge of their strength and their response to exercise is as illogical as it is dangerous.

Functional training . . . was a natural outgrowth of muscle re-education. Functional achievement for the polio patient required new and different techniques in both physical and occupational therapy, and new and different orthotic devices . . . Literally hundreds of . . . functional orthotic devices all developed from our experience with polio.

As we learned how to save the lives of patients with severe and extensive damage to the nervous system, knowledge and experience gained from polio were immediately applicable to the care of the paraplegic, the hemiplegic, the quadriplegic and even the severely brain-damaged patient.[4]

Dr. Bennett continued, "I am convinced that it was through contact with patients who had polio that physiatrists first were established as clinicians with the special interest, essential training and recognized competence in handling those conditions that require carefully prescribed activity."[4]

Changes in the management of poliomyelitis were paralleled by the rapid development of new tools for patients with respiratory impairment and paralysis. Mechanical respirators of several types were introduced, improved, and functionally refined. The large tank-type negative-pressure respirators ("iron lungs") became the standard device and in many instances proved to be life-saving supportive equipment. These devices were stockpiled by the National Foundation for Infantile Paralysis in a number of cities during epidemic years and were made available to hospitals, treatment centers, and patients at home. Other devices included cuirass-type respirators that could be used in wheelchairs and beds, rocking beds, and abdominal pressure belts called pneumobelts. Phrenic nerve stimulators for respiratory paralysis were successfully used in several centers. These phrenic nerve stimulators were later used for selected high-cervical-level traumatic quadriplegic patients.

Spinal Cord Injury and Cerebrovascular Accident

Active interest in rehabilitation of patients with spinal cord injuries evolved in the 1940s, both in England and the United States. Dr. Ludwig Guttmann founded the Stoke-Mandeville National Spinal Cord Injury Center in 1943 in Aylesbury.[16] By 1965 there were seven other national centers in Great Britain. In 1946 Guttmann described some of the problems in management of those patients.[15] In the United States, the first large and comprehensive spinal cord injury center was established at the Hines Veterans Administration Hospital in suburban Chicago. Extensive developments and progress in this area are well documented in several standard textbooks and reference articles.

An in-depth analysis of needs of hemiplegics for expanding rehabilitation services was made in the challenging 1973 Zeiter lecture given by Dr. Kottke.[25]

Summary of the History of Physical Medicine and Rehabilitation

A historical perspective of the specialty of physical medicine and rehabilitation as seen from the late 1980s shows the first glimmers of a new specialty originating in the 1920s. At first, and during the 1930s, there was grouping for a sound base and direction and the seeking of more physician manpower; in the 1940s, the specialty was seen emerging from a physical treatment base to the larger concept incorporating total rehabilitation. Since 1947, growth in residency training and certification of specialists was the significant thrust. Since 1960, there has been increasing recognition of the specialty by the medical community and the public with its growing awareness of needs for more rehabilitation services for the vast numbers of disabled, handicapped, and aging people.

The developments to date indicate growing and active specialty organizations, most notably the following:

American Congress of Rehabilitation Medicine—65 years old with 3,200 members, comprising many medical and allied health professionals
American Academy of Physical Medicine and Rehabilitation—50 years old with 2,500 fellows, associates, and junior members
American Board of Physical Medicine and Rehabilitation—40 years old with over 2,750 certified diplomates
Association of Academic Physiatrists—20 years old with 500 members

International Rehabilitation Medicine Association—17 years old with 450 members

The scientific programs and exhibits at the annual Academy–Congress meetings, plus publications in the *Archives of Physical Medicine and Rehabilitation,* reveal increasing research productivity as well as growing involvement in other areas such as sports medicine, pediatric rehabilitation, and geriatrics.

All of these observations indicate a vital and maturing medical specialty. We see a specialty that is still understaffed, but with multiple opportunities for quality physiatrists in academic settings as well as in clinical practice in many cities and states, some of which have real and perceived deficiencies in providing adequate rehabilitation services.

Epidemiology of Disability

During the past 50 years, medicine and surgery have prevented the deaths of countless people who were critically ill. However, many of these people were left with major disabilities. Multiple sample surveys have estimated that between 5% and 10% of the total population fall into this category of disability. These disabled people have greatly increased costs for maintenance in addition to the costs of medical care required because of the continuing disability. The costs for dependency resulting from such disabilities have a negative effect on the economy, whether those costs are paid by private or by public funds. In either case, dependency consumes resources without enhancing productivity or quality of life for the patient.

What is the economic cost of dependency? Currently in the United States, 10 million people receive disability payments for assistance in maintaining themselves. This is approximately 11% of the gross national product being devoted to disability payments made to about 5% of the population.[51] In 1982, workers' compensation costs were estimated to be $13.8 billion and Social Security costs were $23.1 billion.[43, 52] More than 10% of the population have physical disabilities that limit normal daily activity, self-care, or employment. From 3% to 5% of the population need rehabilitation service at some time.[26] The total federal disability-related expenditures for this working age population were $63 billion in 1977 and have been increasing about 35% per year.

Current Academic Status of Physical Medicine and Rehabilitation

Physical medicine and rehabilitation is one of the projected shortage medical specialties. The American Board of Physical Medicine and Rehabilitation has certified over 2,700 diplomates, 1,500 of them since 1977. The Graduate Medical Education National Advisory Committee (GMENAC) projects a need for an additional 1,800 physiatrists by 1990.[21] The GMENAC information has probably been somewhat responsible for the increase in physical medicine and rehabilitation resident positions and for the greater percentage of American medical graduates in physical medicine and rehabilitation (see Fig. 1-2). In 1985, there were 819 resident slots offered and 795 (97%) filled. There has been an 8.7% increase in resident slots filled in the past year and a 30% increase in the past 5 years. Seventy percent of physical medicine and rehabilitation trainees in the academic year 1985–86 were American medical graduates.

However, the GMENAC data do not seem to have an effect on curriculum planning within medical schools.[6] The specialty is taught in only 68 of the 124 accredited American medical schools. Only 56 of those 68 medical schools in which physical medicine is taught have separate physical medicine and rehabilitation departments. This number has been fairly constant for the past 10 years without increased exposure of the specialty and treatment approach and modalities to medical students. The concept of rehabilitation has become a philosophy of medical responsibility. The American public has accepted this philosophy and seeks its application as the accepted standard of care. However, this concept has not been incorporated into medical practice as taught by many medical schools. This lack of growth of physical medicine and rehabilitation departments may reflect a low priority and lack of understanding within medical schools and/or inadequate funding.

The major bottleneck to balancing the supply and demand for physiatrists is the marked shortage of academic physiatrists.[8] In 1985, there were 442 faculty physiatrists at the primary facilities of the training programs and 470 at the affiliated facilities. From the results of Lane's survey, only 28 of the 71 programs report a faculty of more than five members.[32] According to Dr. Gordon Martin, executive director of the American Board of Physical Medicine and Rehabilitation, the results of a recent survey indicate that these 68 programs project a need, at their programs alone, for an additional 110 academic physiatrists within the next 3 years without expansion into other medical schools.[33]

Finding qualified academic physiatrists who are willing to chair a department of rehabilitation medicine is another significant problem.[8] Considering the excellent quality of residents entering the physical medicine and rehabilitation specialty, these academic shortages should be corrected within the next decade. Until that time, the trend for departments or sections of rehabilitation medicine to be categorized administratively under "rehabilitation related specialties" such as neurology, neurosurgery, orthopedics, or rheumatology will continue. For this academic shortage to be corrected, the specialty must produce academically qualified physiatrists who develop a research base.

At present, residents completing training in physical medicine and rehabilitation can usually choose the city of their choice for their private practice. This is fine for private practitioners but has hurt academic programs. Physiatry is well accepted in the private sector but, unfortunately, has some problems with recognition in academic institutions. Unlike the other specialties, residents in physical medicine and rehabilitation can enter academics without fellowship training. The lack of fellowship training, due to a lack of fellowship training positions and the ready availability of faculty positions, has deprived academic physiatrists of the opportunity to learn grant writing techniques, experimental design, and statistical analysis and to develop within their area of interest the specific techniques necessary for a lifetime of productive research.[8] Many, if not most, academic physiatrists either do not publish papers or jump from one clinical area to another and lack a constant theme to their research.[8]

For physical medicine and rehabilitation to survive as a viable clinical academic discipline, it must develop a stronger research base. As part of training, every resident who expresses an interest in research and an academic career should be given specific time during the residency to learn basic research techniques, whether in the areas of biophysics, biomechanics, neuroscience, or physiology. Selected residents with strong research credentials should be given special training pathways with emphasis on training for academic careers. All physical medicine and rehabilitation residency programs should offer journal clubs and research seminars in which the residents can develop skills in analyzing the literature and evaluating the methodology, results, and conclusions. The graduating residents should be encouraged to participate in a fellowship program to learn these skills. These fellowships should be for at least 2 years. Fellow-

ships offered through the National Institute for Disability and Rehabilitation Research, the Physical Medicine and Rehabilitation Educational Research Foundation, or other sources must be greatly expanded. A significant number of qualified mentors either within the specialty or other basic science and/or clinical departments must also be developed. The field must actively recruit graduates from the master's degree and doctorate programs, especially those with majors in neurosciences.

A high proportion of physical medicine and rehabilitation faculty spend an inordinate amount of their time doing clinical work, which detracts from the quality and quantity of their research. Perhaps the comprehensive nature of our clinical approach makes it difficult for physiatrists to concentrate in one research area and on one basic question. Many academic physiatrists consider our field to be primarily clinical and not appropriate for basic science research. Yet, before our academic work is acknowledged to be commensurate with that of other specialties, and in order for physiatrists to acquire the national stature necessary to avoid repeated crises within medical schools, it is imperative that we make basic science research as much a part of every physical medicine and rehabilitation department as the clinical science component.[8, 10, 19, 34, 50] It is critical, in order to better understand the nature and impact of disabilities, that the field develop a solid scientific base through both basic and applied research.

Academic Training Trends

It is impossible to predict the future, but one must try, since it is critical for short- and long-term planning. Patient outcome, competition, and cost-effectiveness will be the major determinants in physician and allied health professional selection for rehabilitation teams. The physiatry training programs will emphasize primary care for the disabled, but the specific services through which the residents rotate most likely will be thematically based on specific patient–client groups such as spinal cord injury, head injury, and amputee. Fellowship programs will be developed at specific training sites with the goal of developing academic physiatrists within these thematic groups. Unfortunately, funding of graduate education probably will be cut back even for shortage specialties. If the federal government decreases graduate medical education funding, and if the individual states and the third party providers cannot, or will not, absorb the cost, then we can anticipate a return to a preceptorship system in which the trainees perform a specified amount of clinical work/service in return for their specialized training.

Practice Trends

Health and medical care are undergoing evaluation and change in the United States that inevitably will affect the delivery of rehabilitation services. The driving force is the economics of health care.[51] In 1984, spending on health and medical care in the United States reached $450 billion per year, or about $2,000 per person. Hence, in predicting the future of rehabilitation medicine, one must consider costs and cost-effectiveness. Cost-effectiveness leads to cost-containment efforts. Public support for rehabilitation services and methodology, although presently strong, probably will be correlated to reliable scientific data that relate treatment to effectiveness and outcome. Unfortunately, much of what is done in rehabilitation treatment has not been analyzed in that light. Social and economic pressures will force alternative cost-effective methods for providing rehabilitation services (*e.g.,* day hospital, inpatient, outpatient, and home health care programs, as well as independent living centers). The trend may be toward ambulatory as opposed to inpatient service. All rehabilitation services must focus on the needs of these market segments (*i.e.,* patients, referring institutions, and third party payers). In predicting the future, one has to take into account finance and legislation, and either of these could drastically alter the future of rehabilitation services.[13]

As is presently occurring, marketing methods will be applied to the practice of rehabilitation medicine. The economics of rehabilitation service's delivery in the 1990s will probably include a reimbursement system based on the prospective payment system instead of a cost-based, retrospective reimbursement. It may also include physician payments.[18] The prospective payment system can limit the total costs, and the payers may not be involved in making decisions about which treatment should be given each patient.[51] This prospective payment system will possibly be based on a catastrophic classification system and will gradually develop into a bidding system based on specific groups of disabilities.[18] Capitation funding with or without additional reimbursement for high-cost services may also be present. Keen, aggressive competition may develop between rehabilitation service providers to obtain their market share for these contracts. Rehabilitation is becoming a big health care business, and there needs to be cooperation between the physicians and the professional management. More nontraditional providers may attempt to enter the rehabilitation market. Primary care providers will try to absorb rehabilitation into their practice.[11] The health care system will probably become more of a market system. Purchasers may select rehabilitation providers based on factors such as outcome, close accessibility of patients to their living environment, quality of service, type of services, and price. Some of the financial risks will be shifted from the purchaser to the provider of rehabilitation services. Unfortunately, health care may be rationed so that a three-level system could evolve: (1) a low-cost, moderate-outcome level for the publicly funded patients; (2) a moderate-cost and moderate-to-good outcome level, funded by private corporations; and (3) a high-cost and moderate-to-excellent outcome system, funded by private paying patients who have the means to purchase health care in excess of that provided by their employers or government.[18, 50]

Even though cost containment will be a major driving force, there must be a counterbalance that ensures the quality of programs and services. Thus, it is important that rehabilitation personnel become active in developing monitors and standards of care. Inpatient rehabilitation for the elderly, or those people with limited potential for full independence, may be treated in skilled nursing facilities and/or intermediate care facilities. Specific geriatric rehabilitation programs will be developed. As indicated earlier, physiatrists may be primary care providers for specific groups of disabled patients with disabilities such as spinal cord injury, head injury, cerebral palsy, muscular dystrophy, and cerebrovascular disease.

Technology will give us the ability to better manage and use information. This information should include specific patient care information, as well as information related to strategic planning, marketing, program evaluation, and finances. It also holds great potential for improving the quality of life for patients with disabilities. Computers will be used for patient information data bases and monitoring therapeutic progress with respect to the specific therapy goals. Rehabilitation engineering will match patient needs with the proper adaptive equipment.

The organization of rehabilitation service delivery in 1990 may be dominated by multihospital chains, either not-for-profit or for-profit.[18] Some insurance companies are buying or planning to operate their own hospital chains.[51] Competition will be keen for controlling the flow of patients. Freestanding rehabilitation hospitals or centers may decline in number and become regionally based for low-to-moderate acuity and higher functional potential of patients and for the purposes of provision of

education and research to advance the field.[18] These freestanding faculties will have to serve their catchment areas carefully. Outpatient services will be expanded, and many more patients will be treated as outpatients instead of inpatients; outpatient services will also become organized from single discipline services to comprehensive rehabilitation services based on increasing consumer need and demand for this type of service integration. Rehabilitation hotels/motels will serve as overnight facilities to keep the cost down for patients traveling to the outpatient service.[18] Home rehabilitation programs and outreach programs with satellite clinics will be expanded, once again avoiding expensive inpatient treatments. Fitness and wellness programs to maintain health for the disabled will be expanded. The future for rehabilitation services looks bright, but the need to document outcomes and to be competitive with respect to cost-effectiveness and efficiency will become key issues.[18]

Rehabilitation medicine encompasses a special body of knowledge and procedural skills to help patients with acute and/or chronic disease maximize their level of independence. The specialty is relatively young but has already proven its clinical practice value and has the ideal training to produce primary care providers for patients with disabilities. The academic aspects of the specialty need further development, and a core research base with ties to basic science must be established. It is an exciting, growing specialty that emphasizes prevention and treatment. It is not organ based; it can be either hospital or nonhospital based; and it treats all age groups, which allows the practitioner the maximum flexibility to develop a challenging dynamic practice.

REFERENCES

1. American Board of Medical Specialties: 50th Anniversary Edition Annual Report & Reference Handbook. Chicago, IL, 1983
2. Bair J, Gray MS (eds): The Occupational Therapy Manager. Rockville, MD, American Occupational Therapy Association, 1985
3. Baruch S: An Epitome of Hydrotherapy for Physicians, Architects and Nurses. Philadelphia, WB Saunders, 1920, reprinted 1950
4. Bennett RL: Editorial: The contribution to physical medicine of our experience with poliomyelitis. Arch Phys Med Rehabil 50:522–524, 1969
5. Blaxter M: The future of rehabilitation services in Great Britain. Int Rehabil Med 2:199–209, 1980
6. Bowman MA, Katzoff JM, Garrison LP Jr, Will J: Estimates of physician requirements for 1990 for specialties of neurology, anesthesiology, nuclear medicine, pathology, physical medicine and rehabilitation, and radiology: Further application of GMENAC methodology. JAMA 250:2623–2637, 1983
7. Coulter JS: History and development of physical medicine. Arch Phys Med Rehabil 28:600–602, 1947
8. DeLisa JA: Compounding the challenge for PM&R in the 1990s. Arch Phys Med Rehabil 66:792–793, 1985
9. Dyer WG: Team Building: Issues and Alternatives. Reading, MA, Addison-Wesley, 1977
10. Fowler WM Jr: Viability of physical medicine and rehabilitation in the 1980s. Arch Phys Med Rehabil 61:1–5, 1982
11. Freeman SA: Sounding board—Megacorporate health care. N Engl J Med 312:579–582, 1985
12. Gaston EH: Developing a motivating organizational climate for effective team functioning. Hosp Community Psychiatry 31:407–412, 1980
13. Gellman W: Projections in the field of physical disability. Rehabil Lit 35:2–9, 1974
14. Given B, Simmons S: Interdisciplinary health care team: Fact or fiction? Nurs Forum 15:116–184, 1977
15. Guttmann L: Problems of physical therapy for persons with traumatic paraplegia. Arch Phys Med Rehabil 27:750–756, 1946
16. Guttmann L: Spinal Cord Injuries: Comprehensive Management & Research. Oxford, Blackwell Scientific Publications, 1973
17. Halstead LS: Team care in chronic illness: Critical review of literature of past 25 years. Arch Phys Med Rehabil 61:507–511, 1976

18. Harvey RF: The future of rehabilitation: Delivery of rehabilitation services in the 1990's. In Maloney FP (ed): A Primer on Management for Rehabilitation Medicine, pp 321–330. Philadelphia, Hanly and Belfus, 1987

19. Herbison GJ: Research ends, setting environment activities, resources, creativity, health. Arch Phys Med Rehabil 65:112–114, 1984

20. Hollander AR: The American Congress of Physical Therapy: Ten years of progress. Arch Phys Med Rehabil 50:223–226, 1969. Reprinted from Arch Phys Ther X-Ray Rad 16:425–528, 1935

21. Honet JC: Manpower planning for physical medicine and rehabilitation: Comments on GMENAC process. Arch Med Rehabil 65:404–407, 1984

22. Johnson EC: The Association of Academic Physiatrists: Personal communication, 1986

23. Knapp ME: The contribution of Sister Elizabeth Kenny to the treatment of poliomyelitis. Arch Phys Med Rehabil 50:535–542, 1969. Abridged form of 1941 article

24. Koepke GH: The American Board of Physical Medicine and Rehabilitation: Past, present and future. Arch Phys Med Rehabil 53:10–13, 1972

25. Kottke FJ: Historic obscura hemiplegiac: Arch Phys Med Rehabil 55:4–13, 1974

26. Kottke FJ: Future Focus of Rehabilitation Medicine. Arch Phys Med Rehabil 61:1–6, 1980

27. Kovacs R: Progress in physical medicine during the past twenty-five years. Arch Phys Med Rehabil 27:473–477, 1946

28. Krusen FH: And now to carry the torch of Aesculapius. Arch Phys Med Rehabil 50:709–712, 1969

29. Krusen FH: The expanding field of physical medicine. Arch Phys Med Rehabil 27:201–202, 1946

30. Krusen FH: Historical development in physical medicine and rehabilitation during the last forty years. Arch Phys Med Rehabil 50:1–5, 1969

31. Krusen FH: Physical Medicine: The Employment of Physical Agents for Diagnosis and Therapy, chaps 1 and 2. Philadelphia, WB Saunders, 1941

32. Krusen FH, Overholser W et al: Exhibit of physical medicine: Physical therapy, occupational therapy and rehabilitation: Committee report. Arch Phys Med 27:491–498, 1946

33. Lane ME: Preparing for 1990s: A challenge to specialty of PM&R. Arch Phys Med Rehabil 65:740–741, 1984

34. Lehmann JF: Rehabilitation medicine: Past, present and future. Arch Phys Med Rehabil 63:291–297, 1982

35. Longest BB Jr: Management Practices for the Health Professional, 3rd ed, pp 99–158. Reston, VA, Reston Publishing Company, 1984

36. Lundberg LB: What is leadership. J Nurs Admin 12:32–33, 1982

37. Martin G: Physical medicine and rehabilitation residencies in the mid 80s: A report from the American Board of PM&R. Assoc Acad Physiatrist Newsletter 3(4):6–7, 1985

38. Martin GM, Gullickson G Jr, Gerken C: Graduate medical education and certification in physical medicine and rehabilitation. Arch Phys Med Rehabil 61:291–297, 1980

39. Melvin JL: Interdisciplinary and multidisciplinary activities and ACRM. Arch Phys Med Rehabil 61:379–380, 1980

40. Mock HE: Rehabilitation. Arch Phys Med Rehabil 24:676–677, 1943. Reprinted 50:474–475, 1969

41. Nelson PA: History of the Archives: A journal of ideas and ideals. Arch Phys Rehabil 50:367–405, 1969

42. Nelson PA: History of the once close relationship between electrotherapeutics and radiology. Arch Phys Med Rehabil 54:608–640, 1973

43. Pope M, Frymoger J, Andersson G: Occupational Low Back Pain, p 116. New York, Praeger, 1984

44. Rothberg JS: The rehabilitation team: Future directions. Arch Phys Med Rehabil 62:407–410, 1981

45. Rusk HA: Editorial: The growth and development of rehabilitation medicine. Arch Phys Med Rehabil 50:463–466, 1969

46. Sharf BF (in consultation with Flaherty JA): The Physician's Guide to Better Communication, pp 82–91. Glenview, IL, Scott, Foresman & Co, 1984

47. Stickland BA Jr: Physical medicine in the Army. Arch Phys Med Rehabil 28:229–236, 1947

48. Stillwell GK: Meeting a need. Arch Phys Med Rehabil 50:489–494, 1969

49. Stillwell GK: Whence our academy? Arch Phys Med Rehabil 64:97–100, 1983

50. Stolov WC: Rehabilitation research training. Arch Phys Med Rehabil 65:54–56, 1984

51. Thurow LC: Medicine versus economics. N Engl J Med 313:611–614, 1985

52. Tyson K, Merrill JC: Health Care institutions: Survival in a changing environment. J Med Ed 59:773–782, 1984

APPENDIX 1-1. VITAL FACTS ABOUT SOME MEMBERS OF THE REHABILITATION TEAM

Discipline	Organization	Text	Journal	Certification
Occupational therapist	American Occupational Therapy Association 1383 Piccard Drive Suite 301 Rockville, MD 20850 (301) 948-9626	Hopkins HL, Smith HD (eds): Williard & Spackman's, Occupational Therapy, 6th ed. Philadelphia, JB Lippincott, 1983	American Journal of Occupational Therapy (monthly)	Yes
Physical therapist	U.S. Physical Therapy Association 1803 Avon Lane Arlington Heights, IL 60004 (312) 255-6740	Lehmkuhl LD, Smith LK (eds): Brunnstrom's Clinical Kinesiology, 4th ed. Philadelphia, FA Davis, 1983	Physical Therapy	Yes
		Nelson RM, Currier DP: Clinical Electrotherapy. East Norwalk, CT, Appleton & Lange, 1987		
		Kisher C, Colby LA: Therapeutic Exercise: Foundations & Techniques. Philadelphia, FA Davis, 1985		

(Continued)

APPENDIX 1-1. (*Continued*)

Discipline	Organization	Text	Journal	Certification
Prosthetist/orthotist	American Orthotic and Prosthetic Association 717 Pendleton Street Alexandria, VA 22314 (703) 836-7116	Redford JB (ed): Orthotics Etcetera, 3rd ed. Baltimore, Williams & Wilkins, 1986 American Academy of Orthopaedic Surgeons: Atlas of Limb Prosthetics: Surgical and Prosthetic Principles. St. Louis, CV Mosby, 1981	Orthotic & Prosthetics	Yes
Rehabilitation nurse	Rehabilitation Nursing Institute 2506 Gross Pointe Road Evanston, IL 60201 (312) 475-7300		Rehabilitation Nursing (bimonthly)	Yes
Speech pathologist	American Speech-Language-Hearing Association 10801 Rockville Pike Rockville, MD 20852 (301) 897-5700	Boone DR: Human Communication and its Disorders. Englewood Cliffs, NJ, Prentice-Hall, 1987	Journal of Speech and Hearing Disorders (quarterly)	Yes
Social worker	National Association of Social Workers 7981 Eastern Avenue Silver Spring, MD 20910 (301) 565-0333	Hepworth DH, Larsen JA: Direct Social Work Practice: Theory & Skills, 2nd ed. Chicago, IL, Dorsey Press, 1986	Social Work (bimonthly) Health and Social Work (quarterly)	Yes
Vocational counselor	American Association for Counseling and Development 5999 Stevenson Avenue Suite 307 Alexandria, VA 22304 (703) 829-9800		Journal of Counseling and Development (10 issues per year)	Yes
Child life therapist	Association for the Care of Children's Health 3615 Wisconsin Avenue Washington, DC 20016 (202) 244-1801 (202) 244-8922	Thomas RH, Stanford G: Child Life in Hospitals: Theory and Practice. Springfield, IL, Charles C Thomas, 1981	Journal of the Association for the Care of Children's Health (quarterly)	No
Corrective therapist	American Corrective Therapy Association 259-08 148 Road Rosedale, NY 11422 (718) 276-0721		American Corrective Therapy Journal	Yes
Horticultural therapist	National Council for Therapy and Rehabilitation through Horticulture (NCTRH) 9220 Wightman Road Suite 300 Gaithersburg, MD 20879 (301) 948-3010		Journal of Therapeutic Horticulture (annually)	No
Music therapist	National Association of Music Therapists 505 11th Street, SE Washington, DC 20003 (202) 543-6864		Journal of Music Therapy (quarterly)	Yes
Recreation therapist	National Association of Recreation Therapists 3101 Park Center Drive Alexandria, VA 22303 (703) 820-4940		Therapeutic Recreation Journal (quarterly)	Yes
Dance therapist	American Dance Therapy Association 2000 Century Plaza Suite 108 Columbia, MD 21044 (301) 997-4040		American Journal of Dance Therapy (annually)	No

2

Clinical Evaluation

Rolland P. Erickson

Malcolm C. McPhee

OVERVIEW

As with other branches of medicine, the cornerstone of rehabilitation medicine is a meticulous and germane patient evaluation. Therapeutic intervention must be based on proper patient assessment. The disability cannot be isolated from preexisting and concurrent medical problems. Although the rehabilitation evaluation encompasses all elements of the general medical history and physical examination, its scope is more comprehensive; thus the rehabilitation evaluation provides a unique perspective.

The Rehabilitation Evaluation Is an Evaluation of Function

Medical diagnosis concentrates on the historical clues and physical findings that lead the examiner to the correct identification of disease. Once the medical diagnosis is established, the rehabilitation physician must then ascertain the functional consequences of disease that constitute the rehabiliation diagnosis. An adept functional assessment requires that the examiner have a clear understanding of the distinctions among disease, impairment, disability, and handicap.

Disease. Be it illness or trauma, disease is a pathological condition of the body with a unique set of symptoms and signs. Although disease often leads to functional deficit, functional deficit is not a necessary result.

> M.B. lost his right eye because of malignancy as a toddler. Despite initial difficulties with depth perception, and after much training and practice, he completed a college degree on a basketball scholarship and was a skilled outside shooter.
> *Comment:* Initially, visual deficits resulted in functional deficiency, which M.B. later overcame.

Impairment. Most disease does result in impairment. As defined by the World Health Organization (WHO), impairment is "any loss or abnormality of psychological, physical, or anatomical structure or function."[23]

> A.W. was a 36-year-old businessman with complete T6 paraplegia after a motor vehicle accident, and his paraplegia resulted in spastic paralysis of his lower extremities.

> *Comment:* A.W.'s medical diagnosis (disease) was T6 paraplegia. His impairments included lower extremity paralysis.

Disability. When an impairment prohibits one from accomplishing a task required for personal independence, disability is created. According to WHO, disability is "any restriction or lack (resulting from an impairment) of an ability to perform an activity in the manner or within the range considered normal for a human being."[23] To assess the status of the abilities needed by all people, rehabilitation professionals apply various classifications of activities of daily living (ADL) to the impaired person. These activities are the endeavors that we accomplish on a daily basis in order to maintain personal independence. Our abilities to eat, bathe, groom, toilet, move about, and communicate, all have an impact on our capacity to live independently. When we cannot accomplish some or all of these activities, independence is compromised or lost.

> Because of A.W.'s paraplegia, he was unable to ambulate or operate the foot pedals on his automobile.
> *Comment:* His disabilities included an inability to ambulate or drive an autombile.

Handicap. When a disability (or impairment) keeps a person from performing duties within the social milieu, it results in a handicap. According to WHO, "A handicap is a disadvantage for a given individual, resulting from an impairment or a disability, that limits or prevents the fulfillment of a role that is normal (depending on age, sex, and social and culture factors) for that individual."[23]

> A.W. was a traveling salesman. After the accident, it seemed apparent to his employer that his inability to ambulate or drive would keep him from returning to work.
> *Comment:* As a traveling salesman, A.W. was expected to visit his clients. Consequently, by not fulfilling work-related expectations, a handicap was produced.

For rehabilitation to be successful, during the evaluation process the rehabilitation professional must identify and differentiate the disease process, impairments, disabilities, and handicaps faced by the patient so that remedial strategies can be instituted.

With the completion of comprehensive inpatient rehabilitation, A.W. gained no function in his lower extremities. Yet with training in transfers and use of a wheelchair, he achieved wheelchair mobility. His automobile was fitted with hand controls. After he drove his employer to lunch at a restaurant, the employer realized that A.W. could fulfill his job-related expectations, and A.W. returned to work.

Comment: This elementary example shows that despite a lack of improvement in impairments, A.W.'s disabilities and handicaps were reduced. However, this result can be accomplished only through a diligent evaluation of the patient, to identify not only the disease and resulting impairments but also the disabilities and handicaps that necessarily follow.

Our discussion has centered on the identification of functional deficits as a necessary step toward remedy. If the disease cannot be challenged directly through medical or surgical means, measures are used to minimize the impairment. For example, a weak muscle can be strengthened or a hearing impairment can be minimized through an electronic aid. With chronic disorders, disease and impairment are not reducible, hence intervention must address the disability and the handicap. The identification of intact functional capabilities is essential to successful rehabilitation. When intact capabilities can be augmented and adapted to new uses, functional independence can be enhanced.

A.W. had gained much enjoyment and self-esteem as a competitive runner before his spinal cord injury. During and after inpatient rehabilitation, he vigorously pursued a cardiovascular and upper extremity conditioning program. After obtaining an ultra-lightweight sport wheelchair, he resumed competitive athletics as a wheelchair racer, winning several regional races.

Comment: A.W.'s intact capabilities included normal arm strength, a competitive spirit, and self-discipline. Through augmentation and adaptation, he regained enjoyment and self-esteem in his athletic endeavors.

Despite best efforts, the physician is occasionally unable to ascertain the specific disease responsible for a patient's constellation of historical, physical, and laboratory findings. Medical management must then be symptomatic. Although highly desirable, the diagnosis of disease is not a necessary prerequisite to the identification and subsequent management of functional loss. The rehabilitation physician will then attempt to characterize historically the temporal nature of the disease process in an effort to determine expectations of future disease activity based on past activity.

F.Z., a 62-year-old woman, presented with difficulty climbing stairs. Questioning revealed that she and her husband had been in the habit of taking a 30-minute evening walk for many years but 2 years previously fatigue began to limit her to no more than a few blocks. During the previous year she had had difficulty rising from low seating, and 6 months previously she reluctantly quit taking the walks. During the preceding few weeks she had found that climbing stairs was a burden and had started taking showers because she needed assistance getting out of the bathtub.

F.Z. reported no sensory deficits. Physical examination revealed hypotonic muscle stretch reflexes and predominantly proximal muscle weakness. Electrodiagnostic studies and muscle biopsy demonstrated a noninflammatory myopathy; however, further extensive evaluation failed to determine a cause. She was provided with a bath bench, toilet seat riser, lightweight folding wheelchair for long distance mobility, and a cane for short distances. She was instructed in safe ambulation with a cane, operation of the wheelchair, energy conservation techniques, and the proper placement of bathroom safety bars. Safe automobile operation was documented, and she was provided with a parking sticker for handicapped people. The philosophy of rehabilitation medicine concerning her potentially progressive muscle weakness was discussed with her, and she was given supportive counseling.

When F.Z. returned for a follow-up examination 1 month later, muscle testing showed only slight progression of her weakness and her functional capabilities had not changed. Another follow-up examination was scheduled for 6 weeks later.

Comment: Although a specific diagnosis of disease was not established, rehabilitation intervention specific to F.Z.'s functional losses was accomplished. Such extrapolations are not always accurate; however, serial evaluations performed at regular follow-up intervals allow the rehabiliatation physician to identify and minimize future functional loss.

The Rehabilitation Evaluation Is a Comprehensive Evaluation

Unlike some medical specialities, rehabilitation medicine is not limited to a single organ system. Attention to the whole person is a rehabilitation absolute. In that the goal of a rehabilitation physician is to restore handicapped people to the fullest possible physical, mental, social, and economic independence, one must analyze a diverse aggregate of information to achieve the stated goal. Consequently, the person must be evaluated in relation not only to the disease but also to the way in which the disease affects and is affected by the person's family and social environment, vocational responsibilities and economic state, avocational interests, hopes, and dreams.

C.C., a 63-year-old piano tuner, had a left cerebral infarction manifested only as minimal dominant right hand dysfunction. Despite demonstrating discrete digit function in the involved hand on physical examination, he was psychologically devastated to find that he could no longer accomplish the fine but elegant motor patterns necessary to perform his profession.

B.D., a 63-year-old corporate attorney, had a left cerebral infarction resulting in severe spastic weakness of his nondominant upper extremity. He accomplished some paperwork every day during his inpatient rehabilitation and returned to full-time employment shortly after dismissal.

Comment: For each person, the degree of impairment has little or no relationship to the severity of resultant disabilities and handicaps.

The Rehabilitation Evaluation Is an Interdisciplinary Evaluation

Although in most of this chapter we address the history and physical examination as they relate to the rehabiliatation evaluation, they are only a part of the comprehensive rehabilitation assessment. This statement is not meant to deprecate the usefulness of these traditional physician's tools. The patient interview and physical examination are of critical importance and serve as the basis for further evaluation; yet, by their nature, they are also limited. Speech and language disorders can inhibit communication. Subjective interpretation of the facts by the patient and family (when present) can cloud the objective assessment of function. Performance is not optimally assessed by interview.

For example, inquiry about ambulation skills during the interview may identify a potential problem, but they can be objectively and reliably assessed only by having the physician and physical therapist observe the patient during ambulation in various situations. Likewise, the occupational therapist must assess the performance of activities of daily living and the rehabilitation nurse must assess the safety and judgment of the patient while in the ward. The speech therapist furnishes a measured assessment of language function and, through special communication skills, may obtain information from the patient that was missed during the interview. The rehabilitation psychologist provides a quantified and standardized assessment of cognitive and perceptual function and a skilled assessment of the patient's current psychological state. Through interaction with the patient's family and employer, the social worker can provide useful information that is otherwise unavailable regarding the patient's social support system and economic resources. The concept of the rehabilitation team applies not only to evaluation of the patient but also to the ongoing management of the patient.

SETTING AND PURPOSE

Because of the expanding scope of rehabilitation medicine, the evaluation setting can be diverse. A necessary corollary to the setting is the purpose of the evaluation. Both the setting and the purpose will have an impact on the format and extent of the evaluation. Traditionally, the inpatient rehabilitation unit has been the optimal setting for a comprehensive evaluation by the entire rehabilitation team. However, in these days of increasing medical costs and intervention by the government and other third party payers, creativity is being used to accomplish comprehensive rehabilitation evaluations in the clinic and elsewhere in the community (Table 2-1).

HISTORY

Ordinarily, the history is obtained through an interview of the patient by the physician. If communication disorders and cognitive deficits are encountered during the rehabilitation evaluation, additional and collaborative information must be obtained from significant others accompanying the patient. The spouse and family members are valuable resources. The physician may also find it necessary to interview other caregivers, such as paid attendants, the public health nurse, and the home health agency aide.

The major components of the history are the chief complaint, history of the present illness, functional history, past medical history, review of systems, patient profile, and family history.

Chief Complaint

In assessing the chief complaint the intent is to document the patient's primary concern in his or her own words. The complaint often is an impairment (in the form of a symptom) that implies a certain disease or group of diseases. The complaint of "chest pain when I walk up a flight of stairs" suggests cardiac disease, and a report that "my hands ache and go numb when I drive" hints at carpal tunnel syndrome.

Of equal importance is recognition that the chief complaint, when lost function is expressed, may also be the first implication of a disability or handicap. The homemaker's report that "my balance has been getting worse and I've fallen several times" may be related to disease involving the vestibular system and to the disability created by unsafe ambulation. Similarly, the farmer's declaration that "I can no longer climb up onto my tractor" not

Table 2-1
The Rehabilitation Evaluation: Setting and Purpose

Setting	Purpose
Hospital	
Inpatient rehabilitation unit	Comprehensive evaluation by team
Off-service consultation	Assessment by physician of potential for rehabilitation benefit
Clinic	
General rehabilitation clinic	Comprehensive evaluation by team
	Assessment by physician of potential for rehabilitation benefit
	Limited evaluation of specific musculoskeletal disorder
Special clinic	Limited evaluation of specific disease group (*e.g.,* muscular dystrophy, sports injury)
Day rehabilitation program	Comprehensive evaluation by team
Impairment/disability clinic	Evaluation determined by requirements of referring agency (*e.g.,* workers' compensation, Social Security)
Community	
Nursing home	Comprehensive evaluation by team
	Limited assessment by selected members of rehabilitation team
	Assessment by physician of potential for rehabilitation benefit
School	Limited evaluation of physical disability
	Limited evaluation for participation in sports
Transitional Living Facilities	Comprehensive evaluation by team
	Limited assessment of specific problem

only suggests a neuromuscular or orthopedic disease but also conveys to the physician that the disorder has resulted in a handicap by virtue of the inability to accomplish vocational expectations.

History of the Present Illness

The history of the present illness is obtained when the patient tells the story of the medical predicament. It is safe to state that all physicians at some time during their years of medical education have been admonished to "listen to your patients for they will tell you their diagnosis." Few maxims hold greater truth. When necessary, the patient should be asked to define the specific words he or she uses. It is often surprising to find out what "numbness" or "weakness" really means to some patients. At other times, specific questions relating to a particular symptom may help focus the interview. Through these techniques, the patient is gently guided by the physician to follow a chronological sequence and to describe fully the symptoms and their consequences. Above all, the patient should be allowed to tell the story. More than one complaint may be elicited during the interview, and the physician should characterize each problem in an orderly fashion (Table 2-2).[6]

A complete list of current medications should be obtained.

Table 2-2
Analysis of Symptoms

1. Date of onset
2. Character and severity
3. Location and extension
4. Time relationships
5. Associated complaints
6. Aggravating and alleviating factors
7. Previous treatment and effects
8. Progress, noting remissions and exacerbations

(Department of Neurology and Department of Physiology and Biophysics, Mayo Clinic and Mayo Foundation: Clinical Examinations in Neurology, 5th ed. Philadelphia, WB Saunders, 1981. By permission of Mayo Foundation)

Polypharmacy is commonly encountered in people with chronic disease, at times with striking adverse effects. Side-effects to medications can further impede cognition, psychological state, vascular reflexes, balance, bowel and bladder control, muscle tone, and coordination already impaired by the present illness or injury.

The history of the present illness should include a record of handedness, so important in many areas of rehabilitation.

Functional History

The rehabilitation evaluation of chronic disease often reveals lost function. Through the functional history, the physician must characterize the disabilities that have resulted from disease and identify remaining capabilities. It is considered part of the history of the present illness by some physicians and a separate segment of the patient interview by others. In that the examiner must know not only the functional status associated with the present illness but also the level of function at one or more times before the present illness, we prefer to consider it separately

Although the specific organization of the activities of daily living is somewhat variable, the following elements of personal independence remain constant: communication, eating, grooming, bathing, toileting, dressing, bed activities, transfers, and mobility.

Within each activity are several recognizable levels of function.

Levels of Function

INDEPENDENT. The patient is able to accomplish a task without equipment or assistance from another person.

INDEPENDENT WITH AIDS. The patient is able to accomplish a task with one or more adaptive aids but without assistance from another person. To be classified at this level, the patient must also be able to obtain, don, and doff the equipment without help. It is important to list the specific aids needed to perform the task and describe their use. This functional level is demonstrated by a patient with a common peroneal neuropathy who ambulates safely only when wearing an ankle–foot orthosis but can get the orthosis, put it on, and take it off without assistance.

REQUIRES ASSISTANCE. The patient is able to accomplish a portion of a task independently but needs assistance from another person to obtain, don, or doff adaptive aids or to complete the task itself. When assistance is required, it is essential to describe the assistance and the person usually providing the assistance. Assistance may be further classified as follows.

Standby Assistance. A task is generally accomplished independently but another person must monitor the performance of the task. The assistant ensures that the task is performed completely and safely and is ready, if needed, to provide verbal or physical cues. Such is the case in which a patient with cerebellar dysfunction is able to ambulate independently but requires another person to "spot" so as to prevent the occasional fall or a patient with a head injury has the physical skills to dress but is in need of occasional verbal reminders to sequence the correct and most efficient motor activities.

Physical Assistance. A task can be accomplished only if another person provides physical help at some point during the completion. Examples include a hemiparetic patient who eats independently once the meal is "set up" (the assistant puts the food on a scoop plate, cuts the meat, opens the beverage carton, and butters the bread) or who dresses independently but needs assistance with buttons, shoes, and socks.

Clean communication among rehabilitation team members concerning ambulation and transfers is occasionally facilitated by using an additional category of physical assistance. A *one-person assist* means that one assistant is needed, whereas a *two-person assist* implies the need for two assistants for task completion. A large man with Guillian-Barré syndrome may be able to contribute significantly to his transfers yet may still require two assistants for the transfer to be safe for both the patient and the assistants.

DEPENDENT (TOTAL ASSISTANCE). The patient is unable to provide any useful physical effort to perform a task. Such would be the level of hygiene function for a patient with C3 tetraplegia who is respirator dependent. However, many people with severe physical disabilities can efficiently direct the assistant in the performance of their activities of daily living.

Communication

In that a major component of rehabilitation is education, communication is critical. The interviewer must assess the patient's communication options. In the clinical situation, this is an aspect of the evaluation in which the distinction between history and physical examination blurs. It is difficult to interact with the patient in a meaningful way without coincidentally examining his or her ability to communicate; significant speech and language deficiencies become obvious. But, for purposes of discussion, certain facets of the assessment relate more specifically to the history and will be discussed here. Additional facets are presented below in the section on the physical examination.

Speech pathology has provided clinicians with numerous classification systems for speech and language disorders (see Chapter 6). From a functional view, the elements of communication hinge on four abilities: listening, reading, speaking, and writing.[4] By assessing these factors, one can determine a patient's communication abilities.

Representative questions are as follows: Do you have difficulty hearing? Do you use a hearing aid? Do you have difficulty reading? Do you need glasses to read? Do others find it hard to understand what you say? Do you have problems putting your thoughts into words? Do you have difficulty finding words? Can you write? Can you type? Do you use any communication aids?

Eating

The abilities to present solid food and liquids to the mouth, to chew, and to swallow are basic skills taken for granted by able-bodied people. Yet, in those with neurological, orthopedic, or oncologic disorders, these tasks can be formidable. When dysfunctional, eating can be associated with far-reaching consequences such as malnutrition, aspiration pneumonitis, and depression. As in the assessment of other skills for activities of daily living, inquiries about eating function should be specific and methodical.

Representative questions include the following: Can you eat without help? Do you have difficulty opening containers or pouring liquids? Can you cut meat? Do you have difficulty handling a fork (knife, spoon)? Do you have problems bringing food (beverages) to your mouth? Do you have problems chewing? Do you have difficulty swallowing solids (liquids)? Do you ever choke? Do you regurgitate food (liquids) through your nose?

Patients with nasogastric or gastrostomy tubes should be asked who helps them prepare and administer the feedings. The type, quantity, and schedule of feedings should be recorded.

Grooming

Grooming may not be considered as important as feeding. Yet, the inability to make oneself attractive and presentable to oneself and others can have injurious effects on one's body image and self-esteem, social sphere, and vocational options. Consequently, grooming skills should be of real concern to the rehabilitation team.

Representative questions are as follows: Can you brush your teeth without help? Can you remove and replace your dentures without help? Do you have problems fixing or combing your hair? Can you apply your makeup independently? Do you have problems shaving? Can you apply deodorant without assistance?

Bathing

The ability to maintain cleanliness also has far-reaching psychosocial implications. In addition, deficits in cleaning can result in skin maceration and ulceration, skin and systemic infections, and the spread of disease to others. Independency in bathing should be sought.

Representative questions include the following: Can you take a tub bath (shower) without assistance? Do you feel safe in the tub (shower)? Do you use a bath bench (shower chair)? Can you accomplish a sponge bath without help? Are there parts of your body you cannot reach?

For patients with sensory deficits, bathing is also a convenient time for skin inspection and inquiry about the patient's inspection habits should be made. For patients using a wheelchair, architectural barriers to bathroom entry should be determined.

Toileting

To the cognitively intact person, incontinence of stool or urine can be the most psychologically devastating deficit of personal independence. Ineffective bowel or bladder control has an adverse impact on self-esteem, body image, and sexuality and often prevents the sufferer from employment and social relationships. Dignity may even prohibit the person from venturing from the house for fear of an accident. Soiling of skin and clothing often results in ulceration, infection, and urological complications. The rehabilitation physician should vigorously pursue toileting dependency with sensitivity.

Representative questions are as follows: Can you use the toilet without assistance? Do you need help with clothing before or after using the toilet? Do you need help with cleaning after a bowel movement?

For patients with indwelling urinary catheters, usual management of the catheter and leg bag should be understood. If bladder emptying is accomplished by intermittent catheterization, the examiner should learn who performs the catheterization and have a clear understanding of the technique used.

For patients who have had ostomies for urine or feces, the examiner should determine who cares for the ostomy and ask to have the technique described.

In that feminine hygiene is generally performed while on or near the toilet, at this point in the interview it may be convenient to inquire about problems with sanitary napkin and tampon use.

Dressing

We dress to go out into the world—to be employed in the workplace, to dine in a restaurant, to be entertained in a public place, and to visit friends. Even within one's home, convention dictates that we dress to entertain anyone except close friends and family. We dress for protection, warmth, self-esteem, and pleasure. Dependency in dressing obviously results in a severe limitation to personal independence and should be investigated thoroughly during the rehabilitation interview.

Representative questions are as follows: Do you dress daily? What articles of clothing do your regularly wear? Do you require assistance putting on or taking off your underwear (shirt, slacks, skirt, dress, coat, stockings, panty hose, shoes, tie, coat)? Do you need help with buttons (zippers, hooks, snaps, shoelaces)? Do you use clothing modifications?

Bed Activities

The most basic stage of functional mobility is independence in bed activities. The importance of this functional level should not be underestimated. If a person cannot turn from side to side to redistribute pressure and periodically expose skin to the air, he or she is at high risk to develop pressure sores over bony prominences and skin maceration from heat and occlusion. For the person who cannot stand upright to dress, bridging (lifting the hips off the bed in the supine position) will allow the donning of underwear and slacks. Independence is likewise enhanced by an ability to move between a recumbent and a sitting position. Sitting balance is required to accomplish many other activities of daily living, including transfers.

Representative questions include the following: Can you turn onto your front (back, sides) without assistance? Can you lift your hips off the bed when supine? Do you need help to sit (lie)? Do you have difficulty maintaining a seated position? Can you operate the bed controls (with an electric hospital bed)?

Transfers

The second stage of functional mobility is independence in transfers. Skills to move between a wheelchair and the bed, toilet, bath bench or shower chair, standard seating, and car seat often serve as precursors to independence in other areas. Although a male patient can use a urinal to void without transferring, a female patient cannot be independent in bladder care without the ability to transfer to the toilet and will probably require an indwelling catheter. Travel by airplane or train is difficult without the ability to transfer from the wheelchair to other seating. Bathing or showering is not independent without the ability to move to the bath bench or shower chair. The inability to transfer to a car seat precludes the use of a motor vehicle with standard seating. Also included in this category is the ability to move from a seated position to a standing position. Low seats without arm supports present a much greater problem than straight-backed chairs with arm supports.

Representative questions are as follows: Can you move between the bed (toilet, bath bench, shower chair, standard seating, car seat) and the wheelchair without assistance? Can you get out of bed without difficulty? Do you require assistance to stand from low (high) seats? Can you get on and off the toilet without help?

Wheelchair Mobility

The next level of mobility to be assessed is operation of a wheelchair. Although wheelchair independence is more prone to inhibition by architectural barriers than walking, it provides excellent mobility for the nonwalking person. With today's manual wheelchairs of lightweight materials and efficient engineering, the energy expenditure of wheeling on flat ground is only slightly higher than that of walking. With the addition of a motorized drive, battery power, and controls for speed and direction a person without the upper extremity strength necessary to propel a manual wheelchair can still maintain significant independence in mobility.

Quantification of manual wheelchair skills can be accomplished in several ways. A person may report in feet, yards, meters, or city blocks the distance he or she is able to traverse before resting. Alternatively, the number of minutes one can continuously propel the chair can be specified or the environment in which one is able to use the chair can be described (within a single room, around the house, or throughout the community).

Representative questions for manual wheelchair use include the following: Do you propel a wheelchair? Do you need help to lock the wheelchair brakes before transfers? Do you require assistance to cross high-pile carpets (rough ground, inclines)? How far (how many minutes) can you wheel before you must rest? Can you independently move about your living room (bedroom, kitchen)? Do you go shopping (to restaurants, to friends' homes)? With any of these functional levels of wheelchair mobility, the patient should be asked what keeps him or her going farther and whether help is needed to lift the wheelchair into an automobile.

Ambulation

The final level of mobility is ambulation. In the narrow sense of the word, ambulation is walking, and we have used this sense to simplify the following discussion. Yet, within the sphere of rehabilitation, ambulation often is any useful means of movement from one place to another. In the view of many rehabilitation professionals, the bilateral above-knee amputee ambulates with a manual wheelchair, the patient with C4 tetraplegia ambulates with a motorized wheelchair, and a polio victim in a third-world country might ambulate by crawling. To some, driving a motor vehicle also is a form of ambulation. Ambulation ability can be quantified in the same ways as wheelchair mobility. A person may report the distance he or she is able to walk, the duration between necessary rest periods, or the scope of the environment within which he or she walks.

Representative questions are as follows: Do you walk unaided? Do you use a cane (crutches, walker) to walk? How far (how many minutes) can you walk before you must rest? What stops you from going farther? Do you feel unsteady or fall? Can you go upstairs (downstairs) unassisted? Do you go shopping (to restaurants, to friends' homes)? Can you use public transportation (bus, subway) without assistance?

Operation of a Motor Vehicle

In the perceptions of many patients, full independence in mobility is not attained until one is able to accomplish independent operation of a motor vehicle. Although driving skills are by no means a necessity to an urban dweller with readily available public transportation, they are of great advantage to a person living in a suburban or rural environment. Driving skills should always be assessed in patients of driving age.

Representative questions include the following: Do you have a valid driver's license? Do you own a car? Do you drive your car to go shopping (to restaurants, to friends' homes)? Do you drive in heavy traffic or over long distances? Do you use hand controls or other automobile modifications? Have you experienced any motor vehicle accidents or received any citations for improper operation of a motor vehicle since your illness (injury)?

Past Medical History

The past medical history is a record of significant illness, trauma, and health maintenance experienced by a patient during life. The effects of certain past conditions will continue to affect the present level of function. Identification of these conditions affords the rehabilitation physician the opportunity to better characterize the patient's baseline functional level before the present disorder. The examiner must take special care to decipher whether the patient's diagnostic terms accurately represent the true diagnoses. Although many past conditions associated with significant immobilization, deconditioning, and disability are themselves amenable to rehabilitation measures, they will tend to define the goals for future rehabilitation efforts.

> P.B., a 66-year-old woman, was referred for rehabilitation after right above-knee amputation due to vascular disease. The past history was significant for a right cerebral infarction 7 years earlier. Despite comprehensive rehabilitation after the stroke, she was able to ambulate only 1 block with a quadripod cane and ankle–foot orthosis because of spastic left hemiparesis.
>
> *Comment:* After prosthetic fitting and training, most people in P.B.'s age group with an above-knee amputation regain ambulation skills, although many will require a cane or other gait aid. However, in that she had significant ambulation disability due to the left hemiparesis that occurred before amputation, rehabilitation goals included a wheelchair prescription (with consideration of a hemi-chair if she could not accomplish wheeling with the left arm) and training in wheelchair activities. Even though ambulation beyond a few yards was not feasible, a preparatory prosthesis with manual knee lock was provided on a trial basis to determine whether it aided transfers. In this example, ambulation disability was dictated more by previous impairments than by impairments associated with the present illness.

All elements of the standard past medical history should be completed; however, a history of neurological, cardiopulmonary, or musculoskeletal disease should usher in special concern from the rehabilitation physician. Psychiatric disorders are also of special interest to the rehabilitation physician and are discussed below in the section on the psychological and psychiatric history.

Neurological Disorders

Most frequently encountered in older populations but possibly present in any age group, a past history of neurological disease can have a tremendous impact on the rehabilitation outcome of an unrelated present illness. Whether congenital or acquired, preexisting cognitive impairment places restrictions on educationally oriented rehabilitation intervention. Disorders with sensory manifestations such as loss of touch, pain, or joint position and afflictions characterized by perceptual dysfunction retard the patient's ability to monitor performance during the acquisition of new functional skills. These maladies also render the patient more likely to be unresponsive to soft tissue injury from prolonged or excessive skin surface pressures during periods of immobility. When they are coupled with preexisting visual or auditory impairment, function is further encumbered. Likewise, a residual motor deficit can inhibit new motor learning through spasticity, weakness, or decreased endurance. A diligent search for antecedent neurological disease is a fundamental part of the rehabilitation evaluation.

Cardiopulmonary Disorders

In patients with motor disabilities, activities of daily living are accomplished with higher than normal energy cost. When preexisting cardiopulmonary disorders limit the capacity to tolerate the greater energy expenditures imposed on the patient by the motor disability, further functional deficits follow. (This is also the case with many forms of hematological, renal, and hepatic dysfunctions.) The physician is encouraged to gather as much cardiopulmonary data as needed to estimate cardiac reserve accurately. Only when disease of the cardiopulmonary system is identified can rehabilitation be tailored and medical intervention be initiated to maximize cardiac reserve.

Musculoskeletal Disorders

Weakness, joint ankylosis, or instability from previous trauma or arthritis, amputation, and other musculoskeletal dysfunctions can all deleteriously affect functional capacity. A search for such disorders is a necessary prerequisite to a complete rehabilitation evaluation.

Review of Systems

The systems are reviewed to screen for clues to disease not otherwise identified in the history of the present illness and the past medical history. A thorough review should always be completed. Many diseases have potential for adverse effects on rehabilitation outcome. However, as described previously, certain disorders are of special interest to the rehabilitation physician. This part of the evaluation considers constitutional, head and neck, respiratory, cardiovascular, gastrointestinal, genitourinary, neurological, and musculoskeletal symptoms.

Constitutional Symptoms

Of particular interest are suggestions of infection and nutritional deficiency. Fatigue can be a prominent complaint in patients with multiple sclerosis.

Head and Neck Symptoms

Vision, hearing, and swallowing deficits must be identified.

Respiratory Symptoms

Any pulmonary condition that inhibits the delivery of oxygen to the tissues will adversely affect endurance. Symptoms such as dyspnea, cough, sputum, hemoptysis, wheezing, and pleuritic chest pain should be sought.

Cardiovascular Symptoms

The manifestations of heart disease restrict cardiac reserve and endurance. When identified, many can be ameliorated through medical management. Identification of arrhythmias is important for the prevention of recurrent strokes of embolic cause. The presence of chest pain, dyspena, orthopnea, palpitations, and lightheadedness should be determined. Peripheral vascular disease is the leading cause of amputation. The potential for ulceration and gangrene from bed rest, orthoses, pressure garments, and other rehabilitation equipment can be minimized if peripheral disease is recognized. The patient should be asked about claudication, foot ulcers, and varicosities.

Gastrointestinal Symptoms

Almost any form of gastrointestinal disease can result in nutritional deficiency, a particularly insidious condition that limits rehabilitation efforts more frequently than previously realized.[18] Bowel control is of special interest in patients with neurological disorders. Questions about incontinence, bowel care techniques, and laxatives should be asked.

Genitourinary Symptoms

Manifestations of neurogenic bladder must be sought. Questions about specific fluid intake and voiding schedules, specific bladder emptying techniques, urgency, frequency, incontinence, retention and incomplete emptying, sensation of fullness and voiding, dysuria, pyuria, infections, flank pain, hematuria, and stones should be asked. For female patients, a menstrual and pregnancy history should be obtained and inquiries about dyspareunia, vaginal and clitoral sensation, and orgasm should be made. Male patients should be asked about erection, ejaculation, progeny, and pain during intercourse.

Neurological Symptoms

Because of the high prevalence of neurological disorders in patients in a rehabilitation program, a methodical neurological review should always be performed. The following items should be addressed: smell; diplopia, blurred vision, field cuts; imbalance, vertigo, tinnitus; weakness, tremors, involuntary movements, convulsions, depressed level of consciousness, ataxia; loss of touch, pain, temperature, dysesthesias, hyperpathia; and changes in memory and "thinking." Chewing, swallowing, hearing, reading, and speaking may be addressed in either the functional history or the review of the systems.

Inquiry about psychological and psychiatric issues can be made either during the review of symptoms or, as we choose, when obtaining the psychosocial history for the patient profile.

Musculoskeletal Symptoms

The musculoskeletal review must also be extremely thorough because of the high frequency of musculoskeletal dysfunction in patients in a rehabilitation program. Inquiry is made about muscle pain, weakness, fasciculation, atrophy, hypertrophy; skeletal deformities and fractures; and limited joint motion, joint stiffness, joint pain, and swelling of soft tissues and joints.

Patient Profile

The patient profile provides the interviewer with information about the patient's present and past psychological state, social milieu, and vocational background.

Personal History

Psychological and Psychiatric History. In that any present illness accompanied by functional loss is of itself psychologically challenging, a quiescent major psychiatric disturbance can resurface during such stressful times to hinder or halt rehabilitation efforts. When the examiner is able to identify a history of psychiatric dysfunction, the necessary support systems to lessen the chances of recrudescence can be applied prophylactically during the rehabilitation process. The examiner is encouraged to seek a history of previous psychiatric hospitalization, psychotropic pharmacological intervention, or psychotherapy. The patient should be screened for past or current anxiety, depression and other mood changes, sleep disturbances, delusions, hallucinations, obsessive and phobic ideas, and past major and minor psychiatric illness. A review of the patient's prior and current responses to stress often helps us to understand and modify behavioral responses to catastrophic illness or trauma. Therefore, it is important to know the patient's emotional responses to previous illness and family troubles and how the stress of the current illness is being dealt with. Tests to clarify psychological symptoms or a personality disturbance may be requested from a clinical psychologist if initial screening results suggest abnormality.

LIFE-STYLE. Leisure activities can promote both physical and emotional health. The patient's leisure habits should be reviewed to identify special rehabilitation measures that might return independence in these activities. Examples of questions to consider include the following: What sort of interests does the patient have?[20] Does the patient most enjoy physical endeavors, sports, the outdoors, and mechanical avocations (motor oriented)? Is the patient more interested in intellectual pursuits (symbol oriented)? Is the most pleasure derived from social interactions, organizations, and group functions (interpersonally oriented)? Has the patient been actively pursuing these interests? The work-oriented person without avocational interests before the present illness will need recreational counseling during rehabilitation.

DIET. Inadequate nutrition may inhibit rehabilitation efforts. In addition, even after initial myocardial and cerebrovascular events due to atherosclerosis, some secondary prevention can be accomplished through dietary manipulation. The patient's ability to prepare meals and snacks, usual dietary habits, and special diets should be determined.

ALCOHOL AND DRUGS. Drug, alcohol, and nicotine use must be assessed. Patients with cognitive, perceptual, and motor deficits can be further impaired to a dangerous degree through substance abuse. Drugs and alcohol are frequent factors in the cause of head and spinal cord injury. Identification of abuse and dependency provides the opportunity to modify future behaviors through counseling. The CAGE questionnaire[9] is a brief but

---

Table 2-3
The CAGE Questionnaire

1. Have you ever felt you ought to Cut down on your drinking?
2. Have people Annoyed you by criticizing your drinking?
3. Have you ever felt bad or Guilty about your drinking?
4. Have you ever had a drink first thing in the morning to steady your nerves or get rid of a hangover (Eye-opener)?

(Ewing JA: Detecting alcoholism: The CAGE questionnaire. JAMA 252:1905–1907, 1984. Copyright © 1984, American Medical Association)

---

useful screening vehicle for the identification of alcohol abuse and dependency (Table 2-3); a single affirmative answer should initiate further investigation.

Social History

FAMILY. Catastrophic illness in a family member places enormous stress on the rest of the family. When the family is already facing other problems with interaction, health, or substance abuse, the potential for disintegration of the family unit is greater. This is unfortunate because the availability of a sturdy system of family and friends can be as predictive of disposition as functional outcome. The patient's marriage history and status should be determined. Other family members who live at home and their names and ages should be sought. The established roles of each member should be clearly understood (that is, who handles the finances, the cooking, the cleaning, and the discipline). Determine whether other family members live nearby. For all potential assistants, inquire about their willingness and ability to participate in the care of the family member and about their work (school) schedule to ascertain potential availability.

Home. The patient's home design should be reviewed for architectural barriers. Determine whether the patient owns or rents, the location of the home (urban, suburban, or rural), the distance between the home and rehabilitation services, the number of steps into the home, presence of or room for entry ramps, and the accessibility of the kitchen, bath, bedroom, and living room.

Vocational History

EDUCATION AND TRAINING. Although the level of education does not predict intellectual function, the educational level achieved by the patient may suggest intellectual skills that the rehabilitation team could take advantage of during convalescence. In addition, when coupled with the assessment of physical function, the educational background will dictate future educational and training needs. The years of education completed by the patient and whether high school, undergraduate, or graduate degrees were obtained are determined and the patient's performance reviewed. The acquisition of special skills, licenses, and certifications is noted. Future vocational goals are always important to address but are of particular concern with adolescent patients. Discussion of these goals will indicate the need for and type of interest, aptitude, and skills testing and vocational counseling appropriate for the patient.

WORK HISTORY. An understanding of the patient's work experience can also determine whether further education and training will be necessary. In addition, it provides an idea of the patient's motivation, reliability, and self-discipline. The duration and type of previous jobs and the reason for job changes are recorded. Not only titles but also actual job descriptions must be obtained, and the patient should be asked about architectural barriers at the workplace. These principles apply equally to the patient who is a homeworker. The evaluator must define the specific work expectations relating to meal preparation, shopping, home maintenance, cleaning, child rearing, and discipline. In addition the patient should be asked where the clothes washing is done and whether architectural barriers prevent the patient from reaching appliances or areas in the home and yard.

FINANCES. The physician should have a basic understanding of the patient's income, investment, and insurance resources, disability classifications, and debts.

Family History

The family history is used to decipher threads of hereditary disease within the family and to assess the health of people within the patient's home support system. Knowledge of the health and fitness of the spouse and other family members may be eminently important in dismissal planning.

PHYSICAL EXAMINATION

The physical examination performed by the rehabilitation physician shares much with the general medical examination. Of necessity, it is a well-practiced art. Through perceptions gleaned from observation, palpation, percussion, and auscultation, the examining physician seeks physical findings to support and formulate the diagnosis further and to screen for other conditions not suggested by the history.

The physical examination also is different from the general medical examination. After investigating the physical findings that help to establish the medical diagnosis, the rehabilitation physician still has two principal tasks. The first task is to scrutinize the patient for physical findings to define the disabilities and handicaps that emanate from the disease. The second task is to identify remaining physical, psychological, and intellectual strengths to serve as the base from which to reestablish functional independence. In this characterization, rehabilitation medicine places special emphasis on the orthopedic and neurological examinations, and functional assessment becomes an integral part of the examination.

Severe motor, cognitive, and communication impairments make it difficult or impossible for some patients to follow through with directions from the physician and place limitations on certain traditional physical examination maneuvers. Creativity is often required to accomplish the examination. Particularly expert examination skills are necessary in such situations.

We assume that the reader has developed competence in the performance of the general medical examination.[5] In the following discussion, priority is placed on the aspects of the physical examination that have special relevance to rehabilitation medicine. The major segments of the physical examination in rehabilitation medicine are the vital signs and general appearance, integument and lymphatics, head, eyes, ears, nose, mouth and throat, neck, chest, heart and peripheral vascular system, abdomen, genitourinary system and rectum, musculoskeletal system, neurological examination, and functional examination.

Vital Signs and General Appearance

The recording of blood pressure, pulse, temperature, weight, and general observations is important. The identification of hypertension may be meaningful to the secondary prevention of stroke and myocardial infarction. Supine, sitting, and standing blood pressures should be obtained to rule out orthostasis in any patient with unexplained falls, lightheadedness, or dizziness. Tachycardia can be the initial manifestation of sepsis in a patient with high-level tetraplegia or can suggest pulmonary embolism in an immobilized patient. Initial weight recordings are invaluable to identify and follow up malnutrition, obesity, and fluid and electrolyte disorders common to various forms of brain injury. A notation is made if patients are hostile, tense, agitated or if their behavior is uncooperative, inappropriate, or preoccupied. The gestalt of a patient at initial contact can reveal problems not recognized at close scrutiny.

Integument and Lymphatics

Skin disorders are frequently encountered in rehabilitation medicine. Prolonged pressure in patients with peripheral vascular disease, sensory disorders, immobility, and altered consciousness often results in damage to skin and underlying tissues. Many diseases common to disabled people, and their treatments, render the skin more prone to trauma and infection. Skin problems that are only bothersome to able-bodied people can be devastating to those with disabilities when these problems prevent the use of prostheses, orthoses, and other devices. Workers providing rehabilitation services to patients with cancer often confront lymphedema in the extremities after proximal node excision and irradiation.

The skin is inspected in good light. If the skin is considered as each separate body region is examined, the entire body surface can be studied without total exposure of the patient. In particular, the skin over bony prominences and in contact with prosthetic and orthotic devices is examined for lichenification, erythema, or breakdown. Intertriginous areas are inspected for maceration and ulceration, the distal lower extremities in patients with vascular disease examined for pigmentation, hair loss, and breakdown, and the hands and feet in insensate patients observed for unrecognized trauma. All common lymph node sites are palpated for enlargement and tenderness, and areas of edema are palpated for pitting.

Head

The head is inspected for signs of past or present trauma. Gentle palpation is performed for evidence of previous trauma or neurosurgical procedures, shunt pumps, and other craniofacial abnormalities. Auscultation for bruits is done when considering vascular malformations.

Eyes

Unrecognized acuity errors can hamper rehabilitation efforts, especially in patients needing good eyesight to compensate for disorders of other sensory systems. With the patient's usual eyewear in place, far and near vision is tested using standard charts. If charts are not available, the patient's vision is compared with the examiner's vision by object identification and description for far vision and with reading material of several print sizes for near vision. Findings are substantiated with refraction when circumstances permit. A funduscopic examination is performed; if dilation agents are necessary, one of short duration is used and notation is made in the patient's chart of the time of administration and the name of the preparation. Evidence of erythema and inflammation of the globe or conjunctiva is searched for; aphasic patients and those with altered consciousness may not adequately express the pain of acute glaucoma or the discomfort of conjunctivitis. The eyes of comatose patients are inspected for inadequate lid closure; corneal ulcerations from deficient lubrication should be prevented.

Ears

Unrecognized hearing impairment may also limit rehabilitation efforts. Hearing acuity is checked with the "watch test" or by having the patient repeat words presented with a whispered voice. If a unilateral hearing deficit is identified, Weber and Rinne tests are used to determine whether it is a nerve or conductive loss. Findings are substantiated with an audiogram. An otoscopic examination is performed. If otorrhea is present in head-injured patients, the presence of sugar, which would indicate cerebrospinal fluid, is checked for by using Benedict's solution.

Nose

A routine examination of the nose generally suffices. If clear or blood-tinged drainage is noted in head-injured patients, the presence of cerebrospinal fluid is sought.

Mouth and Throat

The oral and pharyngeal mucosa is inspected for poor hygiene and infections (*e.g.,* candidiasis in patients taking corticosteroids and broad-spectrum antibiotics), the teeth for disrepair, and the gums for gingivitis or hypertrophy. Dentures are checked for fit and maintenance needs. In patients with arthritis or trauma, the temporomandibular joints are inspected and palpated for crepitation, tenderness, swelling, or limited motion. Any of these problems can threaten food intake and result in poor nutrition.

Neck

A routine examination of the neck generally suffices. One should be sure to listen for carotid bruits in patients with atherosclerosis and cerebrovascular disorders. In patients with musculoskeletal disorders, range of motion is assessed. However, neck motion is not checked in patients with recent trauma or chronic polyarthritides until radiographic studies have ruled out fracture or instability.

Chest

Tolerance to exercise is significantly affected by pulmonary function. For the patient in whom exercise tolerance is already compromised by neurological or musculoskeletal disease, the examiner must rigorously search for pulmonary dysfunction to minimize the deficit. The standard medical maneuvers are usually sufficient; however, certain aspects of the chest examination merit mention.

The chest wall is inspected to note the rate, amplitude, and rhythm of breathing. The presence of cough, hiccups, labored breathing, accessory muscle activity, and chest wall deformities is noted. Rheumatologic disorders such as the late stages of HLA-B27 arthropathies and scleroderma restrict respiratory excursion and lead to shallow, tachypneic respirations. Likewise, restrictive pulmonary disease with hypoventilation is common in muscular dystrophy and other congenital diseases of the motor unit, severe kyphoscoliosis, and chronic spinal cord injuries. Tachypnea and tachycardia may be the only readily apparent manifestations of pulmonary embolism, pneumonia, or sepsis in patients with high-level spinal cord injuries. The finding of a barrel chest may lead the examiner to document obstructive pulmonary disease so that medical management can minimize its effect on function.

The patient is instructed to cough and notation is made of the force and efficiency of this action. If the cough is weak, the patient is assisted by exerting manual pressure over the abdomen coincidentally with the cough attempt to observe the effect. The chest wall is palpated for tenderness, deformity, and transmitted sounds. During the acute care of a head-injured patient, rib fractures can be missed. Percussion is done to document diaphragmatic level and excursion. Auscultation is performed to characterize breath sounds and identify wheezes, rubs, rhonchi, and rales. Pneumonitis can be especially insidious in the immunosuppressed patient.

When pulmonary disease is suggested, it is documented with function tests and determination of blood gas levels. If the patient has a tracheostomy, the skin around the opening, is examined, the type of apparatus is recorded, and cuff leaks are noted. Any opportunity to screen for breast malignancy in both men and women should not be wasted.

Heart and Peripheral Vascular System

Like pulmonary disease, cardiovascular dysfunction can adversely affect exercise tolerance already encumbered by neurological or musculoskeletal disease. When cardiovascular disorders are identified, intervention can relieve or reduce the deleterious effects on exercise tolerance and general health. Secondary prevention of embolic stroke is contingent on the identification of arrhythmias, valvular disease, and congenital anomalies. The general medical cardiac examination will suffice.

In the clinical situation, the peripheral circulation is usually assessed during scrutiny of the extremities. When bracing is contemplated, one should always search for the pallor and cool dystrophic skin of arterial occlusive disease; inappropriate devices may lead to skin breakdown and subsequent amputation. Deep venous thrombosis is a major risk to patients immobilized by other conditions. When venous stasis and incompetency complicate the situation, the risk is greater. A search is made for varicose and incompetent veins. Bedside Doppler studies should be used whenever necessary to help delineate arterial or venous concerns. Evaluation is done to determine the presence of Raynaud's phenomenon.

Abdomen

In many patients, the general medical examination of the abdomen will be all that is necessary to screen for abnormality and assess gastrointestinal complaints. Again, however, special situations warrant mention. In patients with widespread spasticity, such as occurs with multiple sclerosis and myelopathy, inspection and auscultation are done before attempting palpation and percussion. Manipulation of the abdominal wall often results in a wave of increased tone that will temporarily render the remainder of the abdominal examination difficult or impossible to accomplish. Vigorous abdominal palpation in patients with disordered peristalsis from certain central nervous system diseases may initiate regurgitation of stomach contents. Such patients are examined gently when they are in the semireclined position.

Genitourinary System and Rectum

The genitalia should be examined during any comprehensive evaluation. However, a thorough examination of the male and female genitalia is particularly necessary to evaluate patients with disorders of continence, micturition, and sexual function. In the presence of incontinence in either sex and in male patients using an external collecting device such as the condom catheter, maceration and ulceration can result. Examination of the penile skin in male patients, the periurethral mucosa in female patients, and all intertriginous perineal areas for maceration and ulceration is performed. The scrotal contents are palpated for orchitis and epididymitis in male patients with indwelling catheters. Incontinence from neurogenic causes is common in the rehabilitation population; however, the examiner should not miss a cystocele or other remediable structural cause for the incontinence. Patients with chronic indwelling catheters should be checked for external urethral meatal ulceration and male patients for penile fistulas. Whenever urinary retention is suspected, the physical examination should be followed by an in-and-out catheterization to measure the amount of residual urine.

The rehabilitation assessment is not completed without digital examination of the rectum, anus, anal tone, and perinal sensation. In any patient with suspected central nervous system, autonomic, or pelvic disease, the bulbocavernosus reflex is evaluated. This is accomplished by firmly compressing the glans of the penis or clitoris with one hand while inserting the index finger of the other hand into the anus to monitor sphincter tone. Sphincter tone is increased with many upper motor lesions and decreased or absent with neurogenic disease of or peripheral to the sacral cord (S2–S4).

Musculoskeletal System

Disorders of the musculoskeletal system are a major portion of the pathological conditions addressed by the rehabilitation physician. The examiner must possess expert skills in the evaluation of all musculoskeletal components; while attending to each body region, the bone, joint, cartilage, ligament, tendon, and muscle should be assessed in an orderly fashion. To accomplish this task, full familiarity with surface landmarks and the underlying anatomy is needed.

Assignment of many examination components to the musculoskeletal and neurological examinations is an arbitrary exercise in that neuromusculoskeletal function is so integrated. For discussion, examination of the musculoskeletal system is divided into inspection, palpation, range-of-motion assessment, joint stability assessment, and muscle strength testing.

Inspection

Inspection is done for scoliosis, abnormal kyphosis, and lordosis; joint deformity, amputation, absence and asymmetry of body parts (leg-length discrepancy); soft tissue swelling, mass, scar, and defect; and muscle fasciculations, atrophy, hypertrophy, and rupture. At times, the dysfunction is subtle and decipherable only through careful observation of the patient. While proceeding with the examination, notation is made of any wary and tentative movements of the patient in pain, of the exaggerated and inconsistent conduct of the malingerer, and of the bizarre behavior of the hysterical patient.

Palpation

Localized abnormalities identified through inspection and body regions of concern to the patient should be palpated to ascertain the structural origin of tenderness and deformity. For any such abnormality, it is important to first determine whether the basic consistency is that of soft tissue or bone and whether it is of normal anatomical structure. For soft tissue abnormalities, an attempt is made to identify them further as pitting or nonpitting edema, synovitis, or a mass.

All skeletal elements near areas of hemorrhage and ecchymosis in patients with altered consciousness are palpated. The elderly patient with traumatic subdural hematoma may have experienced an extremity fracture associated with a fall. During the critical care of a motorcyclist with a head injury, an incidental fracture may have been missed. Likewise, any in-hospital fall by a confused patient warrants a search for occult bony trauma.

Range-of-Motion Assessment

Human joint motion is measured during clinical evaluation by many health care professionals for various reasons including initial evaluation, evaluation of treatment procedure, feedback to a patient, assessment of work capacity, or research studies. Of the different methods available, we prefer to regard the anatomical position as the baseline (zero starting point) when identifying a starting point for measuring the range of motion (ROM) of a joint. If rotation is being measured, the midway point between the normal rotation range is chosen as the zero starting point. The technique of measurement was published in detail by Norkin and White.[19]

Considerable variation exists among people when range-of-motion measurements are compared. Factors such as age, sex, conditioning, obesity, and genetics can influence the normal range of motion. A publication of the American Academy of Orthopaedic Surgeons[1] includes average ranges of joint motion for the joints of the human body.

When the patient does not assist the examiner while the joint is taken through a range of motion, the measurement is a passive range of motion. If the patient performs the range of motion without assistance from the examiner, then the range is an active range of motion. If comparisons are made between active and passive ranges of motion, the starting position, stabilization, goniometer, alignment, and type of goniometer should be the same.

Different methods of recording the results of the range-of-motion measurements are available. Graphic recordings are often helpful if feedback to the patient or to a third party is needed. Sometimes the lag between the patient's range and a normal range is of special interest to the examiner, such as when the surgeon wants to follow up finger motion as a guide to recovery after a hand operation.

The goniometer position, starting position, and average range of motion of the more commonly measured joints are shown in Figures 2-1 through 2-26.

(Text continues on page 43)

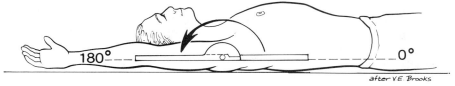

Figure 2-1.   Shoulder flexion. (Courtesy of Dr. J. F. Lehmann)

Starting position

Supine
Arm at side with
    hand pronated

Measurement

Sagittal plane
Substitution to avoid:
    Arching back
    Rotating trunk
Goniometer:
    Axis lateral to joint and just
        below acromion
    Shaft parallel to midaxillary
        line of trunk
    Shaft parallel to midline of
        humerus

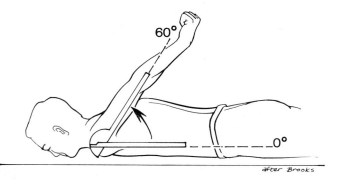

Figure 2-2.   Shoulder hyperextension. (Courtesy of Dr. J. F. Lehmann)

Starting position

Prone
Arm at side with hand
    pronated

Measurement

Sagittal plane
Substitution to avoid:
    Lifting shoulder from table
    Rotating trunk
Goniometer: same as in Figure
    2-1

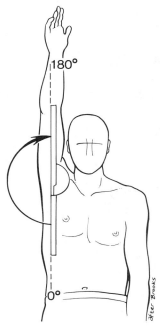

Figure 2-3.   Shoulder abduction. (Courtesy of Dr. J. F. Lehmann)

Starting position

Supine
Arm at side

Measurement

Frontal plane (must externally
    rotate shoulder to obtain
    maximum)
Substitution to avoid:
    Lateral motion of trunk
    Rotating trunk
Goniometer:
    Axis anterior to joint and in
        line with acromion
    Shaft parallel to midline of
        trunk
    Shaft parallel to midline of
        humerus

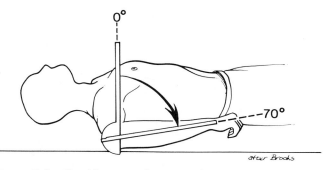

Figure 2-4. Shoulder internal rotation. (Courtesy of Dr. J. F. Lehmann)

Starting position	Measurement

Supine
Arm abducted to 90°
  and elbow off table
Elbow flexed to 90°
  and hand pronated
Forearm perpendicular
  to floor
	Transverse plane
	Substitution to avoid:
	  Protracting shoulder
	  Rotating trunk
	  Changing angle at shoulder
	    or elbow
	Goniometer:
	  Axis through longitudinal axis
	    of humerus
	  Shaft perpendicualr to floor
	  Shaft parallel to midline or
	    forearm

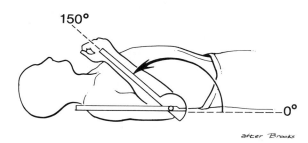

Figure 2-6. Elbow flexion. (Courtesy of Dr. J. F. Lehmann)

Starting position	Measurement

Supine
Arm at side with elbow
  straight
Hand supinated
	Sagittal plane
	Goniometer:
	  Axis lateral to joint and
	    through epicondyles of
	    humerus
	  Shaft parallel to midline of
	    humerus
	  Shaft parallel to midline of
	    forearm

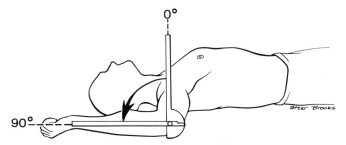

Figure 2-5. Shoulder external rotation. (Courtesy of Dr. J. F. Lehmann)

Starting position	Measurement

Same as in Figure 2-4	Transverse plane
	Substitution to avoid:
	  Arching back
	  Rotating trunk
	  Changing angle at shoulder
	    or elbow
	Goniometer: same as in Figure
	  2-4

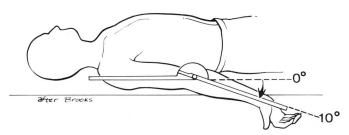

Figure 2-7. Elbow "hyperextension." Demonstration of the method of measuring excessive mobility past the "normal" starting position. (Courtesy of Dr. J. F. Lehmann)

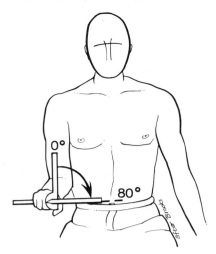

Figure 2-8.   Forearm pronation. (Courtesy of Dr. J. F. Lehmann)

Starting position	Measurement
Sitting (or standing)	Transverse plane
Arm at side with elbow held close to trunk	Substitution to avoid:
	Rotating trunk
Elbow bent to 90°	Moving arm
Forearm in neutral position between pronation and supination	Changing angle at elbow
	Angulating wrist
	Goniometer:
Wrist in neutral position	Axis through longitudinal axis of forearm
Pencil held securely in mid-palmar crease	Shaft parallel to midline of humerus
	Shaft parallel to pencil (on thumb side)

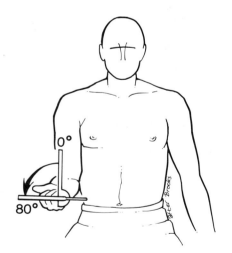

Figure 2-9.   Forearm supination. (Courtesy of Dr. J. F. Lehmann)

Starting position	Measurement
Same as Figure 2-8	Same as Figure 2-8

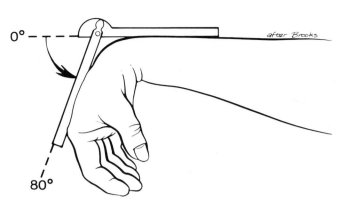

Figure 2-10.   Wrist flexion. (Courtesy of Dr. J. F. Lehmann)

Starting position	Measurement
Elbow bent	Sagittal plane
Forearm and wrist in neutral position	Goniometer:
	Axis over dorsum of wrist (in line with third metacarpal bone)
	Shaft on mid dorsum of forearm
	Shaft on mid dorsum of hand

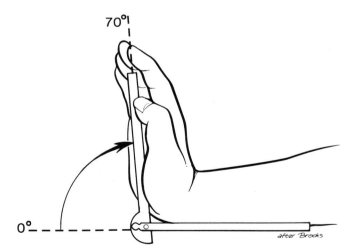

Figure 2-11.   Wrist extension. (Courtesy of Dr. J. F. Lehmann)

Starting position	Measurement
Same as in Figure 2-10	Sagittal plane
	Goniometer:
	Axis on ventral surface of wrist (in line with third metacarpal bone)
	Shaft on midventral surface of forearm
	Shaft on midpalmar surface of hand

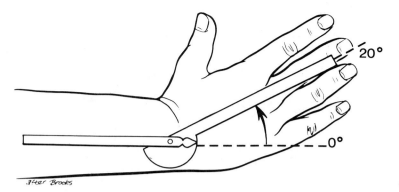

Figure 2-12. Wrist radial deviation. (Courtesy of Dr. J. F. Lehmann)

Starting position

Forearm pronated
Wrist in neutral position

Measurement

Frontal plane
Goniometer:
    Axis over dorsum of wrist
        centered at midcarpal bone
    Shaft on mid dorsum of forearm
    Shaft on shaft of third meta-
        carpal bone

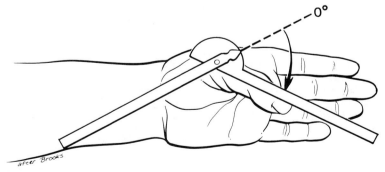

Figure 2-13. Wrist ulnar deviation. (Courtesy of Dr. J. F. Lehmann)

Starting position

Same as in Figure 2-12

Measurement

Same as in Figure 2-12

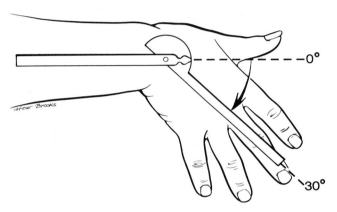

Figure 2-14. First metacarpophalangeal flexion. (Courtesy of Dr. J. F. Lehmann)

Starting position

Elbow slightly flexed
Hand supinated
Fingers and thumb extended

Measurement

Frontal plane
Goniometer:
    Axis on lateral aspect of
        metacarpophalangeal joint
    Shaft parallel to midline of first
        metacarpal bone
    Shaft parallel to midline of
        proximal phalanx

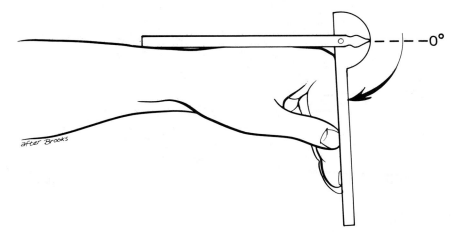

Figure 2-15.   Second, third, and fourth metacarpophalangeal flexion. (Courtesy of Dr. J. F. Lehmann)

Starting position

Elbow flexed
Hand pronated
Wrist in neutral position

Measurement

Sagittal plane
Goniometer:
   Axis on mid dorsum of joint
   Shaft on mid dorsum of metacarpal bone
   Shaft on mid dorsum of proximal phalanx

Figure 2-16.   First interphalangeal flexion. (Courtesy of Dr. J. F. Lehmann)

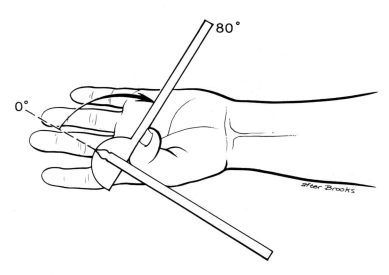

Starting position

Elbow flexed
Forearm supinated
Interphalangeal joint
   extended

Measurement

Frontal plane
Goniometer:
   Axis on lateral aspect of interphalangeal
     joint
   Shaft parallel to midline of proximal
     phalanx
   Shaft parallel to midline of distal phalanx

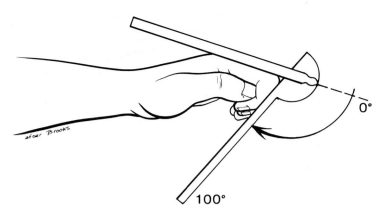

Figure 2-17. Second, third, and fourth interphalangeal flexion. (Courtesy of Dr. J. F. Lehmann)

Starting position

Elbow flexed
Forearm pronated
Interphalangeal joint extended

Measurement

Sagittal plane
Goniometer:
    Axis over dorsal aspect of joint
    Shaft over mid dorsum of proximal phalanx
    Shaft over mid dorsum of more distal phalanx

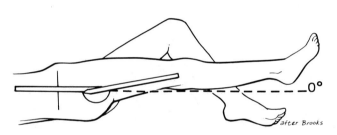

Figure 2-18. Hip extension. See Figure 2-19. (Courtesy of Dr. J. F. Lehmann)

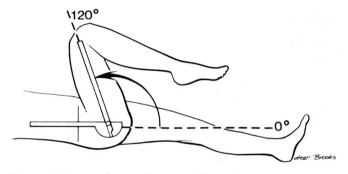

Figure 2-20. Hip flexion. (Courtesy of Dr. J. F. Lehmann)

Starting position

Lying on side or supine (may flex lower knee slightly for support)

Measurement

Sagittal plane
Relocate greater trochanter and redraw C–D, as described in Figure 2-19
Goniometer placement is the same as in Figure 2-19

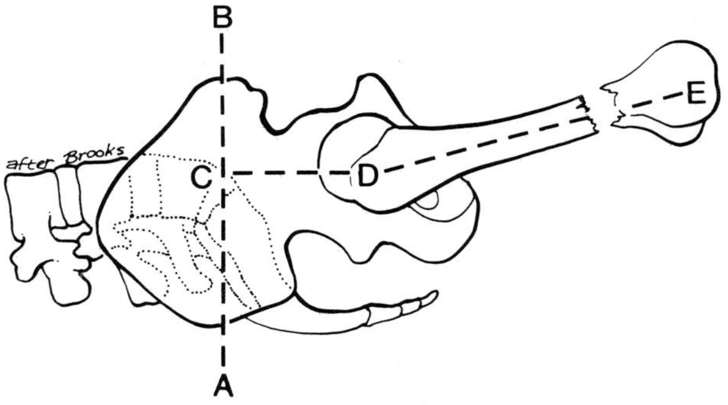

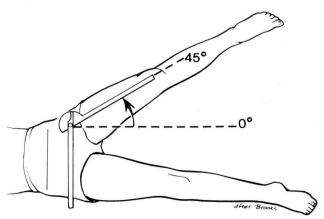

Figure 2-19. Hip extension. (Courtesy of Dr. J. F. Lehmann)

Starting position

Lying on side (or supine)
Lower leg bent for support

Measurement

Saggital plane
Draw line from anterior-superior to posterior-superior iliac spines (B–A)
Drop a perpendicular to the greater trochanter (C–D)
Center axis of goniometer at greater trochanter (D)
Shaft along perpendicular (C–D)
Shaft along shaft of femur (D–E)

Figure 2-21. Hip abduction. (Courtesy of Dr. J. F. Lehmann)

Figure 2-22. Hip abduction. (Courtesy of Dr. J. F. Lehmann)

Starting position	Measurement
Supine	Frontal plane
Leg extended and in neutral position	Mark both anterior-superior iliac spines, and draw a line between them
	Goniometer:
	Axis over hip joint
	Shaft parallel to line between spines of ilium
	Shaft along shaft of femur

Figure 2-23. Hip internal rotation (*left*) and hip external rotation (*right*). (Courtesy of Dr. J. F. Lehmann)

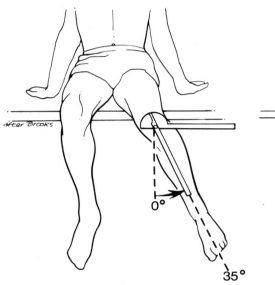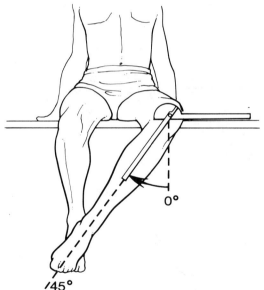

Starting position	Measurement
(Prone)	Transverse plane
Sitting or supine (indicate which position on record)	Substitution to avoid:
Knee flexed to 90°	Rotating trunk
	Lifting thigh from table
	Goniometer:
	Axis through longitudinal axis of femur
	Shaft parallel to table
	Shaft parallel to lower part of leg

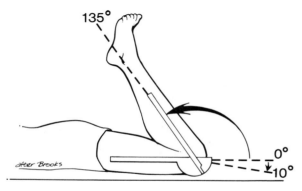

Figure 2-24. Knee flexion. Small arrow indicates hyperextension. (Courtesy of Dr. J. F. Lehmann)

Starting position	Measurement

Prone (or supine with hip flexed if rectus femoris limits motion)	Sagittal plane
	Goniometer:
	   Axis through knee joint
	   Shaft along mid thigh
	   Shaft along fibula

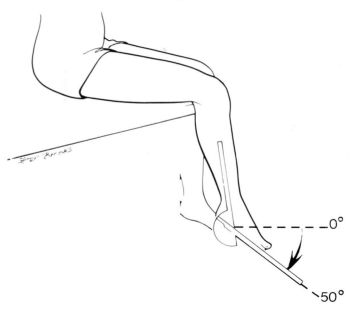

Figure 2-26. Ankle plantar flexion. (Courtesy of Dr. J. F. Lehmann)

Starting position	Measurement
Same as in Figure 2-25	Same as in Figure 2-25

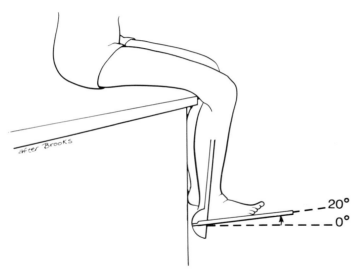

Figure 2-25. Ankle dorsiflexion. (Courtesy of Dr. J. F. Lehmann)

Starting position	Measurement

Sitting
Knee flexed to 90°
Foot at 90° angle to leg
	Sagittal plane
	Goniometer:
	   Axis on sole of foot
	   Shaft along fibula
	   Shaft along fifth metatarsal
	     bone

Joint Stability Assessment

Joint stability is the capacity of the structural elements of a joint to resist forces of inappropriate vector. It is determined by the degree of bony congruity, cartilaginous and capsular integrity, ligament and muscle strength, and the forces required of the joint. For example, the ball-and-socket arrangement of the hip joint is inherently stable because of bony congruity, whereas the glenohumeral joint must rely on musculoligamentous support because of the incongruity of the spherical humeral head in relation to the flat glenoid fossa.

Joint stability is often compromised by disorders common to rehabilitation medicine. Inflammatory synovitis associated with polyarthritis weakens the joint capsule and surrounding ligaments, and the resulting pain inhibits muscle contraction. This inhibition renders the involved joint susceptible to trauma from normal and abnormal forces and leads to joint instability. Instability of extremity and spinal joints is common in traumatic and neurogenic conditions.

Excessive joint motion is often identified during the range-of-motion assessment. However, several specialized physical examination maneuvers (such as Larson's test, Lachman's test, and the pivot-shift test) provide the examiner with tools to assess individual joint integrity. Although a discussion of each of these tests is beyond the scope of this chapter, excellent texts are available.[2, 5, 12]

The stability of each joint is assessed in an orderly fashion. A routine series of individual joint maneuvers is used as part of the general examination and additional tests are performed as necessary to identify more subtle instability when suggested by the history or general examination.

If joint instability is recognized or suspected by physical examination, radiographic studies are often helpful for quantifying the extent of instability. At times, flexion–extension views of the spine and stressed joint views of extremity joints can be helpful; however, these should never be considered until the physical examination and nonstressed films have determined such maneuvers to be safe.

Muscle Strength Testing

Manual muscle testing provides an important means of assessing strength but can also be viewed as a means of assessing weakness. The examiner needs to keep in mind many factors that can affect the effort that a patient is willing to put into the testing.

Such factors are age, sex, pain, fatigue, low motivation, fear, misunderstanding of the test, and the presence of lower or upper motor neuron disease.

Lower motor neuron diseases will result in patterns of motor loss that depend on the location of the disease. For example, a peripheral neuropathy shows a pattern of weakness in the muscles supplied by the affected nerve, or the residual weakness in poliomyelitis is often scattered. The flaccid characteristic of a paretic muscle or muscle group in lower motor neuron disease allows the testing procedure to be uncomplicated by the spasticity or rigidity of upper motor neuron disease. Knowledge of the appearance of the muscle surface when a muscle undergoes atrophy from lower motor neuron disease can also be helpful to the clinician. If the joint crossed by the muscle being tested is unstable owing to a chronic flaccid state, the grade of weakness may be much more difficult to estimate.

Upper motor neuron diseases frequently result in spastic muscles, which make manual testing challenging. For example, the antagonist muscle may be spastic and resist the action of the muscle being tested, or contractures may have developed, complicating the testing by limiting the range of motion available.

For a detailed discussion of the technique of manual muscle testing, the reader is referred to the publications of Kendall and McCreary[14] or Daniels and Worthingham.[3] The anatomical basis for manual muscle testing of the major groups of muscles follows:[6]

Outline of Anatomical Information Required for Tests of Strength of Specific Muscles.   In the following descriptions of the tests, the name of each muscle is followed in parentheses by the corresponding peripheral nerve and spinal segmental supply. There is considerable variability in segmental supply, particularly to certain muscles, as given by different authorities. Furthermore, there is some anatomical variation both in the plexuses and in the peripheral nerves. The segments listed cannot, therefore, be regarded as absolute. The principal and usual supply is underlined. Under ACTION are listed only the principal and important secondary or accessory functions—those particularly useful in testing and those that may cause confusion by substituting for the activity of other muscles. In the description of the test itself the position and movement given first refer to the patient unless otherwise clearly stated. In some instances the movement is adequately indicated by the action of the muscle and, hence, is omitted here. The term *resistance,* unless otherwise specifically stated, refers to the pressure applied by the examiner, and this is in the direction opposite to that of the movement. For brevity and uniformity in description of the tests, the method of testing in which the patient initiates action against the resistance of the examiner is given except when the other method is distinctly more applicable. However, *this concession to uniformity and brevity of description is not meant to imply a preference for the method of testing in which the patient initiates action.* The location of the belly of the muscle and its tendon is often given in order to stress the importance of observation and palpation in identifying the function of that particular muscle. Only those participating muscles are listed that have a definite action in the movement being tested and that may substitute at least in part for the muscle being discussed.

TRAPEZIUS
(Spinal accessory nerve) (Figs. 2-27 and 2-28)
The following text is reprinted from *Clinical Examinations in Neurology* with their permission of the editors. We feel it is an excellent summary and appreciate their contributions.

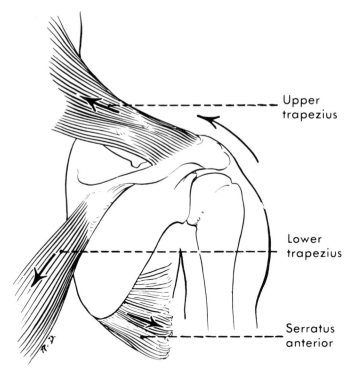

Figure 2-27.   Upward rotators of scapula. (Hollinshead WH: Functional Anatomy of the Limbs and Back: A Text for Students of Physical Therapy and Others Interested in the Locomotor Apparatus, 3rd ed. Philadelphia, WB Saunders, 1969)

Action
Elevation, retraction (adduction), and rotation (lateral angle upward) of scapula, providing fixation of scapula during many movements of arm.

Test
Elevation (shrugging) of shoulder against resistance tests upper portion, which is readily visible.

Bracing shoulder (backward movement and adduction of scapula) tests chiefly middle portion.

Abduction of arm against resistance intensifies winging of scapula.

In isolated trapezius palsy with the shoulder girdle at rest, the scapula is displaced downward and laterally and is rotated so that the superior angle is farther from the spine than the inferior angle. The lateral displacement is due in part to the unopposed action of the serratus anterior. The vertebral border, particularly at the inferior angle, is flared. These changes are accentuated when the arm is abducted from the side against resistance. On flexion (forward elevation) of the arm, however, the flaring of the inferior angle virtually disappears. These features are important in distinguishing trapezius palsy from serratus anterior palsy, which produces an equally characteristic winging of the scapula but in which movement of the arm in these two planes has the opposite effect. Atrophy of the trapezius is evident chiefly in the upper portion.

Participating Muscles:
• Elevation: levator scapulae (third and fourth cervical nerves and dorsal scapular nerve, C3–C5)
• Retraction: rhomboids
• Upward rotation: serratus anterior

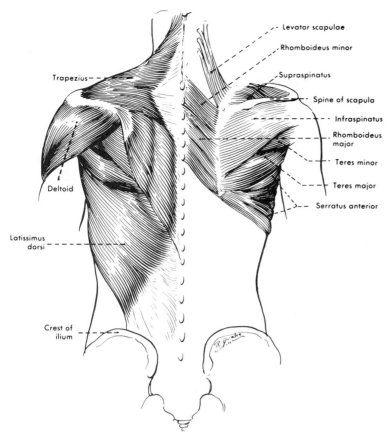

Levator scapulae
Rhomboideus minor
Supraspinatus
Spine of scapula
Infraspinatus
Rhomboideus major
Teres minor
Teres major
Serratus anterior
Trapezius
Deltoid
Latissimus dorsi
Crest of ilium

Figure 2-28. Musculature of shoulder from behind. (Hollinshead WH: Functional Anatomy of the Limbs and Back: A Text for Students of Physical Therapy and Others Interested in the Locomotor Apparatus, 3rd ed. Philadelphia, WB Saunders, 1969).

RHOMBOIDS
(Dorsal scapular nerve from anterior ramus, <u>C5</u>) (Fig. 2-28)

Action
Retraction (adduction) of scapula and elevation of its vertebral border.

Test
Hand is on hip; arm is held backward and medially. Examiner attempts to force elbow laterally and forward, observing and palpating muscle bellies medial to scapula.

Participating muscles: trapezius; levator scapulae: elevation of medial border of scapula

SERRATUS ANTERIOR
(Long thoracic nerve from anterior rami, <u>C5</u>–<u>C7</u>) (Fig. 2-27)

Action
Protraction (lateral and forward movement) of scapula, keeping it closely applied to thorax.

Assistance in upward rotation of scapula.

Test
Outstretched arm is thrust forward against wall or against resistance by examiner.

Isolated palsy results in comparatively little change in the appearance of the shoulder girdle at rest. There is, however, slight winging of the inferior angle of the scapula and slight shift medially toward the spine. When the outstretched arm is thrust forward, the entire scapula, particularly its inferior angle, shifts backward away from the thorax, producing the characteristic wing effect. Abduction of the arm laterally, however, produces comparatively little winging, demonstrating again an important difference from the manifestations of paralysis of the trapezius.

SUPRASPINATUS
(Suprascapular nerve from upper trunk of brachial plexus, C4, <u>C5</u>, C6) (Fig. 2-29)

Action
Initiation of abduction of arm from side of body.

Test
Above action is tested against resistance.

Atrophy may be detected just above the spine of the scapula, but the trapezius overlies the supraspinatus and atrophy of either muscle will produce a depression in this area. Scapular fixation is important in this test.

Participating Muscle: deltoid

INFRASPINATUS
(Suprascapular nerve from upper trunk of brachial plexus, C4, <u>C5</u>, C6) (Fig. 2-30)

Action
Lateral (external) rotation of arm at shoulder.

Test
Elbow is at side and flexed 90°. Patient resists examiner's attempt to push the hand medially toward the abdomen.

The muscle is palpable, and atrophy may be visible below the spine of the scapula.

Participating Muscles: teres minor (axillary nerve); deltoid—posterior fibers

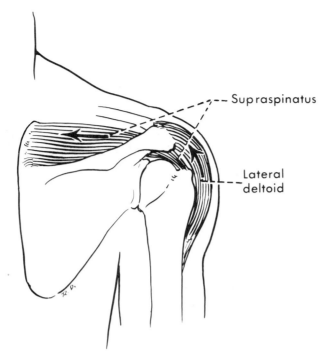

Figure 2-29. Abductors of humerus. (Hollinshead WH: Functional Anatomy of the Limbs and Back: A Text for Students of Physical Therapy and Others Interested in the Locomotor Apparatus, 3rd ed. Philadelphia, WB Saunders, 1969)

Figure 2-30. Chief external rotators of humerus. (Hollinshead WH: Functional Anatomy of the Limbs and Back: A Text for Students of Physical Therapy and Others Interested in the Locomotor Apparatus, 3rd ed. Philadelphia, WB Saunders, 1969)

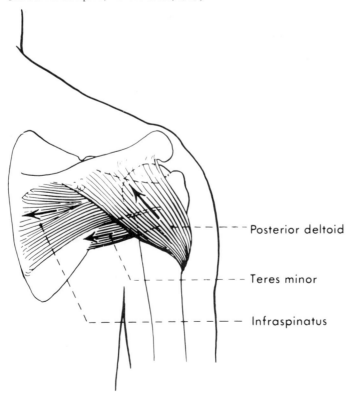

PECTORALIS MAJOR
(Fig. 2-31)
- **Clavicular portion (lateral pectoral nerve from lateral cord of plexus, C5, C6, C7)**
- **Sternal portion (medial pectoral nerve from medial cord of plexus, lateral pectoral nerve, C6, C7, C8, T1)**

Action
Adduction and medial rotation of arm. Clavicular portion—assistance in flexion of arm.

Test
Arm is in front of body. Patient resists attempt by examiner to force it laterally.
The two portions of the muscle are visible and palpable.

LATISSIMUS DORSI
(Thoracodorsal nerve from posterior cord of plexus, C6, C7, C8) (Fig. 2-32)

Action
Adduction, extension, and medial rotation of arm.

Test
Arm is in abduction to horizontal position. Downward and backward movement against resistance is applied under elbow.
The muscle should be observed and palpated in and below the posterior axillary fold. When the patient coughs, a brisk contraction of the normal latissimus dorsi can be felt at the inferior angle of the scapula.

TERES MAJOR
(Lower subscapular nerve from posterior cord plexus, C5–C7) (Fig. 2-32A)

Action and **Test** are the same as for latissimus dorsi.
The muscle is visible and palpable at the lower lateral border of the scapula.

DELTOID
(Axillary nerve from posterior cord of plexus, C5, C6) (Figs. 2-31 and 2-32C)

Action
Abduction of arm.
Flexion (forward movement) and medial rotation of arm—anterior fibers.
Extension (backward movement) and lateral rotation of arm—posterior fibers.

Test
Arm is in abduction almost to horizontal. Patient resists effort of examiner to depress elbow.
Paralysis of the deltoid leads to conspicuous atrophy and serious disability, since the other muscles that participate in abduction of the arm (the supraspinatus, trapezius, and serratus anterior—the last two by rotating the scapula) cannot compensate for lack of function of the deltoid.
Flexion and extension of the arm is tested against resistance.
Participating Muscles:
- Abduction: given above.
- Flexion: pectoralis major—clavicular portion; biceps
- Extension: latissimus dorsi; teres major

SUBSCAPULARIS
(Upper and lower subscapular nerves from posterior cord of plexus, C5, C6, C7) (Fig. 2-32B)

Action
Medial (internal) rotation of arm at shoulder.

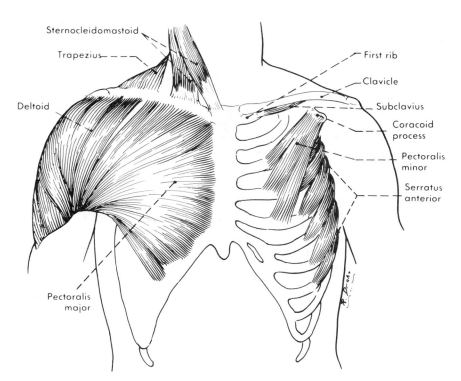

Figure 2-31. Muscles of pectoral region. (Hollinshead WH: Functional Anatomy of the Limbs and Back: A Text for Students of Physical Therapy and Others Interested in the Locomotor Apparatus, 3rd ed. Philadelphia, WB Saunders, 1969)

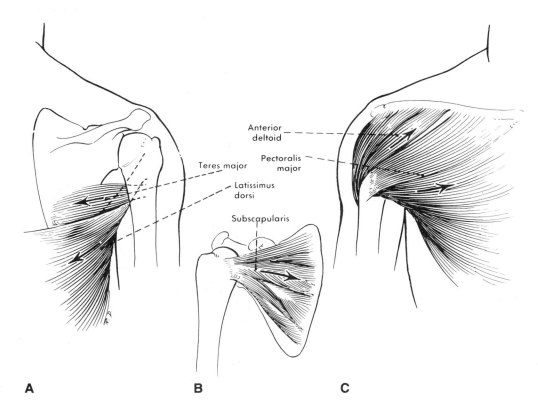

Figure 2-32. Chief internal rotators of humerus. (Hollinshead WH: Functional Anatomy of the Limbs and Back: A Text for Students of Physical Therapy and Others Interested in the Locomotor Apparatus, 3rd ed. Philadelphia, WB Saunders, 1969)

A   **B**   **C**

Test

Elbow is at side and flexed 90°. Patient resists examiner's attempt to pull the hand laterally.

Since this muscle is not accessible to observation or palpation, it is necessary to gauge the activity of other muscles that produce this movement. The pectoralis major is the most powerful medial rotator of the arm; hence, paralysis of the subscapularis alone results in relatively little weakness of this movement.

Participating Muscles: pectoralis major; deltoid—anterior fibers; teres major; latissimus dorsi

BICEPS; BRACHIALIS
(Musculocutaneous nerve from lateral cord of plexus, C5, C6) (Fig. 2-33)

Action
Biceps: flexion and supination of forearm and assistance in flexion of arm at shoulder.
Brachialis: flexion of forearm at elbow

Test
Flexion of forearm is tested against resistance. Forearm should be in supination to decrease participation of brachioradialis.

TRICEPS
(Radial nerve, which is continuation of posterior cord of plexus, C6, C7, C8) (Fig. 2-34)

Action
Extension of forearm at elbow.

Test
Forearm is in flexion to varying degree. Patient resists effort of examiner to flex forearm farther. Slight weakness is more easily detected when starting with forearm almost completely flexed.

BRACHIORADIALIS
(Radial nerve, C5, C6) (Fig. 2-35)

Action
Flexion of forearm at elbow.

Test
Flexion of forearm is tested against resistance with forearm midway between pronation and supination.
The belly of the muscle stands out prominently on the upper surface of the forearm, tending to bridge the angle between the forearm and arm.
Participating Muscles: biceps; brachialis

SUPINATOR
(Posterior interosseous nerve from radial nerve, C5–C7) (Fig. 2-35)

Action
Supination of forearm.

Test
Forearm is in full extension and supination. Patient attempts to maintain supination while examiner attempts to pronate forearm and palpates biceps.

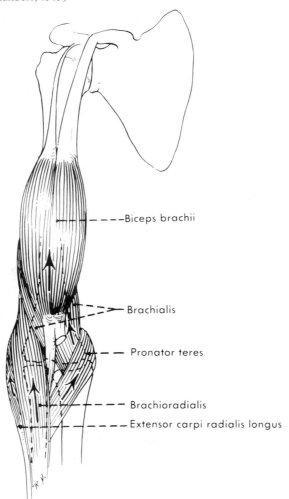

Figure 2-33.   Flexors of elbow. (Hollinshead WH: Functional Anatomy of the Limbs and Back: A Text for Students of Physical Therapy and Others Interested in the Locomotor Apparatus, 3rd ed. Philadelphia, WB Saunders, 1969)

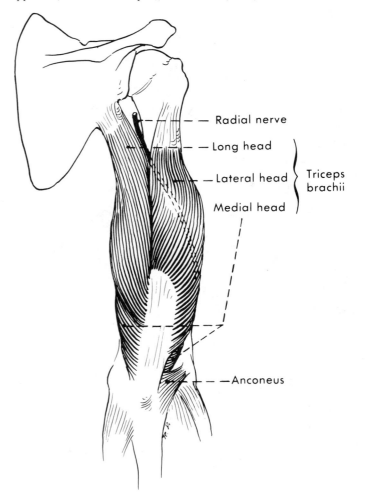

Figure 2-34.   Muscles of extensor (posterior) surface of right arm. (Hollinshead WH: Functional Anatomy of the Limbs and Back: A Text for Students of Physical Therapy and Others Interested in the Locomotor Apparatus, 3rd ed. Philadelphia, WB Saunders, 1969)

Resistance to pronation by the intact supinator can usually be felt before there is appreciable contraction of the biceps.

EXTENSOR CARPI RADIALIS LONGUS
(Radial nerve, C6, C7, C8) (Fig. 2-36)

Action
Extension (dorsiflexion) and radial abduction of hand at wrist.

Test
Forearm is in almost complete pronation. Dorsiflexion of wrist is tested against resistance applied to dorsum of hand downward and toward ulnar side.

The tendon is palpable just above its insertion into the base of the second metacarpal bone. The fingers and thumb should be relaxed and somewhat flexed to minimize participation of the extensors of the digits.

EXTENSOR CARPI RADIALIS BREVIS
(Posterior interosseous nerve from radial nerve, C6, C7, C8) (Fig. 2-36)

Action
Extension (dorsiflexion) of hand at wrist.

Test
Forearm is in complete pronation. Dorsiflexion of wrist is tested against resistance applied to dorsum of hand straight downward.

The tendon is palpable just proximal to the base of the third metacarpal bone. The fingers and thumb should be relaxed and somewhat flexed to minimize participation of the extensors of the digits.

EXTENSOR CARPI ULNARIS
(Posterior interosseous nerve from radial nerve, C7, C8) (Fig. 2-36)

Action
Extension (dorsiflexion) and ulnar deviation of hand at wrist.

Test
Forearm is in pronation. Dorsiflexion and ulnar deviation of wrist are tested against resistance applied to dorsum of hand downward and toward radial side.

The tendon is palpable just below or above the distal end of the ulna. The fingers should be relaxed and somewhat flexed in order to minimize participation of the extensors of the digits.

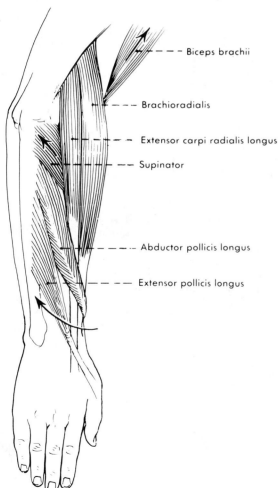

Figure 2-35. Chief supinators of forearm. (Modified from Hollinshead WH: Functional Anatomy of the Limbs and Back: A Text for Students of Physical Therapy and Others Interested in the Locomotor Apparatus, 3rd ed. Philadelphia, WB Saunders, 1969)

Biceps brachii

Brachioradialis

Extensor carpi radialis longus

Supinator

Abductor pollicis longus

Extensor pollicis longus

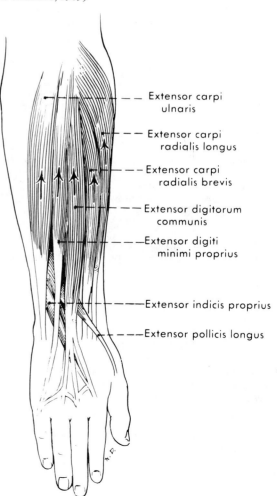

Figure 2-36. Chief extensors of wrist. (Hollinshead WH: Functional Anatomy of the Limbs and Back: A Text for Students of Physical Therapy and Others Interested in the Locomotor Apparatus, 3rd ed. Philadelphia, WB Saunders, 1969)

Extensor carpi ulnaris

Extensor carpi radialis longus

Extensor carpi radialis brevis

Extensor digitorum communis

Extensor digiti minimi proprius

Extensor indicis proprius

Extensor pollicis longus

EXTENSOR DIGITORUM
(Posterior interosseous nerve from radial nerve, C6, C7, C8) (Fig. 2-36)

Action
Extension of fingers, principally at metacarpophalangeal joints.
Assistance in extension (dorsiflexion) of wrist.

Test
Forearm is in pronation. Wrist is stabilized in straight position. Extension of fingers at metacarpophalangeal joints is tested against resistance applied to proximal phalanges.

The distal portions of the fingers may be somewhat relaxed and in slight flexion. The tendons are visible and palpable over the dorsum of the hand.

Extension at the interphalangeal joints is a function primarily of the interossei (ulnar nerve) and lumbricals (median and ulnar nerves).

The extensor digiti quinti and extensor indicis (posterior interosseous nerve, C7, C8), proper extensors of the little and index fingers, respectively, can be tested individually while the other fingers are in flexion to minimize the action of the common extensor. In a thin person's hand the tendons can usually be identified.

ABDUCTOR POLLICIS LONGUS
(Posterior interosseous nerve from radial nerve, C7, C8) (Fig. 2-35)

Action
Radial abduction of thumb (in same plane as that of palm, in contradistinction to palmar abduction, which is movement perpendicular to plane of palm).
Assistance in radial abduction and flexion of hand at wrist.

Test
Hand is on edge (forearm midway between pronation and supination).
Radial abduction of thumb is tested against resistance applied to metacarpal.
The tendon is palpable just above its insertion into the base of the metacarpal bone and forms the anterior (volar) boundary of the "anatomic snuffbox."
Participating Muscle: extensor pollicis brevis

EXTENSOR POLLICIS BREVIS
(Posterior interosseous nerve from radial nerve, C7, C8)

Action
Extension of proximal phalanx of thumb.
Assistance in radial abduction and extension of metacarpal of thumb.

Test
Hand is on edge. Wrist and particularly metacarpal of thumb are stabilized by examiner. Extension of proximal phalanx is tested against resistance applied to that phalanx, while distal phalanx is in flexion to minimize action of extensor pollicis longus.
At the wrist the tendon lies just posterior (dorsal) to the tendon of the abductor pollicis longus.
Participating Muscle: extensor pollicis longus

EXTENSOR POLLICIS LONGUS
(Posterior interosseous nerve from radial nerve, C7, C8) (Fig. 2-36)

Action
Extension of all parts of thumb but specifically extension of distal phalanx.
Assistance in adduction of thumb.

Test
Hand is on edge. Wrist, metacarpal, and proximal phalanx of thumb are stabilized by examiner with thumb close to palm at its radial border. Extension of distal phalanx is tested against resistance.
If the patient is permitted to flex the wrist or abduct the thumb away from the palm, some extension of the phalanges results simply from lengthening the path of the extensor tendon. At the wrist the tendon forms the posterior (dorsal) boundary of the "anatomic snuffbox."

The characteristic result of radial nerve palsy is wristdrop. Extension of the fingers at the interphalangeal joints is still possible by virtue of the action of the interossei and lumbricals, but extension of the thumb is lost.

The next group of muscles examined is that supplied by the median nerve, which is formed by the union of its lateral root, from the lateral cord of the brachial plexus, and its medial root, from the medial cord of the plexus. Then the muscles supplied by the ulnar nerve (arising from the medial cord of the brachial plexus) are tested. However, for convenience in order of examination, some of the muscles in the ulnar group are tested with the median group.

PRONATOR TERES
(Median nerve, C6, C7) (Fig. 2-37)

Action
Pronation of forearm.

Test
Elbow is at side of trunk, forearm is in flexion to right angle, and arm is in lateral rotation at shoulder to eliminate effect of gravity, which, in most positions, favors pronation. Pronation of forearm is tested against resistance, starting from a position of moderate supination.
Participating Muscle: pronator quadratus (anterior interosseous branch of median nerve, C7, C8, T1)

FLEXOR CARPI RADIALIS
(Median nerve, C6, C7) (Figs. 2-37 and 2-38)

Action
Flexion (palmar flexion) of hand at wrist.
Assistance in radial abduction of hand.

Test
Flexion of hand is tested against resistance applied to palm. Fingers should be relaxed to minimize participation of their flexors.
The tendon is the more lateral (radial) one of the two conspicuous tendons on the volar aspect of the wrist.
In complete median nerve palsy, flexion of the wrist is considerably weakened but can still be performed by the flexor carpi ulnaris (ulnar nerve) assisted to some extent by the abductor pollicis longus (radial nerve). In this event, ulnar deviation of the hand usually accompanies flexion.

PALMARIS LONGUS
(Median nerve, C7, C8, T1) (Figs. 2-37 and 2-38)

Action
Flexion of hand at wrist.

Test
Same as for flexor carpi radialis. The tendon is palpable at the ulnar side of the tendon of the flexor carpi radialis.

FLEXOR CARPI ULNARIS
(Ulnar nerve, C7, C8, T1) (Fig. 2-38)

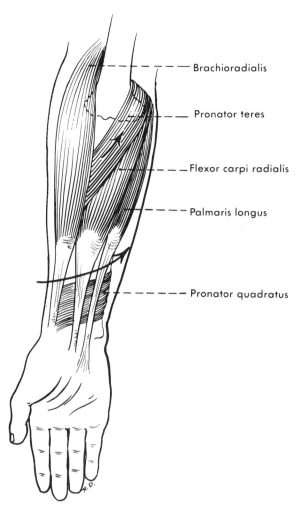

Figure 2-37. Pronators of forearm. (Hollinshead WH: Functional Anatomy of the Limbs and Back: A Text for Students of Physical Therapy and Others Interested in the Locomotor Apparatus, 3rd ed. Philadelphia, WB Saunders, 1969)

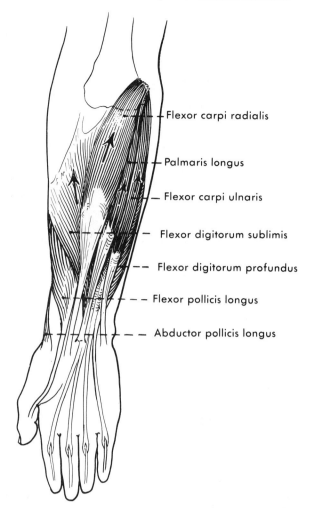

Figure 2-38. Chief flexors of wrist. (Hollinshead WH: Functional Anatomy of the Limbs and Back: A Text for Students of Physical Therapy and Others Interested in the Locomotor Apparatus, 3rd ed. Philadelphia, WB Saunders, 1969)

Action
Flexion and ulnar deviation of hand at wrist.
Fixation of pisiform bone during contraction of abductor digiti quinti.

Test
Flexion and ulnar deviation of hand are tested against resistance applied to ulnar side of palm in direction of extension and radial abduction. Fingers should be relaxed.
The tendon is palpable proximal to the pisiform bone.

FLEXOR DIGITORUM SUBLIMIS
(Median nerve, C7, <u>C8</u>, <u>T1</u>) (Fig. 2-38)

Action
Flexion of middle phalanges of fingers at first interphalangeal joints primarily; flexion of proximal phalanges at metacarpophalangeal joints secondarily.
Assistance in flexion of hand at wrist.

Test
Wrist is in neutral position; proximal phalanges are stabilized. Flexion of middle phalanx of each finger is tested against resistance applied to that phalanx, with the distal phalanx relaxed.

FLEXOR DIGITORUM PROFUNDUS
(Fig. 2-38)

- **Radial portion: usually to digits II and III (median nerve and its anterior interosseous branch C7, C8, T1)**
- **<u>Ulnar portion: usually to digits IV and V (ulnar nerve, C7, <u>C8</u>, <u>T1</u>)**

Action
Flexion of distal phalanges of fingers specifically; flexion of other phalanges secondarily.
Assistance in flexion of hand at wrist.

Test
Flexion of distal phalanges is tested against resistance with proximal and middle phalanges stabilized in extension.
With middle and distal phalanges folded over edge of examiner's hand, patient resists attempt by examiner to extend distal phalanges.

FLEXOR POLLICIS LONGUS
(Anterior interosseous branch of median nerve, C7, <u>C8</u>, <u>T1</u>) (Fig. 2-38)

Action
Flexion of thumb, particularly distal phalanx.
Assistance in ulnar adduction of thumb.

Test
Flexion of distal phalanx is tested against resistance with thumb in position of palmar adduction and with stabilization of metacarpal and proximal phalanx.

ABDUCTOR POLLICIS BREVIS
(Median nerve, C8, T1) (Fig. 2-39)

Action
Palmar abduction of thumb (perpendicular to plane of palm).
Assistance in opposition and in flexion of proximal phalanx of thumb.

Test
Palmar abduction of thumb is tested against resistance applied at metacarpophalangeal joint.
The muscle is readily visible and palpable in the thenar eminence.
Participating Muscle: flexor pollicis brevis (superficial head)

OPPONENS POLLICIS
(Median nerve, C8, T1) (Fig. 2-39)

Action
Movement of first metacarpal across palm, rotating it into opposition.

Test
Thumb is in opposition. Examiner attempts to rotate and draw thumb back to its usual position.
Participating Muscles: abductor pollicis brevis; flexor pollicis brevis

FLEXOR POLLICIS BREVIS
Superficial head (median nerve, C8, T1); deep head (ulnar nerve, C8, T1) (Fig. 2-39)

Figure 2-39. Short muscles of the thumb and little finger. (Hollinshead WH: Functional Anatomy of the Limbs and Back: A Text for Students of Physical Therapy and Others Interested in the Locomotor Apparatus, 3rd ed. Philadelphia, WB Saunders, 1969)

Action
Flexion of proximal phalanx of thumb.
Assistance in opposition, ulnar adduction (entire muscle), and palmar abduction (superficial head) of thumb.

Test
Thumb is in position of palmar adduction with stabilization of metacarpal. Flexion of proximal phalanx is tested against resistance applied to that phalanx while distal phalanx is as relaxed as possible.
Participating Muscles: flexor pollicis longus; abductor pollicis brevis; adductor pollicis

Severe median nerve palsy produces the "simian" hand, wherein the thumb tends to lie in the same plane as the palm with the volar surface facing more anteriorly than normal. Atrophy of the muscles of the thenar eminence is usually conspicuous.

Three muscles supplied, at least in part, by the ulnar nerve have already been described: flexor carpi ulnaris, flexor digitorum profundus, and flexor pollicis brevis. The remaining muscles supplied by this nerve follow.

HYPOTHENAR MUSCLES
(Ulnar nerve, C8, T1)

Action
Abductor digiti quinti and flexor digiti quinti: abduction and flexion (proximal phalanx) of little finger.
Opponens digiti quinti: opposition of little finger toward thumb.
All three muscles: palmar elevation of head of fifth metacarpal, helping to cup palm.

Test
Action usually tested is abduction of little finger (against resistance).
The abductor digiti quinti is readily observed and palpated at the ulnar border of the palm. Opposition of the thumb and little finger can be tested together by gauging the force required

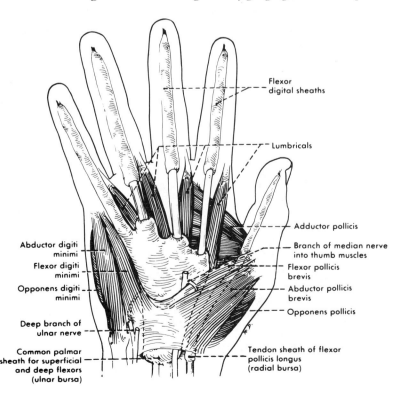

Flexor digital sheaths

Lumbricals

Adductor pollicis

Branch of median nerve into thumb muscles

Flexor pollicis brevis

Abductor pollicis brevis

Opponens pollicis

Tendon sheath of flexor pollicis longus (radial bursa)

Abductor digiti minimi

Flexor digiti minimi

Opponens digiti minimi

Deep branch of ulnar nerve

Common palmar sheath for superficial and deep flexors (ulnar bursa) to separate the tips of the two digits when opposed, or by attempting to withdraw a piece of paper clasped between the tips of the digits.

INTEROSSEI
(Ulnar nerve, C8, <u>T1</u>) (Figs. 2-40 and 2-41)

Action

Dorsal: abduction of index, middle, and ring fingers from middle line of middle finger (double action on middle finger—both radial and ulnar abduction, radial abduction of index finger, ulnar abduction of ring finger).

First dorsal: adduction (especially palmar adduction) of thumb.

Palmar: adduction of index, ring, and little fingers toward middle finger.

Both sets: flexion of metacarpophalangeal joints and simultaneous extension of interphalangeal jonts.

Test

Abduction and adduction of individual fingers are tested against resistance with fingers extended. Adduction can be tested by retention of a slip of paper between fingers, and between thumb and index finger, as examiner attempts to withdraw it.

Ability of patient is tested to flex proximal phalanges and simultaneously extend distal phalanges.

Extension of middle phalanges of fingers against resistance while examiner stabilizes proximal phalanges in hyperextension.

The long extensors of the fingers (radial nerve) and the lumbri-cal muscles (median and ulnar nerves) assist in extension of the middle and distal phalanges. The first dorsal interosseous is readily observed and palpated in the space between the index finger and the thumb.

ADDUCTOR POLLICIS
(Ulnar nerve, C8, <u>T1</u>)

Action

Adduction of thumb in both ulnar and palmar directions (in plane of palm and perpendicular to palm, respectively).

Assistance in flexion of proximal phalanx.

Test

Adduction in each plane is tested against resistance by retention of slip of paper between thumb and radial border of hand and between thumb and palm, without flexion of distal phalanx.

It is often possible to palpate the edge of the adductor pollicis just volar to the proximal part of the first dorsal interosseous.

Participating Muscles:

- Ulnar adduction: first dorsal interosseous; flexor pollicis longus; extensor pollicis longus; flexor pollicis brevis
- Palmar adduction: first dorsal interosseous particularly; extensor pollicis longus

The muscles of the neck and trunk may be examined in groups in most instances.

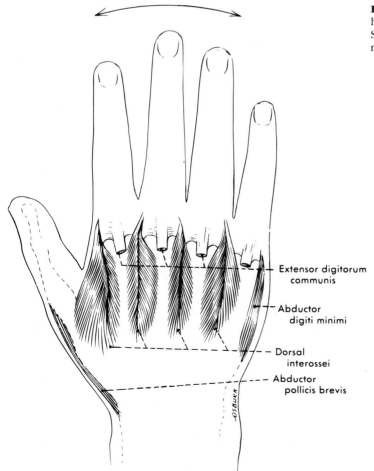

Figure 2-40. Dorsal view of chief abductors of digits. (Hollinshead WH: Functional Anatomy of the Limbs and Back: A Text for Students of Physical Therapy and Others Interested in the Locomotor Apparatus, 3rd ed. Philadelphia, WB Saunders, 1969)

Extensor digitorum communis

Abductor digiti minimi

Dorsal interossei

Abductor pollicis brevis

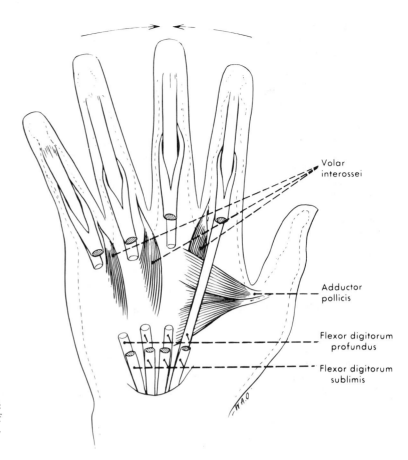

Figure 2-41. Chief adductors of digits. (Hollinshead WH: Functional Anatomy of the Limbs and Back: A Text for Students of Physical Therapy and Others Interested in the Locomotor Apparatus, 3rd ed. Philadelphia, WB Saunders, 1969)

FLEXORS OF NECK
(Cervical nerves, C1–C6)

Test

In sitting or supine position flexion of neck, with chin on chest, is tested against resistance applied to forehead.

EXTENSORS OF NECK
(Cervical nerves, C1–T1)

Test

In sitting or prone position extension of neck is tested against resistance applied to occiput.

DIAPHRAGM
(Phrenic nerves, C3, C4, C5)

Action

Abdominal respiration (inspiration), as distinguished from thoracic respiration (inspiration), which is produced principally by the intercostal muscles.

Test

Patient is observed for protrusion of upper portion of abdomen during deep inspiration when thoracic cage is splinted.

Patient is observed for ability to sniff.

Litten's sign (successive retraction of lower intercostal spaces during inspiration) is sought.

Diaphragmatic movements are observed fluoroscopically.

Weakness of the diaphragm should be suspected in diseas of the spinal cord when the deltoid or biceps is paralyzed, since these muscles are supplied by neurons situated very near those innervating the diaphragm.

INTERCOSTAL MUSCLES
(Intercostal nerves, T1–T11)

Action

Expansion of thorax anteroposteriorly and transversely, producing thoracic inspiration.

Test

Observation and palpation of expansion of thoracic cage during deep inspiration are done while maintaining pressure against thorax.

Observation for asymmetry of movement of thorax, particularly during deep inspiration, is done.

Other more general tests of function of the respiratory muscles are as follows:

- Observation of patient for rapid shallow respiration, flaring of alae nasi, and use of accessory muscles of respiration
- Ability of patient to repeat three or four numbers without pausing for breath
- Ability of patient to hold breath for 15 seconds

ANTERIOR ABDOMINAL MUSCLES
Upper (T6–T9); lower (T10–L1)

Test

Supine: flexion of neck is tested against resistance applied to forehead by examiner.

Contraction of the abdominal muscles can be observed and palpated. Upward movement of the umbilicus is associated with weakness of the lower abdominal muscles (Beevor's sign).

Supine: hands on occiput. Flexion of trunk by anterior abdominal muscles followed by flexion of pelvis on thighs by hip flexors (chiefly iliopsoas) to reach sitting position is tested. Examiner holds legs down.

Completion of this test excludes significant weakness of either the abdominal muscles or the flexors of the hips. Weak abdominal muscles, in the presence of strong hip flexors, result in hyperextension of the lumbar spine during attempts to elevate the legs or rise to a sitting position.

EXTENSORS OF BACK

Test

In prone position with hands clasped over buttocks, the head and shoulders are elevated off the table while the examiner holds legs down.

The gluteal and hamstring muscles fix the pelvis on the thigh.

ILIOPSOAS
Psoas major (lumbar plexus, L1, L2, L3, L4); iliacus (femoral nerve, L2, L3, L4) (Fig. 2-42)

Action
Flexion of thigh at hip.

Figure 2-42. More superficial muscles of anterior aspect of thigh. (Hollinshead WH: Functional Anatomy of the Limbs and Back: A Text for Students of Physical Therapy and Others Interested in the Locomotor Apparatus, 3rd ed. Philadelphia, WB Saunders, 1969)

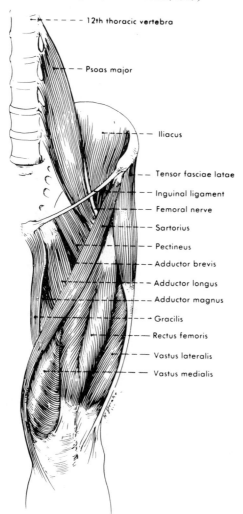

- 12th thoracic vertebra
- Psoas major
- Iliacus
- Tensor fasciae latae
- Inguinal ligament
- Femoral nerve
- Sartorius
- Pectineus
- Adductor brevis
- Adductor longus
- Adductor magnus
- Gracilis
- Rectus femoris
- Vastus lateralis
- Vastus medialis

Test
Sitting: flexion of thigh is tested by raising knee against resistance by examiner.

Supine: flexion of thigh is tested by raising extended leg off table and maintaining it against downward pressure by examiner applied just above knee.

Participating Muscles: rectus femoris and sartorius (both—femoral nerve, L2–L4); tensor fasciae latae (superior gluteal nerve, L4, L5, S1)

ADDUCTOR MAGNUS, LONGUS, BREVIS
(Obturator nerve, L2, L3, L4; part of adductor magnus is supplied by sciatic nerve, L5, and functions with hamstrings) (Fig. 2-42)

Action
Principally adduction of thigh.

Test
Sitting or supine: knees are held together while examiner attempts to separate them.

The two legs can also be tested separately and the muscles palpated.

Participating Muscles: gluteus maximus; gracilis (obturator nerve, L2–L4)

ABDUCTORS OF THIGH
(Superior gluteal nerve, L4, L5, S1) (Fig. 2-43)
- **Gluteus medius and gluteus minimus principally**
- **Tensor fasciae latae to a lesser extent**

Figure 2-43. Abductors of thigh. (Hollinshead WH: Functional Anatomy of the Limbs and Back: A Text for Students of Physical Therapy and Others Interested in the Locomotor Apparatus, 3rd ed. Philadelphia, WB Saunders, 1969)

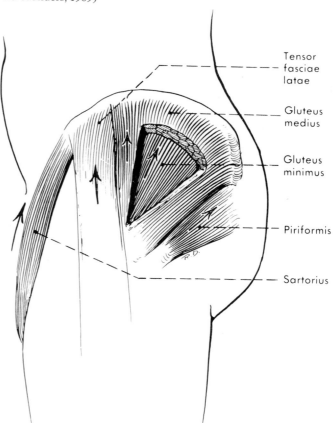

- Tensor fasciae latae
- Gluteus medius
- Gluteus minimus
- Piriformis
- Sartorius

Action

Abduction and medial rotation of thigh.

Tensor fasciae latae assists in flexion of thigh at hip.

Test

Sitting: knees are separated against resistance by examiner.

In this position the gluteus maximus and some of the other lateral rotators of the thigh function as abductors, hence diminishing the accuracy of the test.

Supine: same test as above, but more exact.

Lying on opposite site: hip is abducted (upward movement) while examiner presses downward on lower leg and stabilizes pelvis.

The tensor fasciae latae and to a lesser extent the gluteus medius can be palpated.

MEDIAL ROTATORS OF THIGH
(Same as abductors)

Test

Sitting or prone: knee is flexed to 90°. Medial rotation of thigh is tested against resistance applied by examiner at knee and ankle in an attempt to rotate thigh laterally.

LATERAL ROTATORS OF THIGH
(L4, L5, S1, S2) (Fig. 2-44)
- **Gluteus maximus (inferior gluteal nerve, L5, S1, S2) chiefly.**
- **Obturator internus and gemellus superior (nerve to obturator internus, L5, S1, S2).**
- **Quadratus femoris and gemellus inferior (nerve to quadratus femoris, L4, L5, S1).**

Test

Sitting or prone: knee is flexed to 90°. Lateral rotation of thigh is tested against attempt by examiner to rotate thigh medially.

The gluteus maximus is the muscle principally tested and can be observed and palpated in the prone position.

GLUTEUS MAXIMUS
(Inferior gluteal nerve, L5, S1, S2) (Fig. 2-44)

Action

Extension of thigh at hip.

Lateral rotation of thigh.

Assistance in adduction of thigh.

Test

Sitting or supine: starting with thigh slightly raised, extension (downward movement) of thigh is tested against resistance by examiner applied under distal part of thigh.

This is a rather crude test and the muscle cannot be observed or readily palpated.

Prone: knee is well flexed to minimize participation of hamstrings. Extension of thigh is tested by raising knee from table against downward pressure by examiner applied to distal part of thigh.

The muscle is accessible to observation and palpation in this position.

QUADRICEPS FEMORIS
(Femoral nerve, L2, L3, L4) (Fig. 2-45)

Action

Extension of leg at knee.

Rectus femoris assists in flexion of thigh at hip.

Test

Sitting or supine: lower leg is in moderate extension. Maintenance of extension is tested against effort of examiner to flex leg at knee.

Atrophy is easily noted.

HAMSTRINGS
(Sciatic nerve, L4, L5, S1, S2) (Fig. 2-46)
- **Biceps femoris: external hamstring (L5, S1, S2)**
- **Semitendinosus**
- **Semimembranosus**

Figure 2-44. Posteriorly placed external rotators of thigh. (Hollinshead WH: Functional Anatomy of the Limbs and Back: A Text for Students of Physical Therapy and Others Interested in the Locomotor Apparatus, 3rd ed. Philadelphia, WB Saunders, 1969)

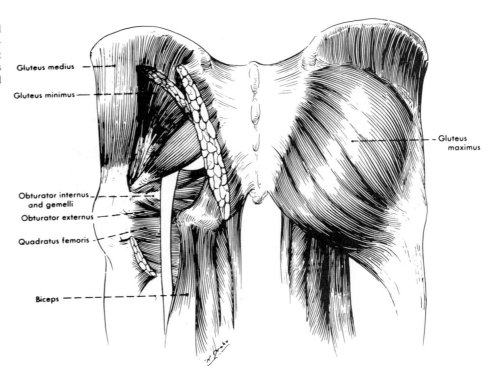

Gluteus medius

Gluteus minimus

Obturator internus and gemelli

Obturator externus

Quadratus femoris

Biceps

Gluteus maximus

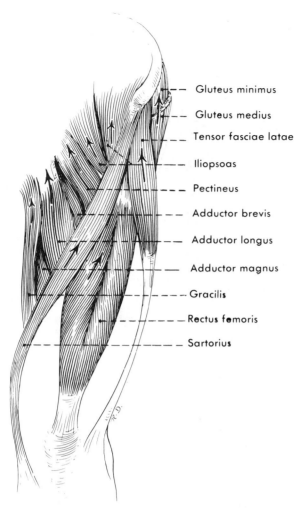

Figure 2-45. Flexors of thigh. (Hollinshead WH: Functional Anatomy of the Limbs and Back: A Text for Students of Physical Therapy and Others Interested in the Locomotor Apparatus, 3rd ed. Philadelphia, WB Saunders, 1969)

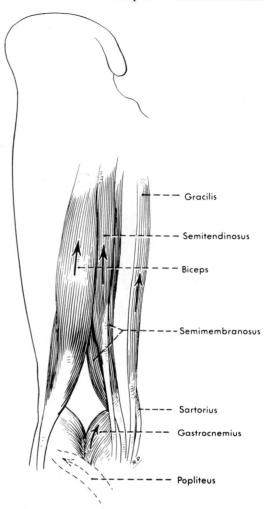

Figure 2-46. Flexors of knee. (Hollinshead WH: Functional Anatomy of the Limbs and Back: A Text for Students of Physical Therapy and Others Interested in the Locomotor Apparatus, 3rd ed. Philadelphia, WB Saunders, 1969)

Action
Flexion of leg at knee.
All but short head of biceps femoris assist in extension of thigh at hip.

Test
Sitting: flexion of lower leg is tested against resistance.
Prone: knee is partly flexed. Further flexion is tested against resistance. Observation and palpation of the muscles and tendons are important for proper interpretation.

TIBIALIS ANTERIOR
(Deep peroneal nerve, L4, L5, S1) (Figs. 2-47, 2-48, and 2-49)

Action
Dorsiflexion and inversion (particularly in dorsiflexed position) of foot.

Test
Dorsiflexion of foot is tested against resistance applied to dorsum of foot downward and toward eversion.
The belly of the muscle just lateral to the shin and the tendon medially on the dorsal aspect of the ankle should be observed and palpated. Atrophy is conspicuous.

Participating Muscles:
- Dorsiflexion: extensor hallucis longus; extensor digitorum longus
- Inversion: tibialis posterior

EXTENSOR HALLUCIS LONGUS
(Deep peroneal nerve, L4, L5, S1) (Fig. 2-48)

Action
Extension of great toe and dorsiflexion of foot.

Test
Extension of great toe is tested against resistance while foot is stabilized in neutral position.
The tendon is palpable between the tendons of the tibialis anterior and the extensor digitorum longus.

EXTENSOR DIGITORUM LONGUS
(Deep peroneal nerve, L4, L5, S1) (Figs. 2-47 and 2-48)

Action
Extension of lateral four toes and dorsiflexion of foot.

Test
Test is similar to that for action of extensor hallucis longus.
The tendons are visible and palpable on the dorsal aspect of the

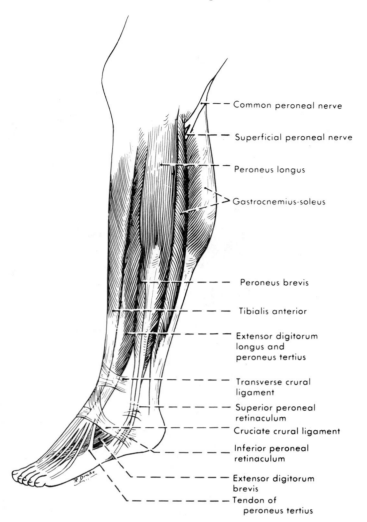

Figure 2-47. Lateral muscles of leg. (Hollinshead WH: Functional Anatomy of the Limbs and Back: A Text for Students of Physical Therapy and Others Interested in the Locomotor Apparatus, 3rd ed. Philadelphia, WB Saunders, 1969)

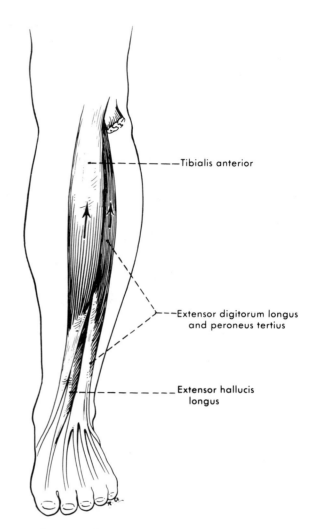

Figure 2-48. Dorsiflexors of foot. (Hollinshead WH: Functional Anatomy of the Limbs and Back: A Text for Students of Physical Therapy and Others Interested in the Locomotor Apparatus, 3rd ed. Philadelphia, WB Saunders, 1969)

ankle and foot lateral to the tendon of the extensor hallucis longus.

EXTENSOR DIGITORUM BREVIS
(Deep peroneal nerve, L4, <u>L5</u>, <u>S1</u>) (Fig. 2-47)

Action
Assists in extension of all toes except little toe.

Test
Belly of muscle is observed and palpated on lateral aspect of dorsum of foot.

PERONEUS LONGUS, BREVIS
(Superficial peroneal nerve, L4, <u>L5</u>, <u>S1</u>) (Fig. 2-49)

Action
Eversion of foot.
Assistance in plantar flexion of foot.

Test
Foot is in plantar flexion. Eversion is tested against resistance applied by examiner to lateral border of foot.
The tendons are palpable just above and behind the external

malleolus. Atrophy may be visible over the anterolateral aspect of the lower leg.

GASTROCNEMIUS; SOLEUS
(Tibial nerve, L5, <u>S1</u>, <u>S2</u>) (Fig. 2-50)

Action
Plantar flexion of foot.
The gastrocnemius also flexes the knee and cannot act effectively in plantar flexion of the foot when the knee is well flexed.

Test
Knee is extended to test both muscles. Knee is flexed to test principally soleus. Plantar flexion of foot is tested against resistance.
The muscles and tendon should be observed and palpated. Atrophy is readily visible. The gastrocnemius and soleus are very strong muscles, and leverage in testing favors the patient rather than the examiner. For this reason slight weakness is difficult to detect by resisting flexion of the ankle or by pressing against the flexed foot in the direction of extension. Consequently, it is advisable to test the strength of these muscles against the weight of the patient's body. The

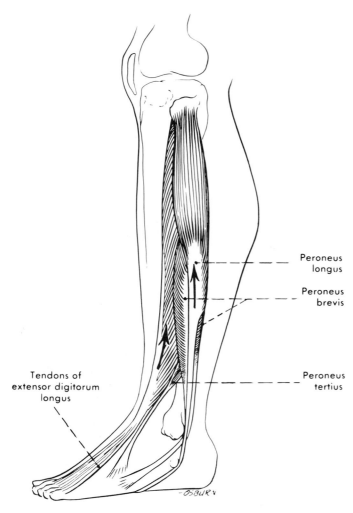

Figure 2-49. Evertors of foot. (Hollinshead WH: Functional Anatomy of the Limbs and Back: A Text for Students of Physical Therapy and Others Interested in the Locomotor Apparatus, 3rd ed. Philadelphia, WB Saunders, 1969)

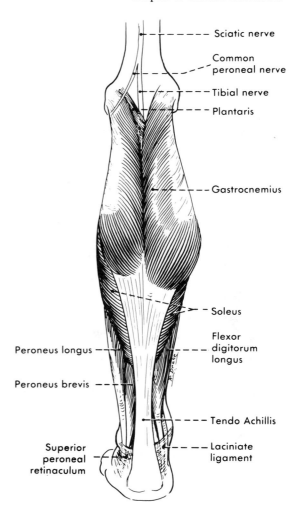

Figure 2-50. Musculature of calf of leg, first layer. (Hollinshead WH: Functional Anatomy of the Limbs and Back: A Text for Students of Physical Therapy and Others Interested in the Locomotor Apparatus, 3rd ed. Philadelphia, WB Saunders, 1969)

patient stands on one foot and flexes the foot so as to lift himself or herself directly and fully upward. Sometimes it is necessary for the examiner to hold the patient steady as this test is performed.

Participating Muscles: long flexors of toes; tibialis posterior and peroneus longus and brevis (particularly near extreme plantar flexion)

TIBIALIS POSTERIOR
(Posterior tibial nerve, L5, S1) (Fig. 2-51)

Action
Inversion of foot.
Assistance in plantar flexion of foot.

Test
Foot is in complete plantar flexion. Inversion is tested against resistance applied to medial border of foot and directed toward eversion and slightly toward dorsiflexion.

This maneuver virtually eliminates participation of the tibialis anterior in inversion. The toes should be relaxed to prevent participation of the long flexors of the toes.

LONG FLEXORS OF TOES
(Posterior tibial nerve, L5, S1, S2)
- **Flexor digitorum longus**
- **Flexor hallucis longus**

Action
Plantar flexion of toes, especially at distal interphalangeal joints. Assistance in plantar flexion and inversion of foot.

Test
Foot is stabilized in neutral position. Plantar flexion of toes is tested against resistance applied particularly to distal phalanges.

INTRINSIC MUSCLES OF FOOT
These include virtually all muscles except extensor digitorum brevis (medial and lateral plantar nerves from posterior tibial nerve, L5, S1, S1)

Action
Somewhat comparable to that of intrinsic muscles of hand. Many people have very poor individual function of these muscles.

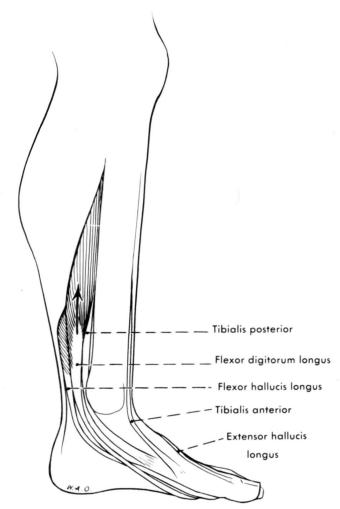

Tibialis posterior

Flexor digitorum longus

Flexor hallucis longus

Tibialis anterior

Extensor hallucis longus

Figure 2-51. Invertors of foot. (Hollinshead WH: Functional Anatomy of the Limbs and Back: A Text for Students of Physical Therapy and Others Interested in the Locomotor Apparatus, 3rd ed. Philadelphia, WB Saunders, 1969)

Test

Cupping sole of foot is adequate test for most clinical purposes.

Neurological Examination

With the exception of the musculoskeletal examination, no other component of the standard physical examination is more important to the rehabilitation assessment than the neurological examination. Although often conducted to identify disease, the neurological examination provides the rehabilitation physician with the opportunity to identify both the neurological impairments to be addressed and the residual abilities to be used in maximizing the functional outcome of the patient.

Although it is customary to record the results of the neurological examination in a separate portion of the examination report, the examination is rarely performed all at one time. The examiner often finds it convenient to integrate the appropriate portions of the neurological examination into the assessment of a specific region of the body. For example, cranial nerve assessment is often performed with other components of the head and neck examination because the patient is positioned appropriately for both. For purposes of discussion, the neurological

examination is addressed separately and is divided into assessments of mental status, speech and language function, cranial nerves, reflexes, central motor integration, sensation, and perception. Muscle strength is discussed in the section on examination of the musculoskeletal system. The assessment of complex motor activities is discussed in the section on the functional examination. The reader is referred to *Clinical Examinations in Neurology*[6] for a comprehensive discussion of the neurological evaluation.

Mental Status

LEVEL OF CONSCIOUSNESS. Before performing a formal mental status examination, the patient's level of consciousness is determined. Qualitative terms such as "drowsy," "lethargic," and "stuporous" are useful in a descriptive sense, but they suffer from a lack of precise definition. "Stuporous" to one examiner may be "lethargic" to another. A definitive classification of mental status requires a standardized approach.[10, 16, 21] In the Glasgow Coma Scale,[13] the examiner classifies the patient's eye, motor, and verbal responses to verbal or physical stimuli according to a numerical scale that is quantifiable and reproducible (Table 2-4). Such a standardized scale is necessary to assess changes over time and to facilitate communication among physicians, nurses, therapists, and family. In patients with traumatic brain injury, other aspects of the neurological assessment such as pupillary responses, ocular movements, and respiration will provide information about the cause of altered consciousness but do not quantifiably relate in a statistical sense to eventual outcome.

COGNITIVE EVALUATION. With the conscious patient, assessment of mental status begins when the physician enters the room, and it continues throughout the examination. However, as with the assessment of the level of consciousness, a formal approach to the mental status examination is beneficial to identify and quantify specific impairments and residual capacity, to recognize subtle temporal changes, and to facilitate communication among caregivers. Excellent systems[12, 13] have been developed to assess intellectual performance in specific populations.

Table 2-4
Glasgow Coma Scale*

Eye Opening		
Spontaneous	E	4
To speech	E	3
To pain	E	2
Nil	E	1
Best Motor Response		
Obeys	M	6
Localizes	M	5
Withdraws	M	4
Abnormal flexion	M	3
Extensor response	M	2
Nil	M	1
Verbal Response		
Orientated	V	5
Confused conversation	V	4
Inappropriate words	V	3
Incomprehensible sounds	V	2
Nil	V	1

*Coma score (E + M + V) = 3 to 15
(Jennett B, Teasdale G: Management of Head Injuries. Philadelphia, FA Davis, 1981)

Although some systems include perceptual testing, speech and language assessment, or an inventory of thought processing and other systems do not, certain components of the evaluation remain constant.

Orientation. The patient is asked to report his or her name, address, and telephone number and the building (hospital, clinic), city, state, year, month, and day.

Attention. Attention is assessed with digit repetition; the patient is asked to repeat a series of random numbers. Two numbers are used initially (e.g., "4, 9"); if the patient answers correctly, increase the sequence by one digit until the patient either repeats seven digits correctly or makes a mistake. Note the number of digits repeated correctly.

Recall. Three numbers or three objects are listed and the patient is asked to remember them because he or she will be asked to repeat them later. A response from the patient is requested in 5 minutes and the number of correct responses is recorded. If all responses are correct, recall responses are obtained at 10 and 15 minutes.

General Fund of Information. Questions are asked appropriate to the patient's age, cultural interests, and educational background. For example, the names of the past five presidents (or other country leaders), the current vice president, and the home-state governor can be requested or inquiries can be made for information about current events and other nearly universal subjects (world wars and basic scientific principles).

Calculations. The patient is asked to count by 7s and the last correct response is recorded. Arithmetic calculations of increasing difficulty are presented.

Proverbs. An explanation of three common proverbs is requested. The patient is assessed as to whether he or she abstracts the principle from the adage or explains it in concrete terms.

Similarities. The patient is requested to describe what is common to an orange and an apple, a desk and a bookcase, and a cup and a fork. The number of correct responses is recorded.

Judgment. The patient is presented with three problems (smelling smoke in a movie theater, finding a stamped and addressed envelope on the sidewalk, and finding a friend in an unfamiliar city) and asked how to handle the situations.

Speech and Language Function

As with the assessment of mental status, analysis of communicative function occurs throughout the entire examination. The patient should be evaluated for the presence and extent of aphasia, apraxia, and dysarthria, and residual communicative skills should be identified. At times, effort is required to discriminate among the disorders of aphasia, apraxia of speech, and the language dysfunction associated with a more generalized cognitive deficit. Expert assessment of speech production and language processing can be a valuable tool for the diagnosis of neurological disease (see Chapter 6). But, as described in the preceding section, assessment of the four basic elements of communication provides a practical framework for functional evaluation.

LISTENING. After first determining that the patient does not have a significant hearing loss, had spoken your language before the onset of disease, and has the requisite motor and visual skills, the patient's auditory comprehension is tested, noting his or her ability to follow specific directions without gestures from the examiner. Often, it is useful to characterize the degree of impairment using stepped commands. First, the patient's ability to follow "one-step commands" is assessed by asking him or her to perform three different single motor activities such as "take off your glasses," "touch your nose," and "open the book." Each command should be given separately and a prolonged pause should be allowed to observe the response. These responses are rated and notation made of whether the patient requires pantomime of the activity before performing the task. If two of the three responses are correct, the patient's skill is assessed at following "two-step commands" such as "touch your nose, then take off your glasses," "point to the window, then close the book," and "touch my hand, then touch your knee." If the patient can follow "two-step commands," then "three-step commands" are assessed in a similar fashion. A simple object such as a toothbrush is held up and the patient is asked to demonstrate its use. This request is repeated at least two times with different objects. If speech is functional, a short phrase is spoken and the patient is asked to repeat it. The response is observed for perseveration and jargon.

READING. It is important to be sure the patient had reading skills before onset of the neurological disorder. The patient is asked to read a short written command and perform the activity; the patient can also try two- and three-step commands. If writing is otherwise functional, the patient is asked to read aloud what he or she has written.

SPEAKING. If auditory comprehension is adequate, language production is tested in the following ways. An object is indicated and the patient is asked to name it and to state its function; at least three objects are used. The patient is asked to report his or her name, home town, telephone number, or other simple verifiable fact. A picture can be shown and the patient asked to describe it. Tests for phonation and resonance deficits are performed by asking the patient to say a prolonged "aaah" and observing for force and steadiness of pitch and tone. The patient is asked to say "pa-pa-pa" to test lip closure, "ta-ta-ta" to test tongue function, and "ka-ka-ka" to test speed, regulatory, and posterior pharyngeal function. If reading is otherwise functional, the patient is asked to read aloud a short passage with various vowels and consonants to assess articulation further.

WRITING. The patient is asked to write his or her name, address, and telephone number and to write a brief paragraph.

Cranial Nerves

CRANIAL NERVE I (OLFACTORY). Olfactory function is evaluated routinely. Deficits are common after head trauma.

CRANIAL NERVE II (OPTIC). Visual field testing of each eye is performed individually, using a temporary patch over the contralateral side. It is best to test each quadrant diagonally to identify quadrantanopias. Although visual double simultaneous stimulation may be more correctly classified under cortical sensation, it is convenient to assess for extinction during visual field testing, once full fields have been ensured. Visual acuity is discussed in the section on eye examination.

CRANIAL NERVES III (OCULOMOTOR), IV (TROCHLEAR), AND VI (ABDUCENS). Visual pathways are assessed by evaluating pupil size, pupillary reactions, and extraocular movements. Strabismus is evaluated by testing corneal light reflections.

CRANIAL NERVE V (TRIGEMINAL).   The muscles of mastication and facial sensation are tested.

CRANIAL NERVE VIII (VESTIBULAR/AUDITORY).   Nystagmus is sought. Auditory function (cranial nerve VIII) is discussed in the section on ear examination.

CRANIAL NERVES VII (FACIAL), IX (GLOSSOPHARYNGEAL), X (VAGUS), AND XII (HYPOGLOSSAL).   Isolating individual cranial nerve function emanating from the lower part of the brain stem is difficult. Cranial nerves are often grouped by function. Taste (nerves VII, IX, and X), muscles of facial expression (nerve VII) and articulation (nerves VII, IX, X, and XII), and swallowing function (nerves IX, X, and XII) are evaluated.

CRANIAL NERVE XI (ACCESSORY).   Sternocleidomastoid and trapezius function is frequently assessed during manual muscle testing.

Brain stem- and visual-evoked responses, electromyography and other forms of electrodiagnostic testing, and swallowing videofluoroscopy are often necessary for better delineation of dysfunction of cranial nerves and their brain stem interactions.

Reflexes

MUSCLE STRETCH REFLEXES.   After the patient is relaxed, muscle stretch reflexes are tested. Commonly, the biceps (C5–C6), triceps (C6–C8), brachioradialis (C5–C6), quadriceps (L2–L4), and triceps surae (L5, S1–S2) are tested. The masseter (cranial nerve V), internal hamstring (L4–L5, S1–S2), and external hamstring (L5, S1–S2) reflexes are tested in selected cases. The patient is observed for clonus.

SUPERFICIAL REFLEXES.   Segmental reflexes are often helpful for localizing the lesion. The corneal (cranial nerves V and VII), gag (cranial nerves IX and X), anal (S3–S5), and plantar (L5, S1–S2) reflexes are tested. At times, it is useful to include the epigastric (T6–T9), midabdominal (T9–T11), hypogastric (T11–T12, L1), and cremasteric (L1–L2) reflexes.

PATHOLOGIC REFLEXES.   Elicitation of the Babinski reflex is attempted. In questionable cases, the confirmatory Chaddock, Oppenheim, and Stransky reflexes are tested.

Central Motor Integration

MUSCLE TONE.   Spasticity, rigidity, and hypotonicity are sought by assessing the patient's resistance to passive movement, pendulousness, and ability to posturally fixate.

COORDINATION.   Coordination in the upper extremities is assessed using the finger–nose, finger–nose–finger, and knee-pat tests. Coordination in the lower extremities is evaluated with the toe–finger and heel–knee–shin test.

ALTERNATE MOTION RATE.   The tongue-wiggle, finger-wiggle, and foot-pat tests are used to identify subtle spasticity, rigidity, and incoordination.

INVOLUNTARY MOVEMENTS.   Tremors, chorea, athetosis, ballismus, dystonia, myoclonus, asterixis, and tics are observed for and described.

APRAXIA.   Apraxia is a failure of motor planning and execution without deficits of strength, coordination, or sensation (although deficits of strength, coordination, and sensation are often also present because of the extent of the lesion). Automatic motor activities are observed while the patient manipulates a pen or pencil, handles clothing, and moves about the examination room; then the patient's ability to perform some of the same maneuvers on command is assessed. The patient is asked to touch his or her nose, drink from a glass, put a pencil in the glass, strike a match and blow it out, and use scissors. The patient is asked to perform these activities without the objects and with each hand. Inefficient or fumbling movements or failure to accomplish the task is noted. Dressing apraxia is assessed by asking the patient to put on a coat. To assess for more subtle deficits, one sleeve of the coat is first turned inside out. Constructional apraxia is evaluated by asking the patient to copy a geometric design or draw the face of a clock.

Sensation

SUPERFICIAL SENSATION.   Light touch is tested with a wisp of cotton, superficial pain with a single-use pin, and temperature with two test tubes, one with hot and the other with cold tap water. Abnormal findings are recorded on a drawing of the human figure and compared with standard charts of spinal dermatomes and peripheral nerves.[6]

DEEP SENSATION.   The evaluation of joint position sense is started with distal hand and foot joints and moved proximally until normal sensation is identified. Testing for deep pain in the upper extremities is done by hyperextension of small finger joints and in the lower extremities by firm compression of the calf muscles or Achilles' tendon. Vibration sense is often evaluated, but its isolated absence does not result in functional deficit.

CORTICAL SENSATION.   If superficial and deep sensations are intact, two-point discrimination, graphesthesia, stereognosis, and double simultaneous stimulation are evaluated.

Perception

Disorders of perception are most common with lesions of the nondominant parietal lobe but can also occur with lesions on the dominant side. The reader is referred to Chapter 29 for an in-depth discussion of perceptual disorders.

AGNOSIA.   Agnosia is a failure to recognize familiar objects despite intact vision, hearing, sensation, and language function (although language is often also deficient because of the extent of the lesion). Pictures of common objects or the objects are shown and the patient is asked to identify them and to describe their components. Agnosia of body parts is assessed by asking the patient to identify his or her (or the examiner's) arm, finger, or eye. Unilateral environmental neglect is screened for by observing ambulation or wheelchair operation for difficulty clearing corners and doorjambs, extinction on double simultaneous stimulation, and failure to scan the complete page width when asked to read a passage or to cross out all the occurrences of the letter "E." Body scheme agnosias are evaluated by searching for denial of obvious physical impairments when the patient is asked to describe them.

RIGHT-LEFT DISORIENTATION.   If agnosia of body parts is not present, the patient is asked to indicate various body parts on the right and left sides.

OTHER PERCEPTUAL TESTS.   If perceptual deficits are identified with the maneuvers described above, additional deficits are tested for, such as geographic and spatial orientation and figure–ground relationships. Comprehensive, formal, quantitative testing of perception by a psychologist and an occupational therapist is warranted if any deficits are found during the physical examination.

Functional Examination

Once impairments have been identified, the consequences of these impairments on the function of the patient must be appraised. Prediction of functional status should not be attempted from the history and physical examination; instead, function is examined. For a comprehensive assessment, the patient must be evaluated by individual rehabilitation team members in settings where the activities are actually performed. Bathing skills should be observed by the rehabilitation nurse in the bathroom while the patient attempts to bathe; eating skills should be analyzed by the occupational therapist while the patient eats a meal; and car transfer skills should be assessed by the physical therapist with use of the patient's car. Each team member will use unique skills to contribute to a comprehensive determination of functional status. Many functional evaluative processes cannot be accomplished at a single point. Safety and judgment can be assessed only from observation of the patient in varying situations within both the rehabilitation environment and the community.

However, the rehabilitation physician in many instances must glean a basic view of functional status at the time of the initial evaluation. For instance, in the clinic the physician may be consulted to determine a patient's need for rehabilitation services. It is unlikely that the physician will be able to observe the patient during a meal, in the bathroom, or transferring from the car. In such cases, the physician must use creativity to place the patient in situations that are similar to those of daily life. Examples are given below.

Components of the communication assessment were discussed in the sections on the history and physical examination and will not be repeated here.

Eating

The patient is requested to use examining equipment in place of feeding utensils to demonstrate proficiency in bringing food to the mouth. The patient is provided with a glass of water and asked to drink (if aspiration has not already been identified).

Grooming

The patient is asked to comb hair and mimic the activities of brushing teeth or putting on makeup.

Bathing

Observation of the patient is done while he or she mimics the activities of bathing. It is important to note if any body parts cannot be reached by the patient, in particular whether the patient can reach the back, scalp, and the axilla and arm contralateral to hemiparesis.

Toileting

The patient must have adequate unsupported sitting balance, must have the requisite wrist and hand motion to reach the perineum adequately, must be able to handle tissue paper, and must be able to rise from low seating.

Dressing

The patient is observed during undressing before the examination and dressing after completion of the examination. It is wise to explain the purpose of the observation and to be accompanied by a nurse or aide.

Bed Activities

During the physical examination, notation is made of whether the patient has difficulty moving between the seated and the supine position, can roll from front to back and back to front, and can raise the pelvis off the examining table while in the supine position.

Transfers

The patient is observed rising from seating with and without armrests and moving between bed and chair.

Wheelchair Mobility

The patient is asked to demonstrate wheeling straight ahead and turning (on carpeted and noncarpeted floors, if available), locking the brakes, and manipulating the leg rests.

Ambulation

To adequately recognize disturbances of gait, the examiner must be able to view body parts. If the examining room is secluded, the assessment is performed while the patient is wearing underwear. If privacy is not possible, the patient should have access to washable or paper shorts. Assuming that the examiner does not already have knowledge of the patient's ambulation skills, it is wise to provide the patient with a safety belt before gait is assessed. If specific gait abnormalities are to be discerned, both the individual components and the composite activity must be studied. The patient is observed from the front, the back, and the sides. If the patient experiences pain during ambulation, the temporal relationship to the gait cycle is noted. The analysis must be approached in an orderly fashion. One routine for gait analysis is outlined in Table 2-5.[15, 20]

Table 2-5
Gait Analysis

Standing Balance
Observe for steadiness of position. Push the patient off balance and note the patient's attempts to regain balanced posture.

Individual Body Part Movements during Walking
Observe for fixed or abnormal postures and inadequate, excessive, or asymmetrical movements of body parts.
Head and trunk: listing or tilting; shoulder dipping, elevation, depression, protraction, and retraction
Arm swing: protective positioning or posturing
Pelvis and hip: hip hiking, dropping (Trendelenburg), or lateral thrust
Knee: genu valgum, varum, or recurvatum
Foot and ankle: excessive inversion or eversion

Gait Cycle Factors
Cadence: rate, symmetry, fluidity, and consistency
Stride width: narrow or broad base; knee and ankle clearance
Stride length: shortened, lengthened, or asymmetrical
Stance phase: normal heel strike, foot flat, push-off; knee stability during all components of stance; coordination of knee and ankle movements
Swing phase: adequate and synchronized knee and ankle dorsiflexion during swing; abduction or circumduction

FUNCTIONAL STATUS				
NAME *John Doe* *3-418-448* Ⓛ *Hemiparesis*				
ACTIVITY	Independent	Independent with aids	Requires Assistance	Dependent
Listening		*aid - Ⓛ ear*		
Reading			*verbal cues to scan Ⓛ*	
Speaking	*dysarthria*			
Writing	✓			
Eating			*set up meal; needs rocker knife; scoop plate*	
Grooming			*verbal cues for Ⓛ body shave Ⓛ face*	
Bathing			*verbal cues for Ⓛ body wash Ⓡ trunk*	
Toileting		*bladder with urinal*	*1 person assist for transfer to commode*	
Dressing			*1 person assist lower body; fasteners*	
Bed Activities		*hospital bed with bed rails*		
Transfers			*verbal cues; lock brakes protect Ⓛ arm & judgement*	
Wheel Chair			*verbal cues to scan Ⓛ unlock wc brakes*	
Ambulation				✓
Driving				✓
If the activity is Independent or Dependent, mark with a check If the activity is Independent with Aids, list the aids needed If the activity Requires Assistance, describe the assistance and list the aids needed				

Figure 2-52. Sample functional status record.

Operation of a Motor Vehicle

Driving is best assessed in an automobile. However, the examiner can gain some information about the patient's motor abilities to drive by requesting the patient to demonstrate the motions of operating the pedals and hand controls.

Quantitation of Function

Several scales can be used to document and quantify functional status in activities of daily living. These are extremely useful to assess a patient's rehabilitation progress (see Chapter 9). When validated and standardized, they become essential tools for analysis of rehabilitation outcome for a series of patients participating in a specific intervention program. When these scales are used by multiple rehabilitation centers to share data, significant information can be obtained to advance the state of the art and assess the cost versus benefit of rehabilitation. The reader is encouraged to develop expertise in the use of these valuable tools.

However, in that the data collection for most validated functional scales requires additional time because of interdisciplinary input, the initial documentation of functional status by the physician must be practical and complete. One such system is shown in Figure 2-52. Findings from both the history and the physical examination should be used to define functional status.

SUMMARY AND PROBLEM LIST

Once the history is obtained, the physical examination has been performed, and the results recorded, the rehabilitation physician summarizes the findings, constructs a problem list, and formulates a plan.

A summary of findings has often been an inconsistent component of the written record. Often of two or three sentences in length, the summary can provide the reader with a succinct and memory-jogging description of significant findings in the history and examination.

For the management of chronic diseases, rehabilitation medicine must commonly address a myriad of physical, psychological, social, and vocational problems. Weed's problem-ori-

Table 2-6
Example of Summary, Problem List, and Plan

Summary

55-year-old male carpenter with left hearing deficit and poorly treated hypertension; 4 days following sudden moderate left-side spastic hemiparesis, moderate sensory deficits, left neglect, nocturnal bladder incontinence, dysarthria. He is alert, oriented, and normotensive; left hip and knee motor function is returning; high serum cholesterol level. He is divorced, lives alone, and has no close family. CT scan of head shows moderate right subcortical infarction. Ischemia is not shown on ECG.

Medical Problems/Plans

1. Right hemisphere infarction with motor, sensory, perceptual, speech deficits: monitor neuromuscular fx, maintain ROM, control spasticity (air splint, positioning, consider meds) motor re-ed, patient ed/risk factors
2. Hypertension: maintain below 140/90 mm Hg with propranolol, 40 mg qid po
3. Hypercholesterolemia: low fat diet, patient ed/diet and food preparation
4. Urinary incontinence: check residual urine volume, culture specimens; treat urosepsis. If residual volume is low, offer urinal frequently, +/− nocturnal condom cath. If residual volumes are high, begin 1800-ml fluid intake schedule, q6h cath, urodynamics, bladder retraining.

Rehabilitation Problems/Plans

1. Communication deficits: speech pathologist for evaluation and therapy
2. Left neglect: OT for perceptual testing, retraining, and compensation; verbal clues to scan left; RN and RT to reinforce OT
3. Left sensory deficits: monitor skin, patient ed/insensate skin care
4. Self-care deficits: OT for upper extremity ROM, re-ed, strengthening, ADL retraining, adaptive aids
5. Safety and judgment deficits: 4 bed rails, RN to monitor closely at night, verbal clues, physical spotting
6. Transfer deficits: PT for retraining, left WC brake extension
7. Mobility deficits: PT for lower extremity ROM, re-ed, strengthening, gait retraining, gait aids
8. Driving dependency: retesting and retraining if improvement
9. Community reentry/poor support system: assess home for architectural barriers, assess home health services, identify additional social support
10. Reactive depression: psychological support
11. Vocational issues: consider prevocational counseling and testing

ented medical record[22] has been applied to the management of patients undergoing rehabilitation.[7,8,11,17] Although use of the problem list itself is the essential factor, a consensus as to the organization and use of the entire system in the rehabilitation setting has proved challenging. The recommendation of Grabois[11] that medical and rehabilitation problems be separately listed is beneficial. In addition, it may be helpful to delineate individual plans for each problem at the conclusion of the workup (Table 2-6).

REFERENCES

1. Committee for the Study of Joint Motion, American Academy of Orthopaedic Surgeons: Joint Motion: Method of Measuring and Recording. Chicago, American Academy of Orthopaedic Surgeons, 1965
2. D'Ambrosia RD (ed): Musculoskeletal Disorders: Regional Examination and Differential Diagnosis, 2nd ed. Philadelphia, JB Lippincott, 1986
3. Daniels L, Worthingham C: Muscle Testing: Techniques of Manual Examination, 3rd ed. Philadelphia, WB Saunders, 1972
4. Darley FL: Treatment of acquired aphasia. Adv Neurol 7:111–145, 1975
5. DeGowin EL, DeGowin RL: Bedside Diagnostic Examination, 4th ed. New York, Macmillan, 1981
6. Department of Neurology and Department of Physiology and Biophysics, Mayo Clinic and Mayo Foundation: Clinical Examinations in Neurology, 5th ed. Philadelphia, WB Saunders, 1981
7. Dinsdale SM, Gent M, Kline G, Milner R: Problem oriented medical records: Their impact on staff communication, attitudes and decision making. Arch Phys Med Rehabil 56:269–274, 1975
8. Dinsdale SM, Mossman PL, Gullickson G Jr, Anderson TP: The problem-oriented medical record in rehabilitation. Arch Phys Med Rehabil 51:488–492, 1970
9. Ewing JA: Detecting alcoholism: The CAGE questionnaire. JAMA 252:1905–1907, 1984
10. Folstein MF, Folstein SE, McHugh PR: "Mini-mental state": A practical method for grading the cognitive state of patients for the clinician. J Psychiatr Res 12:189–198, 1975
11. Grabois M: The problem-oriented medical record: Modification and simplification for rehabilitation medicine. South Med J 70:1383–1385, 1977
12. Hoppenfeld S: Physical Examination of the Spine and Extremities. New York, Appleton-Century-Crofts, 1976
13. Jennett B, Teasdale G: Management of Head Injuries. Philadelphia, FA Davis, 1981
14. Kendall FP, McCreary EK: Muscles: Testing and Function, 3rd ed. Baltimore, Williams & Wilkins, 1983
15. Lehmann JF: Gait analysis: Diagnosis and management. In Kottke FJ, Stillwell GK, Lehmann JF (eds): Krusen's Handbook of Physical Medicine and Rehabilitation, 3rd ed, pp 86–101. Philadelphia, WB Saunders, 1982
16. Levin HS, O'Donnell VM, Grossman RG: The Galveston orientation and amnesia test: A practical scale to assess cognition after head injury. J Nerv Ment Dis 167:675–684, 1979
17. Milhous RL: The problem-oriented medical record in rehabilitation management and training. Arch Phys Med Rehabil 53:182–185, 1972
18. Newmark SR, Sublett D, Black J, Geller R: Nutritional assessment in a rehabilitation unit. Arch Phys Med Rehabil 62:279–282, 1981
19. Norkin CC, White DJ: Measurement of Joint Motion: A Guide to Goniometry. Philadelphia, FA Davis, 1985
20. Stolov WC: Evaluation of the patient. In Kottke FJ, Stillwell GK, Lehmann JF (eds): Krusen's Handbook of Physical Medicine and Rehabilitation, 3rd ed, pp 1–18. Philadelphia, WB Saunders, 1982
21. Strub RL, Black FW: The Mental Status Examination in Neurology, 2nd ed. Philadelphia, FA Davis, 1985
22. Weed LL: Medical Records, Medical Education, and Patient Care: The Problem-Oriented Record as a Basic Tool. Cleveland, OH, The Press of Case Western Reserve University, 1971
23. World Health Organization: International Classification of Impairments, Disabilities, and Handicaps: A Manual of Classification Relating to the Consequences of Disease. Geneva, World Health Organization, 1980

3

Psychological Aspects of Rehabilitation

Daniel E. Rohe

In this chapter the direct and indirect services routinely offered by the rehabilitation psychologists working in a primary health care setting are described. Direct services include assessment, with both nonstandardized and standardized techniques, and psychotherapeutic interventions, including individual therapy, applied behavioral modification, and social skills training. Frequently encountered psychological measures in the domains of personality, intellectual ability, academic achievement, neuropsychological assessment, and chemical use are briefly discussed. The practical importance of these measures for rehabilitation planning is stressed. Indirect services include consultation with team members, staff training and development, and research planning and implementation.

Also provided is an overview of psychological theories explaining the process of adjustment to disability. The major focus of this section is critical examination of "stage theory" in relation to disability adjustment. This is followed by description of two models, the behavioral model and the coping skills model.

A guiding criterion in making decisions about the type and depth of topics covered involved identification of information deemed both practical and useful to the physiatrist working in applied settings. Where coverage of a topic is limited, references are provided to guide further exploration. Some topics of particular relevance, such as vocational evaluation, sexual dysfunction, and interventions with patients who have specific disabilities, are covered in Chapters 4 and 27, and in other parts of the book.

DIRECT SERVICES

Assessment

Nonstandardized Assessment (the Clinical Interview)

The psychologist's first contact with a patient is often pivotal in the development of a therapeutic relationship. This contact often occurs before transfer to the rehabilitation unit. The psychologist may stop in the patient's room before the initial interview and explain the role of the psychologist. The patient's expectations of meeting with the psychologist are largely determined by previous exposure to mental health professionals, communications from the physician, and preliminary explanations from the psychologist. The patient's willingness to interact meaningfully with the psychologist can be strongly influenced by the physician. Physiatrists who view rehabilitation as predominantly a process of "applied physical medicine" are less likely to communicate the importance of working with the psychologist. At the introduction, the psychologist will state that comprehensive rehabilitation includes help with problematic thoughts and feelings occasioned by the disability. Frequently, patients are relieved to discover that contact with the psychologist is a *routine* part of comprehensive rehabilitation.

The initial interview usually lasts at least 1 hour and sometimes longer. Patients with cognitive impairment may be seen only long enough for a general idea to be gained of their information-processing capacity and emotional state. Further assessment will await improvement in their cognitive status or contact with an informed family member. The length of the initial interview with noncognitively impaired patients depends on the complexity of the medical or social issues. There are two major goals for the initial interview. First, a comprehensive history of the patient's social background is obtained. Frequently asked biographical questions are listed in Table 3-1. These data provide insight into previous learning experiences that may affect rehabilitation-related attitudes and behaviors. Second, the psychologist attempts to understand the disability as the patient sees it. The foundation for a meaningful therapeutic relationship is in part laid through taking sufficient time to elicit the patient's perspective. The patient often faces a medical situation that he or she does not fully comprehend. Anxiety and fear often block the effective reception and communication of information between the patient and other rehabilitation team members, especially physicians. The opportunity to have one's perspective, including cognitive and emotional aspects, aired in a supportive and clarifying manner is often therapeutic in itself.

Information gained during the initial interview is usually shared judiciously with other team members. The psychologist occupies an unusually difficult position vis-à-vis other team members. Although a team member, the psychologist also has the professional responsibility of maintaining the confidentiality of the therapeutic relationship. The patient may confide information that is personally sensitive and inappropriate to share with other team members. If directly asked by other team members about such information, the psychologist may have to explain

Table 3-1
Psychosocial Information Sought During Initial Interview

1. Data on Family of Origin
   a. Names, ages, occupations, marital status, and residence of parents and siblings
   b. Religious training
   c. Stability of family during early development
   d. History of major mental disorder in immediate and extended family, including a history of chemical dependency, suicide, or psychiatric hospitalization
2. Relevant Patient Information
   a. Educational background and history of school achievement
   b. Patient's current occupation and previous vocational history
   c. Previous and current avocational activities
   d. History of adjustment to structured social environments, such as school, work, and military service
   e. Previous social adjustment, including any previous arrests, chemical dependency treatment, or psychiatric diagnosis
   f. Previous learning associated with hospitals and health care
   g. Preinjury stresses the patient was coping with at the time of injury
   h. Most difficult loss the patient has had to adjust to previously; success in that task
   i. Previous association with people having disabilities
3. Family Structure
   a. Names and ages of and quality of relationship with spouse and children
   b. Background of dating and sexual relationship with current spouse
   c. Marital adjustment
4. Understanding the Patient's Perspective
   a. The patient's understanding of the cause and probable course of the disability
   b. The patient's initial thoughts at the onset of the disability (if traumatic)
   c. The patient's most pressing immediate concern
   d. How well does the patient think he or she is coping with the situation?
   e. The patient's perception of how the disability will change life-style, including relationships, vocational future, and self-concept
   f. The patient's understanding of the behavioral expectations in the rehabilitation unit compared with those in the acute care unit of the hospital
   g. To what degree was the patient's sense of self-esteem related to physique or physical skills?
   h. The patient's comfort in meeting with a psychologist
   i. What techniques has the patient used successfully in the past to cope with stressful events?
   j. What techniques does the patient use to get and maintain a sense of control over the environment?

that the information is confidential. Usually the patient is informed that any information considered sensitive by the psychologist or so indicated by the patient will not be communicated to others. General information of a less sensitive nature is dictated and typed in the form of an initial interview note. Subsequent therapeutic contacts are recorded in the hospital chart or summarized periodically. The frequency of these contacts depends on such factors as the goals established during the initial interview, the current degree of psychological distress, the potential for behavioral decompensation, and overall staffing levels.

Standardized Assessment

Given the time-consuming and subjective nature of clinical interviews, rehabilitation psychologists use standardized tests[97] to speed assessment and enhance interventions. This section describes a select number of either extremely helpful or frequently encountered psychological instruments. Standardized measures of personality, intellectual ability, and academic achievement are briefly discussed. The domains of neuropsychological and chemical use assessment are covered in more detail because of their particular relevance in rehabilitation settings.

PERSONALITY. A personality test conventionally refers to a measure of personal characteristics, such as emotional status, interpersonal relations, motivation, interests, and attitudes. Currently, there are several hundred personality tests. Personality inventory development has generally involved one or more methods, including content validation, empirical criterion keying, factor analysis, and personality theory. Frequently, a measure uses several of the above-mentioned techniques. Personality measurement has generated controversy over two issues. The first concerns the stability of personality traits across situations as opposed to the situational specificity of behavior.[44] The second issue is, to what degree does a given personality characteristic reflect merely a transitory state rather than a stable underlying trait? Anastasi[2] provided a thorough overview of these issues and of other psychological measurement concepts, including norms, item analysis, reliability, and validity. Two personality inventories frequently encountered by physiatrists are the *Minnesota Multiphasic Personality Inventory* and the *Millon Clinical Multiaxial Inventory.*

Minnesota Multiphasic Personality Inventory (MMPI). The *MMPI* is the most widely used and thoroughly researched objective measure of personality.[30, 58] The inventory consists of statements describing thoughts, feelings, ideas, attitudes, physical and emotional symptoms, and previous life experiences. In general, the material included on the *MMPI* is usually covered in a clinical interview; however, factors of privacy, time savings, and the clinical relevance of the items have ensured its acceptance in health care settings.

The *MMPI* was originally designed to yield information about personality factors related to the major psychiatric syndromes. The 550 true-or-false questions are grouped into 10 clinical scales (Table 3-2) that, despite obsolete psychiatric titles, continue to reflect important aspects of personality. The items composing each scale were determined statistically. An item was included only if a carefully diagnosed group of patients (*e.g.,* those hospitalized for depression) answered that question in a statistically different manner from other carefully diagnosed groups of patients (*e.g.,* schizophrenics) and from a normal control group. This system of item selection (empirical criterion keying) led to the inclusion of both "obvious" and "subtle" items. The subtle items make faking less easy with the *MMPI* than with other personality measures. The empirical nature of the inventory has permitted construction of additional special scales. For example, there are scales to help predict rehabilitation motivation, headache proneness, and tendencies toward the development of alcoholism.[31] Additionally, there are extensive *MMPI* norms on patients with specific diagnoses, such as multiple sclerosis and spinal cord injury.[130]

The ten clinical scales are interpreted with the aid of four "validity" scales (see Table 3-2). These scales provide information on the client's response style, such as literacy, level of cooperation, tendency toward malingering, task comprehension, and use of denial or defensiveness. Norms from the original control group are reported as standard scores with a mean of 50 and a standard deviation of 10. A score of 70 or greater is traditionally considered suggestive of a pathologic level of the trait in question.

Table 3-2
Brief Description of the Minnesota Multiphasic Personality Inventory Validity and Clinical Scales

Number	Name	No. of Items	Elevated Scores Suggest
Q	Cannot say	550	That a large number of items have not been answered, a possible indication that the patient is resentful or is uncomfortable with ambiguity
L	L scale	15	An effort to create the impression of being a person with high moral, social, and ethical values
F	F scale	64	That the whole questionnaire has been invalidated by some factor, such as lack of comprehension, poor reading ability, mental confusion, a deliberate desire to fake psychiatric difficulty, random marking of responses, or scoring errors
K	K scale	30	A self-view of being well adjusted, capable, and confident, which, at higher scale elevations, is likely to be a denial of the true state of affairs
1	Hypochondriasis	33	Undue concern with bodily states and preoccupation with possible symptoms of physical illness
2	Depression	60	Depression, sadness, pessimism, guilt, passivity, and a tendency to give up hope easily
3	Hysteria	60	Psychological immaturity, self-centeredness, superficial relationships, and frequent use of denial in everyday life
4	Psychopathic deviate	50	Assertiveness and nonconformity at moderate elevations; angry rebelliousness and noncompliance with social mores at extreme levels
5	Masculinity–femininity	60	The degree of identification with roles traditionally assigned to the sex opposite that of the respondent
6	Paranoia	40	Interpersonal oversensitivity and irritability about motives or behavior of others, and, at extreme elevations, suspicious thinking similar to that of people with paranoid personality traits
7	Psychasthenia	48	General feelings of anxiety, with excessive rumination about personal inadequacies
8	Schizophrenia	78	Feelings of detachment from the social realm, extending to frank mental confusion and interpersonal aversiveness
9	Hypomania	46	Talkativeness, distractability, physical restlessness, and, at times, impatience, irritability, or rapid mood swings
0	Social introversion	20	Social introversion and a lack of desire to be with others

A variety of criticisms have been leveled at the *MMPI,* some deserved, others not. A major criticism is of the outdated and nonrepresentative original normal sample. This criticism has been muted by Colligan and colleagues,[22] who have established new norms for the *MMPI.* Their large random sample of 1,408 normal subjects, subdivided by sex and age, was studied to assess the validity of the original norms. The resulting data supported the need for new norms. These norms are available through the Mayo Clinic computerized *MMPI* scoring service.[23]

The *MMPI* requires a sixth-grade reading level and is not suitable for children. Norms are available for adolescents beginning at age 15. The test requires between 1½ and 2 hours for completion. Although many computerized scoring services are available, interpretation by an experienced psychologist is necessary. A variety of factors, including race, socioeconomic status, unique family circumstances, and a strong ethnic background, may distort the *MMPI* profile.

Millon Clinical Multiaxial Inventory (MCMI). The *MCMI*[93] was constructed to emulate the *MMPI* but capitalize on advances in psychopathology, diagnosis, and test construction. The inventory is intended for use as a clinical screening instrument in patients thought to have a significant personality disorder. Millon encourages professionals working with physically ill behavioral medicine or rehabilitation patients to use a companion inventory, the *Millon Behavioral Health Inventory.*[95] However, research on this inventory lags behind that for the *MCMI*; consequently, the *MCMI* is described here.

The *MCMI* requires about 30 minutes for one to respond to the 175 true or false items. The items are written at an eighth-grade reading level. The inventory is appropriate for testing people age 17 or older. The 20 clinical scales are composed of 16 to 47 overlapping items. They are divided into three categories that reflect persistent personality features, levels of pathological severity, and current symptom states. In addition to the clinical scales, there are correction scales to identify problems with denial and confusion.

Each clinical scale serves as an operational measure of a syndrome derived from Millon's theory of personality.[91, 92] Millon was a member of the committee that developed the nosologic format for the *Diagnostic and Statistical Manual (DSM-III)* of the American Psychiatric Association.[94] He stated that the *MCMI* is the only clinically oriented personality inventory reflective of *DSM-III* diagnostic categories. The norms for the *MCMI* were originally derived from 297 subjects drawn from colleges, personnel offices, and industrial settings. The subjects were almost equally divided between men and women, and their ages were from 18 to 66 years. The criterion group contained 1,591 subjects primarily drawn from mental health outpatient settings. They were selected to ensure a balance of subjects in the major syndrome categories. Reliability and validity data support use of the test as a diagnostic instrument. Although additional data will determine the *MCMI*'s ultimate acceptance, Millon has done a thorough and careful job of initial test construction and validation.

Strong-Campbell Interest Inventory (SCII). The *SCII* is traditionally considered a measure of vocational interests; however, recent publications have supported its use as a valid measure of personality.[25] The *SCII* is the combined-sex edition of the *Strong Vocational Interest Blank.* First published in 1927, it is one of the most thoroughly researched, highly respected, and frequently used psychological tests. The *SCII* asks the respondent to indicate liking, indifference, or dislike for occupations, school subjects, activities, amusements, and types of people. Two subsections ask for preferences between two occupational activities and the self-rated possession of 13 personal characteristics. The test contains 325 items, requires 45 to 50 minutes to complete, and is written at an eighth-grade reading level.[14]

The *General Occupational Themes,* which form one of the three types of scales on the *SCII,* are based on trait theory derived by John Holland.[66] Holland drew on factor analytic studies of personality and Guilford's factor analysis of human interests to produce a typology of six basic personality types. These types are titled realistic, investigative, artistic, social, enterprising, and conventional. Rohe and Athelstan[114] administered the *SCII* to a national sample of patients with spinal cord injury. Unlike previous researchers, they found unique personality characteristics in patients having spinal cord injury of traumatic onset. These characteristics included an interest in activities requiring physical interaction with things, such as machinery, and a lack of interest in activities that require intense or complex interaction with either data or people. Malec,[87] using the *Eyesenck Personality Inventory* with patients having spinal cord injury of traumatic onset, discovered a pattern of personality characteristics congruent with that found in Rohe and Athelstan's study. These studies suggest that when a disability is of traumatic onset and secondary to the person's behavior, earlier statements in the literature about the lack of relationship between disability and personality characteristics are inaccurate. The previous literature either used measures oriented toward pathologic conditions (*e.g., MMPI*) or studied people whose disability was not the result of trauma associated with their behavior. An additional study sought to determine if personality characteirstics in patients having spinal cord injury would change after years of living with the disability. The data conclusively showed that overall personality characteristics remained constant over an average of 10 years.[115]

In summary, the *MMPI, MCMI,* and *SCII* are three measures of personality frequently used with rehabilitation patients. These measures can help answer pressing diagnostic and management questions. For example, the *MMPI* has been used successfully to diagnose psychopathologic conditions expressed in the form of physical disability, so-called conversion disorders. Additionally, a patient's unwillingness to comply with requested medical interventions or the structure imposed by the hospital environment can be discerned by personality measures. Knowledge of such personality characteristics can help prevent ill-advised interventions and create a treatment environment designed to minimize difficulties with patient compliance.

INTELLECTUAL ABILITY. Intellectual ability tests characteristically provide a single summary score that serves as a global index of a person's general problem-solving ability. The score generated from the intellectual ability test is usually validated against a broad criterion, such as scholastic achievement or occupational success. Such tests are usually constructed of a number of subtests that sample facets of intellectual functioning. However, these measures are usually weighted on tasks requiring verbal ability. The degree to which general problem-solving ability is present may have a significant impact on the type and complexity of medical and vocational rehabilitation goals established. The intellectual ability test also serves as the cornerstone of neuropsychological assessment. The two most frequently encountered measures of intellectual ability are the *Stanford-Binet Intelligence Scale* and the *Wechsler Adult Intelligence Scale, Revised (WAIS-R).*[137] The remainder of this discussion is focused on the *WAIS-R.*

The *WAIS-R* is the revised version of the *Wechsler Adult Intelligence Scale* originally published in 1955. The revised version was standardized on a normative sample of 1,880 "normal adults" from nine age groups. They were carefully chosen to be representative of the United States population as determined by census data. In addition to careful standardization, which included minority group members, the new form altered or eliminated test items that had become obsolete because of societal changes. The *WAIS-R* must be administered by a trained examiner and requires an average of 1½ hours for completion.

The *WAIS-R* comprises 11 subtests. Six subtests are used in the computation of the so-called verbal IQ, and five subtests determine the performance IQ. These subtests and what they purport to measure are included in Table 3-3 and are numbered in their order of administration. The subject's score on some subtests is based on both accuracy and speed. These timed subtests are arithmetic, picture arrangement, block design, object assembly, and digit symbol. All subtest scores are corrected for age and standardized with a mean of 10 and a standard deviation of 3. The full-scale IQ is determined by averaging scores obtained from the verbal and performance IQs.

Cohen[20] and subsequent investigators have consistently found three factors that account for most of the test's variance. A reduced number of *WAIS-R* subtests constitute these factors and are sometimes administered to reduce testing time. The name of the factor scores and the subtests used to compute them are verbal comprehension (information, vocabulary, comprehension, similarities), freedom from distractability (digit span, arithmetic), and perceptual organization (block design, object assembly). As with the traditional IQ scores, factor scores have a mean of 100 and a standard deviation of 15. They are sometimes reported in lieu of the traditional IQ scores.

Because of the surplus meaning attached to IQ scores, psychologists usually convert both IQ scores and discussions about them into either percentiles or classifications (Table 3-4). When the physician is confronted with questions about test results from patients, the use of either percentiles or classifications is recommended.

In summary, the *WAIS-R* is the most frequently used measure of general intellectual ability. Measures of intellectual ability help the physiatrist set appropriate expectations about the rate and complexity of learning legitimately expected from the patient. They also serve as the cornerstone for determining the presence of organic brain dysfunction and provide guidance for postdismissal vocational planning.

ACADEMIC ACHIEVEMENT. A frequently overlooked but nonetheless important aspect of standardized psychological testing within rehabilitation settings is the assessment of academic achievement. Reading and mathematics achievement are of particular concern not only during inpatient rehabilitation but also for longer-range educational and vocational planning. The patient's reading level is a potential limiting factor in tasks ranging from filling out hospital menus to incorporating ideas presented in patient education materials. The average reading level in the United States is roughly at the sixth grade. Patient education materials, however, often reflect the reading levels of the professionals who devise them. As the patient's reading level falls below the national average, progressively greater reliance on oral instruction and audiovisual materials becomes necessary. Patients are often expected to use mathematics when recording fluid intake and taking correct dosages of medications. Two frequently used measures of reading and mathematical achievement are the *Wide Range Achievement Test, Revised,* and the *Woodcock-Johnson Psycho-Educational Battery.*

Wide Range Achievement Test, Revised (WRAT-R). The WRAT-R is the current edition of the *Wide Range Achievement Test.*[70, 71] The test provides two levels of difficulty for each of three types of academic achievement: reading, spelling, and arithmetic. Level 2, used with subjects aged 12 years through adulthood, is most relevant to adult rehabilitation patients. The level 2 reading subtest requires the subject to recognize and correctly

Table 3-3
The Eleven Subtests of the Wechsler Adult Intelligence Scale, Revised

No.	Title	No. of Items	Task	Measures
Verbal Scale				
1	Information	29	Answer oral questions about diverse information acquired through living in the United States	Retention of long-term general knowledge
3	Digit span		Listen to and orally repeat increasingly long lists of numbers, with separate lists presented in forward and reverse directions	Ability to attend; immediate auditory recall
5	Vocabulary	35	Define the meaning of words presented both orally and visually	Verbal and general mental ability
7	Arithmetic	14	Solve arithmetic problems presented in a story format without using pencil or paper	Concentration and freedom from distractability
9	Comprehension	16	Explain what should be done under certain circumstances and why certain social conventions are followed; interpret proverbs	Common sense, abstract reasoning, and social judgment
11	Similarities	14	Explain the way in which two things are alike	Verbal concept formation
Performance Scale				
2	Picture completion	20	Determine which part is missing from a picture of an object or scene	Visual recognition, remote memory, and general information
4	Picture arrangement	10	Arrange sets of cards containing cartoon-like drawings so that they tell a story	Social judgment, sequential thinking, foresight, and planning
6	Block design	9	Reproduce a two-dimensional design on a card by using 1-inch blocks whose sides are red, white, or red and white	Visuospatial organizing ability
8	Object assembly	4	Properly arrange four cut-up cardboard figures of familiar objects	Visual concept formation and visuospatial reasoning
10	Digit symbol		In a timed code substitution task, pair nine symbols with nine digits	Concentration and psychomotor speed

Table 3-4
IQ Scores, Percentile Ranges, and Classifications for the Wechsler Adult Intelligence Scale, Revised

IQ Score	Percentile Range	Classification
130 and above	98 or greater	Very superior
120–129	91 to 97	Superior
110–119	74 to 89	High average
90–109	25 to 73	Average
80–89	9 to 23	Low average
70–79	2 to 8	Borderline
50–69	Below the 2nd	Mild mental retardation
35–49	Below the 1st	Moderate mental retardation
20–34	Below the 1st	Severe mental retardation
Below 20	Below the 1st	Profound mental retardation

pronounce individual words ranging from "milk" to "synecdoche." The spelling test requires correct spelling of words presented by the examiner separately and in the context of a sentence. The level of difficulty ranges from "cat" to "iridescence." Finally, the mathematics test ranges in difficulty from simple counting to performing advanced algebra problems. The test can be completed in roughly 30 minutes, and results are presented in the form of standard scores, percentiles, and grade equivalents. Although the test has adequate reliability and norms, critics highlight that the correct pronunciation of individual words represents a limited index of reading comprehension.

Woodcock-Johnson Psycho-Educational Battery (W-J). The W-J[142, 143] contains 27 subtests subdivided into three domains: cognitive ability (12 subtests), academic achievement (10 subtests), and interests (5 subtests). Although the major concern here is with the measures of academic achievement, the entire battery has received critical acclaim for ease of administration, reliability, validity, and normative sampling procedures.[26, 73] The W-J is appropriate for patients 3 to 80 years of age.

The academic achievement subtests are grouped into four clusters: reading, mathematics, written language, and knowledge. Reading achievement is determined by the average of the scores of three subtests that can be completed in roughly 15 minutes. These three subtests assess sight-word vocabulary, phonetic analysis, and passage comprehension. Thus, the resulting score reflects multiple aspects of reading, not just correct word pronunciation. Achievement scores are reported in the form of age- and grade-normed percentiles and reading ranges (from easy to difficult). Mathematics achievement is based on two subtests consisting of story problems and calculations and requires about 20 minutes for completion. The two remaining achievement clusters are of less relevance to inpatient rehabilitation but may be of use for postdismissal planning.

In summary, both the *WRAT-R* and the *W-J* provide insight

into the patient's current level of academic achievement. This information aids in determining the most appropriate manner of instructing the newly disabled person. Those with low reading and mathematical achievement levels may require special care when patient education is provided. This information is invaluable at the time of postdismissal educational and vocational planning.

NEUROPSYCHOLOGICAL ASSESSMENT. People with cognitive dysfunction form one of the largest groups receiving rehabilitation services. For many, the deficits are transient, and for some, cognitive deficits are permanent and not only will complicate the learning of independent living skills but also will determine future living arrangements, social interactions, and vocational prospects. In both situations, the psychologist is frequently asked to clarify the nature and type of cognitive deficits. This section provides information on two helpful screening tests of cognitive status. Both tests can be readily used by the physician to determine the need or readiness for more extensive neuropsychological assessment. The goals of neuropsychological assessment and two frequently encountered test batteries, the *Halstead-Reitan Neuropsychological Battery* and the *Luria-Nebraska Neuropsychological Battery,* are described.

Screening Measures of Cognitive Status. The physician frequently encounters patients of doubtful potential for appropriate involvement in a rehabilitation program. A question that often arises is whether the patient shows evidence of organic brain dysfunction. A dementia screening test that can be used readily, covers a variety of cognitive domains, and shows good reliability and validity is potentially worthwhile to the physician faced with practical treatment decisions. At present, more than a dozen scales designed to assess the presence of dementia are available.[75] Although each has particular strengths, many do not offer the diversity of content or wide applicability needed for use with a general rehabilitation population. Lezak[81] divided mental status scales into three groups: lengthy scales with multiple content, abbreviated scales with one or two items per cognitive area, and short scales of ten items or fewer. Lengthy scales often require 1 hour to administer and may not provide enough information to warrant the time required. Short scales tend to focus on orientation questions, ignoring the diversity of cognitive abilities.

The *Mini-Mental State*[47] has diverse content, is easily learned, and requires only 5 to 10 minutes for administration. Although it has no abstraction items, a useful measure of delayed verbal memory is included. A standardization sample of 63 elderly (mean age, 73.9 years) normal control subjects provides the normative comparison group. Elderly control subjects score in the range of 24.6 to 27.6 out of a possible 30 points. Senile elderly patient groups obtain scores in the range of 9.6 to 12.2 points. The scores of the control subjects and the senile patients do not overlap.

Although the *Mini-Mental State* is useful for answering the question of *whether* to refer for neuropsychological assessment, the physician must decide *when* to refer for testing, particularly if the patient has a closed head injury or slowly resolving coma. Teasdale and Jennett[132] devised the well-known *Glasgow Coma Scale,* which evaluates three components of wakefulness: eye opening, motor response, and verbal response. This scale is useful for classifying the severity of head injury in the acute stage but is not designed to guide the appropriate timing of psychological assessment.

The *Galveston Orientation and Amnesia Test (GOAT),* developed by Levin and co-workers,[79] assesses amnesia and disorientation after head injury. The scale consists of 10 questions that focus on temporal orientation, recall of biographical data, and memory for recent events. The patient can obtain a maximum of 100 points; the final score is computed by subtraction of the number of error points. The *GOAT* was standardized on a group of 50 young adults (median age, 23) who had recovered from mild closed head injury, usually consisting of a momentary loss of consciousness. Scores below those received by all members of the control group (<65) are designated impaired, scores between 66 and 75 are designated borderline, and those above 75 are considered normal. The greatest scoring difficulty would appear to occur when points are assigned for the patient's accuracy in recalling events before trauma. Post-traumatic amnesia is defined as the time during which the *GOAT* score is 75 or less. Validity data were generated by a comparison of the length of the post-traumatic amnesia with the variables of initial neurologic impairment and scores on the *Glasgow Outcome Scale.* In both cases, the *GOAT* score readily discriminated according to the severity of head injury. Scaling recovery of cognitive function in the noncomatose patient permits meaningful discussion with the family and rehabilitation team members. Most importantly, attempts at more involved neuropsychological assessment usually prove nonproductive until the patient consistently obtains scores of 70 or greater. Once a score of 70 is achieved, neuropsychological test data usually are reliable for further rehabilitation and postdismissal planning.

The Goals of Neuropsychological Assessment. The field of neuropsychological assessment has come full circle since 1935, when Ward Halstead[9] established his laboratory. Halstead observed the behavior of patients with brain damage and then developed psychological tests to measure the characteristics that he observed. Thus, the initial goal of assessment was a better understanding of brain–behavior relationships, particularly in patients with brain impairments. Since Halstead's assessment methods were designed to capture a broad range of complex human behaviors, they quickly proved their worth, when used by experienced clinicians, of reliably and validly diagnosing brain damage and localizing malfunctioning regions of the brain. Their use as a neurodiagnostic instrument gained prominence and is now routine. Their diagnostic validity has been shown to be equal to that of neurodiagnostic techniques in use prior to the introduction of computed tomography and magnetic resonance imaging.[46] As brain imaging technology has improved, however, the importance of neuropsychological assessment has begun to return to the original goal of describing brain–behavior relationships.

The next and final stage in the field of neuropsychological assessment will ultimately be the development of remediation and rehabilitation procedures for patients with brain damage.[15, 33, 118] Unfortunately, most neuropsychological tests were designed with diagnosis, not remediation, as their major goal. The tests are not constructed to provide crisp discriminations about which cognitive abilities in what combinations are minimally necessary for survival in complex environments.[62] Heaton and Pendleton,[64] in a comprehensive review of the neuropsychological literature, lamented that prediction of everyday functioning is a largely ignored topic of research in a field still dominated by diagnostic issues.

Ultimately, new neuropsychological measures may have to be constructed. The normative comparison groups will include cognitively impaired patients who demonstrate appropriate adaptational skills in their home and work environments. If the brain-injured subject could score sufficiently high on combinations of these measures, one could then have faith that this person would be able to function adequately outside a sheltered environment. Traditionally, measurement has focused on the patient and not on the unique environment to which he or she will return. Recently, there has been increased recognition of the inherent limits in neuropsychological assessment. Optimal prediction about the satisfactory matching of people with environments will require new approaches to the measurement of environments.[140]

Halstead-Reitan Neuropsychological Battery.   The *Halstead-Reitan Neuropsychological Battery* consists of three batteries (child, intermediate, and adult).[110] The focus here is on the adult version, which consists of Halstead's original five tests (seven variables) selected for their ability to distinguish people who have frontal lobe dysfunction. Halstead's first graduate student, Ralph Reitan, established his own laboratory and added measures of aphasia, sensory-perceptual integrity, grip strength, and sequential visual scanning, collectively entitled "Allied Procedures." In addition to the *Halstead-Reitan Battery,* a complete battery usually includes the *WAIS-R* and a measure of personality, (*e.g.,* the *MMPI*).

The *Halstead Impairment Index,* computed only for the adult version, is based on the five tests and seven computed values. The index is a summary value computed by dividing the number of test scores in the impaired range by 7. Boll[9] provided a thorough description of the *Halstead-Reitan Battery* and stressed that the impairment index is not by itself a meaningful indicator of brain damage. Rather, the index should be seen as a summary score and be placed in the context of other test data analyzed by inferential methods. Reitan[109] described these inferential methods as follows:

Level of performance. The individual's score is compared with that of a criterion group, and the normality or abnormality of the score is determined. In addition, statements describing the amount or degree of a specific attribute can be provided.
Pattern of performance. Variations of scores within and between tests within the battery can be analyzed for specific strengths and weaknesses.
Specific behavioral deficits or pathognomonic signs. Behaviors occurring only with brain damage, for example, anomia, hemianopsia, and hemiplegia, can be detected.
Comparison of performance of the right and left sides of the body. Measures of motor, sensory, and sensory-perceptual functions from one side of the body are compared with those of the opposite side. Significant discrepancies are likely to reflect brain dysfunction and can help rule out competing explanations of poor performance on more complex neuropsychological tests.

In rehabilitation, as opposed to general medicine, the issue of diagnosing brain damage is of reduced importance. Brain damage is frequently the criterion for entry to a rehabilitation unit. Rehabilitation team members are more concerned with the degree to which the patient will be able to understand and profit from rehabilitation services. A lengthy test battery may not be physically possible because of recent onset of impairment. In these cases, the neuropsychologist attempts to flexibly administer portions of the standard Halstead-Reitan Battery or use tests that place fewer demands on the patient. Before dismissal from the hospital or immediately thereafter, a more nearly complete battery of neuropsychological tests may be administered to more fully assess current cognitive function and to provide guidance on the need for supervision or the ability to return to work.

Although the *Halstead-Reitan Battery* can validly and reliably diagnose the presence and type of brain dysfunction, it is not without its limitations and critics. For example, Halstead's origi-

nal cutting scores were based on the performance of a young sample, with age-graded norms becoming available only recently.[63] Patients with minimal education may spuriously score in the impaired range. Finally, the battery's ability to consistently localize lesions and discriminate psychiatric from organically impaired patients remains problematic.

Luria-Nebraska Neuropsychological Battery.   A.R. Luria[84–86] is the preeminent Russian neuropsychologist whose writings and methods for analyzing brain dysfunction have contributed much to the understanding of brain–behavior relationships. His assessment procedures were clinical and had the advantage of comprehensiveness, short administration time, and an orientation toward the practical issue of rehabilitation. Unfortunately, his clinical methods did not lend themselves to standardized administration, and hence only Luria could ultimately judge their reliability and validity.

Golden and associates,[56] borrowing from the work of Christensen,[16] devised a standardized and objectively scored measure of Luria's investigation. The *Luria-Nebraska Battery* has a total of 269 items divided into 14 clinical scales. Performance on each item is scored from 0, representing no impairment, to 2, representing severe impairment. Total administration time was designed to be a maximum of $2^1/_2$ hours to accommodate patients having brain impairment. Corrections for age and level of education are provided in the manual.

Although the *Luria-Nebraska Battery* appears to be capable of detecting brain damage at better than chance rates, many neuropsychologists have been critical of its value.[81] The criticisms involve issues of diagnostic unreliability, confounding of scale content, insufficient scale length, and difficulty in examining gradations of impairment.

Perhaps the ultimate usefulness of the instrument will be its ability to systematically observe qualitative aspects of the patient's behavior, especially integrated motor performance.

CHEMICAL USE ASSESSMENT. Background.   In the early 1970s, rehabilitation discovered its failure to assess and intervene in the domain of sexuality. The issue of chemical abuse among people with disabilities appears to be at a stage of discovery similar to that of sexuality years ago. A recent literature review on chemical abuse and physical disability revealed few relevant articles.[116] This gap in the literature reflects a failure to adequately address this issue. At present, physicians seldom receive training in the assessment of and intervention in chemical abuse problems. Throughout this section, alcohol and drug abuse are considered jointly. The focus of discussion, however, is on alcohol, the most frequently abused drug.

The importance of alcohol screening is related to both the drug's impact on bodily functions and the associated behavioral aberrations occasioned by its excessive use. Eckardt and co-workers[41] reviewed the detrimental effect of alcohol on most organs, especially the liver, pancreas, and heart. Alcohol ingestion may potentiate the action of prescribed medications, most notably central nervous system (CNS) depressants. This potentiation of action is of particular importance for rehabilitation patients. For example, medications that control blood clot formation and reduce spasticity are frequently used with rehabilitation patients. Alcohol may decrease blood clotting activity and act in an additive manner with muscle relaxants such as diazepam (Valium) and baclofen. In addition, altered consciousness may result in less vigilance in health-compromising situations. If alcohol is ingested in the form of beer, the large fluid volume could seriously compromise a bladder-retraining program.[13]

The cognitive and behavioral aberrations associated with

drug intoxication often result in the onset of a disability. Rohe and DePompolo[116] cited evidence that vehicular crashes and falls, especially while the person is under the influence of alcohol, account for a large proportion of admissions to rehabilitation units. Retrospective chart reviews of patients with central nervous system trauma have shown that alcohol often was present at the time of injury. Fullerton and colleagues[51] found that 50% of their sample of patients admitted to drinking before their injury. Basford[4] found that in 68% of patients with spinal cord injury who had blood screening tests at the time of emergency department admission, blood alcohol test results were positive. O'Donnell and associates[103] found that an identical percentage (68%) of their sample had strong evidence of alcohol or drug use at the time of their injury. In a study from Norway, a country with strict laws governing drinking while driving, Edna[42] found that 32% of 244 patients admitted to the hospital with traumatic head injury were intoxicated. In a prospective study, Rimel[113] found that 72% of 1,330 consecutive patients admitted for CNS trauma had a positive blood alcohol level. Fifty-five percent were legally intoxicated, with blood alcohol levels of 1000 μg/ml or higher. All these data suggest that patients admitted to rehabilitation units with traumatic CNS injuries are not a random sample of the drinking public. Failure to assess this population and to intervene represents a missed opportunity at reducing future medical, social, and personal costs.

It is hoped that the screening for chemical health of all rehabilitation patients will become standard practice. For this to occur, the administration of rehabilitation facilities will have to require that drug screening be standard policy and that rehabilitation professionals, especially physiatrists, have necessary screening skills. Unfortunately, although most representatives of physical medicine and rehabilitation training programs indicated concern about alcohol or drug abuse problems in their patients, only 22% reported that staff were provided education on the issue.[116]

Screening for Chemical Dependency. Individual attitudes about alcohol use, like attitudes about sexuality, are diverse and strongly held and determine the perception of another person's use. Unless one first examines personally held attitudes and values about alcohol use, perceptions of another's use may be highly biased. The two most frequent problems encountered during screening are viewing alcohol as a moral problem and judging the deviance of the patient's drinking through comparison with the interviewer's personal pattern of use. Weinberg[138] stated that the most important aspects of interviewing about alcohol use are getting a detailed history; demonstrating nonjudgmental acceptance; asking direct, specific, and factual questions; maintaining persistence; never discussing alibis; and titrating hostility.

One measure designed to aid in the process of accurate and reliable assessment of alcohol use is the *Self-Administered Alcoholism Screening Test (SAAST)*. Developed by Swenson and Morse,[129] it is a modified version of the *Michigan Alcoholism Screening Test.*[120] The *SAAST* comprises 35 items presented in a yes–no format. A score of 7 to 9 suggests possible alcohol dependence. A score of 10 or greater suggests probable dependence. An advantage of the *SAAST* is its ability to be administered in a structured interview or independently.

Hurt and co-workers[67] reported *SAAST* data on more than 1,000 consecutive patients receiving general medical examinations. They found that 5.4% of the sample gave responses to the *SAAST* that suggested the possible or probable presence of alcohol dependence. Accompanying medical chart reviews revealed a false-negative rate of 6.7%. The study found that subjects scoring 10 or greater are admitting to symptoms of alcohol dependence whether or not they acknowledge being dependent. The study concluded that the *SAAST* is an effective tool for the detection of alcohol dependence in a general medical setting.

In summary, the field of rehabilitation is beginning to discover its responsibility in the screening and treatment of chemical abuse and dependency. Research data suggest that patients with traumatic CNS injuries have a high probability of chemical use. Physiatrists have a responsibility for learning the skills needed for systematic screening of their patients. This intervention, early in the rehabilitation process, is a crucial aspect of prevention of future medical complications.

Psychotherapeutic Interventions

Individual Psychotherapy

Psychotherapy is a frequently misunderstood aspect of psychological services. Some general aspects of all psychotherapy are described here, and forms of therapy frequently provided by an inpatient rehabilitation unit are explained.

What is psychotherapy? Strupp[128] noted that no single definition has found universal acceptance. Part of the reason may be that there are more than 130 varieties of psychotherapy. Interestingly, psychotherapy research has yet to show that any specific variety is clearly superior. Instead, effectiveness seems related to the degree of training in and enthusiasm for the theory and methods espoused by the particular therapy. Data suggest that psychotherapy does produce measurable change in patients. This change, however, can be negative as well as positive. The principle "above all do no harm" is as important in psychotherapy as it is in medicine. Inadequately trained therapists are thus a source of concern in a field lacking firm boundaries.

Psychotherapy is a generic term denoting psychological interventions that ameliorate a wide variety of emotional and behavioral difficulties. Psychotherapy can be defined as an interpersonal process whose goal is modification of problematic affect, behavior, or cognition. The three basic assumptions underlying psychotherapy are as follows: (1) The person seeking services desires change; (2) dysfunctional affect, behavior, or cognition is learned and amenable to change; and (3) the process is a collaborative endeavor that assumes active client participation. Psychotherapeutic intervention is thus contraindicated in patients on whom it must be forced or in those with significant communication or learning impediments. Additionally, if the difficulties are due to factors solely in the patient's environment (long hospitalization, unpleasant medical interventions, prejudice, nonunderstanding staff), the focus of the psychotherapist's intervention may shift from the patient to the environment.

The qualities of effective therapists have been studied and delineated. Therapeutic effectiveness initially depends on good assessment skills. Knowing when and how to intervene and, conversely, when to do nothing is fundamental to the process. Effective therapists are able to instill trust, confidence, and hope in their clients. Regardless of the particular school of therapy, effective therapists have been shown to communicate the specific attitudinal qualities of genuineness, unconditional positive regard, and empathy. As opposed to mere friendship, the therapist provides an atmosphere of acceptance, respect, understanding, warmth, and help in conjunction with deliberate efforts to avoid criticizing, judging, or reacting emotionally with the patient. The creation of this atmosphere results in a framework unmatched by any other human relationship, one conducive to therapeutic change.

Most people living in rehabilitation units are faced with discovering and coping with permanent physical, cognitive, and social losses. This discovery is often accompanied by significant levels of anger, anxiety, dysphoria, grief, and fear. Clinical experience suggests that the patient population can be divided into thirds according to the severity of their reactions. One third of the patients cope extremely well through use of previously established skills and the support of significant others. Another third have greater difficulties but through rather minimal psychotherapeutic intervention are able to successfully manage the crisis. The final third have significant difficulties in coping. They frequently have histories of difficulties in adjustment, such as chemical abuse, major mental disorder, and inability to tolerate structured living environments. This group is of paramount concern to the rehabilitation psychologist and consumes large amounts of professional time.

Because of the pressing practical problems faced by rehabilitation inpatients and the relatively short period of hospitalization, rehabilitation psychologists tend to use time-limited forms of therapy, also known as brief therapy.[12] *Brief therapy* is a general term denoting therapies with different foci, goals, and tactics. Nonetheless, certain elements characterize brief therapy. These include a small number of sessions (6 to 10) and limited, focused, and readily attainable goals. These goals often include amelioration of the most disabling symptoms, reestablishment of previous levels of functioning, and development of enhanced coping skills. The sessions are focused on concrete content and the "here and now." Rehabilitation psychologists frequently apply techniques termed *cognitive-behavioral*. As summarized by Turk and associates[134]

Even though cognitive-behavioral techniques are implemented in diverse ways, some common elements can be identified. Interventions are usually active, time-limited, and fairly structured, with the underlying assumption that affect and behavior are largely determined by the way in which the individual construes the world. Therapy is designed to help the patient identify, reality-test, and correct maladaptive, distorted conceptualizations and dysfunctional beliefs. The patient is assisted in recognizing the connections among cognition, affect, and behavior, together with their joint consequences, and is encouraged to become aware and monitor the role that negative thoughts and images play in the maintenance of maladaptive behavior.

Behavioral Management and Operant Conditioning Techniques

Medical rehabilitation involves a coordinated effort to slow, stop, or reverse the loss of a person's functional abilities. The ultimate criterion of success is the degree to which the patient is able to maintain or improve functional performance. Thus, in medical rehabilitation, in contrast to other areas of medicine, there is a strong and systematic interaction between the medical and the behavioral sciences. Although the physiatrist would not be expected to devise or implement a detailed behavioral modification program, knowledge of the laws of behavior is essential when problems are conceptualized.

This section discusses the three types of learning: observational learning; classic, or respondent, conditioning; and operant conditioning or behavior modification. Because of their relevance to rehabilitation, the principles underlying behavior modification are discussed in detail. Included are the topics of token economies, behavioral contracting, and misconceptions about behavior modification. The following material is drawn from the writings of Martin and Pear,[88] Reynolds,[111] Kazdin,[74] and Fordyce.[49]

THREE TYPES OF LEARNING. Observational Learning. Observational learning, also known as modeling, occurs when a person observes a model's behavior but makes no overt response and receives no direct consequences. The behavior is learned through watching a model without actually performing the behavior. In modeling, a critical distinction is made between learning and performance. The only requirement for learning by modeling is observation of the model. Performance of the learned response, however, depends on the response consequences or incentives connected with the response. Thus, although rehabilitation professionals can effectively use observational learning when instructing patients about desired responses, the principles of behavior modification operate to determine if the observed behavior is actually performed. The likelihood of spontaneously emulating a model depends on a variety of factors, including whether the model is rewarded after the behavior, the similarity of the model to the observer, and the prestige, status, and expertise of the model.

Classic Conditioning. Classic, or respondent, conditioning is the process of repeatedly pairing a neutral stimulus with stimuli that automatically elicit respondent behavior. Some examples of respondents are salivation in response to food in the mouth, muscle flexion in response to pain, and accelerated heart rate in response to loud, unexpected noise. Thus, respondents are responses associated with the organism's glands, reflexes, and smooth muscle. Respondent conditioning does not involve the learning of new behavior but rather involves the capacity of a previously neutral stimulus to elicit a respondent. Respondent behavior is innate, part of the inherited structure of the organism. In respondent conditioning, stimuli that precede the behavior elicit the response. The resulting behavior is stereotyped and rather invariant across species, whereas in operant conditioning, behavior is emitted without any apparent prior stimulus.

The principles of respondent conditioning are used in the treatment of phobias and compulsions. For example, the relatively well-known therapeutic procedure of systematic desensitization involves pairing subjective states of deep muscle relaxation with graded approximations of the stimuli identified as eliciting the pathological anxiety or fear response. Respondent conditioning techniques have been applied to enuresis, excessive eating, smoking, drinking, and deviant sexual behavior.

Operant Conditioning. Operant conditioning is a process by which the frequency of a bit of behavior is modified by the consequences of the behavior. Such behaviors are termed *operants* because they are emitted responses that operate on the environment. Operants are behaviors involving the striated muscles. Most behaviors occurring in everyday life, including those in rehabilitation units, are operants. When an operant is followed by a positive consequence (reinforcer), its frequency increases. Behavior that results in the termination of an aversive stimulus (*e.g.,* turning off an alarm clock) is said to be negatively reinforced. When an operant is followed by a negative consequence (punisher), its frequency decreases. Operants no longer followed by reinforcers decrease in frequency and eventually disappear, a process known as extinction. An additional method of decreasing an undesirable behavior is to reinforce an alternative behavior, one that is incompatible with undesirable behavior. In simple terms, rehabilitation is the process of reinforcing disability-appropriate behaviors and extinguishing (or punishing) disability-inappropriate behaviors.

Environmental events that regularly precede and accompany operants are said to "set the occasion" on which the operant has been reinforced. These environmental stimuli, also known as discriminative stimuli, signal the availability of reinforcement should the previously reinforced behavior occur. Examples of such stimuli in everyday life are a doorbell ringing, a traffic light turning green, and an "open" sign on the front door of a business. Discriminative stimuli are important, because their presence increases the likelihood that a previously reinforced behavior will be emitted.

The speed, amount, and schedule of reinforcement are major determinants of the effectiveness of reinforcement. If possible, the reinforcer should be delivered immediately after the response to maximize the effect of reinforcement. The greater the amount of the reinforcer, the more frequent the response. Schedules of reinforcement have a major impact on the rate of emission of a behavior; they are succinctly described by Reynolds.[111] When one is increasing a low-frequency behavior, it is best to reinforce each occurrence of the behavior. Once the behavior is established, the frequency can be maintained with less frequent (intermittent) reinforcement. The steps for setting up a behavioral modification program are presented in Table 3-5.

TYPES OF REINFORCERS. There are three types of reinforcers. Primary or unconditioned reinforcers are present at birth. They include food, water, sexual stimulation, rest after activity and activity after rest, a band of temperatures, air, and cessation of aversive stimuli. Conditioned reinforcers are stimuli that have been repeatedly paired with primary reinforcers. They are idiosyncratic and are based on the learning history of the person. Generalized reinforcers are stimuli that have been paired with two or more conditioned reinforcers. The prime example of a generalized reinforcer is money; however, verbal responses such as "thank you," "correct," and "great" also are in this category. In addition to the three types of reinforcers, there is an important principle, the Premack principle, which states that any high-frequency behavior can be used to reinforce a low-frequency behavior. This means that such high-frequency behaviors as staying in bed, watching television, and talking with nurses can be used as reinforcers.

TOKEN ECONOMIES. A token economy refers to a reinforcement system based on tokens. The tokens (frequently poker chips) function as generalized reinforcers and can be exchanged at agreed-on rates for back-up reinforcers, such as food, activities, and privileges. The behaviors to be changed (target behaviors) are specified along with the number of tokens earned for their performance. The stipulations of the economy are usually written in the form of a contract, and a "reinforcement menu," which indicates exchange rates and back-up reinforcers, is displayed in a prominent place. Token economies have been used extensively in special education and psychiatric settings. They can be useful with troublesome rehabilitation patients for such behaviors as arriving at therapy sessions late, lack of compliance with fluid

schedules, and failure to perform activities of daily living. As with behavioral contracts, ethical considerations and the success of the program mandate full involvement of the patient in the initial design of the program.

BEHAVIORAL CONTRACTS. Behavioral contracts, also known as contingency contracts, are written agreements between people who desire a change in behavior (rehabilitation team members) and those whose behavior is to be changed (patients). The contract precisely indicates the relationship between behaviors and their consequences. The contract serves four important functions. First, it ensures that the rehabilitation team and the patient agree on goals and procedures. Second, since the goals are specified behaviorally, evidence is readily available regarding fulfillment of the contract. Third, the patient has a clear picture of what behaviors are expected if he or she is to remain in the rehabilitation program. Fourth, the signing of a document functions as a powerful indicator of commitment and helps ensure compliance with the agreement.

COMMON MISCONCEPTIONS ABOUT BEHAVIOR MODIFICATION. Behavior modification has aroused the ire of some people, usually because of a misunderstanding of its underlying principles. Kazdin[74] presented a succinct overview of common objections, two of which are iterated here. A frequent objection is that use of tangible reinforcers is the same as bribery. Bribery can be differentiated from reinforcement, because bribery is used to increase behavior that is considered illegal or immoral and usually involves delivery of the payoff before performance of the behavior, not, as in behavior modification, after. Bribery and reinforcement share the similarity of being ways of influencing behavior, but that is where the similarity ends.

A second objection is that behavior modification is "coercive." Although behavior modification is inherently controlling and designed to alter behavior, multiple safeguards prevent its misapplication. These safeguards include involving the patient when contingencies are negotiated, constructing programs that rely on positive reinforcement rather than negative reinforcement or punishment, and making response requirements for reinforcement lenient at the beginning of the program. The use of behavioral modification in rehabilitation units requires careful training of staff. A limiting factor in many inpatient rehabilitation units is the lack of stability in team membership, especially where shifts in nursing personnel occur frequently.

Social Skills Training

CHANGES IN SOCIAL INTERACTION AFTER DISABILITY. Although only a limited number of the recently disabled may profit from psychotherapy, most can benefit from social skills training. Research on the social psychology of disability is plentiful[3, 32, 34, 55, 112, 125, 131, 145] and underscores the social disadvantages encountered by the disabled, especially the recently disabled. Richardson[112] summarized the literature and found consistently negative public attitudes toward the disabled. He noted that when first encountering a disabled person, the nondisabled experience heightened emotional arousal, anxiety, and feelings of ambivalence. These learned but somewhat involuntary reactions usually result in formal and distorted social interactions.

Often, the nondisabled focus solely on the disability and ignore personal characteristics normally used to evaluate people and establish relationships. The disabled also suffer from the societal norm to be kind to the disabled, which results in a dearth of honest feedback and decreased accuracy in social perception.[61] Consequently, the physically disabled often learn to discount praise and pay close attention to criticism. The factors

---

Table 3-5
Steps in Setting Up a Behavioral Modification Program

1. Define the behavior to be increased or decreased.
2. Define units of that behavior that can be readily measured, such as the beginning or end of a movement cycle.
3. Record the rate of occurrence of the behavior (movement cycle or time).
4. Identify potentially effective and readily controlled reinforcers.
5. Determine a schedule of reinforcement.
6. Implement and modify the program on the basis of outcomes obtained.

mentioned above suggest that social interactions between the disabled and the nondisabled are complex, ambiguous, and unpredictable. Interventions that ameliorate difficulties with social interaction might help reduce emotional distress, speed the slow process of community reintegration,[19] and reduce the risk of future medical problems.[102]

SOCIAL SKILLS: TYPES AND METHODS OF ASSESSMENT. *Social skills* is an inexact term used to describe a wide range of behavior thought necessary for effective social functioning.[24, 27] Dunn and Herman[40] listed three types of social skills: general, general disability-related, and specific disability-related (Table 3-6). Patients with onset of disability before adolescence may require intensive remedial help with the development of general social skills. Patients with onset of disability after adolescence enter the social arena with various competencies in general social skills. However, those with onset after adolescence experience social situations for which they have no previous socialization experiences, hence the importance for training to handle these situations. General social skills can be assessed through a variety of means, including paper and pencil tests, behavioral assessment, and observational techniques.

A social skill frequently identified as a problem is assertiveness; hence, it is used here to illustrate three assessment methods. Three well-known paper and pencil measures of assertiveness are the *Personal Relations Inventory,*[83] the *Rathus Assertiveness Schedule,*[107] and the *Gambrill Assertion Inventory.*[52] As an example, the *Gambrill Assertion Inventory* presents the sub-

ject with 40 situations described by a short phrase, for example, "turn off a talkative friend." The subject then rates his or her degree of discomfort for each situation on a five-point scale ranging from "none" to "very much." Next, the subject rates his or her response probability for each situation on a five-point scale ranging from "always do it" to "never do it." Normative data allow comparisons with the general population and with those having assertiveness difficulties. A measure of assertiveness more relevant to disability is the *Spinal Cord Injury Assertion Questionnaire.*[37] The format of this questionnaire is similar to that of the *Gambrill Assertion Inventory,* but social situations that are potential problems for wheelchair users are described.

Behavioral measures help clarify the frequently found discrepancy between what people say they do and what they actually do. Behavioral measures offer direct and quantifiable data on both verbal and nonverbal aspects of social interactions. Such measures might include checklists or rating scales that permit counting responses, measuring length of time spent interacting, and so on. For example, studies using behavioral measures have shown that disabled people receive less frequent offers of help from strangers than do the nondisabled. However, if help is offered to the disabled, it tends to be overly solicitous.[106, 127] Hastorf and associates[61] found that strangers were more willing to work on a cooperative project if the disabled partner assertively acknowledged the handicap at the beginning of the interaction. Finally, behavioral measures have been used during evaluation of the efficacy of assertion training with disabled people.[39, 54, 96, 99]

Observational techniques can be used by the person, significant others, or staff members. Generally, this type of assessment is less objective than that provided by behavioral measures. Nonetheless, reduced precision is counterbalanced by the opportunity to observe qualitative aspects of the social skill in a natural setting. Several research projects (*e.g.,* Longitudinal Functional Assessment System and Rehabilitation Indicators Project) use observational techniques in the form of diaries, self-reports, and environmental surveys. Thorough descriptions of methods of assessing social skills can be found in a variety of publications.[28, 40, 65] The reader is encouraged to consult relevant social skill training manuals for intervention techniques.[6, 141] Two social skills training programs designed for wheelchair users are described by Hobart (unpublished data) and Dunn.[37, 38]

Table 3-6
General, General Disability, and Disability-Specific Social Skills

A. General social skills
  1. Listening
  2. Positive and negative assertion
  3. Self-disclosure
  4. Receiving compliments
  5. Confrontation
  6. Touching
  7. Conversation
  8. Maximizing physical attractiveness
  9. Meeting new people
  10. Use of humor
  11. Heterosocial skills
B. General disability-related social skills
  1. Acknowledgment of the disability
  2. Asking for help
  3. Acknowledgment of unstated attitudes (making the implicit explicit)
  4. Refusing undesired help
  5. Managing unwelcome social advances
  6. Dealing with staring
  7. Handling unwanted questions
C. Disability-specific social skills
  1. Facilitating communication
  2. Overcoming early deficits in socialization
  3. Managing bowel and bladder problems
  4. Handling reactions to deformity and disfigurement
  5. Disclosing nonvisible disabilities
  6. Dealing with reactions to prostheses

(Dunn ME: Social skills and rehabilitation. In Caplan B [ed]: Rehabilitation Psychology Desk Reference, pp 345–381. Rockville, MD, Aspen Publishers, 1987) By permission of the publisher.

INDIRECT SERVICES

The rehabilitation psychologist's overall aim is to enhance the quality of rehabilitation outcomes for patients. Indirect services in the form of maximizing team interaction skills, staff development, administration, and research provide avenues for enhancing patient outcomes that are as important as those of direct patient services.

The rehabilitation team is a unique structure in the delivery of health care resources. Nowhere else are so many professionals with diverse backgrounds of training expected to communicate in a clear, timely, and comprehensive manner. This communication may become tenuous because of different professional terminologies, overlap in roles, and pressures of productivity in a competitive health care environment.[117] The psychologist can enhance patient outcomes by facilitating cohesion of the rehabilitation team. This task can be accomplished through a variety of methods, including chairing committees to improve interdisciplinary cooperation and leading staff meetings to clarify overlap in professional roles.[1] The rehabilitation psychologist's knowledge of normal and abnormal behavior is frequently called on for staff inservice training. Although some inservice topics focus on patient variables, such as practical management suggestions and brain–behavior relationships, other topics include personal concerns of the staff, such as job stress and communication skills. The psychologist's interpersonal skills often lead to selection for administrative positions.

Rehabilitation psychologists trained at the doctoral level are usually the only team members with specific expertise in research design and statistical methods. As such, they are often consulted by other team members interested in conducting research. They frequently find themselves coordinating experimental investigations, serving as a liaison, or directing research committees. They are also found in a variety of local, state, and national organizations whose function is to promote high quality rehabilitation or social justice for the physically disabled. Finally, the research expertise of psychologists is used through their presence on editorial boards of numerous rehabilitation-related publications.

PSYCHOLOGICAL ADJUSTMENT TO DISABILITY

This section is divided into three parts. The first part provides a brief overview of theories of adjustment to disability. This is followed by a critical analysis of the popularly held but unsubstantiated belief that disabled people go through stages of adjustment to disability. Finally, two disability adjustment models, selected for their heuristic value, are described. These are the behavioral model and the coping skills model.

Overview of Theories of Adjustment to Disability

Theories of adjustment to disability can be grouped along an internal to external continuum.[124] On one end are theories that emphasize internal cognitive events, termed *mentalistic theories,* and on the other end are theories that emphasize events external to the individual, termed *social theories* or *behavioral theories.* The middle of the continuum contains integrative theories that attempt to meld the internal (mentalistic) aspects with the external (social and environmental) determinants.

Before formal theorizing about adjustment to disability, most people believed that the primary source of suffering connected with disability was the disability itself. Hence, removal or amelioration of the disability would presumably reduce distress. However, practice demonstrated that after removal of a disability, some people continued to remain incapacitated. The search for explanations shifted to the then-contemporary principles of dynamic psychology and focused on internal events such as motivation. Patients' difficulties in adjusting to disability were conceptualized in psychodynamic terms, and their incapacitation was transformed into problems of mental health.[72]

As time progressed, it became increasingly clear that dynamic psychology models, especially the classic psychoanalytic model with its emphasis on disease, provided insufficient explanatory power. Professionals came to recognize that physical and social barriers, barriers external to the patient, produce the major source of adjustment problems. Emphasis on sociological concepts such as "sick role"[105] and "illness behavior"[90] ensued. These sociological theories added to the understanding of adjustment to disability on a societal level.[76] However, when individual behavior is of concern, the emphasis of learning theory on the sensitivity of behavior to its consequences provides significant explanatory power. The behavioral model of adjustment to disability is described more fully in a later section.

Theories that attempt to take into account the internal events of the person and the external demands of the environment are called "integrative field theories."[124] Integrative field theories grew out of Lewin's[80] concept of "life space." These theories state that behavior is a joint function of the person and his environment ($B = f[P, E]$). Myerson,[100] Trieschmann,[133] and Wright[144] applied Lewin's basic formulation to problems encountered by the physically disabled. For example, Trieschmann discussed the "educational model of rehabilitation," in which behavior is the joint function of personal, organic, and environmental variables, designated by the formula $B = f(P \times O \times E)$. Her acknowledgment of organic variables highlights the concept that behavior is fundamentally dependent on and limited by the physical capacities of the person.

A popular method of conceptualizing adjustment to disability is through stage theory. The next section draws on the work of Silver and Wortman[126] and Trieschmann[133] and focuses on the basic tenets of stage theory. The validity and impact of these tenets on the practice of rehabilitation are examined.

The Validity of Stage Theory

Stage theory states that people undergoing a life crisis follow a predictable, orderly path of emotional response. Shontz[122, 123] is the major contributor to the application of stage theory to adjustment to disability. Stage theory appears both explicitly and implicitly in a wide variety of rehabilitation-related literature, including that on cancer,[59] hemodialysis,[5, 108] spinal cord injury,[10, 21, 139] and amputation.[104] Additional writers who make implicit or explicit reference to a stage model of adjustment to disability are Dembo and associates,[34] Gunther,[60] and Siller.[125] Unfortunately, these studies are merely descriptive and are based on interview data or anecdotal reports.

Most stage theories set up a series of three to five steps beginning with shock and ending with some form of adaptation. Three commonly held assumptions appear to underlie stage theory formulations applied to the disabled. First, people respond to the onset of disability in specific and predictable ways. Second, they go through a series of stages over time. Finally, they eventually accept or resolve their emotional crises. Each of these assumptions warrants careful scrutiny.

Are There Universal Responses to Disability Onset?

Both Gunther[60] and Shontz[122, 123] indicated that once the crisis of disability is realized, virtually all people experience shock. Unfortunately, the vast majority of studies report retrospective accounts of initial feelings and behavior. In one such study, Parkes[104] interviewed widows and amputees after their losses. Initial feelings of shock and numbness were reported by roughly 50% of the sample. Tyhurst[136] observed disaster victims and described three types of reactions. One group reacted with classic signs of shock, another group appeared cool and collected during the acute situation, and a third group responded with reactions of paralyzing anxiety and hysterical crying. Shock was a predominant but far from universal reaction. Silver and Wortman's[126] literature review concluded that there is little evidence supporting the belief that people react in specific and predictable ways to undesirable life events. Although some patterns are evident, individual variation is inevitably present.

Do Emotional Responses Follow a Pattern After Injury?

The concept that people follow a predictable pattern of emotional response after the onset of a disability is widely held. References to stage models of emotional response occur in the professional literature of nurses,[43, 146] social workers,[139] clergymen,[101] health care professionals,[8] and psychologists.[60, 122, 123, 125]

Silver and Wortman[126] were unable to discover any studies specifically testing stage theory by measurement of affective states over time. Four related studies, all conducted on patients with spinal cord injury, failed to support stage theory. Dunn[36] studied seven psychological variables during three phases of rehabilitation. He was unable to discover a pattern of change in emotions over time; rather, variability among the patients was the norm. McDaniel and Sexton[89] assessed psychological status over four points in time from ratings by rehabilitation team members. Ratings of negative mood states remained relatively constant over the length of the study and were independent of staff ratings of the patient's degree of acceptance of loss. Dinardo,[35] in a cross-sectional study, found that the degree of depression experienced by his subjects was independent of the time that had elapsed since their injury. Finally, Lawson,[77] in a longitudinal study, used a variety of methods to assess the presence of depression. He found no period of at least a week when any of his patients scored consistently in the depressive range on any of the measures. His results suggest that patients with spinal cord injury do not experience a stage of depression during initial rehabilitation.

In summary, although there is much popular and professional literature attesting to the veracity of stages of adjustment to disability, the empirical data do not support such a contention. Silver and Wortman[126] summarized the available data by stating: "Perhaps the most striking feature of available research, considered as a whole, is the variability in the nature and sequence of people's emotional reactions and coping mechanisms as they attempt to resolve their crises." Wright[144] noted: "The process of acceptance of loss is not accomplished once and for all, nor does it march through fixed stages to ultimate acceptance."

Is a Final Stage of Resolution Reached?

Do people who have suffered a major undesirable life event eventually reach a final stage of resolution or acceptance of their disability? The findings across studies suggest that a large minority of people continue to suffer years after a traumatic life event. The unquestioned expectation of resolution or acceptance appears unwarranted for such traumatic life events as severe burns, spinal cord injury, cancer, death of a spouse, and rape.[126] For example, Shadish and associates[121] studied a cross-sectional sample of patients with spinal cord injury. They found that those who had been disabled for as long as 38 years continued to think about and miss physically impossible activities.

Given the lack of support for three common assumptions underlying stage theory, one must look to alternative explanations of why such beliefs permeate clinical folklore and descriptive writing in the area. Although numerous hypotheses could be considered, two come readily to mind. First, professionals working with the recently disabled often encounter unpredictable and emotionally charged situations. One way to help neutralize fears occasioned by such situations is to label the patient as being in a particular stage. This may help transform potentially threatening and seemingly unpredictable behavior into meaningful and predictable categories. A negative outcome of such conceptualizing may be the well-documented tendency for rehabilitation personnel to overdiagnose psychopathological conditions in patients.[53] This interpretation of behavior may also result in the staff inappropriately distancing themselves from the patient by negating the necessity for careful listening. A second reason for the popularity of stage theory may be the enticing belief that all patients eventually resolve the negative effect occasioned by their disability and achieve a final stage of adjustment or resolution. Such a belief has intrinsic appeal to health care professionals, who strive to maximize functional abilities and enhance quality of life.

Models of Adjustment to Disability

The Behavioral Model of Adjustment to Disability

The behavioral model of disability adjustment emphasizes the importance of external factors in determining a person's adjustment. In this model there is reduced interest in the patient's cognitions and a primary focus on observable behaviors. The most frequently cited proponent of this model is Fordyce,[48, 49] and much of what follows is culled from his writings. Additional applications of the behavioral model to rehabilitation problems can be found in the works of Ince[68, 69] and Berni and Fordyce.[7] In the behavioral model of adjustment to disability, the newly disabled face four tasks. The patient must remain in the rehabilitation environment, eliminate disability-incongruent behaviors, acquire disability-congruent behaviors, and maintain the output of disability-congruent behaviors.

The onset of physical disability and entry into the rehabilitation environment represent punishment to most people. In learning theory, punishment is defined as the loss of access to positive reinforcers or the response-contingent onset of aversive stimuli. Thus, the newly disabled find themselves initially operating under a pattern of punishment. Two types of behavior follow the onset of aversive stimuli. The first is escape or avoidance, and the second is aggression. Escape or avoidance behavior is frequently seen in the rehabilitation setting in the form of daydreaming, verbal disclaimers of disability, unauthorized forays off the medical unit, and refusal to participate in scheduled treatments. Aggressive behaviors may consist of either rebellious and capricious behavior or verbal and sometimes physical attack. If avoidant or aggressive behaviors are not understood and dealt with therapeutically, rehabilitation may either never begin or end prematurely.

The intervention strategy for these problems involves the discovery and, if possible, reduction of aversive aspects of the rehabilitation environment. This is accompanied by reinforcement of approximations to active participation in the rehabilitation program. Selecting and systematically graphing a mutually agreed on indicator of rehabilitation progress can help the patient focus on tangible improvements. Patient reactions of hostility are common and should be tolerated within limits. These reactions should never be dealt with through counterhostility, which only increases the probability that the environment, including the treatment staff, will become conditioned aversive stimuli. Systematically ignoring unwanted behavior and establishing therapeutic rapport enhance the probability that the patient will remain in the rehabilitation environment.

The reduction of disability-inappropriate behaviors and the acquisition of disability-congruent behaviors is synonymous with the concept of "adjustment to disability." Disability-inappropriate behaviors are decreased by withdrawal of reinforcers after their occurrence, a process known as extinction. Paradoxically, the laws of behavior demonstrate that withdrawal of reinforcers initially results in a temporary increase in the rate of behavior. This is true for both verbal and performance behaviors.

The patient's verbal behavior is likely to change more slowly than performance behavior. Statements indicating a belief in the eventual return of physical function may require years to extinguish; the staff should neither reinforce nor punish unrealistic verbalizations. Rather, a verbal response suggesting benign neutrality tempered with doubt is least likely to offend the patient. These statements of patients are more frequent at the onset of rehabilitation and possibly reflect the beginning of extinction.

Detailed explanations of anticipated recovery of functional abilities help decrease unrealistic patient or family verbalizations and keep everyone focused on achievable functional goals. This is especially important for family members, who may erroneously believe that the proper way to help the disabled family member cope is through agreeing with unrealistic fantasies about eventual recovery of function.

Difficulties in the acquisition of disability-congruent behaviors are usually considered to be problems in motivation. Learning theory eschews this formulation because it relies on an inference about the internal state of the person. Usually, this label is applied to people who have failed to reach expected levels of performance set by the rehabilitation staff. In learning theory, the problem is that of adjusting contingencies to increase the rate of desired behavior or reduce the rate of behaviors competing with the desired behavior. Unfortunately, most disability-congruent behaviors are initially of low frequency, strength, and value. The steps in changing this situation include establishing reinforcing relationships with the treatment staff, enhancing long-term reinforcers for disability-congruent behaviors, and introducing contingency management interventions that promote the acquisition of disability-congruent behaviors.

Maintaining the output of disability-appropriate behaviors is the final and most important step in adjustment to disability. Rehabilitation is unsuccessful if the behaviors learned in the rehabilitation unit cannot be transferred to the patient's actual living environment. Although the patient may demonstrate the ability to perform a task, the probability of its occurrence depends on contingencies operating in the living environment. Disability-congruent behaviors, such as propelling a wheelchair, maintaining a fluid schedule, and using gait aids, are unlikely to be reinforcing in themselves.

Two strategies for improving generalization are bringing disability-congruent behaviors under the control of reinforcers occurring naturally in the environment and reprogramming the patient's home environment to deliver appropriate reinforcement contingently. The first strategy is promoted through interventions designed to reengage the patient in meaningful vocational and avocational activities after dismissal. Hence, vocational counseling and therapeutic recreation are important as part of inpatient rehabilitation. Gradual and systematic rehearsal of newly learned skills in the home environment during weekend visits is an additional method encouraging generalization. The second strategy is promoted through such interventions as home modifications, assigning a family member to monitor and reinforce home therapy programs, and contracting with the patient for continued compliance. Unfortunately, powerful contingencies may be operating to prevent generalization. For example, the patient may receive reinforcers in the form of increased attention or financial rewards from litigation, a condition also known as secondary gain. Inability to control sources of secondary gain may prevent generalization of disability-congruent behaviors to the home environment. Family interventions are critical to prevent these problems.

The Coping Skills Model

The coping skills model,[98] which emphasizes both cognitive and behavioral factors, is based on the crisis theory originally formulated by Lindemann.[82] Crisis theory asserts that people require a sense of social and psychological equilibrium. After a traumatic event, a state of crisis and disorganization occurs. At the time of the crisis, a person's characteristic patterns of behavior are ineffectual in establishing equilibrium. This state of disequilibrium is always temporary, and a new balance is achieved within days to weeks. The coping skills model comprises seven major adaptive tasks and seven major coping skills. Space limitations permit elaboration of only the coping skills.

The coping skill of *denying or minimizing the seriousness* of a crisis may be directed at the illness or its significance. This skill helps reduce negative emotions to manageable levels. This reduction enhances the mental clarity needed for quick and effective action in emergency situations. The likelihood of implementing a greater range of coping responses is also increased.

The second coping skill consists of *seeking relevant information*. Often, emotional distress is occasioned by a misunderstanding of medical diagnoses and procedures. Understanding often reduces anxiety and provides predictability and a sense of control. The act of gathering information gives the patient and family a concrete task and the accompanying feeling of purposefulness. One longitudinal study of people with chronic illness showed that information-seeking has salubrious effects on adjustment.[45]

Requesting reassurance and emotional support is the third coping skill. The literature shows that perceived social support, adjustment during a crisis, and improved health outcomes are interrelated.[29, 57, 119] Component parts of social support are perceiving that one is cared for, being encouraged to openly express beliefs and feelings, and being provided material aid. Social support may enhance coping by reducing counterproductive emotional states, building self-esteem, and increasing receptivity to new information. Cobb[17, 18] suggested that social support enhances health outcome either directly through neuroendocrine pathways or indirectly through increased patient compliance. He cited evidence showing that patients who receive social support are more likely to stay in treatment and follow their physicians' recommendations. Turner[135] found a reliable association between social support and psychological well-being, especially during stressful circumstances.

Learning specific illness-related procedures reaffirms personal competence and enhances self-esteem, which is often undermined by physical disability. Bulman and Wortman[11] asked social workers and nurses on a rehabilitation unit to define good and poor coping in patients with spinal cord injury. Both groups agreed that good coping included the willingness to learn physical skills that would minimize disability. Conversely, the definition of poor coping included an unwillingness to improve the condition or attend physical therapy.

The fifth coping skill is *setting concrete limited goals*. Limited goal-setting breaks a large task into small and more readily mastered components. As each component is mastered, self-reinforcement accrues and sets the stage for further learning. Limited goal-setting decreases feelings of being overwhelmed and enhances the opportunity to achieve something considered meaningful.

Rehearsing alternative outcomes is the sixth coping skill. Activities such as mental rehearsal, anticipation, discussions with significant others, and incorporation of medical information are involved in this skill. Here, the patient considers possible outcomes and determines the most fruitful manner of handling each. Recalling previous periods of stress and how these were successfully managed is an example of this coping skill. The patient engages in behaviors that alleviate feelings of anxiety, tension, fear, and uncertainty. A cognitive road map is delineated to provide guidance on how any of a variety of possible future stressors will be minimized.

The last coping skill is *finding a general purpose or pattern of meaning* in the course of events. Physical disability is a crisis that can destroy a person's belief that the world is a predictable, meaningful, and understandable place. There appears to be a compelling psychological need to believe that the world is just[78] and to make sense out of a crisis experience. Some theorists[50] claim that the search for meaning is a basic human motivation. One study supports the belief that finding meaning is important to long-term adjustment to disability. Bulman and Wortman[11] studied 29 subjects with spinal cord injury. All subjects reported having asked the question, "Why me?" The authors concluded that "the ability to perceive an orderly relationship between one's behaviors and one's outcomes is important for effective coping."

SUMMARY

In this chapter an overview of direct and indirect services offered by the rehabilitation psychologist and theories of adjustment to disability has been presented. Although the rehabilitation psychologist provides a wide variety of direct and indirect services, certain skills are particularly relevant to rehabilitation. These are training in the standardized measurement of human attributes, behavior modification, and research. Inpatient rehabilitation is a setting in which people under high levels of physical and emotional distress are asked to learn. Many of these people not only are emotionally upset but also have brain injuries that further impair learning efficiency. Standardized measures of personality, intellectual ability, academic achievement, neuropsychological integrity, and chemical health provide a valid and reliable base on which to set rehabilitation goals.

Rehabilitation is specifically concerned with the behavior and functional performance of a person. Rehabilitation team members provide diverse interventions to ensure that the person can physically perform specific activities. Whether this person will actually do so is determined by contingencies in the rehabilitation unit and, more importantly, in the home environment. The rehabilitation psychologist's behavioral modification skills permit the careful assessment and harnessing of these contingencies in the service of the patient.

Progress in any scientific activity depends on research of high quality. Such research is of particular concern for rehabilitation because outcomes are determined by an unusually large and complex set of physical and social variables. Doctoral-level psychologists are usually the only rehabilitation team members with training in research. Traditionally, this training follows the clinician–researcher model, which stresses the asking of practical research questions relevant to clinical problems. These clinical problems may consist of the evaluation of entire rehabilitation service delivery systems.

Theories of adjustment to disability are numerous and can be grouped along a continuum stressing internal cognitive events on the one end and external social and behavioral events on the other. Stage theory is a widely held but largely unsubstantiated model that stresses internal events. Alternative models worth considering are the behavioral model and the coping skills model.

REFERENCES

1. Ackermann L, Campbell D, Hall J, Hawkins H: Role clarification: A procedure for enhancing interdisciplinary collaboration on the rehab team (abstr). Arch Phys Med Rehabil 64:514, 1983
2. Anastasi A: Psychological Testing, 5th ed. New York, Macmillan, 1982
3. Asch A: The experience of disability: A challenge for psychology. Am Psychol 39:529–536, 1984
4. Basford JR, cited in Rohe DE, DePompolo RW: Substance abuse policies in rehabilitation medicine departments. Arch Phys Med Rehabil 66:701–703, 1985
5. Beard BH: Fear of death and fear of life: The dilemma in chronic renal failure, hemodialysis, and kidney transplantation. Arch Gen Psychiatry 21:373–380, 1969
6. Bellack AS, Hersen M: Introduction to Clinical Psychology. New York, Oxford University Press, 1980
7. Berni R, Fordyce WE (eds): Behavior Modification and the Nursing Process, 2nd ed. St Louis, CV Mosby, 1977
8. Bernstein L, Bernstein RS, Dana RH: Interviewing: A Guide for Health Professionals, 2nd ed. New York, Appleton-Century-Crofts, 1974
9. Boll TJ: The Halstead-Reitan Neuropsychology Battery. In Filskov SB, Boll TJ (eds): Handbook of Clinical Neuropsychology, pp 577–607. New York, John Wiley & Sons, 1981
10. Bray GP: Rehabilitation of spinal cord injured: A family approach. J Appl Rehabil Counseling 9:70–78, 1978
11. Bulman RJ, Wortman CB: Attributions of blame and coping in the "real world": Severe accident victims react to their lot. J Pers Soc Psychol 35:351–363, 1977
12. Butcher JN, Koss MP: Research on brief and crisis-oriented therapies. In Garfield SL, Bergin AE (eds): Handbook of Psychotherapy and Behavior Change: An Empirical Analysis, 2nd ed, pp 725–767. New York, John Wiley & Sons, 1978
13. Cameron JS, Halla-Poe D: Alcohol and Spinal Cord Injury. Minneapolis, Brad Thompson Publishing Company, 1985
14. Campbell DP: Manual for the SVIB-SCII, 2nd ed. Stanford, CA, Stanford University Press, 1977
15. Caplan B: Neuropsychology in rehabilitation: Its role in evaluation and intervention. Arch Phys Med Rehabil 63:362–366, 1982
16. Christensen A-L: Luria's Neuropsychological Investigation. New York, Spectrum Publishers, 1975
17. Cobb S: Social support as a moderator of life stress. Psychosom Med 38:300–314, 1976
18. Cobb S: Cited by Garber J, Seligman MEP (eds): Human Helplessness: Theory and Applications. New York, Academic Press, 1980
19. Cogswell BE: Self-socialization: Readjustment of paraplegics in the community. J Rehabil 34:11–13; 35:40, 1968
20. Cohen J: A factor-analytically based rationale for the Wechsler Adult Intelligence Scale. J Consult Psychol 21:451–457, 1957
21. Cohn N: Understanding the process of adjustment to disability. J Rehabil 27:16–18, 1961
22. Colligan RC, Osborne D, Swenson WM, Offord KP (eds): The MMPI: A Contemporary Normative Study. New York, Praeger, 1983
23. Colligan RC, Osborne D, Swenson WM, Offord KP: The aging MMPI: Development of contemporary norms. Mayo Clin Proc 59:377–390, 1984
24. Conger JC, Farrell AD: Behavioral components of heterosocial skills. Behav Ther 12:41–55, 1981
25. Costa PT Jr, McCrae RR, Holland JL: Personality and vocational interests in an adult sample. J Appl Psychol 69:390–400, 1984
26. Cummings JA: Review of Woodcock-Johnson Psycho-Educational Battery. In Mitchell JV Jr (ed): The Ninth Mental Measurements Yearbook, vols 1 and 2, pp 1759–1762. Lincoln, University of Nebraska Press, 1985
27. Curran JP: Skills training as an approach to the treatment of heterosexual-social anxiety: A review. Psychol Bull 84:140–157, 1977
28. Curran JP, Monti PM (eds): Social Skills Training: A Practical Handbook for Assessment and Treatment. New York, Guilford Press, 1982
29. Cutrona C, Russell D, Rose J: Social support and adaptation to stress by the elderly. Psychol Aging 1:47–54, 1986
30. Dahlstrom WG, Welsh GS, Dahlstrom LE (eds): An MMPI Handbook, Vol 1, Clinical Interpretation, rev ed. Minneapolis, University of Minnesota Press, 1972
31. Dahlstrom WG, Welsh GS, Dahlstrom LE (eds): An MMPI Handbook, Vol 2, Research Applications, rev ed. Minneapolis, University of Minnesota Press, 1975
32. Davis F: Deviance disavowal: The management of strained interaction by the visibly handicapped. Soc Probl 9:120–132, 1961
33. Dean RS (ed): Rehabilitation (special issue). Bulletin of the National Academy of Neuropsychologists, vol 2, Autumn 1982, pp 1–15
34. Dembo T, Leviton GL, Wright BA: Adjustment to misfortune: A problem of social-psychological rehabilitation. Rehabil Psychol 22:1–100, 1975

35. Dinardo QE: Psychological adjustment to spinal cord injury. Dissertation Abstracts International 32, Sec B:4206, 1972

36. Dunn D, cited in Trieschmann RB: Spinal Cord Injuries: Psychological, Social and Vocational Adjustment. New York, Pergamon Press, 1980

37. Dunn M: Social discomfort in the patient with spinal cord injury. Arch Phys Med Rehabil 58:257–260, 1977

38. Dunn M, cited in Dunn ME: Social skills and rehabilitation. In Caplan B (ed): Rehabilitation Psychology Desk Reference, pp 345–381. Rockville, MD, Aspen Systems Corporation, 1987

39. Dunn ME, Van Horn E, Herman SH: Social skills and spinal cord injury: A comparison of three training procedures. Behav Ther 12:153–164, 1981

40. Dunn ME, Herman SH: Cited in Dunn ME: Social skills and rehabilitation. In Caplan B (ed): Rehabilitation Psychology Desk Reference, pp 345–381. Rockville, MD, Aspen Systems Corporation, 1987

41. Eckardt MJ, Harford TC, Kaelber CT et al: Health hazards associated with alcohol consumption. JAMA 246:648–666, 1981

42. Edna T-H: Alcohol influence and head injury. Acta Chir Scand 148:209–212, 1982

43. Engel GL: Grief and grieving. Am J Nurs 64(September):93–98, 1964

44. Epstein S, O'Brien EJ: The person-situation debate in historical and current perspective. Psychol Bull 98:513–537, 1985

45. Felton BJ, Revenson TA: Coping with chronic illness: A study of illness controllability and the influence of coping strategies on psychological adjustment. J Consult Clin Psychol 52:343–353, 1984

46. Filskov SB, Goldstein SG: Diagnostic validity of the Halstead-Reitan neuropsychological battery. J Consult Clin Psychol 42:382–388, 1974

47. Folstein MF, Folstein SE, McHugh PR: Mini-mental state: A practical method for grading the cognitive state of patients for the clinician. J Psychiatr Res 12:189–198, 1975

48. Fordyce WE (ed): Behavioral Methods for Chronic Pain and Illness. St Louis, CV Mosby Company, 1976

49. Fordyce WE: Psychological assessment and management. In Kottke FJ, Stillwell GK, Lehmann JF (eds): Krusen's Handbook of Physical Medicine and Rehabilitation, 3rd ed, pp 124–150. Philadelphia, WB Saunders, 1982

50. Frankl VE: Man's Search for Meaning: An Introduction to Logotherapy. New York, Washington Square Press, 1963

51. Fullerton DT, Harvey RF, Klein MH, Howell T: Psychiatric disorders in patients with spinal cord injuries. Arch Gen Psychiatry 38:1369–1371, 1981

52. Gambrill ED, Richey CA: An assertion inventory for use in assessment and research. Behav Ther 6:550–561, 1975

53. Gans JS: Depression diagnosis in a rehabilitation hospital. Arch Phys Med Rehabil 62:386–389, 1981

54. Ginsburg ML: Assertion with the wheelchair-bound: Measurement and training. Dissertation Abstracts International 39, Sec B:5552, 1979

55. Goffman E: Stigma: Notes on the Management of Spoiled Identity. Englewood Cliffs, NJ, Prentice-Hall, 1963

56. Golden CJ, Hammeke TA, Purisch AD: The Luria-Nebraska Battery Manual. Los Angeles, Western Psychological Services, 1980

57. Gottlieb BH: Social support as a focus for integrative research in psychology. Am Psychol 38:278–287, 1983

58. Greene RL (ed): The MMPI: An Interpretive Manual. New York, Grune & Stratton, 1980

59. Gullo SV, Cherico DJ, Shadick R, cited in Garber J, Seligman MEP (eds): Human Helplessness: Theory and Applications. New York, Academic Press, 1980

60. Gunther MS: Emotional aspects. In Ruge D (ed): Spinal Cord Injuries, pp 93–108. Springfield, IL, Charles C Thomas, 1979

61. Hastorf AH, Northcraft GB, Picciotto SR: Helping the handicapped: How realistic is the performance feedback received by the physically handicapped? Pers Soc Psychol Bull 5:373–376, 1979

62. Heaton RK, Chelune GJ, Lehman RAW: Using neuropsychological and personality tests to assess the likelihood of patient employment. J Nerv Ment Dis 166:408–416, 1978

63. Heaton RK, Grant I, Matthews CG: Differences in neuropsychological test performance associated with age, education, and sex. In Grant I, Adams KM (eds): Neuropsychological Assessment of Neu-

ropsychiatric Disorders, pp 100–120. New York, Oxford University Press, 1986

64. Heaton RK, Pendleton MG: Use of neuropsychological tests to predict adult patients' everyday functioning. J Consult Clin Psychol 49:807–821, 1981

65. Hersen M, Bellack AS: Assessment of social skills. In Ciminero AR, Calhoun KS, Adams HE (eds): Handbook of Behavioral Assessment. New York, John Wiley & Sons, 1977

66. Holland JL: The Psychology of Vocational Choice: A Theory of Personality Types and Model Environments. Waltham, MA, Blaisdell Publishers, 1966

67. Hurt RD, Morse RM, Swenson WM: Diagnosis of alcoholism with a self-administered alcoholism screening test: Results with 1,002 consecutive patients receiving general examinations. Mayo Clin Proc 55:365–370, 1980

68. Ince LP (ed): Behavior Modification in Rehabilitation Medicine. Springfield, IL, Charles C Thomas, 1976

69. Ince LP (ed): Behavioral Psychology in Rehabilitation Medicine: Clinical Applications. Baltimore, Williams & Wilkins, 1980

70. Jastak S, Wilkinson GS: Wide-Range Achievement Test Administration Manual. Wilmington, DE, Jastak Associates, 1984

71. Jastak S, Wilkinson GS: Wide-Range Achievement Test Diagnostic and Technical Manual. Wilmington, DE, Jastak Associates, 1984

72. Kahana RJ, Bibring GL: Personality types in medical management. In Zinberg NE (ed): Psychiatry and Medical Practice in a General Hospital, pp 108–123. New York, International Universities Press, 1964

73. Kaufman AS: Review of Woodcock-Johnson psycho-educational battery. In Mitchell JV Jr (ed): The Ninth Mental Measurements Yearbook, vols 1 and 2, pp 1762–1765. Lincoln, University of Nebraska Press, 1985

74. Kazdin AE: Behavior Modification in Applied Settings, rev ed. Homewood, IL, Dorsey Press, 1980

75. Kochansky GE: Psychiatric rating scales for assessing psychopathology in the elderly: A critical review. In Raskin A, Jarvik LF (eds): Psychiatric Symptoms and Cognitive Loss in the Elderly: Evaluation and Assessment Techniques. Washington, Hemisphere, 1979

76. Kutner B: The social psychology of disability. In Neff WS (ed): Rehabilitation Psychology, pp 143–167. Washington DC, American Psychological Association, 1971

77. Lawson NC: Depression after spinal cord injury: A multimeasure longitudinal study. Dissertation Abstracts International 37 Sec B:1439, 1976

78. Lerner MJ: The Belief in a Just World: A Fundamental Delusion. New York, Plenum Press, 1980

79. Levin HS, O'Donnell VM, Grossman RG: The Galveston Orientation and Amnesia Test: A practical scale to assess cognition after head injury. J Nerv Ment Dis 167:675–684, 1979

80. Lewin K: Principles of Topological Psychology. Heider F, Heider GM (trans). New York, McGraw-Hill, 1936

81. Lezak MD (ed): Neuropsychological Assessment, 2nd ed. New York, Oxford University Press, 1983

82. Lindemann E: Symptomatology and management of acute grief. Am J Psychiatry 101:141–148, 1944

83. Lorr M, More WW: Four dimensions of assertiveness. Multivariate Behav Res 15:127–138, 1980

84. Luria AR: Restoration of Function After Brain Injury. Zangwill OL (trans). Oxford, Pergamon Press, 1963

85. Luria AR: The Working Brain: An Introduction to Neuropsychology. Haigh B (trans). New York, Basic Books, 1973

86. Luria AR (ed): Higher Cortical Functions in Man, 2nd ed. New York, Basic Books, 1980

87. Malec J: Personality factors associated with severe traumatic disability. Rehabil Psychol 30:165–172, 1985

88. Martin G, Pear J: Behavior Modification: What It Is and How To Do It, 2nd ed. Englewood Cliffs, NJ, Prentice-Hall, 1983

89. McDaniel JW, Sexton AW: Psychoendocrine studies of patients with spinal cord lesions. J Abnorm Psychol 76:117–122, 1970

90. Mechanic D: The concept of illness behavior. J Chronic Dis 15:189–194, 1962

91. Millon T: Modern Psychopathology: A Biosocial Approach to Maladaptive Learning and Functioning. Philadelphia, WB Saunders, 1969

92. Millon T (ed): Disorders of Personality: DSM-III, Axis II. New York, John Wiley & Sons, 1981
93. Millon T: Millon Clinical Multiaxial Inventory Manual, 3rd ed. Minneapolis, Interpretative Scoring Systems, 1983
94. Millon T: The DSM-III: An insider's perspective. Am Psychol 38:804–814, 1983
95. Millon T, Green CJ, Meagher RB Jr: Millon Behavioral Health Inventory Manual, 3rd ed. Minneapolis, National Computer Systems, 1982
96. Mischel MH: Assertion training with handicapped persons. J Counseling Psychol 25:238–241, 1978
97. Mitchell JV Jr: The Ninth Mental Measurements Yearbook, vols 1 and 2. Lincoln, University of Nebraska Press, 1985
98. Moos RH, Tsu VD (eds): Coping With Physical Illness, pp 3–21. New York, Plenum Medical Book Company, 1977
99. Morgan B, Leung P: Effects of assertion training on acceptance of disability by physically disabled university students. J Counseling Psychol 27:209–212, 1980
100. Myerson L: Somatopsychology of physical disability. In Cruickshank WM (ed): Psychology of Exceptional Children and Youth, 2nd ed, pp 1–52. Englewood Cliffs, NJ, Prentice-Hall, 1963
101. Nighswonger CA: Ministry to the dying as a learning encounter. J Thanatol 1:101–108, 1971
102. Norris-Baker C: Behavioral discriminators of health outcomes in spinal cord injury (abstr). Arch Phys Med Rehabil 63:503, 1982
103. O'Donnell JJ, Cooper JE, Gessner JE et al: Alcohol, drugs and spinal cord injury. Alcohol Health Res World 1981/1982, pp 27–29
104. Parkes CM: Components of the reaction to loss of a limb, spouse or home. J Psychosom Res 16:343–349, 1972
105. Parsons T: Definitions of health and illness in the light of American values and social structure. In Jaco EG (ed): Patients, Physicians and Illness: A Sourcebook in Behavioral Science and Health, 2nd ed, pp 99–117. New York, Free Press, 1972
106. Piliavin IM, Piliavin JA, Rodin J: Costs, diffusion, and the stigmatized victim. J Pers Soc Psychol 32:429–438, 1975
107. Rathus SA: A 30-item schedule for assessing assertive behavior. Behav Ther 4:398–406, 1973
108. Reichsman F, Levy NB: Problems in adaptation to maintenance hemodialysis: A four-year study of 25 patients. Arch Intern Med 130:859–865, 1972
109. Reitan RM: A research program on the psychological effects of brain lesions in human beings. In Ellis NR (ed): International Review of Research in Mental Retardation, vol 1, pp 153–218. New York, Academic Press, 1966
110. Reitan RM: Theoretical and methodological bases of the Halstead-Reitan Neuropsychological Test Battery. In Grant I, Adams KM (eds): Neuropsychological Assessment of Neuropsychiatric Disorders, pp 3–30. New York, Oxford University Press, 1986
111. Reynolds GS: A Primer of Operant Conditioning, rev ed. Glenview, IL, Scott, Foresman & Co, 1975
112. Richardson SA: Attitudes and behavior toward the physically handicapped. Birth Defects 12:15–34, 1976
113. Rimel RW: A prospective study of patients with central nervous system trauma. J Neurosurg Nurs 13:132–141, 1981
114. Rohe DE, Athelstan GT: Vocational interests of persons with spinal cord injury. J Counseling Psychol 29:283–291, 1982
115. Rohe DE, Athelstan GT: Change in vocational interests after spinal cord injury. Rehabil Psychol 30:131–143, 1985
116. Rohe DE, DePompolo RW: Substance abuse policies in rehabilitation medicine departments. Arch Phys Med Rehabil 66:701–703, 1985
117. Rothberg JS: The rehabilitation team: Future direction. Arch Phys Med Rehabil 62:407–410, 1981
118. Satz P, Fletcher JM: Emergent trends in neuropsychology: An overview. J Consult Clin Psychol 49:851–865, 1981
119. Schaefer C, Coyne JC, Lazarus RS: The health-related functions of social support. J Behav Med 4:381–406, 1981
120. Selzer ML: The Michigan Alcoholism Screening Test: The quest for a new diagnostic instrument. Am J Psychiatry 127:1653–1658, 1971
121. Shadish WR Jr, Hickman D, Arrick MC: Psychological problems of spinal cord injury patients: Emotional distress as a function of time and locus of control. J Consult Clin Psychol 49:297–299, 1981
122. Shontz FC: Reactions to crisis. Volta Rev 67:364–370, 1965
123. Shontz FC: The Psychological Aspects of Physical Illness and Disability. New York, Macmillan, 1975
124. Shontz FC: Psychological adjustment to physical disability: Trends in theories. Arch Phys Med Rehabil 59:251–254, 1978
125. Siller J: Psychological situation of the disabled with spinal cord injuries. Rehabil Lit 30:290–296, 1969
126. Silver RL, Wortman CB: Coping with undesirable life events. In Garber J, Seligman MEP (eds): Human Helplessness: Theory and Applications, pp 279–340. New York, Academic Press, 1980
127. Soble SL, Strickland LH: Physical stigma, interaction, and compliance. Bull Psychonomic Soc 4:130–132, 1974
128. Strupp HH: Psychotherapy research and practice: An overview. In Garfield SL, Bergin AE (eds): Handbook of Psychotherapy and Behavior Change: An Empirical Analysis, 2nd ed, pp 3–22. New York, John Wiley & Sons, 1978
129. Swenson WM, Morse RM: The use of a self-administered alcoholism screening test (SAAST) in a medical center. Mayo Clin Proc 50:204–208, 1975
130. Swenson WM, Pearson JS, Osborne D: An MMPI Source Book: Basic Item, Scale, and Pattern Data on 50,000 Medical Patients. Minneapolis, University of Minnesota Press, 1973
131. Tajfel H: Social psychology of intergroup relations. Annu Rev Psychol 33:1–39, 1982
132. Teasdale G, Jennett B: Assessment of coma and impaired consciousness: A practical scale. Lancet 2:81–83, 1974
133. Trieschmann RB: Spinal Cord Injuries: Psychological, Social and Vocational Adjustment. New York, Pergamon Press, 1980
134. Turk DC, Meichenbaum D, Genest M: Pain and Behavioral Medicine: A Cognitive-Behavioral Perspective. New York, Guilford Press, 1983
135. Turner RJ: Social support as a contingency in psychological well-being. J Health Soc Behav 22:357–367, 1981
136. Tyhurst JS: Individual reactions to community disaster: The natural history of psychiatric phenomena. Am J Psychiatry 107:764–769, 1951
137. The Wechsler Adult Intelligence Test, rev manual. New York, Psychological Corporation, 1983
138. Weinberg JR: Interview techniques for diagnosing alcoholism. Am Fam Physician 9(March):107–115, 1974
139. Weller DJ, Miller PM: Emotional reactions of patient, family, and staff in acute-care period of spinal cord injury: I and II. Soc Work Health Care 2(a):369–377, 1977; 3(b):7–17, 1977
140. Wicker AW: Nature and assessment of behavior settings: Recent contributions from the ecological perspective. In McReynolds P (ed): Advances in Psychological Assessment, vol 2. San Francisco, Josey-Bass, 1981
141. Wilkinson J, Canter S: Social Skills Training Manual. New York, John Wiley & Sons, 1982
142. Woodcock RW: Development and Standardization of the Woodcock-Johnson Psycho-Educational Battery. Hingham, MA, Teaching Resources, 1978
143. Woodcock RW, Johnson MB: Woodcock-Johnson Psycho-Educational Battery. Hingham, MA, Teaching Resources, 1977
144. Wright BA (ed): Physical Disability, A Psychosocial Approach, 2nd ed. New York, Harper & Row, 1983
145. Yuker HE, Block JR, Young JH: The Measurement of Attitudes Toward Disabled Persons. Albertson, NY, Human Resources Center, 1966
146. Zahourek R, Jensen JS: Grieving and the loss of the newborn. Am J Nurs 73:836–839, 1973

4

Vocational Evaluation and Rehabilitation

Deborah J. Davis

Liina Paasuke

Since the late 1970s the field of vocational evaluation has grown dramatically. New terminology is continually being introduced into the literature, including such concepts as work capacity evaluation, functional assessment, and work hardening/reconditioning. Emphasis on job analysis methods, use of job site accommodations, and use of technology in the rehabilitation process have created new roles for rehabilitation professionals in vocational rehabilitation.

From a historical perspective, Pruitt[23] indicates that vocational evaluation has emerged from many fields: "Psychology, vocational and industrial education, occupational therapy, military, medicine, and the workshop movement have all contributed to some extent to the field of work evaluation."

The process of vocational evaluation uses information from many sources regarding a person's physical, psychological, social, cognitive, and perceptual abilities. The most unique aspect of vocational (or work) evaluation is the emphasis on the use of real or simulated work as the primary medium for evaluation. This approach differs from earlier efforts in the field of vocational rehabilitation in which paper and pencil tasks along with medical diagnoses and evaluation were used to determine a patient's capacity for vocational training or placement. With the focus on direct observation of the person's performance in a real, simulated, or accommodated environment, the evaluator is likely to get critical and accurate information that will directly and specifically apply to an employment situation.

Another specific definition of vocational evaluation is offered by the Vocational Evaluation and Work Adjustment Association (VEWAA), a division of the National Rehabilitation Association: Work evaluation is "the process of finding out what strengths and weaknesses and limitations of an individual are in terms of optional functional outcome and developing proposals for alternative service plans."[30]

It is clear that an individualized approach to the process of work evaluation is critical. There is no one type of assessment or standardized method of evaluation that can accomplish goals for everyone. Many authors of work evaluation literature recommend a question and answer type of approach as the most appropriate for the initial stages of work evaluation services. It is important to use appropriate referral background, initial interview, techniques, and objectives for work evaluation services. The Commission on Accreditation of Rehabilitation Facilities (CARF) Standards for vocational evaluation emphasize the importance also, of an individually written evaluation plan. The plan usually will identify the questions that need to be answered by the evaluation process, will indicate what type of testing or evaluation methods will be used to answer the questions, and frequently will indicate which staff will provide specific services in carrying out the plan. Also included in such a plan is a method for a review process and renewed planning outline.

An approach to vocational rehabilitation that focused on the needs of the severely handicapped population was developed and widely published in the mid 1970s by Kalisankar Mallik, Sheldon Yaspeh, and James Mueller through their work at the Job Development Laboratory at George Washington University Medical Center. The concept of functional abilities and limitations was established to describe such physical entities as visual limitations, reach, grasp, carrying, lifting, endurance, and so on in relation to specific physical and cognitive work demands. Thus, it became clear that with a new approach to information gathering in the evaluation process, the focus of vocational evaluation could be on critical job demands, the accommodation of the work environment, and the performance capacity of the person in contrast to a broad diagnostic listing of medical information that was difficult for employers and rehabilitation practitioners to use. One of the most limiting factors in returning a person with a handicapping condition to work is defining his or her functional abilities and capacity. In order to do this one must use environmental information (*i.e.,* the actual physical work environment) as well as the physical, cognitive, and social demands of the job. Research at Syracuse University by Faste produced a system for analyzing environmental and equipment design features that is problematic for persons with disabilities. The system is referred to as the "Enabler." According to Mueller, "Faste's Enabler system is based on the premise that any disability can be described in terms of functional limitations. The Enabler simplifies consideration of the vast range of variations in the abilities of disabled persons. Faste illustrated that, although most information concerning the disabled population is cloaked in medical jargon, the range of possible functional limitations can form a basis for the understanding of human factors—or ergonomics—of this population."[21]

It is important to understand and view the field of vocational assessment as a critical one in the overall vocational rehabilitation process. The work of medical practitioners and vocational rehabilitation personnel becomes the task of defining a person's functional capacities and abilities. The use of real or simulated work, the the renewed emphasis on improving physical capacity evaluation techniques, as well as analyzing the work environment for the physical, cognitive, and social demands of the job provides new opportunity for implementation of vocational assessment. This emphasis is perceived as a positive one, providing substantial and real data to the person with a disability to explore his or her capacities and abilities in relation to the real work world. If the vocational evaluation process is appropriately provided, the person will have gained new information that will help in the perception of personal strengths and weaknesses in relation to goals for continuation and/or redirection of his or her life from a vocational perspective.

The skilled evaluator will explore all relevant data and emphasize a person's abilities for vocational rehabilitation recommendations and placement. The assistance, cooperation, understanding, and support of the physician and other medical team members during this process cannot be overemphasized.

SETTINGS

Vocational assessment takes place in many settings across the country. The more traditional settings are the community rehabilitation facilities that are accredited by the Commission on Association of Rehabilitation Facility (CARF), as well as approved by state vocational rehabilitation agencies. Services usually provided include work evaluation, community work adjustment programs, sheltered employment, and assistance with job placement programs. In the more recent past, however, many medical facilities across the country and freestanding private organizations have established work evaluation programs. The impact of diagnosis-related groups (DRGs) on the medical setting is encouraging growth of community-based support services in an effort to provide different types of revenue for a medical setting. A particular focus of these medically related or independent/private organizations is usually work hardening programs and physical capacity evaluation programs. Other settings in which vocational evaluation takes place include community colleges, universities, centers for independent living, and other community-based organizations.

PROFESSIONAL STAFF

Vocational evaluation services are most commonly provided by certified work evaluators who meet the criteria established by VEWAA, vocational rehabilitation counselors, and occupational therapists who all have the long-term historical basis in service provision in the area of vocational assessment. Work hardening programs, functional capacity assessment, and other types of community work-related programs include staffing by occupational and physical therapists, exercise physiologists, vocational evaluators, rehabilitation counselors, psychologists, social workers in some settings, as well as rehabilitation nurses. The training level of each of these groups of professionals is varied, but each profession has its own standards of practice and professional training. However, the most commonly accepted professional groups include practitioners associated with the National Rehabilitation Association, Vocational Evaluation and Work Adjustment Association, American Occupational Therapy Association, American Physical Therapy Association, and others affiliated with the above professions. Almost all professionals have a minimum of training at the bachelor degree level that focuses on a combination of liberal arts, social, and physical science training, as well as specialty training in the professional area. Rehabilita-

tion nurses have an associate's degree as the minimum training level. A new group of professionals being recognized and developed across the country are broadly defined as rehabilitation engineers. This group is, by definition, an interdisciplinary group that focuses on the design, assessment, and use of technology to meet the special needs of people with disabilities. Professional groups most commonly affiliated with rehabilitation engineering include industrial, biomechanical, electrical, and mechanical engineers, as well as various occupational therapists and vocational rehabilitation counselors. The development and integration of rehabilitation engineering services provides a great deal of promise for the overall field of vocational rehabilitation.

EVALUATION PROCESS

A successful vocational evaluation program will develop many questions regarding the potential vocational capacity of a person, as well as provide many answers. The vocational evaluation program must be a carefully planned and enacted service, in order to place the prospective employee in the most beneficial circumstances and provide the most positive outcome from the services. Because every person has different needs and abilities, it is also recognized that everyone has specific and unique strengths and functional limitations. Without careful focus on each person's needs in the process of vocational evaluation, a very negative outcome could occur that limits a person's vocational opportunities and future. The evaluator must take careful referral information and establish some type of intake methodology to plan the evaluation and assess the needs of the prospective employee. The evaluator must be sure to provide the necessary resources and information to establish a well-organized vocational evaluation plan. It is commonly known that the more specific the referral questions are, the more specific the work evaluation process can be. Initially, specific information will need to be available regarding the person's work history, vocational interests, vocational needs, abilities, functional limitations, prior employment, and educational experiences. Three general levels of consideration for the overall vocational evaluation program are (1) can the patient return to his or her former occupation? (2) what are the transferrable skills that this patient can use? (3) what training needs exist to facilitate successful integration or reemployment? Appropriate instrumentation may be used to help better define the patient's vocational interests, vocational aptitudes, intelligence, and physical skills.

The vocational rehabilitation literature supports the assessment of environmental needs as a major consideration during the vocational evaluation process because it may be purely environmental limitations, such as narrowed doorways, that prohibit a person from successful job opportunities. Thus, the vocational evaluation process must include specific information about work environments and actual job demands in order to appropriately meet the needs of people with physical limitations. This focus of assessment is particularly necessary for vocational rehabilitation planning for the severely physically disabled. Without consideration of the environmental demands, it is very unlikely that the person with a severe physical disability will experience successful vocational return.

The vocational evaluation process can be a very positive learning opportunity for the disabled person, as well as all rehabilitation service providers, in helping him or her plan to meet future goals. With the process of planning and providing questions to be answered, the person can gain useful insight into particular strengths and weaknesses and plan accordingly. The positive evaluation will pay attention not only to the current goals and needs of the person but also explore options for future vocational success. Many vocational rehabilitation agencies and state laws have requirements that rehabilitation services need only provide entry level skills and placement for the person. Because of the increasing cost of living in this country, however, it is a narrow perspective. The skilled vocational evaluator will help the patient take a look at immediate needs and perhaps the earliest placement but will also facilitate long-term vocational planning.

It is important that the evaluation plan and documentation of service include limitations of assessment procedures. It is well known, for example, that commercial work samples represent some areas of work in some communities but that the norms that are used may not represent any true relation to the patient or to people in the local work force. Thus, limitations should be carefully stated. The same goes particularly for the use of paper and pencil tests of the work evaluation process, as well as physical capacity evaluations. Such is particularly true for lifting evaluations, static physical capacity evaluations, or those activities that are not based on the particular job demands for which the person is being considered.

INTELLIGENCE, APTITUDE, ACHIEVEMENT, AND INTEREST TESTING

Psychological testing has a strong traditional role in vocational rehabilitation. Used to help determine or describe a person's strengths and weaknesses, psychological testing can be a valuable tool in vocational evaluation. As a paper and pencil task most frequently, however, psychological testing is best used in conjunction with additional sources of information that are based on direct observation of performance in a real or simulated work environment. According to Dr. Karl Botterbusch, "Regardless of the time period, all vocational evaluations need to include an assessment of physical, intellectual, social, personal and behavior factors that comprise the uniqueness of each individual."[5] Four common types of psychological measures used in vocational assessment include intelligence tests, achievement tests, aptitude tests, and interest assessments.

Intelligence Testing

Definitions of intelligence vary among the most learned professionals but generally reflect a person's capacity for problem solving, memory, verbal, and nonverbal communication skills. The *Weschler Adult Intelligence Scale (WAIS)* is the most widely used intelligence test. Intelligence tests are used in vocational rehabilitation to help predict a person's capacity for success in training, educational, or job placement activities.

Achievement Testing

Achievement tests are standardized assessments used to define a person's current level of knowledge and skills. The sources are normally described in grade level equivalence for such areas as reading, math, written communication, and spelling. People who cannot read, do math, or write can be easily discouraged or embarrassed during the vocational evaluation process. The vocational evaluator must determine a person's literacy level so that evaluations are given within his or her ability range. Nonreading aptitude tests are available as well as those that require reading literacy. Well-known standardized assessments include the *Wide Range Achievement Tests (WRAT)* and the *Basic Occupational Literacy Test (BOLT)*.

As with intelligence tests, achievement tests are used to help determine a person's abilities for training or placement activities.

Aptitude Testing

"Aptitude testing is used to determine a person's ability to learn, or develop skills in specific areas of performance or work."[5] Job descriptions in occupational literature published by the United States Department of Labor use a series of 11 aptitudes that relate to specific jobs. These include such aptitudes as general learning ability, motor coordination, and numerical and spatial aptitudes. The most widely used aptitude test is the *General Aptitude Test Battery (GATB)*. Evaluators must be formally trained to administer this test battery through the federal and state employment services.

Interest Inventories

Interest inventories play an important role in vocational rehabilitation. Interest inventories are most often used for vocational exploration with the patient who has limited exposure to work or does not have a clear career goal. They are used to assist a person in defining likes and dislikes in relation to the world of work or various types of vocational groupings (*i.e.*, data, people, or things).

Well-known and widely used interest inventories include the *Strong-Campbell Vocational Interest Inventory* and *Holland's Self-Directed Search*. Interest inventories are available for different vocational skill levels (*i.e.*, professional, blue collar, sheltered workshops) as well as reading and nonreading versions.

FUNCTIONAL ASSESSMENT

Functional assessment is a term used by medical and rehabilitation professionals to describe an evaluation process of a person's abilities and behavior in various activities of life. Halpern provided a new description with an additional element, that of inclusion "of measurement of purposeful behavior in interaction with the environment, which is interpreted according to the assessment's intended uses."[12] Examples of new functional assessments for vocational rehabilitation include the *Available Motions Inventory* and the *Work Simulator*. The *Available Motions Inventory* was developed by the Rehabilitation Engineering Center at Wichita State University, which "evaluates the upper extremity capabilities of individuals with neuromuscular impairments. Results of the evaluation are applied to planning appropriate modifications of a variety of light benchwork tasks performed in an industrial setting."[16] It has excellent application for the evaluation of severely disabled population. The *Work Simulator* was developed by John Engolitcheff and the Baltimore Therapeutic Company. This treatment and evaluation unit uses single base instruments and over 100 attachments to simulate repetitive upper limb motions with varying degrees of resistance over time. Data are gathered regarding work output of the person to compare progress and effort over time. This equipment is very expensive to lease or purchase but provides a high volume of clinical information and direct application to vocational placement. It is most frequently used in the assessment of the industrially injured person. Researchers in medicine, engineering, education, and vocational rehabilitation are identifying new assessment techniques in an attempt to quantify a person's abilities from physical, psychological, perceptual, cognitive, and social perspectives. Although rehabilitation professionals have employed functional assessment techniques for many years, the outcomes tended to be expressed in medical terms, (*i.e.,* a diagnostic focus). The increasing demand of consumers and the raised consciousness of people working in the medical and rehabilitation fields require that assessments address not only the capacities of the person but also the limitations of the environment. This is a dramatic switch. New work in the field has been able to demonstrate the critical role that environment plays in facilitating behavior.

WORK HARDENING/RECONDITIONING

Work hardening is a component of work capacity evaluation. Guidelines for work hardening programs by the American Occupational Therapy Association and the Vocational Evaluation and Work Adjustment Association define work hardening as "an individualized work oriented treatment process involving the client in simulated or actual work tasks, that are structured and graded to progressively increase physical tolerance, stamina, endurance, and productivity with the eventual goal of improved employability."[1] Other standards include definition of professionals who have specific training knowledge and skills to interpret medical information and physical functioning, with the optimal service providers being an occupational therapist and vocational evaluator, along with a multiple disciplinary team. Additional standards include screening or initial review standards, referral standards, evaluation standards, and an individual program outline including exploration of four domains of physical function: (1) biomedical, (2) psychophysical, (3) metabolic cardiovascular, and (4) psychosocial. Goals for work hardening programs, as stated in the standards, will maximize productivity, physical tolerance, endurance and stamina, functional ability, self-confidence, and worker traits and attitudes conducive to employment. These goals also include a process of maximizing and exploring the use of job modifications and adaptive techniques, as well as the use of symptom control techniques, including work simplification, body mechanics, positioning, relaxation, and self-pacing.

Other professionals who provide service in work hardening programs include physicians, physical therapists, exercise physiologists, and rehabilitation counselors. Communication regarding case management issues and related services should occur with other treating rehabilitation professionals, including rehabilitation nurses, psychologists, industrial medicine staff, and industrial personnel staff, to name a few. Settings in which work hardening programs can be found include inpatient and outpatient medical facilities, freestanding rehabilitation facilities, industrial work centers, industrial medicine-transitional work centers, as well as many others.

WORK CAPACITY EVALUATION

Work capacity evaluation is "a process of measuring and developing an individual's capacity to dependably sustain performance in response to broadly defined work demands."[17] Another similar term frequently used in the literature is functional capacity evaluation.

As in other areas of vocational assessment, work capacity evaluation uses simulated work tasks to determine current work tolerance and potential for improvement of work tolerance. The work simulation tasks are classified according to the known job demands of the patient's employer and Department of Labor Standards for job classifications. The evaluation environment is

intended to simulate the real work environment with careful attention paid to productivity, attendance, safety, time utilization, and behavior. A major goal is to decrease focus on the person as a "patient" and to encourage new or regained identity as an "employee."

The work capacity evaluation is an interdisciplinary process. According to Matheson, "Combining elements of vocational evaluation, ergonomics, kinesiology, and industrial psychology, a new discipline has emerged which can be conceptually described as occurring at the interface between medical rehabilitation and vocational rehabilitation."[17]

In Matheson's system for work capacity evaluation, the services are divided into two separate components: work tolerance screening and work hardening. Work tolerance screening is "an intensive evaluation of an individual's ability to sustain work performance, exploring the physiological demands of work."[17] The evaluation is meant to serve as a baseline measurement of the person's performance capacity. Dependent on the outcome, further services may be needed to prepare the person for vocational placement.

JOB SITE ANALYSIS

Job site analysis is critical to the successful return to work for people with disabilities. "Job analysis can be defined as the investigation and collecting of information concerning work tasks."[22] According to the *International Classification of Impairment, Disability, and Handicap Manual* published by the World Health Organization, a person is only considered physically "handicapped" if the physical environment does not meet his or her needs.[31] Thus, careful analysis of the work environment is needed to determine the extent to which the environment creates limitations for successful return to work.

Job site analysis is most commonly performed to evaluate for wheelchair accessibility and mobility. Obviously, a person must be able to enter a building to be able to work in it. Other critical factors in return to work for mobility-impaired people include analysis of the location of the actual work station, use and location of elevators, use of safety procedures, analysis of restrooms, cafeteria, and parking facilities, as well as any other physical barriers. Limitations of access to any of these areas can prohibit a successful return to work.

Other purposes for job site analysis are to identify environmental and social conditions for people with functional limitations other than mobility. Needs of those with hearing, vision, lifting, reaching, and cognition limitations and/or other emotional or physical problems must be accommodated in the workplace. Limitations of the work environment need to be analyzed and recorded with specific recommendations made to eliminate barriers that impede return to work. If the worksite evaluator cannot define options for improvement of the worksite, then a referral should be made to the appropriate professionals within the industry to assist the employer.

Worksite analysis is one of the most complex components of vocational rehabilitation. The rehabilitation professional must be cognizant of state and national standards for accessibility, occupational safety and health standards, business practices and organizational structure, roles of labor and management, along with employer needs in order to best represent the employee with a disability. The "team" in the workplace may be made of different members than the rehabilitation provider is most familiar with. It is the responsibility of the worksite evaluator to develop necessary verbal and written communication skills, professional knowledge and behaviors, and flexibility in new situations to meet the job demands.

JOB ACCOMMODATIONS

The Rehabilitation Act of 1973 includes sections relating to job accommodations. These sections state that employers throughout the country are required to provide "reasonable accommodation" for handicapped applicants and employees, as well as for special disabled veterans. More specifically, the law states that employees who do contractual business with the federal government are required by the United States Department of Labor to "make reasonable accommodations to the known limitations of qualified applicants and employees, except where the employer demonstrates factors involving cost, business necessity, and safety impose an undue hardship upon the company." Conceptually, a "job accommodation is an attempt to make, or an actual adjustment made, to a job, the procedure or methods in which the job is performed, or rearrangement or architectural changes in the work environment for the purpose of increasing efficiency, effectiveness, employee morale, safety, and a return on investment."[6]

The Work Environment and Technology Committee of the President's Committee of Employment of the Handicapped, in proceedings from the joint seminar with the Institute of Industrial Engineers published by the Arkansas Rehabilitation Research and Training Center entitled "Designing Jobs for Handicapped Workers," indicates that there are generally four types of accommodation: (1) accommodation to facilities and equipment design, (2) job design, (3) training, and (4) ongoing support. Facilities and equipment design is perceived as the hardware aspect of the job, including special tools, special jigs, fixtures, or other mechanical and/or electrical equipment design. The work environment itself may require modification to provide wheelchair access or better environmental labeling for a person who has a visual impairment. Facility accommodations may be the building of a ramp to allow a person in a wheelchair to access the environment, enlarged bathroom stalls or raised desks for a wheelchair, or a special sound device in an entryway in an office area to accommodate a blind employee. Job design changes are also referred to as "job restructuring" in various sections of rehabilitation literature. This refers to analyzing the task demands of a job and paying special attention to which job tasks are critical to the performance of the job. It may also include flexible work times, such as a 2-hour lunch break and an altered work shift of 4 hours in the morning and 4 hours of work later, to accommodate a person who has a physical limitation of endurance. Different types of work methods or processes may be used, such as exchanging duties among receptionists in an office area so that less walking is required by one but more filing is required by another, to accommodate an employee with special needs. It is this area of job accommodation that is accomplished with low, or no, cost. Training focuses on the person rather than on the equipment or the job itself. Training may provide new or expanded job skills so that new duties can be assumed. Employers generally have valued employees who have dedicated a number of years to the company and are familiar with the business and the operation procedures, and a new investment in training may simply enhance the performance of the person, as well as enhance the commitment of the person to the employer. Ongoing support is defined as various types of supports or assistance needed for an employee's specific limitations. These limitations may be in the form of visual impairment, in which the employer may allow a reader to be provided to the employee, or in providing a translation or sign language instructor for the hearing impaired. In some cases, co-employees may be taught to provide this ongoing support in methods such as teaching sign language for communication with co-workers and/or providing for safety exit from a building in the case of an emergency.

The concept of reasonable accommodation is frequently a difficult one for business and rehabilitation providers to perceive, but the intent is to avoid the undue hardship on an employer in order to provide accommodations. From a positive perspective, the main idea behind the concept of reasonable accommodations is to give a qualified person a job to do despite the presence of a limitation. If the environment is looked at from a supportive perspective instead of a limiting perspective, then most employers are better able to use the qualifications of the worker. The accommodation procedure must be individualized. This is very critical in the delivery of services in that even two people with the same medical diagnosis may have different amounts of types of limitations, and they may benefit from different types of accommodations. It is most critical for the individual employee to be the primary decision maker in what types of accommodations are necessary or as to the satisfactory conclusion of accommodations. The most promising part of accommodations is the new awareness that it is basically good business. "For a relatively minimal cost, or no cost, persons with a handicapping condition can be productive, valuable, and independent employees."[4] The use of reasonable accommodations and job accommodations in the work environment "permit[s] an organization to take full advantage of the unique talents, abilities, training, and interests of its workers."[4]

JOB ACCOMMODATIONS NETWORK

The President's Committee on Employment of the Handicapped (PCEH) is an organization that is made up of volunteers from the employment, business, and rehabilitation service sectors across the country. One particular group, the Employers Group of the PCEH, became acutely aware of the lack of information to employers throughout the country about job accommodations and the process of job accommodation. Thus, a pilot project was initiated in 1985 called the Job Accommodations Network. This service is supported by the National Institute of Disability Research and the Rehabilitation Services Administration. Collaborative efforts were also achieved with the West Virginia Research and Training Center at West Virginia University and with private industry. The primary mission of the Job Accommodations Network is to provide employers across the country resources and specific information about possible job accommodations to facilitate hiring and retraining of employees with disabilities. Professionals and consumers may call for information as well. The center of the network provides a data base that stores data about job accommodations that have been field tested and proven to work by other employers. The data base also provides information on job accommodations, including the names and addresses of people and organizations involved in the modification of work environments for the disabled. A human factors–rehabilitation engineering resource consultant is available during normal business hours, 5 days a week. A form called the Employer's Accommodation Input Questionnaire is filled out and includes such information as the name of the company, nature of the disability, job title and descriptions, and functional limitations. The Job Accommodations Network represents the most comprehensive resource for job accommodation currently available in the United States. Its work enhances the ability of employers to perform reasonable job accommodations for qualified handicapped people, and in doing so, should result in a substantial increase in job opportunities for the handicapped, nationally and internationally. There is no charge to employers or others for use of this network. The only request is a commitment to send in forms and information about successful accommodations that the business organization has made.

An additional resource for job accommodations is ABLEDATA, a computerized information bank for aids and devices for people with disabilities. This system contains more than 10,000 commercially available aids. Information is provided on products, as well as any consumer feedback on product evaluations. Custom searches are available for a fee through NARIC, the National Rehabilitation Information Center.

JOB SEEKING SKILLS

When the disabled person has completed his or her medical rehabilitation, has made a successful transition back into the community, and has completed vocational counseling and training preparation, he or she is ready to begin the job placement phase of vocational rehabilitation. The preceeding statement assumes that the person has chosen a realistic vocational objective that is compatible with his or her capabilities, is well prepared, and has selected a vocation that is available in the open job market. This process for the person with a disability is most frequently accomplished through the assistance of a state or private rehabilitation agency. Experience increasingly shows that often the job does not go to the most experienced or most skilled worker but to the persons who can locate employers; knows his or her skills, strengths, abilities, and limitations; can communicate in written form to employers; and interviews well.[11]

The disabled job seeker must ultimately accept responsibility for his or her own ability to obtain and maintain employment. The medical team and vocational rehabilitation team can provide extensive support and technical assistance toward this goal, but in the end, the prospective employee must be able to convince the employer that he or she has the ability to be productive and an asset to the company. Each job seeker must be comfortable in dealing with his or her disability in the work environment. The importance of the development of these skills cannot be overemphasized. Citing results from a study at the Minneapolis Rehabilitation Center, Wright indicated the extent to which people possess deficiencies in job seeking skills: "Eighty percent of the clients did not look for work frequently enough, 85 percent could not explain skills to their employers, 40 percent had poor personal appearance or inappropriate mannerisms, and 90 percent could not explain their handicapping conditions."[24]

This is not to say that direct job development by the counselor is not vital. Rather, it is helpful to view job placement activities on a continuum. As Twomey indicates the *Placement of the Severely Handicapped*,[29] at one end of the continuum the person places himself or herself with no counselor assistance other than development of job seeking skills. At the other end, the counselor assumes all placement responsibility. Most job seekers are able to assume some responsibility in locating employment but also need counselor assistance in varying degrees. Skills and personality traits of the job seeker, as well as the nature of the disability, dictate the extent of counselor involvement. In cases of severe disability in which it would be difficult for the person to initiate the employer contact and be interviewed (*i.e.,* cases of severe communication disability or spasticity), counselor involvement will be much greater. Some people, for example, those with high level quadriplegia, will need environmental accommodations to initiate participation in job seeking activity. Examples of this include use of an environmental control unit, an electric page turner, speaker phone, clerical back-up support, and/or use of attendant care. By taking ownership of the search, however, the disabled person learns lifelong job search skills that he or she may well need to use again in the future.

In order to be successful in the job search, employment readiness must be ascertained, the job search must be structured, and the disability dynamics involved in the process (*i.e.,* résumés, applications, and interviews) must be addressed. We will now examine each of these areas. Since it is most likely that the state vocational agency or private rehabilitation agency will be responsible for coordinating the vocational rehabilitation process, let us first address the role of the state agency.

ROLE OF THE STATE AGENCY

The role of the state vocational rehabilitation agency is to provide overall case management and coordination of service delivery toward the goal of assisting people with handicapping conditions to obtain, or maintain, employment. A major impetus for the expansion of these services is based on Title V of the Rehabilitation Act of 1973, as amended. Sections 503 and 504 impact directly on employment. Section 503 requires employers in the private sector to have an affirmative action plan if they do more than $2,500 of business annually with the federal government as a contractor or subcontractor. Section 504 is directed at nonprofit organizations such as hospitals, universities, and state and local governments who receive grants from the federal government.

In order to initiate the state agency's role, the applicant's eligibility for services must be determined. This is based on the functional limitations that stem from the handicapping condition and negatively impact on the applicant's ability to obtain or maintain employment. This handicapping condition can be either physical, cognitive, or emotional and results in significant interference with employment. However, the handicapping condition cannot be so severe that the applicant is not feasible for employment. When eligibility has been determined, services are then focused on the following areas: assessment and vocational goal determination, vocational preparation, placement, and follow-up.

Assessment and Vocational Goal Determination

Medical information is obtained and translated into functional limitations that impact employment. The job seeker's physical capacities are evaluated to determine current work tolerance and function and how these factors might be increased through work hardening services, work adjustment services, or accommodations at the worksite. Work experience is assessed for transferrable skills, and previous work adjustment, aptitudes, and interests are explored in relation to the local job market. Assessment of the person's psychological readiness, educational background, family and community supports, as well as the practical issues of transportation, child care, and economic disincentives and benefits is essential as well. At the conclusion of this assessment, a feasible vocational objective compatible or modifiable to the person's capabilities is determined.

Vocational Preparation

Once the vocational objective has been determined, the barriers to employment are identified and services are designed to overcome these barriers. If the objective is to return to work with a previous employer in a modified or alternate position, the services provided will be consultation with that employer regarding accommodations and facilitating the person's transition back to work. Regardless of the objective, other services in this phase may include coordination or provision of medical treatment, adaptive aids, counseling, job training, and/or work adjustment training.

Placement and Follow-up Services

The placement phase involves training the prospective employee in job seeking skills and how to market himself or herself to best advantage, providing direct job development services to facilitate placement, and when employment is achieved, providing follow up for a minimum of 60 days to ensure successful employment retention. After this 60-day period, the counselor can become reinvolved at any point by request of the employee or the employer.

Therefore, the vocational rehabilitation counselor takes a holistic approach toward rehabilitation case management, since almost any factor can seriously affect the person's employability (*e.g.,* medical stability, psychological issues, a problem with family or community support systems, or resources). The vocational rehabilitation program is funded by both state and federal sources. The average length of time a person is involved in the program is 2 years. In cases of severe traumatic or developmental disability, time in the program may well be 5 to 6 years. The counselor has an average caseload size of 100 and has an annual case service budget from which to authorize service delivery, which is dependent on the nature of the caseload and current appropriation levels. The role of the state agency is thus to provide a bridge from disability to employment reintegration into the community.

EMPLOYMENT READINESS

In order for the job placement and retention process to be successful, the job seeker's employment readiness must be verified. These factors may have changed or evolved since the initial evaluation phase of vocational rehabilitation. If problems are encountered in any of the following areas, it must be determined if further action can be taken to ameliorate them and enhance employment readiness. If these employment readiness factors are not addressed, they could sabotage much of the person's and the counselor's placement activity.

Medical Stability

Has the person's condition remained sufficiently stable so as not to interfere with work? Have there been any medication changes that would affect performance? Is the job seeker sufficiently educated regarding his or her condition to take the initiative and responsibility in appropriately managing the condition (*e.g.,* in the case of the spinal cord injury, is the person managing his or her pressure relief adequately throughout the day)?[7]

Endurance and Scheduling

Does the person have sufficient physical tolerance to work full or part time? What has his or her general activity level been? If attendant care is needed for dressing and other daily living activities, is it reliable and can it be scheduled to enable the person to get to work on time? What are the person's energy patterns? If he or she is independent in dressing, for example, is this so exhausting and time consuming that it will affect the ability to work? Is the job seeker willing to make trade-offs necessary to work? Have provisions been made for assistance in home management activities needed to save energy for work?

Support Systems

Does the person have family support in returning to employment? Are family members willing to make the necessary adjustments required? Are there conflicts that would interfere with the job seeker's employment?

Pyschological Readiness

Is the person motivated to work? Can he or she adjust to the pressures of working? Does he or she have adequately developed social skills so that interaction with co-workers will be comfortable? In cases of visible disability, is the job seeker sufficiently comfortable in discussing his or her disability as appropriate and asking for help as needed or declining unwanted help? The person must be able to initiate this discussion.[15] Will he or she be able to "stick with employment" through the difficult initial transition stage?"

The prospective employee should be reasonably well adjusted prior to seeking employment, both in terms of the disability and the general work adjustment issues (*e.g.,* ability to take supervision, attendance). As Creney[15] states in his article "Considerations of Employment for Spinal Cord Injured":

It has been said that return to work is a result of good adjustment rather than a factor of achieving it. It may not be appropriate for a maladjusted person to take a job in the hopes that it will help him or her adjust. This person should be well adjusted prior to employment. It is crucial not to push a person into taking a job. It is important that the individual feel he got himself employed, after receiving the necessary therapy, guidance and counseling.

Transportation

Does the job seeker have reliable transportation? In what geographic area is it reasonable to seek work? If wheelchair accessible transportation is needed, this must be planned for in advance. If a modified van is necessary, the costs are high since the modifications alone may cost $10,000 or more, depending on the person's needs. Accessible public transportation may be available, but since it services many needs in the community, careful planning may be needed to make sure it is available when needed. The importance of transportation is self-evident. In a study of spinal cord–injured veterans, it was found that of those unable to drive, 16% obtained employment; of those able to drive, 58% became employed.[9]

Economic Disincentives

The issue of economic disincentives must be clearly dealt with since it can have many ramifications. The costs of basic survival, particularly for the severely disabled, are high.[8] There is the cost of attendant care, medications, medical follow-up, adaptive equipment, and transportation in addition to the average housing, food, and family needs to be considered. Higher salaries are required to meet these needs. Is the person sufficiently skilled to compete for these jobs? Frequently, the person is in the forced position of changing careers and of earning entry level wages until further experience is gained. If the applicant becomes employed, he or she loses government benefits such as attendant care assistance. There have been some attempts at providing support toward employment per Social Security Disability regulation as well as Supplemental Security Income program changes.[27] The Social Security Disability Income (SSDI) program provides for a nine-month trial work period, whereby earnings do not affect benefits, for deduction of some work-related expenses, and for temporary extension of Medicare benefits. The Supplemental Security Income (SSI) program allows for simplification of program administration and allows for recipients to help their disability elegibility while they work. Dependent on income with this program, Medicaid benefits may continue; also, clients may be reinstated to the SSI program without a new application if their income drops.[27] Financial disincentives for employment are clearly a major barrier to employment productivity of the severely disabled.[28] On occasion, the person and family may well be better off, financially, to remain on supported benefits. If so, the family must make the clear decisions on the trade-offs involved in working and the value employment has within their family system. The applicant must also know what salary he or she requires and how much negotiation he or she is willing to do on this issue.

Dress

Does the applicant have appropriate dress for interviewing and for employment? If necessary, is it adapted (*i.e.,* Velcro closures) to enhance maximum independence in toileting at work? If assistance is needed, how will this be arranged for? Is all of the person's adaptive equipment in working order?

Realistic Expectations

Does the person have realistic expectations regarding the labor market and marketability of his or her skills?

THE EMPLOYMENT SEARCH

Once it has been determined that a person is indeed ready to return to work, he or she must develop the employment skills that will be required for success in the job search. Specific instruction on development of employment search skills increases the job seeker's ability to compete much more successfully for employment. Instruction relating to the application of reading, writing, and communication skills to common tasks required in the job search is highly beneficial. These tasks include identifying and following up on job leads, résumé writing, application completion, interviewing skills, and job-related social skills.[18] The Job Club or Jobs Skills Training program has been found to be a particularly successful strategy to foster the development of these skills.[24] This is a structured approach that is performance based and that teaches these skills to a group of the job-ready disabled. Participation is expected on a daily basis and focuses on behavior and provides specific instruction on identifying and using transferable skills, finding job leads, organizing the job search, meeting employer expectations, completing job applications, developing a résumé, and interviewing successfully.[13] This learning is facilitated by modeling of appropriate behaviors, role play, and reinforcement. The person uses this forum to develop job leads via telephone, prepare for the interview, and follow up on the interview. Ongoing coaching, supervision, and peer support is provided. Since many employer contacts may be required before one secured employment, this support is necessary to increase the job seeker's confidence and to help reduce the stress involved in the job search (*e.g.,* coping

with rejections). It extends the person's information network since all clients are aware of types of employment sought by their peers and thus may be able to provide additional leads. In addition, the information network should include other disabled people who are currently working since they can also be a productive source of job leads and information.[10] The Job Club approach enables a person to engage in intensive job search activity on a daily basis. This type of close supervision could not be provided by a single counselor, owing to caseload size and demands, and it supplements the job development activity done by the counselor.

Since the program simulates work activity in many ways, it also provides an excellent training ground for related problems to surface and be resolved before they interfere with actual employment. It requires interaction with supervision and co-workers. It provides opportunity to perfect skills in scouting out accessibility in the community, making arrangements, asking for help, and using adaptive aids. According to Azorin,[2] a leader in this field, the Job Club approach was more than 90% successful in obtaining employment for all of the specific populations with severe job finding problems, that is, 92% successful for those with physical problems, 94% for those with mental problems, and 90% successful for Department of Vocational Rehabilitation clients.

INFORMATION INTERVIEWING

The specific purpose of information interviewing is to obtain facts about actual job requirements. It serves as an opportunity for a job seeker to obtain information about the informal job demands as opposed to the formal job demands commonly listed in the occupational literature. Since job descriptions vary from place to place, information interviewing allows a job seeker to obtain a balanced view of selected jobs for comparison purposes. A counselor will generally encourage a person to talk to several people doing the same job.

Best used as a tool early in the job search, information interviewing requires good organizational skills and time management skills. A step up from role playing job interviewing, information interviewing is an opportunity for a person to practice communication skills with employers and to develop interviewing experience in a nonthreatening environment. To select an employer to interview, the person must develop contacts in the real work world. A job seeker has to research job listings through such organizations as college placement officers, chambers of commerce, public libraries, and literature such as trade journals and manufacturing guides.

EMPLOYMENT SKILLS

Job Applications

Job applicants need to have experience in completing a variety of applications. As stressed in the literature available through state employment services, they need to complete the application neatly and accurately, following instructions. No blanks are to be left. Names, addresses, and dates can be verified ahead of time, be written on a small file card, and be brought along to be copied onto the form. The application can also be taken home and completed, if necessary. Employment or professional references should be used, rather than personal ones, and permissions should be obtained prior to their use. The specific job title or job category should be used as the job applied for. Description of work experience should be skill specific. For example, rather than stating "office work," the prospective employee should cite skills such as typing 50 wpm, filing, and using a word processor. Similarly, machines used and tasks completed should be listed. The opportunity should be taken to stress positive work habits and emphasize skills or accomplishments in the "extra information" sections.

The disabled job seeker may or may not choose to disclose the nature of the disability on the application. Legally, the only question that can be asked is, "Do you have any condition (or disability) that would interfere with your ability to perform (the tasks of) this job?" If the disability does impact on performance of the employment, or is obvious, the description of the disability should be as brief as possible and medical terminology should be avoided.[14] This is also true in relation to the résumé and the interview. For example, rather than stating a diagnosis of multiple sclerosis, it would be better to state, "I walk slower or have difficulty in picking up small objects," or, "I use a wheelchair to get around," and then the interview should reaffirm the person's ability to do the job. Another option would be to indicate that the job seeker would like to discuss this question in the interview. All communications or interactions with the employer need to remain focused on skills and abilities not on disability issues.[20] To state the obvious, the job seeker should also be applying for jobs that would be within his or her performance capability. Applications asking illegal questions still abound. Although legally correct, a blanket refusal to answer the question is rarely productive. If left blank, the employer can assume the question was carelessly missed or that the "applicant is hiding something." The questions need to be addressed in some way.

The Résumé

Since the résumé is typically the first contact with employers, it needs to be well organized, concise, and easy to read. The résumé is frequently not read thoroughly but is skimmed to determine who will be interviewed. The best résumés are written by those who know what type of job they are seeking, since they are geared to specify the type of job sought. In many cases, if there are several jobs under consideration, several résumés may be required. If at all possible, the résumé should be kept to one page in length.

In brief, there are basically two types of résumés: the chronological résumé, and the functional résumé.[19] The chronological résumé is organized according to the dates of employment, beginning with the most recent employer. It emphasizes a steady employment record but also gaps in employment. If a career change is involved, it highlights experience only in similar positions. It is traditional and thus many employers prefer it. The

functional résumé is organized to emphasize the qualifications or skills or experience of the applicant without the inclusion of dates. It stresses selected skills such as "writing," "administration," and "sales promotion" and lists related accomplishments. A combination may also be effective, if kept concise. The standard subdivisions in the résumé are listed below:

Objective: This specifies the type of job sought and helps the employer to identify where this is available in the organization.

Experience: This describes work experience, either functionally or chronologically with the employer's needs in mind. Again, this should be skill specific. Recent volunteer or extracurricular experience can also be included for recent graduates or for applicants reentering the job market.

Education: All relevant schools and degrees should be listed.

Grade point average can be included, if impressive. Major subjects areas should also be listed.

Honors: Any of the applicant's awards or recent special recognitions should be listed.

Personal Information: It is no longer advised to include personal information such as age or marital status. However, it can be particularly useful for the disabled job seeker to indicate participation in civic activities or hobbies (*e.g.,* wheelchair or other sports that may counteract general stereotypes or indicate ability or acceptance of responsibility).

References: It can be indicated that references are available on request. This list should be available during the interview.

Again, there is no legal requirement for the disability to be disclosed on the résumé. However, it can be mentioned in this section to avoid "surprise" during the interview. It can be stated indirectly in a positive way. For example, in reference again to wheelchair sports or statements such as, "I am a peer counselor for persons with epilepsy," "I have participated in the Special Olympics in 1983 and 1984," or "I qualify for the Affirmative Action Program under Section 503 of the Rehabilitation Act of 1973."[14]

JOB INTERVIEWING

All of the skills discussed so far lead up to the climax of the job seeking process—the interview.

Preparation begins with researching the business as much as possible so that one's skills can be related to the employer's needs and that appropriate questions can be asked during the interview. The applicant is taught where this information can be found. Sources include directories and reports available through public libraries, chambers of commerce, college placement offices, local business organizations, and newspapers. It is also permissible to request this information directly from the company through the secretary or receptionist. Preferably, the person then needs to become familiar with the address, parking, and accessibility of the business. This should be done ahead of time so as not to increase the stress of the interview situation.

The applicant should dress appropriately for the interview. The type of attire required is specific to the type of job the person is applying for and the nature of the business. If it is a professional, sales, or clerical position, a neutral colored suit would be appropriate for either a man or a woman. For a sales or clerical position, a woman might also wear a skirt and blouse, or a dress with a jacket. Dress should be business-like and conservative. Women should avoid frilly, low cut, or short outfits, as well as excessive jewelry or perfume. Men should avoid loud ties or shirts. The employer will be seeking someone to fit the "corporate image." If it is an assembly, janitorial, servicing, or other blue collar job, good slacks and a matching sports shirt or similarly a casual skirt and blouse is appropriate attire. It is most important for the person to be well groomed and the clothing to be clean and well pressed. Once hired, the employee can observe the dress code of the company and dress accordingly. During the interview, however, it is best to err toward the conservative.

The applicant should arrive at the interview early to allow unexpected parking and other problems. The "interview" begins in the waiting area, since frequently secretarial input may also be obtained. The first 5 to 10 minutes of the interview are the most critical since employers often formulate hiring decisions on their first impressions. The person's enthusiasm for work must be apparent through voice tone and nonverbal cues—good eye contact, posture, and an attentive stance. The person's preparation needs to be evident in his or her concise, skill-oriented statements, use of examples, explanation of disability, and relevant questions. There are many interview styles: some are very structured, others are open ended. It is important to avoid yes/no answers and to be able to elaborate on personal skills. The job seeker needs to be able to take control of the open-ended interview. For example, the employer may request the applicant to tell the employer about himself or herself. The prospective employee should keep the discussion focused on his or her skills, education, and experience. When the interview is closing, the applicant needs to be aware of techniques to be able to request permission to personally check back with the interviewer for the interview results. This "call back closing" holds the interviewer more accountable since he or she will need to speak directly with the applicant. A thank you letter should then be sent for the interview. Role-playing strategies are effective in developing these job interviewing skills.

This technique is especially effective in becoming comfortable in handling disability concerns in the interview. According to survey results provided by Ruffner in 1981,[25] employers are more interested in a person's abilities to sell himself or herself and to meet the demands of the job, than in their disabilities. At the same time, applicants do need to be able to manage the effects of stigma, that is, not overreacting and not "bustling at condescending attitudes."[26]

The disabled person needs to be able to take the initiative in discussing the disability, especially if it is visible. In taking this initiative, the applicant can control the discussion, clear up misconception, and allay any employer apprehensions. This can be an effective strategy. It cannot be assumed that the interviewer knows anything about the disability. A functional definition of the disability adds to the job seeker's professionalism. Again, medical terminology should be avoided. For example, a person with a congenital handicap might say, "I've had this problem all my life and I've learned to do most things that other people can do. I can (give examples of tasks that are quite difficult), but, of course, I cannot move refrigerators." If possible, skills can be demonstrated. For example, prosthetic hook dexterity could be demonstrated by picking up an object from the table. For each physical problem, the client should be aware of the employer's possible reaction and make a reassuring statement. For example, if the applicant uses a wheelchair or crutches, the employer might assume that the person might often be late for work or absent. Statements such as these could be made: "Most people think that my condition would prevent me from getting to work every day. I know that an employer has to be able to depend on his employees coming in on time every day and I have dependable transportation and drive myself. I am a reliable worker." Educating the interviewer on the employment-related consequences of the disability is another aspect of marketing himself or herself.[20]

Another strategy in handling a stereotyped question is to focus on the assumed intent of the question. For example, an unusually blunt question might be "Are you crippled?" The question could be construed as "Will your mobility impairment permit you to do this job?" and answered accordingly.

In summary then, disabled job seekers must be prepared to experience a wide range of interview styles and questions. They must be prepared for any question and not lose their composure. They must be practiced in their responses and must be prepared to initiate discussion of the disability as appropriate. The interview should be followed by a thank-you letter expressing appreciation for the interview and reemphasizing skills and interest.

A remaining issue is asking for job accommodations. It is usually best to wait until a job offer is made, or at least until the second interview, to make this request, particularly if the accommodation is costly.[14] It can be addressed earlier if the interviewer appears to be concerned with it. The accommodation should be presented as good business, not charity or a legal dictate. Prospective employees should definitely know what they will need to function productively on the job, use their own adaptive equipment if at all possible, be aware of resources that can help, and attempt to keep the accommodations as simple and cost effective as possible. This area is not well defined legally, and frequently success in this area depends on each applicant's negotiating skills. In many states there are also incentive programs for employers to "hire the handicapped." Applicants must be effective in presenting these programs. These skills can again be developed through the Job Club approach.

STRESS MANAGEMENT

Seeking employment in today's competitive job market is very stressful, whether one is disabled or not. The disability factor escalates the stress even more as job seekers must deal directly with societal disability stereotypes and education of the employer community and instances of discrimination. If an applicant is in the job market for the first time after trauma, it is a direct confrontation with the reality of the disability and thus the person can feel very vulnerable to rejection. For many, self-concept is closely associated with work and rejection is threatening. It is essential for the disabled person to have an outlet for this stress. This can be provided by a personal or vocational counselor and supported by the physician and other medical rehabilitation personnel. The Job Club approach can also be effective, since job seekers can obtain peer support and see that they are not alone with their frustrations. Therapy is indicated if the stress results in alcohol or drug abuse, other self-destructive behavior, or severe family conflict. Family counseling may also be indicated; the person's spouse or parent may think that the job seeker is not "trying hard enough" or the issue may serve as a "test" or a scapegoat for other family conflicts.

The disabled person can also be encouraged to manage stress through a number of other self-help techniques, including deep breathing, visualization, or progressive relaxation exercises. Instruction can be provided individually or in groups by qualified professionals.

JOB PLACEMENT

Development of job seeking skills is the foundation of successful job placement but is only one aspect of it. In addition to working with job seekers so that they are ready, willing, and able, the vocational rehabilitation professional must also work with prospective employers on these same issues. This process involves a multidimensional approach and includes all of these areas: (1) marketing the concept of employment, (2) marketing the specific client, and (3) follow-up.

Marketing the Concept

Marketing has been a central concept in the business community for years. Marketing of social programs and services is relatively new. This approach requires that vocational rehabilitation redefine its image and scope of services. As Carthell and Boone[7] indicated, "No matter how fine a product vocational rehabilitation can deliver, if the market is not ready, if it shys away from our product, it won't buy it. The rehabilitation philosophy should expand itself to deal with the employer community as a client." Comprehensive services are needed to meet client needs. Thus, the marketing program involves identifying need and developing and implementing operational activities that promote the product (*i.e.,* the entire spectrum of rehabilitation services). Individual client placement falls into the definition of selling, once the groundwork has been laid for its reception by the customer (employer). Marketing involves laying that groundwork and trying to have what the customer wants. It is getting to know and interact with businesses on their own turf. It involves top levels of management in vocational rehabilitation agencies making contact with and communicating with top levels of management in business and organized labor. This results in increased visibility in the business community. Active participation in business and community organizations is essential to this strategy.

The goal of these interactions is to establish increased credibility as a service provider as well as to erase negative employer perceptions of both vocational rehabilitation agencies and their clients.[3] The focus is not just on job placement of individual clients but on a whole package of services tailored to the individual employer's needs. These services could include (1) recruitment services—referral of qualified applicants based on knowledge of the employer's current and future personnel needs and internal processes; (2) consultant services in the same areas of affirmative action assistance, job modification and accommodation, and accessibility awareness training programs; (3) troubled employee assistance programming in which the rehabilitation agency works directly with an injured or disabled worker referred by the employer in order to maintain employment with that employer; and (4) support and follow-up services for agency clients placed with that employer. The "employer account system" is an example of this marketing approach. This system involves a mutually beneficial ongoing relationship of the rehabilitation agency with a major employer (more than 100 employees). Thus, the rehabilitation professional's role is not just "selling" that employer an employee, but he or she is "on call" to provide additional consultant services per employer request. This approach systematically builds links with the business community, which also results in a more reliable barometer of business trends and personnel needs. This, in turn, is of great assistance in performing job market analysis and subsequent employment planning with clients, to ensure that services are based on the actual job market in the community.

Another goal of marketing the concept is to help dispel employer misconceptions both of rehabilitation agencies and of disabled workers. Again, as indicated by Carthell and Boone,[7] most businesses are emersed in a myriad of government regulations and requirements. They are defensive about having to assume the burden of proof when personal practices are questioned. Even though rehabilitation agencies provide many legitimate services that result in direct benefit to employers, they are frequently viewed as "just another bureaucratic agency" ready to impose guilt, unreasonable demands, and bureaucratic processes on them. In addition to these misconceptions, many employers object to hiring the handicapped worker on what they believe are reasonable grounds and reflect concerns around increased cost or risk in the areas of insurance rates, physical modifications, safety, job performance, and job stability.

If this groundwork is laid appropriately, the business climate will be greatly improved toward employment consideration of handicapped applicants whether they apply directly or are represented by a professional. In addition, if allies are cultivated in the business community, they can be very effective in advocating for the concept with their colleagues.

Marketing the Client

The rehabilitation professional who undertakes direct job development on behalf of a client must be well versed in the needs of the local community's job market so that he or she will know what jobs are available. The professional must also thoroughly know the assets, liabilities, and needs of the client and have helped the person to achieve job ready status as previously discussed. As Knorr states, "The goal of the intervention is to assure the client a fair interview."[15]

Precontact research on the employer's needs is essential. If the contact is based on actual need, the employer will be much more receptive. The employer is advised of logical reasons for hiring the handicapped, and financial incentives are explained. These incentives include tax credits, on-the-job training opportunities, limitations of liability in workers' compensation situations, and deviated wage opportunities as applicable. The employer's personnel needs are discussed, a plant tour arranged, and job descriptions obtained so that the counselor can proceed with clear understanding of the actual work environment requirements. This step can increase credibility with the employer. If a potentially feasible job can be identified, the client's résumé can be reviewed. The same employer approach taught to clients, holds true for the professional as well. Elaborate medical terminology needs to be avoided; evaluation results need to be relayed in the employer's terminology and focused on behavioral descriptions of how work performance requirements can be met.[29] If the employer is receptive, a job analysis of the potential job requirements can be done as necessary. If the job is determined feasible, the counselor may accompany the applicant on the interview if necessary. If the applicant is hired, job accommodations may need to be negotiated and adequate follow-up services provided.

This process is modified somewhat when the situation calls for assisting a person to return to work after injury or disability. In this case, the client already has established a "track record" with that employer. The initial role here is to determine whether that employment record is positive or negative and how receptive that employer is toward working with the rehabilitation professional to return the client to employment. The employer's concerns regarding the specific disability can be addressed. Job analysis can be done of the person's former position, as well as potential alternates and recommendations for modifications made, if feasible. Awareness training may also need to be addressed with co-workers. If organized labor is involved, seniority and contractual requirements need to be addressed. If placement is successful, strong follow-up services are again essential.

Follow-up Services

The provision of follow-up services after placement is critical to both the employee and the employer. The goal of these services is to maintain the client successfully on the job. Follow-up services may continue an extended time period with severely disabled clients. Based on the counselor's knowledge of, and rapport with, the client, intervention may be needed to help solve problems the employee may be having that affect work performance or work relationships. There may be a need to help solve personal problems off the job that may affect attendance or performance. Other needs on the job may be addressed with counseling or modifications at the work site. It is also essential that an employee who is not able to function successfully be terminated. Providing assistance during the "exit" interview to the employer can also help to maintain the employer relationship. Additional services can then be initiated for the client to achieve a more successful placement.[7]

As illustrated by the preceding discussion, job placement is a multidimensional process requiring knowledge of a disabled person's capabilities and limitations, community resources, and the physical, cognitive, social, and environmental demands of the job. It also requires visibility and credibility with the local business and industrial community.

REFERENCES

1. American Occupational Therapy Association and Vocational Evaluation and Work Adjustment Association: Guidelines for Work Hardening Programs. Washington, DC, 1986
2. Azorin NH, Besalel VA: Job Club Counselors Manual, Baltimore, University Park Press, 1980
3. Bartels E: Marketing Vocational Rehabilitation. J Rehabil 51:62–64, 1985
4. Berkeley Planning Associates: A Study of Accommodation Provided to Handicapped Employees by Federal Contractors, Final Report, vols I and II. Berkeley, CA, 1982
5. Botterbusch KF: A Comparison of Commercial Vocational Evaluation Systems. Menomonie, WI, Materials Development Center, 1983
6. Bowe F: Reasonable Accommodation Handbook. Washington, DC, National Center for Barrier Free Environment, 1983
7. Carthell D, Boone L: Marketing An Approach to Placement: Report of Study Group of the Ninth Institute on Rehabilitation Issues, University of Wisconsin, 1982
8. Crewe NM, Athelstan GT, Bower AS: Employment After Spinal Cord Injury: A Handbook For Counselors. University of Minnesota Medical Rehabilitation Research and Training Center, Rehabilitation Services Administration Grant #16P-56810 (5-17), 1978
9. El Ghatit A, Hanson R: Variables associated with obtaining and sustaining employment among spinal cord injured males, follow-up study of 760 veterans. J Chronic Dis 31:363–369, 1978
10. Finch E: Job hunting. Disabled USA 4:9–10, 1981
11. Goodman J, Hoppin J, Kent R: Opening Doors: A Practical Guide for Job Hunting. Michigan State Board of Education Vocational Technical Education Service Grant #8002, Oakland University, 1984
12. Halpern AS, Fuhrer MJ: Functional Assessment in Rehabilitation. Baltimore, Paul H Brooks, 1984
13. Kauss P, Soto AM: Job club and transferable skills: Models for placement of severely handicapped. Am Rehabil 6:7–11, 1981
14. Lobodinski J, McFadden D, Markowicz A: Marketing Your Abilities: A Guide for the Disabled Job Seekers. Washington, D.C., Mainstream, 1984
15. Lott J, Owens J, Wilson W (eds): A Holistic Approach for Employment for Persons with Spinal Cord Injury. Virginia Department of Rehabilitation Services, Woodrow Wilson Rehabilitation Center, 1982
16. Malzahn D: Functional Evaluation for Task Modification Using the Available Motions Inventory. In Halpern AS, Fuhrer MJ: Functional Assessment in Rehabilitation. Baltimore, Paul H Brooks, 1984
17. Matheson L: Work Capacity Evaluation: Interdisciplinary Approach to Industrial Rehabilitation. Anaheim, CA, Employment and Rehabilitation Institute of California, 1984
18. Mathews RM, Faucett SB: Assisting in the job search: A behavioral assessment in training strategy. J Rehabil 51:31–35, 1985
19. Michigan Employment Security: Guide to Preparing a Resume, publication #2806, 1980
20. Michigan Department of Education and Michigan Rehabilitation Services: Job Seeking Skills Facilitators Manual. Unpublished Counselors Training Manual, 1976
21. Mueller J: Work Place Accommodations, Access Information Bulletin. Washington, DC, National Center for Barrier Free Environment, 1981
22. Priest JW, Roessler RT: Job analysis and workplace design resources for rehabilitation. Rehabil Lit 44:7–8, 1983
23. Pruitt WA: Vocational (Work) Evaluation. Menomonie, WI, Walt Pruitt Associates, 1977
24. Roessler RT: Self-starting in the job market: The continuing need for job seeking skills training in rehabilitation. J Appl Rehabil Counseling 16:22–25, 1985
25. Ruffner R: Just where's the barrier? Disabled USA 4:3–6, 9–10, 1981
26. Schneider C, Anderson W: Attitudes toward the stigmatized: Some insights from recent research. Rehabil Counseling Bull 23:299–314, 1980
27. Social Security Administration, a Summary Guide to Social Security Income Work Incentives for the Disabled and Blind. Publication 64–030, July 1987
28. Trieschmann R: Variables associated with productivity following spinal cord injuries. In Spinal Cord Injuries: Psychological, Social, and Vocational Adjustment. New York, Pergamon Press, 1980
29. Twomey W: Placement of the Severely Handicapped. RSA Research and Training Center Grant #45-P-810633-01. Washington, DC, 1975
30. Vocational Evaluation and Work Adjustment Association, Vocational Evaluation Project Final Report (special edition of VEWAA Bulletin, vol 8). Menomonie, WI, Materials Development Center, 1975
31. World Health Organization: International Classification of Impairments, Disabilities, and Handicaps. Geneva, 1980

5

Self-Care: Evaluation and Management

Charles H. Christiansen

Richard K. Schwartz

Karin J. Barnes

OVERVIEW

Self-care tasks are those daily and routine activities necessary for living. Included are those personal care activities appropriate to the age, gender, and environment of each person, such as dressing, eating, bathing, grooming, use of the toilet, and mobility within the home. Other important activities of daily living (ADL) are those that Lawton described as instrumental activities.[61] These include food preparation, laundry, housekeeping, shopping, the ability to use the telephone, use of transportation, medication use, and financial management. Child care is also a responsibility in the daily routine of many people. Additionally, participation in leisure and recreational activities can be viewed as instrumental ADL important for the psychosocial and physical well being of a person.

Determining a person's ability to perform self-care tasks is one component in the assessment of overall functional status. The term *function* has been defined in many ways within the medical and health literature, however, it is used here to represent the normal or characteristic performance of a person as a participant in the social system. This differs from more limited definitions of function, which refer to the state of organs or body parts, and hence is consistent with both the sociological view of health as advanced by Parsons[81] as well as contemporary (behavioral-ecological) viewpoints of the rehabilitation process.

Functional status has been described as encompassing four distinct performance dimensions of the patient: physical, mental, emotional, and social. Although it may be tempting to view self-care tasks as requiring only sensorimotor abilities, the ability to perform basic ADL relates to psychological and social dimensions of function as well.

Impairment, Disability, and Handicap: A Distinction Among Misused Terms

In this chapter, the terms *disability* and *dysfunction* refer to any deviation from the normal or characteristic ability of a person to perform tasks of living. This is distinguished from aberrations in organs or body systems, which are defined as *impairments*. In keeping with the terminology and conceptual scheme advanced by the World Health Organization, impairments can lead to dysfunction, which in turn may create conditions perceived as handicapping to a person in the performance of social roles. In this context, the distinctions among impairment, disability, and handicap form a hierarchy with several levels of person–environment interaction. For example, limitation in wrist range of motion (ROM) is an impairment that *may* affect a person's ability to hold a glass. Inasmuch as drinking can be accomplished without holding a glass (*e.g.,* through a straw) the stated impairment may not result in disability. If performance of the task is difficult or not possible, a *disability* is present. If the inability to perform tasks results in social disadvantage, the condition is viewed as a *handicap*. It is important to appreciate that the distinctions among impairment, disability, and handicap are related to the extent to which the effect of physical dysfunction is apparent within broader dimensions of the person's environment. This underscores the importance of viewing functional performance in an environmental context (Fig. 5-1).

Function as an Interaction of Person and Environment

Function, whether one is measuring at the level of impairment, disability, or handicap, involves a relevant environmental condition. Thus, an impairment in muscle function can be assessed using electromyography (EMG). Even at this organic level, function requires an interaction of the body and a relevant environmental condition (the EMG machine). Similarly, disability is concerned with performance of the whole body in relation to the physical environment and is measured through performance of tasks such as dressing or maneuvering a wheelchair. Note that the objects required for performance are part of the environment and interact with the person as part of task completion. As suggested earlier, at the highest level of behavior and environmental interaction, one is concerned with handicap. The extent of handicap is related to the person's environmental interaction in a sociocultural context and can be influenced by conditions in the immediate home or work environment or by more remote factors such as political or economic conditions.

Given that function cannot be properly assessed outside a relevant environmental context, it should not be surprising that research has shown that functional performance following reha-

	Impairment ↓	Disability ↓	Handicap ↓
Level	Organic dysfunction	Difficulty with tasks	Social disadvantage
Impact	Skill deficit	Task performance deficit	Role deficit

Figure 5-1. World Health Organization terminology.

bilitation is highly dependent on various environmental factors. These can include the type of living setting and family resources of the rehabilitant, as well as such factors as age, gender, or marital status.

This chapter is devoted to a review of principles and methods for assessing and managing the self-care needs of patients with disabilities. While attention will be devoted to evaluation and management strategies pertaining to specific types of impairment, an overall emphasis will be placed on the importance of involving the patient in the decision-making process regarding the management of self-care activities. The social, cultural, and physical factors in the environment that influence rehabilitation success will be discussed as related to the planning of self-care treatment.

IMPORTANCE OF ACTIVITIES OF DAILY LIVING

Importance to the Person

The degree to which one is successful in performing self-care tasks is, in part, an indication of the person's success in adapting to the social environment. Self-esteem, or the value accorded oneself, is determined by how well self-evaluation matches the values perceived as being important in the social environment.[86] Self-esteem is based on a person's history of successes and failures during interaction with family, significant others, and society at large. Perceived success in social relationships is influenced, among other things, by the level of dependency on other people. Since the ability to perform self-care tasks contributes to one's level of independence, it can have a direct affect on one's self-esteem.

The importance of independence in self-care is made obvious at a very young age. As a child becomes independent in self-care tasks, such as using eating utensils, it is an indication that the child can participate in wider social arenas with the accompanying personal and social privileges of those situations. For children, the accomplishment of self-care tasks has considerable value in their daily routine. However, as self-care skills are learned, their perceived importance is decreased and other social, educational, and vocational activities replace them in importance. Independence in daily living skills allows for freedom to perform the work and leisure tasks that become meaningful to the person. Nevertheless, the ability to successfully perform these skills is a requirement for perceived success in most social environments.

Usually, self-care activities are taken for granted by the person and society unless successful performance is constrained. Difficulty in performing self-care tasks and dependency on others for their completion can have a devastating effect on a person's psychological, social, and financial well-being. Depression, diminished self-confidence, and lack of motivation can result from the inability of the rehabilitation patient to perform these tasks while successful performance can lead to increased self-concept.[1,67,93] A study of elderly patients found that a relationship existed between self-concept and functional independence and that people who were dependent in ADL scored lower in self-concept.[1]

A study of the self-concept of 71 patients who had spinal cord injuries showed that the subjects who believed they were as physically independent as possible had a more positive self-concept than did subjects who felt less independent than their capability.[38] Another study of 100 spinal cord–injured patients found that the perception of control over one's life decisions was strongly associated with feelings of well-being.[19] These two studies indicate that an important goal of rehabilitation should be to help patients learn to take control over decisions related to daily living, since this may contribute positively to their sense of well-being.

Importance to the Family

The family is a social system in which the members have numerous roles that are performed within established expectations and reciprocities.[93] When a member of the family is no longer able to perform expected activities, the balance in role delineation may be upset and the family's daily routine at home and outside the home may be altered. Switzer[98] suggests that damage to the family processes may weaken the family's total capacity to function, thus jeopardizing positive feelings between family members.

A disabled family member has the potential to upset usual family patterns. Some former roles may be retained, but frequently the physical and social limitations of the disabled member require changes in role performance of all family members.[93] The family must adjust their expectations of the member who is disabled as well as adjusting to changes in the total family dynamics and the physical and social environment.[23]

The care of the family member with a disability may cause changes in the family routine and create stress for the family member who provides it. Jones and Vetter[49] found that the curtailment of the caretaker's social life as a result of the time needed to provide self-care assistance was more stressful than the actual tasks they performed. Their study showed that levels of depression and anxiety among caretakers were higher than that typically found among members of the general population.

Home management is important for the maintenance, emotional stability, and economic productivity of the family unit.[103] Homemaking tasks include meal preparation, cleaning, shopping, organization of objects and time, and, in some households, child care. When these tasks and activities are performed easily and regularly, the family is able to perform other social and economic activities with little or no concern for these tasks. When a family member is unable to perform these tasks due to disability, the emotional, social, and financial structure of the family may change. Duties that were considered important may no longer be accomplished or may be accomplished less capably than before. Thus, other family members must assume the tasks of the person who used to perform them and some tasks may be deferred. For example, floors may no longer be cleaned on a daily basis but cleaned only when another family member is able to do it around other obligations. Additionally, people outside the family may have to assume homemaking roles, which may result in a financial and or social burden.

It should be clear that the family has a considerable influence on the treatment outcome of the disabled patient.[9, 120] A stable and supportive family unit can be of great assistance, while those families that are functioning poorly can impede the patient's rehabilitation.[9, 85] In some cases, failure of rehabilitation can be traced to a lack of family involvement in the rehabilitation process.[86] This suggests that the family should be involved in all aspects of rehabilitation, including evaluation and the setting of rehabilitation goals and treatment strategies.

Importance to Society

A primary source of adjustment difficulties for people having physical disabilities comes from societal treatment of them as socially inferior.[111] The common belief that strength, independence, and appearance are important aspects of self-worth is very damaging to people with disabilities. Interaction within a social group is dependent on the ability to perform at the group's expected level; otherwise, the person will not be included as a significant group member.[94]

Kielhofner[57] contends that society expects adults to be independent in self-care, yet devalues self-care tasks because their accomplishment does not directly contribute a meaningful commodity to the societal group. Self-care tasks are not publicly valued in the same manner as gainful employment. Ironically, they assume importance principally when one's inability to perform them leads to a label of "handicapped." Bartels[8] suggests that when a person is independent in living skills society's view of what it means to be disabled is drastically changed. Independence in ADL helps to refute the idea that a person with a disability may be a financial or social burden to society. Bartels notes that a concept basic to the independent living philosophy is that a disability becomes a barrier to achievement only when it is perceived to be one by others or the environment makes it so.

THE DOMAIN OF SELF-CARE AND INDEPENDENT LIVING

Traditional View of the Treatment of Self-Care Deficits

The traditional treatment approach with people who have difficulty performing self-care tasks has focused on the patient within the hospital or rehabilitation center environment. Typically, self-care intervention has started with instruction in procedures to regain dressing, grooming, hygiene, and eating skills.[27] More recently, the use of adaptive devices and the training of homemaking skills have been recognized as important goals.[118] In pursuit of these goals, treatment sessions have been conducted within the patient's hospital room or in occupational therapy simulation clinics.[119] The treatment approach has involved directly teaching the patient functional skills or the use of adaptive devices so that adaptive skills could be performed at home following discharge.

Unfortunately, training of functional skills in the hospital does not guarantee skill generalization to the patient's home. DiJoseph[24] notes that many patients may perform well in an occupational therapy clinic but that such learned adaptive behavior may not transfer to the patient's room or, more importantly, to the home. Environmental and psychosocial factors that directly influence task performance may be too varied between settings for the patient to generalize the learned skills. Additionally, a patient may become dependent on the staff for self-care performance or lack the opportunity to perform new skills on a regular basis. Consequently, the patient may not perform competently following discharge and/or may lack the confidence and motivation to attempt performance.

Contemporary Views of the Treatment of Self-Care Deficits

In the 1970s, the emphasis on the location of rehabilitation services was expanded in order to focus on the needs of the patient in the home and community.[113] A concern for the disabled person's rights and abilities in the community became an issue as reflected in legislation regarding education, housing, and vocational and medical needs and in an increased consumer advocacy movement.[77] Treatment in the community allowed the medical professions to reach more patients who might not be able to get to the hospital.[113] A rise in the number of home health treatments was seen. Between 1974 and 1982 Medicare payments for home health services increased nearly tenfold while total Medicare expenditures increased only a third as much.[96] Environmental factors began to be viewed as important in determining degrees of independence for people with disabilities.[114] Evaluation and treatment could be conducted in a more natural environment to maximize the patient's independent abilities.[8] Treatment focus began to be changed to the needs of the patient in his home, work, and community. Community skills such as banking, shopping, and going to restaurants began to be addressed by health care professionals.[77]

Treatment in the patient's home environment can be more beneficial than in the hospital setting.[42] The therapist can see each problem with greater knowledge and sensitivity and problems can be more rapidly solved than in isolated, hospital-based therapy clinics. The environment can be evaluated in terms of architectural, transportation, and communication barriers and how these affect the patient's daily living skills. Colvin and Korn[17] described a major city program in which architectural barriers were removed from the homes of people with disabilities. It was proposed that if these barriers were removed and the patient was provided with environmental control devices, they could derive greater benefit from home care programs and be able to participate more fully in self-care and home activities. The participants in this project contended that the environmental modifications made an improvement in their personal and family lives and that they felt safer and more independent.

In addition to the expansion into the home and community, the use of high technology and computerized devices has entered into the field of rehabilitation. These developments have the potential to assist the patient to gain environmental control for self-care and vocational and recreational pursuits. With the aid of computers and environmental control devices, some patients who previously required institutional care have the potential to remain at home.[91]

A Proposed Approach: Management of Options for Self-Care Tasks

The approach to self-care deficits and independent living skills has broadened in the past decade, owing principally to improved treatment procedures and technology as well as increased emphasis on the patient in their environmental setting. However, the goals of intervention are too frequently determined without significant input from the patient and family. This occurs despite the reality that treatment can fail if the goals of the rehabilitation team and the family are not congruent.

When goals are set in collaboration with the patient, the motivation to learn and maintain a skill is better than if the goals are determined by caregivers. Burke[13] notes that motivation comes from self-initiated and self-guided behavior. Each self-care behavior should be evaluated to see if the patient is motivated to learn and maintain it. In a study by Chiou and Burnett,[15] stroke patients' views of the importance of self-care skills were compared with those of their occupational therapists and physical therapists. The results showed that the patients and therapists viewed the importance of specific self-care items differently. This suggests that treatment goals and procedures should be individualized and that patients should not be viewed as members of diagnostic groups with predetermined needs.

Decker and Schultz[19] contend that an important aspect of occupational therapy should be to help improve the patient's perception of self-control over their physical and psychological environment. Their study of middle-aged patients with spinal cord injuries showed that subjects with a high level of life satisfaction had a high correlation with perception of feeling in control of one's life.

The role of the rehabilitation caregiver must change from that of a professional who decides the treatment goals for the patient to that of one who can provide the patient with knowledge about the rehabilitation options available for the attainment of the desired degree of self-care functioning. The therapist's role is to provide the necessary information and treatment to allow patients to make successful choices about their independence in self-care activities since these relate to their total social and physical environment. Through a wide range of treatment options, the therapist will be available to participate in the attainment of patients' individualized goals. The therapist can explain these options to the patient so that a choice about how to accomplish tasks to the desired degree of independence can be made.

One of the first options the occupational therapist and patient should explore concerning the performance of any self-care task is whether the task is necessary or desired by the patient. There may be self-care tasks that were done premorbidly that now the patient may no longer choose to perform. For example, a woman, with hemiplegia who formerly rolled her hair on rollers on a daily basis may decide to have it cut in an easier-to-manage style rather than learn to use rollers with one hand. This type of decision should be based on the patient's desires.

In some instances, training procedures can be used to regain a desired skill. Following a cardiovascular accident (CVA), for example, the therapist may be able to retrain the patient to perform the task as it was performed premorbidly if there is sufficient return of voluntary movement. In some instances, of course, the patient may no longer have the perceptual or physical capability to perform a task as before. However, he or she may be able to learn to accomplish the task using different movement patterns or with different body parts.

Environmental changes represent an additional array of intervention options that the patient and therapist can explore as a means of gaining independence in self-care. In some instances simply rearranging the physical environment may allow the disabled person to perform tasks independently. For example, moving dishes to lower shelves so that the patient can reach them from a wheelchair would represent a modification of the environment requiring only simple rearrangement. Structural changes in the physical environment may also be necessary. These can include major changes such as the reconstruction of

rooms to accommodate wheelchair movement or less extensive modifications such as replacing round doorknobs with lever handles for a person who has weak grasp.

Adaptive equipment and devices can be used to assist in the satisfactory performance of a desired task. Adaptive equipment and devices can range from simple, inexpensive articles, such as bathtub seats, to the use of expensive equipment such as computers for environmental control and communication. The therapist's role is to inform the patient of the existence, cost, and appropriate use of these devices.

Finally, assistance from other people for the partial or total completion of a desired task is another option available to the patient. Assistance may come from spouses, friends, or paid personal care attendants. The role of the therapist in this case must be to instruct the patient and the attendant on optimal approaches to working together for the completion of identified self-care tasks.

Collectively, the personal and environmental intervention options described in this section form the basis for collaborative decision making and treatment planning. It should be borne in mind that neither diagnosis alone nor the extent of impairment can serve as an adequate basis for planning self-care intervention. Together, the rehabilitation team and the patient must determine those approaches that represent the most realistic and achievable goals based on the patient's abilities, values, and personal social circumstances. Only in this way will optimal results be achieved following discharge (Fig. 5-2).

ASSESSMENT OF INDEPENDENT FUNCTIONING IN SELF-CARE

The Purposes of Self-Care Assessment

Assessment at any level has as its ultimate purpose the ability to make informed decisions. Scales and instruments designed to assess the ability of the patient to perform self-care tasks may assist in treatment or discharge planning by describing or documenting current abilities or monitoring changes in functional status. More global scales, which may include self-care components, are used to provide information on the effectiveness of rehabilitation programs, thus playing an important role in program evaluation.

Lawton[61] has noted that formalized assessment of the patient's functioning yields a comprehensive picture of the strengths as well as the weaknesses of a patient and can provide objective evidence of clinical impressions. By providing a documented baseline of the patient's level of functioning, the formalized assessment facilitates communication with other members of the treatment team.

Vash[105] has suggested that because decisions made on the basis of assessment have the greatest ultimate impact on the patients themselves, results of assessments should be shared with them. In so doing, patients enter into the decision-making process and become "consultants" to their own care. Patient involvement in decision making regarding their treatment is viewed as an important dimension of the rehabilitation process and will be emphasized elsewhere in this chapter.

The Development of Self-Care Assessment Tools

Assessment of the patient's ability to function independently has been conducted in medical rehabilitation for nearly 40 years. In an early review of the problems of measurement and evaluation

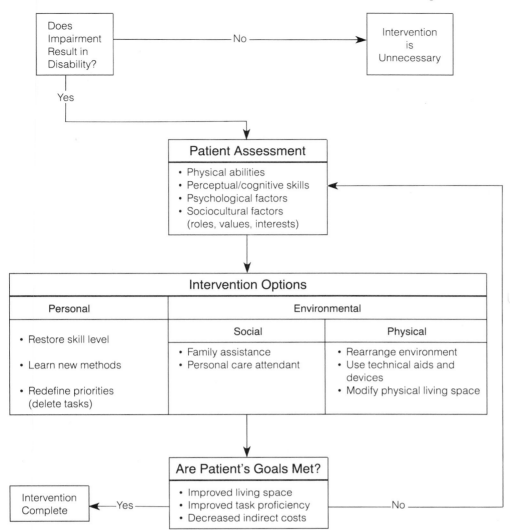

Figure 5-2.   Decision-making for self-care intervention.

in rehabilitation published in 1962, Kelman and Willner[56] found that poorly conceptualized outcome criteria, lack of standardization, disagreement about methods, multidimensional scales, and the influence of the setting on performance were barriers to effective measurement.

Today, although there has been increased agreement about which abilities to measure, many of the problems noted above remain.[47, 52, 53] Moreover, it is common for facilities to develop *ad hoc* measures to fit their particular situations without consideration of the necessary properties of acceptable measures of functional status. This creates difficulties, since the instruments are usually not well developed and thus have questionable validity for clinical management or program evaluation.

Capability Versus Characteristic Behavior

It was noted earlier that function cannot be considered in isolation from its environmental context. This is made especially clear by the distinction between capability and actual behavior. Alexander and Fuhrer[2] have noted this distinction as it pertains to measures of functional ability. Measures of capability represent what the patient *can do* while measures of actual behavior indicate what the patient *does do.*

Most self-care assessments in use during the past 30 years have been designed to measure what the patient is capable of doing within the rehabilitation environment. An assessment of actual behavior, however, must take place in the daily living environment in which the person performs the tasks. This helps to explain why some studies have shown an apparent decline in patient function following discharge from the rehabilitation setting. Awareness of the distinction between capability and actual behavior and their relationship to the patient's environment has had an important impact on the development of new approaches to the assessment of self-care abilities.

The Criterion Problem in Functional Outcome

Frey[31] and Keith[54] have noted that increased emphasis on accountability and the need for determining the benefit–cost ratios of rehabilitation have revealed ambiguities regarding the definition of rehabilitation success. For example, gains in self-care ability, while important to the patient, may not be perceived as beneficial within a system that perceives employability as the sole criterion of success. This has created additional pressure for the development of assessment devices that consider post-discharge function.

Fortunately, the increased attention to these issues has resulted in increased research, which has encouraged the refinement or development and validation of several scales that assess self-care performance. Some of these scales possess characteristics suitable for program evaluation and research as well as clinical decision making. The need remains, however, for greater awareness of the problems associated with functional assessment and the importance of using instruments that possess necessary measurement characteristics.

Desirable Attributes to Self-Care Assessment Scales

Although both practical and technical problems related to the assessment process have precluded the development of an ideal self-care assessment tool, the following checklist highlights those characteristics that such an instrument should possess:

- *It should be standardized.* In order to be standardized, a scale must have explicitly stated procedures for administration and scoring, performance data from a normal population (preferably of varying ages), information regarding the measurement properties of the scale (such as its computed reliability), and a statement of the necessary qualifications of the examiner. Very few self-care scales presently in use meet these guidelines for standardization. It is probably not possible to develop standardized scales that are useful both as measures of capability as well as actual functioning, since the environmental context so important to patient functioning will not be comparable in the administration across the different settings.
- *It should be scalable.* Scaling procedures serve to quantify a person's responses to a defined set of tasks so that they are distributed along a continuum of performance. In order for an assessment device to be considered a true scale, it must be established that the tasks performed will cumulatively yield a score or descriptor that represents increasing capability (or independence). A commonly reported index of scalability is Guttman's scalogram analysis.[40]
- *It should be reliable.* An acceptable scale should provide a *reliable* measure of the patient's level of performance tasks. Reliability refers to a scale's accuracy and consistency in providing information, regardless of the time, setting, or person performing the assessment. Scales that have carefully defined methods and scoring criteria are likely to be more sensitive and consistent and present a more accurate picture of the patient than those that do not.
- *It should be valid.* A scale cannot be valid if it is not reliable. Validity is related to theoretical as well as methodological issues and is therefore dependent on a number of factors. These include the extent to which the scores on the assessment are related to some external criterion, the degree to which the instrument contains items or tasks that represent the domain of interest, and the relationship of the instrument to other measures that collectively support various theoretical assumptions. To the extent that observations of a scale's relationship with other measures and its corroboration with clinical expectations are demonstrated, the scale can be said to demonstrate evidence of its validity. Kaufert[52] notes that a number of factors make it difficult to establish the validity of functional ability indices. Specifically, he notes that the impact of aids, adaptations, and helpers must be considered in measuring functional independence. Moreover, such factors as situational conditions, the patient's level of motivation, the professional perspective of the rater, and the role expectations of the patient can compromise efforts at establishing the validity of these scales. Since there is no standard index for indicating validity, the clinician and researcher should consider these factors in determining the overall merit of a particular scale.
- *It should be comprehensive.* Self-care assessments are more

useful if they determine performance levels for all basic ADL skills and are applicable to every diagnosis. Since patients universally have the requirement to perform (or have performed for them) basic self-care tasks, broad applicability is appropriate and facilitates comparison of research findings among differing patient groups. To the extent that instrumental ADL can be assessed, a scale becomes more useful as a measure of independence in postdischarge settings.
- *It should be performance based.* This characteristic eliminates those scales that are based on patient interviews or reports of professional caregivers. Although studies have indicated that a patient's self-assessment of performance and observations by professionals can be reliable, these methods sacrifice important qualitative information that can be derived from observation of the patient during performance-based assessment. Performance-based scales should not emphasize speed, since speed is irrelevant if a patient cannot perform the task. Moreover, treatment is aimed frequently at improving the quality of movement or impulsivity demonstrated by patients with central nervous system dysfunction. In these cases, performance is often improved if tasks are accomplished more slowly or deliberately.[58] However, time is an issue in performance, since it becomes impractical to perform some tasks independently if the amount of time required for completion is disproportionate to the value of the activity as perceived by the patient or significant other.
- *It should be practical.* The extent to which a scale is designed to facilitate decision making and research is an important consideration in instrument selection. The number of items should be sufficient to permit reliability while requiring a reasonable length of time (30 to 45 minutes) for administration. To the extent possible, items should not require equipment that would unduly limit locations where the scale could be administered. Scoring sheets should contain clear explanations of criteria and should be designed to permit accurate recording as well as coding for data processing. Terminology should be readily understandable, with abilities expressed using everyday language. Finally, the meaning of obtained scores should clearly convey a patient's level of functional independence to caregivers as well as to members of the patient's family.

Widely Used Self-Care Scales

While dozens of instruments designed to assess self-care performance have been reported in the literature, consensus has not been achieved for use of a single scale. However, a handful of scales have demonstrated sufficient validity and frequency in the literature to warrant their review here. It may be instructive, therefore, to describe the composition, measurement properties, and scoring of these scales and to summarize the literature with respect to their use with varying patient populations and evidence of validity. The scales to be reviewed in this section are the *PULSES Profile,*[74] the *Katz Index of ADL,*[50] the *Barthel Index,*[68] the *Kenny Self-Care Evaluation,*[87] and the *Klein-Bell ADL Scale.*[58] They are reviewed here in the order of their development and appearance in the literature.

The PULSES Profile

The *PULSES Profile,* published by Moskowitz and McCann in 1957, has been described as the first major formalized functional assessment instrument to be widely used in American medical rehabilitation settings.[39] The instrument evolved out of a perceived need for a more structured approach to functional assessment and represented an adaptation of a military classification system used by U.S. and Canadian armed forces in the 1940s to classify the overall physical status of military personnel. PULSES is an acronym formed of initials representing the subsections comprising the overall instrument, which is of the global variety. These subsections are designed to measure, respectively, Physical condition, performance using the Upper extremities, mobility as permitted by Lower extremity function, communication and Sensory performance, bowel and bladder or Excretory performance, and psychosocial Status. Within each section, numerical grades ranging from 1 to 4 (from no abnormalities to severe abnormalities limiting independence) are assigned based on the patients functional ability as assessed by an examining physician.

The original *PULSES Profile* had notable weaknesses, including a lack of specifically defined criteria and an underlying assumption that impairment equates with disability. The profile was modified by Granger and associates[35] in 1975 to include a scoring system and improved rating criteria. Studies since that time have added to evidence of its utility in classifying independent status in a wide variety of patient samples.[36, 72, 73] Research suggests that the *PULSES Profile* appears to be more useful in detecting change prior to discharge and is most effective in those situations in which substantial changes in functional status are likely to occur, such as in a patient with CVA or spinal cord injury.

The Katz Index of ADL

The *Index of Independence in Activities of Daily Living*[51] was developed to study results of treatment and prognosis in the elderly and chronically ill. Development of the index was based on observations of a larger number of activities performed by a group of patients with fracture of the hip.

The index is based on an evaluation of the functional independence of patients in bathing, dressing, going to the toilet, transfers, continence, and feeding (Fig. 5-3). Using three descriptors for rating independence in each of six subscales, the rater is able to derive an overall grade of independence with the aid of specific rating criteria. Depending on the determined level of independence, a patient is graded as "A, B, C, D, E, F, G, or Other" (Fig. 5-4). According to the scale, a patient graded as "A" would be functioning independently in all six functions while a patient graded as "G" would be dependent in all rated functions. Patients graded as "Other" are dependent in at least two functions but not classifiable as C, D, E, or F. Through observations over a definite period of time, the observer determines whether the patient is assisted or whether the patient functions on his or her own when performing the six activities. Assistance is classified as active personal assistance, directive assistance, or supervision.

In studies of the index with over 1,000 patients, the scale was found to result in an ordered pattern, so that a person able to perform a given activity independently also would be able to perform all activities performed by people graded at lower levels. This hierarchical structure correctly classifies the functional ability of patients 86% of the time and is the characteristic that makes this index a true Guttman scale.

The *Katz Index of ADL* has been used as a tool to accumulate information about recovery following CVA[5, 32] and the need for care among patients with rheumatoid arthritis[51] and as an instrument to study information about the dynamics of disability in the aging process.[50] More recently, Brorsson and Asberg[11] used the scale in a study of internal medicine patients in a general hospital in Sweden. Their study found a high degree of interrater reliability as well as high coefficients of scalability, which was interpreted as an index of its construct validity.

The Barthel Index

In 1965, Mahoney and Barthel published a weighted scale for measuring basic ADL with chronically disabled patients. Described as "a simple index of independence to score the ability of a patient with a neuromuscular or musculoskeletal disorder to

care for himself," the *Barthel Index* included ten items, including feeding, transfers, personal grooming and hygiene, bathing, toileting, walking, negotiating stairs, and controlling bowel and bladder (Fig. 5-5). Items are scored differentially according to a weighted scoring system that assigns points based on independent or assisted performance. For example, a person who needs human assistance in eating would receive 5 points while independence in eating would be awarded 10 points. A patient with a maximum score of 100 points is defined as continent, able to feed and dress himself or herself, walk at least a block, and climb and descend stairs. The authors were careful to note that a maximum score did not necessarily signify independence, since instrumental ADL such as cooking, housekeeping, and socialization are not assessed. The stability (test–retest reliability) of the *Barthel Index* has been reported by Granger and colleagues[36] as .89, while interrater reliability coefficients were above .95.

The *Barthel Index* is perhaps the most widely studied of published self-care assessments. Several studies have shown that the scale is sensitive to change over time, that it is a significant predictor of rehabilitation outcome, and that it relates significantly with other measures of patient status.

For example, Wade[107] found that scores on the *Barthel Index* were positively correlated with functional status 6 months later in a sample of 83 patients with CVA. Similarly, the initial *Barthel Index* score was found to be the most reliable predictor of final rehabilitation outcome in a 31-month study of 41 stroke patients conducted by Hertanu and colleagues.[45] That study concluded that the *Barthel Index* was a more reliable predictor of rehabilitation outcome than estimates based on computed tomography showing the extent of lesion following CVA. The *Barthel Index* has also been found to correlate significantly with type of discharge and shorter length of stay for patients with CVA,[37, 117] and independent living outcome for patients with spinal cord injury.[22]

In a study of 307 randomly selected severely disabled patients at ten comprehensive medical rehabilitation centers, the *Barthel Index* and the *PULSES Profile* were used to determine functional changes over time. The investigators found that scores for the two instruments were highly correlated, with coefficients ranging from .74 to .80 for point of measurement[35] and .61 to .74 for difference scores. A more recent study of patients with dysvascular amputations[79] has also shown a correspondence between scores on the *Barthel Index* and the *PULSES Profile* (Fig. 5-3).

The Kenny Index of ADL

The *Kenny Index of ADL* was developed at the Sister Kenny Rehabilitation Institute in Minneapolis in the mid 1960s.[87] This scale measures six categories of self-care, including bed movement, transfers, locomotion, dressing, personal hygiene, and feeding. Seventeen items are assessed, with scoring based on a five-point scale ranging from 0 (completely dependent) to 4 (independent). The average score for items within each of the six categories are summed, yielding a total possible score of 24 points, indicating maximum independence on the ADL skills assessed.

In initial studies of the scale's validity, scores on the *Kenny Index of ADL* were found to relate significantly to both the number of bed/wheelchair/commode transfers performed on a rehabilitation unit and the amount of time required for those transfers. Although the *Kenny Index of ADL* has not been studied as widely as most other scales reported in this section, there is adequate evidence that the scale is sensitive to changes in patient functioning and that it can be used to document rehabilitation progress. One comparative study[25] found the *Kenny Index of ADL* to be more sensitive to change than either the *Barthel Index* or the *Katz Index of ADL*.

Index of Independence in Activities of Daily Living: Evaluation Form

Name: _____ Date of Evaluation: _____

For each area of functioning listed below, check description that applies. (The word "assistance" means supervision, direction or personal assistance)

Bathing—either sponge bath, tub bath, or shower.

☐ Receives no assistance (gets in and out of tub by self if tub is usual means of bathing)

☐ Receives assistance in bathing only one part of the body (such as back or a leg)

☐ Receives assistance in bathing more than one part of the body (or not bathed)

Dressing—gets clothes from closets and drawers, including underclothes, outer garments and using fasteners (including braces if worn).

☐ Gets clothes and gets completely dressed without assistance.

☐ Gets clothes and gets dressed except for assistance in tying shoes.

☐ Receives assistance in getting clothes or in getting dressed, or stays partly or completely undressed.

Toileting—going to the "toilet room" for bowel and urine elimination; cleaning self after elimination, and arranging clothes.

☐ Goes to "toilet room," cleans self, and arranges clothes without assistance (may use object for support such as cane, walker, or wheelchair and may manage night bedpan or commode, emptying same in morning.)

☐ Receives assistance in going to "toilet room" or in cleansing self or in arranging clothes after elimination or in use of night bedpan or commode.

☐ Doesn't go to room termed "toilet" for the elimination process.

Transfer

☐ Moves in and out of bed as well as in and out of chair without assistance (may be using object for support such as cane or walker)

☐ Moves in or out of bed or chair with assistance

☐ Doesn't get out of bed

Continence

☐ Controls urination and bowel movement completely by self

☐ Has occasional "accidents"

☐ Supervision helps keep urine or bowel control; catheter is used, or patient is incontinent.

Feeding

☐ Feeds self without assistance

☐ Feeds self except for getting assistance in cutting meat or buttering bread

☐ Receives assistance in feeding or is fed partly or completely by using tubes or intravenous fluids

Figure 5-3. *Katz Index of ADL* evaluation form. From Katz S, Ford AB, Moskowitz RW et al: Studies of illness in the aged. The index of ADL: A standardized measure of biological and psychosocial function. JAMA 185(12):914–919, 1963. Copyright 1963 by the American Medical Association.

The Index of Independence in Activities of Daily Living is based on an evaluation of the functional independence of patients in bathing, dressing, going to toilet, transferring, continence, and feeding.

A—Independent in feeding, continence, transferring, going to toilet, dressing and bathing

B—Independent in all but one of these functions

C—Independent in all but bathing and one additional function

D—Independent in all but bathing, dressing, and one additional function

E—Independent in all but bathing, dressing, going to toilet, and one additional function

F—Independent in all but bathing, dressing, going to toilet, transferring, and one additional function

G—Dependent in all six functions

Other—Dependent in at least two functions but not classifiable as C, D, E, or F.

Figure 5-4. *Katz Index of ADL* scoring summary. From Katz S, Ford AB, Moskowitz RW et al: The index of ADL: A standardized measure of biological and psychosocial function. JAMA 182(12):914–919, 1963. Copyright 1963 by the American Medical Association.

	With Help	Independent
1. Feeding (If food needs to be cut up = help)	5	10
2. Moving from wheelchair to bed and return (includes sitting up in bed)	5–10	15
3. Personal toilet (wash face, comb hair, shave, clean teeth)	0	5
4. Getting on and off toilet (handling clothes, wipe, flush)	5	10
5. Bathing self	0	5
6. Walking on level surface (or, if unable to walk, propel wheelchair)	10	15
(*score only if unable to walk)	0*	5*
7. Ascend and descend stairs	5	10
8. Dressing (includes tying shoes, fastening fasteners)	5	10
9. Controlling bowels	5	10
10. Controlling bladder	5	10

A patient scoring 100 BI is continent, feeds himself, dresses himself, gets up out of bed and chairs, bathes himself, walks at least a block, and can ascend and descend stairs. This does not mean that he is able to live alone: he may not be able to cook, keep house, and meet the public, but he is able to get along without attendant care.

Figure 5-5. *Barthel Index* items and scoring weights. From Mahony FI, Barthel DW: Functional evaluation: The Barthel index. Maryland State Medical Journal 14(2):61–65, 1965.

The Klein-Bell ADL Scale

A more recently developed scale that seems to show promise is the *Klein-Bell ADL scale.* Developed by Ronald Klein, a psychologist, and Beverly Bell, an occupational therapist, this scale was specifically designed to address some of the shortcomings of earlier scales. The scale consists of 170 items in six categories: dressing, elimination, mobility, bathing/hygiene, eating, and communication. A percentage score is computed, based on the number of ADL skills a patient can perform independently. Thus, people able to perform at the 100% level are usually able to perform all self-care skills during the day and have no attendant care needs.

The scale developers reported a 92% level of agreement among raters in a study of the scale's reliability. This was considered to represent a conservative estimate of the scale's reliability since the raters were not trained extensively in its use.[58]

In a follow-up study of 14 patients who had been rated on the *Klein-Bell ADL Scale* just prior to discharge, a significant inverse relationship was found between the score at discharge and the number of hours per week of assistance received 5 to 10 months after discharge ($r = -.86$, $p<.01$). These data suggest that the obtained score on the *Klein-Bell ADL Scale* was a valid predictor of independence in self-care.[58]

Comparisons Among Self-Care Scales

A comparison of the self-care scales reviewed in this section reveals that each (1) focuses on basic ADL, (2) is based on professional observation and judgment, (3) derives an interpretable score that can be used in studies of prediction, and (4) has some evidence of reliability and predictive validity. Of the five scales reviewed, the *Klein-Bell ADL Scale* is the most comprehensive and appears to be the most sensitive to changes in patient status. Only the *Katz Index of ADL,* and to a lesser extent, the *Klein-Bell ADL Scale* derive scores that are readily interpretable in terms of the specific tasks which a patient is able to perform independently. A graphic comparison of the important characteristics of each of these self-care scales is provided in Table 5-1.

Table 5-1
Self-Care Scale Comparison

PULSES (Moskowitz and McCann 1957)	*Index of ADL* (Katz and co-workers, 1963)	*Barthel Index* (Mahoney and Barthel, 1965)	*Kenny* (Schoening and co-workers, 1965)	*Klein-Bell* (Klein and Bell 1982)
Domain/Tasks Assessed • Physical condition • Upper extremity • Lower extremity • Sensory components • Excretory (bowel and bladder) • Status of patient (mental and physical)	• Bathing • Dressing • Going to toilet • Transfer • Continence • Feeding	• Feeding • Wheelchair transfer • Grooming • Toilet transfer • Bathing • Level walking • Stairs • Dressing • Bowel control • Bladder control	• Bed • Transfers • Locomotion (walking, stairs, wheelchair) • Dressing • Personal hygiene (incl. bowel/bladder) • Feeding	• Dressing • Elimination • Mobility (incl. transfers) • Bathing/hygiene • Eating • Communication
Scoring Numerical 4-point scale. Range 0–24. Adapted version relates upper and lower extremity function to ADL tasks and mobility.	Ordinal ranking A–G based on descending levels of independence.	Adapted version is based on weighted numerical scale yielding mobility and self-care score. Range 0–100	Overall score derived from rating (0–4) among all items within each category. Range 0–24	Items scored 0–3. Overall score derived from rating 170 items in above categories. Percentage score is computed.
Reliability/Validity Reported coefficients: Test–retest .87 Interrater >.95 Evidence of predictive and concurrent validity	Coefficient of scalability = .89. Some evidence of predictive and concurrent validity	Reported test–retest reliability .89, interrater reliability >.95. Evidence of predictive and concurrent validity	Formal reliability coefficients have not been reported; some evidence of predictive and concurrent validity	Authors report 92% agreement among three pairs of raters in early study; some evidence of predictive and concurrent validity
Strengths/Limitations Widely used among varying patient populations Lacks subscore detail in discrete ADL variables	Derived score yields specific information about patient's functional independence.	Comprehensive and widely used in United States. Adapted versions permit distinction between levels of independence.	Sensitive to patient change in overall function; has not been extensively validated	One of the most sensitive and carefully designed scales; has not been extensively validated

Several published studies have reported concurrent use of various combinations of the *PULSES Profile, Barthel Index, Katz Index of ADL,* and the *Kenny Index of ADL.*[25, 39] In general, the scales have correlated significantly with one another, providing evidence of their concurrent validity.

Unfortunately, most of these scales possess shortcomings that can be only incompletely addressed here. With the exception of the *Klein-Bell ADL Scale,* their value as reliable assessment instruments hinges on careful adherence to rating criteria by informed raters, and they do not readily serve as precise guides to treatment planning. Moreover, in each scale, the scope of assessed functioning is limited to basic ADLs (including mobility and communication) that collectively represent a limited, albeit important, portion of the overall domain of independent living tasks. Perhaps most importantly, however, the scales were designed to assess capability rather than actual performance, thus limiting their relevance as tools for measuring important rehabilitation outcome.

In part due to recognition of the shortcomings of existing functional assessments, two projects have been funded by the federal government in an attempt to develop improved measures of rehabilitation for both process and outcome purposes that would have the potential for widespread adoption throughout the country. These projects, described below, are the Rehabilita-

tion Indicators Project and the Functional Independence Measure project, both based in New York State.

Rehabilitation Indicators Project

Between 1974 and 1982, a federally funded project at New York University's Institute of Rehabilitation Medicine sought to develop instruments that would sensitively describe the impact of rehabilitation on client functioning and provide a detailed and systematic view of the benefits of rehabilitation. The instruments that were developed under the aegis of this project are collectively referred to as rehabilitation indicator instruments (RI).[12]

The RI instruments have the common characteristic of generating moderately to highly detailed functional assessment data that provide descriptive profiles of client functioning. The instruments are designed so that detailed data can be collapsed into broad indicators for predictive and diagnostic purposes.

In comparison with other measures of functional assessment, the RI instruments have the capability of providing detail for professionals desiring more exact pictures of the needs of clients, while also permitting information on a broader scale. The terminology used in the assessments incorporates lay language as much as possible to facilitate communication.

One of the strongest characteristics of the RI assessment tools is overall flexibility. By incorporating levels of measurement ranging from individual skills (as reflected in skill indicators) to activity clusters (referred to as activity pattern indicators), the instruments can be used to serve a wide range of purposes, ranging from clinical management to outcome evaluation. Additionally, client data can be gathered in different ways, ranging from direct observation to self or professional staff report. Because the instruments evolved from a model in which rehabilitation is viewed as a process dependent on the service system, the person receiving care, and the characteristics of the environment, their design reflects these factors and their inherent complexities.

The flexibility of the RI instruments, while increasing their use as tools for different purposes and settings, restricts attempts to determine their reliability under varying types of administration. This characteristic also precludes any attempt to standardize the various scales, especially the self-care items assessed through the activity pattern indicators. Despite these limitations, the authors believe that the practical benefits derived from having a flexible instrument are more important than the lack of comparability incurred through lack of standardization.

The Functional Independence Measure

In 1983, the National Institute of Handicapped Research and the United States Department of Education awarded a grant to the Department of Rehabilitation Medicine at the School of Medicine, State University of New York, to develop a uniform data system (UDS) for describing and communicating about disability. A national task force met and, under the auspices of this grant, reviewed extant published and unpublished measures of functional independence. This review permitted the identification of items for the *functional independence measure (FIM),*[37] which were then validated at 25 rehabilitation facilities throughout the country. The *FIM* currently consists of 18 items organized under six categories of function, including self-care activities (eating, grooming, bathing, upper body dressing, lower body dressing, and toileting); sphincter control (bowel and bladder management); mobility (transfers for toilet, tub or shower, and bed, chair, wheelchair); locomotion (walking, wheelchair, and stairs); communication (including comprehension and expression); and social cognition (including problem solving, social interaction, and memory). Patients are assessed on each item with either a four-point or a seven-point scale.

Preliminary data, based on 250 patients and 891 clinician assessments performed by therapists, physicians, and nurses reflected good interrater reliability, ranging from $r = .86$ at admission to $r = .88$ on discharge. A study of the *FIM's* domain or content validity reported satisfactory findings.

Although still early in its development, the design of the *FIM* reflects an appreciation of the multidimensional nature of factors related to rehabilitation success and should represent a useful step toward the development of a standardized outcome scale that has application to most types of rehabilitation settings for the purpose of gathering functional outcome data. It may be less useful as an instrument for planning treatment intervention.

Important Factors in Informal Assessment

In the foregoing sections, an historical and conceptual review of *structured* approaches to measuring functional independence in self-care has been provided. A complete analysis of patient assessment in this area, however, must consider other factors that may have an important relationship to the degree of functional independence achieved following rehabilitation. These factors have not been included in traditional assessment instruments, and with few exceptions, may be given insufficient attention in a consideration of the patient's rehabilitation program. These factors include (1) the patient's ability to manage devices that extend independence through environmental control, (2) the family resources available to the patient in the environment to which he or she is to be discharged, (3) the amount of time (or energy) required to perform tasks independently, and (4) the degree of safety with which patients are able to perform tasks.

Developments in high technology for independent living have made it possible (and important) to assess people with severe disability in terms of their available movements and physical resources for controlling switches to activate environmental control units (ECUs). Currently, and paradoxically, these devices are more likely to extend the patient's ability to perform instrumental ADL more proficiently than self-care tasks.

The inability to perform self-care tasks independently, of course, does not dictate discharge to institutional care if human resources are available in an alternative environment. Frequently, the patient can, and does, rely extensively on the assistance of spouse, other family members, or friends to assist with self-care tasks. It can be argued that the presence of these resources, although commonly determined by the social worker in planning discharge, should be given early consideration in planning rehabilitation intervention.

Additional considerations include the amount of time and energy required to perform the task independently versus the value of the task as perceived by the patient. It cannot be assumed, given competing requirements for time and energy, that all patients view the independent performance of all self-care tasks with the same degree of importance. Thus, the motivation to complete the task independently following discharge is likely to be a function of the alternatives available for task completion, the importance of the task to the patient, and the amount of time and energy required to perform the task independently in the face of competing demands. Additionally, the degree of safety with which a task is performed may be of obvious importance to the practitioner but may not be apparent to the patient or those caregivers in the environment who may be providing assistance with self-care tasks. It is therefore important that training in self-care assistance be provided as a part of the rehabilitation effort and that the ability of helpers to render this assistance in a safe and effective manner be assessed before the patient is discharged.

Significance to the Patient as a Consideration in Assessment

No discussion of self-care assessment is complete without a consideration of the values that may be reflected in the process. Although assessment is a judgmental process, it should not be unnecessarily value laden. In fact, the ubiquitous rehabilitation goal of independent functioning itself reflects a societal value not shared to the same extent by all cultures. Given that there are profound differences in the cultural heritages and life experiences of patients, it is also true that they bring differing sets of values toward independence and self-care to the rehabilitation setting. Effective management of the patient requires an appreciation for these differences. It may therefore be important for assessment to include methods for determining premorbid activity patterns and leisure interests as well as values and attitudes toward assistance. Characteristic methods for performing basic and instrumental ADL, as well as the characteristic aspects of the environment in which these have been performed, may also be important information in planning successful intervention strategies for management of self-care and other ADL.

Self-Care Assessment in Children: Special Considerations

Information presented to this point has been based on self-care assessment as it pertains to the adult. It is worth noting, however, that self-care assessment of the pediatric patient requires a number of special considerations. These pertain to incorporating developmental milestones into the structure of the assessment, interacting with the child during the assessment process, and reporting information to parents. While very little has been published in this area, the reader is referred to work accomplished at the Children's Hospital at Stanford University[16] for more specific information.

MANAGEMENT OF SELF-CARE SKILLS

The assessment process characterizes the strengths and weakness of each patient in relation to self-care independence skills. The management process uses this description to develop options that will enable the patient to become more independent in self-care activities. Experience has shown that patients offered a number of options become active and responsible participants in their own rehabilitation. Medical management of self-care can be viewed as an information management process. The practitioner attempts to develop a comprehensive listing of training methods, devices, environmental modifications, and human resources. From these a subset is selected to maximize patient functioning within the constraints of limited time, money, and patient potential for improvement. Most, if not all, of such options fall into one of three goal categories: to improve living space, to minimize indirect costs of self-care/independence, or to decrease the time and/or energy required to perform self-care tasks.

Improve Living Space

People with disabilities usually want the same freedom they enjoyed prior to their illness or accident. They wish to select their own living conditions and/or companions. Rehabilitation professionals should respect the choices of patients and recognize their needs rather than to opt for safe, secure, inexpensive, and/or convenient options when discharge is being considered. The growth of the independent living movement among the disabled in the United States has been described by De Jong[20, 21] and by Neistadt and Marques.[77] Self-care training must be structured toward maximizing the potential of patients to live where they choose and with whom they choose. Neistadt and Marques[77] described a program in which independent living skills are taught in addition to traditional self-care skills to institutionalized mentally handicapped adults. They suggest that such programs should not focus narrowly on the patient's strengths and weaknesses but should focus on a larger community in which the patient desires to live. Adaptive community skills such as "banking, budgeting, consumer advocacy, personal health care, and attendant management" are important training areas often neglected by "traditional" therapy programs. In addition to conceptualizing self-care goals in the context of the community, Levine[63]

urges therapists to "enter the patient's world" and to "adapt treatment to suit the patient's needs." Cultural and ethnic considerations of life-style should provide a framework in which the patient defines preferences and needs.

Minimize Indirect Costs

Physicians and therapists who rely on hospital billing departments and social workers to handle financial arrangements may not be aware of economic constraints on a patient. All too often the self-care options presented to a patient are based on the availability of equipment and not on the ability of the patient to afford such items. In order to realistically plan self-care remediation strategies, there must be some attempt to gather data regarding available resources and to use this to determine which options are feasible for the patient. The philosophy that should guide selection should be "least expensive–simplest" to effect the largest conservation of resources with the least modification/adaptation of performance and/or tools that can still permit independent self-care.

Decrease Time Required for Performance

Time is precious. It is perhaps the most neglected of resources for the physically disabled. All too often rehabilitation professionals train patients to perform self-care tasks without considering whether it is worth the patient's time to do so. Not one of us would spend 20 minutes each morning just to put on our shoes and socks; yet we might ask a patient to do this regardless of what it means to the patient to have to spend his or her time on such a task. The conservation of time should be a goal of all self-care training. As Shillam and associates[92] reported in their study of the role of occupational therapy in bathing independence for the disabled, decreasing the time it takes to perform routine self-care is important not only to the patient but also to family members and other caregivers.

Frank[30] has written that "In medicine and in the allied health fields such as occupational therapy, despite the probabilities that might bear on a given case, the goal of rehabilitation is to achieve a result that is actual, against an indeterminate field of possibility." In our experience, results do not emerge from a field of "indeterminate possibility" but rather from defined listings of options that have been considered not only with respect to a given self-care goal but also with respect to living space, costs, and the time required for performance.

AN OVERVIEW OF APPROACHES

The context of self-care rehabilitation is one in which options are tailored to the economic, social, and time requirements of the patient. These options can include a variety of training approaches, adaptive devices, environmental modifications, and/or personal attendants.

Training

Self-care rehabilitation is a learning process by which patients must adapt to the effects of illness, accident, or birth defect as they affect the demands of everyday life. It must be recognized, however, that the initial acquisition of skills by those who are developmentally or congenitally disabled is a markedly different learning process from the reacquisition of self-care skills by those who have previously been independent at such tasks prior to becoming disabled. When the goals of training are to develop skills in a person with a congenital condition the training process is termed *habilitation*. When the therapist seeks to restore normal function for a person with an acquired disability, the training process is termed *restorative*. In those instances in which there is either a poor prognosis for development of self-care skills or the patient has failed to benefit from habilitation or restorative training, the approach is termed *compensatory* training.

Developmental or Habilitation Training

Practice is an important aspect of all motor training. Cross[18] defines practice as "performance of any overt or covert act one or more times with a view to fixating or improving the spatial and temporal organization of the same or any other act." Mere repetition of activity is not therapeutic training. The occupational therapist or other self-care trainer must provide task structuring, feedback, and strategic suggestions for improvement of performance. The patient must learn to monitor and correct performance errors. Over time desirable behaviors must be systematically rewarded and undesirable behaviors ignored or extinguished.[88]

When children learn self-care tasks initially, they do so over extended periods of time. Most often operant conditioning is provided in which successive approximations toward each goal (feeding, bowel and bladder control, grooming, dressing, and bathing) are rewarded. This incremental learning process is termed *shaping*. Practice usually occurs only at the time(s) each day that a task is appropriate. Children are encouraged to do what they can to help—sometimes starting a task that the adult will need to finish and sometimes completing a task that only the adult can initiate. When practice occurs only as needed it is said to be "distributed" over time as opposed to "amassed" or repeated over and over successively. When one does an entire self-care activity as a unit it is called "whole task" practice. If one practices only a part of a task such as fastening and undoing buttons but not dressing, it is called "partial task" practice. If one learns a task in its natural sequence it is called "forward chaining" and if one learns tasks in the reverse of natural sequence (last step first and first step last) this is referred to as "reverse chaining." In this terminology of motor learning, the way in which a child normally learns self-care is described as distributed, whole task, forward or reverse chaining.[18, 88]

Trombly[102] has reported that there is a demonstrated sequence of self-care independence that is supported by child development and anthropological observations. Feeding, grooming, continence, transfers, undressing, dressing, and bathing usually occur in order. Even such limited information as this may be useful in habilitation training. Using a distributed practice schedule (*i.e.,* teaching, self-care activities only during those times they would normally be performed) is critical for the person unfamiliar with the concept of the task. Part of self-care training is learning the appropriate times and natural sequences of daily activities. The patient who is relearning a task often retains an appreciation of when it is to be performed, but the patient being habilitated needs to learn not only the skills but also the context appropriate to each task. Jarman and co-workers[46] have demonstrated that this approach can be effective in training multiply-handicapped children to perform their morning care routines. Walker and Vogelsburg[110] similarly demonstrated the effectiveness of structured practice with a nonambulatory, severely handicapped woman who was taught to be mobility independent. Habilitation in self-care not only teaches specific tasks, but it also fosters the attitudes and values that sustain one's motivation to do these tasks independently. The

assumption that all patients should be trained to perform similar tasks using the same practice schedules, reinforcement schedules, and task structuring is one that should be challenged vigorously.[89] Learning and relearning may be related phenomena, but they are different. Failure to appreciate this may lead to inappropriate selection of activities for self-care training.

Restorative Training

For the patient with an acquired disability, relearning self-care independence is a distinctly different process than for the habilitation patient. First, there is a loss of self-esteem and sense of failure and frustration when one is unable to perform those tasks that are often taken for granted by the nondisabled. Initial learning is usually motivated by intrinsic rewards of increased competency at self-care tasks[112] as well as by the positive social reinforcement of parents and other caregivers. In learning a task, negative reinforcement (*i.e.,* avoiding unpleasant experiences or consequences) such as avoiding embarrassment over having to ask for assistance for feeding or toileting may be far more effective than positive social reinforcement. The therapist who tries to use social praise to reinforce practice of toileting skills will find that it is not effective. In fact, it will probably be viewed as demeaning to praise an adult in a situation reminiscent of a childhood experience.

For the person who is not previously adept at self-care, the context and timing of practice are more important than for the adult seeking to regain skills. Simulation may be effective as a training method using partial task practice on just those components of activity that are deficient. This may be a better choice than whole-task distributed practice. Using partial-task training and moderately massed practice, skill components can be retrained. Restoration of skills often involves a patient who may make considerable contributions to the therapy process based on his or her previous knowledge and understanding of how the task was performed.

Such patients can monitor their own errors and often use appropriate strategies to minimize deficits. In this case the treatment session is used to develop a practice strategy and the patient practices self-care at each opportunity whether or not the therapist is present. Problems occurring between treatments are discussed, and possible solutions can be practices during the next treatment session.

Although many physically disabled adults with acquired deficits may not fit the above description, there is one category of patient that clearly does not benefit from this approach. This category includes patients with closed head injury or CVA who also have significant cognitive and/or perceptual deficits. As Bjornby and Reinvang[10] have pointed out, such conditions as apraxia may significantly influence the effects of self-care training and may in fact need to be remediated prior to or in conjunction with remediation of self-care dependency. For such patients and for those whom other approaches have failed to produce results, compensatory training should be considered.

Compensatory Training

When habilitation or relearning fails or is inappropriate, other options remain available. Often a skill that one would like to perform in a normal manner can successfully be accomplished some other way. The individual with bilateral above-elbow amputations may not do well at feeding using prostheses but may perhaps develop superior toe prehension and use the feet rather than the hands to eat, write, and manipulate tools. Adaptive equipment may substitute for lost or impaired abilities that limit function. The use of such devices will be discussed in the next section. Regardless of how one approaches compensatory training, the philosophical principle that should guide therapy is that there are many approaches to accomplishing the same task. Creative alterations in task performance may allow people to do something for themselves that under other circumstances they would be dependent on another to perform. It is characteristic of compensatory training that it is the end-result of patient activity (whether it is clean teeth or tied shoelaces) and not the method used to perform the task that is important.

Devices

In the past 20 years there has been an unprecedented increase in the numbers and kinds of devices available to assist the disabled person. It has become virtually impossible for rehabilitation professionals to be aware of, or have access to, information on all such devices. Research suggests that there are nearly 2,000 sources of such equipment worldwide, offering an estimated 25,000 to 30,000 products for sale. The typical occupational or physical therapist, speech pathologist, or physician may have 20 to 50 catalogs readily available for finding some devices but remains unaware of vast numbers of other specific items that could benefit patients. One solution to this problem is to use computerized listings or "databases" of such devices, catalogued according to their areas of application. The most comprehensive resource to date is the *ABLEDATA* data base of the National Rehabilitation Information Center at the Catholic University of America in Washington, DC.

Taylor and associates[101] have described a growing specialty of occupational therapy in which therapists become evaluators and providers of increasingly numerous and complex aids to independence. Their call for an expanded role of rehabilitation therapists in providing technical aids to independence was issued at approximately the same time that Newrick and Langton-Hewer[78] published findings that over two-thirds of a group of 42 patients with motor neuron disease could have benefited from aids to independence that had never been prescribed.

Systems and Devices for the Disabled

To determine which systems or devices each person needs, an array of equipment must be available (Figs. 5-6 through 5-9). A

Figure 5-6. Use of rocker knife and cutting board.

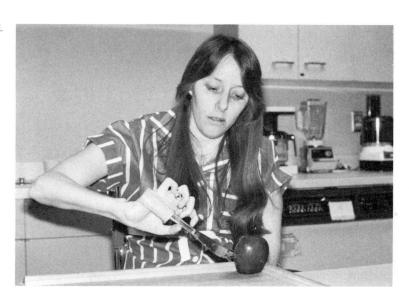

Figure 5-7. Use of bilateral cup holder.

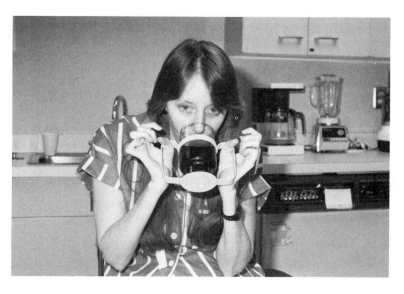

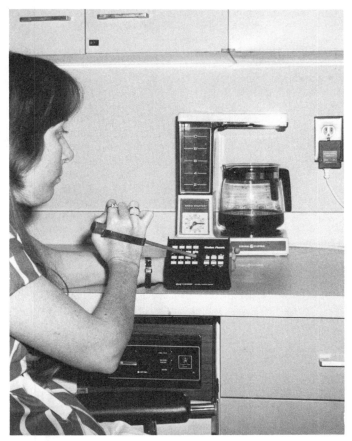

Figure 5-8. Use of environmental control device.

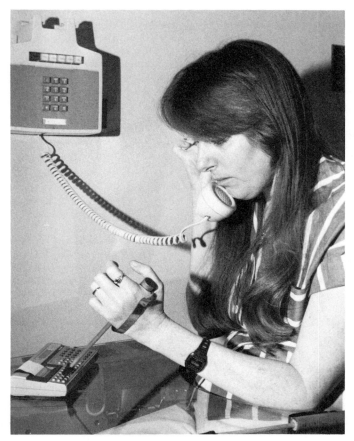

Figure 5-9. Use of pocket size communications computer.

comprehensive team evaluation leads to a list of possible solutions for each identified problem, providing ample information for the patient to make the ultimate decision in the selection of equipment. In every instance, the goal of assessment is to find the simplest, least expensive device to best meet the needs of the patient.[90]

The use of devices or adaptive equipment has its special mission in the application of technology to increase the disabled person's independence. High technology devices and systems are characterized by sophisticated electronic components. These include computers, robots, speech synthesizers, and environmental control systems. Symington[99] has provided an excellent review of the role of environmental control devices in fostering independent living.

Low technology items are simple mechanical aids, such as built-up handles for an arthritic person or shoelaces that can be tied with one hand. Such low technology items are far more numerous than high technology devices, yet they are less well known to many disabled people. The technology of remote control has become increasingly available to our society. For a person unable to reach a light switch, radio, television, thermostat, door lock, or curtain cord, an environmental control system can provide an important new degree of independence. Ultrasonic or infrared signals, sent from a command center, allow a person to "reach" a variety of electronically activated appliances.

The use and acceptance of adaptive devices for self-care is not always related to function or independence. Stein and Walley[95] reported that 60% of the upper extremity amputees fitted with myoelectric versus conventional prostheses preferred the myoelectric ones even though they wore them fewer hours per day and were twice as slow at tasks as with the conventional prostheses. Presumably, cosmesis was a major consideration unrelated to self-care independence that influenced the choice of device by these amputees.

It must be remembered that devices are not always a solution reserved for cases that have failed to respond to other measures. Often adaptive equipment is needed during one stage of recovery and can later be replaced by more normal tools and/or approaches. Haworth[43] studied the use of devices and aids to independence by 163 patients with total hip replacement and clearly showed that patients used devices for ambulation, safety, dressing, and toileting and stopped using them when they were able to manage without such aids.

Environmental Modifications

Both training and devices for self-care independence must be appropriate to the living space of the patient. Modifications of living spaces and the architectural barriers they often impose may greatly enhance independent function in ADL. Such modifications as are needed may range from minimal in the case of rearrangement of furniture to extensive, when apartments or homes must be specially designed for the disabled. Intermediate to these extremes are the cases in which modifications or additions to existing space and equipment may be used to enhance function. In a study of 545 patients with rheumatoid arthritis and 170 patients with ankylosing spondylitis, Urb'anek and colleagues[104] found that environmental conditions such as narrow apartment space negatively influenced the activity of the rheumatoid disease process itself. Liang and co-workers[64] have pointed out the inadequacies of the US health care system in meeting the needs of the estimated 1 million homebound patients in the United States. They describe how many of them could be helped by modifications of their home environment and/or occupational and physical therapy. Unfortunately our health care system tends to place emphasis on acute illness while neglecting important considerations for chronic conditions.

Rearrange Existing Living Space

Many simple modifications that can improve self-care can be suggested by the occupational therapist or other practitioner during the course of a predischarge home visit. When upper extremity ROM is limited, pots, pans, cosmetics, canned goods, and other essential daily living items can be placed out on counters rather than kept in their traditional places, which are often difficult or impossible to reach. For the patient with a visual field deficit such as homonymous hemianopsia, moving the bed and furniture into the patient's intact visual field when viewed from the doorway may make it easier and safer to move around the room. Of course, the view and placement of objects relative to the bed must also be strategically considered for the same reasons. Removal of throw rugs and other common obstacles for the mobility impaired may make a nighttime trip to the bathroom considerably safer.

Modify Existing Living Space

The range of possibilities for modification of living space to meet the needs of disabled people is extensive. Examples of common modifications include widening doorways, adding ramps, converting dens or family rooms into a wheelchair-accessible bedroom, and adding tub rails, toilet rails, and other safety equipment in the bathroom. Several extensive studies have focused solely on the design and modification of bathrooms with respect to both disabled and nondisabled people.[69, 106] Lowman and Klinger[66] have presented many ideas for environmental adaptations cataloged by self-care skill category and by patient deficits. Resources, such as the American National Standards Institute's *Specifications for Making Buildings and Facilities Accessible to and Usable by Physically Handicapped People*[3] give explicit guidelines for many common problems. Unfortunately, lack of information is not usually what prevents patients and caregivers from effecting changes in living space. Expense, and for those who rent, ownership are often barriers to change. Lack of support by third party payers in the reimbursement of environmental modifications is particularly frustrating. Some health care providers have attacked these problems directly by developing partnerships between governmental and community agencies to fund programs designed to eliminate architectural barriers within the home. Colvin and Korn[17] have described one such partnership in New York City between United Cerebral Palsy of New York, Inc, the Mayor's Office for the Handicapped, and the Department of Housing Preservation and Development. This project was found to both be cost effective and to improve the quality of life for those served by it.

Design New Components in Living Space

The most extensive and expensive of options is to redesign or renovate existing living space. Yet for many of the most severely disabled people the only alternative to making such modifications is institutionalization. Everett and Colignon[28] have discussed architectural and self-care needs in relation to independent living for severely disabled people. They suggest that such needs are part of a complex set of interrelated prob-

lems for disabled people and that public policy must be developed to support programs that will provide extensive architectural intervention for these patients. However, architectural renovations alone may not solve the problem. To renovate an apartment for a person with high-level quadriplegia by adding a roll-in shower stall, rerouting pipes to allow wheelchair access to sinks, and performing other changes may not make the person more independent if he or she lacks transportation, has no job, or is unable to communicate. Major modifications of living space must be subject to cost–benefit analysis and justified with respect to the overall level of functioning they permit. Such considerations include, but go beyond, independence in self-care.

Use of Personal Care Attendants

For many of the more severely disabled, there is no combination of training, devices, or environmental modifications that will enable them to function independently in self-care. For such people to live independently outside an institution they must depend on attendants to assist them. Many such attendants are relatives of the disabled person who serve without compensation. Others are paid employees hired to perform essential activities that their disabled employer cannot perform without assistance. Part of the rehabilitation process for people who are going to require attendant care is that they learn to recruit, hire, supervise, and, if necessary, terminate personal care attendants.

Recruitment of Personal Care Attendants

There are a number of excellent manuals and guides to attendant care;[60, 71, 84] however, the availability and quality of personal care attendants varies greatly from one community to the next. One source of attendants is through home health care agencies, many of which provide pre-employment screening and placement on a fee basis. Nurse placement services and agencies specializing in unskilled and/or temporary help are also possible sources of attendants. Classified advertising in local newspapers, announcements strategically place on bulletin boards at colleges, universities, religious institutions, and supermarkets can also be effective. Often, the most difficult task for the patient is that of defining the tasks that require assistance, the degree of assistance that is desired, and the hours of the day when these tasks need to be performed. Since hours, pay, and working schedules (often attendants are needed 7 days per week) are often not competitive with other types of employment, turnover among attendants is high. The occupational therapist or other appropriately trained health care professional can often assist the patient in writing the job description for a personal care attendant and in some cases may work with the patient to be an effective supervisor.

Guidelines for the Appropriate Use of Care Attendants

An important and difficult aspect of working with a care attendant is to be able to define all of the self-care and daily living activities that will require assistance. Many tasks, such as brushing one's teeth, dressing, and grooming, are performed on a daily basis. Other tasks such as washing one's hair or having a bowel movement may be performed less frequently but still quite regularly. Still other tasks such as doing the laundry or changing the bed are even less frequent but are still performed regularly. Finally, there will be tasks such as mending torn clothing or washing windows that are infrequent and not performed on a regular basis. This listing must then be categorized into three distinct classes of activities: those that the patients can perform alone, those that the patient can perform with some assistance, and those that can only be performed by the personal care attendant. The attendant who wants to totally care for the patient or is too impatient to wait for the patient to assist with a task is as harmful as the attendant who neglects the patient. When rehabilitation personnel assist the patient to have a realistic and comprehensive understanding of their self-care strengths and limitations, more effective use of care attendants is possible.

Major Self-Care Considerations by Functional Limitation

The single most important concept in self-care rehabilitation is that neither the type of disability nor the severity can be used to predict how independent a given patient will be. Pressures from new Medicare reimbursement guidelines and the accompanying need for medical care cost containment tends to foster the notion that with controlled studies one can identify factors that predict rehabilitation outcomes. The intent of such efforts is to shift resources toward those believed to have better chances at independence and away from those with less likelihood of functioning independently. That this is a misguided approach is supported by studies such as those by Neill and associates[76] who studied 100 men with coronary disease. They found that there was little or no relationship between actual physical limitations and the activities performed by those patients.

Patient perceptions and not cardiac symptoms accounted for the patterns of independence/dependence in household and social activities. Limited capacity for exertion, which is used by many occupational and physical therapists to recommend appropriate activities, is in fact not a determinant of the activities those cardiac patients performed as part of their daily routine. Is it useful then, to discuss self-care considerations by functional limitations? If the goal is to become aware of special problems or issues unique to a particular disability and not to predict outcomes, then the answer is clearly affirmative.

Cognitive-Perceptual Deficits and Self-Care

There are a number of principles that can be applied to the patient with cognitive and/or perceptual deficits. Right-sided brain damage is associated with visual perceptual and visual search disorders that often make self-care training more difficult.[103] Anstine and Issacs[7] found that problems with dressing were more common in subjects with right hemispheric damage. Gordon and co-workers[34] investigated 78 patients with right-sided brain damage and showed that patients given a comprehensive perceptual remediation program did better at such tasks on discharge than the controls not given this program. Following discharge, the controls tended to show improvement while the experimental group had plateaued. This suggests that rehabilitation training may accelerate recovery of perceptual abilities but is not a *sine qua non* for improvements. Dudgeon and colleagues[26] found that among patients with right-sided brain damage those with defective optokinetic nystagmus (OKN) reflexes showed less improvement in upper extremity dressing skill than those with normal OKN but that both groups showed improvement over time. The OKN deficit group had an average 40% longer hospitalization and a higher incidence of nursing home placement at discharge.

Panikoff[80] described the course of functional recovery from head injury over a 2-year period for 80 head-injured adults. That study found that the longer the period of coma the greater the disability and dependency at 1 year and 2 years after injury. The majority of patients, however, continued to show improvement in ADL and other skills over the 2-year period. Goldkamp[33] studied

53 patients with cerebral palsy for periods of 6 to 25 years and found that the only variable that appeared to influence ADL independence directly was intelligence. Bjornby and Reinvang[10] investigated the relationship of apraxia to ADL skills in 120 persons with right-sided hemiplegia following left-sided CVA. They found that apraxia variables were significant predictors of dependency and that even those less severely involved patients who showed progress in the hospital setting regressed in ADL function after returning home. Their conclusion was that these patients have difficulty in transferring skills learned in the clinic to the home environment and that such patients might best be treated in their own homes.

It appears that cognitive-perceptual limitations may make self-care rehabilitation training more difficult. Patients with such limitations can and do make progress, albeit more slowly than similar patients without such deficits.

Upper Extremity Impairment

Unilateral upper extremity impairment is most often compensated for by use of the uninvolved extremity. When disability affects the preferred hand there will be a need to transfer skill to the other hand. This may or may not require coordination and dexterity training. Bilateral upper extremity weakness, loss of motion, and amputations are more serious threats to self-care independence. For such people, orthotic and prosthetic devices are often useful. In some cases teeth are used for prehension privately whereas the prosthesis may be used publicly. Often cosmesis is as much or more a consideration than function in the selection of a prosthesis.[95]

Lower Extremity Impairment

Mobility and transfer limitations are the most significant self-care problems for lower extremity disabled people including those with hip fractures, amputations, arthritis, and paraplegia. Often wheelchairs and other ambulation aids are needed for independent mobility. Bathroom safety equipment, dressing aids such as extended handle shoehorns, and raised seats are often useful items that may be used either temporarily or permanently. Rearrangement of living space to permit wheelchair access or access using other mobility aids is often necessary. Ramps, chairlifts, and additional railings may be needed if stairs are present. For the person dependent on a wheelchair, it may also be helpful to consider rearrangement of shelves, drawers, and closet space to permit items that are used frequently to be reached from the wheelchair. Narang and associates[75] reported that of 500 lower extremity amputees that they studied, 55% were totally independent in all self-care, 40% required only additional aids to independence for self-care, and 5% were confined to wheelchairs and/or not totally independent. Haworth[43] investigated the patterns of usage of aids to independence in 163 patients following total hip replacement. Findings suggested that aids were used only as long as needed for bathroom safety, dressing, and toileting and that patients discarded them when they could manage independently.

Upper and Lower Extremity Impairment

People with quadriparesis or quadriplegia from traumatic spinal cord injury, cerebral palsy, muscular dystrophy, multiple sclerosis, or amyotrophic lateral sclerosis, must rely on a wide range of options for self-care independence. In most cases there will be a need for attendant care, assistive devices, and modifications of living space. Such people often require high technology devices such as environmental controls, augmentative communications, and other microprocessor-based systems to be fully independent in their own home.[91] DeJong and colleagues[22] have reported that independence for patients with spinal cord injury is a complex and interdependent process in which severity of injury, transportation, education, marital status, and economic disincentives all play a role. A concerted effort to address such issues (including a broader definition of self-care training) appears to be needed to enable such patients to live more productively and in less restrictive environments.

Hemiparesis

Considerations of cognitive and perceptual deficits have been discussed earlier. Perhaps the most important finding that has been emerging recently is that the side of the lesion may predict a pattern of problems but does not predict self-care outcomes. Mills and DiGenio[70] compared 50 right hemispheric CVA patients to 52 left hemispheric CVA patients and found that there was no significant difference in ADL independence between the two groups. Wade and co-workers[108] studied 162 consecutive acute CVAs and found that neither sex nor side of weakness influenced functional recovery *per se* but that patients with left hemispheric CVA attended rehabilitation therapies longer so that they appeared to have made better functional gains at discharge.

The differences between left- and right-sided brain damage do not affect prognosis for self-care independence directly. Instead it appears that patients with left-sided brain damage are easier to train, receive more training, and progress more rapidly. Patients with right-sided damage tend to be more difficult to train, take longer to train, and tend to receive less training. The suggestion that cannot be ignored is that the attitudes and skills of therapists and the economics of medical rehabilitation may be biased toward those with left-sided brain damage. As Dudgeon and colleagues[26] have suggested, the availability of more sensitive tests to predict the patterns of self-care difficulties that may be encountered is needed. Therapists and physicians need to be aware of the implications of their decisions regarding intensity and duration of training for right- versus left-sided brain-damaged patients. They especially need to remember that both groups show gains over time in self-care and that the hospital discharge prognosis for ADL independence is not necessarily the long-term self-care prognosis.

Limitations in Joint Range of Motion

Problems of limited ROM that result in difficulty reaching common ADL items are best addressed by rearrangement of living space. As Urb'anek and co-workers[104] have shown, the home environment, both in its physical dimensions and with respect to support of the family, is significantly related to independence. A home visit by an occupational therapist or other health care provider can suggest safety equipment for the bathroom, removal of obstacles that could contribute to falls, and other adaptive devices that are needed. With respect to training, an emphasis on compensatory training regarding work simplification and energy conservation techniques is needed.

OUTCOME ISSUES

Self-Care Follow-up Studies

A number of follow-up studies have been conducted in an effort to determine the self-care or overall functional status of patients following discharge from medical rehabilitation programs. Because of the equivocal nature of some of the studies or the lack of

comparison among patients, settings, outcome criteria, and assessment methods, it is difficult to generalize results in a manner that provides useful information to practitioners or program planners. By far, the majority of these studies have involved patients who required rehabilitation for spinal cord injury or CVA.[4, 6, 44, 59]

Rogers and Figone[85] assessed the extent of use of self-care skills learned during rehabilitation as well as the orthotic devices provided to support function in 35 patients with traumatic cervical cord injury 1 to 4 years following discharge from a rehabilitation unit. They found that the level of self-care achieved during rehabilitation was maintained by the majority of patients at follow-up. Both improvement as well as regression in function occurred variably among the rehabilitants, reflecting a reordering of time and energy based on personal priorities and other situational factors. The authors suggested that disuse of skills, caused by mobility barriers to important places where skills are normally performed, such as bathrooms, might help explain some regression in function. Moreover, the authors questioned whether rehabilitation training goals of dressing independence for those with spinal cord injury at level C6–7 were realistic, given the impracticality of such activities for rehabilitants in community living.

In other research, Woolsey[115] studied the rehabilitation outcome of 100 patients with recent spinal cord injury. All patients with lesions at level C6 and below were able to attain functional goals of eating and drinking, grooming, and wheelchair mobility. Attainment of goals for bowel and bladder care, transfers to and from the wheelchair, and pressure sore relief were less successful at higher levels of injury.

In one of the few published follow-up studies that has considered medical, personal, and environmental factors in predicting independent living among people with spinal cord injury, DeJong and associates[22] found that the severity of a person's disability was not a significant predictor of living arrangement status. However, the presence of transportation barriers, educational and marital status, economic disincentives, the severity of disability as measured by the *Barthel Index,* and unmet occupational therapy needs explained 63% of the variance in independent living outcomes.

Carey and Posavac[14] described a study of the outcome of rehabilitation for 53 patients with a diagnosis of CVA. Eighty-three percent of the patients were termed "ADL program successes" because they improved during their hospitalization on ADL functions. The study found an apparent relationship between earlier admission and ADL improvement. Additionally, patients with left hemiplegia achieved less functional gain in ADL at discharge than right hemiplegics, which was attributed to the presence of perceptual sequelae. When a follow-up interview was conducted 18 weeks after discharge, patients living at home showed a small overall gain in ADL function but no difference between right and left hemiplegics was noted. Moreover, 75% of the patients perceived that they had made functional gains since discharge.

These findings were consistent with those of Anderson and colleagues,[5] who studied 250 patients 2 to 12 years following rehabilitation for stroke. Nearly two-thirds of the rehabilitants had progressed in rehabilitation status, 72% were generally independent in self-care, and 82% were ambulatory. A positive relationship was found between rehabilitation status at follow-up and living at home as well as having an accepting attitude toward their disability. These relationships were corroborated in a study by Sussett and colleagues[97] based on 475 subjects with varying diagnoses.

Collectively, data from outcome studies show that gains made during rehabilitation are retained and that in some cases independent functioning may increase. They also suggest the importance of early intervention as well as the value of discharge to a home setting where the patient has the support of understanding family members and friends. Motivational factors, environmental barriers, depression, and concomitant medical problems have been identified as factors mitigating against favorable outcomes in follow-up studies.

Costs and Benefits of Increasing Functional Independence

Johnston and Keith[48] have provided an excellent comprehensive overview of cost–benefit studies in medical rehabilitation with a number of diagnoses. Although many studies support the efficacy of programs for patients with spinal cord injury, some data suggest that patients with intermediate severity may show the most favorable ratio of functional improvement to cost. Cost-benefit studies of stroke rehabilitation are more equivocal, although, on balance, the evidence seems to support the value of rehabilitation in promoting functional independence and reducing the necessity for institutional care, at least for patients with stroke of lower to intermediate severity.[29, 62, 65]

If cost-effectiveness studies are to effectively guide the formulation of public policy, alternative approaches to care must be considered. Outpatient treatment, home health care services, and rehabilitation in day care and extended care facilities have all been shown to produce effective results in promoting functional independence for some patients at a cost that is less than care at traditional, institutionally based, comprehensive rehabilitation facilities.[41, 82, 100]

SUMMARY

Assessment and management strategies for promoting independence in self-care represent, from the patient's standpoint, one of the most practical and important aspects of medical rehabilitation. As a rehabilitation goal, independence in self-care has been approached all too frequently from the narrow perspective of the professional and the rehabilitation setting. In this chapter, we have presented a decision process for managing options in which the patient and the professional collaborate in determining goals and methods for managing these important life tasks following discharge. In this decision-making process, the patient's preferences, experiences, and postdischarge living environment assume at least as much importance as the diagnosis or physical limitations. Moreover, such factors as costs of time and energy must enter into decisions about the value of various options for independence.

These options include determining if the task is feasible, if retraining or new training is desirable, if the environment needs to be altered, if assistance needs to be provided through other people, or if adaptive equipment and devices, including high technology, may be useful.

Technological developments to permit independent function will continue to offer promise for the future. However, in the meantime, we feel confident that the participation of the patient in determining self-care goals will ultimately represent an equally important achievement in independent living.

REFERENCES

1. Aitken MJ: Self-concept and functional independence in the hospitalized elderly. Am J Occup Ther 36:243–250, 1982
2. Alexander JL, Fuhrer MJ: Functional assessment of individuals with physical impairments. In Halpern AS, Fuhrer MJ: Functional Assessment in Rehabilitation. Baltimore, Paul H. Brookes, 1984
3. American National Standards Institute (ANSI): Specifications for Making Buildings and Facilities Accessible to and Usable by Physically Handicapped People. New York, 1980
4. Anderson E, Anderson TP, Kottke FJ: Stroke rehabilitation: Maintenance of achieved gains. Arch Phys Med Rehabil 58:345–352, 1977
5. Anderson TP, Boureston N, Greenberg FR, Hilyard VG: Predictive factors in stroke rehabilitation. Arch Phys Med Rehabil 55:545–553, 1974
6. Andrews K, Brocklehurst JC, Richards B, Laycock PJ: The recovery of the severely disabled stroke patient. Rheumatol Rehabil 18:43–48, 1979
7. Anstine LA, Isaacs LI: Diagnostic, Predictive and Operational Significance of Self-Care (Dressing) Problems in Hemiplegia Rehabilitation. Boston, Boston University Medical Center University Hospital, 1971
8. Bartels EC: A contemporary framework for independent living rehabilitation. Rehabil Lit 46:325–327, 1985
9. Bishop DS, Baldwin LM, Epstein NB, Keitner G: Assessment of family functioning. In Halpern AS, Fuhrer MJ: Functional Assessment in Rehabilitation. Baltimore, Paul H. Brookes, 1984
10. Bjornby ER, Reinvang IR: Acquiring and maintaining self-care skills after stroke: The predictive value of apraxia. Scand J Rehabil Med 17:75–80, 1985
11. Brorsson B, Asberg KH: Katz index of independence in ADL: Reliability and validity in short-term care. Scand J Rehabil Med 16:125–132, 1984
12. Brown M, Gordon WA, Diller L: Rehabilitation indicators. In Halpern AS, Fuhrer MJ: Functional Assessment in Rehabilitation. Baltimore, Paul H Brookes, 1984
13. Burke JP: A clinical perspective on motivation: Pawn versus origin. Am J Occup Ther 31:254–258, 1977
14. Carey RG, Posavac EJ: Program evaluation of a physical medicine and rehabilitation unit: A new approach. Arch Phys Med Rehabil 59:330–337, 1978
15. Chiou IL, Burnett CN: Values of activities of daily living: A survey of stroke patients and their home therapists. Phys Ther 65:901–906, 1985
16. Coley IL: Pediatric Assessment of Self-Care Activities. St. Louis, CV Mosby, 1978
17. Colvin ME, Korn TL: Eliminating barriers to the disabled. Am J Occup Ther 38:748–753, 1984
18. Cross KW: Role of practice in perceptual-motor learning. Am J Phys Med 46:487–510, 1967
19. Decker SD, Schulz R: Correlates of life satisfaction and depression in middle-aged and elderly spinal-injured persons. Am J Occup Ther 39:740–745, 1985
20. DeJong G: Disability, home care, and relative responsibility: A legal perspective, p 43. Medford, MA, Tufts University Medical Rehabilitation Research and Training Center, 1978
21. DeJong G: Meeting the personal care needs of severely disabled citizens in Massachusetts: Report number two, p 239. Waltham, MA, Brandeis University Levinson Policy Distribution, 1977
22. DeJong G, Branch LG, Corcoran PJ: Independent living outcomes in spinal cord injury: Multivariate analyses. Arch Phys Med Rehabil 65:66–73, 1984
23. Deutsch CP, Goldston JA: Family factors in home adjustment of the severely disabled. Marriage Family Living: 312–316, 1960
24. DiJoseph LM: Independence through activity: Mind, body, and environment interaction in therapy. Am J Occup Ther 36:740–744, 1982
25. Donaldson SW, Wagner CC, Gresham GE: A unified ADL form. Arch Phys Med Rehabil 54:175–180, 1973
26. Dudgeon BJ, DeLisa JA, Miller RM: Optokinetic nystagmus and upper extremity dressing independence after stroke. Arch Phys Med Rehabil 66:164–167, 1985
27. Edgerton WM: Activities in occupational therapy. In Willard H, Spackman C (eds): Principles of Occupational Therapy. Philadelphia, JB Lippincott, 1954
28. Everett TH, Collignon FC: Cost and policy considerations in improving the capacity for independent living of the most severely handicapped. Berkeley, CA, Berkeley Planning Associates, 1975

29. Feigenson JS: Stroke rehabilitation: Effectiveness, benefits and cost: Some practical considerations. Stroke 10:1–4, 1979

30. Frank G: Life history model of adaptation to disability: The case of a congenital amputee. Soc Sci Med 19:639–645, 1984

31. Frey WD: Functional assessment in the 80s: A conceptual enigma, a technical challenge. In Halpern AS, Fuhrer MJ (eds): Functional Assessment in Rehabilitation. Baltimore, Paul H Brookes, 1984

32. Gibson CJ: Epidemiology and patterns of care of stroke patients. Arch Phys Med Rehabil 55:398–403, 1974

33. Goldkamp O: Treatment effectiveness in cerebral palsy. Arch Phys Med Rehabil 65:232–234, 1984

34. Gordon WA, Hibbard MR, Egelko S et al: Perceptual remediation in patients with right brain damage: A comprehensive program. Arch Phys Med Rehabil 66:353–359, 1985

35. Granger CV, Albrecht GL, Hamilton BB: Outcome of comprehensive medical rehabilitation: Measurement by Pulses Profile and the Barthel Index. Arch Phys Med Rehabil 60:145–154, 1979

36. Granger CV, Dewis LS, Peters NC et al: Stroke rehabilitation: Analysis of repeated Barthel index measures. Arch Phys Med Rehabil 60:14–17, 1979

37. Granger CV, Hamilton BB, Sherwin FS: Guide for Use of the Uniform Data Set for Medical Rehabilitation. Buffalo, NY, Uniform Data System for Medical Rehabilitation, 1986

38. Green BC, Pratt CC, Grigsby TE: Self-concept among persons with long-term spinal cord injury. Arch Phys Med Rehab 65:751–754, 1984

39. Gresham GE, Labi MLC: Functional assessment instruments currently available for documenting outcomes in rehabilitation medicine. In Granger CV, Gresham GE (eds): Functional Assessment in Rehabilitation Medicine. Baltimore, Williams & Wilkins, 1984

40. Guttman L: The basis of scalogram analysis. In Stouffer SA et al (eds): Measurement and Prediction. Princeton, NJ, Princeton University Press, 1950

41. Hammond J: Home health care cost effectiveness: Overview of literature. Public Health Rep 94:305–311, 1979

42. Hasselkus BR, Kiernat JM: Independent living for the elderly. Am J Occup Ther 27:181–188, 1973

43. Haworth RJ: Use of aids during the first three months after total hip replacement. Br J Rheumatol 22:29–25, 1983

44. Henley S, Pettit S, Todd-Pokropek A, Tupper A: Who goes home? Predictive factors in stroke recovery. J Neurol Neurosurg Psychiatry 48:1–6, 1985

45. Hertanu JS, Demopoulos JT, Yang WC et al: Stroke rehabilitation: Correlation and prognostic value of computerized tomography and sequential functional assessments. Arch Phys Med Rehabil 65:505–508, 1984

46. Jarman PH, Iwata BA, Lorentzson AM: Development of morning self-care routines in multiply handicapped persons. Appl Res Ment Retard 4:113–122, 1983

47. Jette AM: Health status indicators: Their utility in chronic disease evaluation research. J Chronic Dis 33:567–579, 1979

48. Johnston MV, Keith RA: Cost benefits of medical rehabilitation: Review and critique. Arch Phys Med Rehabil 64:147–154, 1983

49. Jones DA, Vetter NJ: A survey of those who care for the elderly and home: Their problems and their needs. Soc Sci Med 19:511–514, 1984

50. Katz S, Downs T, Cash H, Grotz R: Progress in development of the Index of ADL. Gerontologist 10:20–30, 1970

51. Katz S, Ford AB, Moskowitz RW et al: Studies of illness in the aged: The Index of ADL: A standardized measure of biological and psychosocial function. JAMA 185:914–919, 1963

52. Kaufert JM: Functional ability indices: Measurement problems in assessing their validity. Arch Phys Med Rehabil 64:260–267, 1983

53. Keith RA: Functional assessment measures in medical rehabilitation: Current status. Arch Phys Med Rehabil 65:74–78, 1984

54. Keith RA: Functional assessment in program evaluation for rehabilitation medicine. In Granger CV, Gresham GE (eds): Functional Assessment in Rehabilitation Medicine. Baltimore, Williams & Wilkins, 1984

55. Kelly CR, Rose DL: Grading the rehabilitation effort. J Kans Med Soc 72:154–156, 1971

56. Kelman HR, Willner A: Problems in measurement and evaluation of rehabilitation. Arch Phys Med Rehabil 43:172–181, 1962

57. Kielhofner G: Occupation. In Hopkins HL, Smith DH (eds): Willard and Spackman's Occupational Therapy, 6th ed. Philadelphia, JB Lippincott, 1983

58. Klein RM, Bell B: Self-care skills: Behavioral measurement with Klein-Bell ADL scale. Arch Phys Med Rehabil 63:335–338, 1982

59. Kotila M, Waltimo O, Niemi ML et al: The profile of recovery from stoke and factors influencing outcome. Stroke 15:1037–1044, 1984

60. Larson MR, Snobl DE: Attendant Care Manual. Marshall, MN, Southwest Minnesota State University, 1977

61. Lawton MP: The functional assessment of elderly people. J Am Geriatr Soc 14:465–481, 1971

62. Lehmann JF, Delateur BJ, Fowler RS Jr et al: Stroke: Does rehabilitation affect outcome? Arch Phys Med Rehabil 56:375–382, 1975

63. Levine RE: The cultural aspects of home care delivery. Am J Occup Ther 38:734–738, 1984

64. Liang MH, Gell V, Partridge A, Eaton H: Management of functional disability in homebound patients. J Fam Pract 17:429–435, 1983

65. Lind K: Synthesis of studies on stroke rehabilitation. J Chronic Dis 35:133–149, 1982

66. Lowman E, Klinger JL: Aids to Independent Living. New York, McGraw-Hill, 1969

67. Malick MH, Almasy B: Assessment and evaluation—life work tasks. In Hopkins HL, Smith HD: Willard and Spackman's Occupational Therapy, 6th ed, pp 189–205. Philadelphia, JB Lippincott, 1983

68. Mahoney FL, Barthel DW: Functional evaluation: The Barthel Index. Md St Med J 14:61–65, 1965

69. Malassigne PM et al: Design of bathrooms, bedroom fixtures and controls for the able bodied and disabled: Annual report. Blacksburg, Virginia Polytechnic Institute and State University College of Architecture and Urban Studies, 1977

70. Mills VM, DiGenio M: Functional differences in patients with left or right cerebrovascular accidents. Phys Ther 63:481–488, 1983

71. Morrione B: Hiring and supervising personal service providers: A guide. Richmond, Virginia Institute for Information Studies, 1980

72. Moskowitz E, Fuhn ER, Peters ME et al: Aged infirm residents in a custodial institution. JAMA 169:2009–2012, 1959

73. Moskowitz E, Lightbody FEH, Freitag NS: Long-term follow-up of the post stroke patient. Arch Phys Med Rehabil 53:167–172, 1972

74. Moskowitz E, McCann CB: Classification of disability in the chronically ill and aging. J Chronic Dis 5:342–346, 1957

75. Narang IC, Mathur BP, Singh P, Jape VS: Functional capabilities of lower limb amputees. Prosthet Orthot Int 8:43–41, 1984

76. Neill WA, Branch LG, DeJong G et al: Cardiac disability: The impact of coronary heart disease on patients daily activities. Arch Intern Med 145:1642–1647, 1985

77. Neistadt ME, Marques K: An independent living skills training program. Am J Occup Ther 38:671–676, 1984

78. Newrick PG, Langton-Hewer R: Motor neuron disease: Can we do better? A study of 42 patients. Br Med J (Clin Res) 289:539–542, 1984

79. O'Toole DMK, Goldberg RT, Ryan B: Functional changes in vascular amputee patients: Evaluation by Barthel Index, Pulses Profile and Escrow Scale. Arch Phys Med Rehabil 66:508–511, 1985

80. Panikoff LB: Recovery trends of functional skills in the head-injured adult. Am J Occup Ther 37:735–743, 1983

81. Parsons T: Definitions of health and illness in the light of American values and social structure. In Jaco EG (ed): Patients, Physicians and Illness, pp 165–187. Glencoe, IL, Free Press, 1958

82. Redford JB, Bronstrom A, Gough KM: Reactivation programs cut nursing care costs in extended care facilities. Dimens Health Serv 51:14–17, 1974

83. Rice FP: The adolescent: Development, relationships and culture, 2nd ed. Boston, Allyn & Bacon, 1978

84. Roberts S, Sydow N: Consumer's Guide to Attendant Care. Madison, Wisconsin, Access for Independence, 1981

85. Rogers JC, Figone JJ: Traumatic quadriplegia: Follow-up study of self-care skills. Arch Phys Med Rehabil 61:316–321, 1980

86. Rohrer K, Adelman B, Puckett J et al: Rehabilitation in spinal cord injury: Use of a patient–family group. Arch Phys Med Rehab 61:225–229, 1980

87. Schoening HA, Anderegg L, Bergstrom D et al: Numerical scoring of self-care status of patients. Arch Phys Med Rehabil 46:689–697, 1965

88. Schoening HA, Iversen IA: Numerical scoring of self-care status: A

study of the Kenny self-care evaluation. Arch Phys Med Rehabil 49:221–229, 1968

89. Schwartz RK: Therapy as Learning. Dubuque, IA, Kendall-Hunt, 1985

90. Schwartz RK, Tynan MP: The Freedom Center. San Antonio, University of Texas Health Science Center, 1985

91. Seplowitz C: Technology and occupational therapy in the rehabilitation of the bedridden quadriplegic. Am J Occup Ther 38:743–747, 1984

92. Shillam LL, Beeman C, Loshin PM: Effects of occupational therapy intervention on bathing independence of disabled persons. Am J Occup Ther 37:744–748, 1983

93. Slatter SB, Sussman MB, Stroud MW: Participation in household activities as prognostic factor for rehabilitation. Arch Phys Med Rehab 50:605–610, 1970

94. Spencer EA: Functional restoration—theory, principles and techniques. In Hopkins HL, Smith HD: Willard and Spackman's Occupational Therapy, 6th ed. Philadelphia, JB Lippincott, 1983

95. Stein RB, Walley M: Functional comparison of upper extremity amputees using myoelectric and conventional prostheses. Arch Phys Med Rehabil 64:2443–2448, 1983

96. Steinhauer MJ: Nationally speaking-occupational therapy and home health care. Am J Occup Ther 38:715–716, 1984

97 Susset V, Vobecky J, Black R: Disability outcome and self-assessment of disabled persons: An analysis of 506 cases. Arch Phys Med Rehabil 60:50–56, 1979

98. Switzer ME: Foreward. In Rehabilitation of the Physically Handicapped in Homemaking Activities: Proceedings of a Workshop, Highland Park, IL. US Department of Health, Education and Welfare, 1963

99. Symington DC et al: Independence through environmental control systems. Canada, Canadian Rehabilitation Council for the Disabled, 1980

100. Tamura H, Lauer LW, Sanborn FA: Estimating "reasonable cost" of Medicaid patient care using a patient-mix index. Health Serv Res 20:27–42, 1985

101. Taylor SJ, Trefler E, Nwaobi O: Occupational therapy and rehabilitation engineering: Delivering technology to the severely physically disabled. Occup Ther Health Care 1:143–154, 1984

102. Trombly CA: Activities of daily living. In Trombly CA (ed.): Occupational Therapy for Physical Dysfunction, 2nd ed. Baltimore, Williams & Wilkins, 1984

103. Tsai LJ, Howe RH, Lien IN: Visuospatial deficits in stroke patients and their relationship to dressing performance. Taiwan I Hsueh Hui Tsa Chih 82:353–359, 1983

104. Urb'anek T, Si'tajov'a H, Hud'akov'a G: Problems of rheumatoid arthritis and ankylosing spondylitis patients in their labor and life environments. Czech Med 7:78–89, 1984

105. Vash CL: Evaluation from the client's point of view. In Halpern AS, Fuhrer MJ: Functional Assessment in Rehabilitation. Baltimore, Paul H. Brookes, 1984

106. Virginia Polytechnic Institute and State University College of Architecture and Urban Studies: Design of Bathrooms, Bathroom Fixtures and Controls for the Able Bodied and Disabled: Final Report. Blackburg, 1980

107. Wade DT, Skilbeck CE, Hewer RL: Predicting Barthel ADL score at six months after an acute stroke. Arch Phys Med Rehabil 64:24–28, 1983

108. Wade DT, Hewer RL, Wood VA: Stroke: Influence of patient's sex and side of weakness on outcome. Arch Phys Med Rehabil 65:513–516, 1984

109. Wade DT, Wood VA, Hewer RL: Recovery after stroke—the first 3 months. J Neurosurg Psychiatry 48:7–13, 1985

110. Walker RI, Vogelsberg RT: Increasing independent mobility skills for a woman who was severely handicapped and nonambulatory. Appl Res Ment Retard 6:173–183, 1985

111. Weinberg N: Physically disabled people assess the quality of their lives. Rehab Lit 45:12–15, 1984

112. White RW: Motivation reconsidered: The concept of competence. Psychol Rev 66:297–333, 1959

113. Wiemer RB, West WL: Occupational therapy in community health care. Am J Occup Ther 24:323–328, 1970

114. Williams GH: The movement for independent living: An evaluation and critique. Soc Sci Med 17:1003–1010, 1983

115. Woolsey RM: Rehabilitation outcome following spinal cord injury. Arch Neurol 42:116–119, 1985

116. World Health Organization: International classification of impairments, disabilities and handicaps. Geneva, 1980

117. Wylie CM, White BK: A measure of disability. Arch Environ Health 8:834–839, 1964

118. Zimmerman ME: Occupational Therapy in the ADL program. In Willard HS, Spackman CS (eds): Occupational Therapy, 3rd ed. Philadelphia, JB Lippincott, 1963

119. Zimmerman ME: Homemaking training units for rehabilitation centers. Am J Occup Ther 20:226–235, 1966

120. Zisserman L: The modern family and rehabilitation of the handicapped: A macrosociological view. Am J Occup Ther 35:14–20, 1981

6

Speech, Language, Swallowing, and Auditory Rehabilitation

Robert M. Miller

Michael E. Groher

Kathryn M. Yorkston

Thomas S. Rees

Speech and language are dynamic, multidimensional behaviors that are constantly influenced by physiological, psychological, and environmental factors. Speech uses anatomical structures and physiological reflexes that are common to both respiration and swallowing. Language is intimately related to cognition and the integration of sensory modalities, most commonly the auditory sense. Because of the complexity of human communication, a number of specialists are involved in studying and treating components of these communication behaviors and the disease states that impair their function.

An introduction to the processes of human communication, a description of disorders that are recognized at each level of the process, and a rationale for the evaluation and rehabilitation procedures that are employed for each condition are presented in this chapter. Because of the complexity of these behaviors, the discussion is limited to the major areas of acquired dysfunction found in an adult population. The major divisions include (1) normal processes for human speech and language, (2) motor speech disorders, (3) laryngectomee rehabilitation, (3) language and intellectual disorders, (4) swallowing evaluation and management, and (5) auditory evaluation and the management of hearing loss.

NORMAL PROCESSES

The process of human speech is accomplished through the systems of cerebration, respiration, phonation, and articulation. Neural organization by the brain programs and sequences the physical processes. The resonating cavities of the pharynx, mouth, and nose influence the acoustic product.

Respiration. Two forms of respiration are recognized: chemical and mechanical. Chemical respiration is concerned with the exchange of oxygen and carbon dioxide to and from the blood while mechanical respiration is concerned with the movement of tidal air in and out of the lungs. The expiration of air through the vocal mechanism, the larynx, is the "power plant" for audible speech. Inhalation is an active process that is accomplished by the contraction of the diaphragm, which increases the vertical diameter of the thorax. The decrease in pressure within the thoracic cavity allows air to flow into the lungs. Other notable muscles of inhalation are the costal elevators, serratus muscles, and certain muscles of the neck and back that elevate the ribs.

Unlike inhalation, exhalation is more passive. Tissue elasticity and gravity contribute to this act as the diaphragm returns to its relaxed position. The abdominal muscles and intercostals can provide force to exhalation or help to control prolonged exhalation for speech.

Phonation. Energy, in the form of exhaled air, passes from the lungs into the subglottic region where the vocal cords are capable of modifying the air stream. Complete closure can result in a Valsalva effect, whereas close approximation increases subglottic pressure and creates a vibratory separation–apposition cycle that results in audible sound energy or voice production. Vocal intensity is increased by raising the level of subglottic pressure. Higher pitch is achieved primarily by increasing the length and tension of the vocal cords and by increasing subglottic air pressure and elevating the larynx. A normal voice is therefore the product of a controlled exhalation of air, steady maintenance of subglottic air pressures, and delicately balanced vocal cords capable of producing regular air pulsations.

Resonation. The raw vocal tone is modified and amplified by resonation within the pharyngeal, oral, and nasal cavities, which are referred to collectively as the vocal tract. The shape of the vocal tract is altered by changing the tension of the pharyngeal walls, by raising or depressing the larynx, by modifying the position of the jaw, tongue, and lips, and by occluding or lowering the soft palate. The innumerable configurations of vocal tract shape provide the human voice with a tremendous variety of potential qualities.

Articulation. The physical event that lends meaning to the resonating voice is articulation. The coordinated action of the tongue, lips, jaw, and soft palate produce the meaningful sounds of speech called phonemes. These organs may shape the vocal tract to produce vowels or voiced consonants, or they may relax, compress, or momentarily stop the air stream as it passes through the oral cavity to produce unvoiced consonants.

Cerebration. Thought transformed into symbols and communicated by speech, writing, or gestural sign is considered language. A broad area of associational cortex in the left hemisphere of the brain is responsible for the symbolization of our thoughts into words or language. The words are organized into a meaningful arrangement, called grammar or syntax, and eventually transmitted either through the physical efforts previously described for speech or by gesture or writing. The brain, more specifically the left frontal cortex, is responsible for organizing and patterning the muscle actions of respiration, phonation, and articulation in order to produce recognizable speech.

COMMUNICATION PATHOLOGY

A pathological condition that affects any organ involved in the process of speech or language influences the final product en mass. At times the pathology is limited to a single speech or language organ and the dysfunction can be detected in only one component of the process (*e.g.,* an isolated voice or articulation impairment). More commonly, however, the pathology of a single organ influences other elements of the communication process in ways that are predictable considering the integrated nature of speech and language. For example, severe obstructive pulmonary disease does not just impair the respiratory support for speech, but one can also detect alterations in vocal pitch, vocal intensity, and phrasing modifications owing to compensations for an impaired ability to sustain air flow. Certain disease states, involving organs that are not directly involved in speech or language, can affect the final communication product in a more diffuse manner. Some endocrine disorders, such as hypothyroidism, can influence voice quality as an isolated component of speech and also lead to language confusion and impaired memory. Considering the complexity and interactive nature of the speech and language processes, whenever one evaluates or treats a patient with a communication disorder, some consideration must be given to overall human physiology as well as the dynamic speech and language systems.

Dysarthria

Definitions and Differential Diagnosis

The dysarthrias are a group of motor speech disorders characterized by slow, weak, imprecise, and/or uncoordinated movements of speech musculature. Rather than a single neurological disorder, the dysarthrias vary along a number of dimensions. The neuroanatomical site of lesion can be either the central or peripheral nervous system or both, including the cerebrum, cerebellum, brain stem, and cranial nerves. One or a combination of pathophysiological processes may be involved, including spasticity, flaccidity, ataxia, tremor, rigidity, and chorea. A number of diagnoses may be associated with dysarthria, including cerebral palsy, parkinsonism, multiple sclerosis, amyotrophic lateral sclerosis, brain stem stroke, and bilateral cortical strokes. All or several speech subsystems may be involved to varying degrees, including the respiratory, phonatory, velopharyngeal, and oral articulatory subsystems.

As a first step, differential diagnosis involves distinguishing the dysarthrias from other neurogenic communication disorders. The dysarthrias are distinct from aphasia in that language function (word retrieval, and comprehension of both verbal and written language) is preserved in dysarthria but impaired in aphasia. Although both apraxia and dysarthria are considered motor speech disorders, they can be distinguished on the basis of several clinical features. In apraxia, automatic (nonspeech) movements are intact, while in dysarthria they are not. Highly

consistent articulatory errors are characteristic of dysarthria while inconsistent errors are a hallmark of apraxia. Finally, in most dysarthrias, all speech subsystems (including respiration and phonation) are involved; in apraxia, respiratory or phonatory involvement is rare. It should be recognized that patients can have elements of both dysarthria and apraxia, particularly those with bilateral brain damage.

Differential diagnosis among the dysarthrias is an area that has received more systematic attention than any other aspect of the disorder. Information related to the various dysarthrias is summarized in Table 6-1.[60] In studies carried out at the Mayo Clinic the perceptual features of the speech of seven groups of dysarthric patients were examined.[15, 16] These groups contained patients who were unequivocally diagnosed as having one of the following conditions: pseudobulbar palsy, bulbar palsy, amyotrophic lateral sclerosis, cerebellar lesions, parkinsonism, dystonia, and choreoathetosis. Speech samples were rated along 38 dimensions, which described pitch characteristics, loudness, vocal quality, respiration, prosody, articulation, and general impression dimensions. Results of this study indicated that each of the seven neurological disorders could be characterized by a unique set of clusters of deviant speech dimensions and that no two disorders had the same set of clusters. Thus, differential diagnosis among the dysarthrias can be made in part on the basis that one type of dysarthria sounds different from others. However, single features, such as imprecise consonants or nasal emission, may not be sufficient to distinguish one type of dysarthria from another. Instead, differential diagnosis is made on the basis of clusters of features reflecting underlying pathophysiology and the examination of the musculature. The following are perceptual descriptions of the unique features of selected types of dysarthria:[14]

Pseudobulbar Palsy.   Speech is slow and labored, the articulation is rather consistently imprecise, especially on more complicated groups of consonant sounds. Pitch is low and monotonous. Voice quality is harsh and often strained or strangled.

Bulbar Palsy.   Hypernasality is associated with nasal emission of air during speech. Inhalation is often audible and exhalation breathy. Air wastage is manifest in shortness of phrases. Articulation is often imprecise because (1) consonants may be weak through failure to impound sufficient intraoral breath pressure due to velopharyngeal incompetence and/or (2) there may be immobility of tongue and lips due to impairment of the hypoglossal and facial nerves, which prevents normal production of vowels and consonants.

Amyotrophic Lateral Sclerosis.   The combined spastic and flaccid dysarthria in this disorder causes progressive deterioration of speech. In an earlier stage, either spastic or flaccid speech and nonspeech signs predominate; in an advanced stage, both sets of features described above are present. Slow rate, low pitch, hoarse and strained-strangled quality, highly defective articulation, marked hypernasality, and nasal emission combine to make the speaker struggle to produce short, barely intelligible phrases.

Cerebellar Disorders.   In ataxic dysarthria one of the following patterns may appear: (1) intermittent disintegration of articulation, together with dysrhythmia and irregularities of pitch and loudness in performing tests of oral diadochokinetic rate; and (2) altered prosody, involving prolongation of sounds, equalization of syllabic stress (by undue stress on usually unstressed words and syllables), and prolongation of intervals between syllables and words.

Table 6-1
*Summary of the Etiologies, Neuropathologies, and Neuromuscular Deficits
Characteristic of the Common Dysarthrias*

Type	Example	Location of Neuropathology	Neuromuscular Deficit
Flaccid	Bulbar palsy	Lower motor neuron	Muscular weakness; hypotonia
Spastic	Pseudobulbar palsy	Upper motor neuron	Reduced range, force, speed; hypertonia
Ataxic	Cerebellar ataxia	Cerebellum (or tracts)	Hypotonia; reduced speed; inaccurate range, timing, direction
Hypokinetic	Parkinsonism	Extrapyramidal system	Markedly reduced range; variable speed of repetitive movements; movement arrests; rigidity
Hyperkinetic			
Quick	Chorea Myoclonus Gilles de la Tourett's syndrome	Extrapyramidal system	Quick, unsustained, random, involuntary movements
Slow	Athetosis Dyskinesias Dystonia	Extrapyramidal system	Sustained, distorted movements and postures; slowness; variable hypertonus
Tremors	Organic voice tremor	Extrapyramidal system	Involuntary, rhythmic, purposeless, oscillatory movements
Mixed	Amyotrophic lateral sclerosis Multiple sclerosis Wilson's disease	Multiple motor systems	Muscular weakness, limited range and speed

(Adapted from Rosenbek JC, LaPointe LL: The dysarthrias: Description, diagnosis and treatment. In Johns DF [ed]: Clinical Management of Neurogenic Communication Disorders, pp 97–152. Boston, Little, Brown & Co, 1985)

Parkinsonism. In hypokinetic dysarthria, vocal emphasis, peaks and valleys of pitch, and variations of loudness are flattened, resulting in monotony. Short rushes of speech are separated by illogically placed pauses, the rate being variable and often accelerated. Consonant articulation in contextual speech and syllable repetition is blurred as muscles fail to go through their complete excursion. Difficulty initiating articulation is shown by repetition of initial sounds and inappropriate silences. The voice is often breathy, and loudness is reduced, at times to inaudibility.

Dystonia. Involuntary body and facial movements cause unpredictable voice stoppages, disintegration of articulation, excessive variations of loudness, and distortion of vowels. Perhaps in anticipation of these interruptions, normal prosody is altered by slowing of rate, reduction in variations of pitch and loudness, prolongation of interword intervals, and interposition of inappropriate silences.

Choreathetosis. The involuntary movements that alter the normal breathing cycle result in sudden exhalatory gusts of breath, bursts of loudness, elevations of pitch, and disintegration of articulation. The overall loudness level may be increased. Anticipated breakdowns are managed by varying the rate, introducing and prolonging pauses, and equalizing stress on all syllables and words.

Assessment of the Dysarthrias

Wood distinguished between the terms *impairment* and *disability* when describing chronic disorders.[75] Impairment re-

fers to "any loss or abnormality of psychological, physiological, or anatomical structure or function." Disability, on the other hand, refers to "any restriction or lack (resulting from impairment) of the ability to perform any activity in the manner or within the range considered normal for the human being." When considering a dysarthric speaker, the impairment would include the movement deficits seen in the respiratory, phonatory, velopharyngeal, and oral articulatory subsystems. The disability resulting from the motor speech impairment is characterized by reduced speech intelligibility, rate, and naturalness. When assessing a dysarthric speaker both the impairment and the overall disability must be considered.

ASSESSING THE IMPAIRMENT. During the assessment of the impairment, focus is placed on the speech production process. The clinician seeks to understand how the weakness, slowness, discoordination, or abnormal tone of the speech musculature has influenced points or places along the speech mechanism, including respiratory, phonatory, velopharyngeal, or oral articulatory subsystems.[51] A number of perceptual or instrumental tools are available for measuring speech performance. The perceptual tools are those that rely on the trained eyes and ears of the clinician while instrumental approaches to assessment include devices that provide information about the acoustic, aerodynamic movement, or myoelectric aspects of speech. Before proceeding with a more detailed description of the assessment of the various speech subsystems, a word of caution is warranted. Viewing speech as a series of isolated points or components would seriously oversimplify a complex process. In dysarthria, the impairment is almost never restricted to a single dimension. Rather, impairments of varying levels of severity may occur at numerous points, all of which are interdependent. For example, consider the function of the muscles and structures of respiration as a pump to provide breath support for speech. The adequacy of respiratory support may be influenced by the efficiency of all of the "upstream" valves. For example, inadequate laryngeal, velopharyngeal, or oral articulatory valving interacts with poor respiratory support to create a cumulative negative effect.

Assessment of the respiratory subsystem begins with perceptual measures including ratings of the number of words produced per breath and the loudness of samples of connected speech or visual observations of the presence of clavicular breathing. Instrumental approaches to the measurement of respiratory function may include acoustic measures of vocal intensity and utterance durations. Aerodynamically, respiratory performance may be assessed by estimating the subglottal air pressure generated by the speaker.[36, 52] Respiratory inductive plethysmography (commercially available as the Respitrace) is an instrumental means of obtaining information about the movements of the rib cage and abdomen during breathing and speech.

Assessment of the phonatory or laryngeal subsystem typically begins with perceptual ratings of pitch characteristics (pitch level, pitch breaks, monopitch, voice tremor), loudness (monoloudness, excess loudness, and variation of volume), and voice quality (harsh voice, hoarseness, wet voice, breathiness, and strained-strangled voice). Acoustically, vocal fundamental frequency and intensity can be measured in the clinical setting. Aerodynamically, measures of laryngeal resistance can be obtained.[68]

Assessment of the velopharyngeal mechanism can be made with perceptual judgments of hypernasality or occurrence of nasal air emission. Nasalization also can be measured acoustically. Precise inferences can be made about the timing of velopharyngeal closure by obtaining simultaneous aerodynamic measures of air pressure and air flow during selected speech samples.[34] Movement of the velopharyngeal mechanism can be observed through cineradiographic techniques.

Assessment of oral articulation can be made perceptually by rating consonant and vowel precision. Although movements also can be inferred using cineradiographic technique and myoelectric activity with EMG recordings, these techniques are not used in routine clinical practice.

ASSESSMENT OF THE DISABILITY. The overall speech disability observed in dysarthric speakers may be characterized by abnormalities in speech intelligibility, rate, and naturalness. Of these measures of disability, intelligibility has received the most attention in the clinical literature for a number of reasons. First, measures of speech intelligibility when accompanied by measures of speaking rate provide a useful index of the severity of the disorder. Second, reduced speech intelligibility and speaking rate is a nearly universal characteristic of dysarthria, regardless of the underlying neuromotor impairment. Finally, intelligibility appears to be closely related to other aspects of the impairment, including measures of information conveyed,[5] movement rates, sounds produced recognizably, and judgments of speech handicap.[57, 58]

Despite the importance of intelligibility, care must be taken when clinically measuring this aspect of dysarthria. Research literature contains numerous examples of how intelligibility scores can be changed depending on the speakers' task, the transmission system, and the judges' task.[77, 79] Standard tools are available for measuring sentence and single word intelligibility and speaking rate using reading or imitation tasks.[79] These measures are used clinically as an index of severity of the disability in order to monitor change over time, and as a measure of the effectiveness of specific intervention techniques such as rate control or palatal lift fitting.

Treatment Considerations

Decisions about the management of dysarthric speakers are twofold. The first level involves the most general decisions about goals of treatment, and the second involves the selection of specific treatment approaches in order to achieve those goals. General goals of treatment vary with the severity of the disability and with the natural course of the disorder.[78]

For severely involved speakers, whose intelligibility is so poor that they are unable to communicate verbally in some or all situations, the general goal of treatment involves establishing a functional means of communication using augmentative approaches. The term *communication augmentation* refers to any device designed to augment, supplement, or replace verbal communication for someone who is not an independent verbal communicator. Systems range from communication boards and books to computer-based systems that employ speech synthesis.[6] The selection of an appropriate augmentation system necessitates a thorough evaluation of the person's communication needs. These needs may vary considerably since some people need a system for survival communication while others manage basic communication well but need assistance in education or vocational communication. Concurrent with the needs assessment, physical and cognitive capabilities are assessed. This assessment tests cognition, language, memory, physical control, vision, and hearing. Due to the person's limited response options, these tests must be carefully selected or modified for the individual. Once the capabilities have been ascertained, system components can be selected and an appropriate system developed.

For those moderately involved speakers who are able to use speech as their sole means of communication, but who are not completely intelligible, the general goal of treatment involves maximizing intelligibility. The term *compensated intelligibility*[60] aptly describes the goal of this phase of intervention. Achieving compensated intelligibility may take a variety of forms depending on the speaker and the nature of the underlying impairment. For example, it may include an effort to control speaking rate for some people with coordination problems.[76] It may also involve prosthetically managing a severely impaired velopharyngeal mechanism through the use of a palatal lift.[25] A palatal lift is a dental retainer with a shelf attached to elevate the soft palate to the height necessary to reduce hypernasality and nasal air emission. An appropriately fitted palatal lift will allow certain dysarthric speakers to better produce speech sounds that require the build up of oral air pressure, such as \p\, \t\, and \d\. In other cases, maximizing intelligibility involves teaching dysarthric speakers to emphasize speech sounds in the final position of words, to control the number of words per breath, and to stress important words in a sentence.

For the mildly involved dysarthric speaker, whose speech is characterized as intelligible but less efficient and less natural than normal, treatment planning must first determine whether there is a handicap. For some speakers, these mild reductions in speech efficiency pose no problems. However, for other mildly involved speakers, treatment is warranted. The general goals of treatment for dysarthric people with mild disabilities include maximizing communication efficiency while maintaining intelligibility and maximizing speech naturalness. Maximizing naturalness is accomplished by teaching appropriate phrasing, stressing patterning and intonation.

Treatment approaches for patients with progressive disorders such as parkinsonism, multiple sclerosis, and amyotrophic lateral sclerosis are different from those used with the recovering dysarthric speaker. Initially, the patients are encouraged to maximize the functional communication level by paying specific attention to the clarity and precision of their speech. At some point, the patients will need to modify their speaking patterns by controlling rate and consonant emphasis and reducing the number of words per breath. Some patients with progressive dysarthria make the adjustment in their speech pattern without specific treatment; others may need to practice these modifications with a speech pathologist or trained family member before the changes become habitual. In severe cases, a communication augmentation system may be considered. These systems usually are chosen or designed to accommodate the life-style of the patient while serving their communication needs over the longest period of time.

Laryngectomee Rehabilitation

Cancer of the larynx may be treated by a single treatment modality or a combination of modalities. Surgery, irradiation, and chemotherapy are all used to treat this condition, and the decision may be made on the basis of the extent of the tumor, the presence of diseased lymph nodes, and the general health of the patient including vitality of specific organs and physiological systems. Even within the surgical modality several options are available. In general terms, some tumors that are limited to the region above the glottis may be treated by supraglottic laryngectomy, lesions lateralized to one side may be treated with hemilaryngectomy, and tumors that involve the glottic area with one mobile arytenoid may be dealt with by a subtotal laryngectomy.[56] In each of these conservation operations the patient's laryngeal tumor is removed yet voice is maintained. Postoperative rehabilitation usually centers more on training compensations for swallowing than voice restoration.

Total laryngectomy remains a common procedure for the treatment of laryngeal cancer. In addition to the obvious need for speech rehabilitation, these patients require education regarding tracheostoma care and adjustment to tracheostoma breathing. For example, the patient must adjust to the relatively dry air entering the lungs without benefit of mucosal humidification from the nose, mouth, and pharynx. Humidifiers and moist stomal covers often are required to prevent crusting and the formation of mucus plugs, especially in the first few postoperative months. Shower bibs, neck wear, and stoma filters may be obtained to assist the patient in adjusting to neck breathing and the changes in appearance.

Speech Options

There are several options available to patients for speaking. External prosthetic devices, specifically electrolarynxes and pneumatic external reeds, offer most patients an opportunity to speak within days following surgery. A tracheal-esophageal puncture (TEP) with insertion of a small one-way valved prosthesis enables some laryngectomees to produce esophageal vibratory voice. A third option, which is satisfactorily attained by a relatively small percentage of patients, is learned esophageal speech.

ELECTROLARYNX. Commercially available electrolarynxes are designed to introduce vibratory sound either directly into the oral cavity via a catheter or indirectly through the neck tissues. In each case, the tone resonates within the oral and pharyngeal cavities and is modified by the dynamic process of articulation to form audible, intelligible words. Often an intraoral electrolarynx can be used within 2 or 3 days following surgery

and provides the patient with a means of communication. Speech therapy that is begun early can prevent the problem of trismus that is so common in head and neck surgical patients who do not use their jaw muscles in speech or mastication for almost 2 weeks after surgery. Intraoral devices can be used long term for patients with necks that are unsuitable for sound transmission, usually because of pain, edema, or scar tissue. Experience suggests that good speech is slower to develop using an intraoral device; therefore, one must be careful to help the patient avoid early frustration associated with not being immediately understood. Although most electrolarynxes designed for neck placement can be easily converted for intraoral use, they are intended to transmit the vibration through the submandibular or neck tissue into the oral and pharyngeal cavities. Patients usually can begin to use neck-held instruments when they are allowed to take nutrition by mouth. In patients with a suitable neck, intelligible speech can be achieved after one or two practice sessions.

PNEUMATIC REEDS. Another type of external voice prosthesis is the pneumatic reed. This device is placed over the tracheostoma to allow exhaled air to pass across a reed to produce a tone that is carried into the mouth much like an intraoral electrolarynx. Although these devices are inexpensive and capable of producing a "pleasant" quality of voice, they are somewhat cumbersome and conspicuous to use and have not gained wide popularity.

TRACHEAL-ESOPHAGEAL PUNCTURE (TEP). TEP procedures have been used since 1980 as a relatively simple procedure for voice restoration.[64] The TEP can be performed either as a primary procedure at laryngectomy[32] or almost any time during the postoperative period. A small one-way valved voice prosthesis is inserted through the TEP (Fig. 6-1) to allow the

Figure 6-1. A one-way valved voice prosthesis can be placed in a surgically created tracheal-esophageal fistula to allow pulmonary air to be shunted into the esophagus for esophageal voice production.

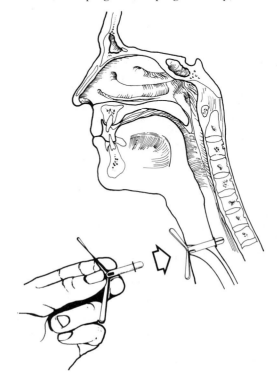

patient to shunt pulmonary air into the esophagus without having esophageal contents enter the TEP. Air passing through the prosthesis and up the esophagus vibrates the pharyngoesophageal segment to produce an esophageal voice. The prosthesis is not the source of the voice, however, the speech outcome is dependent on the size and the design of the prosthesis chosen for the patient. Early speech success following TEP and voice prosthesis fitting has been reported at almost 90%,[65, 73] with reports of long-term success (follow-up from 1 to 3½ years) at between 64% and 83%.[66, 74] Success is largely dependent on patient selection, and in some cases success can be enhanced by surgical techniques such as pharyngeal plexus neurectomy or cricopharyngeal myotomy performed to prevent a pharyngoesophageal segment spasm.[67] Other factors to consider in patient selection are motivation, intellect, dexterity, eyesight, stoma size and sensitivity, hand hygiene, surgical risk, and cost.

ESOPHAGEAL SPEECH. Esophageal speech is accomplished by training the patient to move air from the oral and pharyngeal cavities into the esophagus by injection or suction methods, to hold the air in this esophageal reservoir, and then to release it in a controlled manner through the pharyngoesophageal segment. This method of voice production uses the same anatomical vibratory site as the TEP technique but is accomplished without the necessity of occluding the tracheostoma. Since the volume of air maintained in the esophagus is much less than the pulmonary capacity used by the TEP speaker, the reservoir must be constantly replenished. Many accomplished esophageal speakers can speak clearly and effortlessly; however, up to 75% of laryngectomy patients are unable to learn this technique.[24, 61] Failure may be due to pharyngoesophageal segment tightness, scarring, nerve damage, or learning disorders.

Language Disturbance

An understanding of the mechanisms responsible for the processing and formulation of language is critical to good rehabilitation practice. Success in rehabilitation is dependent on a patient learning a new skill. Learning this new skill is dependent on how well the clinician and patient communicate. The success of this interaction is crucial to the speed, efficiency, and retention of newly learned behavioral patterns. Loss or disruption of available learning (communication) input and output modalities can impede this process unless compensations are made. The necessary compensations are achieved with an understanding of how to assess the patient's language strengths and weaknesses and how these modalities compare with nonlanguage learning modalities. A description of the learning strengths and liabilities of patients with those language disorders frequently associated with cortical and subcortical disease, both focal and diffuse, is presented in this section.

Aphasia

Aphasia is a disorder of both the expression and reception of propositional language secondary to cortical or subcortical disease, usually in the left hemisphere. It interferes with the ability to manipulate the meaning (semantics) and/or order (syntax) of words and gesture. There are three important points to emphasize in this definition.

First, use of the term *aphasia* implies there is impairment in both receptive and expressive language modalities. Expression may be more severely involved than reception, while reception appears grossly intact. However, if the testing instrument is sensitive to subtle change in language behavior, pathology can be identified in the more intact modality. Second, aphasia, by itself, is consistent only with focal (usually left hemisphere) disease. Aphasic symptoms may be part of diffuse pathology; however, these patients evidence more than disruptions in their ability to manipulate linguistic symbols, such as disorientation. Prognosis and recovery for this group is markedly different from those who evidence aphasia alone. And finally, while it is well known that aphasic disturbances primarily are a consequence of cortical disease, identification and classification of more atypical aphasic syndromes are now associated with subcortical infarction and hemorrhage.

LANGUAGE CHARACTERISTICS. Comprehension impairment of spoken language includes deficits of auditory perception and auditory retention. Auditory imperceptions are characterized by a tendency to confuse words that are similar in either meaning or sound. These confusions create a distorted message resulting in errors of comprehension. Most aphasics will experience more errors in comprehension as the length of the auditory input increases. In general, the speed of auditory input, combined with increased length, leads to errors in auditory retention. Additionally, sentence length predisposes a more difficult syntax and vocabulary, interacting to make comprehension more liable to error. It has been demonstrated that some aphasics retain more information from the beginning of an utterance, while others retain information from the end.[9] Evaluation of this aspect of the patient's auditory capacity is especially important if rehabilitation is to succeed. Deficits in the comprehension of graphic material (reading) also are impaired. The impairment often is more pronounced than the severity level of linguistic deficits in other modalities.

Expressively, patients might evidence anomia, agrammatism, paragrammatism, or paraphasias or produce jargon, stereotypic, or echolalic language patterns. Although most aphasics display an overall reduction in word classes available for production, they show particular deficits in the retrieval of nouns (anomia). Because nouns carry a large part of the meaning during an intended message, the language of the anomic patient is described as "empty" since sentences often lack a subject or referent. In their attempts to retrieve words, aphasics make "paraphasic" language errors. When the substitution for the intended word is from the same word class, such as "chair" for "table," it is a "semantic paraphasia." The substitution of like sounds or syllables, such as "flair" for "chair" is classified as a "phonemic paraphasia." A final class of paraphasic error is the "neologism." These productions are words that are attempts at the target that bear no phonemic or semantic relationship to that target, such as "I want to brush my ploker." Patients who find word retrieval difficult, but who do not produce paraphasic language errors in their search for the intended word, often "circumlocute," or talk around the intended noun, such as "I wear it on my wrist" instead of "watch."

"Agrammatism" is a form of expressive deficit characterized by reliance on nouns and verbs (content words) to the exclusion of articles, verb auxiliaries, pronouns, and prepositions (function words). Agrammatic productions often are described as telegraphic. "Paragrammatic" language is characterized by a misuse, rather than an omission of grammatical elements.

Patients whose expressive output is largely incomprehensible, even though the utterance is well articulated and excessive (press for speech), display a form of expressive deficit called "jargon." Concentrations of neologisms are called "neologistic jargon" and may be associated with stereotypes such as "blam, blam, blam" substituted for all attempts at verbalization. A preponderance of unrelated semantic paraphasias is "semantic jargon." Finally, some patients evidence "echolalia" typified by the patient echoing in response the same utterance he or she has just heard.

Expressive graphic output usually is impaired in aphasia, as is the ability to use gestures as a substitute form of expression.[22] A summary of the terminology used to describe expressive language deficits in aphasia is presented in Table 6-2.

CLASSIFICATION OF APHASIC SYNDROMES. Historically there have been many attempts to place pathologic language symptoms into homogeneous groups permitting reference to specific aphasic subtypes. The emergence of the Boston classification system[26] is an attempt to standardize the terminology. The Boston classification system begins with a broad classification of disorders into those in which expressive skills are predominantly fluent and those that are predominantly nonfluent. Although such a distinction might be a useful clinical distinction, it often can be difficult to make, as in the case of a conduction aphasic (fluent aphasia) who may have long pauses and expressive struggle (nonfluency) during speech. The eight major types of aphasia in the Boston system are the more common forms of Broca's aphasia and Wernicke's aphasia, anomia, conduction, and global and the lesser appearing transcortical types (Table 6-3). Each of these syndromes is correlated with a specific localized cortical lesion.[4,38]

Improvements in brain imaging have made it possible to correlate disturbances in language with lesions in the corpus striatum and thalamus. The data are still incomplete, but most of the syndromes described differ from those associated with confirmed cortical disease. Although some characteristics show patterns consistent with site, not every investigator describes the same speech and language deficits from identical lesions.

Preliminary evidence suggests that the speech and language disorders are confined to left hemispheric subcortical structures.[70] There is the suggestion that the causative factor, infarct versus hemorrhage, at the same site may produce differential effects. Lesion size also may be important. Lesions involving the putamen and caudate with anterosuperior extension into the capsule have reportedly produced more dysarthric (with reduced vocal volume) and effortful speech.[49,50] Grammar and comprehension were unaffected. Paraphasia and poor comprehension were associated most with a posterior extension of the lesion. A combination of anterior and posterior capsular lesions resulted in global aphasia. Patients with anterior capsular lesions have been found to have articulation disturbances consistent with buccofacial apraxia, plus disturbances of comprehension.[12]

Linguistic deficits secondary to thalamic hemorrhage also have been reported.[1,47] A great deal of variation is observed in language performance, with some patients having almost normal language performance and others demonstrating marked paraphasia and periods of fluctuating unconsciousness.[47] These fluctuations may be more related to the role of the thalamus in arousal and selective attention as prerequisites to communication than to actual deficits of language.[1]

Although most studies confirm the notion that the symptoms associated with subcortical disease may be transitory, patients seen in our clinic who evidence attentional and arousal deficits beyond the acute stage of illness have not been able to learn compensations for their communication failures in spite of comprehension skills that approach normalcy.

DIFFERENTIATION FROM OTHER DISORDERS. Aphasia, particularly in the acute stages, may be difficult to differentiate from other disorders that compromise communication. Accurate differentiation is necessary since each communication disorder will

Table 6-2
Summary of the Terminology Used to Describe Expressive Disorders of Aphasia

Term	Definition
Agrammatism	The absence of recognized grammatical elements during speech attempts
Anomia	Difficulty retrieving nouns
Circumlocution	Attempts at word retrieval end in descriptions or associations related to the word
Echolalia	An accurate repetition of a preceding utterance when repetition is not required
Empty speech	A fluent utterance that lacks substantive parts of language, such as nouns and verbs
Jargon	Mostly incomprehensible, but well-articulated language
Neologistic jargon	Mostly incomprehensible, some words are partially recognizable, others are contrived or "new"
Paragrammatism	Misuse of grammatical elements, usually during fluent utterances
Phonemic paraphasia	"Flair" for "chair," also called literal paraphasia
Press for speech	Excessively lengthy, often incomprehensible well-articulated language
Semantic jargon	A combination of unrelated semantic and phonemic paraphasia, together with recognizable words
Semantic paraphasia	"Table" for "chair," also called nominal paraphasia
Stereotypes	Nonsensical repetition of similar syllables for all communicative attempts, such as "dee, dee, dee"
Telegraphic speech	Language similar to a telegram, mostly nouns and verbs

Table 6-3
Summary of the Boston Classification System of Aphasia

Type	Language Characteristics
Nonfluent	
Broca's	Telegraphic, agrammatic expression often associated with apraxia; good comprehension except on more abstract tasks
Transcortical motor	Limited language output; fair naming; intact repetition; fair comprehension
Global	Severe expressive and receptive reduction in language
Mixed transcortical	Severe reduction in expression and reception; repetition intact
Fluent	
Anomia	Word-finding difficulty without other serious linguistic deficits
Conduction	Phonemic paraphasic errors; good comprehension; fluency in bursts; deficits in repetition of low probability phrases
Wernicke's	Phonemic and semantic paraphasias; poor comprehension
Transcortical sensory	Fluent neologistic language; poor comprehension; intact repetition

require separate treatment and management approaches. It should be noted that aphasia may occur in conjunction with other syndromes. A comparison of linguistic and nonlinguistic behaviors among disorders that commonly interfere with communication is provided in Table 6-4.

Agnosia. Agnosia is the inability to interpret or recognize information in one given sensory modality when the end organ is intact. For instance, a patient with auditory agnosia would have normal hearing thresholds but cannot interpret speech signals at the cortical level. Therefore, auditory comprehension will be severely compromised. Patients with agnosia can be differentiated from those with aphasia because they only will be impaired in one modality. For instance, the patient with auditory agnosia who has severe comprehension deficits will be able to read the same words through the intact visual modality.

Apraxia. In its pure form, oral apraxia is the motor counterpart of agnosia. Lesions in the premotor cortex are a frequent finding.[13] Apraxia of speech is characterized by effortful and dysprosodic productions resulting in errors of ommission, substitution, and repetition. There is debate over apraxia as a pure motor or linguistic (phonemic) disturbance.[10, 33, 43] Patients have difficulty programming the positioning of the speech musculature and sequencing the movements necessary for speech. Apraxia occurs in the absence of significant weakness and incoordination of muscles, with automatic and reflexive movements undisturbed. It is seen by some as a distinct condition that often co-exists and complicates aphasia, while others regard the characteristics as part of the nonfluent Broca's aphasia. Apraxia of speech carries a negative prognosis for recovery if there is a moderate to severe aphasia in tandem. When it occurs without the concomitant language disturbance, therapy can focus on retraining the patient's ability to program sound patterns, to shift from one sound to another, and to use preserved melodic and rhythm patterns to facilitate speech.

Dementia. Although specific expressive and receptive language disturbances can present as part of dementia, the aphasic patient rarely evidences other cognitive deficits seen in diffuse disease, such as poor memory, inability to learn, poor judgment, disorientation, and inattention to self-care. The distinction between those patients with language deficits secondary to aphasia and those with diffuse disease is particularly relevant in rehabilitation, since the prognosis for retraining specific skills and developing independence is more favorable for the aphasic.

Confusion. Confused language is characterized by reduced recognition; understanding of, and responsiveness to, the environment; faulty memory; unclear thinking; and disorientation.[13] It is often associated with head trauma. It is differentiated, in part, from the language disorders of dementia because the prognosis for recovery after traumatic injury is more favorable.

TESTS FOR APHASIA. Tests for aphasia measure the patient's receptive and expressive language capacities by sampling different levels of abstraction through systematically controlled channels. For instance, an examination of the visual input system (reception) might begin with a concrete task such as copying or matching and proceed to more difficult tasks such as the reading of sentences for comprehension. Tests of expression might range from simple repetition, to naming, to providing definitions. Most test batteries currently in use attempt to provide a representative sample from which one can make inferences about performance in similar linguistic situations. Although most tests of aphasia do sample linguistic competencies, they are not equipped to measure the least and most severe disorders. Therefore, in selected cases, the examination will have to be supplemented by other specialized formal and nonformal measures.

The Minnesota Test for Differential Diagnosis of Aphasia. The *Minnesota Test for Differential Diagnosis of Aphasia (MTDDA)*[62] is the most comprehensive test battery, taking an average of 3

Table 6-4
Aphasia Differentiated from Other Cortical and Subcortical Speech and Language Disorders

Characteristic	Agnosia	Aphasia	Apraxia	Confusion	Dementia	Dysarthria	Subcortical aphasia
Auditory comprehension	+/−	+/−	+	+/−	+/−	+/−	+/−
Auditory memory	+	+/−	+	−	−	+	+/−
Visual memory	+	+	+	−	−	+	+/−
Naming	+	+/−	+	+/−	−	+	+/−
Reading/writing	+/−	−	+	−	−	+	+/−
Generalized cognitive deficits	+	+	+	−	−	+	+/−
Inappropriate behaviors	+	+	+	−	−	+	+/−
Disturbance of attention	+	+	+	−	−	+	−
Learn well	+	+	+	+/−	−	+	+/−
Disorder confined to one input/output modality	−	+	−	+/−	+/−	+	+
Regular errors of speech output	+	+	+	+	+	−	+/−
Irregular errors of speech output	+	+	−	+	+	+	+/−

In acute stages: +, usually unimpaired; −, usually impaired; +/−, patient dependent.

hours to administer. The test has 47 subtests and is particularly useful in recognizing and classifying deficits of auditory comprehension. Means and standard deviations are available for each subtest and patients can be rated from 0 to 6 in each major area of performance (comprehension, reading, expression, and writing). Because of the length of the test it must be given in multiple sessions. Scoring is cumbersome, and subtest instructions for the examiner are not always clear. Patients can be classified into groups by aphasia type, on which a prognosis for recovery is based.

The Boston Diagnostic Aphasia Examination. The *Boston Diagnostic Aphasia Examination (BDAE)*[26] provides the examiner with 27 subtests and an additional group of non–language-based subtests as part of a battery to evaluate parietal lobe dysfunction. It is particularly valuable as a classification tool since it assesses deficiencies in language consistent with the Boston schema of aphasia classification. The examiner rates the patient's conversational speech and auditory comprehension on a seven-point scale. This scale is used for patient classification and is tied to lesion site. Test scores are summarized by modality and are presented as percentiles compared with a large sample of patients.

The Western Aphasia Battery. The *Western Aphasia Battery (WAB)*[37] is a modification and expansion of the *Boston Diagnostic Aphasia Examination*. Subtest scores provide the information used in classification. Auditory and expressive modality scores yield an aphasia quotient (AQ) that is calculated taking spontaneous recovery into account. An AQ score below 93.8 is consistent with aphasia. The patient is assigned a performance quotient (PQ) on the basis of tests of reading, writing, drawing, calculation, block design, and portions of the *Raven's Progressive Matrices*. A summary of cognitive function (CQ) combines the PQ and AQ scores. This summary score is useful in assessing patients with cognitive deficits following traumatic injury.

The Porch Index of Communicative Ability. The *Porch Index of Communicative Ability (PICA)*[59] contains 18 subtests and uses ten common objects to elicit patient responses. Examiners must be trained a minimum of 40 hours and then meet reliability criteria before using the test. The uniqueness of this battery is its 16-point scoring scale. Every response on each subtest is scored from 1 to 16 based on the completeness, accuracy, promptness, responsiveness, and efficiency of the patient's response. Percentile scores by modality can be compared with scores of patients with bilateral and left hemisphere damage. Modality and/or overall test scores can be used to predict recovery. The test is particularly useful in planning programmed treatment and research. It is not particularly sensitive to patients with mild or severe linguistic deficits since it assesses a narrow range of verbal functions.

The Token Test. The *Token Test*[18] is designed to detect subtle auditory comprehension disorders and often is administered to patients who reach ceiling levels on standardized aphasia batteries. Using 20 tokens with two shapes, two sizes, and five colors, the patient is asked through nonredundant language to manipulate them. The five sections (62 total items) increase in difficulty by length and linguistic complexity. Normative data do not come with the test but must be obtained from the literature.[53, 69] Test interpretation can be difficult because patients can make errors due to pure linguistic auditory comprehension problems or auditory memory deficits. A more standardized version (the *Revised Token Test*) is also available.[44] A version in which the examiner moves the tokens and the patient describes what he has seen is the *Reporters Test*.[19]

The Reading Comprehension Battery. The *Reading Comprehension Battery*[39] comprises ten subtests that are used to assess reading skills in greater detail than most standardized aphasia batteries. Subtests include comprehension of morphosyntactic structure, functional reading, synonym recognition, and sentence and paragraph comprehension.

APPROACHES TO TREATMENT. Aphasia treatment should be patient dependent, maximizing communicative strengths in actual interactive situations. To think that aphasics behave alike, regardless of similar classification, is, in part, why statistical analyses of the attempts to demonstrate remediation's effectiveness are less than encouraging. Besides building on the patient's communicative strengths, remediation should be directed toward helping the patient, family, and friends accept the person's liabilities.

Traditionally, the focus of aphasia remediation has been on the stimulation–facilitation approach in which the patient and clinician interact within a stimulus–response framework on tasks that are thought to be related to communication. Although this approach may be most beneficial for the more severely impaired, its relevance in helping the patient solve everyday communicative needs remains questionable. The notion that the clinician's role should be guided toward helping the patient adjust to his or her own particular environment presupposes that family, friends, and employers will receive as much remediation as the patient since they will have to learn how to enhance the patient's communicative competencies. To accomplish this, the speech pathologist must analyze the patient's communicative strengths and weaknesses, then objectify and teach the pragmatics of communication to the language-impaired person and his or her significant others.

In general, patients who evidence diffuse cortical signs in addition to their linguistic deficits, those with unilateral multilobe disease especially secondary to hemorrhage, and those with a severe reduction of test scores after the first month will not be candidates for direct daily speech and language remediation. Monthly reassessment of these patients either with standardized or nonformal testing instruments is necessary to identify any emerging communicative strengths so that they may be further enhanced with treatment. This reassessment should continue until 6 months after the insult and then in 2-month intervals up to 1 year. Treatment with globally involved patients should focus on their ability to learn a new task in a prescribed amount of time. Such tasks usually do not require a great deal of complex processing such as matching picture to object, object to object, or word to object. Data should be kept on the patient's accuracy and processing time as measures of change. Learning success provides prognostic information for further daily remediation in using direct approaches to treatment.

Training in communicative interaction must focus on the following:

- Appropriate rates of auditory presentation and the importance of pause times
- Differences between concrete and abstract language
- Use of redundancy to improve comprehension
- How to carry the load of a conversation while still involving the patient
- Making use of contextual cues in order to comprehend what the patient may be communicating
- How to verify messages from the patient
- How to combine gesture and oral language to facilitate communication
- Allowing the appropriate amount of time for a patient to formulate a response before restimulation (questioning or repeating).

The training modules should be divided into four parts: (1) direct work with the patient and clinician, (2) demonstrations of pragmatics with the family, (3) patient–family interactions critiqued by the clinician, and (4) environmental control training.

Environmental controls are similar to environmental language stimulation described by Lubinski.[42] The patient's environment should be evaluated to determine how it might be manipulated in order to enhance communicative skills and to compensate for deficits. These manipulations should focus on ways to control for distractions, to provide favorable seating and lighting when possible, to control the number of speakers, to suggest the time of day when the patient's performance is best, to control daily situations so that the patient has a need to communicate, and to provide adequate reinforcement for communication. Other environmental controls that enhance communication because they allow for linguistic predictability include the design of a daily regimented schedule and keeping items in the environment such as chairs, utensils, and food items in familiar places. Although these controls may be needed to maximize communicative effectiveness, patients who react favorably to such controls should have them removed at prescribed times, forcing them to use their language in reaction to less predictable situations. These encounters, if positive, can lead to significant improvement in communication.

Communication Impairment Following Right Hemisphere Damage

It is well known that the right hemisphere plays a major role in a person's ability to initiate planned action, make judgments from perceptual integration, and remember information that must be visually coded. In some, neglect or denial of the environment makes these deficits more pronounced and harder to manage. It is easy to overlook these deficits because of the patient's stronger communication skills. Typically the verbal performance is so strong that one might question the reasons for the poor visual motor skills (Fig. 6-2). Evidence suggests that even though the patient with right hemisphere damage may suffer more from visual than linguistic deficits, there is also evidence of affective and extraverbal communication impairment.

The right hemisphere's role in affective aspects of communication is just beginning to be explored. Affective aspects, such as the lack of facial expression while speaking, failure to maintain eye contact, failure to use gesture, and a lack of vocal inflection have all been described in the patient with right hemisphere damage.[63] Loss of inflectional patterns that signal anger or frustration is not surprising when one is reminded of the role the right hemisphere plays in decoding and recalling melodies. It is important that the clinician recognize the possibility of such a pathologic process since loss of these affective cues often are mistaken for the functional states of rudeness or unconcern for another's feelings.

Additional problems with extraverbal aspects of communication also help to explain the "difficulty-to-get-along-with" personality of the patient with right hemisphere damage. Extraverbal skills include behaviors such as appreciation of humor and figurative language and the use of pragmatics such as the ability to maintain a conversational topic and turn-taking during conversation. These patients have difficulty in organizing information and they fail to make use of contextual cues.[48] Failure to recognize these cues results in many conversational irrelevancies and poor monitoring of rate and amount of expressive language as they stray from, or completely lose, the thread of the conversation. Failure to recognize humor and metaphorical language structures may be translated behaviorally into a noncaring, depressed personality. Problems orienting to incoming visual and

Figure 6-2. Comparison of the learning strengths and weaknesses of patients with right and left hemisphere pathology and dementia. (Reprinted with permission from DeLisa JA et al: Stroke rehabilitation. Part I. Cognitive deficits and prediction of outcome, pp 208–214. American Family Physician, November 1982)

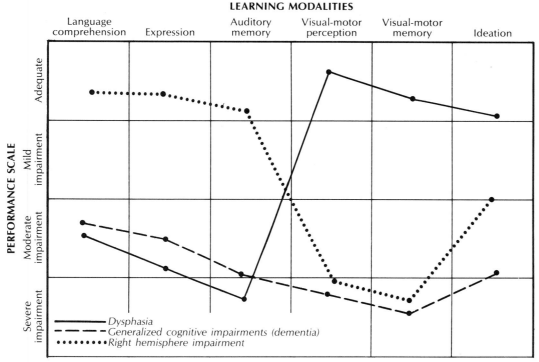

LEARNING MODALITIES

FIGURE   The comparative learning strengths and weaknesses of patients with left (aphasia), right, and bilateral (dementia) brain damage (adapted from Delisa et al., American Family Physician, 1982).

auditory information, long known as a right hemisphere function, make it difficult for these patients to get the point of discourse, leading to further frustration on the sender's part.

ASSESSMENT. Previous to the *Clinical Management of Right Hemisphere Dysfunction*[11] no formal assessment tool was available for the systematic evaluation of the communication skills of the patient with right hemisphere damage. The test offers a scoring system in the assessment of the use of pragmatics, nonverbal skills such as eye contact and facial gestures, interpretation of metaphorical language, memory skills, writing, visual scanning and tracking, and an analysis of conversation including topic maintenance, verbosity, and reference. Approaches to treatment based on the analysis are presented.

Informal assessment tools are described by West and colleagues.[72] Their battery includes a screening of basic language skills, an analysis of single word responses to part–whole tasks, oral opposites, written opposites, oral analogies, and printed analogies. Other sections include interpretation of idioms and proverbs, effects of imagery, and evaluation of the patient's ability to appreciate humor.

TREATMENT. Treatment should concentrate on three broad areas. First, the clinician should use the patient's stronger language capabilities to compensate for poor visuomotor skills. Unable to learn new motor patterns by demonstration, some patients with right hemisphere damage can be taught through intact auditory or graphic channels. Second, the communication specialist should develop tasks that help the patient: (1) attend to contextual cues in an effort to reduce verbosity and improve topic maintenance, (2) retell stories in a fashion that highlights the main points, and (3) produce language that follows a logical sequence. Although these tasks appear related to the impairment, there are no data supporting the success or failure using such strategies. Third, counseling the patient's family on how the loss of pragmatic and affective language can affect their perception of the patient's personality must not be underestimated. Rehabilitation successes in other areas will be diminished or lost if the patient's family does not make the adjustment to a new personality and the reasons it is manifest.

Communication Impairment Following Traumatic Injury

Patients with language impairment from traumatic injury may display a combination of disorientation, aphasic, and memory deficits. Acutely, disorders of perception and behavior mask the severity of deficits, and chronically they may interfere with rehabilitation. Their specific difficulty with attention and arousal, lack of insight, and failure to self-correct make rehabilitation challenging. The combination of these disturbances has become synonymous with the description that these patients display "generalized deficits of cognition," and the treatment offered is thus labeled "cognitive rehabilitation." This designation highlights the importance of recognizing the significance of their diffuse disease manifested by both right (perceptual) and left (linguistic) pathology, as well as deficits in memory, problem solving, and other behaviors that depend on bilateral cooperation. In this way, the language of confusion that is often associated with diffuse traumatic brain injury is different from aphasia and focal disease.

Typically, these patients are young and recovery of linguistic deficits as measured by standardized aphasia batteries is good. However, higher-level language difficulties not assessed by traditional means may persist. Recovery of concrete language skills generally precedes return of orientation and memory independent of length of coma.[28] It is difficult to separate communicative

recovery from cognitive recovery. The return of communication is hierarchical, beginning with restoration of those prelinguistic skills of internal and external attention, followed by discrimination, seriation, recovery of memory, categorization, association, and analysis and synthesis.[31]

Specific linguistic deficits in diffuse traumatic brain injury include problems retrieving auditory and visual information; anomia; decreased auditory comprehension, especially for longer and more syntactically complex utterances; reduced reading comprehension; and difficulty integrating, analyzing, and synthesizing through all modalities. Their expressive language lacks relevancy but is marked by verbosity, confabulation, and circumlocution. At 6 months after the insult, many patients are able to make their needs known but continue to have ideational perseverations, incomplete thought content in expression, and poor verbal reasoning capacities. These cognitive deficits were categorized by Hagen and associates based on recovery through eight stages.[30] Stage one represents patients who are unaware of any external input; stage four (confused-agitated) represents that in which the patient responds primarily to internal confusion with inappropriate verbalizations and confabulation; and stage eight (purposeful and appropriate) is when the patient now can communicate more efficiently by integrating past, present, and future. Social, emotional, and intellectual capabilities remain impaired for more complex language manipulations.

ASSESSMENT. Since these patients often evidence deficits of language, perception, and memory, all should be evaluated with available measures. Because linguistic skills recover quickly, most standardized aphasia batteries are insensitive to change after 6 months, and the clinician must develop methods of analyzing expressive and receptive discourse. Such measures should include an analysis of relevance, auditory analysis and synthesis, expressive integration, serial discrimination and expression, and problem-solving skills that rely on linguistic processing.

TREATMENT. The traumatically brain injured are usually under 30 years of age, display generalized cognitive deficits, recover language at a fast rate, improve for a longer period of time, and often have a chance to return to the work force.[29] These circumstances suggest that treatment strategies with this population may differ from those with impairment from vascular etiologies. Although the patient may benefit from more traditional rehabilitative techniques, especially in the acute stages, he or she will need additional concentration on tasks that improve orientation and memory, help in developing selective attention and discrimination, and eventually must be involved in receptive and expressive language tasks that emphasize analysis and synthesis. Remediation should be directed toward helping the patient retain specific pieces of information gathered from progressively longer utterances. The patient should receive practice in shifting topics without significant delay. Success in job performance and psychosocial adjustment depends on how well the patient can perform on these more abstract linguistic tasks.

Since the loss of memory with its consequences on learning and orientation is a significant finding in this group, tasks must be designed to compensate for memory deficits. Of critical importance to this end is the structuring of the patient's environment so that predictability will reinforce recall and retention. Pneumonic training aids, together with the patient's written or auditory recording of daily events, will help solidify this aspect of rehabilitation.

Disturbances of attention, memory, and nonlanguage problem solving lend themselves to applications of computerized remediation. Computerized programs are particularly useful in treatment of the head-injured patient because of the computer's ability to control stimuli in a repeatable format, helping to focus attention on selected linguistic parameters. Furthermore, the ease of response makes the computer nonthreatening and reinforcing. There are a number of computer-based programs that highlight the skills important in cognitive training. Some, like those designed by Hartley Courseware, focus on aspects of vigilance and attention needed as prerequisites to learning. Other more generic software that was not specifically designed for this population, but can be easily adapted, include offerings from Developmental Learning Materials and Psychological Software Service. These materials are designed to improve problem-solving skills through linguistic and nonlinguistic manipulations. A series of more linguistically based programs that can be adapted for the high level patient are available from Aspen Publishers.

Language Deficits and Dementia

Patients with dementia may evidence specific language deficits as part of generalized intellectual impairment. Wertz[71] characterized the linguistic performance of these patients as a deterioration of capacities in all communication modalities that is consistent with the deterioration of all other mental functions. Since dementia usually results from progressive diffuse pathology, patients rarely improve and it is difficult to identify any learning strengths. The learning strengths and weaknesses of patients with dementia compared with those with right and left cortical disease are presented in Figure 6-2.

Only recently has there been evidence to show that language may be a barometer of change in charting the deterioration in dementia.[2] Knowledge of these changes may be useful in family counseling and subsequent management of the communication disorder.

Language changes can be divided into early, middle, and late stages. Most notable in the early stage is a mild lexical naming deficit.[3] Syntax and phonology remain intact. Analysis of discourse reveals some unnecessary elaboration of content, topic digression, and some difficulty with comprehension of syntactically complex sentences. Repetition is difficult on only low probability items.[55] The patient may complain of some difficulty with reading and writing. In middle-stage disease, naming errors are frequent. Discourse errors are marked by the use of indefinite terms, incomplete phrases, lack of relevance, and general unconcern for their inability to communicate. Comprehension deficits may now be obvious and interfere with conversation. The patient begins to avoid situations that require reading and writing. In the late stages most discourse is full of neologistic jargon with echolalia. Syntax and morphological errors are frequent. Repetition is poor, and there is a dramatic loss of vocabulary. Pragmatics in discourse are lost, and only the most basic comprehension skills remain. Patients become noncommunicative and mute as the disease progresses to termination.

ASSESSMENT. Assessment of linguistic skills usually is informal but should be accomplished at regular intervals to chart progression. Obler[54] suggests the following categories for evaluation: (1) orientation; (2) naming (confrontation and responsive); (3) analysis of discourse; (4) comprehension; (5) repetition; (6) verbal fluency; (7) idioms and proverbs; (8) sentence construction; (9) number facts; (10) automatic speech; and (11) reading and writing. Tests that assess memory, due to its close relationship to linguistic ability, also need to be administered at regular intervals.

TREATMENT. Treatment for patients with communication disorders secondary to dementia should be supportive. Treatment goals should include environmental controls and family education. Environmental structure provides orientation and

reinforces memory that, in turn, will improve the accuracy of linguistic attempts. Interactions with the patient should be structured to reduce any demands beyond the limits of the cognitive system as established by psychometric evaluation. Frequent measures of linguistic function are part of the treatment and are necessary so that family and friends can be informed about how much to expect receptively and expressively from the patient. This knowledge will reduce frustration for both the patient and family. Some patients retain skills longer than others, and knowledge of the best input and expected output modalities is useful in management. Because dementia often results in diminution of all linguistic modalities, performance may be strengthened through multiple channels such as through the combination of gestural, written, and verbal language. This strategy is a process that needs to be demonstrated and taught to family members.

Although the evidence that certain medications facilitate memory in patients with dementia remains controversial, there are no data to support the notion that these facilitative drugs enhance language.

Swallowing Management

Physiology of Swallowing

Swallowing is a multistage sequence that, when normally elicited, momentarily blocks the opening to the respiratory tract as food or beverage is passed through the pharynx, a cavity common to both respiration and deglutition, and into the esophagus. Swallowing can occur either by willful cortical initiation or by a reflex elicited independently from higher brain centers. The reflex of swallowing is stimulated through the sensory modalities of texture, temperature (hot or cold), and pressure.

At rest, the mucous membranes of the oral structures and the pharynx are moist. Respiration usually occurs through the nostrils and the nasopharynx. The lips are either closed or slightly parted. In the event of a completely dry oral cavity and pharynx, initiation of a swallow will be very difficult or impossible. When respiration cannot be accomplished through the nose and nasopharynx, swallowing becomes somewhat uncomfortable and initiation is delayed. With the mouth open, swallowing is possible but extremely difficult to initiate. A normal swallow is accomplished, therefore, with the oral cavity moist, the nasal passages open, and the mouth closed.

ORAL PHASE. The oral phase begins with the oral preparation of the bolus. The manner in which a bolus is prepared for swallowing varies depending on the consistency of the material.

Liquid taken into the mouth generally is held between the tongue and anterior hard palate with the lips sealed to prevent leakage out of the mouth. Because liquids are not cohesive, they are held for only an instant before the base of the tongue and palatopharyngeal regions are stimulated, eliciting one or more complete swallows.

Soft foods may be held immediately between the tongue and anterior hard palate or lateralized for mastication before it is returned to a midline position before swallowing. If the food falls apart in the mouth, it will act like a fluid and stimulate swallowing; however, if thick and sticky, the bolus may adhere to the hard palate and require precise tongue control to compress it into the hypopharynx.

Solids require mastication. The sensations of temperature, texture, and pressure are picked up in the mouth by receptors for the fifth cranial nerve located in the gums and hard palate. The stimulation of these receptors results in a reflexive relaxation of the muscles that keep the jaw shut, the masseter and temporalis. As the jaw relaxes open a stretch reflex of these muscles occurs, resulting in muscle contraction and jaw closure, thus restimulation, relaxation and jaw opening, stretch reflex, and rebound closure. This reflexive cycle continues as the food is manipulated by the lateral tongue to keep it between the teeth while the rotary grinding action of the jaw prepares a cohesive bolus. Saliva is milked from the salivary glands and helps break down the food and stimulate the taste buds. The taste buds, located throughout the tongue, palate, and epiglottis are innervated by the seventh and ninth cranial nerves. It is believed that when these receptors are stimulated a further release of saliva occurs and this eventually leads to swallowing.

Once the bolus is adequately prepared, the tongue is elevated to occlude the anterior oral cavity and compresses the prepared bolus posteriorly toward the oropharynx. The palatopharyngeal folds contract to form a medial slit, allowing only the properly masticated food to pass over the base of the tongue. The levator and tensor veli palatine muscles help to elevate the soft palate and block the nasopharyngeal port.

PHARYNGEAL PHASE   When sensory stimuli travel to the medullary reticular formation, or swallowing center, a complex motor sequence is elicited to propel a bolus through the pharynx, away from the airway, and into the esophagus. The key motor elements consist of posterior movement of the tongue and a pharyngeal constricting wave; laryngeal elevation and tilting with the epiglottis turning under and vocal cords closing to halt respiration and protect the airway; and relaxation of the crico-pharyngeal muscle, which acts as the upper esophageal sphincter, to allow the bolus to pass out of the pharynx and into the esophagus.

ESOPHAGEAL PHASE   The pharyngeal constricting wave that carried the bolus into the esophagus is continued throughout the esophagus as a primary peristaltic wave that strips the bolus through the lower esophageal sphincter and into the stomach. This primary peristaltic wave may be assisted by gravity and by secondary peristaltic waves, which arise locally within the esophagus just above the bolus and progress down over the lower sphincter.

Evaluation of Swallowing

When dysphagia is recognized or a complaint about swallowing is registered, a special examination is often required. Such an examination should consist of the following: a complete medical history, a description of the complaint including details of associated symptoms, a physical examination of the peripheral deglutitory motor and sensory system, and motion radiographic studies. A procedural outline is illustrated in Figure 6-3.

HISTORY.   Data should be compiled from a review of the patient's general health history. Special attention should be paid to the patient's neurological history, which might suggest con-

Figure 6-3. Procedural outline for examination for dysphagia

```
                        Dysphagia Examination

History:


    Medications:


Description of problem:
    Frequency:
    Duration:
    Exacerbating factors:
    Associated symptoms:
        Obstruction:              Pain:
        Nasal regurgitation:      Pneumonia:
        Mouth odor:               Speech/voice change:
        Aspiration:               Weight loss:
        Heartburn (reflux):       Appetite change:

Examination:
    Mental status:



    Weight:                       Gag Reflexes:
    Speech:                       Tongue:
        Voice:                    Indirect Laryngoscopy:
        Articulation:                 Pooling:
    Muscles of Face:                  Function:
    Muscles of Mastication:       Test Swallow:
    Pathological Reflexes:            Delay:
    Oral Mucosa:                      Cough:
    Dentition:                        Oral retention:
```

tributing factors such as stroke, head trauma, central nervous system infections, and demyelinating diseases, all of which are known to impair swallowing. All prior operations should be noted, especially those involving the head and neck. All current prescription and nonprescription medications should be listed. Those that have side-effects of sedation, muscle weakness, drying of mucous membranes, disorientation, or dyskinesia may contribute to dysphagia.

DESCRIPTION OF THE PROBLEM. In many instances the subjective description of the problem gives the examiner clues to the cause of the swallowing problem. The subjective data should include a general statement describing the swallowing complaints. Pertinent details should include statements related to the duration, frequency, and exacerbating factors influencing the problem. It is most important to find out the relative influence of liquids, semi-solids, and solids on the swallowing complaint.

Symptoms associated with swallowing should be noted. In the case of dysphagia for solids, a feeling of obstruction or blockage is common. Failure of the cricopharyngeal muscle to relax, incomplete elevation of the larynx with retention in the vallecula or pyriform sinuses, pharyngoesophageal diverticuli, tumors, strictures, and esophageal dysmotility are some of the reasons for the sensation of obstruction.

Nasal regurgitation is a symptom associated with weakness or incompetence of the palatopharyngeal mechanism. It may also be found in some patients with obstruction in the hypopharynx or cervical esophagus. Unusual mouth odors, particularly when found in combination with obstruction, may suggest a pharyngoesophageal diverticulum. Mouth odor may also be associated with mastication problems, poor hygiene, oral retention of food, tumors, and infections.

Aspiration of food or liquid into the "windpipe" is a common complaint of patients with neurological impairment of the swallowing muscles. Gastroesophageal reflux and the sensation of heartburn also should be noted since this may suggest some incompetence of the gastroesophageal sphincter. Reflux of stomach contents, especially at night, can lead to aspiration pneumonia. Any complaint of pain (odynophagia) associated with swallowing should be explored. Instances of aspiration pneumonia should be recorded as a measure of severity.

Since the anatomical and neuromuscular systems used for speech and swallowing are common, any speech or voice changes should be described. Weight loss may be associated with impaired nutritional intake and can reflect an underlying disease process interfering with swallowing. Any change in appetite or eating habits also should be recorded.

CLINICAL EXAMINATION. The examination begins with an assessment of mental status and the patient's ability to cooperate. When the patient's orientation is in doubt, questions regarding person, time, and place should be posed. A screening of language functions (following spoken commands, expressing thoughts), memory, and visual-motor-perceptual function is helpful.

The muscles of the face, mouth, and neck are examined beginning with the muscles of facial expression. The examination should compare movement of the two sides of the face for signs of weakness. The masseter and temporalis can be palpated as the patient bites and chews. Movement of the lower jaw in a lateral plane assesses the function of the pterygoids.

The presence of any brain stem level primitive reflexes associated with chewing and swallowing, such as the suck or bite, should be noted. These pathological reflexes often are found in patients with bilateral hemispheric or frontal lobe damage.

The examination proceeds to the inspection of the intraoral mucosa. Careful attention should be paid to the presence of lesions, oral debris, abnormal movement, and dryness. Palpation with a gloved hand on the floor of the mouth, gumlines, tonsillar fossa, and tongue serves to help rule out neoplastic growth. Any atrophy and fasciculations of the tongue should be noted. Tongue strength can be assessed by placing fingers against the outer cheek and resisting the patient's tongue as it is pushed into the inner cheek. Each side of the palate should be stimulated separately with resulting gag reflexes observed in the contraction of the velum and pharyngeal muscles. The reflexes should be compared for symmetry.

Mirror or fiberoptic laryngoscopy should be used in most instances as part of the evaluation of swallowing.[45] The examiner should observe the base of the tongue, vallecula and epiglottis, pyriform sinuses, false cords, true cords, and infraglottic area. Pooling of debris, especially in the vallecula and pyriform sinuses, should be noted. The vocal cords should be observed during phonation, as well as during quiet breathing.

Testing the adequacy of a swallow brings a certain degree of risk for aspiration. It is advisable to initially use a substance that is relatively safe if partially aspirated and to ensure that the patient is able to cough to protect the airway in case of aspiration. A spoonful of crushed ice will provide a good medium for eliciting the chewing reflex because of its texture and cold stimulation to the receptors in the gums. The examiner should observe the chewing action and feel for the laryngeal elevation to indicate that a swallow has occurred. Once it has been determined that the patient adequately elevates the larynx and that there is an adequate protective cough, other substances with varying textures and consistencies can be tried. Solids such as canned peaches also will elicit a chewing reflex and allow the examiner to feel for laryngeal elevation. Any signs of coughing, aspiration, or nasal regurgitation should be noted. The mouth should be inspected for oral retention, and a repeat indirect laryngoscopy should be performed to inspect the vallecula, pyriform sinuses, and laryngeal cavity for evidence of pooling or aspiration.

MOTION RADIOGRAPHY. Videotaped or cineradiography of swallowing is needed when the peripheral examination does not completely explain the problem, or the examination suggests the dysfunction is in the cricopharyngeus, esophagus, or gastroesophageal junction. While spot films may be valuable to detect morphological changes in the pharynx or esophagus, they are not useful in studying the dynamics of swallowing. A complete examination should be conducted with a small amount of barium (3 to 5 ml) to avoid obliterating structures. Both a lateral and an anteroposterior view should be obtained with the patient in an upright posture. The oral and pharyngeal stages of swallowing should be studied with the camera focused superiorly on the hard palate and inferiorly on the cervical esophagus. Many clinicians recommend using a variety of textures (thin barium, paste, and a cookie).[41] The examination should include a study of the esophagus and gastroesophageal junction performed with the patient in a prone position when aspiration is not a problem.

Management of Swallowing Impairment

Once the patient's swallowing has been described, the impairment identified, and the compensatory strengths recognized, a recommendation is made to feed the patient by mouth or manage nutrition by an alternative route such as feeding tube. When oral feeding is recommended, a plan is needed that will minimize the patient's risk for aspiration. Each plan must be individualized and is based on what is known about the normal physiology of swallowing, the specific swallowing phase disturbance, and the cause of the disorder when known.

MECHANICAL DISORDERS. Disruptions in the transmission of food and beverage from the anterior oral cavity into the pharynx, whether due to acute inflammations of oral mucosa, trauma to the oral region, tumors, or surgical alterations in the mouth may be described as mechanical disturbances of swallowing. Additionally, patients who have undergone surgical alterations in the pharynx and larynx may experience difficulties in the passage of oral contents into the esophagus.

A type of mechanical disorder is found in the patient with partial or total glossectomy. If pharyngeal sensation and motor function in the pharynx, cricopharyngeus, and larynx is preserved, a special feeding spoon with a plunger to propel food into the posterior oral cavity can be used.[23] A cohesive bolus of soft food can be placed toward the tongue base. Liquids can be placed into the posterior oral cavity by using a syringe and length of tubing that will reach the uvula.[21]

Complications to swallowing for many surgical head and neck cancer patients are caused by radiation therapy. Xerostomia, or dry mouth, results from destruction of the salivary glands and other moisture producing cells in the mucous lining. Artificial saliva used just prior to meals or lemon–glycerin swabs used to clean out oral debris can be helpful for some patients, although others complain they increase dryness.[23] The diet of these patients should emphasize foods lubricated with sauces, gravies, and butter.[21] Mucosal pain associated with irradiation can be managed in part by the use of topical anesthetics, however, patients with impaired pharyngeal swallowing will have a greater aspiration risk because of the reduction in sensation.

Patients who have undergone a supraglottic laryngectomy are at high risk for aspiration because of the loss of the epiglottis and altered sensation. Aspiration can be minimized by training the patient to inhale before swallowing, to swallow, to cough gently while exhaling, and to re-swallow. This procedure ensures that the patient has an adequate amount of air in the lungs to cough out debris that has penetrated the unprotected laryngeal region.

PARALYSIS OF SWALLOWING. Diseases that affect the lower motoneurons may result in paralysis of the swallowing musculature and often interfere with sensation in the mouth, palate, pharynx, and larynx. Amyotrophic lateral sclerosis, myasthenia gravis, brain stem stroke, botulism, and diphtheritic polyneuropathy are conditions that can cause paralysis of swallowing.

In those conditions that are considered to be progressive, and examination indicates oral intake is reasonably safe, management centers on minimizing aspiration risks and preventing the secondary complications associated with dehydration and malnutrition. The posture should be adjusted to keep the patient upright with the neck flexed and chin down toward the chest. This keeps the airway partially blocked by the epiglottis. The patient should increase concentration on eating and swallowing. Some can be trained in the double swallow technique described for the patient with a supraglottic laryngectomy. Care providers should be taught assistive coughing techniques but should also be instructed to recognize that the patient must be allowed every opportunity to clear material with an unassisted cough. The diet should be adjusted to provide foods that hold together as cohesive boluses. Dry and sticky food should be avoided, and the patient must be discouraged from washing down a partially swallowed bite of food.

In those patients with potentially improving conditions, the same principles of management apply; however, exercise may hasten recovery of some motor functions. For example, a patient may be instructed to swallow a feeding tube as a means of stimulating contraction of the tongue and pharyngeal muscle bundles. Not only does this provide a mechanism for strengthen-ing muscles needed for swallowing with a retrievable bolus, it also provides a route for self-administered nutrition.[46] Vocal cord adduction may be strengthened by performing Valsalva maneuvers for exercise.

Some patients with specific muscle weakness can be assisted in swallowing and airway protection by surgical intervention. For example, injection of a paralyzed vocal cord with Teflon or Gelfoam may improve glottic function. Cricopharyngeal myotomy, a surgical procedure to slit the cricopharyngeal muscle in order to facilitate its opening during the swallow, may be beneficial to patients with radiographically demonstrated impairments in this sphincter. When the dysfunction is due to an acute neurologic condition such as post-stroke or head trauma, the myotomy should not be performed within the first 6 months.[7] In the event of persistent aspiration, surgical closure of the glottis and tracheostomy can be considered. Some techniques are potentially reversible should the patient recover function,[40] while others, including total laryngectomy, are permanent. An alternative form of communication becomes the primary consideration.

PSEUDOBULBAR IMPAIRMENT OF SWALLOWING. In pseudobulbar (or supranuclear) impairments, there are frequently both motor and mental components to the swallowing problem. The active swallowing muscles usually are spastic, with diminished speed and delayed initiation of motion. Unlike patients with paralysis of swallowing, the patients with pseudobulbar impairment generally retain reflexes associated with airway protection, such as the gag, cough, and laryngeal elevation. The voluntary initiation of swallowing and coughing often is impaired, but each can be elicited by sensory stimulation.

Perceptual-motor impairments, judgment deficits, and language disorders are common in these patients. These deficits are the major factor either impairing swallowing and the feeding process or complicating the motor impairment. Behaviorally, these deficits are (1) failure to chew and swallow due to impaired awareness and/or distractability; (2) taking excessively large bites or rapid eating due to impaired judgment and/or vision-perception; (3) retaining food in the mouth between bites and ignoring food on one side of the tray due to unilateral sensory neglect; and (4) failure to appreciate the importance of eating, which may mistakenly be attributed to depression or lack of motivation in patients with various forms of motor planning impairments.

Pseudobulbar swallowing impairments are the result of bilateral upper motoneuron involvement. Any process that impairs the cognitive processes can result in pseudobulbar-like swallowing difficulties. Management of the condition is similar in many respects to the principles described for the patient with paralysis of swallowing. Placing patients in an upright posture with the neck flexed, providing foods that maintain a cohesive bolus, and ensuring that they are in an optimal state of nutrition and hydration are very important considerations. Maintenance of good oral hygiene is a necessity. A patient's oral mucosa must be moist before swallowing can occur. Additional attention should be paid to selecting foods that stimulate receptors associated with swallowing. Temperature, texture, and taste are all important qualities for eliciting a swallow. Foods should be pleasant in appearance and aroma. Items that are sticky, dry, tough to chew, or fall apart in the mouth are to be avoided.

Each patient with pseudobulbar swallowing difficulty must be individually evaluated in order to determine the nature and extent of the cognitive impairment. Once this has been ascertained, an individualized plan can be established to control for the intellectual deficits. For example, the patient with language deficits might require an environment for eating that is free of distracting conversation. Patients with motor planning deficits may need verbal cues in order to begin eating and to maintain the process. Patients with impaired perception, judgment, or neglect require close, quiet supervision and monitoring. Most patients with pseudobulbar swallowing problems respond best in quiet settings with a minimum of short verbal instructions.

Auditory Rehabilitation

Two million people in the United States are either totally deaf or lack sufficient hearing to understand speech. Another 12 million have a serious hearing impairment. Some degree of hearing loss is present in 20 million Americans, or nearly 1 in 10. With increasing life expectancy as well as increasing noise exposure, the number of Americans who will suffer the effects of hearing loss will become even greater. The effect of hearing impairment on a person's life may be critical owing to the communication problems it may cause or exacerbate.

Standard Hearing Evaluation

The standard tests used in the assessment of hearing include air and bone conduction pure tone audiometry and speech audiometry. The measurement of hearing sensitivity involves obtaining thresholds for various pure tone and speech stimuli. In clinical audiological practice, the term *threshold* is used to refer to the intensity (loudness) level at which responses occur 50% of the time a signal is presented; at least three responses at this level usually are considered to constitute threshold.

The graph used to record hearing test results is called an audiogram (Fig. 6-4). The frequency (pitch) scale along the abscissa is measured in hertz (Hz), or cycles per second (cps). Even though the young normal adult ear is capable of hearing frequencies as low as 20 Hz to as high as 20,000 Hz, the frequencies used in clinical hearing measurement include only those

from 250 Hz up to 8000 Hz. The most critical frequencies for the reception and understanding of speech are 500, 1000, 2000, and 3000 Hz.

The intensity scale on the ordinate of the audiogram is measured in units called decibels (dB) and covers a range from −10 dB hearing level (very faint) up to 110 dB (very loud). The 0 dB hearing level for each frequency represents the average hearing sensitivity for a young, normal adult.

PURE TONE AUDIOMETRY. Pure tone air conduction audiometry provides information regarding the degree of hearing impairment as well as the configuration of the hearing loss. Thresholds are obtained for the various audiometric frequencies for each ear separately using earphones. Air conduction evaluation measures the responsiveness of the auditory system from the external auditory canal, through the middle ear mechanism to the cochlea and associated neural pathways to the brain. Therefore, a hearing impairment shown by pure tone air conduction may be due to a disorder anywhere in the auditory system.

Pure tone bone conduction audiometry provides information concerning the general anatomical location of a hearing disorder. A small vibrator placed on the mastoid process behind the ear to be tested conducts sound vibrations directly to the cochlea. Thresholds are obtained for the frequencies 250 through 4000 Hz. Since sound transmission by bone conduction bypasses the outer and middle ear, bone conduction results reflect the sensitivity of the sensorineural system only. The use of a masking noise in the nontest ear often is necessary to ensure that the bone conduction responses are not being perceived in the nontest ear.

SPEECH AUDIOMETRY. In addition to pure tone threshold measurements, the basic audiological evaluation includes the measurement of threshold sensitivity for speech and the deter-

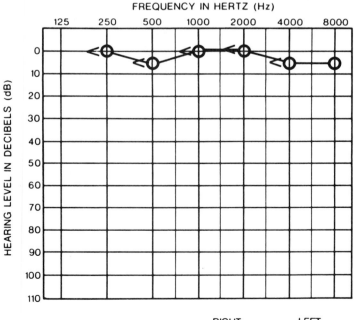

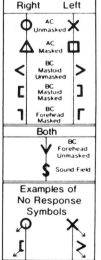

Figure 6-4. Audiogram of a normal ear.

mination of speech recognition (discrimination) abilities. The speech reception threshold (SRT) serves primarily as a reliability check on the pure tone threshold levels. Familiar two-syllable words are presented to each ear separately through earphones. The softest intensity level at which the patient can correctly repeat 50% of the words is defined as the SRT. The SRT should agree within ± 10 dB with the pure tone average (PTA) threshold levels of 500, 1000, and 2000 Hz.

The handicap of a hearing loss may be reflected in an impairment in the ability to understand speech even when speech is sufficiently loud (reduction in speech clarity). The assessment of speech discrimination analyzes the patient's ability to understand speech when presented at a comfortably loud level; it is not a threshold test. Standardized word lists of 25 or 50 phonetically balanced single-syllable words are presented to each ear separately at levels well above the SRT. These words are repeated back by the patient and the percentage of correct responses is the speech discrimination score.

The assessment of speech discrimination is viewed as one of the most important components of the audiological evaluation, since it uses meaningful stimuli (speech) instead of non-meaningful stimuli (pure tones). Speech discrimination performance provides information relative to the extent of the communication handicap caused by the hearing loss.

Audiometric Test Interpretation

DEGREE OF HEARING LOSS. The use of the threshold results obtained using pure tone air conduction assessment provide quantitative information regarding the amount of hearing loss present. Classification systems have been devised in an effort to relate the amount of air conduction hearing loss to the expected degree of handicap imposed by a hearing loss. One system uses the PTA to estimate the hearing loss category (from no impairment to profound impairment) and the expected difficulties

anticipated in the understanding of speech. Other classification systems have most often used PTAs of 0 to 25 dB hearing level as "normal."[17, 27] These classifications have been challenged since a 20 to 25 dB hearing level in children may have deleterious effects on language development and academic skills.[8, 20] In fact, any type of audiometric classification system must be interpreted with some caution since they are primarily based only on pure tone air conduction thresholds alone and do not incorporate the effects of speech discrimination difficulties, etiological factors, or hearing loss configuration.

LOCATION OF AUDITORY IMPAIRMENT. The general anatomical area of a hearing impairment can be determined by comparing air conduction thresholds and bone conduction thresholds. A conductive hearing loss is present when air conduction results demonstrate a hearing loss but bone conduction results are within the normal range (Fig. 6-5). The difference between the air and bone conduction thresholds reflects the amount of conductive hearing involvement and is called the air–bone gap. A conductive hearing loss could be due to any obstruction in the sound-conducting mechanism of the ear from the external auditory canal (*e.g.,* cerumen impaction or foreign body) through the middle ear (*e.g.,* middle ear effusion or otosclerosis). On the basis of the audiometric results alone, the specific etiology or location cannot be predicted. Although otoscopic evidence of a cerumen impaction, tympanic membrane perforation, or serous otitis could account for a conductive hearing loss, there are conductive pathological processes that present in patients with normal otoscopic examinations, such as otosclerosis or ossicular discontinuity.

Patients with pure conductive hearing loss demonstrate normal speech discrimination scores (92 to 100%) since the sensorineural system is normal. Speech only needs to be presented at a louder level than normal to compensate for the conductive deficit.

Figure 6-5. This audiogram demonstrates a mild conductive hearing loss. Note that the air conduction thresholds reveal a hearing impairment of 40 dB but the bone conduction responses are within the normal range. Therefore, an air–bone gap of 35 dB is present. Speech discrimination is normal since no sensorineural involvement is present.

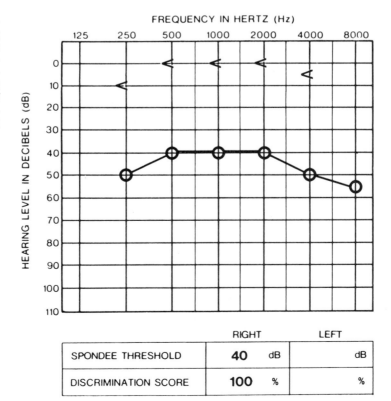

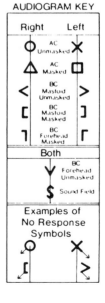

	RIGHT		LEFT	
SPONDEE THRESHOLD	**40**	dB		dB
DISCRIMINATION SCORE	**100**	%		%

When a hearing loss is present and air conduction and bone conduction results are identical, the impairment is called a sensorineural hearing loss (Fig. 6-6). The hearing disorder could be located in the cochlea, the associated neural pathways (retrocochlear system), or both.

Speech discrimination resulting from sensorineural hearing loss can provide some important diagnostic clues. In general, cochlear lesions demonstrate speech discrimination scores that are compatible with the degree of hearing loss. The greater the hearing loss in cochlear disorders, the poorer the speech discrimination. On the other hand, retrocochlear disorders often yield speech discrimination scores disproportionately poorer than would be expected from the pure tone thresholds. That is, a sensorineural hearing loss of 40 dB with a 72% speech discrimination score would be consistent with cochlear involvement, while a similar amount of hearing loss with only 10% speech discrimination would suggest the possibility of retrocochlear involvement.

A loss in hearing sensitivity for bone conduction with a greater loss for air conduction represents a mixed hearing loss (Fig. 6-7). Speech discrimination performance will reflect the amount and etiology of the sensorineural involvement.

SITE-OF-LESION EVALUATION. The basic audiological test battery of pure tone air conduction, bone conduction, SRT, and speech discrimination assessment represents the minimum audiological protocol for evaluating patients with hearing impairment. In the event of an asymmetrical sensorineural hearing loss, or clinical suspicion of eighth nerve or central auditory involvement, special audiological procedures to define the site of impairment are available. The site-of-lesion battery includes tests to determine the presence of loudness recruitment (a cochlear phenomenon), abnormal auditory adaptation (a retrocochlear sign), and speech discrimination "rollover" (a retrocochlear sign). The evaluation of the integrity of the stapedius reflex by

immittance measurement is considered a powerful tool in differentiating between cochlear and retrocochlear involvement. Some abnormality in the acoustic reflex (*e.g.,* elevated reflexes, absent reflexes, or reflex decay) is related to an eighth nerve tumor in a very high number of cases. The electrophysiological analysis of auditory evoked potentials using auditory brain stem response (ABR) audiometry provides one of the most accurate procedures in the diagnosis of acoustic tumors. Electrocochleography (ECoG) also is available for measuring the electrophysiologic activity originating within the cochlea and can supplement information provided by ABR audiometry.

MEASURES FOR SPECIAL POPULATIONS. If a patient cannot respond appropriately to conventional tests, as in the case of the newborn, infant, or mentally handicapped patient, other audiological techniques are indicated. The field of pediatric audiology has many behavioral approaches available to assess the auditory capabilities of these special populations. Reliable and valid measures of hearing sensitivity can be obtained using innovative audiological methods in infants as young as 6 months, and the presence or absence of significant hearing impairment can be determined in newborns by behavioral observation audiometry. When behavioral measures prove unsuccessful or when additional documentation is needed, the use of ABR audiometry is indicated.

The assessment of the patient who is suspected of manifesting functional (exaggerated) hearing loss requires the use of special test procedures developed specifically for this purpose. ABR audiometry may provide additional information.

Management of Hearing Impairment

The management of the person with hearing loss begins with a complete otolaryngological evaluation. Although hearing loss most often occurs alone, it may be one manifestation of a

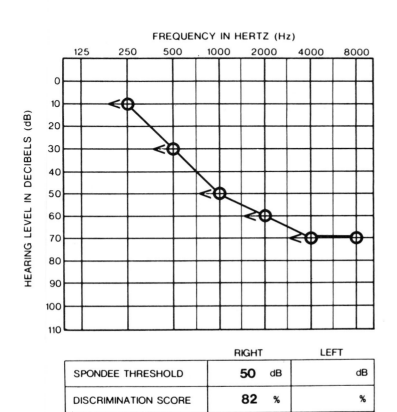

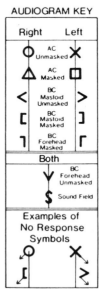

Figure 6-6. This audiogram demonstrates a sensorineural hearing loss, since both the air conduction and the bone conduction thresholds are similarly depressed. Speech discrimination at a comfortable level is relatively good in this illustration (82%) but is reduced from normal performance.

	RIGHT		LEFT	
SPONDEE THRESHOLD	**50**	dB		dB
DISCRIMINATION SCORE	**82**	%		%

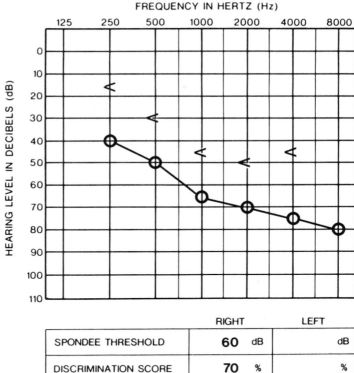

FREQUENCY IN HERTZ (Hz)

Figure 6-7. This audiogram demonstrates a mixed hearing loss. Although both the air conduction and the bone conduction thresholds are reduced, a greater impairment is evident for air conduction. Speech discrimination is reduced (70%), reflecting the sensorineural component of the loss.

	RIGHT		LEFT	
SPONDEE THRESHOLD	60	dB		dB
DISCRIMINATION SCORE	70	%		%

syndrome or a part of a more generalized disease process. As with any symptom or clinical finding, treatment should be based on the underlying pathophysiology. A specific diagnosis should be sought with the objective of reversal of the hearing loss or prevention of additional impairment.

The otological evaluation begins with a thorough history and includes questions relative to the time of onset, whether the loss was sudden or gradual, and if associated symptoms are present (*e.g.,* tinnitus, vertigo, discharge, aural fullness, or pain). In addition, questioning should focus on family history of hearing loss, noise exposure, head trauma, and ototoxic drug use. Following the case history, physical examination with special attention to the head and neck region is completed. The otoscopic examination should include otomicroscopic evaluation and pneumo-otoscopy to assess tympanic membrane mobility. The standard audiological evaluation is administered and any special audiological tests are recommended. The use of associated neurological, laboratory, radiological studies also may be ordered.

Only after the otolaryngological assessment has been completed and a diagnosis established should rehabilitation of the hearing loss be initiated. Too frequently, patients with hearing loss are approached for rehabilitation without antecedent medical evaluation. Many hearing-impaired patients are fitted with hearing aids without medical evaluation of their hearing loss. Neither hearing aid dispensers nor audiologists have the appropriate training to diagnose the cause of hearing loss.

MEDICAL-SURGICAL REHABILITATION. Medical or surgical treatment of hearing loss most often is available for people with impairments of the conductive auditory system. When hearing loss originates in the external auditory canal, it usually is related to a mechanical obstruction in the form of cerumen or foreign body; cerumen impaction is the most common cause of conductive hearing loss. Removal of the obstruction will restore or improve hearing. Infections of the lining of the external canal

(otitis externa) can be treated with topical antibiotics. Hearing impairment originating in the middle ear system may be treated with surgery. Surgical procedures such as myringoplasty (repair of tympanic membrane perforation), tympanoplasty (ossicular reconstruction), stapedectomy (for otosclerosis), and myringotomy with placement of tubes (for middle ear effusion) often can correct the conductive hearing loss. The amount of conductive hearing loss often determines if surgical treatment would be helpful. The otologist bases a surgical recommendation on the size of the air–bone gap and the possibility that closure of the gap would significantly improve hearing. Even in cases of mixed hearing loss, surgical correction of the conductive component may enable the patient to use a less powerful hearing aid or require an aid only on a limited basis.

Otological surgery sometimes is required for treatment of life-threatening disease and not for hearing improvement. Pathological conditions such as cholesteatoma, glomus tumor, or chronic middle ear disease necessitate surgery. In addition, otoneurosurgery is necessary for sensorineural impairment caused by eighth nerve tumors. Hearing preservation is possible in some patients, but the primary goal is the treatment of the disease.

Otological treatment of congenital or hereditary sensorineural hearing loss, noise-induced hearing loss, presbycusis, and most other types of sensorineural impairments is not possible at this time. Prevention of some types of sensorineural hearing loss, most notably noise-induced impairment, is certainly possible. Perhaps the greatest advances in the surgical rehabilitation of sensorineural impairments is now available with the development of the cochlear implant for profound hearing loss.

HEARING AID AMPLIFICATION. The most important rehabilitative avenue for hearing impairment is the hearing aid. Appropriate amplification improves receptive communicative functioning for patients with nontreatable auditory disorders.

A hearing aid is a miniature amplifier of sound, designed to increase the intensity of sound and to deliver it to the hearing-impaired ear with minimal distortion. Although the physical appearance of hearing aids may vary considerably, all electro-acoustic hearing aids have the following basic components: (1) an input microphone to convert airborne sound to electrical energy; (2) an amplifier to increase the strength of the electrical signal; (3) an output receiver to convert the amplified signal back into acoustic energy; (4) a battery to provide the power for the aid; and (5) a volume control to permit the user to adjust the loudness of the sound.

Behind-the-Ear (BTE) Aid. The components of the BTE aid are fit into a curved case that rests behind the pinna. Amplified sound is conducted through a short length of plastic tubing to an earmold placed into the ear canal. Critical to the successful fitting of a BTE hearing aid is the custom-made earmold. The earmold must fit properly in order to achieve a satisfactory acoustical response.

Eyeglass Hearing Aid. The components of the eyeglass hearing aid are all fit within the temple bow of an eyeglass frame. These aids are electroacoustically similar to BTE aids. Although very popular in the 1950s, eyeglass aids are seldom fitted today owing to difficulties in the adjustment of these aids with eyeglass frames. Part-time eyeglass or hearing aid wearers are annoyed when both are in the same unit.

In-the-Ear (ITE) Hearing Aid. The ITE aid is a self-contained hearing aid and earmold unit that fits entirely into the concha of the external ear. ITE aids of the 1960s through 1970s were generally of poor quality and performance, lacking adequate acoustic gain and frequency response for many types of hearing losses. The development of integrated circuits has resulted in improved electroacoustic characteristics, making these aids the instruments of choice for many patients. ITE aids have the advantages of cosmetic appeal, ease of insertion and adjustment, as well as reported superior speech discrimination and sound localization abilities when compared with other hearing aids. The ITE aid is typically custom-fitted for the specific amplification requirements of each patient. ITE aid fitting is usually contraindicated in patients with hearing losses greater than 70 dB and when the loss configuration has a very precipitous drop between octave frequencies.

In-the-Canal (ITC) Hearing Aid. A relatively recent development in ITE aids is the ITC aid, which fits entirely within the external auditory canal. At this time, these aids are appropriate only for people with mild hearing loss; however, with continued improvements in the miniaturization of electronic components, the ITC aid may be the aid of the future. People with dexterity problems often find considerable difficulties in inserting and adjusting these aids.

Body Hearing Aid. The body or pocket hearing aid houses the microphone and amplifier into a case worn at chest level, with a long wire connected to an external receiver fit into an earmold. This aid is considerably larger than other hearing aids and is regarded as the most powerful of all hearing aid devices. Body aids fulfill a need for people with severe hearing loss (90 dB), as well as those who cannot manipulate other types of aids due to dexterity problems or other physical limitations.

Contralateral Routing of Signals (CROS) Hearing Aid System. Harford and Berry in 1965[35] provided a means of assisting unilaterally hearing-impaired people by developing the CROS system. An aid containing a microphone is placed on the poor ear side and sound is routed to an aid on the better ear using FM transmission. The aid on the poor ear acts as an FM transmitter to send the sound to the receiver aid on the better ear side. A modification of the CROS system is the BI-CROS aid, which is intended for patients with bilateral hearing loss whose poorer ear is not suitable for amplification. In addition to the CROS side pick-up, sound is also amplified to the better hearing ear.

Special Features. Special features serve to increase the fitting flexibility of each aid and provide options for specific hearing loss requirements or personal needs. "Telephone circuits" ("T" coil) are available in all hearing aid types, with the exception of the ITC aid. A magnetic induction coil inside the aid picks up signals directly from the receiver of the telephone, bypassing the external microphone. The volume control of the hearing aid can increase the loudness of the telephone message without amplifying background noise. Although some newer telephones do not generate an adequate magnetic field for "T" coil use, a special device is available to connect to the telephone to restore efficient use of the "T" coil. Telephone circuits also can be used in auditoriums and classrooms where induction loop amplification systems are installed. Due to the size requirements for "T" coils, the best circuits are found in body style, BTE, and eyeglass hearing aids.

Many hearing aids incorporate controls for dispenser adjustment of the aid's power, tone, and other acoustic variables. These internal adjustments increase the fitting applications, since a particular aid can be made suitable for a wide range of hearing loss requirements and configurations. Some hearing aids also have user-operated tone controls, which permit the user to change the tone response. This is helpful in situations with background noise, since the adjustment of the tone control can reduce the low frequency amplification of the aid, decreasing noise interference.

Some hearing aid manufacturers offer input microphones with directional properties. Rather than amplifying all sounds in a 360° radius in a similar manner, directional microphones decrease the loudness of sound from the rear and produce a relative enhancement of sounds from the front of the aid.

DETERMINATION OF HEARING AID CANDIDACY. Although there are no universally accepted techniques for the successful selection and fitting of a hearing aid, the prospective candidate should receive a hearing aid evaluation (HAE) performed by a clinical audiologist. During the HAE, the patient is evaluated with several electroacoustically appropriate hearing aids. Tests are administered through a loudspeaker in a sound-treated room to determine which hearing aid(s) best suit the patient's acoustical and psychological needs. Speech recognition tests are sometimes given both in quiet and with competing background noise to determine which hearing aid(s) provides the patient with the best discrimination improvement. Many questions need to be answered during the HAE: Is the patient a hearing aid candidate? Which type of aid (BTE, ITE) would be best suited? Do the patient's hearing loss and personal needs require any specific hearing aid options? What type of earmold should be made? Should the patient have one or two aids?

Attention is directed not only to the audiological test results but also to the expectations of the patient. The patient needs to be counseled regarding the advantages and disadvantages of hearing aid use. Critical to successful hearing aid use are factors unrelated to the audiological assessment. Lack of motivation, negative attitudes, family pressure, denial of hearing difficulties, and other psychological factors can result in an unsuccessful hearing aid fitting.

SPEECH READING AND AUDITORY TRAINING. Speech reading is the use of visual cues in the recognition of speech and incorporates the interpretation of facial expressions, body movements, and gestures. Everyone uses speech reading to some extent, although usually we are not conscious of the importance of visual input in helping us to recognize what is being said. Training in speech reading consists of teaching systematic observation. Many hearing-impaired people, particularly those with a gradually progressive hearing loss, develop this skill through necessity.

The use of speech reading alone cannot be the sole rehabilitative approach in providing the hearing-impaired patient with complete understanding of speech. Although a considerable amount of the speech signal can be visually perceived, only about one-third of English speech sounds are clearly visible. Certain sounds (\f\ and \th\) are relatively easy to see on the lips, others (\k\ and \g\) are not visible, and some (\p\ and \b\) are indistinguishable.

Speech reading usually is taught in conjunction with a program of auditory training. Auditory training teaches the patient to make the most effective use of minimal auditory cues. The combination of visual input and auditory input is superior to either one alone in understanding speech.

ASSISTIVE DEVICES.   Despite the substantial improvements in hearing aid design and application, few patients can achieve normal auditory receptive functioning with hearing aid use alone. The levels of noise and interference found in many public places render speech recognition of the desired message unintelligible to the hearing-impaired person. The amplification of unwanted sounds (other talkers in a crowd, ventilation hum, or background music) to an ear with sensorineural hearing loss interferes with the reception and comprehension of the desired message.

The use of assistive listening devices (ALDs) can make the difference between satisfactory and unsatisfactory communication in adverse listening situations. The primary difference between ALDs and hearing aids are that ALDs are designed to help in only selected listening environments. With ALDs, a microphone is placed close to the desired sound source (e.g., television, theater stage, speaker's podium) and sound is transmitted to the hearing-impaired listener. Transmission methods include infrared, audio loop, FM radio, or direct audio input (Fig. 6-8). The direct transmisson of the sound to the listener's hearing aid or receiver unit improves the "signal-to-noise ratio." The key to success is the direct electronic coupling reaching from the microphone at the desired sound source to the ear of the listener. Some churches, theaters, and classrooms are now equipped with ALDs.

Amplified telephones, low frequency doorbells and telephone ringers, and closed-captioned TV decoders are helpful in everyday activities. Flashing alarm clocks, alarm bed vibrators,

Figure 6-8.   Assistive listening devices (ALDs) provide assistance in selected environments by transmitting sound directly to the hearing-impaired listener. (Courtesy of Phonic Ear, Mill Valley, CA)

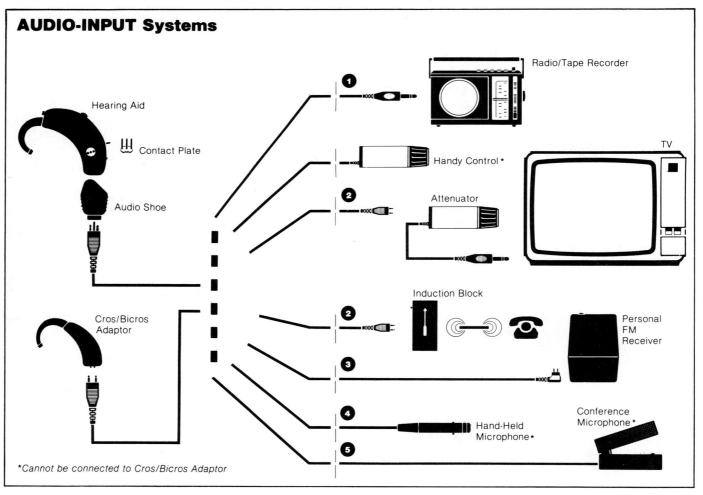

AUDIO-INPUT Systems

Hearing Aid

Contact Plate

Audio Shoe

Cros/Bicros Adaptor

① Radio/Tape Recorder

Handy Control *

② Attenuator

TV

Induction Block

② Personal FM Receiver

③

④ Hand-Held Microphone *

⑤ Conference Microphone *

*Cannot be connected to Cros/Bicros Adaptor

How The Device Produces Hearing Sensation Step-By-Step

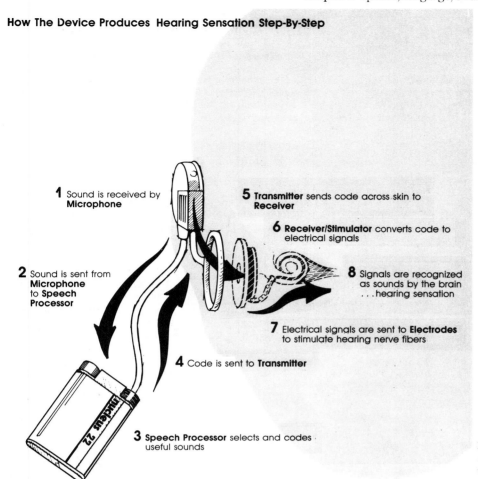

1 Sound is received by **Microphone**

2 Sound is sent from **Microphone** to **Speech Processor**

3 Speech Processor selects and codes useful sounds

4 Code is sent to **Transmitter**

5 Transmitter sends code across skin to **Receiver**

6 Receiver/Stimulator converts code to electrical signals

7 Electrical signals are sent to **Electrodes** to stimulate hearing nerve fibers

8 Signals are recognized as sounds by the brain ...hearing sensation

Figure 6-9. Schematic diagram of cochlear implant system. (Courtesy of Cochlear Corporation, Englewood, CO)

and flashing smoke detectors help to alert the deaf person. Telephone communication for these severely hearing-impaired persons is possible with the use of telephone devices for the deaf. These systems use a typed message for transmission and a written readout either to an LED display and/or printer.

COCHLEAR IMPLANT. The cochlear implant is an auditory prosthesis designed to provide hearing for the profoundly deaf by electrically stimulating residual eighth nerve neurons in the cochlea (Fig. 6-9). Prospective implant candidates first must undergo an extensive audiological evaluation to document that powerful hearing aids would not be of help. If they are a suitable candidate, an electrode wire or electrode array is surgically implanted into the cochlea, connected to an internal coil placed under the skin behind the ear, and aligned with an external coil placed behind the ear. Following a period of healing, the patient is fitted with a microphone and stimulator/signal processor unit. The microphone, usually worn at ear level, picks up sound and transmits the sound to a signal processor unit that resembles a body-type hearing aid. The processor converts the sound to electrical signals that are transmitted to the external coil, through the skin to the internal coil, and to the electrode(s) in the cochlea. Current flows between the active electrode(s) and a ground electrode placed in the eustachian tube, stimulating remaining nerve fibers and producing a sensation of sound.

The cochlear implant, unlike a hearing aid, does not change the electrical impulses back into amplified sounds. Rather, sound is changed into electrical impulses that are delivered directly to the cochlea. Sounds perceived with a cochlear implant are en-

tirely different than sounds heard with a hearing aid. Patients with cochlear implants have described the sounds they hear as buzzes, whistles, or metallic sounds; only rarely are sounds described as "speechlike." Although the implant does allow the profoundly deaf person to "detect" speech, this does not imply the ability to "discriminate" (understand) speech. Electrical stimulation does provide considerable loudness and timing information to the patient, aiding in speech reading. In addition, the implant can help to provide the user with an awareness of environmental sounds. For those people in whom hearing aids cannot be of any help, the awareness of environmental sounds is of benefit, not only for removing the isolation of deafness but also for safety factors.

TACTILE AIDS. For those profoundly deaf patients who are not candidates for cochlear implants, and receive no help from hearing aids, tactile devices are available. These devices convert sound into vibrations to provide the patient with awareness of sound.

REFERENCES

1. Alexander MP, LoVerme SR: Aphasia after left hemisphere intracerebral hemorrhage. Neurology 30:1193–1202, 1980
2. Bayles K: Language function in senile dementia. Brain Lang 16:265–280, 1982
3. Bayles K, Tomeda C: Confrontation naming impairment in dementia. Brain Lang 19:98–114, 1983

4. Benson DF, Sheramata WA, Bauchard R et al: Conduction aphasia: A clinicopathological study. Arch Neurol 28:339–346, 1973

5. Beukelman DR, Yorkston KM: The relationship between information transfer and speech intelligibility of dysarthric speakers. J Commun Disord 12:189–196, 1979

6. Beukelman DR, Yorkston KM, Dowden PA: Communication Augmentation: A Casebook of Clinical Management. San Diego, College-Hill Press, 1985

7. Blakelay W, Garety E, Smith D: Section of the cricopharyngeus muscle for dysphagia. Arch Surg 96:745–760, 1968

8. Brandes PJ, Ehinger DM: The effects of early middle ear pathology on auditory perception and academic achievement. J Speech Hearing Dis 46:301–306, 1981

9. Brookshire RH: Recognition of auditory sequences by aphasic, right hemisphere damaged and non-brain damaged subjects. J Commun Disord 8:51–59, 1975

10. Buckingham HW: Explanation in apraxia with consequences for the concept of apraxia of speech. Brain Lang 8:202–226, 1979

11. Burns MS, Halper AS, Mogil SI: Clinical Management of Right Hemisphere Dysfunction. Rockville, MD, Aspen Publishers, 1985

12. Damasio A, Damasio H, Rizzo M, et al: Aphasia with non-hemorrhagic lesions in the basal ganglia and internal capsule. Arch Neurol 39:15–20, 1982

13. Darley FL: Aphasia. Philadelphia, WB Saunders, 1982

14. Darley FL, Aronson AE, Brown JE: Motor speech signs in neurologic disease. Med Clin North Am 52:835–844, 1968

15. Darley FL, Aronson AE, Brown JE: Differential diagnostic patterns of dysarthria. J Speech Hearing Res 12:246–269, 1969

16. Darley FL, Aronson AE, Brown JE: Clusters of deviant speech dimensions in the dysarthrias. J Speech Hearing Res 12:462–496, 1969

17. Davis H: Hearing handicap, standards for hearing, and medicolegal rules. In Davis H, Silverman SR (eds): Hearing and Deafness, 3rd ed, pp 253–279. New York, Holt, Rinehart & Winston, 1970

18. DeRenz E, Vignolo LA: The token test: A sensitive test to detect receptive disturbances in aphasia. Brain 85:665–678, 1962

19. DeRenz E, Ferrai C: The reporter's test: A sensitive test to detect expressive disturbances in aphasics. Cortex 14:279–293, 1978

20. Downs MP: The expanding imperatives of early identification. In Bess FH (ed): Childhood Deafness: Causation, Assessment and Management, pp 95–106. New York, Grune & Stratton, 1977

21. Dudgeon BJ, DeLisa JA, Miller RM: Head and neck cancer, a rehabilitation approach. Am J Occup Ther 34:243–251, 1980

22. Duffy RJ, Duffy JR, Pearson KL: Pantomime recognition in aphasics. J Speech Hearing Res 18:115–132, 1975

23. Fleming SM: Treatment of mechanical swallowing disorders. In Groher M (ed): Dysphagia: Diagnosis and Management, pp 157–172. Boston, Butterworths, 1984

24. Gates GA, Ryan W, Cooper JC et al: Current status of laryngectomy rehabilitation: I. Results of therapy. Am J Otolaryngol 3:1–7, 1982

25. Gonzalez J, Aronson A: Palatal lift prosthesis for treatment of anatomic and neurologic palatopharyngeal insufficiency. Cleft Palate J 7:91–104, 1970

26. Goodglass H, Kaplan E: The Assessment of Aphasia and Related Disorders. Philadelphia, Lea & Febiger, 1983

27. Goodman A: Reference zero levels for pure-tone audiometer. ASHA 7:262–263, 1965

28. Groher M: Language and memory disorders following closed head trauma. J Speech Hearing Disord 20:212–220, 1977

29. Groher M: Communication disorders. In Rosenthal M, Griffith ER, Miller JD (eds): Rehabilitation of the Head Injured Adult, pp 155–165. Philadelphia, FA Davis, 1983

30. Hagen C, Malkmus D, Durham E: Levels of cognitive functioning. In Rehabilitation of the Head Injured Adult, pp 26–37. Downey, CA, Professional Staff Association, 1979

31. Hagen C, Malkmus D, Burditt G: Intervention strategies for language disorders secondary to head trauma. Short Course Abstract, American Speech and Hearing Association Convention, Atlanta, GA, 1979

32. Hamaker RC, Singer MI, Blom ED, Daniels HA: Primary voice restoration at laryngectomy. Arch Otolaryngol 111:182–186, 1985

33. Hardison D, Marquardt TP, Peterson HA: Effects of selected linguistic variables on apraxia of speech. J Speech Hearing Res 20:334–343, 1977

34. Hardy JC, Netsell R, Schweiger JW, Morris HL: Management of ve-lopharyngeal dysfunction in cerebral palsy. J Speech Hearing Disord 34:123–137, 1969

35. Harford E, Barry J: A rehabilitative approach to the problem of unilateral hearing impairment: The contralateral routing of signals (CROS). J Speech Hearing Disord 30:121–138, 1965

36. Hixon TJ: Respiratory function in speech. In Minifie FD, Hixon TJ, Williams F (eds): Normal Aspects of Speech, Hearing, and Language. Englewood Cliffs, NJ, Prentice-Hall, 1973

37. Kertesz A: The Western Aphasia Battery. New York, Grune & Stratton, 1982

38. Kertesz A, Black SE: Cerebrovascular disease and aphasia. In Darby JK (ed): Speech and Language Evaluation in Neurology: Adult Disorders. Orlando, FL, Grune & Stratton, 1985

39. LaPoint LL, Horner J: Reading Comprehension Battery. Tigard OR, CC Publications, 1979

40. Lindemann RC: Diverting the paralyzed larynx: A reversible procedure for intractable aspiration. Laryngoscope 85:157–180, 1975

41. Logemann J: Evaluation and Treatment of Swallowing Disorders. San Diego, College-Hill Press, 1983

42. Lubinski R: Environmental language intervention. In Chapey R (ed): Language Intervention Strategies in Adult Aphasia, pp 233–245. Baltimore, Williams & Wilkins, 1981

43. Martin AD: Some objections to the term apraxia of speech. J Speech Hearing Disord 39:53–64, 1974

44. McNeil MR, Prescott TE: Revised Token Test. Baltimore, University Park Press, 1978

45. Miller RM: Evaluation of swallowing disorders. In Groher M (ed): Dysphagia: Diagnosis and Management, pp 85–108. Boston, Butterworths, 1984

46. Miller RM, Groher M: General treatment of swallowing disorders. In Groher M (ed): Dysphagia: Diagnosis and Management, pp 113–131. Boston, Butterworths, 1984

47. Mohr JP, Watters WC, Duncan GW: Thalamic hemorrhage and aphasia. Brain Lang 2:3–17, 1975

48. Myers PS: Right hemisphere impairment. In Holland A (ed): Language Disorders in Adults, pp 177–208. San Diego, College-Hill Press, 1984

49. Naeser MA: CT scan lesion size and lesion locus in cortical and subcortical aphasias. In Kertesz A (ed): Localization in Neuropsychology, pp 63–119. New York, Academic Press, 1983

50. Naeser MA, Alexander MP, Helm-Estrabrooks N et al: Aphasia with predominantly subcortical lesion sites: Description of three capsular/putaminal aphasia syndromes. Arch Neurol 39:2–14, 1982

51. Netsell R: Speech physiology. In Minifie FD, Hixon TJ, Williams F (eds): Normal Aspects of Speech, Hearing, and Language. Englewood Cliffs, NJ, Prentice-Hall, 1973

52. Netsell R, Hixon TJ: A noninvasive method of clinically estimating subglottal air pressure. J Speech Hearing Disord 43:326–350, 1978

53. Noll JD, Randolph SR: Auditory semantic, syntactic, and retention errors made by aphasic subjects on the token test. J Commun Disord 11:543–553, 1978

54. Obler L: Language in Age and Dementia. Short Course Abstract. American Speech, Langauge, Hearing Association, Washington, DC, 1985

55. Obler L, Albert MR: Language in the senile patient and the elderly patient. In Sarno M (ed): Acquired Aphasia, pp 395–408. New York, Academic Press, 1981

56. Pearson BW, Woods RD, Hartman DE: Extended hemilaryngectomy for T3 glottic carcinoma with preservation of speech and swallowing. Laryngoscope 90:1950–1961, 1980

57. Platt LJ, Andrews G, Young M, Neilson PD: The measurement of speech impairment of adults with cerebral palsy. Folia Phoniatr 30:30–58, 1978

58. Platt LJ, Andrews G, Young M, Quinn P: Dysarthria of adult cerebral palsy: Intelligibility and articulatory impairment. J Speech Hearing Res 23:28–40, 1980

59. Porch BE: The Porch Index of Communicative Ability. Palo Alto, CA, Consulting Psychology Press, 1967

60. Rosenbek JC, LaPointe LL: The dysarthrias: Description, diagnosis and treatment. In Johns DF (ed): Clinical Management of Neurogenic Communication Disorders, pp 97–152. Boston, Little, Brown & Co, 1985

61. Schaefer SD, Johns DF: Attaining functional esophageal speech. Arch Otolaryngol 108:647–649, 1982

62. Schuell H: The Minnesota Test for the Differential Diagnosis of Aphasia. Minneapolis, University of Minnesota Press, 1965

63. Simmons N: Interaction between communication and neurologic disorders. In Darby JK (ed): Speech and Language Evaluation in Neurology: Adult Disorders. Orlando, FL, Grune & Stratton, 1985

64. Singer MI, Blom ED: An endoscopic technique for restoration of voice after laryngectomy. Ann Otol Rhinol Laryngol 89:529–533, 1980

65. Singer MI, Blom ED, Hamaker RC: Further experience with voice restoration after total laryngectomy. Ann Otol Rhinol Laryngol 90:498–502, 1981

66. Singer MI, Blom ED, Hamaker RC: Vocal rehabilitation after laryngectomy. Otolaryngol Clin North Am 18:605–611, 1985

67. Singer MI, Blom ED, Hamaker RC: Pharyngeal plexus neurectomy for alaryngeal speech rehabilitation. Laryngoscope 96:50–54, 1986

68. Smitheran J, Hixon TJ: A clinical method for estimating laryngeal airway resistance during vowel production. J Speech Hearing Disord 46:138–146, 1981

69. Swisher LP, Sarno MT: Token test scores of three matched patient groups: left brain damaged with aphasia; right brain damaged without aphasia; non-brain damaged. Cortex 5:264–273, 1969

70. Wallesch G, Kornhuber H, Brunner R et al: Lesions of the basal ganglia, thalamus, and deep white matter: Differential effects on language functions. Brain Lang 20:286–304, 1983

71. Wertz RT: Neuropathologies of speech and language: An introduction to patient management. In Johns DF (ed): Clinical Management of Neurogenic Communication Disorders. Boston, Little, Brown & Co, 1978

72. West JF, Leader BJ, Costagliola C: Screening Battery Assessing Cognition in Patients with Right Cerebrovascular Accidents. Piper presented to New York State Speech and Hearing Association, New York, NY, 1982

73. Wetmore SJ, Johns ME, Baker SR: The Singer-Blom voice restoration procedure. Arch Otolaryngol 107:674–676, 1981

74. Wetmore SJ, Krueger K, Wesson K, Blessing ML: Long-term results of the Blom-Singer speech rehabilitation procedures. Arch Otolaryngol 111:106–109, 1985

75. Wood PHN: Appreciating the consequences of disease—the classification of impairments, disabilities and handicaps. WHO Chron 34:376–380, 1980

76. Yorkston KM, Beukelman DR: Ataxic dysarthria: Treatment sequences based on intelligibility and prosodic considerations. J Speech Hearing Disord 46:398–404, 1981

77. Yorkston KM, Beukelman DR: Assessment of Intelligibility of Dysarthric Speech. Tigard, OR, CC Publications, 1981

78. Yorkston KM, Beukelman DR, Bell K: Clinical Management of Dysarthric Speakers. San Diego, College-Hill Press, 1987

79. Yorkston KM, Beukelman DR, Traynor CD: Computerized Assessment of Intelligibility of Dysarthric Speech. Tigard, OR, CC Publications, 1984

7

Disability Evaluation

Ron M. Koppenhoefer

Disability is becoming an increasingly significant health and social problem. In Nagi's text *Disability and Rehabilitation,*[14] published in 1969, it was reported that 1964 statistics showed that workers' compensation costs were slightly greater than 2.7 billion dollars. It was also noted that Social Security programs (Title II, Title XVI) cost 1.3 billion dollars. The cost of disability has risen dramatically since then. In 1982, workers' compensation costs were estimated to be 13.8 billion dollars[15] and Social Security costs were 23.1 billion dollars.[19]

Part of the increase in cost of the above programs is related to a gradual change in the concept of compensable injury or disability. Workers' compensation laws have their origin in the 1884 German Capital Sickness and Accident Law. Massachusetts, in the early 1900s, was the first state to extend legal protection to occupational disease. By 1930, most states had passed laws recognizing occupational disease. These early laws did not provide the employee or the employer the right to sue for liability, and injuries without a specific accident were not covered. These laws were meant instead to provide economic protection for workers with specific injuries that placed them at a disadvantage in the work force. The concept of compensable injury has gradually evolved to the point where some states are expanding the definition of injury to include repetitive physical trauma, stress-related diseases (*i.e.,* coronary heart disease, hypertension, stroke), and neuropsychiatric illness.

DEFINITIONS

It is important for physicians to understand basic terminology necessary to evaluating and responding to questions about disability and impairment. Basic definitions have to be understood and used correctly to avoid misunderstandings between physicians and the various third party agencies or individuals who request information or examinations.

Impairment, in the past, was a term that had been used interchangeably with disability. However, the word has its own definition and it differs radically from disability. Medical impairment has been defined as "an alteration of health status assessed by medical means."[1] The alterations that are present are measurable in terms of objective criteria such as decreased range of motion, motor and sensory loss, loss of a body part, and individ-

ual organ or organ systems dysfunction. Impairment is an objective medical opinion that does not take into consideration a person's educational, vocational, or social experience.

Disability has been defined by numerous authors and agencies. Definitions have ranged from a "term to denote a physical defect or impairment and the resulting social and economic status of the affected individual"[9] to "a complex, imprecise concept, compounded by changing social values and ideologies of vested interest groups."[11] The Social Security Administration defines disability as "inability to engage in any substantial gainful activity by reason of a medically determinable physical or mental impairment which can be expected to result in death or has lasted or can be expected to last for a continued period of not less than 12 months."[17] Disability takes into consideration not only the physical or mental impairment of a person but also limitations placed on that person as a result of education, training, or society.

Impairment and *disability* can be used with various modifiers. These modifiers are used to denote degree (partial, total) and duration (temporary, permanent). The degree of partial impairment and disability is usually determined by using well-established formulas that have been developed by agencies and authors, such as the American Medical Association,[1] the Social Security Administration,[17] Kessler,[9] and McBride.[13]

PURPOSE OF EXAMINATIONS

Before a physician begins to perform an impairment or disability evaluation, he or she must be aware of the needs of the party requesting the examination. Insurance companies, plaintiff and defendant attorneys, and government agencies have specific purposes for the examinations they request and ask specific information of the examiner. Ludwig[11] estimates that there are currently 85 separate public and private programs dealing with workers' compensation, each with its own criteria for determining compensation awards. In addition, Social Security has two programs for disability: Title II (Trust Fund contributed into by workers) and Title XVI (supplemental security income based on financial need, age 65 or older, or blindness). Requests for evaluation from any of these agencies require that the physician give a clinical assessment of the patient's impairment generally or how that impairment relates to his or her occupational requirements.

The physician must also be sure to examine only those people whose impairments fall within his or her specialty area. This then ensures for him or her the ability to examine the pathological process, to have knowledge of the treatment whether it be surgical or nonsurgical, and to know the expected outcome of the treatment as well as expected complications.

The physician, besides being familiar with the physical limitations discovered in the examination, must also understand the disability process. Cailliet[3] states that the "evaluation is not of the disability, it is evaluation of a patient who is disabled." The psychological and societal factors that contribute to a person's disability must be considered. The following reviews illustrate this point:

Ludwig[11] believes that disability encompasses four major elements:

1. Disease—the basic pathological process
2. Impairment—physical, mental limitations in function
3. Sick role—socially sanctioned state that grants a person relief from social, personal, and vocational responsibilities for duration of the illness
4. Illness behavior—coping patterns in response to distress or disease that are shaped by psychological, social, and cultural factors

Because of the above factors, a person being examined for an existing impairment or disability is a complex individual. The physical examination can often be modified by these factors to the point at which limitations or impairments are difficult to assess.

Hirschfeld and Behan[8] studied and reviewed approximately 300 cases of industrial injuries and accidents. Their findings indicated that physical injury often resulted from a definable psychological process. The psychological events preceding the injury were called "an accident process." This "process" caused the "death of the person as a worker when the state of conflict and anxiety within the worker makes him commit or find an injury-producing act." The resultant injury causes a physical disorder, which then replaces the psychological disorder. The physical disorder, with its pain and incapacity, continues the accident process. The accident or injury solves the worker's preexisting life problems, and the injured worker continues to prove his incapacity for work by preserving his symptomatology.

Weinstein[18] uses the term *disability process* to expand on the work of Hirschfeld and Behan. The disability process can be caused not only by a work-related accident but also by a nonindustrial illness. Weinstein believed that if a person's self-esteem is elevated by the disability process, a change from this situation was unlikely; if self-esteem was lowered, the change was actively sought by the person. The person's self-esteem was actively being modified by societal and government reinforcement in the cases Weinstein studied.

EXAMINATIONS

The physician must first explain the purpose of the examination to the patient. It is necessary to inform the patient that the results of the examination will be sent to the third party (attorney, agency) requesting the examination. This understanding is critical in removing the examination and information gained from the examination from the realm of the traditional physician–patient relationship.

A complete medical history is mandatory for a disability or impairment examination. The history should include, but not be limited to, a careful investigation of the action or illness that caused the impairment, activities that have an effect on the impairment, subjective limitations, review of past medical treatments, a complete occupational history, and psychosocial factors affecting the impairment. The medical history must look for conditions that could influence the severity of the impairment. These conditions can be preexisting (*e.g.,* congenital, past fractures), or concurrent (*e.g.,* diabetes mellitus, hypertension).

The occupational history should include the worker's past and present occupations and past educational experiences. Job descriptions from the employer should be reviewed, but the physician must realize that these are often inaccurate in regard to actual physical requirements needed for the job. The job descriptions must be used for reference with additional information from the employee being examined.

Frymoyer and Mooney[5] separated occupational musculoskeletal injuries into four categories: postural stress, cumulative trauma, sudden stress overload, and environmental exposures.

1. Postural stress can be separated into dynamic (*e.g.,* chronic elevation of the shoulders can cause shoulder pain) and static postures such as sitting (*e.g.,* driving has been associated with increased incidence of back pain).
2. Cumulative trauma has been implicated in causing tenosynovitis and epicondylitis. Two-thirds of these cases involve the upper extremities. Spinal structures are particularly susceptible to prolonged vibrational stress such as that which occurs when driving or riding in vehicles. This has been implicated in increased incidence of lumbar, cervical disk herniations in commuters and truck drivers.[6]
3. Sudden stress overload usually occurs during specific lifting or bending episodes that require a force that is beyond the person's physical capacity.
4. Environmental factors such as chronic lead exposure can cause muscle weakness and joint pain.[2]

It is also important for the examiner to obtain from the person any feelings of his or her restrictions. A person should be asked why he or she can't return to work. Often, simple modifications in the job can allow the person to return to work. These modifications can usually be brought out by the answer to the above question.

The physical examination has to fully evaluate the impairment. It should substantiate or disprove the patient's subjective symptomatology. The examination has to document, through direct and indirect observations, the physical signs and limitations that relate to the subjective symptomatology and thus the physical impairment. The signs elicited and measured can then be used to determine the degree of impairment or the limits of the worker.

During the course of the examination, the physician has to search for evidence of consistency. Consistency should be present between formal and informal examinations and observations. Formal examinations are the actual testing for range of motion, manual muscle strength, and observation of gait. Informal testing and observation should include, but not be limited to, the following: watching the person dress and undress if appropriate, movements during transitional activities such as getting on and off the examining table, sitting to stand, and observing gait pattern on entering and leaving the examining room and office suite. The range of motion and strength observed during formal and informal sessions should be consistent for true impairment to exist.

A person should also be examined for evidence of physical activities not contained in the history. The examination should include inspecting the hands for evidence of callus or dirt under the nailbeds; feet should be inspected for evidence of callus formation that is consistent with his gait pattern; shoes should be inspected, if appropriate, for wear consistent with gait deviations observed. Clothing should be evaluated for its inappropriateness for the subjective complaints, such as pullover blouses or shirts worn by people with longstanding shoulder complaints.

The physical examination must evaluate each component of the structure or structures that may contribute to the impairment. An adequate joint examination should evaluate active and passive range of motion, stability, length and angulation of adjoining bones, evidence for active or chronic synovitis, arcs of motion that do or do not cause pain, and associated muscle tone and atrophy. Neurological examination should include coordination, strength, sensation, muscle tone, atrophy, and reflexes.

In some cases, the physicial examination can be supplemented by laboratory testing. It is important to remember that laboratory testing results usually depend on the person's compliance with the testing procedure used. Testing can be related to physiological parameters such as pulmonary function studies, treadmill testing, or function tests such as the *Minnesota Rate or Manipulation and Tapping Test.*[7]

Chaffin[4] has shown that the frequency and severity rates of musculoskeletal problems are about three times greater for workers who are placed in jobs that require physical exertions above those demonstrated in isometric strength tests. Lifting can be measured by isometric or isokinetic testing. Isometric testing has been standardized by Chaffin and his associates[4] for use in preemployment evaluations. The lifting test consists of measurements of a 5-second force applied to a load cell with equipment that can be adjusted for height, lifting position, and pushing and pulling. The test has been standardized for arm, leg, and dorsal lifting for the general population and has a coefficient variation between test and retest of approximately 13%. Isokinetic testing has been standardized in a series of articles by Smith,[16] Mayer,[12] and Kishino.[10] The isokinetic technique allows the patient to apply maximum effort against a device that only moves at a fixed velocity regardless of force applied. The velocity is usually set at speeds of 18, 30, and 36 inches per second.

IMPAIRMENT RATING

There are numerous guides available to the physician for use after completing his or her assessment of the patient. All of the guides have limitations, but they can serve as an excellent reference for the physician. The guides available range from the *American Medical Association Guides to the Evaluation of Permanent Impairment*[1] to books by the Social Security Administration and by individual physicians such as McBride[13] and Kessler.[9]

McBride[13] developed his own medical disability rating system. His system uses two major components of disability that classify the permanent physical impairment:

1. Disabling physical impairments
   a. Anatomical and physiological mass, tissue damage
   b. Clinical manifestations resulting from the mass tissue and structural damage (*e.g.,* pain, tenderness, fatigue)
   c. Restrictions on work restoration (*e.g.,* ability to climb, squat, walk)
   d. Restrictions related to work conditions: uneven ground, environmental restrictions
   e. Intangible or reactionary interferences to recovery: degenerative changes that are difficult to predict tolerance, tissue restriction secondary to age, obesity

2. Disabling functional deficiencies
   a. Quickness of action
   b. Coordination, skill
   c. Strength, stability
   d. Security, confidence
   e. Endurance

McBride rates each of the ten subunits independently for its degree of severity. An average is taken of all the ratings that becomes the rating given for the physical impairment. The impairment is then rated by the following scale: negligible, 0; mild, 5; minor, 10; mediocre, 20; moderate, 30; substantial, 40; severe, 50; quite severe, 60; very severe, 70; extremely severe, 80; profoundly severe, 100.

The Social Security Administration lists impairments for every body system. If an applicant's impairment meets his or her set of symptoms, signs, or laboratory findings, a presumption is made in the absence of work that the applicant meets the Social Security definition of disability.

The *Americal Medical Association Guides to the Evaluation of Permanent Impairment* is a comprehensive publication that entails ratings of all organ systems. It was initially published in 1971 and was revised in 1984. Its purpose is to "provide a structure to set a medical criteria that comprise a reference with which to establish well-formulated medical ratings of permanent impairment." The following case studies illustrate use of this publication:

R.J. is a 19-year-old male college student who was involved in a diving accident that caused a traumatic C5–C6 dislocation. This injury resulted in immediate C6 quadriplegia. He was initially treated by surgical stabilization and he wore a 4-poster surgical collar for 3 months. He underwent an extensive rehabilitation program from which he was discharged to his home environment.

Currently, he denies any pain or discomfort. He is dependent in ADL activities for his lower extremities and transfers. He is independent for his upper extremity ADL activities and oral hygiene.

His mobility is limited to the use of an electric wheelchair but he is independent for pressure relief. His neurogenic bladder is being treated with intermittent catheterization on which he is totally dependent. His neurogenic bowel is dependent on suppository and rectal stimulation by an aide.

Review of systems indicates that recent x-rays of the cervical spine revealed a C5–C6 dislocation to be surgically stable. A recent intravenous pyelogram was within normal limits and a cystometric examination revealed evidence of an uninhibited neurogenic bladder. Reflex erections are possible but no ejaculation has been noted. Currently he takes Ditropan, 5 mg po tid; Bactrim DS, one tablet daily; and Lioresal, 10 mg po tid.

He is a college student majoring in English. He is able to type with the use of a tenodesis splint 15 wpm and is able to keep up with his class work by using dictating equipment.

PHYSICAL EXAMINATION

Vital signs were stable with pulse rate 85/min, blood pressure $^{100}/_{70}$ mm Hg, and respirations 18/min. The lungs were clear to auscultation and percussion. Cardiovascular examination revealed the regular rhythm with no extra sounds or murmurs. Peripheral pulses were symmetrical. Extremity examination revealed full passive range of his lower extremities with mild spasticity. No acute synovitis was noted involving the joints. Passive range of motion involving his upper extremities was full. The back examination revealed no evidence of structural or positional scoliosis. Skin was intact.

Neurological examination revealed positive Babinski's and Hoffman's reflexes. Unsustained clonus was found involving both heel cords. Increased tone was found in the lower extremities and in the upper extremities, particularly involving the finger flexors. Sensation was absent to all modalities distal to the C6 dermatome. Bulbocavernous reflex was present, and sphincter tone was increased. Manual muscle testing revealed normal strength of the neck flexors and extensors. Deltoid, biceps, supraspinatus, infraspinatus, and brachioradialis function was judged to be in the good range. Extensor carpi radialis brevis and pronator teres function was judged to be in the fair-plus range. Wrist and finger flexors, finger extensors, and hand intrinsic musculature were zero. Grasping activities revealed good tenodesis effect involving the wrist extensors. With the opponens splint, the patient had a fair-plus pinch.

In the *American Medical Association Guides*[1] the common impairments associated with spinal cord disorders or injuries are divided into six sections:

1. Station and gait
2. Use of upper extremities
3. Respiration
4. Urinary bladder function
5. Anal/rectal function
6. Sexual function

Station and gait is defined as the ability to stand and walk. Since the patient R.J. cannot stand without an orthosis or the help of others, he would be rated as a 65% impairment to the whole person. His upper extremities can be used with difficulty for self-care activities so he would get a rating of approximately 60% in that area. Respiratory function in the *Guides* is limited to the person's ability to perform the act of breathing. He is capable of spontaneous respiration and has no difficulty in ADL that require extra exertion; therefore, he would have a 0% impairment in this category. His neurogenic bladder will qualify for a 20% impairment. His anal/rectal function would qualify for a 15% impairment. His sexual dysfunction would be applicable for a 22% impairment.

In the *Guides* there is a table for the use of combining impairment ratings for a person. By using this table, R.J. would have a 93% impairment to the body as a whole based on his spinal cord injury.

B.J. is a 35-year-old man who slipped on wet stairs, causing him to strike his buttocks and fall the entire flight of eight steps. This incident, which occurred on August 13, caused him severe back pain. He was taken to a local hospital by the paramedics and x-ray films were taken that revealed evidence of a 50% compression fracture of the vertebral body of L4. He was treated with bed rest for 2 weeks and was placed in a Jewett orthosis. Neurologically, he denied any sort of weakness involving his lower extremities, numbness, tingling, or loss of bowel, bladder, or sexual function. Four months after his injury, he denies having any back pain. He is able to work as an accountant without any discomfort. His hobbies, which include playing golf, cause him no difficulties.

Review of systems is basically unremarkable regarding past illnesses. He has had no surgical procedures.

PHYSICAL EXAMINATION

His gait was normal. Range of motion of the lumbosacral spine was full in all planes without any hesitation. No paravertebral tenderness or spasm was identified in the standing or supine position. Neurological examination of the lower extremities revealed deep tendon reflexes to be symmetrical at 2+, strength was normal; sensation was intact in all modalities. No atrophy or fasciculations were noted. Muscle tone was normal.

X-ray films of the lumbosacral spine revealed an old 50% compression fracture of the vertebral body L4. Disc spaces were slightly narrowed between L4–L5. No other osseous lesions were identified.

According to the *American Medical Association Guides*[1], the patient B.J. would have a 6% impairment to the whole body based on his 50% compression fracture. If he sustained neurological loss or loss of motion, his impairment rating would be higher on the severity of these losses.

A.B. is a 39-year-old woman who is referred for evaluation from her company, W. W. Widget. The company wants to know whether her current right arm complaints are job related.

A.B.'s chief complaint at the current time is right hand numbness. The numbness started in the right hand approximately 6 weeks ago. She describes her numbness as involving her entire hand but mainly localized to the right thumb and index and ring fingers. The numbness occurs at night when sleeping and in the morning when she drives her car to work. The numbness seems to disappear after shaking her hand, and there is no radiation of the numbness into her arm or neck area. There is no history of swelling of her right hand. She denies any type of neck pain, muscle weakness, or hand weakness. Her doctor has been treating her for arthritis with Motrin. No physical therapy or splints have been given.

Her review of systems is basically unremarkable. She is right-hand dominant. She has two children, birth weights 6 and 7 pounds. During pregnancy she had no numbness of her hands. There is no history of diabetes, arthritis, or muscle weakness. There is no history of trauma to the neck or hand.

She has worked for the W. W. Widget Company for the past 3 years. For the past 3 months she was transferred from her normal secretarial job to her job in the factory. Her current factory job consists of assembly line work in which she uses her right hand for repetitive gripping activities. She grips widgets that weigh approximately one-half pound and are 6 inches to 2 inches in size. She grasps the widgets with her right hand and uses both hands to stack them in the carton.

PHYSICAL EXAMINATION

Her height was 5 feet, 6 inches and her weight was 120 pounds. Range of motion of the cervical spine was full on an active and passive basis. Range of motion of the upper extremity joints was full on an active and passive basis. Inspection of the right upper extremity joints revealed no evidence of warmth, redness, or synovial thickening. The right hand was noted to be well calloused.

Neurological examination of the right upper extremity revealed deep tendon reflexes to be 1+; there were positive Tinel and Phalen signs over the right median nerve. Decreased sensation was confined to the right palmar area in the thenar eminence and involving the first, second, and third digits on the palmar side. Decreased strength was found involving thumb opposition (good strength). The rest of the muscle strength of the right arm was judged to be in the normal range. Coordination was intact. No atrophy or fasciculations were found. Palpation of the shoulder girdle area, rotator cuff insertion, bicipital tendons, common extensor tendon, and abductor pollicis longus, and extensor pollicis brevis tendons caused no discomfort. Resisted motions of the right upper extremity revealed pain on finger flexion against resistance. Vascular examination of the upper extremities revealed pulses to be symmetrical.

Capillary filling was normal. Adson's test was normal. Shoulder depression caused no obliteration of the radial pulse.

Electromyographic examination of the right arm revealed positive waves, fibrillations, and complex motor units (polyphasic) confined to the right median innervated thenar musculature. Nerve conduction studies revealed prolongation of the right median latencies with the right motor latency being 4.8 msec and sensory latency being 4.2 msec. Ulnar latencies were within normal limits with the ulnar motor latency being 3.2 msec and ulnar sensory latency being 3.0 msec. Motor velocities over the right median and ulnar nerves were within normal limits at 55 meters/sec. Ulnar velocity in the across-elbow segment was normal at 58 meters/sec.

Based on the physical examination and electrodiagnostic studies, A.B. was diagnosed as having right carpal tunnel syndrome related to her occupation as an assembler. There was no evidence on today's examination to substantiate the diagnosis of arthritis.

At this time, she is able to return to work with avoidance of repetitive grasping and lifting with her right hand. However, activities such as typing with this repetitive finger flexion could also be contraindicated with increase in her symptomatology.

The case of A.B. illustrates the point that examinations are undertaken to evaluate and answer specific questions. The physician should avoid the temptation to suggest treatment in his or her formal report if this question is not asked. However, in cases in which the diagnosis or treatment is not appropriate, the referring party can be contacted by phone to discuss these issues.

EXPERT WITNESS

An expert witness is usually qualified by the court as an expert because of his or her knowledge, training, or education. He or she can form a definite opinion based on medical or scientific theory and express an opinion with reasonable medical certainty (in civil cases, reasonable certainty is defined as at least 51% probable). The testimony must be based on the specific facts of the case and not on personal views. The expert cannot have any personal interest (financial or otherwise) in the outcome of the litigation.

The guidelines to follow when serving as an expert witness include the following:

1. Answer questions simply, never volunteer information.
2. Never guess at answers: "I don't know" is an acceptable answer.
3. If a question is not understood, ask for it to be repeated or rephrased.
4. Avoid citing any one book as authoritative; it is a reference text and is "one of many."
5. Never lose your temper or display agitation during the deposition.
6. Remain in control; pace answers to remain in control.
7. An expert is being paid for time, not testimony.

REFERENCES

1. American Medical Association: Guides to the Evaluation of Permanent Impairment, 2nd ed. Chicago, 1984
2. Baker EL Jr, Landrigan PJ, Barbour AG et al: Occupational lead poisoning in the United States: Clinical and biochemical findings related to blood lead levels. Br J Indust Med 36:314–322, 1979
3. Cailliet R: Disability evaluation: A physiatric method. South Med J 62:1380–1382, 1969
4. Chaffin DB: Preemployment strength testing: An updated position. J Occup Med 20:403–408, 1978
5. Frymoyer JW, Mooney V: Current concepts review occupational orthopaedics. Bone Joint Surg 68A:469–474, 1986
6. Frymoyer JW, Pope MH: Risk factors in low back pain: An epidemiological survey. J Bone Joint Surg 65A:213–218, 1983
7. Gloss, DS, Wardle MG: Reliability and validity of American Medical Association's guide to ratings of permanent impairment. JAMA 248:2292–2296, 1982
8. Hirschfeld AH, Behan RC: Accident process. JAMA 186:113–119, 1963
9. Kessler H: Disability Determination and Evaluation. Philadelphia, Lea & Febiger, 1970
10. Kishino ND, Mayer TG, Gatchel RJ et al: Quantification of lumbar function. Spine 10:921–927, 1985
11. Ludwig AM: The Disabled Society. Am J Psychother 35:5–15, 1981
12. Mayer TG, Smith SS, Kondraoke G et al: Quantification of lumbar function. Spine 10:765–772, 1985
13. McBride ED: Disability Evaluation and Principles of Treatment of Compensable Injuries. Philadelphia, JB Lippincott, 1963
14. Nagi S: Disability and Rehabilitation. Columbus, Ohio State University Press, 1969
15. Pope MH, Frymoyer JW, Andersson GBJ: Occupational Low Back Pain, p 116. New York Praeger Press, 1984
16. Smith SS, Mayer TG, Gatchel RJ, Becker TJ: Quantification of lumber function Spine 10:757–764, 1985
17. Social Security Administration: Disability Evaluation Under Social Security: A Handbook for Physicians, 1979
18. Weinstein MR: The concept of the disability process. Psychosomatics 19:94–97, 1978
19. Ziporyn T: Disability evaluation: A fledgling science. JAMA 190:873–874, 1983

8

Writing Therapy Referrals and Treatment Plans and the Interdisciplinary Team

Donald M. Currie

Rebecca A. Marburger

The concept of rehabilitation is simple: to help a person with limitations caused by some impairment to function optimally in his or her environment. However, several factors make the practice of rehabilitation more complex. Many patients have multiple medical problems with complex interactions among these problems. For example, a person with spastic paraplegia due to a spinal cord injury may develop a urinary tract infection with increased spasticity as the first symptom. A physician unfamiliar with this urological cause of the neurological symptom (increased spasticity) might look for a neurological lesion first, or increase the dosage of antispasticity medication. The physician might miss the urinary tract infection until it becomes more serious. A more catastrophic example might involve an anesthesiologist who is unaware that the use of succinylcholine in general anesthesia for a person with a spinal cord injury can cause hyperkalemia resulting in a fatal cardiac arrest.[2]

Psychosocial, vocational, and educational problems may contribute to the complexity. For example, consider the following case study:

Mr. A. had a cerebrovascular accident (CVA) with right hemiparesis and mild aphasia. Prior to his CVA, he had well-controlled diabetes mellitus with mild coronary artery disease, peripheral vascular disease, and peripheral neuropathy. These problems had little effect on his sedentary life-style as a successful businessman. His job requires frequent telephone communications with his clients. He has a stylish split-level home landscaped with six steps from the driveway to the front entrance. His bedroom is on the second level. Now the increased exercise demands of hemiplegic ambulation may stress his cardiovascular system and the landscaping becomes an architectural barrier to entering his home. The stairs are a barrier to his bedroom, and his aphasia interferes with using the telephone, making it impossible for him to work at his present job.

Multiple caregivers are the rule in rehabilitation (Fig. 8-1). Mr. A. has a neurologist, an internist treating the diabetes and coronary artery disease, a physical therapist, an occupational therapist, a speech pathologist, a social worker, a neuropsychologist, and multiple nurses. If he needs an orthosis to walk, an orthotist joins the team to fabricate and fit it. If he needs a crutch or walker, a company that sells durable medical equipment becomes involved. If he still needs treatment after he is discharged from the hospital, he may need the services of a home health care agency. He has health insurance with one insurance company and disability insurance with another. He needs the services of a vocational rehabilitation counselor. How will all these caregivers and agencies communicate and coordinate with each other so that they work together as a team in the patient's best interest? Without coordination they will act as independent agents. They might send the patient confusing mixed messages about the management of one problem while another problem goes untreated because each caregiver thought another was supposed to address that issue.

The person with a disability needs someone to act as a case manager to help bring all the caregivers together as a team. This case manager should be a professional who understands all the individual problems and the possible interactions among them. Medical knowledge is necessary to manage the medical problems or to refer the patient to the appropriate specialist. This case manager should be familiar with the resources available to help a disabled person. Such resources include health professionals with different capabilities from various disciplines and agencies that provide services. Team management skills are required to ensure that all people and agencies who may be able to help the disabled person work together as an efficient coordinated team.

Physicians have medical skills and knowledge and the legal authority to prescribe treatment, but many lack training about the capabilities of allied health care professionals and agencies who can help a person with a disability. Many physicians have had little training in team management.

Allied health care professionals have extensive knowledge and skills within their own disciplines. They may be familiar with the capabilities of closely related allied health care professionals but be unfamiliar with other disciplines. They lack extensive medical training but may have knowledge of circumscribed areas of medicine and surgery related to their practice. Some have excellent training in team management and organization.

Physiatrists, physicians specializing in physical medicine and rehabilitation, receive formal training in management of the medical, surgical, and psychiatric problems of the disabled. These specialists also learn about resources and capabilities of allied health care professionals and agencies for the disabled. They are trained to lead and participate on the rehabilitation team. Not all of these skills may be necessary to carry out the rehabilitation of a person with a limited and straightforward

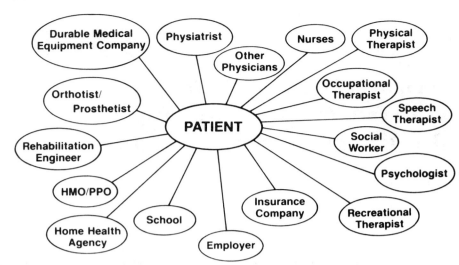

Figure 8-1. Multiple caregivers in rehabilitation.

disability: a physician from another specialty or an allied health care professional may have all the necessary skills. However, for more complex problems, the physiatrist brings together the unique combination of knowledge and skills necessary to manage the disabled patient and lead the team of physicians, allied health care professionals, and agencies who participate in the complex process known as rehabilitation. This concept differs from the traditional medical model of the physician's role, but it is what is needed from the physician who desires to care for patients with complex disabilities.

THERAPY REFERRALS

A prescription is a written formula for the preparation and administration of any treatment. A prescribing physician specifies a treatment (often a drug) with exact instructions regarding dosage, route and frequency of administration, and duration of treatment. The assumption is that the physician has the most complete understanding of all the variables that may affect the outcome, including patient factors, pathophysiology of diagnostic possibilities, and treatment options. Therefore, the prescribing physician is justified in having complete control over the treatment. This assumption is often not valid when a physician needs the help of an allied health care professional associated with disability treatment. The physician does understand the patient's medical problems and the medical and surgical treatments necessary to alleviate them better than any other member of the treatment team. He or she can see the patient's problems from the broadest perspective. However, allied health care professionals have more extensive knowledge of indications for and use of certain evaluation instruments, techniques, and treatment modalities within their areas of expertise. Allied health care professionals usually actually administer the treatment, sometimes using skills in which they are trained and the physician is not. The implications of the word "prescribe" do not fit this situation.

Thus, it is more accurate to say that the treating physician wants a consultation from an allied health care professional. The allied health care professional can evaluate areas within his or her expertise, provide recommendations for further evaluation, and suggest treatment options. The treating physician needs to take these recommendations and apply them to a given patient just as he or she would the recommendations of a physician consultant. The treating physician will decide to follow some of the advice but may decide against other recommendations. These decisions are made by considering the broad perspective of the patient's problems, needs, and goals using his or her best judgment. When the choice is made not to follow a physician consultant's advice, the sensitive physician informs the consultant and explains the rationale for taking another course of action in accordance with good medical etiquette. Nonphysician consultants should be shown the same courtesy. Although written referrals are essential, the need for two-way communication is so great at this step that verbal communication is usually needed before final decisions are made.[8]

In this context, the physician's role is similar to a chief executive officer in a business. The attending physician knows the whole picture. The consultant knows some of the components better than the attending physician. The attending physician must trust the expertise of the allied health care professional consultants. They must trust the physician's ability to make wise and fair decisions based on his or her broader perspective. On a well-functioning team, there is trust, but not blind trust. Team members can discuss alternative treatment plans, defend their suggestions, and appeal decisions with which they differ. Any professional participating on a team must be able to defend his or her viewpoint without being defensive. Consultants should be able to defend their recommendations rationally and logically so that any other team member can understand why a specific treatment or evaluation method is being recommended over the alternatives. The attending physician should also be able to defend the rationale for giving a higher or lower priority to a certain problem, treatment goal, or treatment strategy. If the team members can discuss differences of opinion rationally and defend their points clearly and respectfully, consensus can usually be achieved. In those instances in which differences of opinion remain even after team members have tried to persuade dissenting team members to change, the attending physician must break the deadlock. Such deadlocks occur infrequently on the best teams. When they do occur, mature team members will display professionalism by supporting the decision of the leader without trying to undermine the decision. Only with leaders and team members skilled in group process who are sensitive and attentive to each others messages and respectful of each other can this ideal be approached, so that disagreements can be resolved constructively.

The Choice of the Allied Health Care Professional

One of the attending physiatrist's first decisions is to choose the appropriate team member to whom the patient should be referred. This decision is a matching problem: whose capabilities best match the needs of the patient in any given problem area? A correct decision requires that the physiatrist knows the training, experience, interests, capabilities, resources, and limitations of each team member (see Chapter 1 for a description of members of the rehabilitation team). The health care professional chosen helps develop the treatment plan.

The Referral: What Does the Therapist Need From the Referring Physician?

By law the therapist needs a written referral (Table 8-1). For simple problems, or even for more complex problems in which team members know each other well, a written referral may be all that is necessary. For complex problems, written communication must be supplemented by verbal communication to allow for feedback.[6, 8]

The written referral must include all medical diagnoses that may be relevant to the therapist's treatment. Any precautions the therapist must heed because of the patient's medical condition or treatment should be indicated. Examples of such precautions might be, "Watch for orthostatic hypotension: patient has been at

Table 8-1
Criteria for Therapy Referrals

Criteria that MUST be included on all therapy referrals
1. Diagnosis for which treatment is being requested
2. Goals of treatments: What the patient should be able to do after treatment that he or she cannot do now. Goals may be revised after consultation with therapist. Broad long-term goals and more specific short-term goals should be included.
3. Discipline of therapist to whom referral is directed.
4. Precautions: Other diagnoses or problems that could interfere with treatment or could require emergency medical care and drugs that could interact with therapy, or monitoring of therapy, are the most common precautions.
5. Date when physician plans to reevaluate patient

Criteria that *may* be included on a therapy referral
1. Time estimated to be necessary for each goal to be achieved
2. Request for evaluation using generic or specific evaluation instruments
3. Specific treatment modalities
4. Frequency of treatment
5. Duration of treatment: number of sessions, length of sessions, number of days, weeks, or months to continue treatment
6. Criteria for discontinuation of treatment

A new referral is necessary when
1. There is a change in the patient's condition: surgical procedures, major medical complications, transfer of service, admission to or discharge from hospital, and achievement of goals of treatment are the most common changes.
2. There is a change in the goals of treatment.
3. There is a change in the specific treatment being requested.
4. There is an institutional or third party payer rule that requires a new referral after a patient has been on active treatment for a certain duration, usually 30 or 60 days.

bed rest for 4 weeks." or "Patient on propranolol: heart rate will not increase normally in response to exercise."

The treatment goals may be the most important part of the referral. The written goals communicate to the entire team what the patient should be able to do after treatment that he or she cannot do presently. It is often a good idea to develop these goals after verbal consultation with the specific therapist. Goals should include an estimate of the treatment duration necessary to achieve each goal. They should be considered relevant by the patient. Goal-setting is discussed more extensively below in the section on the treatment plan.

The frequency and duration of treatment need to be written. These parameters are often best determined after discussion with the specific therapist. The physician may face a dilemma because he or she may not be in the best position to determine the ideal treatment frequency and duration or the best treatment activities and modalities but is required to include them in the "prescription." In fact many patients show day-to-day or hour-to-hour variability in their responsiveness to therapy. The solution to this dilemma is to request a detailed therapist evaluation in the initial referral. After the evaluation, the physician and therapist can decide the details of the treatment and agree on the amount of autonomy the therapist should have, and when the therapist should inform the physician of changes in the patient's condition, or in the treatment plan, before proceeding.

There is difference of opinion about the ideal degree of detail and specificity for treatment activities and modalities that should be written on the therapy referral. On any team, such differences of opinion should be discussed openly until consensus can be reached. Unresolved differences in this area can hamper effective team rehabilitation and lead to conflict. Incompatibilities between the team leader and team members in this area increase the risk that informal organization will work against rather than support the team's efforts.[6]

THE TREATMENT PLAN

The treatment plan is the strategy that will be used to help a disabled person reach his or her treatment goals. It may be thought of as a branching document with greater detail in the higher order branches (Fig. 8-2). It should be problem oriented, although sometimes a single therapeutic activity may be intended to effect progress toward solving more than one problem. The treatment plan guides the treatment program or activities, the actual implementation phase.

Evaluation

Evaluation is the initial step. During evaluation the patient's problems are identified and systematically catalogued as a problem list. The patient's strengths and resources are also documented. Evaluation is usually done by multiple team members. There is a hierarchical organization to the evaluation. The broadest evaluation is done by the physician. More detailed component evaluations of individual problems are done by the appropriate team members. Usually the more in-depth evaluations amplify and supplement, but do not contradict, the general evaluation. In those unusual cases in which the in-depth evaluation by the allied health care professional reveals unexpected results that contradict the general evaluation, this new information must be communicated to the rest of the team, since it will usually require modification of treatment goals. Examples of such discrepancies occur more often with children or uncooperative

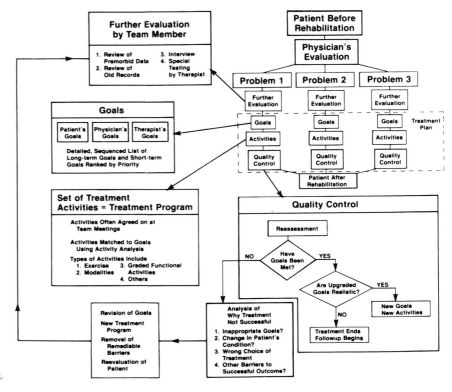

Figure 8-2. Treatment planning.

patients. For example, when the physician initially examines a 2- or 3-year-old boy who cries, clings to his mother, refuses to speak, and is otherwise uncooperative, the child's abilities may be overestimated or underestimated. After the child relaxes and begins to perform in his customary way in the therapy environment, the therapist's evaluation provides a clearer measure of the child's true abilities.

Goals*

After evaluation, treatment goals are developed for each problem. There is a hierarchy to the formulation of treatment goals similar to that for evaluation.

The physiatrist's goals tend to be more general and long term, while those of the therapists include ones that are more specific and short term. These specific goals still relate to the general goals. Reaching the specific and short-term goals should result in reaching the general and long-term ones. Defining short-term goals in terms of measurable functional outcome provides clarification for the patient and the rehabilitation team. For example, the functional significance of the goal, "increasing sitting balance," may be clarified as "improve sitting balance to allow unsupported sitting at the bedside." Once this has been achieved, the next short-term goal may be, "improve sitting balance to allow upper extremity dressing at the bedside." Short-term goals defined in this manner create a clear picture of progress and function gained. Any discrepancies or problems in

*The terms *goals* and *objective* are commonly used interchangeably, as they are here in this chapter. Some health care professionals distinguish between these terms just as educators do. In educational usage, a goal is broader than an objective and does not necessarily state the desired outcome in measurable behavioral terms. An objective is a statement, in measurable behavioral terms, of what a learner or patient should be able to do after a learning experience or treatment.

sequencing of goals can be addressed more easily during formal or informal team meetings.

The patient's goals must not be forgotten when setting goals. Lack of progress may result from unexpressed conflicts between a patient's goals and those of the team, or from a patient's failure to understand the goals. Premorbid values, level of function, and personality influence a patient's goals. For example, a woman has always had a maid keep her house. She intends to continue to use a maid now that she has become disabled. To her, housekeeping is a ridiculous goal. Teaching her how to direct a maid despite her disability might be a goal acceptable to her. Alternatively, explaining to her that some of the movements and skills used in keeping house can be applied to gardening, an activity that really interests her, might also persuade her to accept this goal as relevant to her rehabilitation.

Patients with denial of their disability or unrealistic expectations of what rehabilitation can accomplish may have goals that seem reasonable to them but are not realistic to the team. A paraplegic man whose only goal is to walk may reject all other goals in physical therapy. Counseling by his physician, physical therapist, or psychologist to inform him about different levels of ambulation and about the sequence of intermediate steps necessary before walking is possible might improve cooperation. If the level of paraplegia or other medical considerations make walking an unrealistic goal, the patient must be skillfully informed.

Of course, the patient's future plans influence his or her goals. While housekeeping was not accepted as a goal by the woman who had used a maid, it might be incorporated readily by a man whose post-rehabilitation plans include housekeeping.

Treatment Activities and Activity Analysis

Consider the patient who has had a CVA and desires to return to work. Returning to work is a broad goal shared by the patient and the health care team. Various team members can offer different activities to help him attain this goal. The occupational therapist may focus on the tasks of computer and telephone operation. The physical therapist may emphasize trunk stability and mobility skills necessary to perform these tasks and to move about in the office environment. The speech pathologist may employ treatment techniques to help him compensate for the aphasia or even use an augmentative communication device such as a telecommunication device for the deaf (TDD) system to allow him to send written messages over the phone. The recreational therapist may involve the patient in social activities that will enhance his self-image and improve his business and other interpersonal relationships. This example reinforces the fact that a patient's broad goal is multifaceted and is achieved by meeting several goals through engagement of well-defined activities.

Activity analysis is a process first defined by occupational therapists but now used by other health care professionals.[4] It is essential to match the patient's needs, interests, and abilities with the activities that effect growth and changes.[5, 11] The activity is analyzed from several aspects (Table 8-2). Often the most obvious is the motor component. What motions are required? How much coordination and balance are needed? Is it unilateral or bilateral? Second, one considers the sensory and perceptual components required for the task, such as vision, touch, kinesthesia, hearing, visual figure–ground discrimination, and motor planning ability. Cognitive aspects such as reading, seriation, problem solving, logic, and communication are then considered. Next, one analyzes the psychosocial characteristics. Is the activity performed in a group? Is is an outlet for aggression? Does it require active or passive participation? Finally, practical issues of the activity such as cost and space required are considered. Several methods for activity analysis have been pub-

---

Table 8-2
Conceptual Framework for the Generic Approach to Activity Analysis

I. Sensory Integration
  A. Sensory input
    1. Vestibular
    2. Proprioceptive
    3. Tactile
    4. Visual
    5. Auditory
    6. Olfactory
    7. Gustatory
  B. Opportunity for integration
    1. Reflexes
    2. Multiple stimulation
    3. Sensory discrimination required
    4. Adaptive response required
    5. New response required
    6. Subcortical versus cortical response encouraged
II. Motor Function
  A. Functional capacity required
    1. Gross motor
    2. Fine motor
    3. Strength
    4. Endurance
    5. Range of motion
    6. Coordination
    7. Basic posture required and postural changes necessary
  B. Types of motions
    1. Passive (*e.g.*, patting, stroking)
    2. Active
    3. Aggressive
    4. Rhythmic
    5. Repetitious
III. Cognitive Function
  A. Attention
  B. Memory
    1. Representation
      a. Exocept (motor)
      b. Image
      c. Endocept
      d. Concept
    2. Duration
  C. Orientation
  D. Thought processes
    1. Level of cognitive development required
    2. Creativity required or possible

E. Need for abstract versus concrete thinking
F. Intelligence
    1. Complexity
    2. Number of steps
    3. Directions—demonstrated, pictorial, verbal, written
    4. New learning required
    5. Rate of learning required
    6. The ability of the task to be broken down into component parts (steps)
G. Factual information
    1. General knowledge required
    2. General knowledge to be gained from the activity
H. Problem solving required
 I. Symbolic potential
    1. Universal
    2. Cultural
    3. Idiosyncratic
    4. Potential for facilitating the production of symbols
    5. Similarity to symbolic objects or interactions used in normal development or a part of daily life
    6. Potential for being symbolic of real environmental interactions
    7. Unconscious needs that can be expressed or gratified
IV. Psychological Function
  A. Dynamic states
    1. Needs—expression, satisfaction
    2. Emotional expression permitted or encouraged
    3. Values inherent in activity or able to be expressed
    4. Interests that might be satisfied
    5. Motivation—intrinsic, extrinsic rewards
  B. Intrapsychic dynamics
    1. Potential for the expression of psychodynamics
    2. Defense mechanisms—extent to which they are encouraged
  C. Reality testing
    1. External limits
    2. Readily defined way of using tools and materials
    3. Clearly defined end result—able to be measured against objective criteria
    4. Extent to which sharing of ideas and feelings is possible or encouraged
    5. Extent of feedback available
  D. Insight
    1. Opportunity to experience the effects of one's actions on the environment
    2. Time for thinking about motives and actions

(Continued)

Table 8-2 (*Continued*)
Conceptual Framework for the Generic Approach to Activity Analysis

IV. Psychological Function
  E. Object relations
    1. Possibility for investing libidinal or aggressive energy
    2. Suitability of objects for need satisfaction (people and things)
  F. Self-concept
    1. Sexual identity
      a. Traditional masculine or feminine connotation of the activity
      b. Opportunity for symbolic expression of a sexual nature
      c. Opportunity to interact with members of the same and opposite sex
    2. Body image—opportunity to become aware of one's body
    3. Assets and limitations
      a. Variety of different kinds of skills required
      b. Opportunity for feedback
    4. Self-esteem—likelihood of being enhanced
  G. Self-discipline
    1. Volition—availability of choices
    2. Self-control—required versus external limits
    3. Self-responsibility and direction—extent to which this is possible
    4. Dealing with adversity
      a. Possibility of success or failure
      b. Degree of frustration probable
      c. Degree of anxiety probable
  H. Concept of others
    1. Degree of trust required
    2. Interaction with a possible authority figure required
    3. Degree of interaction with peers
V. Social Interaction
  A. Interpretation of situations—degree to which this is required
  B. Social skills
    1. Communication
      a. Amount required
      b. Degree of verbal versus nonverbal
    2. Dyadic interaction
      a. Degree of interaction with another person required or possible
      b. Degree of structure
      c. Variety of one-to-one relationships possible
    3. Group interaction
      a. Type of group—parallel, project, egocentric-cooperative, cooperative, mature
      b. Need for instrumental versus expressive roles
      c. Degree of structure
  C. Structured social interplay
    1. Cooperation
    2. Competition
    3. Compromise
    4. Negotiating
    5. Assertiveness
VI. Occupational Performances
  A. Relevance to social roles
    1. Family interaction
    2. Activities of daily living
    3. School/work
      a. Work habits—task, interpersonal
      b. Preparation for vocational choice
      c. Relationship to a particular occupation
    4. Play/leisure/recreation
      a. Type of play
      b. Complexity of rules
      c. Possibility as a shared recreational activity
      d. Possibility as a hobby
      e. Possibility for the formation of friendships

  B. Temporal adaptation
    1. Past, present, or future related
    2. Related to a time-specific activity of the day, week, or season
    3. Facilitates the ordering of events in time
    4. Time imposed by the structure of the activity, participation of another person
    5. Involves the coordination of more than one social role
VII. Age
  A. Extent to which activity is age specific
  B. Relevance to age-specific developmental tasks
    1. Those that have been mastered
    2. Those for which it may facilitate mastery
  C. Adaptation to loss
    1. Facilitate mourning
    2. Promote involvement in realistic problem solving
    3. Promote engagement in old or new interests and interpersonal relationships
VIII. Cultural Implications
  A. Ethnic groups
    1. Meaning
    2. Relevance
  B. Socioeconomic group
    1. Meaning
    2. Relevance
    3. Affordability in the community
    4. Educational level necessary
IX. Social Implications
  A. Extent to which members of the individual's social network are or can be involved in the activity
  B. Extent to which family members are or can be involved in the activity
    1. Opportunities for family members to learn about the client's current level of function
    2. Opportunities to explore new ways of communicating and interacting
  C. Implications of the activity relative to the sick role
    1. Dependency versus independence
    2. Passive versus active
    3. Extent to which the activity will help the individual cope with chronic illness or disability
  D. Community resources—extent to which use of community resources is facilitated
    1. Actual participation
    2. Skills necessary for participation
  E. Physical environment
    1. Typical environment in which the activity takes place
    2. Extent to which the activity helps in adjustment to the demands of the physical environment
X. Other Considerations
  A. Place on continuum of simulated to real
  B. Time
    1. Length of total activity
    2. Length of each stage or step
    3. Delays inherent in the process
    4. Sequential ordering of stages linked with time
  C. Extent to which activity can be broken down into parts and number of steps
  D. Equipment and materials needed
  E. Space required
  F. Noise involved
  G. Dirt—are the materials to be used dirty or do they create dirt
  H. Cost of the activity
    1. Equipment and materials
    2. Therapist's time in preparation

(Modified from Mosey A: Psychosocial Components of Occupational Therapy. New York, Raven Press, 1986)

lished.[1,3,5,7,9–11] An example of one format is displayed in Figure 8-3. This activity analysis analyzes digging and planting a garden plot. At first glance, gardening may not appear to be "therapeutic." However, it may be used as an activity to meet the following goals: increase range of motion, strength, and coordination in both upper extremities; improve sitting and standing balance; improve motor planning; enhance self-esteem; improve language and social skills (if required to purchase seeds at a store); and provide proprioceptive and kinesthetic input. Figure 8-3 also includes a column to describe how the activity may be graded. This information is very important to the therapist in formulating a treatment plan, since it determines how the activity may be adapted to meet a patient's changing needs. For instance if one goal of rehabilitation was to increase upper extremity strength, the therapist would first have the patient use lightweight tools with a lightweight, low resistance soil such as peat and then progress towards using heavier tools and more resistive soils. Later, the therapist may choose to have the patient add wrist weights.

When a task involves finer detail or the patient presents a complex level of functioning it is necessary to use other methods to detail the activity's components. A model for analyzing the biomechanics of a specific task is described in Figure 8-4. This activity analysis breaks down the activity into components that

Figure 8-3. Sample of activity analysis form for one specific activity. (Hopkins H, Smith H (eds): Willard and Spackman's Occupational Therapy, 6th ed., p 299. Philadelphia, JB Lippincott, 1983)

ACTIVITY ANALYSIS   *Activity:* digging and planting a garden plot

---

Time Requirement (average range for successful completion): one hour.

Average no. of sessions required to complete: one, but may be done in several short sessions, if needed.

Brief Description (including criteria for determining success):

Garden plot 5' × 5'. Requires digging with spade, raking to remove stones, marking out three rows, planting seeds or small plants.

Success may be determined by the extent to which all the ground is turned over and stone free, and the planting is completed.

Characteristics of Activity	Input	Skills	How can activity be graded?
Physical:			
Gross motor	X	X	The preparation of the 5' × 5' plot in advance will determine the amount of physical work required. A new area will require far more effort than a previously dug area.
Fine Motor	X	X	
Strength	X	X	
Rhythm	X	X	
Repetition	X	X	The nature of the seeds or plants will determine how much fine motor skill is required.
Coordination		X	
Passive			
Active		X	
Sensory:			
Tactile	X	X	The kinds of tools provided, the kinds of seeds or plants; their relative size, texture, fragility, fragrance. Use of hose or can to water.
Visual	X	X	
Auditory	X		
Olfactory	X		
Gustatory			
Perceptual:			
Tactile	X	X	The kinds of tools, seeds or plants; the amount of lifting, bending, stooping.
Visual space	X	X	
Visual form	X	X	
Vestibular	X	X	

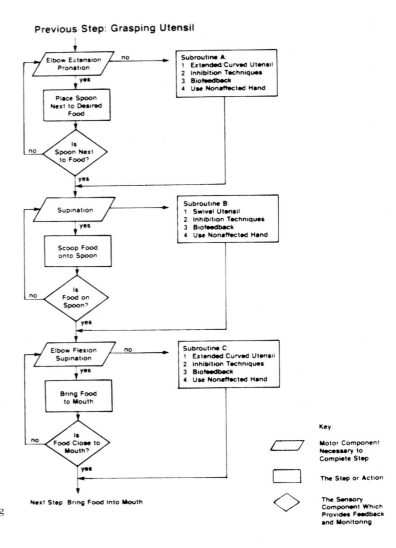

Figure 8-4. Activity analysis for three steps required for eating with a utensil.

may be graded and treated separately and then combined together to meet patient goals. For the purpose of this illustration one segment of the activity of eating is analyzed. The desired action, to scoop food onto a spoon and bring it to the mouth, is effected by upper extremity movements guided by sensory feedback. The sensory component provides continuous monitoring until the step is completed. An able-bodied person will progress to the next step. However, a patient with a set of motor, sensory, cognitive, or psychosocial limitations may need to learn a "subroutine." This subroutine may be viewed as the set of therapeutic activities selected to remediate the patient's limitations. Depending on the discipline of the health care professional, the activities will vary, but the set of activities will later be combined together to restore the function of feeding oneself. Limited elbow motion due to the presence of synergistic patterns may prevent a person with hemiparesis from scooping food onto a utensil or bringing it to his or her mouth. The subroutine or therapeutic activities may consist of inhibition techniques, a temporary extended-handle utensil in occupational therapy, and biofeedback training. The utensil with an extended handle may provide a temporary solution to allow the patient to proceed to the next step of taking the food into the mouth. The alternative measure of training the patient to use the nondominant hand would also allow the person to eat.

The use of activity analysis to help select a treatment activity has several advantages. One of the most important is that an activity that reflects the patient's own goal can be used for treatment (see Fig. 8-2). The activity becomes relevant and purposeful for functional restoration. The patient may be more motivated to participate actively in rehabilitation that involves an activity that is of interest. A second advantage is that it is easier to define treatment systematically. This will facilitate justifying both continued referral and third party payment.

Quality Control

The physician team leader is accountable for the patient outcome. Therefore, he or she has the main responsibility for quality control of the treatment programs, although this function cannot be accomplished adequately without the participation of the entire team. This control function is best built into the treatment plan as a system of closed loops (see Fig. 8-2). These closed loops provide for frequent monitoring of the patient's progress, resulting in a dynamic treatment plan. It responds to changes in the patient's condition with appropriate changes of goals and treatment programs. The ideal way to build this control function into the treatment plan is for the physician leader and other health care professionals on the team to discuss how to do it and develop the closed loops that represent this quality control mechanism together during team meetings. If a member of the team makes changes that may affect other members, he or she must communicate these changes to the other team members.

How to Choose the Appropriate Therapist

In any strategic planning the best result is obtained by applying the available resources correctly so as to be able to accomplish each task at an acceptable level of performance and thus resolve each problem. In rehabilitation, the most important resources are the therapists who carry out the treatments. Each therapist has much more to offer than simply carrying out prescribed treatments. Within their areas of expertise all of the health care professionals on the rehabilitation team can perform specialized evaluation, often using test instruments that have been standardized for a certain type of patient or disability. All of the health care professionals have skills in designing treatment plans and in applying treatment modalities and techniques to specific problems. All can monitor progress or lack of progress toward treatment goals using effective measurement instruments. Rehabilitation professionals have expertise in patient and family education and can design home therapy programs. For children, they can design treatment activities and programs that can be carried out by schoolteachers, including coaches and adaptive physical education teachers. They are trained to be able to communicate all of this information using either technical or "lay" language to other health care professionals, employers, teachers, family members, or disabled people with learning problems.

The problem list can be used as a guide for choosing the correct therapist to whom to refer a new patient. For medical and medically related problems, the most important member of the team is often the rehabilitation nurse.

The physical therapist, occupational therapist, and speech pathologist are most often appropriate for treatment of physical impairments. Often these impairments are not medical problems, but they interfere with a person's ability to move, communicate, or carry out the activities of daily living (ADL), such as dressing, feeding oneself, emptying the bowel or bladder, or carrying out other personal hygiene skills.

Figure 8-5 can be used to choose which therapist is most appropriate. This figure is organized to clarify near and overlapping areas of expertise. For example, both occupational therapists and speech pathologists specialize in the evaluation and

Figure 8-5. Choosing a physical therapist, occupational therapist, or speech therapist.

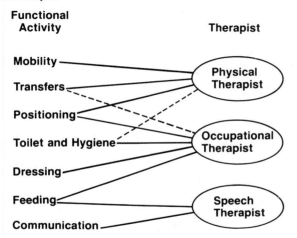

treatment of dysphagia. The choice of the best therapist to treat dysphagia in a given patient depends on many factors. For example, on a given team, the occupational therapist might have more training and experience in treating swallowing problems in one diagnostic category, or the occupational therapist might already have a heavy patient load or need to use all of his or her treatment time to work on another problem at a time when the speech pathologist is not particularly busy. They may be equally qualified to manage swallowing problems, but in this case the speech pathologist may be the logical choice. On a good team, the decisions about which team members will address which problems are decided at staff conferences at which these issues are discussed in a collaborative, not competitive, atmosphere. In any case the most important step to help the patient achieve success may be to instruct the nursing staff and family members to follow through with the same feeding techniques that are being used in the therapy sessions. Overlapping expertise can be an advantage, and the cooperation necessary to make it an advantage rather than a point of conflict is more likely to occur when the therapists know and respect each other's skills. Interdisciplinary inservice training sessions in which one member of the team shares his or her expertise with all the others can help create the proper milieu.

The overlapping skills of physical therapists and occupational therapists cause some of the most common selection problems. Unfortunately, neither title—physical therapist (PT) or occupational therapist (OT)—conveys an accurate picture of the therapist's area of expertise. Perhaps there would be less confusion if PTs were called movement specialists and OTs were called functional activity specialists.

The choice is relatively easy for mobility training (PT) or feeding and dressing skills training (OT). More difficult choices arise in choosing which therapist addresses transfers, positioning, and hygiene skills for a given patient. The choice also tends to be less clear with pediatric patients and with selection or training in the use of adaptive equipment. There is overlapping expertise in the application of certain treatment modalities. For certain specialized categories of rehabilitation, such as in cardiac, cancer, chronic pain, or psychiatric rehabilitation, there is more variability of training and expertise between PTs and OTs than with more common physical disability categories.

When activities or exercises involve the lower extremities, the PT usually treats; but when the upper extremities are involved, the choice is more difficult. It is helpful to choose the therapist according to whether the goal of the therapy is to achieve actual functional tasks (OT) or body movements *per se* (PT). One exception takes place when an OT breaks down a functional activity into component tasks, some of which involve strengthening muscles or increasing the range of motion or coordination of a movement.

Another example of division of labor is transfer training. PTs generally help a patient learn the prerequisite skills necessary to perform transfers, such as adequate strength and range of motion of the upper and lower extremities, sitting balance, and mobility in bed. They teach patients to move their body to and from objects of various heights, such as from wheelchairs to an elevated therapy mat or to the floor. They teach the patient how to use any equipment necessary to transfer safely (*e.g.,* sliding boards and removable wheelchair armrests). Then the labor is usually divided depending on whether the goal is a gross mobility function or the performance of a hygiene activity. According to this scheme, car transfers would be taught more often by a PT and toilet and bathtub transfers by an OT.

Both PTs and OTs can subspecialize in the treatment of children. Motor development is studied in depth because it is so intimately tied to social and cognitive development in infants. The acquisition of language, as an important part of cognitive development, is also studied. Most disabled children under a developmental age of about 2 years can be treated equally effectively by either a pediatric PT or OT regardless of the diagnosis. If many goals are being worked on at once, it is often practical for a child to be treated by both a PT and an OT. When this is done, communication about who is doing what becomes especially important. Home programs often become especially important at this age because children have short and unpredictable attention spans and parents can treat them briefly several times per day whenever the child is attentive and cooperative enough to participate. Treating three or four children together with their parents in a small group led by one or two therapists may be more economical than individual treatments. Group treatments have the added benefit of improving socialization among the children, a common treatment goal for disabled children, and facilitating communication between the therapists. As home programs are reviewed, monitored, and revised during these group sessions, parents may learn from each other and support each other emotionally. Of course, the therapists must be skilled in group leadership in order to be able to direct interactions between parents and children constructively.

Both PTs and OTs teach patients to use adaptive equipment. OTs select and train patients to use adaptive ADL equipment. Most of these items are used in eating, dressing, and hygiene activities or in specific occupational or recreational tasks.

PTs usually select and train patients to use mobility equipment, such as crutches and other walking aids. Both disciplines receive training about the selection, adaptation, and maintenance of wheelchairs, although training in their use for mobility is generally done by PTs. Body positioning aids are selected and fabricated by some PTs and OTs with a great deal of local and individual variation in expertise and training. However, splinting of body parts is nearly always done by OTs, regardless of which extremity is affected, with more complex orthoses fabricated by orthotists (see Chapter 1). Regardless of which team member selects and tests patients in the use of adaptive equipment, a prescription from a physician is necessary for reimbursement by third party providers.

PTs are usually more thoroughly trained in the physiology and use of modalities for heating, cooling, edema control, and pain control. PTs have a more extensive background in exercise physiology and kinesiology than do OTs. Functional electrical stimulation of the lower extremities is usually used by PTs, while OTs may use this modality in the upper extremities.

There is individual and local variation in the work of PTs and OTs in special rehabilitation programs such as cardiac and cancer rehabilitation. Because of their more extensive training in the treatment of psychological disorders, OTs are often chosen to treat patients whose diagnosis has psychological components, such as substance abuse or eating disorders.

Prescriptions for Devices and Equipment

Despite an abundance of devices and varieties of adaptive equipment available to help disabled people, there is a problem getting the right equipment to disabled consumers. Physicians must prescribe devices before third party payers will consider payment. However, most physicians lack training about what items are available and about how to select the correct items for their patients. Physicians are understandably hesitant to prescribe unfamiliar devices, especially costly ones. They are accustomed to having extensive, reliable, and readily available evaluation data about safety and efficacy before prescribing drugs.

These kinds of evaluation date are often difficult to find or nonexistent for rehabilitation devices and equipment.

There are also barriers to getting a device from the idea stage through the design and development stage to become commercially available at a reasonable price. There are difficulties marketing rehabilitation devices so that prospective users, prescribers, and third party payers have access to them. Another potential problem is the small size of the market for most rehabilitation equipment as well as the lack of stability and small size of many of the companies who manufacture and distribute it.

A well-organized approach to prescribing devices and training patients to use them is necessary in order to overcome or minimize these barriers. Educational and continuing education programs for all rehabilitation professionals must be improved in these areas. Qualified rehabilitation engineers should be available as consultants to the rehabilitation team. All team members should be able to match available technology to their patients' needs using resources such as catalogues, scientific literature, and computerized data bases of rehabilitation equipment. Physicians must trust other team members' knowledge about devices in their areas of expertise and be able to add medical expertise and knowledge of the scientific method to the process. All team members must be able to accept the others' different and complementary expertise and constructive suggestions and criticisms. In these ways, the prescription and use of rehabilitation devices can be scientifically based as much as possible.

Causes and Consequences of Lack of Evaluation Data

The lack of valid evaluation data for new adaptive equipment and other rehabilitation devices has many causes. There is low level of public and private funding for research and development, and scientifically valid evaluation is costly. The low priority for device evaluation probably results from a perceived lack of need for evaluation.

Many inventors and developers have excellent engineering skills and are highly motivated to help disabled people but lack the scientific and clinical background to carry out adequate product evaluation.

Furthermore, there are inevitable difficulties and inherent conflicts of interest when the inventor or developer of a device tries to evaluate it, no matter how impartial and objective he or she attempts to be. Yet there are few agencies or clinicians willing or able to carry out adequate objective evaluations of devices developed by others, probably because so little funding is available for this type of research.

A subtle factor that has not been sufficiently appreciated is that manufacturers, users, regulators, third party payers, and clinician prescribers need very different types of "evaluation" data and have very different channels of communication. Manufacturers need informal small-scale evaluations to demonstrate efficacy "anecdotally." They need the information quickly to be able to "tool up" to manufacture a device and get it from the idea phase to the market as soon as possible. They often communicate verbally over the phone and may not even need written evaluative information. Regulators need engineering evaluations to demonstrate safety and protect the consumer. Communication is through bureaucratic governmental channels. Users would profit most from comparative evaluations of similar products, similar to the reports circulated for able-bodied persons in consumer publications such as *Consumer Reports*. Users communicate via disability-oriented consumer publications and formal and informal networking. Third party payers require evidence of safety and efficacy and cost comparison for similar devices. They tend to communicate through trade-oriented insurance networks and meetings. Clinician prescribers need scientifically valid clinical evidence of safety and efficacy, similar to what is now available for drugs. They communicate through professional journals and meetings. One has the impression that currently all these groups, to a greater or lesser extent, continue to develop, market, and prescribe devices on the basis of what "seems logical" rather than on the basis of sound objective data.

If a newly invented device has only one or two costly prototypes, evaluation with a large number of users is tedious and time consuming. This problem may be compounded if the targeted group of users, and thus potential research subjects, is small. The problem is even more complex for devices that must be fitted to the user.

Many devices require both technical and clinical evaluation expertise, but researchers with both these skill are rare. Teams of clinicians and biomedical engineers could be developed to fill this gap, but there is currently no economic incentive to develop such teams.

The effects of insufficient evaluation data have not been studied. Logically, one can surmise that the consequences would include reluctance of clinician prescribers to prescribe new products, a failure of third party payers to fund good devices because of lack of evidence of safety and efficacy, and an increased risk of injury to consumers using inadequately evaluated devices. Because of the diverse channels of communication of those who need evaluation data, there may be a "reinvention of the wheel" phenomenon in which "new" devices are redeveloped without the benefit of others' experience. Good ideas may die between the idea phase and delivery to consumers.

Categories of Devices

Devices may be organized into categories similar to those used for the functional skills noted in the section on how to choose the appropriate therapist. There are devices for mobility, transfer skills, body positioning, hygiene, dressing, feeding, and communication. In addition, there are devices for special uses, such as for vocation and recreation. Whatever the use, the goal of having a patient use a device is increased independence—enabling the person to do something important to him or her that was difficult, impossible, or slower without the device.

Mobility devices may be subdivided into walking aids, wheeled mobility devices, and community mobility devices, such as automobile or van modifications or devices that facilitate the use of public transportation by people with disabilities.

WALKING AIDS. Walking aids can improve the speed or safety of ambulation. Almost all walking aids improve balance by enlarging the base of support. The factors of safety, speed, energy consumption, skill required, convenience, and cost often have to be balanced against each other. For example, a walker may enable an elderly, weak, deconditioned person to walk safely with much less danger of falling, but is slow and inconvenient to transport and store when not in use. It may be easy to use on level ground but requires more skill to use safely on stairs or rough ground. A cane may be safer than using no other walking aid and is inexpensive, easy to store, and relatively maintenance free but may be too unstable for some patients. Its apparent ease of use is deceptive: considerable training may be necessary to teach some patients to use a cane correctly and safely, especially to negotiate barriers and obstacles. Prostheses, orthoses related to mobility, and functional electrical stimulation are specialized walking aids and are discussed in Chapters 15, 16, and 17.

WHEELED MOBILITY AIDS. Wheelchairs are discussed in Chapter 19. Manual wheelchairs are used far more frequently than electrically-powered ones. Manual wheelchairs are easier to transport than electrically-powered ones. Prescribing physicians need to know that most users of electric wheelchairs also need a manual wheelchair, even if they are unable to propel it independently. The manual chair can be pushed by friends and attendants and provide mobility when the specialized equipment necessary to transport an electrically powered chair is impractical. Electric carts steered with handlebars are practical alternatives for some mobility impaired people, and some are easy enough to dissemble and lift that an able-bodied assistant can put them in the trunk of a car. They may be especially useful to people who travel by airplane. The prescriber also needs to recall that any wheelchair also serves as a positioning aid for its user.

Although standing mobility devices have been used experimentally and a few are commercially available, none are in common use. Standing mobility does not seem to have significant practical functional value for many mobility impaired people, and none of the devices available are easily transportable. Most of those who use these devices use them for brief intervals during vocational activities and use a wheelchair at other times.

Automobile adaptations and driving aids, also discussed in Chapter 19, may be thought of as an extension of the concept of wheeled mobility.

TRANSFER AIDS. Transfers may be defined as changes in body position or moving the body from one place to an adjacent location, such as from a wheelchair to the seat of an automobile. Transfer devices may be as simple as a sliding board. More complex devices, such as van lifts, are available. Motorized or manually powered devices to suspend a disabled person by a sling or straps may allow an assistant to transfer a disabled person without having to lift his or her body weight.

POSITIONING AIDS. Positioning aids also vary widely, from pillows and bolsters used to position a bedfast patient, to standing devices for paralyzed patients, to specialized seating systems for a person with extensive deformities, paralysis, or movement disorders. Comfort, control of individual body segments, ease of use, including getting the user into and out of the device, ability to function while using the device, and possible effects on skin integrity are a few of the factors that need to be considered before prescribing positioning aids.

ADL EQUIPMENT. Equipment used for toileting and other hygiene skills, feeding, and dressing is classified as ADL equipment. Thousands of items are presently available in this category, and new items are constantly developed and marketed. Experimental investigation along lines as varied as robotics, environmental control systems, and the use of animals to help disabled people forecasts new advances that may occur in the near future to allow the disabled greater independence in their self-care. Although matching a disabled person's needs to what is available is always difficult for the prescriber, it is especially problematic for this category. Catalogues and computerized data bases, such as ABLEDATA, are essential (Appendices 8-1 and 8-2). A physician's prescription is usually necessary for third party payers to fund this equipment. Teamwork is especially important for the disabled consumer to be best served. If a complex environmental control system is being considered, the rehabilitation engineer can be a valuable addition to the usual treatment team. All team members need to stay up to date with what is available in their field and share their expertise with the physician who must write the prescription. The physician must trust the expertise of team members with more specialized knowledge. A systematic approach to prescription of these devices is discussed in Chapter 19.

COMMUNICATION DEVICES.   The use of devices to augment and supplement the ability to communicate represents an entire field in itself. The prescribing physician must work together with a speech pathologist to prescribe appropriate communication devices. An occupational therapy consultant can also be most useful for the selection of the optimal switching mechanisms and controlled movements by the patient, and for optimal positioning of a patient to use a communication device.

DEVICES FOR SPECIAL FUNCTIONS.   Prescription of devices for specialized needs related to vocation, school, or recreational applications must be individualized. Computer data bases for products should be consulted whenever such needs arise.

Equipment Pools

The science of rehabilitation is not so highly developed that one can predict which device will be most effective for a given patient. In most cases trial and error is necessary to determine what device best meets a disabled person's needs. Few, if any, rehabilitation centers are large enough to have samples of most devices for patients to try out. Yet it is unwise to purchase equipment for a patient until it has been tried. There are partial solutions to this dilemma. It is mutually advantageous for rehabilitation professionals to maintain professional business relationships with vendors of devices and equipment so that devices can be borrowed for a trial before prescription and purchase. Facilities can share equipment formally or informally. A few states and organizations maintain pools of more expensive items of equipment. Items can be borrowed by rehabilitation professionals for patient trials. Money-back guarantees should be requested when it is not possible for a potential user to try equipment before purchase.

Elements of a Prescription for a Device

The prescription for a device should be detailed enough so that it can be filled exactly (Table 8-3). It should include model numbers, and any options must be specified clearly. In addition to these requirements, most third party payers require the patient's diagnosis, the justification for prescribing the device, and the duration of use expected. The justification must explain why the patient needs the device. For inexpensive devices or when the reason is obvious, a brief phrase on the prescription such as "patient cannot walk safely without the device," is all that is necessary. For more expensive devices, or when the justification is not obvious, an explanatory letter to accompany the prescription is necessary. Sometimes obtaining advance clearance from the third party payer is needed. When this is necessary, it is helpful to request that funds be encumbered for training the patient to use the device after he or she has received it.

Almost all devices require training for successful use. Although few data are available to substantiate the claim that training reduces the phenomenon of rejection of rehabilitation devices the claim seems logical.

Table 8-3
Elements of a Prescription for a Device

1. Name of device with model numbers
2. All accessories, sizes, and modifications
3. Diagnosis
4. Justification (may need letter)
5. Duration of use

COST: HOW ARE THERAPY AND REHABILITATION EQUIPMENT PAID FOR?

Many rehabilitation services and devices, like other medical services, are paid for by a third party payer rather than by the user. With medical costs rising, third party payers want evidence that the services and products they pay for will accomplish their intended purposes and are cost effective. A statement by a recognized authority that a patient needs a certain service or device may suffice in some cases. However, more objective evidence of a patient's need and of the efficacy of a service or device is sometimes being demanded by third party payers.

One kind of evidence that a service is needed relates directly to writing treatment plans. This is the quality control aspect of the treatment plan in which there is objective monitoring of improvement, or lack of improvement. Although objectively measured progress in an individual case is not sufficient to prove efficacy (because improvement might have occurred with no treatment), such progress at least represents circumstantial evidence that a patient benefitted from treatment and may still need more treatment to make further progress. This kind of evidence implies that there be an accurate way to measure a person's functional status before and after treatment. Thus, this kind of objective measurement of treatment outcome and functional status becomes very important for financial as well as therapeutic reasons. Since most third party payers will pay for a treatment trial period, it is usually possible to demonstrate need in this way.

For a device, a third party payer wants proof that a device will really improve the patient's function enough to be worth the cost. Usually the best evidence is for the patient to try the device under the supervision of a therapist. The therapist determines what the patient can do with the device that he or she could not do without it. If the device itself cannot be used or is not available for a period of trial usage, sometimes demonstration that a similar device accomplishes the purpose will suffice as evidence.

Third party payers would like to have evidence that rehabilitation therapy techniques and devices accomplish their intended purpose in controlled clinical evaluations. Unfortunately, such evidence is often not available. All rehabilitation professionals need to do or support research that proves or disproves the efficacy and safety of therapy, techniques, and devices. If they do not, a time may come during periods of austerity when third party payers will refuse to pay and patients who are not wealthy will not be able to obtain needed services or devices.

Third party payers may not be knowledgeable about various forms of therapy and devices and may refuse to pay because of lack of knowledge of evidence that a treatment is effective, even when such evidence does exist. Providing the third party payer with information in the form of brochures, copies of articles, or explanatory letters of why a therapy or device is being recommended may persuade a payer to reverse its decision after the payer has initially denied payment. Most companies have an appeals process for such cases. Therefore, when payment is denied, the prescriber should follow the appeals process carefully in order to have the best chance of obtaining a reversal of an initial ruling not to pay.

When usual third party payers refuse to pay for therapy or equipment believed to be necessary by the rehabilitation team, funding can sometimes still be found through charitable organizations. This type of funding may be easier to obtain for tangible equipment than for intangible therapy services because of the public relations value to the charitable organization of photographs of the needy disabled person using the equipment. Being able to use such charitable donations for tax allowance may also be a stimulus that encourages a company to provide a service or device for a needy person. Thus it may be important for rehabilitation professionals from all disciplines to be aware of and support legislation allowing such tax allowances to businesses or charitable organizations.

REFERENCES

1. Allen C: Occupational Therapy for Psychiatric Diseases: Measurement and Management of Cognitive Disabilities. Boston, Little, Brown & Co, 1985
2. Brooke MM, Donovan WH, Stolov WC: Paraplegia: Succinylcholine-induced hyperkalemia and cardiac arrest. Arch Phys Med Rehabil 59:306–309, 1978
3. Cynkin S: Occupational Therapy: Toward Health Through Activities. Boston, Little, Brown & Co, 1979
4. Hinojosa J et al: Purposeful activities. Am J Occup Ther 37:805–806, 1983
5. Hopkins H, Smith H: Willard and Spackman's Occupational Therapy, 6th ed. Philadelphia, JB Lippincott, 1983
6. Longest BB Jr: Management Practices for the Health Professional, 3rd ed. Reston, VA, Reston Publishing Company, 1984
7. Mosey A: Psychosocial Components of Occupational Therapy. New York, Raven Press, 1986
8. Sharf BF (in consultation with Flaherty JA): The Physician's Guide to Better Communication. Glenview, ILL, Scott, Foresman & Co, 1984
9. Trombley C: Occupational Therapy for Physical Dysfunction, 2nd ed. Baltimore, Williams & Wilkins, 1983
10. Trombley C, Quintana LA: Activity analysis: Electromyographic and electrogoniometric verification. Occup Ther J Res 3: 1983
11. Willard H, Spackman C: Occupational Therapy, 4th ed, pp 161–182. Philadelphia, JB Lippincott, 1971

APPENDIX 8-1. MAJOR SOURCES OF ADL DEVICES

The Burdick Corporation
15 Plumb Street
Milton, Wisconsin 53563
(800) 356-0701

Cleo Living Aids
3957 Mayfield Road
Cleveland Heights, Ohio 44121
(800) 321-0595

Lumex
100 Stence Street
Bay Shore, New York 11706
(800) 645-5272

ABLEWARE Maddak, Inc.
Pequannock, New Jersey 07440-1993
(201) 694-0500
Telex: 219359

J.A. Preston Company
60 Page Road
Clifton, New Jersey 07012
(800) 631-7277
(800) 221-2425

Sears Catalogue of Medical Supplies
1409 S. Lamar
Dallas, Texas 75295
(800) 323-3274

APPENDIX 8-2. DATA BASES AND MAJOR ACCESS SYSTEMS FOR REHABILITATION

Data Bases

ABLEDATA and REHABDATA

Listings of available products and literature to service people with disabilities; REHABDATA includes materials from NIDRR and RSA.

The National Rehabilitation Information Center (NARIC), 4407 Eighth Street, NE, Washington, DC 20017. Tel: (800) 34-NARIC or (202) 635-5826.

Accent on Information

Information on rehabilitation aids and devices, disability service organizations, and publications. They publish a buyers' guide annually.

Accent on Information, P.O. Box 700, Bloomington, Illinois 61701.

CTG (Closing the Gap) Solutions

Focuses on computer services and applications for the disabled.

Closing the Gap, P.O. Box 68, Henderson, Minnesota 56044. Tel: (612) 248-3294.

ODPHP (Office of Disease Prevention and Health Promotion)

Health information center publishes HEALTH FINDERS bulletins with a more medical orientation than the above databases.

ODPHP Health Information Center, P.O. Box 1133, Washington, DC 20013-1133. Tel: (800) 336-4797.

THE SOURCE BOOK OF PATIENT EDUCATION MATERIALS FOR PHYSICAL MEDICINE AND REHABILITATION

Extremely complete resource for patient education materials for people with any disability; over 700 pages long.

The Center for Disability and Rehabilitation, Commanche County Memorial Hospital, P.O. Box 129, Lawton, Oklahoma 73502.

Major Access Systems

One can subscribe to most of the above data bases through electronic mail via the following major access systems.

BRS Information Technologies, 1200 Route 7, Lathen, New York 12110. Tel: (800) 345-4BRS.

COMPU SERVE, P.O. Box 20212, 5000 Arlington Center Blvd., Columbus, Ohio 43220. Tel: (800) 848-8199.

Dialog Information Services, 3460 Hillview Avenue, Palo Alto, CA 94304. Tel: (800) 227-1927.

9

Functional Outcome:
Assessment and Evaluation

William D. Frey

Functional outcome assessment and evaluation have received intensive study over the past decade as the health care community continues to seek a better understanding of disablement. The immediacy of these efforts is based on conflicting research reports of the effectiveness of rehabilitation programs and services.[3, 4] However, long-range concerns include the development of useful approaches to planning and evaluating rehabilitation services and to determining the economic and human implications of alternative resource allocations.[15, 18, 20, 39]

Substantial confusion over the meaning of disablement is a major problem which has confounded efforts to resolve these issues.[10] Today's assessment strategies tend to reflect the interests of individual disciplines rather than a broad, common goal orientation that is needed to develop a unified knowledge base for evaluating rehabilitation effectiveness. The reasons for this situation are complex, having much to do with our changing concepts of rehabilitation care, with the multiplicity of professional disciplines involved in the total rehabilitation process, and with the far-reaching nature of permanent or progressive impairments. In discussing this complexity, the information in this chapter is intended to create greater awareness of the unique and pivotal role of outcome assessment in rehabilitation service evaluation, to explain where research progress has been impeded, to recommend solutions to the development of constructive outcome assessments, and to comment on several new initiatives in outcome assessment.

THE PROBLEM OF DISABLEMENT IN HEALTH CARE SERVICE DELIVERY

A new cause for disablement has arisen out of our improved medical abilities to arrest pathological conditions before they result in death. In cancer treatment, for example, recent developments have extended the lives of patients whose diseases were once considered deadly forms of cancer. However, researchers have noted that these patients are left with complications associated with general functioning, including weakness, psychological problems, difficulty in daily living tasks, and pain.[27] Over time, these limitations can become permanently disabling and lead to a reduced quality of life.

Similar problems with disablement occur in people with other diseases, trauma, or acute infections associated with the advance of medical technology over the past 50 years. For example, patients with deadly forms of heart disease can receive artificial hearts and those suffering from diabetes are now able to control their condition with new drugs. Moreover, swift evacuation procedures and advanced life support are preserving the lives of vehicular accident victims. When added, these developments form a new and rapidly growing population of people who are "well" from a traditional medical point of view but who are leaving the health care system incapable of returning to previous levels of functioning.

Understanding the consequences of disease in terms of disablement and its resulting effects on normal life roles is developing as a major health care issue.[14, 30, 37] David Rogers, Executive Director of the Robert Wood Johnson Foundation, stressed its importance in his 1981 Annual Report, suggesting that finding answers to what medicine can do to reduce disability and dependency is the primary health care goal for this decade.[37]

One reason for Rogers' concerns is the sheer magnitude of the growing numbers of people who are leaving the health care system with disabilities. This population has been variously assessed to include approximately 35 million people.[23] Brock and his colleagues[5] note that since the prevalence of disablement increases with age, the increasing size of the elderly population will have a dramatic influence on future use of the health care service system. In 1980, the elderly population represented 11.3% of the total US population; by the year 2000 that percentage is projected to nearly double. The demographic imperative is heightened by Williams' observation that two of three older people will die as a disabled person. The long-term implications are inescapable.[44]

A more immediate concern for disablement issues, however, is the nagging absence of a systematically developed body of knowledge from which health care professionals can draw to make useful clinical decisions. Rehabilitation research literature is notorious for conflicting data about the effectiveness of treatments and programs. As expected, conflicting reports are often the result of poor research procedures, as noted by Ostrow and co-workers[34] and Lind.[28] Ostrow and co-workers, for example, noted in their review of 80 research articles on the topic of stroke rehabilitation outcomes that only 14 articles had any useful research validity.

However, poor research methodology is not the sole reason for this situation. The nature of disablement also presents its own unique set of issues. These issues include the often conflicting goals and outcomes of the multiple disciplines that are a part of the rehabilitation process, as well as the complex interaction between rehabilitation outcomes and personal variables such as age, gender, education, and intelligence. These two issues, when combined with traditional measurement problems in health care research, have created important barriers to the development of a satisfactory rehabilitation research data base.

TERMINOLOGY

Prior to the discussion of outcome assessment issues in rehabilitation, definitions of the terms *assessment, measurement,* and *evaluation* provide clarification. Too often these terms are used interchangeably, leading to unnecessary confusion in the communication of assessment information. Correct references can facilitate greater understanding of, and respect for, outcome assessment in medical rehabilitation.

Assessment refers to multiple methods of gathering and organizing information on factors that are relevant to particular decision-making processes. In this context, assessment means "to sit beside" or "to assist the judge." Assessment stops short of making judgments about the information. Decisions are made on the basis of assessments and evaluations, but these decisions are not considered part of the assessment process. The key terms are *gathering* and *organizing* information. Outcome assessment in medical rehabilitation would be improved significantly if we could standardize our assessment practices to "gather and organize" outcome data in consistent ways.

Measurement refers to the process of assigning numbers to people (or objects) for the purpose of indicating differences among them in the degree to which they possess the characteristic being measured.[11] A person's ability to perform activities of daily living (ADL), for example, can be "measured" in terms of levels of independence, pain, or speed, among other things. We typically take many measurements during the rehabilitation assessment process.

Evaluation is a broader term encompassing both assessment and measurement. It is a step closer to decision making, referring to the act of making judgments about merit based on

measurements and assessments. Decisions are the courses of action resulting from judgments about merit.

ROLES AND PURPOSES OF OUTCOME ASSESSMENT

Outcomes play a central role in the development and delivery of effective medical rehabilitation services. They are inextricably tied to rehabilitation goals, serving as the focus for clinical decision making, evaluation of treatment effectiveness, communication, and institutional and program planning. The general role of outcome assessment in human service delivery is clarified in Figure 9-1 using acute medicine as the example. As noted, assessment strategies relate directly to taxonomies that are typically standard within a given field. In the case of acute care medicine, all assessment methods are designed to correspond to particular diseases, treatment choices and procedures, or morbidity states as they appear in the various taxonomies. Thus, assessment *leads to* classification decisions, or more practically, clinical treatment decisions. Research data bases in medicine are built on data that are classified within one or more categories. Based on these classifications, descriptions of diseases, treatments, or results of treatments (outcomes) can be made.

Clinical Decision Making

Physical medicine and rehabilitation places its primary focus of assessment on the clinical decision-making process. As in other medical services, patient needs are first evaluated (measured and assessed) and linked to services; then as reevaluation determines progress, services are reduced.

Melvin[30] links assessment to the rehabilitation process, pointing out that medical rehabilitation care entails reiteration of three basic steps. The first step requires an assessment of abilities and limitations that are relevant to the particular roles expected of the person, estimation of the future status that is achievable by the person after appropriate intervention, and estimation of the time required to reach the goals identified by the rehabilitation team.

The second step encompasses the selection and initiation of treatment regimens involving the wide variety of disciplines that impinge on the rehabilitation process. Such regimens might be organized and operated by department, such as occupational

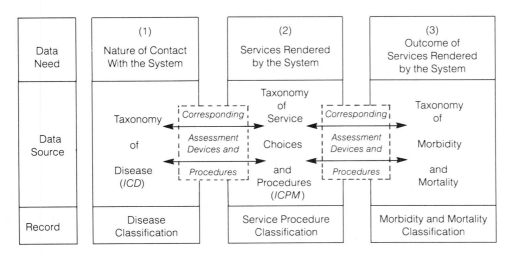

Figure 9-1. Demonstration of relationships among data needs, assessment, and classification systems as applied to a medical model. (*ICD,* International Classification of Diseases; *ICPM,* International Classification of Procedures in Medicine) (Frey WD: Functional assessment in the '80s: A conceptual enigma, a technical challenge. From Halpern AS, Fuhrer MJ [eds]: Functional Assessment in Rehabilitation, pp 11–43. Baltimore, Paul H Brookes Publishing Company. [P.O. Box 10624, Baltimore, MD 21285-0624], 1984).

therapy, speech, and physical therapy. Others might be more tightly controlled by a single office where departments do not exist. The third step concerns evaluation of progress toward the specified goals (and subsequent readjustment of goals), treatment strategies, and timeliness. Reiteration continues until "no significant difference remains between estimates of future potential functional status and current functional status."[30]

Melvin's description highlights the clinical role of assessment. Its importance is emphasized in establishing needs through a determination of the patient's functional status. Referring to Figure 9-1, it can be seen that assessment also leads to selection of specific treatment strategies, serves as the vehicle for monitoring progress, and, finally, serves as a basis for making discharge decisions.

Prediction of Rehabilitation Outcome

Planning and implementing effective rehabilitation programs also presume a solid understanding of the course, duration, and outcomes associated with particular impairments or disabling conditions. Such understanding comes through epidemiological and clinical research. In the best of situations, the rehabilitation team makes its predictions from an assessment of the patient's functional status within a framework that charts the most likely course of events for anyone in that particular population.[39] The framework against which individual patient assessments are compared is built over time from reasearch that carefully documents the relationships between patient characteristics (predictor variables), the types and duration of rehabilitation services, and patient outcomes. When strong associations among patient characteristics, treatments, and outcomes can be made, the framework takes on its appropriate predictive value for clinical decision making.

More broadly, however, predictive value affects institutional planning and reimbursement for services. The goals of providing efficient and effective services have, until recently, been a luxury in medical rehabilitation. This situation may be rapidly coming to an end as medical rehabilitation takes on an increasing role in the medical treatment plan. Consistent with Rogers' prediction, noted earlier, the issues of disablement have received substantial consideration from the health care community during the past 6 years, and as a result many changes in treatment patterns are now emerging. One example is the closer bond that is developing between the traditional health care community and the rehabilitation community. Referrals to rehabilitation units have dramatically increased, signaling a heightened role in the medical treatment plan. In response, the estimated 300 rehabilitation units in hospitals around the country more than doubled between 1985 and 1986 to 630 units.[48]

In a climate of steadily increasing health care costs, the use of assessment information may evolve as the next logical step to determine prospective payments.[14, 18, 30] As in conventional medical treatment in which diagnosis forms the basis for diagnosis-related groups (DRGs) of patients, for example, functional assessment information may well serve a similar role. When specific diagnoses, or comprehensive assessments of patient needs, lead to a predictable consumption of medical resources and when previous costs for treating specific impairment conditions are documented and reasonably consistent, then costs for new patients can be projected.

Even though the basis for developing a prospective payment system exists, its realization in rehabilitation may be years away. Fuhrer[14] notes that as long as assessment practices remain unstandardized, the basis for a useful prospective payment system in rehabilitation will not exist. Thus, without a consistent basis for determining patient needs and outcomes, the predictability of rehabilitation efforts will remain inconclusive.

Unfortunately, the possibility of establishing a prospective payment system based on diagnostic categories alone, however inappropriate in rehabilitation, does exist as economic pressures increase. Arguments against standardizing assessment practices in favor of holding off the introduction of such a system are counterproductive, especially since the possibility of a system based on the alternative (*i.e.*, diagnostic categories) would be disastrous for rehabilitation.[14]

Communication

Less direct, but dramatic in its importance, assessment results structure and facilitate communication about patient status and needs among the long list of people involved in the rehabilitation process (including the patient). The parameters of these discussions are defined through the content and focus of the particular assessment device(s). Therefore, the assessment component takes on an enormous role in the communication of goals and in the communication of progress toward those goals.

It has been well documented that confusion over the content and focus of assessment devices has led to isolation of the various disciplines concerned with the rehabilitation process.[13, 25, 39, 40] The tendency has been for various hospital departments to be extraordinarily provincial as they create their own assessment devices and to use them in their isolated settings. As a patient's rehabilitation program progresses, this fragmentation becomes a barrier to the integration of services needed to facilitate the overall rehabilitation process. Without a common focus and common terminology, goals and outcomes assume the focus of each individual department, and the rehabilitation process therefore lacks unification. Development in communication systems, such as the Uniform Data System for Medical Rehabilitation,[16] the Minimal Record of Disability for Multiple Sclerosis,[20] and the Patient Evaluation Conference System,[18] are intended to bring consistency to the types of data that are collected and analyzed. All three projects are discussed later in this chapter.

Several authors also point to the clinical value of reporting assessment results to the patient.[1, 12, 41, 42] Providing patients with such information strengthens the rehabilitation process through greater collaborative efforts between patient and service provider as well as by broadening the decision-making responsibility. Of course, these positive uses of assessment information are only secondary to the higher priority issue of respect for the patient's dignity, rights, and personal responsibilities that come with receiving assessment results.

Program Evaluation

Assessment also plays an integral role in program evaluation. Medical rehabilitation efforts in this area are primarily directed at accountability and institutional planning issues. As defined earlier, assessment is concerned with data gathering methodology, and program evaluation with making judgments about the merit of measured outcomes. The judgments resulting from comparisons among patient needs, goals, and outcomes are used to demonstrate accountability and to facilitate research and institutional planning.

From a practical point of view, program evaluations are used to judge the merit of particular treatments in facilitating desired improvements in patient functioning. Two important points about this statement bear comment. First, *merit* is a judgment of the effectiveness of the treatment regimen. Merit depends on one's understanding of the program goals as well as the measured progress toward those goals. One cannot judge effectiveness when confusion exists over the goals identified for patients by the rehabilitation team, or when the reliability and validity of the progress measure cannot be confirmed.

A second issue of program evaluation concerns the implication of the treatment strategy in bringing about, *facilitating* the measured effect. Brown and associates[6] comment on the importance of making direct associations between treatment and outcome. Rehabilitationists need to be reasonably sure that the measured outcomes are true results of treatment and not artifacts of some other process, such as maturation. A review of seven "high quality" research articles by Lind[28] led to the conclusion that spontaneous recovery may account for the majority of improved functioning in stroke patients. Lind goes on to suggest that there is limited value in rehabilitation science for stroke patients. This view of rehabilitation effectiveness can be easily contradicted with literature supporting stroke rehabilitation.[3, 33] The point is made, however, that rigorous studies on effectiveness are lacking.

Accountability is more formally addressed in quality assurance studies. Where practical program evaluation has implications for improved treatment/services and greater efficiency of programming, quality assurance studies are directed toward consumer protection and accreditation. Both of these concepts are also closely linked to reimbursement mechanisms. Quality assurance studies review program inputs (including standards for facilities, equipment, and staff), processes (availability of particular service strategies), and outcomes (documentation of treatment results).

Melvin,[30] in his discussion of the relationship between functional assessment and the quality of care review, suggests that three general areas are covered in the four most common types of reviews.* The three areas include (1) program comprehensiveness, (2) program effectiveness, and (3) program efficiency. *Comprehensiveness* refers to whether the program addresses the full range of individual needs specified in the rehabilitation program. Each need should be traceable to a particular intervention strategy. Typically expressed in terms of levels of dependence–independence, a comprehensive plan also addresses the intensity of institutional care required by the patient. For example, Melvin notes that hospital care is a necessity in cases in which bowel or bladder management are uncontrolled. Finally, comprehensiveness requires an estimation of future potential of the patient.

Effectiveness establishes incremental change in the patient's condition in the direction expected. An important ingredient to documenting patient progress, as noted above, is the validation of the treatment strategy (through research) in promoting change. Without this validation it is nearly impossible to rely on outcome status as an indicator of effectiveness.

Program *efficiency* refers to a comparison between program outcomes and program costs. It is generally recognized that efficient programs are those achieving the best outcomes at the lowest possible cost. Program comparisons are only possible when outcomes are carefully specified and consistent across programs and when cost-accounting practices are the same.

Efficiency measures are useful in a variety of ways, including program and manpower planning as well as cost–benefit analy-

*For a discussion of the four types of quality of care review formats, the reader is referred to Melvin,[30] who presents descriptions of the utilization review, audit, PSRO or peer review organization criteria, and program evaluation.

sis. Such measures can assist in making judgments about alternative methods of service delivery. An example would be deciding whether to move a patient with a particular functional status from the hospital to home. Can the same or better outcomes be achieved in the lower cost setting of the home, or are greater benefits produced by remaining in the hospital where intensive services are available? Another example might question whether 5 hours per week of peer group counseling could enhance or move the rehabilitation process along at a faster rate than no peer group counseling at all, or whether the outcomes would, in fact, remain the same. These kinds of questions are answerable when efficiency can be established. The important point among efficiency measures is that outcomes are quantifiable and valid indicators of change explained by treatments and not by time alone or some other process. Costs that are tied to programs with unclear goals and outcomes provide little useful information to program planners, researchers, or clinicians.

FACTORS AFFECTING OUTCOME ASSESSMENT

In a general sense, outcomes are those changes—good, bad, intended, or unintended—that are caused by, or closely associated with, program interventions.[6] Human service delivery makes the assumption that outcomes reflect all of the potential results that can accrue owing to the provision of particular services. Effectivness of those services can be determined only when the potential outcomes are specified and accurately assessed in light of clearly elaborated rehabilitation goals.[15, 22, 46]

Goal Orientation

Because the goals of medical rehabilitation are so closely tied to outcome assessment, confusion over them has played a major role in the development of assessment strategies (instruments) that are inconsistent across programs. This confusion has led to the conduct of studies that evaluate treatment strategies with dissimilar outcomes. Chin[7] points out that a lack of standard outcome measures has left physical and occupational therapists with some confusion over the use of various treatment procedures. One issue is the choice between optimizing residual body functioning (*e.g.,* range of motion, muscle strength, repetitive movement tolerance) or maximizing recovery from disability (*e.g.,* improving performance in spite of residual disability). Improvement of residual body function requires application of physical agents (*e.g.,* heat, light, electricity) and facilitation exercises. Recovery from disability, on the other hand, requires restoration through compensation using special aids or equipment, training the unaffected side (as in hemiplegia), or preventing contractures.

The two approaches can be contradictory and counterproductive. A consistent body of knowledge would allow therapists to make decisions about the appropriate combinations of treatment to meet patient needs. Typically, those studies looking at residual body function measure outcome in terms of range of motion, pounds of strength, number of repetitive movements, and so on. For obvious reasons, these outcomes are clearly inappropriate for comparison with studies that concentrate on compensation approaches and that deemphasize residual functioning.

In her analysis of the efficacy of occupational therapy in the treatment of stroke, Merrill[31] also pointed to the lack of comparable outcome measures as a probable cause of inconclusive research results. In two studies examining the ability of hemisphere stroke patients to perform dressing tasks, she notes that one study found patients with right hemisphere damage more frequently had difficulty in learning to dress. The second study found that neither left- nor right-hemisphere–injured patients could be differentiated on the basis of dressing performance. Merrill concludes that since the two studies employed vastly different "dressing" tasks, when taken together, no conclusive results could be gleaned from them.

Frey's[13] analysis of the historical development of functional assessment in rehabilitation concludes that the multiple goal orientations are partly due to the development of medical rehabilitation concepts over the past 65 years and to the addition of numerous medically related disciplines to the rehabilitation process. These multiple goal orientations are also a result of the broad, far-reaching goals expressed by many programs today.

Early rehabilitation efforts (1920 to 1940) were narrowly focused on the exact quantification of residual function following injury, primarily for purposes of attaching a "cash" value to the impairment. Most assessment activity at that time concerned the measurement of residual physical functioning in quantitive units such as degrees for range in motion, pounds to capture muscle strength, and tolerance toward repetitious use of an affected limb.

As the concept of holistic medicine became prominent in the late 1930s, rehabilitation adopted a new focus. The holistic philosophy emphasized a basic interdependence among traditionally recognized components of behavior, postulating that all behavior represents a coordinated response including all biological, learning, and environmental resources of the person. Thus, behavior was considered unique to each individual and a result of physical and mental capacities, as well as personal experience. Subsequent outcome assessment instruments then began to focus on composite body movements, or "things people do." Measurement of activities and behaviors such as walking, moving about, lifting, and eating were expressed in terms of the amount of assistance required to complete tasks (independence) or level of performance (satisfactory/unsatisfactory, complete/incomplete).

More recently, outcome assessment activity has made another transition adding a more global perspective with a focus still on the patient but within the context of a given environment. This view represents a different kind of experience for the person with a chronic disability. Consistent with a psychosocial model, this perspective entails the patient's interaction with specific environments. Alexander and Fuhrer,[1] point out three distinct principles of rehabilitation embracing this perspective:

1. The primary concern of rehabilitation is the disadvantage (handicap) placed on the person by society.
2. Rehabilitation should be an educational process, providing assistance to people in adapting to their own environments.
3. Rehabilitation efforts should be directed at improving opportunities to pursue activities consistent with the person's goals.

Outcome assessments having this global perspective are more concerned with behavior patterns in daily living and a resumption of normal social roles, rather than with the performance of specific tasks or residual function of body parts. Some examples of outcomes reflecting these views are how patients cope with daily living, including how they use their time, and how often they participate in activities considered a part of the normal social role (e.g., work activities or the use of leisure time). These outcomes are measured in terms of job retention, numbers of daily/weekly social contacts, and distance traveled in a wheelchair.

Person Variables

Understanding disablement also requires acknowledgement of the complex interaction between person variables and rehabilitation outcomes. In cases of temporary impairment, such as severe ankle sprain, torn ligament, or minor stroke, the rehabilitation process is self-limiting. Treatment strategies are directly related to the injury.[35] The intended outcomes include relief of symptoms, such as pain or swelling; restoration of muscle strength, balance, and range of motion; prevention of maladaptive behaviors; and improved functional ability. These problems typically result in temporarily altered daily routines in order to compensate for reduced functional abilities. However, people with these kinds of problems can fulfill normal life roles and nearly maintain previous life-styles.

Rehabilitation is a much more complex process for people with permanent or progressive impairments, such as spinal cord injury, stroke, or multiple sclerosis. The consequences of these conditions can affect nearly every sphere of the person's life, including physical, emotional, or social aspects.[47] Depending on personal circumstances, permanent impairment can result in a loss of ability to perform normal daily tasks. These tasks may include things like personal hygiene, shopping for groceries, or getting to work or church. Over time, inabilities to independently perform these "daily duties" can lead to generalized failure in performing social roles, such as maintaining economic levels commensurate with preinjury standards (e.g., keeping a job) or maintaining social obligations and relationships.

These possibilities are inextricably tied to the immense variety in personal variables that comprise individual situations. Hence, the consequences of impairment are nearly always unique to the patient; and person variables such as age, education, and intelligence will strongly influence outcome assessment results. The lives of three people having the same precise impairment can be affected in vastly different ways and to greater or lessor extents. A bricklayer aged 52 with a spinal cord injury that remains after recovery from a fall may be unable to return to work because of the inability to meet certain job requirements, namely, the need for continuous and coordinated movement of the trunk and lower and upper limbs. This situation may in turn lead to unemployment and ultimately to a loss of earning power and economic self-sufficiency. In a 52-year-old draftsman, the same spinal cord injury may have no affect whatsoever on job performance because continuous trunk and body movements are not requirements of the job, thereby allowing the person to return to work after recovery and thus maintain his or her previous earning power and standard of living. For a third person the spinal cord injury may also completely disrupt job performance. However, the particular skills associated with the job, plus the fact that the person is college educated and only 34 years old, may lead to a reasonable transition into another job. These latter two cases will cause substantial disruption of the patients' personal life albeit in different ways, but the impairment may not have quite the far-reaching effects of the case in which earning power is completely lost.

Medical rehabilitation, then, for these people becomes a long-term process of adaption to limited functional abilities in light of personal situations and attributes. The process involves learning new strategies for completing daily tasks, improving physical skills and abilities, learning new methods and requirements for personal care and health maintenance, and learning how to cope with physical and psychological barriers posed by the community. The amount and types of efforts required on the part of the rehabilitation team are completely dependent on the complex interactions between the extent of the impairment, the patient's personal characteristics and experiences, and the environment in which the patient chooses to reside.

Poor Measurement Properties of Outcome Assessment Instruments

Comparability among outcome assessments is further hampered by the weak or conflicting measurement properties of many assessment devices. Keith[25] refers to a lack of attention to the scalability of criterion measures, reliability, validity, and standardization.* Scalability, for example, addresses the quantification of a criterion measure. Some commonly used criterion measures are *independence, pain,* and *quality of performance.*

Keith[25] notes that a set of numbers and labels are typically assigned to a listing of possible outcome alternatives without much regard to whether the alternatives reflect equal distances between them. Arbitrary scale values such as "almost always," "often," "sometimes," "frequently," and "practically never" will negatively affect scale reliability since these terms are open to a sizable number of interpretations. At the same time scale validity can be affected if the meaning attached to differences between such general terms is unclear. One could ask the question whether the pain that exists "almost always" is as detrimental to functioning as pain that is reported as occurring "often." One might also ask whether a pain program can assert its success if patients report gains between these two categories.

Even among programs that embrace similar interpretations of rehabilitation goals, the procedures used to assess patient outcomes vary considerably. A program may assess the complex task of feeding with only a single assessment item. One popular ADL assessment device has only two ways to categorize feeding behavior, "Independent: gets food from plate or its equivalent into mouth." and "Dependent: assistance in act of feeding; does not eat at all or parenteral feeding." Another program may employ procedures that consider several component eating tasks, including cutting meat or other foods, getting food from plate to mouth, masticating, and swallowing. The criterion for determining functioning on this latter scale is also independence. However, several additional categories describe the type of dependence, such as requires use of aids, requires assistance from another person, requires both aids and assistance, or performs task alone.

These differences in the *levels of measurement* and in the *criteria* used to scale each measure may seem insignificant on the surface. However, problems are created when goals and outcomes are viewed differently or when attempts are made to compare effectiveness across programs or treatments that employ dissimilar assessment methodology. In these situations, outcome research is compromised, resulting in additional interferences in the orderly development of rehabilitation knowledge.

Kaufert[24] provides an excellent analysis of several validity issues related to the use of alternate assessment scales. His results tell us much about problems with our current methods of outcome assessment in rehabilitation. The four areas studied were (1) the impact of aids, adaptations, and helpers; (2) situational and motivational variables; (3) professional perspectives of

the rater (home nurses versus physicians); and (4) role expectations of the patient.

Kaufert's results indicate that trichotomous rather than dichotomous scale items more adequately controlled the compensatory effects of aids, adaptations, and personal assistants. Test–retest comparisons also revealed that variability due to client motivation and "test situation" was reduced by having primary care staff complete follow-up ratings in patients' homes. Apparently, assessment in the home environment provides the patient with a valid referent for test performance whereas hospital-based assessments may be too artificial.

Comparisons were also made between self-ratings by patients and those ratings by physicians and home visiting nurses. The general results suggested that differences do exist in the clinical perspectives of physicians and visiting nurses. Nurse ratings showed higher proportions of matches with patient ratings of complex mobility functions such as self-help, shopping, and using public transport. Physicians' proportional ratings were higher on just one assessment item, bed transfer. Kaufert concludes that these differences support the notion that familiarity with the patients' home environment leads to a better match with the client's understanding of those ratings.

Lastly, it was noted that systematic variation occurred in self-reported and clinically rated performances of males and females. It was suggested that ratings are also affected by culturally determined role expectations of males and females.

REQUIREMENTS FOR OUTCOME ASSESSMENT

The specification of functional outcomes in rehabilitation first requires a complete understanding of rehabilitation goals. Too often rehabilitation professionals have narrowed their focus to address only those patient needs relating to their individual disciplines, rather than viewing their work as contributing to a larger combined goal. The example provided by Merrill[31] and discussed previously is a classic case in point. One stroke research project interpreted dressing skills in terms of specific disciplinary outcomes. The other study addressed a more general level of functioning. Unfortunately, the two studies are not comparable owing to the different professional perspectives.

Individual professions can frequently respond to the many rehabilitation needs of people with transient conditions such as ankle sprain or minor stroke. However, the fact that these professionals view their work as "rehabilitation" in isolation may suggest that their view is generalized to the needs of patients with permanent or progressive impairments. In fact, rehabilitation of these people requires a long-range, coordinated, and inter-disciplinary involvement of many professionals, including physiatrists; psychologists; speech, occupational, or physical therapists; specialty nurses; vocational counselors; or any of the myriad of practitioners of the acute care subdisciplines.

Each discipline must contribute expertise in comprehensive rehabilitative settings in a way that moves the patient toward common rehabilitation goals and expected outcomes. Given that many rehabilitation disciplines have overlapping roles, the need for a coordinated and unified program becomes even more imperative. This situation requires that rehabilitation professionals recognize the most salient aspects of their contribution to a given rehabilitation effort. It also requires that they recognize the limitations of their individual disciplines in responding to the needs of people with permanent or progressive impairments.

For these reasons, it is useful to recognize a broad goal orientation for rehabilitation. Such an orientation should reflect the comprehensive needs of patients, taking into account the far-

---

*The issues and difficulties associated with the development of satisfactory outcome assessment devices in medical rehabilitation are well documented in recent literature.[6, 9, 13, 18, 21, 22, 24, 25] A general review of assessment issues is discussed here. However, a complete analysis would be beyond the scope of this chapter. Therefore, the reader is referred to these resources for more extensive discussions about the variety of conceptual and measurement issues in outcome assessment.

reaching consequences of disablement, and it should encompass the wider range of human services available to respond to those needs. Alexander and Fuhrer[1] suggest that these goals include the following:

1. To limit the effects of impairment.
2. To prevent loss of health associated with various impairment conditions.
3. To reestablish behavioral functioning and independence.

This last goal encompasses community integration and adjustment where rehabilitation effort is directed toward improving the relationship between the patient's abilities and the demands of his or her chosen environments. A major emphasis is focused over and above improving physical functioning and on the person's need to learn (new) strategies for coping with the demands of daily life. These needs are evidenced in the strong growth of peer support groups, independent living centers, and special interest organizations (*e.g.,* the National Stroke Association and the Traumatic Brain Injury Association).

The three goals also encompass a broad range of experiences that are potential consequences of disease or trauma. These goals correspond to the conceptual framework emphasized by the World Health Organization[46] and presented by Wood.[45] Wood details his model in the International Classification of Impairments, Disabilities, and Handicaps (ICIDH), and he suggests that four planes of experience are associated with illness and can explain disablement processes. These planes are represented in Table 9-1 as serious injury/disease, impairment, disability, and handicap.

Wood describes the first plane of experience as representing a chain of causal circumstances (disease or injury) that results in changes to the structure or functioning of the body (the pathology). These changes are often accompanied by certain signs and symptoms, but not always. The second plane represents the "exteriorization" of the changes in functioning. This stage is the point at which the patient first becomes aware of the impending consequences of the disease. *Impairment,* the term referring to this stage, includes "any loss or abnormality of psychological, physiological, or anatomical structure or func-

tion."[45] Impairments can occur at the organ, body part, or system level. We most often think in terms of groups such as skeletal, neurological, and sensory impairments. Other impairment types include intellectual, psychological, language, visceral, disfiguring, and so on.

The third plane of experience is the performance or behavior that may be affected by the impairment. Wood labels this "objectification" of the impairment as *disability* and defines it as "any restriction or lack of ability to perform an activity in the manner or within the range considered normal for the human being."[45] Whereas impairments are concerned with functions of organs, body parts, or body systems, disabilities represent integrated (holistic) functioning of the entire person that is brought to bear on the completion of tasks, skills, or other human behaviors. Some examples would include personal care disabilities (such as hygiene, dressing, and eating), locomotor disabilities (ambulation, lifting, and transfers), and body disposition disabilities (reaching, kneeling, and crouching).

A fourth plane is experienced when impairment or disability places the person at a disadvantage relative to others. Wood refers to this experience as a *handicap,* designating society's level of recognition of these entities. The patient experiences a "socialization" of the disease, referring to a "disadvantage, resulting from the fulfillment of a role that is normal (depending on age, sex, and social or cultural factors) for that individual."[45] Introduced as a social phenomenon, handicaps are those disadvantages that result from being unable to conform to social and cultural expectations. There are several dimensions to handicap. Some of the more commonly recognized ones include occupation of time (vocational status), physical independence, and social integration. Type of living arrangement after discharge from the rehabilitation unit is a typical outcome of rehabilitation service that is associated with handicap.

It is important to recognize that these four planes of experience provide a framework for understanding the phenomenon of disablement. However, they only represent the universe of potential consequences to "ill health." Although presented by Wood as a unidimensional model, one plane is not necessarily dependent on a prior plane for the experience to occur. Impairments do not necessarily result in (cause) disabilities or hand-

---

Table 9-1
Four Planes of Experience Associated With Serious Injury or Disease

Serious Injury/Disease	Impairment	Disability	Handicap
Definition			
Disruption of normal body processes	Any loss or abnormality or psychological, physiological or anatomical structure or function	Any restriction or lack (resulting from an impairment) of ability to perform an activity in the manner or within the range considered normal for a human.	A disadvantage for a given person (resulting from an impairment or a disability) that limits or prevents the fulfillment of a role that is normal (depending on age, sex, social, cultural factors) for that person
Type of Loss or Abnormality			
Active pathological process	Structure or function of individual parts of human body	Compound and integrated activities, tasks, skills, behaviors	A complex survival role that is appropriate (based on age, sex, social and cultural factors) for a person
Type of Manifestation			
Coincident symptomatology	Organ or mechanism	Person's activities, tasks, skills, behaviors	Attitudes and responses of people experiencing a handicap and not experiencing a handicap

Adapted from Bettinghaus CO: International Standards for a System of Disability Classification. Paper presented at the Annual Meeting of the American Psychological Association, Montreal, 1980. Data from: World Health Organization: Classification of Impairments, Disabilities, and Handicaps. Geneva, World Health Organization, 1980.

icaps. Disfigurement, for example, may not be associated with any *disability;* yet it can easily result in a serious handicap in that the person is placed at a social disadvantage. Similarly, a person with the inactive presence of the human immunodeficiency virus may not show any signs of impairment or disability while it remains in its dormant stage. However, on acknowledgement of the carrier virus through routine testing, the person may be placed at a serious social and vocational disadvantage if the information becomes widely known.

In some ways, disabilities or handicaps may result in additional impairments. Schumacher[38] suggests that it is entirely possible for an elderly person who is isolated over a long period of time (either by living alone or in an institution) to gradually lose cognitive faculties related to memory and orientation. Perhaps the lack of intellectual stimulation and sensory input resulting from an externally imposed restriction (handicap) leads to a newly recognized mental impairment. Similarly, a child with cerebral palsy who cannot sit independently and who does not receive proper postural support may indeed develop a scoliosis.

These examples, and there are many like them, simply point out the multidimensional and complex nature of disablement. Given this context, one should not emphasize the causal progression of the four planes of experience—disease to impairment, impairment to disability, and disability to handicap. Instead, emphasis should be placed on the categorical nature of the *potential* consequences of disease. Together they describe DISABLEMENT. Alone, each becomes a domain of possible outcomes of the disablement experience. Combined with the variety of appropriate assessment scales, these four planes of experience form the basis for measuring progress toward the three goals mentioned earlier.

The implication that a medical model is associated with the consequences of disease is not intended. In fact, disablement represents psychosocial and environmental perspectives, taking on a more global view of the person living in the context of specific environments. Outcomes having this psychosocial/environmental focus are more concerned with behavioral patterns in daily living rather than with performance of specific tasks or residual function of body parts alone. Disease may cause impairments, but, as noted earlier, impairments are only one set of many factors that lead to disability. Subsequent handicaps are further complicated by an even larger number of factors such as age, intelligence, gender, and so forth.

The Wood model, which only explains the consequences of a disease experience, is immensely useful for categorizing potential rehabilitation outcomes and then tying these outcomes to useful assessments. The three consequences of the disease experience—impairment, disability, and handicap—provide the basis for a classification system of functional outcomes. These categories in turn will help to clarify the focus of the many diverse assessment devices already available. They also provide a conceptual understanding of the focus for various rehabilitation activities. For example, efforts to prevent further impairment and increase body functioning through application of physical agents and exercise are directed toward the site of impairment. Education and training efforts typically focus on either reduction in disability or movement toward higher levels of independence.

Both Duckworth[10] and Granger[15] have presented functional assessment frameworks based on the concepts of the ICIDH. Their works also reflect the need for a broader goal orientation encompassing all the possible consequences/outcomes of disablement. Duckworth emphasizes that the overloaded meaning of the concept of "disability" has led to the need for clarification of the term. He carefully dissects various meanings that have developed in recent years, leading to the conclusion that the con-

cepts of impairment, disability, and handicap express multiple meanings rather well.

Granger has attempted to develop the ICIDH concepts a bit further by molding the framework into a functional assessment model. His model extends the conditions and key terms used by Wood in the development of the ICIDH to include corresponding levels of analysis and interventions. Essentially, Granger suggests that impairments are documented (his term is "analysis") using diagnostic descriptors, disabilities via performance descriptors, and handicaps by role descriptors. The corresponding interventions for impairments become medical restorative therapy; those for disabilities include adaptive equipment and reduction of physical and attitudinal barriers; and those for handicap include supportive services and social policy changes.[15]

Granger concludes his model by suggesting that functional assessment becomes the process that (1) facilitates a comprehensive analysis of pathology, impairment, disability, and handicap; (2) facilitates identification of "discordances between diagnoses, performances (behaviors) and social roles.";[15] (3) facilitates identification of outcomes in social roles that are interrupted by functional limitations resulting from impairment, and (4) facilitates development of a rehabilitation service/treatment strategy.

It is unfortunate that after bringing the ICIDH model to the point of connecting it to a useful functional assessment model, Granger implies the development of instrumentation is an open-ended task to be left to the interests of individual rehabilitation departments and programs. The model neither accounts for the inconsistencies in the levels of measurement and criteria noted earlier in many functional assessment instruments nor does it specify rehabilitation outcomes with sufficient definitional clarity. Without a further step specifying actual indicators of rehabilitation outcomes, the Granger model is only a framework of domains representing the possible experiences of people who are disabled.

Rehabilitation Outcomes Associated With Impairment

In order to facilitate the outcomes assessment process, the Granger model requires expansion in the area he labels "analysis." Table 9-2 represents a comprehensive picture of this expansion, including the three planes of experience, analysis of outcomes, and types of interventions. The disease plane is purposely left out of the chart since outcomes in medicine are relatively clear.

Analysis of outcomes associated with the impairment plane require documentation of the type of impairment as well as the functional limitations imposed by the impairment. Representative domains for type of impairments include skeletal, intellectual, ocular, and so on. Functional limitations have been categorized in many ways by a variety of groups, including the Department of Labor, specialists in ergonomics, and vocational specialists. However, the system employed in the *ERTOMIS* Assessment Method[32] is both comprehensive and representative of the many other systems that are currently available.

Each elemental function associated with various impairments (or disabilities) can be measured in terms of physical characteristics such as range of motion (degrees) and strength (pounds). Measurement of these physical characteristics is not considered outcome assessment but rather *primary assessment*. There is no misunderstanding that the focus of specific rehabilitation efforts may be purposely directed toward increasing range

Table 9-2
Model for Outcome Assessment

	Disability ⟷ Handicap ⟷ Impairment		
	Disability	**Handicap**	**Impairment**
1. Planes of Experience			
2. Analysis of Outcomes			
A. *Areas of Assessment (Domains for Documentation)*	1. Locomotor 2. Personal care 3. Body disposition 4. Dexterity 5. Behavioral 6. Communication 7. Situational 8. Particular skill areas 9. Other activity restrictions	1. Economic self-sufficiency 2. Occupation 3. Mobility 4. Physical independence 5. Social integration 6. Orientation 7. Other	a. Type of impairment 1. Skeletal 2. Intellectual 3. Neurological 4. Psychological 5. Aural 6. Ocular 7. Visceral 8. Disfiguring 9. Generalized, sensory, other b. Functional limitations imposed by impairment 1. Body parts 2. Sensory organs 4. Psychological/behavioral 5. Communication 6. Environmental tolerance 7. Other
B. *Primary Assessment Criteria*	Examples include: 1. Questionnaire 2. Performance Test 3. Inventory of Skills	Examples include: 1. Miles traveled in wheelchair 2. # of social contacts 3. Vocational status	Examples include: a. Range in motion b. Pain c. Strength d. Repetitive motion
C. *Outcome Classification*	a. Dependence/Independence • no difficulty in performance • difficulty in performance • aided performance • assisted performance • dependent performance • augmented performance • complete inability b. Quality of performance • normal • diminished/reduced • lack of performance	a. Financial status/level of support needed b. Customary social role (employment, homemaker, student, etc.) c. Living arrangement d. Level of personal assistance required e. Type/frequency of social activity	a. Categorical assignment using impairment codes in ICIDH b. General functional ability* • full function • restricted/reduced function • no function
3. Intervention†	Adaptive equipment and environmental modification	Social service and social policy	Medical and restoration therapy

*Adapted from Mittelsten Scheid E: An assessment system that matches abilities with job requirements to facilitate reintegration of disabled people into employment. In Habeck RV, Frey WD, Galvin DE et al (eds): Economics and Equity in Employment of People with Disabilities: An International Perspective, pp 77–80. East Lansing, Michigan State University, University Center for International Rehabilitation, 1985.

†Adapted from Granger CV, Gresham GE: Functional Assessment in Rehabilitation Medicine. Baltimore, Williams & Wilkins, 1984.

of motion, increasing muscle strength, or decreasing pain. However, the *outcome* of these efforts is a generalized functional ability simply measured in terms of full, restricted (high/low), or no ability. Successful rehabilitation efforts should, by contrast, be reflected in increased general functional ability. Primary assessment issues such as pain, range of motion, muscle strength, and flexibility are the specifics that are addressed by physiatrists and therapists in order to produce greater functional ability.

A framework that emphasizes levels of general functional ability also facilitates rehabilitation team efforts. Each professional (physiatrist, psychologist, physical therapist, occupational therapist) brings primary assessment data to bear on ratings of general functional ability. These general ratings can be discussed and understood in the context of interdisciplinary team efforts. Subsequent discussions facilitate communication and present a united effort as team members are able to resolve disagreements on the patient's general functional ability. It should be noted, however, that communication is also enhanced, even when there is no team effort, for instance, with third party payers or when a patient is referred to outside professionals.

Rehabilitation Outcomes Associated With Disability

Entirely different sets of entities and outcomes are associated with disabilities. The generally accepted categories are noted in Table 9-2 along with several appropriate outcome criteria. One immediately noticeable difference between the outcomes for disability and those for impairment is the focus on behavioral functioning. The medical rehabilitation effort can be directed toward improvements at the sight of abnormal body functioning (impairment) or more generally with behavioral tasks. A focus that includes disability also requires a shift in the focus of treatment. Newly emphasized are education and training activities that take into account the wide variety of personal factors (such as motivation, gender, age, and education) and environmental factors (such as specific home or community settings) that influence behavioral functioning/performance.

There are two outcome areas of interest to rehabilitation that are also associated with behavioral functioning. The first of these represents the type of *dependence* required, if any, by the person to perform various tasks. A common set of scale points includes normal ability, difficulty in performance, aided performance, assisted/dependent performance, and unable to perform. This model, for example, has been employed in the ICIDH system.[45] A second outcome of interest concerns the *quality of performance* as affected by issues such as pain, speed, or confidence. The focus of this latter criterion is on the patient's ability to perform a task within a range that considers success, not necessarily within a range considered "normal." A stroke patient may be able to dial a telephone properly, but it may take two or three attempts to do it with accuracy or the patient may take more time than the telephone company allows before automatically cutting off the line. This is not success. The task is affected by other factors, including speed, pain, or confidence, and so forth.

One scale currently under development[8] defines performance capacity (*i.e.,* the ability to personally achieve success on a task) in terms of the following categories:

1. *Normal capacity* (patient performs task with satisfactory completion)
2. *Diminished capacity* (patient performs task but satisfactory completion is somewhat affected by problems with pain, speed, confidence, and so on

3. *Reduced capacity* (patient performs task but satisfactory completion is seriously affected by problems with pain, speed, confidence, and so on
4. *Incapacity* (patient cannot perform task with satisfactory completion)

Elderly blind clients of the Michigan Commission for the Blind are asked a series of questions related to the disability domains listed in Table 9-2. More precisely, these clients are asked if they have difficulty performing the particular task. Based on their response, follow-up questions attempt to determine which of the four categories best reflects the client's ability to complete the task. The interviewer then selects the appropriate rating. In cases in which the task is performed by another person (such as grocery shopping or the receipt of meals-on-wheels program), the client is asked how well it could be done if needed. Probing the client stops when a category becomes clearly appropriate or when the interviewer determines that no accurate rating can be made.

Assessments that are less direct may be used to determine rehabilitation outcomes. These assessments, labeled here as primary assessments, can include a wide variety of measures focusing on different levels of complexity. The comparison of studies by Merrill[31] looking at dressing behavior provides a good example of how taking an additional step to specify outcomes from primary assessments could have avoided some of the confusion brought about by the use of individual assessment inventories. Had the researchers applied the primary assessment data to the two outcomes recommended here (dependence and quality of performance) and had they used the domains listed in the "Dressing" section of the ICIDH, then comparable research results would have been possible.

Patient progress and "incremental" gains are important evaluation concepts in rehabilitation. However, some concern has been voiced over the ability of a dependence–independence criterion to measure these concepts. The question is whether a valid scale can be constructed to reflect levels of independece. A patient, for example, may be able to complete a particular task with success but with extreme difficulty. Typically, this person would receive a "difficulty in performance" rating on the independence criterion (see Table 9-2). The rehabilitation team recommending an aid or device to assist in improving the quality of the performance will not be able to document "progress" on a scale of independence because the patient now performs the task at a more dependent level—with an aid. So while the performance capacity improves substantially with the use of an aid, the independence outcome measure shows greater dependence rather than less dependence.

This dependence–independence issue with respect to incremental change is precisely the problem raised earlier about scalability and the need for a unidimensional construct that can reflect change in both positive and negative directions. One solution may be to categorize the type of dependence but not scale it. A combination of descriptive categories of levels of independence and a scaled measure of performance capacity would improve our understanding of disability-related outcomes and the effects of particular treatment strategies on them.

Rehabilitation Outcomes Associated With Handicap

A third set of outcomes is needed at the level of handicap that considers the performance of normal life roles and community integration. Categories that are commonly addressed, including physical independence and social integration, are listed in Table 9-2 along with several possible outcome criteria. It is evident that the experience of handicap as it appears in the Wood model is the least well developed of the three planes of experience following disease. However, pioneering efforts are underway to explore this area further. The ICIDH manual does recommend a set of experimental scales associated with each handicap category.[45] Another set of scales, called the *Environmental Status Scale,* is included as part of the *Minimal Record of Disability for Multiple Sclerosis,* developed by the International Federation of Multiple Sclerosis Societies.[20] A number of other researchers have also presented concepts related to experimentation in the handicap domain.[29, 36, 43]

Standard procedures for assessing rehabilitation outcomes require the development of a useful rehabilitation data base. In order to facilitate this task, we must place stronger emphasis on the differences between primary assessments and outcome assessments. The distinctions allow us to gain an understanding of useful procedures that help to develop a consistent rehabilitation data base. For example, primary assessments are completed by professionals representing various disciplines in the rehabilitation process. These measures are detailed analyses of the various component characteristics eventually leading to outcomes. A physiatrist, consequently, may be immediately preoccupied with pain or lack of feeling in one arm of a patient. The primary assessment (measurements) of pain may help to adjust specific treatment strategies. With the same patient, the physical therapist may instead focus on restoration of muscle strength. Primary assessments would include measures of improving muscle strength or arm rotation. Together the physiatrist and physical therapist can use their individual primary assessments to determine overall arm functioning. By contrast, consensus is required on the outcome of general functional ability of the affected arm. Thus, the goals and context are the same (*i.e.,* they focus solely on impairment in this case), but the points of view taken by each professional are different, as they should be. A similar example could include expanded interest in the disability plane of experience. Here the therapist may emphasize use of the affected arm in completing personal care tasks. The outcome of interest now shifts to independence and level of performance.

In the handicap area, primary assessments may involve many questions and concepts including distance traveled in a wheelchair, activity participation, or means for getting to/from these activities. The outcome assessment will require bringing all of these primary assessments together in order to establish a composite image of mobility.

Applications of Functional Outcome Assessment Systems

Pressures to improve accountability practices, increase effectiveness, and reduce costs related to the treatment of disablement have continued to mount in rehabilitation. At the same time, documenting the effectiveness of rehabilitation efforts continues to be an enigma for the field. However, several significant developments have been made in recent years in the standardization of disablement information collection. Among these developments are the *Minimal Record of Disability for Multiple Sclerosis,* the *Patient Evaluation Conference System,* and the *Uniform Data System for Medical Rehabilitation.* Interestingly, as described below, each of these developments have come through different approaches to the problems of functional outcome assessment.

Minimal Record of Disability for Multiple Sclerosis

The first project, begun in 1979, focused on disablement as it related to the particular disease processes associated with multiple sclerosis (MS). Developed by the International Federation of Multiple Sclerosis Societies,[20] the *Minimal Record of Disability (MRD)* creates a comprehensive profile of patients with MS. Its development represents a significant step forward in the process of constructing a consistent rehabilitation data base in this area.

The primary goal of the *MRD* project is to improve communication among clinicians, researchers, and patients about care for people with MS. It was anticipated that planning and evaluation of services to people with MS would be improved with a better understanding of the implications of alternative service deliveries. The requirements for the system set by the organizing committee suggested that the *MRD* provide a simple, comprehensive, and standardized profile to those professionals involved in the treatment and management of MS.

The *MRD* contains five sections, including the following:

1. Demographic information
2. *Neurological Functional Systems of Kurtzke (NFS)*
3. *Disability Status Scale (DSS)*
4. *Incapacity Status Scale (ISS)*
5. *Environmental Status Scale (ESS)*

Each section is standardized and contains instructions for the administration and rating as well as coding of information.

The *MRD* was originally designed to match the framework of the ICIDH. However, the usage of the terms *impairment, disability,* and *handicap* sometimes becomes confusing when trying to understand the five scales. The *Neurological Functional Systems of Kurtzke* and the *Disability Status Scale* correspond to the medical status of the disease and to impairment. An alternative method for determining medical status is offered by the *MRD* using the *Standard Neurological Examination.* These scales are concerned with signs and symptoms associated with neurological dysfunction. Two examples from the *Neurological Functional Systems of Kurtzke* include the following:

PYRAMIDAL FUNCTIONS

0—Normal
1—Abnormal signs without disability
2—Minimal disability
3—Mild to moderate paraparesis
4—Marked paresis or hemiparesis
5—Paraplegia, hemiplegia, or marked quadriparesis
6—Quadriplegia
9—Unknown

CEREBELLAR FUNCTIONS

0—Normal
1—Abnormal signs without disability
2—Mild ataxia
3—Moderate truncal or limb ataxia or hemiparesis
4—Severe ataxia in all limbs
5—Unable to perform coordinated movements due to ataxia
9—Unknown

The *Incapacity Status Scale (ISS)* corresponds to the disability section of the ICIDH concerning restrictions or lack of ability in behavioral performance. The domains addressed in the *ISS* are similar to the general areas covered in the ICIDH, but they do not always offer the same detail. For example, feeding is addressed in just one item in the *ISS;* by contrast, the ICIDH breaks feeding behavior into several categories. The criterion for measuring disability is a rating of the level of independence in performing set tasks. Quality of performance is not assessed.

The *Environmental Status Scale* corresponds rather closely to the "Handicap" section of the ICIDH. The areas that are addressed include work, financial status, home living modification, personal independence, transportation, social activity, and community service needs. Each item contains its own scale according to customary roles. For example, the financial scale includes the following categories:

0—No MS-related financial problems
1—Family maintains usual financial standard without external support
2—Family maintains usual financial standard with aid of some external financial support
3—Family maintains usual financial standard by receiving basic disability pension as defined in location of residence
4—Family maintains usual financial standard only because it is receiving all available financial assistance
5—Family is unable to maintain usual financial standard despite receipt of all available financial assistance.

The *MRD* clearly provides a significant addition to functional outcome assessment efforts. The data collection system is comprehensive in that it addresses all of the potential planes of experience related to MS and it sets a standard for information collection. Over time the data will form the basis for better understanding of the implications of MS. Two limitations in the system are its inconsistent use of some terminology and lack of an outcome for level of performance within the disability scale (*ISS*). Moreover, the *MRD* uses the term *disability* in a loose way referring to all aspects of the profile. The medical impairment sections are both labeled with the term *disability,* thereby increasing confusion of the underlying ICIDH framework. Although it is recognized that *disablement* is probably a most acceptable term to use in referring to the combined planes of experience associated with disease, it becomes counterproductive to apply the term *disability* to each specific plane.

The second limitation concerns the measurement (or assessment) of disability using the *ISS*. The criterion applied to the various categories is a scale of independence. Unfortunately, this scaling implies greater or lesser levels of dependence. As noted earlier, this distinction can be quite confusing when attempting to understand the meaning of movement in one direction or another on the scale. Movement from having difficulty walking to the use of a cane may, in fact, create greater independence by allowing the person to attempt walking more often because of increased confidence when using the cane. Yet scoring of independence using the *ISS* reflects a person who is now more dependent because an aid is used. It may clarify matters if the dependence–independence criterion were simply used as descriptive categories rather than as a change scale. In addition, it would be helpful to add an outcome that clarifies a level of performance in ability to complete the various tasks, such as that described earlier in the section on outcomes of disability.

The Patient Evaluation Conference System (PECS)

The second project addressing functional outcomes concerns a response to functional assessment problems by a university-related rehabilitation medicine unit. The *Patient Evaluation Conference System (PECS)* establishes an interdisciplinary method for assessing behavior functioning of patients. The pri-mary objectives for developing the scale were to improve communication among staff, students, and patients as well as to improve documentation of patient needs, goals of individual programs, and outcomes.

In developing the *PECS,* Harvey and Jellinek[18] have listed the requirements for a useful functional assessment system. They present five system needs, including the following:

1. Development of a scale sensitive enough to record small changes (gains) in functional performance
2. A broad inventory of functional performance areas, including medical, physical, psychological, social, and vocational
3. A system having a common scale value to show changes in levels of dependence
4. A system that documents both status and goals in a clear manner
5. A system that can be easily understood by the wide variety of people concerned in the individual rehabilitation process, incuding patients, professionals, students, families, peer reviewers, and third party payers.

The resulting assessment device contains two general sections, one that addresses medical restoration and a second addressing psychosocial concerns. The medical restoration section is divided into rehabilitation departments (rehabilitation medicine, nursing, physical therapy, occupational therapy, communication disorders, pharmacy, dietary, and orthotics). Rehabilitation objectives are reflected within the tasks performed by departments. Nursing, for example, addresses bowel, urinary, and skin programs. Physical therapy is concerned only with transfers, ambulation, and wheelchair mobility. Occupational therapy addresses eating, dressing/personal care, and homemaking skills. The psychosocial section of the *PECS* similarly includes psychological, social, and vocational aspects of the total rehabilitation program.

Each department fills out a *PECS* worksheet that is designed specifically for that department. Prior to each rehabilitation conference, forms are collected and compiled onto a *PECS* master form. The consolidated form serves as a tool for overall patient evaluation and planning.

Additional *PECS* design features facilitate communication; all items are rated using a common seven-point scale (1–7) to determine level of independence. A zero point indicates an area was not assessed. In addition, all ratings are general, reflecting a judgment of performance based on individual disciplinary assessments. The occupational therapist, for example, could assess the patient's ability to feed himself or herself by any of a number of measurement strategies. Following these measurements, a general judgment of feeding ability is assessed. These positive characteristics make the *PECS* highly relevant to comprehensive rehabilitation programs in which professionals from multiple disciplines must meet to plan an individual program or just to communicate with each other during the rehabilitation process.

Another feature of the *PECS* effectively addresses the need to set patient goals. *PECS* administration requires a goal for level of independence be set for each appropriate outcome. As noted earlier, goal setting aids clinical decision-making and program evaluation efforts.

The *PECS* has reasonably good measurement data. Harvey and Jellinek[18] report interrater reliability statistics within disciplines ranging from .68 to .80. These data suggest that any two raters within the same professional orientation will most likely agree on the patient's level of independence. Additionally, the authors report that feedback from the various departments suggests that *PECS* has good content validity. Unfortunately, no information is provided about criterion-related validity for the

PECS. As noted before, however, the scalability of a dependence–independence criterion remains debatable.

Overall, the *PECS* appears to address the majority of areas recommended by the World Health Organization in the ICIDH.[46] In addition, the system facilitates communication and documentation of patient progress using criteria that encourages communication across discipines.

Uniform Data System for Medical Rehabilitation

A most important step forward in rehabilitation data base development is the *Uniform Data System for Medical Rehabilitation*. Coordinated through the State University of New York at Buffalo, (Buffalo General Hospital), the project is a multi-organizational effort to develop a standard rehabilitation information data base. The task force created to develop the system is composed of rehabilitation experts from the American Congress of Rehabilitation Medicine, the American Academy of Physical Medicine and Rehabilitation, the American Spinal Injury Association, and the Model Spinal Injury Association, among others. Since its inception in 1983, the Task Force has obtained recognition and support from many of the multidisciplinary organizations in rehabilitation, including, among others, the National Association of Rehabilitation Facilities and the American Occupational Therapy Association.

The purpose, as stated in the project abstract, is to improve effectiveness and efficiency of rehabilitation service for disabled persons by developing and making accessible to service providers, researchers, and educators an operational data system with commonly understood terms and uniform measures of demographic characteristics, impairment, disability, handicap, outcome, and cost of rehabilitation care for disabled individuals in the United States.[2]

The *Uniform Data System for Medical Rehabilitation* monitors the patient's functional status from admission through discharge to a 3-month to 6-month followup. Together, the data from these three points in time provide information about severity of disability, patient progress, program effectiveness, and efficiency.[9] Currently, the system requests standardized information on 22 items, including admission and discharge dates, functional status, payment sources, and diagnosis (Table 9-3).

The system does have limitations, however, in its current stage of development. First, only two items are clearly related to outcomes in the handicapped domain: living arrangement and vocational status (employment/homemaker/student). Whether additional outcomes, such as economic self-sufficiency, social integration, or other "occupation of time" will be added later is not yet clear. A second limitation to the system concerns the lack of an impairment category as defined in the ICIDH. The system currently addresses diagnostic categories and impairment groups. However, the impairment groups are simply generalized diagnostic labels. For example, stroke is an impairment group label for ICD−9 categories such as spastic hemiplegia, subarachnoid hemorrhage, and occlusion of cerebral arteries. Better descriptors of actual impairments would give the system greater flexibility in describing the full range of consequences experienced by people with disabilites. Much can be accomplished if the *Uniform Data System for Medical Rehabilitation* becomes accepted practice across the majority of medical rehabilitation programs, primarily because the system provides a consistent set of characteristics for describing human services directed at the reduction of disability and dependency. Its major steps forward are in the explication of a wide variety of factors related to rehabilitation outcomes and, more generally, to the data needs for human services evaluation described earlier.

To date, the system reports excellent interrater reliability on the Functional Independence Measure (the system's functional status item) across multiple disciplines and at the three assessment points. Validity data, also very positive, consisted of an assessment of items by the clinicians who participated in the reliability study. Basically, they felt that none of the items were difficult to evaluate, all items were necessary, and no new items should be added. Sixty-four hospitals in 22 states currently participate in the *Uniform Data System for Medical Rehabilitation* service, which provides quarterly and annual reports of each program's data in comparison to aggregated regional and national data. Additionally, the developers estimate that over 100 inpatient rehabilitation facilities currently use the Uniform Data Set, even though all may not subscribe to its services.

SUMMARY

Human services evaluation requires a clear understanding of four types of information; (1) the overall goal of the system, (2) the reasons why people come in contact with the system (needs), (3) the range of possible responses to those contacts (treatments), and (4) the outcome(s) of the contact. When corresponding data are reliable and valid, it is possible to answer questions about experiences of the system. These experiences can relate to individual contacts, to institutional planning and evaluation, or to the nature of problems addressed by the system.

Questions that focus on individual contacts with the system are mostly concerned with day-to-day operation and clinical decision making. Such questions might include the following: What are specific patient needs? How are these needs best addressed? Are patient needs being reduced by particular treatments? Is it time to stop treatment?

A different set of questions leads to efficient human service planning. What are the needs currently being presented? In what

---

Table 9-3
Items Comprising the Uniform Data System for Medical Rehabilitation

1. Rehabilitation facility code
2. Patient number
3. Admission Date
4. Discharge date
5. Program interruptions (up to 3)
6. Admission classn
7. Zip code
8. Birthdate
9. Sex
10. Race/ethnicity
11. English language ability of patient
12. Marital status
13. Living arrangement (setting and people)
14. Vocational status
15. Followup (date, information source, method, health maintenance, and therapy
16. Impairment group
17. Date of onset
18. Principal diagnosis
19. Other diagnoses (up to 7)
20. Payment source
21. Charges (total dollars)
22. Functional independence measure (18 items)

*Admission class has three codes referring to first time admission, short-term (10 days) admission, or readmission.

ways is the system responding to a particular set of needs? Is the system successful in responding to all needs or only certain needs? Whether answers pertain to a specific program, institution (hospital), or agency, the information is useful for making decisions about reducing or increasing manpower, for establishing new directions for services, or for determining the cost benefits of particular services. The information also serves documentation needs for accountability and communication with appropriate referent groups (*e.g.,* third party payers, quality assurance committees, private boards, and legislators).

When data are aggregated in consistent ways across institutions, programs, and agencies, a picture emerges as to the nature of the problems addressed by the system. This aspect, typically referred to as epidemiology in health care, helps to determine exactly the kinds of needs addressed or, more importantly, what needs are not effectively addressed by the system. How extensive are those needs? Is there a particular characteristic of the people presenting certain needs, such as their gender, where they live, or their age, that can clarify the nature of the problem? Do the needs present a new problem for the system? Are services effectively reducing needs? Which treatments are least/most effective for certain problems? All of these questions assist in our understanding of problems confronting people in our society.

The conditions giving rise to disablement are partly medical and partly situational, the latter including personal characteristics and environmental conditions. Thus disablement represents a collection of needs cutting across numerous human service systems, including medical health care, mental health, education, and a variety of social services. Together with the increasing presence of disability and dependency in our society, this combination of factors creating disablement has resulted in responses from a multitude of disciplines and agencies, some of which include medicine, nursing, physical therapy, occupational therapy, biomedical engineering, psychology, social work, education, and computer sciences.

The consequences of this multidisciplinary concern for disablement issues are simply understood by our inability to collect consistent data that are requirements for human service systems. With so many disciplines and agencies addressing the needs of people with disability, the goals for rehabilitation become unclear and ever changing, depending on the perspective of the service being provided. Unfortunately, there is no commonly understood goal toward which the multiple disciplines can work to achieve interdisciplinary outcomes. Therefore, the corresponding data needs concerning the nature of contacts with the system, services rendered, and outcomes all tend to reflect the individual disciplines involved in the rehabilitation process.

Over the past 10 years there has been a recognition of these problems relating to disablement. More recently attempts have been initiated to correct system deficiencies, through projects such as the *Minimal Record of Disability for Multiple Sclerosis,* and *Patient Evaluation Conference System,* and the *Uniform Data System for Medical Rehabilitation.*

However, greater understanding and cooperation is needed before a truly comprehensive data base for rehabilitation can be developed and effectiveness of services proven on a wider scale. First, we all must recognize the need to communicate across disciplines in a consistent fashion, for when we fail to do so, we fail to serve the greater purposes of communication in human service delivery. Second, there is need for greater respect for the importance of consistent data collection in rehabilitation for the purposes of planning, evaluation, and better understanding of disablement. The time has come for widespread cooperation among the multiple disciplines interested in relieving the problems of disability and dependency that can come through efforts such as the *Uniform Data System for Medical Rehabilitation.*

Such cooperation can lead away from confusing multidisciplinary efforts to more unified interdisciplinary efforts.

Third, a better understanding is required of the planes of experience encompassed by disablement. Agreement on the meanings of terms such as *diagnosis, impairment, disability,* and *handicap* to describe these planes would facilitate our communication efforts greatly.

Last, we need to clarify the meaning of outcomes and attach those meanings to useful human service paradigms. For example, reintegration into society of a person with a newly acquired spinal cord injury should involve a single human service paradigm that moves the patient from acute care to maximum independence and complete empowerment over personal rights and responsibilities.

REFERENCES

1. Alexander JL, Fuhrer MJ: Functional assessment of individuals with physical impairments. In Fuhrer MJ, Halpern AS (eds): Functional Assessment in Rehabilitation, pp 45–59. Baltimore, Paul H Brookes, 1984
2. American Congress of Rehabilitation Medicine/American Academy of Physical Medicine and Rehabilitation: Annual meeting, Boston, October 21–26, 1984
3. Anderson TP, Anderson E, Arndts L et al: Stroke rehabilitation: Evaluation of its quality by assessing patient outcomes. Arch Phys Med Rehabil 59:170–175, 1978.
4. Basmajian JV: Series editor's foreward. In Granger CV, Gresham GE (eds): Functional Assessment in Rehabilitation Medicine. Baltimore, Williams & Wilkins, 1984
5. Brock DB, Freeman DH, Lemke JH et al: Demographic characteristics. In Cornoni-Huntley J, Brock DB, Ostfeld AM et al (eds): Established Populations for Epidemiologic Studies of the Elderly, pp 11–32. National Institute on Aging, Information Center Silver Springs, MD, 1987
6. Brown M, Diller L, Gordon WA: Functional assessment and outcome measurement: An integrative review. Annu Rev Rehabil 3:93–120, 1982
7. Chin PL: Physical techniques in stroke rehabilitation. J R Coll Physicians Lond 3:165–169, 1982.
8. Crews J, Frey WD: Independent Living for the Older & Multiply Handicapped Blind, National State of the Art. Michigan Commission for the Blind, Saginaw, MI, unpublished
9. Data Management Service: Guide for Use of the Uniform Data Set For Medical Rehabilitation. The Buffalo General Hospital, State University of New York, Buffalo, New York, 1987
10. Duckworth D: The needs for a standard terminology and classification of disablement. In Granger CV, Gresham GE (eds): Functional Assessment in Rehabilitation Medicine, pp1–13. Baltimore, Williams & Wilkins, 1984
11. Ebel RL: Essentials of Educational Measurement. Englewood Cliffs, NJ, Prentice-Hall, 1972
12. Eisenberg M: Disability as stigma. In Duval RJ, Eisenberg M, Griggins C (eds): Disabled People as Second-Class Citizens, pp 3–12. New York, Springer Publishing, 1982
13. Frey WE: Functional assessment in the '80s: A conceptual enigma, a technical challenge. In Fuhrer MJ, Halpern AS (eds): Functional Assessment in Rehabilitation, pp 11–43. Baltimore, Paul H Brookes, 1984
14. Fuhrer MJ, Halpern, AS: Functional Assessment in Rehabilitation, pp 1–9. Baltimore, Paul H Brookes, 1984
15. Granger CV, Gresham GE (eds): Functional Assessment in Rehabilitation Medicine. Baltimore, Williams & Wilkins, 1984
16. Granger CV, Hamilton BB, Sherwin FS et al: A uniform national data system for medical rehabilitation. In Fuhrer MJ (ed): Rehabilitation Outcomes. Baltimore, Paul H Brookes, 1986
17. Gresham GE, Labi MGC: Functional assessment instruments currently available for documenting outcomes in rehabilitation. In Granger CV, Gresham GE (eds): Functional Assessment in Rehabilitation Medicine, pp 65–85. Baltimore, Williams & Wilkins, 1984

18. Harvey RF, Jellinek HM: Functional performance assessment: A program approach. Arch Phys Med Rehabil 62:456–461, 1981
19. Indicies Inc: Functional limitations: A state of the art review. US Department of Health, Education, and Welfare, Rehabilitation Services Administration, grant No. 13-P-59220/3-01, 1979
20. International Federation of Multiple Sclerosis Societies: Minimal Record of Disability for Multiple Sclerosis. New York, National Multiple Sclerosis Society, 1985
21. Jette AM: Functional capacity evaluation: An empirical approach. Arch Phys Med Rehabil 61:85–89, 1980
22. Jette AM: Concepts of health and methodological issues in functional assessment. In Granger CV, Gresham GE (eds): Functional Assessment in Rehabilitation Medicine, pp 46–64. Baltimore, Williams & Wilkins, 1984
23. Joe T: Foreward. In Granger CV, Gresham GE (eds): Functional Assessment in Rehabilitation Medicine. Baltimore, Williams & Wilkins, 1984
24. Kaufert JM: Functional ability indices: Measurement problems in assessing their validity. Arch Phys Med Rehabil 62:260–267, 1983
25. Keith RA: Functional assessment measures in medical rehabilitation: Current status. Arch Phys Med Rehabil 65:74–78, 1984
26. Klein RM, Bell B: Self-care skills: Behavioral measurement with Klein-Bell scale. Arch Phys Med Rehabil 63:335, 1982
27. Lehman JF, deLateur BJ, DeLisa JA et al: Cancer rehabilitation: Assessment of need, development, and evaluation of a model of care. Arch Phys Med Rehabil 59:410–419, 1978
28. Lind K: A synthesis of studies on stroke rehabilitation. J Chronic Dis 35:133–149, 1982
29. Livneh H: Person-Environment congruence: A rehabilitation perspective. Int J Rehabil Res 10:3–45, 1987
30. Melvin JL: The relationship of functional assessment to quality of care review. In Granger CV, Gresham GE (eds): Functional Assessment in Rehabilitation Medicine, pp 140–153. Baltimore, Williams & Wilkins, 1984
31. Merrill SC: The efficacy of occupational therapy in the treatment of stroke: A qualitative synthesis. In Lieberman D, Merrill SC, Ostrow PC (eds): Outcomes of Stroke Rehabilitation, pp 119–129. Rockville, Maryland, American Occupational Therapy Association, 1985
32. Mittelsten Scheid E: An assessment system that matches abilities with job requirements to facilitate reintegration of disabled people into employment. In Habeck RV, Frey WD, Galvin DE et al (eds): Economics and Equity in Employment of People With Disabilities: An International Perspective, pp 77–80. East Lansing, Michigan State University, University Center for International Rehabilitation, 1985
33. National Stroke Association: The Road Ahead: A Stroke Recovery Guide. Colorado, National Stroke Association, 1986
34. Ostrow PC, Lieberman D, Merrill SC (eds): Outcomes of Stroke Rehabilitation. Rockville, Maryland, American Occupational Therapy Association, 1985
35. Partridge CJ: The effectiveness of physiotherapy; A classification for evaluation. Physiotherapy 66:153–155, 1980
36. Rintala DH, Alexander JL, Buck EL et al: Self-observation and report technique (SORT). In Fuhrer MJ, Halpern AS (eds): Functional Assessment in Rehabilitation, pp 205–221. Baltimore, Paul H Brookes, 1984
37. Rogers DE: The Robert Wood Johnson Foundation Annual Report, p 4. Princeton, NJ, Robert Wood Johnson Foundation, 1981
38. Schumacher K: The International Classification of Impairments, Disabilities and Handicaps (ICIDH): Relevance to Physical Therapy and Rehabilitation. Paper presented to the World Congress of Physical Therapy, Sydney, Australia, 1987
39. Susset V, Raymond PM: Prognosis and prediction: From patient to policy. In Granger CV, Gresham GE (eds): Functional Assessment in Rehabilitation Medicine, pp 324-342. Baltimore, Williams & Wilkins, 1984
40. US Department of Education: Annual Report of the National Council on the Handicapped. Washington, DC, National Institute of Handicapped Research, 1982
41. Vash CL: The Psychology of Disability. New York, Springer Publishing, 1981
42. Vash CL: Evaluation from the client's point of view. In Halpern AS, Fuhrer MJ (eds): Functional Assessment in Rehabilitation, pp 253–267. Baltimore, Paul H Brookes, 1984
43. Willems EP, Alexander JL: Behavioral indicators of client progress after spinal cord injury: An ecological-contextual approach. In Green CJ, Meagher RB, Millon T (eds): Handbook of Health Care Clinical Psychology. New York, Plenum Press, 1982
44. Williams TF: Foreword, In Coroni-Huntley J, Brock DB, Ostfeld AM et al (eds): Established Populations for Epidemiologic Studies of the Elderly. Rockville, Maryland, National Institute on Aging, 1987
45. Wood PHN: Appreciating the consequences of disease: The classification of impairments, disabilities, and handicaps. WHO Chron 34:376–382, 1980
46. World Health Organization: Classification of Impairments, Disabilities, and Handicaps. Geneva, World Health Organization, 1980
47. Wright GN: Total Rehabilitation. Boston, Little, Brown & Co, 1980
48. Zollar C: Personal Communication. National Association of Rehabilitation Facilities, November, 1987

Part 2

Diagnostic and Management Methods

10

Neural Aspects of Motor Function as a Basis of Early and Post-Acute Rehabilitation

Paul Bach-y-Rita

Jo-Anne C. Lazarus

Michael G. Boyeson

Richard Balliet

Theodore A. Myers

Some recovery of motor function takes place after a central nervous system lesion. In this chapter we will explore the neural mechanisms that are or may be related to such recovery. Rather than a comprehensive review of neuroanatomy, neurophysiology, and neurochemistry, we will emphasize data that are particularly important to an understanding of physiological mechanisms of recovery of function and to the role of rehabilitation in obtaining the maximum possible recovery.

NEURAL ASPECTS OF MOTOR FUNCTION SPECIFICALLY RELEVANT TO REHABILITATION

Neuroanatomy

Hierarchical Organization of the Brain

The nervous system develops in a hierarchical sequence both in regard to phylogeny and to ontogeny, although, as will be discussed below, functional organization appears to be based on other organizational modes as well. The central nervous system (CNS) includes the archi-, paleo-, and neomammalian components. The oldest, or archi, portion is the central core; the autonomic and reticular systems of the neuraxis and the archi cerebellovestibular system are included in this component, while protopathic or protective systems make up the paleomammalian portion. The newest, or neomammalian, part of the brain is the epicritic or exploratory component of the CNS. The archi systems have neuronal processes that, in general, project bilaterally. These are also highly multisynaptic. A large portion of paleo system pathways cross (decussate) and thus exert their major influences contralaterally; this system has fewer multisynaptic connections.

The neocerebral systems, which constitute 90% of the mass of the human brain, appear to give humans laterality; they have direct fiber systems between lower and higher centers and vice versa, and are the last to develop full functional capabilities, often years after birth. They are the most subject to damage, because of their exposed location and the fact that the blood vessels supplying these structures are principally terminal branches, thus allowing little opportunity for collateral circulation.[136]

Integrative Structures

Integration is a major activity of the CNS. Long interneurons comprise the majority of both the ascending and descending fibers in the white matter. Thus, many pyramidal tract fibers originate from interneurons with integrative functions. Some synapse on other interneurons before synapsing on α and γ motoneurons. Many play a role in modifying incoming sensory information or in relaying information to subcortical nuclear areas. Most, but not all, pathways have many collaterals. As the phylogenetic scale is ascended the numbers of commissural neurons increase. These commissural interneurons, which transmit information from one side to the other, play a role in bilateral coordination such as in dressing.[136]

Clinical and Experimental Evidence for Ipsilateral Pathways

Although motor control is primarily contralateral, some ipsilateral control can be demonstrated. In 1933, Bucy and Fulton[32] demonstrated in primates ipsilateral control from the precentral cortex. They further showed that one motor area is capable of integrating movements of all four extremities, ipsilateral as well as contralateral. Ipsilateral control has been reported in hemispherectomy cases: Gardner[75] noted that a considerable amount of motor control, including walking, returned in a patient following hemispherectomy, and Glees,[82] following a review of his research and the animal and clinical hemispherectomy studies of others, reported that intellectual function and sensory and motor control for the whole body could be subserved by the remaining hemisphere. In some cases bimanual function was obtained.

Some "hemiplegic" patients have been shown to have ipsilateral deficits. Jebson and co-workers[103] noted ipsilateral hand deficits including slowness of writing, eating, and emptying and filling cans. The neuroanatomist Brodal,[29] following his recovery from a stroke, noted that ipsilateral defects are not usually described in a clinical examination because they are not looked for. In patients with right hemisphere lesions, significant ipsilateral deficits were reported in two gross motor tests requiring proximal limb speed and coordination: hand–arm tap and directed reaching. Most of the patients were unaware of the ipsilateral deficits[124]; the authors suggested that their results were not surprising since anatomical data demonstrated ipsilateral control of proximal limb muscles. Several research groups, including that of Brinkman and Kuypers,[28] had shown that although each half of the brain has control over arm, hand, and finger movements contralaterally, proximal arm movements can be controlled ipsilaterally as well.

Neurophysiology

Three levels of neuromuscular organization—spinal level, brain stem level, and cortical and subcortical movement control—will be discussed with reference to CNS damage. Significant interaction also occurs within the various levels of the CNS; thus, a brief discussion on action systems is presented that attempts to integrate the various levels within a distributed control viewpoint. In addition, the importance of inhibitory mechanisms in functional motor control is addressed.

Spinal Level Neuromuscular Organization

PATTERNS OF MUSCLE FIBER ACTIVATION. Muscular action is the result of the activation of functional elements called motor units. A motor unit consists of a single motoneuron and all of the muscle fibers that it innervates. The ratio of muscle fibers to motoneurons determines the delicacy or level of refinement of the movement that the motor units produce. However, overt movement of a limb is not typically produced by a single motor unit. Even very small movements of an individual finger require at least the recruitment of several motor units in order to be visible to the naked eye. In cases such as movement of the eye or index finger in which finely controlled movements are possible, an extremely low ratio of muscle fibers to motoneurons exists (e.g., 3 : 1), allowing rapid, coordinated movements to be executed. For grosser movements such as trunk posturing and limb movements, a single motoneuron may innervate hundreds of muscle fibers.[57] In incomplete spinal cord injuries resulting in paraplegia or quadriplegia, reliance on observation alone may preclude finding functional motor units in a seemingly paralyzed limb. Technical high-resolution equipment such as needle and surface electrode electromyography may assist the physician and/or therapist in determining the potential for recovery of function through therapy.

Motor units are typically recruited in a systematic smallest-to-largest order. Orderly recruitment of motor units due to the size principle[95] results in the ability to regulate force. In addition to controlling the number of motor units, the firing rate or frequency of each motor unit recruited is also regulated; the greater the firing rate, the greater the force developed. Evidence by Broman and colleagues[30] has suggested that smooth control of muscle output results from the interaction of motor unit recruitment and firing rate, an increase in the former having an inhibitory influence on the latter. Such a mechanism allows for smooth control of muscle output by the peripheral circuitry, thus reducing the amount of input required by the CNS. Inputs to the motor units are both sensory and motor. The descending motor pathways provide efferent input for the execution of movement. The γ motor system via muscle spindles also provides a short-loop input to motor units on stretch of the muscle spindles. Other sensory inputs, such as the Golgi tendon organs, provide inhibitory input to the motor unit. Through interneurons, the active motor unit interacts with antagonist motor units by way of reciprocal inhibition.

Damage to the CNS may result in a loss of motor units and/or diminished muscle tension feedback, leaving the system with a limited ability to produce or regulate force. Recent work has demonstrated substantial disorders in recruitment of motor units in patients with certain neurological disorders (i.e., parkinsonism,[134] post-acute polymyositis[133]), resulting in neuromuscular dysfunction. As such, therapeutic exercises should be performed in a manner that perpetuates slow (tonic) muscle control associated with low-threshold motor units.[11] Moreover, an example of "deordering" in normal humans has been reviewed by Desmedt.[49] When the first dorsal interosseous was used as a synergist with the thumb in a functional pinch rather than as a prime mover, large rather than small motor units were involved. Hence, differential recruitment may be task dependent, emphasizing the need for careful selection of functional tasks in rehabilitation.

SENSORY MECHANISMS REGULATING MOVEMENT. Rather than describe the various sensory organs in the periphery related to movement (i.e., muscle spindles, Golgi tendon organs) as independent structures, their functions will be described within the context of the stretch reflex, demonstrating how sensory mechanisms interrelate with the motor system in an organized systematic way. If the patellar tendon is tapped, as is done during a neurological examination, the muscle spindles respond to this stretch by increasing their firing rate. The impulses are sent to the spinal cord via IA afferent fibers, where they establish contact directly with the α motoneurons that innervate the quadriceps. These motoneurons, in turn, increase their firing rate, which serves to contract the main, extrafusal muscle fibers, thus extending the leg at the knee joint. Contraction of the extrafusal muscle fibers serves to decrease the stretch on the muscle spindles, causing a decrease in the rate of spindle afferent firing. Muscle spindles can contract by activity in the γ motoneurons, and, integral with this process, they function as sensory receptors. The γ activation during α activation (α–γ coactivation) causes the muscle spindle to contract, disallowing it to slacken, providing a follow-up servomechanism and indirect control over muscle contraction.

While muscle spindles monitor the length of the muscle fibers, Golgi tendon organs situated at the junction of the muscle fibers and tendon respond primarily to tension or force exerted by the active contraction of muscle fibers. Impulses from Golgi tendon organ afferents synapse on interneurons, which are inhibitory to the motoneurons of the muscle of origin, thus decreasing activity in the contracting muscle. This serves to reduce or "dampen" the stretch reflex. In addition to agonist excitation, a patellar tendon tap results in inhibition of the antagonist (hamstring). This is accomplished via primary spindle afferents, which synapse on interneurons that have an inhibitory effect on motoneurons of the antagonist muscle.

The entire monosynaptic stretch reflex provides automatic compensation for unexpected changes in the load acting on a muscle as well as some postural adjustments. The strength of the contraction for a given tap force is the gain of the reflex. Cerebrovascular accidents (i.e., stroke and traumatic brain injury) can result in a reduced sensory threshold and an elevated response to a given stimulus so that the gains of the tendon reflexes are elevated.[189] Thus the muscles are said to be hyperreflexive. This response parallels that seen in young infants as a result of unmyelinated areas of the cerebral cortex. The recovery of motor function following stroke,[11] in terms of reflexive activity, closely resembles the developmental sequence in early stages of life. This has become the basis for some types of therapeutic intervention (i.e., Brunnstrom, Bobath).

SPINAL LEVEL MOVEMENT CONTROL. The assumption has been made that reflexes, or "co-ordinative structures,"[54] underlie normal motor function. However, two camps have emerged regarding the relationship of innate or primitive reflexes and the development of voluntary motor behavior.[191] One position is that reflexes must be dissolved or extinguished before voluntary motor control becomes possible.[131] This view is unattractive in that it implies an inherent antagonism between reflexes and voluntary motor actions. It is often interpreted too literally, leading to the conclusion that the neural mechanisms subserving the reflexes "disappear" from the nervous system with maturation. As we know, the predominance of reflex-like behavior following CNS damage precludes this conclusion. The alternate position states that with increasing age, primitive reflexes are modulated by higher centers to serve as subassemblies[177] or elements[54] of voluntary movement. Critics of this hypothesis often cite the lack of evidence for a direct connection between reflex behavior and voluntary motor control, as well as for the apparent "hard-wired" nature of the reflex response. It is clear, however, from studies such as that of Thelen and Fisher[172] that one must consider many factors before denying the relationship between reflex behavior and voluntary motor control. For instance, these researchers demonstrated that the disappearance of neonatal stepping could be explained as a result of increasing leg mass simply by placing the child vertically in water, thereby reducing leg mass and demonstrating the reflex, and that the retention of this reflex with practice[194] may be simply an exercise effect.

The dynamic properties of reflexes demonstrated in a series of studies by Forssberg and his colleagues[69, 70] provide evidence against reflexes being immutable or simple stimulus–response linking systems. During various phases of the step cycle, tactile stimuli were applied to the dorsum of the paw of chronic spinal cats. During the swing phase, a stimulation evoked a flexion response with a concomitant crossed extension, whereas during the stance phase it induced an increased ipsilateral extension. The organization of such responses is such that the animal is allowed to respond appropriately in accordance with changing states in the environment. The underlying mechanism (or mechanisms) cannot be as simplistic as previously believed. Additionally, from a motor development perspective, reflexes continue to be modified through the life span as a natural phenomenon. The early appearance of subcortical and spinal reflexes (e.g., Babinski) in infancy, subsequent suppression throughout childhood and adulthood, and the often reappearance during aging and insult exemplifies the modification of their expression by higher inhibitory control centers.

Brain Stem Movement Control

Brain stem reflexes such as the asymmetrical tonic neck reflex (ATNR), the symmetrical tonic neck reflex (STNR), and the tonic labyrinthine reflex (TLR), and the positive and negative supporting reactions serve to maintain posture for righting, walking, and various other body positions. Their centers are located in the red nucleus and parts of the basal ganglia (caudal level). The vestibular apparatus, located in the inner ear area, sends sensory impulses to the brain stem (as well as cerebellum), which in turn synapse on neurons used to contract muscles associated with both modifiable movements (e.g., postural control) and preprogrammed movements (e.g., saccadic eye movements). Damage to the brain stem results in disequilibrium or inappropriate postural responses during voluntary displacement of a limb or some external perturbation. However, evidence from decorticate animal studies[176] demonstrates that, by providing passive limb, trunk, and neck movements 10 to 14 times per day, contractures could be avoided and the ability of the animal to right itself, sit, stand, and walk alone could be demonstrated.

The interaction of brain stem reflexes with spinal level reflexes has been demonstrated. Todor[173] replicated a Hayes and Sullivan[93] study demonstrating the effects of the ATNR on the stretch reflex in normal adults. By separating the various components of the reflex (i.e., neural time representing the time from tendon contact to electromyographic (EMG) onset, and motor time representing the time from EMG onset to movement onset) Todor was able to show that head turning served to increase or reduce the latency of the motor component significantly over control conditions (head in midline). This suggests that the ATNR serves to bias the motoneuron pool toward facilitation or inhibition, enhancing or attenuating the parameters of the response of a low level reflex. This effect is probably minimal in a normal population but may be enhanced in clinical populations.

Brain stem reflexes not only interact with lower level systems (spinal reflexes) but have also been shown to interact with higher level cortical systems during voluntary movement. Hellebrandt and Waterland[94] have demonstrated the effect of the ATNR on the performance of a unilateral continuous wrist flexion or wrist extension task in normal adults. When the head turn is congruent with task requirements (i.e., head toward/wrist extension; head away/wrist flexion), the decrement in performance due to fatigue is minimized, demonstrating a neural bias as a direct result of head position. Another function, then, of brain stem reflexes, albeit minimal in normal adults, is to bias the nervous system during the performance of volitional actions. Such a bias may be enhanced in neurological populations. Furthermore, the interactive process is bidirectional in that brain stem mechanisms can also be altered through cortical involvement. The human vestibulo-ocular response (VOR) is considered a primitive reflex. Yet, Melvill-Jones and Gonshor[130] have demonstrated that it is possible to change the human VOR by inducing vision reversal with prism goggles during head rotation. In addition, McKinley and Peterson[126] describe voluntary control of the VOR by normal subjects.

Balliet and Nakayama[19] were able to train normal subjects to make voluntary cyclotorsional eye movements (rotations around the visual axis of the eye) of up to 30°. Without this specialized training, these movements can only occur as a reflexive action (e.g., counterrotations of the eyes during lateral head tilt). In addition, Balliet and Nakayama[18] found that these learned movements, which were independent of vestibular or visual stimulation, could by themselves induce quantitatively identical sensations as actual head and body rotations of the same magnitudes. (See section on information processing in neuromuscular retraining for more details.)

Because of the highly integrative nature of the nervous system, seemingly hard-wired subsystems may have the potential to be modified. Although, in normal populations, reflexive movements may not always be readily apparent on observation, they serve to coordinate movement in an organized fashion. The interactive nature of brain stem mechanisms with other CNS levels suggests that rehabilitation should focus on reflexive behavior as an integral component of retraining voluntary movement.

Cortical and Subcortical Movement Control

The cerebral cortex in humans is highly specialized for fine control, particularly in movements involving the fingers and mouth (as in speech). However, even with the development of this phylogenetically young structure, the control of voluntary movement is not restricted to cortical involvement. Subcortical structures such as the basal ganglia, cerebellum, and thalamus play a crucial role in most movements that are volitional. Wing's[189] modification of Allen and Tsukahara's model[3] (Fig. 10-1) for depicting pathways involved in the planning, execution, and control of voluntary movement is extremely helpful in viewing and explaining the interaction between various levels of the nervous system.

ASSOCIATION CORTEX. The idea for movement finds its expression as neural activity in the prefrontal (association) cortex. This structure occupies approximately one third of the entire neocortex in humans.[73] Several experiments by Kornhuber and his associates[46, 47, 97, 110] have revealed that a readiness potential (a slowly rising negative potential) occurs bilaterally over the prefrontal cortex approximately 800 msec prior to the onset of muscle activity and subsequent voluntary movement of the finger or arm. This readiness or *Bereitschaftspotential* has come to represent the mobilization of cortical areas involved in the initiation, evaluation, and control of the ensuing movement.[46]

More recently, Fuster[73] has summarized evidence from lesion data in monkeys, neuroelectrical data in humans and monkeys, and clinical data in humans to argue more specifically for a critical role of the prefrontal cortex in the temporal organization of goal-directed behavioral sequences. At least in terms of cognitive functions, the association cortex appears to regulate the processes of memory and anticipation of events that are delayed in time but related to each other in some way. For example, in a delayed-response task, a cue (white-light illumination of a left or right response button) is given and then, after a delay, during which time the monkey must remember the cue, both response buttons are illuminated simultaneously. The animal's response is to press the button on the side of the cue for a reward. In this task, the second event is contingent on the first event. By characterizing the patterns of discharge of prefrontal neurons during the performance of this task, Fuster and his colleagues were able to identify various areas of the prefrontal cortex associated with the presentation of the cue, the delay, and the response alternatives. Most importantly, an elevated discharge in some prefrontal cells (particularly in the cortex of the dorsolateral prefrontal convexity) is apparent during the delay, representing memory for the cue or a "looking back" to the cue in order to retain information

related to the overall plan of the response. Other prefrontal cells show a gradual increase of firing in apparent anticipation of the choice, a sort of "looking forward" to the coming motor act, or preparation for a response associated with the goal.

The contingent negative variation (CNV), a prefrontal field potential, or expectancy wave[183] exemplifies the cortical activity associated with the idea (planning and preparation) for voluntary movement. Gevins and associates[79] have documented left prefrontal activity (movement-related cortical potentials) just prior to the execution of an accurate index finger isometric contraction of either the left or the right hand. In addition, cerebral blood flow studies[151–153] and other metabolic data[101] support the temporal preparatory function of the prefrontal cortex.

Motor disorders of prefrontal function are difficult to specify since they are neither sensory nor motor in a strict sense. Teuber[171] identified the problems associated with prefrontal lesions as lacking the ability to properly anticipate the consequences of movements and, thus, unable to adjust sensory receptors to anticipated changes in sensory input resulting from the movements. In this regard, prefrontal lesions produce more of an action disorder, more specifically affecting perception as a component of motor action. Traditionally, such a disorder has been referred to as a general motor planning disorder.

LATERAL CEREBELLUM. Output from the association cortex travels through the basal ganglia and/or the lateral cerebellum prior to reaching the motor cortex for execution. The cerebellum acts as an integrative center, handling highly digested sensory information from the association cortex. Based on learning and prior experience, the lateral cerebellum is necessary for preprogramming the duration of rapid, ballistic (open-loop) movements prior to their initiation.[108] As such, it plays an important role in the acquisition of motor skills.[31] In particular, fine control of the hand and fingers in highly skilled dextrous actions occurs because of the connections between the lateral cerebellum, ventrolateral thalamus, and premotor and motor cortex. These connections provide the cerebellum with access to the fast, highly myelinated corticospinal tract that controls more distal movements of the arms and fingers. Following cerebellar lesions, recovery may involve substituting slower closed-loop control for the faster cerebellar control of movements.

Figure 10-1. Hypothetical relations between brain structure and voluntary movement control. (Wing AM: Disorders of movement. In Smith MM, Wing AM [eds]: The Psychology of Human Movement, pp 269–296. London, Academic Press, 1984.)

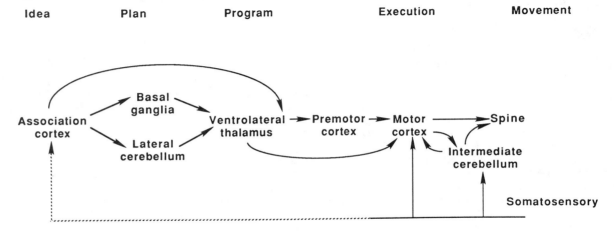

BASAL GANGLIA. The other primary subcortical structures involved in the regulation of movement are the basal ganglia. These masses of neurons, which are clustered into large nuclei (caudate nucleus, putamen, globus pallidus, subthalamic nucleus, and the substantia nigra), receive input from the reticular formation and the prefrontal cortex and send signals to the motor cortex via the ventrolateral thalamus as well as to subcortical structures. Kornhuber[108] refers to the basal ganglia as a ramp generator, serving to generate in particular, but not solely, slow, controlled movements. Damage to the basal ganglia (substantia nigra) in parkinsonism, for example, usually results in a release of inhibition such that the following symptoms emerge: resting tremor, muscular rigidity (cogwheel phenomenon), involuntary movements (akathisia), postural disorders, righting disorders, locomotor disorders (e.g., festination or speeded walking), speech disturbances, and akinesia.[122] Hallett and Khoshbin[92] argue for an activational or energizing component of programming by the basal ganglia, such as the failure of patients with parkinsonism to increase the level of EMG for larger amplitude movements although the relative timing of EMG bursts was within the normal range.

Another, more diffuse, basal ganglia disorder is Huntington's chorea. A progressive degenerative disease, it often involves dysfunction of several integrated neural systems, including the cortex, caudate nucleus, globus pallidus, and thalamus. The disease is characterized by choreiform movements or rapid, involuntary jerks of the limbs. As the normal ramp generator function of the basal ganglia is disturbed, slow, controlled movements are disrupted. However, experiments in subhuman primates[99] have shown that motor control following basal ganglia damage can sometimes be recovered by providing monkeys with the additional sensory input of external visual guidance during movement in place of their own internal guidance. This sensory substitution mechanism has also been observed clinically in patients with parkinsonism. Although they appear to be able to perform visually guided movements fairly well, internally generated movements are greatly impaired. Since the basal ganglia is critical in generating movements on the basis of internally guided memory processes, damage may require a shift to other modes of control, especially to control that uses continuous sensory information.

THALAMUS. The current understanding of the function of the ventrolateral thalamus is that it acts as a relay center between subcortical structures (cerebellum, basal ganglia) and cortical structures (premotor cortex, motor cortex, sensory cortex). In addition, it is thought to play a role in sensorimotor integration.

PREMOTOR CORTEX. The remaining structure involved in the programming of voluntary movement just prior to movement execution is the premotor cortex (part of the larger prefrontal cortex). Anterior to the motor strip, the premotor cortex receives input from subcortical structures via the thalamus and from the association cortex. The premotor cortex (PMC) is bilaterally organized. Unilateral damage produces proximal disturbances of interlimb coordination with a slight increase in muscle tone and reflex responses.[72] Bilateral damage produces severe instability of stance and gait.[72] The primary role of the premotor cortex appears to be the preparation of motor acts involving the setting of postural tone and the timing of subsequent motor sequences. Since the indirect corticoreticulospinal tract originates from the PMC, receiving polysensory input that is largely visual, it also provides visual guidance during such tasks as reaching.

MOTOR CORTEX. When information arrives at the motor cortex, which acts as a final relay station for previous inputs occurring in other cortical and subcortical areas, it is highly digested and organized for execution of the motor act. Representation in the motor strip is not proportional to muscle size but rather to the fine coordination required for the movement. The pyramidal tract originates in the motor cortex with some monosynaptic (in addition to multisynaptic) connections to distal motoneurons on the opposite side of the body, allowing for extremely fast neural transmission and thus rapid movement. Pyramidal tract neurons (PTN) are summing points in a transcortical loop; thus performance of the action results in decreased discharge of PTN, while failure to produce the action results in increased discharge.[58]

There are strong intrahemispheric projections within adjacent regions of the motor strip as well as to the premotor and supplementary motor areas and somatosensory cortex.[55] Between the two cerebral hemispheres, there exist connections between homotopic areas of the motor cortex (with the exception of the fingers and feet) and some nonhomotopic areas of the motor cortex. Additionally, there exist motor cortex projections to the contralateral premotor area and a few fibers to the contralateral sensory area. These connections may help facilitate reorganization of control following insult. Cortical focus for a particular movement has a fringe that in part controls the motoneurons involved in more than one movement[148]; thus, recovery may also include a shift in control to other intact cortical (and/or subcortical) areas.

INTERMEDIATE CEREBELLUM. As well as sending signals down the spinal cord for movement execution, the signals from the motor cortex are continually being monitored and updated via closed-loop connections with the intermediate cerebellum. This part of the cerebellum plays an important role in the ongoing control and monitoring of movement. As part of a dynamic cerebral-cerebellar feedback loop, this subcortical structure (cerebellum), when damaged, results in disequilibrium, tremor during voluntary movement, disturbances in timing and coordination (ataxia), and overactive reflexes. Although it has often been assumed that voluntary modification of the functions of the cerebellum is probably impossible, Balliet and co-workers[15] have demonstrated systematic improvement in the ability to walk without upper extremity weight bearing as a result of specific therapeutic techniques in patients with cerebellar ataxia.

SOMATOSENSORY CORTEX. Somatosensory feedback during the execution of a movement allows for continuous guidance of precise limb movements. Afferent signals continually update the cerebellum, motor cortex, and association cortex. Although deafferented monkeys were able to climb, reach, and grasp in several studies by Taub and Berman,[169, 170] the quality of the control of movement was poor, suggesting that feedback is necessary for fine tuning of movements. In most cases, movements that were performed well were highly overlearned skills or relatively gross motor activities. Similarly, Marsden and co-workers[121] concluded from a review of deafferentation studies that somatosensory feedback is required in order to learn and refine certain higher level motor programs for fine coordination, while other more primitive motor programs are already available within the immature nervous system (i.e., motor programs for relatively gross motor activities such as walking and reaching) without the aid of somatosensory feedback. Additionally, they concluded that such feedback is used to provide for control of a constant motor output, for load compensation, and for the signals necessary to detect and correct errors in program execution. For example, a patient with severe sensory loss due to peripheral nerve lesions (reported by Rothwell and associates[157]) was able to perform finger–thumb opposition, however, he had difficulty maintaining muscle tension while holding an object unless he continually monitored the grasp with vision. This further supports the role of somatosensory feedback in monitoring and updating the quality (*e.g.,* force parameter) of movement.

What neurophysiological changes occur following elimination of somatosensory feedback (through injury) that affect subsequent motor control and rehabilitation? Although regeneration of the nerve has been found to occur following peripheral nerve division and suturing in monkeys, marked misrepresentations of the peripheral sensory fields in the cortex have also been consistently found.[144] Wynn Parry[193] and Dellon[48] have reported successful sensory education in numerous clinical populations. In patients with peripheral nerve injuries, specific sensory retraining appears to provide the patient with the proper conditions to learn recoding of mismatched nerve fibers to new corresponding, functionally specific, receptors in the brain.[48] Sensory retraining is currently being investigated by Balliet and Knight[16] in patients with CNS damage (somatosensory cortex) as well.

Distributed Movement Control and Action Systems

A complementary interface between the study of normal motor control and the study of pathological motor behavior is conspicuously absent from the literature. One of the reasons for these fields of research being carried out in a parallel rather than interactive fashion is the lack of a common theoretical framework. In particular, at least two problems arise in motor control research that cannot be addressed by the traditional theories (*i.e.,* open-loop theory,[111] closed-loop theory[1]). First, these theories cannot, in themselves, account for the large number of degrees of freedom of the human motor system. Degrees of freedom refers to the number of independent ways of moving. For any given joint, degrees of freedom equals the number of axes about which the joint can rotate. A second problem arises from the assumption of a one-to-one mapping of motor program to movement. If this were the case, as suggested by these theories, the human system would have to have an endless reservoir for storage.

Common to both lines of research (clinical and nonclinical) contemporary views of CNS organization depict the system as a hierarchy (*i.e.,* higher centers controlling lower centers in a unidirectional fashion). Although this may be true from a structural viewpoint (as described earlier in this chapter), such an organization defies the emergency of functional plasticity. If it is assumed that the locus of control for all motor behaviors resides only in higher cortical centers and that the flow of information is only in one direction (*i.e.,* top–down or central to peripheral), a patient with upper motor neuron dysfunction should not be able to demonstrate functional recovery post-acutely (more than 2 years from the time of injury). However, this is clearly not the case since there is clinical evidence for functional motor recovery in various neurological populations many years after injury.[11, 17, 20]

Due to the inability of traditional hierarchical theories to account for this discrepancy, one trend has been to model the function of the nervous system as a *distributed control* system.[7, 106] The fact that the locus of control can reside anywhere in this model "reduces the vulnerability of the system to potential insults and help(s) preserve its behavioral stability."[106] Such a model gives support to the theories of brain plasticity.

Correspondingly, various levels of the nervous system not only substantially interact with each other but also are intricately related to changes in the environment. Kelso and Tuller[106] outline a coalitional model of movement control in which actions are not considered independent of the context in which they take place. A coalitional model involves distributed control but manages to deal with the degrees of freedom problem through context-dependent actions; that is, actions are minimally organized relative to the context within which they operate. Evidence for the context-dependent nature of reflexes, for example, has been demonstrated by several investigators.[69, 70, 138, 139]

In conjunction with the hypothesis of a distributed control system, many motor control researchers are viewing the motor system primarily as one mechanism underlying an integrated *action system.*[7, 74, 150] As Reed[150] points out, both the peripheralist and centralist theories of motor control have been refuted by experimental data and theoretical reflection. Motor equivalence, or the fact that the same goal can be realized by various movements, demonstrates that the central program theory is untenable. For example, if a specific motor program was set up to control a specific behavior (*e.g.,* pick up the pen), how is it that one is able to perform this act in various ways from numerous postures and still achieve the same goal? Similarly, the notion of bilateral transfer[80] of conditioned reflexes (the conditioning paradigm being performed on one side only) suggests that there is some central contribution to what was thought to be solely a peripheral response. The divisions of sensory and motor, afferent and efferent, and central and peripheral are simply convenient ways of viewing the total system but are misleading in terms of actual function. An action system approach better describes what is now known to be true of human motor behavior. Evidence that reflexes and other triggered responses are adaptable to external conditions and experience or learning attests to the extremely complex integration of the sensorimotor system.

In the study of action systems, the components of action are not "mechanisms" *per se* (as in reflexes, pattern generators, and so on) but rather "movements" and "postures," which are themselves relations and changes of relations between organism and environment.[150] Thus, action systems are differentiated by their function. Motor acts do not take place irrespective of the environment. Instead they are derived from the organism's perception of that environment and involve the functional utilization of energy reserves. In effect, the damaged nervous system not only suffers from structural abnormalities but also suffers from a severing of the functional relationships between the components of action. As Bernstein[22] has noted, specific disorders of coordination are always accompanied by more general disorders of tonus or postural organization. An action system viewpoint supports such an observation.

Underlying the components of action are various neurophysiological mechanisms that allow for the expression of movements and postures. Reflexes, oscillators, and servomechanisms[74] are examples of the organization of muscles into "functional units" that can be individually controlled. This serves to decrease the degrees of freedom and, in turn, reduce the requirements for a more detailed high-level central controller, making the human motor system more economical. Relatively low level reflexes and other involuntary responses (*e.g.,* spinal control of the locomotor step cycle, brain stem–spinal equilibrium response) can control various parameters of movement while higher levels serve to integrate the various subcomponents without having to directly designate all parameters.

An example of a functional unit that requires regulation under various conditions can be found in the motor development literature. A strong bilateral interaction between the two upper limbs often manifests itself overtly as associated or mirror movement.[37, 68, 175, 192] This neural constraint or synergy may be beneficial for symmetrical tasks, but it also requires inhibition or regulation for asymmetrical tasks. Similarly, a strong bilateral interaction may be advantageous at a young age in terms of controlling simple voluntary movement, but it requires modification for more complex unimanual and bimanual control as the system matures. Further examples of associated movement can be found in the clinical literature.[37, 195] CNS-damaged patients often show excessive associated movements demonstrating the inability of higher centers to inhibit the effect of lower level neuromotor synergies. Abnormal patterns and synergies emerge that are often perpetuated unless appropriate therapy is introduced. The focus of therapy should include the use as well as the modification of these synergistic patterns in order to perform functional movements. Since there are multiple combinations of potential interaction between the components of action, and their functional relationships have been drastically altered or disorganized, one input (*e.g.,* a single therapeutic technique) is not likely to adequately address this multifaceted problem. Rehabilitation should focus on multiple stimuli in an attempt to re-educate the components of action, eventually establishing adaptable and generalized representation.

Inhibitory Mechanisms

In the rehabilitation of motor function, an implicit assumption is that observed functional improvement reflects refinement in the neural control, coordination, and complexity of movement. The manner in which this occurs is due, in part, to the ability to generate, excite, or plan the appropriate movement patterns or sequences of action. However, inhibitory processes in the learning (or relearning) of motor acts play an equal, if not more important, role. The CNS response to injury and the compensatory motor behavior that may evolve often reflect the use of previous, but now inappropriate, motor programs. Prior learned responses do not cease to influence behavior. As in neuromotor development, movement patterns that are appropriate at a young age need to be suppressed, inhibited, or incorporated into new response patterns that serve the needs of the older child.[174] Similarly, patients with CNS damage, particularly after acute injury with a multitude of compensatory activity, need to actively inhibit or incorporate ineffectual patterns into new motor response patterns.

Knowledge of the development of inhibition and the complex interactions between excitation and inhibition can assist in the understanding of the progressive changes in functional ability that occur during therapy. As suggested by Todor and Lazarus,[174] a given movement pattern may dominate or be preeminent for two reasons: (1) the nervous system is structured in a way that facilitates this movement or (2) there is a learned movement pattern that due to use or practice is more easily elicited. Early in rehabilitation following nervous system insult, the former explanation predominates; that is, the structural damage resulting from injury facilitates a particular motor response. However, much later in recovery (several years or longer) it is likely that the latter explanation (learned or overlearned movement patterns) plays an increasingly greater role in the production of a particular motor response. Easily elicited, but inappropriate movement patterns, prevent the person from learning more effective and more complex movement patterns. Accordingly, at this point in time, recovery of function requires inhibition or modulation of these innate response tendencies.

Not only is it necessary to inhibit learned patterns of response but also other components of action such as "associated reactions." The terms *motor overflow, associated movement, synkinetic movement, and associated reaction* all represent to some degree a form of involuntary movement that accompanies an intended motor act. Associated movements, for example, occur in young children as a normal, developmental phenomenon[38, 68, 192] and abound in clinical populations with CNS dysfunction.[37, 195] Lazarus[112] demonstrated that normal children ranging in age from 6 through 16 years were able to voluntarily inhibit the intensity of associated movement in the contralateral limb during a unimanual task when attention was drawn to that limb through enhanced (auditory) feedback. Lazarus concluded that the primary limitation in spontaneous inhibition of associated movement was not neural immaturity but rather ineffectual allocation of attentional resources. Since cognitive processes appear to be involved in the regulation of associated movement, as indicated in the Lazarus study and in other studies,[37] therapeutic techniques that emphasize relaxation and inhibition may have substantial benefit for motor control.[17, 20]

A further example of the role of inhibitory mechanisms in motor skill development is the time course of primitive and postural reflexes. As mentioned previously in the section on spinal level movement control, two prevailing views exist on the relationship of innate or primitive reflexes to the emergence of voluntary motor behavior. However, the fact that under certain conditions primitive reflexes have been demonstrated to influence (bias the motoneuron pool toward facilitation or inhibition) the adult nervous system[93, 94] supports a model positing the development of an inhibitory mechanism.

Primitive and postural reflexes often reemerge in normal aging[102, 145] and in CNS dysfunction.[34, 182] Overt ATNR posturing in clinical populations supports the view that, in normal adults, cortical inhibitory mechanisms influence activity of the α motoneuron pools, reducing the number of motoneurons brought to discharge threshold by head turning alone.[174] In addition, hyperactive stretch reflexes (*e.g.,* repetitive response or clonus) in populations with upper motor neuron disease demonstrate an excitatory imbalance or lack of inhibitory control.[2] The inhibition or control of primitive reflexes has been demonstrated to be crucial for the emergence of motor competence in both normal[35] and mentally retarded[135] populations. Again, rather than imply that reflexes are structurally dissolved or extinguished, the implication is that they are inhibited or modified by higher control centers.

At the synaptic level, Bliss and colleagues[23] suggested that a great majority of pathways, examined following conditioning experiments in isolated cortical slabs, must have contained synaptic functions that were less likely to transmit excitation the more often the pathway was used. Creutzfeldt[43] noted that each cortical neuron is inhibited by its neighbors (over a distance of 300 to 400 mm) and that the individual cortical connections are essentially and dominantly inhibitory. Such a network organization allows for parallel processing of information and prevents mass excitation of cortical neurons. The importance of inhibition becomes increasingly clearer when viewed in context with excitation. In 1906, Sherrington[164] emphasized the role of excitation–inhibition balance in the integrative action of the nervous system. Alterations in the balance of excitation and inhibition may play a role in the "unmasking" of preexisting but functionally depressed pathways.[9, 10] Unmasking as a potential mechanism of brain plasticity involved in recovery of function will be discussed in the section on neuroplasticity.

Neurotransmitters

Neurotransmitters are endogenous pharmacological agents; their manipulation can lead to enhanced recovery of function when they are an integral part of a therapy program for motor dysfunction. The catecholamine norepinephrine has shown the most promise for augmenting the recovery of motor function in brain-injured patients. Other neurotransmitters relevant to rehabilitation have been discussed in the *Syllabus* of the American Academy of Physical Medicine and Rehabilitation.[5]

Biochemistry of Norepinephrine

The major precursor of the catecholamines is tyrosine. Tyrosine is lipophilic and crosses the blood–brain barrier easily. Three important catecholamines are formed from it: dopamine, norepinephrine, and epinephrine. Storage of catecholamines in vesicles protects them from enzymatic inactivation. As will be discussed later, release of catecholamines, particularly norepinephrine, is in part mediated directly by presynaptic α_2-receptors, also termed *autoreceptors*. Rates of neuron firing, influenced by somatic α_2-receptors, indirectly affect norepinephrine release. Pharmacological agents that may directly cause the release or block the reuptake of catecholamines include amphetamine, cocaine, and the tricyclic antidepressants.[27,39]

The Locus Coeruleus System

The locus coeruleus (LC) is the major ascending source of norepinephrine to the forebrain areas. Four ascending tracts arise from the LC: Three run in the medial forebrain bundle to the cerebral cortex and subcortical structures; the fourth tract goes to the cerebellar cortex.[27] The cerebral cortical tracts from the LC run in a rostrocaudal direction and have a medial portion and a lateral portion.[137] The medial part curves over the corpus callosum and forms arborizations in the cingulate gyrus. The lateral part curves through the frontal cortex and arborizes in the dorsolateral cortex. This continuous dense sheet of tangential-longitudinal LC axons results in a high density of norepinephrine fibers throughout the deep cortical layers. This provides a tangential component to an otherwise radially oriented cortex, forming a three-dimensional network of intersecting and interacting neurons. Thus, this projection is furnished with the unique capacity to modulate neuronal activity synchronously throughout a vast expense of neocortex crossing cytoarchitectural and functional boundaries.[137] Due to the widespread distribution of the LC, injury to most brain areas results in concomitant damage to the LC. For example, a very small lesion in the frontal cortex can lead to widespread norepinephrine deprivation in remote areas of the cerebral cortex (*e.g.,* in the cerebellum).[24]

Norepinephrine requires membrane receptors to exert its effect on target cells. Norepinephrine receptors are either α or β; with regard to recovery of motor function, α-receptors of the LC system appear to be of prime importance. α_2-receptors cover the soma, dendrites, and axons of LC cells; they function as axoaxonic, axodendritic or axosomatic autoreceptors, or as free autoreceptors responsive to interstitial norepinephrine.[39] An α_2-agonist causes presynaptic inhibition, which results in decreased norepinephrine release from LC cell axons. An α_2-antagonist causes presynaptic excitation, which results in increased norepinephrine release from LC axons.[39] α_1-Receptors are postsynaptic, covering the target cells of the LC system. An α_1-agonist causes postsynaptic excitation, which simulates a norepinephrine effect on the target cell. An α_1-antagonist causes postsynaptic inhibition, which opposes the effect of norepinephrine on the target cell.

The cerebral cortex acts primarily as an inhibitory system, decreasing the nonselective motor activity and reflexes initiated by spinal cord and brain stem centers. The LC system, through its extensive arborizations, is an ideal system for modulating sensorimotor information. It does not modulate sensory-specific information but seems to increase sensorimotor signal-to-noise ratio via a neurohumoral or field effect mechanism.[137] Some of the target cells of the LC are cortical inhibitory neurons. The effect of α-receptor agonists or antagonists can either increase or decrease the activity of these inhibitory neurons. Therefore, cortical activity can be modulated via LC system activity, and this activity can be altered by various pharmacological agents.

LC and Learning

Lesions of the LC nuclei or tracts result in learning deficits. It is believed that the norepinephrine system is responsible for facilitation of learning, reinforcement, and the consolidation of memory, and there is evidence that norepinephrine system activation plus reinforcement results in persistent changes in synaptic activity.[27] In one particular study in which norepinephrine levels were reduced to less than 15% of control values by treatment with a norepinephrine-specific neurotoxin, acquisition of one- and two-way avoidance learning was significantly impaired. Treatment with desipramine blocked norepinephrine neuron degeneration and allowed the learning of avoidance-acquisition.[141] Bilateral LC lesions also result in decreased forebrain norepinephrine levels and decreased food–reward learning.[6]

LC and Cerebral Metabolism

Because of the widespread ramifications of the LC, damage to a small number of ascending tracts of the LC can result in retrograde inhibition of LC nuclei activity. This reversible retrograde reaction is considered to be due to a metabolic shift from neurotransmitter synthesis to structural protein synthesis within the LC neurons for repair purposes. The remote effects of retrograde LC inhibition may explain the cortical metabolic changes that occur after a relatively small cortical or subcortical injury (remote functional depression).[156] Cerebral oxidative metabolism appears to be diffusely reduced after a focal cortical injury.[64] This can be measured in experimental animals by the use of 2-deoxyglucose or staining for α-GPDH (an oxidative enzyme). Unilateral sensorimotor cortex ablation results in decreased oxidative metabolism in the cerebral cortex and LC. Amphetamine reverses this effect, and the reversal lasts at least 24 hours, much longer than the half-life of the single-dose of amphetamine. Haloperidol, an α_1-antagonist in addition to its well-known dopamine blocking capacity, magnifies the decrease in oxidative metabolism compared with findings in injured controls. Unilateral lesions of the LC alone result in no change in oxidative metabolism; if this is followed in 2 weeks by a motor cortex lesion, the decrease in cerebral oxidative metabolism occurs much more rapidly than when the LC is intact. Amphetamine reverses this effect, and haloperidol blocks the amphetamine-induced reversal. Apomorphine, a dopamine agonist, has no effect.[64]

Neuropharmacological Modification of Motor Recovery

Those drugs that affect cerebral metabolic parameters also facilitate or retard motor recovery. Norepinephrine agonists accelerate recovery of motor function, and antagonists retard or reinstate motor deficits. Unilateral ablation of the motor cortex

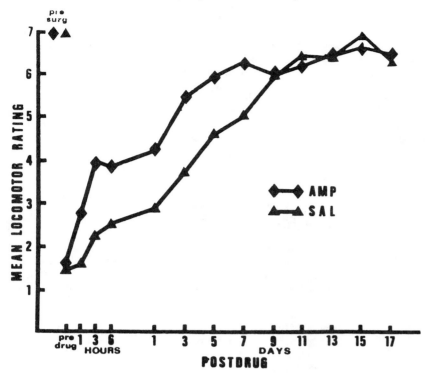

Figure 10-2. The effect of a single injection of amphetamine (*AMP*) or saline (*SAL*) given 24 hours after injury on locomotor ability on a beam walking task for rats with unilateral sensorimotor cortex ablation.

results in the inability of rats or cats to walk on a beam. Spontaneous recovery of this ability occurs in 9 to 14 days in rats and in approximately 28 days in cats. Rats given amphetamine and "rehabilitation" (attempting to walk on a beam 24 hours after injury) show an improved ability within 1 hour of administration, and this improvement is maintained over days and weeks (Fig. 10-2).[61] Amphetamine alone, without rehabilitation, has no significant effect. Cats given amphetamine 10 days after injury, in conjunction with "rehabilitation," also show an immediate increase in the ability to perform beam-walking.[100] A single dose of amphetamine can result in the permanent acceleration of motor function recovery; an additive effect with additional doses is also seen when given at appropriate intervals. Even with delayed administration (*e.g.,* 10 days after injury in a cat model) a positive effect still results, consistent with a mechanism *independent* of any general "arousing" effect amphetamine might have.[60, 61, 100] A pilot study investigating the effect of amphetamine on recovery of motor function in stroke patients found that a single dose of amphetamine, combined with physical therapy, increased recovery of function compared with results in stroke patients receiving physical therapy alone. Long-term studies are in progress at this time.[44]

Certain drugs would appear to be contraindicated in patients with cortical damage, at least in the early phase of recovery. Minor tranquilizers, the benzodiazepines, directly decrease the firing rate of the LC neurons.[40, 159] Major tranquilizers, the antipsychotics, directly antagonize α_1-receptors. Haloperidol, an α_1-antagonist, decreases the rate of recovery of motor function although it will not actually reinstate deficits once recovery has occurred. Phenoxybenzamine, a very potent α_1-antagonist, has been shown to actually reinstate motor deficits even months after injury/recovery in rats and cats (Fig. 10-3).[24] In an animal model, phenoxybenzamine increased the incidence, severity, and mortality secondary to stroke.[125] α_2-Agonists, such as clonidine, may indirectly have this same general effect via presynaptic inhibi-

Figure 10-3. The effect of 10 mg/kg of phenoxybenzamine given intraperitoneally on beam walking in recovered brain-injured and sham control animals.

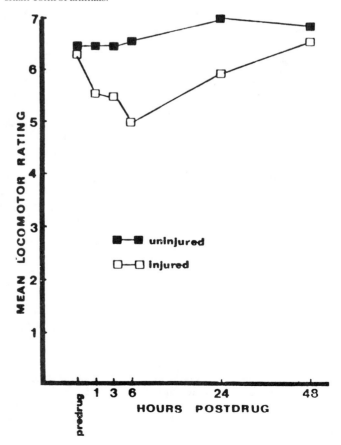

tion. Lithium has undesirable effects on norepinephrine concentration, increasing reuptake and decreasing release. These effects lessen the capacity of the LC/norepinephrine system to facilitate and maximize motor function recovery in the early phase of recovery. For treating agitation in the early phase of recovery, drugs such as propranolol appear to have a less detrimental effect on the recovery of motor function. β-Receptor agonists/antagonists have not been shown to play a role in the recovery of function following cortical injury, supporting the use of propranolol for the treatment of agitated/aggressive behavior in brain-injured patients.[24, 91]

Role of the Cerebellum in Recovery From Cortical Injury

Cerebellar LC innervation is relatively small compared with the cerebral innervation. Individual norepinephrine cells in the LC innervate both cortices, however, allowing simultaneous modulation of cerebral and cerebellar activity.[142] Cerebellar norepinephrine deafferentation in animals results in impaired acquisition of motor skills and impaired ability to coordinate and "choreograph" the movements necessary to perform locomotor tasks.[184] Boyeson and his collaborators demonstrated that direct infusion of norepinephrine into the cerebellum of rats with a sensorimotor cortex injury immediately restores their ability to walk on a beam.[26] Additionally, when the cerebellum is destroyed, enhanced recovery of motor function via norepinephrine agonists fails to take place, demonstrating the primary importance of the cerebellum in recovery from sensorimotor cortex injury.[24]

Conclusions on the Locus Coeruleus

There are diverse afferent inputs to the LC, and ascending LC neurons project diffusely into most areas of the brain. Without being primarily or directly responsible for motor function or learning, the LC system modulates cerebral and cerebellar activity, enhancing cortical function. Following cortical injury, stimulation of the LC/norepinephrine system "enables" functionally depressed areas involved in the learning and performance of motor functions to resume activity and aid functional recovery.

With its capacity for increasing the rate and amount of recovery of function, amphetamine may become a routine component of comprehensive brain-injury rehabilitation treatment programs. Its use would augment, not replace, traditional therapy. One possibility is the use of amphetamine in combination with propranolol: amphetamine increases LC/norepinephrine system effectiveness; propranolol blocks the cardiovascular side-effects of amphetamine, prevents agitated/aggressive behavior, and appears to have no detrimental effect on recovery of function.

Brain Metabolic Correlates of Motor Activity

The neural aspects of recovery of function have been inadequately studied and many questions still remain. There exists only fragmented information on how, where, or why recovery takes place in the brain. Recent advances in brain imaging techniques offer the potential to supply anatomical, morphological, and physiological information indicating changes associated with recovery of function after neurological damage. The combination of computed tomography (CT), magnetic resonance imaging (MRI), positron emission tomography (PET), as well as electroencephalogram event-related potentials (ERP) and evoked potentials (EP) may provide new windows into the functions of the living brain.

For example, in 1980, the first of several important studies was conducted by Kennedy and colleagues.[107] In this study, PET, using the 2-[^{14}C] deoxyglucose method, was employed to evaluate local metabolic responses in brain activity in monkeys as related to motor performance. Motor, somatosensory, and cerebellar regions were studied during the performance of a task that required a bar-pressing response. Rates of glucose utilization were measured at various levels of the neuraxis in four working and four inactive monkeys. Right–left differences were not found in any structure in the inactive animals. In working animals, however, up to 50% laterality was found in the following structures: laminae I through IX of the cervical cord, the cuneate nucleus, the lateral reticular nucleus, crus II of the cerebellum, the red nucleus, the ventral posterolateral nucleus of the thalamus, part of the globus pallidus, and discrete portions of the posterior parietal, somatosensory, primary, premotor, and supplementary motor cortices. It was concluded that during repetitive arm and hand movements more energy is expended in somatosensory monitoring and cerebellar control systems than in the primary motor system.

In a more recent brain metabolism study in humans, metabolic changes during motor acts were monitored by Mazziotta and associates.[123] PET and the application of F-18 fluorodeoxyglucose were used to measure the cerebral glucose metabolic responses in complex motor tasks. Normal subjects demonstrated significant increases in local cerebral metabolic rate for glucose versus controls in the sensorimotor cortical strip contralateral to the moving hand as well as bilateral activations of the striatum. Their results suggest that patients with Huntington's disease may use neural reorganization to perform overlearned tasks (writing) that are typically used for novel tasks (finger sequences) in normal subjects.

Neuroplasticity

The capacity of the brain to recover from diverse injuries has prompted researchers to postulate that the brain is capable of a great degree of "plasticity." If there were clear deficits that never recovered following a brain injury, one hypothesis where structure equals function could be offered to explain the functional deficits. The main problem with such a hypothesis is that considerable recovery can and does take place following a brain injury. As a consequence of "sparing" of function, numerous hypotheses have been generated to explain recovery from brain injury. New growth of neural processes could conceivably underlie some of the observable recovery.

Sprouting

The idea that new growth or sprouting may serve a functional purpose in recovery suggested that recovery of function may have a physiological and anatomical basis. Sprouting is the growth of a cell body to another cell as a consequence of normal growth, a vacancy at a particular site, or a return to a particular site. Although the largest and best body of evidence for sprouting in the CNS derives from studies on nonmammalian species, studies have demonstrated that sprouting occurs in mammals with greater frequency than previously thought possible.[119] In the CNS, however, several criteria must be met before any functional significance is ascribed to the new growth. First, the sprouts should return to the original denervated area. Second, the sprouts must form functional synaptic connections in the denervated area. Third, following demonstration that the first two events occur, the behavioral recovery must coincide in time with the functional sprouting. Finally, it must be demonstrated that if the first three criteria are met, a subsequent resectioning of the new sprouts must result in a reinstatement of the original deficit. If these four criteria are met, then a very strong argument can be made for sprouting being the basis of recovery of function following an injury. Since regenerative sprouting (the severed axon regrowing to original point) probably does not occur to a great extent in CNS[21, 104] only collateral sprouting will be discussed.

Collateral sprouting is different than regenerative sprouting in that collateral sprouts are new axonal processes that have budded off an uninjured axon and grow into the tissue vacated by degenerated axons. Evidence for collateral sprouting following partial denervation of an area in the CNS has been clearly established in a number of studies.[89, 116, 117] Goodman and Horel[89] reported collateral sprouting following unilateral visual cortex injuries. At a later point in time they bilaterally removed the eyes of rats to trace the degeneration of the tracts in order to detect collateral sprouts. Subsequent to the eye removal, a stain for degenerating myelin fibers from the retina indicated that as a consequence of the unilateral ablation, collateral sprouts had formed in the lateral geniculate nucleus and pretectal nucleus. Since the occipital input to these regions had been removed, the retinal projections that normally project to the same region sprouted into the denervated regions normally occupied by the occipital inputs. Although such sprouting may serve a useful function, others have reported maladaptive consequences of sprouting.[161, 168]

The previous studies indicate that sprouting does indeed occur in the CNS and that the sprouting can proceed into partially denervated areas. However, efforts to find a behavioral recovery that correlates with axonal sprouting in mammals have not met with success. Lesions of the entorhinal cortex have been found to result in subsequent sprouting of the commissural projection into the deafferentated molecular layer of the dentate gyrus,[118, 120] with physiologically functional synaptic connections.[186] Following the entorhinal cortex lesions, animals also display a behavioral deficit (spontaneous alternation) that recovers by 10 to 12 days after injury.[115, 186] In this regard, Loesche and Steward[115] severed the dorsal psalterium in rats (the route of the new sprouts) and found that the spontaneous alternation deficit was reinstated, although Ramirez[149] and others[160] have not been able to replicate the finding. Ramirez[149] additionally demonstrated that rats with bilateral lesions of the entorhinal cortex would recover spontaneous alternation by 30 days after injury if given massed trials. Since all afferent inputs are severed by the bilateral lesions, sprouting does not appear to be involved in the recovery from spontaneous alternation.

Clearly much work needs to be done before definitive conclusions can be reached on the role of sprouting in recovery of function. What is presently clear, however, is that sprouting does occur in response to injury and seems to form viable synapses. Sprouting may simply reflect a vestigial response characteristic of a neonatal system that persists into adulthood, or it may represent a continuous synaptic turnover process throughout life.[41] However, once a nerve is functionally mature, marked sprouting may occur simply in response to a vacancy in denervated tissue with the new connections providing little restitution of a lost function.

Denervation Supersensitivity

The concept of denervation supersensitivity, described by Cannon and Rosenblueth,[33] elegantly provided a mechanism for recovery of function. In essence, denervation supersensitivity results in a permanent increase in a neuron's responsiveness to diminished input. The postsynaptic receptor sites may become more sensitive to a neurotransmitter through alterations of the receptor site or adenylate cyclase,[50, 51] or the receptors may actually increase in numbers.[85, 178]

An extensive literature exists demonstrating supersensitivity in the peripheral nervous system,[33, 56] and data have been established for the CNS. Ungerstedt[178, 179] demonstrated a 40% increase in binding sites for tritiated haloperidol following a unilateral lesion of the nigrostriatal pathway. The increase in binding sites occurred in the denervated striatum from 1 to 10 weeks postoperatively. Behaviorally, animals lesioned in the nigrostriatal pathway prior to the development of the supersensitivity rotate toward the side of the lesion when challenged with dopamine agonists. Following a period of time and the concurrent development of supersensitivity, animals injected with a dopamine agonist turn in a direction opposite the lesion, indicating that the damaged striatum had become supersensitive.[42, 83] In a similar fashion, supersensitivity has been demonstrated in serotonergic[140] and noradrenergic systems.[51, 162] These studies represent good support for a possible role of supersensitivity in recovery of function, although as Stavrky[168] points out, in some cases denervation supersensitivity may actually be deleterious to recovery of function. For example, when one afferent system that is normally antagonistic to another is removed, the deficit could be exaggerated by the supersensitivity.

Both sprouting and denervation supersensitivity represent reorganization processes in the CNS, and as such may provide a substrate for vicariation models of recovery function. Vicariation models propose that over time remaining tissue takes over the function originally subserved by the lost tissue. To the extent that collateral sprouting and denervation supersensitivity accurately reflect restitution of function, these processes could conceivably support vicariation approaches to recovery of function. Indeed, if our current state of knowledge allowed us to predict where and when sprouting and supersensitivity occurred and its relationship to functional recovery, vicariation theories could be entertained as a viable mechanism of recovery.[87, 115] However, the evidence to support vicariation models is weak.[25, 65] Without knowing the relationships between sprouting, supersensitivity, or other physiological reorganizations with the behavioral events the hypotheses intend to explain, vicariation hypotheses infinitely regress to other purported circuits to explain recovery of function. For example, if successive removal of more tissue thought to be involved in recovery results in continuing recovery of behavior, one keeps postulating a different circuit to explain the recovery.

Behavioral Compensation

Damaged tissue is lost forever following experimentally induced brain injury. The varying degrees of recovery of function that occur are related both to the extent and to the location of the injury. These two observations have led to a host of interpretations concerning the nature of recovery of function. In 1930, Foerster[67] and Goldstein[88] opposed each other on this issue. Foerster maintained that for recovery to occur, the brain over time had to structurally reorganize, while Goldstein contended that the functional characteristics of the lost tissue were permanently lost and that recovery reflected a new behavioral strategy that compensated for the lost tissue and function. Goldstein contended that what looked like true recovery of function (*i.e.,* the regaining of the exact behavior following brain injury) was really an inability on the part of the experimenter to detect the difference. For example, rats learn mazes more quickly with an intact visual system, although they are capable of learning the maze without a visual system by predominately using olfactory cues.[98] Examples of the way animals[77, 86] and humans[76, 78] can compensate for injury are abundant, and therefore, behavioral compensation models have wide appeal.[45, 166]

In essence, behavioral compensation approaches to recovery of function state that following brain injury, recovery of function does not entail recovery of the behavior observed pre-injury but rather the development of a new and sometimes abnormal behavior that is used to attenuate a permanent deficiency that occurs after injury. Thus a patient may use different groups of muscles, stimulus cues, and cognitive strategies to compensate for behavior deficits after injury. Stated as such, behavioral compensation models do not allow for distinctions between losses of functions and preferences for alternative behaviors. An animal may opt to use an alternate strategy without having lost the ability to recover the original strategy. Sprouting and denervation supersensitivity may be easily visualized as compensatory acts in aiding recovery from deficits, or if maladaptive, forcing a compensatory shift from one strategy to another. However, recovery of function may also involve noncompensatory motor programs as well. Although it is difficult to train animals not to compensate and to only use the affected muscle groups, this ability has been demonstrated in humans by several research groups. Noncompensatory motor control of the affected muscles can be specifically retrained in humans even many years after trauma (see section on information processing in neuromuscular retraining). Although there is no doubt that the brain-injured patient can learn new compensatory or noncompensatory functional motor control, this alone provides little insight into the actual neural mechanisms underlying recovery of function.

Unmasking

Wall and his colleagues[132, 181] have found that the receptive field capacity (a homunculus representation) in the thalamus changes as partial deafferentation is induced in the nucleus gracilis. When the areas are deafferented, stimulation of fibers projecting to gracile or thalamic nucleus reveal an enlarged somatotopic representation of the intact inputs compared with normal animals.[181] The above findings represent the "unmasking" of quiescent neuronal connections that are inhibited in the normal state.[9, 10, 53] Such inhibition is readily demonstrated in the development of muscle control in children[143] and in the inhibition of neonatal reflexes.[130]

Inhibition may also play a role in actively suppressing recovery of function.[167] Following right occipital-temporal cortical lesions in cats, a total hemianopia occurs in the left visual fields that lasts at least for 1 year following the injury. However, if the left superior colliculus is subsequently lesioned in the same animal, it results in an immediate restitution from the left visual field deficits. These results indicate that following the cortical injury the contralateral colliculus is exhibiting a tonic inhibition of the opposite colliculus. In confirmation of this crossed tectal inhibitory influence, the same but slower restitution of function is achieved when the commissure of the superior colliculus is cut following the cortical injury.

Diaschisis is a form of unmasking that is probably more important in the acute period after an injury. Von Monakow,[180] in an effort to account for recovery of function, suggested that remote structures connected to the site of injury are temporarily depressed and that a dissipation of this functional shock parallels and produces the recovery of function. Explicit in the proposal is that the lost tissue is not mediating the recovery from symptoms; rather the recovery occurs by dissipation of depression in remote brain areas connected to the site of injury. Thus the hypothesis, unlike vicariation proposals, is not burdened with postulating how functional reorganization might be reflected in the recovery process; recovery simply occurs with the dissipation of diaschisis.

Diaschisis as proposed by von Monakow at the turn of the century is merely a description of clinical observations and lacks any explanatory power since no mechanisms were offered through which the alleviation of diaschisis could operate. However, the concept has recently been resurrected and correlated with specific changes in neurotransmitter functioning in the CNS. Feeney and Hovda[62] demonstrated that following unilateral ablation of the frontal cortex in cats, the permanently lost tactile placing in the contralateral forelimb can be temporarily restored by amphetamine as early as 4 days after injury. This drug-dependent restoration of placing increased in frequency at 9 and 15 days after injury, with no further change in response to the drug after 15 days. Since amphetamine stimulates catecholamines and the effect is blocked by the catecholamine antagonist haloperidol, these researchers interpreted the results in terms of a catecholamine diaschisis. More direct evidence of diaschisis stems from recordings of sensorimotor cortex following unilateral sensorimotor cortex injury of the hindlimb area in the rat. Evoked potentials in the adjacent forelimb cortical area are initially depressed following injury to the hindpaw area but return to normal values over a 9- to 15-day period.[114] Complementary results for stimulation of motor cortex have been reported in rats and cats. A transient increase in thresholds to elicit forelimb movements from areas anterior and adjacent to injured hindlimb sensorimotor cortex revealed a similar recovery period that was consistent with the evoked potential data.[25, 81]

Age Factors

The age at which an injury occurs may influence the rate and level of recovery. Indeed, many clinical and laboratory findings have indicated that greater sparing of dysfunction is observed with infants rather than with adults. The sparing may be due to multiple factors such as differential maturation of some neural systems compared with others at the time of injury, the location and extent of the injury, and environmental conditions. However, it has also been found that often the sparing is less in infants compared with adults,[129, 147] suggesting that it may not always be best to have a brain injury early in life.

Although little research has directly addressed the issue of differential maturation of some neural systems compared with others, it would seem logical to expect differential effects. For example, while motor deficits have been noted in animals from day 14 after birth to adult following either lateral hypothalamic or medial forebrain bundle damage, no deficits are noted when injury occurs 1 to 5 days after birth.[4, 66] These results have been correlated with less somatic and dendritic growth in affected neurons in the early time period of injury compared with adults.[127, 128] At the younger age, the lateral hypothalamic neurons appeared equally stimulated by all forms of sensory stimulation, contrasted to adults in whom specific sensory stimulation was necessary to activate specific neurons.[4, 66] This suggests, at least in cases of hypothalamic injury, that the infant was developmentally more nonspecific in neural responsibility and as a consequence perhaps more neuroplastic in response to the injury by shifting functional requirements among "uncommitted" neurons.

The area and extent of an injury in relation to the time of the injury also affects subsequent recovery of function. For example, Hicks and d'Amato[96] demonstrated that early cerebral hemispherectomy results in considerable sparing of function compared with comparable adult lesions and that the bases for the sparing may be reflected in the emergence of an aberrant corticospinal projection in young animals. Neuronal remodeling also occurs after early cerebellar injury when compared with late cerebellar injury.[36, 113] However, in some cases, it appears that early cerebellar cortical injury can also result in more severe deficits than those observed in adult injury.[90]

Environmental Variables

Environmental variables have clearly been shown to be involved in not only influencing normal neural development but also in effecting recovery from brain injury. In this context, it becomes apparent that the rehabilitation setting may play an important role in facilitating recovery from injury. The subsequent reduction in hospital time would therefore pay financial and emotional dividends to the patient and family.

Numerous studies have shown that the environment can affect neural and behavioral development in animals. Changes in environmental conditions have been shown to change an organism's response to neurological damage.[158, 165, 187] Environmentally "enriched" living conditions have been shown to increase brain size,[154] changes in cell structure,[84] and CNS biochemistry[188] in animals and in some cases provide protection if enriched before injury.[52] The animal literature has been interpreted for clinical rehabilitation by Rosenzweig.[155] For example, "overtraining" on a task appears to protect an animal from some of the subsequent deficits following CNS injury. Although this is an uncontrolled variable in a clinical setting, the point to be made is that preinjury environments can adversely affect recovery from CNS damage. Therefore the structure of the environment after injury is important to a clinical setting in the rehabilitation of brain-injured patients. Schwartz[163] demonstrated that following postnatal injury in rats, rearing in an enriched environment facilitated subsequent recovery to the point at which the animals actually outperformed uninjured normal controls. The same sparing of function phenomena holds for adult animals as well.[105] Extrapolation of these findings to a rehabilitation setting would suggest that a "sterile" hospital setting may limit the functional reorganization capacity of the patients[190] and that the findings should extend beyond the hospital setting.[8]

INFORMATION PROCESSING IN NEUROMUSCULAR RETRAINING

The Late Post-Acute Patient: An Essentially Unserved Population

Most professionals in rehabilitation agree that the *acute* or early stage of rehabilitation in patients with nonprogressive neurological disease consists of the time that the patient is initially treated on an inpatient basis. This period may be a matter of days or as long as a year. There is less agreement as to how long patients should be continued on a *post-acute* outpatient (or sometimes inpatient) basis. Most clinicians today would consider additional treatment of post-acute patients for up to 1 or 2 years. These can be considered *early post-acute* patients. Patients who have residual dysfunction after more than 2 years from the time of their injury can be considered *late post-acute* patients. In this section late post-acute rehabilitation will be discussed; earlier rehabilitation is discussed in Chapters 29–44 of this book.

Typically, late post-acute patients have been thought to have a permanent neuromuscular disability. Attempts are seldom made to obtain significant increases in motor performance in the late post-acute stage. A major factor contributing to this situation has been the traditional belief that the speed of recovery usually dramatically slows or stops at 1 to 2 years after injury.

An early group to demonstrate late recovery was Franz and co-workers.[71] In 1915, they reported that, with specific training, brain-injured patients could obtain significant functional recovery as late as 20 years after injury. From their results and the results of other human and animal studies, they concluded

> the possibility that conclusions regarding the permanency of paralysis from cerebral accidents were neither accurate or scientifically grounded, and that more attention should be paid to possible improvement in these cases. Lesions of the motor cortex or the upper part of the pyramidal tract in man do not [necessarily] abolish function, but put the function in abeyance until such time as the appropriate condition is present for production of movement. We should probably not [always] speak of permanent paralyses, but of uncared-for paralyses. This we say because many of the conditions which we have met appear to resemble . . . phenomena of disuse, rather than actual inabilities.

Few additional studies were published until the late 1960s and early 1970s when various clinical studies reported the successful treatment of late post-acute neurological patients including traumatic brain injury, stroke, and facial paralysis (reviewed by Bach-y-Rita and Balliet[11] and Balliet[13]). However, these results have been only slowly applied to clinical services.

The Optimization of Sensory Information

Neurological patients often have deficits in information processing. Information processing, in this case, refers to aspects of cognition including processes such as perception, memory, and judgment. Of primary concern is the optimization of sensory information that can be made available in the (re)training of functional abilities. Fundamentally, the rehabilitation potential of acute or post-acute patients depends not only on the extent of the lesion but also on the reestablishment of information input to the sensory association areas of the brain that direct or redirect motor programming. Optimal neural adaptation or plasticity of motor control reprogramming depends on the optimization of sensory information.[11]

In rehabilitation, this (re)training approach has not received the high priority that it has in other fields, such as experimental and cognitive psychology, higher education, music, and certain sports. The application of learning theory to these fields has basically consisted of maximizing motivation through various methods of individualized instruction and active participation by the trainee. This philosophy has been in response to the belief that the responsibility for increased functional success is ultimately that of the trainee and not that of the trainer. Consequently, persistence, discipline, and exact compliance with instructions on the part of the trainee are considered to be essential. For example, in cognitive psychology, as it relates to attention and arousal, the following factors have been found to be significant in the modification of a trainee's performance[59]:

reinforcement and incentives, task characteristics, intrinsic versus extrinsic motivation, anxiety, worry, emotionality and failure, sleep deprivation, vigilance, selective attention, and external noise. Only in recent years has the field of clinical rehabilitation attempted to address such factors. A series of factors have been found to be critical in obtaining maximum recovery: these include the appropriate environment and other issues such as motivation and family support (reviewed by Bach-y-Rita[8, 9]).

Recovery of function may be a discontinuous process. Research has demonstrated that learning occurs in alternating stages of acquisition and consolidation. During each consolidation stage, no progress is apparent, but each stage is necessary before another step of progress can be taken. It is important to determine if intermittent progress is a characteristic of recovery from brain damage. If shown to be so, we would have to alter our concept of "plateau" (currently defined as the final level of function), which would then be identified as a consolidation stage between two stages of acquisition (progress in functional capacities).

Signal to Noise Ratio (S/N) and the Reduction of Noise

The previous discussions can be included under one primary concept that is actually an acoustical electrical engineering relationship. This extremely simple relationship can be considered basic to the neuromuscular retraining of neurological patients.[11] It is written as follows:

$$E = S/N$$

where E equals the potential effectiveness or the power of a signal S, S equals any information that is to be processed, and N equals any internal or external noise that may be present at the same instant in time. No information can be conveyed when N is greater than or equal to S. Only minimal information can be conveyed under conditions when N is less than S and both numbers are similar. The most effective situation is when N is very low and S is relatively high.

This concept has been expanded to include more complex equations, such as the prediction of articulation in various speech disorders in the field of speech pathology and audiology[146]; however, it has not been applied to the assessment of the comparative effectiveness of rehabilitation procedures. One reason for this has been that there appears to be too many unknown factors in the required equation. Another reason has involved the fact that even if one knew what all the factors were, there is currently no method available to quantify or to equate their importance to the individual patient. Despite these problems, it is possible to qualify certain factors potentially affecting patient rehabilitation (some of these have been discussed previously in detail by Bach-y-Rita and Balliet[11]).

Although it is clear that only the best therapy methods (high signal) should be involved in retraining, many potential noise factors (high noise) that could reduce the effectiveness of these methods are usually not adequately controlled in a clinical setting. The following are illustrative of a few of the possible qualitative factors that can affect any method of (re)training:

Immediate Optimization of Sensory Feedback Information

During the time that a particular training method is providing immediate and relatively short-term sensory information, environmental noise factors that might inhibit performance must correspondingly be controlled and minimized. In order to facilitate the attention and concentration of the trainee as well as the trainer, training areas that are auditorily and visually isolated should be available. We do not expect a child to learn to play the piano in the middle of an orchestra; similarly, we should not expect a patient to acquire adequate training in the middle of a crowded gym area. Potentially compromising attentional as well as arousal factors should not only be minimized in the formal training area but also outside of the training area, such as under conditions in which self-training is performed in the home.

Slow Process of Reaching Long-term Goals

Neuromuscular reprogramming (particularly late post-acute) is usually a relatively slow process requiring the achievement of successive short-term goals. More comprehensive long-term goals may take many years to achieve. The expectation that the functional gains must occur quickly can lead to a sense of disappointment, depression, and reduced motivation in both trainer and trainee. This internal "noise" can nullify possible training effects. If a person who is learning to play the piano is unrealistically expected to master the task within a few months (or even 1 or 2 years), he will rapidly become discouraged from an apparent lack of progress. Similarly a post-acute neurological patient, who does not have spontaneous recovery effecting rapid gains should not be expected to acquire new motor control in only a few months. This unrealistic expectation of the therapist and the patient will eventuate in frustration, disappointment, and early termination of the therapy program. Instead it is more realistic to expect these training experiences to take many years to achieve.

Another unrealistic expectation is that patients should train using methods that are relatively fast or intense. Instead, fast movements should be reserved for only the final stages of retraining, with repetitions being conducted in a manner that is not tedious. Each training trial should stand alone as a unique training experience in the mind of the trainee. For example, it is well known that in sports ranging from pole vaulting to golf it is better to perform the desired response slowly and carefully than it is to perform the same response rapidly and incorrectly many times over. Kottke[109] noted that "a person cannot monitor a control activity to cause isolated contraction as a prime mover and maintain relaxation of all other muscles unless activity is slow. If the activity is rapid or against increased resistance the increased effort causes irradiation of impulses transcerebrally [noise] and through internuncial synapses to produce cocontraction of other muscles." Desired motor acts should be performed in a manner that reinforces alertness and attention through the use of different therapy modalities to achieve short-term goals. In this manner the ability to perform more difficult motor control sequences may eventually become functionally automatic and generalizable.

Retraining Conducted Away From Primary Trainer

The majority of (re)training can be conducted by the trainee without the trainer present (e.g., home training) if it is conducted under the same rigorous conditions that occurred in the trainer's presence. This may or may not include the use of a secondary or nonprofessional trainer who is trained by the primary trainer to supervise certain sequences. Students who are learning to play an instrument or to become a ballerina train mainly on their own or with the help of a secondary trainer; however, rehabilitation has traditionally not relied on strict home programs. Outpatient programs that rely primarily on very specific home programs that may involve the help of significant others can be effectively and economically used in the treatment of patients. Such methods provide more exposure to conditions that optimize the generalization of appropriate motor patterns.

Psychosocial Issues

Intervening human factors such as fear of new situations, secondary gains, as well as significant stress associated with potential occupational or family situations can delay or stop progress during (re)training. These potential (noise) problems must be resolved before full functional abilities can be obtained. When such issues are primarily related to changes in function, they may be best handled by the trainer; more serious issues should be addressed by other professionals (*e.g.*, psychologist, social worker).

Optimizing Sensory Information in Training Paradigms

Laboratory and clinical studies in both the basic sciences and in the therapies that use some or all of the previous principles have demonstrated success in (re)training various motor performance tasks involving late post-acute patients. A laboratory example of motor control training was reported by Balliet and Nakayama in 1978.[18, 19] Previous to this work, it was thought that cyclotorsional eye movements (a motor response of the eye made around the visual axis) could only occur as an involuntary response or reflex. These movements include the counterrotation of the eye during lateral head tilt, rotary nystagmus induced by large rotating field, and disjunctive cyclotorsions that occur during ordinary convergence. Using a visual-feedback procedure, normal humans were trained to make conjugate and voluntary cyclotorsional eye movements of 20° and up to 30° in magnitude (Fig. 10-4). Over a period of a few months, these eye movements could eventually be made in the absence of any feedback device and included torsional slow pursuit and the saccadic tracking of rotating objects. Therefore, the torsional oculomotor system is not "hard-wired" and can be brought under voluntary control, demonstrating neuroplasticity.

Balliet and Nakayama systematically optimized their training strategies through the evaluation of previous failures and the replication of previous research to determine optimal signal–noise conditions. On the basis of this analysis their methods included the following:

1. The development of a simple subjective method involving afterimages to provide instantaneous and a highly accurate (0.1°) visual feedback to the subject. This allowed for a strong short-term feedback "signal" to be presented and reduced potential internal noise factors associated with a lack of selective attention. Also, in order to encourage concentration, discipline, and persistence, a dark, sound-deadened room where only the feedback stimulus was available was used to reduce external "noise" factors.
2. Volitional torsional responses were slowly and systematically shaped over a period of months. Small movements of only 0.2° were trained at first. Once these were learned, the outer limits of movement were extended at the average rate of only 0.8°/hour/day of training until 20° to 30° of voluntary torsion were eventually obtained. Both subjective and objective measures

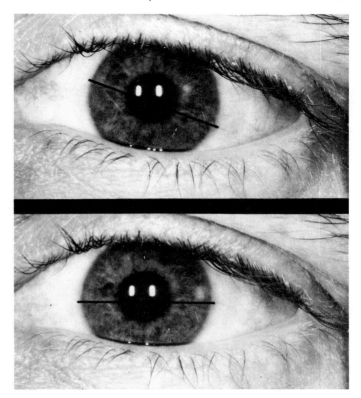

Figure 10-4. Before (*top*) and after (*bottom*) photographs of a 20° cyclotorsional eye movement. Bars drawn on photographs intersect limbal-scleral blood vessels. Note: the light spot on each iris is a photographic artifact. (Balliet R, Nakayama K: Training of voluntary torsion. Invest Ophthalmol Vis Sci 17:303–314, 1978)

of angular rotation and the amount of time that eccentricities could be held (fixated) were recorded. These measures not only provided accurate sensory information (signal) to the subject but also potentially reduced internal noise factors associated with anxiety, worry, and fear of failure.
3. Initially, the training apparatus was set up so that subjects could train themselves on the instrument. Only periodic supervision was required by the experimenter. It was not possible at the time to practice outside the laboratory because the apparatus was half the size of a small room. Once movements were large enough to perceive, practice was conducted at home without any feedback.
4. During initial training, subjects experienced severe changes in egocentric orientation (illusion of body tilt), stomach nausea, headaches, body fatigue, eyelid tremors, and hallucinations.[18] Subjects were encouraged to discuss these sensations and perceptions with the examiner as well as with other subjects. These changes in egocentric localization were also subjectively measured.[18] These measurements helped both the trainees and the trainers better understand these problems, to fear them much less, and to eventually work through them until they no longer persisted, thus reducing internal "noise" factors.

One of the clinical examples of the application of optimization strategies has been the treatment of certain patients with postsurgical facial paralysis. Since the face is not only our primary means of expression but also the primary mechanism by

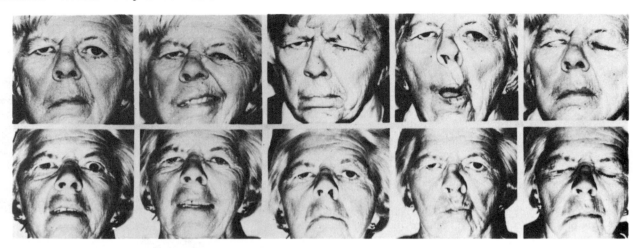

Figure 10-5. Therapeutic EMG sensory feedback with mirror exercises for facial reanimation. *Top:* before training; *bottom:* after training. *From left to right:* resting tone, smile, frown, pucker, and eye closure. A 64-year-old female had an excision of a right acoustic neuroma through a right posterior craniotomy resulting in a complete (0%) right facial paralysis. A right partial tarsorrhaphy was performed to protect the cornea. Three years after surgery, stimulation of the facial nerve with electrodes over the nasalis caused no evoked response. Needle EMG examination found evidence of mild membrane irritability in the form of occasional fibrillation potentials and positive waves in all right facial muscles sampled. No motor unit recruitment was found in either the mentalis orbicularis oris, orbicularis nasalis, or frontalis. Denervation of the right seventh cranial nerve with no apparent evidence of of reinnervation was concluded.

> After 3 months (three 1-hour per day sessions per week) of surface electrode EMG, muscle control of approximately 30% on the Janssen scale[16] was established, both in the ocular and oral areas of the face. However, stimulation of the facial nerve caused no evoked response. Needle EMG examination demonstrated prolonged insertional activity in all right facial muscles examined. Fibrillation and potentials and positive sharp waves were not seen. Volitional nascent motor unit potentials were seen throughout the investigated muscles. Some motor units were 4000 μV in amplitude with poor to fair recruitment patterns with firing rates of 40 to 50/sec, with early innervation apparent. After 8 months of therapy the patient was rated as having an overall functional score of 77% function, with the greatest decrement being in the area of the frontalis (30%). Although some muscle weakness was noted with fatigue, she had essentially no dyskinesis or synkinesis. Even though drops were no longer required to maintain the right cornea's tearfilm the patient decided not to reverse the previous tarsorrhaphy procedure. Two years later it was found that she had not regressed and that she was still performing some of her exercises, approximately 30 minutes per week to maintain overall facial muscle tone. (Balliet R, Shinn JB, Bach-y-Rita P: Facial paralysis rehabilitation: Retraining selective muscle control. Int Rehabil Med 4:67–74, 1982)

which we are judged, the quality of life of these people is usually drastically affected by this chronic condition. Although surgical techniques for the patient with facial paralysis have evolved over the past few decades, residual function after such procedures usually included dyskinesia, synkinesia, and mass action. The brain apparently cannot spontaneously relearn functional motor control after these procedures; it must be specifically retrained to reacquire these abilities.

The exact method by which facial retraining is conducted is particularly important. The two methods that have most frequently been used for many decades have been relatively passive electrical stimulation and the relatively active technique of gross exercises such as "try hard to smile." However, it has recently been found that electrical stimulation is ineffective[185] and that both methods are potentially contraindicated.[12, 13] Currently, the most successful method of training facial reanimation in post-surgical facial paralysis patients involves the relatively recent use of therapeutic EMG sensory feedback in combination with specific mirror exercises (Fig. 10-5; reviewed by Balliet[12, 13] and Balliet and co-workers[20]).

Using surface electrodes this method provides very specific information that allows the patient to permanently relearn how to use specific groups of muscles essential to normal facial expression. Patients actively participate in intense, detailed mo-

tor control assessment and subsequent retraining. Some of the more significant signal–noise factors involved in this therapy are the following[13]:

1. Recent advances in electronics, microprocessors, and overall design have allowed surface electrode EMG equipment to be developed for everyday clinical use. This equipment is now of very high quality, is extremely "user friendly," and is relatively low in price. The EMG acts as a sensory facilitator or substitution device providing immediate visual and auditory information. This relatively short-term information increases both the patient's and the therapist's proprioceptive inputs to very specific areas of the face until through long-term goals the patient can reacquire sufficient motor control and associated sensibility. At this point, EMG is no longer required and a mirror can suffice in providing the visual feedback necessary and reinforcing the motor control of specific muscle groups. All of these procedures act to increase specific motor patterns (signal) while deconditioning inappropriate motor patterns (noise), such as synkinesia and mass action.

2. Patients are informed that it is realistic to expect that significant functional gains could take a few months or up to several years to obtain. The specific planning of such long-term goals is facilitated by the extensive use of Polaroid photographs and

video tape assessments. These included both voluntary and involuntary motor control of individual muscle groups. In this manner, long-term "signal" input to both patient and therapist is provided. The recording of small gains in function apparently helps lower anxiety and reduce internal noise associated with fears of failure. External noise factors are controlled through the use of one-to-one therapist trainee ratios and rooms that were quiet, well lit, and fully equipped.

3. Retraining procedures using specialized instruction in the clinic are rapidly supplemented or replaced by very specific mirror exercises that can be conducted by the patient at home, in the car (with the rearview mirror at stop lights), or in a quiet place with a hand-held mirror. The average ratio of nonsupervised self-training to supervised clinical instruction is about 20 : 1.[14]

4. The majority of the facial paralysis patients, including even those with mild facial palsies, tend to keep their faces relatively immobile and expressionless so as to not accentuate their paralysis. Unfortunately, this common compensatory strategy not only inhibits the potential for increased neuromuscular function but also inhibits the patient's natural affect and personality. Therefore, therapists also counsel patients in certain psychosocial adjustments as they relate to retraining,[13] including the following:

   a. Reactions of friends and family who, since the onset of the paralysis, were no longer friends or who have remained supportive.

   b. Positive and negative experiences associated with the patient's facial paralysis (*e.g.,* surgery, experiences with strangers, or work-related problems).

   c. Availability of patient advocacy groups that can provide additional information and help find local support groups (*e.g.,* the Acoustic Neuroma Association of America in Carlisle, Pennsylvania, and the Acoustic Neuroma Association of Canada in Edmonton, Alberta).

SUMMARY

Dramatic changes have occurred over the past 20 years in our understanding of the neural bases of rehabilitation. The field of rehabilitation medicine is beginning to develop a solid scientific foundation. This chapter has concentrated on the following: motor and sensory mechanisms regulating movement; concepts of organization of actions; the role of neurotransmitters in recovery from brain damage; neuroplasticity; and theoretical and management concepts for the early and late post-acute patient. Topics that have been minimally discussed in this chapter but that merit greater attention include learning theory, the role of environments (including home and therapeutic environments) in recovery of function, and the relation of mental activity to physiological functions. To be successful, this scientific base must be developed without losing a strong humanistic, patient service orientation: Rehabilitation medicine must continue to emphasize the art of rehabilitation medicine while developing its science.

REFERENCES

1. Adams JA: A closed loop theory of motor learning. J Motor Behav 3:111–149, 1971
2. Adams RD: Motor paralysis. In Wintrobe MM, Thorn GW, Adams RD et al (eds): Harrison's Principles of Internal Medicine, 7th ed, pp 78–85. New York, McGraw-Hill, 1974
3. Allen GI, Tsukahara N: Cerebrocerebellar communication systems. Physiol Rev 54:957–1006, 1974
4. Almli CR, McMullen NT, Golden GT: Infant rates: Hypothalamic unit activity. Brain Res Bull 1:543–552, 1976
5. American Academy of Physical Medicine and Rehabilitation: Syllabus: Rehabilitation in Brain Disorders. Chicago, 1985
6. Anlezark GM, Crow TJ, Greenway AP: Impaired learning and decreased cortical norepinephrine after bilateral locus coeruleus lesions. Science 181:682–684, 1973
7. Arbib MA: Perceptual structures and distributed motor control. In Brooks VB (ed): Handbook of Physiology, vol III, Motor Control. Bethesda, MD, American Physiological Society, 1980
8. Bach-y-Rita P (ed): Recovery of function: Theoretical Considerations for Brain Injury Rehabilitation. Baltimore, University Park Press, 1980
9. Bach-y-Rita P: Brain plasticity as a basis for the development of rehabilitation procedures for hemiplegia. Scand J Rehabil Med 13:73–83, 1981
10. Bach-y-Rita P: Central nervous system lesions: Sprouting and unmasking in rehabilitation. Arch Phys Med Rehabil 62:413–417, 1981
11. Bach-y-Rita P: Balliet R: Recovery from stroke. In Duncan PW, Badke MB (eds): Motor Deficits Following Stroke. Chicago, Year Book Publishers, 1986
12. Balliet R: Motor control strategies in the retraining of facial paralysis. In Portmann M (ed): Proceedings of the Vth International Symposium on the Facial Nerve. Paris, Masson, 1985
13. Balliet R: Facial paralysis and other neuromuscular dysfunctions of the peripheral nervous system. In Payton OD (ed): Manual of Physical Therapy Techniques. New York, Churchill Livingstone (in press)
14. Balliet R: Unpublished data, University of Wisconsin Medical School, Madison, Wisconsin, 1986
15. Balliet R, Harbst K, Kim D, Vanderwilt RS: Retraining of functional gait through the reduction of upper extremity weight bearing in chronic cerebellar ataxia. Int Rehabil Med 8:148–153, 1987
16. Balliet R, Knight R: Sensory rehabilitation of the hand after central nervous system (CNS) injury. University of Wisconsin Medical School, Madison, Wisconsin, 1986
17. Balliet R, Levy B, Blood KMT: Upper extremity sensory feedback therapy in chronic cerebrovascular accident patients with impaired expressive aphasia and auditory comprehension. Arch Phys Med Rehabil 67:304–310, 1986
18. Balliet R, Nakayama K: Egocentric orientation is influenced by trained voluntary cyclorotary eye movements. Nature 257:214–215, 1978
19. Balliet R, Nakayama K: Training of voluntary torsion. Invest Ophthalmol Vis Sci 17:303–314, 1978
20. Balliet R, Shinn JB, Bach-y-Rita P: Facial paralysis rehabilitation: Retraining selective muscle control. Int Rehabil Med 4:67–74, 1982
21. Bernstein JJ, Bernstein ME: Neuronal alternation and reinnervation following axonal regeneration and sprouting in mammalian spinal cord. Brain Behav Evol 8:135–161, 1973
22. Bernstein N: The Co-ordination and Regulation of Movements. New York, Pergamon Press, 1967
23. Bliss TVP, Burns BD, Uttley AM: Factors affecting the conductivity of pathways in the cerebral cortex. J Physiol 195:339–367, 1968
24. Boyeson MG, Feeney DM: The role of norepinephrine in recovery from brain injury. Neurosci Abstr 10:68, 1984
25. Boyeson MG, Feeney DM, Linn RT et al: Motor cortex organization after focal injury in the rat. Neurosci Abstr 6:221, 1980
26. Boyeson MG, Krobert KA, Hughes JM: Norepinephrine infusions into the cerebellum faciiltate recovery from sensorimotor cortex injury. Neurosci Abstr 12:1120, 1986
27. Bradford HF: Chemical Neurobiology. New York, WH Freeman, 1985

28. Brinkman J, Kuypers HGJM: Cerebral control of contralateral and ipsilateral arm, hand and finger movements in the split-brain rhesus monkey. Brain 96:653–674, 1973

29. Brodal A: Self-observations and neuroanatomical considerations after a stroke. Brain 96:675–694, 1973

30. Broman H, DeLuca CJ, Mambrito B: Motor unit recruitment and firing rates interaction in the control of human muscles. Brain Res 337:311–319, 1985

31. Brooks VB, Thach WT: Cerebellar control of posture and movement. In Brooks VB (ed): Handbook of Physiology, Section 1, The Nervous System, Vol II, Motor Control, Part 2. Bethesda, MD, American Physiological Society, 1981

32. Bucy PC, Fulton JF: Ipsilateral representation in the motor and premotor cortex of monkeys. Brain 56:318–342, 1933

33. Cannon WB, Rosenblueth A: The Supersensitivity of Denervated Structures. New York, Macmillan, 1949

34. Capute AJ, Acardo PJ, Vining EPG et al: Primitive reflex profile. Phys Ther 58:1061–1065, 1978

35. Capute AJ, Shapiro BK, Accardo PJ et al: Motor functions: Associated primitive reflex profiles. Dev Med Child Neurol 24:662–669, 1982

36. Castro AJ, Smith DE: Plasticity of spinovestibular projections in response to hemicerebellectomy in newborn rats. Neurosci Lett 12:69–74, 1979

37. Cohen HJS, Taft LT, Mahadeviah MS, Birch HG: Developmental changes in overflow in normal and aberrantly functioning children. J Pediatr 71:39–47, 1967

38. Connolly KJ, Stratton P: Developmental changes in associated movements. Dev Med Child Neuro 10:49–56, 1968

39. Cooper JR, Bloom FE, Roth RH: The Biochemical Basis of Neuropharmacology. New York, Oxford University Press, 1982

40. Corrodi H, Fuxe K, Lidbrink P, Olson L: Minor tranquilizers, stress, and central catecholamine neurons. Brain Res 29:1–16, 1971

41. Cotman CW, Nadler JV: Reactive synaptogenesis in the hippocampus. In Cotman CW (ed): Neuronal Plasticity, pp 227–271. New York, Raven Press, 1978

42. Creese I, Burt D, Snyder S: Dopamine receptor binding enhancement accompanies lesion-induced behavioral supersensitivity. Science 197:596–598, 1977

43. Creutzfeldt O: Some problems of cortical organization in the light of ideas of the classical "Hirnpathologie" and of modern neurophysiology. In Zulch KJ, Creutzfeldt O, Galbraith GC (eds): Cerebral Localization, pp 217–226. Berlin, Springer, 1975

44. Crisostomo EA, Davis JN, Feeney DM, Duncan PW: Amphetamine with physical therapy facilitates recovery of motor function in stroke patients. Proceedings of the 15th Princeton Cerebrovascular Conference, New York, Raven Press (in press)

45. Davis N, LeVere TE: Recovery of function after brain damage: The question of individual behaviors or functionality. Exp Neurol 75:68–78, 1982

46. Deecke L, Grozinger B, Kornhuber HH: Voluntary finger movement in man: Cerebral potentials and theory. Biol Cybernet 23:99–119, 1976

47. Deecke L, Scheid P, Kornhuber HH: Distribution of readiness potential, pre-motion positivity, and motor potential of the human cerebral cortex preceding voluntary finger movements. Exp Brain Res 7:158–168, 1969

48. Dellon AL: Evaluation of Sensibility and Re-education of Sensation in the Hand. Baltimore, Williams & Wilkins, 1981

49. Desmedt JE: Size principle of motoneuron recruitment and the calibration of muscle force and speed in man. In Desmedt JE (ed): Motor Control Mechanisms in Health and Disease, pp 227–251. New York, Raven Press, 1983

50. Dismukes RK, Daly JW: Adaptive responses of brain cyclic AMP-generating systems to alteration in synaptic input. J Cyclic Nucleotide Res 2:231–236, 1976

51. Dismukes RH, Ghosh P, Daly JW: Altered responsiveness of adenosine 3,5'-monophosphate-generating system in rat cortical slices after lesions of the medial forebrain bundle. Exp Neurol 49:725–735, 1975

52. Donovick PJ, Burright RG, Swidler MA: Presurgical rearing environment alters exploration, fluid consumption, and learning of septal lesioned and control rats. Physiol Behav 11:543–553, 1973

53. Dostrovsky JO, Millar J, Wall PD: The immediate shift of afferent drive of dorsal column nucleus cells following deafferentation: A comparison of acute and chronic deafferentation in gracile nucleus and spinal cord. Exp Neurol 52:480–495, 1976

54. Easton TA: On the normal use of reflexes. Am Sci 60:591–599, 1972

55. Eccles JC: The Understanding of the Brain. New York, McGraw-Hill, 1977

56. Emmelin N: Supersensitivity following pharmacological denervation. Pharm Rev 13:17–37, 1961

57. Evarts EV: Brain mechanisms of movement. Sci Am 241:164–179, 1979

58. Evarts EV: Brain control of movement: Possible mechanisms of functional reorganization. In Bach-y-Rita P (ed): Recovery of Function: Theoretical Considerations for Brain Injury Rehabilitation, pp 173–186. Baltimore, University Park Press, 1980

59. Eysenck MW: Attention and Arousal: Cognition and Performance. Berlin, Springer-Verlag, 1982

60. Feeney DM, Gonzalez A, Law WA: Amphetamine restores locomotor function after motor cortex injury in the rat. Proc West Pharmacol Soc 24:15–17, 1981

61. Feeney DM, Gonzalez A, Law WA: Amphetamine, haloperidol, and experience interact to affect rate of recovery after a motor cortex injury. Science 217:855–857, 1982

62. Feeney DM, Hovda DA: Amphetamine and apomorphine restore tactile placing after motor cortex injury in the cat. Psychopharmacology 79:67–71, 1983

63. Feeney DM, Hovda DA, Salo AA: Phenoxybenzamine reinstates all motor and sensory deficits in cats fully recovered from sensorimotor cortex ablations. Fed Am Soc Exp Biol 42:1157, 1983

64. Feeney DM, Sutton RL, Boyeson MG et al: The locus coeruleus and cerebral metabolism: Recovery of function after cortical injury. Phys Psych 13:197–203, 1985

65. Finger S, Stein DG: Brain Damage and Recovery: Research and Clinical Perspectives, pp 287–302. Orlando, FL, Academic Press, 1982

66. Fisher RS, Almli CR: Postnatal development of sensory influences on lateral hypothalamic neurons in the rat. Dev Brain Res 12:55–75, 1984

67. Foerster O: Restitution der Motilitat Restitution der Sensibitat. Symposium on Restitution of Function After Lesions in the Nervous System 115:248–314, 1930

68. Fog E, Fog M: Cerebral inhibition examined by associated movements. In Bax M, MacKeith RC (eds): Minimal Cerebral Dysfunction, pp 52–57. London, Spastics Society/Heinemann, 1963

69. Forssberg H, Grillner S, Rossignol S: Phase dependent reflex reversal during walking in chronic spinal cats. Brain Res 85:103–107, 1975

70. Forssberg H, Grillner S, Rossignol S: Phasic gain control of reflexes from the dorsum of the paw during spinal locomotion. Brain Res 132:121–139, 1977

71. Franz S, Scheetz M, Wilson A: The possibility of recovery of motor function in long-standing hemiplegia. JAMA 65:2150–2154, 1915

72. Freund HJ: Premotor areas in man. Trends Neurosci 7:481–483, 1984

73. Fuster JM: The prefrontal cortex, mediator of cross-temporal contingencies. Human Neurobiol 4:169–179, 1985

74. Gallistel CR: The organization of action: A new synthesis. Behav Br Sci 4:609–650, 1981

75. Gardner WJ: Removal of the right cerebral hemisphere for infiltrating glioma. JAMA 101:823–826, 1933

76. Gazzaniga MS: Cerebral mechanisms involved in ipsilateral eye–hand use in split-brain monkeys. Exp Neurol 10:148–155, 1964

77. Gentile AM, Green S, Nieburgs A et al: Disruption and recovery of locomotor and manipulatory behavior following cortical lesions in rats. Behav Biol 22:417–455, 1978

78. Geschwind N: Late changes in the nervous system: An overview. In

Stein DG, Rosen JJ, Butters N (eds): Plasticity and Recovery of Function in the Central Nervous System, pp 467–508. New York, Academic Press, 1974

79. Gevins AS, Morgan NH, Bressler SL et al: Human neuroelectric patterns predict performance accuracy. Science 235:580–584, 1987

80. Gibson JJ, Hudson L: Bilateral transfer of the conditioned knee-jerk. J Exp Psychol 18:774–783, 1935

81. Glassman RB: Recovery following sensorimotor cortical damage: Evoked potentials, brain stimulation and motor control. Exp Neurol 33:16–29, 1971

82. Glees P: Functional reorganization following hemispherectomy in man and after small experimental lesions in primates. In Bach-y-Rita P (ed): Recovery of Function: Theoretical Considerations for Brain Injury Rehabilitation, pp 106–126. Baltimore, University Park Press, 1980

83. Glick SD, Jerussi TP, Fleisher IN: Turning in circles: The neuropharmacology of rotation. Life Sci 18:889–896, 1976

84. Globus A, Rosenzweig MR, Bennett EL, Diamond MC: Effects of differential experience on dendritic spine counts in rat cerebral cortex. J Comp Physiol Psychol 82:175–181, 1973

85. Gmegy ME, Costa E: Catecholamine receptor supersensitivity and subsensitivity in the central nervous system. In Youdin MBH, Lovenberg W, Sharman DF, Lagnado JR (eds): Essays in Neurochemistry. London, John Wiley & Sons, 1980

86. Goldberger ME: Restitution of function in the CNS: The pathological grasp in *Macaca Mulatta*. Exp Brain Res 15:79–96, 1972

87. Goldman PS, Galkin TW: Prenatal removal of frontal association cortex in the fetal rhesus monkey: Anatomical and functional consequences in postnatal life. Brain Res 152:451–485, 1978

88. Goldstein K: Die Restitution bei schadigungen der Hirnrinde. Symposium on Restitution of Function After Lesions in the Nervous System 116:2–26, 1930

89. Goodman DC, Bogdasarian RS, Horel JA: Sprouting of optic tract projections in the brain stem of the rat. J Comp Neurol 127:71–88, 1966

90. Gramsbergen A, Paassen JI: Early cerebellar hemispherectomy in the rat. In Finger S, Almi CR: Early Brain Damage, pp 155–175. Orlando, FL, Academic Press, 1984

91. Greendyke RM, Schuster DB, Wooton JA: Propranolol in the treatment of assaultive patients with organic brain disease. J Clin Psychopharm 4:282–285, 1984

92. Hallett M, Khoshbin S: A physiological mechanism of bradykinesia. Brain 103:301–314, 1980

93. Hayes KC, Sullivan J: Tonic neck reflex influence on tendon and Hoffman reflex in man. Electromyogr Clin Neurophysiol 16:251–261, 1976

94. Hellebrandt FA, Waterland JC: Indirect learning: Influence of unimanual exercise on related muscle groups of the same and the opposite side. Am J Phys Med 41:45–55, 1962

95. Henneman E, Somjen G, Carpenter DO: Functional significance of cell size in spinal motoneurons. J Neurophysiol 28:560–580, 1965

96. Hicks SP, d'Amato CJ: Motor-sensory and visual behavior after hemispherectomy in newborn and mature rats. Exp Neurol 29:416–438, 1970

97. Hink F, Deecke L, Kornhuber HH: Force uncertainty of voluntary movement and human movement-related potentials. Biol Psych 16:197–210, 1983

98. Honzik CH: The sensory basis of maze learning in rats. Comp Psych Monogr 13:1–113, 1936

99. Hore J, Meyer-Lohmann J, Brooks VB: Basal ganglia cooling disables learned arm movements of monkeys in the absence of visual guidance. Science 195:584–586, 1977

100. Hovda DA, Feeney DM: Amphetamine with experience promotes recovery of locomotor function after unilateral frontal cortex injury in the cat. Brain Res 298:358–361, 1984

101. Ingvar DH: "Memory of the future": An essay on the temporal organization of conscious awareness. Hum Neurobiol 4:127–136, 1985

102. Jacobs L, Gossman MD: Three primitive reflexes in normal adults. Neurology 30:184–188, 1980

103. Jebson RH, Griffith ER, Long EW, Fowler R: Function of "normal" hand in stroke patients. Arch Phys Med Rehab 51:170–181, 1971

104. Kao CC: Spinal Cord Reconstruction. Raven Press, New York, 1983

105. Kelche CR, Will BE: Effets de l'environnement sur la restauration fonctionnelle après lesions hippocampiques chez des rats adultes. Physiol Behav 21:935–941, 1978

106. Kelso JAS, Tuller B: Toward a theory of apractic syndromes. Brain Lang 12:224–245, 1981

107. Kennedy C, Miyaoka S, Suda S et al: Local metabolic responses in brain accompanying motor activity. Trans Am Neurol Assoc 105:13-17, 1980

108. Kornhuber HH: Cerebral cortex, cerebellum, and basal ganglia: An introduction to their motor functions. In Evarts EV (ed): Central Processing of Sensory Input Leading to Motor Output, pp 267–280. Boston, MIT Press, 1975

109. Kottke F: The neurophysiology of motor function. In Kottke F, Stillwell GK, Lehmann JF (eds): Krusen's Handbook of Physical Medicine and Rehabilitation, pp 218–253. Philadelphia, WB Saunders, 1982

110. Kristeva R, Keller E, Deecke L, Kornhuber HH: Cerebral potentials proceding unilateral and simultaneous bilateral finger movements. Electroencephalogr Clin Neurophysiol 47:229–238, 1979

111. Lashley KS: The accuracy of movement in the absence of excitation from the moving organ. Am J Physiol 43:169–194, 1917

112. Lazarus JC: Age differences and cognitive involvement in the regulation of associated movement, dissertation. University of Michigan, 1986

113. Leong SK: Plasticity of cerebellar efferents after neonatal lesions in albino rats. Neurosci Lett 7:281–289, 1978

114. Linn RT, Feeney DM, Boyeson MG et al: Enhanced somatosensory evoked potentials adjacent to focal injury of rat cortex. Neurosci Abstr 7:283, 1981

115. Loesche J, Steward O: Behavioral correlates of denervation and reinnervation of the hippocampal formation of the rat: Recovery of alternation performance following unilateral entorhinal cortex lesions. Brain Res Bull 2:31–39, 1977

116. Lund RD, Lund JS: Reorganization of the retinotectal pathway in rats after neonatal retinal lesions. Exp Neurol 40:377–390, 1973

117. Lynch G, Matthews D, Mosko S et al: Induced acetylcholinesterase-rich layer in rat dentate gyrus following entorhinal lesions. Brain Res 42:311–318, 1972

118. Lynch G, Mosko S, Parks T, Cotman CW: Relocation and hyperdevelopment of the dentate commissural system after entorhinal lesions in immature rats. Brain Res 50:174–178, 1973

119. Lynch G, Smith RL, Cotman CW: Recovery of function following brain damage: A consideration of some neural mechanisms. In Buerger AA, Tobis JS (eds): Neurophysiologic Aspects of Rehabilitation Medicine, pp 280–298. Springfield, IL, Charles C Thomas, 1980

120. Lynch G, Stanfield B, Parks T, Cotman CW: Evidence for selective post-lesion axonal growth in the dentate gyrus of the rat. Brain Res 69:1–11, 1974

121. Marsden CD, Rothwell JC, Day BL: The use of peripheral feedback in the control of movement. Trends Neurosci 7:253–257, 1984

122. Martin JP: The Basal Ganglia and Posture. London, Ritman, 1967

123. Mazziotta JC, Wapenski J, Phelps M: Cerebral metabolic responses to complex motor tasks: Normal subjects versus patients with Huntington's disease. Neurosci Abstr 10:523, 1984

124. McClanahan M, Vigano S: Evaluation of sensory motor function of the "uninvolved" upper extremity of patients with unilateral brain damage from stroke, thesis. Division of Physical Therapy, Stanford University, Stanford, CA, 1978

125. McGraw CP, Pashyan AG, Wendall OT: Cerebral infarction in the Mongolian gerbil exacerbated by phenoxybenzamine treatment. Stroke 7:485–488, 1976

126. McKinley PA, Peterson BW: Voluntary modulation of the vestibulo-ocular reflex in humans and its relation to smooth pursuit. Exp Brain Res 60:454–464, 1985

127. McMullen NT, Almli CR: Neuronal development in the medial

forebrain bundle: A Golgi study of preoptic and hypothalamic neurons in the rat. Fed Proc 38:1397, 1979

128. McMullen NT, Almli CR: Cell types within the medial forebrain bundle: A Golgi study of preoptic and hypothalamic neurons in the rat. Am J Anat 161:323–340, 1981

129. Meisel RL, Lumia AR, Sachs BD: Disruption of copulatory behavior of male rats by olfactory bulbectomy at two, but not ten, days of age. Exp Neurol 77:612–624, 1982

130. Melvill-Jones G, Gonshor A: Goal-directed flexibility in the vestibulo-ocular reflex arc. In Lennerstrand G, Bach-y-Rita P (eds): Basic Mechanisms of Ocular Motility and Their Clinical Implications, pp 227–245. Oxford, Pergamon Press, 1975

131. Milani-Comparetti A, Gidoni EA: Pattern analysis of motor development and its disorder. Dev Med Child Neurol 9:625–630, 1967

132. Millar J, Basbaum AI, Wall PD: Restructuring of the somatotopic map and appearance of abnormal neuronal activity in the gracile nucleus after partial deafferentation. Exp Neurol 50:658–672, 1976

133. Milner-Brown HS, Fisher MA, Weiner WJ: Electrical properties of motor units in parkinsonism and a possible relationship with bradykinesia. J Neurol Neurosurg Psychiatry 42:35–41, 1979

134. Milner-Brown HS, Stein RB, Lee RG, Brown WF: Motor unit recruitment in patients with neuromuscular disorders. In Desmedt JE (ed): Motor Unit Types, Recruitment and Plasticity in Health and Disease: Progress in Clinical Neurophysiology, vol 9, pp 305–318. Basel, Karger, 1981

135. Molnar GE: Analysis of motor disorder in retarded infants and young children. Am J Ment Defic 83:213–222, 1978

136. Moore J: Neuroanatomical considerations relating to recovery of function following brain injury. In Bach-y-Rita P (ed): Recovery of Function: Theoretical Considerations for Brain Injury Rehabilitation, pp 9–90. Baltimore, University Park Press, 1980

137. Morrison JH, Molliver ME, Grzanna R: Noradrenergic innervation of cerebral cortex: Widespread effects of local cortical lesions. Science 205:313–316, 1979

138. Nashner LM: Adapting reflexes controlling the human posture. Exp Brain Res 26:59–72, 1976

139. Nashner LM, Cordo PJ: Relation of automatic postural responses and reaction-time voluntary movements of human leg muscles. Exp Brain Res 43:395–405, 1981

140. Nygren LG, Fuxe K, Jonsson G, Olson L: Functional regeneration of 5-hydroxytryptamine-induced degeneration. Brain Res 78:377–394, 1974

141. Ogren SO, Acher T, Ross SB: Evidence for a role of the locus coeruleus noradrenaline system in learning. Neurosci Lett 20:351–356, 1980

142. Olson L, Fuxe K: On the projections from the locus coeruleus noradrenoline neurons: The cerebellar innervation. Brain Res 28:165–171, 1971

143. Paillard J: The patterning of skilled movements. In Handbook of Physiology, vol 3, pp 1697–1708. Baltimore, Williams & Wilkins, 1960

144. Paul RL, Goodman H, Merzenick M: Alterations in mechanoreceptor input to Brodmann's area 1 and 3 of the post-central hand area of *Macaca mulatta* after nerve section and regeneration. Brain Res 39:1–19, 1972

145. Paulson G, Gottlieb G: Developmental reflexes: The reappearance of foetal and neonatal reflexes in aged patients. Brain 92:37–52, 1968

146. Pavlovic CV, Studebaker GA: An evaluation of some assumptions underlying the articulation index. J Acoustic Soc Am 75:1606–1612, 1984

147. Perry VH, Cowey A: A sensitive period for ganglion cell degeneration and the formation of aberrant retinofugal connections following tectal lesions in rats. Neurosci 7:583–594, 1982

148. Phillips CG, Porter R: Corticospinal Neurones: Their Role in Movement, p 450. London, Academic Press, 1977

149. Ramirez J: Behavioral correlates of entorhinal cortex lesions, thesis, Clark University, Worcester, MA, 1980

150. Reed ES: An outline of a theory of action systems. J Motor Behav 14:98–134, 1982

151. Roland PE: Metabolic measurements of the working frontal cortex in man. Trends Neurosci 7:430–435, 1984

152. Roland PE, Larsen B, Lassen NA, Skinhoj E: Supplementary motor area and other areas in organization of voluntary movements in man. J Neurophysiol 43:118–136, 1980

153. Roland PE, Skinhoj E, Lassen NA, Larsen B: Different cortical areas in man in organization of voluntary movements in extrapersonal space. J Neurophysiol 43:137–150, 1980

154. Rosenzweig MR: Responsiveness of brain size to individual experience: Behavioral and evolutionary implications. In Hahn ME, Jensen C, Dudek BC (eds): Development and Evolution of Brain Size, pp 263–194. New York, Academic Press, 1979

155. Rosenzweig MR: Animal models for effects of brain lesions and for rehabilitation. In Bach-y-Rita P (ed): Recovery of Function: Theoretical Considerations for Brain Injury Rehabilitation, pp 127–172. Baltimore, University Park Press, 1980

156. Ross RA, John TH, Reis DJ: Reversible changes in the accumulation and activities of tyrosine hydroxylase and dopamine-beta-hydroxylase in neurons of nucleus locus coeruleus during the retrograde reaction. Brain Res 92:57–72, 1975

157. Rothwell JC, Traub MM, Day BL et al: Manual motor performance in a deafferented man. Brain 105:515–542, 1982

158. Salz R: Effects of part time "mothering" on IQ and SQ of young institutionalized children. Chil Dev 9:166–170, 1973

159. Sanghera MK, German DC: The effects of benzodiazepine and nonbenzodiazepine anxiolytics on locus coeruleus unit activity. J Neural Transm 57:267–279, 1983

160. Scheff SW, Cotman CW: Recovery of spontaneous alternation following lesions of the entorhinal cortex in adult rats: Possible correlation to axonal sprouting. Behav Biol 21:286–293, 1977

161. Schneider GE: Is it really better to have your brain lesion early? A revision of the "Kennard Principle." Neuropsychologia 17:557–583, 1979

162. Schwartz JC, Costentin J, Martres MP et al: Modulation of receptor mechanisms in the CNS: Hyper- and hyposensitivity to catecholamines. Neuropharmacology 17:665–686, 1978

163. Schwartz S: Effect of neonatal cortical lesions and early environmental factors on adult rat behavior. J Comp Physiol Psychol 57:72–77, 1964

164. Sherrington C: The Integrative Action of the Nervous System. New Haven, Yale University Press, 1947 (1st edition, 1906)

165. Skeels HM: Adult status of children with contrasting early life experiences. Monogr Soc Res Child Devel, No. 31, 1966

166. Sperry RW: Effect of crossing nerves to antagonistic limb muscles in the monkey. Arch Neurol Psychiatry 58:452–473, 1947

167. Sprague JM: Interaction of cortex and superior colliculus in mediation of visually guided behavior in the cat. Science 153:1544–1547, 1966

168. Stavrky GW: Supersensitivity Following Lesions of the Nervous System. Toronto, Canada, University of Toronto Press, 1961

169. Taub E: Movements in nonhuman primates deprived of somatosensory feedback. Exerc Sports Sci Rev 4:335–374, 1976

170. Taub E, Berman AJ: Movement and learning in the absence of sensory feedback. In Freedman SJ (ed): The Neuropsychology of Spatially Oriented Behavior, pp 174–192. Homewood, IL, Dorsey Press, 1968

171. Teuber HL: The frontal lobes and their functions: Further observations on rodents, carnivores, subhuman primates, and man. Int J Neurol 5:282–300, 1966

172. Thelen E, Fisher DM: Newborn stepping: An explanation for a "disappearing" reflex. Dev Psych 18:760–775, 1982

173. Todor JI: Unpublished data. University of Michigan, Ann Arbor, MI, 1980

174. Todor JI, Lazarus JC: Inhibitory influences on the emergence of motor competence in childhood. In Zaichowsky LD, Fuchs CZ (eds): The Psychology of Motor Behavior: Development Control,

Learning and Performance. Ithaca, NY, Mouvement Publications, 1986

175. Todor JI, Lazarus JC: Exertion level and the intensity of associated movements. Dev Med Child Neurol 28:205–212, 1986

176. Travis AM, Woolsey CN: Motor performance of monkeys after bilateral partial and total cerebral decortication. Am J Phys Med 35:273–310, 1956

177. Twitchell TE: Normal motor development. Am Phys Ther Assoc 45:419–423, 1965

178. Ungerstedt U: Striatal dopamine release after amphetamine or nerve degeneration revealed by rotational behavior. Acta Physiol Scand Suppl 367:49–68, 1971

179. Ungerstedt U, Arbuthnott GW: Quantitative recording of rotational behavior in rats after 6-hydroxydopamine lesions of the nigrostriatal dopamine system. Brain Res 24:485–493, 1970

180. Von Monakow C: In Pribram K (ed): Brain and Behavior. Harris G (trans). Baltimore, Penquin Books, 1969

181. Wall PD, Egger MD: Formation of new connexions in adult rat brains after partial deafferentation. Nature 232:542–545, 1971

182. Walshe FMR: On certain tonic or postural reflexes in hemiplegia, with special reference to the so-called "associated movements." Brain 46:1–37, 1923

183. Walter W, Cooper R, Aldridge V et al: Contingent negative variation: An electric sign of sensorimotor association and expectancy in the human brain. Nature 203:380–384, 1964

184. Watson M, McElligott JG: Cerebellar norepinephrine depletion and impaired acquisition of specific locomotor tasks in rats. Brain Res 296:129–138, 1984

185. Waxman B: Electrotherapy for treatment of facial nerve paralysis (Bell's palsy). In Health Technology Assessment Reports, vol 3, pp 27–35. National Center for Health Services Research, Rockville, MD Health Care Technology Assessment, 1984

186. West JR, Deadwyler SA, Cotman CW, Lynch GS: An experimental test of diaschisis. Behav Biol 18:419–425, 1976

187. White B, Held R: Plasticity of sensorimotor development in the human infant. In Rosenblith J, Allinsmith W (eds): The Causes of Behavior: Readings in Child Development in Educational Psychology, pp 60–70. Boston, Allyn & Bacon, 1966

188. Will BE, Rosenzweig MR, Bennett EL et al: Relatively brief environmental enrichment aids recovery of learning capacity and alters brain measures after postweaning brain lesions in rats. J Comp Physiol Psychol 91:33–50, 1977

189. Wing AM: Disorders of movement. In Smith MM, Wing AM (eds): The Psychology of Human Movement, pp 269–296. London, Academic Press, 1984

190. Wolff PH: Normal variation in human maturation. In Connolly KT, Prechtl HFR (eds): Maturation and Development: Biological and Psychological Perspectives (Clinics in Developmental Medicine No. 77/78). London, Heinemann Medical Books, 1981

191. Wolff PH: Theoretical issues in the development of motor skills. In Lewis M, Taft LT (eds): Developmental Disabilities: Theory, Assessment, and Intervention, pp 117–134. New York, Spectrum, 1982

192. Wolff PH, Gunnoe CE, Cohen C: Associated movements as a measure of developmental age. Dev Med Child Neurol 25:417–429, 1983

193. Wynn Parry CB: Sensory rehabilitation of the hand. Aust NZ J Surg 50:224–227, 1980

194. Zelazo PR: The development of walking: New findings and old assumptions. J Motor Behav 15:99–137, 1983

195. Zulch KJ, Muller N: Associated movements in man. In Vinken J, Bruyn GW (eds): Handbook of Clinical Neurology, vol 1, pp 404–426. Amsterdam, North Holland, 1969

11

Electrodiagnostic Evaluation of the Peripheral Nervous System

Richard D. Ball

Electrodiagnostic testing of the peripheral nervous system is an adjunct to the history, physical examination, and other laboratory studies in the overall evaluation of neuromuscular disease. Neuromuscular disorders may involve the motor unit (anterior horn cell body/axon, neuromuscular junction, and associated muscle cells), sensory neurons, and related cells (*e.g.,* the Schwann cell). While the nature of neurological dysfunction in a specific disease process may be suggested by symptoms and/or signs obtained during the physical examination, electrodiagnostic studies frequently provide additional information that can be obtained in no other manner. The widespread use of electrodiagnostic testing is based on several facts:

* When used appropriately, it can result in markedly improved diagnostic accuracy.
* It can provide quantitative/semiquantitative data regarding the severity and/or prognosis of a disease process.
* It is a relatively objective measure of neurological function.

The process of performing electrodiagnostic studies consists of the following basic steps:

1. Evaluating the patient by history/physical examination and arriving at a preliminary differential diagnosis
2. Using this differential diagnosis to select the proper electrodiagnostic tests to perform
3. Performing the selected tests in a technically competent manner
4. Properly interpreting the results obtained so as to identify the most likely diagnose(s) and exclude unlikely diagnoses.

Although these steps seem simple at first glance, the ability to perform them rests on a thorough understanding of a large and complex body of information about the underlying clinical, physiological, and electrical phenomena. Principles and concepts of a general nature will be emphasized here rather than specific information that may relate to only a small part of the overall process. The information in this chapter refers exclusively to the peripheral nervous system; electrodiagnostic testing of the central nervous system is discussed in Chapter 12.

Although the functional status of the peripheral motor or sensory systems can usually be determined from the history and physical examination, the underlying cause of sensorimotor dys-function frequently cannot be established in this manner. For example, it may be difficult to decide whether proximal muscle weakness is due to dysfunction of the neuromuscular junction or due to a myopathy. Since rational management requires specific diagnoses, the clinician needs information not only on a patient's overall neuromuscular function but also on the specific status of the various physiological and anatomical components of the peripheral nervous system, including the following:

* Motor neurons
* The neuromuscular junction
* Sensory neurons
* Schwann cells/myelin sheath
* The muscle cell (myocyte)

The task of the electrodiagnostician is therefore to determine the isolated electrical properties of these physiological and anatomical components and correlate abnormal electrical properties with the pathological processes present in specific disease categories; that is, are the electrodiagnostic abnormalities consistent with the following:

1. Anterior horn cell disease
2. Polyneuropathy
   (Axonal versus demyelinating, sensory, motor, sensorimotor)
3. Mononeuropathy
4. Mononeuropathy multiplex syndrome
5. Plexopathy
6. Radiculopathy or polyradiculopathy
7. Polyradiculoneuropathy (*e.g.,* Guillain Barré syndrome)
8. Neuromuscular junction disorder
9. Myopathic process

In order to perform electrodiagnostic testing accurately and efficiently, a structured approach is necessary. The number of electrodiagnostic tests that could be performed on any one patient is large, the time required may be considerable, and the patient frequently experiences discomfort during the examination. For this reason, the electrodiagnostician must make an effort to obtain the correct answer with a minimum number of individual tests. Most clinicians approach problems by taking a history, performing a physical examination, obtaining results of laboratory studies, and then analyzing the results according to the following questions with respect to involvement of the peripheral nervous system.

1. Does the disorder appear to involve the anterior horn cells, sensory neurons, nerve roots, peripheral nerve, neuromuscular junction, or muscle?
2. What is the distribution of abnormalities likely to be? Is the problem diffuse and generalized (*e.g.,* a myopathy or toxic polyneuropathy), multifocal (*e.g.,* a mononeuritis multiplex syndrome), or localized to the distribution of specific roots, plexi, or peripheral nerves?
3. What is the temporal course of the disorder? Is it acute, subacute, chronic, stable, improving, fluctuating, or progressing? How long have the symptoms been present?

The differential diagnosis synthesized from the answers to these questions allows the electrodiagnostician to decide which tests are most likely to lead directly to the most probable diagnosis.

OVERVIEW OF BASIC ELECTRODIAGNOSTIC TESTS

A discussion of specific electrodiagnostic tests is provided later in this chapter, but first an overview is provided of the most commonly used techniques and the general properties of the peripheral nervous system that are evaluated by these tests. Detailed descriptions of electronic theory and the relevant electronic equipment have been well covered in standard electronic and electromyography (EMG) texts.[8, 62] A basic understanding of nerve and muscle physiology is assumed.

Sensory Nerve Conduction Studies

Standard sensory nerve conduction studies are performed by stimulating a nerve at one point and measuring the whole nerve action potential at some other point (Fig. 11-1A). Since the whole nerve action potential is simply the sum of the action potentials from all axons in the nerve, we are therefore concerned with how the integrity of the peripheral sensory axon action potential is affected by various disease processes. From this standpoint, the anatomical characteristics of peripheral sensory neurons make it useful to divide clinical sensory dysfunction into preganglionic and postganglionic categories based on whether failure of sensory function is the result of a pathological process distal or proximal to the sensory neuron cell body. Preganglionic disorders (*e.g.,* radiculopathies, cauda equina lesions, or posterior column disease) do not significantly damage the sensory cell body in the dorsal root ganglion and leave the distal axon intact. Sensory electrodiagnostic studies in these disorders are normal even though clinical sensory function may be markedly abnormal. "Postganglionic" disorders are those disorders that damage the sensory cell body/axon or the associated Schwann cell and result either directly or indirectly in axonal dysfunction. Sensory electrical studies in these disorders may be abnormal if the damage is severe enough.

Information obtained from sensory nerve conduction studies includes the sensory nerve action potential (SNAP) conduction velocity along various segments of the sensory nerve, and the amplitude/shape of the SNAP. Analysis of the SNAP amplitude, shape, distal latency, and conduction velocity can provide specific information regarding the number, type, and state of myelination of sensory axons functioning in various segments of the nerve.

Motor Nerve Conduction Studies

Motor nerve conduction studies are performed by stimulating motor nerves and recording the resulting compound muscle action potential (CMAP) from the muscle (Fig. 11-1B). The results of motor nerve conduction studies may be affected by any process that damages the anterior horn cell body or axon, associated Schwann cells, the neuromuscular junction, or the muscle cell. In contrast to the sensory neurons, where peripheral lesions could be preganglionic or postganglionic, all peripheral lesions of motor axons occur distal to the cell body, thereby possibly affecting axonal function. This anatomical difference between sensory and motor neurons is helpful to the electromyographer in differentiating lesions that cause both motor and sensory dysfunction, since lesions proximal to the dorsal root ganglion (*e.g.,* radiculopathies) frequently produce abnormal motor studies with concomitantly normal sensory studies while lesions distal to the dorsal root ganglion can affect both motor and sensory electrical function.

As in sensory nerve conduction studies, the major results obtained are the nerve conduction velocity in various nerve segments and the amplitude/shape of the CMAP. Although the interpretation of the motor nerve conduction velocity and CMAP shape is similar to that of sensory nerves, the interpretation of CMAP amplitude is markedly different. The SNAP amplitude of a sensory nerve is dependent primarily on the number of functioning large myelinated axons present. The CMAP amplitude, on the other hand, is dependent primarily on the number and density of innervated muscle fibers, not the number of axons innervating them. These two parameters do not always correlate highly with one another. Abnormal neuromuscular junction or muscle cell function, never a factor in sensory studies, may also produce abnormalities in the CMAP amplitude.

Information obtained from motor nerve conduction studies includes the motor nerve action potential conduction velocity along various segments of the motor axons and the amplitude/shape of the CMAP. Analysis of the CMAP amplitude/shape, distal latency, and motor nerve conduction velocity can provide specific information regarding the state of myelination of motor axons functioning in various segments of the nerve, the number/density of innervated/functioning muscle fibers, the function of the neuromuscular junction, and the muscle cell itself.

Late Responses

Standard sensory and motor nerve conduction studies are usually performed on distal segments of the nerves, that is, those portions physically located in the extremities. It is difficult to evaluate nerve conduction velocity in extremely proximal segments of peripheral nerve (the proximal plexi and roots) owing to technical problems associated with selectively stimulating nerves and nerve roots close to the spine. When there is a need to examine these portions of the peripheral nerves, a class of nerve conduction studies known as "late responses" are usually used. These studies, so called because the response occurs much later after the stimulus than the direct muscle response, include the H reflex and the F response (Fig. 11-2). For the time being, these nerve conduction studies can be categorized by the fact that they are the result of a distally initiated nerve action potential (sensory axon for H reflex, motor axon for F response) that travels proximally, initiating a motor neuron action potential at the level of the spinal cord, which in turn is conducted distally and recorded via the muscle response. The major value of these studies is that they involve conduction over proximal portions of the nerve that are difficult to study with standard techniques.

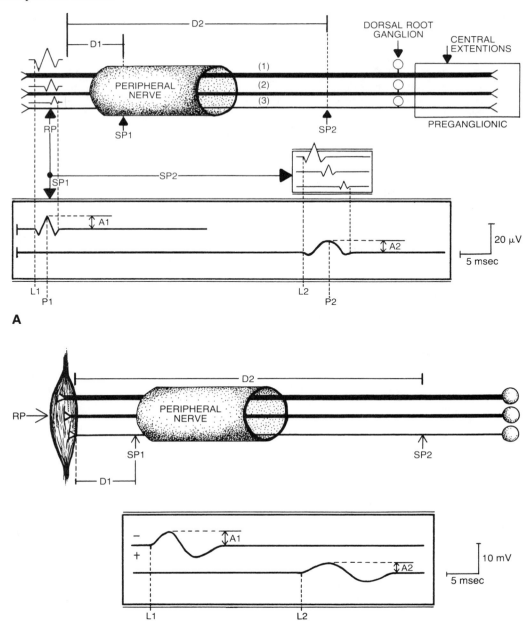

Figure 11-1. Determination of latencies, nerve conduction velocities, and evoked response amplitudes.[29,60] (*A*) Sensory nerves; Key: *RP*, recording point; *SP1*, stimulus point one; *SP2*, stimulus point two; *D1*, distance from *SP1* to *RP*; *D2*, distance from *SP2* to *RP*; *L1*, latency one—time required for fastest conducting fibers to travel distance *D1*; *P1*, peak latency of sensory nerve action potential (SNAP) obtained with stimulation at *SP1*; *L2*, latency two—the time required for fastest conducting fibers to travel distance *D2*; *P2*, peak latency of SNAP obtained with stimulation at *SP2*; *A1*, amplitude of SNAP obtained with stimulation at *SP1*; *A2*, amplitude of SNAP obtained with stimulation at *SP2*. The latencies are a function of the length of nerve and the average action potential conduction velocity between the stimulation and recording sites. The "distal" latency is the latency obtained from the most distal point of stimulation of the nerve. In an analogous fashion, the "proximal" latency is the latency obtained with the proximal stimulation point. The average conduction velocity of the nerve segment between the stimulation points is calculated as follows:

$$\text{Conduction velocity} = \frac{(\text{Distance}_2 - \text{distance}_1)}{(\text{Latency}_2 - \text{latency}_1)}$$

In general, the latencies used to calculate sensory (and motor) nerve conduction velocities are measured from the time of the stimulus to the earliest part of the evoked response. Note that this technique measures only the responses of the most rapidly conducting nerve axons. When the SNAP distal latency is used in isolation, the distal sensory latency is taken as the time from the stimulus to the peak of the negative deflection of the potential (*P1*), not the leading edge of the response (*L1*). The

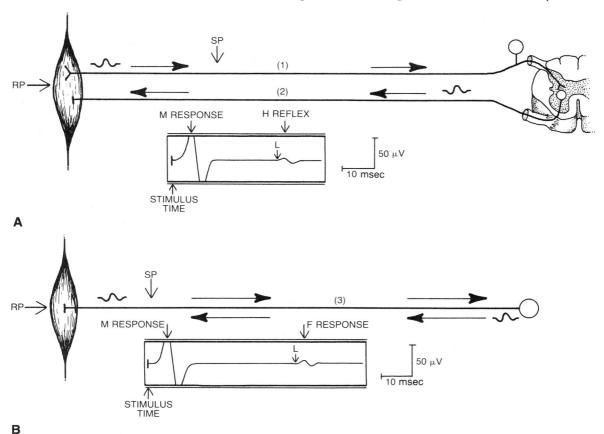

Figure 11-2. Late responses. (*A*) H reflex. A distal stimulus-initiated action potential travels ortho-dromically along an IA-afferent sensory axon (*1*) involved in the monosynaptic stretch reflex. On reaching the synapse in the spinal cord, the afferent discharge results in firing of the associated motor neuron (*2*) and a subsequent evoked response in the muscle fibers innervated by that motor neuron. (*B*) F response. A distal stimulus-initiated action potential travels antidromically along the motor axon (*3*) to the motor neuron cell body where a recurrent discharge is initiated in the same cell. This action potential travels orthodromically and results in an evoked response in the muscle fibers innervated by that motor neuron. (*SP,* stimulus point; *RP,* recording point; *L,* latency)

Conduction in proximal nerves can also be studied by the use of direct stimulation of the nerve root using monopolar stimulation electrodes.[4]

Repetitive Stimulation

Standard motor nerve conduction studies involve single stimuli delivered to the nerve at a relatively low frequency (once every several seconds). This does not functionally stress the neuro-muscular junction unless severe abnormalities are present. On the other hand, repetitive stimulation of a motor nerve at higher frequencies (2 to 50 Hz) can unmask mild to moderate neuro-muscular junction dysfunction. When disorders of the neuro-muscular junction such as myasthenia gravis, Eaton-Lambert syn-drome, and others are suspected, repetitive stimulation of motor nerves must be included in the evaluation. Repetitive stimulation may also be used to evaluate other disorders (*e.g.,* myocyte disorders such as myotonic dystrophy) or disorders in which neuromuscular junction transmission may be secondarily abnor-mal (*e.g.,* rapidly progressive motor neuron disease with exten-sive denervation/reinnervation). Repetitive stimulation repre-sents a technique that is easily done but frequently underused.

Needle Electrode Examination

The needle electrode examination is performed by inserting a small recording electrode into skeletal muscle and recording the electrical activity present at rest and during voluntary activation

action potentials from large (*1*), medium (*2*), and small (*3*) myelinated axons are shown. These are intended to represent populations of axons with these size characteristics. Note the change in the SNAP shape and amplitude due to temporal dispersion as the distance over which the action potentials are conducted increases (see text). (*B*) Motor nerves: Key: *RP, D1, D2, L1, L2, SP1,* and *SP2* are defined in a manner identical to those for sensory nerve conduction studies above. Note that the compound motor evoked response (CMAP) is recorded from muscle, not nerve. Three motor units are shown in the diagram, representing motor neurons with (*1*) large, (*2*) medium, and (*3*) small myelinated axons. Temporal dispersion is illustrated in a manner analogous to that for sensory nerves.

of the muscle. The recording surface of the electrode is small (150 to 600 μ in diameter, depending on electrode type), and as a result, a very small volume of muscle is examined. The action potentials and other electrical phenomena related to individual muscle fibers/motor units are identifiable during these recordings. Specifically, the needle electrode examination evaluates the following muscle characteristics:

1. Insertional activity: Electrical activity present as the electrode is passed through muscle cells
2. Spontaneous activity: Electrical activity present when the muscle is at rest and the electrode is not being moved
3. Motor unit action potential (MUAP) shape and amplitude
4. Motor unit recruitment patterns

The needle electrode examination of these items provides close-range evaluation of the electrical characteristics of individual muscle fibers and motor units and can provide information regarding the state of innervation/integrity of individual muscle fibers and the anatomical organization of motor units (e.g., the number and density of muscle fibers in a motor unit). Analysis of motor unit recruitment patterns provides information on the number and functional status of the anterior horn cells innervating a muscle.

Most of the information provided by the needle electrode examination is complementary to that provided by motor nerve conduction studies. CMAP amplitudes obtained during motor nerve conduction studies are a function of the number and functional status of innervated muscle fibers present. As such, the CMAP amplitude is a gross property of the muscle and is insensitive to processes that affect only a small percentage of the total muscle fibers; for example, a process that denervates 5% of the muscle fibers will probably not produce a detectable change in the CMAP even though abnormalities may be present on needle electrode examination. Additionally, CMAP amplitude measurements do not provide any information on how the muscle fibers are innervated, only that they *are* innervated. All other factors being equal, a muscle with 100 normal motor units might have essentially the same CMAP amplitude as a muscle that has lost 80% of its motor neurons and now has 20 markedly abnormal motor units possessing five times the normal number of muscle fibers. Lastly, needle electrode examination may identify abnormal electrical events that for one reason or another may not be detected during routine motor nerve conduction studies.

In almost all cases, a complete electrodiagnostic study will require both nerve conduction studies and a needle electrode examination.

Single Fiber Electromyography

Certain electrodiagnostic techniques, while not in widespread use, may be of substantial value in some situations. One of the most important of these techniques is that of single fiber electromyography (SFEMG), a technique for evaluating the performance of the neuromuscular junction. SFEMG is much more sensitive than motor nerve repetitive stimulation in detecting the abnormalities that occur in primary disorders of the neuromuscular junction (e.g., myasthenia gravis, Lambert-Eaton syndrome). In situations in which a primary disorder of the neuromuscular junction is suspected, and repetitive stimulation studies are normal, SFEMG will confirm the diagnosis in many cases.[13, 43, 49, 51, 76, 77, 81]

Neuromuscular junction transmission may also be abnormal where immature neuromuscular junctions are present as a result of ongoing denervation/reinnervation (e.g., in motor neu-

ron disease). SFEMG may provide diagnostically and prognostically useful information in these settings by documenting abnormal neuromuscular junction function consistent with denervation/reinnervation when routine studies are equivocal. SFEMG may also be used to estimate motor unit muscle fiber density, another measurement that may be abnormal in myopathies and neuropathies when the results of routine electrodiagnosis are equivocal.[43, 77, 81] A major drawback to the routine use of SFEMG is the need for special equipment/expertise.

The electrodiagnostic tests described above form the basis for almost all routinely performed electrodiagnostic studies. The reader should understand this section well before proceeding to more advanced sections of this chapter.

NERVE CONDUCTION STUDIES

Basic Techniques and Terminology

Sensory and motor nerve conduction studies involve the analysis of the properties listed below. Discussion of these properties will be organized depending on whether the principles underlying that respective property of motor and sensory nerve conduction studies are similar or different.

Conduction velocity: Determined primarily by axonal diameter and the state of axonal myelination. The factors underlying normal and abnormal nerve conduction velocities are essentially identical for both motor and sensory nerves and will be discussed together.

Distal latency (see Fig 11-1): An index of conduction velocity in the most distal portion of the nerve.

Temporal dispersion: (Fig. 11-3A): Similar for motor and sensory nerve conduction studies.

Conduction block (Fig. 11-3B): Similar for motor and sensory nerve conduction studies.

Evoked response amplitude: Physiological factors underlying sensory (SNAP) and motor (CMAP) evoked response amplitudes differ significantly and will be discussed separately for motor and sensory nerve conduction studies.

Nerve Conduction Velocities

Interpreting nerve conduction velocity studies requires knowledge of several facts about axonal action potential propagation. This discussion is restricted to myelinated axons since these are the axons that determine the conduction velocity of motor and sensory nerves. The same physiological principles determine motor and sensory nerve conduction velocities, since it is the conduction velocity of the nerve axon that determines this property in both cases. These properties may be listed as follows:

1. Axonal action potential conduction velocity is related to axonal diameter in a roughly linear fashion, although this relationship is complex when comparing a wide range of axonal diameters.[57, 88]
2. Nerve conduction studies are performed in a manner such that the fastest conducting axons determine the conduction velocity (see Fig. 11-1A).
3. Conduction velocities may be abnormally low owing to processes that
   a. Directly affect the conduction velocities of large myelinated fibers (e.g., demyelination). Demyelinating processes may result in conduction velocities ranging from

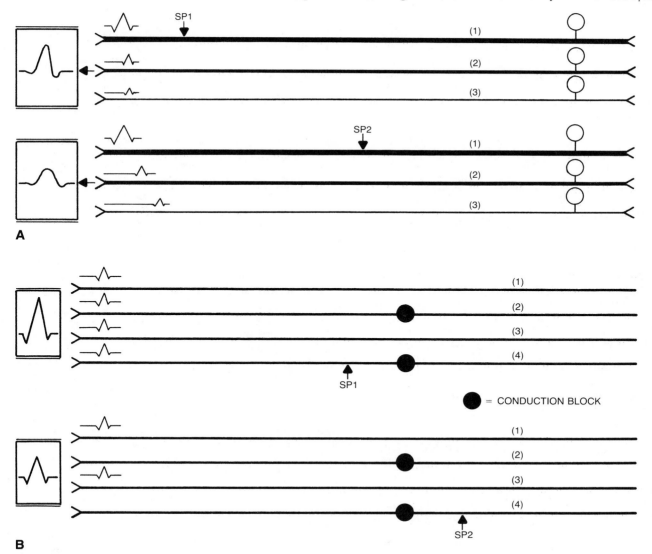

Figure 11-3. Temporal dispersion and conduction block. (*A*) Temporal dispersion. Three myelinated sensory axons with fast (*1*), medium (*2*), and slow (*3*) action potential conduction velocities are shown, representing populations of axons with these characteristics. These fast, medium, and slow conducting action potential populations form the leading edge, mid portion, and trailing edge of the evoked response. When action potentials are simultaneously initiated in all three axons close to the recording electrode, the time difference between arrival of the fast and slow conducting action potentials is minimal and the evoked response has a relatively short duration and high amplitude. When action potentials are simultaneously initiated in all three axons "far" from the recording electrode, the time difference between arrival of the fast and slow conducting action potentials is exaggerated and the evoked response has a longer duration and lower amplitude. Temporal dispersion in motor nerves is similar to that in sensory nerves. (*B*) Conduction block. Conduction block is the result of any process (*e.g.,* focal demyelination) that prevents an action potential from propagating past a given point while permitting the distal axon to conduct relatively normally. In the figure, axons (*2*) and (*4*) have conduction block at the point indicated. When the nerve is stimulated between the point of conduction block and the recording electrode (*SP1*), all axons conduct and the evoked response amplitude is maximal. If the stimulus is moved proximally on the nerve such that the point of conduction block lies between the stimulus and the recording electrodes (*SP2*), the contributions of axons with conduction block will be eliminated and the resultant evoked response will have a diminished amplitude relative to the evoked response obtained with distal stimulation. (*SP1, SP2,* stimulus points 1, 2)

low normal (40 to 50 meters/sec) to as low as 5 to 10 meters/sec, depending on the severity and nature of the underlying process.

   b. Result in a loss of the majority of large myelinated fibers, leaving the smaller, slower conducting axons to determine the conduction velocity. Loss of faster conducting axons does not result in markedly decreased conduction velocities since conduction velocities usually cannot be determined reliably with routine techniques (for technical reasons) when all medium and large myelinated fibers are lost. The loss of faster conducting axons can explain decreases in conduction velocity down to approximately 80% of the lower limit of normal. (Lower limit of normal = 40 to 50 meters/sec, depending on the nerve.) The relationship of evoked response amplitude to conduction velocity with loss of large myelinated axons is important and will be discussed subsequently.

4. The conduction velocity of peripheral nerve tends to decrease in a proximodistal manner. This phenomenon is small and not of major importance until the last few centimeters of terminal nerve are reached. The nerve conduction velocity of the terminal nerve branches decreases, probably to as low as 5 to 10 meters/sec, owing in part to marked decreases in the diameter of terminal axons. Since nerve conduction velocities along a nerve are heterogeneous, *average* nerve conduction velocities over specific segments of the nerve are calculated, rather than determining the exact conduction velocity at specific points. For nerve segments proximal to the last 5 to 10 cm of a nerve, the average conduction velocity (distance traveled divided by time required) is a reasonably accurate estimate of the range of conduction velocities present (see Fig. 11-1). This is not true for the distal few centimeters of a nerve in which the conduction velocity drops progressively and rapidly as the action potential propagates more distally. Normal conduction velocity behavior of distal nerve is therefore best characterized by determining the time required for an action potential to travel a standardized distance. This is termed a *distal latency,* with values ranging from 2.5 to 6.5 msec. These data are usually not converted into a conduction velocity since it has little meaning in this form. In the case of motor nerves, the time delay at the neuromuscular junction is also included in the distal latency, introducing a small, but additional error if an action potential "conduction velocity" is calculated by dividing distance traveled by time required.

5. The conduction velocity or nerve decreases significantly with decreased temperature, and distal latencies become correspondingly prolonged. Most laboratories use a surface temperature of 32°C as standard for determining normal values. Since nerve temperature in the deep tissues of normal limbs is relatively well maintained, conduction velocities in proximal nerve are usually affected only when ambient temperatures are extremely low or when limbs are markedly atrophic. Distal limb temperatures (*e.g.,* finger temperature) are markedly affected by low environmental temperatures and patients must frequently be warmed to 32°C before accurate studies can be performed. As an approximation, conduction velocities drop by 1.5 to 2.5 meters/sec/°C and distal latencies become prolonged by 0.1 to 0.3 msec/°C. Nerve evoked response amplitudes tend to increase with decreased temperature, primarily owing to decreased temporal dispersion.[10, 48, 55]

6. Conduction velocities in newborns are approximately half those in mature adults and are even lower in premature infants. Conduction velocities reach approximately 80% of adult values at 1 year of age and reach adult values at 3 to 5 years of age.[47, 55]

7. Conduction velocities tend to decrease slightly after 30 to 40 years of age, with the maximum decrement being approximately 10 meters/sec at ages 60 to 80.[14, 86]

8. Nerve conduction velocities are estimated either by calculating an average conduction velocity over a specific nerve segment or by determining the time (latency) required for the nerve action potential to travel a specified distance. Decreased nerve conduction velocities or increased latencies may indicate demyelination, loss of large, rapidly conducting myelinated axons, or substandard nerve temperatures.

   Theoretically, metabolic abnormalities of the axon could reduce conduction velocities in the absence of demyelination or loss of large myelinated axons.[17] The importance of this phenomenon in routine clinical applications is unknown.

   There are no known pathological conditions in which conduction velocities are increased. When this appears to occur, it is generally due to technical error or an anatomical anomaly.

Temporal Dispersion

   All peripheral nerves contain myelinated axons that are heterogeneous with respect to size and conduction velocity. When a nerve is stimulated supramaximally, an axonal action potential is simultaneously initiated in each axon. If the recording electrode is near the point of stimulation, action potentials from rapidly and slowly conducting axons arrive at the electrode nearly simultaneously and the recorded nerve action potential has a relatively high amplitude and short duration (see discussion of amplitude). If the recording electrode is moved farther from the point of stimulation, the time difference between arrival of the action potentials from the faster conducting axons and the action potentials from slowly conducting axons increases (see Fig. 11-3A). The nerve action potential recorded at the longer distance will therefore have a relatively lower amplitude and longer duration than the nerve action potential recorded closer to the stimulus. This phenomenon is referred to as *temporal dispersion.* Temporal dispersion in both sensory and motor nerves is the result of heterogeneity of axonal conduction velocities. Some temporal dispersion is normal, but it is markedly increased in disease processes causing multifocal demyelination (*e.g.,* Guillain-Barré syndrome). Under these circumstances, axons are demyelinated in an uneven manner with some axons relatively spared and some heavily involved, resulting in a wide range of conduction velocities. Processes that cause diffuse demyelination (*e.g.,* Charcot-Marie-Tooth disease) affect most axons to approximately the same extent, causing much smaller increases in temporal dispersion than multifocal processes, even though the conduction velocity may be comparably decreased. As a generalization, short duration, acquired processes such as Guillain-Barré syndrome produce multifocal demyelination whereas chronic/inherited disorders such as Charcot-Marie-Tooth disease result in diffuse demyelination.[59, 65, 66] This leads to the generalization that marked temporal dispersion of sensory or motor evoked responses suggests an acquired, relatively short duration, multifocal process.

Conduction Block

   Owing to saltatory conduction along the nodes of Ranvier, myelinated nerve has a relative high conduction velocity (40 to 80 meters/sec) as compared with unmyelinated nerve (1 to 5 meters/sec). Damage to Schwann cells and secondary demyelination therefore can cause a significant reduction in the conduction velocity in the affected nerve. If Schwann cell/axonal damage is severe enough, action potentials may not propagate past the damaged region, a condition known as conduction block (see Fig. 11-3B).[9] Action potential conduction distal to the conduction block is frequently normal, especially when the block is due to focal damage (e.g., an ulnar pressure neuropathy at the elbow). The presence of conduction block is suggested when the amplitude of a motor or sensory evoked response drops abnormally when the stimulus site is moved more proximally on the nerve, that is, when the test is performed in a manner that requires axonal conduction across the damaged region.

The amplitude of a sensory or motor evoked response may be affected by either temporal dispersion or by conduction block. It would be of value to be able to absolutely distinguish the two phenomena, and many attempts to do this have been made. Perhaps the most common approach to this problem has been to make use of the fact that the area of an evoked response (integration of the area under the curve) is affected much less by temporal dispersion than is the amplitude or duration. This has led to the assumption that temporal dispersion does not decrease the area of an evoked response while conduction block does, and the two phenomena can be distinguished in this manner. This is only partially true, and low degrees of conduction block are difficult to identify in the presence of abnormal temporal dispersion. Conduction block is best identified when the ratio of proximal/distal evoked response amplitudes drops significantly (<0.7 to 0.8) without significant changes in the ratio of proximal/distal evoked response durations (<1.2).[67]

In the presence of conduction block, nerve conduction velocities tend to be underestimated since larger, faster conducting axons are usually more susceptible. The distal latency obtained by stimulation distal to the block is determined by the faster conducting axons, while the proximal latency obtained by stimulation proximal to the block is determined by slower conducting fibers. The *calculated* conduction velocity is then somewhat lower than the *true* conduction velocity of the slower conducting axons.

Conduction block may be seen with focal compressive entrapment neuropathies (e.g., carpal tunnel syndrome) or diffuse/multifocal lesions (e.g., Guillain-Barré syndrome). Other causes of altered proximal/distal evoked response amplitude ratios such as anomalous innervation and temporal dispersion must be excluded. Conduction block, when unequivocally present, documents either focal or multifocal demyelination of the nerve in question. Conduction block may be the predominant abnormality in some demyelinating conditions.

Temporal Course of Nerve Conduction Velocity Abnormalities

Demyelinating neurological lesions (and all other types) should be analyzed with respect to their stage. Is the process

- Acute (days to weeks in duration)?
- Subacute (weeks to months in duration)?
- Chronic (months to years in duration, active)?
- Old (months to years since onset, inactive)?

Several situations may exist in demyelinating processes, depending on the stage and type of disease process. If a demyelinating process is diffuse (favoring a chronic or old process), that is, all axons are involved to a similar extent, then the predominant finding will be that of slowed conduction velocity with relatively minimal to moderate temporal dispersion of the evoked response. On the other hand, a multifocal demyelinating process such as early Guillain-Barré syndrome may leave some axons in

the nerve relatively uninvolved while others are severely involved. This may result in several different electrodiagnostic pictures with time. If all axons are involved, but still conducting action potentials, conduction velocities will generally be reduced with significant temporal dispersion of the evoked response. However, if a significant number of the large, myelinated fibers are minimally affected, the conduction velocity may be normal or near normal, with the dominant abnormality being temporal dispersion and/or conduction block. As discussed, nerve conduction velocities may be underestimated in the presence of conduction block. Nerve conduction studies may be essentially normal in the presence of significant clinical sensory and/or motor dysfunction if the majority of conduction block is occurring proximally at the root level. If most of the large myelinated fibers are heavily involved, conduction velocities will be markedly reduced. When evaluating an evolving process, the examiner should be prepared to find any of the above patterns.

Decreased conduction velocities do not necessarily correlate with clinical motor function since nonfunctioning axons have no effect on measured whole nerve conduction velocity and axonal conduction velocity *per se* has no effect on the force of muscle contraction. Even if conduction velocities are markedly reduced, significant motor dysfunction may not be present if all axons in a nerve are conducting. Sensory function (e.g., vibration and/or light touch sense) may be abnormal under the same circumstances. A patient may present with severe weakness and sensory dysfunction secondary to conduction block in a high percentage of axons. The remaining axons may be minimally demyelinated, resulting in only moderately decreased conduction velocities. As time goes on, the relatively unaffected axons may become more involved while conduction block in severely involved axons begins to resolve. Whole nerve conduction velocities may therefore actually decrease while the patient's clinical function is improving owing to resolution of conduction block in axons that were initially nonconducting. Motor nerve evoked response amplitudes may be normal in the presence of severe weakness, with or without slowing of conduction velocity, if the dominant abnormality is conduction block at the root level.

Sensory Nerve Conduction Studies

Physiological Factors Determining SNAP Amplitude and Conduction Velocity

The sensory nerve action potential (SNAP) measured in routine electrodiagnostic studies is a complex function of the sum of the longitudinal currents produced by action potentials of individual sensory nerve axons within the nerve and normally ranges from 2 to 100 μV depending on the nerve.[44] The nerve axon evoked response can be modeled as shown in Figure 11-4. The amplitude of the recorded action potential is proportional to the total current that the underlying nerve action potential longitudinal currents can drive through the tissues separating the recording electrodes. This current is a complex function of the nerve axon diameter, the metabolic condition of these cells, cell density (cells/mm²), and the electrical properties of surrounding tissue. In most cases, abnormally low SNAPs are due to a loss of functioning axons and subsequent decrease in functioning axonal density. Theoretically, abnormal metabolic states can diminish the currents produced by the axons and result in decreased SNAP amplitudes, despite normal fiber density. A detailed discussion of the relationship between the action potential and axonal population of sensory nerve is presented by Lambert and Dyck.[57]

At this point, a review of several properties of nerve axons is in order:

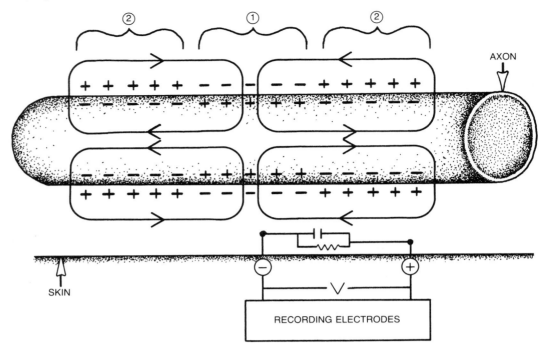

Figure 11-4. Longitudinal current. The extracellular surface region of an axon that is conducting an action potential (*1*) is electrically negative with respect to other portions of the surface of the axon. (*2*). Likewise, the active intracellular interior of the axon is positive relative to areas of the axon cytoplasm that are not conducting an action potential. The net effect of this situation is that a positive (conventional) longitudinal current loop is set up on both sides of the active region of the axon where intracellular current flows away from the active region and extracellular current flow is toward the active region.[44] Conventional electrodiagnostic studies detect the voltage (*V*) produced by this extracellular current loop roughly according to Ohm's law, $V = IZ$, where I is the current/cm^2 conducted through and Z is the impedance (resistance + 1/capacitance) of the tissue separating the recording electrodes. All other factors being equal, the total current (and hence amplitude of the recorded evoked response) is proportional to the *density* of axons (or muscle cells) within the pickup radius of the recording electrodes. The CMAP can be analyzed in an analogous fashion.

1. Axonal conduction velocity is roughly linearly related to axonal diameter.
2. The longitudinal current and the amplitude of the axonal action potential is approximately proportional to the square of the fiber diameter.
3. The evoked response amplitude recorded from a whole nerve is proportional to the density and type of axons present, all other factors being equal.

A myelinated axon with a diameter of 10 μ would therefore have an action potential approximately four times larger and would conduct at a velocity roughly two times faster than a myelinated fiber with diameter of 5 μ. In normal sensory nerve, there are approximately three times as many unmyelinated as myelinated axons present, with unmyelinated axons ranging from 0.3 to 1.5 μ in diameter. Approximately 30% of the myelinated axons have diameters greater than 8 μ, with a range of 2 to 22 μ. From these data, it can therefore be concluded that both the SNAP amplitude *and* the conduction velocity are determined primarily by the large-diameter myelinated axons and that small-diameter myelinated and unmyelinated nerve fibers make a minimal contribution to the SNAP amplitude and temporal dispersion and essentially no contribution to SNAP conduction velocity. A process such as amyloidosis that involves primarily small unmyelinated fibers could completely eliminate the action potentials of these fibers without the results of conventional sensory nerve conduction studies becoming abnormal.

Temporal Course of Sensory Nerve Conduction Abnormalities

The specific electrodiagnostic findings in a disease may depend highly on the stage of the disease process. Major interpretive errors can be made if this is not taken into account. For this reason, the sensory nerve conduction changes that occur at different times after axonal transection are reviewed. The stages of demyelinating lesions have been reviewed previously.

After a sensory axon has been transected, the segment of nerve distal to the transection point will initially conduct in a normal fashion, with normal conduction velocity and evoked response amplitude. Individual axons within the nerve will cease to conduct action potentials over the next 5 to 10 days, resulting in a progressive loss in SNAP amplitude over time as fewer and fewer axons are functioning. The SNAP amplitude would diminish after 2 to 4 days, and no SNAP would be present after 7 to 11 days.[92]

The presence of a SNAP is generally taken to indicate that at least some sensory axons are intact and functioning in a given nerve. If the time interval between axonal injury and subsequent testing is less than 7 to 11 days, a detectable SNAP does not prove axonal continuity.

Normal and Abnormal Sensory Nerve Conduction Studies

Conventional sensory nerve conduction studies provide an evoked response amplitude (proportional to diameter, number, and density of functioning axons), a distal latency (a function of average distal nerve conduction velocity), segmental conduction velocities (a function of axonal diameter and state of myelination), and SNAP conformation (a function of temporal dispersion and conduction block). Abnormalities may occur in any one of these measurements, either in isolation or combination.

PROLONGED DISTAL LATENCY. Prolonged distal latency may occur with the following:[9, 17]

1. Low distal limb temperatures
2. Generalized or focal/multifocal processes resulting in demyelination in the distal segment of the nerve
3. Generalized or focal/multifocal processes causing a loss of large, myelinated fibers
4. Processes causing a severe reduction in axonal diameters

Examples of generalized/multifocal processes would include Guillain-Barré syndrome and other polyneuropathies, while focal processes would include the carpal tunnel syndrome. When a loss of large, myelinated fibers or severe stenosis is the underlying basis for a prolonged distal latency, a decreased evoked response amplitude is seen as well. Since it is the large, myelinated, rapidly conducting fibers that also produce most of the evoked response amplitude, loss of these axons must necessarily result in a low SNAP amplitude in conjunction with the prolonged distal latency. Axonal stenosis, frequently seen in distal polyneuropathies, produces decreased SNAP amplitudes directly and is frequently associated with loss of axons, further decreasing the SNAP amplitude.[17] Distal axonal stenosis may be the earliest manifestation of a generalized process.

DECREASED CONDUCTION VELOCITY. Decreased conduction velocity may be seen with the following:[9, 17, 57]

1. Diffuse demyelination
2. Loss of large, myelinated fibers
3. Focal or multifocal demyelination
4. Marked axonal stenosis

From an etiological standpoint, it is important to determine how much conduction velocity decreases and whether it is associated with temporal dispersion/conduction block. Conduction velocities may be mildly decreased secondary to loss of the faster conducting axons without any significant demyelination occurring. It is generally held that this can be responsible for conduction velocities down to, but not lower than, approximately 80% of the lower limit of normal.[17] This explanation for decreased conduction velocities is *only* valid when the SNAP amplitude is markedly diminished as well (10 to 30% of the lower limit of normal). As discussed previously, it is the large, myelinated, rapidly conducting fibers that also produce most of the evoked response amplitude.[17] If the majority of these axons is lost, both the SNAP amplitude and conduction velocity must necessarily decrease. If the SNAP amplitude is not markedly reduced, and temperature is not a factor, conduction velocities less than the lower limit of normal are most consistent with demyelination. The interpretation of reduced conduction velocities is therefore

dependent on the associated SNAP amplitude. When the SNAP is not markedly reduced, mild demyelination can produce conduction velocities ranging from 80 to 100% of the lower limit of normal.[17] This type of demyelination is present in many conditions and is relatively nonspecific.[9] Markedly decreased conduction velocities (*e.g.,* 20 to 80% of the lower limit of normal) are seen in conditions in which demyelination is the *predominant* feature of the disease and suggest a relatively small group of disorders: Guillain-Barré syndrome,[1] Charcot-Marie-Tooth Disease (hereditary sensorimotor neuropathy [HSMN] type I), Déjèrine-Sottas disease (HSMN, type III), chronic inflammatory demyelinating polyneuropathy (CIDP), diphtheria, metachromatic leukodystrophy, and some dysimmune neuropathies such as those associated with paraproteinemias,[45] lymphomas, systemic lupus erythematosus, and Castleman's disease.

For technical reasons, it frequently is impossible to determine sensory nerve conduction velocities when the above abnormalities are present, forcing the electrodiagnostician to rely on analysis of motor nerve conduction studies to evaluate the presence or absence of demyelination. Motor nerves demonstrate essentially the same relationships between CMAP amplitude, loss of large IA myelinated axons, and axonal conduction velocity as do sensory nerves, although for slightly different underlying reasons.

DECREASED SNAP AMPLITUDE. Decreased SNAP amplitude may be seen with the following:

1. Temporal dispersion
2. Conduction block
3. Severe axonal stenosis
4. Significant loss of large, myelinated axons
5. Technical factors such as poor electrode placement, significant swelling of soft tissue surrounding the nerve, or submaximal stimulation.

When the decreased evoked response amplitude is secondary to severe axonal stenosis, loss of large myelinated axons, or demyelinated/temporal dispersion without conduction block, the distal latency should be prolonged as well. Increased distal latencies may also be associated with conduction block since processes causing conduction block may also cause loss of large myelinated axons and focal demyelination, as in the carpal tunnel syndrome.

INCREASED TEMPORAL DISPERSION. Increased temporal dispersion is noted primarily in multifocal disorders in which some axons within a nerve may have only minimal demyelination and demonstrate only mild decreases in conduction velocity, while other axons are more significantly involved and conduction velocities are much slower. This is a feature of certain phases of acquired disorders such as acute inflammatory demyelinating polyneuropathy (AIDP, Guillain-Barré syndrome), early chronic inflammatory demyelinating polyneuropathy (CIDP), and other polyneuropathies.[1] Long-standing disorders, such as hereditary sensorimotor neuropathy (HSMN type I, Charcot-Marie-Tooth disease) or long-standing CIDP, will generally involve all axons within a nerve to a similar degree, producing marked slowing of the nerve conduction velocity with a much lesser degree of temporal dispersion.[59, 65, 66]

Motor Nerve Conduction Studies

The underlying determinants of motor nerve conduction studies are very similar to those for sensory nerve conduction studies, with the important difference that it is the compound muscle action potential (CMAP) that is being measured after motor nerve stimulation, not the nerve action potential. The neuromuscular junction is also involved in producing the evoked response, thereby making motor nerve conduction studies a simultaneous test of nerve, neuromuscular junction, and muscle cell function. One can apply all the logic developed for sensory nerve conduction studies when analyzing conduction velocity, distal latency, temporal dispersion, and conduction block, but different principles must be used to analyze CMAP amplitude. Normal CMAP amplitudes for commonly studied muscles range from 2 to 25 mV depending on the muscle.

Physical Factors Affecting CMAP Amplitude

One difference between sensory and motor nerve conduction studies is related to the physical size of the electrically active tissues. Owing to the relatively small size of nerves, surface electrodes used in standard sensory conduction studies record action potentials from essentially all axons in the nerve. This is not always the case with CMAPs since many muscle fibers may be too far from the recording electrode for their longitudinal currents and resultant action potentials to be significant (see Fig. 11-4). In the case of small muscles, such as those of the hands and feet that are used in most routine nerve conduction studies, the electrical activity of most of the muscle fibers in the muscle will be recorded by the electrode. For a large muscle such as the quadriceps, most of the muscle fibers in the muscle are too far from the recording electrode to make a significant contribution to the recorded potential and the recording electrode therefore only measures action potentials from a small fraction of the total number of muscle fibers. The resultant CMAP is therefore proportional to the longitudinal current produced by the muscle fibers within the pickup range of the electrode, not the total number of fibers in the muscle. All other factors being identical, this longitudinal current is primarily a function of the muscle fiber density (fibers/cm^2). The CMAP amplitude changes observed with pathological processes that affect the number of innervated muscle fibers (e.g., denervation or segmental necrosis of muscle fibers) will therefore be minimal unless the *density* of *innervated* muscle fibers *within the recording range* of the electrode is altered.[57]

Motor Neuron Numbers and CMAP Amplitude

The amplitude of the potential is a function of the number and density of innervated muscle fibers, not the number of axons innervating them. In an old lesion, such as might be seen with old poliomyelitis, relatively few axons might survive, but the motor evoked response amplitude may be normal if all the originally denervated muscle fibers are reinnervated. In an acute lesion in which reinnervation has not had time to occur, the evoked response amplitude is roughly proportional to the number of functioning axons.

Disuse Atrophy and CMAP Amplitude

The longitudinal current and resulting action potential amplitude of a muscle fiber, as is the case for nerve axons, is proportional to the square of the diameter of the fiber; that is, larger muscle cells produce larger action potentials. Muscle atrophy, with the concomitant reduction in fiber diameters, does not generally produce major reductions in CMAP amplitude since atrophy is offset to a large degree by an increase in fiber density. Although good studies of this problem are lacking, it is generally believed that disuse atrophy cannot easily explain CMAP amplitude decreases below 70 to 80% of the lower limit of normal.

Metabolic Impairment and CMAP Amplitude

If a muscle cell is metabolically impaired, as may occur in some myopathies (e.g., hypokalemic and hyperkalemic periodic paralysis), transmembrane/longitudinal currents and the resulting action potential/CMAP may be diminished or even absent.

Anomalous Innervation and CMAP Amplitude

Since the ratio of proximal/distal CMAP amplitudes is of major importance (see sections on conduction block, temporal dispersion), other phenomena that affect CMAP proximal/distal amplitude ratios must be discussed. One of these phenomena is the presence of anomalous motor innervation (e.g., an accessory peroneal nerve or the Martin-Gruber anastomosis). When an accessory peroneal nerve is present, it passes behind the lateral malleolus and may innervate some or all of the extensor digitorum brevis. It is not stimulated when peroneal nerve conduction studies are carried out in standard fashion, where the distal stimulation point is over the deep peroneal nerve on the anterior ankle. The amplitude of the CMAP obtained by distal stimulation will be lower than the CMAP obtained with proximal stimulation. The presence of this anomaly may be detected by stimulating behind the lateral malleolus and recording from the extensor digitorum brevis.

The Martin-Gruber anastomosis (Fig. 11-5) occurs when motor axons innervating normally ulnar innervated intrinsic hand muscles pass in the proximal median nerve and "crossover" to the ulnar nerve in the forearm. When ulnar nerve conduction studies are performed, the CMAP obtained with distal stimulation is larger than the CMAP obtained with proximal stimulation since the axons that crossover in the forearm are stimulated at the wrist but not at the elbow. This may be mistakenly interpreted as indicating conduction block in the forearm if the Martin-Gruber anastomosis is not detected. The reverse may occur when studying the median nerve; that is, higher median CMAP amplitudes are obtained when stimulating at the elbow, since ulnar bound axons involved in the crossover and innervating muscles of the thenar eminence will be stimulated at the elbow but not at the wrist. The median-ulnar crossover should be suspected when the above pattern of median/ulnar distal/proximal CMAP amplitude ratios is obtained. The anastomosis can usually be confirmed by stimulating the median nerve at the elbow and recording from normally ulnar-innervated intrinsic hand muscles. Details on variations of the Martin-Gruber crossover are provided by Gutmann and co-workers[39] and Stevens.[82]

Normal/Abnormal Findings in Motor Nerve Conduction Studies

PROLONGED DISTAL LATENCIES. Distal motor latencies may be interpreted in essentially the same fashion as distal sensory latencies. The relationship between prolonged distal latencies and evoked response amplitude remains the same, although for slightly different reasons.

DECREASED EVOKED RESPONSE AMPLITUDES. Decreased CMAP amplitudes may be seen primarily with the following:

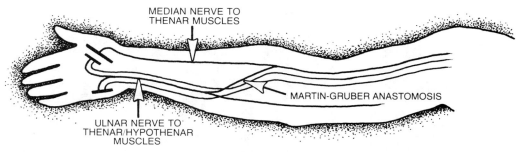

Figure 11-5. The Martin-Gruber anastomosis is present when motor axons that normally enter the ulnar nerve in the brachial plexus travel instead in the median nerve until the level of the forearm, where they then "crossover" into the ulnar nerve. This creates a situation in which these fibers are stimulated in the median nerve at the elbow but in the ulnar nerve at the wrist. Ulnar nerve CMAP amplitudes may therefore appear to drop with stimulation at the elbow relative to the wrist since more axons are stimulated at the wrist. This may mimic conduction block and cause confusion if not identified. The median CMAP amplitude is usually higher with stimulation at the elbow than at the wrist.

1. Disorders that decrease the density of functionally innervated muscle fibers within the pickup radius of the electrode: anterior horn cell disease, neuropathies, neuromuscular junction disorders, muscle fiber segmental necrosis
2. Disorders that affect the action potential current generating capacity of the muscle fiber: myopathies
3. Temporal dispersion
4. Conduction block
5. Anomalous innervation
6. Technical factors such as poor electrode placement, massive soft tissue swelling at the electrode site, or submaximal stimulation

The number of motor axons innervating a muscle may be markedly reduced, but the CMAP can be normal if all muscle fibers have been reinnervated (*e.g.,* as can occur in old poliomyelitis). CMAP amplitudes are therefore more likely to be decreased in acute lesions in which reinnervation has not had time to occur, as opposed to old or chronic lesions in which enough motor axons have survived to carry out full reinnervation of denervated muscle fibers.

DECREASED CONDUCTION VELOCITIES. Decreased conduction velocities in motor nerves can be interpreted according to the same principles as can conduction velocities in sensory nerves.

INCREASED TEMPORAL DISPERSION. Increased temporal dispersion may be interpreted in the same manner as for sensory conduction studies. In the absence of crossovers or conduction block, which might alter the ratio of distal to proximal amplitudes, a proximal/distal CMAP amplitude ratio of 0.7 or lower in conjunction with a proximal/distal CMAP duration ratio greater than approximately 1.2 can be taken as presumptive evidence of temporal dispersion due to demyelination.[2] If crossovers or conduction block are present, then the proximal/distal CMAP amplitude ratio may be of little value and the identification of temporal dispersion must be made on the basis of the proximal/distal CMAP duration ratio alone. Proximal to distal CMAP *area* ratios may be of value in distinguishing temporal dispersion from conduction block as discussed previously.

REPETITIVE FIRING. Repetitive firing is an infrequently seen phenomenon in which a single stimulus to a motor nerve results in a second peak in addition to the primary response. The second peak is usually superimposed on the trailing edge of the primary peak and is usually of significantly lower amplitude. Repetitive firing is seen with anti-acetylcholinesterase toxicity and in an extremely rare disorder of the neuromuscular junction, hereditary acetylcholinesterase deficiency.[36] It should be specifically sought when myasthenics on large doses of anti-acetylcholinesterase medications are being evaluated for an acute exacerbation and it is unclear whether the correct diagnosis is myasthenic crisis or cholinergic crisis.

TEMPORAL COURSE OF CMAP AMPLITUDE ABNORMALITIES. Temporal evolution of abnormalities in motor nerve conduction studies may be analyzed according to the same principles as sensory nerve conduction studies with one exception. When a motor axon is transected, neuromuscular transmission fails well before failure of axonal action potential propagation. As an approximation, complete neuromuscular junction transmission failure occurs by 3 to 7 days, while axonal conduction may persist for an additional 3 to 7 days. Since it is the axon potential that is recorded directly in sensory conduction studies, the SNAP can be recorded for 1 to 3 days after CMAPs become unobtainable secondary to failure of neuromuscular transmission.

Late Responses

H Reflex

The H reflex (H response) represents the electrical analog of the muscle stretch reflex minus the involvement of the muscle spindle. This reflex is obtained by distal stimulation of IA afferent fibers from muscle spindles, which in turn conduct into the spinal cord, initiating the monosynaptic stretch reflex and evoking a motor response in the muscle involved (see Fig. 11-2A). Although it occurs normally in a few other muscles, the only H reflex routinely used for clinical purposes is that involved in the ankle jerk reflex and recorded from the gastrocsoleus muscles. The widespread presence of the H reflex in muscles in which it does not frequently occur suggests hyperreflexia as a result of upper motor neuron pathology.

In most applications, only the latency of the H reflex is used since the factors influencing the amplitude are complex and not easily interpreted. The H reflex therefore provides information related to conduction velocity and differs from standard nerve conduction studies in that it involves the proximal portion of the plexi and roots that are difficult to study directly. This fact allows the H reflex to detect demyelination when pathology is limited to the proximal portions of the nerves and roots, a situation in which the results of standard conduction studies will usually be normal. This situation is frequently encountered in evaluating patients with probable Guillain-Barré syndrome. The H reflex may also prove useful for evaluating focal radicular disease at the S1 level.[6, 89] It is not a sensitive index of focal radiculopathies at other levels or of lesions such as plexopathies unless they heavily involve S1 axons. Kimura[53] has provided a detailed discussion of the H reflex.

F Response

The F response (F wave) is produced by a stimulus-initiated action potential traveling proximally along the motor axon to the body of the anterior horn cell, triggering a secondary discharge of the same anterior horn cell (see Fig. 11-2*B*). This produces an action potential that travels distally and evokes a muscle action potential.[52] The F response, like the H reflex, is useful primarily as a long pathway nerve conduction study that examines proximal segments of the nerve, plexi, and roots. It differs from the H reflex in that it can be elicited from almost all muscles and is therefore of more general applicability. It is a multiroot level response and requires that only a small percentage of the axons be intact. It is therefore not sensitive to processes affecting a single root level or plexus branch and has relatively little applicability in the study of focal radiculopathies or plexopathies. Although the F response may be abnormal with severe radiculopathies or plexopathies, it usually provides little additional information since there are almost always many other electrodiagnostic abnormalities in this setting.[3]

EVALUATION OF THE NEUROMUSCULAR JUNCTION

Motor nerve conduction studies analyze the behavior of nerve, neuromuscular junction, and muscle fiber. With the exception of myotonic disorders and the periodic paralyses, the ability of the nerve axon and the muscle fiber to produce normal action potentials is not stressed with short bursts of repetitive stimulation at frequencies below 50 Hz. (Fifty Hertz is chosen here because is represents a common practical upper limit for stimulation frequencies in electrodiagnostic studies, not because it represents any intrinsic property of nerve or muscle.) However, repetitive stimulation of motor nerves at frequencies ranging from 2 to 50 Hz may produce clear-cut abnormalities when dysfunction of the neuromuscular junction exists, even when the results of standard motor nerve conduction studies are normal.[13, 23, 49, 61, 71, 76] For this reason, repetitive stimulation of motor nerves should be included in any electrodiagnostic evaluation in which a disorder of the neuromuscular junction may exist, such as in myasthenia gravis, the Eaton-Lambert syndrome, or drug/botulism toxicity.

Neuromuscular transmission may also be abnormal in immature neuromuscular junctions present as a result of denervation/reinnervation. Although this is usually a nonspecific finding, it may be useful for prognosticating in neuropathic conditions such as motor neuron disease, in which the presence of abnormal results with repetitive stimulation suggests large amounts of denervation/reinnervation and implies a poorer prognosis than if the results of repetitive stimulation were normal. Abnormal neuromuscular transmission may rarely be seen as a nonspecific finding with direct muscle cell damage as can be seen with inflammatory myopathies.

Basic Mechanisms and Pharmacology of Acetylcholine Synthesis, Storage, and Release in the Normal Functioning of Motor Neurons

Acetylcholine is synthesized within the nerve terminal from choline and acetyl CoA by the enzyme choline-O-acetyl transferase. It is then transported into synaptic vesicles. Current information indicates that the acetylcholine in the nerve terminal can be grossly divided into two major functional pools. The first of these pools is commonly referred to as the "immediately available" pool and constitutes a small percentage of the total acetylcholine in the nerve terminal. This is the acetylcholine that is biologically available for immediate release into the synaptic cleft during synaptic transmission. The majority of acetylcholine is in the "reserve" pool and must be first transported into the "immediately available" pool before it can be used. This phenomena of transfer to the immediately available pool is referred to as "mobilization." When a resting nerve terminal begins to fire repetitively, the size of the immediately available pool is transiently decreased until mobilization from the reserve pool occurs.

When an action potential invades the presynaptic nerve terminal, the membrane permeability to calcium increases, leading to markedly increased intracellular calcium concentrations. The increased intracellular calcium concentrations trigger, in some as yet poorly understood manner, the release of acetylcholine from the nerve terminal into the synaptic cleft. The major facts about acetylcholine release are summarized as follows:

1. Acetylcholine release is dependent on the fourth power of the the extracellular calcium concentration.
2. Acetylcholine release is antagonized by hypocalcemia or hypermagnesemia.
3. Acetylcholine is released in discrete quanta, which appear to correspond to the contents of the synaptic vesicles.
4. The number of acetylcholine quanta (M) released by a single nerve action potential can be modeled with the following equation:[63]

$$M = P \times N$$

where N is the number of acetylcholine quanta in the "immediately available" pool, and P is the probability of release. The probability of release, P, is directly related to the intracellular calcium concentration and other factors such as magnesium concentrations, presence of certain antibiotics, and other molecules that are known to affect acetylcholine release.

Acetylcholine diffuses across the synaptic cleft to bind to the postsynaptic acetylcholine receptors, resulting in an increased sodium influx into the muscle cell. This generates the miniature end plate potentials (MEPP), which sum with other MEPPs to yield the net end plate potential (EPP). The EPP will initiate a muscle cell action potential if it is suprathreshold. All other things being equal, the amplitude of the muscle cell EPP is proportional to the amount of acetylcholine released by the presynaptic nerve terminal and the number of functional postsynaptic acetylcholine receptors. Decreases in either the amount of acetylcholine released or in the number of *functional* postsynaptic acetylcholine receptors will decrease the probability of the resultant EPP being suprathreshold. Acetylcholine bound to postsynaptic acetylcholine receptors is in rapid equilibrium with free acetylcholine and is rapidly hydrolyzed to choline and acetic acid by the acetylcholinesterase enzyme bound to the postsynaptic membrane. Free choline is then taken up by the nerve terminal to complete the cycle.

Effects of Repetitive Stimulation on Acetylcholine Release by the Presynaptic Nerve Terminal

The "immediately available" pool of acetylcholine in the nerve terminal is relatively small and must be replenished by mobilization from the reserve pool during repetitive firing of the nerve terminal. When a resting nerve terminal is stimulated repetitively at 2 to 5 Hz, the rate of mobilization initially lags behind the rate of release of acetylcholine from the immediately available pool, resulting in a transient decrease in the size of the immediately available pool. Since the number of acetylcholine quanta released per nerve stimulus is proportional to the size of the immediately available pool ($M = P \times N$), this means that the actual number of acetylcholine quanta released by a single nerve impulse will progressively decrease with 2 to 5 Hz repetitive stimulation until mobilization can restore the initial size of the immediately available pool. This increased rate of mobilization from the reserve pool takes 500 to 2000 msec to occur. The net result of this phenomenon is that when a nerve is repetitively stimulated at 2 to 3 Hz, the amount of acetylcholine released drops successively during the first three to five stimuli before returning to baseline. This is usually of no significance to the normal individual, in that two to three times as much acetylcholine is released as is necessary to result in a suprathreshold postsynaptic endplate potential. However, if the amount of acetylcholine initially released is barely sufficient to result in a suprathreshold EPP (for whatever reason), this transient drop in the amount of acetylcholine released may actually result in subthreshold EPPs during the initial three to five stimuli at 2 to 3 Hz. When observed at the single fiber level, an "all or none" phenomenon would be seen (i.e., a normal muscle cell action potential or no potential at all). When simultaneously observing a large number of muscle fibers in a muscle, as is done with standard motor nerve conduction studies, a certain percentage of muscle fibers would fail to fire. This will manifest itself as a "decrement" in the CMAP amplitude recorded during several of the initial stimuli at 2 to 5 Hz (Fig. 11-6). The majority of the decrement will occur between the first and second stimuli. This "decrement" serves as the basis for electrodiagnostic testing of the neuromuscular junction by this technique. Normal subjects demonstrate less than a 5% decrement with repetitive stimulation when technical artifacts such as electrode or stimulator movement are eliminated.

Acetylcholine release is facilitated (increased probability of release) by high rates of stimulation (e.g., 20 to 50 Hz) or by the functional equivalent, maximal exercise. This phenomenon may outweigh the decrease in the amount of acetylcholine release caused by a decrease in the immediately available pool size. It is then possible that no failure of neuromuscular transmission may be observed at 20 to 50 Hz, while clear failure may occur at 2 to 3 Hz. It is for this reason that repetitive stimulation testing at 2 to 3 Hz is included in the evaluation of diseases of the neuromuscular junction such as myasthenia gravis. Stimulation frequencies of 20 to 50 Hz are still used in eliciting facilitation and in the evaluation of the Eaton-Lambert syndrome and botulism.[24, 25]

Facilitation by relatively high stimulation frequencies is believed to occur because higher intracellular calcium concentrations (resulting in increased acetylcholine release) can be achieved with high frequencies (20 to 50 Hz) than with frequencies in the 2 to 3 Hz range. This is also the explanation for why a decrement observed on repetitive stimulation in myasthenia gravis will be eliminated (i.e., repaired) by having the patient exercise vigorously for 5 to 10 seconds prior to repetitive stimulation.

In the myasthenic syndrome (Lambert-Eaton syndrome), a presynaptic defect of neuromuscular transmission results in failure of neuromuscular transmission in rested neuromuscular junctions. This is evidenced in standard nerve conduction studies by a reduced CMAP amplitude. If low CMAP amplitudes are due to the Lambert-Eaton syndrome, a marked increment (> 100%) in the CMAP amplitude will be seen with high-frequency stimulation (20 to 50 Hz), or after maximal exercise. This increment is also believed to be due to increased presynaptic nerve terminal calcium concentrations.

Single Fiber Electromyography

Single fiber EMG is an extremely powerful tool for the evaluation of the neuromuscular junction.[77, 81] It is performed by positioning an electrode with a very small recording surface (25 μ diameter) such that it simultaneously records the single fiber action potentials (SFAPs) from two or more muscle fibers within the same motor unit. The interpotential interval between these two SFAPs is then measured and analyzed (Fig. 11-7). It has been well established that the duration of this interpotential interval (1 to 4 msec) is not constant from one firing of the motor unit to the next but has a variation averaging 10 to 60 μsec. This variability occurs primarily in the time required for neuromuscular transmission to occur and is related to the time at which the muscle cell EPP reaches threshold value (see Fig. 11-7). If the EPP amplitude is high, the muscle fiber threshold is reached early in the EPP and the time of threshold occurrence relative to the

Figure 11-6. Repetitive stimulation of a motor nerve at 2 Hz. (A) In the normal person, the amplitude of the CMAP shows no significant decrement (<5%). (B) When impaired neuromuscular transmission is present, a decrement greater than approximately 5% may be seen during the first few (one to four) stimuli.

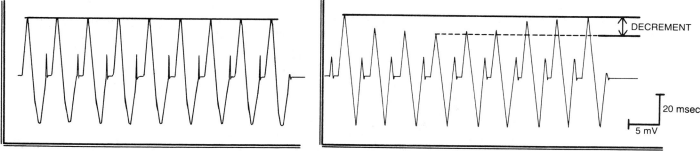

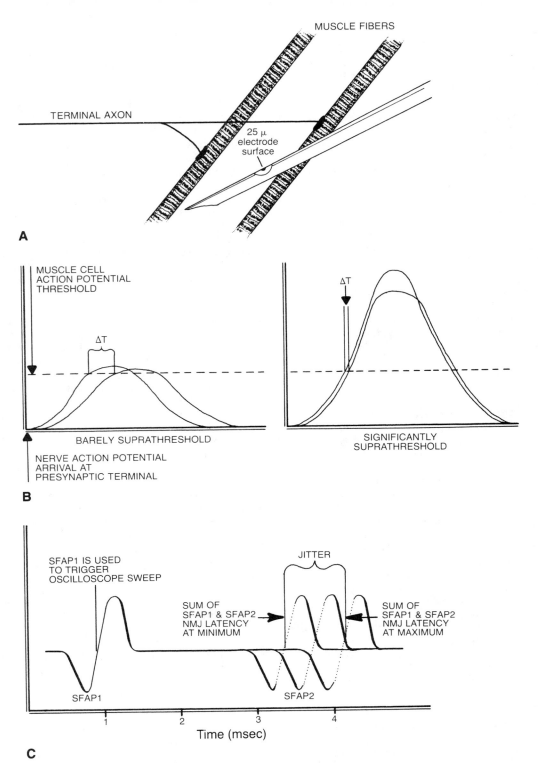

Figure 11-7. Jitter. (*A*) Fiber/electrode position. The recording electrode is positioned such that the SFAPs from two or more single muscle fibers from the same motor unit are recorded simultaneously. (*B*) Muscle cell end plate potential (EPP). Two barely suprathreshold and two significantly suprathreshold EPPs are shown. The neuromuscular junction (NMJ) latency is defined as the elapsed time from the arrival of the nerve action potential at the synaptic terminal to the time that the postsynaptic EPP reaches the threshold for an action potential. Note that the neuromuscular junction latency is relatively independent of EPP amplitude when the EPP is well above the threshold value, while the neuromuscular junction latency varies significantly when the EPP is barely suprathreshold. (*C*) Jitter. The "interpotential interval" (IPI) is the difference in time between the arrival of the first and second SFAPs at the recording electrode site. The variability in the IPI has been shown to be due primarily to variability in the neuromuscular latency of the two fibers involved, which in turn is affected by the factors outlined in (*B*) above. The variability in the IPI is termed the *jitter* and is increased when neuromuscular function is abnormal.

arrival of the action potential at the nerve terminal does not vary much from one firing to the next. If the EPP amplitude is low and variable, as is the case in many disorders of the neuromuscular junction, then threshold values are reached near the peak of the EPP where the time of occurrence relative to the arrival of the nerve action potential may vary widely. This variability is known as the "neuromuscular jitter." If the EPP is barely threshold, failure may intermittently occur, a phenomenon known as "blocking." If an abnormal decrement of the CMAP amplitude is observed on repetitive stimulation, blocking must be present on SFEMG. However, jitter may be markedly increased even when there is no overt failure of neuromuscular transmission. The SFEMG is therefore a much more sensitive technique, albeit more difficult, for diagnosing disorders of the neuromuscular junction than is repetitive stimulation. Patients who have normal standard repetitive stimulation studies but who are strongly suspected of having a disorder of neuromuscular junction function should have SFEMG studies.

Single fiber EMG also has the ability to provide an indirect estimate of motor unit fiber density (*i.e.*, the number of muscle fibers per unit cross-sectional area belonging to a single motor unit). This is done by randomly inserting the SFEMG electrode next to single muscle fibers and counting the number of additional SFAPs that can be recorded in that location. Normal values range from 1.3 to 1.7, depending on the muscle. This parameter will frequently be abnormal in many disease processes that result in anatomical reorganization of the motor (*e.g.*, motor neuron disease or some myopathies).

THE NEEDLE ELECTRODE EXAMINATION

The needle electrode examination comprises the remaining major component of the electrodiagnostic evaluation. Although nerve conduction studies provide information primarily on the numbers and physiological state of functioning nerve axons and muscle fibers, the needle electrode examination provides additional information on the physiological state of individual muscle fibers, the anatomical organization of the motor unit, motor unit recruitment properties, and other motor unit phenomenon (*e.g.*, fasciculations).

Basic Physiology and Pathophysiology

Before discussing pathophysiology, some basic definitions and concepts will be reviewed. Subsequent sections will discuss each topic in more detail.

Insertional Activity

As the needle electrode is passed through muscle fibers, the tip is alternately exposed to and detects the extracellular poten-

tial (approximately 0 mV) and the intracellular potential (approximately -70 mV). Additionally, the muscle cell transmembrane potential may be destabilized enough by the passage of the electrode to generate a muscle membrane action potential, adding to the electrical activity detected by the electrode. Since insertional activity is usually evaluated at an amplifier gain setting of 50 to 100 μV per division (500 to 1000 μV from the top to the bottom of the screen on most EMG machines), the potential changes encountered by the needle electrode (10,000 to 50,000 μV) are sufficient to cause the trace on the oscilloscope to deflect off of the screen. Depending on the low-frequency response of the amplifier, this insertional activity should return to baseline in 500 to 1000 msec or less. In normal muscle, there should be near electrical silence after electrode movement ceases. The primary value of insertional activity is that it tells the electromyographer when the needle electrode is actually in muscle tissue. Markedly decreased insertional activity (as seen when minimal electric potential changes are detected when the electrode is moved) indicates that either the electrode is not in muscle or that the muscle has undergone severe atrophy and replacement by nonelectrically active tissues such as fat or connective tissue. This finding is common in the intrinsic muscles of the feet in the presence of a severe polyneuropathy, or in any muscle after long-standing, severe denervation.

Spontaneous Activity

Normal muscle should be virtually electrically silent when the patient is relaxed and the electrode is not being moved. Persistent electrical activity after the needle electrode has stopped moving may be related to the following:

1. Voluntary motor unit activity secondary to poor relaxation
2. Normal electrical events (*e.g.*, motor end plate noise or nerve potentials, detected because of fortuitous placement of the electrode)
3. A state of the motor unit associated with abnormal nerve and/or muscle membrane stability
   a. Abnormal muscle fiber states. The most common form of this type of spontaneous activity is the presence of "positive sharp waves" and/or "fibrillation potentials" (Fig. 11-8). Although muscle fiber spontaneous activity may be seen with other conditions (*e.g.*, acid maltase deficiency), the most common etiology is the marked membrane electrical instability that results when a muscle fiber (or segment of a fiber) loses its innervation. A large amount of electrophysiologic data suggests that fibrillation potentials are relatively normal SFAPs recorded remote from the point of generation of the action potential. Positive sharp waves (see Fig. 11-8) also are believed to represent SFAPs. Positive sharp waves are thought to occur when the electrode is in contact with the damaged muscle fiber and the action potential is blocked at this site or the repolarization phase

Figure 11-8. Spontaneous activity.

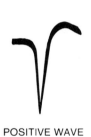

POSITIVE WAVE

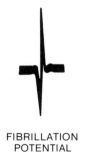

FIBRILLATION POTENTIAL

50 μV

5 msec

of the action potential is markedly slowed. Fibrillation potentials, on the other hand, are believed to represent a normally conducted action potential recorded at a distance from the muscle fiber.

The length of time required for positive sharp waves and fibrillation potentials to appear in a denervated muscle is proportional to the length of nerve remaining in continuity with the muscle. For example, if a nerve root is severed at the spinal foramen, spontaneous activity may appear in the paraspinous muscles 1 to 2 weeks before it appears in distal muscles of the extremities. Likewise, if the median nerve is cut at the wrist, spontaneous activity will appear earlier than if the lesion is located in the axilla. It is generally believed that spontaneous activity may take as long as 3 weeks to appear in distal muscles when the lesion is proximal at the root level. These factors should be considered when examining an evolving lesion.

The presence of spontaneous activity is related to the stage of a pathological process. It may take weeks to begin following an insult and may then resolve completely if all of the muscle fibers are reinnervated. This should be considered when attempting to decide whether the absence of spontaneous activity mitigates against a particular diagnosis (*e.g.,* the electrodiagnostic examination may have been performed either before or after spontaneous activity was present).

b. Fasciculations: Spontaneous, repetitive single discharges of individual motor units. Fasciculations may be seen in motor neuron disease, polyneuropathies, radiculopathies, and benign idiopathic conditions.

c. Complex repetitive discharge (CRDs); also known as high-frequency discharges or iterative discharges): A relatively nonspecific abnormality noted in a wide range of disorders such as polyneuropathies, radiculopathies, and inflammatory myopathies. CRDs are usually associated with chronic disorders.

d. Myotonic discharges: Associated with myotonic disorders, myotonic dystrophy, myotonia congenita, paramyotonia congenita,[84] and hyperkalemic periodic paralysis.

e. Myokymia: Grouped repetitive discharges most often associated with postirradiation nerve damage, old neurogenic lesions, and multiple sclerosis.

f. Neuromyotonia Associated with continuous motor unit activity syndromes.

A more detailed discussion of the characteristics and significance of the types of spontaneous activity listed in *b*

through *f* is beyond the scope of this discussion, and the reader is referred elsewhere.[21, 28, 54]

Motor Unit Action Potential Configuration

The motor unit action potential (MUAP) represents the summation of single fiber action potentials (SFAPs) from the muscle fibers in a given motor unit. Because the origin of the MUAP is complex, an extensive discussion will be devoted toward analyzing it. Many types of motor unit pathology will produce characteristic changes in the duration, amplitude, polyphasia, and variability of amplitude of the MUAP (Fig. 11-9).

Recruitment

Recruitment refers to the pattern in which motor units are activated. The force produced by a muscle can be controlled by changing either the actual number of active motor units and/or by changing the firing frequency of individual motor units.[31] As the motor unit discharge frequency increases, muscle fibers develop increasing force up to a plateau known as the "maximum tetanic tension" (Po).[72] In humans, motor units are capable of discharging from a minimum of 2 to 3 Hz up to 30 to 60 Hz (or even as high as 100 Hz and above under special circumstances). The general scheme used by spinal cord mechanisms is to recruit "low threshold" motor units and increase force output by increasing their discharge frequency slightly, while simultaneously recruiting additional motor units with slightly higher thresholds. The frequency at which a motor unit starts firing is referred to as its "onset frequency," and the frequency at which the next motor unit is recruited is referred to as the "recruitment frequency" of the preceding unit.[70] In conditions in which there is substantial axonal loss, as in a severe radiculopathy or polyneuropathy, onset and/or recruitment frequencies of the initial motor unit pool are increased. This situation, however, is referred to as "decreased recruitment," since a given level of force is produced by *fewer* MUAPs firing at higher average rates relative to the normal situation.

When a myopathy is suspected, the other "recruitment abnormality" that must be considered is "rapid recruitment." To refer to this condition as an abnormality of recruitment is misleading, however, because the pattern of recruitment of individual MUAPs is essentially normal. The abnormality noted in a myopathy is that a larger number of motor units must be recruited or activated to produce a given force output. Evaluating rapid recruitment, therefore, requires knowledge of the force

Figure 11-9. Schematic motor unit action potential (MUAP) characteristics are labeled. This MUAP has four major phases (three baseline crossings plus one). Note that both of the major positive (downward) deflections are serrated.

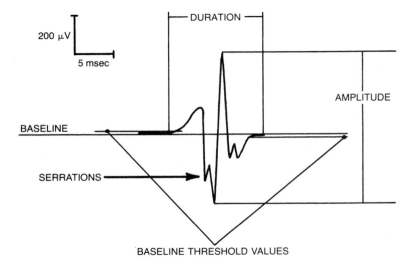

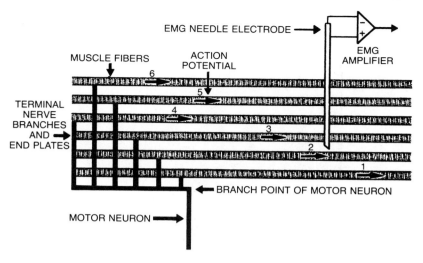

Figure 11-10. Schematic representation of motor unit action potential (MUAP) generation and recording by concentric needle electrode. The neuronal action potential diverges at the branch point of the motor neuron to asynchronously initiate muscle fiber action potentials. The muscle fiber action potentials then travel toward the electrode position at approximately 4 meters/sec. Location of the respective muscle fiber action potentials at a single point in time is shown by the numbered arrows.

produced in addition to the recruitment information obtained from the needle electrode in the muscle. This is not true in the case of decreased recruitment, which can be identified using only the information present on the screen of the EMG machine.

Analysis of MUAP Electrophysiology

The motor unit electrophysiology necessary for an in-depth understanding of the EMG needle electrode examination is discussed in the following section. A mechanistic approach is taken using relatively simple models. Thus, a few comments on biological models are in order. In all cases involving modeling of biological phenomena, there is a tradeoff between accuracy and simplicity; that is, the more accurate a model of a given phenomenon, the more complex and less easily understood it is. Simplicity, as opposed to complexity, will be emphasized in the following discussion. More detailed descriptions are provided by Boyd and co-workers[5] and Griep and associates.[38]

*Modeling of the MUAP**

The motor unit can be considered to consist of approximately 150 infinitely long, parallel muscle fibers arranged in a cylindrical fashion (Fig. 11-10). Between these muscle fibers are fibers belonging to other motor units. The number of muscle fibers per unit cross-sectional area is defined as the "fiber density." Do not confuse this with the fiber density as determined by SFEMG. They are different, although they both measure the same motor unit characteristic. An innervation zone is then selected for the fibers where the anterior horn cell divides to provide innervation to each individual muscle fiber. Lastly, the electrode is positioned a "significant distance" away from the innervation zone. The term *significant distance* refers to a point where motor end plate events related to the initiation of the muscle SFAP are not detected by the electrode; all that the electrode detects is the muscle fiber action potential moving toward it. This arrangement represents the majority of electrode positions used by the clinical electromyographer.

The anterior horn cell action potential travels down the axon to the point where the axon branches to supply all the individual muscle fibers (see Fig. 11-10). At this point, the individual action

potentials of the terminal nerve branches are synchronized. Because the lengths of the terminal nerve branches to the individual muscle fibers are not identical, and because the conduction velocities probably are not identical in each terminal nerve branch, all muscle fibers in the motor unit are not activated simultaneously. The action potentials of fibers closest to the branch point of the motor nerve will be initiated before the muscle fibers that are farthest away from the motor neuron branch point. Owing to the anatomical spread of motor end plates, not all muscle fiber action potentials start exactly in the same location. The action potentials of some muscle fibers therefore have a head start in reaching the electrode. After each individual muscle fiber is activated, their action potentials travel down the muscle fibers at 2 to 4 meters/sec toward the electrode position. Additionally, because the conduction velocities of individual muscle fibers are not identical, by the time the group of SFAPs reaches the electrode position there will be a difference of approximately 4 msec or less between the time of arrival of the earliest and latest SFAP in a given area of a normal motor unit.[81] What the EMG machine displays is the net sum of these individual SFAPs passing by the recording electrode.

It has been previously stated that the MUAP is the summation of the SFAPs in that motor unit and it has been shown how a group of SFAPs pass the electrode position in a spread-out (temporally dispersed) fashion. The relative position of the electrode and a given muscle fiber has a major effect on the contribution of that SFAP to the overall MUAP as well.

The potential represented in Figure 11-11*A* is an approximation of the SFAP under the recording conditions used by the clinical electromyographer. An in-depth discussion of this potential is provided by the Stalberg and Trontelj;[81] and Rosenfalck.[74].

The action potential consists of an initial positive deflection and a terminal negative deflection. The positive and negative deflections are usually of approximately equal amplitude and duration, depending on the exact electrode position.

The middle portion of the potential, extending from the positive peak to the negative peak, is the "major deflection" of the potential, and its slope is related to what is called the "rise time" of the potential. The higher the slope of the major deflection, the shorter the rise time of the potential. This is a function of the distance from the electrode to the single fiber.

The absolute amplitude of the SFAP is approximately proportional to the square of the diameter of the muscle fiber. For a given electrode position, a 100μ diameter muscle fiber will produce an action potential roughly four times larger than a 50μ fiber.

---

*Familiarity with the basic definitions and anatomy of skeletal muscle motor units is assumed. Details regarding normal values for MUAP duration, polyphasia, and amplitude are presented elsewhere.[11, 15, 16, 50, 75]

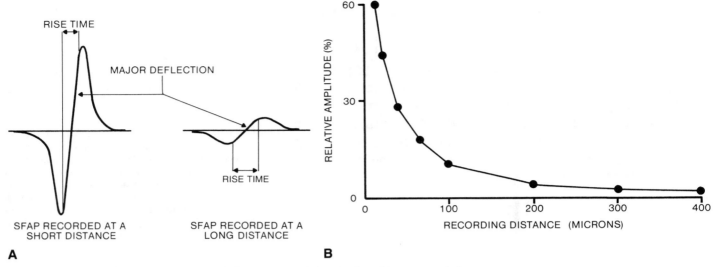

Figure 11-11. Single fiber action potential characteristics. (*A*) Examples of SFAPs recorded near and far away from the single fiber. The rise time progressively increases and the peak-to-peak amplitude falls exponentially (*B*) as the distance from the muscle fiber to the recording electrode increases. This occurs over a relatively short distance. The rise time is usually defined as the time required for a potential to change from 10% to 90% of its maximum value.

Examining the effect of electrode distance on the SFAP configuration, there are several major points (Fig. 11-11*B*):

1. The peak-to-peak amplitude of the action potential decreases exponentially as the distance from the electrode to the single fiber increases.
2. The amplitude of the leading and trailing edges of the SFAP falls off much less rapidly than the peak-to-peak amplitudes as the electrode–fiber distance increases.
3. The slope of the major deflection decreases markedly (*i.e.,* the rise time increases considerably) as the electrode–fiber distance increases.

From these observations the following conclusions can be made regarding the effects of fiber–electrode distance on the contribution of individual single fibers to the observed MUAP:

1. The appearance of the MUAP will be dominated by those fibers very close to the electrode because of the exponential fall-off of single fiber peak-to-peak action potential amplitude with increasing distance from the electrode. Extremely high amplitudes can be obtained by being very close to a single fiber. In this situation, however, the high amplitude will be associated with a very short rise time of the major deflection of the potential, and the amplitude observed will be critically dependent on electrode position (*e.g.,* minor adjustments in electrode position will cause major changes in the peak-to-peak amplitude of the MUAP). This is the major reason why it is difficult to clinically quantitate MUAP amplitude, since variable fiber–electrode distances produce marked variations in the observed peak-to-peak amplitude. A wide range of MUAP amplitudes can therefore be obtained from a given motor unit simply by altering electrode position.
2. Fibers that are remote from the electrode will contribute significantly more to the duration than they do to the peak-to-peak amplitude, primarily because of the manner in which duration is determined (see Fig. 11-9). Although a few close fibers (one to ten) may dominate MUAP amplitude, there are

many more muscle fibers (150 to 1,500) that are remote from the electrode, making low-amplitude contributions (<10 to 50 μV) to the initial, middle, and trailing edges of the MUAP. Since average MUAP peak-to-peak amplitudes will be in the range of 400 to 2,000 μV for most electrode types, these low-amplitude contributions to overall peak-to-peak amplitude will not be significant. The low-amplitude contribution to the measured MUAP duration does, however, make a significant difference. Since MUAP duration is defined as the difference in time between the initial deviation from baseline by a threshold amount (*e.g.,* 5 to 10 μV) and the time where it falls below the threshold value in returning to the baseline, small contributions to the amplitude in the leading and trailing regions of the MUAP will increase the measured duration.

Factors Influencing MUAP Duration, Polyphasia, and Amplitude

Using the above information regarding the anatomical and physiological factors that determine the MUAP configuration, we will refine our understanding as follows:

DURATION. The duration of the MUAP is determined by several factors:

1. The difference in arrival time between the earliest and latest SFAPS. Early and late SFAPS from muscle fibers *close* to the electrode have a major influence on duration.
2. The absolute number of muscle fibers in a motor unit. This is directly correlated with duration, since even distant early- and late-arriving muscle fibers will contribute a few microvolts to the leading and trailing edges of the MUAP, respectively, keeping the MUAP amplitude above the threshold values for determining duration.
3. Increased fiber density. All other parameters being equal, this will increase the measured MUAP duration, since the SFAPS from more muscle fibers at the leading and trailing edges of

the MUAP make a detectable contribution to the potential detected by the electrode.

AMPLITUDE. The amplitude of the MUAP is determined by the number of muscle fibers "very close" to the electrode. This in turn is a function of muscle fiber density and electrode position. When MUAP amplitude is dominated by a single fiber, the rise time of the major deflection is extremely short and the MUAP amplitude changes drastically with minor changes in electrode position.

MUAP POLYPHASIA. MUAP polyphasia is a difficult concept to define rigorously, and, in fact, there is no completely satisfactory method of measuring polyphasia. One definition of polyphasia states that the number of MUAP phases is equal to the number of baseline zero crossings plus one, with MUAPs having greater than four phases being considered "polyphasic" (see Fig. 11-9). Although simple and convenient, this definition is also inadequate. The other definition of polyphasia is based on the number of slope reversals, known as "serrations," in the MUAP. The serration definition, which is a more general index of polyphasia, is preferable, since pathological processes of interest may produce serrations without crossing the baseline.

Using the model developed so far, one can consider the MUAP that results if all SFAPS reach the electrode simultaneously. The resultant MUAP will resemble a large SFAP, and there will be no polyphasia.

The other extreme of polyphasia can be illustrated by considering a motor unit with ten muscle fibers located equidistant from the electrode. The arrival time of each SFAP will be chosen so that sequential SFAPs reach the electrode as the previous SFAP has almost passed by. (Line up ten SFAPs "head to tail.") The resultant MUAP will have 20 phases, as determined by baseline crossings, plus 1 with no serrations. Sometimes, an SFAP will arrive late so that it is completely separated from the main MUAP. This is referred to as a "satellite" potential or "linked potential" (LP), and usually suggests reinnervation with immature, slowly conducting terminal nerve branches. If the arrival times of the SFAPs are moved closer together, the resultant MUAP becomes serrated with fewer baseline crossings but remains highly polyphasic. From these illustrations, it can be concluded that MUAP polyphasia is produced primarily by temporal dispersion of SFAPs from muscle fibers close to the electrode when there is enough temporal separation between SFAPs that they retain their individual identities.

MUAP Recruitment

As discussed previously, the spinal cord modulates the force developed by a muscle by controlling both the number of motor units firing and the rate at which the motor units are firing. Excellent discussions of motor unit recruitment can be found elsewhere.[19, 20, 31, 42] Now consider the case of a "ramp" contraction when the force developed by a muscle is gradually and slowly increased from zero up to a moderate level. (This may be 10% to 20% of a maximum voluntary contraction [MVC] for a normal muscle and up to 100% of an MVC in a weak muscle.) This is the only type of contraction that is routinely of interest to the electromyographer performing the needle electrode examination. In a ramp contraction, motor units are recruited at their onset frequency and their rate of firing is increased (rate modulation) until the recruitment frequency is reached and an additional motor unit is recruited. Different muscles use recruitment and rate modulation to varying degrees.[31] Disregarding the effects of inhibitory reflexes and other influences not covered

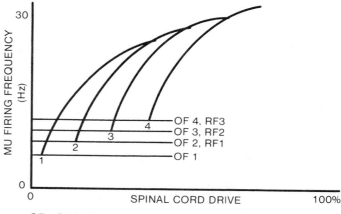

Figure 11-12. Recruitment. Schematicized representation of the discharge characteristics of the first four motor units recruited as the strength of the contraction increases. The electromyographer is generally focusing on the onset and recruitment frequencies of the first few motor units. In this model of recruitment, if motor unit 2 is lost for some reason, the onset frequency of unit 2 and the recruitment frequency of unit 1 are replaced by the onset frequency of unit 3 and the recruitment frequency of unit 2. The average firing frequency of all motor units will be increaased for the number of motor units that have been recruited.

here, recruitment will be discussed using the model in Figure 11-12. Detailed discussions of recruitment are provided by Burke,[19, 20] Henneman,[42] and De Luca.[31]

MUAP unit recruitment and modulation of firing rates are done by spinal cord–level mechanisms that receive their input from the corticospinal tracts as well as other neuronal systems. The intensity of this input signal is referred to as spinal cord "drive"; that is, a weak contraction has a low drive to the spinal cord mechanisms controlling a given muscle, while a strong contraction has a high "drive."

Each motor neuron belonging to a given muscle "pool" possesses properties that determine the probability of firing at any given level of spinal cord drive. For example, the first unit recruited has a probability of firing at almost any nonzero spinal cord motor drive level, while the last motor unit recruited has almost no probability of firing until spinal cord motor drive reaches its highest levels. Low-threshold units are generally type I, fatigue-resistant units, while high-threshold units tend to be type II, rapidly fatigable motor units.[19, 20]

Increased spinal cord motor drive will first cause a motor unit to start discharging at its onset frequency when its recruitment threshold is reached. The discharge rate will continue to increase with increasing motor drive until a plateau value is reached.

Decreased Recruitment

Now consider the first six motor units normally recruited in a muscle and damage the motor neurons belonging to motor units 2, 4, and 6 without affecting units 1, 3 and 5. Assume that this does not alter the recruitment properties of units 1, 3 and 5. When spinal cord drive increases to the level attained when the first six motor units were recruited, only units 1, 3, and 5 will be firing and less force will be developed, since the contributions of units 2, 4, and 6 will be missing. As the spinal cord drive is increased from zero, unit 1 is recruited normally, but the recruitment frequency for unit 1 is now the frequency at which unit 3 is recruited, not unit 2 as was the case previously; that is, unit 1 is firing more rapidly than normal when the next unit is recruited. A similar situation occurs for subsequent motor units recruited. Lastly, to achieve the previous force levels, spinal cord drive must increase to produce a higher percentage of maximum voluntary contraction, resulting in higher overall firing frequencies for each motor unit and perhaps the recruitment of additional motor units. Muscles with both normal and subnormal strength may demonstrate decreased motor unit recruitment. There may be a significant decrease in the number of functioning anterior horn cells innervating a muscle, producing decreased motor unit recruitment, but if all of the muscle fibers are reinnervated by functional axons, strength may be normal. This is frequently seen in old poliomyelitis. The presence of decreased recruitment therefore indicates that a significant percentage of the motor neurons and/or their axons originally innervating a muscle are nonfunctional. This may be due to irreversible causes (*e.g.,* motor neuron death) or reversible causes, (*e.g.,* demyelination and conduction block of the axon). Decreased recruitment may therefore be reversible.

In summary, then, these are the major features of decreased recruitment:

1. Elevated recruitment and/or onset frequencies
2. Higher average firing rates of individual motor units for the number of motor units recruited

This latter condition is the condition most often recognized in clinical practice since recruitment and onset frequencies are usually elevated by very small amounts that must be evaluated on a statistical basis unless axonal loss is extremely severe. It is most easily appreciated since motor units will be observed firing at high rates that would normally be obscured by the concomitant firing of other motor units. No knowledge of force production is necessary to identify the above conditions.

Unless the decrease in numbers of motor units is so severe that the majority of units are recruited under the conditions used, this technique of examining recruitment involves only the first few motor units recruited, thereby ignoring a large part of the motor unit pool. Much effort has gone into examining late motor unit recruitment, but these techniques have limitations and are not routinely used. Note that the model assumes that axonal loss is randomly distributed over all types of motor units (early and late recruited units).

One feature of this recruitment model is that for decreased recruitment to occur, a large number of motor neurons must be nonfunctional, meaning that a loss of 5 to 20% of motor units or possibly even more will probably not be detectable. Recruitment analysis is a relatively *insensitive* indicator of the extent of neuronal damage and demonstrates unequivocal abnormalities only when a large percentage of motor neurons is nonfunctional.

Abnormalities Detected by Needle Electrode Examination

The motor unit changes described in subsequent paragraphs are artificially separated according to the underlying mechanism. Many real-life situations will have several of these mechanisms operating simultaneously, producing abnormalities that are the sum of the individual phenomena. Partial loss refers to the loss of a percentage of the motor neurons innervating a given muscle.

Significant Partial and Permanent Axonal/Motor Neuron Loss (Discrete Insult, No Continuing Axonal Loss), With Surviving Axons

Partial and permanent axonal/motor neuron loss may be seen in partial nerve transection (axonotmetic lesion), acute poliomyelitis, some cases of Guillain-Barré syndrome, radiculopathy, plexopathy, and other lesions producing partial axonal disruption. The common factor in each of these situations is that a significant number of muscle fibers is denervated and the remaining motor neurons are capable of sprouting to reinnervate these muscle fibers. The findings here may be arbitrarily classified according to time course.

INITIAL FINDINGS. Decreased recruitment will be present immediately when axonal loss occurs, but the axonal loss must be extensive for decreased recruitment to be detected. After an appropriate time interval (1 to 3 weeks) has elapsed, spontaneous activity will be present in the form of positive sharp waves and fibrillations. Spontaneous activity may be present even if only a small percentage of axons are lost (*e.g.,* 2 to 3%).

INTERMEDIATE FINDINGS. Remaining motor units "pick up" additional muscle fibers by axonal sprouting, producing increased fiber density and increased MUAP amplitude, duration, and polyphasia. Additionally, conduction velocities in immature nerve terminals are slow, resulting in increased temporal dispersion and leading to increased duration, polyphasia, and possibly "satellite" or "linked" potentials. The magnitude of the motor unit abnormalities will increase as more and more muscle fibers are added to each motor unit. Spontaneous activity may disappear if all muscle fibers are reinnervated.

LATE FINDINGS. As the previous processes advance, it is hypothesized that maturation of terminal nerves and subsequent increases in conduction velocity will partially offset the increases in duration and polyphasia caused by increased fiber density, while the addition of more muscle fibers to the motor unit and increased conduction velocity of maturing new terminal nerve branches both contribute to increased MUAP amplitude (more SFAPs arriving at the electrode position in a more synchronous manner). This may explain why in cases of old, recovered motor neuron lesions, as seen in old poliomyelitis, increased MUAP amplitude is the dominant abnormality, whereas increased polyphasia is less prominent. Remodeling of motor units may also contribute to this process (*e.g.,* a single muscle fiber contributing to increased MUAP polyphasia and duration as a result of being innervated by a long, slowly conducting terminal nerve branch may be transiently denervated and become part of another motor unit where it does not contribute significantly to increased duration or polyphasia.

The extent of the changes seen will be proportional to the number of motor units denervated. As the percentage of motor units denervated increases, more muscle fibers will have to be picked up by fewer remaining functional motor units and the average percent increase in the number of muscle fibers per motor unit will be larger. Spontaneous activity may or may not be present, depending on whether all muscle fibers have been reinnervated.

DISCUSSION. If it is hypothesized that a motor unit must increase its number of muscle fibers by 5 to 20% before MUAP changes can be unequivocally detected (possibly an underestimate), spontaneous activity should be seen at some point after injury; that is, that many muscle fibers probably cannot be acutely denervated without spontaneous activity being present at some time. Spontaneous activity will resolve if all denervated fibers are reinnervated. Minor injuries (approximately 5% of fibers denervated) will probably not be detectable through MUAP configuration changes, although spontaneous activity should be present at some time.

Although quantitative data are lacking, it is generally believed that depending on the nature and extent of the pathological insult, somewhere between a minimum of 4 to 12 weeks is required for enough reinnervation to occur to produce detectable MUAP changes. If the electromyographer finds unequivocal MUAP changes 1 day after an acute partial nerve transection, these cannot be due to the lesion in question; they must be the result of some previous lesion.

Severe or Complete Neuronal Loss With Reinnervation

If the majority of axons innervating a muscle are disrupted, and enough time has passed to allow some reinnervation to occur, a different picture is obtained. In this case, the majority of MUAPs will be newly created by neurons regrowing into the denervated muscle, rather than by modification of preexisting motor units. The MUAP will have few muscle fibers initially and will subsequently add more muscle fibers until large numbers belong to each motor unit. Owing to the low number of muscle fibers present in early units formed in this manner, as well as to the temporal dispersion produced by slow conduction velocities in immature nerve sprouts, the resultant MUAPs typically have a long duration and low amplitude and are very polyphasic. This type of motor unit is known in the older literature as a "nascent" motor unit. There will also be a short period in which the motor unit has so few fibers that the duration may be short. As additional muscle fibers are added, these MUAPs will eventually evolve into the long-duration, high-amplitude polyphasic MUAPs characteristic of neurogenic injuries that will evolve as described in the previous section. Profuse spontaneous activity should be present within 1 to 3 weeks after the injury and should persist for long periods of time.

Partial Axonal Loss With Surviving Axons, With or Without Discrete Injury, With Ongoing Axonal Loss and Reinnervation

Partial axonal loss with surviving axons is seen in most axonal neuropathies, motor neuron disease, and some radiculopathies/plexopathies/compressive neuropathies. The electrodiagnostic findings relative to MUAP configuration changes here are similar to those discussed previously, except that the number of denervated muscle fibers at any one time may be small, and these few fibers may be reinnervated before they develop detectable spontaneous activity. Therefore, one may see MUAP changes without evidence of spontaneous activity. In these cases, SFEMG may demonstrate the increased jitter of immature neuromuscular junctions associated with denervation and subsequent reinnervation. With very slowly progressive lesions, as seen in some cases of motor neuron disease, markedly increased amplitude with less prominent polyphasia may be the predominant feature for the same reasons postulated in previous paragraphs.

It can be hypothesized that as axons are lost in the above manner, decreased motor unit recruitment should accompany the development of MUAP changes. MUAP changes are probably more easily detected than decreased recruitment, so that the detection of the former is not invariably linked to the unequivocal detection of the latter.

Demyelination of Terminal Nerve Branches

Demyelination of terminal nerve branches is seen in acute demyelinating neuropathic processes, such as Guillain-Barré syndrome, chronic inflammatory demyelinating polyneuropathies, and neuropathies such as hereditary motor sensory neuropathies I, III, and IV. It is frequently accompanied by axonal loss.

This phenomenon will increase MUAP duration and polyphasia while possibly decreasing MUAP amplitude if no axonal loss and reinnervation are involved. That is, arrival time differences at the electrode between first and last fibers increase, producing increased polyphasia and duration while the decreased synchrony of SFAP arrival actually decreases MUAP amplitude. Conduction block in terminal nerve sprouts may also contribute to decreased MUAP amplitude. If there is accompanying axonal loss (frequently seen) and enough time has elapsed for reinnervation to occur, MUAP amplitude will increase, producing the classic finding associated with neurogenic lesions as described previously.

Processes Producing Severe Atrophy of Muscle Fibers Without Segmental Necrosis of Muscle Fibers

Processes producing severe muscle fiber atrophy are seen in myopathies (e.g., corticosteroid myopathies) in which relatively little actual necrosis of muscle fibers occurs. The predominant underlying process is a decrease in muscle fiber diameter, as well as possible metabolic dysfunction, resulting in a decrease in the SFAP amplitude. This leads to decreased MUAP duration and amplitude with no or minimal increases in polyphasia. Spontaneous activity is not usually seen in these conditions.

Acute Processes Involving Random Segmental Necrosis and Atrophy of Muscle Fibers or Random Denervation of Individual Muscle Fibers

Segmental necrosis may be seen in inflammatory and other myopathies. Since muscle fibers are innervated only at one location, any lesion that anatomically interrupts the muscle fibers produces for all practical purposes two muscle fibers, one that is innervated and one that is not. If the segmental necrosis is extensive and some segments of the muscle fiber are far away from the innervation zone, these muscle segments may never be reinnervated. The result will be chronic spontaneous activity. Some myopathic processes, such as polymyositis, also damage terminal nerve branches, and may produce a completely denervated muscle fiber. Extensive damage to the neuromuscular junction by botulism toxin may produce similar results. Spontaneous activity is therefore common at some stage of these disorders.

The MUAP lesions seen in this type of process are similar to those described in the previous section, except that the actual loss of muscle fibers results in even greater decreases in MUAP duration and amplitude, and the presence of reinnervation can increase MUAP polyphasia. "Fiber splitting" seen in some myopathies may also contribute to polyphasia.

Chronic/Old Myopathies With Segmental Necrosis

Reinnervation of denervated muscle segments/fibers may occur, producing changes similar to those discussed for various neuropathic processes. Additionally, if many muscle fibers are not reinnervated and atrophy/degenerate, it is hypothesized that the interfiber distances between muscle fibers belonging to a given motor unit may decrease, resulting in higher muscle fiber density. These factors may produce long-duration, moderately high-amplitude, polyphasic MUAPs in chronic myopathies. In some cases, this may produce confusion when trying to differentiate chronic neuropathic from chronic myopathic processes.

Abnormal Neuromuscular Transmission of the Type Seen in Myasthenia Gravis

By the criteria and techniques applied in routine clinical examinations, the MUAP seen with myasthenia gravis–type neuromuscular junction dysfunction has an essentially normal configuration except for moment-to-moment variability in amplitude. This variability in amplitude is secondary to the intermittent failure of neuromuscular transmission in individual muscle fibers and therefore can be seen in any disorder in which neuromuscular transmission is abnormal. When examining moment-to-moment variability, one must make sure that superimposition of other MUAPs is excluded and that electrode position is absolutely constant. If these precautions are observed, normal MUAPs will have almost no variability in amplitude (<1%).

If the defect in neuromuscular transmission is so severe that transmission is continuously failing in a large percentage of the neuromuscular junctions in each motor unit, short-duration, low-amplitude, polyphasic MUAPs may result. This should not be interpreted as suggesting a superimposed myopathic process.

Abnormal Neuromuscular Transmission of the Type Seen in the Lambert-Eaton Syndrome

As in myasthenia gravis, the MUAP seen in the Lambert-Eaton syndrome has significant moment-to-moment variability in amplitude. The characteristic feature of MUAPs in the Lambert-Eaton syndrome is that the amplitude is relatively low at low firing frequencies and increases to near normal levels as the motor unit firing rate increases.

Short-duration, low-amplitude, polyphasic MUAPs may be seen in the Lambert-Eaton syndrome for the same reasons given above for myasthenia gravis and should be interpreted in a similar manner.

ELECTRODIAGNOSTIC FINDINGS IN NEUROMUSCULAR DISORDERS

The basic electrodiagnostic abnormalities observed in various neuromuscular disorders are summarized in this section. The text by Brown and Boulton[8] is highly recommended and should be considered a major reference for this information. Summaries of typical electrodiagnostic findings in neuromuscular diseases are listed in Tables 11-1 through 11-4.

Motor Neuron Disease

The reader is referred to the monograph by Daube[26, 27] for a comprehensive discussion of the electrodiagnostic abnormalities in motor neuron disease.

Sensory Nerve Conduction Studies. Sensory nerve connection studies are essentially normal. The presence of significant electrodiagnostic sensory abnormalities suggests either a different or an additional diagnosis.

Late Responses. F response and H reflex latencies are generally normal.

Repetitive Stimulation. A small decrement may be present if extensive denervation-reinnervation is occurring. The presence of a decrement is a negative prognostic factor, signifying relatively rapid motor neuron loss.

Motor Nerve Conduction Studies. The results of motor nerve conduction studies are either normal or demonstrate low evoked response amplitudes. Significant conduction block and/or temporal dispersion is not generally present, although evoked responses may appear dispersed when amplitudes are markedly reduced. Conduction velocities may be mildly decreased if the evoked response amplitude is very low. Low motor evoked response amplitudes are associated with a poor overall prognosis.

Needle Electrode Examination. Spontaneous activity may be present and is a negative prognostic factor in that it signifies either very rapid axonal loss or loss of a large percentage (>30%[26, 27]) of the original motor neurons. The MUAP abnormal-

Table 11-1
Typical Effects of Repetitive Stimulation on Motor Evoked Response Amplitudes in Several Commonly Encountered Neuromuscular Disorders

Disorder	Single Response (Normal range: 5–20 mV)	2 Hz Stimulation, Rested Muscle (Normal: Decrement <5%–8%)	20–50 Hz Stimulation or 2 Hz Stimulation Immediately Post Exercise (Normal: May increment <20%–50%)	2 Hz Stimulation 2–4 Minutes Post Exercise (Normal: Decrement <5%–8%)
Myasthenia gravis	Normal or low Usually >80% Lower limit or normal	Normal, mild, or marked decrement 0–60%	Decrement partially or completely repaired	Decrement may increase or appear (Decrement may be present only under these conditions)
Myasthenic syndrome	Low 5%–90% Lower limit of normal	>5%–8% Decrement	Marked increment 100%–2000% of baseline response	Decrement may increase
Botulism	Normal or low	Normal or >5%–8% Decrement	No change (severe cases) or increment (mild cases)	Facilitation may persist

ities noted are those associated with progressive chronic motor neuron loss. The dominant abnormality is the presence of MUAPs with moderately to markedly increased amplitude and lesser degrees of increased polyphasia and duration. Late in the disease process, low-amplitude, short-duration, polyphasic MUAPs may occur along with the larger MUAPs as individual motor units degenerate and possess only a few muscle fibers.

Discussion. The electrodiagnostic abnormalities of advanced motor neuron disease are usually marked and widespread, involving all four extremities and possibly bulbar mus-

cles. Early motor neuron disease, however, can present in a radicular or peripheral nerve distribution, making it difficult in some cases to differentiate motor neuron disease from other neurological disorders such as syringomyelia, radiculopathy, polyradiculopathy, or neuropathies (when sensory abnormalities are not prominent). Previous neurological disease resulting in the loss of significant numbers of motor neurons (*e.g.,* old poliomyelitis, may also mimic motor neuron disease electrodiagnostically. Electrodiagnostic studies should generally not be considered as supporting the diagnosis of motor neuron disease unless abnormalities are present in three or more extremities

Table 11-2
Typical Electrodiagnostic Results of Motor Nerve Conduction Studies in Commonly Encountered Neuromuscular Disorders

Disorder	Distal Latency	Conduction Velocity	Evoked Response Amplitude	Temporal Dispersion	Conduction Block	Late Responses
Motor neuron disease						
Mild	Usually normal	Usually normal	Usually normal	Usually normal	None	Usually normal
Advanced	Normal or slightly prolonged	Normal or mildly decreased	Usually decreased	Usually normal	None	Normal or mildly prolonged
Entrapment neuropathy						
Mild	Prolonged if across lesion	Slow across lesion	Usually normal	Usually normal	Normal to mild	normal
Severe	Prolonged if across lesion	Slow across lesion	Usually decreased	Normal or slightly increased	Mild to marked	May be mildly prolonged if lesion is proximal to stimulus site
Radiculopathy	Normal	Usually normal	Normal unless severe	Normal	None (distally)	May be slightly prolonged if severe
Neuromuscular junction disorders	Normal	Normal	Normal or decreased	Normal	None	Normal
Myopathies	Normal	Normal	Normal or decreased	Normal	None	Normal

Table 11-3
Typical Electrodiagnostic Results of Motor Nerve Conduction Studies in Polyneuropathies

Disorder	Distal Latency	Conduction Velocity	Evoked Response amplitude	Temporal Dispersion	Conduction Block	Late Responses
Axonal polyneuropathy						
Mild	Normal or slightly prolonged	Normal or slightly decreased	Usually normal	Usually normal	Usually none	Normal or slightly prolonged
Severe	Normal or prolonged	Usually slightly decreased	Usually decreased (may be marked)	Normal or slightly increased	None to minimal	May be mildly prolonged or absent
Demyelinating polyneuropathy						
Mild	Usually prolonged	Usually decreased	Normal or decreased	Normal to marked*	None to mild	Normal to prolonged or absent
Severe	Usually prolonged (may be marked)	Usually decreased (may be marked)	Usually decreased	Normal to marked*	Mild to marked	Usually prolonged or absent

* Temporal dispersion may be prominent in acquired demyelinating polyneuropathies whereas it is less marked in congenital/hereditary polyneuropathies.

Table 11-4
Typical Electrodiagnostic Results of Sensory Nerve Conduction Studies in Commonly Encountered Neuromuscular Disorders

Disorder	Distal Latency	Conduction Velocity	Evoked Response Amplitude	Temporal Dispersion	Conduction Block
Motor neuron disease					
Mild	Normal	Normal	Normal	Normal	None
Advanced	Normal	Normal	Normal	Normal	None
Polyneuropathy					
Axonal					
Mild	Normal or prolonged	Normal or slightly low	Normal or decreased	Normal or slightly increased	None to slight
Severe	Usually prolonged	Usually slightly low	Decreased or absent	Normal or slightly increased	None to slight
Demyelinating					
Mild	Usually prolonged	Usually decreased	Normal or decreased	Usually increased	None to moderate
Severe	Prolonged (may be marked)	Decreased (may be marked)	Decreased or absent	Usually increased (may be marked)	None to marked
Entrapment neuropathy					
Mild	Prolonged if across lesion	Slow across lesion	Normal or low	Usually normal to mildly increased	Normal or slight
Severe	Prolonged if across lesion	Slow across lesion	Low or absent	Normal to moderately increased	Slight to marked
Radiculopathy	Normal	Normal	Normal	Normal	None
Neuromuscular junction disorders	Normal	Normal	Normal	Normal	None
Myopathies	Normal	Normal	Normal	Normal	None

and/or bulbar muscles and previous neurological disease resulting in the loss of anterior horn cells has been ruled out. Even with these criteria, old poliomyelitis or multiple radiculopathies secondary to bony spine disease involving both cervical and lumbosacral regions may be difficult to differentiate from motor neuron disease.

When evaluating possible motor neuron disease in the childhood/adolescent years (*e.g.,* Werdnig-Hoffman or Kukelberg-Welander disease), the differential diagnosis discussed above is much less of a factor, since superimposed diseases are less frequently present.

Polyneuropathies

There are many different hereditary and acquired etiologies of peripheral nerve dysfunction that affect distal/proximal and motor/sensory components of the peripheral nervous system in a differential fashion, and which may or may not produce significant demyelination. Different disease processes may also vary widely in their temporal course. Consequently, many different motor/sensory, axonal/demyelinating, anatomical, and temporal patterns of electrodiagnostic abnormalities can be seen. The specifics of individual disease processes are discussed elsewhere.[32, 33, 64, 65, 78, 79] Only general patterns are discussed here.

Sensory Nerve Conduction Studies.   Electrodiagnostic sensory abnormalities may include prolonged distal latencies, abnormal conduction velocities, conduction block, temporal dispersion, and decreased evoked response amplitudes. Significant temporal dispersion suggests an acquired multifocal demyelinating polyneuropathy (see Table 11-4).

F Response.   The F response, if obtainable, is usually moderately to markedly prolonged in neuropathies in which de-

myelination is prominent and is normal to mildly prolonged in other neuropathies. It is frequently unobtainable when the neuropathy is severe, irrespective of the underlying mechanism.

H Reflex.   The H reflex follows a pattern similar to that observed for the F response.

Repetitive Stimulation.   A small decrement may be present if large amounts of denervation/reinnervation are present.

Motor Nerve Conduction Studies.   As in sensory nerve conduction studies, electrodiagnostic motor nerve conduction study abnormalities may include prolonged distal latencies, abnormal conduction velocities, conduction block, temporal dispersion, and decreased evoked response amplitudes (see Table 11-3). Significant temporal dispersion suggests an acquired multifocal demyelinating polyneuropathy.[59, 65, 66] In many neuropathies, temporal dispersion and conduction block must be determined solely from motor nerve conduction studies since the proximal sensory response may not be detectable.

Needle Electrode Examination.   *Spontaneous Activity.* If axonal loss is occurring at a significant rate and sufficient time has elapsed, spontaneous activity will usually be present. If the rate of axonal loss is low and reinnervation is occurring rapidly, axonal loss may occur without detectable spontaneous activity.

MUAPs. If a substantial percentage of the axons supplying a muscle have been lost and the denervated muscle fibers have been added to remaining motor units, MUAP amplitude, duration, and polyphasia will increase in proportion to the number of muscle fibers added to the average motor unit.

Motor Unit Recruitment. Motor unit recruitment will be decreased if a substantial percentage of the motor axons are lost. For technical reasons, MUAP conformation changes will probably be detectable before recruitment abnormalities are unequivocally present.

Entrapment Neuropathies

The most common entrapment neuropathies are those of the median nerve at the wrist,[82] the ulnar nerve at the elbow,[56] and the peroneal nerve at the fibular head,[92] although many other variants occur.[30, 68, 80, 85] Hallett[41] and Wilbourn[92] have provided excellent discussions of the general pathophysiology underlying entrapment neuropathies.

Sensory Nerve Conduction Studies. Abnormalities noted on sensory nerve conduction studies include slowing of the SNAP across the lesion, mild temporal dispersion, and decreased evoked response amplitudes secondary to either temporal dispersion, conduction block, or axonotmesis.

F Response. F response latencies may be prolonged if the stimulus is applied distal to the lesion. F response latencies are usually very insensitive in detecting entrapment neuropathies owing to the long length of normal nerve included in the conduction pathway. They are not routinely used in the detection of uncomplicated entrapment neuropathies.

Motor Nerve Conduction Studies. As is the case for sensory nerve, abnormalities noted include slowing of the nerve action potential across the lesion, mild temporal dispersion, and decreased evoked response amplitudes secondary to either conduction block or axonotmesis.

Needle Electrode Examination. If axonotmesis has occurred and sufficient time has elapsed, spontaneous activity may be detected on needle electrode examination. If a large percentage of axons are nonconducting for any reason, motor unit recruitment may be decreased. If significant permanent axonal loss has occurred with subsequent reinnervation, increases in MUAP duration, polyphasia, and amplitude will be observed.

Mononeuropathy Multiplex Syndromes and Plexopathies

Mononeuropathy multiplex syndromes are characterized by multifocal lesions of peripheral nerves and are associated with systemic disorders such as diabetes, vasculitis, amyloidosis, direct tumor involvement, and paraneoplastic syndromes.[69, 91] Aside from the anatomical distribution of abnormalities, plexopathies share the same electrodiagnostic features as the mononeuropathy multiplex syndromes in that they are both lesions of peripheral nerves that result in primarily axonal damage of both motor and sensory fibers. Mononeuropathy multiplex syndromes can be distributed bilaterally distally and proximally throughout the body and have a predilection for associated entrapment neuropathies, while plexopathies tend to be localized to the proximal portions of the peripheral nerve structures innervating the limbs and trunk. A plexopathy may, in fact, be part of a mononeuropathy multiplex syndrome, and the differential diagnosis are similar (see Tables 11-2 through 11-4).

Sensory Nerve Conduction Studies. The lesion(s) in these disease categories are distal to both the motor and sensory cell bodies and result in either axonal disruption or abnormal axonal conduction. A major distinguishing point between radiculopathies and plexopathies is that sensory studies are usually normal in the former and frequently abnormal in the latter. This distinction may be important clinically and is subject to the following qualifications. Sensory nerve conduction studies will be abnormal in the presence of axonal disruption if the sensory axons of

the nerve being studied pass through the involved area and are interrupted. The appropriate sensory nerve must therefore be studied. If an L4 radiculopathy/plexopathy is suspected on the basis of electrodiagnostic and clinical evidence, the sural nerve (involving predominantly the S1 level) cannot be used to distinguish an L4 radiculopathy from a plexopathy involving primarily L4 muscles. While this seems obvious, it is a mistake frequently made.

Sensory nerve conduction studies will only be abnormal if a large enough percentage of the sensory axons are damaged. A lesion that eliminates conduction in 10% of the sensory axons will produce a loss of SNAP amplitude that may not be unequivocally detectable. Axonotmesis in that many motor axons will probably produce easily detectable spontaneous activity after an appropriate time interval. The presence of a "normal" sensory response may therefore be seen in a plexopathy in which spontaneous activity is present, even when the appropriate sensory nerve is studied.

Late Responses. Late response latencies may be prolonged or absent.

Repetitive Stimulation. A small decrement may be present if significant denervation/reinnervation is present.

Motor Nerve Conduction Studies. Motor nerve conduction abnormalities are similar to those seen in axonal polyneuropathies and entrapment neuropathies with the exception of the anatomical distribution.

Needle Electrode Examination. Abnormalities noted on needle electrode examination are those associated with axonal dysfunction as listed for radiculopathies and neuropathies.

Radiculopathy and Polyradiculopathy

A radiculopathy may occur with extensive bony spine disease, intervertebral disk disease, carcinomatous/lymphomatous meningitis, other mass lesions, and some metabolic/inflammatory disorders.[34, 90] Cord level lesions (*e.g.,* syringomyelia, intramedullary mass lesions) that damage anterior horn cells are difficult to distinguish electrodiagnostically from radiculopathies and should always be considered if clinically appropriate. One of the primary features of radiculopathies and polyradiculopathies is that damage to the nerve root usually occurs proximal to the sensory neuronal cell body. Electrodiagnostic abnormalities are therefore restricted to the motor unit unless a secondary process (*e.g.,* a sensorimotor polyneuropathy) is present. Typical findings in radiculopathies/polyradiculopathies are discussed both in terms of severity of neuronal damage and chronology of electrodiagnostic abnormalities.

Sensory Nerve Conduction Studies. Sensory nerve conduction studies are almost always normal. In rare cases, the dorsal root ganglia may be damaged, producing sensory abnormalities.

F Wave. F wave latencies are usually normal unless the radiculopathy is severe and/or multilevel. The F wave usually provides little additional information since there are generally significant abnormalities on the needle electrode examination and/or motor nerve conduction studies by the time that F wave latencies become abnormal.[3]

H Reflex. The H reflex may be abnormally prolonged in S1 radiculopathies and may assist in making the diagnosis under some circumstances.[34, 89] Prolongation or absence of the H reflex correlates well with a diminished or absent ankle reflex in radicular disease (although not necessarily in polyneuropathies).

Repetitive Stimulation. A small decrement may be present if extensive denervation and reinnervation is present.

Motor Nerve Conduction Studies. Motor nerve conduction studies are usually normal in radiculopathies unless a large percentage of the axons innervating the muscle being tested have been anatomically interrupted (axonotmesis). When this occurs under acute conditions, the amplitude of the motor evoked response is normal initially and decreases to its nadir 3 to 7 days after injury. Motor nerve conduction velocities and temporal dispersion are usually normal unless the motor evoked response amplitude is markedly decreased. If the lesion is chronic or old, and the majority of the originally denervated muscle fibers have been reinnervated by surviving axons, the motor evoked response amplitude may be normal in spite of significant permanent axonal loss. High-amplitude, long-duration, polyphasic MUAPs should be present on needle electrode examination in this situation. If axonal loss is severe and permanent, CMAP amplitudes may remain low, in which case spontaneous activity should persist for long periods of time, or even permanently. Lesions of the nerve root producing only conduction block (neurapraxia) do not affect the results of standard nerve conduction studies since the nerve is stimulated distal to the conduction block.

Needle Electrode Examination. *Spontaneous Activity.* In acute or short-duration radiculopathies (<1 to 3 months), abnormalities on needle electrode examination are primarily the following:

1. The presence of spontaneous activity (if axonotmesis has occurred and sufficient time has elapsed).
2. Decreased motor unit recruitment (if a large enough percentage of the axons are not conducting action potentials for any reason).

Spontaneous activity will be the most sensitive indicator of neuronal damage if axonal interruption occurs, since a small percentage of motor axonal loss (2 to 3%) will probably be detectable.

Spontaneous activity may require 1 to 2 weeks to appear in the proximal muscles (paraspinal muscles) and 2 to 3 weeks to appear in distal muscles. Spontaneous activity is therefore not of significant value in evaluating radiculopathies in the acute setting in which symptoms have been present only a few days.

Spontaneous activity may resolve earlier in proximal muscles than in distal muscles. The electrodiagnostician may therefore observe a pattern in which spontaneous activity may be present only in proximal muscles, present in both proximal and distal muscles, or present in distal muscles only, depending on the timing of the examination with respect to the injury. No spontaneous activity may be detected at any time if anatomical axonal interruption does not occur or if reinnervation is rapid.

The presence of spontaneous activity in a muscle is often taken to indicate ongoing denervation, a conclusion that is incorrect in many cases. It is known that spontaneous activity can persist for many years when major axonal loss has left a muscle with relatively few functioning axons. This usually occurs in the setting of severe old poliomyelitis, near-complete peripheral nerve lesions, and so on, and probably reflects the inability of the remaining motor neurons to reinnervate the denervated muscle fibers. The situation is much less clear in settings in which only a small percentage of the axons have been damaged, as is the case with most radiculopathies. If the following conditions are present:

1. The patient has no superimposed neurological disease that would affect the ability of motor neurons to sprout and reinnervate denervated muscle fibers.
2. The majority of the original motor neurons are intact and functioning. The number of muscle fibers per motor unit will therefore not be excessively large and the ability of the motor neuron to innervate additional muscle fibers is not impaired.
3. The mechanism underlying spontaneous activity is denervation.

It is unlikely that significant numbers of muscle fibers could remain denervated for long periods of time in the absence of recent injury. Under these conditions, the presence of spontaneous activity strongly favors the conclusion that denervation has occurred within the past several weeks or months. This logical framework is useful when analyzing the significance of spontaneous activity in the muscles of patients who present with symptoms of short duration (weeks) and a history of neurological injury in the remote past. This logic does not assist in deciding whether denervation is actually occurring at the moment of the electrodiagnostic examination.

It is often difficult to determine the significance of spontaneous activity in the paraspinal muscles following laminectomies. Spontaneous activity in this setting may be the result of direct surgical damage to muscle fibers/intramuscular nerve branches, or it may be secondary to axonotmesis produced by a new radiculopathy. Although it has been proposed that spontaneous activity located more than 3 cm from the scar is usually not the result of surgical trauma,[89] this assumption should be made with reservation since the location and size of the surface wound does not always identify the location and extent of the surgical trauma. Damage to nerves innervating the paraspinal muscles may also result in spontaneous activity remote from the surgical scar. This discussion may be qualified by considering the surgeon and surgical technique. In the hands of a careful surgeon, a one-level microdiskectomy using an operating microscope is unlikely to produce major damage to paraspinal muscles or muscular nerve branches as compared with a wide laminectomy/fusion involving multiple levels and extensive periosteal stripping.

Spontaneous activity in the paraspinal muscles after laminectomy should be analyzed as follows:

1. When examining a postlaminectomy patient for the first time, or if no accurate records regarding previous studies after laminectomy are available, spontaneous activity in the paraspinal muscles should be attributed to surgical trauma, particularly if low amplitude. This assumption may be modified by considering the surgeon and surgical technique.
2. When performing electrodiagnostic studies on a postlaminectomy patient, the posterior myotomes should be carefully searched and the spontaneous activity present described accurately. An evaluation for initial documentation should take place at least 1 month after surgery.
3. Subsequent studies should attempt to document an interval increase in the distribution or amount of spontaneous activity present in the paraspinal muscles before deciding that abnormalities noted are relevant with respect to the current clinical complaints.

Motor Unit Recruitment. Decreased motor unit recruitment will be present immediately on injury if the percentage of nonconducting axons innervating that muscle is large enough. Abnormalities of motor unit recruitment may resolve completely if secondary to conduction block or may be permanent if axonotmesis occurs and the axons are permanently lost.

MUAP Configuration. If a significant percentage of the motor axons supplying a muscle are permanently lost, and enough time has elapsed (>1 to 3 months) so that the muscle fibers originally innervated by those axons are added to other motor units, the amplitude, duration, and polyphasia of the remaining motor units will increase. This may occur with either old (inactive) or chronic (active) lesions and is primarily dependent on the total percentage of axons lost.

Anatomical Distribution of Abnormalities. Many tables exist that list the predominant root level supply of commonly studied muscles of the trunk and limbs.[22, 46, 89] Since the axons supplying a given muscle are topographically localized in the nerve root, damage may occur to the axons innervating any or all of the muscles supplied by that root. On this basis alone, electrodiagnostic abnormalities may be present in only one or a few of the muscles supplied by a given nerve root and, in fact, may not even involve the entire muscle. Lastly, reinnervation is significantly more efficient in proximal muscles, with the result that persistent abnormalities may be noted only in distal muscles innervated by that root. When combining these phenomena with the time course of abnormalities discussed previously, it should be clear that marked variations in the pattern of electrodiagnostic abnormalities may occur with radiculopathies. It is only in the severe radiculopathy that a majority of the axons in the nerve root are damaged, producing unequivocal, long-standing abnormalities in multiple anterior and posterior myotome muscles predominantly innervated by that root.

Polyradiculoneuropathy

The term *polyradiculoneuropathy* generally designates a disease process that affects peripheral nerve but in contrast to generalized polyneuropathies demonstrates an additional predilection for the nerve roots themselves. Many of these disorders appear to be immunological, vasculitic, or toxic in origin, and this particular anatomical distribution is believed to reflect the relative permeability of the blood–nerve barrier at the point where the nerve roots enter the subarachnoid space, providing access to injurious agents. Acutely presenting polyradiculoneuropathies are usually considered to fall under the differential diagnosis of the Guillain-Barré syndrome. The majority, although not all, of these acute disorders have demyelination as a predominant feature and are therefore classified as acute inflammatory demyelinating polyradiculoneuropathies. Classification of chronic polyradiculoneuropathies is poorly defined, and for this discussion will be taken to refer to chronic inflammatory demyelinating polyradiculoneuropathies (CIDP). The reference by Albers provides an excellent discussion of the clinical and electrodiagnostic features of the inflammatory demyelinating polyradiculoneuropathies.[1]

Sensory Nerve Conduction Studies. Electrodiagnostic sensory abnormalities may include prolonged distal latencies, abnormal conduction velocities, conduction block, temporal dispersion, and decreased evoked response amplitudes. One peculiarity of these disorders is the frequent relative preservation of the sural sensory evoked response while median and sometimes ulnar sensory evoked responses are significantly abnormal.[1] Extreme prolongation of distal latencies and slowing of nerve conduction velocities may be present. It is frequently impossible to determine sensory conduction velocities since temporal dispersion and conduction block make the proximal sensory response undetectable (see Table 11-4).

F Response. The F response, if obtainable, may be moderately to markedly prolonged when demyelination is prominent. It is one of the most important studies where Guillain-Barré syndrome is suspected since all nerve involvement may be proximal or at the root level, resulting in normal peripheral nerve conduction studies. F response latencies may be markedly prolonged under these conditions when other portions of the electrodiagnostic studies are within normal limits. The F response latency may be normal in Guillain-Barré syndrome if conduction block is the dominant abnormality and those axons that are conducting the F response are conducting relatively normally. The F response is usually unobtainable when the neuropathy is severe.

H Reflex. The H reflex follows a pattern similar to that observed for the F response.

Repetitive Stimulation. A small decrement may be present if large amounts of denervation/reinnervation are present.

Motor Nerve Conduction Studies. Electrodiagnostic motor abnormalities may include prolonged distal latencies, abnormal conduction velocities, conduction block, temporal dispersion, and decreased evoked response amplitudes as is seen with sensory nerves. Abnormalities may be marked, with distal latencies two to three times the upper limit of normal and nerve conduction velocities of 20 to 30% of the lower limit of normal. Motor nerve conduction studies are usually the only way that conduction block and temporal dispersion can be identified since it is common for the proximal sensory response to be undetectable. Conduction block and temporal dispersion may occur in the presence of normal conduction velocities. Low nerve conduction velocities are not a negative prognostic factor since the prognosis for demyelinating lesions is much better than that for lesions involving axonal loss. Distal CMAP amplitudes determined after the disease has stabilized correlate directly with prognosis (see Table 11-3).

Needle Electrode Examination. *Spontaneous Activity.* If significant axonal loss has occurred and sufficient time has elapsed, spontaneous activity will usually be present. In the case of an acute presentation, spontaneous activity will not be present at the time of the initial diagnostic evaluation. If the rate of axonal loss is low and reinnervation is occurring rapidly, axonal loss may occur without detectable spontaneous activity. All other factors being equal, the presence of significant amounts of spontaneous activity is a negative prognostic factor since it signifies axonal loss.

MUAPs. If a substantial percentage of the axons supplying a muscle have been lost and the denervated muscle fibers have been added to remaining motor units, MUAP amplitude, duration, and polyphasia will increase in proportion to the number of muscle fibers added to the average motor unit. Again, in the acute presentation, MUAPs will usually be normal unless some antecedent neurological insult has occurred in the remote past. Mild increases in polyphasia and duration may be present early if demyelination affects the terminal nerve branches.

Motor Unit Recruitment. Motor unit recruitment will be decreased if a substantial percentage of the motor axons are nonconducting. In an acute presentation, decreased motor unit recruitment may be the only abnormality noted during the electrodiagnostic examination if the lesions are predominantly those of conduction block at the nerve root level.

Neuromuscular Junction Disorders

The electrodiagnostic abnormalities noted in disorders of the neuromuscular junction are described in Tables 11-1 through 11-4 and in selected texts.[43, 71, 76, 77]

Sensory Nerve Conduction Studies.   Normal.

F Response.   Normal.

H Reflex.   Normal.

Repetitive Stimulation.   See section on evaluation of the neuromuscular junction and Table 11-1.

Motor Nerve Conduction Studies.   See Table 11-2.

Needle Electrode Examination.   See section on abnormalities detected by needle electrode examination.

Primary Muscle Disorders

Attempting to discuss general abnormalities in "myopathies" is difficult since the term represents a large group of diseases, including inflammatory muscle disease, the various muscular dystrophies, myotonic disorders, periodic paralysis, and myopathies secondary to enzyme deficiencies and endocrine, parasitic, and toxic etiologies. As might be expected, the clinical and electrodiagnostic characteristics of these disorders vary widely.[7, 28, 37, 58, 87]

Sensory Nerve Conduction Studies.   Normal.

Late Responses.   F response and H reflex latencies are generally normal.

Repetitive Stimulation.   The results of repetitive stimulation are usually normal. A mild decrement may be present if neuromuscular junctions are abnormal as a result of primary muscle cell dysfunction. Decrements may also be present in myotonic disorders as a result of abnormal muscle fiber membrane function and the resulting inability to repetitively generate normal muscle cell action potentials.

Motor Nerve Conduction Studies.   The results of motor nerve conduction studies are usually normal with the exception of the evoked response amplitude, which may be decreased.

Needle Electrode Examination.   The abnormalities noted on the needle electrode examination in primary muscle diseases depend highly on the disease process and as such are discussed by group.

Muscular Dystrophies. The muscular dystrophies include a large number of disorders with widely varying characteristics. Abnormalities on needle electrode examination may be distal, proximal, and/or craniopharyngeal; spontaneous activity may or may not be present; and MUAP changes may vary widely, ranging from near normal to short duration, low amplitude MUAPs to moderately high duration, normal/high amplitude MUAPs, depending on the disease and its stage. While MUAP polyphasia is usually increased, it may not be prominent. Details are provided in the works of Daube[28] and Buchthal.[18]

Acquired Inflammatory Myopathies. The untreated, acquired inflammatory myopathies are usually characterized by the presence of spontaneous activity, decreased MUAP amplitude and duration with increased polyphasia, and rapid motor unit recruitment. Treatment with steroids or other immunosuppressant drugs may suppress spontaneous activity. The MUAPs in chronic acquired inflammatory myopathies may evolve into moderately high amplitude, long-duration, polyphasic MUAPs.

Endocrine Myopathies. Endocrine myopathies (*e.g.,* steroid, hypo/hyperthyroid, hyperparathyroid, and other myopathies) generally demonstrate MUAPs that either are normal or demonstrate minimally decreased amplitude and duration. Motor unit recruitment is usually rapid in proportion to clinical weakness. Fibrillations and positive waves are not generally a feature of these disorders, although increased insertional activity, short myotonic discharges, doublets, fasciculations, and other poorly defined irregular spontaneous discharges may be seen in disorders such as hypothyroidism and hyperparathyroidism.

Toxic Myopathies. Toxic myopathies, such as those seen with alcoholic myopathy,[40] may present with findings similar to those seen with inflammatory myopathies if muscle fiber damage is severe enough. Most toxic myopathies (*e.g.,* those seen with chloroquine, pentazocine, and clofibrate) are significantly milder and present as electrodiagnostic abnormalities similar to those observed in endocrine myopathies.

Inherited Myopathies. Inherited myopathies generally demonstrate decreased MUAP amplitude and duration, increased polyphasia, and rapid motor unit recruitment. Spontaneous activity may be profuse (*e.g.,* acid maltase deficiency) or absent (*e.g.,* fiber type disproportion).

Periodic Paralysis. The characteristic feature of the periodic paralyses is the impaired ability of the muscle cell membrane to generate a normal action potential.[12] This results in electrical silence with paralytic attacks, during which insertional activity is decreased, voluntary MUAPs are absent, and no CMAP can be elicited by stimulation of the motor nerve. Lesser degrees of abnormalities are noted during milder attacks, which produce weakness, not paralysis. Depending on the degree of impairment of muscle fiber action potential generation, MUAPs may range from normal to low amplitude/short duration. In hyperkalemic periodic paralysis, fibrillations and myotonic discharges may be seen between attacks, although they disappear during an attack. Hypokalemic periodic paralysis does not demonstrate spontaneous activity but may demonstrate an abnormal drop (>50%) in the CMAP amplitude after exercise or in response to intra-arterial injection of epinephrine.[35]

Myotonic Disorders. The myotonic disorders include myotonic dystrophy, myotonia congenita, and paramyotonia congenita.[73, 83] The hallmark of these disorders is the myotonic discharge,[12] a repetitive discharge of single muscle fibers that varies widely in frequency and amplitude, giving rise to what is usually described as a "dive bomber" sound. Firing rates vary from 2 to 100 Hz. Myotonic discharges are not absolutely specific for the myotonic disorders and can also be seen in hyperkalemic periodic paralysis, acid maltase deficiency, hypothyroid myopathy, myotubular myopathy, and inflammatory myopathies.

INTERPRETATION OF ELECTRODIAGNOSTIC RESULTS

Analysis of results obtained during the electrodiagnostic evaluation is one of the most challenging aspects of the overall process. The following scheme is one approach to this problem. As presented, it assumes that no technical errors have been made (*e.g.,* low distal limb temperatures resulting in prolonged distal latencies). The raw data obtained during the examination should be reviewed and its major features summarized.

Nerve Conduction Study Analysis

A summary of the typical nerve conduction study abnormalities found in commonly encountered neuromuscular disorders is provided in Tables 11-1 through 11-4.

1. Were all of the necessary tests performed? A negative examination is frequently the result of neglecting a key test. Review the initial differential diagnosis as well as any abnormal results obtained during the examination to decide this.
2. If nerve conduction studies are abnormal, determine the distribution of abnormalities. Are abnormalities symmetrical or asymmetrical, focal or diffuse/multifocal, distal or proximal?
3. Are abnormalities sensory, motor, or both?
4. If CMAP amplitudes are generally low, was the patient tested for a defect in neuromuscular transmission?
5. If obtained, were F response or H reflex latencies disproportionately prolonged relative to distal nerve conduction velocities, suggesting proximal demyelination?
6. Is abnormal temporal dispersion present in evoked responses following proximal and distal stimulation, suggesting multifocal demyelination?
7. Is there evidence of conduction block in any nerve tested, suggesting a focal lesion in between the stimulus sites?
8. Is there evidence of significant demyelination as evidenced by markedly reduced conduction velocities?

Needle Electrode Results Analysis

The following questions should be asked for insertional activity, spontaneous activity, MUAP abnormalities, and recruitment abnormalities.

1. Were the appropriate muscles examined?
2. Are abnormalities symmetrical or asymmetrical, focal or diffuse/multifocal, distal or proximal? Do they follow the distribution of a specific peripheral nerve, plexus, or root?
3. What type and stage of disease process is suggested by the abnormalities?
4. Can abnormalities noted on motor nerve conduction studies be verified on needle electrode examination? Processes of pathological significance that produce an abnormality of CMAP amplitude usually produce abnormalities on needle electrode examination, although this is not necessarily true for those processes resulting in only motor nerve conduction velocity abnormalities.

Conclusion

Final Diagnosis

The results of this analysis should allow identification of the most likely underlying pathological process, such as, sensory, motor, or sensorimotor polyneuropathy, mononeuropathy, multiple mononeuropathies (mononeuropathy multiplex), polyradiculoneuropathy (as can be seen with Guillain-Barré syndrome), motor neuron disease, (poly)radiculopathy, plexopathy, disordered neuromuscular transmission, or myopathic processes. In some cases it is necessary to invoke multiple diagnoses to explain all electrodiagnostic abnormalities. Examples of this might include a polyneuropathy with superimposed entrapment neuropathies (*e.g.,* carpal tunnel syndrome).

Etiologies

The summary should guide the referring clinician in further evaluation of the patient by including a differential diagnosis of etiologies that could produce the electrodiagnostic findings noted on the examination.

Relationship to Clinical Complaints

When electrodiagnostic abnormalities are present, but the electrodiagnostician does not believe that they are likely to be the basis of the patient's clinical complaint, some statement should be made to this effect. This can avoid confusion in the mind of the nonelectromyographer who reads the report.

Dating of Pathological Processes

When possible, the electrodiagnostic findings should be classified as being consistent with acute, subacute, chronic, or old pathological processes. This information is frequently of value in interpreting the electrodiagnostic results when the duration of clinical symptoms and the estimated age of the electrodiagnostic abnormalities do not correlate well with one another, (*e.g.,* the presence of marked increase in MUAP duration, polyphasia, and amplitude is not consistent with a process of 1 week's duration). In this particular case, the significance of electrodiagnostic abnormalities would be diminished in explaining the major clinical complaint, or the differential diagnosis might be considerably shortened.

Progression and Prognosis

When the diagnosis is relatively certain, some statement should be made regarding prognosis and progression of the disease, if possible. Considerable confusion often occurs in this area, and considerable attention is therefore devoted to this topic.

Electrodiagnostic data may be used in certain conditions to estimate the prognosis for recovery of neurological function or for estimating the rate of progression of a disease. This must be done on a disease-by-disease basis. Diseases for which this may be done include motor neuron disease, peripheral nerve injury, acquired polyneuropathies, myasthenia gravis, inflammatory myopathies, inflammatory demyelinating polyneuropathies, and others.

The electrodiagnostic examination is often misused when it comes to establishing whether a given disease process is ongoing or not. When using electrodiagnostic findings in isolation, progressive/ongoing processes can only be evaluated by demonstrating an interval change between two serial electrodiagnostic studies. Even under these circumstances, the only conclusion that can be drawn is that the event responsible for the interval change occurred shortly before the first examination or between the two examinations, not that progression is occurring at the time of the second examination. As an example, the presence of spontaneous activity is often interpreted as being diagnostic of ongoing denervation. This is incorrect since under certain conditions spontaneous activity may persist for years after the insult that was responsible. An example of this would be a complete and rapid transection of the median nerve at the wrist. An electrodiagnostic study performed 1 hour after nerve transection will not demonstrate spontaneous activity, while repeat studies 1 month later will demonstrate marked spontaneous activity. Although denervation occurred only transiently, spontaneous activity will be recorded from distal median innervated muscles for months to years; that is, profuse spontaneous activity will be present even though there is no ongoing denervation. Under the proper circumstances (see discussion of radiculopathy in previous section), the presence of spontaneous activity suggests that a recent neurological insult has occurred, although it is still not possible to state that injury is occurring at the time of the electrodiagnostic examination. Similar analyses can be made of most types of electrodiagnostic abnormalities, including demyelination, increased neuromuscular jitter, abnormal decrements on repetitive stimulation, low motor/sensory evoked response amplitudes, pathological MUAP changes, and motor unit recruitment abnormalities.

Fibrillation potential amplitude may be useful as an indicator of the age of a lesion. The presence of large numbers of very low amplitude fibrillation potentials (5 to 25 μV), as occur when denervated muscle fibers undergo severe atrophy with time, signify an event that occurred in the remote past. Large amplitude fibrillation potentials (100 to 200 μV) suggest a recent or ongoing event.

These limitations of the electrodiagnostic examination must be kept in mind when making a statement as to whether a disease process is ongoing. The electromyographer must learn to integrate historical, clinical, and electrodiagnostic data to estimate the probability that a disorder is ongoing at the time of evaluation. To do this, the electrodiagnostician must have a thorough understanding of the clinical presentation and course and electrodiagnostic abnormalities associated with the disease under consideration (*e.g.,* the presence of spontaneous activity may be useful in determining the recent course of an inflammatory myopathy and may assist in gauging the effectiveness of recent therapy, while the same findings may be of no value in deciding whether a radiculopathy of recent onset is currently active). Statements regarding ongoing progression of a disease process may have considerable practical significance regarding medical or surgical management and should be made with care.

Improbable Diagnoses

Finally, a statement should be made regarding diagnoses that are virtually excluded by the electrodiagnostic results. In many cases, it is a trivial task to eliminate a particular diagnosis by electrodiagnostic criteria when it is impossible to do so on the basis of clinical or other laboratory data.

REFERENCES

1. Albers JW: The nonhereditary acute and chronic inflammatory demyelinating polyneuropathies. In Brown WF, Boulton CF (eds): Clinical Electromyography. Wolbourn, MA, Butterworth (in press)
2. Albers JW, Donofrio PD, McGonagle TK et al: Sequential electrodiagnostic abnormalities in acute inflammatory demyelinating polyradiculoneuropathy. Muscle Nerve 8:528–539, 1985
3. Aminoff MF, Goodin DS, Parry GJ et al: Electrophysiologic evaluation of lumbosacral radiculopathies: Electromyography, late responses, and somatosensory evoked potentials. Neurology 35:1514–1518, 1985
4. Berger AR, Busis NA, Logigian EL et al: Cervical root stimulation in the diagnosis of radiculopathy. Neurology 37:329–332, 1987
5. Boyd CD, Lawrence PD, Bratty PJA: On modeling the single motor unit action potential. IEEE Trans Biomed Engin BME-25:326–243, 1978
6. Braddom R, Johnson EW: Standardization of "H" reflex and diagnostic use in S1 radiculopathy. Arch Phys Med Rehabil 55:161, 1974
7. Brooke MH: A Clinician's Guide to Muscle Disease, 2nd ed. Baltimore, Williams & Wilkins, 1986
8. Brown WF, Boulton CF: Clinical Electromyography. Boston, Butterworth, 1987
9. Brown WF: Conduction in Abnormal Nerve. In the Physiological and Technical Basis of Electromyography, pp 37–94. Boston, Butterworth, 1984
10. Brown WF: The normal transmembrane potential and impulse conduction. In The Physiological and Technical Basis of Electromyography, pp 95–168. Boston, Butterworth, 1984
11. Brown WF: Electromyography—Normal. In The Physiological and Technical Basis of Electromyography, pp 287–338. Boston, Butterworth, 1984
12. Brown WF: Normal and abnormal spontaneous activity in muscle. In The Physiological and Technical Basis of Electromyography, pp 339–368. Boston, Butterworth, 1984
13. Brown WF: Neuromuscular transmission—Normal and abnormal. In The Physiological and Technical Basis of Electromyography, pp 369–428. Boston, Butterworth, 1984
14. Brown WF, The recording of conducted electrical potentials in nerve trunks and conduction in human motor and sensory fibers. In The Physiological and Technical Basis of Electromyography, pp 95–168. Boston, Butterworth, 1984
15. Buchthal F, Guld C, Rosenfalck P: Action potential parameters in normal human muscle and their dependence on physical variables. Acta Physiol Scand 32:200–218, 1954
16. Buchthal F: An Introduction to Electromyography. Copenhagen, Scandinavian University Books, 1957
17. Buchthal F, Rosenfalck A, Behse F: Sensory potentials of normal and diseased nerves. In Dyck PJ, Thomas PK, Lambert EH, Bunge R (eds): Peripheral Neuropathy, 2nd ed, pp 981–1015. Philadelphia, WB Saunders, 1985
18. Buchthal F: Electromyography in the diagnosis of muscle disease. In Aminoff MJ (ed): Electrodiagnosis. Neurologic Clinics, vol 3, pp 573–598. Philadelphia, WB Saunders, 1985
19. Burke RE: Motor units in mammalian muscle. In Sumner AJ (ed): The Physiology of Peripheral Nerve Disease, pp 133–194. Philadelphia, WB Saunders, 1980
20. Burke RE: Motor units: Anatomy, Physiology, and functional organization. In Brookhart JM, Mountcastle VB (eds): Handbook of Physiology, Section 1, The Nervous System, Vol II, Motor Control, Part 1. Baltimore, Williams & Wilkins, 1981
21. Chu-Andrews J, Johnson RJ: Electrodiagnosis: An Anatomical and Clinical Approach, pp 213–217. Philadelphia, JB Lippincott, 1986
22. Chu-Andrews J, Johnson RJ: Electrodiagnosis: An Anatomical and Clinical Approach, pp 253–254. Philadelphia, JB Lippincott, 1986
23. Chu-Andrews J, Johnson RJ: Electrodiagnosis: An Anatomical and Clinical Approach, pp 258–263. Philadelphia, JB Lippincott, 1986
24. Cornblath DR, Sfladky JT, Sumner AJ: Clinical electrophysiology of infantile botulism. Muscle Nerve 6:448–452, 1983
25. Cornblath DR: Disorders of neuromuscular transmission in children. Muscle Nerve 9:606–611, 1986
26. Daube JR: EMG in Motor Neuron Diseases, Minimonograph #18. American Association of Electromyography Electrodiagnosis, 1982
27. Daube JR: Electrophysiologic studies in the diagnosis and prognosis of motor neuron disease. In Aminoff MJ (ed): Electrodiagnosis. Neurologic Clinics, vol 3, pp 473–494. Philadelphia, WB Saunders, 1985
28. Daube JR: Electrodiagnosis of Muscle Disorders. In Engel AG, Baker BQ (eds): Myology. New York, McGraw-Hill, 1986
29. DeLisa JA, MacKenzie K, Baran EM: Manual of Nerve Conduction Velocity and Somatosensory Evoked Potentials, 2nd ed. New York, Raven Press, 1987
30. DeLisa JA, Saeed MA: The tarsal tunnel syndrome. Muscle Nerve 6:664–670, 1983
31. DeLuca CJ: Control properties of motor units. In Basmajian JV, De Luca CJ: Muscles Alive: Their Functions Revealed by Electromyography, pp 125–167. Baltimore, Williams & Wilkins, 1985
32. Dyck PJ, Lambert EH, Thomas PK, Bunge R (eds): Peripheral Neuropathy. Philadelphia, WB Saunders, 1984
33. Dyck PJ, Thomas PK, Asbury AK et al: Diabetic Neuropathy. Philadelphia, WB Saunders, 1987
34. Eisen A: Electrodiagnosis of radiculopathies. In Aminoff MJ (ed): Electrodiagnosis. Neurologic Clinics, vol 3, pp 494–510. Philadelphia, WB Saunders, 1985
35. Engel AG, Lambert EH, Rosevear JW, Tauxe WN: Clinical and electromyographic studies in a patient with primary hypokalemic periodic paralysis. Am J Med 38:626, 1965
36. Engle AG, Lambert EH, Gomez MR: A new myasthenic syndrome with end-plate acetylcholinesterase deficiency, small nerve terminals, and reduced acetylcholine release. Ann Neurol 1:315–330, 1977

37. Engle AG, Baker BQ (eds): Myology. New York, McGraw-Hill, 1986
38. Griep PAM, Boon KL, Stegeman DF: A study of the motor unit action potential by means of computer simulation. Biol Cybernetics 30:221–230, 1978
39. Gutmann L, Gutierrez A, Riggs JE: The contribution of median-ulnar communications in diagnosis of mild carpal tunnel syndrome. Muscle Nerve 9:319–321, 1986
40. Haller RG: Experimental acute alcoholic myopathy: A histochemical study. Muscle Nerve 8:106–203, 1985
41. Hallett M: Electrophysiologic approaches to the diagnosis of entrapment neuropathies. In Aminoff MJ (ed): Electrodiagnosis. Neurologic Clinics, vol 3, pp 531–542. Philadelphia, WB Saunders, 1985
42. Henneman E, Mendell LM: Functional organization of the motoneuron pool and its inputs. In Brookhart JM, Mountcastle VB (eds): Handbook of Physiology, Section 1, The Nervous System, Volume II, Motor Control, Part 1. Baltimore, Williams & Wilkins, 1981
43. Jablecki CK: Electrodiagnostic evaluation of patients with myasthenia gravis and related disorders. In Aminoff MJ (ed): Electrodiagnosis. Neurologic Clinics, vol 3, pp 557–572. Philadelphia, WB Saunders, 1985
44. Junge D: Electrical recordings from neurons and single muscle fibers. In Nerve and Muscle Excitation, 2nd ed, pp 1–16, Sinauer Associates, 1981
45. Kelly JJ: The electrodiagnostic findings in peripheral neuropathy associated with monoclonal gammopathy. Muscle Nerve 6:504–509, 1983
46. Kimura J: Anatomic basis for localization. In Kimura J: Electrodiagnosis in Diseases of Nerve and Muscle, pp 3–25. Philadelphia, FA Davis, 1983
47. Kimura J: Anatomy and Physiology of Peripheral Nerve. In Electrodiagnosis in Diseases of Nerve and Muscle: Principles and Practice, pp 59–81. Philadelphia, FA Davis, 1983
48. Kimura J: Principles of Nerve Conduction Studies. In Electrodiagnosis in Diseases of Nerve and Muscle: Principles and Practice, pp 83–104. Philadelphia, FA Davis, 1983
49. Kimura J: Techniques of repetitive nerve stimulation. In Electrodiagnosis in Diseases of Nerve and Muscle: Principles and Practice, pp 189–206. Philadelphia, FA Davis, 1983
50. Kimura J: Techniques and normal findings. In Electrodiagnosis in Diseases of Nerve and Muscle: Principles and Practice, pp 235–257. Philadelphia, FA Davis, 1983
51. Kimura J: Single fiber electromyography. In Electrodiagnosis in Disease of Nerve and Muscle: Principles and Practice, pp 305–318, Philadelphia, FA Davis, 1983
52. Kimura J: The F wave. In Electrodiagnosis in Diseases of Nerve and Muscle: Principles and Practice, pp 353–378. Philadelphia, FA Davis, 1983
53. Kimura J: The H reflex and other late responses. In Electrodiagnosis in Diseases of Nerve and Muscle: Principles and Practice, pp 379–398, Philadelphia, FA Davis, 1983
54. Kimura J: Neuromuscular diseases characterized by abnormal muscle activity. In Electrodiagnosis in Diseases of Nerve and Muscle: Principles and Practice, pp 549–565. Philadelphia, FA Davis, 1983
55. Kimura J: Nerve Conduction Studies and Electromyography. In Dyck PJ, Thomas PK, Lambert EH, Peripheral Neuropathy, 2nd ed, 2, pp 919–966. Philadelphia, WB Saunders, 1984
56. Kincaid JC, Phillips LH, Daube JR: The evaluation of suspected ulnar neuropathy at the elbow. Arch Neurol 43:44–47, 1986
57. Lambert EH, Dyck PJ: Compound action potentials of sural nerve in vitro in peripheral neuropathy, pp 1030–1044. In Dyck PJ, Thomas PK, Lambert EH, Bunge R (eds): Peripheral Neuropathy, 2nd ed. Philadelphia, WB Saunders, 1984
58. Layzer RB: Neuromuscular Manifestations of Neuromuscular Disease. Philadelphia, FA Davis, 1985
59. Lewis RA, Sumner AJ: Electrodiagnostic distinctions between chronic acquired and familial demyelinating neuropathies. Neurology 30:371, 1980
60. Ma DM, Liveson JA: Nerve Conduction Handbook. Philadelphia, FA Davis, 1983
61. MacLean I: Neuromuscular junction, In Johnson EW (ed): Practical Electromyography, pp 91–109. Baltimore, Williams & Wilkins, 1980
62. Malmstadt HV, Enke CG, Crouch SR: Electronics and Instrumentation for Scientists. Reading, MA, Benjamin/Cummings, 1981
63. McArdle JJ: Overview of the Physiology of the Neuromuscular Junction. In Brumback RA, Gerst J (eds): The Neuromuscular Junction, pp 65–120, Mount Kisco, NY, Futura, 1984
64. McLeod JG, Evans WA: Peripheral neuropathy in spinocerebellar degenerations. Muscle Nerve 4:51–61, 1981
65. Miller RG: Hereditary and acquired neuropathies: Electrophysiologic aspects. In Aminoff MJ (ed): Electrodiagnosis. Neurologic Clinics, vol 3, pp 543–556. Philadelphia, WB Saunders, 1985
66. Miller RG, Gutmann L, Lewis TA, Sumner A: Acquired versus familial demyelinative neuropathies in children. Muscle Nerve 8:205–210, 1985
67. Olney RK, Miller RG: Conduction block in compression neuropathy: Recognition and quantification. Muscle Nerve 7:662–667, 1984
68. Omer GE, Spinner M (eds): Management of Peripheral Nerve Problems. Philadelphia, WB Saunders, 1980
69. Parry GJG: AAEE Case Report #11: Mononeuropathy multiplex. Muscle Nerve 8:493–498, 1985
70. Pettijan JH: Motor unit control. In Desmedt JE (ed): Motor Unit Types, Recruitment and Plasticity in Health and Disease. Basel, Karger, 1981
71. Pickett JB: Neuromuscular Transmission. In Sumner AJ (ed): The Physiology of Peripheral Nerve Disease, pp 239–264. Philadelphia, WB Saunders, 1980
72. Podolsky RJ: Force generation and shortening in skeletal muscle. In Peachey L (ed): Handbook of Physiology. Section 10, Skeletal Muscle. Baltimore, Williams & Wilkins, 1983
73. Ricker R, Rudel R, Lehmann-Horn F, Kuther G: Muscle stiffness and electrical activity in paramyotonia congenita. Muscle Nerve 9:299–305, 1986
74. Rosenfalck P: Intra- and extracellular potential fields of active nerve and muscle fibers. Acta Physiol Scand S321:1–168, 1969
75. Sacco G, Buchtal F, Rosenfalck P: Motor unit potentials at different ages. Arch Neurol 6:366–373, 1962
76. Sanders DB: Acquired myasthenia gravis. In Brumback RA, Gerst J (eds): The Neuromuscular Junction, pp 257–294. Mount Kisco, NY, Futura, 1984
77. Sanders DB, Howard JF: AAEE Minimonograph 25: Single fiber electromyography in myasthenia gravis. Muscle Nerve 9:809–819, 1986
78. Schaumberg HH, Spencer PS, Thomas PK: Disorders of Peripheral Nerves. Philadelphia, FA Davis, 1983
79. Sheilds RW: Alcoholic polyneuropathy. Muscle Nerve 8:183–187, 1985
80. Spinner M: Injuries to the Major Branches of Peripheral Nerves in the Forearm. Philadelphia, WB Saunders, 1978
81. Stalberg E, Trontelj JV: Single Fiber Electromyography. Old Woking, Surrey, Mervalle Press, 1979
82. Stevens JC: The electrodiagnosis of carpal tunnel syndrome. Muscle & Nerve 10:99–113, 1987
83. Streib EW: Paramyotonia congenita: Successful treatment with tocainide: Clinical and electrophysiologic findings in seven patients. Muscle Nerve 10:155–162, 1987
84. Subramony SH, Malhotra CP, Mishra SK: Distinguishing paramyotonia congenita and myotonia congenita by electromyography. Muscle Nerve 6:374–379, 1983
85. Sunderland S: Nerves and Nerve Injuries. Edinburgh, Churchill Livingstone, 1978
86. Wagman IH, Lesse H: Maximum conduction velocities of motor fibers of ulnar nerve in human subjects of various ages and sizes. J Neurophysiol 15:235, 1952
87. Walton JN: Disorders of Voluntary Muscle, 4th ed. London, Churchill Livingstone, 1981
88. Waxman SG: Determinants of conduction velocity in myelinated nerve fibers. Muscle Nerve 3:141–150, 1980
89. Weingarten HP, Mikolich LM, Johnson EW: Radiculopathies. In Johnson EW (ed): Practical Electromyography, pp 91–109. Baltimore, Williams & Wilkins, 1980
90. Wilbourn AJ: The value and limitations of electromyographic examination in the diagnosis of lumbosacral radiculopathy. In Hardy RW (ed): Lumbar Disc Disease, pp 65–109. New York, Raven Press, 1982
91. Wilbourn AJ: Electrodiagnosis of Plexopathies. In Aminoff MJ (ed): Electrodiagnosis. Neurologic Clinics, vol 3, pp 511–531, Philadelphia, WB Saunders, 1985
92. Wilbourn AJ: Common peroneal mononeuropathy at the fibular head. Muscle Nerve 9:825–836, 1986

12

Central Nervous System Electrophysiology

Jeffrey L. Cole

Alfred P. Pavot

Gary Goldberg

Neil I. Spielholz

Central nervous system (CNS) electrophysiology can be used in the practice of rehabilitation medicine to understand the physiological basis of disability due to CNS impairment. Not only can it be used to define a particular disease process or injury, but it can also help to determine what remains viable. These new tools yield quantitative, objective information that effectively extends the range of the clinical examination. Sensory pathways originating in almost any part of the body can be studied. Additionally, the processes that prepare and control movement can be examined. The information derived from the available test protocols is unique in that it is generally related to physiological activation of relevant neural tissue. It is therefore complementary to imaging studies that define anatomy and structural pathology.

In rehabilitation medicine, a wide range of disease processes producing CNS damage is encountered. In cerebrovascular accident (CVA) and traumatic brain injury, these diagnostic studies can be applied to define the degree of CNS disruption, the specific areas of involvement, and the prognosis for functional recovery. In the treatment of spinal cord injury, these studies have been used to define and document the level and extent of injury. As a research tool in management of spinal cord injury, they can help define injury states and assess therapeutic interventions.

The first observations of electrical activity recorded from the brain were made by Richard Caton in 1875 when he reported detection of electrical currents from electrodes placed on the skull or exposed brains of rabbits and monkeys.[12, 16] In 1929, Hans Berger published "On the Electroencephalogram of Man,"[10] documenting his recordings of electrical current flow on the scalp in humans using recording galvanometers that represented the "state of the art" of his time in electrical potential recording. Although his colleagues were initially skeptical, the discovery of alpha blocking with eye opening was accepted following a historical demonstration before the Physiology Society in London in 1935. Subsequent developments, including the application of a wide range of signal analysis methods and the acquisition of clinicopathological correlation, set the format for clinical electroencephalography (EEG) as it is now applied and gave practitioners a powerful tool for investigating the pathophysiology of the CNS.[78, 92]

In many ways, subsequent advances were dependent on applications of the "state of the art" in available instrumentation. The first reported use of photographic averaging of the EEG by superposition was by Dawson in 1947.[25] This technique was used to improve the ability to resolve synchronized responses to a specific event. The "giant" somatosensory evoked potentials (SEP) associated with some forms of myoclonus were observed serendipitously using this method, thus allowing the recording of the first event-related cerebral responses to peripheral nerve stimulation and initiating an entire new area of electrophysiological investigation.[26]

With the advent of electronic averaging and low-noise amplifiers, the ability to record an evoked potential (EP) became more accessible. As digital computer technology has been applied to this endeavor, and as advances in integrated circuit technology have produced precipitous drops in the costs associated with digital signal processing, these recording methods have moved out of the research laboratory and are now widely available and routinely employed clinically.

This chapter on CNS electrophysiology will primarily provide an overview of the use of EP studies in clinical rehabilitation practice. A review of the basic issue of electrophysiological recording is followed by sections on specific recording paradigms used clinically. How these studies can be applied to specific clinical problems encountered in the practice of rehabilitation medicine is then examined. In the final section the question of how this approach could be applied to investigate the physiological correlates of brain plasticity is discussed (see Chapter 10).[6]

The interested reader is encouraged to delve more deeply using the references provided. There can be no substitute for extensive reading and experience performing the procedures. A minimum of 6 months of intensively supervised training in a recognized facility is also necessary to acquire the prerequisite knowledge and technical facility needed for proficiency in performing and accurately interpreting EP studies. The use of rote pattern recognition can lead to serious errors and is discouraged. As in all electrodiagnostic work, the results cannot be interpreted in isolation from the clinical context. The physician must review the relevant clinical history and perform a focused physical examination prior to planning the studies. The interpretation must address the specific clinical questions prompting the referral, and the results should be correlated with other available laboratory and radiological information before any conclusions can be drawn regarding specific pathology. Some of the relevant basic science, applications, interpretation, and technical pitfalls of the different testing methods will also be reviewed in this chapter.

BASIC ISSUES IN CNS ELECTROPHYSIOLOGY

Basic Aspects of Bioelectrical Field Generation

The cellular membranes of excitable cells (*e.g.,* neurons, muscle cells) are capable of dynamic changes in their resistance to the flow of various ionic species. These changes in membrane ionic permeability allow changes in the movement of ions down their concentration gradients between the extracellular and intracellular spaces, which, in turn, induce widespread ionic movement throughout the extracellular space surrounding the active cells. These events alter the distribution of electrical potential throughout this space, and these changes in potential are detectable at the body's surface. There are dynamic changes in ionic current flowing across excitable membranes during the transmission of action potentials as well as with the generation of postsynaptic potentials (PSP). These ionic movements are usually related to transient conformational changes in channel proteins embedded in the cellular membrane. Such transient ionic flows may be produced by voltage-sensitive transitions in membrane conductance, as in sodium channel activation supporting the conduction of an action potential, or they may be due to chemically mediated changes in postsynaptic membrane conductance, produced through the presynaptic release of a neurotransmitter that activates specific receptors on the outer surface of the postsynaptic membrane. Transmembrane ionic currents can be defined precisely in basic cellular studies by using intracellular electrodes and recording the transmembrane voltages directly. With the use of a special voltage or "patch" clamping technique, it is possible to record the specific ionic currents and brief changes in membrane conductance due to brief ionic channel "openings," which are the ultimate determinants of the bioelectrical phenomena. The potential differences induced by these ionic flows in the surrounding space can be recorded by electrodes placed in the extracellular space adjacent to the active cell. With one electrode fixed in space, it is possible to move the other electrode around throughout the extracellular space to define the spatial distribution of the electrical potential, the *potential field.* The cell or group of cells giving rise to the transmembrane current flows that produce the extracellular potential field is called the *source* or *generator* of the field and, under specific conditions, may be sampled at large distances or from the surface of the body overlying the generator (Fig. 12-1).

Extracellular potential fields can be generated by transmembrane currents associated with the transmission of action potentials or with synaptic activity. Postsynaptic potentials can be either excitatory or inhibitory. However, when a potential is recorded extracellularly at some distance, it is not possible to conclude if the generator is excitatory or inhibitory (Fig. 12-2). For an electrode located at the scalp, excitation deep in the cortex cannot be distinguished from inhibition that appears superficially, and vice versa.

The recorded scalp potentials result from the superposition of the electrical potential fields produced by such sources within the brain. Since the total net electrical charge throughout the brain is zero, only pairs of *separated* positive and negative charges can give rise to the observed potential fields. A separated pair of electrical charges is called a *dipole* and is represented by a vector whose magnitude is given by the product of the separated amount of charge multiplied by the distance of separation and whose direction is determined by the orientation of an imaginary line drawn between the separated point charges. The activity of a source can thus be modeled electrically as a dipole or set of dipoles whose general orientation in space will influence the configuration of the potential distribution in the volume conductor. A radially oriented dipole will produce a distribution with a maximum potential directly overlying the dipole location, with the amplitude of the potential falling off as the electrode moves away from this point. A tangentially oriented dipole gives rise to a polarity reversal in the surface distribution with a positive peak on one end and a negative peak on the other. The site of the dipole is located beneath the "zero crossing" between these extrema. Obliquely oriented dipoles give rise to distributions that are effectively hybrids of these two types of field.[40]

The exact manner in which the potential field distributes and how the scalp potentials can be used to make inferences about the generator characteristics depend on many different factors. These are related to the geometry and electrical properties of the surrounding tissues, plus the internal geometry of the cells comprising the generator and the location of the recording electrodes with respect to the generator. The process by which the source activity can be recorded by remote electrodes when the source exists in an electrically conductive medium is called *volume conduction.* It is necessary to understand this process in order to make inferences about the activity and location of the source and to recognize that the recorded remote activity is an *interactive* phenomenon that reflects properties of the source, the extracellular environment, as well as the various important relationships between the two. The surrounding tissue factors can be quite complex in view of the fact that the electrical properties are nonhomogeneous and the geometry of surrounding structures may be quite irregular. In some instances, components of the EP reflect changes in the volume conductor geometry or in the relative orientation of the propagating activity, both of which are not indicative of functional neural activity.[63, 108] This issue is extremely important to recognize when one is attempting to infer information about relevant neural activity from scalp-recorded EP components.

The internal geometry of the generator is important in determining the two main types of field generators or activity ("open" or "closed") and whether extracellular fields will be recordable at a distance from the generator (Fig. 12-3). If the internal structure is spatially regular, then when the responding population of cells is synchronously activated, the potential fields generated by each individual cell will spatially summate throughout the extracellular space. This is called an *open field generator.* If the cells are not all oriented in the same direction, then spatial cancellation at a distance can result. Such structures, such as deep nuclei, may make relatively little contribution to the extracellular potential field outside the immediate vicinity of the source. Penetrating electrodes must be inserted to detect their activity. This is referred to as a *closed field generator.*

When the source of the activity is relatively close to the recording electrodes, as when a scalp electrode is recording activity directly over a cortical generator, this is called a *near-field recording.* Such fields are characterized by large spatial gradients because there is less "spread" of the extracellular activity through the volume conductor between the site of generation and the site of recording. When sampling a near field, electrodes may be spaced relatively close together on the surface to define the spatial gradient, as in a *bipolar recording,* or they can be placed close to the source with the other electrode placed at a relatively inactive distant site often called the reference site, as in *monopolar recording.* This differentiation is only a relative one and can be misleading, since, in fact, there is no ideal "inactive" reference site. All electrode locations may be in a position to detect significant activity so that all surface recording systems are

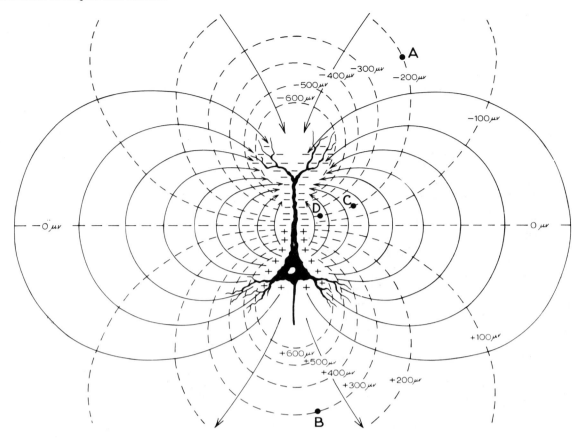

Figure 12-1. Dipole modeling of generators. The fundamental dipole of the cortex is the pyramidal cell. A dipolar field is generated when the cellular membrane receives synaptic input to the dendritic tree. This creates a net relative negativity or positivity superficially in the apical dendrites that generates a potential difference between the cell body and basal dendrites and the apical dendrites. For example, superficial excitatory input, as illustrated here, causes a relative negativity of the apical dendrites and positivity in the cell body and basal dendrites. The transient dipolar field causes a current to flow through the volume conductor and is recorded as a voltage on the scalp. This resultant surface potential (*dashed lines*) represents the linear summation of the individual cellular generators and will depend on synchronization of generator activation as well as on the geometry of both the generators and the volume conductor. Current flows are shown as solid lines. (Gloor P: Neuronal generators and the problem of localization in electroencephalography: Application of volume conductor theory to electroencephalography. J Clin Neurophysiol 2:327–345, 1985)

really bipolar. When there is a deflection in the recorded potential, then it is important to recognize that *both* electrodes may be contributing to the recorded component.

When the generator site is quite far from the accessible surface, the type of field is called a *far field*. In this case the amplitudes of the activity are quite low because of the resistive attenuation along the pathway between generator and electrode, and many trials must be averaged to define the waveform. There is also a larger "spread" of the source-induced current throughout the volume conductor, and the spatial gradients of the field are low, requiring widely spaced electrodes for recording.

In recording far fields, "stationary peaks" are frequently observed in the field (*i.e.,* peaks that do not propagate or move about). Kimura and colleagues[63] have demonstrated that some of these components may be produced by the passage of transmitted activity across a discontinuous junction at which the geometry of the volume conductor rapidly changes.[62] Thus caution is extremely important in assigning functional significance to such components of the EP. The presence of these components can also distort the structure of components related to actual functional source activity.

Both action potentials and PSPs can generate extracellular potential fields that could contribute to the EP recording. Although afferent neurograms can be readily attributed to summation of action potentials, the cortical surface and scalp EP near fields are dominated primarily by temporally and spatially summated excitatory and inhibitory synaptic activity from a responding population of cortical neurons with relatively minimal contribution from synchronized action potentials. This is probably because the rapid voltage transient associated with the action potential requires a greater degree of synchronization for temporal summation to occur because of its short duration, whereas the more prolonged and spatially more distributed fields due to PSPs can more readily summate with synchronous activation.

When activity is recorded without the application of specific stimuli, this is referred to a "background" or "spontaneous" activity and is the usual mode for recording the EEG. When segments of the data are captured with the application of a discrete stimulus, this is referred to as evoked activity or sensory EP and, depending on the rate of stimulation, may be either a *transient* or a *steady-state* response. With the transient EP, the rate of stimulation is slow enough that the response to one

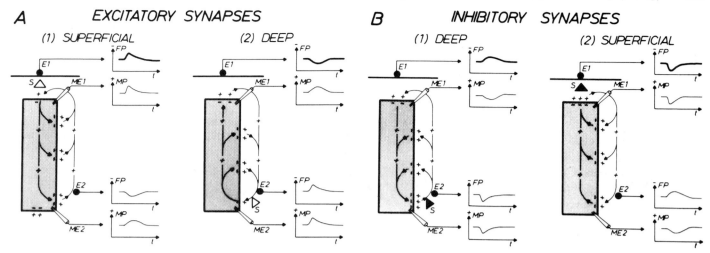

Figure 12-2. Relating cellular potential changes to extracellular field potentials (EFP). (*A1*) Superficial excitatory synaptic activation produces depolarization superficially. The extracellular electrode at the surface records a transient negativity associated with a positivity at depth. (*A2*) Activation of a deep excitatory synapse sets up a pattern of current flow opposite to that in *A1*. The EFP at the cortical surface now shows a positive deflection associated with a negativity at depth. (*B1*) An inhibitory postsynaptic potential is generated at depth in the neuronal element. The current flow is such that the EFP at the surface is negative with the EFP at the depth being a positive deflection. (*B2*) With activation of a superficial inhibitory synapse, the current flows in the opposite direction compared with *B1*. Thus, the surface EFP is now a positive deflection, while the EFP recorded at depth is a negativity. It is, thus, not readily determined from scalp recordings alone whether the underlying process giving rise to a deflection is inhibitory or excitatory. (Speckmann E-J, Elger CE: Neurophysiological basis of the EEG and of DC potentials. In Niedermeyer E, Lopes da Silva F [eds]: Electroencephalography: Basic Principles, Clinical Applications, and Related Fields. Baltimore, Urban & Schwarzenberg, 1982)

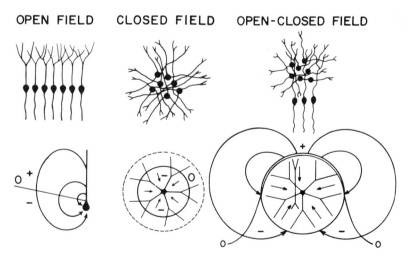

Figure 12-3. The effect of source geometry on field potential recording. Current flow and potential field produced by synchronous depolarization of the cell bodies of a row of neurons with parallel orientation (open field), with the cell bodies clustered and dendrites spreading radially (closed field), and with a combination of radial and parallel elements. (Allison T, Wood CC, McCarthy G: The central nervous system. In Coles MGH, Donchin E, Porges SW [eds]: Psychophysiology: Systems, Processes and Applications. New York, Guilford Press, 1986; adapted from Lorente de No R: Action potential of the motor neurons of the hypoglossus nucleus. J Cell Comp Physiol 29: 207–287, 1947)

stimulus is complete before the next arrives. With the steady-state EP, the rate is high enough that the response to one stimulus interacts with the response to the next. Depending on the stimulation rate, the steady-state response can show reduction or augmentation with response overlap. The primary emphasis in this chapter will be on the transient EP. However, in a more general sense, the event of interest in the recording paradigm need not be a discrete sensory stimulus but can be some form of repeating, neurally relevant occurrence. These events may be seen as involving a discrete informational or energy transfer in either direction between the subject and the surrounding environment and may range from the beginning of a spontaneous

movement associated with the recording of a readiness potential to the absence of an expected stimulus associated with the recording of a so-called emitted potential (P300). In this broader context, one refers to the bioelectrical activity associated with such an occurrence as an event-related potential (ERP) (Fig 12-4).

It is clear from this brief consideration of basic issues in CNS electrophysiology that the ability to perform clinical studies requires a broad familiarity with a wide range of issues including both anatomical and physiological considerations as well as the basic physics of electrical field theory in addition to the technical aspects of instrumentation and recording methods. EP studies

Figure 12-4. Recording paradigm common to all stimulus-evoked potentials. (*A*) Discrete repeating structured stimuli are applied to a receptor field or peripheral nerve of the relevant part of the nervous system being studied to give rise to an electrophysiological signal. This series of synchronous afferent volleys traverses the chosen input pathway to its primary cortical region to be recorded as a somatosensory evoked potential (*SEP*). Signals theoretically can be recorded from the receptors themselves (*e.g.,* as an electroretinogram [*ERG*], electrocochleogram [*EcoG*]) or along its peripheral or subcortical course as well while a particular event of interest recurs. This event could be the application of a particular sensory stimulus or the start of a motor response. Latency information obtained by comparing components in these signals can be used to characterize the rate of transmission along the pathway. (*B*) The relevant part of the nervous system being studied gives rise to its "baseline" activity plus an electrophysiological signal in response to the particular event of interest. This latter response occurs synchronously to the stimulus, generating a time-locked, stable potential to each occurrence of the event, which is then extracted from background signal and noise through an averaging process. (*C*) Synchronized frames of data that surround the point in time at which the event of interest (*e.g.,* shock, flash, sound) happened are captured and averaged together to extract the signal components consistently related to the triggering event of interest.

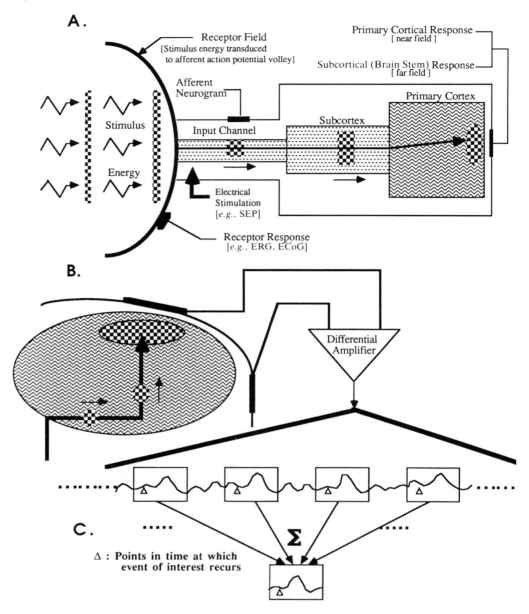

must always be interpreted in the context of a thorough understanding of the general principles of neurophysiological recording.

The Recorded Evoked Potential

The recorded surface potential obtained between a particular pair of electrodes is a spatial and temporal sampling of the summated activity of all bioelectrical generators potentially contributing to the recording. Selective activation of particular structures (*e.g.,* peripheral nerve, retina, cochlea, cortex) the clinician wishes to examine can be produced by the application of specific provoking stimuli. The selected stimulus is applied repeatedly at a particular rate, and the signal is extracted by signal averaging (see Fig. 12-4). However, it becomes extremely important to distinguish activation of the target structure from bioelectrical activity produced by other generators. Among these many possible sources of bioelectrical "interference" are cardiac (electrocardiogram) and skeletal muscle (electromyogram) signals, the

ongoing "background" EEG, and corneoretinal signals produced by eye movement (electro-oculogram). Additional artifacts and "noise" may arise at the skin–electrode interface and from within the instrumentation. Further possible sources of electrical interference involve radiated noise from the surrounding environment. The most troublesome of this latter group is interference from electrical power lines producing alternating fields at a frequency of about 60 Hz. Interference can also be generated by other electrically powered devices such as motors, lights, and telephones. To ensure the best and most reliable information it is necessary to maximize the contribution of the desired signal being produced by the bioelectrical source one is attempting to isolate and to minimize the effect of all other contaminating sources.

The physician must be aware of and able to recognize and limit the effects of all interfering activity. Noise from skeletal muscle can be reduced by ensuring the patient is relaxed and as comfortable as possible throughout the test. Facial and scalp electromyographic (EMG) activity can be reduced by having the patient relax the jaw and allow the mouth to drop open. A towel roll can be used to support the head and reduce contraction of the neck musculature. It is difficult to completely eliminate interference because of eye movement and blinking. These artifacts, however, are usually very large signals that can be dealt with by using a rejection filter based on an amplitude criterion. When the amplitude of the recorded potential exceeds the window, the recorded activity does not contribute to the ongoing averaging. This is often referred to as an automatic artifact reject feature in EP instrumentation. It is sometimes useful to listen to the input activity over an audio amplifier or to observe the "raw" input activity on an oscilloscope that can allow the recognition of intermittent periods of artifactual activity. The averaging process can then be manually "paused" during these intervals.

When reporting the results of the study, certain minimum standards should be followed. The report should include the relevant aspects of the history and physical examination and the reason for the referral. The signals used for the data analysis and interpretation must be recorded showing at least two superimposed waveforms obtained by repeating the study. This test–retest protocol is used to document the reproducibility of the results obtained. A printout of the signals should be attached to the written report. The stimulus and recording parameters employed should be included, as well as a brief description of the technique. Interpretation should be based on statistical comparisons to normative measures using standard methods for determining deviation from the mean for normally distributed variables. Most authorities recommend a conservative interpretation in which abnormality is concluded only when the patient measurement lies beyond a range of 2.5 to 3 SD from the mean. To improve sensitivity, it may be necessary to correct for subject variables such as age, sex, and height.

New methods for recording and displaying EP data are described in the literature on a regular basis. Computer-based digital signal acquisition and processing combined with color display graphics offer a myriad of different ways to examine the signal data and to attempt to extract and display useful information. Techniques for topographic mapping of scalp potential fields[29, 31] and dipole source localization methods[118] will eventually become important clinical tools, although their application is now primarily limited to research questions. A wide variety of analysis techniques have been applied to time-varying brain signals.[38, 74] It is important to remember that the ability to apply these methods requires a basic understanding of the power and limitations of the method and cannot take one beyond the basic issues involved in recording and interpreting the data. None of these techniques has received broad-based acceptance in the clinic although many serve as important and useful research tools. A complete examination of this range of data processing and display methods is beyond the scope of this chapter. However, it is quite possible that these approaches that apply emerging technology to the problem of extracting useful information from electrophysiological signals may, through carefully planned research, yield important tools for the assessment of function in the CNS that take the field beyond the basic techniques to be reviewed here.

Electrode Placement

In an effort to standardize methods for EEG study comparison, a system for scalp electrode location and nomenclature was devised that became known as the International Ten-Twenty System.[55] This system allows for uniform electrode positioning relative to fixed landmarks no matter what the size of the subject's skull. This is accomplished with the use of percentages of an easily reproducible measurement rather than by fixed distances,

so that the spacing on the scalp is maintained proportional to head size. In adults, these scalp sites correlate with specific brain structures (Fig. 12-5), which are consistent from patient to patient and cover all significant cortical areas. In infants, there is larger variation between the skull landmarks and the underlying cortical structures. All the electrode sites are derived by measuring distances from four landmarks (Fig. 12-6) on the skull: the nasion, the left and right preauricular points, and the inion. The standard electrode sites are derived from these four reference points using measurement protocols that are available in any EEG technology textbook.[20] This system, therefore, is an ideal starting point to designate scalp sites for EP studies.

The Ten-Twenty System was developed to answer EEG needs for an easily reproducible scheme for applying scalp electrodes, but in EP studies its rigidity is not desirable. For example, a common practice in EP studies is to place an electrode "behind" a designated site and use a prime (') mark for each centimeter distance away. This evolved because these subtle electrode shifts were found to maximize the averaged evoked amplitude or improve the separation or identification of certain "peaks." There is, as yet, no standardized nomenclature for most noncephalic sites that are used as references and for subcortical information derivations. Also, the EEG "O" site is often labeled "Oz" when used in SEP and VEP studies. Although these necessary adaptations described above are common practices for EP studies, they are not permitted for EEG recordings.

Evoked Potential Instrumentation

Electrodes

The instrumentation consists of many linked components. As we move from the patient to the equipment, the first connection is a skin-electrode interface. The electrode site should be

Figure 12-5. Anatomical correlation of the brain lobes, central sulcus, Sylvian fissure, and the midline electrode positions.

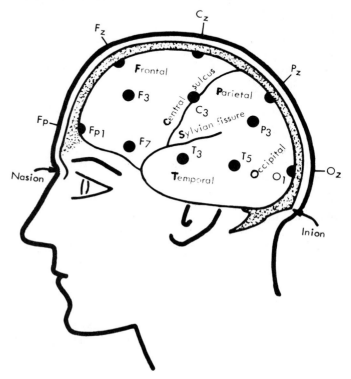

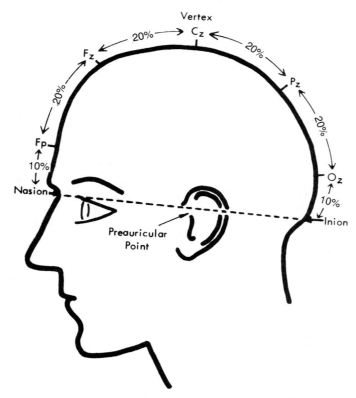

Figure 12-6. Reference point landmarks on the skull (nasion, right and left preauricular points, and inion) as shown from the left lateral view. The relative percentages of distance between electrode sites are shown along the midline measurement from nasion to inion.

lightly abraded, a coupling electrolyte used, and the electrode well fixed in place so no movement occurs during the testing and a constant low impedance is maintained. The interface so formed has characteristics that vary significantly with the type of electrode (cup, disk, intradermal pin, Ag/AgCl, surface clip, etc.) applied. This is because the interface formed behaves electrically like a resistor and capacitor wired in parellel to each other, allowing alternating and direct current signals to cross this interface. This should be checked with an AC impedance meter. For surface electrodes, this should be less than 5 kilo-ohms to ensure good recordings. Interdermal pin or clip-type surface electrodes have inherently higher impedances, which cannot be reduced because of the nature and size of the skin-electrode interface. To ensure good readings, patients are advised to wash their scalp and hair the morning of the test and not to apply any conditioners, lotions or similar hair dressings because the salts in sweat and conditioning agents can produce bridging between the electrodes. It is also good practice to soak regular surface electrodes thoroughly in a disinfectant, and pin or needle electrodes and surface electrodes used in the genital areas should be soaked in a 2% solution of glutaraldehyde, bleach, or equivalent disinfectant, and then can be processed for regular gas or "high-vac" sterilization.

Amplifiers

Amplifiers used for electrophysiological studies are typically high-gain differential amplifiers with high-input impedance, low noise, and the ability to attenuate greatly the amplitude of the common-mode signal via the ground electrode. The amplifier's gain setting is selected so that the displayed signal will fill the majority of the screen without wandering out of range too often. Another way of estimating the gain setting with an amplitude limiter or reject system is when 5 to 10% of the sweeps are rejected.

Filters

The signal one is trying to record has its electrical energy within a specific limited frequency range. Filters are used to limit interference due to noise sources whose frequency range does not overlap greatly with that of the EP signal's frequency. The filter setting determines the "cutoff" or break frequency, which is the frequency at which a specific degree of amplitude attenuation is obtained. The filter's characteristics also include the rate at which power attenuation occurs near the cutoff frequency. It is generally better to use wide-band recording to minimize their distorting effect and to keep the settings equal from one recording to the next. Proper use of our filters is a necessity to attain efficient EP acquisition, and the application of new filtering techniques is allowing "single sweep" EP recordings on a clinical level to speed analysis as well as to look at rapid stimulus-to-stimulus changes. Whatever the approach, the key is normal data standardization so that the study is set up in an identical manner each time it is performed.

Digitalization and the Averaging Process

A natural bioelectrical signal is a continuously varying voltage, called an *analog signal*. To facilitate the averaging process, this signal is first converted to digital form. The captured waveform is digitized by separating the amplitude into discrete levels of voltage and is quantized by sampling the signal at regular discrete points in time at a particular rate, called the *sampling rate*. The total amplitude scale of the input range, not the input signal, is divided into a set number of discrete intervals determined by the number of binary digits, or *bits,* available in the converter. Thus an 8-bit digitizer divides the voltage scale into 256 divisions, while a 10-bit digitizer gains better resolution by dividing the range into 1,024 divisions. The horizontal resolution on the time axis is determined by the sampling rate. The higher the sampling rate, the more accurately the signal is represented in the time domain and the more memory required for storing a signal over a given time window. For accurate clinical use, the time sampling rate should be between three and five times the highest frequency of the desired EP signal. This generally is about three times the recommended upper filter setting for that study.

The improved signal-to-noise ratio due to the averaging process is directly related to the number of sweeps averaged, and the noise reduction is proportional to the square root of the total number of sweeps counted. Overaveraging can increase the relative contribution of the stimulus-dependent and regularly occurring noises and will tend to reduce the recorded EP amplitude. Averaging a large number of sweeps should never be a substitute for inadequate skin-electrode preparation, changes in stimulation or recording parameters between runs, or other unacceptable practices.

Recording Guidelines

The various common problem areas are listed in Table 12-1 by the type of interference encountered or its presumed source, and some methods are suggested to correct or at least minimize them. Routine recording parameters for a variety of CNS electrodiagnostic studies are presented in Table 12-2.

Table 12-1
Methods to Maximize the Desired Response and Minimize the "Noise"

Signals Entering the Electrodes	Electrical Characteristics	Methodologies to Improve Overall Recorded Signal
Stimulus-evoked bioelectrical potentials (the desired signal)	Low amplitude Selective/specific bandwidth or groups of frequencies	Electrode selection and placement to maximize the desired signal amplitude Appreciably enhanced by stimulus "time-locked" averaging techniques Low electrode impedance (2000–5000 ohms) Appropriate filter settings (band-pass control selection)
Bioelectrical noise from neural generators not related to the stimulus	Relatively high amplitudes Usually low frequencies	Reduced appreciably by averaging techniques Reduced by combining: a. Good recording techniques b. Appropriate patient management and positioning for relaxation (and comfort) during the examination c. Positioning and appropraite stimulus intensity to minimize synchronous movement artifacts at the stimulation point d. Amplitude gating (reject control) of the input signal e. Band-pass control (lmited by frequency overlaps of the desired signal and bioelectrical and system noises) selection f. Electrode placement to minimize bioelectrical background noises g. Firm electrode fixation to prevent movement artifact (can be as much as 5-mV potentials) h. Skin preparation
Bioelectrical noise not related to the neural generators (*e.g.,* myogenic potentials, volume conduction)	High amplitudes Usually low frequenices (30–300 Hz)	
Electromagnetic noise (system and environment)	Usually high frequency with variable amplitudes but can be present at low frequencies (less than 10 Hz and line current 60 Hz) with high amplitudes	Suitable selection of electronic components (*e.g.,* high input impedance, low peak-to-peak noise level, high common mode rejection ratio, high gain amplifiers) Appropriate maintenance and calibration of equipment Reduce man-made (*e.g.,* fluorescent lights, motors) electrical noise Good patient grounding and elimination of ground loops Balanced electrode impedances (greater than 1000 ohms) Minimize electrode and cable movement and cable lengths

Reprinted from Cole, JL: Equipment parameter determinants in evoked potential studies. Bull Am Soc Clin Evoked Potentials 3(1):3–9, 1984, with permission.

SPECIFIC PARADIGMS

Brain Stem Auditory Evoked Potentials

Some of the earliest EPs recorded from the human brain were related to auditory stimulation.[24] It was not until Jewett and his colleagues[56-58] and Sohmer and Feinmesser[102, 103] began looking at the very early components of the scalp potential that the more robust elements of the response were defined. These early components normally observed in the first 10 msec after the stimulus are the *brain-stem auditory evoked potential (BAEP).* This study has been applied in a wide range of clinical situations for both audiological assessment as well as for site-of-lesion neurodiagnostic assessment. These are far-field components with amplitudes that are generally a fraction of a microvolt.

The response consists of a series of seven deflections labeled with Roman numerals in accordance with the Jewett system (Fig. 12-7). These deflections are recorded as positive at the vertex with reference to the earlobe on the side being stimulated. A number of variations of the normal waveform have been described including a bifid wave I and absence of wave IV. Wave V is usually identified by the large negative deflection that immediately follows it.

The broad clinical application of the BAEP has been possible because of the reproducibility and robustness of the response, the apparent anatomical specificity of the various components, and their general resistance to a wide variety of physiological stresses. The study can be used to investigate the integrity of brain-stem transmission of auditory impulses and has also been used to examine hearing thresholds in patients in whom conventional audiometry is not possible. The study can thus be useful in selected cases for the investigation of hearing loss. The BAEP is also a sensitive diagnostic examination that can, for example, be used for early detection of tumors of the cerebellopontine angle and posterior fossa.

Relevant Anatomy

The BAEP has been recorded from a broad range of different animals, and there have been a number of animal studies attempting to localize the generators of the BAEP components. These studies have linked the generation of these components to different structures in the brain-stem auditory pathway (Fig. 12-8), and a brief review of transmission through this pathway may be of value.

When a traveling wave of air vibration is of sufficient magnitude to induce movement of the tympanic membrane, the process of "sound perception" begins. The vibrating membrane transmits this mechanical energy through the auditory ossicles of the middle ear to the basilar membrane of the cochlea. The organ of Corti lies in the membranous cochlea and is the sensory organ of hearing. It is a two and one-quarter turn coil formed around a central bony axis or modiolus. An osseous spiral lamina projects from the modiolus into the cochlea. The afferent fibers of the auditory nerve pierce the small canals of the spiral lamina, which connect with the spiral canal containing the spiral gan-

Table 12-2
Evoked Potential Recording Parameters: General Guidelines for Select Studies

	Auditory Evoked Potentials	Visual Evoked Potentials	Upper Extremity SEP	Lower Extremity & Pudendal SEP	Electro-spinogram (ESG)	Cognitive Evoked Potentials
Amplifier						
Sensitivity	0.5–2.0 µV/div	5–10 µV/div	2.0–5.0 µV/div	5–10 µV/div	0.5–5.0 µV/div	2.0–5.0 µV/div
Sweep speed	1 msec/div	20–40 msec/div	5 msec/div	10 sec/div (120 msec/div intra-operatively)	5–10 msec/div	50–100 msec/div
Filters						
Low (high pass)	80–160 Hz	0.8–1.0 Hz	2–20 Hz (non-cephalic reference) or 16–32 Hz (cephalic reference)	8–16 Hz (16–64 Hz intra-operatively)	20 or 200 Hz	0.1–0.3 HZ
High (low pass)	2500–3600 Hz	80–100 Hz	1600–2000 Hz	1000–2000 Hz	1000–3000 Hz	70–100 Hz
Stimulator						
Repetition rate	10 pps	2 reversals/sec	3–8 pps	1–3 pps	1–4 pps (0.3 intra-operatively)	0.5–1.0 stim./sec
Duration	0.1 msec (100 Hz–8 kHz)		0.05–0.2 msec	0.05–0.2 msec		0.05–0.2 msec
Stimulus intensity	60–65 above hearing thres-hold; noise 38 db below click level	Constant lumens output; max-imum (100%) contrast	5 mA above minimal thumb abduction twitch	5 mA above min-imal hallux abductor/flexor (maximum stimulator voltage intraoperatively) Pudendal stimulation at three times threshold level	10 mA above minimal toe flexion	Variable; may be used as a "target" parameter
Averager						
No. sweeps for good S/N ratio	1000	100–500	500–1000	100–500	100–1000	100–500
Electrode Placements	C$_z$–active, A$_1$/M$_1$ or A$_2$/M$_2$ reference; opposite ear ground	O$_z$ (occasionally O$_1$ or O$_2$)–C$_z$ or F$_z$; midline ground	C$_3$/C$_3'$ or C$_4$/C$_4'$ to contralateral noncephalic reference or F$_z$ (& Erb's pt marker)	C$_z$–F$_z$ (use ESG as proof of entry and marker)	L1–T11 vertebral level (midline at interspinous ligament)	C$_z$–active; joined A$_1$–A$_2$ or M$_1$–M$_2$ reference; mid-line ground

(Adapted from Cole, JL: Equipment parameter determinants in evoked potential studies. Bull Am Soc Clin Evoked Potentials 3(1):3–9, 1984, with permission.)

glion that contains the bipolar cells that are the first order neurons of the auditory pathway. The axons of these cells consti-tute the cochlear nerve, and their distal extent connects with the sensory hair cells where the transduction from mechanical en-ergy to electrophysiological signaling occurs. The proximal axons of the cells of the spiral ganglion enter the brain stem as the cochlear division of the eighth cranial nerve to reach the dorsal and ventral cochlear nuclei.

The central auditory system contains rhomboencephalic, mesencephalic, diencephalic, and telencephalic components. The BAEP provides information primarily about the first two of these. The rhomboencephalic components of the pathway in-clude the ventral and dorsal cochlear nuclei, the lateral and medial nuclei of the superior olivary complex, the trapezoid body, and the lateral lemniscus. The mesencephalic component is represented by the inferior colliculus. The cochlear nuclei (CN) give rise to two separate transverse bundles of fibers that run through the trapezoid body (from the ventral CN) and the dorsal acoustic striae (from the dorsal CN). The trapezoid body

reaches the lateral part of the pons and turns rostral to become the lateral lemniscus. Some of these fibers also reach cells in the superior olivary complex. Fibers in the dorsal acoustic stria pass over into the lateral lemniscus in the vicinity of the superior olivary complex. The fibers of the lateral lemniscus then ascend to the inferior colliculus (IC). Brain-stem transmission may be either multisynaptic or direct from CN to IC. There are also both ipsilateral and contralateral projections, although the bulk of the fibers cross the midline at the lower pontine level. From the IC, transmission continues to the diencephalic component, the me-dial geniculate nucleus. The last segment of the pathway is from this level to the primary auditory cortex in the superior temporal cortex in the floor of the lateral sulcus.

Because of the complexity of the anatomical pathway, it is difficult to assume a simple serial model of transmission with sequential activation of sources in the pathway. In actuality, scalp components probably represent propagated activity in parallel pathways with overlapping sources. Clinicopathological correla-tion, however, suggests that a general guideline regarding source

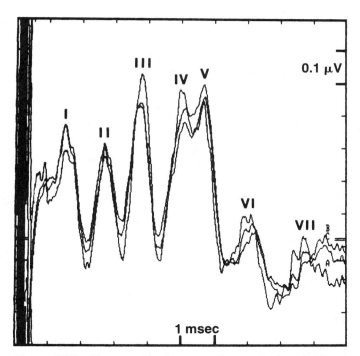

Figure 12-7. The normal brain-stem auditory evoked potential typically contains seven waves, which are designated as peaks I through VII. They are recorded as a series of high-frequency vertex (C_z) positive far-field potentials during the first 10 msec after a discrete stimulus. When the stimulus and recording parameters are adequately controlled (See Table 12-2), the waves I, III, and V are reliably correlated with the known pathway and various pathological conditions and lesions.

activity is possible with the interval between component I and III related to transmission from the cochlear nerve through to the approximate level of the superior olivary complex in midpons, while the interval between waves III and V related to transmission from midpons through to the level of the IC. The exact localization of the sources for each of the scalp components of the BAEP remains controversial because of the complexity of brain-stem auditory transmission. It is possible that the recorded components observed reflect the synchronization of nerve impulses transmitted through the auditory brain-stem system rather than specific spatial generator sites.

Indications

ADULTS. In testing adults, the BAEP has been helpful in the investigation of a variety of audiological problems. These include patients with unexplained "central" impairment on audiometric testing. The tests can also be employed to check for the presence of significant sudden onset unilateral hearing loss. They can detect the presence of demyelinating disease or acoustic neuroma. The BAEP has also been used for intraoperative monitoring during surgery in the region of the cerebellopontine angle and posterior fossa as well as for monitoring the integrity of patients in barbiturate-induced coma. The tests have been used with varying degrees of success to assess brain-stem function in patients who are in coma or who appear to be "brain dead."

CHILDREN. Audiometry using the BAEP, sometimes called objective audiometry, can be used in infants and newborns to detect the presence of hearing loss at an early age. Infants in neonatal intensive care units are at relative high risk of either brain-stem neurological or audiological deficit. These patients

can be screened by performing a BAEP with both high- and low-intensity clicks. Other children at risk include those with a known family history of genetic disease with associated hearing loss, children with orofacial dysmorphic syndromes, term infants who have had significant hypoxic episodes, newborns with congenital infections or infants with bacterial meningitis, and infants or children who have required treatment with ototoxic drugs. Detection of hearing loss at an early stage is important since aural rehabilitation can be successful if a detected partial hearing loss is compensated and if therapy begins early. A follow-up examination 1 to 3 months after the initial examination is usually necessary to confirm any detected abnormality. The BAEP may have particular use in assessing children with delayed language development or severe behavior difficulties. With the institution of a program of corrective augmentation and aural rehabilitation, the early detection of significant hearing loss made possible by the application of objective audiometry (*i.e.,* audiometric examination using the BAEP) can make a very significant difference in the eventual outcome.[37] These studies may also be helpful in assessing young patients with hypoxic or traumatic encephalopathies for whom prognostic considerations are foremost.

Procedure and Test Parameters

A physical examination of the cranial nerves as well as an otoscopic examination of the external auditory canal and the tympanic membrane should precede the test, along with the taking of a focused history. The clinical question being addressed should be carefully determined: Is the primary concern neurological, audiometric, or both? The patient is then positioned supine on a bed or in a reclining chair with good support for the head to help ensure relaxation of scalp and neck muscles. Auditory stimuli may be delivered by way of audiometric headphones or through tubal insert phone (TIPs). The TIPs have the advantage of sealing the external auditory canal and also introducing a fixed delay between the stimulus artifact and the waveform. Electrodes are placed at the vertex (C_z) and on each earlobe or on the skin overlying the mastoid process. It is critical in performing the study to be able to recognize the wave I component. On occasion this may be difficult for technical reasons. The use of a subdermal electrode placed in the skin of the outer aspects of the external auditory meatus has been recommended when wave I cannot be readily recorded. A ground electrode is placed at the F_z or F_{pz} position, or the contralateral earlobe or mastoid site may be used if a single-channel recording is performed. With a single-channel recording, C_z is routed to the noninverting input while the ipsilateral earlobe is connected to the inverting input. With two-channel recording, C_z is referenced to one earlobe/mastoid site on the first channel and the other earlobe/mastoid site on the second channel. Some authors have found an earlobe-to-earlobe recording useful for defining wave I.

Stimulation is usually provided by a click of about 0.1 msec in duration at a rate of about 10 per second, although factors of 60 should be avoided to prevent synchronization with line frequency. In forming the average, 1,500 to 2,000 sweeps are collected with each run and a retest protocol is employed until the superimposed waveforms demonstrate good reproducibility of the recorded structure.

It is an accepted convention that sound intensity is expressed as a ratio with respect to a reference level. In a cooperative subject, the behavioral threshold or sensation level (SL) can be determined using the staircase method with the threshold determined by the average of the ascending and descending threshold levels. A fixed increase (usually about 75 dB) is then added to threshold reference to arrive at the test level. The stimulus intensity referred to sensation level is denoted as dB SL.

Anatophysiological Processes	Waves Produced

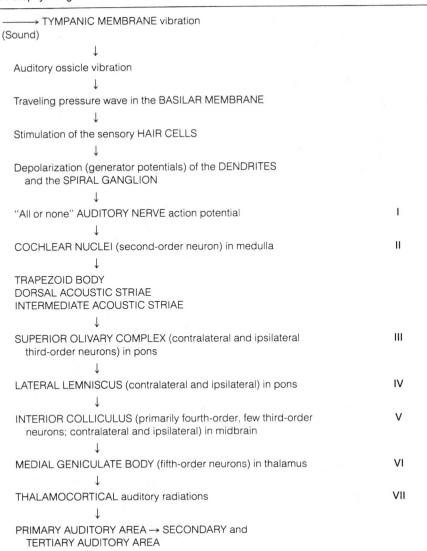

$\longrightarrow$ TYMPANIC MEMBRANE vibration
(Sound)

$\downarrow$

Auditory ossicle vibration

$\downarrow$

Traveling pressure wave in the BASILAR MEMBRANE

$\downarrow$

Stimulation of the sensory HAIR CELLS

$\downarrow$

Depolarization (generator potentials) of the DENDRITES
and the SPIRAL GANGLION

$\downarrow$

"All or none" AUDITORY NERVE action potential   I

$\downarrow$

COCHLEAR NUCLEI (second-order neuron) in medulla   II

$\downarrow$

TRAPEZOID BODY
DORSAL ACOUSTIC STRIAE
INTERMEDIATE ACOUSTIC STRIAE

$\downarrow$

SUPERIOR OLIVARY COMPLEX (contralateral and ipsilateral   III
third-order neurons) in pons

$\downarrow$

LATERAL LEMNISCUS (contralateral and ipsilateral) in pons   IV

$\downarrow$

INTERIOR COLLICULUS (primarily fourth-order, few third-order   V
neurons; contralateral and ipsilateral) in midbrain

$\downarrow$

MEDIAL GENICULATE BODY (fifth-order neurons) in thalamus   VI

$\downarrow$

THALAMOCORTICAL auditory radiations   VII

$\downarrow$

PRIMARY AUDITORY AREA $\rightarrow$ SECONDARY and
TERTIARY AUDITORY AREA

Figure 12-8.   Schematic auditory pathway correlated with far-field recording peaks.

In subjects who cannot indicate reliable behavioral responses, a fixed intensity is measured either in sound pressure level (denoted dB sPL) or with respect to an average click threshold for a group of normal young adult subjects determined under standardized conditions (denoted dB nHL). EP instruments may be calibrated using either of these scales. It should be noted that, for the purposes of neurological investigation, if interpeak latencies are employed as the measured parameters, sensitivity to stimulus intensity is very much reduced since these measures are relatively stable across a wide range of stimulus intensities. A "masking" stimulation of white noise is frequently applied to the contralateral ear to minimize the effects of "cross-talk" due to bony transmission of the unilateral stimulus.

The click may be produced by either rarefaction or condensation, depending on the polarity of the pulse applied to the transducer. Rarefaction tends to produce a shorter latency peak than does condensation, and wave I tends to be seen better with rarefaction clicks. Most authors recommend the initial use of rarefaction with condensation clicks employed to clarify findings obtained with rarefaction. Alternating polarity can also be employed to reduce the stimulus artifact, but this can lead to some distortion of wave I and the electrocochleogram because of the superposition of different wave structures.

Clinical Interpretation

A set of normal adult values (N = 63) is presented in Table 12-3 for the absolute peak and interpeak latencies using 10 click per second rarefaction stimuli at 60 to 65 dB SL, "white noise" masking of the contralateral ear at 30 dB below the stimulus level, with a filter of 100 to 3000 Hz, measured after 1,000 sweeps were averaged on each run. Normal values should be established for each laboratory using similar recording parameters as well as any additional testing conditions needed. On comparing multiple runs, the intertrial latency differences for absolute peak latencies should not exceed 0.25 msec.

Interpeak latencies are the most useful measures since they are relatively stable with changes in click intensity. Side-to-side comparison of the interpeak latencies can also be used to improve sensitivity with unilateral impairment. The I–III interpeak latencies have shown excellent correlation with documented lesions in the peripheral auditory mechanism, auditory nerve, and lower pons level lesions. The I–V latency difference, also known as the auditory brain-stem transmission time, has had widespread application in brain-stem, thalamic, and cortical structure injuries when the I–III interpeak latencies are normal. Additionally, there can be diffuse involvement both in the I–III and III–V interpeak central conduction times in multiple sclerosis and demyelinating diseases. The BAEP can be of some assistance in assessing the relative integrity of brain-stem structures in the presence of diffuse brain damage due to traumatic brain injury. Although severe impairment of the BAEP is generally a poor prognostic sign in the stable patient with traumatic brain injury, the presence of preserved responses does not necessarily correlate with a good recovery because of the possibility of a normal BAEP in a patient with severe diffuse cerebral damage. The BAEP may not always be contributory in such patients because of damage to the auditory nerve or peripheral auditory apparatus, which precludes the use of the BAEP as a probe of brain-stem circuitry.

Various techniques may be employed to help identify individual waves and to clarify the waveform. Slowing down the stimulation rate can give a better relative amplitude to wave V and also augment and separate waves I and III. Clarification of components can sometimes be improved by reducing stimulus intensity. Wave V is most resistant to the effects of continuing to reduce the stimulus intensity and can be isolated through a reduction in stimulus intensity.

The BAEP provides the clinician with a tool that can be applied to test the integrity of the peripheral and brain-stem central auditory mechanisms and can also be used to assess transmission through the brain-stem. An extensive literature has now developed around the application of the BAEP to a variety of different audiological and neurological problems, and the interested reader is invited to examine this literature and more detailed reviews and monographs devoted to this topic. The BAEP is a useful test of auditory function particularly for patients who cannot be tested by conventional audiometric methods. Longer latency responses can be used to examine central transmission to the cortical level. This tool may prove valuable to the physiatrist in specific clinical situations in which the assessment of auditory and/or brain-stem function becomes important in planning and implementing rehabilitation programs.

Visual Evoked Potentials

Relevant Anatomy

Light energy enters the eye and impinges on the retinal photoreceptors and generates an electrophysiological signal that is processed by the retinal layers and transmitted by the ganglion cell layer into the optic nerve. The optic nerve is really a piece of brain bathed in cerebrospinal fluid and is composed of about 1.2 million fibers that transmit action potentials intracranially to the optic chiasm from which the optic tracts emerge and convey impulses to the lateral geniculate body. From here, the signals continue, after thalamic processing, the primary visual cortex through the optic radiation. The visual evoked potential (VEP) to pattern shift stimulation is generally thought to arise in primary visual cortex. Although it is possible to record a response to a diffuse light flash, the use of a checkerboard reversal or "pattern shift" has the advantage that the luminance of the stimulus remains constant throughout and the response is therefore less variable (Fig. 12-9).

Test Procedures

Electrodes are placed over the occipital region in the midline and at fixed distances to the left and right of the midline. These references are generally referred to an electrode on the

Table 12-3
Sample Brain-Stem Auditory Evoked Potential Normal Values

Jewett Peak Latencies	Interpeak Latency Differences
I = 1.35–2.08 msec	I–III = 1.93–2.30 msec
II = 2.54–3.22 msec	I–IV/V = 3.60–4.20 msec
III = 3.58–4.30 msec	I–V = 3.75–4.38 msec
IV = 5.00–5.60 msec	III–IV/V = 1.50–2.10 msec
IV/V = 5.25–6.00 msec	III–V = 1.74–2.18 msec
V = 5.32–6.16 msec	
VI = 7.05–7.78 msec	
VII = 8.70–9.45 msec	

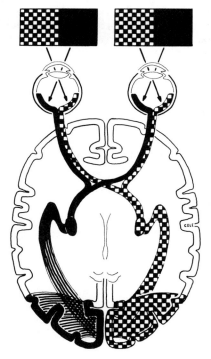

Figure 12-9. Basic anatomy and simplified visual pathways. The monitor at the top shows a left hemifield pattern stimulus and a blank signal on the right half of the screen. The left stimulus is transmitted to the medial right occipital lobe's primary visual cortex, and the "blank" signal is transmitted to the left occipital lobe primary cortex. Then both signals are transmitted to the secondary areas where integration and perception occur. In this situation the "pattern reversal" refers to the switching of light and dark components of the checkerboard on the left, not to a left-to-right reversal of the pattern and the blank half-screens.

vertex, although some prefer to use a midfrontal site as a reference. In some cases, an electrode placed at the midline parietal site, P_z, is also of value when a component at the midoccipital site is not readily discerned. An alternative reference site is linked earlobes. A signal is generally collected by averaging approximately 100 trials, and the averager is set for a sweep duration of 300 to 500 msec. If there is any question about the response, the study should be repeated and the individual results superimposed until a trend in the data can be confidently recognized or until it is certain that the response is missing. Visual acuity should be checked as part of the examination, and the subject should wear glasses, if needed, for the test. It is important to ensure that a well-focused image of the pattern appears on the retinal surface. It is also important to know if a field defect is present.

With the electrodes placed, the subject is moved in front of a screen (usually a TV monitor) on which the reversing pattern is displayed. The subject is positioned 70 to 100 cm from the screen, and the check size is adjusted to produce an effective visual angle of 10 to 30 minutes of arc. This can be computed using Table 12-4, assuming that the subject is seated 1 meter from the screen. The amplitude of the VEP is generally related by an inverse U curve to the check size. This relationship can be explored using multiple check sizes.[76] Each eye is tested independently, and the pattern is reversed at a rate of about 2 per second. The subject must maintain focused attention on the center of the screen and should be monitored by the examiner to ensure that attentive gaze is maintained on the center of the presented pattern.

The evoked response has a triphasic structure, with the second major peak, at a latency of about 100 msec, having the greatest reliability and being most useful for clinical measurement purposes (Fig. 12-10). It is a large occipitally positive component generally referred to as the P_{100} component. The most important aspect is its latency.[46]

Other important measurements that can be obtained include the intereye latency difference of the P_{100} and the ratio of amplitudes between the two sides where the amplitude may be defined as either peak to peak or baseline to peak. Loss of visual acuity may attenuate the P_{100} but should have no significant effect on the latency. The P_{100} latency will change systematically with a number of stimulus factors, including stimulus luminance, contrast, field size, and check size. Latencies also depend on the type of stimulator used. Subject factors such as age and gender can also influence the result. It is important that laboratory standards

for this study be obtained once specific recording parameters are chosen.

Clinical Indications and Interpretation

The VEP is particularly useful in complementing the neuro-ophthalmological examination when clinical problems are mild enough that the findings on clinical examination are either equivocal or suggestive. In such instances, the VEP can be of value in detecting the presence of and/or confirming a lesion of the anterior optic pathway. These studies are highly sensitive in

Table 12-4
Degrees of Visual Stimulation

Checkerboard Check Sizes in Millimeters	Visual Angle in Minutes of Arc with 1 Meter From Eyes to Screen
2.00	6.88
(2.91)	(10.00)
3.00	10.31
4.00	13.75
5.00	17.19
(5.82)	(20.00)
6.00	20.63
7.00	24.06
8.00	27.50
(8.73)	(30.00)
9.00	30.94
10.00	34.38
(11.64)	(40.00)
12.00	41.25
14.00	48.13
16.00	55.01
18.00	61.88
20.00	68.76

For any other check size there are simplified formula (for "minutes of arc" and "millimeter" units) to obtain the visual arc from the measured check size (angle = 3.438 × check size) or the check size to be used for a desired stimulation angle (check size = 0.291 × visual arc angle). The patient must be positioned with the screen producing the checkerboard pattern 1 meter away at eye level. Most tests are usually started with 20 or 25 minutes of retinal arc representation and compared with standardized data for the arc stimulation used.

Figure 12-10. Normal visual evoked potentials recorded at the O_1, O_z, and O_2 electrode sites in response to full-field, left-hemifield and right-hemifield pattern-reversal stimuli to both eyes. The full-field response from O_z (*middle left*) is labeled to show typical peak nomenclatures.

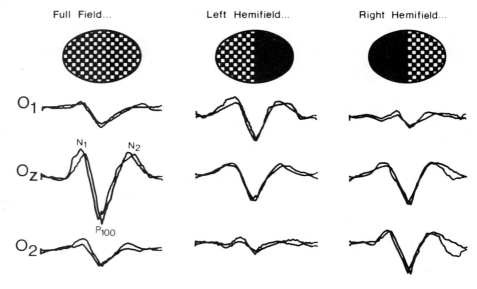

the detection of small demyelinating lesions due to optic neuritis or multiple sclerosis. Abnormal findings, however, are not specific for a particular etiology but, rather, indicate a lesion that must be further delineated through other studies.

The most common indication for performing VEP studies involves examination of optic nerve transmission in suspected multiple sclerosis or in optic neuritis.[48] The hallmark finding is a delay in P_{100} latency that may or not be symmetrical. The test can also be helpful in differentiating acute transverse myelitis from multiple sclerosis.[11, 93] Other diseases of white matter that may cause central conduction delay with involvement of the optic nerve can produce similar results. Compressive lesions of the optic nerves and chiasm tend to lead to loss of amplitude and a change in structure of the EP as opposed to an increase in latency.[47] This test can be of some value in patients with conversion symptoms involving factitious visual loss. When a normal VEP is found in spite of moderately impaired to poor visual acuity, there is reason to suspect that vision is better than it appears with subjective testing.[51] The VEP may just as readily be employed to detect an organic lesion of the optic nerve in a patient suspected of "feigning" visual loss.

Somatosensory Evoked Potentials

Many disabling neural diseases are associated with significant somatic sensory impairments as well as loss of motor function. The ability to open a physiological window on these CNS functions can provide the physiatrist with important information for understanding the physiological basis of the dysfunction observed clinically. A link between the manifest behavior and the underlying physiology may thus be sought and exploited for the purposes of gaining insight and improving care. Consider the following case.[7, 51]:

> A 17-year-old woman was admitted to the rehabilitation hospital with a diagnosis of traumatic paraplegia. Several aspects of her history and examination, however, raised questions regarding the actual extent and severity of her injury in that it appeared to be disproportionate to the motor impairment. Although voluntary strength in the legs was very limited, tendon reflexes and muscle tone were normal and it was difficult to define a clear "sensory level." She was referred for testing of somatosensory evoked potentials (SEPs), which were found to be entirely normal. The results of the study were carefully explained to her and a confident prediction was made that her condition would improve. She subsequently made a rapid and complete recovery with physical therapy and supportive counseling.

This brief example demonstrates that electrophysiological testing can be used to obtain objective evidence that either confirms or conflicts with subjective examination findings. These studies are particularly useful in subjects in whom a bedside sensory examination is either unreliable or not possible. They also help to quantitate and localize the somatosensory impairment.

The SEP study can be viewed in a simplistic but useful sense as the central equivalent of the peripheral sensory nerve action potential study. With the SEP technique the afferent impulses produced by electrical stimulation of a peripheral nerve are traced along their proximal route through to the spinal cord and from there to the brain stem and cerebrum. Since the SEP pathways can involve some of the longest axons in the body, the SEP tends to be more useful than visual and auditory studies for detecting impairment at various anatomical levels, including peripheral nerve, plexus, root, and spinal cord.

Relevant Anatomy

In performing the SEP study the peripheral receptors in the skin are commonly bypassed by the application of electrical stimulation over the peripheral nerve, producing a highly coherent but unphysiological afferent volley. It is possible to demonstrate cortical SEP recordings with mechanical tapping of the skin or muscle stretch,[89] but the advantages of employing electrical stimulation include the fact that it permits the synchronous activation of a large proportion of the low-threshold, large-diameter fibers, which produces a highly coherent transmission. When a mixed nerve such as the median or tibial nerve is stimulated, this coherent volley of action potentials is conducted along the peripheral processes of these fibers that, for the most part, convey the epicritical sensations of discriminative tactile and proprioceptive information. The volley then continues along the central processes of these cells to travel rostrally in the ipsilateral dorsal column of the spinal cord to synapse at the cervicomedullary junction in the dorsal column nuclei. Second-order cells at this level give rise to fibers that continue rostral transmission, crossing through the internal arcuate fibers in the lower medulla and continuing to the ventroposterolateral nucleus of the thalamus via the medial lemniscus. From the thalamus, third-order neurons convey the activity to the region of the contralateral primary somatosensory cortex that corresponds to the part being stimulated. Thus, tibial nerve stimulation at the ankle activates medial regions of the contralateral hemisphere, producing a focus of activity that is usually recorded best around the vertex, while median nerve stimulation at the wrist produces a focus of activation located over the contralateral centroparietal convexity.

Testing Procedures and General Considerations

For good quality studies, it is important to have a comfortable, relaxed subject. In a very anxious subject, it is possible to use a mild sedative, but this is usually not necessary. The use of a sedative can also make it difficult to interpret the response beyond the initial cortical complex. Upper limb studies are performed with the patient supine, resting comfortably with the head and neck supported on an examination table or reclining chair. Lower limb studies with spinal recordings are best performed with the subject prone with a pillow under the hips to help relax the paraspinal muscles.

The particular paradigm is chosen (*i.e.*, the nerve being stimulated and sites recorded) to address the clinical problem being considered, and recording electrodes are carefully placed. Generally, bipolar, near-field recording techniques should be employed to avoid the confusion regarding generators that may be introduced with far-field recording using noncephalic references. One compromise is to use the earlobes as a reference site. The skin over the ground and stimulation electrode sites should be prepared in the same way as that for the recording electrode sites. This helps to reduce the size of the stimulus artifact. Bipolar electrodes are placed over the peripheral nerve, and the stimulus current is adjusted until the sensory threshold is detected. The current is then increased two to three times the threshold level or until there is a moderately brisk contraction of the distal muscle being innervated by the stimulated nerve. When stimulating a sensory nerve, the current is adjusted to be a fixed multiple of the threshold. The patient is allowed to accommodate to the stimulation before data acquisition is initiated. The patient is instructed to open the mouth and relax the jaw and temple muscles of the face and to try to minimize swallowing, yawning, talking, or moving about while the signals are being recorded. The stimulation can be applied in blocks to each side or can be alternated from side to side in a single block to improve side-to-side comparison. Yamada and co-workers[120] suggest the use of simultaneous bilateral stimulation as an efficient screening mechanism that facilitates side-to-side comparison.

For all lower extremity and pudendal nerve studies, the electrode sets should include a vertex site referenced to a frontal (F_{pz} or F_z) site for primary clinical interpretation. For upper extremity studies, one channel records from the contralateral hemisphere's lateral central site, often displaced 2 cm posterior to the standard site to place the site closer to primary somatosensory cortex, referenced to either a frontal or an earlobe site. Averaging begins with the stimulation rate between 0.5 and 5 per second, depending on the selected protocol. Averages are collected of 500 to 1,000 sweeps, and a retest is performed with the results superimposed for the purpose of documenting reproducibility.

Components are identified as either present or absent, and latencies and amplitudes are measured and compared with reference laboratory normal values from healthy matched volunteer subjects from whom data were obtained using an identical protocol. Distances between recording electrodes can be measured and peripheral and central conduction velocities computed. Sensitivity can be improved if certain significant subject variables such as age and height can be "regressed out" using standard linear regression methods.

An example of a four-channel tibial nerve SEP is shown in Figure 12-11 with stimulation at the level of the medial malleolus. The time base is 80 msec with a 10% prestimulus period. The waveforms are shown with the negative polarity upward. The bottom recording is obtained from electrodes placed over the nerve at the level of the popliteal fossa. The next channel up shows the L1 level electrospinogram, recorded over the spinous

process and referenced to the iliac crest contralateral to the stimulation side. The third channel from the bottom shows the cortical response obtained in the midline, and the top channel displays the cortical SEP recorded from lateralized central electrodes. Absolute and interpeak latencies are shown for this typical normal set of data. The time between the peak of the lumbar potential and the peak of the cortical response is sometimes referred to as the spinal transit time, although it actually involves transmission through spinal cord and brain from the root entry level.

In the upper extremity, the most common technique involves stimulation of the median nerve at the wrist. A typical normal study is shown in Figure 12-12. This demonstrates proximal progression of the afferent volley from the peripheral arm stimulation site to the primary somatosensory cortex. The time base is 55 msec with a 10% prestimulus period. Two major interpeak latencies can generally be measured: that between the Erb's point potential and the cervical spine peak (P/N_{13}) and that between the cervical spine and the contralateral cortex. This last measurement is called the central somatosensory conduction time and is a measure of the time required for the stimulation to traverse the brain from the base of the brain stem to the cortex. This measurement may be of clinical value because it is readily measured and has a relatively small range of normal variation.[15, 53]

Anatomical and Clinical Correlation

The exact generators of the different components of the cervical and cortical SEPs with upper extremity stimulation have not been clearly defined, and significant controversy remains.

Figure 12-11. Normal four-channel posterior tibial nerve SEP study. Traces are each average of 1,000 sweeps with two averages superimposed. Time-base is 8 msec/division. Channel 1 (*bottom traces*): Afferent neurogram recorded over the ipsilateral popliteal fossa; scale = 5 μV/div. Channel 2: Lumbar potential (electrospinogram) recorded at the level of the L1 vertebral body as monopolar response referenced to the contralateral iliac crest; scale = 2 μV/division. Channel 3: Standard lower extremity midline recording from active electrode at C_z'' (negative grid 2 cm dorsal to vertex) referenced to F_z (positive grid) site; scale = 1.5 μV/division. Channel 4 (*top traces*): Active recording from C_4' referenced to C_3', scale = 3 μV/division.

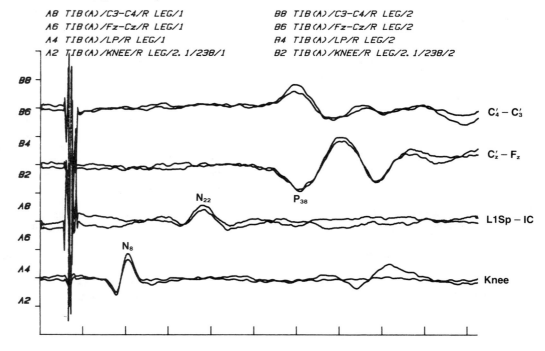

A8 TIB(A)/C3-C4/R LEG/1	B8 TIB(A)/C3-C4/R LEG/2
A6 TIB(A)/Fz-Cz/R LEG/1	B6 TIB(A)/Fz-Cz/R LEG/2
A4 TIB(A)/LP/R LEG/1	B4 TIB(A)/LP/R LEG/2
A2 TIB(A)/KNEE/R LEG/2. 1/238/1	B2 TIB(A)/KNEE/R LEG/2. 1/238/2

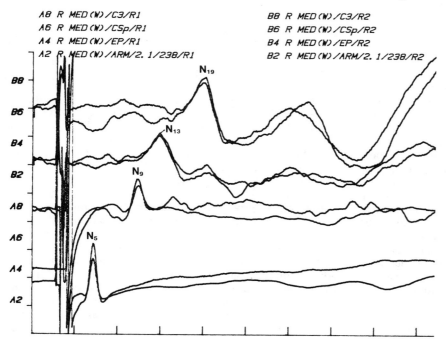

A8 R MED(W)/C3/R1 B8 R MED(W)/C3/R2
A6 R MED(W)/CSp/R1 B6 R MED(W)/CSp/R2
A4 R MED(W)/EP/R1 B4 R MED(W)/EP/R2
A2 R MED(W)/ARM/2.1/238/R1 B2 R MED(W)/ARM/2.1/238/R2

Figure 12-12. Normal median nerve SEP study demonstrating the normal components of the afferent volley with a four-channel system. The traces shown each represent an average of 500 sweeps with two averages superimposed. Time base is 5.5 msec/division. Channel 1 (*bottom*): Afferent neurogram recorded over the ipsilateral median nerve at the elbow level; scale = 10 µV/division. Channel 2: Afferent neurogram from the shoulder level recorded over the ipsilateral clavicle (Erb's point) area and referenced to the contralateral mid clavicle; scale = 5 µV/division. Channel 3: Cervical spinal level potentials recorded over C2 vertebral spinous process, referenced to a mid-frontal (F_z site) electrode; scale = 2 µV/division. Channel 4 (*top traces*): C_3' or C_4' responses from the contralateral hemisphere central (relative to the side of stimulation) to a cephalic reference at the F_z site; scale = 1 µV/division.

The N_{11} component of the cervical record is thought to be generated by the cervical roots and by transmission up the dorsal columns, while the P/N_{13} may be a compound PSP generated locally by a focal "stationary" source in the spinal cord interneurons with a horizontally oriented anterior-posterior dipole.[30] The dorsal column nuclei may also be contributing to this component. At the cortical level, some investigators contend that there is a single tangentially oriented dipole in the posterior central sulcus dominating the response and explaining the polarity reversal across the central sulcus.[2, 119] Others believe there is a separate frontal generator in primary and supplementary motor cortices that can be distinguished from the postcentral generator in the primary somatosensory cortex.[29, 72] Corticographic recordings have been reported to support this latter idea,[83] and there are reports of retention of a precentral SEP component following complete removal of the postcentral gyrus.[101]

Animal studies with stimulation of lower extremity mixed nerves indicate that the large-diameter peripheral nerve fibers and dorsal columns contribute primarily to waveform components seen in the early response, while the small diameter fibers and anterolateral columns contribute to later components seen beyond 70 msec after application of the stimulus. In patients with dissociated sensory loss, abnormal SEP components are seen on the side with proprioceptive impairment, whereas little change, if any, occurs in association with loss of pain and temperature sensation alone.[39, 49] Consistent with this information is the animal work of Cusick and colleagues,[23] who demonstrated that SEP cortical components were abolished with complete lesions limited to the dorsal columns in monkeys. The tibial nerve SEP can thus be viewed as a sort of "test of continuity" of transmission through the lemniscal system from periphery through spinal cord to cortex.

Principles of Interpretation

As a test of the quality of transmission through a given pathway, the SEP is generally employed by attempting to detect the arrival of the test volley at different levels in the pathway. In the periphery and over the cauda equina, this involves establishing the presence of an afferent neurogram. Over central sites, a specific component is identified as being linked with arrival of the volley at a particular structure in the CNS route. With the peak latencies of these critical components, interpeak latencies or "conduction times" can be measured between these components and used to indicate the rate and effectiveness of transmission through different segments of the afferent pathway. Loss of proximal components that are reliably obtained in normal subjects would indicate a block or severe dispersion of conduction, while significant delay in transmission would be reflected in a prolonged conduction time across the affected segment. Abnormality may thus be characterized as loss of expected components, prolonged central conduction times (absolute), abnormal asymmetries in conduction times, or abnormal amplitude ratios between sides. It should be noted that, with measurement of an afferent neurogram, peripheral nerve conduction velocities can also be measured and the tests can be particularly useful for examining the proximal segments of the peripheral nerves.[3]

Other SEP Paradigms

Various peripheral nerves and alternative stimulation methods can be selected to look at different root levels or to investigate proximal nerve lesions. Lower extremity studies give access to transmission through the lumbar and thoracic spinal cord, while stimulation of upper extremity nerves can be used to focus on transmission through the brachial plexus and cervical spinal cord. Specific mixed or cutaneous nerves can be stimulated and employed to focus on a specific root level or proximal nerve segment.[32–35, 44]

The SEP can also be modified for better assessment and anatomical localization of root impairment by using direct stimulation of the skin in a particular dermatomal distribution. In the dermatomal SEP, cortical responses are evaluated with electrical stimulation of a particular dermatome, typically either the L5 region on the medial dorsum of the foot in the first web space, or the S1 region along the lateral aspect of the foot.[61] These studies may be of some value in radiculopathy that is limited primarily to sensory fibers and in patients who have equivocal nondiagnostic EMG findings.[5, 60]

Other specialized stimulation studies include examinations of the sacral roots and cord as well as pelvic peripheral nerve function using pudendal stimulation methods. The pudendal nerve SEP, when combined with the electrical bulbocavernosus reflex and select EMG evaluations of sacral root function, can be used to evaluate the sacral spinal cord, sacral plexus, and pelvic nerves. These studies are particularly useful in the assessment of urological and gynecological dysfunction.[43, 45]

Detailed studies of spinal cord transmission can be performed using specialized approaches to recording the electrospinogram with either surface electrodes placed in a chain along the back with lower extremity stimulation or with monopolar needle electrodes inserted into the interspinous ligament at various levels.[18] The electrospinogram is important in lower extremity studies for marking the entry of the afferent volley along the root and into the spinal cord and its subsequent rostral transmission. Using multiple level recordings, segmental conduction velocities along the cord can be calculated to evaluate the impact of local pathology on spinal cord transmission. These studies can also be usefully employed to detect radicular pathology.

It is also possible to perform SEP studies with trigeminal nerve stimulation.[9] This paradigm has proven of some value in examining patients with trigeminal neuralgia.

Of all the clinical neurophysiological studies of CNS function, the SEP is probably of the greatest general value and one of the more flexible approaches available in that the basic paradigm can be adjusted sufficiently to address a broad range of clinical questions. It is probably the most commonly performed type of clinical evoked potential study, although questions remain regarding the proper indications for referral.[4] They are also the studies that are the most natural extensions of the traditional electrodiagnostic domains of electromyography and nerve conduction studies. For this reason, it is most probable that the SEP will be one study in which most physiatrists have their greatest interest. Because of the growing and diverse applications of these methods, a detailed consideration cannot be attempted here. The interested reader is encouraged to explore other sources[17, 59, 79, 81, 104, 121] and to survey the relevant literature.

Transcranial Cortical Stimulation and Movement-Related Cortical Potentials

While the SEP techniques allow evaluation of transmission through the dorsal column pathway, they cannot provide direct information about the condition of efferent central conduction pathways transmitting impulses from the output regions of the cortex along the anterior and lateral corticospinal tracts to the motor neuron pools in the ventral horn of the spinal cord. To be able to look at efferent transmission, there would appear to be two possible options: (1) activate a proximal output region by external means and track the efferent volley out to the periphery or (2) look for electrophysiological correlates of self-generated movement. Two separate paradigms allow these approaches to be pursued using emerging methods that are now becoming accessible to the clinical neurophysiologist.

Transcranial Motor Cortex Stimulation

It has been known since the past century that certain regions of the cerebral cortex are uniquely responsive to the application of electrical stimulation in that movements of the limbs can be elicited with direct application of stimulating current to the cortex. The classic "motor strip" of the precentral gyrus was identified by this characteristic. Until recently, this type of demonstration was restricted to situations in which the cortical surface was exposed, for example, in laboratory animals or in human patients undergoing surgical exploration of the cortical surface. Merton and his colleagues,[73] however, demonstrated that it is possible to stimulate the human precentral motor cortex and the spinal cord transcutaneously with surface electrodes placed on the scalp or over the spine, thus producing brief contralateral limb movements. These evoked movements could be recorded as compound muscle action potentials (CMAPs) in the muscles of the arms or legs by placing surface recording electrodes over the responding muscles. They were able to do this using brief high-voltage stimuli produced by a purpose-built stimulator and applied to the skin's surface through bipolar stimulating electrodes overlying the neural tissue to be stimulated. Alternative methods that have since emerged include a unipolar technique that employs generally available electrophysiological stimulators[94, 95] and the use of a high-current magnetic field stimulator[8] that has the advantage of avoiding the discomfort associated with electrical stimulation by directly inducing stimulus currents at the stimulation site rather than causing such currents to have to pass through the resistive load of the intervening structures. Using these methods for stimulating central efferent structures (presumably, primary motor cortex), an efferent volley is generated that travels out to peripheral muscle where a CMAP is evoked. When this CMAP is recorded, it is possible to measure the latency or propagation time of the central efferent volley from the moment of stimulus application to the onset of the CMAP using methods similar to those commonly employed in performing motor conduction studies. By subtracting latencies obtained from stimulating cervical spinal cord from that obtained by stimulating the cortex through the scalp, it is possible to compute a central efferent conduction time.

This stimulation method is currently undergoing clinical testing to determine its general safety and what specific contraindications may exist. At this point, this method is still considered experimental in the United States and clinical testing is limited to approved centers involved in this evaluation. In a way, this paradigm could be viewed as the proximal extension of the motor nerve conduction study familiar to the electromyographer. The muscle contractions produced are entirely involuntary and are produced by the external application of energy in the form of either an electrical potential or a magnetic field. In effect, this test can be viewed as the inverse of the SEP in which we are now involved in a test of continuity of efferent central pathways. It should be remembered, however, that the "single cable" model of the CNS applied in the interpretation is a highly oversimplified one and that, in fact, the outflow from the cortex travels to many different subcortical regions other than the spinal cord.

A clinical example drawn from the literature is shown in Figure 12-13. This method shows promise in rehabilitation medicine in areas such as the assessment of spinal cord function in the presence of a traumatic injury. An excellent introductory source for this general area is the January 1987 issue of the journal, *Neurosurgery,* in which the proceedings of a meeting on "Motor System Evoked Potential Monitoring" were published.

The transcranial stimulation technique plays a role complementary to that of the SEP in that it can provide information about the functional integrity of the descending motor pathways producing movement in the intact human subject. It is likely that this technique will receive an increasing amount of attention as we learn more about it as it becomes more widely available for clinical use.

CORTICAL STIMULATION

A.

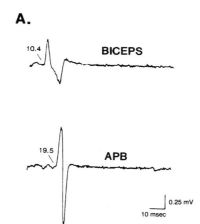

B.

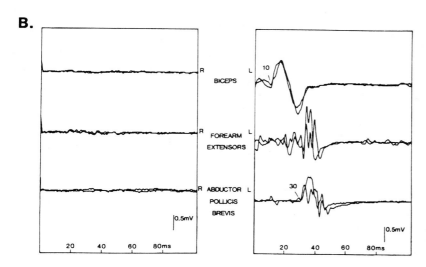

Figure 12-13. Compound muscle action potential recorded from biceps and thenar eminence following transcranial cortical stimulation. (*A*) Surface EMG responses recorded at the biceps and abductor pollicis brevis (*APB*) after stimulation of contralateral motor cortex by a transcranial current produced by a brief, high-current stimulus. (*B*) Compound muscle action potentials produced by transcranial cortical stimulation in a patient who sustained a C3–C4 fracture dislocation and cervical spinal cord injury. Clinically, the patient improved on the left but had a residual paralysis of the right arm and leg. These studies show absent responses from the right arm with left motor cortex stimulation and delayed motor responses in the left APB following right motor cortex stimulation. (Data reproduced from Thompson PD et al: Examination of motor function in lesions of the spinal cord by stimulation of the motor cortex. Ann Neurol 21:389–396, 1987)

Movement-Associated Cortical Potentials ("Readiness" Potential)

While the production of skeletal muscle contraction with transcranial stimulation of the motor cortex can be used to examine transmission of efferent impulses, the "movement" thus produced is not initiated through normal internal processes and, effectively, bypasses the voluntary mechanism. An alternative approach is necessary to allow examination of these volitional processes through which a movement is prepared and executed by an active, behaving subject. This approach involves capturing the ongoing EEG signal before, as well as after, a self-generated voluntary movement occurs. In this case, the event of interest about which the averaging process is centered is the onset of *self-generated* EMG in the moving limb. This technique involves the continuous storage and updating of the EEG data in a "circular buffer." This process is then interrupted when the occurrence of a movement is detected and the data in the buffer are captured in a preset time window that precedes and follows the trigger event. In this paradigm, EEG data are recorded with a high-pass filter cut-off set down to 0.01 Hz so that slow changes can be registered. When 100 to 200 frames of these data are averaged together a slow negative drift of the scalp potential can be identi-

fied, particularly in the central regions. The change from baseline begins up to a second or more before the peripheral EMG appears.[27, 28, 99, 100, 111, 114] This potential is variably referred to as the readiness potential, Bereitschaftspotential, human motor potential or movement-associated cortical potential. The recording in Figure 12-14 shows a typical, normal readiness potential associated with a brief flexion movement of the interphalangeal joint of the right thumb. The traces shown were recorded from the vertex (C_z) and the site overlying the contralateral hand region of the primary motor cortex (C_3). One sees a ramplike increase in negativity that begins almost a full second before the EMG onset in primary acting muscle.

The readiness potential presumably reflects processes involved in the preparation and execution of a self-generated voluntary act.[65] It can be recorded in advance of vocalization and saccadic eye movements as well as movements of the hands and feet, and it can be used to examine the normal physiology of movement preparation within different volitional contexts.[70] Furthermore, the study of the readiness potential and the related contingent negative variation (CNV)[117] may be able to provide insights into disorders of voluntary action and impairments of motor learning, anticipation, and adaptive behavior. The ability to prepare, execute, and control voluntary goal-directed action,

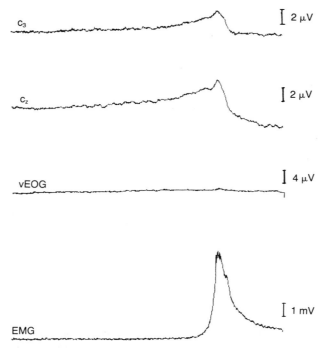

Figure 12-14. Normal movement-related cortical potential (MRCP): average formed from 500 sweeps; three seconds prior to movement and 1 second following rapid flexion of interphalangeal joint of the right thumb; band pass: 0.01–100 Hz; gain: 20,000. Channel 1: Averaged EEG recorded from the C_3 electrode. Channel 2: MRCP recorded at C_z overlying the supplementary motor area. Channel 3: Vertical electro-oculogram (vEOG). Channel 4: Rectified surface electromyogram (EMG) recorded from electrodes placed over the motor point of the flexor pollicis longus.

as well as the ability to learn new motor skills, are key elements of daily adaptive function. The readiness potential and the CNV may be applied to the examination of how voluntary action and anticipatory learning are normally organized by brain structures and how these critical processes are affected by different disabling conditions. This noninvasive, physiologically produced information could help to provide direction to the development of compensatory and adaptational strategies for improving functionality, where "function" is conceptualized as actively adaptive and volitional.

Cognitive Event-Related Potential (ERP) Studies

The SEP, BAEP, and, to an extent, the VEP are *obligatory* responses to specific external stimuli and, therefore, fall under the general classification of "exogenous" evoked potentials—EPs whose components depend primarily on the physical characteristics of the external stimulus (*e.g.,* intensity, rate, modality). Exogenous EPs are stimulus specific and receptor and pathway specific, and they do not require particular cooperation or active participation by the subject (except for some ability to fix gaze in the VEP). They also do not vary with the manner in which the subject may be attributing significance to the stimuli or with the subject-relevant contextual information contained in the stimulus. It is for these reasons that the exogenous EPs have found clinical utility: they are robustly insensitive to the psychological state of the subject and are more dependent on the integrity of

input transmission through afferent pathways. However, these studies leave the psychophysiological domain,[19] in which active cognition is considered, essentially unexplored.

A second major category of EP is the "endogenous" group. In contrast to the characteristics of exogenous EPs, endogenous EPs are stimulus nonspecific; are not linked to specific receptors or input pathways; and require that the subject actively participate in the procedure by attending to stimuli and making decisions about them according to certain instructions. The components of the response can be shown to vary with the relevance and detected information of the stimulus in an information-processing context.

These endogenous potentials, or cognitive event-related potentials (ERPs), can be elicited when the subject detects a significant change, designated a "target," appearing in an ongoing stimulus pattern. The subject actively recognizes the target, implying that the stimulus has been attended and actively processed leading to a cognitive decision about the nature of the stimulus. The ERP is nonspecific since it does not matter very much in which modality the stimulus was presented. These components can even be elicited by the absence of an expected stimulus.[87]

A commonly employed ERP is the P_3 or P_{300} component. This is a "decision" potential that occurs hundreds of milliseconds after the stimulus has been applied and probably reflects the completion of a stimulus-processing phase whose conclusion is a particular decision about the stimulus.

The most common way the P_{300} is recorded clinically is using the so-called auditory "oddball" stimulus paradigm. Electrodes are typically placed along the midline at the F_z, C_z, and P_z sites with linked ears used as a reference. Each run consists of 100 stimuli presented binaurally at a slow rate of less than 1 per second. Amplifier filters are set to record slow changes in the EEG typically between 0.1 and 70 Hz. The stimuli are tone pips produced with a controlled pitch. Eighty to 90% of the stimuli in the presented sequence are "frequents," or *nontarget stimuli,* presented at one pitch, for example, 1000 Hz. The remaining 10% to 20% are "rares," or *targets,* presented at a second pitch of, for example, 2000 Hz. The targets are distributed randomly throughout the sequence. The physical characteristics of the tone pips are identical except for pitch. The subject is given the task of concentrating on detecting the target stimuli and counting them or pressing a button each time a rare is heard. Conversely, the nontargets are to be ignored. Responses evoked by rares are averaged separately from those evoked by frequents. The P_{300} is then seen as a large vertex-positive deflection seen at 300 to 400 msec latency in the response to rares, which is not seen in the response to frequents. A typical result is shown in Figure 12-15.

Factors Influencing the P_{300} Component

Several experimental and subject factors can influence the latency and amplitude of the P_{300} component.

LATENCY EFFECTS. Three factors in particular have been shown to affect the peak latency of the P_{300}. These are the ease with which the target and the nontarget can be discriminated, the age of the subject, and the presence of a dementing condition.

Task Difficulty. The easier it is to discriminate between target and nontarget, the shorter the latency of the P_{300}. For example, although it is fairly easy to discriminate pitches of 2000 Hz from those of 1000 Hz, it is somewhat more difficult to distinguish 1100 Hz form 1000 Hz. Since this second pair are not too dissimilar, a longer period of time is involved in reaching a decision about which of the two tones has just been heard. This is

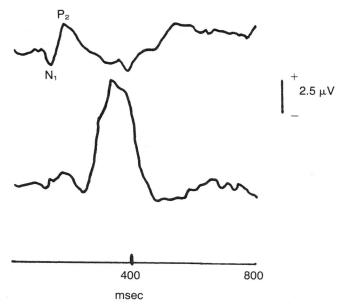

+

2.5 μV

−

400   800

msec

Figure 12-15. Vertex event-related potentials recorded from a normal 55-year-old subject. (*Top*) Averaged response to frequent 1000 Hz tones showing typical N_1–P_2 complex or "auditory potential." (*Bottom*) Response to 2000 Hz rare tones after subtracting the averaged response to the frequent tones. This "difference" potential accentuates the P_{300} by reducing components that were common to both, including N_1 and P_2.

reflected in a longer average latency compared with the easier discrimination task. The detailed physiological mechanism and anatomical substrate for this dependence of the P_{300} latency is not known.

Age. For a given discrimination task, the P_{300} latency increases progressively with age. Indeed, latencies may approach 400 msec in normal people in their eighth decade. Several studies have examined the details of this relationship. In some studies, a linear relationship has been found between P_{300} latency and age. In one study, P_{300} latency was found to increase at a rate of 1.1 msec/yr in adults[110] while in another study, P_{300} latency was shown to increase at a rate of 1.8 msec/yr for subjects over 15 years of age, while, between the ages of 6 and 15, P_{300} latency steadily decreased at a rate of 18.4 msec/yr.[42] In another study, however, the increase in P_{300} latency after the age 15 and particularly above age 45 was found to be exponential.[14] Regardless of whether the increase in P_{300} latency with age is linear or exponential, the trend is quite consistent. This phenomenon appears to reflect an age-dependent prolongation of processing time required to make a decision about a stimulus.

Dementia. Dementing illnesses can produce marked increases in the age-corrected P_{300} latency. However, although it has been possible to distinguish between *populations* of demented and normal patients, it can be difficult to make a definitive statement in an individual patient about the presence of organic dementia based on the P_{300} latency alone. This is because of the inherent variability of the measurement, which can give rise to an unacceptable number of false-positives and false-negatives.

AMPLITUDE EFFECTS. A number of factors appear to selectively affect the amplitude of the P_{300} component.

Expectancy. The "frequents," or nontarget stimuli in the test sequence, produce what is essentially a flat response in the

P_{300} latency region. The infrequent "rares" produce a large response. It appears that the amplitude of the response is inversely related to the subjective probability of the triggering event. The rares are less expected so that when they occur the event carries a greater deal of information. Generally, the more expected a stimulus, or the greater its subjective probability (*i.e.,* the perceived chances of its occurrence), the lower will be the P_{300} amplitude.[106]

Attention to Stimulus. The ERP generally requires that the subject attend and participate actively in the test paradigm. This is actually not entirely true since, if the difference in probability and structure is great enough between the frequents and the rares, subjects who are purposefully distracted and not attending to the stimulus sequence still generate P_{300}s although they are smaller in amplitude and of longer latency than is observed with active concentration on the task.[88, 107] The P_{300} cannot be completely suppressed voluntarily when an unpredictable stimulus is perceived or appreciated via an intact sensory pathway. In situations in which malingering or hysteria may be a factor, the P_{300} can still be detected.

Age. The P_{300} amplitude decreases with age at a rate of about 0.2 μV/yr. The overall behavior of the component is to become smaller and later with increasing age.

Conclusions

In general, factors that tend to increase latency tend to produce concomitant decreases in amplitude. Thus, ERP amplitudes are generally lower and latencies longer in the aged and the demented or when the experimenter increases the difficulty of the task. In order to perform clinical studies with an ERP paradigm it is imperative that an age-matched control data base be obtained with the same test paradigm for comparison purposes.

The application of ERPs in the practice of rehabilitation medicine is in its infancy. ERPs may be applied to assess the physiological correlates of cognitive deficits in patients with brain damage. Some initial attempts have been made to correlate P_{300} changes with memory deficits in patients who have sustained a head injury.[82, 84] These studies show some promise for this application and may prove to be useful in documenting the physiological substrate of memory dysfunction following traumatic brain injury.[41] In another report,[113] patients with a CVA resulting in either aphasia or aprosodia were shown to differ significantly from normal matched controls and from each other using three different auditory tasks that required different forms of stimulus processing accessing the affected processing systems. It is possible that ERP methods may be employed clinically to assess and document deficits in cognitive function in patients with brain damage and may be useful in developing new methods for performing cognitive retraining.[41]

CLINICAL APPLICATIONS IN REHABILITATION MEDICINE

Cerebrovascular Accident

EP studies have been used for almost 20 years to evaluate patients with cerebrovascular lesions. Liberson, in 1966, studied aphasic subjects using SEPs and noted that the preservation of a normal SEP was frequently accompanied by subsequent clinical improvement.[69] The quest for a good predictor of outcome in CVA has been addressed by a number of researchers.[1, 50, 116] Specific clinical signs available at the first encounter such as age, presence of visual field impairment, and incontinence are used in various combinations as possible prognostic indices.

Characterization of the structural abnormality seen on computed tomography or magnetic resonance imaging failed to adequately predict outcome. A possible relationship between evoked potential studies and stroke outcome has been sought by a number of investigators. Liberson[69] noted a correlation between SEP and outcome in aphasia in 15 patients with left hemispheric lesions. In the 10 patients in whom the median nerve SEP was markedly impaired over the damaged hemisphere, the aphasic impairment was severe in 8 and moderate in 2. In 4 of the 5 patients with normal SEP studies, the aphasia was mild. Vredeveld[115] reported on 89 hemiplegic patients and found that absence of the N_{19} cortical component was inevitably accompanied by a poor outcome. La Joie and associates[66] reported the correlation of median nerve SEP and right arm return of motor function in 68 right hemiplegic patients seen consecutively at a rehabilitation center. In 42 patients with absent SEP, only 1 showed some functional gain, while more than 36% of the patients with normal or mildly diminished SEPs showed some functional gain at discharge.

Ignacio and co-workers[54, 85] reported on the relationship between the SEP and functional outcome in 130 patients following an acute CVA using the method of bilateral simultaneous median nerve stimulation with comparison of the recordings obtained from C_3 and C_4 referenced to F_z. The SEPs were graded in the manner demonstrated in Figures 12-16 through 12-19 on a four-point scale. Functional recovery was graded on three parameters: return of function in the affected hand, self-care activities, and ambulation.

A significant correlation was found between the CNS studies and the degree of functional recovery (Table 12-5). Patients with a grade I or II showed significant return of function in the affected hand and were able to perform self-care activities independently or with minimal assistance. They were generally more likely to ambulate independently. As a result, most of these patients were able to return home and function reasonably well in the home environment. Grade IV patients, on the other hand, did uniformly poorly. None regained useful function of the affected hand, and none regained independence in self-care activities or in ambulation. Half of these patients required placement in a nursing home because of their poor functional status. Patients with grade III responses fell between these two groups in terms of their functional outcome.

EPs, and in particular the SEP, appear to hold promise for the problem of establishing a prognosis for functional outcome in stroke and may also be particularly helpful in assessing the sensory status of patients who are difficult to examine at the bedside due to aphasia.[64]

Spinal Cord Injury

In most cases of civilian spinal cord injury, the cord is acutely contused or compressed but not physically transected. The actual extent of physiological impairment accompanying the injury can vary widely. One of the challenges in caring for patients with spinal cord injury is predicting outcome. Two types of patients demonstrate a tendency to recover function: (1) those patients whose lesion is clinically incomplete on initial presentation and (2) those patients whose lesion is initially clinically complete but who start to regain some sensory or motor function within the first few days. Patients who retain even a limited degree of sensory function are frequently those who have a subsequent return of voluntary motion.[109]

If the SEP is recordable with tibial or peroneal nerve stimulation in the leg when the study is performed within 24 to 48 hours following spinal cord injury, this is usually associated with some degree of clinical improvement.[86, 96, 97, 105] It would appear

Figure 12-16. Normal SEP—grade I. Note the similarity between the two tracings (C_4F_z—right parietal; C_3F_z—left parietal). The difference in N_{19}–P_{24} and P_{24}–N_{30} peak-to-peak amplitude is less than 25% between right and left.

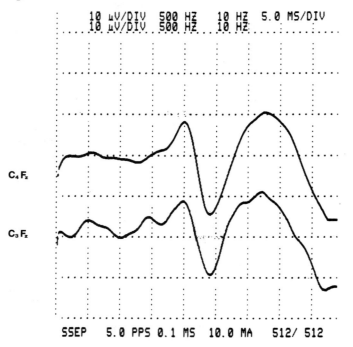

Figure 12-17. Abnormal SEP—grade II. Although the tracings are symmetrical, there is a difference in the N_{19}–P_{24} and P_{24}–N_{30} peak-to-peak amplitude—the one on the right tracing being approximately 30% less than the left. ($C_4 F_z$—right parietal; $C_3 F_z$—left parietal).

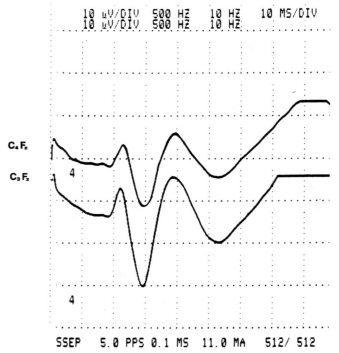

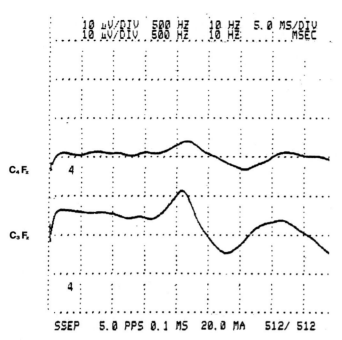

Figure 12-18. Abnormal SEP—grade III. Note the assymetry between the two tracings ($C_4 F_z$—right parietal; $C_3 F_z$—left parietal) with relative increase in latency in the P_{24} and N_{30} potentials on the right. The N_{19}–P_{24} and P_{24}–N_{30} peak-to-peak amplitude shows a diminution of approximately 70% compared with the left.

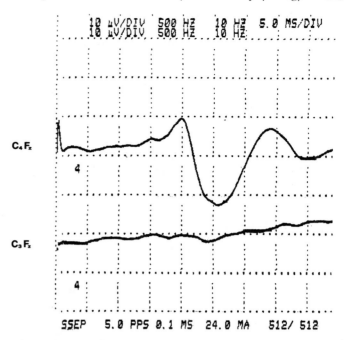

Figure 12-19. Abnormal SEP—grade IV. Note the marked asymmetry between the two tracings ($C_4 F_z$—right parietal; $C_3 F_z$—left parietal). The N_{19}, P_{24}, N_{30} potentials are not discernible in the $C_3 F_z$ recording. This type of SEP is usually accompanied by a poor prognosis for functional outcome.

that the presence of a cortical SEP with stimulation of a leg nerve soon after spinal cord injury is generally a good sign that at least some recovery may be expected. It is also true, however, that an absent SEP is not necessarily ominous if there is clinical evidence that the lesion is incomplete; in this case, a careful clinical examination of sensation may actually be more sensitive than the SEP. This is probably because the SEP is really testing a limited

contribution to the spinal population of transmitting fibers and also tests only one submodality of somatic sensation. The clinician can also, of course, assess motor function below the level of the lesion, which the SEP cannot do. The use of transcranial motor cortex or spinal stimulation may be of some value in this regard. Of course, in the patient who is unconscious or uncooperative, the SEP may be the only reliable test of lower extremity sensation available to the clinician.

Traumatic Brain Injury

In severe traumatic brain injury, the magnitude and degree of impairment can vary tremendously from one case to the next and numerous attempts have been made to predict the long-term outcome during the early phases following presentation. The basic clinical standard for the assessment of these patients is the *Glasgow Coma Scale*. This assessment can be combined with a variety of other pieces of data to try to develop prognostic indices. EP studies can be used to improve the prognostic power of such indices. Multimodality evoked potentials (MEPs) can be used to assess the extent to which individual sensory systems are able to respond to specific inputs in the comatose patient or in the patient who has been placed in a protective induced coma. The addition of MEPs to a prognostic index has been shown to improve the accuracy and confidence limits of outcome predictions.[75] The value of performing these studies can be improved by performing them serially and looking for dynamic trends in the measured parameters.[77] Measurement of the central somatosensory conduction time in severe traumatic brain injury also appears to be of some value in predicting outcome.[52] Rappaport[91] has reviewed his own work and that of his co-workers in this area. In their work, a correlation was found between the degree of abnormality of EP patterns and the severity of the disability outcome. Rappaport suggests that the VEP and SEP

Table 12-5
Functional Outcome According to SEP Grades

Outcome	SEP Grades			
	I	II	III	IV
Hand function				
Excellent	100%	20%	0	0
Fair	0	65%	21.5%	0
Poor	0	14%	78.5%	100%
Activities of daily living				
Excellent	100%	80%	0	0
Good	0	20%	47%	0
Fair	0	0	21%	9%
Poor	0	0	32%	91%
Gait and mobility				
Independent	70%	40%	0	0
Independent but requiring assistive device	30%	33%	10%	0
Ambulating short distance with assistive device but relying on wheelchair for mobility	0	27%	47.5%	25%
Wheelchair bound	0	0	42.5%	75%

studies that examine cortical function correlate better with long-term outcome than the BAEP. He also reports that EP studies performed up to a year after the injury can provide useful information on the status and eventual outcome for individual patients.

Multiple Sclerosis

Multiple sclerosis (MS) is a disease characterized by patchy demyelination, which can involve any part of the central nervous system (CNS), going through stages of activity followed by inactivity, producing neuromuscular deficits based on the areas of involvement. Until recently, the diagnosis of MS was based almost exclusively on clinical findings and was often a diagnosis of exclusion. The EEG or EMG was typically normal or showed only nonspecific changes, while lymphocytosis was usually noted in the cerebrospinal fluid (CSF). More recently, increased immunoglobulin (IgG) has been found in 60 to 75% of MS patients. Oligoclonic bands in the CSF added another helpful test, although their presence is not uniquely associated with MS. About a decade ago, several workers noted that pattern shift VEPs were abnormal in patients with optic neuritis. Since this condition is one of the frequent and early manifestations of MS, VEP soon proved to be a very useful tool in the diagnosis. Also, BAER and SEP studies were abnormal in a high percentage of patients. Most recently, the addition of magnetic resonance imaging (MRI) has significantly enhanced the diagnosis of CNS lesions because of its ability to distinguish between tissues having different fluid contents and densities, thus allowing MS plaque visualization. Concomitantly, the effect of these lesions can be shown electrophysiologically.

The VEP abnormalities associated with MS are most often related to optic neuritis, affecting one or both eyes, with one eye usually affected more than the other. The principal VEP changes with MS are (1) prolonged P100 latency; (2) interocular latency differences; (3) relative amplitude diminution; (4) dispersion or change in duration of the P100 potential; and (5) waveform morphology changes. The mean for P100 is prolonged 10–30 msec but the most sensitive indicator of optic nerve dysfunction is the interocular latency difference. The P100 potential amplitude is affected by various technical factors, plus such factors as visual acuity, refractory errors, medial opacities, retinal disease, patient's concentration, direction of gaze, luminance, and so forth. With full-field stimulation, a total amplitude less than 3 uV should be considered suspicious, and a side to side amplitude difference greater than 50% may be considered abnormal. The P100 shape is often abnormal in MS patients, especially if they have visual symptoms. It is common to see latency prolongation with relapses associated with visual impairment, but if the relapse is not accompanied by any residual visual loss, the VEP remains unchanged. MS associated incidence of VEP abnormalities ranges from 47–96%. Decreases in the check size and hyperthermia increases the test's sensitivity and incidence of VEP abnormalities.

The BAER has been found to be abnormal in 30% of possible MS patients, 41% of probable MS patients, and 67% of definite MS patients. The principal abnormalities are (1) absence of waves, especially Peak V; (2) marked diminution of amplitude of the waves; (3) increased interpeak latency differences; and (4) reversal of I/V amplitude ratio. Any of the waves, or any combination of them, may be prolonged, attenuated, or abolished, with the most commonly involved being Peak V, followed by Peak III. Exacerbations and acute changes in clinical course usually do not show a high correlation with the BAER. In view of the great variability in different individuals, one must be very careful in interpreting an abnormality solely on the basis of amplitude. Interpeak latency prolongation is one of the most frequent findings in MS with the III–V difference generally more frequently involved than the I–III. Changes in the I/V amplitude ratio (the ratio of amplitude of wave I divided by the amplitude of wave V) are suggestive of a conduction defect rostral to lower pons.

SEP studies in MS patients show that abnormalities can be documented in a higher percentage (58% overall) than BAER or VEP changes. The abnormalities include (1) peak latency prolongation; (2) prolongation of interpotential latency; (3) diminution of amplitude; (4) absence of common peaks; and (5) change in morphology. Prolongation of the absolute peak or interpeak latencies is among the most commonly found abnormalities, being present in 54% of upper extremity studies and 64% of lower limb studies. As MS or its sequelae may affect peripheral nerves, the spinal cord, or the central nervous system, SEP changes will show various combinations of abnormalities. A marked diminution of amplitude typically affecting several, rather than a single, potential is a common finding in MS. As the latencies prolong, peaks are dispersed, amplitudes are effectively reduced, and the normal wave pattern is distorted. The waves may lose their pointed apex or, because of their low amplitude and latency shifts, are hard to visualize and tend to merge into one another. In definite MS, the abnormality rate is 77%, 67% in probable MS, and 49% in possible MS.

Comparison of the relative diagnostic sensitivities suggests that the SEP is abnormal in the largest percentage (over 40%) of cases, the BAER in the least (less than 25%), and the VEP is abnormal in about 37% of such studies. This appears to be primarily a function of the tract's length or amount of white matter pathway being tested and, secondly, of the individual system's susceptibility to demyelination. The principal value of this type of "multimodality" EP complement is that it often helps in suspected MS cases with one area of involvement to uncover involvement of another, and it helps detect abnormalities and corroborate the diagnosis in patients with unsuspected lesions. Motor cortex electrical or magnetic stimulation for the study of central and peripheral conduction in normal subjects and MS patients showed the cord-to-axilla conduction to be normal in both groups, while central conduction, that is, cord-to-cord, was markedly slowed in MS patients. The MRI appears to have revolutionized the diagnosis of MS by detecting demyelinating lesions as small as 3 millimeters in diameter and has been shown to be very effective in revealing multiple lesions in the spinal cord. In that circumstance, it is often superior to EP studies in the probable MS category. In brainstem lesions, however, the BAER is more sensitive than MRI. Also, in optic neuritis secondary to MS, the MRI has usually been normal, whereas VEPs have been abnormal in about 95% of cases. The sensitivity of EP in the most sought diagnostic category, probable MS, was 60% for SEP, 56% for VEP, and 32% for BAER. EP, therefore, remains an excellent diagnostic tool. Progression of the disease has not always borne a direct relationship to the EP abnormalities. Attempts at prognosticating the disease's course using EP studies have not met with significant success, and, bearing in mind the nature of this illness, this is not surprising.

Intraoperative Monitoring

During Spinal Surgery

The EP methods reviewed here can be adapted to provide "on-line" information regarding the status of a particular pathway through the CNS. This becomes particularly useful in the operating room where it is now possible to monitor a pathway that is placed at known risk during an operation. On-line information regarding transmission through this pathway can be examined serially during critical phases of surgery, and the surgeon can be given almost immediate feedback regarding the neurophysiological status of the monitored pathway. If it is apparent that the pathway is failing, this information can be provided to the surgeon, who can then choose to take a course of action directed to normalizing the abnormality detected through monitoring. The effectiveness of this "evasive action" can then be checked through continued monitoring.

Typically, the spinal cord is monitored during procedures in which the spine is instrumented and significant traction will be placed on the spinal cord in the course of the operation (Figs. 12-20 through 12-22). Tibial nerves are usually stimulated, and recordings are obtained from peripheral nerve, lumbar or cervical spine, and scalp. To differentiate between actual spinal cord dysfunction versus a generalized effect on cortical activity (*e.g.*, drop in blood pressure, use of barbiturate anesthetic agents) the SEP with response to median nerve stimulation can be recorded on another channel. If this EP remains unchanged while the tibial SEP deteriorates, this would localize the problem to below the cervical spinal cord. The anesthetic agent being used can have a significant impact on the waveform compared with the baseline study obtained in the awake patient. A second baseline should therefore be established once anesthesia has been induced (see Fig. 12-21). Barbiturate agents should also be avoided whenever possible since they greatly attenuate the cortical response. Some of these problems involving variability of the cortical response can be circumvented if it is possible to record from electrodes placed close to the cord in the epidural space.[80] The peripheral afferent neurogram should also be recorded to ensure that the volley is being properly generated. It should be noted always that the SEP is not testing the full range of tracts in the spinal cord but is rather looking at a rather limited region. Thus, it is theoretically possible for a patient to awaken weak because motor pathways were not specifically studied during surgery. An isolated lesion affecting motor pathways in the anterior and lateral columns could produce weakness without affecting the SEP during the operation. This may occur rarely and has been reported.[68]

During Aortic Surgery

Paraplegia is a recognized complication of surgery on the aorta. Its incidence has been estimated at up to 15% for resection of a thoracoabdominal aneurysm. SEPs can be used to help determine whether spinal cord blood flow remains adequate during cross-clamping of the aorta, or whether a bypass or shunt is required to maintain adequate spinal cord perfusion.[22, 66] Spinal cord ischemia produces detectable changes in the SEP starting after 3 minutes with total loss of all peaks of the evoked potential after about 9 minutes. Maneuvers designed to increase both distal spinal cord blood flow and perfusion via a heparinized shunt, various bypass techniques, or reimplantation of critical intercostal arteries resulted in the reappearance of the SEP. The ability of the SEP to help differentiate critical from noncritical intercostal arteries or to show that a distal shunt or

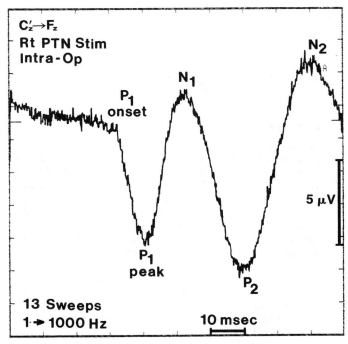

Figure 12-20. During intraoperative studies maximal (transcutaneous) stimulation can yield exceptionally clear averaged responses with very few sweeps. This allows rapid examination of short time intervals during critical surgical events. This SEP trace is typical of unilateral posterior tibial nerve stimulation recorded with narcotic anesthesia during an uneventful Harrington rod placement and distraction.

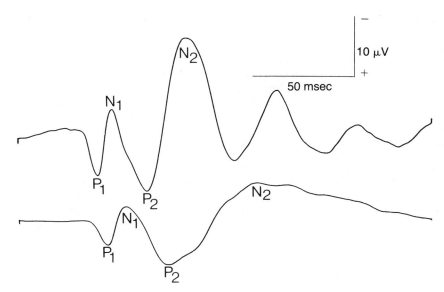

Figure 12-21. Differences in SEP obtained in an adolescent female patient with progressive idiopathic scoliosis when awake (*top*) and when anesthetized (*bottom*). Anesthesia consisted of nitrous oxide, oxygen, narcotic, and muscle relaxant. Two hundred traces were summed in response to simultaneous bilateral stimulation of the posterior tibial nerves at the medial malleoli. During the preoperative study, the patient's SEP was so large it could be discerned in the analog signal. She did not, however, have evidence of myoclonic epilepsy. Note the marked prolongation of N_2 latency and absence of peaks after N_2 when patient was anesthetized. Also, during anesthetia, the earlier peaks (P_1, N_1, and P_2), although still present, are reduced in amplitude and of slightly longer latency than when patient is awake. (Spielholz NI, Engler GL, Merkin H: Spinal cord monitoring during Harrington instrumentation. Bull Am Soc Clin Evoked Potentials 4:12–16, 1986)

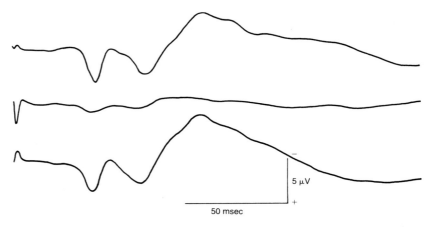

Figure 12-22. A series of recordings demonstrating a patient in whom the SEP disappeared almost completely within a few minutes after distraction. The top trace represents a SEP obtained during predistraction phase. The middle trace shows the SEP markedly reduced approximately 5 minutes after distraction. Subsequent runs over the next 10 minutes showed the same low level of response. The bottom trace shows the SEP return within 3 minutes of rod removal. The SEP was then used to "titrate" how much distraction could be safely tolerated and the patient awoke with no neurological deficit. (Spielholz NI, Engler GL, Merkin H: Spinal cord monitoring during Harrington instrumentation. Bull Am Soc Clin Evoked Potentials 4:12–16, 1986)

bypass is performing adequately represents a very important addition to corrective surgery of the aorta.

During Carotid Endarterectomy

Carotid endarterectomy, which entails temporary clamping of the carotid artery, is occasionally associated with neurological deficits secondary to ischemia of the ipsilateral cerebral hemisphere. A bypass shunt is frequently inserted in those patients who do not have sufficient collateral circulation to sustain the hemisphere during the clamping period. However, shunting is not routinely employed because of complications associated with shunting. The problem becomes how to determine which patients need to have the shunt placed intraoperatively. A number of reports now appear to support the value of SEPs in the early detection of cerebral ischemia in this situation.[71] Nonshunting of patients in whom the SEP disappeared during clamping has been followed by neurological deficits whereas shunting that restored the deteriorated SEP was followed by an uneventful outcome.[98] The intraoperative monitoring technique involved recording the SEP to median nerve stimulation contralateral to the side being operated. Disappearance or marked attenuation of SEP amplitude was used as an indication to shunt. Rapid reestablishment of circulation was frequently associated with the SEP returning to preclamp levels.

EP recording in the operating room adds a new range of possibilities for the application of this technology. The challenge of obtaining technically good, reliable recordings in the electrically hostile environment of the operating room requires careful attention to technique and a thorough understanding of the ways in which noise sources can be minimized. The provision of these services may be a time-consuming and costly endeavor, however, and the application of expensive equipment and personnel involvement should be reserved for situations in which there is a well-documented risk to be countered through monitoring. The ability to dynamically probe and assess CNS function in the anesthetized patient throughout the course of surgery is powerful and may provide a means for reducing the risks of particular surgical complications in a significant number of patients. The future of this endeavor will involve an interesting interplay between a number of forces involved in the shaping of modern health care practices. These include the availability of resources, the ability to demonstrate unequivocal benefit of operating room monitoring in a significant number of instances that would not be otherwise possible, efforts to control the costs of this service, and medicolegal questions. The interested reader is referred to a monograph on the application of EP monitoring in the operating room for a more detailed consideration.[80]

ELECTROPHYSIOLOGY IN NEUROPLASTICITY AND THE ADAPTIVE PROCESS

Functional change and the assessment of disability, a primary domain of rehabilitation medicine, as well as the form of the associated disturbance of physiological processes, are not related in a straightforward way to underlying structural damage. A physiological description, however, is critically important in understanding the process disturbed and the impairment of performance that becomes manifest as a result of the pathology. It is also important in determining how to manage the dysfunction, in identifying adaptive ("recovery") changes, in making important management decisions, and in assessing prognosis.

Physiology is thus a *process-oriented science* that examines the dynamic performance of biological tissues under normal and disturbed conditions. As such, it is the basic science that examines the biological correlates of behavioral performance. Rehabilitation medicine, through applied physiology, is a *process-oriented medical discipline* that is concerned with the impact of pathology on goal-directed behavioral performance. It focuses on understanding the bases of adaptive human performance and the development of practical approaches designed to enhance human functionality based on that understanding.

Rehabilitation is particularly concerned with the dynamic processes associated with *adaptation* and with the general notion of *adaptational biology*.[90] Adaptation is defined here as the dynamic process by which an organism changes in its capacity to survive and function by altering relations with its external, physical, biotic environment or within its internal structures. This approach attempts to establish a link between two apparently disparate and conflicting approaches to biological and medical science. Analytical reductionism, the most widely maintained current approach, argues that all biological processes are structurally predetermined in a continuous causal linkage. The way to understand complex systems is to break them down into their component structures, which are then analyzable as separate entities. Reductionists tend to discount behavioral description, see little to be gained from a holistic approach, and prefer to focus narrowly on a particular compartment of the system rather than on the relations between system components. Decomposition of a complex system, however, can lead to serious misunderstandings of how the system operates because it tends to obscure the complete system dynamics that follow from an understanding of how components interrelate in a functional sense. Whole-organism or "relational" biologists tend to have a broader perspective, trying to understand the behavior of the intact system, and see much more to be gained from a more comprehensive approach emphasizing the interaction of the ecology and physiology of the intact organism. It is this latter perspective, that of the relational biologist, that is of greatest relevance to the functionalist and to the physiatrist, and it is in this context that adaptation and performance can best be studied. Prosser[90] has proposed that adaptational biology should follow an intermediate course—that of seeking "reductionist explanation of holistic phenomena."

Adaptation can occur at multiple levels of organization ranging from the molecular level through that of the behavior of the intact organism.[90] Adaptive change operates across multiple time scales, ranging from the evolutionary time scale across which phylogenetic differentiation (speciation) occurs to the "microgenetic" time scale across which the ongoing adaptive behavior of the individual organism emerges. Adaptational biology, through comparative physiology, is concerned with the developmental and historical processes that shape and constrain the functional capacity of biological systems.

Physiology may be viewed as an important basic science and, specifically in this context, clinical neurophysiology as an important investigative tool for examining adaptive processes. Clinical neurophysiological studies thus become a part of the functional examination, permitting a careful operational analysis of clinical functionality. Some of the current and potential applications of clinical neurophysiology in rehabilitation medicine are guiding the development of individualized programs and assisting in decision making regarding the design of such programs; assessing prognosis for recovery and/or the stage to which recovery has progressed; evaluating the impact of therapy; detecting clinically unsuspected neural system malfunction; evaluating function in patients who may be difficult to evaluate clinically (*e.g.,* children, comatose or aphasic patients) because of problems obtaining reliable subjective reports; monitoring objective changes in patient physiological status; detecting principles of physiological change associated with recovery of function and predicting responsiveness to therapies; helping to guide and assist the development of new rehabilitation methods and to evaluate their effectiveness; and detecting dysfunction in a child early so that an appropriate intervention can occur that may help to reduce subsequent disability.

The phenomenon of motor nerve sprouting in partial nerve injury is an interesting example. Although this may seem out of place in a discussion of CNS physiology, it is quite apparent that the phenomena of fiber sprouting and related synaptic plasticity are ubiquitous throughout the nervous system and are probably quite important in the CNS during development and recovery from injury.[21, 112] Motor nerve sprouting in the adult following injury can be understood as occurring through a process that recapitulates the ontogenetic process through which the initial connective matrix of the nervous system forms and through which the initial innervation of skeletal muscle occurs.[13] This may be one example of how recovery in the adult may occur through a reenactment of developmental processes.[36] Motor nerve sprouting is clearly an adaptive process that has a very important functional result for the subject: it leads to the "recapturing" of denervated muscle fibers, albeit a partial recovery of muscle strength and without as refined a capability for tension control. Patients with poliomyelitis provide a prime example of the extent to which such functional recovery can occur and the far-reaching implications of this "built-in" adaptive process.

A large proportion of long-term disability encountered in clinical practice is related to impairment of the brain and spinal cord. Specialized paradigms have been developed to perform detailed studies of particular CNS subsystems and behavioral functions (Table 12-6). The study of the physiology of motor behavior and the functional disordering of actions or movement can be accomplished using the techniques of (poly)electro-

Table 12-6
Clinical Neurophysiological Methods

Electroencephalography
Resting—eyes opened or closed
Activated
Quantitative analysis
  Spectral analysis
  Feature analysis
  Topographical mapping

Time-Locked Event-Related Brain Potentials
Exogenous potentials
  Auditory and brain-stem evoked
  Electrospinograms
  Intraoperative monitoring
  Somatosensory
  Topographic mapping
  Visual
Endogenous potentials
  Cognitive studies/"event-related" potentials/P_{300}
  Contingent negative variation
  Readiness potential
  N_{100}

Magnetoencephalography
Evoked magnetic fields
Spontaneous fields

Motor Control Analysis Techniques
Electromyographical kinesiology of limb movement—Surface or inserted wire electrode, polyelectromyography, and electrogoniometry
Gait analysis
  Slow motion video
  Spotting systems
  Polyelectromyography
  Floor contact analysis (*e.g.,* multicontact gait mat)
  Reaction force measurement with force plate
  Biomechanical modeling and force-energy analysis
Posturography
Tremor analysis

Peripheral Testing
Electromyography
Nerve conduction studies
  Motor
  Sensory
  Autonomic
Microneurography

Reflex and Long Latency Studies
Blink reflex—R1 and R2
Bulbocavernosus reflex—penile or clitoral
F-wave latency
H-reflex latency and recovery curves
Long latency reflexes—elicited by electrical nerve stimulation (V1, V2, and V3, or C), and elicited by muscle strength (M1, M2, and M3)
Tonic vibration reflex

Transcutaneous Cortical and Spinal Cord Stimulation
Electrical stimulation
Magnetic stimulation

Urodynamic
Cystometry
Nocturnal penile tumescence
Pudendal nerve evoked potentials
Sphincter electromyography
Urethral pressure profile

myographic kinesiology, combined with spotting systems or goniometers for documenting goal-directed limb motion. Such studies are focused on the analysis of particular forms of volitional motor behavior such as walking, usually in the context of a gait analysis laboratory. Electro-oculography can be used to assess eye movement control under a variety of conditions. Motor control analysis can also be used to examine arm movement control particularly in the context of performing functional acts such as reaching to grasp and retrieve an object and eating.

There has been a tremendous proliferation of techniques and methods in clinical neurophysiology over recent years, designed for a variety of different specific clinical problems and contexts. Because of the rapid expansion and the lack of uniformity in nomenclature and technique, an exhaustive listing and review of these methods is not possible in the context of this chapter. In many cases, these methods are being applied in neurological diagnosis. In others, the use of the tests in rehabilitation evaluation and management is quite clear. It must be understood that there is yet a great deal of basic and applied research to be done to fully appreciate the potential research and clinical value of these powerful methods in rehabilitation medicine.

CONCLUSIONS

This has been a necessarily limited introductory examination of some of the established and emerging methods in CNS neurophysiology. Clinical neurophysiology of the CNS offers a unique opportunity to the physiatrist to view impairment through a physiological window that provides a means to assess and quantitate the physiological changes associated with disability. This information could be used to classify patients with CNS dysfunction into different neurophysiological categories according to objective criteria. This could ultimately lead to the development of rational observation-based criteria for the selection of different forms of rehabilitation therapy. Furthermore, these methods offer unique approaches to the assessment of infants and young children, patients in coma or persisting vegetative state, and patients with a communication disorder who could not otherwise be objectively evaluated. Such information may prove useful to the process of developing a prognosis for recovery of function and making difficult determinations about whether a particular patient is a reasonable candidate for intensive medical rehabilitation. As a powerful clinical research tool, these studies may be applied to obtain important insights into the processes of adaptation and recovery of function following brain damage. These studies may prove to be important and sophisticated tools that extend the ability of the physiatrist to assess, evaluate, and understand the physiological basis of patient functionality.

REFERENCES

1. Allen CMC: Predicting the outcome of acute stroke: A prognostic score. J Neurol Neurosurg Psychiatry 47:475–480, 1984
2. Allison T: Scalp and cortical recordings of initial somatosensory cortex activity to median nerve stimulation in man. Ann NY Acad Sci 388:671–678, 1982
3. Aminoff M: Use of somatosensory evoked potentials to evaluate the peripheral nervous system. J Clin Neurophysiol 4:135–144, 1987
4. Aminoff MJ: The clinical role of somatosensory evoked studies: A critical appraisal. Minimonograph #21, American Association of Electromyography and Electrodiagnosis, 1984
5. Aminoff MJ, Goodin DS, Parry GJ et al: Electrophysiologic evaluation of lumbosacral radiculopathies: Electromyography, late responses and somatosensory evoked potentials. Neurology 35:1514–1515, 1985
6. Bach-y-Rita P: Brain plasticity as a basis for the development of rehabilitation procedures for hemiplegia. Scand J Rehabil Med 13:73–83, 1981
7. Baker JHE, Silver JR: Hysterical paraplegia. J Neurol Neurosurg Psychiatry 50:375–382, 1987
8. Barker AT, Jalinous R, Freeston IL: Non-invasive magnetic stimulation of the human motor cortex. Lancet 1:1106–1107, 1985
9. Bennett MH, Jannetta PJ: Trigeminal evoked potentials in humans. Electroencephalogr Clin Neurophysiol 48:517–526, 1980
10. Berger H: Uber das Elektrenkephalogramm des Menschen: I. Arch Psychiatr Nervenkr 87:527–570, 1929
11. Blumhardt LD, Barrett G, Halliday AM: The pattern visual evoked potential in the clinical assessment of undiagnosed spinal cord disease. In Courjon J, Mauguiere F, Revol M (eds): Applications of Evoked Potentials in Neurology, pp 463–471. New York, Raven Press, 1982
12. Brazier MAB: A History of the Electrical Activity of the Brain: The First Half-Century. London, Pitman Medical, 1961
13. Brown MC: Sprouting of motor nerves in adult muscles: A recapitulation of ontogeny. Trends Neurosci 7:10–14, 1984
14. Brown WS, Marsh JT, LaRue A: Exponential electrophysiological aging: P3 latency. Electroencephalogr Clin Neurophysiol 55:277–285, 1983
15. Cant BR, Shaw NA: Central somatosensory conduction time: Method and clinical applications. In Cracco RQ, Bodis-Wollner I (eds): Evoked Potentials, pp 58–67. New York, Alan R Liss, 1986
16. Caton R: The electric currents of the brain. Br Med J 2:278, 1875
17. Chiappa KH: Evoked Potentials in Clinical Medicine. New York, Raven Press, 1983
18. Cole JL, Ducommun EF: Electrospinograms: Evolution and applications as a clinical tool. J Am Soc Clin Evoked Potentials Vol. 5 No. 2, 1987
19. Coles MGH, Donchin E, Proges SW (eds): Psychophysiology: Systems, Processes and Applications. New York, Guilford Press, 1986
20. Cooper R, Osselton JW, Shaw JC: EEG Technology, 3rd ed. Boston, Butterworths, 1980
21. Cotman CW (ed): Synaptic Plasticity. New York, Guilford Press, 1985
22. Cunningham JN Jr, Laschinger JC, Merkin JH et al: Measurement of spinal cord ischemia during operations upon the thoracic aorta: Initial clinical experience. Ann Surg 196:285–296, 1982
23. Cusick JF, Myklebust JB, Larson SJ, Sances A Jr: Spinal cord evaluation by cortical evoked potentials. Arch Neurol 36:140–143, 1979
24. Davis PA: Effects of acoustic stimuli on the waking human brain. J Neurophysiol 2:494–499, 1939
25. Dawson GD: Cerebral responses to electrical stimulation of peripheral nerve in man. J Neurol Neurosurg Psychiatry 10:134–140, 1947
26. Dawson GD: Investigations on a patient subject to myoclonic seizures after sensory stimulation. J Neurol Neurosurg Psychiatry 10:141–149, 1947
27. Deecke L, Grozinger B, Kornhuber HH: Voluntary finger movements in man: Cerebral potentials and theory. Biol Cybernetics 23:99–119, 1976
28. Deecke L, Scheid P, Kornhuber HH: Distribution of the readiness potential, pre-motion positivity, and motor potential of the human cerebral cortex preceding voluntary finger movements. Exp Brain Res 7:158–169, 1969
29. Desmedt JE, Bourguet M: Color imaging of parietal and frontal somatosensory potential fields evoked by stimulation of median or posterior tibial nerve in man. Electroencephalogr Clin Neurophysiol 62:1–17, 1985
30. Desmedt JE, Cheron G: Prevertebral (esophageal) recording of subcortical somatosensory evoked potentials in man: The spinal P13 component and the dual nature of the spinal generators. Electroencephalogr Clin Neurophysiol 52:257–275, 1981
31. Duffy FH (ed): Topographic Mapping of Brain Electrical Activity. Boston, Butterworths, 1986
32. Eisen A: SEP in the evaluation of disorders of the peripheral nervous system. In Cracco RQ, Bodis-Wollner I (eds): Evoked Potentials, pp 409–417. New York, Alan R Liss, 1986
33. Eisen A, Elleker C: Sensory nerve stimulation and evoked cerebral potentials. Neurology 30:1097–1105, 1980

34. Eisen A, Hoirch M: The electrodiagnostic evaluation of spinal root lesions. Spine 8:98–106, 1983

35. Eisen A, Hoirch M, Moll A: Evaluation of radiculopathies by segmental stimulation and somatosensory evoked potentials. Can J Neurol Sci 10:178–182, 1983

36. Finger S, Almli CR: Brain damage and neuroplasticity: Mechanisms of recovery or development? Brain Res Rev 10:177–186, 1985

37. Galambos R, Hicks GE, Wilson MS: The auditory brain stem response reliably predicts hearing loss in graduates of a tertiary intensive care nursery. Ear Hear 5:254–260, 1984

38. Gevins AS: Analysis of the electromagnetic signals of the human brain: Milestones, obstacles and goals. IEEE Trans Biomed Eng 31:833–850, 1984

39. Giblin DR: Somatosensory evoked potentials in healthy subjects and in patients with lesions of the nervous system. Ann NY Acad Sci 112:93–142, 1964

40. Gloor P: Neuronal generators and the problem of localization in electroencephalography: application of volume conductor theory to electroencephalography. J Clin Neurophysiol 2:327–345, 1985

41. Goldberg G, Kwan HC, Murphy JT: A neurophysiologic approach to the assessment of functional prognosis following brain damage. Electromyogr Clin Neurophysiol (in press)

42. Goodin D, Squires K, Henderson B, Starr A: Age-related variation in evoked potentials to auditory stimuli in normal human subjects. Electroencephalogr Clin Neurophysiol 44:447–458, 1978

43. Haldeman S: Pudendal nerve evoked spinal, cortical and bulbocavernous reflex responses: Methods and application. In Cracco RQ, Bodis-Wollner I (eds): Evoked Potentials, pp 68–75. New York, Alan R Liss, 1986

44. Haldeman S: The electrodiagnostic evaluation of nerve root function. Spine 9:42–48, 1984

45. Haldeman S, Bradley WB, Bhatia NN, Johnson BK: Pudendal evoked responses. Arch Neurol 39:280–283, 1982

46. Halliday AM, Barrett G, Carroll WM, Kriss A: Problems in defining the normal limits of the visual evoked potential. In Courjon J, Mauguiere F, Revol M (eds): Clinical Applications of Evoked Potentials in Neurology, pp 1–9. New York, Raven Press, 1982

47. Halliday AM, Halliday E, Kriss A et al: The pattern-evoked potential in compression of the anterior visual pathways. Brain 99:357–374, 1976

48. Halliday AM, McDonald WI, Mushin J: Visual evoked potentials in the diagnosis of multiple sclerosis. Br Med J 4:661–664, 1973

49. Halliday AM, Wakefield GS: Cerebral evoked potentials in patients with dissociated sensory loss. J Neurol Neurosurg Psychiatry 26:211–219, 1963

50. Henley S, Pettit S, Todd-Pivroper AT, Tupper AM: Who goes home: Predictive factors in stroke recovery. J Neurol Neurosurg Psychiatry 48:1–6, 1985

51. Howard JE, Dorfman LJ: Evoked potentials in hysteria and malingering. J Clin Neurophysiol 3:39-49, 1986

52. Hume AL, Cant BR: Central somatosensory conduction after head injury. Ann Neurol 10:411–419, 1981

53. Hume AL, Cant BR: Conduction time in central somatosensory pathways in man. Electroencephalogr Clin Neurophysiol 45:361–375, 1978

54. Ignacio DR, Pavot AP, Kuntavanish A: Somatosensory evoked potentials: Their prognostic value in the management of stroke. Arch Phys Med Rehabil 63:537, 1982

55. Jasper HH: The Ten-Twenty electrode system of the International Federation. Electroencephalogr Clin Neurophysiol 10:371–375, 1958

56. Jewett DL: Averaged volume-conducted potentials to auditory stimuli in the cat. Physiologist 12:262, 1969

57. Jewett DL, Romano MN, Williston JS: Human auditory evoked potentials: Possible brain-stem components detected on the scalp. Science 167:1517–1518, 1970

58. Jewett DL, Williston JS: Auditory evoked far-fields averaged from the scalp in humans. Brain 94:681–696, 1971

59. Jones SJ: Clinical applications of short-latency somatosensory evoked potentials. Ann NY Acad Sci 388:369–386, 1982

60. Katifi HA, Sedgwick EM: Evaluation of the dermatomal somatosensory evoked potential in the diagnosis of lumbo-sacral root compression. J. Neurol Neurosurg Psychiatry 50:1204–1210, 1987

61. Katifi HA, Sedgwick EM: Somatosensory evoked potentials from posterior tibial nerve and lumbosacral dermatomes. Electroencephalogr Clin Neurophysiol 65:249–259, 1986

62. Kimura J, Ishida T, Suzuki S et al: Far-field recording of the junctional potential generated by median nerve volleys at the wrist. Neurology 36:1451–1457, 1986

63. Kimura J, Mitsudome A, Beck DO et al: Stationary peaks from a moving source in far-field recording. Electroencephalogr Clin Neurophysiol 58:351–361, 1984

64. Kussofsky A, Wadell I, Nilsson BY: The relationship between sensory impairment and motor recovery in patients with hemiplegia. Scand J Rehabil Med 14:27–32, 1982

65. Kutas M, Donchin E: Preparation to respond as manifested by movement-related brain potentials. Brain Res 202:95–115, 1980

66. La Joie WJ, Reddy NM, Melvin JL: Somatosensory evoked potentials: Their predictive value in right hemiplegia. Arch Phys Med Rehabil 63:223–226, 1982

67. Laschinger JC, Cunningham JN Jr, Nathan IM et al: Intraoperative identification of vessels critical to spinal cord blood flow: Use of somatosensory evoked potentials. Curr Surg 41:107–109, 1984

68. Lesser RP, Raudzens P, Leuders H et al: Postoperative neurological deficits may occur despite unchanged intraoperative somatosensory evoked potentials. Ann Neurol 19:22–25, 1986

69. Liberson WT: Study of evoked potentials in aphasics. Am J Phys Med 45:135–142, 1966

70. Libet B, Wright EW, Gleason CA: Readiness potentials preceding unrestricted "spontaneous" vs. pre-planned voluntary acts. Electroencephalogr Clin Neurophysiol 54:322–335, 1982

71. Markand ON, Dilley RS, Moorsby SS, Warren C Jr: Monitoring of somatosensory evoked responses during carotid endarterectomy. Arch Neurol 41:375–378, 1984

72. Mauguiere F, Desmedt JE, Courjon J: Astereognosis and dissociated loss of frontal or parietal components of somatosensory evoked potentials in hemispheric lesions. Brain 106:271–311, 1983

73. Mertan PA, Morton HB, Hill DK, Marsden CD: Scope of a technique for electrical stimulation of human brain, spinal cord and muscle. Lancet 2:597–600, 1982

74. Morgan NH, Gevins AS: Wigner distributions of human event-related brain potentials. IEEE Trans Biomed Eng 33:66–70, 1986

75. Narayan RK, Greenberg RP, Miller JD et al: Improved confidence of outcome prediction in severe head injury: A comparative analysis of the clinical examination, multimodality evoked potentials, CT scanning, and intracranial pressure. J Neurosurg 54:571–762, 1981

76. Neima D, Regan D: Pattern visual evoked potentials and spatial vision in retrobulbar neuritis and multiple sclerosis. Arch Neurol 41:198–201, 1984

77. Newlon PG, Greenberg RP, Hyatt MS et al: The dynamics of neuronal dysfunction and recovery following severe head injury assessed with serial multimodality evoked potentials. J Neurosurg 57:168–177, 1982

78. Niedermeyer E, Lopes da Silva F: Electroencephalography: Basic Principles, Clinical Applications and Related Fields. Baltimore, Urban & Schwarzenberg, 1982

79. Nodar RH, Barber C (eds): Evoked Potentials II. Boston, Butterworths, 1984

80. Nuwer MR: Evoked Potential Monitoring in the Operating Room. New York, Raven Press, 1986

81. Oken BS, Chiappa KH: Somatosensory evoked potentials in neurological diagnosis. In Cracco RQ, Bodis-Wollner I (eds): Evoked Potentials, pp 379–389. New York, Alan R Liss, 1986

82. Olbrich HM, Nau HE, Loudman E et al: Evoked potential assessment of mental function during recovery from severe head injury. Surg Neurol 26:112–118, 1986

83. Papakostopoulos D, Crow HJ: Direct recording of somatosensory evoked potentials from the cerebral cortex of man and the difference between precentral and postcentral potentials. In Desmedt JE (ed): Progress in Clinical Neurophysiology, Vol 7, Clinical Uses of Cerebral, Brainstem and Spinal Somatosensory Evoked Potentials, pp 15–26. Basel, Karger, 1980

84. Panpanicolaou AC, Levin HS, Eisenberg HM et al: Evoked potential correlates of posttraumatic amnesia after closed head injury. Neurosurgery 14:676–678, 1984

85. Pavot AP, Ignacio DR, Kuntavanish A, Lightfoote II WE: The prognos-

tic value of somatosensory evoked potentials in cerebrovascular accident. Electromyogr Clin Neurophysiol 26:333–340, 1986

86. Perot PL Jr, Vera CL: Scalp-recorded somatosensory evoked potentials to stimulation of nerves in the lower extremities and evaluation of patients with spinal cord trauma. Ann NY Acad Sci 388:359–368, 1982

87. Picton TW, Hillyard S: Human auditory evoked potentials: II. Effects of attention. Electroencephalogr Clin Neurophysiol 36:191–199, 1974

88. Polich J: Attention, probability and task demands as determinants of P300 latency from auditory stimuli. Electroencephalogr Clin Neurophysiol 63:251–259, 1986

89. Pratt H, Starr A: Somatosensory evoked potentials to natural forms of stimulation. In Cracco RQ, Bodis-Wollner I (eds): Evoked Potentials, pp 28–34. New York, Alan R Liss, 1986

90. Prosser CL: Adaptational Biology: From Molecules to Organisms. New York, John Wiley & Sons, 1986

91. Rappaport M: Brain evoked potentials in coma and the vegetative state. Head Trauma Rehabil 1:15–29, 1986

92. Remond A (ed): Handbook of Electroencephalography and Clinical Neurophysiology. Amsterdam, Elsevier, 1976

93. Ropper AM, Miett R, Chiappa KH: Absence of evoked potential abnormalities in acute transverse myelopathy. Neurology 32:80–82, 1982

94. Rossini PM, DiStefano E, Stanzione P: Nervous impulse propagation along peripheral and central (spinal and intracranial) fast conducting sensory and motor pathways in normals. Electroencephalogr Clin Neurophysiol 60:320–334, 1985

95. Rossini PM, Marciani MG, Caramia M et al: Transcutaneous stimulation of motor cerebral cortex and spine: Noninvasive evaluation of central efferent transmission in normal subjects and patients with multiple sclerosis. In Cracco RQ, Bodis-Wollner I (eds): Frontiers of Clinical Neuroscience, Vol. 3, Evoked Potentials, pp 76–84. New York, Alan R Liss, 1986

96. Rowed DW: Value of somatosensory evoked potentials for prognosis in partial cord injuries. In Tator CH (ed): Early Management of Acute Spinal Cord Injury, pp 167–180. New York, Raven Press, 1982

97. Rowed DW, McLean JAG, Tator CH: Somatosensory evoked potentials in acute spinal cord injury: Prognostic value. Surg Neurol 9:203–210, 1978

98. Russ W, Fraedich G, Hehrlein FW, Hampelmann G: Intraoperative somatosensory evoked potentials as a prognostic factor of neurologic state after carotid endarterectomy. Thorac Cardiovasc Surg 33:392–396, 1985

99. Shibasaki H: Movement-related cortical potentials. In Halliday AM: Evoked Potentials in Clinical Testing. Edinburgh, Churchill Livingstone, 1982

100. Shibasaki H, Barrett G, Halliday E, Halliday AM: Components of the movement-associated cortical potential and their scalp topography. Electroencephalogr Clin Neurophysiol 49:213–226, 1980

101. Slimp JC, Tamas LB, Stolov WC, Wyler AR: Somatosensory evoked potentials after removal of somatosensory cortex in man. Electroencephalogr Clin Neurophysiol 65:111–117, 1986

102. Sohmer H, Feinmesser M: Cochlear action potentials recorded from the external ear in man. Ann Otol Rhinol Laryngol 76:427–435, 1967

103. Sohmer H, Feinmesser M: Cochlear and cortical audiometry. Isr J Med Sci 6:219–223, 1970

104. Spehlmann R: Evoked Potential Primer. Boston, Butterworths, 1985

105. Spielholz NI, Benjamin MV, Engler G, Ransohoff J: Somatosensory evoked potentials and clinical outcome in spinal cord injury. In Popp AJ (ed): Neural Trauma, pp 217–222. New York, Raven Press, 1979

106. Squires KC, Donchin E, Herning RI, McCarthy G: On the influence of task relevance and stimulus probability on event-related potential components. Electroencephalogr Clin Neurophysiol 42:1–14, 1977

107. Squires N, Ollo C: Human evoked potential techniques: Possible applications to neuropsychology. In Hannay J (ed): Experimental Techniques in Human Neuropsychology. New York, Oxford University Press, 1985

108. Stegeman DF, Van Oosterom A, Colon EJ: Far-field evoked potential components induced by a propagating generator: Computational evidence. Electroencephalogr Clin Neurophysiol 67:176–187, 1987

109. Suwanwela C, Alexander E Jr, Davis CH Jr: Prognosis in spinal cord injury with special reference to patients with motor paralysis and sensory preservation. J Neurosurg 19:220–227, 1962

110. Syndulko K, Hansch EC, Cohen SN et al: Long latency event-related potentials in normal aging and dementia. In Courjon J, Mauguiere F, Revol M (eds): Clinical Applications of Evoked Potentials in Neurology, pp 279–285. New York, Raven Press, 1982

111. Tamas LB, Shibasaki H: Cortical potentials associated with movement: A review. J Clin Neurophysiol 2:157–171, 1985

112. Tsukahara N: Synaptic plasticity in the mammalian central nervous system. Ann Rev Neurosci 4:351–379, 1981

113. Twist D, Squires N, Spielholz NI, Silverglide R: Event-related potentials as a measure of hemispheric specialization in aphasic and aprosodic disorders. Proceedings of the Eighth International Conference on Event-Related Potentials of the Brain (EPIC VIII), pp 216–217 (abstr), Stanford, California, 1986

114. Vaughn HG Jr, Costa LD, Ritter W: Topography of the human motor potential. Electroencephalogr Clin Neurophysiol 25:1–10, 1968

115. Vredeveld JW: Predictive somatosensory evoked potentials. Electroencephalogr Clin Neurophysiol 52:340, 1983

116. Wade DT, Skilbeck CE, Hewer RL: Predicting Barthel ADL score at six months after an acute stroke. Arch Phys Med Rehabil 64:24–28, 1983

117. Walter WG, Cooper R, Aldridge VJ et al: Contingent negative variation: An electrical sign of sensorimotor association and expectancy in the human brain. Nature 203:380–384, 1964

118. Wood CC: Application of dipole localization methods to source identification of human evoked potentials. Ann NY Acad Sci 388:139–155, 1982

119. Wood CC, Cohen D, Cuffin BN et al: Electrical sources in human somatosensory cortex: Identification by combined magnetic and potential recordings. Science 227:1051–1053, 1985

120. Yamada T, Dickins QS, Machida M et al: Somatosensory evoked potentials to simultaneous median nerve stimulation in man: Method and clinical application. In Cracco RQ, Bodis-Wollner I (eds): Evoked Potentials, pp 45–57. New York, Alan R Liss, 1986

121. Yamada T, Machida M, Tippin J: Somatosensory evoked potentials. In Owen JH, Davis H (eds): Evoked Potential Testing: Clinical Applications, pp 109–158. New York, Grune & Stratton, 1985

13

Physical Agents and Biofeedback

Jeffrey R. Basford

Superficial physical agents such as heat, cold, light, friction, and pressure have been used in therapy for thousands of years. This century has seen the refinement of these approaches as well as the development of the diathermies and the increasing acceptance of other electromagnetic and biofeedback therapies.

Treatment has never been static; agents that were once widely used are now rarely seen. Others involving lasers and electromagnetic devices are under evaluation. This continuing reassessment and discovery process requires of the clinician to keep an open mind—to avoid the fad, but adopt the improvement.

In this chapter, the emphasis will be on the clinical use, effectiveness, limitations, and safety of physical agents and biofeedback. Relevant biophysics and mechanical features of the equipment will also be briefly reviewed.

HEAT AND COLD

The amount of energy that tissue will gain or lose during treatment depends on the nature of the tissue itself, the treatment modality involved, and the duration of exposure. In addition, the body places physiological limits on the amount of heat and cold it will tolerate. For example, exposure of skin to temperatures above 45 or 46°C is uncomfortable, and prolonged exposure to temperatures above 50°C may cause injury.[59] Temperatures below 13°C are uncomfortable, and if the body is cooled below 28°C death may occur.[59]

Metabolism is temperature dependent; even moderate temperature changes can have significant effects. For example, a temperature elevation of 3°C, such as occurs in an inflamed rheumatoid knee, increases synovial collagenase activity by 300%.[70] Exposing the hands to 45°C temperatures reduces metacarpophalangeal (MCP) joint stiffness 20%. Temperature decreases of 18°C, on the other hand, will increase MCP stiffness by 10 to 20%.[195] Temperature changes of a few degrees alter nerve conduction, and changes of 5 to 7°C significantly alter blood flow[1, 50, 69, 95] and collagen extensibility.[113]

In practice, most heat treatments attempt to warm tissues to between 40 and 45°C. Cold treatments are limited to superficial agents; and although marked decreases in skin and subcutaneous temperatures are possible, the cooling of deeper tissue is usually restricted to a few degrees.

Systemic hyperthermia (fever therapy) was used until well into this century to treat a variety of diseases such as syphilis, gonorrhea, and pelvic inflammatory disease.[92] Interest in regional and local diathermy has recently increased as it becomes apparent that many tumors are sensitive to heat. Although regional and local cancer hyperthermia experiments do not apply directly to routine physical medicine, the techniques and approaches are pertinent and have been widely reported.[11, 12, 47, 77, 161]

Although there are exceptions, the basic therapeutic uses of heat (Table 13-1) are based on analgesia, hyperemia, local and systemic hyperthermia, and reduction of muscle tone. The general contraindications for heat (Table 13-2) are, for the most part, obvious, such as acute trauma, ischemia, and bleeding disorders.

Many of the same indications and contraindications apply to the use of cold modalities (Tables 13-3 and 13-4).

Superficial Heat

All heating modalities warm tissue by one or a combination of three mechanisms: conduction, conversion, and convection. Among the superficial agents, hot packs exemplify conduction effects, heat lamps employ conversion (converting radiant energy to heat) and hydrotherapy convection.

The physical properties of superficial heating modalities differ, but none of these agents are able to overcome the combination of skin tolerance, tissue thermal conductivity, and the body's responses to produce localized temperature elevations of more than a few degrees at depths of a few centimeters.[115] The following paragraphs review characteristics of the more common superficial agents.

Hot Packs

Hot packs, frequently referred to simply as "Hydrocollator" packs, are the best known conductive heating modality. These packs are available in several sizes and typically consist of segmented canvas bags filled with silicon dioxide which, when exposed to moisture, absorbs many times its own weight. It, and the pack, essentially acquire the large heat capacity of water.

Hot packs are suspended on racks in hot (70° to 80°C) water and are only removed from the bath when needed. Packs cool

Table 13-1
General Indications for Heat Modalities

Pain
Muscle spasm
Contracture
Tension myalgia
Production of hyperemia
Acceleration of metabolic processes
Hematoma resolution
Bursitis
Tenosynovitis
"Fibrositis"
Superficial thrombophlebitis
Induction of reflex vasodilation
Collagen vascular diseases

Table 13-2
*General Contraindications and Precautions
for Heat Modalities*

Acute inflammation, trauma, or hemorrhage
Bleeding disorders
Insensitivity
Inability to communicate or respond to pain
Poor thermal regulation (*e.g.,* from neuroleptics)
Areas of malignancy
Edema
Ischemia
Atrophic skin
Scar tissue

Table 13-3
General Indications for Cold Modalities

Acute musculoskeletal trauma
  Edema
  Hemorrhage
  Analgesia
Pain
Muscle spasm
Spasticity
Adjunct in muscle re-education
Reduction of local and systemic metabolic activity

Table 13-4
*General Precautions and Contraindications
for Cold Modalities*

Ischemia
Cold intolerance
Raynaud's phenomenon and disease
Severe cold pressor responses
Cold allergy
Insensitivity

slowly and, when wrapped in six to eight layers of toweling or an insulating cover (Fig. 13-1), can maintain clinically useful temperatures for 30 minutes.

The advantages of hot packs include low cost, minimal maintenance, long life (packs last as long as 5 years; reservoirs up to 30 years), patient acceptance, and ease of use. Although they are a time-consuming modality, hot packs may be used at home if the patient is willing to use the same techniques and follow the same precautions as the therapist.

Hot packs have few risks that are not associated with all heating modalities. However, to avoid scalding, excess water should be drained before use and the covering towels should be checked for dampness.

Kenny packs are wool cloths which are soaked in 60°C water and spun dry before being placed on the patient. The cloths contain little water after being spun and cool rapidly. As a result, they must be replaced several times during a therapy session and produce a cyclic heating pattern. In the past, Kenny packs were favored by many clinicians for polio patients because they were considered to be effective for muscle pain and spasm. Due to equipment requirements, labor intensity, and probably the odor of wet wool, they are now seldom used.

Electric heating pads, hot water bottles, and circulating water heating pads are alternatives to hot packs. Many of these devices do not cool spontaneously, and patients should be cautioned to avoid burns by limiting exposure to 20 minutes. Patients should also be warned that heat use can produce temporary as well as permanent skin mottling (erythema ab igne).

Heat Lamps

Heat lamps are an inexpensive, versatile, and easy way to warm superficial tissues. Ordinary incandescent light bulbs produce large amounts of infrared energy, so that special infrared sources (*e.g.,* quartz, tungsten) are seldom essential.

Heat lamps often use 250-watt bulbs and are usually placed about 40 to 50 cm from the patient. Heating rates and maximum temperatures are controlled by adjusting the distance between the lamp and the patient (*i.e.,* the $1/r^2$ law). Although "bakers" with multiple bulbs and units with special heating elements are available, simple lamps that clamp on furniture are the most frequently used.

The choice of whether to use a heat lamp or hot pack will depend on the patient. If the patient is difficult to position or cannot tolerate pressure, radiant heat is the better option. Similarly if patients feel that radiant heat dries their skin or if they prefer moist heat, the choice is easy. At other times, ease of use and the preference of the physician or therapist dictate the choice. Some find that the cleanliness, ease of use, and reduced laundry costs of heat lamps outweigh most advantages of hot packs.

Hydrotherapy

Whirlpool baths (Fig. 13-2) and Hubbard tanks (Fig. 13-3) are the most common forms of hydrotherapy. These units use pumps to agitate water and they provide convective heating, massage, and gentle debridement. Tanks vary in size from small 120-liter whirlpools designed to treat a single extremity to Hubbard tanks of several thousand liters in which the entire body can be placed.

The temperature of the water depends on how much of the body is immersed, treatment goals, and the patient's condition. In general, 33 to 36°C temperatures are considered "neutral" and are well tolerated. Hubbard tanks can alter body temperatures, so to avoid problems, water temperature in these units is

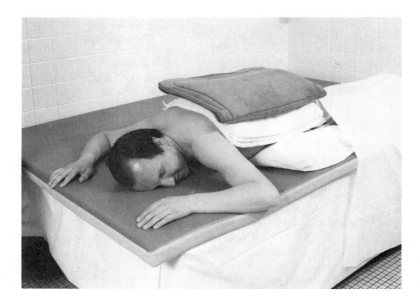

Figure 13-1. Hot pack treatment of the low back. Note that the pack is covered with an insulated wrapper and separated from the patient with several layers of toweling.

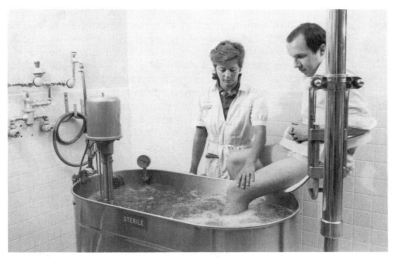

Figure 13-2. Whirlpool treatment of the lower leg. Water temperatures may range from 11° to 43°C depending on the condition and the amount of surface area treated. Entering and leaving the bath is less difficult with a hydraulic chair.

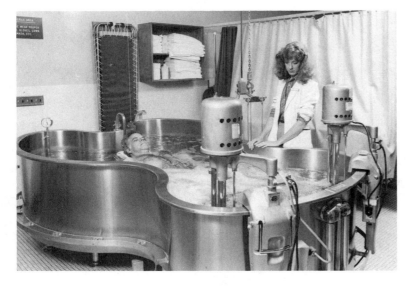

Figure 13-3. Hubbard tank treatment. These tanks are large, expensive to operate, and occupy large amounts of floor space. Nevertheless, they are necessary for the cleansing of large wounds and helpful in treating patients with conditions involving multiple joints.

usually limited to 39°C. Treatment of a single extremity can be more rigorous and, for the healthy patient, temperatures of 43°C to as much as 45 or 46°C are possible. Because the water is in constant motion, no insulating layer of cooler water forms on the surface of the skin. As a result, more vigorous heating occurs than would be the case in stationary water of the same temperature.

Hydrotherapy is well suited for wound and burn treatment for which gentle agitation, heat, and solvent action are needed. Neutral temperatures are chosen and, after the patient is immersed, the agitators are turned on to provide gentle debridement and aid bandage removal. A "sterile" tank should be specified for wound and burn treatment. Although true sterility is not possible, a close-enough approximation is possible to make disease transmission unlikely. If wounds are large, or if there is a significant exposure of internal organs, such as the intestines, sodium chloride may be added to the water (about 10 kg for a Hubbard tank) to improve comfort and lessen the risks of hemolysis and electrolyte imbalance. Povidone-iodine and gentle detergents may also be used according to individual discretion and prejudice.

Hydrotherapy is also effective for mobilization of joints following cast removal and as an adjunct in the treatment of conditions such as rheumatoid arthritis, diffuse tension myalgias, and muscle spasm. It is important to remember that patients may find being lowered into Hubbard tanks frightening, and entry into whirlpools difficult.

Hydrotherapy requires large areas of floor space, is expensive, and consumes vast amounts of hot water. In order to save space and money, therapy departments are reducing the number of Hubbard tanks to a minimum and are using as small a whirlpool as possible for each therapy.

CONTRAST BATHS. The effectiveness of contrast baths is thought to be due to reflex hyperemia produced by the alternating exposure to heat and cold.[192] Temperatures of the baths are usually about 43°C and 16°C. Typically treatments begin with an initial soaking of the hands or feet in the warm bath for about 10 minutes and then proceed to four cycles of alternate 1- to 4-minute cold soaks and 4- to 6-minute warm soaks.

Although a variety of applications are possible, contrast baths are often used in treatment programs for rheumatoid arthritis and reflex sympathetic dystrophy (RSD). Rheumatoid arthritics often benefit, but many will prefer to use simpler warm soaks at home. RSD patients also seem to benefit, but their improvement usually occurs in conjunction with other desensitization and activity programs.

ALTERNATIVE FORMS OF HYDROTHERAPY. Alternative forms of hydrotherapy include saunas, warm springs, cold sprays (douches), and peloid (mud) baths.[119] Many of these are popular in Europe, but are either seldom used in this country or are not found in physical therapy departments.

Hydrotherapy uses water as the heat exchanging medium, but other media are possible. Substances as diverse as pulverized corn cobs and small beads may be heated and "fluidized" by jets of hot air. Treatments are performed in much the same way as standard hydrotherapy. Although these latter devices enjoy some popularity and have been available since the 1970s,[3, 26] the benefits derived from the dry, high temperature and low heat capacity aspects of this approach remain controversial.

Paraffin Baths

Paraffin baths are less commonly used than radiant heat, hot packs, or hydrotherapy. Nonetheless, they continue to have a

definite, albeit limited, role. The typical paraffin bath consists of a container filled with roughly a 1 : 7 mixture of mineral oil and paraffin maintained at 52 to 54°C. Although these temperatures are higher than those associated with water-based therapy, they are well tolerated because (1) the mixture has a low heat capacity and (2) an insulating layer of wax builds up on the treated area.

Two paraffin treatment approaches predominate. One is the *dip* method in which the patient repetitively dips and removes the treated area from the paraffin. A brief pause is made between each dip to allow the paraffin to solidify. After about ten dips, the treated area is covered with a plastic sheet and wrapped with toweling (or an insulating pack) for about 20 minutes (Figs. 13-4 and 13-5). The paraffin is then stripped off and returned to the container. Because the feet have poorer circulation than most parts of the body, a few insulating layers of paraffin may be painted on before the feet are dipped or immersed.[73]

Paraffin dipping initially elevates skin temperatures to about 47°C, but at the end of a 30-minute treatment these temperatures have fallen within a few degrees of baseline. Dipping produces subcutaneous temperature increases of 3°C and intramuscular temperature changes of about 1°C.[2]

An alternative to dipping is *continuous immersion* of the treated part for 20 to 30 minutes. Heating with this approach is more intense than in the dip method, but is easily tolerated because a layer of insulating solidified paraffin forms on the skin. Immersion treatments, like the dip method, also produce maximum skin temperatures of about 47°C. However, at the end of treatment, skin temperature is still significantly elevated (about 41.5°C). Maximum subcutaneous temperatures increase about 5°C, but these elevations are maintained about 2°C higher than those obtained with dipping. Intramuscular temperatures increase about 3°C and also remain higher than those obtained from dipping.[2]

A thermometer should be kept in the reservoir and paraffin temperature checked before each use. A film of solidified wax at the margins of the reservoir is a reassuring sign, since it means that the paraffin is not likely to be much above a therapeutic temperature.

Figure 13-4. Paraffin bath treatment using a dipping technique. An extremity is immersed in the bath approximately ten times with a short pause between each dip. Following the dipping, the extremity is wrapped in an insulating cover for about 20 minutes before the wax is removed.

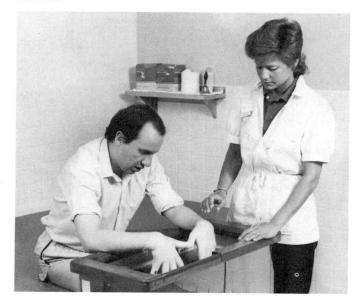

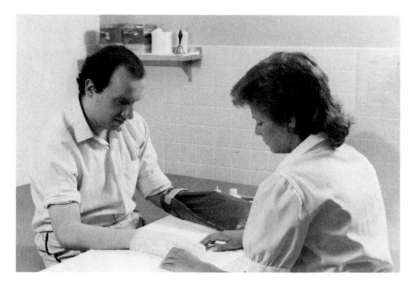

Figure 13-5. Following the paraffin immersions, the left hand is shown placed in a plastic-coated, insulated bag to slow cooling. As an alternative, the hand may be wrapped with toweling and a plastic sheet.

Paraffin is primarily used to treat contractures, particularly for patients with rheumatoid arthritis, hand contractures, or scleroderma. Most treatments are done with the dip or immersion technique, but occasionally paraffin will be brushed on difficult-to-treat areas. The literature is scant, but the treatments, although messy, are frequently helpful.[2]

Some patients will want to continue paraffin treatments at home. Although paraffin-oil mixtures can be heated in a double boiler on a stove, small commercial units are available, which have the advantages of ease of use and lower risk of fire and burns.

Deep-Heat Modalities

Of the three deep-heating modalities discussed here—ultrasound and short wave and microwave diathermy—ultrasound and short wave are used the most often.

Ultrasound

Ultrasound (US) is arbitrarily defined as sound at frequencies above the limits of human hearing (*i.e.,* more than 17,000 Hz). Except for frequency-dependent effects, US is indistinguishable from sound in general: it consists of alternating compressions and rarefactions, it requires a medium for transmission, it transmits energy, and it can be focused, refracted, and reflected. Over the years the biophysical and therapeutic effects of US have been studied in detail. Although arguments are made for a variety of frequencies, practical considerations of focusing, penetration, and standardization have resulted in US treatments in the United States being limited to 0.8 to 1 MHz.

BIOPHYSICS. Therapeutic effects are not ascribed directly to sound itself, but rather to the conversion of sound to other forms of energy. Heat production is the most important and best understood interaction. However, other nonthermal effects may occur depending on the frequency, the tissues involved, and method of treatment. The best known nonthermal effects include cavitation, media motion (streaming and microstreaming), and standing waves. These effects can occur at clinical energies and frequencies,[36, 139, 181, 188] but their significance is unclear. Because nonthermal phenomena are potentially beneficial or harmful, they should be well understood by the clinician.

Cavitation is the production of gas bubbles in a media by high frequency sound or turbulence. Once produced, bubbles may rhythmically oscillate in size (stable cavitation) or may rapidly grow and abruptly collapse (unstable cavitation). Although unstable cavitation seems more obviously capable of producing damage, both forms of cavitation may cause movement of material, mechanical distortion, and alteration of cellular function.[36, 139, 181, 188]

Acoustic streaming refers to the movement of material as a result of pressure asymmetries produced by sound as it passes through a medium. Cellular effects attributed to streaming processes include plasma membrane damage and acceleration of metabolic processes.[48]

Standing waves are produced by the resonant superposition of sound waves. They are formed when regions of high pressure (compression) are juxtaposed at half wavelength intervals with regions of low pressure (rarefaction). (Since sound velocities in soft tissues are about 1500 m/sec,[66] therapeutic US wavelengths are about 1.5 mm.) Quite graphic effects are possible; Dyson and co-workers, for example, observed repetitive bands of red blood cells at half wavelength intervals in the vessels of chick embryo preparations during US exposure.[49]

Sound absorption, and therefore the penetration of sound into tissue, changes with frequency. Although 50% of the energy of a therapeutic US beam can penetrate several centimeters in muscle, penetration decreases by a factor of six between 0.3 and 3.3 MHz.[66] Bone absorption is more rapid and 50% attenuation occurs within a few tenths of a millimeter. Again, frequency dependence is a strong factor, and an eightfold decrease in penetration occurs between 0.8 and 3.5 MHz.[66]

The orientation of an US beam is also important. In muscle about 50% of a therapeutic (in this case 0.87 MHz) US beam will penetrate about 2 cm in a direction perpendicular to the fibers. In a direction parallel to the fibers, the same beam will penetrate about 7 cm.[66] US is poorly absorbed in fat and 50% of a beam will penetrate 7 to 8 cm.[66] In practice, temperature increases of 4 to 5°C may be found at depths of 8 cm.[108]

US diathermy involves interaction of sound with muscle, bone, ligament, cartilage, and fat. Sound discontinuities exist at tissue interfaces, and local changes in sound propagation and absorption may become significant. The most abrupt changes occur where there are the greatest changes in absorption characteristics of the tissues, at bone—soft tissue interfaces. In these regions temperature elevations of more than 5°C may occur.[108, 109] It is important to remember that most absorption occurs far beneath the skin and that maximal heating may be limited by deep tissue factors and not by skin tolerance.

EQUIPMENT. US machines use ceramic and quartz piezoelectric crystals to produce ultrasonic energy. The crystals are bound to metal and this combination serves as the applicator. Each machine has dials to indicate when the applicator is energized, the nominal output power, and, when appropriate, the waveform and frequency. US machines are equipped with timers that turn off the machine at the end of treatment, and may have additional options, such as concurrent electrical stimulation.

US frequency is relatively invariant and is usually within 5% of the manufacturer's specifications.[172] Output power, however may change with the age of the unit as well as during a treatment period. As a result, US output energies routinely vary by 20% or more from specifications. Intensities (power output divided by the active area of the applicator) also are often incorrect.[6, 172] For these reasons, machines should be recalibrated on a routine basis.

TECHNIQUE. US may be the most frequently used diatherapy.[172] Two practical factors should be considered when specifying treatment. The first is that the intensities used in clinical practice (typically between 0.5–2 W/cm^2) can cause injury. The second factor is that applicator sizes (usually 5–10 cm) limit the area that can be treated during a session.

Once US is chosen for treatment, the waveform must be specified. *Continuous wave* ultrasound is delivered as a continuous, unmodulated wave. If an *interrupted waveform* is chosen, the beam is modulated to deliver energy in pulses, with pulse shapes and durations are determined by the characteristics of the machine being used. (Frequently square pulses with a 1 : 5 on-off cycle are used.) Obviously, if the same average energy is used for continuous and interrupted treatments, higher instantaneous intensities occur in the interrupted mode. Thus, although the amount of energy delivered is similar, the interrupted mode may be chosen in an attempt to emphasize nonthermal effects.

Heat is lost from a treated area by conduction through the tissue and by the cooling effect of the local blood supply. Cooling thus takes place over time, and different rates of heating will result in different equilibrium temperatures. This means that a 5-minute treatment at 2 W/cm^2 is not equivalent to 0/.5 W/cm^2 for 20 minutes.

US treatment may be by direct or indirect contact. *Direct* US

involves stroking or, rarely, stationary placement of the applicator on the skin (Fig. 13-6). Applicator movement is usually favored because it allows coverage of larger areas, lessens temperature nonhomogeneities, and reduces the potential for nonthermal effects. Strokes are overlapped and repeated frequently enough to maintain temperature elevations. Typical treatments involve slow (1–2 cm/sec) linear or circular sweeps for 5 to 10 minutes over areas of about 100 cm^2.

The area to be treated should be cleansed to permit an effective skin–applicator coupling. A variety of experiments have been done to determine the most effective coupling media. In general, little practical difference exists between degassed water, commercial gels, and mineral oil for direct applications. Glycerine is somewhat less efficient, but is acceptable.[13, 160, 187] For indirect US applications, degassed water seems the least expensive and most reasonable choice.

Indirect US is usually used to treat irregular surfaces (*e.g.,* ankle, hand) where it is difficult to maintain contact between the applicator and the patient. In these situations the applicator and body part are placed in a container filled with degassed water. The sound head is kept at a distance of 1 cm from the skin and moved over it without touching. Power intensities are comparable with those of direct treatments, but may be slightly higher due to absorption in the water.

Phonophoresis is a variant of direct US in which biologically active substances are combined with the coupling medium, in the hope that the ultrasound will force the active material into tissue and thereby potentiate treatment effectiveness. Penetration depths are not well established, but startling claims of increased cortisol concentrations at depths of several centimeters have been made.[68] Detectable concentrations of lidocaine in rabbit muscle have also been reported following phonophoresis.[148] One clinical study compared the effectiveness of combined lidocaine and corticosteroid phonophoresis with a similar US treatment with an inert coupling agent.[141] Both of the treated groups fared better than control patients who received only sham US treatments. Although the phonophoresis group improved more than the standard US group (88% versus 56%), the difference was not statistically significant. Other clinical studies report success with phonophoretic carbocaine anesthesia during fracture reduction,[32] and with phenylbutazone and chymotrypsin application.[186]

Clinical treatments usually consist of stroking the applicator on the skin. Research protocols, in contrast, may use a stationary treatment to increase data reproducibility. The difference in

Figure 13-6.   Direct contact ultrasound treatment of lateral epicondylitis. Note the use of a coupling agent between the sound head and the skin.

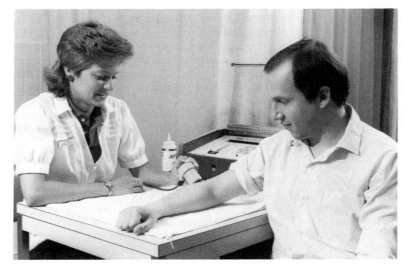

approach can be significant and must be considered when reviewing experimental reports.

INDICATIONS. Tendonitis and Bursitis. Clinical studies, which again tend to be small or poorly controlled, usually find US effective for subacute tendonitis and bursitis. In one investigation 33 patients with bursitis and 27 patients with bicipital tendonitis[51] were treated with a series of daily or three times a week 5-to-8 minute sessions of 1 MHz US at 1.2 to 1.8 W/cm². Good to fair improvement (in terms of decreased pain and increased motion) was found in 88 to 95% of the patients.[51] Two other studies of 47 and 175 patients treated with corticosteroid injections in conjunction with US (5–10 min of up to 3 W/cm² 1 MHz US on a daily or alternate day schedule) found 80 to 90% of the patients had excellent or moderate improvement.[37, 147] Although one of the studies[147] compared different US treatments, neither included untreated controls, so that whether patients would have improved with different or even no treatment is unknown. Findings of effectiveness are not universal. At least one small study found the combination of US with anti-inflammatory medication and range-of-motion (ROM) exercises no more effective in patients with subacromial bursitis than medication and exercise alone.[45]

Degenerative Arthritis. US is often used as an adjunct to superficial heat, posture, and exercise programs for individuals with degenerative arthritis. Treatments usually involve intensities between 0.5 and 2 W/cm² and are limited to 5 to 10 minutes. Since only limited areas can be treated in a session, treatments are restricted to circumscribed areas.

The goals of treatment are reduced pain, increased ROM, speeded healing, and reduction of muscle spasm. Studies tend to find significant improvement with treatment (frequently 70–80%) but are limited by the subjective nature of the complaints and poor controls.[4]

Contractures. Contracture treatment approaches vary, but all include heat and vigorous stretching. Since the distensibility of collagen increases with temperature, a prolonged stretch must be maintained during heating. Stretched connective tissue "sets" as it cools, so that stretching should be maintained until tissue temperature has returned to its baseline.[113]

Lehmann and co-workers found US treatment can produce joint temperature elevations of as much as 8 to 10°C.[109] This same group found temperature elevations of this magnitude effective in increasing tendon extensibility.[113] Controlled studies find US effective in increasing ROM in shoulder periarthritis and hip contracture.[111, 112] US, in fact, is the only modality which can produce significant temperature elevations in the hip joint.[114] Successful treatment of hand contractures and, to a limited extent, Dupuytren's contractures have also been reported.[131]

Herpes Zoster. Treatment of post-herpetic neuralgia pain with cold packs, medication, pressure, and transcutaneous electrical nerve stimulation (TENS) is frequently unsuccessful. Low intensity US with pulsed and continuous 1 to 1.5 MHz and energies of 0.25 to 0.8 W/cm² has also been evaluated. The studies tend to be uncontrolled and the results mixed: some find marked improvement,[61, 81] while other find no benefit.[155] Since there is support for both thermal and possibly nonthermal US effects on nerve conduction,[40, 54, 65] further evaluation needs to be done.

Plantar Warts. In one study[35] 50 patients with plantar warts were treated with weekly 15-minute sessions of indirect US at 0.5 W/cm² at 0.8 or 1 MHz. Of the treated group, 80% were reported

cured and 83% had pain relief. A control group, containing only 5 patients, showed no improvement. Another study[185] found both direct and indirect US treatments effective. The directly treated group, however, fared somewhat better in terms of pain relief (97 versus 88%) and lesion destruction (83 versus 51%). Not all studies find US effective for plantar wart treatment. Another group[27] evaluated US treatment of previously untreated plantar warts in a double blinded, controlled study. No significant benefit was found from weekly 0.8 mW/cm² treatments, and the investigators noted warts resolved in 82% of the treated patients and 87% of the untreated patients. However, this study differed from the others in that the warts were shaved and cleansed with peroxide before each treatment. The effect of differing approaches and patient selection on results is unclear. At present, the effectiveness of US for plantar wart treatment is not established.

Keloids. Keloids have been treated with injection, surgery, and radiation with mixed success. US have also been tried, but, at least, in one small series of six patients, no improvement was noted after a course of 24 0.5 to 0.8 W/cm² treatments.[194]

Trauma. US can increase tissue damage if used too soon after an injury. However, there are limited reports of speeded resolution of injection indurations[144] and hematomas.[149] Other studies found that 5-minute, pulsed 1 W/cm² US significantly reduced "post-partum" perineal pain[57] and that US was significantly more effective than radiant heat, short wave diathermy, or paraffin baths in helping patients with a variety of soft tissue injuries to return to work.[137]

Skin Ulcers. US is periodically reported to promote protein synthesis and to accelerate the healing of skin ulcers. Investigations of this sort are difficult to design and usually use only historical controls. One study[154] reported that 0.5–1 W/cm² US treatments healed 57% of patients with ulcers that had failed to improve with previous treatment.

PRECAUTIONS AND CONTRAINDICATIONS. In addition to the general contraindications of heat (see Table 13-2), US has a number of specific limitations. Fluid-filled cavities such as the eyes and gravid uterus should be avoided due to the risks of cavitation and heat damage. Sonification of the heart, brain, cervical ganglia, tumors, areas of hemorrhage or stasis or ischemia, pacemakers, and infection sites should be avoided for obvious heat, neurophysiological, and mechanical reasons. The spine should not be exposed to high intensities and laminectomy sites should be avoided.[46]

A number of studies have shown that the presence of metal in muscle or next to bone produces no more of a temperature elevation than would be expected if no metal or bone alone was present.[30, 64, 170] These studies were carried out with a limited number of objects and it is possible that some geometries might focus US energies and produce areas of higher heating. Since joint prostheses have abrupt metal–bone, metal–cement, plastic–bone interfaces, treatment over these implants should be avoided.

Short Wave Diathermy

Short wave diathermy (SWD) uses radio waves to heat tissue conversively. These devices can cause electrical interference, and the Federal Communications Commission (FCC) has restricted industrial, scientific and medical (ISM) use to 27.12, 13.56, and 40.68 MHz (wavelengths 11, 22, and 7 meters respectively). In the United States most SWD machines operate at 27.12 MHz.

BIOPHYSICS. Radio waves are attenuated as they pass through tissue, but actual penetration depths depend on tissue composition, applicator choice, and frequency. Inductively coupled applicators produce magnetically induced eddy currents and, as a rule of thumb, temperature elevations are relatively higher in conductive water-rich tissues such as muscle. Capacitively coupled applicators emphasize electric field heating, and maximum temperatures tend to occur in water-poor substances such as fat.[91] At clinical energies, subcutaneous fat temperature elevations may be 15°C; 4 to 6°C elevations may occur in muscle at 4-cm to 5-cm depths.[107]

Some short wave diathermy machines are designed to deliver energy in pulses rather than as a continuous wave. Over time, the same amount of energy may be delivered, but heat buildup is limited by dissipation between pulses. Thus temperature elevation is lessened, and bursts of higher electromagnetic intensity can be tolerated, conditions that emphasize nonthermal effects. Although a number of nonthermal phenomena (e.g., pearl chains) exist, there is no strong evidence that they have significant clinical effects.[106]

TECHNIQUE. A SWD machine is essentially a radio transmitter that is tuned in the same way that any transmitter is tuned: a circuit element (a capacitor or inductor) is adjusted to produce an optimal signal. The patient is part of the circuit and is protected from injury by tuning the circuit (often automatically) for maximum coupling before the power is increased. Once tuning is maximized, patient movements can only reduce heating.

A number of SWD applicators have been developed.[91] In a *capacitive* arrangement, the patient is placed between two plate electrodes to complete a circuit (Fig. 13-7). The patient's tissue serves as a dielectric (a resistive substance) and is heated by the actions of the rapidly alternating electric field.

Inductive applicators use a different approach. The patient is coupled into the SWD circuit by the magnetic field of a coil. The drum, cable, and pad applicators are all basically a coil; either arranged by the therapist or preformed and ready to use (as are the drum and pad types). *Cable* applicators are rubber coated, about 2 cm in diameter, and typically a few meters long. Cables are useful because they are flexible and can be shaped into coils which are wrapped around an extremity or laid over the body. Treated areas must be covered with six to eight layers of toweling and, to prevent short circuits, the cable cannot touch itself. Cables are more difficult to use than many applicators and

are becoming less available. *Drum* applicators consist of coils encased in rigid containers. A number of these coils may then be connected by hinges to allow placement around regions such as the shoulder. *Pad* applicators are manufactured, semi-flexible mats containing a coil that are connected to a SWD machine and placed against the patient. Pads may have dimensions of 0.5 by 0.75 meters and typically are used on the low back.

Rectal and *vaginal* applicators heat capacitively and have been used for vigorous pelvic heating. The probes are inserted carefully (the vaginal probe should lie under the cervix in the posterior fornix) and an external pad is used to complete the circuit. Pelvic temperature can be elevated to 5 to 6°C. Although these probes are now rarely used, treatment indications, often in association with antibiotics, include refractory pelvic inflammatory disease, chronic prostatitis,[197] and pelvic floor myalgia. Despite the fact that temperatures of the same magnitude cannot be achieved by other means, patients are often reluctant to use these invasive probes. As a compromise, external applicators on the sacrum and low abdomen may be substituted.

PRECAUTIONS AND CONTRAINDICATIONS. In addition to the general contraindications of heat (see Table 13-2), there are additional limitations due to the nature of SWD itself. Perspiration is conductive and can result in heating on the skin. As a result, six to eight layers of dry toweling, or an equivalent, should be used to absorb moisture as well as to maintain applicator spacing. Metal can distort electromagnetic fields and produce areas of localized heating; treatment should be done on a nonconductive table and the patient should wear no jewelry. Pacemakers, stimulators, surgical implants, contact lenses, metallic intrauterine devices, and the menstruating or pregnant uterus should not be exposed to SWD. Small metallic surgical clips may not be significantly heated, but many clinicians adopt a rule of no metal when prescribing SWD. Given that the effects of diathermy on immature skeletal development are not well known, treatment of growing children should be avoided.

In general, inductive applicators have higher magnetic leakages and capacitive electrodes have higher electrical leakages. In any event, leakages vary widely, but at distances of 50 to 60 cm they are typically less than 10 mW/cm².[91, 179] The American National Standards Institute (ANSI) guidelines[8] are frequency dependent in this portion of the spectrum (Table 13-5); for example, at 27.12 MHz the exposure is about 1 mW/cm². These standards are on a time-averaged basis, and therapists who use

Figure 13-7. Short wave diathermy treatment using a capacitive plate arrangement. The patient wears no jewelry and lies on a nonconductive table.

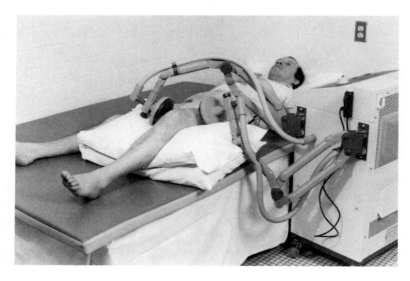

Table 13-5
American National Standards Institute
Guidelines for Radio Frequency Protection

Frequency (MHz)	Intensity (mW/cm²)
0.3–3	100
3–30	$900/(MHz)^2$
30–300	1
300–1500	$(MHz)/300$
1500–100,000	5

SWD intermittently and are rarely close to the equipment would seem to be safely within these limits. Obviously SWD equipment operating instructions should be periodically reviewed.

Microwave

Electromagnetic radiation can be well focused only when the wavelengths of the radiation is comparable to the dimensions of the directing devices. The FCC-approved ISM frequencies for microwaves are 915 and 2456 MHz (wavelengths 33 cm and 12 cm). Reasonable sizes for clinical applicators are between about 15 cm and 30 cm. Thus, microwave frequencies satisfy the wavelength-device requirements, and unlike short waves, can be relatively easily focused.

BIOPHYSICS. Microwaves, in general, do not penetrate tissue as deeply as short wave and ultrasound. Penetration increases at lower frequencies, and deeper heating is reported at 434 MHz than at 915 MHz, and at 915 MHz than at 2450 MHz.[47, 91, 191] Leakage and focusing become more difficult problems with longer wavelengths, and the 434 MHz band has not been allocated for ISM use in the U.S.[91]

Microwave radiation is selectively absorbed by water and should preferentially heat muscle. Fat, however, overlies muscle and absorbs a significant portion of the beam. As an example, at 915 MHz subcutaneous fat temperatures may increase by 10 to 12°C, while 3 to 4 cm deep muscles will be heated only 3 to 4°C.[43]

TECHNIQUE. Microwave diathermy is used primarily to heat relatively superficial muscles and joints. Other uses include speeded resolution of experimental hematomas[110] and local hyperthermia in cancer treatment.[47, 77] Indications for which microwaves would be appropriate are now often treated with superficial heat, SWD, or US.

PRECAUTIONS AND CONTRAINDICATIONS. In addition to the precautions needed for heat in general (see Table 13-2), there may be localized temperature elevations at tissue interfaces. Although newborns have been exposed without complications,[165] the effect of microwaves and heat on bone growth is not well known; treatment of children is best avoided. Because water is selectively heated, treatment over edematous tissue, moist skin, and fluid-filled cavities and blisters can produce unacceptable local heating.[193] Microwaves can produce cataracts,[159] and both patients and therapists should wear protective goggles.

Microwave leakage depends on the applicator, wave mode, shielding, spacing, and a variety of other parameters.[91, 191] Leakage, however, is typically less than 10 mW/cm² at distances 50 to 60 cm from the applicators.[91, 143] According to the ANSI guidelines[8] (see Table 13-5), at 915 MHz a time-averaged exposure of

3 mW/cm² is considered acceptable. At 2450 MHz the guidelines allow 5 mW/cm². Therapists use microwave equipment so intermittently that their exposure in most situations seems acceptable. Obviously, operators should be familiar with the manual of each machine.

Cold (Cryo) Therapy

Cryotherapy, or the use of cold, is restricted to superficial agents which are inexpensive, usually primitive, but effective. Ice and cold water are the usual agents, but vaporizing liquids, refrigerated units, and chemical packs may also be used. Even though treatments are restricted to superficial applications, cold therapy may produce longer-lasting physiological changes than are possible from heat treatments of similar intensities.

BIOPHYSICS. Chilling a limited portion of the body results in a number of local and distant physiological changes. Although there is some controversy,[95] most clinicians feel that there is an initial period of vasoconstriction due to local reflexes and increased sympathetic constrictor tone.[59, 69] Vasoconstriction is thought to continue until subcutaneous temperatures fall to about 15°C. Below 15°C, vessels dilate, probably as a result of contractile mechanism paralysis or blockage of constrictor signals. An oscillating "hunting" pattern of constriction and reactive hyperemia may occur, at least in the digits, as was described by Lewis.[59, 95] At 0°C, skin blood flow may be above normal.[69]

If the cooling agent is ice, skin temperature will initially decrease rapidly and then will more slowly approach an equilibrium temperature of about 12 to 13°C in 10 minutes. Subcutaneous temperatures decline more smoothly and in 10 minutes will fall by 3 to 5°C. Deep muscle temperatures decrease the least, and in 10 minutes may lessen by a degree or less.[106] Chilling for longer periods results in more pronounced effects and intramuscular forearm temperature decreases of 6 to 16°C are reported following periods of 20 minutes to about three hours of vigorous cooling.[1, 71] Vasoconstriction reduces blood flow and the return of cooled tissue to normal temperatures is slower than in heated and hyperemic tissue.

In summary, superficial cold reduces blood flow, decreases metabolic activity, lessens muscle tone, and inhibits spasticity and clonus.[71, 99, 138] Superficial cold also increases gastrointestinal motility,[19] slows nerve conduction, and produces analgesia.[95]

TECHNIQUE. Cryotherapy is used in association with exercise and other therapy approaches. As a result, a lexicon of terms such as *cryokinetics* (cold with exercise) and *cryostretching* (cold with stretching) has developed.

Ice packs, iced compression wraps, and slushes have high heat capacities and cool treated areas rapidly. Treatments tend to be for 20 to 30 minutes. Techniques are straightforward, but if ice packs are used, the skin is often first coated with a thin film of mineral oil and a towel is placed around the pack.

Iced whirlpools cool vigorously and are usually used for 20- to 30-minute periods. Although an athlete may be motivated enough to tolerate them, the average patient finds temperatures below 13 to 15°C uncomfortable. If the feet are exposed to the cold bath, neoprene booties may be used to protect the toes and increase tolerance.

Ice massage consists of rubbing a piece of ice (an ice cube, or water frozen in a small cup) over the painful area. Good analgesia can be obtained in 7 to 10 minutes, and most patients report successive sensations of cold, burning, aching, and numbness. Although chemical and refrigerated agents may have temperatures below 0°C and can produce frostbite, ice treatments for periods of less than 30 to 45 minutes do not seem to cause injury.[71, 98]

Prepackaged chemical ice packs are also available. They may consist of two compartments (*e.g.,* one filled with water, the other with ammonium nitrate), which, when broken and the contents mixed, produce a cooling, endothermic reaction. Although these packs are convenient and pliable, they are small, expensive, and tend to cool poorly.

Cooling can also be produced with evaporative sprays. In the past, ethylene chloride was used, although now less flammable fluoromethanes have been substituted. These sprays produce abrupt temperature changes, but only over a limited area. Currently they are used on a limited basis for "spray and stretch" spasm inhibition[183] and for local skin anesthesia.

INDICATIONS. Trauma. One of the major indications for cryotherapy is acute musculoskeletal trauma. Many studies find that chilling lessens hypoxic damage, limits edema, and reduces compartmental pressures following injury.[18, 142, 166] Although there are reports that cooling does not reduce post-traumatic swelling,[130, 132] ice remains the mainstay of acute soft tissue injury.[98]

Rest, ice, compression, and elevation are the initial steps in treating many musculoskeletal injuries. Ice for 20 minutes per half hour to 30 minutes per 2 hours is, for the first 6 [97, 126] to 24 hours, the common regimen for sprains. If cooling is used, acute sprains, fractures, and other trauma should be cooled and elevated even before initial evaluation is complete.

After the first 48 hours, the choice between cryotherapy and heat therapy is a matter or preference and experience. Some physicians prefer cooling and feel that a combination of icing for 10 to 20 minutes to reduce pain, and active exercising is the most effective way to speed recovery.[96] After the initial period, many physicians will prefer to use heat. Either way, heat and cold are only adjuncts to a progressive mobility and strengthening program.

Chronic Pain. Occasionally patients with chronic musculoskeletal pain will find ice so effective that they will religiously follow a home program. Some research supports these preferences. One study[103] of 117 military patients hospitalized with low back pain showed that a standard exercise program with either hot packs or ice massage produced equally effective results, but there was a nonsignificant tendency for the chronic patients to respond more favorably to the ice regimen. Other investigators have found TENS and ice massage equally effective in patients with chronic low back pain.[134]

Spasticity. After 10 to 20 minutes of vigorous cooling, spastic muscle loses considerable tone[71, 138] and voluntary function may be easier to isolate. As a result, patients with spasticity that limits muscle re-education will often have the involved muscles cooled with ice before therapy.

PRECAUTIONS AND CONTRAINDICATIONS. The major precaution is to avoid tissue damage from too vigorous or prolonged cooling. Pressor responses to cold aggravating cardiovascular disease and the effects of direct and consensual vasoconstriction in ischemic limbs should also be considered. More specific concerns are exacerbation of Raynaud's phenomenon and disease. Cold hypersensitivity and urticaria are conceivably possible but seldom seem to occur during therapy.[71] Because cold reduces local metabolic rates and blood supply, it may also serve to slow wound healing.[126] As is true for all the modalities, risks and benefits of treating an insensate or unresponsive patient must be weighed before beginning treatment.

ULTRAVIOLET THERAPY

Photons in the ultraviolet (UV) spectrum (less than 0.4 microns) are more energetic than those in the visible or infrared regions. Their interaction with tissue can produce nonthermal photochemical reactions, the effects of which form the rationale of UV treatment.

BIOPHYSICS. Although UV is widely used in dermatology and neonatology, its use in physical therapy is now very limited. For this reason the discussion is limited to the facts needed for basic understanding. More detailed information can be found in other sources.[176]

The UV spectrum is arbitrarily divided into a number of portions. In one scheme, the nearest portion extends from the visible spectrum (0.4 microns) to 0.29 microns and is called the *near* UV. The remainder of the spectrum, that is; wavelengths less than 0.29 microns, is then termed the *far* UV. Other classification systems exist, for example, UVA (0.315–0.4 microns), UVB (0.28–0.315 microns), and UVC (0.2–0.28 microns).

"Hot quartz" lamps are now seldom used, and UV therapy is usually given with small, hand-held "cold quartz" lamps. These lamps contain mercury at low pressure in a quartz tube and operate at low temperatures. In distinction to the broad spectrum of the high pressure hot quartz lamps, cold sources produce a narrow band of light at 0.2537 micron.[175] Black light, such as produced by a Wood's lamp, is simply a UV source filtered to eliminate visible radiation.

Dosages are determined by the nature of the tissue treated, UV intensity, source–target separation, and wavelength. It is possible to calculate these parameters and produce a treatment table, but in practice, such calculation is difficult, tedious, and differs for each source. A simpler method has been devised: the time required to produce a minimal erythema is minimal erythemal dose (MED) is determined. Typically a MED is established by exposing small portions of the volar forearm to differing exposure durations. The time that produces a reddening within several hours is defined as 1 MED. Treatment times are then specified in terms of multiples of this number. Although most UV lamps have a MED between 5 and 30 seconds, sources age and it is advisable to determine MED several times a year. (For reference, 2.5 MEDs produce a more pronounced reddening and pain, which persists for a few days; 5 MEDs produce local edema, pain, and desquamation; and 10 MEDs produce blistering.[175])

TECHNIQUE. Once the MED of the device is known, the patient is shielded so that only the area to be treated is exposed, and protective goggles or shields are worn by the therapist and patient. It is important that the treatment distance is the same as that used in the determination of the MED and that a timer is used to limit exposure duration.

INDICATIONS. Currently the major use of UV in physical therapy is the treatment of skin ulcers. UV is highly bacteriocidal to motile bacteria. (Spore-forming bacteria are resistant during the spore stage, but they too are killed when motile.) UV increases vascularization at the margins of wounds and there are a number of reports of UV-accelerated wound healing.[175] A recent animal study, however, found occlusive dressings more effective than UV in healing wounds of superficially wounded pigs.[15]

For fistulas, or mouth wounds, an orofacial probe may be

Table 13-6
Surgical and Obstetric TENS Applications

	Number of Subjects	Experimental Design	Results
General Surgery			
Abdominal surgery[5, 38, 163]	12–50	Randomized, controlled	Up to 77% of patients reported "good or excellent" relief; 50%–67% reported reduction in medication use.
Abdominal and thoracic surgery[78]	213	Randomized	TENS group had less pain, less atelectasis, less ileus, and shorter ICU stays.
Mixed surgery and trauma[156]	20	Uncontrolled; patients with prolonged postoperative and post-traumatic ileus	80% were relieved of protracted ileus within 24 hours.
Orthopedic Surgery			
Total hip replacement[158]	40	Randomized	Reduced medication use in TENS group
Knee surgery[72]	34	Consecutive patients; no controls	Increased ROM; 75%–100% reduction of narcotics
Low back surgery[167]	52	Randomized, controlled	TENS group reduced narcotic consumption 57%.
Podiatric surgery[7]	125	Controlled	TENS groups required fewer narcotics; 74% with TENS noted excellent pain relief compared with 17% of controls.
Obstetrics			
Labor and delivery[10, 162, 173]	35–147	Uncontrolled	78%–88% reported some relief, best relief in first stage; 70% required prudendal or epidural blocks.

used to direct the beam. In general, UV dosages begin with 1 or 2 MED and are kept to less than 5 MED to avoid slowed healing and tissue damage.[175] Success is difficult to evaluate and UV wound treatment is done less frequently than in the past.

PRECAUTIONS AND CONTRAINDICATIONS. Superficial burns and eye exposure are the most likely complications. A person using photosensitizing medication or cosmetics, or who has a fair complexion, scars, or atrophic skin will be overly sensitive to normal dosages. In these individuals, treatment may be deferred, the initial dose reduced, or progression to higher exposures slowed.

TENS

Aristotle, Pliny, and Plutarch all wrote about the ability of electric rays, eels, and catfish to produce numbness.[90] Over the years a bizarre variety of electrical generators have been used with questionable benefit to the patient. Finally this century reliable electrical and electronic equipment has become available, and with it, a new acceptance of electrical analgesia.

Transcutaneous electrical nerve stimulation (TENS) is the most obvious example of electrically based analgesia. Widespread reports of success have ensured acceptance, and TENS, with various degrees of effectiveness, is used to treat a diversity of conditions (Tables 13-6 and 13-7).

BIOPHYSICS. A satisfactory explanation of TENS analgesia does not exist. In 1965 Melzack and Wall[136] published a new theory of pain, the *gate theory*. They stated that afferent nociceptive signals can be blocked at the spinal level before they are transmitted to the brain and perceived as pain.

Table 13-7
Indications for TENS

Acute post-traumatic pain
Post-surgical pain
Post-herpetic neuralgia
Reflex sympathetic dystrophy (RSD)
Childbirth (first stage)
Chronic low back pain
Chronic neck pain
Headache
Post-traumatic spine pain
Osteoarthritis
Rheumatoid arthritis
Brachial plexitis
Diabetic neuropathy
Peripheral nerve injury
Peripheral vascular disease
Raynaud's disease
Phantom limb pain
Postphlebitic syndrome
Dental procedures

The gate theory proposed that cells in the substantia gelatinosa were stimulated by both nociceptive and sensory signals. It was postulated that these cells served as a gate and inhibited the relaying of nociceptive information to the brain if nonpainful sensory afferent signals were also present. Electrical stimulation could provide the sensory afferent signals, and, following some successful trials, TENS became the widely accepted method.

The gate theory, however, did not explain a number of phenomena, such as prolonged analgesia after treatment, distal effects, painless neuropathies, and delayed onset of analgesia. As a result, other theoretical constructs have been advanced, including, for example, that TENS analgesia affects pain perception by altering central nervous system endorphins. Controversy has not prevented TENS use, but has resulted in a large, often arcane, literature.[44, 133, 136, 146]

TECHNIQUE. TENS units are basically simple devices consisting of a power source (often a rechargeable battery), one or more signal generators, and a set of electrodes. Units are small, frequently programmable, and produce a variety of stimuli with currents between 0 and 100 mA, pulse rates between 1 and 200 Hz, and pulse widths from 10 to a few hundred microseconds. Biphasic waveforms are chosen to avoid skin irritation (from electrolysis and iontophoresis associated with unidirectional currents). Asymmetric waves are often favored because they may be the most comfortable.[184] There are numerous manufacturers and a plethora of unproven variations available.

All TENS devices permit adjustment of stimulus intensity (amplitude). Although less expensive units may have fixed frequencies and waveforms, most devices will allow some variation of these parameters. Additional features such as "burst" modes and wave-train modulation may also be available, and in some cases, may be helpful. In all cases, they permit an infinite number of permutations, which are often ignored out of frustration and confusion.

Electrode placement remains more art than science. Frequently, treatment directly over the painful area will be initially evaluated. However, placement over peripheral nerves, acupuncture and trigger points,[135] as well as at locations proximal to, contralateral to, and distal to the pain are also used. Although carbon-impregnated rubber electrodes are inexpensive and sufficient for initial evaluation, many patients find them difficult to keep in place. For these individuals, more expensive self-adhesive electrodes may be more acceptable.

The patient is usually allowed to control the strength of the stimulus. Whether the patient also adjusts the frequency, pulse width, or other parameters will depend on the approach of the clinician as well as the unit's design. In the end, the choice of stimulus parameters and electrodes placement is subjective, and many therapists and physicians prefer to routinely begin with low amplitude–high frequency settings and then try more noxious parameters if the first trial is unsuccessful. It is difficult to predict response[117] and selection is ultimately based on trial and error.

INDICATIONS. Pain is the most common indication for TENS. Success rates vary from lows of about 25% to highs of 80 to 95%[50, 168, 171, 178] and may be affected by the stimulating parameters, electrode placement, conditions treated, chronicity, previous treatment, experimental design, and length of follow-up. TENS evaluations range in quality from well designed prospective, randomized, and controlled studies, to tabulated case reports. Placebo effects (30–35%) are about the same as those found in medication studies.[7, 182] Even when studies are controlled, it is not clear whether the controls should be dummy TENS units or simply a standard treatment.

A number of studies of TENS effectiveness with postoperative and labor pain have been summarized in Table 13-6. As the table shows, pain complaints are reduced about 80% and narcotic usage is lessened. Some studies noted in the table also find TENS use shortens intensive care stays, improves respiratory status, lessens ileus, and improves mobility. It should be noted that about 80% of obstetrical patients experienced reductions of back pain in the first stage of labor. Benefits were less obvious in the second stage, and about 70% of women required additional analgesia.[10, 162, 173]

Most studies of chronic pain find more benefit from TENS than a placebo. Success rates, however, vary widely between 25 and 77%.[50, 58, 80, 94, 102, 121, 129, 182] As the duration of follow-up increases, success rates lessen.[120]

Ebersold and colleagues[50] evaluated the effectiveness of TENS in 155 patients with prolonged post-surgical low back pain, post-traumatic spinal pain, and "mechanical" back pain. Evaluation was carried out at the end of the initial treatment, at 2 months and at 6 months. At the 6-month follow-up, 77% of those with post-surgical back pain, 85% of those with spinal pain, and 65% of those with mechanical back pain reported complete or partial relief of pain. Studies of osteoarthritis, reflex sympathetic dystrophy, peripheral vascular disease, and several scleroderma also show marked benefits, although the studies vary in quality.

Studies have found TENS relieved pain, improved cutaneous perfusion, and increased distal skin temperatures by 6 to 11°C in individuals with scleroderma and diabetic neuropathy. Other interesting observations were that temperature changes were found in untreated limbs, were not blocked by conventional doses of naloxone, persisted after treatment, were larger than those obtained in normal patients,[152] and were more marked in patients who had had sympathectomies. These findings are supplemented by reports of successful TENS use in reflex sympathetic dystrophy.[177]

TENS has also been proposed as a treatment for chronic skin ulcers. Studies of this type are difficult to perform, but one study[82] reported that of 23 patients with chronic ulcers who were treated with low frequency TENS on a three-times-a-day schedule, 20 (87%) healed and thin, atrophic skin gained a more normal appearance.

PRECAUTIONS AND CONTRAINDICATIONS. There are few precautions or contraindications associated with TENS. All patients will report discomfort if the intensity is too high. Skin irritation may occur and can usually be resolved if the electrode positions are shifted or a different conductive gel is used. Occasionally an electrode partially detaches and increases current intensities to uncomfortable levels.

Treatment near the carotid sinus and epiglottis is avoided, as is treatment of individuals with demand pacemakers[53] and dysrhythmias. Caution dictates that at least the low backs, abdomens, and proximal lower extremities of pregnant women should not be treated. Patients with psychogenic pain are frequently unresponsive to TENS,[121] and the use of TENS in these individuals should be judicious. These precautions undoubtedly err on the side of caution. There is, unfortunately, little documentation to support their validity.

IONTOPHORESIS

Iontophoresis is a process in which electrically charged molecules or atoms (ions) are driven into tissue with an electric field. Since electric force is proportional to the voltage, voltage provides the driving force. Iontophoretic currents are a measure of ion flux and therefore of the amount of material moved into the tissues.

BIOPHYSICS. Iontophoresis effectively delivers high concentrations of polar substances into the skin. Although these substances may be found in the systemic circulation following treatment, evidence for penetration much beyond the skin is variable and may depend on the particular substance.[34, 150] Most penetration, in fact, probably occurs at sweat glands and areas of skin breakdown.[74]

TECHNIQUE. Iontophoretic equipment is simple and consists of a direct current power source, two electrodes, and gauze pads moistened with a dilute (often about 1%) solution of the desired substance.[174] The material to be transmitted must be polar, and is placed on a pad under the electrode of the same polarity. Currents used will depend on the area of the active electrode, and may be estimated by multiplying that area by 0.1 to 0.5 mA/cm^2. The size of the inactive electrode is immaterial, but is kept as large as convenient for patient comfort.

INDICATIONS. A wide variety of musculoskeletal conditions have been treated with iontophoresis. The technique, however, is slow and cumbersome and many studies are subjective, inconclusive, and poorly controlled. As a result many physicians are skeptical and feel that most benefits can be obtained more quickly, and more reliably, with an injection.

Iontophoresis is widely used to treat hyperhidrosis of the hands and feet. Although a number of compounds have been used, tap water phoresis is routinely 90% successful. Benefits may persist for months or may be maintained with treatments every 4 to 5 weeks.[74, 157, 169] Treatments may consist of either placing the hand or foot to be treated in a single container with both the anode and cathode, or having one extremity and one electrode in each of two containers. Currents vary with the approach, but are about 10 to 30 mA. The mechanism of action is unclear, but it is felt that the preferential flow of ions along the sweat ducts is significant.

Tooth hypersensitivity is successfully treated with sodium fluoride iontophoresis.[33, 76, 127] Iontophoresis has also been used to introduce antibiotics into avascular tissues such as the eye (gentamycin),[55] burn eschar (penicillin),[67] middle ear (cefoxitin),[153] and ear cartilage (gentamycin).[101] In general, therapeutic concentrations are reported, but the approaches have not been widely adopted.

Case reports and uncontrolled studies report successful treatment of a number of other applications of iontophoresis. Examples include salicylate iontophoresis for persistent postsurgical pain;[62] iodine iontophoresis for reduction of scar tissue and tendon adhesion;[104, 180] acetic acid iontophoresis for resolution of calcium deposits;[87] zinc iontophoresis for the treatment of ischemic ulcers;[39] lidocaine iontophoresis for myringotomies;[116] idoxuridine iontophoresis for treatment of herpes simplex virus and aphthous ulcers.[116] Although there is controversy over the effectiveness of corticosteroid iontophoresis,[34] it has been recommended for a number of conditions including Peyronie's disease,[89] facial pain,[88] and apthous ulcers.[116]

VIBRATION

Vibration is widely used for muscle facilitation and re-education. Although a variety of commercially available vibrators are used, many therapists feel that frequencies in the 150-Hz range and vibration amplitudes of 1.5 mm are the most effective.[20–22] The effects are usually brief, but are often dramatic. At some centers, most patients with upper motor neuron lesions are evaluated for vibrational facilitation at some stage of their rehabilitation.

More recently, a group of investigators has reported roughly 70% success rates in the treatment of acute and chronic musculoskeletal pain and sinusitis.[124, 125] This group also compared the relative effectiveness of TENS, vibration , and aspirin in 60 patients with musculoskeletal pain,[122] and found 80% benefited from at least one of the treatments, with the majority of them feeling that vibration or TENS was at least as effective as aspirin. These experiments were not controlled, but a number a maneuvers were done to assess placebo effects. Best results were found at frequencies between 100 and 200 Hz and with firm contact with the stimulated tissues (perhaps due to improved transmission of the vibratory stimulus to mechanoreceptors and muscle spindles). Pain relief from vibration was not reduced by naloxone.[123]

Another study examined the effect of vibration on wound healing in 120 mice treated with 20 minutes of vibration three times a day over a 6-month period.[105] Compared with wounded animals who did not get vibratory treatment, the treated animals were reported to have significantly less edema, fewer adhesions, and improved lymphatic and venous repair.

LOW ENERGY LASER

Low energy (about 1–50 mW) lasers are promoted as a new, effective way to produce analgesia and accelerate healing. Although they are not approved for these uses in this country, low power laser treatments are done in many countries and are supported by some experimental evidence.

In the United States, treatments typically involve 1- to 5-minute exposures with 1 mW helium neon (HeNe) or gallium aluminum arsenide (GaAlAs) lasers. These energies are too small to elevate tissue temperatures more than 0.1°C. Nevertheless, low energy lasers are reported to stimulate collagen production, alter DNA synthesis, accelerate wound healing, and improve function of damaged nerve tissue.[14] Although studies frequently find wound healing speeded in rabbits and rodents, the changes often occur primarily in the early stages of healing. Healing benefits are more difficult to find in other animals such as pigs and humans.[14, 15] Some studies of osteoarthritis, back pain, headache, and neuropathy find good to excellent local and systemic pain relief in 60 to 80% of the subjects. Other studies, however, find no benefit.[14]

At present there is no accepted mechanism to explain the effects of low energy lasers. In addition the energies, wavelengths, and treatment approaches have not been established. Until theoretical and clinical questions have been addressed, the value of laser treatment will remain unclear. In view of the number of positive reports and the innocuous nature of treatments, further evaluation should be done.

BIOFEEDBACK

Biofeedback (BFB) is a therapeutic approach that uses nonphysiological feedback to facilitate control of physiological processes. The approach does not specify the processes or the conditions to be treated, but some neurological or hormonal pathway must exist. Processes treated may be either volitional or nominally nonvolitional activities, such as gastrointestinal motility, cardiac rhythm, seizure thresholds, blood pressure, and skin temperature. Frequently the distinction is not clear, since, for example, volitional striated muscle contractions can become habitual and unnoticed (*e.g.,* tension myalgia).

BFB of some form is used in almost all therapy: that is, the therapist tells the patient how well the task was done, the patient incorporates the information and attempts to perform more effectively in the next trial. About 25 years ago electronic equipment became simple and small enough that additional feedback approaches became practical. Today a multitude of conditions (Table 13-8) are treated with a variety of electronic and nonelectronic devices (Table 13-9).

Table 13-8
Reported Indications for Biofeedback

Headache (tension and vascular)
Tension myalgia
Urinary incontinence and retention
Fecal incontinence and retention
Insomnia
Relaxation
Dystonia
Anxiety
Muscle re-education following brain, spine, nerve or muscle damage
Shoulder subluxation
Joint contracture with co-contraction
Head control
Raynaud's disease and phenomenon
Gait training
Seizure control
Cardiac dysrhythmia
Elevated intraocular pressure
Hypertension
Orthostatic hypotension
Functional bowel syndrome
Bruxism
Hyperventilation

Table 13-9
Biofeedback Approaches

Electromyography (EMG)
Electroencephalography (EEG)
Electrocardiography (ECG)
Blood pressure
Ventilatory
Skin temperature
Pressure
Goniometry
Skin conductivity

In this section the emphasis will be on the use of biofeedback in physical medicine. Many other applications have been extensively reviewed.[9, 16, 28]

BIOPHYSICS. Specifics of treatment vary with the situation. In general, a signal (*e.g.,* muscle activity) that is normally not perceived by the subject is recorded, amplified, and presented in a responsive and easily detected manner. Feedback is usually audible or visible, but pressure, temperature, position, and other presentations are possible.

Once it is established that a patient can produce at least a minimal amount of the necessary response, training can begin. Approaches differ, but essentially the patient is given a task (*e.g.,* finger temperature elevation) and allowed to find ways to vary the characteristic. Initially minimal goals are set and control is gained by chance, or by nonspecific processes such as emotions and mental imagery. Once the patient is able to produce consistent responses, goals are increased by small increments (*e.g.,* successive small temperature increases). As the patient is able to isolate the change gained, control becomes more specific. If the individual is able to sense the change, the activity itself may provide its own feedback, allowing the feedback device to be omitted altogether.

Duration of treatment benefits is variable and some report that, for example, chronic tension and vascular headache sufferers maintain improvements of 65 to 80% 4 years after treatment.[24] Numerous studies of biofeedback and relaxation approaches to hypertension have been reported.[52] Many of the short-term studies are poorly controlled and report results that may be present at longer term follow-up, but are more difficult to verify.[52, 145] In some cases patients can maintain improvements with little effort; in other situations practice must continue indefinitely if gains are to be maintained.[25, 118]

BFB training requires a motivated subject and a trained therapist, and is often combined with other treatments. Thus it is not surprising that it is difficult to isolate BFB effectiveness. For example, the reduction of headache frequency and medication usage often reported by tension headache patients could be the result of specific BFB effects, or could be due to general relaxation and improved understanding. Evidence supports both views and some experiments find relaxation and autogenic training results comparable with those of BFB.[23, 145, 151] However, experiments with animals, intact humans, and spinal cord injured often find isolated effects without other changes (*e.g.,* blood pressure changes without heart rate changes or increased muscle tension).[28, 140, 151]

It is obvious that the intense efforts involved, physician and therapist expectations, and emphasis on a patient's problem can produce improvements which may not be due to BFB. A further complication in evaluation is the difficulty in designing a blinded study in which neither the patient nor the therapist is able to detect the control. Even in the well-controlled studies, comparison is frequently with no treatment or another behavioral treatment and not with standard medical practice. Nevertheless, biofeedback does help in some situations. The lack of a compelling mechanism(s) limits understanding, but the techniques continue to be used.

INDICATIONS. BFB indications as listed earlier are varied: muscle re-education, relaxation, spasticity, head position, fecal[189] and urinary incontinence, headache, myopia, elevated intraocular pressure,[164] blood pressure, heart rhythm, and seizure control.[151] EMG biofeedback, in particular, is widely used and has some of the broadest and oldest literature. Nevertheless, even in this area, validation is difficult and many studies have flaws that prevent acceptance.

In physical medicine emphasis is on muscle re-education, tension myalgia, relaxation training, digital warming, and bowel and bladder retraining. Although many treatment approaches are possible, only a few will be emphasized here.

Tension Headaches. EMG BFB is widely used to treat tension headaches. Numerous studies dating from the early 1970s show 50 to 80% reductions in headache severity and frequency over several months to 3-year periods.[56, 151] Treatments typically involve several weeks, emphasize frontalis muscle biofeedback, and require home practice. When relaxation and biofeedback are directly compared, improvements are frequently comparable.[16, 28, 31, 42, 56, 100, 151] Whether a common mechanism underlies the two approaches is unknown, but interestingly patients who respond to one approach may be resistant to the other.[151]

Vascular Headaches. EMG biofeedback is not generally felt to be as successful for vascular as for tension headaches. Emphasis, therefore, has been on vascular training with digital warming and blood volume feedback techniques, and improvements of 40 to 80% have been reported.[63, 75, 93, 151] Vascular head-aches are associated with stress; the effects of relaxation as well as the possibility of some control over the headaches influence results.[42, 151]

Tension Myalgia. Tension myalgia, whether in the neck, upper back, jaw, pelvic floor, or elsewhere, is frequently treated with EMG biofeedback programs involving a combination of exercise, posture, and relaxation. Frontalis muscles are often treated, but nuchal, perineal, and shoulder girdle muscles may also be used. As is true for headache sufferers, these patients often improve, but the biofeedback benefits are obscured by the other interventions.[23, 24, 41, 42, 151]

Muscle Re-education. EMG biofeedback for muscle re-education is one of the most developed areas of feedback. Common indications include stroke, head injury, spinal injury, cerebral palsy, peripheral nerve injury, and muscle transfer surgery.[16, 17, 28, 79] Although treated separately, tension myalgia BFB is also essentially muscle re-education.

Treatment often emphasizes multichannel feedback with both visible and aural signals. Often treatment will begin with electromyographic isolation of impaired, but innervated muscle. Following isolation, motor unit recruitment is emphasized with BFB drilling. Further training, and perhaps electrical stimulation, are then used to strengthen and improve control of the involved muscles.

Treatments are intense and may last for 1 to 3 months or more. If progress is to be made, stroke and head-injured patients should exhibit some volitional control within three or four sessions.[28] Once observable movement is possible, the patient is able to begin exercises without augmented BFB, and training may be advanced to different muscle groups. As is true for biofeedback training in general, the staff must be well trained and have a thorough understanding of the pathophysiology involved.

Orthostatic Hypotension. Remarkable success with the treatment of disabling orthostatic hypotension in spinal cord-injured individuals has been reported.[28, 29] This approach uses visible and audible blood pressure feedback information. The patient initially uses imagery and trial and error to find an approach to increase pressure. Once an approach is found, the patient perfects control. Elevations of 40 to 60 mm Hg are obtainable. The effects are thought to be due to increased peripheral resistance, since changes in heart rate and muscle activity do not occur.[28, 29]

Interestingly orthostatic hypotension is usually initially treated with progressive tilt-table elevation. It is possible that the tilt table itself serves as an adversive BFB device and uses the effects of falling blood pressure as feedback. Electronically augmented feedback, then, is merely a more sophisticated feedback regimen reserved for refractory cases.

Raynaud's Disease and Phenomenon. Raynaud's disease, as well as a variety of collagen vascular diseases, including systemic lupus erythematosus (SLE) and progressive systemic sclerosis (PSS), are reported to respond to digital warming and vascular feedback techniques. Dramatic temperature increases of 5 to 11°C are routinely reported.[190, 196] Clinical benefits are more difficult to establish; although 44 to 57% reductions in pain and skin ulcers are reported,[196] other studies find no benefit.[60] Treatment courses often require several months, and benefits gained are largely lost if there is no home program.

Urinary Incontinence and Retention. Stress incontinence, functional urinary retention, and neurogenic bladder dysfunction (due to spinal injury or stroke and head injury) may be treated with biofeedback programs.[128] With the occasional exception of stress incontinence, urological status should be evaluated with renal studies, cystoscopy, and a cystometrogram before a program is begun. Once these results are available, a program is designed to fit the individual patient.

Stress incontinence training at times requires only instructions in a fluid schedule and pelvic floor exercises. However, bladder pressure and pelvic floor feedback may also be needed. In this latter situation, EMG feedback may be obtained from superficial perineal electrodes or from dumbell-shaped anal "plug" electrodes. Pressure data can be recorded with a variety of pelvic and bladder transducers.

Neurogenic and functional urinary retention are difficult to evaluate and treat. Urological evaluation is required to document the status of the urinary system, diagnose the dysfunction, and to delineate the treatment approach. Documentation of a baseline is particularly important if reflux, stones, and high bladder pressure damage are to be avoided. Treatment usually requires concurrent monitoring of bladder pressure, pelvic floor activity, and intra-abdominal pressure (usually inferred from a rectal balloon) with a multichannel cystometrogram–EMG (CMG–EMG) machine.

The emphasis of therapy is on educating the patient to increase bladder pressure, while simultaneously reducing pelvic floor activity and minimizing intra-abdominal pressure. Frequently used maneuvers include tapping to trigger detrusor contractions, crede (pressure), strain, and relaxation.

Medications such as bethanechol, baclofen and oxybutynin may be helpful adjuncts in bladder management. In these cases, effectiveness can be monitored and dosages titrated with serial examinations. The overall success rate neurogenic bladder training programs is 70%.

REFERENCES

1. Abramson DI, Chu LSW, Tuck S Jr et al: Effect of tissue temperature and blood flow on motor nerve conduction velocity. JAMA 198:1082–1088, 1966
2. Abramson DI, Tuck S, Chu LSW, Agustin C: Effect of paraffin bath and hot fomentations on local tissue temperatures. Arch Phys Med Rehab 45:97–94, 1964
3. Alcorn R, Dowser B, Henley EJ, Holloway V: Fluidotherapy and exercise in the management of sickle cell anemia. Phys Ther 64:1520–1522, 1984
4. Aldes JH, Jadeson WJ; Ultrasonic therapy in the treatment of hypertrophic arthritis in elderly patients. Ann West Med Surg 6:545–550, 1952
5. Ali J, Yaffe CS, Serratte C: The effect of transcutaneous electric nerve stimulation on postoperative pain and pulmonary function. Surgery 89:507–512, 1981
6. Allen KGR, Battye CK: Performance of ultrasonic therapy instruments. Physiotherapy 64:174–179, 1978
7. Alm WA, Gold ML, Weil LS: Evaluation of transcutaneous electrical nerve stimulation (TENS) in podiatric surgery. J Am Podiatry Assoc 69:537–542, 1979
8. American National Standards Institute, Inc: Safety Levels with Respect to Human Exposure to Radio Frequency Electromagnetic Fields, 300 kHz to 100 GHz, 1982
9. American Psychiatric Association: Introduction in Biofeedback, p 111. American Psychiatric Association Task Force on Biofeedback. Washington, DC, 1979
10. Augustinsson LE, Bohlin P, Bundsen P et al: Pain relief during delivery by transcutaneous electrical nerve stimulation. Pain 4:59–65, 1977

11. Babbs CF: Biology of local heat therapy for cancer. Med Instrum 16:23–26, 1982

12. Babbs CF, DeWitt DP: Physical principles of local heat therapy for cancer. Med Instrum 15:367–373, 1981

13. Balmaseda MT, Fatehi MT, Koozekanani SH, Lee AL: Ultrasound therapy: A comparative study of different coupling media. Arch Phys Med Rehabil 67:149–152, 1986

14. Basford JR: Low energy laser treatment of pain and wounds: Hype, hope or hokum? Mayo Clin Proc, August 1986

15. Basford JR, Hallman HO, Sheffield CG, Mackey GL: Comparison of cold quartz ultraviolet, low-energy laser, and occlusion in wound healing in a swine model. Arch Phys Med Rehabil 67:151–154, 1986

16. Basmajian JV: Introduction: Principles and Background in Biofeedback—Principles and Practice for Clinicians. Baltimore, Williams & Wilkins, 1979

17. Basmajian JV, Gowland C, Brandstater ME et al: EMG feedback treatment of upper limb in hemiplegic stroke patients: A pilot study. Arch Phys Med Rehabil 63:613–616, 1982

18. Basur RL, Shephard E, Mouzas GL: A cooling method in the treatment of ankle sprains. Practitioner 216:708–711, 1976

19. Bisgard JD, Nye D: The influence of hot and cold application upon gastric and intestinal motor activity. Surg Gynecol Obstet 71:172–180, 1940

20. Bishop B: Vibratory stimulation. Part I. Neurophysiology of motor responses evoked by vibratory stimulation. Phys Ther 54:1273–1282, 1974

21. Bishop B: Vibratory stimulation. Part II. Vibratory stimulation as an evaluation tool. Phys Ther 55:28–34, 1975

22. Bishop B: Vibratory stimulation. Part III. Possible applications of vibration in treatment of motor dysfunctions. Phys Ther 55:139–143, 1975

23. Blanchard EB, Andrasik F, Nef DG et al: Biofeedback and relaxation training with three kinds of headache: Treatment effects and their prediction. J Consult Clin Psych 50:562–575, 1982

24. Blanchard EB, Guarnieri PC, Andrasik F, Neff DF: Two, three and four year prospective follow-up of the behavioral treatment of chronic headache. In Self-Regulation and Health, pp 15–18. Biofeedback Society of America Seventeenth Annual Meeting, March 21–26, 1986

25. Blanchard EB, McCoy GC, Musso A et al: A controlled comparison of thermal biofeedback and relaxation training in the treatment of essential hypertension: Short term and long term outcome. In Self-Regulation and Health, pp 19–22. Biofeedback Society of America Seventeenth Annual Meeting, March 21–26, 1986

26. Borrell RM, Parker R, Henley EJ et al: Comparison of in vivo temperatures produced by hydrotherapy, paraffin wax treatment and fluidotherapy. Phys Ther 60:1273–1276, 1980

27. Braatz JH, McAlistar BR, Broaddus MD: Ultrasound and plantar warts: A double blind study. Milit Med 139:199–201, 1974

28. Brucker BS: Biofeedback. In Rehabilitation in Current Topics in Rehabilitation Psychology. pp 173–199. New York, Grune & Statton, 1984

29. Brucker BS, Ince LP: Biofeedback as an experimental treatment for postural hypotension in a patient with a spinal cord lesion. Arch Phys Med Rehabil 58:49–53, 1977

30. Brunner GD, Lehmann JF, McMillan JA et al: Can ultrasound be used in the presence of surgical metal implants: An experimental approach. Phys Ther 38:823–824, 1958

31. Budzynski TH: Biofeedback strategies in headache treatment. In Biofeedback—Principles and Practice for Clinicians, p 132. Baltimore, Williams & Wilkins, 1979

32. Cameroy BM: Ultrasound enhanced local anesthesia. Am J Orthop 8:47, 1966

33. Carlo GT, Ciancio SG, Seyrek SK: An evaluation of iontophoretic application of fluoride for tooth desensitization. JADA 105:452–454, 1982

34. Chantraine A, Ludy JP, Berger D: Is cortisone iontophoresis possible? Arch Phys Med Rehabil 67:38–40, 1986

35. Cherup N, Urben J, Bender LF: The treatment of plantar warts with ultrasound. Arch Phys Med Rehabil 44:602–604, 1963

36. Coakley WT: Biophysical effects of ultrasound at therapeuatic intensities. Physiotherapy 64:166–169, 1978

37. Coodley EL: Bursitis and post-traumatic lesions: Management with combined use of ultrasound and intra-articular hydrocortisone. Am Practit 11:181–188, 1960

38. Cooperman AM, Hall B, Mikalacki et al: Use of transcutaneous electrical stimulation in the control of postoperative pain. Results of a prospective, randomized, controlled study. Am J Surg 133:185–187, 1977

39. Cornwall MW: Zinc iontophoresis to treat ischemic skin ulcers. Phys Ther 61:359–360, 1981

40. Currier DP, Greathouse D, Swift T: Sensory nerve conduction: Effect of ultrasound. Arch Phys Med Rehabil 59:181–185, 1978

41. Dahlstrom L, Carlsson SG, Gale EN, Jansson TG: Clinical and electromyographic effects of biofeedback training in mandibular dysfunction. Biofeedback Self Regul 9:37–47, 1984

42. Daly EJ, Donn PA, Galliher MJ, Zimmerman JS: Biofeedback applications to migraine and tension headaches: A double-blinded outcome study. Biofeedback Self Regul 8:135–152, 1983

43. DeLateur BJ, Lehmann JF, Stonebridge JB et al: Muscle heating in human subjects with 915 MHz. Microwave contact applicator. Arch Phys Med Rehabil 51:147–151, 1970

44. Dennis SG, Melzack R: Pain-signalling systems in the dorsal and ventral spinal cord. Pain 4:97–132, 1977

45. Downing DS, Weinstein A: Ultrasound therapy of subacromial bursitis. A double blind trial. Phys Ther 66:194–199, 1986

46. Dussick CT, Fritch DJ, Kyraizidan M, Sear RS: Measurement of articular tissues with ultrasound. Am J Phys Med 37:160–165, 1958

47. Dutreix J, Cosset JM, Salama et al: Experimental studies of various heating procedures for clinical application of localized hyper thermia. Biomed Thermology: 585–596, 1982

48. Dyson M: Non-thermal cellular effects of ultrasound. Br J Cancer 45:165–171, 1982

49. Dyson M, Pond JB, Woodward B, Broadbent J: The production of blood cell stasis and endothelial damage in the blood vessels of chick embryos treated with ultrasound in a stationary wave field. Ultrasound Med Biol 1:133–148, 1974

50. Ebersold MJ, Laws ER, Stonnington HH, Stillwell GK: Transcutaneous electrical stimulation for treatment of chronic pain: A preliminary report. Surg Neurol 4:96–99, 1975

51. Echternach JL: Ultrasound. An adjunct treatment for shoulder disabilities. Phys Ther 45:865–869, 1965

52. Eisenberg SE: Biofeedback-aided relaxation for mild hypertension with special attention to the therapist-client relationship. In Self-Regulation and Health, pp 15–18. Biofeedback Society of America Seventeenth Annual Meeting, March 21–26, 1986

53. Eriksson M, Schuller H, Sjolund B: Hazard from transcutaneous nerve stimulation in patients with pacemakers. Lancet 1:1319, 1978

54. Farmer WC: Effect of intensity of ultrasound on conduction of motor axons. Phys Ther 48:1233–1237, 1968

55. Fishman PH, Jay WM, Rissing JP et al: Iontophoresis of gentamicin into aphakic rabbit eyes. Sustained vitreal levels. Invest Opthalmol Vis Sci 25:343–345, 1984

56. Ford MR: Biofeedback treatment for headaches, Raynaud's disease, essential hypertension and irritable bowel syndrome: A review of the long term followup literature. Biofeedback Self Regul 7:521–536, 1982

57. Foulkes J, Yeo B: The application of therapeutic pulsed ultrasound to the traumatised perineum. Br J Clin Prac 34:114–117, 1980

58. Fox EJ, Melack R: Transcutaneous electrical stimulation and acupuncture: Comparison of treatment for low-back pain. Pain 2:141–148, 1976

59. Franchimont P, Juchmes J, Lecomite J: Hydrotherapy—Mechanisms and indications. Pharmacol Ther 20:79–93, 1983

60. Freedman RR, Ianni P, Wenig P: Behavioral treatment of Raynaud's phenomenon in scleroderma. J Behav Med 7:343–353, 1984

61. Garrett AS, Garrett M: Ultrasound therapy for herpes zoster pain. J Coll Gen Prac, 32:709, 711, 1982

62. Garzione JE: Salicylate iontophoresis as an alternative treatment for persistent thigh pain following hip surgery. Phys Ther 58:570–571, 1978

63. Gautheir J, Doyon J, Lacroix, Drolet M: Blood volume pulse biofeedback in the treatment of migraine headache: A controlled evaluation. Biofeedback Self Regul 8:427–442, 1983

64. Gersten JW: Effect of metallic objects on temperature rises produced in tissue by ultrasound. Am J Phys Med 37:75–82, 1958

65. Gersten JW: Non-thermal neuromuscular effects of ultrasound. Am J Phys Med 37:235–237, 1958

66. Goldman DE, Heuter TF: Tabular data of the velocity and absorption of high-frequency sound in mammalian tissues. J Acoust Soc Am 28:35–37, 1956

67. Greminger RF, Elliott RA, Rapperport A: Antibiotic iontophoresis for the management of burned ear chondritis. Plast Reconstr Surg 66:356–360, 1980

68. Griffin JE, Touchstone JC, Liu A: Ultrasonic movement of cortisol into pig tissue. II. Movement into paravertebral nerve. Am J Phys Med 44:20–25, 1965

69. Guyton AC: Muscle blood flow during exercise; Cerebral, splanchnic, and skin blood flows. In Textbook of Medical Physiology, 7th ed. pp 336–346. Philadelphia, WB Saunders, 1986

70. Harris ED, McCroskery PA: The influence of temperature and fibril stability on degradation of cartilage collagen by rheumatoid synovial collagenase. N Engl J Med 290:1–6, 1974

71. Hartviksen K: Ice therapy in spasticity. Acta Neurol Scand 38:79–84, 1962

72. Harvie KW: A major advance in the control of postoperative knee pain. Orthopedics 2:26–27, 1979

73. Helfand AE, Bruno J: Therapeutic modalities and procedures. Part 1. Cold and heat. Clin Podiatry 1:301–313, 1984

74. Hill AC, Baker GF, Jansen GT: Mechanisms of actin of iontophoresis in the treatment of palmar hyperhidrosis. Cutis 28:69–70, 72, 1981

75. Hoelscher TJ, Lichstein KL: Blood volume pulse biofeedback treatment of chronic cluster headache. Biofeedback Self Regul 8:553–541, 1983

76. Holman DJ: Desensitization of dentin by iontophoresis: A review. Gen Dent 30:481–483, 1982

77. Hunt JW: Applications of microwave, ultrasound and radio-frequency heating. Natl Cancer Inst Monogr 61:447–456, 1982

78. Hymes AC, Yonehiro EG, Raab DE et al: Electrical surface stimulation for treatment and prevention of ileus and atelectasis. Surg Forum 25:222–224, 1974

79. Ince LP, Leon MA, Christidia D: Experimental foundations of EMG biofeedback with the upper extremity: A review of the literature. Biofeedback Self Regul 9:371–383, 1984

80. Indeck W, Printy A: Skin application of electrical impulses for relief of pain in chronic orthopaedic conditions. Minn Med 58:305–309, 1975

81. Jones RJ: Treatment of acute herpes zoster using ultrasonic therapy. Report on a series of twelve patients. Physiotherapy 70:94–95, 1975

82. Kaada B: Vasodilation induced by transcutaneoud nerve stimulation in peripheral ischemia (Raynaud's phenomenon and diabetic polyneuropathy) Eur Heart J 3:303–341, 1982

83. Kaada B: Promoted healing of chronic ulceration by transcutaneous nerve stimulation (TNS). VASA 12:262–269, 1983

84. Kaada B, Eielsen O: In search of mediators of skin vasodilation induced by transcutaneous nerve stimulation: I. Failure to block the response by antagonists of endogenous vasodilators. Gen Pharmacol 14:623–633, 1983

85. Kaada B, Eielsen O: In search of mediators of skin vasodilation induced by transcutaneous nerve stimulation: II. Serotonin implicated. Gen Pharmacol 14:635–641, 1983

86. Kaada B, Helle KB: In search of mediators of skin vasodilation induced by transcutaneous nerve stimulation: IV. In vitro bioassay of the vasoinhibitory activity of sera from patients suffering from peripheral ischaemia. Gen Pharmacol 15:115–122, 1984

87. Kahn J: Acetic acid iontophoresis for calcium deposits. Phys Ther 57:658–659, 1977

88. Kahn J: Iontophoresis and ultrasound for post-surgical temporomandibular trismus and paresthesia. Phys Ther 60:307–308, 1980

89. Kahn J: Use of iontophoresis in Peyronie's disease. A case report. Phys Ther 62:995–996, 1982

90. Kane K, Taub A: A history of local electrical analgesia. Pain 1:125–128, 1975

91. Kantor G: Evaluation and survey of microwave and radiofrequency applicators. J Microwave Power 16:135–150, 1981

92. Kendell HW: Fever therapy. In American Medical Association: Handbook of Physical Medicine and Rehabilitation, 1st ed, pp 45–72. Philadelphia, Blakiston, 1950

93. Kewman D, Roberts AH: Skin temperature biofeedback and migraine headaches. A double-blinded study. Biofeedback Self Regul 5:327–345, 1980

94. Kirsch WM, Lewis JA, Simon RH: Experiences with electrical stimulation devices for the control of chronic pain. Med Instrum 9:217–220, 1975

95. Knight KL: Circulatory effects of therapeutic cold applications. In Cryotherapy: Theory, Technique and Physiology, 1st ed, pp 83–100. Chattanooga, Chattanooga Corporation, 1985

96. Knight KL: Cryokinetics in rehabilitation of joint spasms. In Cryotherapy: Theory, Technique and Physiology, 1st ed, p 55. Chattanooga, Chattanooga Corporation, 1985

97. Knight KL: Ice, compression and elevation for initial injury care. In Cryotherapy: Theory, Technique and Physiology, 1st ed, pp 53–54. Chattanooga, Chattanooga Corporation, 1985

98. Knight KL: Ice, compression and elevation in the immediate care of acute traumatic injuries. In Knight: Cryotherapy: Theory, Technique and Physiology, 1st ed, pp 15–26. Chattanooga, Chattanooga Corporation, 1985

99. Knutsson E, Mattsson E: Effects of local cooling on monosynaptic reflexes in man. Scand J Rehab Med 1:126–132, 1969

100. Lacroix JM, Clarke MA, Bock JC, Doxey NCS: Muscle-contraction headaches in multiple-pain patients: Treatment under worsening baseline conditions. Arch Phys Med Rehabili 67:14–18, 1986

101. LaForest NT, Cofrancesco C: Antibiotic iontophoresis in the treatment of ear chondritis. Phys Ther 58:32–34, 1978

102. Laitinen L: Placement des electrodes dans la stimulation transcutanee de la douleur chronique. Neurochirurgie 22:517–526, 1976

103. Landon BR: Heat or cold for the relief of low back pain. Phys Ther 47:1126–1128, 1967

104. Langley PL: Iontophoresis to aid in releasing tendon adhesions. Suggestions from the field. Phys Ther 64:1395, 1984

105. Leduc A, Lievens P, Dewald J: The influence of multidirectional vibrations on wound healing and on regeneration of blood and lymph vessels. Lymphology 14:179–185, 1981

106. Lehmann JF, deLateur BJ: Diathermy and superficial heat and cold therapy. In Krusen's Handbook of Physical Medicine and Rehabilitation, 3rd ed, pp 275–350. Philadelphia, WB Saunders, 1982

107. Lehmann JF, deLateur BJ, Stonebridge JB: Selective heating by shortwave diathermy with a helical coil. Arch Phys Med Rehabil 50:117–123, 1969

108. Lehmann JF, deLateur BJ, Stonebridge JB, Warren CG: Therapeutic temperature distribution produced by ultrasound as modified by dosage and volume of tissue exposed. Arch Phys Med Rehabil 48:662–666, 1967

109. Lehmann JF, deLateur BJ, Warren CG, Stonebridge JB: Heating of joint structures by ultrasound. Arch Phys Med Rehabil 49:28–30, 1968

110. Lehmann JF, Dundore DE, Esselman PC: Microwave diathermy: Effects on experimental muscle hematoma resolution. Arch Phys Med Rehabil 64:127–129, 1983

111. Lehmann JF, Erickson DJ, Martin GM, Krusen FH: Comparison of ultrasonic and microwave diathermy in the physical treatment of periarthritis of the shoulder. Arch Phys Med Rehabil 35:627–634, 1954

112. Lehmann JF, Fordyce WE, Rathbun LA et al: Clinical evaluation of a new approach in the treatment of contracture associated with hip fracture after internal fixation. Arch Phys Med Rehabil 42:95, 1961

113. Lehmann JF, Masock AJ, Warren CG, Koblanski JN: Effect of therapeutic temperatures on tendon extensibility. Arch Phys Med Rehabil 51:481–487, 1970

114. Lehmann JF, McMillan JA, Brunner GD, Blumberg JB: Comparative study of the efficiency of short-wave, microwave and ultrasonic diathermy in heating the hip joint. Arch Phys Med Rehabil 40:510–512, 1959

115. Lehmann JF, Silverman DR, Baum BR et al: Temperature distributions in the human thigh, produced by infrared, hot pack and microwave applications. Arch Phys Med Rehabil 47:291–299, 1966

116. Lekas MD: Iontophoresis treatment. Otolaryngol Head Neck Surg 87:292–298, 1979

117. Leo KC, Dostal WF, Bossen DG et al: Effect of transcutaneous electrical nerve stimulation characteristics on clinical pain. Phys Ther 66:200–205, 1986

118. Libo LM, Arnold GE: Relaxation practice after biofeedback therapy: A long term followup study of utilization and effectiveness. Biofeedback Self Regul 8:217–227, 1983

119. Licht S: Medical Hydrology. Baltimore, Waverly Press, 1963

120. Loeser JD, Black RG, Christman A: Relief of pain by transcutaneous stimulation. J Neurosurg 42:308–314, 1975

121. Long DM, Hagfors N: Electrical stimulation in the nervous system: The current status of electrical stimulation of the nervous system for relief of pain. Pain 1:109–123, 1975

122. Lundeberg T: The pain suppressive effect of vibratory stimulation and transcutaneous electrical nerve stimulation (TENS) as compared to aspirin. Brain Res 294:201–209, 1984

123. Lundeburg T: Naloxone does not reverse the pain-reducing effect of vibratory stimulation. Acta Anaesthesiol Scand 29:212–216, 1985

124. Lundeberg T, Ekblom A, Hannsson P: Relief of sinus pain by vibratory stimulation. Ear Nose Throat J 64:163–167, 1985

125. Lundeberg T, Nodemar R, Ottoson D: Pain alleviation by vibratory stimulation. Pain 20:25–44, 1984

126. Lundgren C, Muren A, Zederfeldt B: Effect of cold-vasoconstriction on wound healing in the rabbit. Acta Chir Scand 118:1–4, 1959

127. Lutins ND, Grecot GW, McFall WT: Effectiveness of sodium fluoride on tooth hypersensitivity with and without iontophoresis. J Peridontol 55:285–288, 1984

128. Maizels M, King LR, Firlit CF: Urodynamic biofeedback: A new approach to treat vesical sphincter dyssynergia. J Urol 122:205–209, 1979

129. Mannheimer C, Lund S, Carlsson CA: The effect of transcutaneous electrical nerve stimulation (TENS) on joint pain in patients with rheumatoid arthritis. Scand J Rheum 7:13–16, 1978

130. Marek J, Jezdinsky J, Ochonsky P: Effects of local cold and heat therapy. Acta Univ Palacki Olomuc Fac Med 66:203–228, 1973

131. Markham DE, Wood MR: Ultrasound for Dupuytren's contracture. Physiotherapy 66:55–58, 1980

132. Matsen FA, Questad K, Matsen AL: The effect of local cooling on postfracture swelling. A controlled study. Clin Orthop 109:201–206, 1975

133. Melzack R: Prolonged relief of pain by brief, intense transcutaneous somatic stimulation. Pain 1:357–373, 1975

134. Melzack R, Jeans ME, Stratford JG, Monks RC: Ice massage and transcutaneous electrical stimulation: Comparison of treatment for low back pain. Pain 9:209–217, 1980

135. Melzack R, Stillwell DM, Fox EJ: Trigger points and acupuncture points for pain: Correlations and implications. Pain 3:3–23, 1977

136. Melzack R, Wall PD: Pain mechanisms: A new theory. Science 150:971–979, 1965

137. Middlemost S, Chatterjee DS: Comparison of ultrasound and thermotherapy for soft tissue injuries. Physiotherapy 64:331–332, 1978

138. Miglietta O: Action of cold on spasticity. Am J Phys Med 52:198–205, 1973

139. Miller DL, Nyborg WL: Platelet aggregation induced by ultrasound under specialized conditions in vitro. Science 205:505–507, 1979

140. Miller NE: A learned visceral response apparently independent of skeletal ones in patients paralyzed by spinal lesions. In Birbaumer N, Kimmel HD (eds): Biofeedback and Self Regulation, pp 287–304. Hillside, NJ; Lawrence Erlbaum Associates, 1979

141. Moll MJ: A new approach to pain: Lidocaine and decadron with ultrasound. USAF Med Serv Dig 30(3):8–11, 1979

142. Moore CD, Cardea JA: Vascular changes in leg trauma. South Med J 70:1285–1286, 1977

143. Moseley H, Davison M: Exposure of physiotherapists to microwave radiation during microwave diathermy treatment. Clin Phys Physiol Meas 2:217–221, 1981

144. Mune O, Thoseth K: Ultrasonic treatment of subcutaneous infiltrations after injections. Acta Orthop Scand 33:347–349, 1963

145. Murdock B and Crider A: Progressive relaxation and autogenic training as adjunctive treatments in essential hypertension. In Self-Regulation and Health, pp 113–116. Biofeedback Society of America Seventeenth Annual Meeting, March 21–26, 1986

146. Nathan PW: The gate-control of theory of pain. A critical review. Brain 99:123–158, 1976

147. Newman MK, Kill M, Frampton G: Effects of ultrasound alone and combined with hydrocortisone injections by needle or hypospray. Am J Phys Med 37:206–209, 1958

148. Novak EJ: Experimental transmission of lidocaine through intact skin by ultrasound. Arch Phys Med Rehabil 45:231–232, 1964

149. Oakley EM: Evidence for effectiveness of ultrasound treatment in physical medicine. Br J Cancer 45:233–237, 1982

150. O'Malley EP, Oester YT: Influence of some physical chemical factors on iontophoresis using radio isotopes. Arch Phys Med Rehabil 36:310–316, 1955

151. Orne MT: Assessment of Biofeedback Therapy: Specific vs Non-specific Effects in Biofeedback, pp 12–33. American Psychiatric Association Task Force on Biofeedback. American Psychiatric Association, Washington, DC, 1979

152. Owens S, Atkinson ER, Lees DE: Thermographic evidence of reduced sympathetic tone with transcutaneous nerve stimulation. Anesthesiology 50:62–65, 1979

153. Passali D, Bellussi L, Masieri S: Transtympanic iontophoresis: Personal experience. Laryngoscope 94:802–806, 1984

154. Paul BJ, Lafratta CW, Dawson AR et al: Use of ultrasound in the treatment of pressure sores in patients with spinal cord injury. Arch Phys Med Rehabil 41:438–440, 1960

155. Payne C: Ultrasound for post-herpetic neuralgia. A study to investigate the results of treatment. Physiotherapy 70:96–97, 1984

156. Perdikis P: Transcutaneous nerve stimulation in the treatment of protracted ileus. S Afr J Surg 15:81–86, 1977

157. Peterson JL, Read SI, Rodman OG: A new device in the treatment of hyperhidrosis by iontophoresis. Cutis 29:82–83, 87–89, 1982

158. Pike PMH: Transcutaneous electrical stimulation. Its use in the management of postoperative pain. Anesthesia 33:165–171, 1978

159. Richardson AW, Duane TD, Hines HM: Experimental lenticular opacities produced by microwave irradiations. Arch Phys Med Rehabil 29:763–769, 1948

160. Reid DC, Cummings GE: Efficiency of ultrasound coupling agents. Physiotherapy 63:255–257, 1977

161. Robinson JE: Review of concepts presented related to the physics of heating: Emphasis on clinical applications. Natl Cancer Inst Mongr. 531–533, 1982

162. Robson JE: Transcutaneous nerve stimulation for pain relief in labour. Anesthesia 34:357–360, 1979

163. Rosenberg M, Curtis L, Bourke DL: Transcutaneous electrical nerve stimulation for the relief of postoperative pain. Pain 5:129–133, 1978

164. Rotberg MH, Surwit RS: Biofeedback techniques in the treatment of visual and ophthalmolgic disorders. A review of the literature. Biofeedback Self Regul 6:375–388, 1981

165. Rubin A, Erdman WJ: Microwave exposure of the human female pelvis during early pregnancy and prior to conception. Am J Phys Med 38:219–220, 1959

166. Schaubel HJ: The local use of ice after orthopedic procedures. Am J Surg 72:711–714, 1946

167. Schuster GD, Infante MC: Pain relief after low back surgery: The efficacy of transcutaneous electrical nerve stimulation. Pain 8:299–302, 1980

168. Shealy CN: The viability of external electrical stimulation as a therapeutic modality. Med Instrum 9:211–212, 1975

169. Shrivastava SN, Singh G: Tap water iontophoresis in palmoplantar hyperhidrosis. Brit J Derm 96:189–195, 1977

170. Skoubo-Kristensen E, Sommer J: Ultrasound influence on internal fixation with a rigid plate in dogs. Arch Phys Med Rehabil 63:371–373, 1982

171. Solomon RA, Viernstein MC, Long DM: Reduction of postoperative pain and narcotic use by transcutaneous electrical nerve stimulation. Surgery 87:142–146, 1980

172. Steward HF, Harris GR, Herman BA et al: Survey of use and performance of ultrasonic therapy equipment in Pinellas County, Florida. Phys Ther 54:707–714, 1974

173. Stewart P: Transcutaneous nerve stimulation as a method of analgesia in labour. Anaesthesia 34:361–364, 1979

174. Stillwell GK: Electrical stimulation and iontophoresis. In Krusen, Kottke, Elwood (eds): Handbook of Physical Medicine and Rehabilitation, pp 374–380. Philadelphia, WB Saunders, 1971

175. Stillwell GK: Ultraviolet therapy. In Krusen, Kottke, Elwood (eds): Handbook of Physical Medicine and Rehabilitation, 2nd ed, pp 363–373. Philadelphia, WB Saunders, 1971

176. Stillwell GK: Ultraviolet therapy. In Kursen's Handbook of Physical

Medicine and Rehabilitation, 3rd ed, pp 351–359. Philadelphia, WB Saunders, 1982

177. Stilz RJ, Carron H, Sanders DB: Case history number 96. Reflex sympathetic dystrophy in a 6-year-old: Successful trstment by transcutaneous nerve stimulation. Anesth Analg 56:438–443, May-June 1977

178. Strassberg–Krainick JU, Thoden U: Influence of transcutaneous nerve stimulation (TNS) on acute pain. J Neurol 217:1–10, 1977

179. Stuchly MA, Repacholi MH, Lecuyer DW, Mann RD: Exposure to the operator and patient during short wave diathermy treatments. Health Physics 42:341–366, 1982

180. Tannebaum M: Iodine iontophoresis in reducing scar tissue. Phys Ther 60:792, 1980

181. Ter Haar GR, Stratford IJ: Evidence for a non-thermal effect of ultrasound. Br J Cancer 45:172–175, 1982

182. Thorsteinsson G, Stonnington HH, Stillwell GK, Elveback LR: The placebo effect of transcutaneous electrical stimulation. Pain 5:31–41, 1978

183. Travell J: Ethyl chloride spray for painful muscle spasm. Arch Phys Med Rehabil 33:291–298, 1952

184. Tyler E, Caldwell C, Ghia JN: Transcutaneous electrical nerve stimulation: An alternative approach to the management of postoperative pain. Anesth Analg 61:449–456, 1982

185. Vaughn DT: Direct method versus underwater method in the treatment of plantar warts with ultrasound. A comparative study. Phys Ther 53:396–397, 1973

186. Wanet G, Dehon N: Etude clinique de l'ultrasonophorese avec un topique associant phenylbutazone et alpha-chymotrypsine. J Belge de Rhumatologie et de Medecine Physique 31:49–58, 1976

187. Warren CG, Koblanski JN, Sigelmann RA: Ultrasound coupling media: Their relative transmissivity. Arch Phys Med 57:218–222, 1976

188. Webster DF, Harvey W, Dyson M, Pond JB: The role of ultrasound induced cavitation in the "in vitro" stimulation of collagen synthesis in human fibroblasts. Ultrasonics 16:34–39, 1980

189. Whitehead WE, Parker L, Bosmajian L et al: Treatment of fecal incontinence in children with spina bifida: Comparison of biofeedback and behavior modification. Arch Phys Med Rehabil 67:218–224, 1986

190. Wilson E, Belar CD, Panush RS, Ettinger MP. Marked digital skin temperature increase mediated by thermal biofeedback in advanced scleroderma. J Rheumatol 10:167–168, 1983

191. Witters DM, Kantor G: An evaluation of microwave diathermy applicators using free space electric field mapping. Phys Med Biol 26:1099–1114, 1981

192. Woodmansey A, Collins DH, Ernst MM: Vascular reactions to the contrast bath in health and in rheumatoid arthritis. Lancet 2:1350–1353, 1938

193. Worden RE, Herrick JF, Wakim KG, Krusen FH: The heating effects of microwaves with and without ischemia. Arch Phys Med Rehabil 29:751–758, 1948

194. Wright ET, Haase KH: Keloids and ultrasound. Arch Phys Med Rehabil 52:280–281, 1971

195. Wright V, Johns RJ: Quantitative and qualitative analysis of joint stiffness in normal subjects and in patients with connective tissue diseases. Ann Rheum Dis 20:36–46, 1961

196. Yocum DE, Hodes R, Sundstrom WR, Cleeland CS: Use of biofeedback training in treatment of Raynaud's disease and phenomenon. J Rheumatol 12:90–93, 1985

197. Zanetic F, Markovic B, Starcevic LJ: Kratkotalasna terapija kao komplementarna terapija hronicnog prostatitisa. Med Arh 35:157–159, 1981

14

Traction, Manipulation, and Massage

Steve R. Geiringer

Cynthia B. Kincaid

James J. Rechtien

The treatment modalities discussed in this chapter date back at least several thousand years. Each has been used, in various forms, throughout the world, having arisen independently in one civilization after another. Traction, manipulation, and massage are all treatments for the relief of painful conditions—sometimes with noticeable immediate effects—that are being sought after by an ever-increasing number of people, particularly manipulation and massage. Despite these favorable common factors, open-armed acceptance within the medical community has not been forthcoming, nor is it expected to be in the near future.

At best, the medical community has mixed emotions about these modalities. A discussion of manipulation, for example, rarely fails to evoke strong feelings. Proponents note that 90 million manipulations are performed yearly in the United States alone,[6] that patients generally feel better after a series of manipulations, and that complications rarely arise and only then because of an unqualified practitioner performing an inappropriate maneuver. Opponents argue that patients who improve with manipulaton would have done so anyway; that complications, although rare, are often grievous and sometimes fatal; that treatments are aimed at the pocketbook and not the pain; and that claims of success, especially concerning visceral, nonmusculoskeletal disorders, are totally unproven.[112]

What has led to the apparently dichotomous thinking among some physiatrists that dismisses manipulation but embraces such other treatments as transcutaneous nerve stimulation, neither of which has been scientifically proven efficacious? One reason may be that the traditional, allopathic medical community looks askance at any modality of treatment not developed by its own members. Traction, manipulation, and massage, described centuries to millenia ago, do not fit into that category. In addition, they are treatments that can be performed by nonphysicians; particularly manipulation and massage. A treatment appears less scientific and perhaps less efficacious if it can be obtained from nonphysicians, even nonlicensed, practitioners. A more acceptable rationale for rejecting these treatments may be their lack of scientific proof of benefit. The principles of traction are the most well established of the three modalities, and are based on objective experimental data. Not surprisingly, use of traction among allopaths is less controversial than use of manipulation.

The use of any treatment should be limited to those condi-

tions that can be reasonably expected to benefit from the physiological effects of that treatment. The macroscopic effects of traction and massage have been well elucidated and offer reliable guidance to indications. This is not yet true for manipulation, and empirical findings and speculation largely sway the clinician's opinion.

TRACTION

Traction is the act of drawing or pulling, or a pulling force.[111] In medicine, forces are applied to the body, generally to stretch a given part or separate two or more parts. In physiatry, traction is generally limited to the cervical or lumbar spine with the hope of relieving pain in or originating from those areas.

To a greater extent than manipulation and massage, traction has benefited from technological advances and from the measurable nature of its effects on the spine. Treatment of long bone fractures led to the development of several traction techniques in the 1800s.[102] Since the days of Hippocrates, attempts at correction of scoliosis have frequently involved traction in one form or another. More recent attempts have included applying traction manually,[30] with free weights and a pulley (the patient supplies the pull with his hands or feet), with motorized equipment,[108] and even by hanging the patient inverted.[87] Other than the advent of gravity traction, a debatably safe procedure, no major advance in the application of traction has occurred in several decades.

To critics who argue that traction is worthless and unproven, it can be pointed out that after proper patient selection, many improve with its use. The few who might see traction as a panacea, ordering it for painful conditions indiscriminately, need to be reminded that specific contraindications for traction do exist, and that no treatment works for all maladies. Above all, the primary reason for not using traction is lack of expertise on the part of the person prescribing it or applying it.

Physiologic Effects

The use of traction should be limited to those conditions that can be reasonably expected to benefit from its documented physiological effects.

Cervical Spine

Motions of the normal cervical spine have been extensively studied.[17, 40, 60, 63, 75] Of particular interest here are the relative motions of the interspaces in flexion and extension. Colachis and Strohm[17] observed the C5–C6 interspace to undergo the greatest movement, followed by the C4–C5 and C6–C7 interspaces. Most observers concur, although C4–C5 is held by some[60, 63] to demonstrate the greatest motion in flexion, or both flexion and extension.

The most reproducible result of traction to the cervical spine is elongation. Cyriax[30] reports applying a force of 300 pounds manually, resulting in a 1-cm increase in cumulative interspace distance. Judovich,[64] using varying weights, concluded that the minimum weight for effecting any vertebral separation is 25 pounds. Greater forces,[79] and in some cases much greater forces,[34] have been used, but most studies have concluded that elongation of 2 mm to 20 mm of the cervical spine is achievable with 25 pounds or greater tractive force. Twenty-five pounds is a reasonable amount, given that about 10 pounds is needed to counterbalance the weight of the head.[60]

It has been postulated, but not proven, that prolonged pull on the cervical spine with adequate force leads to fatigue of the paraspinal muscles.[31]

Lumbar Spine

Once friction is overcome with either adequate force of pull[65] or a split table[34] the major physiological effect of traction on the lumbar spine is also elongation, although this has not been as uniformly reported as with the cervical spine. Those investigators[19, 80, 127] who did report widening of the lumbar interspaces used up to several hundred pounds to cause lengthening up to 30 mm.

Techniques of Applying Traction

Manual

Cyriax[31] has written most extensively about manual application of spinal traction, primarily as an adjunct or precursor to spinal manipulation. Physicians and therapists often use manual traction to the cervical spine on a trial basis to help decide whether a full treatment course might be worthwhile. Practitioners wishing to adopt this method should have sufficient training in the procedure and be attentive to contraindications.

Mechanical

Pull is generally transmitted to the spine by a free weight and pulley system. Adequate pull for the cervical spine is achievable with an appropriate apparatus. Many units for home use consist of a bag filled with 20 or more pounds of water or sand. If a pull of only 20 pounds is possible, the system will likely fail to achieve therapeutic results. With one-half of that weight counterbalancing the head in the sitting position,[60] only a suboptimal 10 pounds of true traction remains. This limitation has led to the development of supine home cervical traction units, which sacrifice only a few pounds of pull to overcome friction. Most, however, are difficult for the patient to set up without assistance.

Home cervical traction usually fails unless a physical therapist intermittently monitors the patient's technique of application. Improper head and neck position, along with inadequate (*i.e.,* not enough) weight, are the two major reasons home traction fails. At the initiation of home traction use, the patient should demonstrate apparatus set-up weekly, and then less frequently after that.

Adequate pull can also be achieved on the lumbar spine with weights and pulleys if the proper apparatus is used. The 5 to 10 pounds of lumbar traction often applied to hospitalized patients serve only to keep the patient in bed.

Motorized

Motorized traction, particularly for the cervical spine, provides continuous or intermittent application of a reproducible force. Most patients tolerate greater forces of pull if given intermittently. Its advantages over home traction also include close therapist monitoring of patient positioning and effect of traction on symptoms. The obvious relative disadvantage is the need to be in the physical therapy clinic or the physician's office. Often the patient is prescribed motorized traction under close supervision early in the treatment course, followed by home traction with decreasingly frequent therapist monitoring.

Gravity

In recent years, manufacturers vociferously supported inversion therapy devices for use at home, although enthusiasm now seems to have waned. Theoretically, body weight while inverted provides sufficient pull to distract lumbar vertebrae, and is a simple, at-home means of treating low back pain. Some contraindications come to mind immediately, such as hypertension, bleeding disorders, and glaucoma. Otherwise asymptomatic low back pain patients, undergoing inversion to the point of tolerance, tend to develop a litany of new complaints related to therapy, including persistent headaches, blurred vision, petechiae, and numerous musculoskeletal complaints.[44] Although back pain might also be relieved, inversion therapy carries too many accompanying risks to be prescribed casually.

Parameters

As with many other areas of physiatric therapeutics, little has been proven about the efficacy of traction. Details concerning the specific parameters, sitting versus supine, continuous versus intermittment, and so on, depend more on the practitioner's own empirical observations than on objective data. Individual physicians should, within the limits of reason and the experiences of others, develop personal guidelines regarding amount of weight, duration of traction, and other parameters. Above all else, the patient should be made comfortable during traction therapy, and monitoring by the physical therapist is essential to ensure that the traction applied is not ineffective or aggravating a painful condition.

Positioning

In cervical traction, the choice of sitting *versus* supine positioning should be based on patient comfort and ability to relax. For most, lying supine seems most effective. Lumbar traction can be accomplished by upright body suspension, but chest discomfort from the harness is often a limiting factor, and therefore the supine position is most commonly chosen. Hip flexion is routinely incorporated in order to cause relative lumbar spine flexion, leading to optimal vertebral separation. No reliable home device for self-application of supine cervical or lumbar traction has yet been devised.

Crue was the first to suggest the importance of neck position in cervical traction.[26, 27] He incorporated 20 to 30° of neck flexion into the traction protocol of 20 patients with neck pain who previously had failed trials of supine cervical traction. Nineteen of the 20 improved. This now seems clearly related to widening of the intervertebral foramina with flexion,[16] with the maximal effect coming at between 20 and 30°. For relief of radicular symptoms, cervical traction is routinely ordered with the neck flexed to within this range. If cervical traction is being used for conditions unrelated to nerve root compression (*e.g.,* muscle spasm), less flexion or even the neutral position might be prescribed. Neck extension during traction should be avoided regardless of the underlying condition.

Continuous Versus Intermittent Traction

The decision to administer traction at a constant level over time or on an intermittent, pulsed basis depends largely on patient comfort and physician preference rather than objective data. According to Cyriax,[31] pull is only transmitted to bones and joints once muscles fatigue, necessitating continuous traction. Most authors, however, feel that more weight can be administered intermittently, since some patients are uncomfortable with even small weights pulling continuously. There are experimental findings[18] suggesting that a constant pull causes no more vertebral separation after 30 or 60 seconds than it does after 7 seconds.

Weight

If cervical traction is done in the sitting position, about 10 pounds is required to counterbalance the patient's head. Amounts less than this may be used initially to condition the patient to the feel of the halter and pull. Colachis and Strohm[18] have shown that 30 pounds of traction to a neck flexed to 24° can cause vertebral separation, particularly posteriorly, but increasing the pull to 50 pounds produced no clear-cut additional separation. This correlated with Judovich's[64] earlier finding that a minimum of 25 pounds was needed before cervical vertebrae separated.

Overcoming friction becomes an important consideration in the lumbar spine. In a widely quoted article[65] Judovich reported that a pull equal to about one-half the weight of a body part is needed to overcome friction; for the lower body this becomes 26% of total body weight. Either this amount of pull needs to be achieved before "true" traction on the spine is accomplished, or a split table[34, 65] must be used. Regardless of whether the effect of traction is overpowered or bypassed, another 25% or more of body weight is then needed to cause vertebral separation. For example, Colachis and Strohm[20] used 50 and 100 pounds of lumbar traction with a split table and measured statistically significant vertebral separation with both weights. Posterior vertebral separation predominated at 50 pounds; anterior and posterior widening occurred at 100 pounds. With tractive forces above 100 pounds, the counterforce, in the form of a chest or axillary harness, is a limiting factor for many patients.

Duration

Colachis and Strohm, having carried out the most extensive and elegant studies on the physiological effects of traction, also reported on the optimal duration of each session.[19] With a pull of 30 pounds, cycling 7 seconds on, 5 seconds off, on cervical spines flexed to 24°, maximal vertebral separation occurred at 25 minutes. Others have applied traction for 10 to 30 minutes,[128] 20 minutes to 8 hours,[79] and to patient tolerance. Lumbar traction with minimal weight is often used for up to many days to ensure

immobilization, without the expectation of any physiological effect from the traction itself. As with other parameters, practitioners need to rely as much on observation and experience as on objective data when deciding how long traction is needed.

Other Modalities

Whether or not paraspinal muscles are primarily involved in the condition being treated with traction, their relaxation is crucial during the procedure. Superficial heat is therefore often used prior to or concomitant with the application of traction, to facilitate muscular relaxation. Other modalities, such as massage or manual stretching, that are best done on relaxed muscles, are more effective immediately following traction.

Indications for Traction

Cervical Spine

Cervical traction has been used for a wide spectrum of painful conditions, based on its physiological effects of vertebral separation, widening of the intervertebral foramina, and possibly muscle relaxation. Generally, if symptoms are felt to be at least partly resultant from radiculopathy or disk herniation, cervical traction can be considered. (An exception to this will be discussed in the following section.) The percentage of patients meeting this criterion clearly depends on the examining physician's philosophy of the origin of soft tissue pain. Cyriax,[30] for example, envisions the herniated or displaced disk as the culprit in most cases of neck pain. In the belief that traction creates a suction force that reduces the herniation, he often uses traction in conjunction with manipulation.

Nerve root compression, whether from disk protrusion or some other cause, may be ameliorated by traction, which widens intervertebral foramina. It should be noted that controversy exists regarding the use of traction in cases of radiculopathy, with or without neurological deficit.[15, 28, 34, 57] Those who believe in the ability of traction to cause muscle relaxation suggest it might be applied to posterior neck muscles that are tight or in spasm, even if from an underlying cause.

Lumbar Spine

Lumbar traction is indicated for generally the same conditions as cervical traction. Low back pain arising from herniated nucleus pulposus, lumbar radiculopathy, or muscle spasm might improve with appropriately applied traction of adequate force. Again, the number of patients for whom lumbar traction is prescribed will be highly correlated with the practitioner's beliefs concerning pain origins. An additional indication for lumbar traction is patient immobilization, as in the acute treatment of lumbar disk herniation.

A critical factor in the use of cervical or lumbar traction, even if it is felt to be indicated, is the physician's and particularly the therapist's time in applying and monitoring the treatment. The patient's interests are not served by writing a prescription for a home cervical traction unit and expecting a pharmacy clerk to explain its use, nor is lumbar traction reliably self-applied by the patient at home. Therapist input therefore becomes critical to the successful use of traction.

The principal reason for traction to fail is inadequate weight with improper neck or body positioning, or a combination of these two. Thirty pounds of pull with the neck in extension might aggravate radicular pain if the patient sits facing away from, rather than toward, the door to which the pulley is attached. However, even with the neck in an appropriate amount of flexion,

10 pounds of traction will neither harm, nor improve, a painful condition.

Contraindications

Inadequate expertise in the application of traction constitutes the single greatest contraindication to its use, because it is the most commonly flouted. A patient should never be provided a home traction unit without first undergoing instruction and monitoring by a physician or therapist. Once the patient learns the proper use of a home cervical traction unit that allows for adequate pull, he or she should still be checked intermittently for proper use and positioning. This might occur weekly at first, and then less frequently over time. Some patients use a home unit on an infrequent, as-needed basis. Should such a patient find that traction becomes ineffective, having a therapist check for proper use should be the first intervention.

Cervical ligamentous instability, as might be seen with rheumatoid arthritis or other conditions, is an absolute contraindication to cervical traction, thereby avoiding atlantoaxial subluxation with spinal cord compromise. Existing disease of the vertebrobasilar arterial system, in combination with traction with the head improperly extended rather than flexed, could lead to compromise of the posterior circulation. In such cases, neck extension must be avoided; preferably, traction should not be used at all. If clinical signs of myelopathy exist, traction must not be used.

Documented or suspected tumor in the region of the spine is an absolute contraindication to use of traction. At least two instances of quadriplegia following traction have been reported[78] in which a previously undetected metastasis of a prostate tumor was present extradurally in the cervical spine. The clinical findings were those of severe neck and shoulder pain with radiographs indicating severe changes of osteoarthritis.

Significant osteopenia rules out the use of traction.

Lumbar traction should not be used on pregnant women.

Old age is only a relative contraindication to the use of traction. The safest route is to avoid traction altogether in the aged, given the likelihood of at least one of the above conditions being present. Should a practitioner wish to prescribe traction for an elderly person, a careful screening process should occur first.

Traction should not be used in the presence of an infectious process of the spine or supporting soft tissues, as with diskitis or tuberculosis. Patients with restrictive lung disease or other breathing disorders should not be subjected to the pull of a chest harness, as is needed with heavy lumbar traction. Extreme anxiety on the part of the patient is a relative contraindication to the use of traction, as muscle relaxation is vital.

Weinberger[122] strongly condemns the use of traction in acute soft tissue injury of the neck, particularly whiplash injuries. He points out that pulling on injured muscles exacerbates, not ameliorates, the microscopic damage already present, and that the time-honored treatment of rest should be prescribed initially. His article highlights the fact that most of what is "known" and written about soft tissue injury, diagnosis, and treatment, including traction, is unproven.

Writing the Referral

The practitioner can no more write, "Cervical traction, please" as a treatment prescription than ask for "Physical therapy for back pain." He or she is obligated to write a detailed, parameter-specific prescription for cervical or lumbar traction. As with other physical therapy referrals, the following patient information is included: age, sex, diagnosis or treatment, precautions to be taken, and patient symptoms for the therapist to be alert for that would signal a need to discontinue traction.

The following specific parameters are those that must be outlined in all traction referrals:

- Body position: sitting, supine, hip/knee flexion
- Neck position: between neutral and 30° of neck flexion
- Mode of applying traction: continuous or intermittent. It might be written to use continuous traction if tolerated, otherwise intermittent.
- Weight: a range is necessary to allow patient acclimation. For example, in sitting cervical traction, 10 to 35 pounds is a reasonable prescription, because it allows the therapist to start with a small weight (just enough to counterbalance the head), yet provides an upper limit that will cause vertebral separation and forminal widening.
- Other modalities (for example, superficial heat for relaxation), to be used prior to or concomitant with traction
- Duration of session: in most instances, 20 minutes
- Frequency and duration of treatment course. For example, 3 to 4 times weekly for 3 to 4 weeks. This needs to be coordinated with the following parameters:

  Interval for return visit to the physician

  Guidelines regarding when to discontinue the traction trial if symptoms are not relieved or, in fact, worsen. Should traction exacerbate the painful condition for which it is prescribed, the decision to end it is not difficult. Less clear-cut is the timing of ending traction if a patient's condition is benefited little or not at all. A reasonable yardstick to use is that if no relief is reported after 4 to 6 sessions, and the technique of application is known to be correct, alternative treatments should be explored.

  Guidelines for monitoring home use of traction. If a supervised trial of cervical traction is successful, a home unit can be prescribed with the proviso that the therapist check the patient for correct head and neck positioning and for use of adequate weight. The monitoring interval will vary depending on the patient, but will likely increase over time.

MANIPULATION

The subject of spinal manipulation therapy rarely fails to evoke strong emotional responses among health care professionals, particularly in the United States and Britain. Since the 1890s, when manipulation became a cornerstone of the therapeutic approach of osteopathy and chiropractic medicine, the subject has produced radically polarized views: proponents note the rapid and continuing growth of manipulation therapy and the ever-increasing public demand, while opponents point to the lack of proof of efficacy and the rare, but occasionally catastrophic, complications. Common sense suggests that a middle ground exists between "it cures nothing" and "it cures everything." Some of this divergence of viewpoint can be explained by the fact that the opposing factions treat each other's failures. The fact that manipulation skills are significantly different from those acquired in allopathic medical schools also serves to reinforce the division between the two camps. In contrast, in continental Europe professional conflict has been relatively absent and the discussion of manipulation,[81] although not uniformly welcomed, has developed in an anger-free, knowledge-seeking environment.

The very definition of spinal manipulative therapy is controversial, but can be summarized as a passive mechanical treatment applied to a specific vertebra or vertebral regions of the spinal column by a physician or therapist; not included are massage, which is applied to soft tissue, traction, which is not specific, and active exercise. This definition has the advantages of clearly stating the relationship of spinal manipulative therapy to other modalities and of including non-thrust techniques, which many physical therapists are now trained to perform.

Osteopaths and chiropractors perform spinal manipulation for a number of different reasons.[92] Most[54] of the 90 million annual chiropractic manipulations performed in the United States, and likely most manipulations by practitioners of other disciplines, are for complaints of musculoskeletal pain in the back and neck. Spinal manipulation is neither chiropractic nor osteopathic per se, but is an application of forces to the muscles, tendons, ligaments, joints and capsules, bones, and cartilage of the veterbral column, the major goal of which is the restoration of normal spinal motion and the elimination of pain secondary to disturbed biomechanics. Most physiatrists see patients who present with problems potentially treatable by spinal manipulation.

Because many of the patients treated by physiatrists will have had or soon will undergo manipulation, all physiatrists at the very least should know the types of manipulation their patients might encounter, along with contraindications. Some will actively refer patients, usually those who have failed inital therapeutic interventions, to practitioners of manipulation, and a few will incorporate manipulation into their own practice of physiatry. This section will provide some of the information the practitioner needs to rationally select one of the above relationships to manipulative therapy.

Choosing Manipulation

Risks and Benefits

Few risks are involved in spinal manipulative therapy, and no complications resulting from isometric or articulatory treatment have been reported. There are reports of complications of thrust manipulation, but the number of reported problems—in the hundreds[71]—is actually quite small considering that at least 90 million manipulations is performed annually in the United States alone. In addition, as will be discussed, most of these complications probably could be avoided.

Of the reported side-effects[113] of spinal manipulative therapy the most common is a transient increase in discomfort[73] for 6 to 72 hours following therapy. Pain should resolve to less than the pretreatment level in a short time and should be less of a problem with each successive treatment. Minor autonomic effects such as increased perspiration and early or increased menses have been reported.

Thrusting has an immediate effect and improvement should be seen within 1 week of initiation of therapy.[91] Isometrics take longer and run concurrent with physical therapy. However, lack of improvement in objective findings after 2 to 4 weeks would suggest the need to reevaluate the diagnosis and the therapeutic plan. Some problems do not resolve despite accurate diagnosis and treatment, but long-term therapy does appear to have some subjective value. This needs to be decided on an individual basis.

Osteopathic and chiropractic proponents of spinal manipulative therapy believe in distant visceral benefits, beyond the systemic benefits produced by good structural and biomechanical efficiency and relief of pain.[92] Distant visceral complications related temporally to manipulation, however, have been documented only twice[48, 105] in the last 100 years, which means the physiatrist is able to evaluate the benefits or detriments of manipulation solely on the musculoskeletal results.

Although benefits of manipulation have not been proven, proponents report excellent results in treating acute musculoskeletal problems, and good results with chronic conditions. Empirically, these outcomes are comparable to those achieved with conventional modalities, which also often carry no proof of efficacy. If nothing else, the great number of patients obtaining manipulative therapy speaks to a perceived benefit, and that number increases yearly.

Applicability to Physiatry

A physiatrist who practices manipulative therapy is able to identify a patient subpopulation likely to benefit from it. This group will include people with structural problems such as pelvic asymmetries and vertebral rotations, and others depending on the physiatrist's familiarity and expertise with palpatory diagnosis. Patients with chronic back pain might be referred for a course of manipulation, in conjunction with epidural injections, transcutaneous nerve stimulator units, psychological counseling and other interventions.

A general physiatric examination must be followed by a segmental examination in areas suggested by symptoms or by a gross examination. The physiatrist looks for tenderness[97] elicited by pressure over vertebral processes or by induced vertebral motion. Passively induced vertebral motion[6] is evaluated for range, symmetry, and the force needed to achieve range. The latter is discussed in the literature as the quality or feel[52, 54] of motion. Combinations of motions of the vertebra, such as flexion and rotation, are examined. Springing[54] of the vertebra and tenderness elicited by local pressure on the interspinous ligament[83] are useful clues to pathology and loss of joint play. Subcutaneous texture changes[54] (edema and fibrosis) noted by palpation and skin rolling[91] are signs of dysfunction, and some manipulators look carefully for segmental autonomic changes such as perspiraton[99] and hyperemic response to light scratch. The ribs, occiput, and pelvis often need inclusion in this part of the examination. Vertebral position, including relative posterior position of the transverse process, can be misleading owing to bony vertebral anomalies. It is useful only for screening. Vertebrae identified by positive findings are considered dysfunctional or pathological and are candidates for manipulation. Such an examination will add 5 to 10 minutes to a initial visit and less than 5 minutes to subsequent visits.

Modes of Practice

Availability of spinal manipulative therapy depends on how the physiatrist chooses to provide treatment.

REFERRAL TO A PHYSICIAN. Physiatrists who wish to use spinal manipulative therapy but not practice it themselves have two alternatives. One is the referral of the patient for concurrent manipulative care to another practitioner. This works well in some cases and in some areas,[12] but potential problems exist. Among these are ultimate control of the patient, accurate assessment of the manipulator's competence, and resentment of a referral to an osteopathic or chiropractic practitioner.

REFERRAL TO A PHYSICAL THERAPIST. The second option is that the physiatrist diagnose the problem to be treated and write a prescription for specific manipulation to be done by a physical therapist.[97] As more physical therapists acquire training in spinal manipulative therapy, this becomes a viable option. In the United States, physical therapists traditionally have been limited to providing isometric and articulatory techniques, and such techniques are successful with many patients. The manipulation can be provided as part of the overall physical therapy program. Even with such a referral pattern, however, the physician must at least acquire palpatory diagnostic skills. He or she must be able to write a specific prescription for the anatomical area to be treated and specific motion to be restored, along with the technique to be used and frequency and length of intervention. More importantly, the physician is then able to monitor progress of the therapy objectively and determine the end point and possible side-efforts or failure of the manipulation. Sequential monitoring of each manipulative intervention can be left to the therapist; this is acceptable given the time course and safety of isometric and articulatory techniques. The acquisition of the minimal diagnostic palpatory skills may take 1 to 2 weeks, and with use, these skills are easily maintained. The time commitment and economic investment are far less in this option than in the provision of manipulative therapy itself.

Most manipulators[6, 113] believe that the restoration of the vertebral joint's normal passive and active ranges of motion (ROM) and resting equilibrium position is the end point of treatment. In this view, spinal manipulative therapy is the vertebral equivalent of peripheral passive range of motion and end stretching. It becomes a natural extension of the physical therapy that physiatrists already prescribe for back problems; it simply addresses individual joints rather than the spine as a whole.

Spinal manipulative therapy differs from peripheral joint therapy in several ways:

Most patients cannot actively perform ROM for specific vertebral joints, so that passive ROM is necessary

Vertebral bones have short lever arms and small normal ROM, making loss of mobility hard to detect compared to peripheral limbs

Loss of a single joint's mobility is usually well compensated for by other vertebrae, so gross spinal motion often remains normal or nearly so

Forceful thrusting maneuvers have been traditionally used in spinal manipulative therapy to restore ROM but this is less commonly done on the larger peripheral joints.

The practice of physician referral of patients to physical therapists for manipulative treatment will likely become more common in the United States, and brings the benefits of spinal manipulative therapy to those patients who have chosen the nonosteopathic, nonchiropractic approach to health care for musculoskeletal problems.

Acquiring Manipulation Skills

Three obstacles exist to the physiatrist performing manipulation himself: (1) acquiring initial skills, (2) maintenance of skills, and (3) economics of manipulation. Thrust-type manipulation, because of the significant forces involved and potential for harm, is best learned on volunteers, not patients, under the close direction of a skilled operator. The minimum initial learning time required is approximately 3 to 6 months.[81, 91] Even 3 months may be too great a commitment for most physiatrists. Because of their inherent safety, isometric or muscle energy and articulatory techniques sufficient for therapy initiation can usually be acquired in 1 to 2 weeks of formal course work. The training time is short because an inappropriate or nonindicated isometric technique, unless repeated very frequently or over a prolonged period, rarely causes detrimental effects. Thus, the operator may begin working with patients early in training and develop improved techniques with time.

Maintenance of skills is relatively easy for a full-time manipulator but may be problematic for the physiatrist whose practice is general in nature or heavily hospital oriented. Manipulative skills, unlike those involved in riding a bicycle, for example, will deteriorate unless frequently used. The actual minimum frequency of use needed to maintain competence or excellence varies considerably from person to person. Clearly, though, the potential user should consider maintenance of skills before investing time and money in the acquisition of these skills.

Closely tied to the frequency of use is the economics of performing this service. Manipulation, if done well, is time consuming.

Although manipulation techniques can be studied by any physician, skillful manipulation is demanding, and not all physicians will derive satisfaction from providing it. Anecdotally, at least, manipulators who do not enjoy performing manipulation will not do it well.

Techniques of Spinal Manipulative Therapy

The discussion here has been limited to those techniques which the physiatrist is most likely to encounter early in his investigation of manipulative therapy.

Thrusting

Thrusting is also known as *impulse*[37] (European) or *high velocity–low amplitude* manipulation.[6, 32, 41, 45, 51, 54, 67, 81, 83–85, 89, 91, 113] In most approaches, the operator diagnoses the pathological vertebral segment by identifying position or motion abnormalities or related tissue changes, including tenderness to palpation or to induced motion. He or she then rotates, sidebends and flexes, or extends the vertebral segments below it, "locking" their facets so that further motion is limited to the vertebra in question. This vertebra is then passively moved to its limit of motion, or its barrier, so that all slack motion is removed by the operator and a small force, localized to the joint in question and in the direction of the restricted motion, is applied to hold this position. A controlled thrust is then applied for a short time (10–100 msec)[131] to the involved vertebra in the direction perceived as limited, and a small motion in the desired direction—either flexion, extension, rotation, or sidebending—occurs as the vertebra traverses the barrier (Fig. 14-1). Often an audible pop[96] or click[70] is produced. The acceleration, and therefore the forces involved, have never been measured but are presumably quite high. Increased passive ROM is the end result.

If the force is applied over a spinous or transverse process, the procedure is termed a *short lever technique*. If the force is applied distant from the vertebra through the locked vertebral column, the procedure is called a *long lever technique*. All thrust techniques can do harm if the forces are misdirected or not well localized to the vertebra or vertebral region involved.

Some manipulators take up slack and apply thrust in a direction opposite the restricted direction.[83] This type of approach, away from the restriction, is called an *indirect technique*. The success of this approach probably implies a facet-locking mechanism, as opposed to a soft tissue restriction source of dysfunction. Other manipulators work with less specificity, but may add traction and direct the thrust at relocating a bulging disk.[32]

Articulatory

Articulatory manipulation[52] is also called *mobilization* (Europe) and *low velocity–high amplitude* (United States) and is very similar to *oscillatory*[85] techniques (New Zealand). The ver-

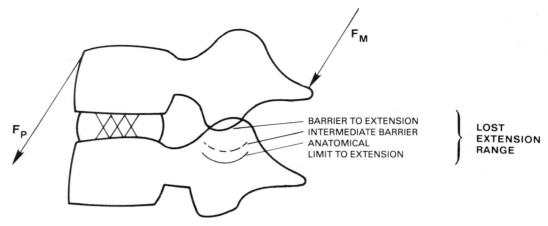

Figure 14-1. In the thrust technique, the patient is relaxed and is not applying force (F_p). The manipulator applies a quick force (F_m) in the direction shown to extend the upper vertebra to the anatomical limit in one motion. In the muscle energy technique, the manipulator applies force (F_m) and the patient contracts muscles with net force (F_p) in the directions shown so that no torque exists around the center of flexion-extension rotation. After 5 seconds, patient and doctor relax and a new extension barrier to passive range of motion nearer the anatomical limit is found. Repeated manipulations will bring succeeding barriers closer to the normal passive anatomical limit.

tebral joint is passively moved in a reduced range defined by its resting position and the pathological limit of motion. The extent of motion and end point of the motion are varied according to a grading scheme, but ultimately the end point and the pathological barrier become the same and the barrier is teased with repeated motion. Ideally, the quality or feel of the induced motion, as well as the quantity of force and excursion, are normalized by this procedure. Occasionally, a small amount of additional force takes the vertebra through its barrier or restriction and this technique blends into thrust. Other variables include frequency of repetition, duration of hold time at the extremes, and velocity of motion.

Oscillatory techniques are similar to articulatory techniques in that there are various grades or magnitudes of pressure applied. But oscillatory techniques apply and remove pressure at a rate of 120 times a minute or more, for 15 to 20 seconds.[96]

Muscle Energy

The nonthrusting technique of muscle energy is also called *isometrics,* and by some Europeans, *mobilization,* and bears a strong relationship to proprioceptive neuromuscular facilitation.[114] It requires the operator to position the patient and remove slack as in thrust procedures. The operator then positions himself or herself to prevent the patient from actively moving the affected vertebra away from its barrier. The patient then exerts small to moderate forces against the resistance offered by the operator for 5 to 10 seconds, and then relaxes. After this isometric maneuver, the operator finds that the barrier has been displaced and he can now move the affected vertebra beyond its original barrier. The procedure is repeated two to three times, with diminishing gains in range being achieved. The procedure, generally painless, often needs to be repeated and generally requires accompanying physical therapy to maintain the corrections that are obtained. The time scale for treatment, normally every other day to every third day, fits in coincidentally with the rest of the usual physical therapy prescription for back pain. Muscle energy techniques have also been used in an indirect approach.

Other Techniques

Other nonthrusting techniques exist and have gained some popularity recently because of their gentleness. In *functional techniques* the operator assists the patient to find a vertebral joint position of ease, away from the barrier.[7] Postural forces and active patient positioning are used and the operator applies only guidance and monitoring. The mechanism of action is not known, but is thought to be related to interference with the spindle system's input to the spinal cord.[7] Since reflex muscle guarding is inhibited,[97] the technique is appropriate for muscle spasm—induced joint dysfunction. *Counterstrain* involves a similar positioning for 90 seconds with slow return to the neutral position, but differs in that the operator monitors pressure with his or her hand over a myofascial trigger point, instead of the vertebra, in order to find the position of greatest relaxation.[8, 62] The trigger point may be distant from the vertebra, even in an anterior myotome. Counterstrain has been applied successfully to situations involving reflex spasm. *Craniosacral* manipulation involves monitoring rhythms in the cerebrospinal fluid.[118] The operator palpates subtle cyclic pressure changes with his or her hands on the patient's skull or sacrum or both and exerts corrective pressure to regions of the skull or sacrum to normalize pressure symmetry and frequency of the cycle. *Myofascial release* is a global approach that involves many of the above modalities, particularly massage-like stretching maneuvers.[121] In general, however, these and the many other possible approaches have a less extensive literature and are perceived as second-level approaches to manipulation.

Indications for Spinal Manipulative Therapy

Spinal manipulative therapy is applicable in all musculoskeletal pain problems of the back, pelvis, and neck in which loss of vertebral function or localized tenderness on induced motion may be a contributing factor, and in which there are no contraindications. All visceral or systemic pathologies must be excluded or at least placed under concurrent care.

Some authors[89] believe that if induced motion of a vertebra does not reproduce a symptom the vertebra should not be manipulated. Others claim that in a many-bodied linkage system such as the spine, restricted motion in one area of the system might cause discomfort in a distant vertebra that has to compensate for this loss of motion. There is no supporting evidence either way.

Related to this issue is the question of prophylaxis. Both the osteopathic and chiropractic professions tend to treat vertebral motion restrictions in asymptomatic patients for several reasons:

Future stress in the form of mechanical use, systemic illness, psychogenic problems, or a loss of compensatory motion in an aging mechanical system will eventually cause problems in the restricted area

Structural normality lessons metabolic demands

There may be visceral effects

Restrictions become fixed by fibrosis or a type of neurological set (engram) if untreated.

The individual physiatrist must decide how much of this philosophy to accept, and weigh against this the obstacles (in terms of third-party pay, etc.), that are involved.

Contraindications

Spinal manipulative techniques differ as to their degree of invasiveness. Because of the higher forces involved, thrust is considered the most invasive, with articulation, isometrics, and functional approaches less invasive. The more invasive the modality the more likely it is to be contraindicated. The literature concerning contraindications to thrusting techniques has been coprehensively reviewed by Kleynhans,[71] and contraindications to articulation are discussed by several authors.[52, 85] Inadequate skill of the manipulator is a major contraindication for all types of manipulation.

Articulation is contraindicated in vertebral malignancy, infection, or inflammation, cauda equina syndrome, myelopathy or spondylosis, multiple adjacent radiculopathies, vertebral bone diseases, vertebral joint instability such as fractures or dislocations, and rheumatoid disease in the cervical region. Thrust is clearly contraindicated in these cases plus the following: the presence of spinal deformity and most anomalies; systemic anticoagulation (either disease-related or pharmacological); severe diabetes; atherosclerosis; severe degenerative joint disease (DJD); vertigo or symptoms and signs of vertebral basilar disease or insufficiency; spondyloarthropathies (psoriatic, ankylosing spondylitis, Reiter's syndrome); inactive rheumatoid disease, ligamentous joint instability or congenital joint laxity, and syndromes such as Marfan's or Ehlers-Danlos; aseptic necrosis; local aneurysm; and osteomalacia and osteoporosis. Spondylolisthesis does not contraindicate manipulation localized to neighboring vertebrae. Excessive ROM in a vertebra joint, termed *hypermobility,* of any etiology is a contraindication to further manipulation of that joint.[47, 67]

Certain patients with a tendency toward obsessional neurosis and fixation on painful anatomical areas probably are poor candidates for thrust.[52] In addition, some authors consider the absence of any pain-free direction of vertebral motion a contraindication to thrust. Pregnancy with known threat of miscarriage is an absolute contraindication to manipulation. The normal low-risk pregnancy is discussed by Grieve,[52] who advises avoiding compressive and rotational thrusting techniques but doing some very conservative mobilization techniques up to the eighth month. Objective radicular signs are a contraindication to articulation or thrust. The question of manipulation for clearly defined root pain without objective findings is controversial; some authors avoid rotational thrust in a side-lying position and some avoid any forceful intervention at all. Isometrics in a nonlateral position would appear to be safe, but there is no firm literature on this or any other contraindication ,to isometrics. Vertebral isometric techniques should not be used if the pathology present would preclude passive ROM, gentle stretching, or isometrics in a peripheral joint with the same pathology. Catastrophic results do not occur from isometric techniques, so that they may be used cautiously in some of the absolute contraindications to thrust and articulation, specifically osteoporosis, severe diabetes, rheumatoid disease away from the cervical area, DJD, and joint laxity. Concurrent active myositis may contraindicate isometrics because of the patient's active muscular contraction.

Complications generally are related to procedures done when contraindicated. We know of no literature specific to isometric manipulative complications nor have we heard anecdotally of any major problems. Nonetheless, the specific issue of cervical manipulation requires comment. The major disasters following manipulation that have received the most attention in the literature are related to cervical thrust manipulation. In almost all cases, the neck was extended[6, 54, 76, 110, 113] during the procedure and the complication was a vascular insult to the basilar system or the cord. No reported cases of permanent problems following isometric cervical manipulation are reported. It seems prudent, however, to exclude from cervical spinal manipulative therapy all patients with objective signs and symptoms referrable either to the vertebrobasilar artery system or cervical spondylosis. Whether patients without signs or symptoms should receive provocative examination, such as those described by Bourdillon[6] and Maigne,[84] is subject to debate. Even if isometric techniques are employed, it seems reasonable to avoid neck extension during treatment if possible.

Severe complications in lumbosacral manipulation are very rare[58, 106] and have been limited to thrust manipulation. Coincidental development of a disk syndrome during a course of manipulation has occurred, but has not "yielded a significant literature." Such a possibility gives emphasis, however, to the need of the physiatrist to examine and document the vertebral dysfunction before and during the performance of spinal manipulative therapy.

Hypotheses of Pathology

Manipulation is basically a mechanical intervention. It is therefore not surprising that most hypotheses offered in explanation of the pathology or the cure involve position and motion of the vertebral body and accompanying disks, ligaments, and muscles. The various hypotheses differ based on whether efficacy is evaluated by measures of pain or palpable findings. It is helpful to realize that various terms refer to the same problem: minor intervertebral derangement (MID), osteopathic lesion, chiropractic subluxation, manipulable lesion, joint blockage, segmental dysfunction, and somatic dysfunction.[10]

Barrier models have been suggested by several authors to explain palpable findings (Fig. 14-2).[51, 67, 69] Normal joints possess an active ROM and a larger passive ROM. A barrier or motion restriction, produced by abnormal muscle contraction, or capsular or ligamentous shortening, forms in one or more directions between the neutral position and the normal limit of active range so that the patient is unable to achieve normal range and the manipulator needs additional force to achieve the normal pas-

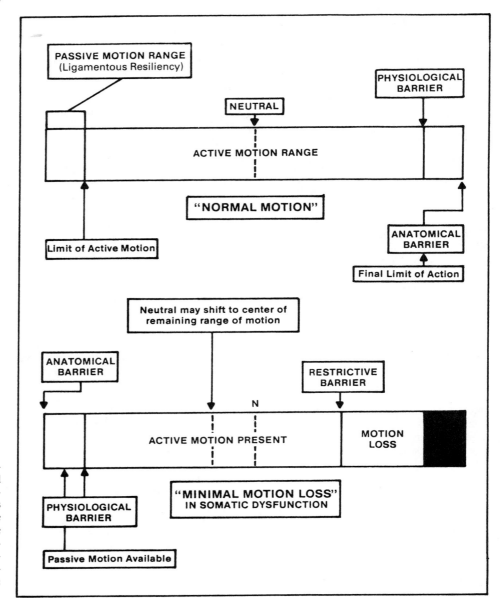

Figure 14-2. A model of barrier or motion restriction. The motion represented may be rotation, sidebending, or flexion-extension. The anatomical barrier consists of cartilage and bony elements whereas the restrictive and physiological barriers are made up of muscular and ligamentous elements. (Modified from Kimberly PE: Formulating a prescription for osteopathic manipulative treatment. J Am Osteopath Assoc 79: 506–513, 1980)

sive range. Force asymmetry may lead to the vertebra finding a new resting position away from anatomical neutral. A variant[36] of this approach considers strain of soft tissue as the basic pathology; the resulting inflammation and edema then start a local vicious cycle with pain and spasm resulting. After time, edematous thickening leads to barrier formation.

In the *facilitated segment model* a vertebral body, chronically malpositioned by contractures or overly active muscle, is assumed to flood the segmentally related area of the cord with inappropriate nonfatiguing proprioceptive impulses, which then spill over and facilitate outgoing motor neurons, gamma efferents, and autonomics in the same vertebral segment of the cord.[72] The visceral afferents can independently facilitate the somatic outflow of a related segment. Thus, pathways are present for interaction between soma and viscera, making palpatory diagnosis of visceral pathology and manipulative influence on the viscera at least within possibility. This interaction also allows abnormal segmental areas that are generally asymptomatic to acquire symptoms from general illness, emotional stress, or distant pathology. Physiatrists familiar with reflex bladder and autonomic hyperreflexia will probably accept the concepts of

somatovisceral reflexes and segmental spillover, but the extent and importance of these effects in a normal individual is still unclear.[21, 109]

Modern extrapolations of this general picture accept the fact that the gamma input is only one of many to the spinal cord, which must therefore respond to a pattern of afferent impulses.[72] Spinal cord vertigo results from conflicting proprioceptive and gamma afferent input information.[74] The possibility of chronicity caused by spinal cord learning similar to cortical engram formation[100] has also been proposed.

This hypothesis has been recently criticized[99] on the basis of the plurisegmental nature of proprioceptive afferents and the complexity and suprasegmental nature of known viscerosomatic pain reflexes. Another model, almost directly opposed to the facilitated segment model, has been proposed that suggests manipulation serves to increase proprioceptive input to the dorsal root. This input competitively prevents pain input from cephalad transmission (*i.e.,* the gate of the gate theory). Thus, manipulation acts like a mechanical transcutaneous electrical nerve stimulation (TENS), although a recent trial did not confirm endorphin release after manipulation.[101]

Distinct from the various neurophysiological hypotheses is the primarily mechanical model of *altered joint play*. All normal voluntary joint motion must be accompanied by some motion in a direction perpendicular or possibly tangential to the plane of the voluntary motion.[66, 91, 125] This joint play, defined as allowable motions in directions other than those of voluntary motion, exists because joint surfaces are not perfectly congruent. Play in the joints is conceptually different from coupling,[123] which involves obligate related voluntary motions such as rotation and side-bending. Loss of this play due to soft tissue restrictions may inhibit voluntary motion. Passive intervention is needed to normalize function, since the lost motion is in an involuntary direction. Pain is not addressed directly by this model but arises from poor mechanical function.

A bulging disk or dislodged disk fragment pressing on the posterior longitudinal ligament can cause pain.[89] One model suggests that manipulation, often accompanied by traction, acts to replace the fragment or to reduce the bulge; pain associated with vertebral motion is relieved as a secondary effect. A modification of this approach[83, 84] suggests that the bulge creates asymmetry and locking or wedging in the facet joints, resulting in loss of motion. According to this particular modification, because further voluntary motion will accentuate the problem, passive intervention is needed. The possibility of asymptomatic dysfunctional joints creating symptoms under stress is part of this model.

McKenzie[89] defines three classes of abnormality: (1) a postural syndrome characterized by intermittent pain associated with postural stress, (2) a dysfunction syndrome characterized by pain and lost vertebral motion similar to the barrier model, and (3) a derangement syndrome which involves disk abnormalities as previously cited.

Numerous hypotheses have been advanced by the chiropractic profession to describe and explain the relationships between altered structure and resultant pathology. These are adequately reviewed by Janse.[61] The deleterious neurophysiological effects resulting from nerve compression caused by vertebral derangement have been conjectured to be a major cause of somaticovisceral complaints. This viewpoint, which has been prominent since the earliest foundations of chiropractic, is perhaps the one most associated with chiropractic by other professionals. However, a number of other speculations including neurodystrophic effects, various combinations of somaticovisceral reflexes, and a proprioceptive input phenomenon similar to the segmental facilitation model have also received attention in the chiropractic literature.

Some European authors[81] believe there is soft material in the vertebral joint spaces, a meniscoid, which can become trapped between the cartilage surfaces and block smooth joint motion until moved by manipulative gapping or repeated mobilization.

Soft tissue pain and palpatory findings, although related to vertebral dysfunction, do not always follow obvious segmental patterns,[6] and attempts[36] to incorporate these findings, called myotendinosis, into the classical picture have been made. The term *spondylogenic reflex* has been coined to describe the suprasegmental organizing process.

There have been admirable efforts[94] to unify the various hypotheses, but with limited success to date.

Hypotheses of Pain Relief

The mechanism by which spinal manipulative techniques relieve pain is not known. Hypotheses focus on different specific actions of the therapy: (1) it addresses vertebral function by restoring vertebral ROM and ease of motion or the vertebra's resting position; (2) it restores normality and symmetry either at the disk or facet level, or both; or (3) it mechanically produces an afferent signal to the cord and directly diminishes pain awareness by a gate effect.

In the first case, the restriction or resistance to motion ultimately arises from restrictive muscle contraction and either shortened or stiffened passive elements such as ligament, capsule, myofascial tissue, or connective tissue of muscle. All forms of manipulation are thought to interfere with abnormal muscular contraction, either by production of afferent stimuli which attenuate a hyperexcitable gamma system, or by elimination of proprioceptive input which stimulates the gamma system. In addition, thrust and possibly articulatory and isometric techniques can stimulate Golgi tendon organ input.[72] Articulatory and isometric techniques may elicit permanent lengthening of collagenous tissue by inducing a permanent set with repeated stretching in the viscoelastic range.[119] Alternatively, repeated deformation of soft tissue by changing the mechanical history of the tissue may normalize its mechanical response to load, that is, soften the material so that deformation occurs at lower load.[59] This functional lengthening of the tissue can be a passive phenomenon, but the time scale of isometric and articulatory treatment (over days) would allow metabolic participation of the tissue. This has not been addressed in the literature to date. Thrust differs from articulatory technique and isometrics in that it has similarities to impact loading. This results in high stress levels and probably very high strain rates in the soft tissues for a very short time. The implication of these high strain rates in short time periods has not been investigated in tissue, but it seems reasonable to speculate that a non-uniform distribution of strain will result which may lead to very localized tissue injury and subsequent healing with permanent elongation.

The net result of either muscle relaxation or collagenous tissue stretch is that the vertebra will regain normal play and active and passive ROM and the forces needed to produce them will be normalized. Pain is reduced secondary to return of function.

In the second instance, facet malposition[83] or malfunction can be directly influenced by passive motion of the joint, or a malpositioned meniscoid[62] can be relocated. A bulging disk is envisioned as being replaced or normalized by a manipulation, often in concert with traction, which relieves compressive stresses on the disk, creates suction and, because of the stretched posterior longitudinal ligament, pushes the bulge anteriorly.[32]

Lastly, there can be no question that proprioceptive input to the cord is altered and this might act by closing the gate on pain[99] or by removing a facilitating input.

It should be clear to the reader that manipulators report success in many, if not most, patients using widely varying techniques and operating under very different assumptions as to the cause of the problem and action of therapy. It would seem that any procedure that induces muscular relaxation or vertebral motion has some chance of success. As most of the postulated actions of manipulation are accomplished by most techniques, success itself provides little feedback as to the validity of the model. There is, as yet, too much "joint play" in our knowledge to discern the pathway to a definitive understanding of back pain or therapy. All, or possibly none, of the hypotheses presented may ultimately be found valid.

Future Directions of Research

No other medical modality has ever had so many practitioners (50,000 osteopaths and chiropractors in the United States alone) and consumers (90 million chiropractic manipulations in the nation annually) and so many critics (a significant proportion of the allopathic medical profession) with so little hard data to support or refute it. Forty-six clinical trials of spinal manipulative therapy have been summarized by Brunarski.[10] Detailed reviews and critiques of selected trials have been done by Evans,[39] Haldeman,[54] and most recently by Tobis and Hoehler,[116] and have been the subject of two international meetings.[10, 11]

The conclusions of the various studies are difficult to compare. For example, Coxhead and co-workers[24] reported no significant differences in their study of manipulation as compared to traction, corset, or exercises, whereas Rasmussen[103] reported that 11 of 12 manipulated patients reported pain relief compared to 3 of 12 patients receiving placebo short wave diathermy. However, to truly understand these conflicting data, one needs to know that Rasmussen[103] eliminated chronic back pain patients from the study, used rotational manipulation in the pain-free direction, studied the effects at 2 weeks post-initiation of therapy, and had favorable but somewhat different results when using the modified Schober test as his criterion for improvement. Coxhead and colleagues[24] studied patients with sciatic pain with or without back pain, using Maitland's technique of manipulation[85] and evaluating the improvement of pain at 4 weeks and 4 months. Thus, criteria for inclusion were different, manipulative technique was different, criteria for improvement were partly different, and timing of the follow-up evaluations was different. These differences between studies are typical and it is not surprising that the results of these studies are equivocal.

In general, the studies vary as to whether pain or motion is used as the entry criterion or improvement criterion, duration of the problem, time of the evaluation, nature of the placebo or control, type and specificity of technique employed, and method of statistical analysis used. With rare exceptions,[46] the studies address a chief complaint of pain without regard to objective findings. Given the plethora of pathological conditions that cause back pain, the perplexity of the results is understandable. The situation is analogous to an attempt to determine whether surgery is a more efficacious therapy than bed rest for a complaint of abdominal pain when neither the etiology of the abdominal pain nor the surgical procedure employed is defined. In addition, designers of studies who are denied the double blind techniques of drug research are confronted with the strong emotional bias of those who must do the manipulation (and are sure it works) and those who must evaluate the results (who are often sure it doesn't). How this dilemma will be resolved is not clear.

Knowledge of small tissue strains, as opposed to injury level deformations, is now being accumulated. Much has been learned in the last 15 years about pain and mechanoreceptors[55, 129] and spinal cord anatomy and physiology.[21, 72] It seems reasonable to expect that our understanding of vertebral mechanics and physiology will expand rapidly in the near future and to hope that the knowledge obtained may lead to better designs of efficacy trials. Until such time, the physiatrist will be forced to evaluate manipulation based on incomplete information and the similarity or dissimilarity between manipulation and other equally unproven techniques of physical medicine.

MASSAGE

Massage is the application of systematic manipulation to the soft tissues of the body for therapeutic purposes. Although various assistive devices and electrical equipment are available for the purpose of delivering massage, use of the hands is considered the most effective method of application because palpation can be used as an assessment as well as a treatment tool.

History

Massage has been used throughout history as a physical means to alleviate pain and discomfort. It was rooted in folk medicine in ancient China as long ago as 1800 B.C. The ancient Egyptians, Buddhists, Persians, and Japanese used massage and movement in the treatment of various diseases and injuries, and massage continued to be a vital part of medical treatment up to the 5th century A.D. Hippocrates viewed massage as a very important therapeutic tool and described qualities, indications, and contra-indications for massage in his *On Articulations.*[56] He indicated that physicians must be experienced in friction as well as other methods of medical treatment. Asclepides,[50] another Greek physician, also had a great influence on the development of massage. He proposed that there were only three therapeutic agents, hydrotherapy, exercise, and friction. More detailed classifications and descriptions of techniques in terms of quality (pressure and direction) and quantity (frequency of treatment) were put in writing by Galen (*ca* A.D. 129–199),[38] who wrote as many as 16 books related to massage exercise. The Greeks, who highly valued physical health, beauty, and athletic powers, used applied massage for athletes both before and after an athletic event. This was termed *apotherapy* and was thought to prepare the musculature prior to the event, then clear the extremities of superfluous material and fluid after strenuous activity.

Throughout the Middle Ages little was written about massage until Pare[98] of France in the 16th century translated and published the ancient literature on frictions along with his own specific application for surgical patients. His work was well recognized and the French terminology for specific massage techniques is still used today.

During the next three centuries, a resurgence of interest and applications of massage spread to other countries. Perhaps the most notable contribution to the reestablishment of massage was by Per Henrik Ling[82] of Sweden, who in 1813 was credited with the establishment of the Central Royal Institute of Gymnastics in Stockholm. Ling organized massage and therapeutic exercise into a system that became known as medical gymnastics. Ling's followers continued his work and by 1860 there were similar institutes in England, France, Austria, Germany, and Russia.

Like many forms of medical treatment, massage has been abused and purported to have curing effects for all diseases at one time or another. It is interesting to note that in 1894, the *British Medical Journal* published several reports which attacked the fraudulent use of massage, calling it scandalous and associating it with quackery and prostitution. Now, almost a century later, massage still has a distinct vulnerability to disreputable practice.

At the turn of the century, massage was slowly being adopted in the United States largely due to the writings and influence of Douglas Graham,[49] a Boston physician, and John Kellogg of Battle Creek.[68] During the subsequent 50 years, several new approaches were identified in the Western world. Both Mennell and Cyriax in England used a specific application of deep friction massage to injured contractile and noncontractile joint structures in both acute and chronic conditions. This method has gained in popularity in the United States in recent years and will be discussed in this section.

Developments in special techniques were also occurring in Germany. Dicke[35] discovered that deep massage over one part of the body could have distinct, observable favorable effects on body parts distant from the part being treated. She called this phenomenon *reflex zone massage* or *Bindegewebsmassage* (known in this country as *connective tissue massage*). This massage approach applies superficial and deep palpation to assess and treat sites of muscle or connective tissue tightness that may be in the same segmental distribution as a site of disability either in peripheral or visceral structures. It is reported that Dicke created her massage system after successfully correcting a severe circulatory disorder in her own lower extremity through massage to the lower back.[115b] Dicke's work in this area is the basis, at least in part, for what we now know as soft tissue mobilization and myofascial release technique. A variation of reflex zone massage was also described by another German physician, Cornelius,[22, 23] who applied deep pressure to specific points, calling this procedure *nerve point massage*. This may have been the first time that the oriental treatment of acupressure or shiatsu was described in Western medical literature.

In the history of massage several significant trends have emerged:

Massage has been used as a therapeutic tool throughout history. Its value has been recognized by multiple and diverse cultures. The physiological foundation in support of the use of massage has progressed from purely empirical to more scientific. Although this century has seen more diverse methods of massage emerge, massage in the United States has not kept pace with its use in other countries.

Modern technology has resulted in an explosion in new medical instrumentation. In many cases, machines have replaced human touch as a means of delivering patient care. However, renewed interest and enthusiasm for manual therapeutic intervention has surfaced in the medical community, perhaps because of increased recognition of the psychological component of human physical contact as a healing modality.

General Principles

Patient Preparation

GENERAL ENVIRONMENTAL CONCERNS. For maximal therapeutic results, massage should be applied in a warm, quiet area, free from distracting stimuli. Rhythmic sound at low volume also tends to reduce unwanted muscle contraction.

POSITION. The patient must be comfortable and relaxed with the part to be treated well supported. If the intent of the treatment is to reduce edema, the extremity must be elevated above the level of the heart to allow the force of gravity to assist in the drainage of excessive fluid. Unless otherwise indicated, the patient should be in a recumbent position in order to promote relaxation; bolsters and pillows may be used as necessary. The therapist must assume a comfortable standing position that will allow easy access to the entire treatment area without undue movement and disruption of treatment. The height of the plinth should be appropriate to allow for good body mechanics of the therapist.

DRAPING. With only the part being treated exposed, the rest of the patient's body should be well covered for warmth as well as modesty. Tight clothing should be loosened, particularly proximal to the treatment area.

MASSAGE MEDIUM. Selection of a massage medium is dependent upon the therapeutic intent of treatment. In cases of muscle tightness and spasm or edema, a medium is necessary to allow the hands to slide smoothly over the skin and to avoid abrasions of the skin and pulling of the hair. Mineral oil, glycerin, coconut oil, cocoa butter, Nivea cream or oil, and powder are all appropriate. Standard hand lotions are absorbed too quickly into the skin, necessitating reapplication part way through treatment. If the treatment objective is to loosen scar tissue of skin, fascia, or subcutaneous tissue, or to prevent or break up adhesions in musculoskeletal tissue, no medium is used so that the therapist's fingers and the patient's skin move as one over underlying structures.

Components of Massage

The components of massage (Table 1) are rhythm and rate, pressure, direction, and duration of the movements to be employed. In addition, frequency of application must also be considered. Components are determined by the specific therapeutic intent of the procedure employed. They must be differentiated

---

Table 14-1
Components of Massage

Therapeutic Intent	Rate and Rhythm	Pressure	Direction	Duration
General relaxation/sedative effect	Slow speed, even rhythm	Light to medium	Trunk—follow direction of muscle fibers Extremities—centripetal	Dependent upon size of area to be treated; full back massage, 10 minutes minimum
Decrease muscle spasm/tightness	Slow speed, even rhythm	Begin light, move to deeper movements, end light	Parallel to direction of muscle fibers, deep circulation over trigger points	Dependent upon size of area to be treated, *e.g.,* low back or neck and upper back, 10 minutes
Reduce edema	Slow speed, even rhythm	Moderate to deep	Centripetal; treat proximal segment first	Dependent upon size of area
Loosen/stretch fascia	Slow to moderate speed, even rhythm	Moderate	All directions	Dependent upon size of area
Prevent or break up adhesions in ligaments, tendons, and muscle	Moderate speed, even rhythm	Heavy	Perpendicular to direction of fibers	15 minutes per involved structure
Stretch scar of skin and subcutaneous tissue	Moderate speed, even rhythm	Moderate to heavy	Circular and all directions	5 minutes minimum

from generalized approaches associated with different schools of thought.

RHYTHM AND RATE. The rhythm of massage movements should be even. Rate may vary, but in general terms, massage given to achieve a relaxation effect or to reduce edema should be slow and may match the patient's respiratory rate. The rate can be faster when applying friction massage to stretch or loosen adhesions in superficial or deep structures.

PRESSURE. The amount of pressure applied is critical to achieving the desired results in any technique. A sedative or relaxation effect is obtained with light to medium pressure. The amount of pressure may vary during the treatment of muscle tightness, starting out light, then deepening over painful areas and finishing light again. In order to have any mechanical effect on adhesions, pressure must be sufficiently strong to both stabilize as well as distort appropriate structures.

DIRECTION. Knowledge of anatomy and kinesiology is imperative when deciding upon the appropriate direction of massage movements. The most commonly employed direction of movement is centripetal (toward the heart) and parallel to the muscle fibers when the objective is relaxation or reduction of edema. When treating fibrotic areas, the movement must apply tractive forces to the involved structures. Pressure must therefore be applied in the direction of restriction. For detection of fibrositic nodules and the prevention and treatment of adhesions in soft tissue, deep friction must be carried out perpendicular to the direction of the affected fibers and specifically applied at the site of pathology.[29]

DURATION AND FREQUENCY. The duration of any massage technique is dependent upon the size of the area to be treated, the pathology involved, and the tolerance of the patient. Frequency of application is the least understood and most controversial of all components. There is wide variation of appropriate frequency reported in the literature.[126a] In general, if the appropriate therapeutic results are achieved, declining frequency over a course of treatment is appropriate.

Effects of Massage

The effects of massage can be best understood as having both physiological and psychological components. In addition, physiological effects can be either mechanical or reflexive in nature. Although they are discussed separately, all effects are highly interactive.

Physiological Effects

MECHANICAL. The mechanical effects of massage applied to the peripheral vascular system have been clearly demonstrated. Applying external pressures to an edematous extremity in the appropriate direction will assist in venous blood return, whereas massage in general will have a substantial effect on improving blood flow to a normal extremity only if the massage is vigorous and of long duration. Wakim and associates,[120] in their study of circulatory changes following massage, concluded that "there is a moderate, consistent and definite increase in circulation after deep stroking and kneading massage to the extremities of subjects who have flaccid paralysis." However, they noted no consistent changes in blood flow in the contralateral extremities. Increases in superficial blood flow are easily observable, as evidenced by hyperemia of the skin following massage. This response could be due to stimulation of mast cells, which produce a histaminelike substance which causes vasodilation of superficial arterioles. Another contributing factor may be the mechanical stimulation of sensory endings, which causes a reflex response mediated by the spinal cord.[1, 126b] These factors demonstrate the interactive nature of the physiological consequences of massage. However, the lymphatic system is passive and solely dependent on external forces such as muscle action to create flow of lymph. Bauer and associates[2] demonstrated that proteins injected into the joints of dogs were removed by the lympathic system and that massage and passive exercise accelerated this process. It is well accepted that compression, whether applied manually or with pneumatic devices, combined with elevation of the part to be treated is effective in treating lymphedema.[132]

Tissue healing and repair processes associated with the musculoskeletal system often create secondary pathology with the formation of adhesions of muscle to fascia, tendon to tendon sheath, or skin to underlying tissue. Friction massage has often been employed successfully in this type of problem. The specific limited approach of cross-fiber light friction massage has often been used to prevent adhesions in the acute stage of injury. Deep friction to break up cross linkages of fibrous material in the subacute and chronic stages of musculoskeletal injury has also been employed with clinical effectiveness.[29] Despite many claims that have been made, there is no evidence that massage will have any effect on obesity, muscle mass, muscle strength, or the rate of atrophy of denervated muscle.[126b]

Percussion massage movements as used in chest physical therapy apply sufficient mechanical forces to the thorax to loosen and mobilize secretions in the lungs. When applied in combination with the forces of gravity, this is an effective means to prevent respiratory complications following surgery as well as to treat pulmonary conditions once they have occurred.[14]

REFLEXIVE. Reflexive effects may be best explained as those related to changes in electrical threshold and activity associated with the neurological system. Modern scientific inquiry has expanded this concept to include the central, autonomic, and peripheral nervous systems as well as the gamma motor system. In addition, massage produces increased perspiration and secretion of the sebaceous glands. Barr and Taslet[1] in their study of the autonomic responses to back massage in normal subjects concluded that an increase of sympathetic activity occurred during massage as measured by delayed increase in systolic blood pressure, increased heart rate, sweat gland activity, peripheral skin temperature, body temperature, and decreased respiration rate. The extensive work of Dicke[35] on her system of connective tissue massage is based entirely on the premise that there are reflex zones close to the surface of the body (specifically in the connective tissue lying between skin and muscle) which, when disrupted, diseased, or shortened, can have a distinct effect on visceral organs. The much reported and observable sedative or general relaxation effects of slowly administered massage are considered a reflex response, but this is difficult to separate from the psychodynamics that may arise from "laying on of the hands."

Recent clinical applications of massage have been based on the purported physiological effects of massage on the gamma motor system. Some emphasis has been placed on stimulating Golgi tendon organs through deep pressure and on changing resting length of muscle spindles through manipulative means.[4] For example, massage has been used as a vehicle to enhance trunk flexion by relaxation of back extensors and other muscles.[95] Massage has also been applied to the hamstring muscle group to achieve recumbent straight leg raising.[25]

Psychological Effects

There is no doubt that patients highly value massage as part of their treatment. There are those patients who have a tendency to become dependent on massage, but they may be exhibiting a dependency on individual attention and contact with another person interested in their welfare and not on the massage itself.

Our current psychological understanding of massage indicates that it is best viewed at three levels:

1. The physical act of touching another individual
2. The symbolic meaning of one person entering into another person's "life space"
3. The specific individualized response based upon values and past experience of the patient

The practitioner must consider the variables at each level with regard to the psychological outcomes of treatment. The mere process of being touched by another human being may produce a withdrawal response in some patients. Within the patient–therapist relationship, trust, mutual respect, and an appreciation for personal sensitivities will maximize the physiological results of treatment. More intrinsically, it is important to recognize that human contact in our society occurs under rather specific circumstances often associated with life stages. Maternal nurturing, previous health care experiences, conflict involving bodily harm, sexual activity, and recreation including contact sports, all may shape the patient's response to massage.

Techniques of Massage

A therapeutic approach is composed of a body of knowledge and associated techniques, which have sufficient commonality to be considered a school of thought. *Technique* is defined as an appropriate method of applying a therapeutic procedure. To be considered a legitimate treatment modality, a therapeutic technique must have an appropriate theoretical rationale. Given the previous review of the historical development of massage, it is not surprising that therapeutic approaches can be conveniently categorized into Eastern and Western traditions. Although there are noteworthy exceptions, the main thrust of the Western tradition is the use of mechanical means for intervention in the musculoskeletal and peripheral vascular systems. The Eastern tradition heavily emphasizes attempts to affect the neurological system. The efficacy of a particular approach to massage is judged differently depending upon the cultural milieu in which it is found. Eastern culture places high value on acceptance of tradition and reported effectiveness over continued use. In contrast, Western physicians demand scientific proof of effectiveness prior to widespread adoption. The theory and practice of the major therapeutic approaches are summarized below.

Western Massage

The four approaches to massage in current use in the Western hemisphere are classical massage, cross-fiber (transverse) friction massage, connective tissue massage, and soft tissue mobilization.

CLASSICAL MASSAGE. The most well known massage movements are those that involve stroking and gliding (effleurage), kneading (petrissage), and percussion (tapotement) to soft tissues of the body. Friction massage may also be included in this category, since it has been a long-standing method for releasing fibrotic tissue. The classical approach is one of blending the various strokes just mentioned to achieve the physiological effects pertinent to the individual patient problem being treated.

Stroking, gliding, and friction movements are particularly helpful in the detection of abnormal tone or a painful area that might require further attention. Stroking has an added effect of muscle relaxation (Fig. 14-3). Kneading consists of alternately compressing and releasing muscle tissue to assist in the removal of unwanted fluid and waste products. This is done in an attempt to simulate muscle pump action. Percussion in the form of sudden forces applied to a body part is most commonly used in chest physical therapy in the United States; clapping with cupped hands is applied to the thorax to loosen and mobilize secretions in the lungs. For maximal effectiveness of percussion, the exact location of congestion must be known and the patient must be positioned correctly to allow gravity to assist in draining the involved segments of the lungs. The value of this treatment in respiratory care is well respected.[14] Percussion in the form of tapping is also useful in desensitizing operative sites in the rehabilitation of amputees. Whenever it is necessary to loosen or break up adhesions of healed scar tissue, friction massage is indicated. This can be applied with the fingertips moving in circular motions with pressure dependent upon the depths of the affected tissue. The intent is to move superficial tissue of the underlying structure, which requires that the therapist's fingers and the patient's skin move as one. Classical massage is perhaps the most widely accepted approach in current practice. Excellent texts are available with detailed descriptions of each of these movements.[115a, 126]

CROSS-FIBER FRICTION MASSAGE. Deep friction massage was promoted first by Storms in the treatment of fibrositic nodules with the strong pressure applied parallel to the muscle fibers.[115a] The specific limited approach of deep friction massage

Figure 14-3. Stroking massage movements in the directions shown can aid in muscle relaxation.

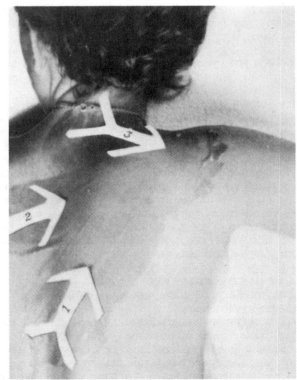

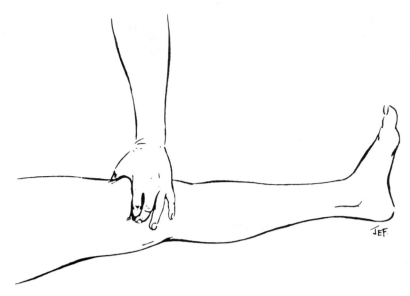

Figure 14-4.   Deep friction massage is applied across the medial collateral ligament with knee in extension. The purpose is to prevent adhesions from forming and limiting movement.

is applied transversely across the fibers of muscle, tendon, or ligament (Fig. 14-4). This technique prevents adhesions in the acute stage and breaks up adhesions in the subacute and chronic stages of injury to these tissues. Cross-fiber friction massage is a component of the approach introduced by Cyriax.[29] The therapeutic focus is to intervene in the body's repair process of contractile and noncontractile tissue to ensure full freedom of movement of the involved structures and the restoration of function. Maximal effectiveness depends on an accurate diagnosis of the exact location of pathology, pressures of sufficient depth and breadth to reach the involved structures, and massage movement applied perpendicular to the long axis of the fibers of the structure under treatment. Although this technique has a reasonable histological basis,[13] there are no data available in the literature which document clinical effectiveness. Nevertheless, cross-fiber friction massage continues to gain popularity in the United States.

CONNECTIVE TISSUE MASSAGE (BINDEGEWEBSMASSAGE). The cutaneovisceral reflex was reported and described in Germany by Dicke during the first part of this century. Specific strokes are applied to reach the connective tissue underlying the skin with the intent of affecting organs whose innervation corresponds to cutaneous dermatomes. This method is applied strictly to facilitate changes in autonomic nervous system activity. Connective tissue massage in the strictest sense is not commonly used in the United States, although, it continues to be popular in Europe. The few studies that have been reported in the literature are contradictory with regard to effect.[42, 88, 107] Its purported influence on the nervous system resembles that of Eastern methods. However, the lack of data to support peripheral manipulation of the nervous system producing visceral effects places this approach in a similar category as various schools of chiropractic.

SOFT TISSUE MOBILIZATION.   Soft tissue mobilization is defined as "the forceful passive movement of the muscle-fascial system element through its restrictive direction beginning with the superficial layers and progressing into depth while taking into accord the relationship of the joints concerned."[53] This approach is unique in two ways. It may be the first system to have originated in the United States, and it also has the therapeutic intent of impacting on the nervous and musculoskeletal systems simultaneously by incorporating movement and joint position

with the basic application of connective tissue massage techniques.

It differs from most approaches to massage in that it places fascia and muscle in an elongated rather than a relaxed or shortened position. This achieves multiple therapeutic outcomes, including surface exposure of the tissue to be treated, elongation of connective tissue, and change in the resting length of muscle. It therefore simultaneously incorporates the principles of massage, manipulation, and therapeutic exercise. Although it is not yet cited in the literature, this approach is being widely disseminated by workshops held throughout the United States.

Eastern

The Eastern view of medicine was shaped by the ancient Chinese cultures, presumably originating from folk medicine. The Eastern concept of human physiology and function is quite divergent from the Western orientation. For example, the Chinese believe that normalization of the flow of life forces along meridians is the key to alleviating disease and disability. Through systematic observation, they identified cutaneous points along meridians that become highly sensitive when illness or dysfunction occurs. Eastern massage specifically targets the cutaneovisceral reflex as the mechanism of intervention, and in this respect it closely resembles connective tissue massage.

ACUPRESSURE.   Travell introduced the concept of trigger points in the treatment of myofascial syndromes in the middle of this century.[117] The term *trigger point* is widely accepted in current practice. Trigger points are considered to be discrete, hypersensitive areas found primarily in muscle but also in other connective tissue. These predictable points on the skin have a measurable decreased resistance to the passage of an electrical current.[86] The histological basis for this phenomenon is hypothesized but not yet known. It is interesting to note that 71% of the time, the locations of acupuncture points correspond with trigger points, motor points, or a superficial peripheral nerve trunk.[86] Acupressure can be considered a noninvasive version of acupuncture; instead of inserting needles at specific points on the body as in acupuncture, sustained deep pressure is applied by the fingertips. The practice of applying an external stimulus to specific points of the body is not new to Western medicine.

Current practice includes treatment of these areas with a variety of modalities including heat, cold, ultrasound, and electrical stimulation. For example, acupuncture points are commonly chosen as electrode placement sites in the application of TENS. There continues to be a slowly growing interest and acceptance of this approach to massage.

REFLEXOLOGY AND AURICULOTHERAPY. Reflexology and auriculotherapy are based again on the cutaneovisceral reflex phenomenon and are in reality specific applications of acupressure. The Chinese believe that the total body is represented cutaneously on the sole of the foot, the ear, the eye, and the palm of the hand.[115a] Reflexology and aurioculotherapy involve the application of deep finger pressure over points that correspond with identified organ dysfunction on the sole of the foot or the ear, respectively. The Japanese equivalent of this treatment is called shiatsu. These approaches are not well accepted or used in current Western medical practice. However, there remains the possibility that the functional organization of the nervous system is distinct from its structural organization and that discrete functional entry points into the nervous system exist.

Indications for Massage

Therapeutic benefits can be expected of massage when it is used appropriately to accomplish the following objectives:

- Reduction of excessive fluids in interstitial spaces or joints
- Increased circulation to paralyzed musculature
- Restoration of tight muscles to normal resting length
- Mobilization of tissues which are abnormally adhered to surrounding structures
- Increased tolerance of tissues to pressure
- Relief of pain
- Specific and general relaxation
- Enhanced psychological well-being

Massage is best used in combination with other modalities designed to reduce pain, promote healing, and restore function.

Contraindications

The use of massage should be limited when its known therapeutic effects would be harmful for a particular patient condition. Adverse reactions can be expected under three different types of circumstances: (1) when massage is medically contraindicated, (2) when the particular technique is inappropriate for the condition being treated, or (3) when an appropriate technique is incorrectly applied. For example, massage is medically contraindicated over malignancies, open wounds, thrombophlebitis, and infected tissues. An inappropriate massage technique can be damaging if applied to calcified soft tissue, skin which has undergone trophic changes, skin grafts, tissue which is acutely inflamed, or during anticoagulant therapy. Nerve damage has been reported[43] when acupressure was applied too vigorously, resulting in peripheral nerve compression from hematoma formation. Judicious attention must be given to the potential consequences of any massage technique prior to its application.

Research Trends in Massage

A paucity of research on massage leaves much to be done to determine its appropriate application and clinical effectiveness. The interaction between psychosocial and physiologic compo-

nents presents a considerable challenge in the pursuit of definitive scientific support of various therapeutic approaches and associated techniques. Like many of the healing arts, the clinical effectiveness of massage may well depend not so much on scientific supportive evidence as on the belief of the practitioner in the value of the approach and his skill in applying it. Nevertheless, recent scientific inquiry appears to fall into the following five categories.

Therapeutic Effects

These studies attempt to define the physiological effects of massage on various biological systems. Examples include the positive effect of massage on enhancing muscle length[25, 95] as well as increased circulation in paralyzed musculature.[120] Massage has been demonstrated to be effective in significantly increasing the excretion of neurohormones in the urine of patients with lymphedema without significant changes in blood composition.[77] In addition, significant changes in sympathetic activity have been demonstrated following massage to the low back.[1]

In general, studies in this category are confined to only one biological system. The effects of massage on multiple biological systems remain obscure. Current trends in this category appear to be directed toward determining the histological basis of specific techniques[13] rather than effects on interacting biological systems.

A recurring theme appearing in the literature related to massage is the call for renewed investigative attention to therapeutic effectiveness.[3, 104, 124] This call should not be taken lightly. In the current socioeconomic climate surrounding health care, the continued use of massage will be threatened unless both therapeutic efficacy and cost effectiveness can be demonstrated.

Application to Specific Pathological Conditions

A major thrust of studies concerning specific pathological conditions has been in the area of psychosomatic phenomena. Massage has been shown to be effective in the treatment of anxiety disorders.[88] No evidence has been found for reduction of symptoms in its application for bronchial asthma.[107] Concurrent attention has been given to musculoskeletal pathology. An important study has shown that massage is capable of increasing plasma levels of myoglobin associated with reduced tension levels in cases of fibrositis.[33] Some preliminary work has been reported on the effects of massage on the reduction of limb pain that was unrelieved by surgical sympathectomy.[42]

Contraindications

Contraindications have received the least amount of research activity. The absence of studies is not surprising as contraindicated procedures cannot be applied to human subjects without risk of adverse effects. Extrapolated approaches using normal subjects are potentially valuable. An example of this methodology is the use of normal subjects exposed to whole body massage with the subsequent determination of increased serum enzyme levels associated with stressed muscle metabolism known to be damaging in patients with dermatomyositis.[42]

Mechanical Versus Manual Techniques

Such studies investigate the outcomes of different massage techniques on a single pathological condition. An outstanding example of this type of study was done on the effects of three different massage techniques, two mechanical and one manual, on edema reduction for post-mastectomy patients.[132] The results indicated that both pneumatic massage with uniform pressure and manual massage produce a statistically significant permanent reduction in edema in this patient population. Pneumatic pressure-wave was not effective. Additional measurements of subjective patient responses by use of a visual analogue scale and self-scoring mood questionnaire were consistent with objective findings. This study demonstrated that both mechanical and manual applications of massage can have similar therapeutic outcomes. In addition, the methodology employed in the above study provides a means of differentiating between the physiological and psychosocial components contributing to massage effectiveness.

Relationship to Other Modalities

Massage is rarely prescribed independent of other therapeutic interventions. The comparative effects of massage and other treatment modalities assessed separately or interactively are therefore important areas for scientific inquiry. Examples of both types of inquiry appear in the literature. For example, TENS was shown to be more effective than gentle mechanical massage in relieving pain in low back syndromes as measured by a standardized pain assessment tool and straight leg raising.[90] An interesting interactive effect of massage applied concurrently with ice demonstrated no effects on relief of delayed muscle soreness following exercise.[130] A major deficiency of such studies is that they are often not designed to show both main effects as well as interactive effects of the treatment modalities employed.

Research on massage has been broad-based, but not of sufficient depth to provide conclusive evidence of its effectiveness. Creative research methodologies need to be employed to better ascertain the relationship between the contributions of psychosocial and physiological factors to the efficacy of massage. Given the limitations of clinical research in today's health care environment, greater attention needs to be given to case study reports and single subject research designs.

REFERENCES

1. Barr J, Taslet N: The influence of back massage on autonomic functions. Phys Ther 50:1679–1691, 1970
2. Bauer N, Short L, Bennet G: The manner of removal of proteins from normal joints. J Exp Med 57:419, 1933
3. Bell A: Massage and the physical therapist. Physiother 406–408, December, 1964
4. Binder MD, Houk JC, Nichols TP et al: Properties and segmental actions of mammalian muscle receptors: An update. Fed Proc 41:2907–2918, 1982
5. Bork K, Korting G, Faust G: Das Verhalten einiger Serumenzyme nach Ganzkorpermuskelmassage. Arch Derm Frosch 240:342–348, 1971
6. Bourdillon JF: Spinal manipulation, 3rd ed. New York, Appleton-Century-Crofts, 1983
7. Bowles CH: Functional technique: A modern perspective. J Am Osteopath Assoc 80:326–331, 1981
8. Brandt B, Jones LH: Some methods of applying counterstrain. J Am Osteopath Assoc 75:786–788, 1976
9. Brodin H, Bang J, Bechgarrd P et al: Manipulation AV Ryggraden, as reported by Nwuga VC: Manipulation of the Spine. Baltimore, Williams & Wilkins, 1974
10. Brunarski DJ: Clinical trials of spinal manipulation: A critical appraisal and review of the literature. J Manipulative Physiol Ther 7:243–249, 1984
11. Buerger AA, Greenman PE (ed): Validation of Spinal Manipulation. Springfield, Charles C Thomas, 1985
12. Cassidy JD, Kirkaldy-Willis WH, McGregor M: Spinal manipulation of chronic low back and leg pain: An observational study. In

13. Buerger AA, Greenman PE (eds): Validation of Spinal Manipulation, pp 119–148. Springfield, Ill, Charles C Thomas, 1985
14. Chamberlain G: Cyriax's friction massage: A review. J Orthop Sp Phys Ther 4:16–22, 1982
15. Cherniak R, Cherniak L, Naimakr A: Respiration in Health and Disease, 2nd ed, p 452. Philadelphia, WB Saunders, 1972
16. Christie BGB: Discussion on the treatment of backache by traction. Proc R Soc Med 48:811–814, 1955
17. Colachis SC, Strohm BR: A study of tractive forces and angle of pull on vertebral interspaces in the cervical spine. Arch Phys Med Rehabil 46:820–830, 1965
18. Colachis SC, Strohm BR: Radiographic studies of cervical spine motion in normal subjects; Flexion and hyperextension. Arch Phys Med Rehabil 46:753–760, 1965
19. Colachis SC, Strohm BR: Relationship of time to varied tractive force with constant angle of pull. Arch Phys Med Rehabil 46:815–819, 1965
20. Colachis SC, Strohm BR: Effect of duration of intermittent cervical traction on vertebral separation. Arch Phys Med Rehabil 47:353–359, 1966
21. Colachis SC, Strohm BR: Effects of intermittent traction on separation of lumbar vertebrae. Arch Phys Med Rehabil 50:251–258, 1969
22. Coote JH: Somatic sources of afferent input as factors in aberrant autonomic sensory and motor function. In Korr IM (ed): Neurobiologic Mechanisms in Manipulative Therapy, pp 91–111. New York, Plenum, 1978
23. Cornelius A: Die Nervenpunktlehr. Leipzig, 1909
24. Cornelius A: Die Nervenpunkte. Munich, JF Lehman, 1933
25. Coxhead CE, Inskip H, Meade PW et al: Multi center trial of physiotherapy in the management of sciatic symptoms. Lancet 1:1065–1068, 1981
26. Crossman L, Chateauvert S, Weisberg J: The effects of massage to the hamstring muscle group on range of motion. J Orthop Sp Phys Ther 6:168–172, 1984
27. Crue BL: Importance of flexion in cervical traction for radiculitis. US Air Force Med J 8:374–380, 1957
28. Crue BL: Importance of flexion in cervical halter traction. Bull Los Angeles Neurol Soc 30:95–98, 1965
29. Cyriax JH: Conservative treatment of lumbar disk lesions. Physiotherapy 50:300–303, 1964
30. Cyriax J: Textbook of Orthopaedic Medicine, 7th ed. Great Britain, Cassell, 1979
31. Cyriax JH: Textbook of Orthopaedic Medicine, Diagnosis of Soft Tissue Lesions, 8th ed. London, Balliere Tindall, 1982
32. Cyriax JH: Textbook of Orthopaedic Medicine, Treatment by Manipulation, Massage and Injection, 10th ed. London, Balliere Tindall, 1982
33. Cyriax J: Textbook of Orthopaedic Medicine, vol II, 2nd ed. London, Bailliere Tindall, 1984
34. Danneskiold B, Christiansen E, Lund B, Anderson R: Regional muscle tension and pain. Scand J Rehab Med 15:17–20, 1982
35. De Seze S, Levernieux J: Pratique rheumatologies des tractions vertebrales. Sem Hop Paris 27:2085–2104, 1951
36. Dicke E: Meine Bindegewebsmassage, Stuttgart, Hippokrates, 1953; 8th ed, 1975
37. Dvorak J: Neurological and biomechanical aspects of back pain. In Buerger AA, Greenman PE (eds): In Validation of Spinal Manipulation, pp 241–266. Springfield, Ill, Charles C Thomas, 1985
38. Dvorak J, Dvorak V, Schneider W (eds): Manual Medicine. Berlin, Springer-Verlag, 1984
39. Ebner M: Connective tissue massage. Physother 64(7):208–210, 1978
40. Evans DP: The design and results of clinical trials of lumbar manipulation: A review. In Buerger AA, Greenman PE (eds): Validation of Spinal Manipulation, pp 228–238. Springfield, Ill, Charles C Thomas, 1985
41. Fielding JW: Cineroentgenography of the normal cervical spine. J Bone Joint Surg 39:1280–1288, 1957
42. Fisk JW: The painful neck and back. Springfield, Ill, Charles C Thomas, 1977
43. Frazer F: Persistent post sympathetic pain treated by connective tissue massage. Physiother 64(7):211–212, 1978

43. Geiringer S, Leonard J: Posterior interosseous palsy after dental treatment: A case report. Arch Phys Med Rehabil 66:711–712, 1985

44. Gianakopoulos G, Waylonis GW, Grant PA et al: Inversion devices: Their role in producing lumbar distraction. Arch Phys Med Rehabil 66:100-102, 1985

45. Gitelman R: A chiropractic approach to biomechanical disorders of the lumbar spine and pelvis. In Haldeman S (ed): Modern Developments in the Principles and Practice of Chiropractic, pp 297–330. Norwalk, Conn, Appleton-Century-Crofts, 1984

46. Godfrey CM, Morgan PP, Schatzken J: A randomized trial of manipulation for low back pain in a medical setting. Spine 9:301–304, 1984

47. Goodridge JP: Muscle energy technique: Definition, explanation, methods of procedure. J Am Osteopath Assoc 81:249–252, 1981

48. Gorman RF: Cardiac arrest after cervical mobilization. Med J Aust 2:169, 1978

49. Graham D: Massage, Manual Treatment and Remedial Movements. Philadelphia, JB Lippincott, 1902

50. Green RM (trans): Asclepides: His life and writings. New Haven, E Licht, 1955

51. Grice AS: A biomechancial approach to cervical and dorsal adjusting. In Haldeman S (ed): Modern Developments in the Principles and Practice of Chiropractic, pp 331–358. Norwalk, Conn, Appleton-Century-Crofts, 1984

52. Grieve GP: Mobilization of the spine, 3rd ed. Edinburgh, Churchill Livingstone, 1979

53. Grodin A: Personal communication with Alan Grodin of the Center for Orthopedic Rehabilitation, Atlanta, Georgia

54. Haldeman S: Spinal manipulative therapy in the management of low back pain. In Finneson BE (ed): Low Back Pain, 2nd ed, pp 245–275. Philadelphia, JB Lippincott, 1980

55. Haldeman S: The neurophysiology of spinal pain syndromes. In Haldeman (ed): Modern Developments in the Principles and Practice of Chiropractic, pp 119–142. Norwalk, Conn, Appleton-Century-Crofts, 1980

56. Hippocrates: Deuvres complete d'hippocrat. Littre E (ed). Paris, 1861

57. Hood LB, Chrisman D: Intermittent pelvic traction in the treatment of the ruptured intervertebral disk. Phys Ther 48:21–30, 1968

58. Hooper J: Low back pain and manipulation paraparesis after treatment of low back pain by physical methods. Med J Aust 1:549–551, 1973

59. Hubbard RP, Chun KJ: Repeated extensions of collagenous tissue—measured responses and medical implications. Proceedings of the Twelfth Annual Northeast Bioengineering Conference, pp 157–160, New Haven, 1986

60. Jackson R: The Cervical Syndrome, 2nd ed. Springfield, Charles C Thomas, 1958

61. Janse J: History of the development of chiropractic concepts; Chiropractic terminology. In Goldstein M (ed): The Research Status of Spinal Manipulative Therapy, pp 25–42. Bethesda, DHEW Publication No (NIH) 76–998, 1975

62. Jones LJ: Strain and counterstrain. Colorado Springs, Am Acad Osteopathy, 1981

63. Jones MD: Cineradiographic studies of the normal cervical spine. Calif Med 93:293–296, 1960

64. Judovich BD: Herniated cervical disk; A new form of traction therapy. Am J Surg 84:646–656, 1952

65. Judovich BD: Lumbar traction therapy—Elimination of physical factors that prevent lumbar stretch. JAMA 159:549–550, 1955

66. Kaltenborn FM: Mobilization of the extremity joints. OSLO, OLAF Norlis, 1980

67. Kappler RE: Direct action techniques. J of Amer Osterpathic Assn. 81:239–243, 1981

68. Kellogg JH: The Art of Massage: Its Physiological Effects and Therapeutic Applications. Battle Creek, 1895; 12th ed, 1919

69. Kimberly PE: Formulating a prescription for osteopathic manipulative treatment. J Am Osteopath Assoc 79:506–513, 1980

70. Kirkaldy-Willis WH: Manipulation. In Kirkaldy-Willis WH (ed): Managing Low Back Pain. New York, Churchill-Livingstone, 1983

71. Kleynhans AM: Complications and contraindications to spinal manipulative therapy. In Haldeman S (ed): Modern Developments in the Principles and Practice of Chiropractic, pp 359–384. Norwalk, Conn, Appleton-Century-Crofts, 1980

72. Korr IM: Neural basis of the osteopathic lesion. J Am Osteopath Assoc 47:191–198, 1947

73. Korr IM: Proprioceptors and somatic dysfunction. J Am Osteopath Assoc 74:638–650, 1985

74. Korr IM: Somatic dysfunction, osteopathic manipulative treatment, and the nervous system: A few facts, some theories, many questions. J Am Osteopath Assoc 86:109–114, 1986

75. Kottke FJ, Mundale MO: Range of mobility of the cervical spine. Arch Phys Med 40:379–382, 1959

76. Krueger BR, Okazaki H: Vertebral-basilar distribution infarction following chiropractic cervical manipulation. Mayo Clinic Proc 55:322–332, 1980

77. Kurz W, Kurz R, Litmanovich Y et al: Effect of manual lymph-drainage massage on blood components and urinary neurohormones in chronic lymphadema. Angiol 32(2):119–27, 1981

78. Laban MM, Meerschaert JR: Quadriplegia following cervical traction in patients with occult epidural prostatic metastasis. Arch Phys Med Rehabil 56:455–458, 1975

79. Lawson GA, Godfrey CM: A report on studies of spinal traction. Med Services J Can 14:762–771, 1958

80. Lehmann JF, Brunner GD: A device for application of heavy lumbar traction; Its mechanical effects. Arch Phys Med Rehabil 39:696–700, 1958

81. Lewitt K: Manipulative Therapy in Rehabilitation of the Motor System. London, Butterworths, 1985

82. Ling PH: The Gymnastic Free Exercise. Georgii (ed). Boston, Tichnor, Reed and Fields, 1853

83. Maigne R: Manipulation of the spine. In Basmajian JV (ed): Manipulation, Traction and Massage, 3rd ed. Baltimore, Williams & Wilkins, 1985

84. Maigne R: Orthopedic Medicine. Springfield, Ill, Charles C Thomas, 1972

85. Maitland GD: Vertebral Manipulation, 4th ed. London, Butterworths, 1977

86. Mannheimer J, Lampe G: Clinical Transcutaneous Nerve Stimulation, p 269. Philadelphia, FA Davis, 1984

87. Mara JR: Gravity inversion. Aches Pains 4:6–12, 1983

88. McKechie A, Wilson F, Watson N, Scott D: Anxiety states: A preliminary report on the value of connective tissue massage. J Psychosom Res 27:125–129, 1983

89. Mckenzie RA: The Lumbar Spine. Walkanae, New Zealand, Spinal Publications, 1981

90. Melzak R, Vetere P, Finch L: Trancutaneous electrical nerve stimulation for low back pain: A comparison of TENS and massage for pain and range of motion. Phys Ther 63:489–493, 1983

91. Mennell JM: Back Pain. Boston, Little, Brown & Co, 1960

92. Miller WD: Treatment of visceral disorders by manipulative therapy. In Goldstein M (ed): The Research Status of Spinal Manipulative Therapy, pp 295–301. Bethesda, DHEW Publication # (NIH) 76–998, 1975

93. Mitchell FL, Moran PS, Pruzzo NA: Evaluation and Treatment Manual of Osteopathic Muscle Energy Technique. Kansas City, Moran & Pruzzo, 1979

94. Neuman HD: A concept of manual medicine. In Buerger AA, Greenman PE (eds): Validation of Spinal Manipulation, pp 267–272. Springfield, Ill, Charles C Thomas, 1985

95. Nordshaw M, Bierman W: The influence of manual massage on muscle relaxation: Effect on trunk flexion. Phys Ther 42:653–657, 1962

96. Nwuga VC: Manipulation of the Spine. Baltimore, Williams & Wilkins, 1976

97. Nyberg R: Role of therapists in spinal manipulation. In Basmajian JV (ed): Manipulation, Traction and Massage, 3rd ed, pp 22–46. Baltimore, Williams & Wilkins, 1985

98. Pare A: Ouevres Completes. Paris, JB Balliere, 1941

99. Paterson JK, Burn L: An Introduction to Medical Manipulation. Lancaster, MTP Press, 1985

100. Patterson MM: Louisa Burns Memorial Lecture 1980: The spinal cord—Active processor not passive transmitter. J Am Osteopath Assoc 80:210–216, 1980

101. Payson SM, Holloway HS: Possible complications of using naloxone as an internal opiate antagonist in the investigation of the role of endorphins in osteopathic manipulative treatment. J AM Osteopath Assoc (suppl) 84:152–156, 1984

102. Peltier LF: A brief history of traction. J Bone Joint Surg (AM) 50:1603–1617, 1968

103. Rasmussen TG: Manipulation in treatment of low back pain (a randomized clinical trial). Manuelle Med 1:8–10, 1978

104. Reiter S, Garrett T, Erickson D: Current trends in the use of therapeutic massage. Phys Ther 49:158–161, 1969

105. Rettig H: Observation of an acute basilar syndrome after chiropractic treatment of the cervical spine. Med Klin 26:1528, 1955

106. Richard J: Disk rupture with cauda equina syndrome after chiropractic adjustment. NY State J Med 67:2496–2498, 1967

107. Robertson A, Gilmore K, Froth P, Antic R: Effects of connective tissue massage in subacute asthma. Med J Aust, Jan 7, 1984

108. Rogoff JB: Motorized intermittent traction. In Basmajian JV (ed): Manipulation, Traction and Massage, 3rd ed, pp 201–207. Baltimore, Williams & Wilkins, 1985

109. Sato A: Physiological studies of the somato-autonomic reflexes. In Haldeman S (ed): Modern Developments in the Principles and Practice of Chiropractic, pp 91–105. Norwalk, Conn, Appleton-Century-Crofts, 1985

110. Sherman DG, Hart RG, Easton JD: Abrupt change in head position and cerebral infarction. Stroke 12(1):2–6, 1981

111. Stedman's Medical Dictionary, 2nd ed, p 1315. Baltimore, Williams & Wilkins, 1972

112. Stillwell GK, deLateur BJ, Geiringer SR et al: Physiatric therapeutics. In Self-Directed Medical Knowledge Program in Physical Medicine and Rehabilitation, syllabus. American Academy of Physical Medicine and Rehabilitation, 1986

113. Stoddard A: Manual of Osteopathic Practice, 2nd ed. New York, Harper & Row, 1969

114. Tanigawa MC: Comparison of the hold relax procedure in passive mobilization on increasing muscle length. Phys Ther 32:725–735, 1972

115. Tappan F: Healing Massage Techniques, pp 7(a), 23(b), 140(c). Reston, Virginia, Reston Publishing, 1980

116. Tobis JS, Hoehler F: Musculoskeletal Manipulation. Springfield, Ill, Charles C Thomas, 1986

117. Travell J: Myofascial Pain and Dysfunction. Baltimore, Williams & Wilkins, 1983

118. Upledger JE, Vredevoogd JD: Craniosacral Therapy. Chicago, Eastland Press, 1983

119. Viidik A: Biomechanical behavior of soft connective tissues. In Akkas N (ed): Progress in Biomechanics, pp 75–113. Alphen Aan Den Rijn, The Netherlands, Sijthoff & Noordhoff, 1979

120. Wakim K, Martin G, Terrier J et al: The effects of massage on the circulation on normal and paralyzed extremities. Arch Phys Med Rehabil 30:135–144, 1949

121. Ward RC: Myofascial Release Concepts and Treatment. East Lansing, Michigan State University, 1985

122. Weinberger LM: Trauma or treatment? The role of intermittent traction in the treatment of cervical soft tissue injuries. J Trauma 16:377–382, 1976

123. White AA, Panjabi MM: Clinical Biomechanics of the Spine. Philadelphia, JB Lippincott, 1978

124. Williams J: Physiotherapy is handling. Physiother 72:66–77, 1986

125. Wolff HD: The theory of joint play. In Greenman P (ed): Concepts and Mechanisms of Neuromuscular Functions. Berlin, Springer-Verlag, 1984

126. Wood E: Beard's Massage, Principles and Techniques, pp 30–35(a), 51–55(b). Philadelphia, WB Saunders, 1974

127. Worden RE, Humphrey TL: Effect of spinal traction on the length of the body. Arch Phys Med Rehabil 45:318–320, 1964

128. Wramner T: Observations on the symptoms and diagnosis of cervical rhizopathia and experience with vertebral traction. Acta Rheumatol Scand 3:108–114, 1957

129. Wyke B: The neurology of low back pain. In Jayson MIV (ed): Lumbar Spine and Back Pain, 2nd ed, pp 265–340. Kent, Pitman Medical, 1980

130. Yackzan L, Adams C, Francis K: The effects of ice massage on delayed muscle soreness. Am J Sports Med 12:159–164, 1984

131. Young K, Hubbard RP, Goodridge J, Rechtien J: Time scale of cervical thrust manipulation (to be published)

132. Zanolla R, Monzeglio C, Balzarini A, Martino G: Evaluation of the Results of Three Different Methods of Postmastectomy Lymphedema Treatment. J Surg Oncol 26:210–213, 1984

15

Functional Neuromuscular Stimulation

Robert J. Weber

Functional neuromuscular stimulation (FNS) is the use of electrical current to produce useful muscle contraction in paralyzed individuals. The methods of control, means, source, and target of stimulation change with the specific application.

FNS systems incorporate knowledge from many fields, including physiology, rehabilitation medicine, engineering, computer science, orthotics, and kinesiology. In addition, research groups have developed and combined components of varying sophistication into their work, so that the scientific merit of individual systems must often be evaluated component by component rather than by the total functional output. Techniques of control and stimulation are progressing rapidly, reflecting the contributions of the numerous investigators in the field. The proper medical application and benefit of these devices remain controversial, since not only technical effectiveness but also patient goals, societal values, and resources must be considered. This chapter will review the development of FNS, its current applications, hardware, and prospects.

HISTORY

Electricity, like many of the physical elements, has a long history of medical use. Man's first exposures to electrical forces were from lightning strikes and natural static electrical sparks. Since lightning was an impractical source of useful electrical force, the only controllable ancient electrical forces were static electricity (*e.g.,* wool and amber) or biological generators such as the torpedo fish, which provides a reliable, if exotic, safe source of electrical energy.

The application of electricity to medicine is recorded from about the beginning of the Christian era. Scribonius Largus, in his work *Compositiones Medicae,* A.D. 46, advocated treatment of gout and headache pain by application of the animal's electrical discharge.[35] Within 30 years, T. Diosconides, a Greek physician, had written of his doubts concerning the efficacy of the headache treatment, but proposed yet other, more exotic applications.[35] A pattern of cyclical popularity of medical electricity developed, which has been frequently repeated: discovery of an electrical "device"; advocation of medical applications (almost always to a chronic and discomforting, but not fatal, illness); a period of vogue followed by contrary opinion and eclipse; new application and eclipse; and finally, loss of interest in the device.

The rise of experimental science in the 18th century set this cycle into ever more rapid motion. Electrostatic generator development evolved through the 17th and early 18th centuries, with attendant attempts at medical application. With the development in 1745 of the Leyden jar, the forerunner of the modern capacitor (consisting of a glass jar lined both inside and out with metal foil), a powerful electrical charge could be accumulated, stored, and discharged at will. This force was capable of producing involuntary contraction of large muscle masses, and its use for treatment of paralysis became prominent in the literature of the day, as recounted by Licht.[44] Kratzenstein, Jallabert, and Deshais were advocates of electrification as a cure for various degrees of paralysis, including hemiplegia; Nollet, Morand, de la Sone, Meunier, and Boucot were unable to substantiate the claims. Perhaps these early advocates of electrical treatment of paralysis were unlucky and chose patients with conversion disorders as their subjects; perhaps they were victims of their own naiveté or of self-deception. Whatever the facts of these reports, it is clear from our perspective that the essential elements for effective application of electricity to medical problems were not yet at hand: no source of sustained electrical power existed, no means of controlling its application was as yet remotely contemplated, and no theoretical construct of neuromuscular physiology existed.

Luigi Galvani introduced the concept of the spontaneous generation of "animal electricity" as the basis of neuromuscular function in 1791, supporting this premise with his famous frog-leg contraction experiment. He produced contraction of a frog's leg by connecting the frog's spinal cord to the leg.[20] Later, Volta demonstrated that the contraction was the result not of animal electricity conducted from the spinal cord, but of an electrical current generated by the contact of the two dissimilar metals employed to form the connection. This led him by 1796 to devise the voltaic pile—an early bimetal battery representing the first source of sustained electrical current (known as *galvanism* and, later, *direct current*).[20] Discoveries in the application of galvanic current which are pertinent to FNS followed, including Grapengiesser's recognition that muscle contraction resulted from the make or break of the electrical circuit and not continuous current flow,[25] the differential effect of the positive and negative poles on nerve stimulation, and the development of applicator electrodes[44] (including increased surface area, saline-metal, and various needle electrodes)—the direct forerunners of current FNS models.

Faraday's 1831 development of the induction generator made available a new stimulating force, *faradic*, or alternating, current. Advocates of galvanic, interrupted galvanic, and faradic current were soon upon the scene proposing numerous medical applications.

In this century, progress in understanding the physiology of excitable membranes accelerated in conjunction with technological progress in electronics, permitting clinical application of electricity to the diagnosis of neuromuscular disease, specifically, the determination of strength–duration curves and of chronaxy. These procedures distinguish lower from upper motor neuron injuries through the difference in electrical excitability between muscle fibers without neuronal connections (denervated, lower motor neuron injury), and those in which the motor neuron is intact (upper motor neuron injuries). Much of the research in electrical stimulation prior to the 1970s was directed toward peripheral nerve or lower motor neuron injuries. Attempts at stimulating denervated muscle proved inherently difficult. Muscle membrane differs fundamentally from that of nerve. It does not respond to short-duration electrical currents at tolerable intensities. Since it doesn't accommodate, or increase, its depolarization threshold in response to slowly changing electrical fields, long-duration stimulation at low intensities can produce depolarization. Rates of 1 Hz can be used but are too slow for effective fusion or functional use. Further, the entire muscle must be stimulated rather than the motor points or nerve (which is absent) in order to produce contraction.[84] These problems are not currently being addressed in FNS applications and will not be further explored in this chapter.

Interest in FNS intensified in the 1960s with the availability of better electronics and with improving understanding of neuromuscular function. FNS systems must substitute for, integrate with, and control or be controlled by elements of both the central nervous system (CNS) and the peripheral neuromuscular system.

PHYSIOLOGY OF RESPONSE

Neuromuscular System

This system is often presented as a hierarchical one in which the signal to initiate movement arises at the cortical level of the brain, is coordinated at lower CNS levels, is transmitted through the peripheral nervous system, and results in shortening of muscle fibers with body motion. Were the control mechanisms strictly hierarchical, the work of developing an effective functional electrical stimulation system in paralyzed individuals would be greatly simplified. However, some of the complexity (and effectiveness) of the system is due to the use of sensory information, both prospectively and on a continuing feedback basis, to control and direct movement. This results in continual changes both in the intended movement and in the actual execution of a specific movement in order to effect appropriate body positioning. The process is further complicated by the fact that specific movements come not from single muscle contractions, but rather from muscles functionally contracting in agonist/antagonist pairings and in complex, multijoint patterns.

Higher Centers

Simply stated, the role of the cortex, cerebellum, and brainstem in movement is to establish goals, activate or relax smoothly and continuously each somatic muscle in the body, consider spatial relationships of body and environment, maintain balance, correct for resistance to body movements, calculate velocities of movement and forces of contraction necessary to accomplish the task, correct for errors at frequent intervals, monitor all "inactive" systems, utilize feedback from the periphery and special senses to modify movement plan, and continuously consider alternate goals. The data-processing requirements for these tasks are staggering and clearly beyond the current capability of FNS to replace. Although poorly understood, this system probably operates indirectly at the actual movement level by modifying built-in movement patterns rather than constructing every movement *de novo*.

An important function of the higher centers is to suppress spinal-level reflex responses. These uncontrolled motor and autonomic behaviors can be triggered by FNS and can obstruct FNS-directed movement and result in subject injuries. Since the brain's planning and analysis functions cannot be replaced, FNS systems must be designed to permit easy and effective control and adjustment of their functions by the user. Although this is currently limited to simple switching control, more complex integration is needed for truly effective systems.

Spinal Cord

The spinal cord contains many of the processing, organizing, and operating subsystems, which are mostly controlled and modified by higher level systems. Thus reflex voiding, deep tendon reflexes, and other simple afferent-efferent synaptic circuits or motor response patterns can be suppressed in humans. Likewise, the cord's autonomic nervous system component, which controls functions such as circulation, digestion, and elimination, is also modulated by higher order signals.

Certain first-order input processing by the cord in normal man leads to actions directed by the cord, such as flexion withdrawal response from unexpected thermal stress. It is now believed that the cord plays an important role in suppressing sensory information flow centrally, thus filtering out low-grade signals which may result in the unnecessary perception of pain if conducted centrally.[41] In spinal cord injuries, these complex subsystems are released and can produce independent motor actions. Attempts to drive the peripheral neuromuscular system with external electrical stimulation can result in triggering automatic spinal responses through direct or indirect afferent signals, producing competitive, augmentative, extraneous, or catastrophic results. There is experimental interest in triggering some of these spinal cord–directed "useful" behaviors such as the flexor response with afferent FNS stimulation as part of FNS gait.[41] A more ambitious approach would be to activate them directly using implanted electrodes on the spinal cord. Current FNS interest lies more in the desire to suppress these reflex spinal level responses, since they often overpower the desired FNS motor behavior or result in undesired responses such as autonomic dysreflexia, spasm, or incontinence.

Peripheral Neuromuscular System

The effector unit of movement is the lower motor neuron, comprised of the neuron body, axon, myoneural junctions, and muscle fibers attached. Activation comes from depolarization of the charged cell membrane, which can be initiated by a number of chemical or mechanical stimuli and by electrical fields. When activated, all muscle fibers of the motor unit contract more or less simultaneously.

There are two types of both motor muscle cells and anterior horn cells. The anterior horn cell types are distinguished by their size and by their firing characteristics, that is, the initial firing rate at which they are recruited and the frequency range in which they usually operate.[32] In normal circumstances, it is this firing characteristic of the anterior horn cell which causes the differentiation of muscle cells into their separate types, type I and type II.[6, 42] Type I muscle fibers are small in diameter and rich in oxidative cytochromes, which given them a red color. They have a slow twitch speed and are specialized for contraction over sustained periods of time. In the normal physiological state, these fibers are the first recruited, fire at relatively lower frequencies, and can maintain contraction for hours.[32] They are normally employed for such endurance tasks as running, bicycling, and usual postural support activities.

Type II muscle fibers have a larger diameter, appear white since they have lower levels of oxidative cytochromes, and contain relatively greater amounts of contractile proteins.[42] They usually fire at higher frequencies and normally are recruited for short bursts of time to produce strong but short-duration contractions.[32] They are the fibers recruited for such heavy tasks as weight lifting.

The intact nervous system differentially recruits the two types of motor units in order to perform specific tasks. In theory, the larger diameter axons are more susceptible to electrical stimulation,[58] but in practical terms, functional electrical stimulation systems are unable to recruit the two types of motor units differentially. This means that with current FNS systems, there is inappropriate recruitment of different fiber types, regardless of the type of task being performed. Thus, whether working to develop endurance or strength, FNS exercise differs somewhat from that occurring with an intact nervous system.[32] There is considerable experimental evidence that cross-reinnervation can cause a change in the histological muscle fiber type of the newly reinnervated muscle fiber.[42] Some animal model studies of sustained exercise have also suggested that motor fiber type conversion can occur based on use, without physically replacing the innervating neuron.[26] It is quite possible that functional electrical stimulation may also lead to a change in the morphological and physiological characteristics of the motor units thus activated.[5, 17, 26, 52, 79, 80, 87]

FNS systems can activate the motor unit by electrical stimulation of neurons, peripheral nerves, or the terminal nerve portion where the myoneural junction is located, known as the *motor point*. To date only the latter two approaches have been employed directly, in addition to indirect (reflex) activation of the neuron.

The Peripheral Afferent System

The afferent, or sensory, nervous system provides us information, some of which we are fully conscious of (temperature, pressure, or touch), and some of which we are not (joint position, tendon position, muscle tension, movement, blood pressure). Advanced FNS systems must substitute artificial systems of feedback reporting for the absent sensory information. To date, joint angle or heel pressure have been used more frequently. In some clinical situations, particularly with cervical level injuries or incomplete injuries, some useful direct sensory information remains available for conscious evaluation and use. As previously mentioned, attempts have been made to use stimulation of the sensory afferents to evoke useful reflex motor response, but this has been of limited practical usefulness.

Paralyzed Muscle Response to Electrical Stimulation

Both nerve and muscle are excitable tissues: they maintain electrically charged (polarized) cell membranes through the expenditure of energy. This electrical potential can be discharged to initiate constructive activity of nerve releasing chemical transmitters and initiating muscle contraction. Depolarization is usually initiated by chemical neurotransmitters such as acetylcholine, but electrical fields can also initiate depolarization. Isolated nerve and muscle cells differ in the way they respond to changing electrical fields, and thus in their response to electrical stimulation.

Electrical current is measured in amperes and is the product of the voltage and the time over which it is applied. When measuring responses in excitable tissues, the minimum intensity of current which produces a response (depolarization) when applied for an extended period of time is termed the *rheobase*. *Chronaxy* is the stimulation time required to produce depolarization of tissue when a stimulation intensity twice that of the rheobase is applied. Both the rheobase and the chronaxy of muscle are higher than that of nerve. Therefore it is necessary to apply much greater electrical currents when stimulating a muscle that has lost its motor neuron (lower motor neuron injuries) than one that has its motor unit intact. Denervated muscle will not respond at all to short-duration stimulation, regardless of the current applied. Not only are high current levels potentially dangerous to the subject when used to generate a large electrical field in the body, but they are intolerably painful in sensate subjects.

Another significant problem encountered in stimulating lower motor neuron type of injuries is that there is no longer a localized point of sensitivity to simulation. When the motor unit is intact, the muscle can be easily activated by either an isolated stimulation to its motor nerve or to the area of muscle where the synaptic connection of nerve to muscle occurs. This so-called motor point is a well-defined area and is quite small in relationship to the overall size of the muscle. In denervated (lower motor neuron) muscle, the electrical field for stimulation must reach all areas of the muscle to produce full contraction, since no localized motor point is present.

This quantitative difference in response between nerve and muscle is important in functional electrical stimulation studies, since paralysis may be either from loss of the ability to activate and control otherwise healthy motor units (as in upper motor neuron paralysis from stroke, spinal cord injury, multiple sclerosis) or from damage to the motor unit (as in lower motor neuron paralysis from peripheral nerve injury, plexus injury, cauda equina injuries, myopathy, anterior horn cell disease, or certain spinal cord injuries in which the anterior horn cells [motor neurons] are destroyed). Because of the limitations cited, only individuals with upper motor neuron paralysis are appropriate for current functional electrical stimulation techniques.

Components of FNS Systems

Conceptually, FNS systems consist of a number of basic elements: a control system, a means of obtaining information about the world and the effect of the FNS on it (feedback), a strategy for interfacing with the body, stimulators to produce the needed electrical current, and electrodes for applying the stimulation to the body. Details of each element vary among current projects in the field. The choice of element design should be based on the goals of the individual FNS project. Factors in design include portability, ability to modify the system easily for experimental purposes, cost, reliability, and maintenance requirements. Systems should be judged both on overall and on individual component effectiveness. As FNS sophistication advances, esthetic considerations will become a more important factor in element design.

Control and Feedback

Control of normal movement in humans is an extremely complex process requiring large-scale integration of cortical, subcortical, and peripheral information. Broken into a crude step-wise representation, the process is as follows:

1. Conception of desire to move
2. Assessment of possibility of completing the move
3. Decision to move
4. Initial elements of motor activation chosen
5. Template for movement formed
6. Calculation and choice of initial forces, including acceleration, of body parts
7. Implementation of movement
8. Assessment of movement template based on feedback from
   Joint position
   Muscle–tendon tension
   Joint acceleration
   Body position (visual, vestibular)
   Resistance encountered
   Cutaneous feedback

The control process is represented diagramatically in Figure 15-1.

The subcortical phases can continue through many cycles independent of cortical input, but there is a periodic reassessment performed and movement goals can be reset, modified, or stopped by conscious decisions.

Current FNS systems permit only very limited motor actions. Furthermore, individuals have access to only one simple action sequence at a time: they can sit–stand–stop, grasp–release, or exercise. Thus, the only planning decision is whether or not to perform the permitted action. When future systems permit access to multiple actions, cortical planning will be essential to combine and sequence these effectively.

Current FNS exercise systems limit cortical reassessment to stopping the exercise. In FNS gait systems, cortical reassessment is frequently required at key branch points in the behavior, such as sit–stand, stand–step, step–step, or grasp–release. This conscious decision-making input control can be exercised through such devices as mechanical switches, myoelectric signals from nonparalyzed muscles, or voice recognition systems. As activity choices increase, nonmechanical control will become more important.

Most recent FNS research and development involve the "pre-movement" phase and the incorporation of feedback assessment into real time movement control. In normal voluntary movements, a conscious assessment presets the forces initially applied by the muscles based on an estimate of the effort required. The normal importance of this preset is demonstrated by the frequent occurrence of industrial lifting injuries when the prelift estimate of the weight of the object to be lifted is grossly wrong. System designers have several options when substituting for the normal premovement process. They can preset the system to a stimulation level high enough to create a near-maximal muscle contraction. This will overpower most resistance and lead to rapid and full joint excursion. This approach may also increase chances for injury owing to sudden soft tissue stress, joint hyperextension, and terminal joint impact. A somewhat less traumatic approach is to increase or "ramp up" the stimulation intensity gradually at a predetermined rate to the desired level. This results in a more physiological muscle activation pattern, but does not itself permit the final muscle contraction level to be appropriate to the need.

Another approach to selecting the appropriate muscle contraction (*i.e.,* stimulation force) is to use an algorithm for determining stimulation intensity; the response to a known test stimulation is compared to a mathematical model of muscle response.[68, 69, 75] To do this, some means of real time monitoring of muscle contraction is required, leading directly to the other major research area in FNS, feedback monitoring.

Current FNS systems are either open-loop or closed-loop systems. *Open-loop systems,* such as the Ljubljana walking system, use high fixed stimulation intensities sufficient to lock weight-bearing joints in extension[37, 38, 40, 41] rather than adjust the stimulation intensity in a real time response to actual muscle contraction and joint movement.

In *closed loop systems,* such as the Wright State walking program, real time measurements of some measure of muscle contraction (joint motion, in this instance) are fed back to modify the intensity of stimulation applied.[60, 63, 65, 72] Feedback is essential for all but the simplest of FNS systems to protect against injury, correct for unanticipated obstacles, and ensure efficient operation, since sustained strong contractions may lead to injury, muscle fatigue, high electrical current drain, and poor coordination of movement.

The most desirable feedback values are tendon tension, joint movement, joint position, and limb position. Tendon tension is particularly desirable, since high values directly predict potential tissue injury, and it can be combined with the stimulation intensity to indicate system efficiency. Tendon tension readings can also be combined with joint movement measurements to indicate where mechanical movement obstruction has been encountered. Unfortunately, no external means of measuring tendon tension exists and no practical implantable method is yet at hand.

Joint motion can be measured by attaching potentiometers externally to the joint. Potentiometers alter electrical flow in proportion to their angular position and thus indicate rotational joint position. This information can be fed back to the FNS system to control the intensity of muscle stimulation. Both absolute position of the joint and rate of change can be calculated and used.

Most reported open-loop systems are controlled by "hardwired" electrical devices; that is, they permit only a few adjustments in their operation, which are accomplished through mechanical controls.[4, 34, 38, 71] It is possible to create hard-wired feedback-controlled stimulation systems which will have a few responses to the feedback information, but a microprocessor-controlled device is much better suited to this task. Microprocessors are the heart of computers, and when provided with appropriate programs, are able to perform extensive calculations on feedback information and make elaborate adjustments in the control parameters to all muscles being stimulated by the FNS system. They operate rapidly enough that these adjustments can be made repeatedly during the course of muscle stimulation

Figure 15-1. Movement Control Process

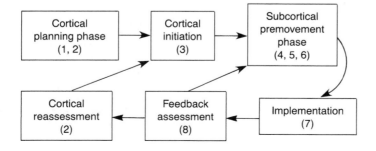

to create a smooth onset–shortening–hold cycle of muscle activation similar to that seen in voluntary muscle contraction.

Microprocessor control of FNS systems has advantages which make it essential for the development of advanced systems:

- Uses feedback information to create smooth, natural muscle contractions
- Sets initial and final stimulation intensities based on the actual load encountered rather than preset high values
- Coordinates multiple simultaneous or sequential tasks and makes changes in all components in real time based on feedback
- Can be programmed to permit real time changes in the sequence of operations in response to conscious commands from the subject
- Employs artificial intelligence programs to adjust the FNS program in response to obstacles, unexpected resistance, and system malfunction
- Coordinates the FNS operations to action of nonparalyzed portions of the body relayed to it by other sources. For example, upper body location information from small gyroscopes could be used to modify a lower extremity walking program to improve balance.

Stimulating Strategies

There are theoretical advantages for FNS stimulation within the CNS. Movements are thought to be stored there in the form of complex patterns rather than as specific muscle contractions; thus, a single stimulus might recruit a fully coordinated motor behavior. Intraoperative cortical stimulation experiments support this concept.

Similarly, simple movement patterns exist within the spinal cord neuronal "hard wiring." There have been attempts to use these integrated movements by indirect triggering through afferent reflex areas.[41] Direct stimulation of the cord might better control such movements, and the potential for such a system in continence management would justify development effort. However, stimulation technology remains inadequate; advances in electrode reliability and survivability in the CNS, ability to isolate stimulation to small numbers of neurons, and feedback control are all required.

All FNS systems to date use one of four approaches: surface stimulation of peripheral nerves, surface stimulation of motor points, percutaneously inserted fine wire electrode motor point stimulation, or cuff electrode stimulation of large peripheral nerves. Future options may include stimulation with implanted electrodes of nerve roots or small branches of motor nerves, and systems which combine several of these stimulation techniques.

Stimulators

The stimulator section of an FNS system produces the electrical discharge responsible for producing muscle contraction. The principal concern in designing a stimulator section is to ensure patient safety from the standpoints of both the electrical shock and the reliability of operation. Electrical safety can be ensured by using a battery-powered system, since this provides isolation from potentially catastrophic sources of electrical current. Operation failure during standing or other situations in which the body is mechanically loaded can result also in significant subject injury. Protection from this is sought through the use of solid-state electronic components with high inherent reliability, back-up circuits, and warning systems. Input and output characteristics of the FNS system are determined by the needs of that particular system.

Stimulating Electrodes

Several types of stimulating electrodes are currently in use, and their choice is sometimes a source of controversy. The ideal electrode system is not yet available, but would fulfill the following requirements:

- Be safe
- Be reliable, that is, never fail when in use
- Produce identical contractions with each use
- Be maintenance-free
- Be noninvasive and unobtrusive
- Be manageable by the subject
- Be inexpensive
- Be specific
- Be permanent
- Be efficient

Three basic electrode types are currently available: surface, percutaneous, and implantable cuff electrodes. The appropriate electrode choice must be based upon the demands and objectives of each experimental situation.

Surface-type electrodes have evolved from the torpedo fish and the saline-soaked cloth over metal pads to the current gel-coated carbonized rubber pads. They can effectively stimulate both superficially located motor points and peripheral nerves.

Skin burns reported from older metal electrodes are not encountered with current commercial systems, which we have used for many years without incident. These electrodes are reliable, are easily applied (often by the subject), and can be left in place for up to several days. Incorporation of the electrode pads and wiring into elasticized garments can sometimes simplify application. Reproducibility of muscle contraction is fairly good during short periods of activity, but requires recalibration with each use. Specificity of stimulation is good only for major functional muscle groups. It is difficult to restrict the stimulation to a small area, and it is impossible to stimulate deep-lying muscles without also stimulating all other muscles in the area. Thus, surface stimulation is well suited to activities requiring contraction of large muscle groups. The ability to change stimulation locations easily is also helpful in experimental studies in which frequent changes in protocol are expected.

Percutaneous electrodes can be inserted using a hypodermic needle as the introducer. These fine-wire electrodes are most often inserted intramuscularly for motor point stimulation, but direct nerve stimulation is also possible with perineural placements. The Cleveland group[50] employs a coiled, Teflon-coated, 76 μm stainless steel wire built up of ten separate 25 μm diameter strands. A hook is fastened at the exposed tip. Because of their smaller stimulation field, many electrodes are required per muscle rather than the three pads per muscle group used in typical rotary-type surface stimulation. Marsolais and Kobetic reported failure rates of 35% at 4 months and 62% at 1 year, mostly from electrode breaking or movement.

Percutaneous electrodes can be left in place for longer periods than surface electrodes, require less stimulating current, and are often better able to isolate the stimulus to a specific muscle. They still must be recalibrated with each use, they require closer supervision by trained personnel, and insertion is tedious. They are susceptible to mechanical failure, and the complication potential is greater than with surface stimulation.

They appear best suited at this time to upper extremity applications in which fine control is sought or in which a specific, poorly accessible muscle is to be activated. Once reliability problems are overcome, applications should expand.

Implantable electrodes theoretically offer the best prospect for a permanent, specific, unobtrusive means of FNS. Typically, such electrodes form a cuff surrounding the nerve and are connected by wires to an induction coil placed subcutaneously at a convenient location.[4] They are activated by an electrical current induced in the subcutaneous coil by an electrical field generated directly over the implanted coil. A cuff electrode suitable for rotary stimulation of three separate subpopulations of axons within a single nerve has been used in animals.[59, 67]

Several obstacles remain to practical use of these stimulators in FNS. Experience gained from diaphragmatic pacing with implanted electrodes indicates that although they are able to remain in place for extended periods, they cannot yet be considered permanent.[29] Second, to take advantage of the specificity of stimulation, these electrodes often must be placed on specific motor nerve branches. These small branches are less accessible than the large nerve trunks (the stimulation of which results in the nonspecific activation of large groups of muscles) that have been used to date. Thus many separate implants are required to produce sophisticated functional systems, making the technique more invasive. If important benefit from large muscle group exercise programs for paralyzed individuals is established, implantable electrodes may prove a practical method of stimulating the few large groups of muscles required for a simple exercise system.

Contraction Strength With FNS

During voluntary exercise, the strength of a contraction is increased in two ways: increasing the number of motor units activated (recruitment) and increasing the firing rates of those motor units which are active (temporal summation). FNS systems employ the same general approach, although they lack the ability to adjust the recruitment order among the motor unit types.

Recruitment is accomplished by increasing the volume of tissue in which the electrical field from the stimulator is sufficient to cause depolarization. The tissue volume of the electrical field is related to the current flowing from the stimulator, which in turn is the product of the electrical voltage and the time over which it is applied. FNS systems usually adjust either voltage or pulse duration to regulate stimulation. Excessive current flow can produce tissue damage through electrical burns, and therefore the total recruitment that can be produced by any given electrode is limited by the amount of electrical current that it can safely disperse. This, in turn, is related both to the surface area of the electrode and the impedance of the electrode–tissue interface, that is, the resistance to electrical current flow in the tissue surrounding the electrode. Recruitment can also be increased by using additional stimulating electrodes, either to activate portions of a very large muscle not reached by the already active electrode array, or to recruit additional muscles which can reinforce the desired movement.

The increase in strength of contraction produced by increasing the frequency of firing is independent of that produced by increasing the volume of the electrical field; therefore, FNS systems can employ a combination of these two factors to regulate the strength of muscle contraction. From a practical standpoint, fatigue of the muscle fibers is a direct result of firing frequency, so a high frequency of stimulation will eventually result in loss of contraction strength. Thus, the strategy employed

for regulating the strength of contraction with an FNS system depends on the functional goal of the system.

If the goal is to ensure muscle contractions for extended periods, then an effective strategy is to fix the firing rate at a frequency that will not result in exhaustion of the muscle in any circumstance in which the FNS system is to be employed. The strength of contraction is then regulated by altering recruitment. If a wide range of contraction strength is required, including some period of maximum contraction, then control of both recruitment and firing frequency may be required. A pre-set program for adjusting the relative portions of each can be used, a technique similar to that used for setting automatic camera exposures. The upper level of frequency permitted in this system can be set at a high level, allowing neuromuscular exhaustion following maximum contraction, or at a relatively lower level, so as not to permit rapid muscle fiber exhaustion. If muscle exhaustion is permitted by the stimulation program, some means must be provided to prevent mechanical injury to the subject when the contraction fails.

FNS APPLICATIONS

There are currently three broad areas of applications studies: exercise studies in which FNS-driven muscles are worked in standardized exercise programs similar to usual athletic conditioning routines; functional movement studies in which daily tasks such as walking, grasping, or mobility are accomplished using FNS-driven muscle as the power source; and physiology of spinal cord injury (SCI) studies in which the indirect effect of FNS on SCI human physiology and on medical complications of SCI is observed. In the long term, the practical effectiveness of the mobility programs will continue to improve with advances in technology, providing more dramatic accomplishments, but the practical justification of FNS, at least for the intermediate term, may well lie in the latter two areas of study.

Liberson[43] reported an attempt to employ electrically induced muscle contraction to improve ambulation in hemiplegics in 1961. His group used tetanic stimulation of the peroneal nerve at the fibular head at rates of 30 to 100 Hz and controlled the activation of the stimulation with a heel switch in the ipsilateral foot. A number of his observations remain pertinent to current investigation: the possibility of discomfort in sensate areas, the limited adaptability or "plasticity" of the system compared to the broad range of motor requirements, the problem of induced spasms in SCI individuals, and the possibility of improved voluntary control for a period after stimulation was discontinued.

This approach was extended by others with positive functional results; however, lightweight plastic orthoses have replaced the FNS units, which required frequent servicing and adjustment. Long and Masciarelli developed a FNS-driven flexor hinge splint for use by a high-level quadriplegic, publishing results in 1963.[47] They used motor point stimulation of the extensor digitorum communis with a 100 μsec duration and 66 Hz interrupted direct current without problems of tolerance or skin injury. The voltage of stimulation was controlled by the subject using a mechanical potentiator mounted to the opposite-side flexor hinge splint. The splint closure was spring-driven.

Exercise Applications

To increase strength or endurance, exercise must be performed against resistance. Although this principle has been empirically applied to athletic training and physical rehabilitation for many years, its application to electrical muscle stimulation studies is quite recent. Efforts to exercise muscle electrically were stymied by the fact that in order to obtain a functionally effective muscle contraction (*i.e.,* observable shortening against resistance), the stimulation frequency had to be set at high rates, often 100 to 300 Hz. This produced the fused tetany response sought, but at these rates myoneural junction failure occurred in seconds due to exhaustion of acetylcholine supplies. Most muscle work obtained was expended overcoming the series elastic component of muscle and tendon, and the contraction ended before conditioning work could be accomplished.[46, 67]

During the 1950s, improved understanding of the normal physiological control mechanisms of the human motor system evolved. Studies demonstrated that motor units are sequentially recruited based on the intrinsic firing rate of their motor neurons, slowest firing first, faster firing in turn. The slower firing units are more resistant to fatigue (high oxidative metabolism, type I), and only in extraordinary circumstances are more than a portion of the units firing simultaneously. Thus, each motor unit is able to fire at sustainable rates that permit recovery of myoneural junction conduction.

Rotary Stimulation System

Studies in muscle physiology also were hindered by the limitations of electrical muscle stimulation. Due to the problem of contraction failure during tetanic stimulation, studies of muscle cellular metabolism relied on data obtained from brief electrically induced twitches rather than from sustained muscle contraction.[58] By 1969, Rack and Westbury overcame this limitation in physiological studies by developing an electrical stimulation system that more closely mimicked voluntary muscle activation.[76] They isolated the spinal motor roots supplying the muscle under study in experimental animals, divided the axons into multiple bundles, and stimulated each bundle in rotation with a single pulse in one bundle followed by a single pulse to the next bundle, repeating the sequence after delivering a pulse to each bundle in turn. Since motor units are continuously contracting in the muscle as a whole (the sum of the frequency of each bundle), a strong contraction similar to that obtainable with voluntary activation is obtained, and yet this *rotary* stimulation technique reduces the frequency of any one axon to a sustainable level.

Lindt and Petrofsky[46] showed that most of the total improvement obtainable from the elaborate multichannel rotary stimulation system could be obtained by dividing the axons into just three bundles, and subsequent systems have been effective using only two alternating groups of motor units.

The rotary stimulation FNS systems have been combined with each of the traditional forms of exercise equipment to permit full training of paralyzed muscle in an SCI subject. In each type of exercise, feedback information from the equipment, such as force and angular movement, is used by the microprocessor to adjust stimulation intensities. Furthermore, the microprocessor monitors both work output of the muscle (from the feedback sensors) and the output of the stimulators (proportional to muscle fatigue, since increased intensity is used to recruit additional motor units through volume conduction spread of the stimulation as fatigue occurs) to determine the advancement of the exercise program.[28, 66, 73] Therefore, these units can be characterized as closed-loop, rotary stimulation, limited artificial intelligence systems.

Isokinetic Knee Trainer

An exercise system using two rotary channels capable of strengthening quadriceps and hamstring muscle groups in a manner analogous to that of a standard knee table has been developed.[31, 73] Graded resistance is applied through a weighted cable run through a pulley system. A single-turn potentiometer provides feedback information regarding knee angular movement. Converted to digital terms, it is fed to the microprocessor controller (Apple II computer), which in turn regulates the output of a two-channel sequential stimulator. Output is of constant duration, 300 μsec pulses at 50 Hz (changeable by software), with voltage varied for recruitment.

The system is software-controlled. The lowest stimulation voltage which will produce trace muscle contraction is determined by trial and error and placed into the program. Similarly, maximum muscle tension from stimulation is determined by a progressive increase in the voltage, and measurement of the resultant isometric pull is made with a strain gauge. That voltage is also placed into the program and is used by the program as the maximal allowed voltage for the exercise period. The desired weights are added and the exercise begun. The program produces a smooth voltage increase over 3 seconds to the level necessary to produce the knee angular movement programmed (60°). Voltage is held and is then slowly reduced over 3 seconds, resulting in a smooth isokinetic type of exercise. The exercise is carried to muscle fatigue, that is, until the programmed movement is not obtained despite applying maximum permitted voltage. The principles of progressive resistive exercise (PRE) are employed:[15] slow repetitive movement of muscle loaded to approximately two-thirds of maximum muscle strength, resulting in a rapid increase in strength.

Similarly a second system, a four-channel isometric exercise system was developed capable of exercising the knee extensors–flexors and ankle dorsiflexors–plantar flexors in SCI individuals still on bed rest.[17, 18] In this instance, strain gauges at the "locked" ankle joint and knee joint of a double upright knee-ankle-foot orthosis provided muscle force measurements. Since maximum force of isometric contraction could not safely be tested, normal values tables based on subject size were used to set upper limit force targets (80% of normal), and stimulation voltage upper limits were set within safe limits from experience. Excellent results based on contraction force and muscle bulk increase were obtained in a newly injured SCI subject.[17]

Bicycle Ergometer System

A third basic system involving dynamic exercise uses a modified bicycle ergometer.[62] Dynamic exercise principally improves endurance by stressing the oxidative muscle systems, but it also produces strength and bulk increase in highly atrophied muscle such as seen in long-standing SCI. Severely deconditioned individuals were preconditioned using the isokinetic knee trainer. The bicycle ergometer system has seen considerable development and is now commercially available. The pedal incorporates a continous 360° potentiometer to provide movement information. Resistance is increased progressively in the usual manner for bicycle ergometers, and pedaling continues to muscle fatigue. Again, minimal effective and maximum voltages for system use must be obtained by trial and error for each session. Pedaling can be accomplished using various muscles singly or in combinations, including glutei, hamstrings, vasti, and gastroc soleus.

Further improvement in the exercise systems has been made by the development of software, which enables the system to compare the results of each lift cycle with expected responses. If fatigue has altered the response between lifts, the program adjusts the stimulation parameters based on algorithms developed from previous exercise studies. This helps ensure that full, effective exercise sessions are delivered. Using this system with three-times-per-week, 15-minute-per-session PRE training, strength increased 50% during a 6-week period in eight long-time SCI subjects. Thigh girth increased 2.7 ± 0.6 cm in the same subjects.[66]

Dynamic exercise using a four-channel (bilateral gluteus maximus, quadriceps) system also showed impressive results. A 15-minute-per-day, three-day-per-week regimen resulted in an endurance increase of 500% in seven subjects during the initial 2 weeks of training. These subjects had previously been trained with the isokinetic system to be able to lift 20 kg using knee extension.[66] Subjects who exercised for extended periods developed muscle mass and endurance improvement comparable to those of able-bodied individuals engaged in exercise.

From these and ongoing studies, it is clear that FNS systems using rotary stimulation techniques coupled with traditional athletic training regimens can produce muscle hypertrophy, strengthening, and endurance increases. Other studies of electrical stimulation in humans[52] and exercise[26] and electrical stimulation in animals have shown that muscle phenotype (fiber type) can be altered in response to prolonged patterns of use. Preliminary information suggests that muscle fiber type can also be altered in humans by FNS.[52]

Ambulation Applications

FNS Applications

By the early 1970s efforts were under way to use multichannel stimulation in SCI subjects[37] to assist in reaching a standing position and to lock the knees, obviating the use of heavier long leg bracing. The Ljubljana group used tetanic stimulation of up to 50 Hz with resultant rapid muscle fatigue and low strength of contraction. Pre-use conditioning stimulation over periods of several months resulted in improved but still marginal muscle contraction strength. All control parameters were preset or manually activated. After 3 months of cycled (4 sec on, 8 sec off) 12-hour-per-day stimulation, no further improvement of muscle contraction performance was obtained.[37] They were able to stimulate bilateral quadriceps and triceps surae, usually with motor point surface electrodes, but the system had limited flexibility of stimulation parameters and they had difficulty maintaining consistent muscle response. As with all studies reported to date, individuals with strong spontaneous or induced spasms were disqualified from the study. Results, while important experimentally, were still not a qualitative improvement over conventional bracing.

By 1978, the Ljubljana group was able to report results of a six-channel stimulating system in hemiplegics.[81] These subjects were able to ambulate prior to entering the study, and FNS was employed for gait correction. The six channels were applied to combinations of ankle dorsiflexors–plantar flexors–evertors, knee flexors–extensors, and hip flexors–extensors–abductors, based on individual subject assessment and trial-and-error adjustment. Timing sequences were individually determined, and each change in a single muscle group stimulation parameter usually required changes in all others. This system, as with their previous units, had no provision for graduated onset and offset of stimulation. It did have the provision for proportional adjustment of all stimulation cycles based on gait speed.

Again, consistent stimulation response was a problem due to poor electrode contact or electrode movement. Stimulation pain frequently prevented the system from completely overpowering unwanted movements. The authors found that it was not possible to produce gait correction by simply stimulating in phase with normal muscle activation patterns. Rather, they developed a system of incremental adjustments in the stimulation pattern, adding one channel at a time, starting with the foot

dorsiflexors and evertors and working proximally. A heel switch was used to set sequential timing. They reported improved goniometric correspondence of impaired as compared to normal side movement patterns and increased (more normal) stance phase time with use of the system. Ankle control, in particular, was improved. These studies reemphasized the problems of stimulating sensate individuals and the problems of obtaining consistent muscle contraction in open-loop FNS systems. At the same time, they demonstrated in these stroke patients that the technical problems of FNS are reduced when some voluntary neuromuscular control is preserved.

Other ambulation studies during this period with SCI subjects were also under way. Brindley[4] used an implanted system with cuff electrodes for stimulation of the femoral nerve or its branches plus the superior and inferior gluteal nerves. The induction receivers were placed subcutaneously in the subcostal area and a six-channel transmitter was used. The continuously stimulated nerves produce a splinting type locking of the knee joints. Muscle fatigue, as with the preceding studies, was encountered. Kralj[40] reported a novel approach to the gait problem. In addition to their usual electrical splint approach, the Ljubljana group attempted to assist the swing phase of gait by triggering a flexion reflex by posterior fossa afferent stimulation. Results with this approach were sometimes helpful, but inconsistent.

Petrofsky's[67] use of microprocessor control in conjunction with the rotary stimulation technique was a fundamental break with previous practice; it was introduced not to mimic previous mechanical stimulation timing systems but to permit real time feedback control of stimulation. It permitted the use of submaximal stimulation intensities calculated from feedback to approximate specific needs for each movement, and it permitted the coordination of multichannel stimulation systems. By breaking down each component of FNS into a series of "software" subroutines, it permitted easy experimental modification of the control system and opened the way for incorporation of artificial intelligence in FNS.

The Wright State University (WSU) group developed six-[71] and later eight-channel walking systems incorporating rotary stimulation and microprocessor control with real time joint position feedback (closed loop). This combination of rotary stimulation and feedback to reduce stimulation intensity to functionally sufficient rather than near-maximal levels resulted in improved endurance. The joint position feedback and variable stimulation intensity improved swing phase control over open-loop (no feedback) systems. The closed-loop system also reduced the problem of inadequate contraction seen in open-loop systems when minor electrode movement decreased the effective stimulation intensity, since the stimulation intensity would increase in response to the joint position feedback information. The use of multiple stimulating electrodes per muscle group as necessitated by the rotary stimulation system and the use of rather large gel-coated surface electrodes also increased the reliability of the system.

Despite its improvements, it is obvious from observing results that, like the previous open-loop systems, this closed-loop system does not provide a practical solution to the problem of ambulation in SCI. Six or eight muscles (compared to the hundreds in normal gait) are insufficient to control the complex, multi-articulated body which must be stabilized and manipulated during walking. More muscles under more reliable and precise control will be required. Such a system requires better feedback systems, some form of "permanent" electrodes, and control programs with elaborate artificial intelligence, along with a solution to the spasticity problem, in order for it to approach the point of general use.

Control Bracing

An interim approach to using FNS for mobility in SCI subjects is to constrain the multi-articular system through the use of control bracing, thus reducing the problems of stability and intercoordination of limb movement. The control brace joints also provide a convenient location to obtain position information for feedback to the stimulator system. The WSU group has had excellent results from combining the Louisiana State University (LSU) control brace system with their multichannel FNS walking system. This combination produces dramatic cosmetic gait improvement. Experimental subjects are able to ambulate for distances of up to several miles and without full-time reliance on other aids such as walkers or canes. Independent stand-up, sit-down, and ambulation can be functionally performed, thus improving mobility in tight space areas such as kitchens. There are still the problems of applying and removing the equipment, electrode function, and system upkeep and reliability.

Other Mobility Applications

Another approach is to use the leg muscle function available from simple FNS systems to power a modified wheelchair or tricycle. Although neither of these approaches currently promises to provide otherwise unavailable functional capabilities, they may have a role in overall fitness or recreational programs for SCI.

Special Needs of Upper Extremity FNS

FNS in the upper extremities differs from FNS in lower extremities in its functional goals and often in the underlying neuropathologic status:

- No weight-bearing is required.
- Areas of sensation are usually present.
- Some voluntary motor function often remains.
- There may be a mixed finding of lower motor neuron loss and upper motor neuron signs and normal function.
- Precise control of FNS movement is more important.

Most upper extremity tasks are divisible into two separate subcomponents: placement/orientation of the hand in space (static or dynamic) and grip-release by the hand. The specific needs for FNS assistance in quadriplegia differ at each level of spinal injury, and the response to FNS for any individual will vary depending on the amount of lower motor neuron (and thus unstimulatable) loss present. Quadriplegia at or above the C4 level is fully dependent on FNS to place the hand and to grip. At C5, some placement assist is required, along with grip control. Below C7, only grip assist is required, while at C6, the need for placement assistance will vary but full grip assistance is required.

Control systems for upper extremity FNS can make greater use of voluntary cortical feedback and decision-making, since by C5 levels, proprioceptive and sensory awareness of limb placement is present, and by C6 levels, some awareness of pinch force may be present. Also, visual monitoring is readily available.

The complexity of stabilizing and controlling the scapulothoracic and scapulohumeral joints with FNS greatly exceeds current capability. The scapulothoracic joint would be particularly difficult to control, but fortunately it remains stable in all but the most proximal or cord injuries. The scapulohumeral joint contains 3° of rotational freedom and gliding motion within the glenoid fossa, presenting a severe control challenge for FNS. Because of this, most research to date has been focused on

injuries sparing at least C5. Off-body robotic assistance using voice control may be a more practical method of prehension assistance at very high SCI levels until complex, fully implantable technology becomes well established.

Injury below C5 leaves intact proximal control of arm placement, allowing performance of many functionally useful tasks with assistive devices. Some tenodesis grip is present, particularly with increasing C6 sparing, but the pinch is usually too weak to lift objects. Principal issues that must be addressed by FNS systems in these subjects are the choice of grip type, management of hand orientation, and control mechanisms.

Because the FNS-driven prehensile function of the hand is ultimately limited by voluntarily controlled hand placement, continuous cortical management of the upper extremity FNS status is more critical than in lower extremity. This task is made easier by the fact that subjects can easily see the hand and because they have at least some proprioceptive and often some sensory feedback of the hand orientation/grip status. Subjects can not only switch grip on and off, but can also regulate grip strength. Increased force is generated by increased intensity (pulse duration, voltage) and frequency of the electrical stimulus. The signal from the subject to activate this increase can be either a discrete, stepwise signal or a proportional one. Stepwise signals consist of an input signal that is repeated (on–off) for each fixed increase or decrease in contraction strength. Proportional control allows the increase or decrease in the contraction to be proportional to the input control.

Both types of input signals can be operated from the electromyography (EMG) output of voluntarily activated muscles or from body movement. More recently, voice recognition control has been introduced.[53] Control of the on–off status of the system is of course necessary and can be done with any of the inputs available. Peckham[57] has emphasized the benefits of a "hold" state in simplifying functional tasks. This permits the subject to signal the system to maintain the current grip force and to disregard signals from the input device until further notice. The subject can then attend to other chores, and the part of the body being used to generate the control signals can be used for other tasks while grip is automatically maintained. This is particularly helpful when proximal muscles are used to control the grip signal and it is necessary to reposition the hand while gripping an object. Using voluntary EMG signals for control input poses difficulties because of the signal to noise—a false signal—problem. This can be reduced by using logic systems in the controller that respond to signal sequences rather than simple on–off threshold inputs. The difficulty with proportional control by EMG signals led the Cleveland group to use mechanical motion of the shoulder or head as their proportional control of the signal source.[56, 57]

Most C6 quadriplegics are able to position objects in the hand, but lack ability to grip and lift all but the lightest. Most gripping tasks are accomplished using lateral (key) grip, in which the thumb pad presses against the lateral side of the index finger, or palmar (three-jaw) grip, in which the thumb pad presses the index and long finger pads. Lateral (key) grip can be produced with FNS activation of opponens pollicis or adductor pollicis and flexor digitorum profundus, and sublimis, and released with the extensor pollicis and extensor digitorum communis (EDC). Palmar grip is generated by the flexor sublimis and profundus and released by the EDC and extensor index activation. Peckham employed these muscles by activating them through percutaneous wire electrodes with good success.[56] The implanted electrodes (three in the forearm flexors, one in each of the other groups) permitted good control of grip force and localization of activation to the desired muscles.

The natural instability of the wrist complicates FNS grip experiments. The Cleveland group[57] has addressed this problem in a way similar to that used by Long[47] in the original FNS grip work by using orthoses to stabilize the wrist or control wrist and finger position. Another approach begun by Nathan[53] is to quantify the contribution to movement in each axis caused by each stimulated muscle. Logic programs in the computer controller then attempt to balance the resultant motion in all planes by adjusting the contraction of many muscles. This approach is far more complex, employing as it does artificial intelligence and requiring adequate feedback data to self-correct motion errors, but still it approaches the very long-term objectives of all FNS programs.

Calculating the motion vectors in each plane (flexion-extension, pronation-supination) resulting from stimulation of forearm muscles has the advantage of permitting control of more complex motions. The grip effect and the pronation-supination effect of FNS-activated forearm muscles can be simultaneously adjusted to ensure both the desired pinch and the desired vertical orientation of the hand. This problem increases in difficulty at each higher level of SCI.

FNS and SCI Physiology

Cardiovascular deconditioning is an established consequence of SCI. Even with upper extremity exercise in paraplegic individuals, maximum cardiac stress is less than that which can be obtained in non-SCI individuals. This is due to the reduced muscle mass that can be activated at any one time, thus reducing maximum rates of oxygen consumption.[3] The spinal level of the SCI greatly affects the cardiac response to exercise. A full exposition of the cardiovascular and metabolic consequences of SCI is outside the scope of this chapter, but has been reviewed in the literature.[7-10] In brief, both cardiac contractility and cardioaccelatory responses to exercise are dependent on stimulation from lower spinal sympathetic centers. These are the source of exercise-induced increases in cardiac output[58] and are entirely lost in lesions above T1. Lower lesions produce proportional blunting of the response to exercise. In addition, these spinal centers control the peripheral redistribution of blood flow and venous return necessary for an efficient response to exercise. This response normally shunts blood from inactive to active muscles, controls blood pressure, and improves venous return to the heart, which in turn increases cardiac output. This, like the cardioregulatory sympathetic function, is progressively compromised with higher thoracic-level SCI. A further problem is that these spinal sympathetic control centers can occasionally produce uncontrolled vasoconstriction and threateningly high blood pressure elevations when they are reflexly triggered (autonomic dysreflexia) by peripheral afferent stimulation.

FNS-driven exercises in SCI subjects have indeed shown some of the anticipated responses.[21, 73] The cardiac acceleration produced as a result of FNS exercise progressively lessens the more cephalad the SCI is located, until it is minimal at quadriplegia levels. Blood pressure response, however, is fairly predictable with lower spinal levels of injury but becomes erratic in quadriplegics. Some quadriplegics who were usually hypotensive have shown rapid systolic and diastolic blood pressure increases in response to low levels of FNS exercise, suggesting a triggering of unmodulated sympathetic outflow to the periphery. The loss of ability to increase cardiac output coupled with this rapid rise in peripheral resistance is sufficient to place some high-level SCI subjects at risk for acute congestive heart failure during FNS. Fortunately, this severe blood pressure response often modulates with further FNS conditioning. A benefit of FNS conditioning is the observed increase in resting blood pressure in previously severely hypotensive quadriplegics. An average resting level increase of greater than 10 mm Hg diastolic has been seen, resulting in fewer problems from orthostatic hypotension.[21]

Loss of bone density is a well known complication of SCI, resulting in increased susceptibility to fracture. Both mineral and bone matrix are lost.[11] FNS exercise studies at WSU in long-standing SCI have shown rapid redevelopment of muscle tissue, but not of bone calcification. Some fractures have been noted in FNS subjects coincidental with increased exercise stress. Extended weightlessness studies conducted on the Skylab orbiting space station in which subjects exercised regularly[89] showed demineralization but not bone matrix loss. There was rapid remineralization upon return from weightlessness. A preliminary study of isometric stimulation shortly post-SCI suggested some ameliorization of calcium loss.[17, 18] More extended studies are required to determine if FNS can modify the osteoporosis/osteopenia of SCI. If not, the cumulative effects of repeated bone trauma may ultimately limit FNS applications.

Body heat loss during exercise is controlled by sweating. Sweating in turn is dependent on the spinal sympathetic outflow and does not occur below the level of an SCI. Quadriplegics have little tolerance for heat stress, but paraplegics—particularly lower level injuries—usually tolerate environmental heat stress well. Human exercise is highly inefficient, with the majority of the work going to generate heat, thus increasing the body thermal load.

In a study of exercise tolerance and environmental temperature, quadriplegic subjects were unable to tolerate 30 minutes of handcrank exercise (25 watts) at room temperatures above 35°C. Thus, when heavy FNS work loads are imposed, care regarding temperature, clothing, and core temperature increase should be observed.

Although it is clear that a conditioning effect occurs in the muscles exercised, it is not yet certain whether the usual beneficial effects of cardiovascular conditioning which occur in the able-bodied population accrue to SCI subjects receiving FNS. Although there are theoretical reasons to hope that some of the other secondary consequences of SCI, such as osteoporosis, spasticity, neurogenic bladder, and pressure ulcers may in some ways be favorably modified by long-term FNS, there is no conclusive evidence yet for this benefit.

REFERENCES

1. Bajd T et al: Standing-up of a healthy subject and a paraplegic patient. J Biomech 15:1–10, 1982
2. Bajd T, Trnkoczy A: Attempts to optimise functional electrical stimulation of antagonistic muscles by mathematical modelling. J Biomech 12:921–928, 1979
3. Bergh U et al: Maximal oxygen uptake during exercise with various combinations of arm and leg work. J Appl Physiol 41:191–196, 1976
4. Brindley GS et al: Electrical splinting of the knee in paraplegia. Paraplegia 16:428–235, 1978–1979
5. Buchegger A et al: Effects of chronic stimulation on the metabolic heterogeneity of the fibre population in rabbit tibialis anterior muscle. J Physiol 40:391–413, 1973
6. Buller AJ, Eccles JC, Eccles RM: Interactions between motor neurons and muscles in respect of the characteristic speeds of their responses. J Physiol 150:417–439, 1960
7. Claus-Walker J, Halstead LS: Metabolic and endocrine changes in spinal cord injury: I. The nervous system before and after transection of the spinal cord. Arch Phys Med Rehabil 62:595–601, 1981
8. Claus-Walker J, Halstead LS: Metabolic and endocrine changes in spinal cord injury: II (section 1). Consequences of partial decentralization of the autonomic nervous system. Arch Phys Med Rehabil 63:569–575, 1982

9. Claus-Walker J, Halstead LS: Metabolic and endocrine changes in spinal cord injury: II (section 2). Partial decentralization of the autonomic nervous system. Arch Phys Med Rehabil 63:576–580, 1982

10. Claus-Walker J, Halstead LS: Metabolic and endocrine changes in spinal cord injury: III. Less quanta of sensory input plus bedrest and illness. Arch Phys Med Rehabil 63:628–631, 1982

11. Claus-Walker J, Halstead LS: Metabolic and endocrine changes in spinal cord injury: IV. Compounded neurologic dysfunctions. Arch Phys Med Rehabil 63:632–638, 1982

12. Crago PE et al: The choice of pulse duration for chronic electrical stimulation via surface, nerve, and intramuscular electrodes. Ann Biomed Eng 2:252–264, 1974

13. Crago PE et al: Closed-loop control of force during electrical stimulation of muscle. IEEE Trans on Biomed Eng 27:306–312, 1980

14. Crago PE et al: Modulation of muscle force by recruitment during intramuscular stimulation. IEEE Trans on Biomed Eng 27:679–684, 1980

15. DeLorme TL, Watkins AL: Progressive Resistance Exercise. New York, Appleton-Century-Crofts, 1951

16. DiRocco P et al: Cardiopulmonary responses during arm work on land and in a water environment of nonambulatory, spinal cord impaired individuals. Paraplegia 23:90–99, 1985

17. Flores JF Jr: Electrically induced isometric exercise as a means of preventing muscle atrophy and bone demineralization. Master's of science thesis, Wright State University, Dayton, OH

18. Flores JF Jr, Petrofsky JS, Weber R: Electrically induced isometric exercise as a means of preventing muscle atrophy and bone demineralization (abstr). Wright State University School of Medicine, Dayton, OH 1985

19. Freyschuss U, Knutsson E: Cardiovascular control in man with transverse cervical cord lesions. Life Sciences 8 (1):421–414, 1969

20. Geddes LA, Hoff HE: IEEE Spectrum 8(12):38–46, 1971

21. Glaser RM: Physiologic aspects of spinal cord injury and functional neuromuscular stimulation. Central Nervous System Trauma 3:49–62, 1986

22. Glaser RM et al: Exercise program for wheelchair activity. Am J Phys Med 60:67–75, 1981

23. Glaser RM et al: Locomotion via paralyzed leg muscles: Feasibility study for a leg-propelled vehicle. J Rehabil R D 20:87–92, 1983

24. Gracanin F, Trnkoczy A: Optimal stimulus parameters for minimum pain in the chronic stimulation of innervated muscle. Arch Phys Med Rehabil 56:243–249, 1975

25. Grapengeisser CJC: Versuche den Galvanismus zur Heilung einiger Krankheitern anzuwenden, Berlin, 1801

26. Green HJ et al: Fiber type specific transformations in the enzyme activity pattern of rat vastus lateralis muscle by prolonged endurance training. Pflügers Arch 299:216–222, 1983

27. Gruner JA: Considerations in designing acceptable neuromuscular stimulation systems for restoring function in paralyzed limbs. Central Nervous System Trauma 3:37–47, 1986

28. Gruner JA et al: A system for evaluation and exercise-conditioning of paralyzed leg muscles. J Rehabil R D 20:21–30, 1983

29. Hambrecht FT: Neural prostheses. Ann Rev Biophys Bioeng 8:239–267, 1979

30. Hambrecht FT, Reswick JB: Functional Electrical Stimulation. New York, Marcel Dekker, 1977

31. Heaton H III et al: Computer controlled exercise guy for building muscle strength. IEEE NAECON Rec: 1172–1177, 1983

32. Henneman E: Recruitment of motoneurons: The size principle. In Desmedt JE (ed): Motor Unit Types, Recruitment and Plasticity in Health and Disease. Basel, S Karger, 1981

33. Holle J et al: Functional electrostimulation of paraplegics. Experimental investigations and first clinical experience with an implantable stimulation device. Orthopedics 7:1145–1155, 1984

34. Isakou E et al: Biomechanical and physiological evaluation of FES-activated paraplegic patients. J Rehabil R D 23(3):9–19, 1986

35. Kellaway P: Bull Hist Med 20:112–137, 1946

36. Kljajic M et al: Quantitative gait evaluation of hemiplegic patients using electrical stimulation orthoses. IEEE Trans on Biomed Eng 22:438–441, 1975

37. Kralj A, Grobelnik S: Functional electrical stimulation—A new hope for paraplegic patients? Bull Prosth Res 10–20:75–102, 1973

38. Kralj A, Vodovnik L: Functional electrical stimulation of the extremities: Part 2. J Med Eng Technol 75–79, March 1977

39. Kralj A et al: Improvement of locomotion in hemiplegic patients with multichannel electrical stimulation. In Human Locomotor Engineering. London, Institution of Mechanical Engineers, 1974

40. Kralj A et al: Electrical stimulation providing functional use of paraplegic patient muscles. Med Prog Technol 7:3–9, 1980

41. Kralj A et al: Gait restoration in paraplegic patients: A feasibility demonstration using multichannel surface electrode FES. J Rehabil R D 20:3–20, 1983

42. Kugelberg E: The motor unit: Morphology and function. In Desmedt JE (ed): Motor Unit Types, Recruitment and Plasticity in Health and Disease. Basel, S Karger, 1981

43. Liberson WT et al: Functional electrotherapy: Stimulation of the peroneal nerve synchronized with the swing phase of the gait of hemiplegic patients. Arch Phys Med Rehabil 101–105, Feb 1961

44. Licht S: Therapeutic Electricity and Ultraviolet Radiation, 2nd ed, pp 1–70, New Haven, Elizabeth Licht, 1967

45. Licht S: Electrodiagnosis and Electromyography, 3rd ed. New Haven, Elizabeth Licht, 1971

46. Lind AR, Petrofsky JS: Isometric tension from rotary stimulation of fast and slow cat muscles. Muscle Nerve 1:213–128, 1978

47. Long C, Masciarelli VD: An electrophysiologic splint for the hand. Arch Phys Med Rehabil 44:499–503, 1963

48. May KP et al: Central hemodynamic responses for electrically stimulated leg exercise of paralyzed individuals. Fed Proc 44:1367, 1985

49. Marsolais EB, Kobetic R: Functional walking in paralyzed patients by means of electrical stimulation. Clin Orthop 175:30–36, 1983

50. Marsolais EB, Kobetic R: Implantation techniques and experience with percutaneous intramuscular electrodes in the lower extremities. J Rehabil R D 23:1–8, 1986

51. Mortimer JT et al: Intramuscular electrical stimulation: Tissue damage. Ann Biomed Eng 8:235–244, 1980

52. Munsat TL et al: Effects of nerve stimulation on human muscle. Arch Neurol 33:608–617, 1976

53. Nathan RH: The development of a computerized upper limb electrical stimulation system. Orthopedics 7:1170–1180, 1984

54. Nilsson S et al: Physical work capacity and the effect of training on subjects with long-standing paraplegia. Scand J Rehabil Med 7:51–56, 1975

55. Peckham PH et al: Alteration in the force and fatigability of skeletal muscle in quadriplegic humans following exercise induced by chronic electrical stimulation. Clin Orthop 114:326–334, 1976

56. Peckham PH et al: Controlled prehension and release in the C5 quadriplegic elicited by functional electrical stimulation of the paralyzed forearm musculature. Ann Biomed Eng 8:369–388, 1980

57. Peckham PH et al: Restoration of key grip and release in the C6 tetraplegic patient through functional electrical stimulation. J Hand Surg 5:462–469, 1980

58. Petrofsky JS: Control of the recruitment and firing frequencies of motor units in electrically stimulated muscles in the cat. Med Biol Eng Comput 16:302–308, 1978

59. Petrofsky JS: Digital analogue hybrid 3-channel sequential stimulator. Med Biol Eng Comput 17:421–424, 1979

60. Petrofsky JS et al: Applications of the Apple as a microprocessor controlled stimulator. Collegiate Microcomputer 1:97–104, 1983

61. Petrofsky JS et al: Outdoor bicycle for exercise in paraplegics and quadriplegics. J Biomed Eng 5:292–296, 1983

62. Petrofsky JS et al: Bicycle ergometer for paralyzed muscle. J Clin Eng 9:13–19, 1984

63. Petrofsky JS et al: Closed loop control for restoration of movement in paralyzed muscle. Orthopedics 7:1289–1302, 1984

64. Petrofsky JS et al: Computer control of walking in the paralyzed man. Abstract presented, at 9th Annual AIAA Mini-symposium, Air Force Institute of Technology, Wright-Patterson AFB, September 13, 1983

65. Petrofsky JS et al: Feedback control system for walking in man. Comp Biol Med 14:135–149, 1984

66. Petrofsky JS et al: Leg exerciser for training of paralyzed muscle by closed loop control. Med Biol Eng Comput 22:298–303, 1984

67. Petrofsky JS et al: Microprocessor controlled stimulation of paralyzed muscle. National Center for Rehabilitation Engineering, Wright State University, Dayton, OH

68. Petrofsky JS, Phillips CA: Constant-velocity contractions in skeletal

muscle by sequential stimulation of muscle efferents. Med Biol Eng Comput 17:583–592, 1979

69. Petrofsky JS, Phillips CA: The influence of recruitment order and fibre composition on the force-velocity relationship and fatigability of skeletal muscles in the cat. Med Biol Eng Comput 18:381–390, 1980

70. Petrofsky JS, Phillips C: Active physical therapy: A modern approach to rehabilitation therapy. J Neurol Orth Surg 4:165–173, 1983

71. Petrofsky JS, Phillips CA: Computer controlled walking in the paralyzed individual. J Neurol Orthop Surg 4:153–164, 1983

72. Petrofsky JS, Phillips CA: Feedback control stimulation to achieve movement in man. Elektroniker 14:53–60, 1985

73. Petrofsky JS, Phillips CA: The use of functional electrical stimulation for rehabilitation of spinal cord injured patients. Central Nervous System Trauma 1:57–73, 1984

74. Phillips CA et al: Functional electrical exercise. A comprehensive approach for physical conditioning of the spinal cord injured patient. Orthopedics 7:1112–1123, 1984

75. Phillips CA, Petrofsky JS: A mathematical approach for functional electrical stimulation in the cat. National Center for Rehabilitation Engineering, Wright State University, Dayton, OH

76. Rack RMH, Westbury DR: The effects of length and stimulus rate on tension in the isometric cat soleus muscle. J Physiol 204:443–460, 1969

77. Rattan SN et al: Skeletal muscle pumping via voluntary and electrical induced contractions. Physiologist 28:363, 1985

78. Riley DA, Allin EF: The effects of inactivity, programmed stimulation, and denervation on the histochemistry of skeletal muscle fiber types. Exp Neurol 40:391–413, 1973

79. Salmons S et al: Ultrastructural aspects of the transformation of muscle fibre type by long term stimulation: Changes in Z discs and mitochondria. J Anat 127:17–31, 1978

80. Salmons S, Vrbova G: The influence of activity on some contractile characteristics of mammalian fast and slow muscles. J Physiol 201:535–549, 1969

81. Stanic U et al: Multichannel electrical stimulation for correction of hemiplegic gait. Scand J Rehabil Med 10:75–92, 1978

82. Stanic U, Trnkoczy A: Closed-loop positioning of hemiplegic patient's joint by means of functional electrical stimulation. IEEE Trans of Biomed Eng 21:365–370m, 1974

83. Stenberg J et al: Hemodynamic response to work with different muscle groups, sitting and supine. J Apply Physiol 22:61–70, 1967

84. Stillwell G: Clinical electric stimulation. In Licht S (ed): Therapeutic Electricity and Ultraviolet Radiation, 2nd ed, pp 111–112. New Haven, Elizabeth Licht, 1967

85. Thrope GB et al: A computer-controlled multichannel stimulation system for laboratory use in functional neuromuscular stimulation. IEEE Trans on Biomed Eng BME-32:363–370m, 1985

86. Vodovnik L et al: Control of a skeletal joint by electrical stimulation of antagonists. Med Bio Eng 5:97–109, 1967

87. Vrbova G: Factors determining the speed of contraction of striated muscle. J Physiol 185:17–18, 1966

88. Wilhere GF et al: Design and evaluation of a digital closed-loop controller for the regulation of muscle force by recruitment modulation. IEEE Trans on Biomed Eng BME-32:668–676, 1985

89. Wronski TJ et al: Alterations in calcium homeostasis and bone during actual and simulated space flight. Med Sci Sports Exerc 15:410–414, 1983

16

Orthotics and Shoes

Kristjan T. Ragnarsson

Orthotics is the systematic pursuit of straightening and improving function of the body or body parts by the application of an orthosis to the outside of the body. The term *orthosis* may refer to a number of devices with a more restricted or specific meaning, such as braces, splints, calipers, and corsets. Depending on the design, an orthosis may totally immobilize a joint or body segment, restrict movement in a given direction, control mobility, assist with movement, or reduce weight-bearing forces. In the presence of weak or paralyzed muscles, orthotic immobilization of a joint or an entire limb provides support. In the presence of unbalanced muscle forces, an orthosis prevents the generation of a deformity or joint contracture. In the presence of inflamed or injured musculoskeletal segments, orthosis reduces pain and allows healing. Extension of an orthosis to a healthy body part can transfer or redistribute the weight-bearing forces, thereby reducing the actual load on a long bone or whole limb. This may help to relieve pain and allow healing of injured parts. The primary principle behind the prescription of an orthosis is the improvement of function.

Before an orthosis is prescribed, the precise functions which it is meant to improve must be determined. The physician needs to know the indications for prescribing a specific orthosis, the anatomy and neuromuscular function, and the functional and biomechanical deficits present. The physician must also thoroughly understand the mechanical principles of orthotic application, the materials used in fabrication, the various designs that are available, and the training that the patient must receive, both before and after receiving the orthosis. Finally, the physician needs to be aware of the cost of the orthosis and the patient's financial means, carefully judging whether the benefits to be obtained will justify the cost.

While the indications for prescribing and using an orthosis may be obvious, contraindications are more subtle. The use of an orthosis should be discontinued when it causes pain, reduces function, worsens posture or gait, causes emotional distress, or when more effective results may be achieved by physical therapy or relatively minor surgical procedures. Allergy to the orthotic materials, restriction of peripheral circulation, or development of pressure sores requires immediate alteration or adjustment of the orthosis. Although an orthosis may significantly improve mobility and self-sufficiency, it also is a visible reminder of a lasting or permanent disability. Cosmetic appearance and comfort of the orthosis are two factors that will ease the patient's adjustment to the disability and facilitate acceptance of the device.

Materials and Mechanics

A wide variety of materials have been used to fabricate orthotic appliances, some of them in use for centuries (metal, rubber, leather, and canvas) while others have been developed more recently (plastics and synthetic fabrics).[8] When selecting the appropriate materials for an orthotic device one needs to carefully consider strength, durability, flexibility, and weight. The orthotic design should be simple, inconspicuous, comfortable, and as cosmetic as possible. It should adhere to the basic principle of distributing forces over a sufficiently large surface area. Parts that are in contact with the body should be accurately contoured and padded.

The choice of orthotic material depends on the clinical purpose and the characteristics of the patient. Traditional orthotic devices employ metals to provide strength and durability with straps and padding made of leather (Fig. 16-1). The metals that are primarily used are steel and aluminum, mostly in alloy forms with various other metals to further increase the strength of the orthosis and to resist corrosion. Although metal orthoses are heavy and are not cosmetic, they are adjustable, which allows them to accommodate for growth and the changing needs of the patient.

Orthoses that are made of plastic (Fig. 16-2) generally are lighter and closer fitting, since they can be molded directly to the body or over a plaster replica of the body part. The close fit of the plastic orthosis provides wider distribution of the corrective forces than is possible with a metal orthosis. Comfort may be increased by adding foam liners on the inside of the orthosis. Based on the weight of the patient, the use of the orthosis, the specific type of plastic employed, and the design or the orthosis, plastic materials generally provide adequate strength and durability. Plastic orthoses are generally not adjustable in length, but some materials allow heating and subsequent molding to accommodate or provide relief at pressure points. Plastic orthoses are usually fitted with metal joints or flexible spring-loaded plastic bars, since durable plastic joints have not yet been developed.

Two major types of plastic materials are used in orthotics: thermosetting and thermoplastic materials. *Thermosetting plas-*

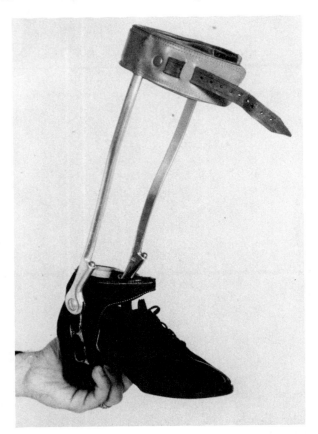

Figure 16-1. Klenzak ankle-foot orthosis with a medial T-strap.

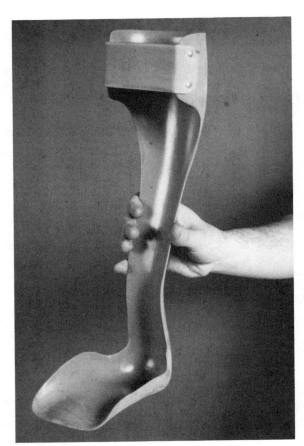

Figure 16-2. Plastic ankle-foot orthosis (shown is a PLSO, plastic leaf spring orthosis).

tics, for example, formaldehyde, epoxy, and polyester resins, are typically used as laminates in a laminated form. They require heat to harden but do not soften with subsequent heating. *Thermoplastics* soften when they are heated. This makes the material moldable. Subsequent heating will soften the material for further molding, and lowering the temperature hardens the material once again. Low temperature thermoplastics, such as Orthoplast and Plastazote, become workable at temperatures that are just below the body temperature. This allows quick fabrication and molding directly on the body. Unfortunately these materials lack strength and durability and are therefore not indicated for long-term use. The high temperature thermoplastics, such as polyethylene, polypropylene, copolymers, ortholene, and vinylpolymers, require heating to 150°F to make them workable. Fabrication of an orthosis made of any of these materials requires an exact plaster replica of the body part. The heated plastic is then applied to the replica for proper molding. These materials are generally strong and durable, and if they are flexible, they have a good "memory," returning to their original position after deformation. The orthosis provides support and may also give a spring-action force. Most plastic orthoses designed for long-term use are made of high temperature thermoplastics.

Terminology

Until recently, the lexicon of terms used to describe orthotics was very confusing. Clinicians used different terms to describe even the most basic device. Devices or parts of an orthosis were given names that might describe their purpose, the body part to which

they were applied, the inventor of the devices, or where they were developed. To facilitate communication and minimize the use of acronyms, a logical, easy-to-use system of standard terminology was developed. This system uses the first letter of the name of each joint which the orthosis crosses in correct sequence, with the letter O (for orthosis) attached at the end. Thus, the more common orthoses would be named AFO (ankle–foot orthosis), KAFO (knee–ankle–foot orthosis), KO (knee orthosis), CO (cervical orthosis), CTLSO (cervicothoracolumbosacral orthosis), and WHO (wrist–hand orthosis). A properly written orthotic prescription does not just state the name of the orthosis. It is also necessary to state the desired function to be obtained, the specific material from which the device is to be made, and the specific design and construction that is to be employed.

UPPER LIMB ORTHOTICS

Biomechanics

The evolution of the upper limb in primates to its current status in humans is a remarkable development. In quadriped animals the forelimbs provide stability, whereas in humans the interaction of the shoulder, elbow, forearm, wrist, and hand provides a great degree of mobility as well as distal prehension with an infinite number of positions and functions. This important development of the upper limb was associated with increased cortical motor and sensory representation of the hand, which allowed for the development of a highly sophisticated feedback system. The shoulder girdle mechanism in humans consists of seven joints, which move in harmony to provide excellent mobility but relatively little stability. Elbow, forearm, and wrist motions rotate, shorten, and lengthen the upper limb to position the hand and to manipulate and move objects toward and away from the body.

In man the hand serves multiple purposes. In communication it adds an affective component to our speech and substitutes for the ineffective sensory systems of blind and deaf people. Its most basic functions, however, are to provide prehension to grasp and manipulate objects and an exquisite sensation to scan the immediate environment. The long and mobile human thumb with its rich sensory innervation is controlled by many muscles both for strength and dexterity. Thumb opposition is unique in the animal kingdom and, when combined with its other motor and sensory functions and extensive cortical representation, it provides the hand with enormous potential. Several basic hand grips are used based on the nature of the task: palmar, tip (three-jaw chuck) and lateral (key) prehensions for precision, and cylindrical, spherical, and hook prehensions for power (Fig. 16-3). For optimal function the hand is best placed in the pronated position with slight extension and ulnar deviation at the wrist, and with the thumb in opposition and the fingers slightly flexed at all joints (the "position of function" in Fig. 16-3).

Any condition which alters the joint range of motion, muscle strength, sensation, and skin integrity will impair the use of the upper limb. Upper limb orthoses are often used as an adjunct to other treatment modalities in order to maintain joint alignment, to assist with movement, and to increase joint mobility, muscle strength, coordination, and function for various tasks. The term *splint* is often used for an upper extremity orthosis, especially one that is ready-made, commercially available, or intended for temporary use only. Custom-made orthoses of durable materials should be prescribed when extended use is anticipated.

Classification

Upper limb orthoses are frequently classified as static or dynamic (functional).

Static Orthoses

Static orthoses have no moving parts and are used to provide rest, protection, support, and correction. The joints are immobilized in the desired position to decrease pain, prevent overstretching, and facilitate healing, as well as to increase function. Through fabrication of serial orthoses a contracted joint may be forced into better alignment. Static orthoses are used in the management of neurological and arthritic disabilities, fractures, joint and soft tissue injuries, burns, and postoperative conditions. Various types of static finger orthoses (FO) can be used to stabilize one or more interphalangeal (IP) joints. *Static hand orthosis* (HO, opponens orthosis) consists of a firm band, which runs from the dorsum of the second metacarpal bone (Fig. 16-4). Proximal to the metacarpophalangeal (MCP) joint of the thumb, a bar is attached which stabilizes the thumb in opposition and slight flexion. Many modifications can be added to the static HO, such as attachments for writing or eating, a C-bar, thumb post, and MCP stop. The C-bar holds the thumb abduction to maintain the web space. A thumb post is useful to completely immobilize the paralyzed thumb for prehension. A MCP stop (lumbrical bar) is a dorsal bar across the proximal phalanges which prevents MCP hyperextension in the presence of weak intrinsic hand muscles and "claw hand" deformity. *Wrist hand orthoses* (WHO) are of various designs and can be placed against the dorsal, palmar, lateral, or medial aspects of the wrist. Some designs provide wrist support only while allowing full freedom of the thumb and fingers, but others may be attached to the basic HO with its various modifications described above. A *resting WHFO* is a static device that immobilizes the wrist, fingers, and thumb in optimal position. *Static elbow orthoses* (EO) are used to maintain or increase elbow range of motion usually by serial applications or by use of turn buckles to increase the force applied to the arm and forearm. *Static shoulder orthoses* are usually made to hold the arm in abduction (airplane splint) to prevent contracture following various kinds of injuries, burns, manipulations, and surgery (Fig. 16-5).

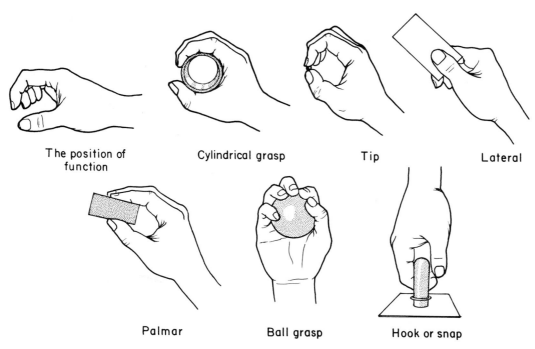

Figure 16-3. The position of optimal function and basic hand grips.

The position of function

Cylindrical grasp

Tip

Lateral

Palmar

Ball grasp

Hook or snap

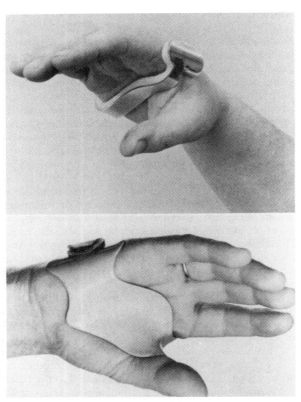

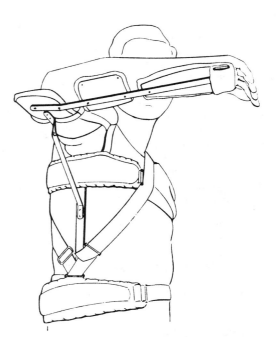

Figure 16-5. Static shoulder orthosis (airplane splint). (Redford JB (ed): Orthotics Etc. Baltimore, Williams & Wilkins, 1980)

Figure 16-4. Static hand orthoses. (American Academy of Orthopedic Surgeons: Atlas Of Orthotics. St Louis, CV Mosby, 1975)

Figure 16-6. Wrist-hand orthosis with (*A*) and without (*B*) dynamic metacarpal phalangeal extension assist.

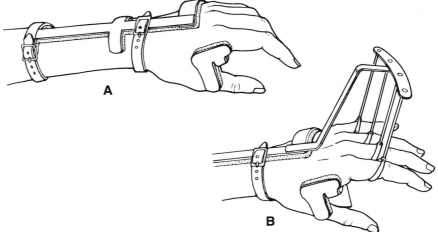

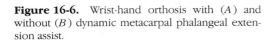

Dynamic Orthoses

Dynamic or functional orthoses allow joint mobility and assist weak or paralyzed muscles by specific forces and directional pull through the use of levers, pulleys, mobile joints, and external power sources, including elastics, springs, batteries, compressed gas, or myoelectric signals. Dynamic flexion and extension of fingers may be obtained by outriggers or hooks attached to a static HO or WHO connected with rubber bands to loops around the fingers. *Dynamic wrist orthoses* (DWO) are rarely used without hand orthoses (DWHO), but as such can be fabricated in many variations. Loss of wrist and finger extension due to radial nerve injury may be managed by a WHO with wrist and MCP extension assistance through rubber bands placed

dorsal to the axis of the wrist and MCP outrigger-elastic-finger-loop mechanism as described above (Fig. 16-6).

Wrist-driven prehension WHO (tenodesis splint) is used for severe paralytic conditions such as C6 quadriplegia (Fig. 16-7). Here the IP joints of the second and third digits and the IP and MCP joints of the thumb are immobilized to obtain a three-jaw chuck prehension either through an adjustable parallelogram of metal bars which transform wrist extension and flexion into finger flexion and extension, respectively, or through external power sources. *Dynamic elbow orthoses* depend on gravity for extension, but for flexion they use elastics, springs, external power sources, or a shoulder harness and cable system (as in an above-elbow prosthesis). These orthoses usually require a hinged elbow joint mechanism with locks for proper position-

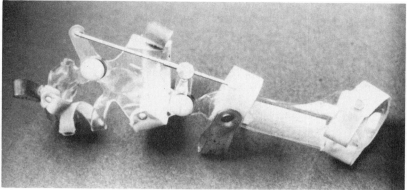

A

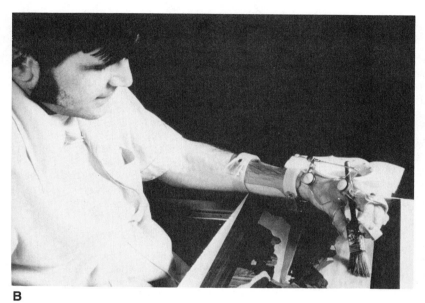

B

Figure 16-7. (*A*) Wrist-driven wrist-hand plastic orthosis (tenodesis splint). (*B*) Orthosis allows a C6 quadriplegic to hold and use a brush.

ing. *Dynamic shoulder orthoses* are rarely used except to give mobile upper limb support, such as a balanced forearm orthosis (BFO). In general, dynamic orthoses are not tolerated as well as static orthoses due to pressure and discomfort from stretching and circulatory disturbances.

Balanced forearm orthoses (also known as linkage feeder, mobile arm support) was initially developed at the Georgia Warm Springs Foundation as an assistive device for polio victims with paralyzed upper extremities.[1] Today, it is mostly used in order to bring the hand toward the head in high quadriplegia and neuromuscular conditions that have resulted in insufficient voluntary strength and endurance of shoulder and elbow muscles (Fig. 16-8). Residual muscle function of the wrist, hand, and fingers with even a weak manual prehension widens the scope of possible use.

This orthosis consists of a resting forearm orthosis (trough) that is attached by a balancing hinge joint to an adjustable ball-bearing swivel arm and bracket. This bracket is secured to a wheelchair, lapboard, or body corset. The design supports the weight of the arm against gravity and reduces the friction of mechanical moveable joints to a minimum. It thus provides movement useful for various functional activities by use of gravity and the minimal need for residual muscle power in neck, trunk, and shoulder girdle. The patient is able to move the arm horizontally in a circle by use of the swivel mechanism. Flexion of the elbow brings the hand up to the mouth or head.

Figure 16-8. Balanced forearm orthosis assists with paralyzed upper arm movement. (Redford JB (ed): Orthotics Etc. Baltimore, Williams & Wilkins, 1980)

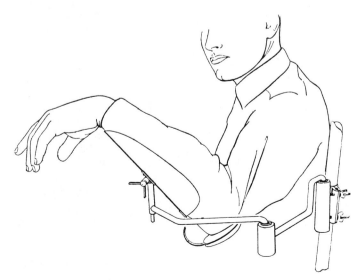

Users of the BFO must have some useful residual muscle strength and coordination, full range of motion of the shoulders and elbow joints, and adequate trunk stability and endurance in the sitting position. The BFO is frequently used in the early phases of rehabilitation when the retraining of weak muscles takes place in order to protect against excessive stretching, fatigue, immobility, and pain, as well as for the therapeutic restoration of joint range of motion, muscle strength, and endurance. When a permanent need exists the BFO may enable the patient to perform numerous functional activities such as feeding, writing, typing, painting, and playing checkers, chess, and other table-top activities. The clinician must ensure that the BFO is properly adjusted for optimal fit and control.

LOWER LIMB ORTHOTICS

Gait

The clinician prescribing lower extremity orthoses needs to have a thorough understanding of normal human locomotion, which can be defined as a forward translation of the body's center of gravity (COG) by bipedal gait. Bipedal gait is a learned activity as evidenced by the fact that congenitally blind children have to be taught to walk on two legs, and that children who have been brought up among animals have been found to walk on all fours. Gait patterns are irregular early in life, but by the age of 7 or 8 children establish a regular rhythmical gait pattern. Although individual differences in gait can be striking, the basic characteristics of normal gait are very similar. To maximize energy-efficient locomotion both the common and individually unique characteristics of gait are adopted to minimize the movement of COG vertically and laterally. Significant deviation from an individual's gait pattern, either willfully or by pathology, will increase the energy expenditure for any distance traveled in a given length of time. Prescription of proper orthoses for pathological gait may make the gait safer and more energy efficient, and the pattern more normal.

Gait Cycle

The *gait cycle* consists of the activity from heel strike of one foot to the next heel strike of the same foot. It is subdivided into the stance phase and the swing phase. The *stance phase,* that is, the period when the foot is in contact with the ground, normally constitutes 60% of the gait cycle. It starts with the heel of one foot striking the ground and ends when the toes of the same foot leave the ground. The stance phase is divided into four parts: the heel strike, foot flat, mid-stance, and push off. Since weight bearing is the major function of the lower extremities, the stance phase usually reveals most clinical problems. The *swing phase,* the period while the foot is off the ground, constitutes the remaining 40% of the gait cycle. It begins when the toes leave the ground and ends with heel strike. The swing phase is divided into acceleration, mid-swing, and deceleration. During normal gait, the period when both legs are in stance phase is referred to as *double support.* It is quite variable in length, being long in slow gait, short in fast gait, and absent altogether during running.

Gait Analysis

Although gait is most commonly analyzed by direct clinical observation, modern technology has provided more sophisticated analysis tools, introducing several bioengineering techniques such as photographic recording, motion pictures, video recording, electromyographic studies, electrogoniometry, and force place studies. Through these techniques, walking has been shown to involve the forward translation of the body's COG through a path that requires minimal energy expenditure according to the formula, Force = Mass × Acceleration. The less the COG is displaced, the smaller the energy expenditure.

Saunders, Inman, and Eberhart[13] described six elementary determinants of gait that reduce the COG displacement. The vertical displacement of COG follows a smooth sinusoidal curve and is considered to be less than 2 inches in normal adults. The six determinants of gait are (1) *pelvic rotation* of 4° to each side occurring at the hip joint. This may be increased with increasing speed of gait. The pelvic rotation increases the length of the supporting leg and thus elevates the lowest point of COG by 3/8″ (less than 1 cm). Thus it allows longer steps without changing COG displacement significantly. (2) *Pelvic tilt* of 5°, a lateral horizontal dip of the pelvis on the swing side, which results in a relative adduction of the stance side (positive Trendelenburg sign) reducing the summit of the COG curve by 3/16″ (less than 1/2 cm). Further lateral tilt of the pelvis is resisted by the iliotibial tract and the hip abductors on the contralateral stance side. (3) *Knee flexion during mid-stance phase* of 15° to 20°, which lowers the summit of the COG curve by 7/16″ (1.2 cm). (4) (5) Certain synchronized movements of the knee, ankle, and foot that allow the knee to remain essentially horizontal during the entire stance phase. Knee flexion is then able to more effectively flatten the pathway of the hips. Put together, these elementary determinants of gait result in a total reduction of COG vertical displacement of 2″, or 1″ (2.5 cm) on each side. (6) *Lateral displacement* of COG of less than 2″ (4.5 cm) toward the stance side occurs as the body is shifted over the weight-bearing leg with each step. The lateral displacement of COG is reduced by relative adduction at the hip joint during stance and a slight valgus between the tibia and the femur, keeping the feet close to the plane of progression. The lateral displacement is increased by a wider pelvis, by walking with the feet more widely separated, and by certain pathological conditions. The normal width of the walking base is 2″ to 4″ as measured between midpoints of heel strike. Cadence, or speed of walking, varies widely, from less than 70 steps per minute in slow walking, 90 to 110 steps during normal walking (approximately 2 1/2 mph), and up to 130 or more steps during fast walking. The average stride length of an adult varies and depends on body height (leg length) and cadence. During normal walking, both stride length and cadence are subconsciously and individually controlled in order to provide the most energy-efficient locomotion possible.

When analyzing gait the clinician needs to determine the position of each lower extremity joint (kinematic analysis) and assess the magnitude and direction of internal (muscles) and external (gravity, floor reaction) forces on each joint during the various phases of gait (Table 16-1) and to observe the movement of the trunk and upper extremities, the type of footwear, and even the person's emotional state.

Analysis of abnormal gait requires an organized and systematic approach. The clinician must observe the general posture and symmetry of all parts of the body both during quiet standing and all phases of the gait cycle. This includes head position, shoulder height, arm swing, trunk movements, balance, width of walking base, stride length, cadence, smoothness of movements, length of stance phase on each side, and the position of each lower extremity joint. A pathological change or loss of one of the elementary determinants of gait may be partly compensated for by the other determinants. Causes of abnormal gait are too many to enumerate them all, but the more common deserve brief description, along with the clinical deviations observed and suggested orthotic intervention.

Table 16-1
Kinematic and Kinetic Analysis of Gait

Gait Cycle	Joint Position	Muscle Action
Hip		
Heel strike	20° flexion	Hip extensors (hamstrings and gluteus) contract to prevent jack-knifing.
Mid-stance	Extension	Abductors contract to prevent excessive pelvic dip.
Push off	5°–15° hyperextension	Iliopsoas Adductors contract to stabilize pelvis.
Acceleration	Extension	Quadriceps followed by iliopsoas contract for flexion.
Mid-swing	20° flexion	Iliopsoas activity tapering off.
Deceleration	20° flexion	Hip extensors decelerate forward motion with lengthening contraction.
Knee		
Heel strike	178° extension	Lengthening contraction of quadriceps (only) to prevent knee from buckling
Mid-stance	20° flexion	
Heel off	Extension	Shortening contraction of quadriceps
Toe off	40° flexion	Results from gastrocnemius action, but primarily from floor reaction force passing behind knee joint
Acceleration	Flexion 40°–65°	Lengthening contraction of quadriceps to prevent excessive heel rise
Mid-swing	Flexion 65°	
Deceleration		Shortening contraction of quadriceps; hamstrings contract to decelerate forward motion.
Ankle		
Heel strike	Neutral	Dorsiflexors contract against gravity to prevent foot slapping.
Foot flat	15° plantarflexion	
Mid-stance	2°–3° dorsiflexion	No muscle action
Heel off	15° dorsiflexion	Plantarflexors contract (gastrocnemius strongest).
Toe off	20° plantarflexion	Plantarflexors contract (flexor hallucis longus strongest)
Swing	Neutral	Dorsiflexors

EFFECTS OF NEUROLOGICAL DYSFUNCTION. Generalized neurological conditions may significantly change gait patterns. *Hemiparesis* due to brain damage often causes weak hip flexion and dorsiflexion of the ankle, which results in impaired forward placement of the impaired limb and inadequate foot clearance during the swing phase of gait. These deficits are partly compensated for by hip hiking and circumduction or by appropriately prescribed AFO. Children with *spastic diplegia* due to cerebral palsy ambulate with a stiff or jerky gait pattern with hips flexed and adducted, knees flexed and in valgus position, and the ankles in equino-valgus position. Initially, a KAFO and appropriate footwear may be indicated, but following appropriate surgery no or minimal orthotic intervention may be necessary. Patients with *ataxia* due to cerebellar or brain-stem disorders walk with abnormal trunk motions, increased width of walking base, and jerky uncoordinated foot placement. Sturdy footwear and gait aids may help them to increase safety and improve the gait pattern. In *Parkinson's disease* several abnormal gait patterns may be observed, such as decrease or loss of arm swing and diagonal trunk motions, short shuffling steps or short accelerating propulsive (festinating) steps. Appropriate footwear and gait aids are useful, but other types of orthotics are not very helpful. *Sensory deficits* due to central or peripheral disorders are usually characterized by incoordinated movements, poor balance, and increased width of walking base. Weighted, sturdy footwear and gait aids are often helpful.

EFFECTS OF LOWER EXTREMITY PARALYSIS. Paralytic conditions of the lower extremities often result in specific gait deviations. Weak dorsiflexion of the ankle results in a steppage gait or "toe drag" during the swing phase of gait because of the excessive leg length caused by the foot-drop. It also results in a foot-slap, which occurs in the early stance phase instead of the normal heel strike. Similar gait deviations may be noted with equinus deformity of the ankle and foot. Spring-loaded AFO may effectively compensate for the weak ankle and foot dorsiflexors. Weak plantar-flexors are evident when there is poor push off at the end of stance phase. This clinical deficit is also seen in those with ankle-foot calcaneous deformities, causing the whole foot to be lifted up at once and carried forward. AFO with a dorsiflexion stop may help to adjust for this deficit. Weakness of the quadriceps muscle may result in buckling or collapse of the knee during mid-stance, but this may be prevented by muscle substitution (hip extensors and gastrocnemius), externally rotating the extremity, supporting the knee manually, or by a KO locking the knee. Weakness of hip extensors, including the hamstrings, if bilateral, may result in the body falling forward (jack-knifing) during walking. This problem can be compensated for by increased lumbar lordosis, manual support at the back of the hip, especially if unilateral, and by use of gait aids such as crutches or canes.

Orthoses with locking mechanisms for the hip are rarely used. Weakness of hip abductors results in a waddling gait with the lateral trunk bending toward the affected side during mid-stance to direct COG over the hip joint. Stance phase is usually decreased in length on the affected side and increased on the good side. Similar gait pattern is noted in those with painful hip conditions (antalgic gait) as the COG is placed over the hip to reduce pull of the abductor muscles and thus decrease the intra-articular pressure. With the added support of a cane held in the opposite hand this gait deviation can be effectively corrected. Weakness of the hip flexors results in poor forward placement of the leg, short steps, and poor clearance of the foot during the swing phase. Hip hiking and pelvic rotation through quadratus lumborum and other trunk muscles help to raise the extremity and move it forward. Excessive voluntary toe rise or prescription of a footlift on the shoe for the opposite side will facilitate clearing of the foot during swing.

LOWER EXTREMITY STRUCTURAL ABNORMALITIES. Numerous lower extremity structural abnormalities will affect the gait. Leg length discrepancy is evident by toe walking on the shorter leg during stance or inadequate clearance of the swing leg for which an appropriate footlift may be prescribed. Fusion of one hip results in compensatory motions of the spine and exaggerated motions of the normal hip during walking, but the exact gait pattern is affected by the position of fusion. Flexion contractures of hip or knee are evident by conspicuous limp due to the leg shortening.

Energy Cost of Locomotion

A normal person walks about 83 meters per minute and expends 0.063 kcal/min/kg and 0.000764 kcal/meter/kg, according to an average of results.[4] This speed of walking is both comfortable and results in minimal energy consumption, that is, the least number of calories spent per meter walked per kilogram of body weight (cal/meter/kg). Any increase or decrease in the speed of walking results in reduced energy efficiency. A person with a physical disability walks more slowly than a nondisabled person in order to avoid excessive increases in energy expenditure per minute, in other words, to keep energy expenditure per minute as close as possible to that of a nondisabled person. The greater the physical disability, the greater are the gait deviations. Thus more energy is expended per meter ambulated and the gait becomes less efficient. A disabled person, like the nondisabled person, will automatically and subconsciously select his or her own most comfortable and most energy-efficient speed of walking. This can be increased with training and prescription of appropriate gait aids and orthosis. It has been shown,[2] for example, that in hemiparetic patients with ankle and foot weakness who ambulate without AFO, the average comfortable walking speed is 41 meters per minute, about half the normal walking speed. The energy expenditure per minute at this speed was 64% greater than for normal controls walking at the same speed. However, when the hemiparetics walked with an AFO there was a significant increase in their speed of walking and a decrease in their energy expenditure.

Numerous studies have shown that patients with thoracic paraplegia require enormous energy expenditure to ambulate with crutches and KAFOs. Generally, therefore, only paraplegics with lumbar lesions and voluntary control of their pelvis and with some intact hip and knee movements ambulate functionally in the community.[5] The energy consumption of paraplegics while ambulating tends to decrease and their speed tends to increase with descending lesion levels. However, energy expenditure tends to be similar for most paraplegics, regardless of the

level of injury, because they select a comfortable level of energy expenditure rather than a specific speed of walking. For the most part, oxygen consumption is three to five times the resting rate, depending on the speed of ambulation. Even after 1 or 2 years of training, only 50% of thoracic paraplegics reach a steady state of energy consumption during ambulation and the speed of ambulation rarely exceeds 15 to 25 meters per minute.

Shoes and Footwear

The basic function of commercial shoes is to protect the feet from rough walking surfaces, the weather, and the environment, and to provide support for the feet during standing and walking. To improve comfort and function special shoes are commercially available for certain unusual or abnormal foot activities, mostly for recreational use and for pathological foot conditions. The clinician frequently fails to appreciate the importance of comfortable and well fitting shoes. Foot problems that could easily be corrected by prescription of proper shoes or shoe modifications frequently interfere with optimum functional performance.

Components

The parts of a shoe (Fig. 16-9) consist of the sole, the heel, the upper, the linings, and reinforcements. Each component is made of a wide variety of materials and designs depending on the quality and specific use of the shoe.

The sole is the bottom part of the shoe. It is divided into the *outer sole,* or the surface that touches the ground, and the *inner sole,* the part closest to the foot to which the upper and the outer sole are attached. Sometimes a compressible filler made of cork or latex separates the inner from the outer sole. It is preferable that both the inner and the outer soles be made of leather of variable thickness. Leather soles best maintain proper fit and are especially indicated if shoe modifications are required. Rubber soles make modifications more difficult and have the additional drawback of eliminating a large ventilating surface, which may result in excessive sweating and skin problems. The greater

Figure 16-9. Shoe components.

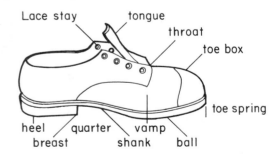

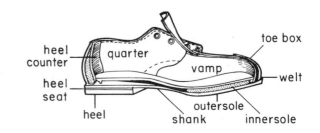

friction coefficient of rubber soles may also cause the shoe to stop short on heel strike, thrusting the foot forward into the forepart of the shoe. The widest part of the sole is at the metatarsal heads and is called *the ball.* The narrowest part of the sole, between the heel and the ball, is called the *shank.* The shank is usually reinforced by a strip of metal, leather, fiberboard, or other firm material. The external *heel seat* is the posterior part of the sole to which the heel is secured. The *toe spring* is the space between the outer sole and the floor. Its purpose is to cause rocker effect during push off and to help reduce wrinkling of the upper.

The heel is attached to the outer sole under the anatomical heel and is made of leather, wood, plastic, rubber, or metal. The heel block which is fastened to the heelseat is made of a firm material, but the plantar surface is usually made of hard rubber. The anterior surface of the heel is called the *breast.* The height of the heel is measured in eighths of an inch at the breast. The height and design of the heel vary greatly. The *flat heel* has a broad base and measures $^6/_8''$ to $1^1/_4''$ in height. A *Thomas heel* is flat and has a medial extension in order to support a weak longitudinal foot arch. A *military heel* has a slightly narrower base and measures $1^1/_4''$ to $1^3/_8''$ in height. A *Cuban heel* has a still narrower base but is higher. Heels up to 2″ to 3″ high exist, but they are mainly used for fashionable appearance rather than for extended walking. Shoes with lower heels, no heels, or negative heels also exist. A *spring heel,* which has a heel base of $^3/_8''$ to $^3/_4''$ and is placed under the outer sole, eliminates the heel breast. This type of heel is common on shoes for infants and children up to age 3. Many athletic shoes including running shoes have no heels, as running is faster without heels. The *negative heel* popularized on the "earth shoe," provided comfort for some people. The clinician needs to be aware that the height of the heel affects foot and ankle positions as well as the general posture of the trunk. Heel height may thus be a factor in certain clinical conditions, such as shortening of gastrocnemius and low back pain. High heels, especially those with a tapered narrow striking point, make the ankle and foot more unstable and thereby contribute to ankle injuries and falls.

The *upper* is that part of the shoe that is above the sole. It is most commonly made of leather, although any soft and durable material may be used. Leather is found to be most comfortable as it allows evaporation and absorption of moisture and molds well to the shape of the foot. The upper consists of the vamp, quarters, and lace stay. The *vamp* is the anterior portion of the upper, which covers the toes and the instep. The *tongue,* a strip of leather lying under the laces, and the *throat,* the opening at the base of the tongue, are parts of the vamp. Anteriorly the vamp has a reinforced *toe box* or toe cap to maintain appearance and to protect the toes against trauma. The *lace stay,* or the portion containing the eyelets for laces, is usually part of the vamp, but it may be part of the quarters.

Two *quarters* make up the posterior part of the shoe. The quarters are usually reinforced by the *heel counter* which stabilizes the foot by supporting the calcaneus, and gives structural stability to the shoe. The counter usually extends anteriorly to the heel breast, but it may extend further forward or upward on specially made shoes. It, like the toe box, is made of firm leather or synthetic material. Laterally, the quarter is cut lower to avoid infringing on the lateral malleolus. Sometimes a band of leather, referred to as a *collar* is stitched to the top of the quarters to reduce pistoning or to prevent the shoe from falling off. The *linings* are made of leather, cotton, or canvas, and should be used in all portions of the shoe that are in contact with the foot to absorb perspiration and smooth the contact area and thus provide added comfort.

Fabrication

Shoes are built around a positive model or replica of the weight-bearing foot, which is called a *last.*[15] The last, which is made of solid rock maple or plastic materials, determines the fit, the walking comfort, the appearance, and the style of the shoe. Usually the last has a slight forefoot inflare. Other common lasts include the broad toe last with a straight medial border that extends from the heel to the toe; the juvenile symmetrical straight last, which can be bisected into nearly equal right and left halves; and the orthopedic last with special features that are designed to accommodate various structural and anatomical problems (*e.g.,* varus, valgus).

During fabrication the insole is nailed to the last, the lining is tucked to the inner sole rim, and the reinforcements (the counter and the toe box) are attached. The upper of the shoe is softened by humidity for easier molding and fitted snugly to the last to adapt to its every detail and then nailed or glued to the inner sole. Finally, the outer sole and heel are attached. The Goodyear welt construction of shoes is a method used in production of high quality shoes in which the upper is sewn to the sole. This method provides a perfectly smooth inner surface, comfort, and a strong shoe that retains its shape and is easy to modify and repair. Unfortunately, these shoes tend to be bulky, heavy, and less flexible.

Types and Styles

There are innumerable shoe types and styles (Fig. 16-10), although basic designs are relatively few. The basic designs are mainly determined by the shape of the upper, especially the design of the toe and the height of the quarters. On *low-quarter shoes,* or the *Oxford,* the quarters extend approximately 1″ below the malleoli and do not restrict ankle or subtalar motions. In *high-quarter shoes* the quarters may cover the malleoli, either just barely, as in the *chukka* shoe, or by 2″ or more as in *boots.* This style prevents piston action during walking, and back and forth sliding of the foot. In addition, it provides mediolateral stability at the ankle and subtalar joints and resistance to plantar flexion. The most common throat style is the *blucher type* in which the lace stay is not directly fastened to the vamp. This style gives a wide opening for the foot for easy insertion and greater adjustability over the midfoot. The *bal type* (Balmoral) throat which has the lace stay attached directly to the vamp does not provide such easy foot access. A *lace-to-toe shoe,* often referred to as a surgical shoe, allows exposure of the entire foot by opening up to the toes. Shoe closure is usually accomplished by cotton laces, which thread through two or more pairs of eyelets, although closure can also be achieved by buckles, zippers, velcro flaps, or elastics.

Fitting

The first requirement of a shoe is that it fits and does not cause pain, skin problems, or deformities. When fitting shoes, each shoe should be judged individually in a full weight-bearing position. The shoe should fit snugly enough not to fall off, but be loose enough to adapt to the size and shape of the foot, which change with climate, ambient temperature, time of day, body position, and weight-bearing (whether the person is lying, sitting, or standing). Since the foot expands with weight-bearing, shoes should be initially carefully tested for fit, not only by standing but by walking or running several steps and stopping short. The real proof of fit, however, is if the shoe is comfortable after hours of continuous wear or walking. An old piece of advice

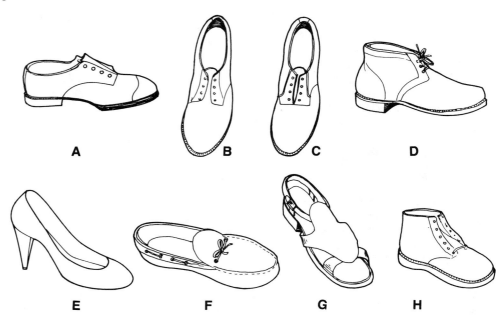

Figure 16-10. Shoe types and styles: (*A*) oxford or low quarter, (*B*) blucher-type Oxford, (*C*) Bal-type Oxford, (*D*) chukka or high quarter, (*E*) pump, (*F*) moccasin, (*G*) sandal, and (*H*) child's.

is to find a comfortable pair of shoes and then take one size larger.

In length the shoes should extend at least ½″ beyond the longest toe, usually the hallux or the second toe. The heel-to-ball distance of the foot and the shoe should be equal. Thus, the first metatarsal joint should be located at the inner curve of the shoe, and on toe dorsiflexion the shoe should bend easily and the toe break should run directly across the ball. In width, the widest part of the shoe, the ball, should coincide with the broadest part of the foot, leaving enough free space between the heads of the first and fifth metatarsal bones and the medial and lateral shoe borders, respectively. The transverse arch of the foot should function normally, weight should be evenly distributed, and no sliding of the forefoot within the shoe should occur. The medial and lateral quarters should not gap and the heel counter should close around the heel bone without bulges, allowing only a small amount of pistoning. Some pistoning is usually unavoidable in a shoe with a rigid sole and heel counter. The height of the vamp should be adequate to prevent pressure or irritation over the toes and the instep. The height of the quarters should be sufficient to hold the shoe securely on the foot. If the quarters are too high they can cause irritation of the malleoli.

Different shoe *sizes* are commercially available to accommodate different size feet. Shoe sizes are marked by numbers to indicate length and by letters to indicate width. The numbers used in the United States and Europe are different, as are the numbers used to indicate the sizes of men's, women's, and children's feet. Sizes often vary from one manufacturer to another. In the United States the smallest shoe would be infant size 000 and the largest a man's size 16. However, most shoe stores only carry men's shoe sizes up to 14 or 15 and women's sizes up to 12 or 13. Larger sizes are available in specialty shoe stores or they may be ordered directly from the manufacturer or be custom-made, at great expense. The shoe widths measured at the ball are available in different sizes ranging from A, which is narrow, to E, which is wide. Each size represents a ¼″ increase in width. Few shoe stores stock shoes of extreme width. Shoe depth is not fabricated in different sizes, although extra depth shoes and shoes with adjustable insoles are available to accommodate foot abnormalities and shoe inserts.

Children's shoes (see Fig. 16-10) are generally of similar design as those for adults. Shoes for infants and children up to age 2 or 3 who have started to stand and walk should be made of soft leather and have a straight medial border, a broad toe, high tops, a firm and snug heel counter, and a low spring-type heel. Soles should be firm and reinforced at the shank. Soft, flexible soles are advantageous for the crawling child, since they bend and do not force the foot into eversion or inversion. To accommodate the growing feet of children older than age 3, it is better to use an adult shoe design with wide, round, or square toe boxes that allow ½″ of space between the shoe and the toes during weight-bearing.

Modifications

Stock shoes may require minor or major modifications by various methods to support the abnormal foot during weight-bearing, to reduce pressure on painful areas, and to limit motion of weak, unstable, or painful joints. For these purposes the clinician may select a special type of shoe, order certain alterations in the construction of the shoe, or apply corrections directly to the foot. The clinician needs to make an accurate diagnosis of the problem, have a clear understanding of why corrections are needed, and write a specific prescription that is best accompanied by a simple drawing in order to clarify the request. Although certain simple external modifications are easily applied to many types of commercial shoes, welt shoes are more suitable to work with, especially for major internal modifications, because the shoe structure is not altered by removing and reattaching the sole to the upper. *"Orthopedic" shoes* are welt shoes made of good leather, with relatively thick soles, a high-wide toe box, extended medial heel counter, rigid wide steel shank, and a Thomas heel. They are the most frequently prescribed shoes for foot problems requiring shoe modification, although they may be regarded as high quality footwear for normal feet. *Extra-depth orthopedic shoes* have been made commercially available relatively recently. They offer removable insoles, which allow the placement of most foot orthoses without compromising fit or comfort. *Moldable shoes* have uppers that are constructed from thermoplastic materials, which can be reshaped when heated to accommodate minor to moderate foot deformities.

A fixed deformity needs accommodation, using the shoe to bring the weight-bearing surface to the foot, whereas a flexible deformity may be actively corrected. Adults usually have relatively fixed deformities requiring passive stabilization, but young children have flexible deformities which may be corrected actively by proper shoe prescription when they are minor or moderate. In more severe cases, serial plaster cast and surgical operations may be required.

INTERNAL. Shoe modifications can be classified as either internal (those that are inserted into the inner surface of the shoe or sandwiched between shoe components) or external (those which are attached to the sole or heel). Internal modifications are mechanically more effective. Although they are generally made of soft materials, they are less well tolerated since they reduce the size of the shoe and distort the inner sole. They may be removable or built in as an integral part of the shoe. Internal shoe corrections include steel shanks, "cookies," scaphoid and metatarsal pads, interior heel lifts and wedges, extended or reinforced heel counters, and protective metal toe boxes. *Steel shanks* can be used to support a weak longitudinal arch, but if this is insufficient a "cookie" made of firm materials such as leather or rubber may be placed along the medial border of the insole at the talonavicular joint. *Scaphoid pads* also provide additional longitudinal arch support, but are made of compressable material. They are prescribed for people who cannot tolerate the firmness of a cookie. The longitudinal arch support of a cookie or scaphoid pad is further improved by insertion of a long medial counter made of rigid leather. *Metatarsal pads,* which are commercially available in many sizes, may be positioned inside the shoe just proximally to the metatarsal heads to protect and reduce pressure on the second, third, and fourth metatarsal heads. A *sesamoid* or a "dancer's" pad is thicker and broader, and extends medially to the proximal part of the first metatarsal head. Thus, it provides greater support for more severe cases of metatarsalgia. *Heel elevations* of more than ¼″ should be placed externally. *Interior heel wedges* of ¹/₁₆″ to ⅛″ in height may be placed on either half of the interior heel.

EXTERNAL. External shoe modifications (Fig. 16-11) include sole and heel wedges, flanges and elevations, metatarsal and rocker bars, and different types of heel designs. *Wedges* are constructed of leather and are positioned under the outer sole or

heel. Sole and heel wedges are usually placed medially but occasionally they are placed laterally in order to shift the body weight from that side of the foot to the other. *Flanges* or "flare-outs" are ¼″ wide medial or lateral extensions of the sole or heel, which provide rotatory stability. A lateral flange provides a lever arm, which ensures a foot flat in the presence of excessive inversion or varus deformity. Such small lateral flanges are seen on most commercially available runner's shoes.

Elevations (lifts) of the sole and heel are prescribed for leg length discrepancies. Leg length discrepancies of less than ½″ do generally not require a shoe modification, but a greater discrepancy should be corrected to make the pelvis level. It may not be necessary or even desirable to provide an elevation in order for the total leg length to be equal on both sides. If an elevation of more than ¼″ is required, these should be applied externally. Elevations up to 1″ in height can be added exclusively to the heel. When an elevation of greater than 1″ is indicated, it has to be applied to both the heel and sole of the shoe. The height of the elevation must be greatest at the heel and taper off from the ball of the shoe to the toe. Elevations greater than 1″ should be made of layered cork or other lightweight materials.

The *metatarsal bar* (anterior heel) is made of leather or rubber and may be attached transversely to the outer sole immediately proximal to the metatarsal heads to relieve pressure on them and to reduce pain. A *rocker bar* is similarly placed but extends distally beyond the metatarsal heads. It also relieves pressure on the metatarsal heads and reduces metatarsal-phalangeal flexion on push off by providing a smooth plantar roll to toe off. It thus may improve gait when painful or paralytic conditions prevent good push off. A *Denver bar* is placed under the metatarsal bones to support the transverse arch extending from the metatarsal heads anteriorly to the tarsal-metatarsal joints posteriorly.

External *heel* modifications are of several kinds. Already mentioned are heel elevations, wedges, and flanges. The *Thomas heel* (Fig. 16-11), or the orthopedic heel, is similar in design and material to the regular flat heel but has an anteromedial extension to provide additional longitudinal arch support. This extension may be of variable length depending on the extent of support required and its effect may be further augmented by a medial wedge, or a Thomas heel wedge. A *reverse Thomas heel* is an anterolateral extension to support a weak lateral longitudinal arch, but this variety is rarely used. Occasionally compressible

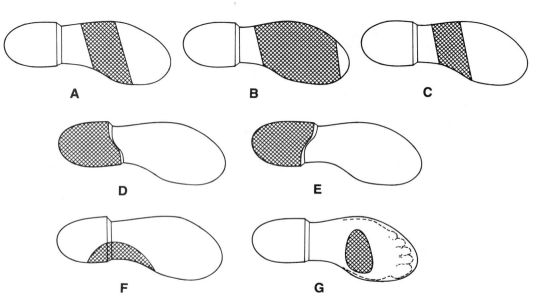

Figure 16-11. Common shoe modifications (plantar views): (*A*) metatarsal bar, (*B*) rocker bar, (*C*) Denver bar, (*D*) Thomas heel, (*E*) reverse Thomas heel, (*F*) scaphoid (navicular) pad insert, and (*G*) metatarsal pad insert.

resilient materials are inserted into the heel (solid ankle cushion heel [SACH]), usually in conjunction with a rocker bar to cushion the heel strike. The result is a simulation of plantar flexion with minimal ankle movement, while the rocker bar provides smooth push off. Thus a more natural gait may be obtained in certain clinical conditions despite relative immobilization of the foot and ankle.

Foot Orthoses

Foot orthoses (FO) are removable foot supports made of variable materials placed inside the shoe to manage different foot symptoms and deformities. They have the advantage over shoe modifications in that they can be transferred from shoe to shoe, may be modified without disturbing the shoe, and are more durable than the modified shoe. Although commercially available arch supports exist, such devices are relatively ineffective. Therefore, custom-made FOs are preferred when maintenance of a specific foot alignment over long periods of time is indicated. The usual clinical indications for FOs are to relieve pressure on areas that are painful, ulcerated, scarred, or calloused; to support weak or flat longitudinal or transverse foot arches; and to control foot position and thus affect the alignment of other lower limb joints.

Soft or *flexible FOs* are made from leather, cork, rubber, soft plastics, and plastic foam. Many of these are commercially available and used for simple problems, but they are a poor choice for more severe conditions. The soft FOs are usually fabricated in full length from heel to toe with increased thickness where weight-bearing is indicated and relief where no or little pressure should occur. Rubber FOs are generally least acceptable because of poor permeability for evaporating perspiration, lack of molding properties, and excessive compression on weight-bearing. Materials that provide best cushioning tend to wear out fast and therefore may require frequent replacement. Numerous kinds of thermoplastic polyethylene foams, such as Plastazote, are available in different densities and thicknesses. They are commonly used for ischemic, insensitive, ulcerated, and arthritic feet. After heating, some of these materials can conveniently be molded directly on the foot, but others with high specific heat require the use of a positive model of the foot. The softer grade materials tend to bottom out early and may require a latex cork backing to prolong usefulness. Some of these materials have a high friction coefficient and may have to be covered on the foot side with softer material to reduce shear.

The *semi-rigid* and *rigid FOs* come in a variety of materials such as leather, cork, and metals, but most commonly they are made of solid plastics, which allow minimal flexibility. Optimal fabrication requires applying a plaster of Paris cast on the patient's feet, removing it, and making a positive replica of the foot on which the orthosis can be accurately molded. These orthoses generally extend from the posterior end of the heel to the metatarsal heads (three-quarter length) and may have medial and lateral flanges. They are molded to provide support under the longitudinal arch and metatarsal area and to provide relief for painful or irritated areas. The most rigid FOs are made of metal, usually steel or duralumin, covered with leather, and molded on a positive cast of the patient's foot (Whitman, Mayer, and Shaffer plates; Boston arch support).

Management of Foot Conditions

Numerous clinical foot problems and deformities are best managed by modification of shoes or fabrication of a foot orthosis. The more common of these conditions are listed in Table 16-2

with the suggested shoe modifications. No single remedy or combination of remedies can serve for all cases and instances. Each case has to be judged individually and other shoe modifications and different interventions considered. It is worth bearing in mind that very frequently a custom-made foot or ankle–foot orthosis may negate the necessity for shoe modification and that surgical operations may be required to obtain optimal correction. Strappings, paddings, and appliances may be applied directly to the foot and toes in order to correct deformities and protect tender areas such as corns, calluses, ulcers, nails, bony outgrowths, and excessive friction or pressure. Prior to padding, excess corns, calluses, and nails are best removed.

The clinician prescribing shoes, shoe modifications, and foot orthoses needs to be thoroughly familiar with the normal anatomy, biomechanics, and development of the foot, diagnosis and management of pathological conditions affecting the foot, as well as the terminology, mechanisms, and manufacture of shoes, their components, and modifications. The clinician needs to educate the patient with foot disorders about foot care and footwear needs. Before and after applying shoe modifications and periodically thereafter, the shoe and the foot should be carefully examined to ensure proper fit, comfort, and mechanics.

Ankle–Foot Orthoses

Ankle–foot orthoses (AFO) are most commonly prescribed for muscle weakness affecting the ankle and subtalar joints,[6] such as weakness of dorsi- and plantar flexors, invertors, and evertors. AFO can also be prescribed for prevention or correction of deformities of the foot and ankle and reduction of weight-bearing forces. Besides having mechanical effects on the ankle, the AFOs also may affect the stability of the knee by varying the degree of plantar or dorsiflexion at the ankle. An ankle fixed in dorsiflexion will provide a flexion force at the knee and thus may help to prevent genu recurvatum; a fixed plantar flexion will provide an extension force, which may help to support a weak knee during the stance phase of gait.

Although traditional metal orthoses are still prescribed, plastic AFOs are more common. They may be fabricated from either thermoplastic or thermosetting materials, depending on the function required. Inexpensive, ready-to-use AFOs are widely available and useful for minor or temporary deficits, but custom-made orthoses molded on a replica of the foot, ankle, and leg are indicated for more severe and permanent deficits. Plastic AFOs are worn inside the shoe and consist of the foot plate, an upright component, and a Velcro calf strap. The shoe which attaches the orthosis to the foot has to have secure closures. Although these orthoses can be changed from shoe to shoe, it is important that all shoes worn have the same heel height in order to provide equal biomechanical effect at the ankle and knee. The foot plate in a custom-made AFO may be accurately molded to provide all the functions of a molded foot orthosis; at the least it should always support the metatarsal and longitudinal foot arches.

The upright components on plastic AFOs vary in design, depending on the desired function, but usually these extend from the foot plate without a joint mechanism to the upper calf approximately 1″ to 2″ below the head of the fibula. A plastic AFO can be fabricated to control plantar flexion, dorsiflexion, inversion, or eversion of the ankle depending on the design, built-in position of the orthosis, thickness of the material used, and location of the trim lines. Plastic leaf spring orthosis (PLSO) is the most commonly prescribed type of AFO (see Fig. 16-2). It substitutes for weakness of ankle dorsiflexors and provides some mediolateral stability. An associated strong tendency for ankle inversion as often seen in hemiplegics may be counteracted by

Table 16-2
Clinical Foot Conditions and Suggested Modifications of the Orthopedic Shoe

Clinical Condition	Objectives of Modifications	Modifications

Limb shortening	Provide symmetric posture
	Improve gait
		Heel elevation:
		   If <1/2″: Internal
		   If >1/2″: External
		Heel and sole elevation
		Rocker bar
		High-quarter shoe

Arthritis, fushion or instability of ankle and subtalar joints	Support and limit joint motion Accommodate deformities Improve gait	High-quarter shoe Reinforced counters Long steel shank Rocker bar SACH heel

Pes plano-valgus	Reduce eversion
	Support longitudinal arch
	Accommodate rigid deformity
		For children:
		   High-quarter shoe with broad heel, long medial counter, and
		   medial heel wedge
		For adults:
		   Thomas heel with medial heel wedge
		   Medial longitudinal arch support with "cookie" or scaphoid pad

Pes equinus (fixed)	Provide heel strike Contain foot in shoe Reduce pressure on metatarsal head Ease putting on of shoe Equalize leg length	High-quarter show, especially for children Heel elevation Heel and sole elevation on other shoe Modified lace stay for wide opening Medial longitudinal arch support Rocker bar, occasionally
Pes varus	Obtain realignment for flexible deformity Accommodate a fixed deformity Increase mecdial and posterior weight bearing on foot	High-quarter shoe Long lateral counter Reverse Thomas heel Lateral sole and heel wedges for flexible deformity Medial wedges for fixed deformities Lateral sole and heel flanges Medial longitudinal arch support
Pes cavus	Distribute weight over entire foot Restore anterior-posterior foot balance Reduce pain and pressure on metatarsal (MT) heads	High-quarter shoe High toe box Lateral heel and sole wedges Metatarsal pads or bars Molded inner sole Medial and lateral longitudinal arch support
Calcaneal spurs	Relieve pressure on painful area	Heel cushion Inner relief in heel and fill with soft sponge Medial longitudinal arch support
Metatarsalgia	Reduce pressure on MT heads Support transverse	Metatarsal or sesamoid pad Metatarsal or rocker bar Inner sole relief

Hallux valgus	Reduce pressure on 1st
	   metatarsophalangeal (MTP) joint and
	   big toe
	Prevent forward foot slide
	Immobilize 1st MTP joint
	Shift weight laterally
		Soft vamp with broad ball and toe
		Relief in vamp with cut-out or balloon patch
		Low heel
		Metatarsal or sesamoid pad
		Medial longitudinal arch support

Hallux rigidus	Reduce pressure and motion of 1st MTP joint Improve push off	Soft vamp Long steel spring in sole Sesamoid pad Metatarsal or rocker bar Medial longitudinal arch support
Hammer toes	Relieve pressure on painful areas Support transverse arch Improve push off	Soft vamp, extra-depth shoe with high toe box or balloon patch Metatarsal pad
Foot shortening (unilateral)	Fit shoe to foot	Extra inner sole and padded tongue for difference of less than one size Shoes of split sizes or custom-made
Foot fractures	Immobilize fractured part	Long steel shank Longitudinal arch support Metatarsal pad Metatarsal or rocker bar

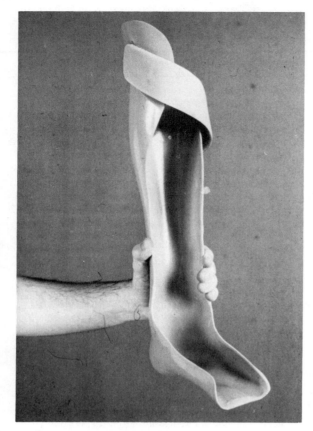

Figure 16-12.   Plastic solid ankle-foot orthosis.

increasing the rigidity of the upright component at the ankle and increasing the lateral support at the calf. Severe spasticity of the ankle may require prescription of a solid ankle plastic AFO (Fig. 16-12). Most ready-to-wear AFOs are of the PLSO or solid ankle varieties. A plastic spiral AFO may be effectively prescribed for concomitant weakness of both dorsi- and plantar flexors of the ankle when spasticity is absent or insignificant.

Metal AFOs usually have both medial and lateral uprights with an ankle joint mechanism. The uprights are attached to the shoe by a stirrup and secured to the calf by a padded leather-covered calf band, leather strap, and a buckle. Sturdy shoes, such as orthopedic shoes, are required for metal orthosis. The stirrups are usually attached directly to the shoe between the sole and the heel, although a foot plate inside the shoe is occasionally used. The upper end of the stirrup connects with the uprights at the ankle joint. A solid stirrup is most commonly used and provides the most rigid and least bulky shoe attachment. The split stirrup allows transfer of the orthosis to any shoe with a flat caliper insertion.

Different ankle joint mechanisms allow fixed, limited, or full dorsiflexion or plantar flexion. Some designs, such as the Klenzak orthosis (see Fig. 16-1), permit assistance of ankle motion in either plantar or dorsiflexion by inclusion of a spring. A plantar flexion stop can induce knee flexion, whereas a dorsiflexion stop uses a knee extension force during the stance phase of gait. The *rough caliper* is a design that attaches uprights without ankle joints to the shoe by a metal plate, but they are easily detachable. Motion occurs where the uprights are inserted into the sole of the shoe at a considerable distance from the axis of the anatomical ankle joint. The round caliper is often prescribed for children with cerebral palsy who have difficulty putting on an

orthosis. *T-straps* (see Fig. 16-1) may be attached to the shoe medially or laterally to control valgus (eversion) or varus (inversion) and are buckled around the contralateral upright to apply a counteracting force.

Knee–Ankle–Foot Orthoses

Knee-ankle-foot orthoses (KAFO) are prescribed in order to provide knee stability for weight-bearing in the presence of severe lower limb weakness due to upper or lower motor neuron lesions.

STANDARD KAFO. Below the knee, the components of the standard KAFO are the same as those of metal AFOs, except that the uprights extend to the knee joint where they join the thigh uprights (Fig. 16-13). Although the anatomical knee joint has a changing axis of rotation, *polycentric designed knee joints* have few clinical applications, since during ambulation the orthotic knee joint is usually locked. A *free knee joint* is indicated when mediolateral instability or genu recurvatum is present but knee extension strength is adequate for weight-bearing.

If knee extensors are weak and buckling occurs, a knee lock is indicated. The *drop-ring lock* is most commonly used. It is placed on the lateral upright bar and drops over the joint when it is fully extended. A *spring-loaded pull rod* may be added to the ring to ease locking and unlocking, especially when the patient is unable to reach the knee. A *cam lock* with a spring-loaded cam which fits into a groove in full extension is easier to release, but gives good stability and may be used in severe spasticity. A *bail lock* (Swiss lock) is a level bow which snaps into locked position on full extension and unlocks automatically when pressed against an object, such as a chair. In the presence of a knee flexion contracture, an adjustable knee joint may be indicated using either a *fan* or *dial lock.*

In the absence of knee flexion spasticity or contracture, a *posteriorly offset knee joint* provides a stable knee during stance, but allows flexion during the swing phase. Even when mechanically locked, the knee would bend on weight-bearing if not stabilized by straps above and below the patella or by a *patellar strap,* a soft leather pad covering the knee cap and fastened with four adjustable straps.

The thigh uprights are connected by a rigid, padded upper thigh band with an anterior soft closure. This band should clear the ischium by 1½″ unless ischial rest is prescribed. Usually, a second rigid lower thigh band is also used with soft anterior straps.

The *Scott-Craig orthosis*[10] eliminates the lower thigh and calf bands which makes it easier to put on and remove (Fig. 16-14). It consists of two uprights with four rigid connections: a posterior rigid upper thigh, bail knee lock, rigid anterior upper tibial band with soft posterior strap, and, at the lower end, a stirrup with a rigid sole plate built into the shoe extending to the metatarsal heads. It is connected to the uprights by double-stop (Becker) ankle joints which are adjusted to the orthosis in 5° of dorsiflexion for optimum balance. The shoe sole is perfectly flat from the heel to the metatarsal bar where it becomes slightly rounded to the toe. Properly adjusted, the orthosis should stand balanced on its own. It is a stable orthosis which biomechanically functions as the standard KAFO.

MODIFIED KAFO. *Plastic laminated thigh–knee–ankle orthoses* (KAFO) may incorporate standard ankle and knee components, but the uprights and bands are made of skin-colored laminated plastic which closely fits the limb and is lightweight (Fig. 16-15). The thigh piece is a quadrilaterally shaped posterior thigh shell with or without an ischial weight-bearing seat closed

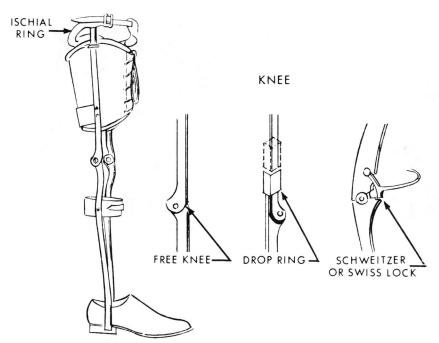

ISCHIAL RING

KNEE

FREE KNEE — DROP RING — SCHWEITZER OR SWISS LOCK

Figure 16-13. Conventional knee-ankle-foot orthosis, with variations of kneelocks. (American Academy of Orthopedic Surgeons: Atlas of Orthotics. St Louis, CV Mosby, 1975)

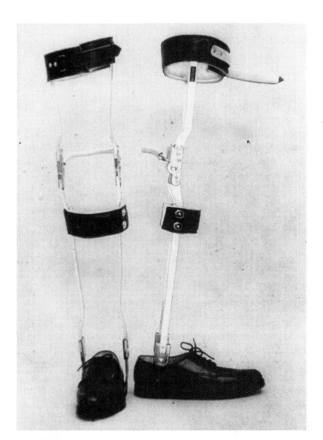

Figure 16-14. The Scott-Craig knee-ankle-knee orthosis.

anteriorly by a plastic band and a Velcro strap. A suprapatellar or pretibial shell provides knee extension force, which eliminates the need for a patellar strap and provides mediolateral knee stability. At the lower end, the uprights are connected to a molded plastic foot plate to be worn inside a shoe.

Plastic laminated supracondylar KAFO[7] is indicated for pa-

tients who lack knee and ankle muscle power but have normal hip extensors, full knee extension, and no spasticity. A molded foot plate and a solid ankle immobilize the foot and ankle in equinus, which produces a knee extension force during stance. Genu recurvatum is controlled by a supracondylar anterior shell and a counteracting popliteal shell posteriorly. The absence of a mechanical knee joint allows free knee flexion during swing phase with better gait pattern and reduced energy cost.

Knee orthoses (KO) are prescribed to prevent genu recurvatum and to provide mediolateral stability. Numerous designs are currently available, a development enhanced by the growing field of sports medicine. Most KOs consist of two uprights, free or adjustable knee joints, and thigh and calf cuffs. The Swedish knee cage (Fig. 16-16) prevents recurvatum, but permits flexion. The recently designed three-way knee stabilizer (TKS) orthosis appears similar and gives good control of structural knee instability in the lateral, medial, and posterior direction and is indicated for genu valgum, varus, and recurvatum. The standard KOs have short lever arms and may not be effective when strong forces are required. They also have a tendency to slip down. In recent years numerous KO designs with longer lever arms and often derotational components have been commercially fabricated and prescribed for advanced physical activities and athletics.

Hip–Knee–Ankle–Foot Orthoses

Hip-knee-ankle-foot orthoses (HKAFO) consist of the same components as described for the standard AFOs and KAFOs with the addition of an attached lockable hip joint and a pelvic band to control movements at the anatomical hip joint. The hip joint usually has a ring-drop lock. The pelvic band, which may be unilateral or bilateral, encompasses the pelvis between the iliac crest and greater trochanter laterally, curves down over the buttocks, and then passes up again over the sacrum. The indications for prescribing a pelvic belt have been controversial, because several studies indicate that it increases lumbar excursion and displacement of gravity during ambulation and thus energy cost may be greater. For most paraplegics, pelvic bands are probably not necessary although they may improve standing balance, especially if spasticity is severe.

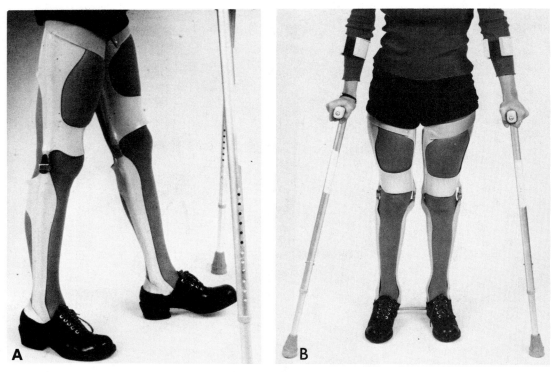

Figure 16-15. Plastic laminated TKA (knee-ankle-foot orthosis) viewed from side and front.

Figure 16-16. Knee orthosis (Swedish knee cage).

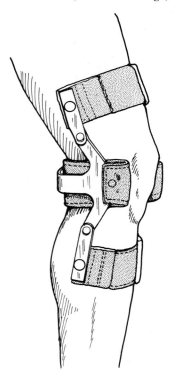

The LSU (Louisiana State University) Reciprocating Gait Orthosis (Fig. 16-17) provides bilateral KAFOs with posterior offset knee joints, knee locks, posterior plastic ankle–foot and thigh pieces, a custom-molded pelvic girdle, and special thrust-bearing hip joints, coupled together with a cable and conduit, and a thoracic extension with Velcro straps.[3,8] The cable-coupling mechanism provides hip stability by preventing simultaneous bilateral hip flexion, yet allows free unilateral hip flexion/extension in a reciprocal fashion when step is attempted. Using two crutches, paraplegics are able to ambulate in a four-point gait pattern. This orthosis has also been tested and used in conjunction with Functional Electrical Stimulation (FES) system to facilitate paraplegic ambulation.

Fracture Orthoses

Orthoses of different designs have been used in the management of fractures.[12] By definition, a plaster of Paris cast applied to a fractured limb is an orthosis that provides rigid immobilization while healing occurs. The term *fracture orthosis,* however, refers to a concept of management based on the hypothesis, which is supported by considerable clinical evidence, that mobilization of adjacent joints does not impede healing of fractures, that functional activity stimulates osteogenesis, and that rigid immobilization of fractures is not a prerequisite for healing. Even when this management concept is applied, all fractures are initially immobilized either by traction or in conventional casts while the acute pain and swelling associated with the injury subsides and early healing takes place. Such immobilization should be maintained for at least 3 weeks but no more than 6 weeks before applying the fracture orthosis. The initial immobilization is done to minimize leg shortening, but the lowest incidence of leg shortening has been found in those patients who have had fracture orthoses applied 2 to 4 weeks post-injury.

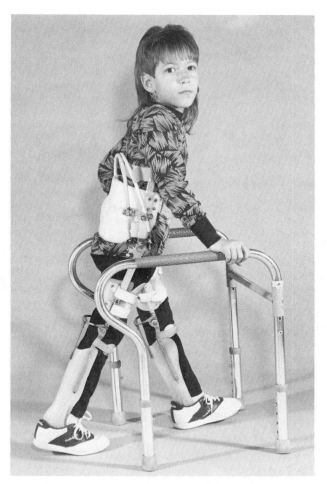

Problems associated with fracture orthoses are increased angulation of the bone and refracturing, both of which are rare. Fracture orthoses have been most often used to treat fractures of the shafts of the tibia and femur when internal fixation is unnecessary, contraindicated, or refused by the patient and when healing is significantly delayed or does not occur. Fracture orthoses are contraindicated when satisfactory alignment of the fracture cannot be obtained or maintained.

Initial efforts to use orthotic devices for lower extremity fractures were inspired by prostheses for lower extremity amputees. Three basic components are required to make a fracture orthosis: a cylinder, foot plate, and joint mechanisms. The cylindrical component closely fits the fractured limb in order to provide a hydraulic mechanism that will promote stability for the bony structures and resist shortening. The vertical load of weight-bearing is offset by lateral and oblique forces from an essentially incompressible fluid chamber that is created by the encasing cylindrical orthotic component. Most proximally on the orthosis, a weight-bearing surface may be provided, such as a patellar tendon bearing or ischial seat, to further reduce the pressure on the fracture site. This mechanism is far less important in the distribution of weight-bearing pressures than the hydraulic mechanism. The cylindrical components are usually made of plaster of Paris or low temperature thermoplastics (orthoplast). The second major component of a fracture orthosis is a foot plate, which is to be worn inside a shoe. The foot plate is usually prefabricated and made of plastic, although custom-

made foot plates are occasionally made. The foot plate is usually attached to the cylindrical component by simple plastic hinges rather than metallic joints. Similar joint mechanisms may be used for the knee, connecting the above- and below-knee pieces.

Appropriately designed and fitted, fracture orthoses allow functional ambulation with progressively increasing weight-bearing. Absence of pain, good callus formation, and lack of gross motion at the fracture site indicates that the fracture is stable. The fracture is considered healed when full weight-bearing is tolerated and x-rays show that the fracture is obliterated with evidence of good callus formation and consolidation.

Fractures of the tibial shaft generally do not require surgical intervention and heal spontaneously. Following 2 to 4 weeks of immobilization in a long leg cast, most patients with closed tibial fractures are ready for active range of motion of the knee and ambulation with increased weight-bearing. Fractures of the distal tibia can be treated with below-knee orthosis with a patellar tendon indentation for weight-bearing (Fig. 16-18). Fractures of the proximal tibia, especially those involving the knee joint, generally require a thigh piece that is connected to the leg portion with a polycentric knee joint. Closed transverse fractures of the mid-femoral shaft are generally best treated with intramedullary nailing, but for some open, severely comminuted, or oblique femoral fractures, management with fracture orthoses may present a better approach.[14] Fractures of the mid- or distal femoral shaft are more successfully managed with fracture orthoses than are fractures of the proximal femoral shaft due to the latter's strong tendency to produce varus angulation and malalignment. The thigh component of the orthosis resembles that of the quadrilateral above-knee prosthesis with an ischial seat and a three-point fixation contour that resists varus angulation

Figure 16-18. Orthosis for fracture of the tibia. (American Academy of Orthopedic Surgeons: Atlas of Orthotics. St Louis, CV Mosby, 1975)

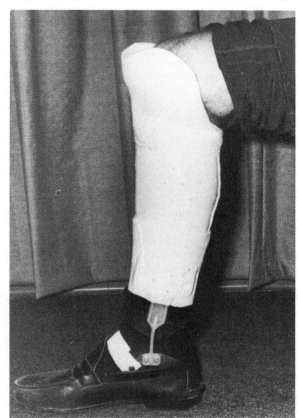

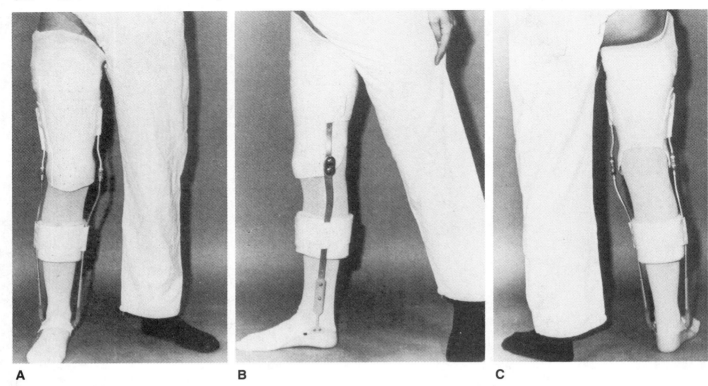

A   B   C

Figure 16-19. Three views of an orthosis for fracture of the distal femur. (American Academy of Orthopedic Surgeons: Atlas of Orthotics. St Louis, CV Mosby, 1975)

(Fig. 16-19). The thigh component is connected to the calf piece by freely moving metal or plastic joints. The calf piece is attached to a foot plate by joints, as seen in the tibial fracture orthosis (see Fig. 16-18).

Occasionally fracture orthoses are used in the management of fractures of the forearm and wrist as a therapeutic alternative to other means of external or internal fixation. A cylindrical forearm component is attached by a joint mechanism to a hand piece. Active use of muscles and joints is encouraged, although weight-bearing is not generally indicated and may not be necessary.

SPINAL ORTHOTICS

The spine, which consists both of rigid (bones) and deformable (disks) units, is both strong and flexible. It provides protection for the spinal cord and nerves as well as good body support and mobility. The spinal column consists of seven cervical, twelve thoracic, and five lumbar vertebrae, the sacrum, and the coccyx. The vertebrae increase in size from the first cervical through the fifth lumbar, after which they decrease in size caudally to the coccyx. Each vertebra above the sacrum typically consists of the body, which functions primarily for the transmission of forces; the lamina and the pedicles, which combine with the body to enclose the spinal canal; one posterior spinous and two transverse processes for the attachment of muscles and ligaments; and the posterior articular processes or facets, which control motions between adjacent vertebrae. The vertebrae articulate posteriorly by two facet joints which are true synovial joints, and anteriorly by the intervertebral disks.

Each disk has a central nucleus pulposus consisting of a gelatinous material spanning 50% to 60% of the diameter of the disk; a surrounding annulus fibrosus made of an inner layer of fibrocartilage and an outer layer of collagen fibers obliquely directed to connect the adjacent vertebrae; and two cartilagenous plates that separate the disks from the vertebral bodies. These plates are the weakest part of the disk-vertebrae complex. They are the first to crack under large compression forces resulting in the leak of nuclear material into the vertebral body.

Several sets of longitudinal ligaments bind the vertebrae together, either in a system that binds all the vertebrae together into one mechanical unit (anterior and posterior longitudinal and supraspinous ligaments) or a system that attaches one vertebra to the next one (interspinous, intertransverse, iliolumbar, and flavum ligaments).

The spine has three basic physiological curves in the anterior/posterior plane—cervical lordosis, thoracic kyphosis, and lumbar lordosis—in order to decrease the effects of vertical compressive forces and to adapt to the upright posture. The intervertebral disks, however, are the main cushioning mechanism against compressive forces. Multiple factors are responsible for proper posture of the spine, but of primary importance is the pelvic or lumbosacral angle, since the entire spine balances on the sacrum as its foundation. The pelvic angle, in turn, is affected by the positions of the main lower extremity joints. The physiological spinal curves and posture may be further affected by heredity, structural abnormalities, habit, and physical conditioning. Although investigators differ in their opinions with regard to the degrees of motion at various levels and segments of the spine, Table 16-3 shows the mean motions of different segments of the spine.

Spinal orthoses can be classified according to the spinal segments involved: cervical orthoses (CO), head cervical orthoses (HCO), thoracolumbosacral orthoses (TLSO), lumbosacral orthoses (LSO) and cervical thoracic lumbosacral orthoses (CTLSO). They may also be classified according to the restriction

Table 16-3
Mean Motion of the Spine (in degrees)

Movement	Cervical	Thoracic	Lumbar
Flexion	60	15	40
Extension	78	15	25
Total flexion-extension	138	30	65
Lateral flexion, right	44	15	20
Lateral flexion, left	44	15	20
Total lateral flexion	88	30	40
Rotation, right	78	40	5
Rotation, left	78	40	5
Total rotation	156	80	10

provided as flexible, semi-rigid, or rigid, or according to the prescription objective as either corrective or supportive.

Cervical and Head Cervical Orthoses

Cervical orthoses (CO) (Fig. 16-20) are prescribed to mechanically restrict motion of the cervical spine and serve as a reminder (through sensory feedback) to limit head and neck motions in the treatment of such neck disorders as soft tissue injury, pain, muscle spasm, nerve root irritation, and bony insta-

bility. Three basic designs exist: collars, poster appliances, and custom-molded devices. Generally COs are more effective in limiting flexion and extension than rotation and lateral tilting.

Soft collars provide little mechanical restriction of motion but serve as a reminder to limit motion through sensory feedback. More rigid collars of various materials and designs provide additional support and restriction.

Poster appliances have rigid adjustable metal uprights, which more effectively restrict flexion and extension. The four-poster cervical orthosis consists of chin and occipital pieces connected by four metal uprights to sternal and back plates. The sternal-occipital-mandibular immobilizer (SOMI) (Fig. 16-21) has one anterior metal poster attached to the sternal piece below and the chin piece above and two posterior uprights to hold the occipital piece. It is lightweight, comfortable, and easily applied. Several types of cervicothoracic orthoses (CTO) exist that encompass more of the trunk than the SOMI. Not only are these more difficult to fit on the patient with cervical spine injuries, it is doubtful that they provide any advantages over the SOMI.

Custom-molded total contact body appliances require that a modified positive cast be made, over which leather or plastic material is molded or laminated. The Thomas-type appliance is one which extends from the chest and shoulders to the chin and mastoid line; the Minerva-type orthosis encloses the occiput posteriorly and sometimes has a band around the forehead. Both of these devices control lateral motions and rotations better than the poster appliances while effectively limiting flexion and extension.

Maximum restriction of cervical spine motions requires the

Figure 16-20. Cervical orthoses: (*A*) cervical collar, (*B*) semi-rigid adjustable cervical collar, (*C*) semi-rigid thermoplastic two-piece cervical collar (Philadelphia collar), and (*D*) cervical multiple poster appliance.

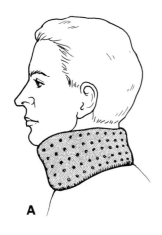

A

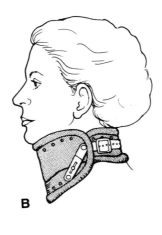

B

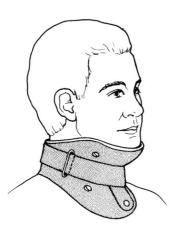

C

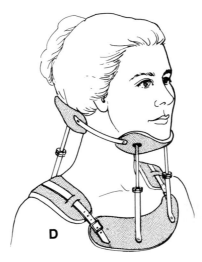

D

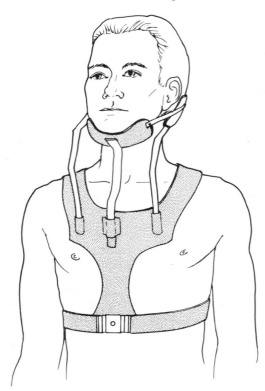

Figure 16-21. Sternal-occipital-mandibular immobilizer (SOMI orthosis).

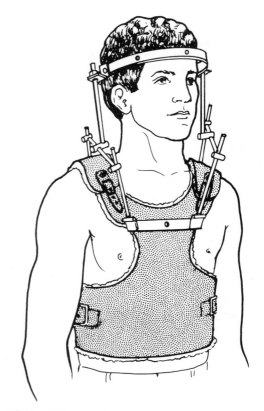

Figure 16-22. Halo orthosis.

Figure 16-23. Thoracolumbosacral orthosis (TLSO).

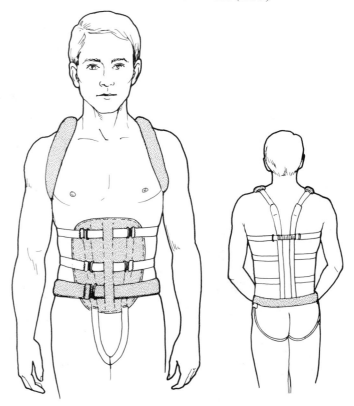

Halo orthosis (Fig. 16-22). A metal Halo ring is fixed to the skull bones with four metal pins. Upright bars are attached to the Halo ring above and below to a rigid plastic thoracic jacket lined with soft material, such as sheepskin. Application and adjustment requires skill and care. Skin problems may arise, both from pin site infection and from pressure over bony prominences under the jacket. This device is generally well tolerated and provides excellent fixation for union of a fractured cervical spine, while allowing the patient to be mobilized out of the bed and to participate in the rehabilitation program. In different designs the upright bars which are attached to the Halo ring may also have a more caudal fixation, such as to the pelvis or the femur, either through a molded pelvic girdle or through skeletal fixation to the pelvis or the femoral shafts, thus obtaining a more extensive restriction of spinal motions.

Lumbosacral and Thoracolumbosacral Orthoses

The *lumbosacral (LSO)* and *thoracolumbosacral orthoses (TLSO)* (Fig. 16-23) are available in numerous designs and are made of diverse materials. They are prescribed for a wide range of common clinical symptoms and conditions, but mostly to reduce pain, compensate for muscle weakness, correct deformities, provide trunk support, and control motion and alignment. The materials used for these types of spinal orthoses are usually combinations of cloth, leather, plaster, metal, plastic and rubber. Each design provides different degrees of spinal rigidity. Commonly these orthoses are referred to as belts, corsets, braces, or jackets, according to design. Trunk support is obtained by raising intra-abdominal pressure and applying the three-point pressure system. Raising the intra-abdominal pressure by substituting a firm orthotic support for weak abdominal muscles reduces the force on the spine by creating a semi-rigid hydropneumatic cylinder surrounding the spinal column. This cylinder both spreads the load and reduces the lumbar lordosis. The three-point pressure system is more important for spinal motion control and realignment than trunk support. Although the three-point pressure system is employed by all spinal orthoses, effectiveness varies considerably depending on design. Sensory feedback is a powerful factor in inhibiting motion and correcting trunk position.

The negative effects of spinal orthotic applications include muscle weakness and atrophy due to reduced functional demands, tightness and contractures due to fibrosis of muscles and connective tissues associated with prolonged spinal immobilization, and psychological dependence on the orthosis. Early institution of an exercise program is therefore important when spinal orthoses are prescribed to prevent these complications.

Corsets, either lumbosacral or thoracolumbosacral, are made of fabrics with adjustable lacing encircling the trunk for abdominal support. They are reinforced with rigid, paraspinal metal stays, which serve as a reminder to limit motion rather than as a means of restricting motion. Corsets are prescribed for various painful back disorders.

Rigid orthoses provide abdominal compression anteriorly and distribute counterforce over an extensive area through a network of posterior paraspinal metal stays. The lumbosacral orthosis (LSO), often called the chairback brace, consists of a pelvic band placed between the greater trochanter and the iliac crest and a thoracic band 1″ below the scapula. The bands are joined together by two paraspinal and two lateral metal uprights and an anterior corset. Thoracolumbosacral orthoses (TLSO) extend the full length of the thoracic spine and provide rigid support to the lumbar spine and the sacrum. The Taylor orthosis is designed similarly. It has long rigid posterior paraspinal metal uprights, which extend to the shoulders where straps are attached, passing over and around the shoulders under the axilla and fastening to the thoracic band. It is designed to limit flexion and extension but has been found to be relatively ineffective in restricting lumbar motion. It is only effective for thoracic spine restriction if the straps are tightly fastened. Variations of the TLSO include the Magnuson, Arnold, and Steindler braces. The Boston brace is a prefabricated molded plastic TLSO with a rear-opening girdle. It extends from the pelvis to the axilla applying corrective pressure to certain areas, but has prebuilt reliefs. It is prescribed for management of lumbar and thoracolumbar scoliotic curves with an apex below T8.

Molded spinal jackets made of plaster of Paris, leather, or plastic provide total body contact and therefore distribute pressure evenly over a wide area. They are commonly prescribed to provide spinal support for fractures of the spine, osteoporosis, spinal metastasis, and generalized muscle weakness.

Hyperextension orthoses (Jewett, Baker, Griswold) use the three-point pressure system by applying pressures anteriorly on the sternum above and on the pelvis or pubis below by means of a firm metal frame, and posteriorly over the mid-back by the use of a pad with adjustable straps (Fig. 16-24). These orthoses provide no abdominal muscle support and although lightweight, may be uncomfortable because the corrective forces are distributed over relatively small areas. They are prescribed to prevent spinal flexion after vertebral compression fractures.

Cervical Thoracic Lumbosacral Orthoses

Cervical thoracic lumbosacral orthosis (CTLSO) primarily refers to the *Milwaukee brace* for scoliosis. It consists of a molded pelvic girdle, with three expandable metal uprights, one anteriorly and two posteriorly, attached above to a steel neck ring,

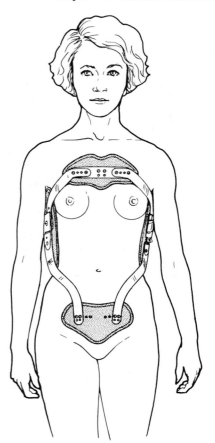

Figure 16-24.   Jewett hyperextension (TLSO) orthosis.

which is inclined 20° anteriorly. Two occipital pads and an anterior throat mold are attached to the ring. Several pads are then properly attached to the uprights to provide the corrective forces for the scoliotic curves at various levels. The scoliotic patients wear this brace for 23 hours per day and are instructed to perform a prescribed exercise program to prevent muscle weakness and to improve mobility of the chest and spine.

GAIT AIDS

Canes

Canes when properly used increase the base of support, decrease loading and demand on the lower limb and skeletal structures, provide additional sensory information, and assist with acceleration and deceleration during locomotion. Canes are prescribed for various disabilities to improve balance, to decrease pain, to reduce weight-bearing forces on injured or inflamed structures, to compensate for weak muscles, and to scan the immediate environment. Pathological conditions affecting the upper limbs may interfere with the use of canes and crutches or warrant prescription of specially designed gait aids.

The total length of a properly measured cane should equal the distance between the upper border of the greater trochanter to the bottom of the heel of the shoe. Standing with the cane the elbow is flexed at 20° to 30° and both shoulders are level. The patient should be instructed in the proper use of the cane: to hold the cane in the hand opposite the affected limb, and to advance the cane and the affected leg together in a three-point gait pattern. When ascending stairs the good leg is advanced first, but when descending, the cane and the affected leg lead.

Canes are most commonly made of hardwood or aluminum but can vary in design (Fig. 16-25 *A, B, C, D,* and *E*). All canes should be fitted with a deeply grooved 1″ to 2″ wide rubber tip for good traction and safety, and the clinician should regularly check these for wear. The common C-handle or crook top cane is inexpensive, but this type of handle may be uncomfortable and difficult to grasp, especially for those with hand problems. Additionally the weight-bearing line falls behind the shaft of the cane, thus reducing its supportive value. A functional handle that fits the grip, conforms to the natural angle of the hand, and is more centered over the shaft of the cane is more comfortable and provides better support. Wide-based canes made of metal provide a wider area of support. These designs consist of three or four short legs attached to a single upright shaft with a molded or wooden handle. Several base widths are available and the length of the shaft is adjustable. Wide-based canes are prescribed for persons with impaired balance, preferably for only temporary use, since these canes are often heavy and awkward in appearance.

Crutches

The indications for prescribing a pair of crutches are similar to those for canes, but the clinical deficits are usually greater. Good strength of the upper limbs usually is required, since persons needing crutches tend to require them more for weight-bearing and propulsion than for balancing or as sensory aids. For effective crutch walking the upper limb joints should have good range of motion and the key muscle groups (*i.e.,* the shoulder flexors and depressors, elbow and wrist extensors, and finger flexors) should be strong.

Axillary crutches (Fig. 16-25F) are the most commonly prescribed crutches in the United States. The wooden axillary crutch is easily adjustable and made of hardwood with two upright shafts connected by a padded axillary piece on top, a hand piece in the middle, and an extension piece below. The extension piece and shafts have numerous holes at regular intervals so the total length of the crutch and the height of the handles may be adjusted. A large soft rubber suction tip is attached to the extension piece to allow total contact with the floor. Metal axillary crutches consist of a single contoured tubular structure, which can be adjusted by telescoping and push-button positions. A functional handle is adjustable in height.

When measuring a person for axillary crutches, the total length of the crutch and the height of the handle are the two main dimensions. The handle height is measured in the same manner as with canes, but the total length of the crutch should be equal to the distance from the anterior fold of the axilla to either a point 6″ anterolaterally from the foot or to the bottom of the heel plus 1″ or 2″.

The popular *Lofstrand crutch* (Fig. 16-25G) consists of a single aluminum tubular shaft, adjustable in length, a molded hand piece, and a forearm piece bent posteriorly just above the

Figure 16-25. Canes, crutches, and walkers: (*A*) C-handle (crook top) cane, (*B*) adjustable aluminum cane, (*C*) functional grip cane, (*D*) wide-base quad cane (adjustable), (*E*) hemi-walker, (*F*) axillary crutch (adjustable, wooden), (*G*) Lofstrand crutch (adjustable, aluminum), (*H*) forearm support (platform) crutch, and (*I*) walker or walkerette.

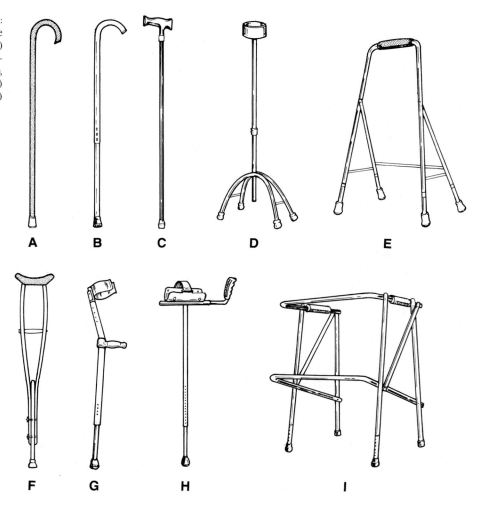

A   B   C   D   E

F   G   H   I

hand piece. The forearm piece, also adjustable in length, extends to 2″ below the elbow, where a forearm cuff with a narrow anterior opening is attached. This crutch is lightweight, easily adjustable, and gives freedom for hand activities, since the hand piece can be released without losing the crutch. However, it requires greater skills than the axillary crutch, good strength of the upper limbs, and adequate trunk balance for safe ambulation.

The *Canadian elbow extensor crutch* (triceps crutch) has a single aluminum upright shaft attached to bilateral uprights, which extend to above the elbow. These are connected by a handle and two half cuffs, one below and one above the elbow. This crutch is rarely prescribed today but may benefit those with triceps weakness.

Forearm support (platform) crutches (Fig. 16-25*H*) may be prescribed when clinical conditions of the forearm, wrist, or hands prevent safe or comfortable weight-bearing, such as in the presence of arthritis of the elbow, wrist, or hand, fractures of forearm or hand, or weakness of triceps or grasp.

Walkers

Walkers provide a wider and more stable base of support than do either canes or crutches (Fig. 16-25*I*). They may be prescribed for patients who require maximum assistance with balance, the elderly, the fearful, and the incoordinated. The patient must have good grasp and arm strength bilaterally. Walkers are conspicuous in appearance and interfere with the development of smooth reciprocal gait patterns. Although they are very useful during rehabilitation, care should be taken that the patient does not become too dependent on the walker. Walkers are available in various sizes, are adjustable in height, and come in different designs, such as folding, rolling, reciprocal, or stair walkers.

REFERENCES

1. Bennett RL: The evolution of the Georgia Warm Springs foundation feeder. Artif Limbs 10:5–9, 1966
2. Corcoran PJ, Jebsen RH, Brengelmann GL, Simons BC: Effects of plastic and leg braces on speed and energy cost of hemiparetic ambulation. Arch Phys Med Rehabil 51:69–77, 1970
3. Douglas R, Larson PF, D'Ambrosia R, McCall RE: The LSU Reciprocation Gait Orthosis. Orthopedics 6:834–839, 1983
4. Fisher SV, Gullickson G Jr: Energy cost of ambulation in health and disability: A literature review. Arch Phys Med Rehabil 51:69–77, 1978
5. Hussey RW, Stauffer ES: Spinal cord injury: Requirements for ambulation. Arch Phys Med Rehabil 54:544–547, 1973
6. Lehmann JF: Biomechanics of ankle foot orthoses: Prescription and design. Arch Phys Med Rehabil 60:200–207, 1979
7. Lehneis HR: New developments in lower limb orthotics through bioengineering. Arch Phys Med Rehabil 53(July):303–310, 1972
8. LSU Reciprocating Gait Orthoses—A Pictorial Description and Application Manual. Chattanooga, Durr-Fillauer Medical, 1983
9. Murphy EG, Burstein AH: Physical properties of materials, including solid mechanics. In Atlas of Orthotics: Biomechanical Principles and Application. St Louis, CV Mosby, 1975
10. O'Daniel WE, Hahn HR: Follow-up usage of the Scott-Craig orthosis in paraplegia. Paraplegia 19:373–378, 1981
11. Pictorial Reference Manual of Orthotics and Prosthetics. American Orthotics and Prosthetic Association, Alexandria, VA, 1986
12. Sarmiento A, Sinclair WF: Fracture orthoses. In Atlas of Orthotics: Biomechanical Principles and Application. St. Louis, CV Mosby, 1975
13. Saunders JBDECM, Inman VT, Eberhart HD: Major determinants in normal and pathological gait. J Bone Joint Surg (Am) 35:343–558, 1953
14. St Pierre RK, Holmes HE, Flemming LL: Cast bracing of femoral fractures. Orthopedics 5(June):739–745, 1982
15. Zamosky I, Licht S, Redford JB: Shoes and their modifications. In Orthotics Etc, pp 368–431. Baltimore, Williams & Wilkins, 1980

17

Prosthetics

James A. Leonard, Jr.

Robert H. Meier, III

The rehabilitation of the individual with limb loss requires the skills of many health care professionals: orthopedic surgeon, general or vascular surgeon, physiatrist, prosthetist, physical therapist, occupational therapist, social worker, psychologist, and vocational counselor. Ideally these health care specialists function together as an integrated team; in particular, teams in regional amputee or prosthetic centers who see a large number of amputees are able to provide, through their combined experience, research, and education, the optimum in prosthetic rehabilitation.[26]

Advances in the care and prosthetic restoration of the amputee have always come from multiple fronts: development in new surgical techniques, improvements in the pre- and postoperative management, advances in prosthetic technology, and better understanding of the psychosocial implications of limb loss. In the last several years, it has been the areas of prosthetic designs, material technologies and fabrication techniques for prosthetic construction, and engineering technologies especially in the field of electronics that have seen the greatest number of advancements. These new developments have not replaced previous technology and techniques, but have been added to the options available to the clinic team in prescribing the most appropriate prosthesis for the individual patient.

If amputee rehabilitation programs are to provide a useful service, they must focus on the individual who has experienced the catastrophic loss. A prosthesis can be fabricated for almost every level of amputation, but it may not meet the amputee's perceived needs. It is the art of assisting the amputee to achieve these needs that is the foundation of amputee rehabilitation. Seldom is the prosthesis the desired replacement of the body part lost. However, tempering expectation with reality is an essential part of the rehabilitation experience. Assuring that the most comfortable, cosmetic, and functional prosthesis has been made available is only a part of working with the amputee. Guidance also most be given in the proper use and care of the prosthesis. The true test of the rehabilitation program is the manner in which the amputee incorporates his or her natural body parts, with or without a prosthesis, into his or her life-style.

ACQUIRED AMPUTATIONS

Incidence and Etiology

The etiology of limb loss and the associated medical conditions are often important considerations when developing a management program for the amputee. Loss of limb is generally divided into two broad categories: acquired and congenital. Congenital deficiencies will be discussed later in this chapter.

The loss of part or all of an extremity as the direct result of trauma or by surgery is known as an *acquired amputation*. Surgical amputations are performed for disease, benign or malignant tumors, and for traumatic injuries to the extremities that have no hope of salvage. The exact number of amputees or amputations performed in the United States is not known. Review of data collected by the National Center for Health Statistics (NCHS) provides estimates of the incidence of amputations. In 1981 there were an estimated 631,000 individuals with major limb loss (excluding loss of fingers or thumb only) in the United States. If individuals with finger or thumb loss are included, the total is 1,715,000.[44] Earlier work by the NCHS in 1977 provides a much more detailed breakdown with respect to the level of amputation, socioeconomic data, age and geographic distribution, and use of a prosthesis.[45,46] In 1984, an estimated 129,000 amputations were performed in acute care, nonfederal hospitals, the majority in the lower extremity. Of the 110,000 lower extremity amputations, 41,000 were toe or partial foot amputations, 32,000 at the below-knee level, and 33,000 above the knee.[43] The 1 : 1 ratio of below-knee to above-knee amputations varies from previous reports by other studies suggesting a ratio of approximately 2 : 1.[18] The studies noting more below-knee amputations may be biased in that these data were generated from prosthetic centers where patients were being actively fit with prostheses. The reader is referred to the work by Sanders for a detailed discussion of lower extremity amputation statistics.[35]

Trauma is the leading cause of acquired amputation in the upper extremity (approximately 75%), occurring primarily in males ages 15 to 45. Disease and tumors are responsible for about equal numbers of the remaining surgical upper extremity amputations. In the lower extremity, disease states account for approximately 75% of all acquired amputations, with complications of diabetes and peripheral vascular disease far and away accounting for most of these, especially in the 60 and over population. Trauma is the next most common cause for lower extremity amputation (20%), followed by tumors (5%). However, among children ages 10 to 20, tumor is the most frequent cause of all amputations (upper and lower extremity).[13, 18, 35]

Amputation Surgery

Amputations frequently occur after extensive medical and surgical effort has been expended to save the involved extremity. In such a setting, amputation surgery may be mistakenly considered by the health care team rendering the acute care to be a course of last resort, in other words, a failure of modern medicine. Amputations may be performed by less experienced members of the surgical team, and the healing and final result of the residual limb may be less than optimum. To provide the best potential for rehabilitation and prosthetic restoration, amputation surgery must be approached as a plastic and reconstructive procedure. Careful attention must be given to the management of the various tissues involved, such as beveling the ends of bones; sharp transection of nerves, which are allowed to retract into proximal soft tissues so that they do not become adherent in scar or remain in a location where they might be traumatized by a prothesis; appropriate myofascial closure of the muscle or myodesis to provide good control of the remaining bone in the residual limb; and appropriate placement of the skin incision line to avoid bony prominences and adherence to underlying bone. Such attention to detail will result in a well-shaped residual limb that can be best fitted with a prosthesis and permit maximum prosthetic function.[12]

When performing an amputation, careful consideration must be given to the level of amputation. In general the approach is to save as much length as is possible. A level must be chosen that will ensure good healing of the surgical incision with adequate full-thickness skin coverage, although skin grafts in nonvascular amputees have been used successfully to preserve length. In patients with vascular disease, noninvasive vascular studies such as ankle–brachial indices, Doppler wave-form analysis, and xenon washout studies are but a few of the techniques available to help predict which levels of lower extremity amputation will successfully heal. Often, however, the final decision in choosing the level of amputation in the vascular patient cannot be made until the time of surgery when the amount of blood flow in the tissues at the level of proposed amputation can actually be observed.[3, 6] Function with a prosthesis following an amputation must also be taken into account when choosing an amputation level. Sometimes a slightly shorter residual limb can be fitted with a more functional and cosmetic prosthesis, making, for example, a long above-elbow amputation preferable to an elbow disarticulation.

In the lower extremity the preferred levels of amputation are toe amputations, ray resections, transmetatarsal amputations, Symes amputation (disarticulation of the foot), below-knee amputation (at a level proximal to the junction of the middle and distal third of the leg), knee disarticulation, above-knee amputation (at a level 8 cm or more proximal to the level of the knee joint so that the femoral condyles are excised), hip disarticulation (short above-knee amputations at or proximal to the greater trochanter are considered functionally as a hip disarticulation), and hemipelvectomy. In the upper extremity the preferred levels are finger or thumb amputation, ray resection, transcarpal resection, wrist disarticulation, below-elbow amputation, elbow disarticulation, above-elbow amputation (6.5 cm or more proximal to the elbow joint), shoulder disarticulation, and forequarter amputation.

PATIENT EVALUATION AND MANAGEMENT

The interaction of the health care team working with the patient to achieve the goal of prosthetic restoration and rehabilitation can be referred to as prosthetic management. Prosthetic management is a process that follows a temporal sequence, which for the sake of convenience, can be divided into three distinct segments: pre-prosthetic management, prosthetic fitting, and prosthetic follow-up care.

Pre-Prosthetic Management

Preoperative

Pre-prosthetic management begins when the decision to perform an amputation is made, when a patient is initially evaluated following a traumatic amputation, or when a child is born with a congenital skeletal deficiency. It ends with the fitting of a provisional or definitive prosthesis. If the patient can be evaluated by members of the preprosthetic team prior to amputation, the optimum of care can be provided. Evaluation should assess and document the patient's range of motion and strength in the involved as well as the noninvolved extremities, mobility and ambulation, activities of daily living and self-care skills, social support, and the patient's reaction to the planned surgery. Ideally the patient should be seen prior to the amputation in order to give him or her information about the rehabilitation and prosthetic restoration process following surgery. This will often help allay some of the fears the patient may have about life after surgery. This is also an excellent time to start therapy programs instructing the patient in the relaxation techniques, range of motion, conditioning exercises, correct positioning of the residual limb, ambulation with gait aids, and activities of daily living that will continue following surgery. The patient is often more able to absorb and comply with a therapy program during the preoperative period than during the early postoperative period when incisional pain, medication, or apprehension may interfere with the ability to follow through with such a program.

Postoperative

Postoperatively the goals of preprosthetic management are healing of the incision, preparation of the residual limb for prosthetic fitting, maintenance of range of motion (especially in the remaining proximal joints of the amputated extremity), independent mobility, independence in self-care and activities of daily living, education regarding prosthetic fitting and care, and support for the adaptation to the changes resulting from the amputation.

The response to amputation has been compared to the grieving process in that the amputee experiences identifiable stages of denial, anger, depression, coping, and acceptance. Not every individual will progress through these stages or ultimately adapt to the loss. The etiology of the amputation may contribute significantly to the patient's response to the limb loss. The ultimate response of the individual to the psychosocial impact of limb loss is determined by many factors, including the individual's character and inner strengths, the quality of the social support systems available to the individual, and the comprehensive care provided by the prosthetic team.[11]

Residual Limb Care

In addition to maintaining range of motion and strength, postoperative treatment includes shaping of the residual limb and reduction of soft tissue volume. Sterile soft dressings commonly used following amputation surgery do little to protect, shape, or shrink the residual limb. At the most, soft dressings provide an environment to promote uneventful wound healing, but may prevent optimal healing because they allow the development of postoperative edema. The shrinking and shaping process can be accomplished in one of several ways, all of which can be used in the early postoperative period without compromise to wound healing if carefully done. Soft dressings such as elastic bandage wraps, elastic stockinette (Compresso-Grip), stump shrinkers, or Una paste casts have been used quite successfully. The use of elastic bandage wraps requires considerable cooperation, skill, and attention on the part of the patient, family, or medical staff because the wraps need to be reapplied frequently and carefully in order to be successful.

With an experienced team, immediate rigid dressing may be the preferred method of amputation wound care. It can be either removable or nonremovable.[8, 48] Ideally, the rigid dressing should be applied immediately postoperatively in the operating room before postoperative edema has a chance to develop. By limiting postoperative swelling, the rigid dressing helps to promote wound healing and limit postoperative pain. Typically a nonremovable rigid dressing is taken off and changed 5 to 10 days postoperatively. A removable rigid dressing may be taken off and replaced whenever the wound needs to be viewed, but must be replaced immediately before edema has a chance to develop. The rigid dressing has the additional advantages of providing some protection for the extremity in case of a fall, and it can serve as a socket to which temporary components can be attached, thus creating a preparatory prosthesis.

The pre-prosthetic phase of management prior to definitive prosthetic fitting can typically last 6 to 10 weeks for the dysvascular lower extremity amputee, a considerably shorter period of time for the traumatic lower extremity amputee, and 3 to 6 weeks for the upper extremity amputee.

Prosthetic Fitting

The prosthetic fitting period of care begins when the residual limb is ready for casting and a prescription has been written for a preparatory or definitive prosthesis. This period continues until the completion of training in the use of the prosthesis. Input from all members of the team, especially the patient, will result in the most appropriate prosthetic prescription. The prosthetic prescription takes into account the needs, objectives, and abilities of the amputee and selects from the available prosthetic designs and components.

Prosthetic fitting presumes that an amputee is a candidate for a prosthesis or wishes to be fitted with a prosthesis. Not all amputees are candidates for prosthetic fitting. There are no hard and fast rules regarding who is or is not a prosthetic candidate, but there are some general guidelines that can be followed. An amputee should have reasonable cardiovascular reserve, adequate healing, skin coverage, range of motion, muscle strength, motor control, and learning ability to achieve useful prosthetic function. Poor candidates for functional prosthetic fitting would be a vascular lower extremity amputee with an open or poorly healed incision, an above-knee amputee with a 45° flexion contracture at the hip, or a below-elbow amputee with a flail elbow and shoulder. Lower extremity amputees who can walk with a walker or crutches without a prosthesis usually possess the necessary balance, strength, and cardiovascular reserve to walk with a prosthesis. Generally bilateral short above-knee amputees over age 45 are considered to be unlikely candidates for full-length prosthetic fitting. Additional medical problems such as severe coronary artery disease, pulmonary disease, severe polyneuropathy, or multiple joint arthritis may result in an amputee who could be fitted with a prosthesis but may not be a functional prosthetic user. In borderline cases, it may be necessary to proceed with actual prosthetic fitting to determine eventual prosthetic function. The use of a less costly preparatory prosthesis is appropriate before making the decision about fitting such an individual with a more costly definitive prosthesis.

Once it is felt that an amputee is a prosthetic candidate, a decision is made regarding the purpose of prosthetic fitting. The prosthesis can be functional, cosmetic, or both. Prostheses which are intended to replace function never totally replace the function of the body part that has been lost. Each prosthetic component provides a different type of functional capability. A prosthesis might be designed to meet specific vocational, recreational, or social needs. It is important that the prosthetic team spend time reviewing the activities of daily living and the vocational and avocational activities for which the prosthesis is to be used. In the case of young children, a prosthesis is often necessary for the attainment of normal developmental milestones.

It is important to consider a passive, cosmetic prosthetic restoration for selected individuals. These cosmetic prostheses can be fabricated to have an amazingly similar appearance to the opposite limb. There are only a few prosthetists in this country who specialize in this art form of prosthetic fabrication.

The next decision is when to fit the prosthesis. For the acquired upper extremity amputee there has been good evidence to suggest that early fitting is extremely important to ensure better functional prosthetic use and return to pre-amputation activity levels and occupation. Malone and colleagues have gone so far as to describe the 30 days following upper extremity amputation as the "golden period," during which prosthetic fitting should occur to ensure good prosthetic outcome.[25] Prosthetic fitting for the upper extremity amputation occurring after this 30-day period has resulted in a significant reduction in prosthetic acceptance and use and a much lower rate of return to previous occupational activity levels. A preparatory prosthesis—either conventional or myoelectric—can be applied immediately in the operating room, but will not achieve a better outcome than early fitting (7–30 days postoperatively). The definitive upper extremity prosthesis should be fit when the residual limb is well healed and shaped and the limb volume has stabilized.

The timing of prosthetic fitting for the lower extremity is more controversial than for the upper extremity. Since the majority of lower extremity amputations in the United States occur as the result of complications of peripheral vascular disease, primary wound healing at the amputation site is of paramount importance. At one time, immediate postoperative fitting of a rigid dressing and pylon prosthesis was advocated to speed prosthetic, functional, and psychological rehabilitation for the lower extremity amputee.[8] Immediate prosthetic fitting with a pylon is no longer recommended for vascular amputees because this technique may jeopardize primary wound healing and may contribute to reamputation at more proximal levels because of compromised wound healing. If properly fabricated and applied, however, an immediate postoperative prosthesis can be safely used for ambulation with partial weight-bearing. Because there are a limited number of individuals with the necessary experience and skill to properly fabricate this type of prosthesis, immediate fitting in the vascular amputee is usually not recommended. Immediate fitting in the younger traumatic amputee has been more successful and is a reasonable method of treatment. For the lower extremity amputee, whether vascular or nonvascular, early preparatory prosthetic fitting is a more accepted form of prosthetic management. Vascular amputees tend to have less complications with provisional prostheses when the socket of the provisional prosthesis is a custom-fabricated thermoplastic or laminated socket rather than a plaster socket.

Prosthetic Fabrication

Considerable progress has occurred in prosthetic fabrication during the past decade. Improved materials, new designs, and better fitting techniques have resulted in prostheses that are lighter and stronger and provide improved comfort, function, and cosmesis.

Preparatory Prosthesis

In the past, a temporary, provisional, or preparatory prosthesis used a socket usually made from plaster bandages (conventional plaster or synthetic plaster). Today, more provisional sockets are being made from thermoplastics (Fig. 17-1). Some of these thermoplastic sockets come ready-made in various sizes to be used as needed. Most thermoplastic sockets, however, are now custom-made because they provide a better fit and are more durable than plaster. Because the plastic must be heated in an oven to 300°F or higher to be moldable, the socket must be formed over a positive mold of the residual limb. The prosthetist must make a cast of the residual limb, modify the resulting positive mold, and then vacuum-form the provisional socket, often over a foam liner. In contrast, the plaster provisional socket can be constructed by a physician, prosthetist, or therapist, but will need several changes and modifications to maintain an adequate fit. Both types of sockets can be used to attach modular prosthetic components as necessary to complete the provisional prosthesis.

Definitive Prosthesis

When the shaping and shrinking process has been completed and the residual limb volume has stabilized, a definitive or permanent prosthesis is made. This process for the upper extremity usually follows these steps:

1. Casting of the residual limb
2. Making of a plaster of Paris positive mold of the residual limb
3. Modification of the plaster positive: removing plaster from the pressure tolerant areas and adding plaster to the pressure-sensitive areas of the residual limb
4. Fabrication of a wax check socket over the modified plaster positive
5. Trial fitting of the wax check socket with modification of the wax socket as necessary to ensure an adequate, comfortable fit
6. Making a new plaster positive mold from the check socket
7. Fabrication of the final plastic socket over the new plaster positive.

For the lower extremity the final prosthetic socket is generally fabricated directly over the modified plaster positive mold (step 3 above) and then fit on the patient with additional modifications being made directly to the definitive socket. More and more prosthetists are using clear check sockets for lower extremity prosthetic fabrication. Instead of the wax check socket (step #4 above), a clear thermoplastic sheet (Lexan, Duroplex, Surlyn) or cone (Orthoglass) is vacuum-formed over the modified positive and then the fit is checked on the patient. Because the check socket is clear, areas of excessive pressure or of noncontact between the socket and residual limb will be seen on direct observation. The fit can be quickly modified to achieve the desired optimum fit of the socket; a new positive can then be made for the fabrication of the definitive socket. Clear thermoplastic check sockets are also being used more frequently in upper extremity prosthetics, either replacing or in addition to the wax check socket (Fig. 17-2). The thermoplastic check socket can be used with a suspension system and other prosthetic components attached to provide a temporary prosthesis. This temporary prosthesis is useful for further evaluating the fit of the socket, the resulting prosthetic function, or for altering placement of other prescribed prosthetic components such as electrodes in a myoelectric prosthesis.

Definitive prosthetic sockets are usually fabricated from thermosetting resins, either polyester or acrylic. In the fabrication of the socket, the resins are drawn under vacuum into a fabric stockinette, usually Dacron or nylon, providing reinforcement to the plastic. Other reinforcing fabric materials such as graphite fibers and Kevlar are available to provide extremely lightweight but strong laminations. Although some prosthetists

Figure 17-1. Synthetic plaster below-elbow postoperative rigid dressing and thermoplastic preparatory prosthesis.

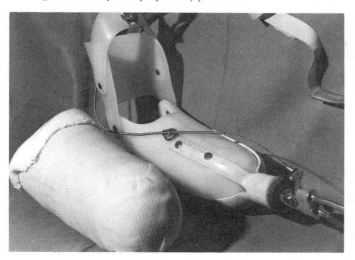

Figure 17-2. (*From left to right*) Plaster positive for a below-elbow residual limb, wax check socket, and clear thermoplastic check socket.

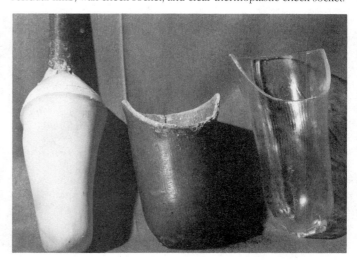

are using thermoplastics and vacuum-forming techniques, the majority of definitive prosthetic sockets in use today are laminated. Wooden sockets, once a mainstay, are now rarely seen.

Prosthetic Construction Design

Prosthetic construction can be either exoskeletal or endoskeletal. Exoskeletal design is the more traditional construction, comprising a rigid plastic lamination over a filler material of wood or foam, which has been shaped to provide the cosmetic appearance of the prosthesis. It is the outer plastic lamination that provides the strength, weight-bearing ability, and durability for the prosthesis.

Endoskeletal design uses internal modular components and tubing to provide strength and weight-bearing capabilities. The cosmetic appearance is provided by shaped foam covers slipped over the metal components. The design of the modular components of the endoskeletal system allows for relatively easy changing of the components or alignment of the prosthesis after final fabrication has been completed. These changes are not easily accomplished with an exoskeletal prosthesis. For proximal level amputations, an endoskeletal prosthesis will be lighter, especially if tungsten modular components are used.

UPPER EXTREMITY PROSTHESES

A prescription for an upper extremity prosthesis must describe the choice of socket and joint components, terminal device, method of suspension, and control system. As previously mentioned, a detailed history of the individual's preferred activities is necessary to make a proper selection of the options available.

An upper extremity prosthesis attempts to replace very complex functions. Part of the normal upper extremity is the hand, which is positioned for functional activities by the coordinated movements of the muscles and joints in the extremity proximal to the hand. Once positioned in space, the hand is able to perform tasks ranging from those requiring fine dexterity with light prehensile forces to gross grasping movements with great prehensile forces, all the while providing multiple levels of sensory feedback to allow modulation of the prehensile activity. The level of dexterity and functional capability is greatest in the dominant upper extremity.

Typical prosthetic replacement for the upper extremity can replace several of the grasping and manipulating functions of the hand and allow movement of proximal prosthetic joints to position the terminal device in space, but it cannot provide for any sensory feedback directly from the terminal device. Prosthetic function in a unilateral upper extremity amputee seldom approaches the level of skill and dexterity equal to that of the dominant upper extremity it has replaced. When the dominant upper extremity has been amputated, the individual amputee usually transfers the role of dominant function to the remaining nonamputated upper extremity, and the prosthesis serves in the role of assisting in bimanual function. In general, the more distal the amputation, the more functional the individual is with the prosthesis because more "normal" control is maintained by the proximal muscles and joints of the extremity.

Upper extremity prostheses can be divided into two groups based on their power source: conventional or body-powered, and externally powered. In North America, externally powered prostheses refer to prostheses that are powered by small electric motors to provide the forces necessary for prehension and joint movement. These electric motors can be controlled by myoelectric signals, switches, or even acoustic signals.[4, 36] Historically, carbon dioxide gas has also served as a source of external power,

primarily in Europe. Many components for both types of prostheses are similar.

Body-Powered Prostheses

All conventional upper extremity prostheses have these component parts: socket, suspension, interposing joints (as needed by the level of amputation), terminal device(s), and a control system.

Partial Hand/Wrist Disarticulation

For partial hand/wrist amputations (phalanges, ray resections, transmetacarpal, or transcarpal), a prosthesis may not be necessary. Surgical reconstruction may be a more appropriate choice of treatment to preserve or enhance function while maintaining sensation in the residual partial hand. Often all that is necessary to restore function for this level of amputation is an opposition post, either fixed or adjustable; which permits prehension of objects while at the same time providing sensory feedback from the skin of the remaining portion of the hand. A cosmetic alternative can be provided for this level of amputation. Often such a prosthesis is discarded in favor of greater function and the use of remaining sensation.

All prostheses for amputation levels proximal to the hand/wrist will have a terminal device, wrist unit, suspension harness, and control system. Terminal devices for body-powered prostheses can be hooks, functional hands, cosmetic hands, or special terminal devices for specific function (bowling ball terminal device, golf club holder, and so on). The most commonly used functional terminal devices (hooks or hands) have voluntary opening, with springs or rubber bands providing prehensile forces. Voluntary closing terminal devices allow the amputee to provide and control a variable prehensile force transmitted through the control cable to the terminal device. Many different voluntary opening hook designs are available for various functional applications, the most commonly prescribed being the Dorrance 5X, 5XA, and 7. Functional prosthetic hands, usually with voluntary opening, are heavier than the hooks and frequently do not provide as much function. Cosmetic hands are lighter than functional hands and can be passively positioned, but provide little if any function. Both types of hands are covered by a cosmetic glove that has been tinted to approximate the appropriate skin color

Wrist units provide a receptacle for connecting the terminal device to the prosthesis and for proper prepositioning of the terminal device for functional activities (supination/pronation for all units, or flexion if the appropriate unit is used). Wrist units control terminal device rotation either by friction or a special locking mechanism. The appropriate wrist unit design can be chosen as needed for the individual amputee. A quick disconnect wrist unit permits an easy interchange of different terminal devices, such as a hook for a hand.

The socket of a conventional upper extremity prosthesis is suspended by a harnessing system (usually a figure-of-eight harness) to which the control cables are attached. A shoulder saddle with a chest strap is an alternative suspension that permits carrying heavier loads with the prosthesis. Socket designs such as a suction socket or a self-suspending socket (Muenster) can provide partial or complete suspension. If the socket provides complete suspension for the prosthesis, then a figure-of-nine harness can be used for the control cable to provide body power for terminal device operation.

A wrist disarticulation spares the distal radial-ulnar articulation and thus preserves full forearm supination/pronation.

Socket designs for this level are tapered and flattened distally to allow the amputee to fully use active supination/pronation, thus avoiding having to preposition the terminal device for functional activities. A special thin wrist unit is used to minimize the overall length of the prosthesis because of the extremely long residual limb. If cosmesis is of importance to the amputee, a long below-elbow amputation may be a more appropriate amputation level. The socket is attached to a triceps pad by flexible elbow hinges and the harness attaches to the triceps pad.

Below-Elbow Amputations

Below-elbow amputations are classified by the length of bony forearm remaining: very short (less than 35%), short (35%–55%) and long (55%–90%). Long below-elbow residual limbs retain from 60° to 120° of supination/pronation and short below-elbow residual limbs retain less than 60°. Flexible elbow hinges are used for these two levels of amputation to attach the socket to the triceps cuff. For very short below-elbow amputation levels, rigid hinges are generally used. This can be accomplished by using external metal joints attached to the socket and cuff, or by directly attaching a modified plastic triceps cuff to the socket itself. With below-elbow amputations, in which range of motion is limited at the elbow, polycentric elbow joints or a split socket with step-up hinges can be used to provide additional flexion. The additional flexion is gained with the use of these elbow hinges, but there is a resultant loss of elbow flexion power and a decrease in the amputee's ability to actively lift weight with the prosthesis.

Elbow Disarticulation

Elbow disarticulation sockets are flat and broad distally to conform to the anatomic configuration of the condyles of the distal humerus. This design provides the amputee with active control of humeral rotation. The length of the socket requires the use of external elbow joints, with a cable-operated locking mechanism on the medial joint. The harness is either a figure-of-eight or a shoulder saddle and chest strap. The control system for this level uses two separate cables: one activates the elbow lock, the other cable is a fair-lead control system which has two functions: it provides power for elbow flexion when the elbow is unlocked, and provides tension when the elbow is locked that will open the terminal device.

Above-Elbow Amputations

Above-elbow amputations are also classified by the length of residual humerus: humeral neck (less than 30%), short above-elbow (30%–50%), and standard above-elbow (50%–90%). In above-elbow amputations with residual limb lengths greater than 35%, usually the proximal trimline of the socket ends approximately 1 cm lateral to the acromion, and the socket is suspended by either figure-of-eight or shoulder saddle and chest strap suspension systems. Sockets for residual limbs shorter than 35% should have the proximal trimline extend 2.5 cm medial to the acromion. This socket design can often be suspended with only a chest strap, but other harness systems can be used if appropriate.

In selecting an elbow unit, if the level of amputation is 4 cm proximal to the level of the epicondyles, then an internal positive-locking elbow unit can be used. An above-elbow residual limb with bony or soft tissue length that extends more distally than this will require a prosthesis similar to those for the elbow disarticulation level; that is, that can maintain an elbow joint center equal to that of the nonamputated side. However, the use of internal elbow joints is preferred. Internal elbow units have a turntable that allows passive positioning of humeral rotation. Elbow spring-lift assist units are also available for internal elbow units to help counterbalance the weight of the forearm and make elbow flexion easier for the amputee. The control system is the same dual control cable system used for the elbow disarticulation level.

Shoulder Disarticulation/Forequarter Amputations

For the more proximal levels of amputation, shoulder disarticulation and forequarter amputation, the socket extends onto the thorax to position and stabilize the prosthesis. The portion of the thorax covered by the socket is more extensive for the forequarter amputation. In some cases an open-frame socket rather than a plastic laminated socket is chosen for these levels to reduce prosthesis weight and to minimize heat buildup by reducing the amount of skin coverage.

Prosthetic components are similar to those for the above-elbow prosthesis with the addition of a shoulder unit, which allows passive positioning of the shoulder joint in flexion-extension and abduction-adduction. These sockets are suspended by chest straps attached anteriorly and posteriorly to the socket. The control system is a triple cable system in which three cables provide distinct functions. One cable, attached to the forearm shell and an axilla loop, provides active elbow flexion when the opposite humerus is flexed. A second cable, attached to the terminal device and the chest strap, provides terminal device opening with chest expansion. A third cable, attached to the elbow lock and a nudge control, locks and unlocks the elbow when the nudge control is depressed by the chin or opposite hand.

The difficulty of providing body-powered control motions of sufficient strength may be a reason for considering externally powered prostheses for these proximal levels of amputations.

It is important to consider a passive, cosmetic prosthetic restoration for selected individuals. These cosmetic prostheses can be fabricated to have an amazingly similar appearance to the opposite limb. There are only a few prosthetists in this country who specialize in this art form of prosthetic fabrication.

Externally Powered Prostheses

In North America, external power for upper extremity prostheses refers to the use of small electic motors incorporated into the prosthesis to control various functions. At the present time reliable external power units are available for terminal device operation, wrist rotation, and elbow flexion-extension.[28] Externally powered prostheses can provide not only greater prehensile forces than the body-powered prostheses, but also proportional prehension. Externally powered prostheses may provide more elbow function, especially in the short above-elbow or more proximal level amputee in whom control motion or strength may be limited.

The electric motors are controlled either by switches or myoelectric signals.

SWITCH-CONTROLLED PROSTHESES. For switch-controlled prostheses, small microswitches are incorporated into either the inside or outside of the prosthetic socket and are operated upon contact by the amputee. Pull switches incorporated into conventional harness and cable control systems that are activated by conventional body control motions are also available to control prosthetic function.

MYOELECTRIC PROSTHESES. Myoelectrically controlled prostheses are currently the most appealing of the externally powered prostheses. In the case of the below-elbow level amputation, the prosthesis has a self-suspending socket that eliminates the need for a harness.

A myoelectrically controlled prosthesis has a set or sets of electrodes imbedded in the prosthetic socket. These electrodes make contact with the skin and detect muscle action potentials from a voluntarily contracting muscle in the residual limb. The detected electrical signal is then amplified and rectified. The final signal is then capable of turning on an electric motor to provide a function (*i.e.,* terminal device operation, wrist rotation, or elbow flexion). Several different systems are available to process myoelectric signals. One system uses two sets of electrodes and amplifiers to control motion, one for a motion in one direction and one for the opposite motion, that is, terminal device opening and terminal device closing. Another system uses one set of electrodes for both motions. In this system it is the strength of voluntary contraction (amplitude of the myoelectric signal) that controls which motion will occur; a weak contraction will close the terminal device and a strong contraction will open the terminal device. This latter system is called a *single-site control system.*[36] The single-site control system allows an amputee with only one good control site (site of a strong reproducible voluntary contraction) in the residual limb to operate a myoelectrically controlled prosthesis. A single-site system will also allow an amputee to use two control sites to power two different functions, as in terminal device operation and wrist rotation.

In some systems the strength of contraction controls the speed of the function controlled. The Liberty Mutual (Boston) elbow is a proportional electric elbow that will flex or extend faster indirect proportion to the increasing amplitude of the contraction within the control muscle. The most sophisticated and expensive of the current myoelectric systems is the Utah elbow developed by Motion Control, Inc. (Fig. 17-3). This system employs microprocessor technology and two sets of electrodes to provide both elbow function and terminal device operation.

This system also allows for a free-swing phase of the elbow joint to approximate a "normal" cosmetic arm swing when walking.

The major resistance to prescription of myoelectrically controlled prostheses have been their cost, reliability, and weight. These systems are expensive because of large research and development costs, limited production, and small consumer market. Thus, no significant reductions in myoelectric component cost should be expected. Reliability was a significant issue when these systems were first introduced. Today, the reliability is much improved, and local prosthetists are now able to make many of the adjustments or repairs necessary to keep the units functioning rather than having to return them to the manufacturer as was done initially. The Utah elbow was designed with field serviceability in mind in that it has a limited number of easily and quickly replaced modular components. Myoelectric prostheses are generally heavier than their equivalent conventional prostheses because of the additional motors, batteries, and electrodes. Myoelectric prostheses are occasionally rejected because of the increased weight, but most amputees are able to accommodate to the increased weight.

Myoelectric prosthetic components are available that may be fitted to a wide range of individuals, from children as young as 3 or 4 years to adults. The majority of myoelectric terminal devices and components have been designed and manufactured for adult sizes in view of the significant costs involved with their production. Most myoelectric terminal devices tend to be hands, but some electric hook designs are also available. Myoelectrically controlled prostheses can and have been fitted immediately postoperation,[24] but it is generally recommended that myoelectric fittings be delayed until the residual limb is completely healed and the limb volume has stabilized sufficiently. Myoelectric prosthetic fitting that has occurred prior to stabilization of the residual limb volume may lead to frustration in the amputee because of poor socket fit and skin electrode contact, both of which occur with reducing limb volume and may necessitate an early replacement of the prosthetic socket. Myoelectric components have been combined with body-powered components to

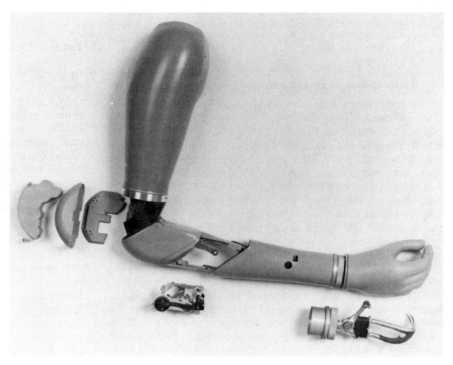

Figure 17-3. Utah elbow system. Shown are the controller electronics, battery, motor, and terminal device options. A myoelectric hand is atatched to the prosthesis. The voluntary opening hook terminal device is available if body power is to be used for terminal device control. (Motion Control, Inc)

result in a "hybrid" prosthesis, which may provide better function for some amputees than either myoelectric or body power control used alone.

Final Prosthetic Evaluation and Controls Training

After the prosthesis has been fabricated, it should be reviewed by the members of the prosthetic team. The prosthesis should be checked to make sure that the fit is comfortable and that the control system is properly adjusted for maximum functional operation. The amputee should then initiate a program of prosthetic training with the therapist. This training should include instruction in how to put on and remove the prosthesis, wearing and care of limb socks, opening and closing of the terminal device, grasping and releasing objects, transferring objects, and prepositioning of the terminal device for functional activities. As skills progress for the basic uses of the prosthesis, activities of daily living, home making, and occupational and recreational activities should be undertaken and simulated in the training sessions. Prosthetic training generally occurs in an outpatient setting. The amputee should be given a home program with specific goals to be achieved between the outpatient training sessions. Upper extremity amputees must be cautioned to frequently remove their prothesis to check for signs of excessive pressure or irritation that may occur with poor socket fit or overuse until skin tolerance increases. Initially the prosthesis should only be worn for 15 to 20 minutes before checking the skin. If no problems are apparent, wearing time is gradually increased. With good skin tolerance, the upper extremity amputee can expect to wear the prosthesis for an entire day within a few days after receiving the prosthesis.

Control training for externally powered prostheses is more complex than for body-powered prostheses. The same goals mentioned for conventional prostheses are appropriate for myoelectrically controlled prostheses. In addition, the amputee must learn to separate, control, and sustain voluntary muscle contractions in the muscles selected to control the powered functions of the prosthesis. As for conventionally powered prostheses, a home program to practice and enhance prosthetic control skills should be outlined in order to achieve independent function.

Adults and older children can be expected to practice specific tasks and routines both in therapy and at home as outlined by the therapist in order to achieve the necessary skills for independent function. The training time in a young child with an upper extremity prosthesis will be significantly longer than for an adult or older child.

In adults, unilateral upper extremity basic training should follow this timetable: below elbow, 5 hours; above elbow, 10 hours; shoulder disarticulation, 15 hours or more. Basic prosthetic training usually occurs in a short period of time when spent under the guidance of a therapist. However, prosthetic learning occurs over a lifetime of use as the amputee continues to be challenged with new bimanual experiences. The amputee becomes the problem-solver and develops new use patterns that are most efficient for his or her activity needs.

Bilateral Upper Extremity Amputations

The bilateral upper extremity amputee is immediately faced with the lost ability to perform almost every activity of daily living. Early restoration of any activity of daily living is important. Providing a utensil cuff, which can be attached to a residual arm, can assist the patient with feeding and tooth brushing.

With the bilateral amputee, early prosthetic fitting should be accomplished even with temporary or preparatory prostheses.

In the bilateral amputee, dominance is usually assumed by the longer residual limb. Special component considerations apply in this case. Wrist flexion units, at least on the dominant side or perhaps bilaterally, will permit midline activities such as shirt buttoning and belt buckling. Also, wrist rotator units, which provide automatic terminal device positioning, provide for easier prosthetic use.

Special toileting techniques must be taught for patient independence. In addition, foot skills should be reviewed and lower extremity mobilizing exercises should be performed.

Upper Extremity Prosthetic Follow-up

The routine follow-up visits to the clinic for a new amputee should occur initially 4 to 6 weeks after receipt of the prosthesis, then at 3 months, then at 6 months, and then at yearly intervals. Additional clinic visits should occur whenever a problem arises. At these follow-up visits the amputee's use and function with the prosthesis should be reviewed, any difficulties or problems resolved, the fit and condition of the prosthesis evaluated, and the condition of the residual limb noted. If necessary, additional therapy may be suggested, repairs to the prosthesis made, medical problems with the residual limb attended to, and a new prosthesis prescribed if indicated. With average use, an upper extremity prosthesis can be expected to be worn for 3 to 5 years before replacement is necessary.

While our emphasis has been on prosthetic restoration, the focus of rehabilitation should remain on the amputee and his desired life-style following limb loss. Many amputees do well without the aid of a prosthesis and should not be viewed to have failed if they do not choose to wear a prosthesis.

LOWER EXTREMITY PROSTHESES

The functions provided by a lower extremity prosthesis are weight-bearing, locomotion, and cosmesis. These functions are less complex and more uniform from amputee to amputee than those an upper extremity prosthesis attempts to replace. Because weight-bearing is a major concern in a lower extremity prosthesis, the distribution of forces at the interface between the skin of the residual limb and the socket of the prosthesis becomes critical. The residual limb-socket interface is often the major source of lower extremity prosthetic fitting problems and the reason for most lower extremity prosthetic modifications. The second major function, locomotion, should allow the amputee to walk with as little variation as possible from normal gait. The cosmetic effect of a lower limb prosthesis should be considered a function of prosthetic use when seated, standing, walking, and running.

The prosthetic prescription must balance the individual amputee's need for stability, safety, mobility, durability, and cosmesis. The availability of prosthetic services must also be considered, since some components require more frequent maintenance than others. A lower extremity prosthetic prescription should describe the construction design, socket type, suspension method, appropriate joint components, and prosthetic foot.

Levels of Prosthesis

Partial Foot Amputations

Partial foot amputations involving the forefoot, such as toe amputations, ray resections, and transmetatarsal amputations, generally require only shoe fillers or shoe modifications. The shoe modifications required may include the addition of a steel spring shank extending to the metatarsal heads, a rocker sole, and padding of the tongue of the shoe to help hold the hindfoot firmly in the shoe. Transtarsal amputations (Chopart, Boyd, Lisfranc) are not recommended as elective levels of amputation, but will occasionally be encountered and will need to be fit with a prosthesis. The best prosthetic option for a hindfoot amputation is the use of a custom prosthetic foot with a self-suspending split socket, which allows a regular low-quarter shoe to be worn.[14] A posterior leaf spring ankle foot orthosis is another alternative.

Syme's Amputations

A Syme's level amputation is the next proximal site of amputation and is preferred to one at the transtarsal level. Preservation of the articular cartilage covered by the heel pad allows for direct end-bearing on the residual limb. This advantage is frequently proposed as the primary reason for choosing this level of amputation, since the amputee can easily stand and walk on the end of the residual limb without wearing a prosthesis.

The distal bulbous end of the leg, which results from the flaring of the tibia and fibula at the malleoli, has led to socket designs that are self-suspending. The classical socket designs have been either a posterior or medially opening Canadian Syme's prosthesis. Both entail removal of a portion of the distal total contact socket wall to allow the bulbous distal residual limb to pass through the narrower portion of the socket. The socket wall is then replaced to provide the necessary suspension. The major disadvantage of this level of amputation is the poor cosmesis of the prosthesis. The distal bulbous end of the residual limb is further accentuated by the prosthesis.

Newer socket designs which incorporate either an expandable air suspension chamber inside the socket or a thin removable expandable inner socket liner provide a more cosmetically acceptable prosthetic design. Because there is no need to remove a section from the socket wall, the structural integrity of these latter two designs is maintained, resulting in a prosthetic socket that can be thinner, lighter, and stronger. The usual prosthetic foot is a Syme's SACH (solid ankle cushion heel) foot. A Syme's S.A.F.E. (stationary attachment flexible endoskeleton) foot is also available. These prosthetic feet are discussed further in the following section.

Below-Knee Amputations

COMPONENTS. The standard socket used for the average below-knee amputee is the total contact patellar tendon bearing (P.T.B.) socket which bears weight over the entire surface of the residual limb, with more weight-bearing borne in the area of the patellar tendon and the tibial flare and reduced weight-bearing over the bony prominences such as the tibial crest, distal end of the tibia, and the head of the fibula. A soft liner can be added to the socket to protect fragile or insensate skin, to reduce sheer forces, or to provide a more comfortable socket for tender residual limbs. Soft liners can be made of closed cell thermoplastic foams, rubber covered with leather, or silicone gels covered with leather.

A supracondylar cuff is the most common form of suspension for a below-knee prosthesis. Alternative options for suspension include thigh corsets with knee joints, waist belt and forkstrap (Y-Strap), supracondylar medial wedge suspension, supracondylar self-suspending socket, and rubber or neoprene sleeve suspension. Ankle rotator units are available for those amputees who require absorption of axial torque, such as golfers or boaters. The selection of a prosthetic foot completes the below-knee prothesis prescription.

PROSTHETIC FEET. The SACH foot is the most commonly used prosthetic foot because it is durable, lightweight, inexpensive, and easily interchanged to accommodate shoes of different heel heights. The presence of a compressible heel and wooden keel in this foot design allow it to simulate the motions of the ankle in normal walking without actual ankle movement occurring. The compressibility of the heel permits the SACH foot to partially accommodate for uneven terrain, but this foot is best suited for flat level surfaces.

A single axis foot permits movement of the foot–ankle complex in one plane. Movement occurs in the plantar flexion–dorsiflexion axis. The movement is controlled by the use of adjustable internal rubber bumpers which provide resistance to dorsiflexion and plantar flexion. This foot is heavier than the SACH foot and the internal components need periodic adjustment or replacement. This foot is not usually used with a below-knee prosthesis, but with prostheses for more proximal amputation levels which require additional knee control or stability.

Multiaxis prosthetic feet are being prescribed more frequently for the amputee who is involved in athletic activities or who walks on uneven terrain. The advantage of the multiaxis foot is that it offers some controlled movement in the normal anatomic planes of the ankle: dorsiflexion–plantar flexion, inversion–eversion, and rotation. A number of different foot designs are available to provide this multiaxial motion. Some of the prosthetic feet accomplish this movement without the use of mechanically moving parts; they rely instead on the inherent flexibility of the materials and design of the foot. The S.A.F.E. and RAX feet are examples. Other multiaxis feet which use mechanical systems to provide this mobility include the Greissinger, Cope's, and McKendrick foot. The additional mechanical components necessary for the movement in these feet add to their overall weight and may require frequent maintenance especially in the very active amputee. For the active amputee, however, the improved balance, coordination, and function provided by these feet generally outweigh the disadvantages of increased weight and more frequent maintenance.

One hydraulic foot–ankle complex, the Mauch C III, is currently available. This unit, although heavy, is the only one which allows free positioning of the unweighted ankle in either plantar flexion or dorsiflexion. Unlike other multiaxis feet, this unit provides a variable resistance to dorsiflexion by using a hydraulic unit, which is activated either as the result of the position of the shank of the prosthesis with relationship to the foot or by active loading of the foot. This feature provides an advantage for ramp and stair climbing not available with other prosthetic feet. The unit also permits adjustable resisted inversion–eversion and axial rotation. The major disadvantage to the hydraulic ankle is its weight and cost compared to other multiaxis foot options.

One of the recent major advances in lower extremity prosthetic component design has been the energy-storing prosthetic foot such as the Flex-Foot (Fig. 17-4), Seattle foot (Fig. 17-5), Stored Energy (STEN) foot (Fig. 17-6), and the Carbon Copy II foot (Fig. 17-7). The design of these feet incorporates the use of resilient, flexible energy-storing materials. Energy is stored in the foot at the time of heel strike as the weight of the body either compresses or flexes the resilient material within the foot and is returned to the amputee at the time of push off as the components of the energy-storing foot return to their normal shape or configuration. Preliminary data indicate that these prosthetic foot designs make prosthetic ambulation more efficient and require less energy consumption by the amputee.[7, 20, 33] The resiliency of these feet makes them particularly suitable for amputees involved in activities requiring running and jumping. The reduction of the mass of the prosthesis with the lightweight Flex-Foot also aids in reducing energy expenditure.

Knee Disarticulation

Knee disarticulation level amputations have some of the same advantages and disadvantages as the Syme's level amputation. This level provides a good, wide, flat surface for endbearing within a prosthesis and an anatomic configuration ideal for a self-suspending socket. The bulbous distal end of a knee disarticulation residual limb presents some of the same cosmetic concerns that are present with the Syme's residual limb. More significantly, however, the knee disarticulation level of amputation presents the problem of trying to maintain equal knee centers of motion between the amputated and nonamputated lower extremities. The development of special knee units, such as the OHC (Orthopedic Hospital Copenhagen) disarticulation knee unit, has resulted in a prosthesis with nearly equal thigh lengths, leg lengths, and knee centers, thereby making knee disarticulation level amputations more cosmetically acceptable.

Above-Knee Amputations

Research following World War II led to the development of the total contact quadrilateral socket. This design replaced the plugfit socket as the standard for the above-knee prosthesis. The quadrilateral socket, until recently, was the only socket design used for above-knee prostheses. Now two new socket designs have been introduced for above-knee prostheses: (1) a narrow medial–lateral socket known by the eponyms NSNA (normal shape, normal alignment) or CAT–CAM (contoured adducted

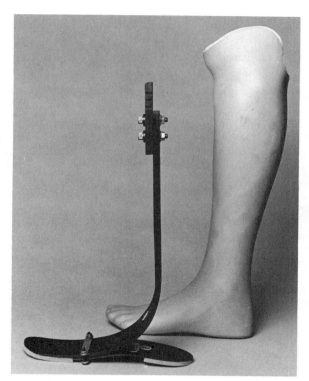

Figure 17-4. Flex-Foot prosthetic foot and shank component with and without cosmetic foam cover. The flexibility of the carbon fiber–epoxy foot and shank gives it the ability to store and return energy. (Flex-Foot, Inc)

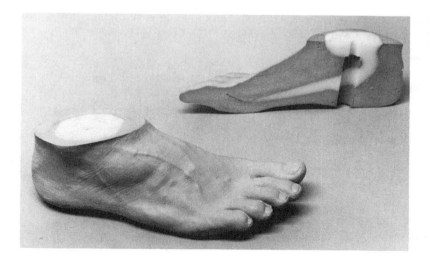

Figure 17-5. Seattle foot. The saggital section demonstrates the flexible keel of this foot. (Model & Instrument Development)

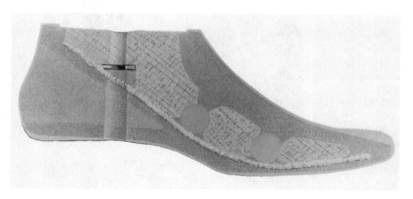

Figure 17-6. STEN foot. The two rubber bumpers placed between the wooden keel of this design compress to store energy and return energy as they expand during ambulation. (Kingsley Manufacturing Company)

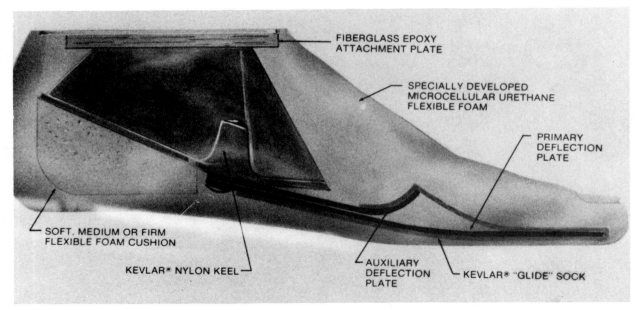

Figure 17-7. Carbon Copy II foot. Construction components permitting energy storage are highlighted. (Ohio Willow Wood Company)

trochanteric–controlled alignment method), and (2) the flexible AK socket variously known as the Scandinavian, Icelandic, or ISNY socket.[16, 22, 34]

The narrow medial-lateral design was developed to provide a more normal anatomical alignment of the femur inside the prosthesis. (Fig. 17-8). It also stabilizes the relationship between the pelvis and the proximal femur, since the ischial tuberosity is controlled inside the socket rather than just sitting on the top of the posterior brim as the tuberosity does in the quadrilateral socket. To control the pelvis, the trimline of the socket is brought more proximal than that of the quadrilateral socket. This higher trimline results in better control of the residual limb, particularly for short above-knee amputations.

The Scandinavian flexible socket has a total contact thermoplastic inner socket supported by a graphite reinforced laminated framework. (Fig. 17-9). Either the traditional quadrilateral socket or the narrow medial–lateral socket shapes can be used with this type of socket design. The socket is flexible because of the characteristics of the thermoplastic material used to form the inner socket. As this material warms to body temperature it becomes even more flexible. The advantages of this type of socket design are threefold: increased comfort because the socket is able to change configurations due to the flexibility of the material; increased proprioceptive feedback and prosthetic control, since the socket wall moves with the contracting muscles in the residual limb; and direct observation of the residual limb–socket interface both in static and dynamic situations because the socket is made of transparent material. Better prosthetic socket fit can be achieved because fitting problems are directly observed and corrected.

Several options are available for suspension of above-knee prostheses, but the use of a suction socket is usually preferred. The use of a suction socket, however, requires a stable residual limb volume. Increase in residual limb volume will prevent the amputee from fitting completely in the socket and a reduction in residual limb volume will result in a loss of suction and suspension, making it impossible for the amputee to wear the prosthesis. A suction socket is worn without a sock on the residual limb. A Silesian belt can be used either as an auxiliary form of suspension with a suction socket or can be used as the primary form of suspension. A standard Silesian belt attaches to the anterior and lateral portions of the proximal prosthetic socket and passes over the opposite iliac crest. A pelvic band and belt with hip joint is a third alternative for suspension of an above-knee prosthesis. Attaching an above-knee prosthesis is easiest with this suspension method. The pelvic band is closely contoured about the anterior iliac crest on the side of the amputation

Figure 17-8. Narrow medial-lateral above-knee socket (NSNA design) viewed from above. The valve seen distally is on the medial aspect of the socket.

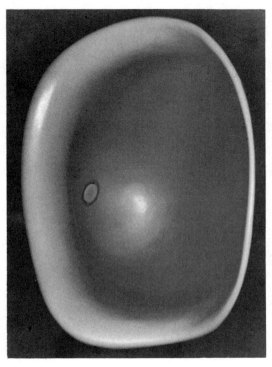

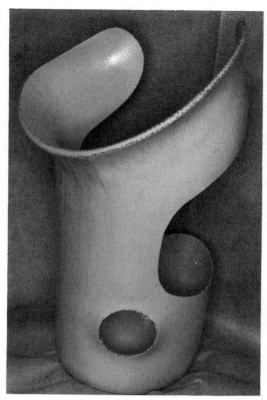

Figure 17-9. Carbon fiber reinforced laminated framework supports a flexible thermoplastic above-knee prosthetic socket.

to discourage rotation of the prosthesis on the residual limb during ambulation. Occasionally an amputee who would be a candidate for a pelvic band and belt suspension will not be able to wear a belt around the waist (*i.e.,* an individual who has a subcutaneous axillary femoral bypass graft which cannot be compressed by a waist belt); he or she will require the use of a shoulder belt or suspender suspension for the prosthesis.

The distal end of the above-knee residual limb should be at least 8 cm proximal to the level of the distal end of the femur and above the condyles of the femur to allow the use of a conventional internal prosthetic knee joint. Several different designs of prosthetic knee joints are available. The purpose of the knee joint of the prosthesis is to allow for knee flexion when sitting and an arc of movement of the shank relative to the thigh of the prosthesis during the swing phase of gait. The knee unit should control the heel rise of the shank and assist or resist the acceleration and deceleration of the shank during swing phase. A constant friction unit is the most commonly used. Hydraulic knee units are available, which can provide either swing phase control or swing and stance phase control for amputees who are very active and change their cadence frequently. For amputees who have difficulty maintaining knee stability during stance, locking knees and safety knees are available.

Thigh rotators are available for individuals who have a need or desire to cross their legs or to be able to sit on the floor. All of the prosthetic feet mentioned in the below-knee amputation section are available for use, as appropriate, with above-knee prostheses.

Hip Disarticulation/Hemipelvectomy

Individuals with less than 5 cm of residual femur are usually fitted as hip disarticulation level amputees. The standard prosthesis for a hip disarticulation is the Canadian hip disarticulation

prosthesis. The socket of this prosthesis encloses the hemipelvis on the side of the amputation and extends around the hemipelvis of the nonamputated side, leaving an opening for the nonamputated lower extremity. There is a flexible anterior wall with an opening that allows for donning of this prosthesis. Weight is borne on the ischial tuberosity of the amputated side. Endoskeletal prosthetic components are preferred for this level of amputation to reduce the overall weight. The endoskeletal hip joint has an extension assist as does the knee unit, which is usually a constant friction knee. A single axis or SACH foot with a soft heel and cosmetic cover completes the prosthetic prescription. If necessary, locking hip or knee joints can be used.

The prosthesis for a hemipelvectomy resembles that for the hip disarticulation except in the interior configuration of the socket. In the hemipelvectomy most of the weight is borne by the soft tissues on the amputated side with some of the weight being borne by the sacrum and the opposite ischial tuberosity.

Final Prosthetic Evaluation and Gait Training

After the prosthetist has statically and dynamically aligned the prosthesis and ensured the fit of the socket, the amputee should be seen for final prosthetic evaluation by the entire clinical team. At this time the prosthesis is evaluated for appropriate fit, alignment, and length. Minor adjustments in alignment and length can be made at the time of this evaluation, prior to the completion of the definitive prosthesis, if the prosthesis is an exoskeletal design and is still on the alignment fixture, or if it is an endoskeletal prosthesis.

Gait Training

After completion of the final prosthetic evaluation, a new amputee will require a period of gait training to learn how to function using the prosthesis. This training is done under the direction of the physical therapist. For the new amputee it may be appropriate to have the initial gait training occur while the prosthesis is still capable of being adjusted, so that minor adjustments in alignment or length may be made as they become apparent through the gait training process. The amputee is instructed in how to put on and take off the prosthesis, how to determine the appropriate ply and number of limb socks to be worn, when and how to check the skin for evidence of irritation, and how to clean and care for the prosthesis. Gait training often occurs on an outpatient basis and may last from 1 week to a month with three to five visits per week. The more proximal levels of amputation require more lengthy gait training.

After the amputee has learned to put on the prosthesis, he or she is initially taught to shift weight onto the prosthesis while working in the parallel bars. Having mastered weight-shifting, a program of progressive ambulation begins in the parallel bars and progresses to the most independent level of ambulation, using a walker, crutches, or cane, or walking unassisted. Following the mastery of ambulation on flat level surfaces, techniques for managing uneven terrain, stairs, ramps, curbs, and falling and getting up off the ground are accomplished. Transfer activities should also be reviewed as part of the gait training.

Wearing tolerance for the prosthesis must gradually be increased. Initially during training the amputee will only wear the prosthesis for 15 to 20 minutes, removing it to check the condition of the skin. As the skin's ability to tolerate increased pressure with weight-bearing increases, the length of wearing time is gradually increased. Several weeks may be required before the amputee is able to wear the prosthesis full time. The amputee should be allowed to take the prosthesis home from therapy when he has demonstrated that he can ambulate safely and independently with or without aids and the therapist is assured that the amputee will check the condition of the residual limb at appropriate intervals.

Gait Analysis

A familiarity with the cycle and determinants of normal gait is necessary to evaluate whether a prosthesis adequately substitutes for the amputed lower extremity during walking. An amputee's gait should be reviewed in a systematic fashion. First, the base of support is observed. Next the symmetry of movement from side to side is evaluated joint by joint for the lower extremities, the trunk, and the upper extremities. The movements should occur in a fluid manner from one part of the cycle to the next. Reports of pain should be noted both with respect to its location and when it occurs during the gait cycle.

Normal gait is a regularly recurring cycle of events that can be identified, quantified, and evaluated. The end result of this cyclical activity is the forward translation of the body. The recurring elements of gait, also known as the *gait cycle,* include the repeating movements of the lower extremity, trunk movements, and upper extremity movements.[42] The series of events begins with the heel strike of one foot and ends with the next heel strike of the same foot. This cycle has classically been divided into a *stance phase,* the time when the foot is in contact with the ground, and a *swing phase* when the foot is not in contact with the ground. Stance phase constitutes 60% of the cycle and is frequently further divided into heel strike, midstance, and push off. Swing phase is the remaining 40% of the cycle and can be divided into toe off, mid-swing, and late swing. Because the swing phase is shorter than the stance phase, there is a period of time when both feet are in contact with the ground. This period of time is called the *period of double support.* As the velocity of walking increases, the period of double support is reduced until there is no double support. Running is defined as ambulation without double support. The distance covered from one heel strike to the next heel strike of the same foot is known as a *stride length.* The distance from heel strike of one foot to heel strike of the opposite foot is a *step length. Stride width* is defined as the distance from the center of one foot during stance to the center

of the other foot during stance. *Cadence* is the number of steps per minute.

Recurring movements are also noted in the trunk and upper extremity throughout the gait cycle. These are often referred to as associative movements. During the gait cycle the pelvis rotates forward on the side that is in swing phase and posteriorly on the side in stance. The shoulders move in the opposite direction to the pelvis during normal gait. The upper extremities swing freely at the shoulders throughout the gait cycle and move in the direction opposite to the ipsilateral lower extremity (*i.e.,* as the right hip flexes the right shoulder extends).

For the purpose of gait analysis, the mass of the body is considered to be concentrated at the body's center of gravity, a point just anterior to the body of the second sacral vertebra. Inman and colleagues have described six major elements or determinants of gait that combine to reduce the movement of the center of gravity in both the vertical and horizontal planes. The six elements are pelvic rotation, pelvic list (tilt), knee flexion in stance phase, foot and ankle motion, synchronized knee and ankle motion, and lateral displacement of the pelvis.[15] The combination of these determinants results in a movement of the center of gravity in a smooth sinusoidal path both vertically and horizontally with an amplitude of about 5 cm in each plane. Muscle activity (work) is required to raise the center of gravity during the gait cycle and by keeping this movement to a minimum, the energy expenditure required to walk is minimized. A normal comfortable walking speed for an adult without an amputation is about 75 to 80 meters per minute (4.5–4.8 km/hr). Walking at this speed requires an energy expenditure of approximately 59 cal/min/kg, which is a minimal energy expenditure per kilogram of body weight to walk 1 meter (Table 17-1). Factors, like an amputation, which interfere with the normal biomechanics of the lower extremities, will alter the energy required to walk[8] (see also Chapter 16). An individual with an amputation using a prosthesis will expend more energy to walk at the same velocity as a normal individual. Moreover the energy expenditure of prosthetic walking increases significantly as the amputation level moves proximally. The lower extremity amputee, rather than maintaining the same walking speed as a nonamputee, reduces his or her gait velocity to achieve an energy expenditure that is nearly equivalent to the nonamputee adult walking at 75 to 80 meters per minutes (Tables 17-2 and 17-3).

Table 17-1
Normal Ambulation

Researcher, Date	Number	Type of Disability and Appliances	Speed in meters/min	Energy Expenditure kcal/min/kg	kcal × 10^{-3}/meters/kg
McDonald, 1961	583	Normals (F)	80	0.067[†]	0.83
		Normals (M)	80	0.061[†]	0.76
Ralston, 1958	19	Normals (M & F)	74[‡]	0.058[†]	0.78
Corcoran, 1970	32	Normals (M & F)	83[‡,§]	0.063[†]	0.76
Waters, 1976	25	Normals (M & F)	82[§]	0.063[†]	0.77
Ganguli, 1973	16	Normals (M)	50[‖]	0.044	0.088[*]
Bobbert, 1960	2	Normals (M)	81[‖]	0.063[#]	0.079[*]
Peizer, 1969	?	Normal (?)	80[**]	0.043[**]	0.57

* Calculated knowing kcal/min and meters/min
† Calculated knowing kcal/meters and meters/min
‡ Most efficient speed of ambulation
§ Speed chosen by subjects
‖ Speed chosen by the researcher (the only speed or a representative speed)
Calculation from author's equation and/or percentage figure
** Approximated from a graph
(SDMKP in PM&R, 2nd ed. Syllabus, AAPM&R, 1986)

Table 17-2
Ambulation of Below-Knee Amputees With Prostheses

Researcher, Date	Number	Type of Disability and Appliances	Speed in meters/min	Energy Expenditure kcal/min/kg	kcal × 10⁻³/meters/kg
Waters, 1976	15	Vascular Syme's	54[‡]	0.055**	1.01[#, **]
Reitemeyer, 1955	2	Below knee	60[§]	0.035[†]	0.58
Ralston, 1971	1	Below knee	49[§]	0.055[§]	1.12
Molen, 1973	54	Traumatic below knee	50[§]	0.060[‖]	1.20
Ganguli, 1973	20	Below knee	50[§]	0.060	1.20
Gonzales, 1974	9	Below knee	64[‡]	0.062[#, **]	0.97*
Waters, 1976	13	Vascular below knee	45[‡]	0.056**	1.25**
Waters, 1976	14	Traumatic below knee	71[‡]	0.074**	1.04**
Gonzales, 1974	?	Bilteral below knee	66[‡]	0.070[#, **]	1.07*

* Calculated knowing kcal/min and meters/min
[†] Calculated knowing kcal/meters and meters/min
[‡] Speed chosen by the subjects
[§] Speed chosen by the researcher (the only speed or a representative speed)
[‖] Calculation from author's equation and/or percentage figure
[#] Approximated from a graph
** Calculated from oxygen consumption
(SDMKP in PM&R, 2nd ed. Syllabus, AAPM&R, 1986)

Table 17-3
Ambulation of Above-Knee Amputees With Prostheses

Researcher, Date	Number	Type of Disability and Appliances	Speed in meters/min	Energy Expenditure kcal/min/kg	kcal × 10⁻³/meters/kg
Muller, 1952	2	Above knee	70[‖]	0.053[†]	0.76[††]
Muller, 1952	1	Above knee	40[‖]	0.023[†]	0.60[††]
Inman, 1961	1	Above knee	62	0.017[†]	1.05[#]
Durnin, 1967	?	Above knee	60[‖]	0.067	1.12*
Bard & Ralston, 1959	6	Above knee	68[‡, §, #]	0.061[#]	0.90[#]
Ganguli, 1974	6	Above knee	50[‖]	0.088	1.76*
Traugh, 1975	9	Above knee	39[§]	0.048[#, **]	1.23*
Ralston, 1971	1	Above knee	49[‖]	0.049	1.01*
Waters, 1976	13	Vascular above knee	36[§]	0.061**	1.25**
Waters, 1976	15	Traumatic above knee	52[§]	0.062**	1.19**
James, 1973	37	Traumatic above knee	51[§]	0.061	1.19
Erdman, 1960	9	Above knee	47[§]	0.035[†]	0.76

* Calculated knowing kcal/min and meters/min
[†] Calculated knowing kcal/meters and meters/min
[‡] Most efficient speed of ambulation
[§] Speed chosen by the subjects
[‖] Speed chosen by the researcher (the only speed or a representative speed)
[#] Approximated from a graph
** Calculated from oxygen consumption
[††] Original data reanalyzed
(SDMKP in PM&R, 2nd ed. Syllabus, AAPM&R, 1986)

Lower Extremity Prosthetic Follow-up

The frequency of follow-up visits for lower extremity amputees is similar to that for upper extremity amputees. During the initial 6 to 18 months, most amputees will experience rapid loss of residual limb volume resulting in a prosthetic socket that will be too large. During this period of time, the return visits to the clinic or prosthetist should occur at intervals frequent enough to ensure that this loss of residual limb volume is being adequately compensated for by the use of additional limb socks or by appropriate modifications of the prosthetic socket. It is not un-usual for a new amputee to require replacement of the prosthetic socket during this time period because of the significant loss of soft tissue volume. At the follow-up clinic visits the condition of the residual limb, the prosthesis, the amputee's gait, and the level of function are reviewed. Appropriate medical treatment, prosthetic modifications, or additional therapy are prescribed as needed. When the residual limb volume has sufficiently stabilized and the amputee is doing well with the prosthesis, yearly visits to the amputee clinic are appropriate. Once the residual limb has stabilized, the average life expectancy for a lower extremity prosthesis before replacement should be 3 to 5 years.

SPECIAL PROSTHETIC ISSUES

Phantom Sensation and Phantom Pain

All individuals with acquired amputations experience some form of *phantom sensation,* which is the awareness of a nonpainful sensation in the amputated part. This sensation is most prominent in the period immediately following amputation and gradually diminishes in intensity over time, but can persist throughout the amputee's entire life. *Phantom pain* is the awareness of pain in the amputated extremity. It may be diffuse throughout the entire amputated extremity or it may be restricted to the distribution of a single peripheral nerve. The occurrence of phantom pain is generally considered to be a significant problem in only 5% or less of the total amputee population, but some authors have noted that phantom pain has been reported by more than three-quarters of all amputees at some time during their life following amputation.[40, 41] In the early postoperative period, phantom pain may be significantly reduced with the use of amitriptyline, 50 to 150 mg at bedtime. Range-of-motion exercises, relaxation exercises, and gentle massage of the residual limb may also help reduce phantom pain. For chronic phantom pain, many therapeutic modalities have been suggested and tried with varying rates of success.[23, 40, 41] Often the treatment modalities employed, either medical or surgical, do not provide long-lasting relief. The various forms of therapy attempted to treat phantom pain have been reviewed by Sherman.[38, 39]

Dermatological Disorders

Numerous problems with the skin on the residual limb can occur such as hyperhydrosis, folliculitis, allergic dermatitis, or breakdown of the skin at the site of adherent scars or split-thickness skin grafts. Skin problems can be minimized by instructing the amputee to carefully wash and dry the residual limb daily and to wear natural fiber limb socks that are absorbent to minimize the moisture inside the socket in order to prevent skin maceration. At times it is appropriate to use nylon or polyamide sheaths between the skin and the limb sock to reduce shear forces that can cause skin breakdown.

Hyperhydrosis can be successfully controlled by using concentrated antiperspirants, such as Drysol, on the residual limb. Folliculitis may require the use of antibiotics, and sebaceous cysts may require surgical drainage or excision. Allergic dermatitis can result from the detergents used to wash the limb socks and may only require the changing of the detergent. In rare cases the dermatitis may result from the materials used to fabricate the prosthetic socket, in which case, a new prosthetic socket needs to be fabricated from nonallergenic materials.

Socket Fit

Both upper and lower extremity amputees can have problems with socket fit. The usual reasons for changes in socket fit are weight gain or weight loss and changes in limb contour. Frequently minor problems in socket fit can be handled by modifications to an existing prosthetic socket or with the use of growth liners. Significant changes in socket fit will require a new prosthetic socket.

One specific problem that can result from poor socket fit for the lower extremity amputee, that is not typically encountered with the upper extremity amputee, is a choke syndrome. This situation results when the prosthetic socket is tight circumferentially in the proximal region and there is no good distal contact between the residual limb and the socket. The proximal constriction results in obstruction of venous outflow producing edema of the distal end of the residual limb where socket contact is not present. Usually this area of edema produces a circular, well-circumscribed margin. If the choke syndrome is allowed to progress, the edema will progress to induration, erythema, breakdown, and drainage. The area of choke is quite tender to palpation and is prone to developing cellulitis if there is an open lesion. If a choke syndrome becomes chronic, the tissues involved on the distal residual limb can become brownish orange as the result of pigments (hemosiderin) from extravasated red blood cells that accumulate in the tissues. This pigmentation is usually permanent, even if the choke syndrome is ultimately resolved. The tissues in a chronic choke syndrome can also take on a verrucous appearance. The appropriate treatment for a choke syndrome is to relieve the proximal constriction and to restore total contact distally between the residual limb and the socket.[21]

Pediatric Limb Loss

The absence of part or all of an extremity at birth is more appropriately referred to as a *congenital skeletal deficiency,* rather than a congenital amputation. The 1984 Annual Summary of health statistics for the United States reports the incidence of these congenital reduction deformities at 309 for 1983, or 4.1 per 10,000 births.[47] When a child is born with an absent or malformed limb, the question "Why?" is always asked, but often no etiology can ever be identified. A few genetically determined syndromes, such as Holt-Oram, Fanconi's syndrome, and thrombocytopenia-absent radius (TAR), have been associated with skeletal deficiencies.[37] Congenital amniotic bands have occasionally been implicated, but no clear understanding of how these occur has been reached. Exposure to teratogenic agents during limb development, such as thalidomide and excessive radiation, has been identified as resulting in limb defects at birth.[5, 37]

Multiple systems for classifying congenital limb deficiencies have been proposed in both Europe and North America, but no one system has been universally accepted. In the United States some form of the Frantz-O'Rahilly system is most commonly used. The ISPO Dundee Classification System was developed by a group of international experts with the hope that it would become the standard for classification of congenital limb deficiencies. The fact that this has not occurred has made data collection for epidemiological and etiological purposes difficult. Classification of congenital limb deficiencies is often further confused when congenital deficiencies are described in the same terms used for acquired amputations, such as "below elbow" or "below knee." The use of similar terminology occurs either because the congenital deficiency appears similar to an acquired amputation or because a congenital skeletal deficiency has undergone a surgical conversion to accommodate appropriate prosthetic restoration. Surgical conversion has been estimated to be necessary in the management of 50% of lower extremity congenital deficiencies and only 8% of upper extremity deficiencies.[3]

When performing amputations in children for disease, tumor, or trauma, or when surgically converting a congenital skeletal deficiency to a level more appropriate for prosthetic fitting, a disarticulation level amputation is preferred rather than an amputation through a long bone when the resulting level of function with a prosthesis will be similar.

Approximately 12% of children with acquired amputations experience a condition known as *bony overgrowth.* Bony overgrowth is the appositional deposition of bone to the end of the amputated long bone. This bone growth results in a spikelike formation at the end of the bone which has a thin cortex and no medullary canal. The bone frequently grows faster than the overlying skin and soft tissues; a bursa may develop over the sharp end, or the bone may actually protrude through the skin with subsequent development of cellulitis and osteomyelitis. Overgrowth is most frequently seen in the humerus, fibula, tibia, and femur, in that order. It has been reported in the congenital limb deficiencies, but rarely. Several treatment approaches have been advocated for the management of this problem, all with limited success. The technique proposed by Marquardt in which the distal end of the bone is capped with a cartilage epiphysis is the best of the surgical options available to manage this problem.[2]

For the child with a congenital skeletal deficiency, the initial prosthesis for the upper extremity is usually fitted when the child has attained independent sitting balance, or at approximately 6 months of age. For the lower extremity, the initial prosthesis may be fitted when the child begins to pull to a stand, which is generally between 9 and 14 months. Young children and infants usually learn to use their prostheses by incorporating them as part of play activities rather than through specific exercises. Prosthetic training periods for children may only last for several minutes at a time because of limited attention span, and they may require much longer periods of free play interspersed between actual training sessions. It is important that parents be instructed in techniques to help their children attain the necessary prosthetic skills because much of the training in the use of the prosthesis will occur in the home rather than in the clinic.

REFERENCES

1. Aitken GT, Frantz CH: Child amputee. Clin Orthop 148:3–8, 1980
2. American Academy of Orthopedic Surgeons: Atlas of Limb Prosthetics: Surgical and Prosthetic Principles. St. Louis, CV Mosby, 1981
3. Banerjee SN (ed): Rehabilitation Management of Amputees. Baltimore, Williams & Wilkins, 1982
4. Barry DT, Leonard JA, Gitter AJ, Ball RD: Acoustic myography as a control signal for an externally powered prosthesis. Arch Phys Med Rehabil 67:267–269, 1986
5. Bender LF: Prostheses and Rehabilitation After Arm Amputation. Springfield, IL, Charles C Thomas, 1974
6. Burgess EM, Matsen FA III: Determining amputation levels in peripheral vascular disease. J Bone Joint Surg (Am) 63:1493–1497, 1981
7. Burgess EM, Poggi DL, Hittenberger DA et al: Development and preliminary evaluation of the VA Seattle foot. J Rehabil 22:75–84, 1985
8. Burgess EM, Romano RL, Zettl JH: The Management of Lower-Extremity Amputations. Washington, DC, US Government Printing Office, 1969
9. Davies EJ, Friz BR, Clippinger FW: Amputees and their prostheses. Artif Limb 14:19–48, Autumn 1980
10. Fisher S, Gullikson G Jr: Energy cost of ambulation in health and disability: Literature review. Arch Phys Med Rehabil 59:124–133, 1978
11. Friedman LW: The Psychological Rehabilitation of the Amputee. Springfield, IL, Charles C Thomas, 1978
12. Friedman LW: The Surgical Rehabilitation of the Amputee. Springfield, IL, Charles C Thomas, 1978
13. Glattly HW: A statistical study of 12,000 new amputees. South Med J 57:1373–1378, 1964
14. Hayhurst DJ: Prosthetic management of a partial-foot amputee. Inter-Clin Info Bull 17:11–15, 1978
15. Inman VT, Ralston HJ, Todd F: Human Walking. Baltimore, Williams & Wilkins, 1981
16. Jendrzejczyk DJ: Flexible Socket Systems. Clin Prosthet Orthot 9:27–31, 1985
17. Karacoloff LA: Lower Extremity Amputation: A Guide to Functional Outcomes in Physical Therapy Management. Rockville, Aspen, 1985
18. Kay HW, Newman JD: Relative incidences of new amputations: Statistical comparisons of 6,000 new amputations. Orthot Prosthet 29:3–16, 1975
19. Kostuik JP (ed): Amputation Surgery and Rehabilitation. New York, Churchill Livingstone, 1981
20. Leonard JA, Trower TA: The application of the flex-foot prosthesis design to the bilateral amputee (abst). Arch Phys Med Rehabil 66:552, 1985
21. Levy SW: Skin Problems of the Amputee. St Louis, Warren H. Green, 1983
22. Long IA: Normal shape–normal alignment (NSNA) above-knee prosthesis. Clin Prosthet Orthot 9:9–14, 1985
23. Lundeberg T: Relief of pain from a phantom limb by peripheral stimulation. J Neurol 232:79–82, 1985
24. Malone JM, Childers SJ, Underwood J et al: Immediate post surgical management of upper extremity amputation: Conventional, electric, and myoelectric prostheses. Orthot Prosthet 35:1–9, 1981
25. Malone JM, Fleming LL, Robenson J et al: Immediate, early, and late postsurgical management of upper-limb amputation. J Rehabil RD 21:33–41, 1984
26. Malone JM, Moore WS, Goldstone J, Malone SJ: Therapeutic and economic impact of a modern amputation program. Ann Surg 189:798–802, 1979
27. Meier RH: Amputations and prosthetic fitting. In Fisher SU, Helm PA (eds): Comprehensive Rehabilitation of Burns, pp 267–310, Baltimore, Williams & Wilkins, 1984
28. Michael JW: Upper-limb powered components and controls: Current concepts. Clin Prosthet Orthot 10:66–77, 1986
29. New York University Postgraduate Medical School: Lower Limb Prosthetics, Prosthetics and Orthotics. New York University, 1982 revision.
30. New York University Postgraduate Medical School: Upper Limb Prosthetics and Orthotics. New York University, 1982 revision.
31. Peiser E, Pirrello T: Principles and practice in upper extremity prostheses. Orthop Clin North Am 3:397–417, 1972
32. Reinstein L: Rehabilitation of the lower extremity cancer amputee. Maryland State Med J 29:85–87, 1980
33. Reswick JB: Evaluation of the seattle foot. J Rehabil RD 23:77–94, 1986
34. Sabolich J: Contoured adducted trochanteric-controlled alignment method (CAT-CAM): Introduction and basic principles. Clin Prosthet Orthot 9:15–26, 1985
35. Sanders GT: Lower Limb Amputations: A Guide to Rehabilitation. Philadelphia, FA Davis, 1986
36. Scott RN (ed): Progress Report No. 17, Myoelectric Control Systems. Fredrickton, University of New Brunswick, 1980
37. Setoguchi Y, Roseufelder R: The Limb Deficient Child, 2nd ed. Springfield, IL, Charles C Thomas, 1982
38. Sherman RA: Published treatments of phantom limb pain. Am J Phys Med 59:232–244, 1980
39. Sherman RA, Sherman CJ, Gail NA: Survey of current phantom limb treatment in the United States. Pain 8:85–99, 1980
40. Sherman RA, Tippens JK: Suggested guidelines for treatment of phantom limb pain. Orthopedics 5:1595–1600, 1982
41. Siegfried J, Zimmermann M: Phantom and Stump Pain. Berlin, Springer-Verlag, 1981
42. Soderberg GL: Kinesiology. Baltimore, Williams & Wilkins, 1986.
43. United States Department of Health & Human Services: Vital and Health Statistics: Detailed Diagnoses and Procedures for Patients Discharged from Short Stay Hospitals, United States, 1984. Series 13, 86:182, 1986
44. United States Department of Health & Human Services: Vital and Health Statistics: Prevalence of Selected Chronic Conditions—United States, 1979–1981. Series 10, 155:29–32, 1986
45. United States Department of Health & Human Services: Vital and Health Statistics: Prevalence of Selected Impairments, United States—1977. Series 10, 134:14–17, 28–29, 1981
46. United States Department of Health & Human Services: Vital and Health Statistics: Use of Special Aids—United States—1977. Series 10, 135:12–13, 15–16, 23–25, 1980
47. United States Department of Health & Human Services: Public Health Service: Reported Morbidity and Mortality in the United States—Annual Summary, 1984. MMWR 3:84, 1986
48. WU Y, Krick H: Removable rigid dressing for below-knee amputees. Clin Prosthet Orthot 11:33–44, 1987

18

Therapeutic Exercise

R. L. Joynt

The term *therapeutic exercise* carries two implications. *Exercise* implies that muscles are being used in some type of exertion causing motion of parts of the body. *Therapeutic* implies that this type of exercise should be part of a program of treatment under medical supervision and appropriately prescribed by a physician, and that improvement of muscle function should result.

Exercise is probably the most commonly used modality in the field of physical medicine and rehabilitation, prescribed in some form in the treatment of most of the conditions encountered. Many of the concepts in exercise physiology are based on studies of normal individuals and athletes, and, therefore, are not necessarily applicable to the sick or disabled.

Exercise as a therapy is based on the hypothesis that an organism adapts to the stresses placed on it. The so-called *overload principle* indicates that greater stress must be applied than that to which an organism or tissue is accustomed in order to have adaptation take place. Conversely, if an organism or tissue is not stressed, it deconditions and loses the ability that it once possessed, and is able to respond only to the decreased amount of stress. The expertise in therapy involves applying and adjusting stress of the appropriate type and amount to result in the adaptations that are desired without producing injury. For example, if an increase in strength is desired, a muscle must repeatedly be required to exert an amount of force greater than that to which it has previously adapted.

BASIC CONCEPTS

Before discussion of exercise and its effects, certain terminology and concepts should be reviewed. Muscle contraction can be described in several ways related to the motion involved. *Isometric* (same measure) exercise is static exercise with muscle contraction but no movement of the load, resulting in no change in the total length of the muscle. *Isotonic* (same tone) exercise is dynamic exercise with a constant load but uncontrolled speed of movement. Movement is through a range as the muscle shortens or lengthens. The term incorrectly suggests that the muscle exerts a constant tension throughout the movement. *Isokinetic* (same motion) exercise is exercise with the movement controlled so that it occurs through a range at a constant angular velocity (number of degrees per second) as the muscle shortens or lengthens, but the load or force exerted may be variable. If a muscle shortens while contracting it is referred to as a *concentric contraction,* and if it lengthens it is called *eccentric.* Eccentric contractions occur during many phases of ambulation as muscle contraction opposes the external forces of gravity and inertia. During most activity, all of the above types of contraction occur in various combinations.

Several terms are used in describing the forces produced by muscle contraction. *Force,* for practical purposes, can be considered a push or pull tending to cause a change in position or direction of motion. *Tension* is the contraction force of a muscle and cannot be measured directly in humans. *Torque* is a force acting with a certain lever arm and tending to cause rotation about an axis. It is the quantity often measured when assessing strength. The amount of torque produced by a given load or force will depend on the length of the lever arm (moment arm) (Fig. 18-1). Measurements of work (force times distance) and power (work performed per unit time, or rate of doing work) are also occasionally used to quantify exercise.

Kinesiological factors are particularly relevant when describing strength. Major considerations are the angle of exertion of muscle tension on the lever arm and the angle of application of the load. If these forces are not being exerted at right angles to the lever arm, the *effective* force is related to the angle at which they act, and must be resolved into components (vectors) acting perpendicular and parallel to the lever arm to demonstrate the actual effects (Fig. 18-2). The perpendicular vectors result in rotation of the lever arm. The vectors parallel to the lever arm will be compressive or distractive at the point of rotation at the joint. Because the moments causing rotation in each direction must be equal in order for the system to be balanced, the distance that the load is placed from the joint or center of rotation determines the force that must be exerted during an exercise program by the muscle to balance the load (see Fig. 18-1). A change in the load or lever arm length will change the amount of muscle tension needed to keep the system balanced.

The speed at which a limb can be moved is related to the lever arm length also. The closer the muscle is inserted to the center of rotation of the joint (*i.e.,* the shorter the lever arm), the

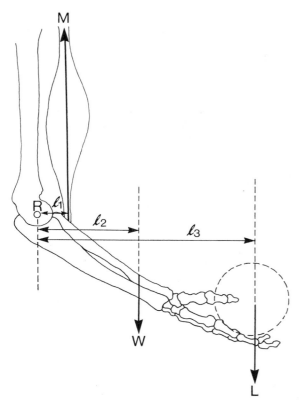

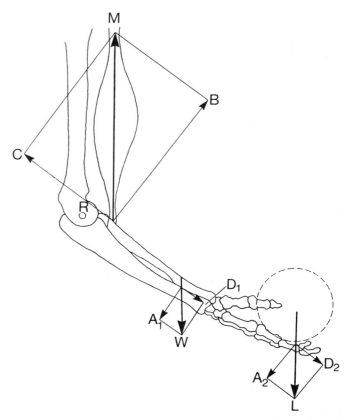

Figure 18-1. Forces acting at the elbow joint. The amount of torque generated $(M \times l_1) = (W \times l_2) + (L \times l_3)$ foot-pounds. M, muscle tension; W, forearm weight; L, load; l_1, muscle lever arm; l_2, forearm lever arm; l_3, load lever arm; R, joint axis of rotation.

Figure 18-2. Resolution of forces at the elbow. M, muscle tension; W, forearm weight; L, load; B, muscle tension vector causing counter-clockwise rotation; C, muscle tension vector causing compressive forces at the joint; A_1 and A_2, forearm and load vectors causing clockwise rotation; D_1 and D_2, forearm and load vectors causing distractive forces at the joint; R, joint axis of rotation.

more movement will occur in a given time with a given amount of muscle shortening. As shown in Figure 18-3, the speed of movement is twice as fast for brachialis shortening as for biceps shortening of an equal amount. It would seem, therefore, that muscles such as the brachialis would be more likely to be used than the biceps in performing rapid movement. Studies, however, have not confirmed this suspicion, although the concept of "spurt" and "shunt" muscle persists.[16] The fact remains that different muscles may be recruited when movements at different speeds are performed.

The ultimate purpose of an exercise program is to improve function or performance. Actual performance depends on a multitude of factors. Certainly the characteristics of the muscle tissue itself (strength, endurance, and contraction speed) are important. Also important are the ability of the nervous system control apparatus to direct and coordinate the movement, and the properties of the lever system itself. Such factors as length of lever arms (bones), range of motion (joints), connective tissue constraints (ligaments, joint capsules), and the methods of muscle attachments to the system (tendons) must be considered when evaluating motion. And finally, there is the psychological or motivational component, which may be more critical than the purely anatomical and physiological factors in determining actual performance.

Motor performance is a combination of the capacities of the peripheral effector organs and the central control system. The limitations placed on the system by heredity, such as a certain mix of muscle fiber types and certain motor control patterns or programs, are to some degree modifiable by training and other environmental factors. These basic anatomical and physiological considerations will be reviewed.

Muscle Anatomy

Muscle can be classified grossly by the way the muscle fibers attach to the tendon. In parallel and fusiform muscles, the fibers run from origin to insertion, approximately parallel to each other. When the muscle contracts, there is a direct relationship between the amount of muscle shortening and the amount of motion produced (see Fig. 18-3). In pennate muscles (Fig. 18-4), muscle fibers are oriented obliquely with respect to their connections to the tendons. Motion produced by muscle shortening in this situation depends, in addition, upon the angle at which the muscle joins the tendon (Fig. 18-4C). In Figure 18-4, the muscle fibers have shortened to 50% of the original length, but the amount of shortening at the insertion is only 37%. More power can be generated by pennate muscles because there are more fibers present in a given cross-section of muscle, and force production is related to the total cross-sectional area.

Histologically, muscle fibers are classified by their reaction to staining for oxidative enzymes, glycolytic enzymes, and myosin adenosine triphosphatase (ATPase) activity. The oxidative and glycolytic enzyme stains reflect the type of metabolism, aerobic or anaerobic, that is predominant. The myosin ATPase activity reflects the twitch speed of the muscle fiber: high alkaline-stable myosin ATPase levels are present in fibers with a fast-twitch speed and low levels are present in slow-twitch fibers. Fast or slow myosin is related to the type and number of light and heavy chains in the myosin molecule. Fast-twitch speed also requires a

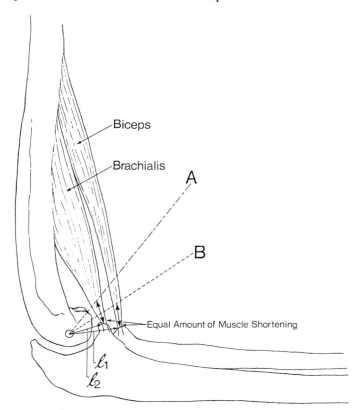

Figure 18-3. The effect of the site of muscle insertion on the movement produced by muscle contraction. l_1, biceps lever arm; l_2, brachialis lever arm; A and B, forearm positions with equal amounts of shortening in the biceps and brachialis muscles.

Figure 18-4. Contraction of pennate muscle. A and B, muscle cross-section in stretched and shortened conditions; C, angle of insertion of the muscle fibers into the tendon.

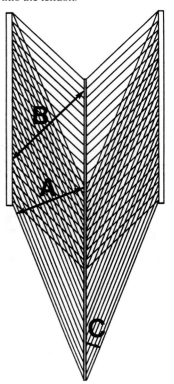

faster release and uptake of calcium by the sarcoplasmic reticulum; as a result, fast-twitch fibers have a highly developed reticular system.

Muscle fibers have been divided into types based on these parameters. The classic type I muscle fibers are high in oxidative enzymes and low in myosin ATPase activity, indicating that they are slow-twitch fibers and resistant to fatigue. Type IIB fibers are high in glycolytic enzymes and myosin ATPase, indicating that they are fast-twitch fibers, their metabolism is anaerobic, and they are easily fatigued. An intermediate group (type IIA) is high in oxidative and glycolytic enzymes and myosin ATPase, indicating that these fibers are fast twitch but relatively fatigue-resistant (Table 18-1). In most human muscles, a mixture of fibers is present. The properties appear to be established by the innervating neuron and can be altered by innervation changes as demonstrated in denervation-reinnervation or cross-innervation situations.[165]

There is considerable controversy concerning the ability of a muscle fiber to change type.[76] The traditional view is that an individual inherits a specific pattern of fast and slow fibers that remains constant throughout life. Studies of twins showed that monozygotic twins showed similar percentages of fast and slow twitch fibers, whereas dizygotic twins did not.[115] Persons who inherit a high number of fast-twitch fibers are considered more likely to be speed and power athletes, whereas those with slow-twitch fibers will tend toward endurance activities. Animal experiments, however, have shown that all the physiological and biochemical parameters can be changed by chronic nerve stimulation[58, 152, 160] and that the twitch speed may be related to the frequency or pattern of electrical stimulation.[58, 164] Chronic low frequency electrical activity seems necessary to maintain slow-twitch fibers.[165] There is also little doubt that the metabolic capacity of fibers can be changed, as evidenced by many studies that have shown oxidative capacity of fibers to increase with training. The ability to change the type of myosin in the fibers by training, however, is still controversial, as is the relative importance of heredity and environment in deciding an individual's muscle fiber composition.[73, 76, 100, 114, 165]

Muscle Physiology

Contraction

Muscle contraction is initiated when a wave of depolarization propagates over the muscle fiber membrane. Low-threshold, early recruited motor units fire at low rates for long periods of time and innervate slow-twitch muscle fibers (type I), whereas high-threshold, late recruited units fire in short, high-frequency bursts and innervate the fast fatiguable fibers (type IIB). Type IIA fibers have an intermediate position. Contraction of a muscle fiber results from the interaction of actin and myosin filaments and is thought to occur by rotation of the myosin head at sites of actin-myosin cross-linkages with a ratchetlike motion, sliding the myosin along the actin (Huxley's sliding filament theory). This process requires energy, which is obtained from adenosine triphosphate (ATP) and manufactured in the mitochondria either anaerobically or aerobically. The anaerobic method produces ATP by converting glycogen to lactate; it is a rapid process and is the main method used in glycolytic (type IIB) fibers. The aerobic method uses oxygen to convert glycogen to pyruvate, but this process is much slower than the anaerobic process. Aerobically, in addition to carbohydrate, other substrates such as fat and protein can be used. The end product of aerobic metabolism is carbon dioxide and water.

Table 18-1
Comparison of Muscle Fiber Types

	Type I (Red)	*Type IIA (Intermediate)*	*Type IIB (White)*
Twitch speed	Slow	Fast	Fast
Myosin ATPase activity	Low	High	High
Metabolism and enzymes	Oxidative	Oxidative and Glycolytic	Glycolytic
Fatigability rate	Slow	Intermediate	Rapid
Mitochondrial number	Many	Many	Few
Myoglobin content	High	High	Low
Capillary density	High	High	Low
Fiber size	Small	Intermediate	Large
Glycogen content	Low	Intermediate	High
Motor unit and neuro-muscular junction size	Small	Intermediate	Large

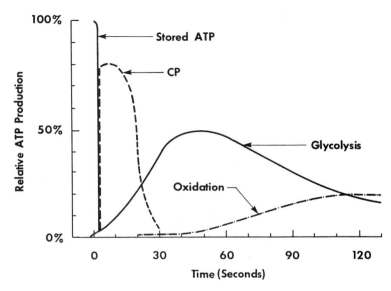

Figure 18-5. ATP sources during muscle contraction. *CP,* creatine phosphate.

During muscle contraction, there appears to be an orderly production and utilization of ATP (Fig. 18-5). A certain amount of stored ATP is immediately available for initiating muscle contraction, but this declines in a matter of several seconds. ATP must then be produced from creatine phosphate, which is converted reasonably rapidly. Within 30 seconds to 3 minutes, however, the stored creatine phosphate will also be exhausted and the muscle must then depend upon other metabolic pathways to produce more ATP. Initially glucose and glycogen can be used. Glycogen production of ATP (glycolysis) probably peaks in 40 to 50 seconds, but glycogen will be depleted in about one hour if the activity continues at approximately 70% of maximum effort. Activities continuing for longer than 60 seconds require aerobic production of ATP. This oxidative production gradually increases over the first one to two minutes and then becomes the major source of ATP. Breakdown of fat and protein, in addition to carbohydrate, is then used for ATP production. Prolonged aerobic work of three hours uses fat to provide 70% of the energy.[20]

Fiber Characteristics

Muscle function can be described in terms of strength, endurance, and speed.

STRENGTH. The tension produced by a muscle is related to the number of motor units firing and the rate of firing. Maximum force is produced when muscle fiber twitches are fused into a tetanic contraction. The firing rate at which this occurs is related to the fiber's contraction speed, and the relationship between force and firing rate is sigmoidal. In absolute terms, muscle strength is related to muscle fiber diameter and is variously quoted as being from 1 to 4 kilograms per square centimeter, or 15 to 60 newtons per square centimeter.[30, 135, 165, 167] Strength is not a function of the muscle fiber type.[114, 165] Muscle fibers with larger diameters (type 2) have more myofibrils and more actin-myosin cross-bridges to produce the contractile force, and muscles with a higher percentage of fast-twitch fibers have been reported to demonstrate greater force development capability.[42, 177] The strength of a whole muscle is related to the cross-sectional area of the muscle when measured perpendicular to the length of the muscle fibers (see Fig. 18-4). The cross-sectional measurement changes with contraction and relaxation.

Strength can be defined in many ways, depending on the specific method of measurement. In general, however, it is defined as the maximum force that is exerted under certain specified conditions. The actual tension exerted by a muscle is not measured directly, but can be calculated if the factors of lever arm lengths and angles of pull are known (see Fig. 18-1). These factors must be considered when strength is being compared between individuals.

Isometric strength is measured by a static apparatus such as a strain gauge. *Isotonic strength* is usually measured by the amount of weight that can be lifted concentrically a specified number of repetitions, and is referred to as the one or ten repetition maximum (1 or 10 RM). It can also be measured eccentrically. *Isokinetic strength* is the peak torque generated during movement at a certain preset rate. The torque developed will vary during movement as the angle changes, but maximum torque generally develops when the muscle is near its resting length. There is no good correlation between the measurements obtained by these different methods.[148]

Measured strength varies with other parameters, such as the velocity at which the load is moved. For concentric contractions, as the angular velocity increases, the ability to produce force decreases (Fig. 18-6); that is, the heavier the weight, the slower it can be moved. As a corollary, as a muscle becomes stronger, it can then move the same weight faster. For eccentric contractions, the reverse is true: as the weight increases, the ability to resist movement decreases and the load moves faster. This relationship between strength and speed is thought possibly to be related to the twitch speed of the muscle fibers. As the rate of movement increases, the slow-twitch fibers are able to contribute progressively less force to the total force development because their contraction time is slow.[150]

A relationship also exists between the muscle fiber length and its tension development ability. A muscle is able to exert maximum contractile force at a length approximating its resting length. As its length becomes longer or shorter, its tension-developing capabilities decrease. This phenomenon is thought to result from the relationship in the sarcomere between the overlapping actin and myosin fibers (Fig. 18-7). Maximum strength is produced when there are a maximum number of actin–myosin cross-bridges available to produce the contraction force (Fig. 18-7, positions 2 to 3). As the muscle lengthens, there are fewer actin–myosin linkages, and as it shortens, the actin fibers are thought to overlap and therefore interfere to some extent with the cross-linkages. However, total tension is higher for a contracting muscle that is longer than its resting length, because total tension is the sum of contractile tension and elastic tension. A phenomenon called *pre-stretching* is well known in athletics—for instance, when a thrower cocks his arm before throwing or a jumper crouches before jumping. This phenomenon is the increased ability of a muscle to develop tension if contraction occurs immediately after the muscle is stretched.[20, 121] Although the physiological reason for this phenomenon is uncertain, there may be some elastic recoil from tissue stretching that is used to assist the shortening process, or there may be some actual backward rotation of the heads of the myosin molecules that stores energy.[8, 26, 36, 114] Another possibility is the potentiation of contraction by the stretch reflex, stimulated by the muscle stretch.

In the assessment of strength and strengthening programs, mechanical factors (such as the length of moment arm and the angle of application of the muscle and load forces) must be balanced against physiological factors (muscle length). The relative importance of each of these factors depends on the specific joint and muscle involved. For example, the biceps produces the greatest torque when the angle between the arm and forearm is appoximately 90°, but the resting length of the biceps occurs when the lever arms are at 180°, suggesting that the mechanical factors are more important in this instance in determining the point of maximum torque.[30]

Clinicians familiar with muscle testing also realize that the apparent strength of a muscle is related to the position of other joints (particularly if two joint muscles are involved), stabilization of the body while testing, and the substitution or addition of other muscles to the one actually being tested.

Age and sex must also be considered in the evaluation of strength. Studies have shown a progressive decrease in strength, particularly after the age of 50.[20, 122] One study reported a 1% per year strength decrease after the age of 20. Biopsy studies from the quadriceps have shown both a decrease in number and in area of type II fibers with aging.[80, 122] In general, males are stronger than females, even after corrections are made for weight and body fat content.[154] Absolute strength increases with body weight, but strength per pound of body weight actually decreases slightly with increasing weight.[20]

ENDURANCE AND FATIGUE. Muscle endurance can be defined as the ability to produce work over time or the ability to persist in or maintain an effort. Endurance can be measured in

Figure 18-6. Relationship between velocity of movement and torque development capability.

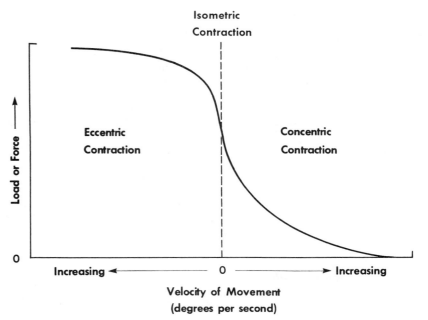

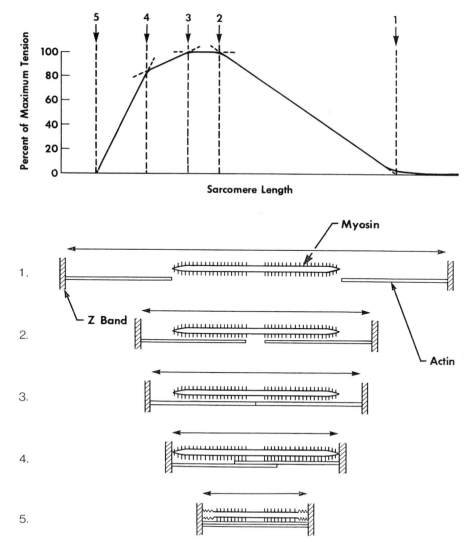

Figure 18-7. Relationship between muscle tension development, sarcomere length, and actin-myosin interaction.

several ways depending on the particular kind of activity studied. *Anaerobic endurance* is measured under simulated anaerobic conditions, with high-intensity or isometric activity decreasing the oxygen availability. *Aerobic endurance* must be measured under conditions that use aerobic metabolism, such as low-intensity dynamic exercise that avoids anaerobic components. *Isotonic endurance* is measured by the number of repetitions with given weight. *Isokinetic endurance* is the number of repetitions at a certain angular velocity before a specified decrease in torque develops. *Isometric endurance* is the time that a certain weight could be maintained in a static position or a certain force exerted against a strain gauge. To compare endurance between individuals, it is most appropriate to use a percentage of the individual's maximum force capability for testing rather than a fixed load, because of the relationship between strength and absolute endurance.

The mathematical relationship between strength and endurance is hyperbolic (Fig. 18-8). At low force levels (less than 15% maximum),[21] endurance would theoretically be infinite, and at high force levels endurance would be zero. The reason for the hyperbolic relationship may be related to the relative contributions from aerobic and anaerobic metabolism.[112] This relationship holds for individual muscles and also for general body exercises such as running, cycling, and work performance generally.[45] It is reasonably obvious that there must also be a relationship between absolute strength and absolute endurance, that is, a muscle whose maximum force capability is 100 pounds can hold a 20-pound weight much longer than a muscle whose maximum capability is 30 pounds. Strength and relative endurance, however, are not correlated; at 50% of maximum ability, the muscle with greater absolute strength does not necessarily perform more repetitions than that with less absolute strength.[13]

Fatigue is the inability to continue to generate further force or the loss of endurance and has been shown to occur at any exercise level greater than 15% of maximum.[21] It can be operationally defined as occurring when a certain percentage decrease from maximum force occurs or further repetitions cannot be performed. Physiological muscle fiber fatigue occurs when there is a failure to maintain twitch or tetanic tension when electrical stimulation frequency and intensity are unchanged. Fatigue can refer to tiredness or inability to continue doing an activity, generally, or more specifically to individual exercising muscles.

Fatigue may occur at many levels in the motor system. Central nervous system fatigue can occur with the loss of motivation or concentration or the onset of pain. Fatigue has not been shown to occur in the conduction mechanism from the brain to the muscle, although it may occur at the neuromuscular junction at very high rates of stimulation (beyond the usual physiological rates) or in patients with neuromuscular junction diseases. De-

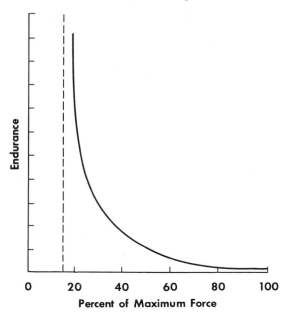

Figure 18-8.   Relationship between strength and endurance.

creased muscle fiber conduction velocity has been reported to be associated with fatigue,[137] but actual failure of conduction has not been observed.

Although failure in the contraction-excitation coupling mechanism is possible, the major source of muscle fatigue appears to be in the contractile process, and fatigue appears to occur because of the failure of the muscle fiber to continue producing, at a sufficient rate, the energy necessary for contraction. Following depletion of ATP and creatine phosphate stores, the body must use stored glycogen and then carbohydrate, fat, or protein to produce energy. Failure to produce further energy could occur because of exhaustion of stored energy forms, the exhaustion of the substrates with which to produce more energy, exhaustion of an enzyme necessary in the energy production process, an inability to deliver oxygen for aerobic ATP production, or an accumulation of metabolites or heat that interferes with one of the energy production processes. Under isometric contraction conditions, the activity must end when anaerobic production stops because oxygen is not available for aerobic energy production. It has been shown that at static contractions greater than 60 to 70% of maximum,[55] the circulation is interrupted, indicating that fatigue obviously occurs more rapidly with isometric than with isotonic contraction.[38]

Lactate has been commonly implicated as the metabolic product responsible for fatigue, but studies show that lactate actually is removed faster at exercise rates of approximately 60% of maximum than at lower intensity exercise levels, so lactate would most effectively be decreased by continuing activity at a 60% level.[20, 74] In addition, correlation of lactate levels with fatigue is not good.[188] The specific cause of fatigue in short-duration maximum work is still uncertain and may be related to any of the above factors. In long-duration endurance activities, there is considerable evidence that substrates are depleted,[130] but whether or not depletion of one substrate in particular results in fatigue is not known.

Because of their largely glycolytic metabolism, type IIB fibers will be the most easily fatigued. Type I fibers with their oxidative capacity will be the most fatigue-resistant. As fiber fatigue occurs, relaxation time increases and the firing rate needed to produce tetanic contraction decreases, so less energy is needed to maintain the contraction.[21]

Recovery from fatigue is reported to occur more rapidly from isotonic than from isometric exertion in the first minute, but by the end of the second minute the recovery is similar.[38]

SPEED.   Speed is an important parameter of motor function but less well investigated than strength and endurance. When rapid muscle contraction is needed, the usual recruitment order of motor units is probably reversed and the fast-twitch units are selectively fired first. In situations of rapid alternating movement, slow-twitch fibers are probably not used and indeed would likely interfere, since the slow contraction time would inhibit the ability to rapidly change movement direction.[58] Strong individuals can obviously develop more rapid movement than weaker individuals because of the relationship between strength and velocity. However, it also appears that strong individuals can move loads of a given percentage of maximum faster than a weaker individual can.[20] Some studies have suggested that the speed of actual muscle contraction is correlated with the fiber type predominating in that muscle; subjects with a higher percentage of fast-twitch fibers were able to achieve higher maximum angular velocities.[42, 104, 114, 180]

Power is an important parameter in athletic events in which speed and force production are both necessary. Power also appears related to the fiber type. Peak power is achieved at approximately 50% of maximum force capability (Fig. 18-9A) and at 50% of maximum velocity (Fig. 18-9B) and varies slightly from muscle to muscle depending on the predominant fiber type in the muscle.[154, 180]

Motor Control

Physiology

Motor control can be used generally to refer to brain control of motor activities, or more specifically to refer to a specific voluntary activity or a specific movement or muscle action under conscious voluntary control. A specific action requires concentration, and very few motor activities can be attended to at the same time. Control has been seen traditionally as a hierarchical system in which the higher centers control the lower centers and specify the general outline of the movement.[87] The lower centers in the brain and brain stem fill in the details, with the final specifics of the action being determined by local spinal cord mechanisms. Sensory feedback to the cerebellum results in modifications of the basic command. Any voluntary activity requires a multitude of secondary actions to provide posture, stabilization, balance, and positioning. Any action therefore requires the activity not only of prime movers, but also of many synergic, fixation, and antagonist muscles.

The centralist theory of motor control states that certain motor patterns such as ambulation appear to be inherited or "hard-wired" into the system, and are stereotyped fixed-action patterns.[166] These patterns are switched on by appropriate motor program generators which involve specific facilitations and inhibitions. A movement can therefore be thought of as the playing of a motor tape[101] that has previously been stored in memory and triggered by a combination of inputs or chosen by the nervous system from the many available. The details of the movement can be varied according to the specific immediate activity and feedback information (*servo regulation*).[87] It is known that locomotion patterns are programmed because neural control signals for locomotion are emitted even in animals paralyzed by curare.[31, 87] It has been suggested, however, that the neuromuscular system is merely a reflex sensorimotor system with neuronal activation occurring as a response to external stimuli (peripheralist theory).[116, 166] To think, however, that motor behavior can be broken

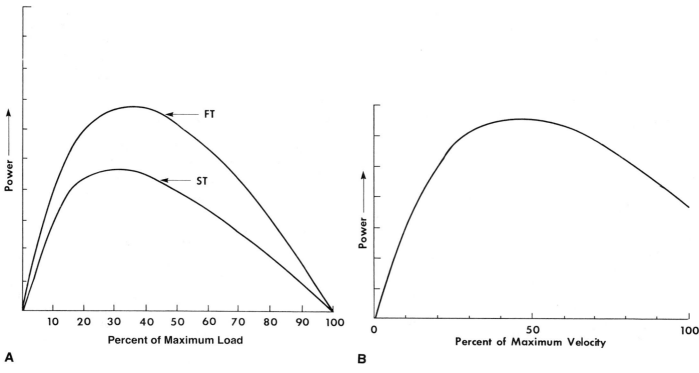

Figure 18-9. (*A*) Relationship between load and power. *FT,* muscles with a high content of fast-twitch fibers; *ST,* muscles with a high content of slow-twitch fibers. (*B*) Relationship between velocity of movement and power.

down into successive reflex components is probably naive. It seems unlikely that motor behavior, other than simple reflex activity, is generated to any extent solely by reflexes;[101] rather, a combination of peripheral and central factors interact.[166]

Control of motor activity can be considered to be present in varying degrees of complexity. The simplest motor activity would be a reflex, such as the stretch reflex, which involves a single synapse. The next level would be an activity controlled by a motor program, with gaps being filled in by reflex actions but with little sensory guidance. As the activity becomes more complicated and requires more concentration, feedback from the actual motor performance would be compared to a sensory engram and constant alterations made as the movement proceeds.[101]

Certain motor tapes or programs would appear to be inherited and genetically determined (such as the ability to roll one's tongue). Others (such as that for bipedal ambulation) appear to be genetically created and stored, possibly in memory in the cerebellum, as sensory tapes, engrams, or memory chips, to allow comparisons with current motor activity.

Motor Learning

Motor learning is accomplished by comparing a performed motor activity to a previously developed and stored sensory pattern. The first step of motor learning, therefore, is to develop the sensory engram, if it is not yet available. This can be done in many ways and using several senses; for example, an individual may start to learn to play tennis by watching a film of expert tennis players. As motor activities progress, there is constant comparison of the actual motor activity to that previously acquired as a sensory pattern, and a motor pattern is then developed. The "feel" of the current movement is compared to the memory of past movements, and adjustments are made in future

movements. As motor learning progresses, the motor activity can proceed with less and less need for comparison to the sensory engram, and eventually the sensory engram can be dispensed with and the activity performed with very little sensory feedback, except for minor modulations related to specific sensory inputs. Motor skill, therefore, is the optimal or automatic use of programmed movements with little need for compensatory adjustments during movement.[31, 171] Studies with animals suggest that when a motor activity is well learned, it can be reproduced quite accurately with complete sensory deafferentation.[101]

The traditional anatomical concept of motor learning suggests that as learning occurs, control is transferred from area 4 to area 6 or other supplementary motor areas.[167] Efferent activity is then passed through extra-pyramidal pathways with the sole role of the cortex being to initiate the specific activity. Monitoring and adjustments occur through sensory feedback and the cerebellum. Others have suggested that as the task is learned and becomes automatic, the main site of control is shifted from the cortex to the cerebellum with reliance upon proprioceptive rather than visual feedback. Motor learning is, then, the shift of attention from the specific elements of the task to the signal that stimulates the cortex to initiate the movement.[167] Motor learning may involve storage of information about γ-loop settings, thereby producing a faster reaction time with improved coordination and performance.

Others feel that motor learning involves learning to control and facilitate reflexes with gradual augmentation and control. A child is reflex-bound until he can dominate his reflexes by specific facilitation and inhibition techniques.[116]

What occurs structurally in the nervous system with learning is an interesting topic of speculation. It has been suggested that the frequent use of synapses stimulates protein synthesis and branching of dendrites to establish additional synapses.[167] An analogy to computer memory may be made. Memory can be thought of as a microchip carrying charges represented by ones or zeros. Learning can then be speculated to be the conversion of random-access memory to read-only memory, which remains after the computer is turned off.

Learning is said to require multiple repetitions. The number of repetitions probably varies with the complexity of the task, but at some time during the learning stage, insight or understanding of the task appears to occur and the rate of improvement of performance suddenly increases.[31]

Coordination

Coordination can be viewed as the whole movement pattern relating to a specific controlled movement. It is the ability to put everything together at the right time, with the right force, and the right speed. It is not generally considered to be under direct cortical control. It does, however, include measures of performance and such things as speed, efficiency, flexibility, adjustability, and timing, therefore involving not only the motor and sensory systems but also cerebral functions such as intelligence, reasoning ability, judgment, alertness, concentration, motivation, and personality. The cerebellum is usually considered to be the structure most intimately involved in skillful motor execution and the source of pathology when incoordination develops.

Controversy exists as to whether or not coordination is an inherited or learned characteristic. There would appear to be the usual mixture of effects. Certain advantages and limitations to coordination may be genetically present (most of us could never be concert pianists no matter how long and hard we practiced). Some suggest that motor learning is highly task-specific; that is, a person who appears to be highly coordinated is one who has many task-specific abilities.[133] Although some transference of these abilities may occur between similar activities, there also appears to be evidence of negative transference between two activities that are similar but not exactly the same, so that learning one activity interferes to some extent with the other, such as tennis with squash.[167]

Many different kinds of tests, usually involving speed and accuracy of performance on a specific set of tasks, have been designed to measure coordination. These measurements, however, are generally quite task-specific, so that results on one task do not necessarily carry over to another. A general test of an individual's coordination is difficult to create.

Constraints to Motion

Connective tissue provides the main structural integrity for various organs and body parts. In the musculoskeletal system, it provides the attachment of the muscle to the bone in the form of tendons, and also provides constraints to joint motion in the form of ligaments and other periarticular tissues that surround the joint. The main load placed on these structures is tension.

Anatomy

Connective tissue is composed of fibers embedded in a ground substance. These fibers, collagen, reticulin, and elastin, are synthesized by fibroblasts and distributed in a ground substance of glycosaminoglycans. This material, which is also synthesized and secreted by fibroblasts, is important in maintaining structural integrity, providing lubrication, and conferring viscoelastic properties. Seven glycosaminoglycans have been identified, including hyaluronic acid and the chondroitin sulfates.

Collagen represents approximately 80% of the dry weight of these connective tissues and provides high tensile strength and stiffness. When loaded, some extensibility is present, but col-

lagen fibers will fracture at 6 to 8% of elongation. Collagen fibers are composed of collagen molecules, which are made up of polypeptide chains combined in a triple helix configuration. Fifty percent of the protein in the polypeptide chains is glycine, proline, and hydroxyproline, with many molecules both cross-linked and end-linked to form the collagen fibers. Five different types of collagen have been identified.

Elastin fibers allow tissue extensibility. With low loads, extensibility is greater than 200% with abrupt rupture at this stage, but elasticity of these fibers decreases with age. Elastin fibers have approximately one-fifth the resistance to stretch of collagen fibers. They are also high in glycine and proline, but have little hydroxyproline and no hydroxyglycine. Reticulin fibers have a structure similar to collagen, but are formed in a network of free branching fibers and appear to provide bulk.

Tendons and ligaments may vary in form, from quite narrow, specific, rope-like bands to broad fascial sheets. The way that a muscle transmits its force to the bony lever system depends on the anatomical configuration of the particular tendon attachment. The specific motion permitted at a given joint is a function of the connective tissue constraints as well as the shape of the bony contact surfaces. A review of joint motions is beyond the scope of this chapter but, in general, joint movement occurs around an axis, and the ligamentous configuration at the joint is set up to best permit this motion and to restrict unwanted motions.

Tendons are composed mostly of collagen fibers (mainly type I) and perform mechanically as pure collagen fibers. Collagen is present with a dense parallel configuration. Tendon strength is proportional to the cross-sectional area, and tendon rupture generally occurs at forces approximately twice that which can be created by contraction of the attached muscle.[145]

Ligaments have a less-consistent orientation of the collagen fibers, depending on the specific ligament. Most ligaments are mainly collagen, but certain ligaments such as the ligamentum nuchae and ligamentum flavum are two-thirds elastin. Ligament strength is also related to its cross-sectional area and is found to decrease with age.

Physiology

Collagen turnover is generally very slow with a half-life of 300 to 500 days. More rapid turnover does occur in growing tissue or during remodeling, healing, and immobilization. Little is known about elastin turnover. Ground substance turnover is rapid (1.7–7 days).

Collagen metabolism has been studied to some extent in healing scars. Fibrin is initially deposited from a clot, and then fibroblasts proliferate and secrete collagen. Measurements performed on healing wounds show that the wound actually produces tension as collagen is laid down.[117] In tendon repairs, strength is gradually gained and has been reported to approach normal by 20 days in experimental studies in dogs.[182] Denervated tissue, however, appears to produce less tension than normal during healing.[117]

Range of Motion

Normal joint motion is determined by the bony contour of a joint and the restraining ligaments and capsule surrounding the joint. In some instances there may normally be constraint by the muscle–tendon unit, but this condition is more commonly pathological. Normal range of motion varies considerably among individuals. The concept that some individuals are "tight" and others "loose" must be kept in mind when deciding whether or not a range is normal for a given individual and a given joint.

LOSS OF MOTION. Range of motion can be lost for many reasons. An injury or abnormality in the articulating surface can block movement. Intra-articular loose bodies (bone or cartilage) and excessive fluid can also prevent full range of joint motion.

A contracture causing loss of motion is generally thought to be produced by soft tissue such as the joint capsule, the muscle–tendon system, or the skin surrounding the joint. Physical causes of contracture most often involve an inflammatory process resulting from disease or trauma, spasticity, or a decrease in motion from pain, paralysis, or externally applied appliances such as casts.

Collagen progressively shortens when not opposed by some stretching force. Independent mobility of the collagen fibers in the tissue is necessary to maintain normal connective tissue mobility.[3] When a joint is kept in one position, the collagen tissue on the more relaxed side of the joint shortens and the position gradually becomes fixed. Many animal studies of joint immobilization show progressive contracture of the joint capsule and periarticular structures, and concomitant encroachment on the joint by intra-articular fibro-fatty connective tissue that eventually obliterates the joint.[59] The areolar connective tissue is reorganized to dense connective tissue within 1 week of immobilization, and if complicated by other factors such as edema, trauma, or circulatory impairment, additional collagen fibers are laid down within 3 days. In one study of immobilization for 9 weeks to produce contractures, connective tissue analysis showed decreased water and glycosaminoglycans, particularly hyaluronic acid, but no change in total collagen and no evidence of collagen synthesis.[3] It was postulated that the loss of ground substance, which normally lubricates the connective tissue fiber interfaces and minimizes the anomalous formation of cross-linkages, permits fibril to fibril friction, adhesion development, and formation of cross-linkages. Range is also maintained by motion, which stimulates proteoglycan synthesis and inhibits cross-linkages.

In addition to changes in the periarticular collagen, the connective tissue in the muscle belly region shortens with immobilization.[175] Immobilization with the muscle in a shortened position also results in a decreased number of sarcomeres in the muscle, and immobilization in a lengthened position results in an increased sarcomere number.[93] The muscle appears to adapt so as to be able to develop maximum tension in the immobilized position. The causative factors appear to be myogenic since the change in length occurs independent of innervation.[72]

Contractures become particularly important when they interfere with a functional activity such as ambulation, self-care, or attendant care, or cause complications such as skin sores. A slight reduction of range may be accommodated for by an increase in range in other areas or a change in posture. This may, however, place unusual stress on tissues that are not able to handle the increased stress. A common example of this problem is a hip flexion contracture that causes increased lumbar lordosis in order to produce realignment of the center of gravity during standing. Because of the ability of other areas to accommodate, the loss of range may not be obvious unless looked for and, when it occurs, may appear to occur suddenly when the accommodations fail. The clinician must be alert to this possibility in conditions that predispose to range losses.

EXERCISE

Effects of Exercise

Exercise has immediate or acute effects as well as chronic, adaptive, or training effects on the local exercised tissue and on the body in general.

Acute Effects

The strenuousness of exercise and its effect on the body as a whole are generally measured in terms of oxygen consumption. This consumption can be related to resting oxygen consumption and described in terms of multiples of the resting level (METS). The systemic effects of exercise depend on such factors as the type of activity, the particular muscles used, and the percentage of maximum force exerted. At the start of exercise, the body makes an anticipatory response of increased heart rate, cardiac output, blood pressure, and vasodilatation, which is likely cerebrally mediated because it occurs before any metabolic demands are made. As the activity itself begins, the heart rate increases rapidly, probably under neural influences, since the rate of increase is greater than that made necessary by the metabolic demands. Systolic blood pressure also increases. Local muscle contraction increases venous return, and local vasodilation increases blood flow to the exercised muscles. The combination of increased venous return and increased heart rate results in an increased cardiac output.

In isotonic exercise, peripheral resistance decreases in the muscles being exercised to increase muscle blood flow. Vasoconstriction occurs in areas unrelated to the exercise, such as in the gastrointestinal regions. With isometric exercise, however, local blood flow to the contracting muscle is decreased in relationship to the force at which the muscle is contracting, but this has little effect on the general peripheral resistance. Blood pressure, however, rises more with isometric exercise than with isotonic, and one study comparing the types of exercise showed that isokinetic exercise in the upper extremity performed at 100% of maximum voluntary contraction actually showed the highest blood pressure times heart rate product.[79] When static and dynamic exercises are performed simultaneously, the cardiovascular effects are additive.[147] Circulation is also shunted to the skin vessels to maintain body temperature.

As exercise continues at a constant rate, a steady state of heart rate, blood pressure, and cardiac output is attained. At this stage, if the exercise is basically aerobic, the oxygen uptake parallels the severity of the exercise and is considered to be a measure of the intensity of the activity. Maximum oxygen uptake is the parameter used to describe an individual's work capacity. At the cessation of the exercise, there is an initial rapid decrease in heart rate and then a slower return to normal. A sudden drop in blood pressure may occur, particularly if the activity is stopped abruptly.

If the exercise is greater than the body's ability to maintain, the heart rate will plateau at a maximum level, stroke volume and arterial blood pressure will decrease slightly, but oxygen consumption will remain constant. Eventually fatigue occurs and the activity ceases.

Other body systems are also involved during exercise. The respiratory rate abruptly increases as exercise starts, possibly controlled by neural inputs originally and then later by the chemical receptors. Respiration is rarely the factor limiting exercise capability unless respiratory disease is present. Certain hormonal changes, such as decreased insulin production and increased glucagon production (possibly to maintain blood glucose levels), have also been observed. In intense exercise, there is an increase in catecholamines. Changes in many other hormones such as growth, adrenocorticotropic, thyroid-simulating, posterior pituitary, adrenal, and androgens have also been observed.

With increasing age, the maximum oxygen uptake, along with the maximum heart rate and maximum stroke volume, decreases and peripheral resistance increases.

Sudden exercise not preceded by an appropriate warm-up has occasionally resulted in electrocardiographic abnormalities.[12] A condition called *post-exercise syncope* is sometimes seen after vigorous exercise.[22] Hypotension appears to result from pooling of blood in the exercised extremities. This stimulates catecholamine release and risks development of dysrhythmia and cardiac ischemia in susceptible individuals.[54] This can be prevented by a gradual reduction in the vigorousness of the activity.

Slightly different systemic effects are produced by arm exercise and leg exercise.[65, 94] With arm exercise, systolic and diastolic blood pressures and heart rate are higher than with leg exercise. Also a higher oxygen uptake occurs with a given work load. Arm exercise produces increased cardiac output mainly because of an increase in heart rate, not stroke volume. Exercise programs involving the arms, therefore, should use work loads 40 to 60% lower than those used for lower extremity exercise to obtain comparable systemic effects.

In the muscle being exercised, there is increased oxygen extraction with a linear increase in oxygen consumption with the severity of the exercise. An increase in carbon dioxide production is also seen and vasodilatation is present in the exercising areas. During isometric contraction, complete occlusion of blood flow will occur at 70% of the maximum voluntary contraction level.[55] Depletion of energy substrates is also evident. Glycogen depletion appears to be related mainly to the work intensity, but the mode of the exercise also appears to be important.[61] In isotonic exercise at all workloads, the slow-twitch fibers are the first to lose glycogen; glycogen depletion in fast-twitch fibers occurs as the exercise continues.[77] In isometric contractions at greater than 20% of maximum, fast-twitch fibers show glycogen depletion; at less than 20% depletion occurs in slow-twitch fibers.[75]

Exercised muscles may also develop soreness,[7] peaking at 48 hours. Soreness is associated with an increase in limb volume and is thought to be related to actual tissue damage,[23, 174] possibly of connective tissue, because increased hydroxyproline excretion has been observed.[1] Eccentric exercise produces a greater effect than concentric and has resulted in myofibrillar damage.[66] Actual muscle necrosis has been reported with very severe exercise.[97]

Training and Detraining Effects

Strengthening programs have little systemic training effect and mainly develop hypertrophy of individual muscle fibers. Unused muscles atrophy and lose strength at rates of from 5% per day[142] to 8% per week.[129] Atrophy has been found to occur in both fiber types, but some authors report a greater effect on slow-twitch fibers,[24, 83] or a change of slow twitch to fast twitch[131] with immobilization such as casting. Immobilization also reduces glycogen and creatine phosphate concentrations[189] and decreases oxidative capacity and capillary density;[129, 165] no decrease in actual fiber number, however, is seen.[35] One study of highly trained endurance athletes showed a decreased number of slow-twitch fibers following detraining.[123] Immobilization causes ligament strength to decrease, compliance to increase, and collagen degradation to increase.[4, 146]

Endurance training programs increase the oxidative capacity of muscle and therefore its ability to use the oxygen being delivered, as reflected in an increased arteriovenous oxygen difference. Endurance exercise programs also have significant training effects on the body as a whole and improve cardiorespiratory fitness. There is a generalized increase in aerobic capacity as measured by the maximum oxygen uptake. This increase in work capacity is related both to the increased ability to use oxygen peripherally in the muscle as well as to the central

cardiovascular adaptations.[39] These programs result in a decreased resting heart rate, although probably no change in maximum heart rate, and, at a given level of exercise, a decreased heart rate and increased stroke volume. There is an increase in maximum cardiac output at higher exertion levels and more rapid return of these changes to resting levels after exertion. Endurance-type exercises appear to produce an increase in left ventricular end diastolic volume and some increase in mass with a small increase in ventricular wall thickness. Isometric exercise, however, tends to produce an increased left ventricular mass and increased ventricular wall thickness, possibly related to the increase in blood pressure and consequent pressure load on the heart that has been noted during isometric tasks. Other exercise adaptations include an increased maximum ventilatory ability, increased blood volume, increased hemoglobin, and decreased hormonal responses to exercise, probably because increased use of fatty acids results in better control of blood glucose.[167] In addition, thermal regulation is improved as sweating begins at a lower temperature and has less salt content.

Bed rest or relative decrease in activity results in deconditioning.[30] This is reflected by changes in the cardiovascular system resulting in decreased work capacity. Significant decreases in aerobic capacity are seen after 1 to 2 weeks of detraining,[154] accompanied by a lower maximum oxygen uptake, lower cardiac output and stroke volume, decreased venous return, and decreased myocardial contractility. In addition, changes such as orthostatic hypotension, decreased blood volume, hormonal changes, and bone loss also occur.[30, 167] When exercise is discontinued, some conditioning effects remain and a complete reversion to pre-exercise levels is not usually seen.

The local effects on the exercised tissue are described in detail in the sections about the specific exercise methods.

Exercise Prescription Considerations

Before prescribing an exercise program, several factors should be considered.

Type of Exercise

One way of describing exercise is by the relative amounts of effort provided by the patient and therapist. If an exercise is done passively (PROM), it implies that all the effort must come from the therapist and none from the patient. The usual reason for using this kind of exercise is that the patient is unable to provide the necessary effort because of paralysis, and range of motion must be maintained. As the patient develops the ability to produce movement, exercise can be done actively, or with some assistance (active-assisted, or AAROM). Assistance can be provided manually by the therapist, by counterbalancing with weights, by gravity, by the buoyancy of water, or by methods to decrease friction such as powder boards and skate boards. Assistance can also be provided by facilitation methods such as reflex techniques, electrical stimulation, or biofeedback. As strength improves, assistance is less necessary and the exercise can be done more actively (AROM) with the progressive addition of resistance, if increased strength is a goal.

Exercises can also be done by engaging in functional activity. Mobility training, activities of daily living, and leisure activities, all involve strength, endurance, control, and range of motion. Activities can be designed by physical, occupational, and recreational therapists to simulate stresses that may be encountered at home or at work. Patients often find it less tedious and more interesting to perform upper extremity strengthening activities by weaving a rug on a loom, or to perform lower extremity exercises by walking or cycling rather than by lifting weights in physical therapy. As these activities are often less well quantified than organized exercise programs, the stress must not be underestimated or injury may result.

Goals and Objectives

In order to appropriately write an exercise prescription, the physician must first have the goals of the program clearly in mind. The general goal of most programs is to improve performance or increase function, but more specific objectives should be developed. Common objectives of exercise programs would include increased strength or endurance, improvement of range of motion, increased control and coordination, and increased ability to appropriately relax muscles. If one of these objectives is important for a patient, exercise therapy may be appropriate. An additional objective often is to increase the general fitness or conditioning of the individual, and this may be either a primary goal or a side-effect of the other parts of the program.

Specific Considerations

With specific objectives in mind, details of the exercise prescription can be formulated. Some components are best specified by the prescribing physician, but others may be left to the discretion of the therapist to be appropriately adjusted as conditions indicate. Communication between the physician and therapist is critical to establish the most appropriate program for each individual. The following factors must be carefully considered.

CLINICAL STATUS. The etiology or clinical diagnosis relating to the motor deficit is of major importance. The strengthening program for weakness related to lower motor neuron disorders is quite different from that related to upper motor neuron problems. The risks of injury from exercise must be considered and are much greater in a recent tendon repair than in a normal muscle–tendon system, for example. Whether or not the etiological process is static or progressive must also be considered, since the program for a young patient with a spinal cord injury from trauma would be different from that of an older patient with a cord injury from cancer.

Secondary diagnoses must also be considered. Acute myocardial infarction, unstable angina, congestive heart failure and other unstable cardiac conditions involving serious dysrhythmias, carditis, dissecting aneurysms, or pulmonary embolism would contraindicate an exercise program.[118] Precautions must also be taken in other related situations such as poorly controlled rhythm problems, gross cardiomegaly or cardiac hypertrophy, vascular disease, or certain acute illnesses such as thyroid, renal, or liver disease.

Decreased cardiovascular responses to exercise and decreased maximum heart rate may occur with increasing age. The strenuousness of the exercise therefore may not be obvious in the aged, and appropriate monitoring of the responses and careful planning to avoid excessive stress may be necessary. All exercises and, in particular, isometric exercises and Valsalva-type activities do increase blood pressure and are best avoided in certain individuals. The differences between arm and leg exercise must also be recognized. If the physician is uncertain about the ability of an individual to sustain the cardiovascular stress of an exercise program, a formal stress test can give exact information regarding the maximum heart rate and blood pressure that can be tolerated.

TIMING. Time factors vary considerably from patient to patient. An initial consideration is when to begin an exercise program. Too early institution of a program may carry with it some risks of injury or interference with healing, whereas therapy begun too late will have prolonged the period of disability and possibly allowed complications to develop. Other timing problems include decisions regarding the number of exercise sessions per week and the amount of rest between sessions, the number of sets of exercises done in a given session and the amount of rest between sets, and the number of repetitions of a given exercise and the amount of rest between each repetition. Balance must be achieved between adequate stress and adequate rest time for adaptation. A related factor is the speed at which the exercise should be performed, that is, the angular velocity of movement of the resistance (recall that speed and force are related). Also to be considered is the total length of each exercise session and the total duration of the exercise program, from the initial session until the decision to terminate or substitute a less intensive maintenance program.

RESISTANCE. The resistance may be given in an isotonic, isometric, or isokinetic manner and many varieties of equipment may be used. The amount of resistance used is important and will depend on the specific goal of the exercise program. Because of the kinesiological factors previously discussed, it is important to standardize factors such as the placement of the weight on the extremity and the angle of the extremity during the exercise in order to have a reproducible amount of effort from session to session.

ENVIRONMENT. Changing environmental conditions may also affect the amount of exertion that is reasonable at a given time. Factors such as temperature, altitude, and humidity must be considered. Also, special care must be shown to the individual who is dehydrated because of debility, environmental temperature, or drug treatment. Individuals exercising outdoors must also be cognizant of wind and other weather effects.

WARM-UP AND COOL-DOWN. Activity preceding and following the actual exercise sessions must also be considered. It is generally recommended that a warm-up period be included to produce a gradual increase in body temperature and circulation. Beginning slowly with low resistance will decrease local injury as well as gradually increase cardiovascular stress, thus minimizing the incidence of cardiovascular problems.[12] The exercise session should end with a cool-down period with a gradual reduction of muscular activity to prevent post-exercise syncope.

SPECIFICITY OF INSTRUCTIONS. It is important for the physician who has made the diagnosis to be specific in the description of what body part is to be exercised. It may be a specific muscle or anatomical structure, a general location such as proximal or distal, or a general region such as an extremity, or even a more generalized total body process. The physician should be as specific as is necessary, given the particular circumstances of the patient and the problem for which the exercise is being prescribed. In many routine situations, relatively nonspecific instructions are adequate. Other situations require that the prescription be extremely specific if the goal which the physician wishes to achieve is to be safely accomplished.

The stated goals and objectives can usually be achieved by many different methods, provided the principle of progressive stress and overload is applied in a reasonable manner. In certain situations, however, and for certain goals, some factors become more important. In requesting therapy, the physician must realize that, having established a diagnosis, it is his or her responsibility to make sure that the instructions to the therapist are adequate to achieve desired goals and to avoid complications or untoward events. The physician should, therefore, include in the prescription any precautions or special instructions that will ensure both the patient's safety and the desired results. Appropriate follow-up is necessary to determine whether or not the goals and objectives are being achieved and to modify the program as needed.

Exercise for Strength

There are several physiological ways for muscles to produce an increase in force. The possibilities include nervous system factors to produce more motor unit firings, and muscle tissue factors to produce more force per motor unit. More motor unit firings can be achieved either through recruitment of additional motor units or through increasing the rate of firing to tetanus of the motor units that are already active. Once a motor unit firing rate reaches a tetanic level, however, there is little evidence that force is increased by a further increase in the firing rate. In fact, the firing rate can actually decrease while the force is maintained.[21] Synchronization of motor unit firing may also be associated with increased force.[138] The production of more force per motor unit could result from more force being produced by each muscle fiber in the motor unit or by an increased number of muscle fibers per motor unit.

Stimulus to Increase Strength

If an increase in strength is desired, it is important to know what factors stimulate the motor system to increase its ability to generate force. The principle of overload obviously applies, but the specific stimulus is more difficult to determine. The most likely stimulus appears to be increased tension in the muscle fiber.[71] There is some evidence that tension may be developed either by muscle contraction or by muscle stretch, since studies have shown that passive stretch is a significant stimulus to muscle fiber growth.[99] This growth, however, may be in fiber length by adding sarcomeres in series.[92] In practice, this principle is manifested in the use of high resistance exercises to increase strength. High resistance requires maximum recruitment of motor units, which requires tension production in the greatest number of muscle fibers.

Studies relating the actual amount of mechanical work to the amount of strength increase show that the greater the amount of work, the greater the increase in strength. An increased number of exercise sessions or an increased number of sets of exercise in a strengthening program, therefore, will increase strength at a greater rate, but the strength increase is not in proportion to the increased amount of work performed. As the time spent performing more work increases, it is progressively less efficient in producing strength increase.[49]

Effects of Strengthening Exercise

Each of the possible methods may play some role in the actual increase in strength that results from exercise. Muscle fiber hypertrophy has been consistently shown to occur with strength training,[165] and appears to result from an increased number of myofibrils in a given muscle fiber,[58] since increased protein synthesis and decreased protein degradation occur.[71] This is evident in all fiber types, but somewhat more so in the fast-twitch than in the slow-twitch fibers.[129, 179] Also reported to accompany strength increase are metabolic changes such as increases in muscle glycogen, creatine phosphate, ATP, ade-

nosine diphosphate, creatine, phosphorylase, phosphofructokinase, and Kreb's cycle enzymes.[30, 129] It is controversial whether or not there is any true fiber type change from slow to fast in man resulting from training.[73, 135, 179] Fiber hypertrophy takes some time to occur and is thought to be recognizable in 6 to 8 weeks. Animal studies, which have increased strength by tetanic stimulation, also show that this increase is seen mainly after 6 weeks.

Some investigators have suggested that the increase in strength may also be related to increased numbers of fibers of both types as, in addition to hypertrophy, some fiber splitting and new fiber formation have been observed in work-stressed animal muscle.[78, 98, 156, 163, 184] Other investigators, however, have been unable to find this increase in fiber number.[73, 165]

An increase of strength without evidence of muscle fiber hypertrophy has also been observed.[151, 190] Also when hypertrophy occurs, the strength increase is not proportional to the increase in fiber area.[103, 105, 129] Muscle fiber ultra studies have suggested that this increase occurs as a result of an increased density of actin and myosin filaments and that the actual number of filaments does increase even though hypertrophy does not occur.[151] Fiber hypertrophy does not appear to be a necessary or consistent consequence of strength training. It is postulated that some of the increase in strength, particularly that occurring early, is the result of neurological mechanisms such as increased recruitment, even though maximal effort has apparently previously been given. An increase in electromyographic activity has been reported following strength training, with the greatest increase occurring in the first several weeks of training.[84] It has also been reported that in a 5-week isometric training program, increased voluntary strength was produced but with no change in electrically-stimulated force.[136] These studies would support the fact that some of the training effect is in motor learning or neural facilitation because of a greater number of motor units firing, an increase in rate of firing, or a more efficient pattern of recruitment.[135, 161] The reason for increased recruitment is somewhat unclear, but it may be related to motor learning or overcoming inhibition. It is seen also in emergency situations or under hypnosis when the strength demonstrated is greater than that normally produced voluntarily. Bypassing of inhibition from Golgi tendon receptors and other receptors may possibly be the cause. An increase in synchronization has also been reported to occur as strength increases, and it is thought to produce an increased rate of tension generation.[138] Studies of strengthening programs in the elderly also have suggested that an increase in strength is mostly from neural factors rather than muscle fiber hypertrophy.[141] The phenomenon of cross-transference of training effects from an exercised area to nonexercised muscles would appear to be another example of neurally mediated strength improvement.[37, 90, 105, 119, 168]

Strength training has no effect on oxidative capacity and indeed may decrease this parameter. In weightlifters, mitochondrial and capillary density are found to be decreased, possibly from a dilution effect because of hypertrophy.[129, 155, 176] This also would increase the diffusion distances and reduce the oxidative capacity per unit area of muscle fiber. Decreased lipid storage is also seen in all fibers.[155]

The rate of strength increase depends on the nature of the exercise and its intensity.[135] There appears to be a limiting strength beyond which one cannot progress. The rate of strength gain depends on the initial state of the muscle and at what point between maximum and minimum on the strength scale an individual is at the onset of the exercise program. As one approaches maximum, the rate of gain tends to decrease. Once the plateau is reached, strength may be maintained by exercise as infrequently as once monthly.[37, 158]

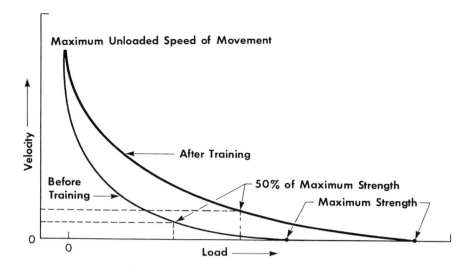

Figure 18-10. The change in the force–velocity relationship with training.

Along with an increase in strength comes an increase in speed, as might be expected because of the force–velocity relationship previously discussed (see Figs. 18-6 and 18-10). Studies also suggest that a weight of the same percentage of maximum can be moved faster after training than it could before. This may result from the greater hypertrophy of fast-twitch fibers by strengthening programs. The maximum velocity with zero load, however, does not change (see Fig. 18-10).

Strength training also affects tissue other than muscle.[20] Changes have been reported in the anterior horn cells[68] and motor end plates.[6] Enzyme changes and enlargement of the nucleolus with training suggest that there is adaptation at the neural cellular level. Muscle connective tissue increases.[165] Bone is strengthened with an increase in mineral and hydroxyproline and an increase in bone density.[25] Cartilage thickens between articulating joints. Tendons and ligaments also appear to increase their strength.[146] Ligaments in dogs have been found to show greater strength, higher hydroxyproline concentrations, and larger diameter fiber bundles after exercise training.[181]

Methods to Increase Strength

Techniques for building muscle strength use a high resistance against which a muscle must work maximally. These techniques involve active muscle contraction, with the amount of resistance determined by the muscle's capability. Physiologically, this probably requires long high-frequency bursts of motor neuronal firing. Resistance to motion can be applied manually by the therapist or through various types of equipment. A strengthening exercise would generally be in one of three forms: isotonic, isometric, or isokinetic.

ISOTONIC EXERCISE. For the most part, isotonic exercise involves movement of a constant weight through a range of motion. The first proponent of organized isotonic exercise appears to have been DeLorme[52] who was responsible for the idea of low repetition, high resistance for strength increase and the reverse program to develop endurance. DeLorme's strengthening program involved the use of progressive resistance (PREs)[53] with ten repetitions at 25%, 50%, 75%, and 100% of the maximum capability for successive efforts. Two minutes of rest were allowed between repetitions and the weight was increased weekly by redetermination of the 10 RM. A theoretical disadvantage of this program was that all the motor units were only recruited with the 100% effort.

The DeLorme regimen was modified in the Oxford program, which uses the reverse schedule, beginning with 100% of the maximum capability. This schedule circumvents the problem with the DeLorme program that often the 100% amount could not be lifted because of fatigue from prior lifts. Theoretically, the Oxford program allows closer to a maximum number of motor units to be recruited with each effort because, with fatigue, less weight can be lifted in a maximum effort. Another method to progressively increase the work is to increase the rate of repetition with the same load.[89] This was felt to be as effective as increasing the amount of weight. Other investigators have described their preferred methods.[20, 30, 45, 121, 135, 154]

Most recommendations currently suggest five to seven repetitions done in three sets per session. Most also recommend using weights that are at a maximum for the number of repetitions, to ensure full activation of all motor units. Most methods have resulted in satisfactory strength gains, with some differences in rates of strength gained because of different intensity, frequency, and duration of the exercise.[135]

Various kinds of weights are available to assist in performing the exercises. Free weights such as dumbbells, bar bells, cuff weights, or improvised weights made from various household goods, all seem to be satisfactory. Special devices to attach the weights such as boots, straps, and cuffs also may be helpful. Pulleys are useful to change the direction of the pull so that exercises can be done in a convenient position. The body itself can be used as resistance by moving the body against gravity in techniques such as push-ups, sit-ups, and chin-ups. These methods have the advantage of simplicity but are also limited in their application to certain body parts.

In general, isotonic exercises have the advantage of being straightforward and requiring relatively simple equipment. They can be time-consuming because weights or equipment must be changed to accommodate different muscles. There is some risk of dropping the weights and causing physical injury. Muscle soreness is relatively common with isotonic exercise. A major theoretical disadvantage is that the weight being used is maximum only at one point in the motion cycle because of the factors of the lever system, muscle length, and angles of muscle attachment and load application, as previously discussed. Theoretically, therefore, proper training occurs only at one point in the motion cycle. Equipment (*e.g.,* Nautilus) that uses cams and pulleys to vary the lever arm length of the load as motion occurs was developed in an attempt to overcome this problem. The system becomes quite involved, with a different configuration of cams designed for each joint being exercised. This system, however, is safe to use, with no free weights that could be dropped.

The equipment also has the capacity for prestretching, which is thought by some to be important. However, the superiority of this method over others in producing strength gains has not been demonstrated.[9, 30] In addition, the considerable cost makes it an option only for institutions such as health clubs and athletic training facilities. Another theoretical disadvantage of isotonic methods is related to the inertia of the weights; it takes more force to start movement than to continue, and once the movement starts, it tends to continue in the same direction. The actual muscle-generated force then varies with the inertial force.

Most isotonic exercise techniques involve concentric exercise, although an eccentric component is obviously present in returning the weight to a starting position. Push-ups, squats, chinning, and sit-ups also have major eccentric components. Studies specifically using eccentric exercise techniques have not shown superior results and so these techniques are rarely used.[107, 132] Eccentric exercise requires less energy consumption and results in less electromyographic activity than an equal amount of concentric work. It does, however, produce more muscle soreness, and studies have shown evidence of significantly more muscle damage, particularly to type II fibers.[66, 143] To perform eccentric exercise without concentric components requires either special equipment or a helper to raise the weight into position for the patient to lower. Safety problems are present because of the heavy weights used. Eccentric exercises for some lower extremity muscles can be performed by walking down a slope or down steps.

ISOMETRIC EXERCISE. Isometric exercise is performed by exertion against an immovable object or by holding an object in a static position. Initial studies suggested that these exercises could be effectively done for a few seconds per day with less than maximum effort,[142] but subsequent studies have modified these recommendations.[135] The principle for developing strength holds true as for other techniques: the maximum number of muscle fibers must be recruited. This can be done by exerting effort of sufficient force and for a long enough period against an immobile object until all the muscle fibers are recruited. Unless maximum effort is obtained, the high-threshold, last-recruited fibers are not used. If exercise is performed by holding a weight in a static position, the weight must be heavy enough and must be held in the position long enough so as to recruit all the muscle fibers. The actual force exerted is probably not critical, but is must be sufficient to fatigue all the muscle fibers. The use of high force levels is the most efficient way to accomplish this. Daily exercise is generally suggested with at least five maximum contractions per session held for several seconds with 2 to 3 minutes recovery between contractions. Strength gains in the range of 5% per week are reported with these methods.[135]

Isometric exercises have the advantage of being easy to perform for most muscles, requiring little time, and resulting in little muscle soreness. If motivation is satisfactory, a near-maximum effort can be obtained and all fibers recruited. Because of the lack of motion, these exercise are useful when joint motion is painful or otherwise contraindicated. However, there is some question about the transference of isometric strength to a dynamic situation,[9, 67, 127, 142] and it has been suggested that the strength gain occurs mainly at the angle at which the exercise was done, implicating neural influences rather than muscle hypertrophy as the cause of the strength increase. It is also said that activities requiring movement are not improved, and these exercises actually may hamper the ability to exert force rapidly.[30, 127]

Another significant problem is the particularly large increase in blood pressure during isometric exercise.[55, 139] The amount of increase is related to the amount of tension developed, and effort greater than 15% of maximum voluntary effort will produce the response.[40, 147] This appears to be caused at least partially by a peripherally originating reflex as it is seen even with sustained contraction of small muscle groups, although to a lesser degree than with large muscles.[34] The response stops as soon as the exercise stops. The increased blood pressure is produced by an increase in heart rate without a change in general peripheral resistance.[55] The increased heart rate produces reduced diastolic filling time and stroke volume actually decreases as muscle tension increases. The effect decreases somewhat with age. Care, however, must be taken in the use of isometric exercise in patients with cardiovascular problems. In addition, isometric exercise has been found to produce ventricular dysrhythmia in a significant percentage of patients with heart disease.[10] Isometric exercise may also be accompanied by a Valsalva maneuver, which also affects the cardiovascular system, although it does not appear to be the major cause of the blood pressure change.

Another disadvantage of isometric exercise is the difficulty in measuring progress without the use of equipment such as a strain gauge. Also, there is no direct feedback and no way to objectively check for maximum exertion or to continually monitor progress. The program tends to be rather uninteresting for the patient, so maintenance of the program may be difficult.

ISOKINETIC EXERCISE. Isokinetic exercise is exercise performed at a constant rate. The equipment permits movement only at a preset angular velocity and accommodates to whatever force is exerted. Theoretically, maximum muscle tension can then be exerted throughout the range of motion. If high tension is the best stimulus for an increase in strength, this should be a better method than isotonic exercise because maximum tension can be exerted at all angles. It also avoids the possible problem of angle specificity found in isometric exercises.

The major controversy with isokinetic exercise is the importance of the rate at which the load is moved. Some investigators have found no difference in strength increase using different rates,[2] but others have indicated that strength gains achieved at one rate of training do not transfer to other rates.[43, 109] This suggests possible selective recruitment of fast- or slow-twitch fibers depending upon the rate of movement, or selective learning of a certain rate pattern. Some evidence of transference of strength from high rate–trained exercises to low rates was seen, but the reverse did not occur.[43] It appears, therefore, that exercising at a slow rate does not necessarily transfer the increase in strength to activities performed at high rates.[153] High rates would appear to be better than low rates. Muscle biopsy performed following fast-rate exercise showed type II fiber hypertrophy, suggesting selective recruitment of type II fibers. The force–velocity relationship, however, suggests that more tension can be exerted at slower rates, making that technique the most desirable from a physiological point of view to stimulate strength development in the maximum number of fibers. A study controlling for both repetitions and time found that those training at slow rates showed more torque improvement at all speeds and suggested that the previously reported relationship to speed may be an artifact of the training protocol.[46] If, however, one is practicing for a high velocity activity, using high velocity training would appear to be most appropriate. Exercise may need to be done at varying rates or at an intermediate rate for best gains at all speeds. It is again likely that the intensity of the contractions is more important than the rate,[20] and that the principle of maximum recruitment should be followed. Recommendations regarding the number of repetitions are similar to those for isotonic exercise: five to seven repetitions in three sets.

Isokinetic exercise has the physiological advantages of maximum effort throughout the range of motion. The equipment

(Cybex, Orthotron) is quite safe because there are no free weights that could cause injury. Also, little soreness has been reported following exercise possibly because of the absence of eccentric contraction. The system can also be accommodated to different patients and some different muscle areas fairly rapidly without the need to change weights or machines, thus reducing the total exercise time. The equipment also provides a print-out of the torque developed throughout the motion that can be used as a graphic record for analysis of the movement, and feedback to the exerciser. However, it cannot give actual muscle-generated force values because it does not take into account the weight of the equipment and the limb, and whether or not movement is with or against gravitational forces.[191] A major disadvantage is the cost of the equipment. In addition, significant blood pressure increases have been noted[79] and accommodation to some muscle groups is difficult.

COMPARISON STUDIES. Several studies have compared the relative effectiveness of isotonic, isometric, and isokinetic exercise, but comparisons are somewhat difficult because of the difficulty in measuring the actual total work performed in each method.[9, 20, 37, 50, 51, 81, 121, 159, 178] All methods have demonstrated an ability to increase strength, with some studies showing slight superiority of one method over another.[149, 153, 178] A more rapid increase in strength with isometric training has been reported,[56, 186] possibly because of the slower learning of the more complicated motions in isotonic and isokinetic exercise. In various cross-over studies, subjects in general did better when tested on the task at which they had trained,[51, 67] suggesting that some of the increase in strength is related to motor learning, but this was not invariable. In one study, isokinetic exercise was shown to result in greater improvement in athletic performance than isotonic.[153] If movement is important, dynamic training would appear best because the muscle adapts to the specific training stress applied.[56] Isometric exercise would appear to be most useful when motion is, for one reason or another, not desired. Isokinetic training is indicated if the activity being trained for requires a specific rate of movement.

The basic principle of strength training is to use resistance and repetitions adequate to require recruitment of all motor units. The more similar the exercise is to the activity being practiced for, the more likely the exercise is to be helpful in that activity. The best exercise to improve performance is likely the task itself.

Electrical Stimulation. Electrical stimulation has been shown by some investigators to be effective in strengthening.[82, 135] This would seem reasonable, since this is merely an external method of producing muscle contraction, which is generally produced internally. Studies in normal subjects have shown variable results in producing increased strength[44, 135, 170] possibly because of the variation in stimulation protocols. Atrophied muscle, however, did show an increase in strength.[62] In one study in postoperative anterior cruciate ligament repairs, electrical stimulation decreased quadriceps atrophy and prevented the usual decrease in succinic dehydrogenase activity.[60] Animal studies have shown the ability to produce an increased force with stimulation parameters in the range of 40 Hz with 1500 five-second tetanic contractions per day. Some clinical studies in neurologically impaired individuals have suggested that prolonged stimulation is necessary for at least several hours per day to produce a significant increase in strength. Muscle stimulation *in vitro* has been shown to retard the rate of protein degradation.[71]

The practicality of stimulating many muscles and of using high intensity current for long periods of time is questionable.[92]

In lower motor neuron lesions, there is some evidence of decreased terminal sprouting with stimulation.[32] Blood pressure should probably be monitored during the stimulation particularly in high spinal–injured patients because of the risk of autonomic hyperreflexia. The role of electrical stimulation in clinical strengthening programs is not yet clear. It may be useful when traditional strengthening methods are not possible because of pain or other causes of low muscle activation.

Problems

The development of increased strength in specific muscles introduces the risk of muscle imbalance if a muscle group is strengthened out of proportion to its antagonists.[18] Imbalance may result in deformity or postural problems (*e.g.*, ball squeezing can strengthen hemiplegic finger flexors, producing further difficulty in opening the hand). Exercising against weak or diseased restraint systems may result in deformity (*e.g.*, strengthening finger flexors in rheumatoid hands can produce ulnar deviation and metacarpophalangeal subluxation).[169]

There is also some risk of increasing the weakness of weak muscles by exercising. This may be caused by overstretching (*e.g.*, overstretching the serratus anterior by performing shoulder abduction exercises without the scapula supported). It may also result from direct over-fatigue of the exercised muscle, as has been reported in polio and muscular dystrophy,[19, 108] although this concern has been disputed.[47, 185]

Exercise for Endurance

Exercises for endurance are often thought of as mainly for cardiovascular conditioning. An increase in local muscle endurance to enable a muscle to continue an activity for a longer time or avoid the early onset of fatigue may, however, be an important goal in itself as well as an accompaniment of general conditioning.

Endurance depends upon the metabolic ability to supply the energy for muscle contraction. Increasing this capability requires an increased metabolic capacity of the individual muscle cell. Metabolic capacity may increase either aerobically or anaerobically. An increased anaerobic capacity would result from an increase in the immediate storage of ATP or creatine phosphate, or an increase in the glycolytic capacity, either by an increase in the amount of glycogen available or an increased ability to convert that glycogen to ATP. Aerobic endurance can be increased by increasing the delivery capacity of oxygen, or by increasing the ability to use oxygen through an increased availability of the substrates or enzymes used to produce energy.

Another possible way to increase endurance would be to reduce energy costs for a given amount of work. This might be accomplished by converting fast-twitch fibers to slow-twitch ones. Because of the slower contraction and relaxation of slow-twitch fibers, a lower frequency of contraction is needed to maintain tension, so less energy is consumed.

Stimulus to Increase Endurance

The overload principle again appears to hold true: a muscle fiber is stimulated to increase its metabolic capabilities by regular exhaustion of those capabilities in the mitochrondria. The stimulus for increasing the anaerobic capacity is exhaustion of the glycolytic system, and for the aerobic capacity, exhaustion of the oxidative system.

The actual stimulus that could cause conversion of fast-twitch to slow-twitch fibers to increase aerobic endurance may be prolonged duration of the active state of the muscle contraction time, since this phenomenon has been observed in animals after chronic electrical stimulation.[58, 160, 167]

Effects of Endurance Exercise

Endurance training has been observed to produce significant metabolic effects within a two- to four-week training period.[30, 58, 167] As previously discussed, the organism as a whole shows an increase in aerobic capacity and this is reflected in the increased aerobic capacity of all muscle fibers exercised, both type I and type II.[100] Type I fibers still continue to show approximately five times the aerobic capacity of the type IIB fibers, as prior to exercise. The increase in muscle oxidative capacity is seen as an increase in myoglobin, oxidative enzymes, mitochondrial density and size, number of capillaries, and lipid content, and a decrease in lactate production with exercise.[100, 110, 155] An increase in glycolytic capacity, mainly of fast-twitch fibers, is also seen.[73] Endurance-trained athletes are found to have a higher percentage of slow-twitch fibers, but whether this represents actual fiber conversion from fast-twitch types is not known.[73] Some reports of apparent fiber type conversion with exercise have been published.[100, 152] Increased aerobic capacity is reflected in an increase in arteriovenous oxygen difference because of the increased ability of the muscle to extract oxygen from the blood. Actual blood flow, however, has not been shown to increase after training.

The increased aerobic capacity is also reflected in the higher utilization of free fatty acids and their mobilization from adipose tissue to produce a glycogen-sparing effect.[20] A higher percentage of energy is therefore produced from fat in trained individuals. An increase in glycogen and ATP stores and glycolytic enzymes in fast-twitch fibers is also generally reported following training.[165] Reports of actual muscle fiber size changes are divergent. An increase[73] and even a decrease have been reported in different studies.[58] A decrease could facilitate a more rapid exchange of metabolites during endurance activities.

It has been suggested that endurance training improves absolute endurance but not relative endurance; that is, the number of repetitions of an activity that can be performed with a given weight is increased, but if the activity is performed at the same percentage of maximum strength capability, the number of repetitions does not change.[172] This suggests that an endurance increase merely reflects a strength increase. However, one study with well-controlled measurements showed that, although high resistance exercise produces the greatest strength increase, there was a decrease in relative endurance, whereas the low resistance exercise group showed an increase in relative endurance; they could do more repetitions with a weight of the same relative size when compared to maximum capability.[5]

Endurance training has also been shown to cause an increase in the strength of tendons and ligaments, and the stability of their attachment sites.[165] One study, however, demonstrated a lack of strength increase using sprint-type exercise and suggested that longer duration endurance exercise was necessary to achieve increased strength.[181]

Methods to Increase Endurance

To increase anaerobic endurance, exercise must be performed that depletes the glycolytic system, which functions in the first one to two minutes of exercise. High resistance, short duration dynamic activities at 80% of maximum are needed.[121] Interval training with intense short duration activity of one to two minutes has been recommended. If the activity is not intense enough, it will not be strictly anaerobic.

To increase aerobic capacity, a muscle's oxidative metabolism must be stressed. The cell's aerobic ability is depleted by prolongd exercise with moderate-rate motor unit firing in order to exhaust the oxidative metabolic processes. For exercise to reach this stage, resistance must be low enough to allow the exercise to continue and high enough to recruit the larger fibers. If too high a resistance is used, the aerobic fibers are not able to continue the activity after the anaerobic late-recruited large fibers tire because the load is too great, so they are not active to the stage of fatigue. If the resistance is too low, the activity may be carried out without ever recruiting the higher threshold fibers, so the aerobic metabolic mechanisms will not be stressed and no adaptation will occur. Less than 60% of maximum effort is necessary in endurance training, and the number of repetitions should be the maximum number that can be done. Exercises in this category are most often isotonic, but could be either of the other types as well. Any of the methods used for strength development can be used to develop endurance, with suitable modification. Equipment such as treadmills and bicycle and arm ergometers, designed to develop general aerobic capacity is often used, as it allows development both of general body and local muscle aerobic capacity.

The actual load and number of repetitions or duration of the exercise is not critical, as long as the exercise is taken to the stage of fatigue.[49] There is an optimal duration of exercise related to size of the load and the specific characteristics of the muscle being exercised, and exercise prolonged past this optimum time will not achieve greater results. Exercises for endurance can be done daily, but 4 or 5 days per week is usually sufficient.[57]

Designing Programs of Exercise for Strength and Endurance

An exercise program must be designed with a particular goal in mind, and a decision made as to whether or not strength or endurance or a combination is most desirable. The principle of specificity of training, or DeLorme's classic low repetition, high resistance exercise for strength, and low resistance, high repetition for endurance,[52] is generally applicable, although there is considerable transferability between the exercise types.[48] The principle of overload continues to hold true, in that if a certain capacity is overloaded, it will adapt to produce the changes necessary to accommodate to the load. The question is not so much of high load or low load, or high repetition or low repetition, but rather of the specific nature of the stress needed, the metabolic system being stressed, and the degree of stress. For specific problems or disabilities, the program should be designed to simulate the specific final functional goal as closely as possible. Most evidence suggests that the closer the training is to the activity being trained for, the better the results.[50, 52] Often, a combination of both strength and endurance is useful. In certain situations, if there has been a specific loss of fibers of a certain type such as with immobilization (loss of type I fibers), exercises designed to stimulate those particular fibers would be indicated. In most programs, it is also generally suggested to include aspects to maintain range of motion and flexibility, and to assist in general cardiovascular conditioning.

There is some evidence that highly specific exercise can cause negative transference or interference with other activities, particularly at the upper levels of performance. For example, a high degree of strength training can interfere to some extent with endurance, since the hypertrophy of the muscle fiber decreases its oxidative metabolic capabilities. Conversely, aerobic training can interfere with strength increase when the upper limits of strength ability are reached.[96] One study showed that running with weights actually resulted in a higher energy cost after training (when the running was done with the weights removed) than before the training.[111]

Exercise for Speed

Speed is a less frequently considered property both of muscle contraction and of the nervous system control mechanism. Fewer studies on speed training have been made than on strength and endurance. An increase in muscle contraction speed is of most interest to athletes involved in sports in which rapid movement is important.

Because of the relationship between strength and speed, an increase in strength also results in an increase in velocity of movement (see Figure 18-10). There is some suggestion that speed can be trained,[114] and several methods have been described to attempt to increase speed performance. These involve attempts at rapid weight movement, such as jumping, or the use of sudden loading with muscle stretch before contraction (plyometric loading). Some trainers use high resistance, high speed isokinetic exercises for athletes whose major need is speed.[41] This is said to selectively cause hypertrophy of type II fibers and avoid hypertrophy of type I. The athlete, therefore, becomes both stronger and faster. Explosive-type training has been reported to result in improvement in parameters of fast force production.[85] Isotonic training will increase the speed of movement against light loads, whereas isometric training increases the speed against high mechanical resistance.[56] These techniques are not as yet widely used.

Speed, usually thought of in terms of quickness or reaction time, is at least in part a function of the control system and is less likely related specifically to actual muscle fiber composition.

Exercise for Control and Coordination

Coordination and control exercises are obviously used in those individuals who, on examination, demonstrate ataxia, incoordination, or lack of control of movement. In some situations, these problems can be related to loss of strength and endurance, so the etiology of the coordination difficulty needs to be carefully evaluated. Most often these exercises are employed in upper motor neuron disorders such as cerebral palsy, brain injury, and stroke, but the principles are also applicable in some lower motor neuron and soft tissue disorders.

Much less is known about the stimuli that increase control and coordination, and about the physiological effects of exercise for control and coordination, than is known about exercises for strength and endurance. Although control and coordination are closely related, they are not the same. *Control* refers specifically to discrete activity with use of specific prime movers in a motion being directly attended to. *Coordination* is the synthesis of the factors necessary to result in a smooth movement pattern and includes many other body areas. The automatic multi-muscle motor patterns that are used to perform activities appear to be developed at a conscious level before they are learned and stored. As previously discussed, what happens physiologically with motor learning as control and coordination develop is speculative.

The goal of control and coordination exercises is to develop sensory engrams and motor programs that can be stored in the brain and then be used for future activities. After central nervous system injury, the process may involve relocation of the programs and engrams in other areas, possibly by collateral growth of intact neurons or substitution of alternate pathways or neurons.[11] When the central nervous system is intact and movement is impaired by lower motor neuron or soft tissue problems, the exercises attempt to reactivate the neuronal pathways that for some reason have been inhibited.

Methods to Increase Control and Coordination

The main method of teaching control and coordination is repetition. If an activity is repeated enough times, the process is learned and stored, and then can be performed with progressively less concentration and effort. Three approaches to training are possible.

1. Practicing the specific task that is to be accomplished. In other words, if walking is the main goal, the patient practices walking by whatever methods and by use of whatever assistive devices are necessary. One should not worry whether the initial efforts are correct or coordinated, as these can be refined as the gross pattern is learned. If walking is not possible, the goal should be reduced to a level which seems achievable (*e.g.,* standing, sitting, or balancing) and this activity practiced until it is mastered sufficiently to proceed to the next level.
2. Breaking the task into sections and practicing the individual sections before putting them together. For example, before walking, the patient would practice each component of the walking activity such as foot placement, leg swing, foot contact, balancing, and weight transfer, and would not walk until each individual component was performed satisfactorily. The more complicated the task, the more it must be broken down into separate sections. When each pattern is performed satisfactorily, then the components can be gradually put together.
3. Performing relatively unrelated activities with the goal of improving general control and coordination before attempting the specific task. For walking, the patient would practice coordination of foot movements, ankle movements, hip movements, reciprocal motions, and various patterns to inhibit or facilitate certain muscle groups, and would not walk until the movements were satisfactory. Other examples would be the attempt to improve hand control for self-care activities by placing pegs in holes and transferring various-size items from one spot to another, or learning to write through the practice of making ovals and shapes rather than practicing the actual letters.

In this regard, it has been suggested that the whole is something different from the sum of its parts and that skills cannot be learned element by element.[88]

Ideally, for appropriate development of control and coordination, certain structures and processes should be present. One would like to have intact motor and sensory control and storage centers and intact pathways connecting the centers to the peripheral effector organs. In particular, sensory feedback is critical, since the creation of a sensory engram is the initial goal to be achieved. Position sense, touch, and pressure should be emphasized when present. If normal sensation is not present, additional feedback methods must be developed, using those senses that are intact. Passive motion may provide initial proprioceptive input when active motion is decreased. Verbal praise for the correct movement reinforces the correct response. Visual feedback is also useful and is to be encouraged. Electromyographic biofeedback may be helpful, since the muscle contraction is reinforced by visual and auditory sensations indicating when the muscle is active and to what extent.[14, 15, 33] This method has been of particular use in tendon transfers,[18] and also is reported to be successful in training with foot drop[17] and to be of help in stroke patients with subluxed shoulders and impaired hand function.[14] If adequate strength, endurance, and range of motion are not present, work on correcting these problems may be required as well, or additional body support provided while the exercise is being done.

Cerebral factors such as mental age, concentration, attention, insight, and motivation may be deficient. It may be necessary, therefore, to decrease the effect of these interfering factors by decreasing the distractions, increasing the interest of the activity, and decreasing the complexity of an activity. It is also important to avoid fatigue or discomfort, and to create a setting with security and a low tension and anxiety potential. In order to develop an accurate sensory engram, the activity must be confined to the specific movement and substitution or overflow avoided. Undesired activity can be decreased by minimizing the amount of voluntary effort, by using satisfactory support and positioning, and by using certain postures and equipment. Some, however, feel that resistance and effort are important to developing proprioceptive feedback.

With these factors in mind, the principal technique used is the identification of the specific movement or task to be achieved and then constant repetition of the activity with correction of mistakes until the appropriate sensory engram and motor pattern is developed.

Additional techniques may be combined with the above to help facilitate movement. Facilitation by use of reflexes, electrical stimulation, or the use of sensory facilitation techniques such as cold, vibration, and skin manipulation may be helpful. Reflexes and postures can also be used to inhibit unwanted motion.

Several individuals have developed systems of therapy to facilitate muscle control and coordination and these systems are based on a variety of neurophysiological principles.[27, 70, 86, 125, 134] Studies comparing these systems to each other and to other methods have generally failed to show superiority of one method over another.[125, 134] They are generally most applicable in upper motor neuron disorders. Fay developed a technique based on the supposition that ontogeny recapitulates phylogeny. This system, which has been popularized by Doman and Delacato, uses pathological reflexes to obtain movement and carries an individual through the various stages of phylogenetic development. Movements are patterned by passive positioning of the trunk and extremities, and it is felt that the patterning will cause brain development at progressive stages. Proficiency at one level of development is required before proceeding to the next level. This system requires extensive numbers of individuals to carry out the patterning techniques and is highly controversial.[134]

A system developed by Brunnstrom uses primitive synergistic patterns in training and attempts to progressively obtain control of the various flexion-extension synergies. These patterns are then used to perform purposeful activity. The Bobaths also use reflexes and patterns extensively and try to use postures that inhibit abnormal patterns that interfere with desired movement. Activation or facilitation of the normal patterns and postures is accentuated and the constant repetition of the normal proprioceptive input, along with the blocking of the abnormal patterns, hopefully results in development of normal movement.

Kabat, along with Knott and Voss, developed a system called proprioceptive neuromuscular facilitation (PNF) based primarily on proprioceptive feedback. This system employs maximum resistance and the most favorable part of the active joint range to facilitate movement and develop proprioception, and uses the irradiation of responses from this effort to activate weaker muscle groups. Stretch reflexes are also employed in training, and diagonal patterns in combinations are thought to be important. The system developed by Rood emphasizes the stimulation of sensory receptors for facilitation and uses stroking and icing of cutaneous receptors to facilitate function of the underlying mus-

cle. Many components of these systems would appear to be useful, while strict adherence to one or another system would not appear to have research support at this time.[125, 134, 192]

Other systems of coordination exercises have been developed for various problems. Frenkel originally developed a series of lower extremity coordination exercises for locomotor ataxia. These exercises are essentially repetitions of slow, precise, lower extremity motions beginning with simple patterns and gradually progressing as control is attained. Upper extremity coordination exercises generally involve the use of various prehension forms such as the three-jaw chuck, power grip, or thumb-index opposition patterns. These various methods are then used to perform certain control activities such as placing pegs in holes, or for functional activities developed by the occupational therapist, or in recreational activities. Coordination activities are also used to develop balance and to precede locomotion. These exercises involve weight shifting, initially with support that is gradually removed as progress is made.

Problems

A major disadvantage of any of the systems for developing control and coordination is the inordinate amount of time that is required. It is said that many millions of repetitions are necessary to establish appropriate patterns and that any errors in correct performance delay the development of the proper patterns. Cerebral palsy children often receive therapy for many years in the hopes of eventually improving motor performance or at least preventing deterioration. Information regarding the number of repetitions necessary and over what period of time it is reasonable to carry out the exercises is lacking.

Another major problem is the lack of precise knowledge about the plasticity and adaptability of the central nervous system. Injury obviously places significant constraints on the ability to function in a manner similar to pre-injury. Just how much the brain is able to regenerate damaged circuits, change memory locations, or adopt alternative strategies is not known.

Exercise for Relaxation

Exercises for relaxation are often used in individuals experiencing pain related to muscle contraction phenomena. Relaxation is also important when muscles are being stretched to increase range. The usual goal of the exercise is to make the individual more aware of the feeling of muscle contraction so that he or she can consciously, and eventually unconsciously, prevent the constant muscle tension. This exercise is often also facilitated by the use of electromyographic biofeedback because the visual and auditory response makes the presence of muscle contraction much more recognizable.[14]

Methods to Increase Relaxation

Exercises should be done in a controlled environment where relaxation is most easily achieved. It is helpful, therefore, to have a quiet, slightly darkened area. A development of awareness of muscle contraction is accomplished by having the patient contract and relax muscles so that the feeling of the muscle contraction is experienced. The electromyographic biofeedback can provide an indication not only as to when a muscle is contracting so that it reinforces the sensory feedback, but also as to how much contraction is occurring. It provides a measure of progress because the electrical activity can be seen to decrease when efforts are successful. Relaxation is also helped by mild passive stretching or the use of pendular exercises.

Exercises can be directed at specific muscles that appear to be creating pain, or they can be of a more generalized nature. Generalized exercises require development of a feeling of general relaxation and are helped by appropriate relaxed postures and methods, such as breathing control or the use of a tank or pool. The success of relaxation exercises in treating pain conditions has not been established.

Exercise for Motion

Range-of-motion exercises may be performed with the objective of preventing loss of range in susceptible individuals in whom a possible cause of range loss is present, or of increasing range in those individuals who have lost range. In individuals who are paralyzed, the exercise is passive, with the therapist moving the joint through the range of motion. In patients who have muscle function, the exercise can be done with some or no assistance from the therapist. Exercises performed actively by the patient accomplish the goals of not only maintaining range but also increasing strength and endurance at the same time.

Maintaining Range of Motion

In a normal individual, joint range is maintained by the movements of daily activities. In athletes, stretching exercises or range maintenance exercises are suggested as part of exercise programs, since there is some evidence that range can be lost during strengthening and endurance exercise programs if it is not specifically maintained. These exercises should use slow prolonged stretch and not ballistic or bouncing methods which stimulate the stretch reflex in antagonists and are more likely to produce injury. Stretching can also be facilitated to some extent by contraction-relaxation techniques in which the muscle is initially stretched and then contracted while it is under stretch.[140] This technique appears to increase the extensibility of the muscle beyond that obtained by stretch alone.

In susceptible individuals, range of motion can readily be lost and must therefore be maintained by appropriate exercises. The joint should be put through its full range of motion two or three times daily so that no connective tissue changes are allowed to develop. This should be done unless there is a specific contraindication in which motion would be disruptive to healing. Even in recent fractures and tendon repairs, properly controlled regular motion appears useful.

METHODS TO MAINTAIN RANGE. Range-of-motion exercises are most often done manually by a therapist, but can be done by aides and nurses or other individuals who can be taught the techniques. As soon as possible, an individual can be taught self range of motion, either passively using another extremity to produce motion, or actively or assisted. Codman's pendulum exercises for the shoulder are an example of a mainly passive exercise with the occasional active use of minimal contraction of muscles around the shoulder. Equipment such as pulleys or shoulder wheels for elevating the arm in shoulder range-of-motion exercises may also facilitate self range-of-motion exercises. Ropes and belts to allow self range of motion in the lower extremities are also useful.

Recently, passive motion equipment has been developed to ensure range of motion following certain injuries or operative procedures to joints.[157] Constant motion in a joint has been found to successfully prevent loss of range and also decrease edema and increase the healing rate in joints. It may also be useful in reducing the incidence of pulmonary emboli. It is important that the motion be carefully controlled.[64]

An important but often overlooked method of maintaining range and preventing contractures is the use of positioning with props or pillows in a bed or chair, or with splints to support certain extremity joints. Positions that encourage contractures should be avoided.

Increasing Range of Motion (Stretching)

When range of motion has been lost and a contracture has developed, more vigorous efforts are needed to reduce the contracture and regain range. Stretching is advocated for use in warm-ups for athletic performances as a preventative for stretch-type injuries.[102]

Connective tissue demonstrates nonlinear properties when stretched.[120] Initially, the tissue stretches with little force as the collagen fibers straighten. This is the period of elastic stretch, and the collagen will return to its original length if the load is removed. Once the fibers are straight, more force is needed to cause further elongation. If the load is maintained, connective tissue will undergo plastic deformation or *creep,* a slow deformation of the tissue which does not recover when the load is removed. This process is greatest in the first 6 to 8 hours, but continues at a slow rate for months if the load is continued.[145] In addition, if soft tissues are stretched to a certain length and the length maintained, the tension in the connective tissue will gradually decrease. This decrease also occurs most in the first 6 to 8 hours, but continues for months as well, such as when an extremity is placed in a cast with some tension on the tight structures. When stretching a contracture, the force needed for stretch is larger for the first stretch than for subsequent ones, possibly because of initial breaking of adhesions or intermolecular cross-linkages.[193] Studies also show that increasing the temperature of the structure being stretched produces significant additional elongation with less tissue damage than when stretch is used alone.[120, 187] A slow rate of application of the stretching force produced more elongation than a rapid rate.[183] High loads produce rapid elongation of collagen, but when the load is removed the tissue returns to its previous length. Lower loads produce slower but greater eventual elongation. These physiological studies suggest that stretch should be of long duration with low force and a gradual increase in the force. The force should be maintained, not relaxed, and the use of heat during the stretch increases the effectiveness.[124]

Stretching of muscle tissue has been shown to result in an increase in the number of sarcomeres in the muscle fibers.[93] Simple passive stretch of muscle has also been shown to reduce the net protein breakdown *in vitro,* and an actual hypertrophy of muscle is described for the first week when stretching denervated muscle.[71] It is postulated that myofilaments are added to the muscle in series.[92]

SPECIFIC CONSIDERATIONS IN STRETCHING. Several factors must be considered when the decision is made to attempt to increase range or reduce a contracture. If the objective of the stretching is to increase function, the main effort must be directed toward those areas where reduction of the contracture will be most helpful. In certain areas major contractures may exist, but reduction of the contracture would not result in an increase in function. On the other hand, minor contractures may occur in areas such as the hip joint in a patient with muscular dystrophy and result in an inability to ambulate. Efforts must therefore be directed where they will do the most good. One must also consider the practicality of attempting to increase the range. Conservative stretching may take considerable time and may interfere with other activities or treatments. If many joints are involved this further complicates the process. A reasonable chance of success with the program should also be expected, that is, the tissue to be stretched will respond and the patient will show functional improvement.

The etiology of the contracture and its duration must also be considered. Range loss from bony abnormality is not conducive to improvement by conservative means and may require surgery. Other loss of range may be most appropriately treated by surgical release of tendons, the use of nerve blocks, motor point blocks, or drugs. The degree of fixed soft tissue contracture is often difficult to determine in a very spastic patient, and only after relief of spasticity is the actual amount of fixed contracture evident. In soft tissue contractures of long duration, the collagen is usually relatively mature and unlikely to respond rapidly or significantly to stretching. Surgery with tendon or soft tissue releases may be more appropriate in these situations.

If a contracture exists that appears amenable to improvement by stretching, and this improvement would appear to result in improved function or ease of care, a decision must be made as to the most appropriate technique to use.

METHODS TO INCREASE RANGE. Stretching may be preceded by other modalities that may improve the results or make the situation safer or more tolerable. Heat has been mentioned as a useful adjunct and, when appropriate, should be chosen and applied in a manner that most effectively reaches the tissue to be stretched. A general warm-up may also facilitate stretching. Analgesics or transcutaneous nerve stimulation are helpful if the stretching appears to be causing discomfort. Antispasticity medications or other muscle relaxants may also facilitate the stretching. In patients with clotting disorders, the prophylactic use of clotting factors may be indicated. Hydrotherapy may aid in relaxation, in addition to having a heating effect.

The principles previously mentioned of slow prolonged stretch with heating apply. The longer that the stretching force is applied, the more quickly the tissue will elongate. Stretch should be continued after heating is stopped. The amount of force applied is a compromise between the force necessary to cause elongation without disrupting the tissue, and the force that can be tolerated by the patient. Consideration must also be given to the pressure problems created on the tissue at the sites of application of the stretching forces. Because of the need for slow prolonged stretch, manual stretching is generally not useful. There are situations, however, where prolonged stretching by equipment is not possible or practical, and manual stretching by the therapist is needed.

Manual stretching is more an art than a science and is recommended to be to, or just past, the point of pain, but not so vigorous that pain persists for longer than 24 hours. The stretch is applied by the therapist and maintained for 15 to 30 seconds and slowly released. The amount of force to be used is variable and only an experienced therapist can judge when a tissue can be stretched farther or when a fixed blockage to stretching is present. The therapist must also be adept at convincing the patient to tolerate a certain degree of discomfort, since discomfort may be necessary to achieve progress. In children, the personality of the therapist is critical in enabling cooperation with stretching.

Manual stretching can also be performed by the patient using another extremity or the body weight, with techniques such as leaning on the hand or stretching the heel cord by standing and leaning toward a wall. Equipment such as pulleys, ropes, belts, and broom handles may also facilitate stretching.

Equipment is often necessary if there is a significant contracture because it can apply force over a long period of time without alteration. Traction devices can be set up with weights, pulleys, or wedges, and the patient positioned to produce a three-point

system of forces to reduce the contracture. Similar force systems can also be set up with braces, either of a static or dynamic type.

Techniques of posturing, use of cold, and facilitation of antagonists may be helpful in spastic patients. A slow stretch to avoid stimulation of the stretch reflex to allow relaxation of the muscle being stretched should always be used. Facilitation by active muscle contraction, either proprioceptive neuromuscular facilitation (PNF) or the contract-relax technique, also appears to be helpful[140] if the tightness is related to muscle tissue. In this situation, the patient participates by actively contracting and relaxing the muscle while it is being stretched. This appears to increase the extensibility of the muscle tissue quickly but may result in more pain.[102] Contraction of antagonist muscles may also be useful to reciprocally inhibit the muscle that is being stretched. This also has the effect of strengthening muscles that are tending to overcome the tightness. These techniques have not been shown by controlled studies to offer significant advantages over traditional stretching methods, however.[128] Most studies of the various methods of reduction of contractures do show the ability to make significant gains, but the amount of gain is highly dependent on the factors previously discussed.[126, 173]

Manipulation is another technique to increase range, by tearing adhesions in some cases, or in others, by restoring joint play (see Chapter 14).

PROBLEMS. The main problem related to stretching is the possible production of tissue injury.[18] Injury generally occurs when too much force is used or when the joint is moved beyond its available range. Loss of sensation predisposes to injury because the patient is not aware that too much stretch is being applied. In addition, tissues weakened from disease or inactivity are more likely to be injured because of their decreased ability to withstand forces. Ballistic stretching (bouncing or intermittent forceful stretching) either by the therapist or by the patient doing self-stretching is not recommended because of the risk of excessive loading and possible injury. This technique may also result in stimulation of the stretch reflex, which acts antagonistically to the direction of the stretch. If injury does occur, the contracture may be increased because of the production of hemorrhage or inflammation, and possible stimulation of heterotopic ossification. Edematous tissue is particularly susceptible to injury with stretching. If pain does occur and does not disappear within 24 hours, the stretching has been too vigorous and should be eased.[173] This pain may also increase muscle spasm.

Another possible complication of stretching is the production of joint subluxation. The knee in particular is subject to this problem because it does not move as a hinge joint but has gliding and rolling components of movement. The usual three-point system of stretching does not take into account this sliding feature and may therefore create joint instability. Also there is some risk of increasing the weakness of weak muscles by overstretching. Prolonged or chronic overstretching can result in an increased number of sarcomeres in the muscle fibers and may produce a muscle of improper length related to the lever system. Stretching may also result in motion in an unwanted segment because another area resists stretching less than the contracted area (e.g., development of a rocker-bottom foot from heel-cord stretching). In addition, stretching of healing tissues, particularly tendons or ligaments, before they gain their normal strength, may result in excessive laxity.

Further Considerations

Equipment

The use of equipment for exercise programs has advantages and disadvantages. In a well-equipped physical therapy department, exercises are often facilitated by the use of equipment that is designed for specific purposes and is easy to use. If a wide range of equipment is available, individuals can often be moved from one piece of equipment to another quickly so the time needed to change exercises is reduced. Equipment may also be a disadvantage when a patient becomes reliant upon it and feels it is indispensable. The patient may stop exercising and not assume responsibility for continuation of the program when discharged from a formal program. The cost of equipment is also a major consideration. Encouragement in the use of community resources such as health clubs and YMCAs may stimulate the patient to continue exercising. Assistance in the development of practical home substitutes for the equipment may also be helpful.

General Problems With Exercise Programs

TIME. If significant progress is to be made toward any of the goals of exercise, a considerable time commitment is necessary. Rarely will an exercise program result in changes in a few days or weeks. The patient, therefore, may become discouraged before results are evident. Occasionally early rapid progress is made, possibly because of neural factors, before major adaptations occur. When the rate of progress later slows, the patient becomes discouraged and may discontinue.

PAIN. Some exercises may involve discomfort. Strengthening exercise results in muscle soreness and this can, at times, be severe. This discomfort may be minimized by beginning with low intensity exercise and encouraging the patient to continue, since pain is usually best relieved by further exercise rather than by rest. Less pain is also experienced as time passes and muscle conditioning occurs. The eccentric phase of exercise should be minimized when possible. Pain may also be a major problem during stretching exercises, but for significant progress, must also be tolerated to some extent.

MEDICAL PROBLEMS. Injuries may occasionally result from exercise. The most common are soft tissue injuries such as strains and sprains, but more serious injuries such as fractures and peripheral nerve injuries or compression syndromes can occur. Attempts must be made to minimize the risk of injury by the use of proper techniques and to treat injuries rapidly when they are recognized.

Cardiovascular problems may arise both during and after exercise and can be minimized by proper warm-up and cool-down periods.

COST. The cost of an exercise program is considerable, as it often requires many weeks or months of treatment. This is often beyond the resources of the individual, unless covered by insurance.

EXERCISE PRESCRIPTION AND FOLLOW-UP. The physician must have definite goals and objectives in mind when the exercise prescription is written and must regularly follow-up and evaluate the progress. If this is not done, the program is unlikely to be successful.

MOTIVATION. Exercise is a process which requires that the patient participate in the treatment. In the standard medical model, patients are used to being treated passively by someone else. They often, therefore, do not understand the need for their participation and the need for the exertion of considerable effort. The doctor and therapist must therefore be convincing in explaining to the patient this need if the program is to be successful.

RESULTS. The eventual goal of an exercise program is to improve performance. The ability to show improved performance in an activity from an exercise not directly related to the activity (*e.g.,* in ambulation by lifting weights) may be difficult.

Exercise in Disease States

MEDICAL DISEASE.[28] In individuals with cardiovascular disease, extra care is necessary during exercise programs that require significant exertion. A more gradual warm-up is necessary to prevent blood pressure changes, and more care during the slow-down period is also indicated to prevent hypotensive episodes. Care in the use of high resistance and isometric exercise[147] and avoidance of the Valsalva maneuver is also suggested, particularly in hypertensives. If there are any questions about the status of the cardiovascular condition, monitoring or prior stress testing is useful. The effect of cardiac drugs on exercise also must be considered.[30, 95]

In diabetes,[106, 113, 162] the increase in utilization of glucose by the exercise must be balanced against the amount of insulin being taken, since hypoglycemia may be a problem. Injection of insulin into an area that will be exercised may increase the insulin absorption rate and cause a greater than usual effect from the insulin.

In asthmatics, there is a risk of precipitating attacks with exercise.[69] It is therefore useful to give medication before exercise and have medications available should they be needed. Patients with chronic obstructive pulmonary disease may experience problems of hypoxia, pulmonary hypertension with resistance to right ventricular output, and air trapping.[29]

ARTHRITIS. In patients with joint pain or deformity, isometric exercise often helps to maintain strength if there is evidence of inflammation and pain in the joint with movement. Maintenance of range of motion, however, is critical. General exercise programs for strength and endurance in persons with arthritis have also been shown to be helpful and have resulted in a better disease outcome.[144]

NEUROMUSCULAR DISEASE. A major concern regarding strengthening exercise in neuromuscular disease is that exercise may increase weakness.[18] In addition, excessive exercise in partially denervated or reinnervating muscles may interfere with reinnervation.[91] It is therefore recommended in diseases with some involvement of the lower motor neuron that the amount of exercise and the change in muscle strength and possibly muscle enzyme levels be carefully monitored to ensure that no adverse effects are being produced.[63, 92]

REFERENCES

1. Abraham WM: Factors in delayed muscle soreness. Med Sci Sports Exerc 9:11–20, 1977
2. Adeyanju K, Crews TR, Meadors WJ: Effects of two speeds of isokinetic training on muscular strength, power and endurance. J Sports Med 23:352–356, 1983
3. Akeson WH, Amiel D, Woo SLY: Immobility effects on synovial joints: The pathomechanics of joint contracture. Biorheology 17:95–110, 1980
4. Amiel D, Akeson WH, Harwood FL, Frank CB: Stress deprivation effect on metabolic turnover of the medial collateral ligament collagen. Clin Orthop 172:265–270, 1983
5. Anderson T, Kearney JT: Effects of three resistance programs on muscular strength and absolute and relative resistance. Res Q Exerc Sport 53:1–7, 1982
6. Appell HJ: Proliferation of motor end-plates induced by increased muscular activity. Int J Sports Med 5:125–129, 1984

7. Armstrong RB: Mechanisms of exercise-induced delayed onset muscle soreness: A brief review. Med Sci Sports Exerc 16:529–538, 1984

8. Asmussen E, Bonde-Petersen F: Storage of elastic energy in skeletal muscles in man. Acta Physiol Scand 91:385–392, 1974

9. Atha J: Strengthening muscle. Exerc Sports Sci Rev 9:1–73, 1981

10. Atkins JM, Matthews OA, Blomquist CG, Mullins CB: Incidence of arrhythmias induced by isometric and dynamic exercise. Brit Heart J 38:465–471, 1976

11. Bach-y-Rita P: Rehabilitation versus passive recovery of motor control following central nervous system lesions. In Desmedt JE (ed): Motor Control Mechanisms in Health and Disease. New York, Raven Press, 1983

12. Barnard RJ, Gardner GW, Diaco HV et al: Cardiovascular responses to sudden strenuous exercise. J Appl Physiol 34:833–837, 1973

13. Barnes WS: The relationship between maximum isokinetic strength and isokinetic endurance. Res Q 51:714–717, 1980

14. Basmajian JV: Biofeedback—Principles and Practice for Clinicians. Baltimore, Williams & Wilkins, 1979

15. Basmajian JV: Biofeedback in rehabilitation: A review of principles and practices. Arch Phys Med Rehabil 62:469–475, 1981

16. Basmajian JV, Deluca CJ: Muscles Alive, 5th ed. Baltimore, Williams & Wilkins, 1985

17. Basmajian JV, Kukulka CG, Narayan MG, Takebe K: Biofeedback treatment of foot-drop after stroke compared with standard techniques. Effects on voluntary control and strength. Arch Phys Med Rehabil 56:231–236, 1975

18. Bennett RL: Use and abuse of certain tools of physical medicine. Arch Phys Med Rehabil 41:485–496, 1960

19. Bennett RL, Knowlton GC: Overwork weakness in partially denervated skeletal muscle. Clin Orthop 12:22–29, 1958

20. Berger RA: Applied Exercise Physiology. Philadelphia, Lea & Febiger, 1982

21. Bigland-Ritchie B, Woods JJ: Changes in muscle contractile properties and neural control during human muscular fatigue. Muscle Nerve 7:691–699, 1984

22. Bjurstedt H, Rosenhamer G, Balldin U, Katkov V: Orthostatic reactions during recovery from exhaustive exercise of short duration. Acta Physiol Scand 119:25–31, 1983

23. Bobbert MF, Hollander AP, Huijing PA: Factors in delayed onset muscular soreness of man. Med Sci Sports Exerc 18:75–81, 1986

24. Booth FW, Gollnick PD: Effects of disuse on the structure and function of skeletal muscle. Med Sci Sports Exerc 15:415–420, 1983

25. Booth FW, Gould EW: Effects of training and disuse on connective tissue. Exerc Sport Sci Rev 3:83–112, 1975

26. Bosco C, Komi PV, Ito A: Prestretch potentiation of human skeletal muscle during ballistic movement. Acta Physiol Scand 111:135–140, 1981

27. Bouman HD (ed): Exploratory and analytical survey of therapeutic exercise. Am J Phys Med 46:711–1047, 1967

28. Bove AA, Lowenthal DT: Exercise Medicine. Physiological Principles and Clinical Application. New York, Academic Press, 1983

29. Braun SR, Fregosi R, Reddan WG: Exercise training in patients with COPD. Postgrad Med 71:163–173, 1982

30. Brooks GA, Fahey TD: Exercise Physiology: Human Bioenergetics and Its Applications. New York, John Wiley & Sons, 1984

31. Brooks VB: The Neural Basis of Motor Control. New York, Oxford University Press, 1986

32. Brown MC, Holland RL: A central role for denervated tissues in causing nerve sprouting. Nature 282:724–726, 1979

33. Brudny J, Korein J, Grynbaum BB et al: EMG biofeedback therapy: Review of treatment of 114 patients. Arch Phys Med Rehabil 57:55–63, 1976

34. Buck JA, Amundsen LR, Nielsen DH: Systolic blood pressure responses during isometric contractions of large and small muscle groups. Med Sci Sports Exerc 12:145–147, 1980

35. Cardenas DD, Stolov WC, Hardy R: Muscle fiber number in immobilization atrophy. Arch Phys Med Rehabil 58:423–426, 1977

36. Cavagna GA, Citterio G: Effect of stretching on the elastic characteristics and the contractile component of frog striated muscle. J Physiol 239:1–14, 1974

37. Clarke DH: Adaptation in strength and muscular endurance resulting from exercise. Exerc Sport Sci Rev 1:73–102, 1973

38. Clarke DH, Stull GA: Strength recovery patterns following isometric and isotonic exercise. J Motor Behavior 1:233–243, 1969

39. Clausen JP, Klausen K, Rasmussen B, Jensen JT: Central and peripheral circulatory change after training of the arms or legs. J Physiol 225:675–682, 11973

40. Coote JH, Hilton SM, Perez-Gonzalez JF: The reflex nature of the pressor response to muscular exercise. J Physiol 215:789–804, 1971

41. Counsilman JE: The importance of speed in exercise. Scholastic Coach 46:94–99, 1976

42. Coyle EF, Costill DL, Lesmes GR: Leg extension power and muscle fiber composition. Med Sci Sports 11:12–15, 1979

43. Coyle EF, Feiring DC, Rotkis TC et al: Specificity of power improvements through slow and fast isokinetic training. J Apply Physiol 51:1437–1442, 1981

44. Currier DP, Lehamn J, Lightfoot P: Electrical stimulation in exercise of the quadriceps femoris muscle. Phys Ther 59:1508–1512, 1979

45. deLateur BJ: Therapeutic exercise to develop strength and endurance. In Kottke FJ, Stillwell GK, Lehmann JF: Krusen's Handbook of Physical Medicine and Rehabilitation, 3rd ed. Philadelphia, WB Saunders, 1982

46. deLateur BJ, Alquist AD, Giaconi RM, Esselman PC: Specificity of velocity of training: Unexpected outcome. Arch Phys Med Rehabil 67:643, 1986

47. deLateur BJ, Giaconi RM: Effect on maximal strength of submaximal exercise in Duchenne muscular dystrophy. Am J Phys Med 58:26–36, 1979

48. deLateur BJ, Lehmann JF, Fordyce WE: A test of the DeLorme axiom. Arch Phys Med Rehabil 49:245–248, 1968

49. deLateur BJ, Lehmann JF, Gianconi R: Mechanical work and fatigue: Their roles in the development of muscle work capacity. Arch Phys Med Rehabil 57:319–324, 1976

50. deLateur B, Lehmann J, Stonebridge J, Warren CG: Isotonic versus isometric exercise: A double shift transfer of training study. Arch Phys Med Rehabil 53:212–216, 1972

51. deLateur BJ, Lehmann JF, Warren CG et al: Comparison of effectiveness of isokinetic and isotonic exercise in quadriceps strengthening. Arch Phys Med Rehabil 53:60–64, 1972

52. DeLorme TL: Heavy resistance exercises. Arch Phys Med Rehabil 27:607–630, 1946

53. DeLorme TL, Watkins AL: Techniques of progressive resistance exercise. Arch Phys Med Rehabil 29:263–273, 1948

54. Dimsdale JE, Hartley LH, Guiney T et al: Postexercise peril. JAMA 251:630–632, 1984

55. Donald KW, Lind AR, McNichol GW et al: Cardiovascular response to sustained (static) contractions. Circ Res XX & XXI (Suppl) 1:15–32, 1967

56. Duchateau J, Hainaut K: Isometric or dynamic training: Diferential effects on mechanical properties of a human muscle. J Appl Physiol 56:296–301, 1984

57. Dudley GA, Abraham WM, Terjung RL: Influence of exercise intensity and duration on biochemical adaptations in skeletal muscle. J Appl Physiol 53:844–850, 1982

58. Edstrom L, Grimby L: Effect of exercise on the motor unit. Muscle Nerve 9:104–126, 1986

59. Enneking WF, Horowitz M: The intraarticular effects of immobilization on the human knee. J Bone Joint Surg 54A:973–985, 1972

60. Eriksson E, Haggmark T: Comparison of isometric muscle training and electrical stimulation supplementing isometric muscle training in the recovery after major knee ligament surgery. Am J Sports Med 7:169–171, 1979

61. Essen B: Glycogen depletion of different fiber types in human skeletal muscle during intermittent and continuous exercise. Acta Physiol Scand 103:446–455, 1978

62. Fournier A, Goldberg M, Green B et al: A medical evaluation of the effects of computer assisted muscle stimulation in paraplegic patients. Orthop 7:1129–1133, 1984

63. Fowler WM, Taylor R: Rehabilitation management of muscular dystrophy and related disorders. The role of exercise. Arch Phys Med Rehabil 63:319–321, 1982

64. Frank C, Akeson WH, Woo SLY et al: Physiology and therapeutic value of passive joint motion. Clin Orthop 185:113–125, 1984

65. Franklin BA, Vander L, Wrisley D, Rubenfine M: Aerobic require-

ments of arm ergometry: Implications for exercise testing and training. Phys Sports Med 11:81–90, 1983

66. Friden J: Muscle soreness after exercise: Implications of morphological changes. Int J Sports Med 5:57–66, 1984

67. Gardner GW: Specificity of strength changes of the exercised and non-exercised limb following isometric training. Res Q 34:98–101, 1963

68. Gerchmann LB, Edgerton VR, Carrow RE: Effects of physical training on the histochemistry and morphology of ventral motor neurons. Exp Neurol 49:790–801, 1975

69. Gerhard H, Schachter EN: Exercise-induced asthma. Postgrad Med 67:91–101, 1980

70. Gillette HE: Systems of Therapy in Cerebral Palsy. Springfield, IL, Charles C Thomas, 1969

71. Goldberg AL, Etlinger JD, Goldspink DF, Jablecki C: Mechanism of work-induced hypertrophy of skeletal muscle. Med Sci Sports 7:185–198, 1975

72. Goldspink G, Tabary C, Tabary JC et al: Effect of denervation on the adaptation of sarcomere number and muscle extensibility to the functional length of the muscle. J Physiol 236:733–742, 1974

73. Gollnick PH: Relationship of strength and endurance with skeletal muscle structure and metabolic potential. Int J Sports Med 3:26–32, 1982

74. Gollnick PD, Hermansen L: Biochemical adaptations to exercise: Anaerobic metabolism. Exerc Sport Sci Rev 1:1–43, 1973

75. Gollnick PD, Karlsson J, Piehl K, Saltin B: Selective glycogen depletion in skeletal muscle fibers of man following sustained contractions. J Physiol 241:59–67, 1974

76. Gollnick PD, Matoba H: The muscle fiber composition of skeletal muscle as a predictor of athletic success. An overview. Am J Sports Med 12:212–217, 1984

77. Gollnick PD, Piehl K, Saltin B: Selective glycogen depletion pattern in human muscle fibers after exercise of varying intensity and at varying pedalling rates. J Physiol 241:45–57, 1974

78. Gonyea W, Sale D, Gonyea F, Milesky A: Exercise induced increases in muscle fiber number. Eur J Appl Physiol 55:137–141, 1986

79. Greer M, Dimick S, Burns S: Heart rate and blood pressure response to several methods of strength training. Phys Ther 64:179–183, 1984

80. Grimby G, Danneskiold-Samsoe B, Hvid K, Saltin B: Morphology and enzymatic capacity in arm and leg muscles in 78–81 year old men and women. Acta Physiol Scand 115:125–134, 1982

81. Grimby G, Gustafsson E, Peterson L, Renstrom P: Quadriceps function and training after knee ligament surgery. Med Sci Sports Exerc 12:70–75, 1980

82. Gruner JA, Glaser RM, Feinberg SD et al: A system for evaluation and exercise-conditioning of paralyzed leg muscles. J Rehabil R & D 20:21–30, 1983

83. Haggmark T, Eriksson E, Jansson E: Muscle fiber type changes in human skeletal muscle after injuries and immobilization. Orthopedics 9:181–185, 1986

84. Hakkinen K, Komi PV: Electromyographic changes during strength training and detraining. Med Sci Sports Exerc 15:455–460, 1983

85. Hakkinen K, Komi PV, Alen M: Effect of explosive type strength on isometric force- and rehabilitation-time, electromyographic and muscle fibre characteristics of leg extensor muscles. Acta Physiol Scand 125:587–600, 1985

86. Harris FA: Facilitation techniques in therapeutic exercise. In Basmajian JV: Therapeutic Exercise, 3rd ed. Baltimore, Williams & Wilkins, 1978

87. Hasan Z, Enoka RM, Stuart DG: The interface between biomechanics and neurophysiology in the study of movement: Some recent approaches. Exerc Sport Sci Rev 13:169–234, 1985

88. Hellebrandt FA: Motor learning reconsidered: A study of change. In Payton OD, Hirt S, Newton RA: Scientific Bases for Neurophysiological Approaches to Therapeutic Exercise, pp 33–45. Philadelphia, FA Davis 1977

89. Hellebrandt FA, Houtz SJ: Methods of muscle training: The influence of pacing. Phys Ther Rev 38:319–322, 1958

90. Hellebrant FA, Parrish AM, Hontz SJ: The influence of unilateral exercise on the contralateral limb. Arch Phys Med Rehabil 18:76–85, 1947

91. Herbison GJ, Jaweed MM, Ditunno JF: Effect of swimming on reinnervation of rat skeletal muscle. J Neurol Neurosurg Psychiatry 37:1247–1251, 1974

92. Herbison GJ, Jaweed MM, Ditunno JF: Exercise therapies in peripheral neuropathies. Arch Phys Med Rehabil 64:201–205, 1983

93. Herring SW, Grimm AF, Grimm BR: Regulation of sarcomere number in skeletal muscle: A comparison of hypotheses. Muscle Nerve 7:161–173, 1984

94. Hershfield S, Kottke FJ, Kubicek WG et al: Relative effects on the heart by muscular work in the upper and lower extremities. Arch Phys Med Rehabil 49:249–257, 1968

95. Hertanu JS, Davis L, Focseneanu M, Lahman L: Cardiac rehabilitation exercise program: Outcome assessment. Arch Phys Med Rehabil 67:431–435, 1986

96. Hickson RC: Interference of strength development by simultaneously training for strength and endurance. Eur J Appl Physiol 45:255–263, 1980

97. Hikida RS, Staron RS, Hagerman FC et al: Muscle fiber necrosis associated with human marathon runners. J Neurol Sci 59:185–203, 1983

98. Ho JW, Roy RR, Tweedle CD et al: Skeletal muscle fiber splitting with weight-lifting exercise in rats. Am J Anat 157:433–440, 1980

99. Holly RG, Barnett JG, Ashmore CR et al: Stretch-induced growth in chicken wing muscles: A new model of stretch hypertrophy. Am J Physiol 238:C62–C71, 1980

100. Howard H, Hoppeler H, Claassen H et al: Influences of endurance training on the ultrastructural composition of the different muscle fiber types in humans. Pflugers Arch 403:369–376, 1985

101. Hoyle G: Muscles and Their Neural Control. New York, John Wiley & Sons, 1983

102. Hubley-Kozey CL, Standish WD: Can stretching prevent athletic injuries? J Musculoskeletal Med 1:25–32, 1984

103. Ikai M, Fukunaga T: A study on training on strength per unit cross-sectional area of muscle by means of ultrasonic measurement. Eur J Appl Physiol 28:173–180, 1970

104. Ivy JL, Withers RT, Brose G et al: Isokinetic contractile properties of the quadriceps with relation to fiber type. Eur J Appl Physiol 47:247–255, 1981

105. Jansson F, Sjodin B, Tesch P: Change in muscle fiber type distribution in man after physical training. Acta Physiol Scand 104:235–237, 1978

106. Jensen MD, Miles JM: The roles of diet and exercise in the management of patients with insulin-dependent diabetes mellitus. Mayo Clin Proc 61:813–819, 1986

107. Johnson BL, Adamczyk JW, Tennoe KO, Stromme SB: A comparison of concentric and eccentric muscle training. Med Sci Sports 8:35–38, 1976

108. Johnson EW, Braddom R: Overwork weakness in facioscapulohumeral muscular dystrophy. Arch Phys Med Rehabil 52:333–336, 1971

109. Kanehisa H, Miyashita M: Specificity of velocity in strength training. Eur J Appl Physiol 52:104–106, 1983

110. Karlsson J, Nordesjo CO, Jorfeldt L, Saltin B: Muscle lactate, ATP and CP levels during exercise after physical training in man. J Appl Physiol 33:199–203, 1972

111. Kennedy C, VanHuss WD, Heusner WW: Reversal of the energy metabolism responses to endurance training by weight loading. Percept Mot Skills 39:847–852, 1974

112. Knuttgen HG: Development of muscular strength and endurance. In Knuttgen HG (ed): Neuromuscular Mechanisms for Therapeutic and Conditioning Exercises. Baltimore, University Park Press, 1976

113. Koivisto VA, Sherwin RS: Exercise in diabetes. Postgrad Med 66:87–95, 1979

114. Komi PV: Physiological and biochemical correlates of muscle function: Effects of muscle structure and stretch-shortening cycle on force and speed. Exerc Sport Sci Rev 12:81–121, 1984

115. Komi PV, Karlsson J: Physical performance, skeletal muscle enzyme activities, and fiber types in monozygous and dizygous twins of both sexes. Acta Physiol Scand 105 (Suppl):462, 1979

116. Kottke FJ: From reflex to skill: The training of coordination. Arch Phys Med Rehabil 61:551–561, 1980

117. Kottke FJ, Pauley DL, Ptak RA: The rationale for prolonged stretching for correction of shortening of connective tissue. Arch Phys Med Rehabil 47:345–352, 1966

118. Kottke TE, Casperson CJ, Hill CS: Exercise in the management and rehabilitation of selected chronic diseases. Prevent Med 13:47–65, 1984

119. Krotkiewski M, Aniansson A, Grimby G et al: The effect of unilateral isokinetic strength training on local adipose and muscle tissue morphology, thickness, and enzymes. Eur J Physiol 42:271–281, 1979

120. LaBan MM: Collagen Tisue: Implications of its response to stress in vitro. Arch Phys Med Rehabil 43:461–466, 1962

121. Lamb DR: Physiology of Exercise. Responses and Adaptations. New York, Macmillan, 1978

122. Larsson L: Morphological and functional characteristics of the ageing skeletal muscle in man. Acta Physiol Scand 104 (Supp):457, 1978

123. Larsson L, Ansved T: Effects of long-term physical detraining on enzyme histochemical and functional skeletal muscle characteristics in man. Muscle Nerve 8:714–722, 1985

124. Lehmann JF, Masock HJ, Warren CG, Koblanski JN: Effect of therapeutic temperatures on tendon extensibility. Arch Phys Med Rehabil 51:481–487, 1970

125. Levitt S: Treatment of Cerebral Palsy and Motor Delay. Oxford, Blackwell Scientific Pub, 1982

126. Light KE, Nuzik S, Personius W, Barstrom A: Low-load prolonged stretch vs high-load brief stretch in treating knee contractures. Phys Ther 64:330–333, 1984

127. Lindh M: Increase of muscle strength from isometric quadriceps exercises at different knee angles. Scand J Rehab Med 11:33–36, 1979

128. Lucas RC, Koslow R: Comparative study of static, dynamic, and proprioceptive neuromuscular facilitation stretching techniques on flexibility. Percept Mot Skills 58:615–618, 1984

129. MacDougall JD, Elder GCB, Sale DG et al: Effects of strength training and immobilization of human muscle fibers. Eur J Appl Physiol 43:25–34, 1980

130. Mahler DA, Loke J: The physiology of endurance exercise. The marathon. Clin Chest Med 5:63–76, 1984

131. Maier A, Crockett JL, Simpson DR et al: Properties of immobilized guinea pig hindlimb muscles. Am J Physiol 231:1520–1526, 1976

132. Mannheimer JS: A comparison of strength gain between concentric and eccentric contractions. Phys Ther 49:1201–1207, 1969

133. Marteniuk RG: Individual differences in motor performance. Exerc Sport Sci Rev 2:103–130, 1974

134. Matthews GE: Pediatric Rehabilitation. Baltimore, Williams & Wilkins, 1985

135. McDonagh MJN, Davies CTM: Adaptive response of mammalian skeletal muscle to exercise with high loads. Eur J Appl Physiol 52:139–155, 1984

136. McDonagh MJN, Hayward CM, Davies CTM: Isometric training in human elbow flexor muscles. J Bone Joint Surg 65-B:355–358, 1983

137. Milner-Brown HS, Miller RG: Muscle membrane excitation and impulse propagation velocity are reduced during muscle fatigue. Muscle Nerve 9:367–374, 1986

138. Milner-Brown HS, Stein RB, Lee RG: Synchronization of human motor units. Possible roles of exercise and supraspinal reflexes. EEG Clin Neurophysiol 38:245–254, 1975

139. Mitchell JH, Wildenthal K: Static (isometric) exercise and the heart: Physiological and clinical considerations. Ann Rev Med 25:369–381, 1974

140. Moore MA, Hutton RS: Electromyographic investigation of muscle stretching techniques. Med Sci Sports Exerc 12:322–329, 1980

141. Moritani T, deVries HA: Neural factors versus hypertrophy in the time course of muscle strength gain. Am J Phys Med 58:115–130, 1979

142. Muller EA: Influence of training and inactivity on muscle strength. Arch Phys Med Rehabil 51:449–462, 1970

143. Newham DJ, Jones DA, Edwards RHT: Plasma creatine kinase changes after eccentric and concentric contractions. Muscle Nerve 9:59–63, 1986

144. Nordemar R, Ekblom B, Zachrisson L, Lundqvist K: Physical training in rheumatoid arthritis. Scand J Rheumatol 10:17–23, 1981

145. Nordin M, Frankel VH: Biomechanics of collagenous tissues. In Frankel VH, Nordin M (eds): Basic Biomechanics of the Skeletal System. Philadelphia, Lea & Febiger, 1980

146. Noyes FR, Keller CS, Grood ES, Butler DL: Advances in the understanding of knee ligament injury, repair, and rehabilitation. Med Sci Sports Exerc 16:427–443, 1984

147. Nutter DO, Schlannt RD, Hurst JW: Isometric exercise and the cardiovascular system. Modern Concepts of Cardiovascular Disease 41:11–15, 1972

148. Osternig LR, Bates BT, James SL: Isokinetic and isometric torque force relationships. Arch Phys Med Rehabil 58:254–257, 1977

149. Parker RH: The effects of mild one-legged isometric or dynamic training. Eur J Appl Physiol 54:262–268, 1985

150. Parker MG, Ruhling RO, Bolen TA et al: Aerobic training and the force-velocity relationship of the human quadriceps femoris muscle. J Sports Med 23:136–147, 1983

151. Penman KA: Human striated muscle ultra structural changes accompanying increased strength without hypertrophy. Res Q 41:418–424, 1970

152. Pette D, Vrbova G: Invited review: Neural control of phenotype expression in mammalian muscle fibers. Muscle Nerve 8:676–686, 1985

153. Pipes TP, Wilmore JH: Isokinetic vs isotonic strength training in adult men. Med Sci Sports 7:262–274, 1975

154. Pollock ML, Wilmore JH, Fox SM: Exercise in Health and Disease. Philadelphia, WB Saunders, 1984

155. Prince FP, Hikida RS, Hagerman FC et al: A morphometric analysis of human muscle fibers with relation to fiber types and adaptations to exercise. J Neurol Sci 49:165–179, 1981

156. Reitsma W: Skeletal muscle hypertrophy after heavy exercise in rats with surgically reduced muscle function. Am J Phys Med 48:237–258, 1969

157. Richardson WJ, Garrett WE: Clinical uses of continuous passive motion. Contemp Orthop 10:75–79, 1985

158. Rose DL, Radzminski SF, Beatty RR: Effect of brief maximal exercise on the strength of the quadriceps femoris. Arch Phys Med Rehabil 38:157–164, 1957

159. Rosentsweig J, Hinson MM: Comparison of isometric, isotonic and isokinetic exercises by electromyography. Arch Phys Med Rehabil 53:249–252, 1972

160. Rubinstein N, Mabuchi K, Pepe F et al: Use of type specific antimyosins to demonstrate the transformation of individual fibers in chronically stimulated rabbit fast muscles. J Cell Biol 79:252–261, 1978

161. Rutherford O, Jones D: The role of learning and coordination in strength training. Eur J Appl Physiol 55:100–105, 1986

162. Sachdeo SK, Schneider SH, Khachadurian AK: Exercise in the treatment of diabetes mellitus. Practical Diabetology 2:1–18, 1983

163. Salleo A, Anastasi G, LaSpada G et al: New muscle fiber production during compensatory hypertrophy. Med Sci Sports Exerc 12:268–273, 1980

164. Salmons S, Hendriksson J: The adaptive response of skeletal muscle to increased use. Muscle Nerve 4:94–105, 1981

165. Saltin B, Gollnick PD: Skeletal muscle adaptability: Significance for metabolism and performance. In Peachey LD, Adrian RH, Geiger SR (eds): Handbook of Physiology. Section 10: Skeletal Muscle, pp 555–631. Bethesda, MD American Physiological Society, 1983

166. Schmidt RA: Past and future issues in motor programming. Res Q Exerc Sport 51:122–140, 1980

167. Shepard RJ: Physiology and Biochemistry of Exercise. New York, Praeger, 1982

168. Slater-Hammel AT: Bilateral effects from muscle activity. Res Q 21:203–209, 1950

169. Smith EM, Juvinall RC, Bender LF et al: Flexor forces and rheumatoid metacarpophalangeal deformity. Clinical implications. JAMA 198:130–134, 1966

170. Stefanovska A, Vodovnik L: Change in muscle force following electrical stimulation. Scand J Rehab Med 17:141–146, 1985

171. Stelmach GE, Larish DD: A new perspective on motor skill automation. Res Q Exerc Sport 51:141–157, 1980

172. Stull GA, Clark DH: High resistance, low-repetition training as a determinant of strength and fatiguability. Res Q 41:189–193, 1970

173. Swezey RL, Weiner SR: Rehabilitation medicine and arthritis. In McCarty DJ (ed): Arthritis and Allied Conditions, pp 697–721. Philadelphia, Lea & Febiger, 1985

174. Talag TS: Residual muscle soreness as influenced by concentric, eccentric and static contraction. Res Q 44:458–469, 1973

175. Tardieu C, Tabary JC, Tabary C, Tardieu G: Adaptation of connective tissue length to immobilization in the lengthened and shortened positions in cat soleus muscle. J Physiol (Paris) 78:214–220, 1982

176. Tesch PA, Thorsson A, Kaiser P: Muscle capillary supply and fiber type characteristics in weight and power lifters. J Appl Physiol 56:35–38, 1984

177. Tesch PA, Wright JE, Vogel JA: The influence of muscle metabolic characteristics on physical performance. Eur J Appl Physiol 54:237–243, 1985

178. Thistle HG, Hislop HJ, Moffroid M, Lowman EW: Isokinetic contraction: A new concept of resistive exercise. Arch Phys Med Rehabil 48:279–282, 1967

179. Thorstensson A: Muscle strength, fibre types and enzyme activities in man. Acta Physiol Scand (Suppl) 443:1–45, 1976

180. Tihanyi J, Apor P, Fekete G: Force-velocity power characteristics and fiber composition in human knee extensor muscles. Eur J Appl Physiol 48:331–343, 1982

181. Tipton CM, Matthes RD, Maynard JA, Carey RA: The influence of physical activity on ligaments and tendons. Med Sci Sports 7:165–175, 1975

182. Urbaniak JR, Cahill JD, Mortenson RA: Tendon suturing methods: Analysis of tensile strengths. In: Am Academy of Orthopedic Surgeons, Symposium on Tendon Surgery in the Hand, pp 70–80. St Louis, CV Mosby, 1975

183. VanBrocklin JD, Ellis DG: A study of the mechanical behavior of toe extensor tendons under applied stress. Arch Phys Med Rehabil 46:369–373, 1965

184. Van Linge B: The response of muscle to strenuous exercise. J Bone Joint Surg 44B:711–721, 1962

185. Vignos PJ: Physical models of rehabilitation in neuromuscular disease. Muscle Nerve 6:323–338, 1983

186. Ward J, Fisk GH: The difference in response of the quadriceps and the biceps brachii muscles to isometric and isotonic exercise. Arch Phys Med Rehabil 45:614–620, 1964

187. Warren CG, Lehmann JF, Koblanski JN: Heat and stretch procedures: An evaluation using rat tail tendon. Arch Phys Med Rehabil 57:122–126, 1976

188. Weltman A, Regan JD: Prior exhaustive exercise and subsequent maximal constant load exercise performance. Int J Sports Med 4:184–189, 1983

189. Wills CA, Caiozzo VJ, Yasukawa DI et al: Effects of immobilization on human skeletal muscle. Orthop Rev 11:57–64, 1982

190. Wilmore JH: Alterations in strength, body composition and anthropomorphic measurements consequent to a 10-week weight training program. Med Sci Sports 6:133–138, 1974

191. Winter DA, Wells RP, Orr GW: Errors in the use of isokinetic dynamometers. Eur J Appl Physiol 46:397–408, 1981

192. Wolf JM (ed): The results of treatment in cerebral palsy. Springfield, Charles C Thomas, 1969

193. Woo SLY, Matthews JV, Akeson WH et al: Connective tissue response to immobility. Arthritis Rheum 18:257–164, 1975

19

Adaptive Systems and Devices for the Disabled

Catherine W. Britell

Samuel R. McFarland

Adaptation of technology to allow an individual to compensate for a disability is a very important part of the rehabilitation process. Whether an assistive device is as simple as a jar opener or as complex as a personal robot, the greater level of independent functioning it allows results in improved self-esteem, more meaningful interaction with others, and practical independent skills.

As a member of the rehabilitation team, the rehabilitation engineer contributes expertise in basic mechanics, biophysics, electronics, and systems analysis, as well as skill in determining feasibility and economics of development of adaptive systems. Familiar with all aspects of a wide range of disabilities, the rehabilitation engineer is able to use his or her unique problem-solving ability to adapt existing technology or devise new systems to solve the problems presented by a disability.

Two of the major goals of technology adaptation are to improve mobility and to facilitate manipulation of the user's environment. Mobility in the home, community, and workplace is a major determinant of self-esteem, of the attitudes of others, and of employability. The old image of the person with a disability as a shut-in is quickly dispelled by the quadriplegic corporate lawyer, psychiatrist, or stockbroker who drives to work and functions superbly in a highly competitive setting. The concept of environmental control has expanded greatly as computers have become inexpensive and available common tools in the home and workplace for communication, data management, systems control, and entertainment. Microprocessors have made it possible to make control functions ever more complex and compact to fit practical space and energy requirements.

Modern technology affords almost limitless possibilities for the accomplishment of isolated tasks, no matter what the disability to be overcome, and it is often tempting to look toward ever more complex devices to solve the problems presented by a disability. As a device becomes more complex, however, its cost increases, as does its potential for malfunction and the necessity of maintenance, adjustment, and repair. Furthermore, as more energy is required to operate a device, it and its operator become less mobile, tied down by cumbersome power sources. Another limitation of technology is acceptance by the user.[4] As an extension of the individual using it, an adaptive device must be aesthetically pleasing and must not interfere with human interaction and communication. By affording greater independence, a complex environmental control device may, for instance, isolate the user by allowing the individual to be without a constant attendant. Fear of this isolation is often a major reason for poor acceptance of environmental control devices. In addition, an individual surrounded by a complex array of switches, motors, and actuators may become quite formidable to others. People may be reluctant to touch him or her or may find it difficult to listen to what he or she has to say because of preoccupation with the devices.

Cost is an important factor when considering devices. Since the major cost is in research and development, it is most economical to use existing technology whenever available. It follows, then, that knowledge of devices and systems available is essential to finding the most cost-effective solution to mobility, control, and communications problems, and the ability to make minor adaptations in existing systems will often be necessary. The line between effective problem-solving and gadgetry must be carefully observed, and the goals of functional independence and meeting the needs of the patient must be kept in sight. In order to do this, rehabilitation engineering as a rehabilitative discipline must be integrated into the entire rehabilitation process. The engineer should be involved early as a member of the rehabilitation team in order to become familiar with the pertinent medical, physical, psychological, social, and vocational issues of the patient and to take part in decision-making regarding the entire rehabilitation process.

PERSONAL MOBILITY

Wheelchairs

The proper wheelchair can often be the major determinant of free community mobility and adequate self-esteem, and should be chosen with the goal of optimizing efficiency and appearance.[7] Wheelchair prescription is most often carried out by the rehabilitation team, with the physical therapist or occupational therapist performing the major part of the evaluation and determining most necessary specifications, incorporating input from the physician, nurse, and vocational rehabilitation specialist. Since most payors require that a physician take overall responsibility for wheelchair prescription, it is imperative that physicians understand the functions, aesthetics, mechanics, and economics of wheelchairs.

Choice of a wheelchair is dictated by the user's size, weight, activity, and level of disability. For a person who spends a significant amount of time in a wheelchair and who depends upon the chair for mobility, it is imperative that the wheelchair be customized, with the features that will maximize mobility for that person.[5]

Everyone in a wheelchair should have every opportunity possible to maintain strength, aerobic fitness, and a rewarding recreational life. To do this, a specialized chair is often necessary, particularly for those in competitive sports. No one chair will be adequate for all sports or for all people participating in the same activity. Also, because of the large number of sports wheelchair manufacturers, it is useful to have one rehabilitation team member evaluate the wide array of chairs from a knowledgeable professional standpoint and advise the patient on the most appropriate choice.

Traditionally, wheelchair design and selection was carried out according to the needs of the professional care-givers and not of the users. As wheelchairs have become more user-friendly, mobility and other capabilities of people with disabilities have improved. It is important to remember that an optimally independent and educated user is often in the best position to make appropriate decisions regarding his or her means of locomotion, which is, after all, an extension of the user.

Manual Wheelchairs

When considering a manual wheelchair, the goal is to find one with the lightest weight that affords appropriate durability (Fig. 19-1). There are many materials available for wheelchair frames, from chrome-plated steel to stainless steel to aluminum to many light, strong alloys. Manual wheelchair frames are generally of two designs: those that fold and those that do not. In general, the nonfolding frames afford greater strength for weight; however, newer folding models may not be significantly heavier or less durable.

Many newer wheelchair frames afford wide flexibility in the placement of wheels, casters, seats, leg rests, and arms. They allow wheelchair modification during the course of rehabilitation for a patient for whom one anticipates a high level of function in the chair.

ADJUSTMENT CAPABILITY. Axles and bearings should afford locomotion with the least possible expenditure of energy. Most good-quality manual wheelchairs afford adjustment capability for the rear axle (Fig. 19-2). Besides bearings, which are most often maximized in good-quality chairs, the important factors which arise from wheel-axle components are axle location and weight distribution, height position, width adjustment, and camber adjustments.

Axle location and weight distribution. Moving the rear axle forward causes the chair to roll easier by shifting the weight more toward the axle of the larger rear wheel. At the same time, the balance is affected so as to make the chair tip backward more

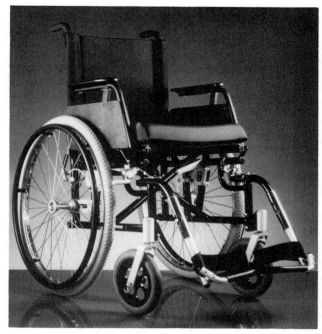

Figure 19-1. A lightweight wheelchair.

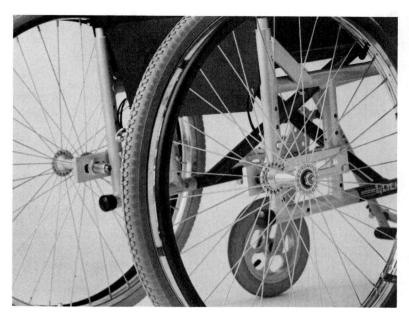

Figure 19-2. An axle plate allows adjustment of rear wheel location to accommodate various needs.

easily. Placing the rear axle farther back will make the chair more stable, but will require more energy for wheeling and make the turning radius larger. In general, a more active person with good trunk stability will have wheels moved more forward, and a person with a higher level disability will require more rear placement. Often, as a person progresses in rehabilitation, wheel placement may be changed.

Height position. Many wheelchairs allow seat height to be modified by raising or lowering the rear axle and caster positions. This is useful in adapting to taller users; however, raising the seat will lessen the overall stability of the chair. In general, seating is most comfortable and stable with the seat tilted backward by 3° to 5°. This will also allow greater stability in the wheelchair for people with poor trunk control without tying them into the chair.

Width adjustments. It is possible on many chairs to space the wheels out laterally to increase mediolateral stability. Obviously, this adds to the overall width of the chair, which becomes a factor in negotiating doorways and tight spaces. It is generally most desirable to have the narrowest chair possible which will allow adequate seat width. Wraparound armrests help to decrease chair width. If a folding chair must be temporarily narrowed to go through a doorway, a crank device may be used to partially fold the chair.

Camber adjustments. *Camber* is the angle between the vertical axis of the wheels and a line perpendicular to the floor. For general uses, having the wheels tilted approximately 7° outward from top to bottom will maximize lateral stability without making the chair too wide. Many chairs allow changes in camber by the addition of camber washers. For some sports uses, an increase in camber is necessary to maximize stability in quick turns or for long reachers.

Connection. A quick-disconnect axle (Fig. 19-3) is very convenient, both with folding and nonfolding chairs, for portability.

Figure 19-3. A quick-disconnect axle.

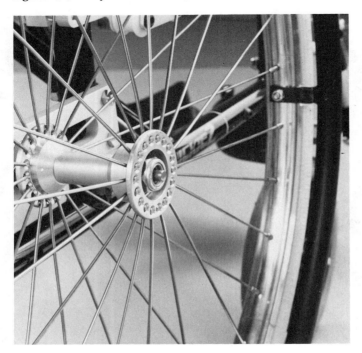

WHEELS. Wheels may have spokes, which are lighter in weight, or "mag-type" solid construction, which is heavier but more durable. Tire type is determined by the terrain and use intended. In general, solid, smooth tires are best on smooth, hard indoor floors, as found in the nursing home. Pneumatic tires will give a smoother ride outdoors on uneven ground, and treads will afford better traction. Flat tires can be minimized by thorn-resistant tubes or by the addition of a latex gel, which takes the place of the air but adds considerable weight.

SUPPORT. Armrests can aid significantly in transfers, weight shifts, reducing ischial pressure by carrying the weight of the arms, and maintaining trunk balance. Those who have marginal pressure management should definitely use sturdy, supporting armrests that are variable in height. Those with poor trunk control, generally above about T6, often need armrests for stability. Armrests may be removable or fixed, and may be adjustable to maximize support. For most users with significant lower extremity dysfunction, removable armrests will greatly facilitate transfers. Those who do weight shifts easily and have no skin problems often choose to dispense with armrests, partly for greater freedom of movement and also significantly for cosmesis.

When wheeling outside, clothing protectors attached to armrests are useful in keeping the clothes from getting dirty or torn, especially if the user's stature is at the limits of the width of the chair. These can be metal sides, which are part of the armrests, or lightweight plastic or fabric triangles laced to the armrest or the back.

Wheelchair back height should be sufficient to support the user in good posture and prevent fatigue over an extended time, while affording as much freedom of movement as possible. In all cases the back should provide good support for the lumbar spine. An adjustable back height is sometimes desirable for the user with varying needs throughout the day. It is very important that the wheelchair back does not force the user into a poor posture. Push handles are a matter of individual taste. At this time, most users prefer not to have these on the chair, since they denote expectations of a certain amount of dependence and are often associated with invalidism. Obviously, if the user spends a significant amount of time being pushed, the handles are a necessity.

The purpose of leg supports and footrests is to afford protection, proper positioning, and maximal balance and weight-bearing. The height of footrests should enable the foot to be supported sufficiently to maintain circulation in the lower extremities and keep the ankle in a neutral position, but should not be so high as to force more weight backward onto the ischial tuberosities and risk pressure ulcers. For someone with significant spasticity, a large foot plate with a proper foot restraint system may be necessary. If wheelchair control is imprecise, or the feet are not clearly visible, foot plates that afford protection from injury may be indicated. Someone with a high degree of mobility, good control, and who readily maintains ankle range of motion may do just as well with a simple bar with webbing or, at most, tubular footrests, which are much lighter. Swing-away and detachable swing-away leg rests, available on many chairs, (Fig. 19-4) often greatly simplify transfers for a highly involved individual. The trade-off is added weight and narrowing of wheelchair choices. Elevating the leg rests is often done in treating lower extremity edema, injury, or a stiff knee, but in the long run, if possible, the problem should be managed in another way, since the elevated leg greatly alters accessibility, turning, balance, and cosmesis.

HAND RIMS AND BRAKES. Hand rims may be of varying sizes and have a number of modifications to aid in gripping, from a simple increase in tubular size to rim projections. For high speeds, a smaller diameter rim which is relatively smooth and is close to the wheel is best. For power and maneuverability, a large rim is indicated. Coatings may increase gripping and improve appearance, but virtually all coatings eventually rub off, discolor the hands, or become rough and may injure the hands. A good pair of leather gloves is often the first and best way to improve gripping of the hand rims. Rim projections are sometimes useful for the person with quadriplegia, and may be varied in spacing and angle. Another means of improving gripping on hand rims is to position them at a distance to the wheel that allows the hands

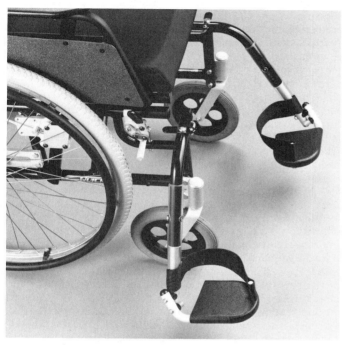

Figure 19-4. Detachable, swing-away footrests.

to use the sidewalls of the tires for increased traction without touching the treads.

Brakes are necessary for almost all users (Fig. 19-5). The only significant variation seen is to position them low for very active people who use a very long pushing stroke and who thus sometimes jam their thumbs on brakes in the traditional position. Brake handles may be extended and positioned for greater ease of setting and releasing. Those who have difficulty maintaining forward momentum going uphill benefit from grade aids, or hill climbers, which are simple spring-loaded teeth which allow the chair to move only forward, and can be selectively activated on uphill grades (Fig. 19-6).

CASTERS. Casters are most often on the front of the chair. In general, a caster that is hard and contacts the ground in a small area (is of small diameter) affords the best turning characteristics (as for basketball and tennis). On the other hand, this kind of caster will get stuck on uneven terrain or soft ground, and so a larger pneumatic caster has greater utility outdoors. For track and field uses, very large diameter casters will minimize bearing friction on the strightaway and turns are most often gentle. Caster placement toward the rear of the chair increases turning ability but decreases stability.

Electrically Powered Wheelchairs

In general, in considering a powered wheelchair, weight is less important and functional characteristics and reliability are of greater concern. The overall goal associated with a choice of a powered chair is greater mobility over a wider range with greater independence. It must be remembered, however, that the decreased portability of the electrically powered chair will complicate community mobility. Powered wheelchairs must be considered in much the same way as environmental controls, taking into account all of the abilities of the user and making maximal use of them to achieve the purpose at hand.

Frame and wheels must be of sufficient strength for the weight of the individual and the use intended. Individual choices

Figure 19-5. Brake options: (*A*) pull-to-lock high brakes, (*B*) push-to-lock high brakes with extension, and (*C*) low brakes.

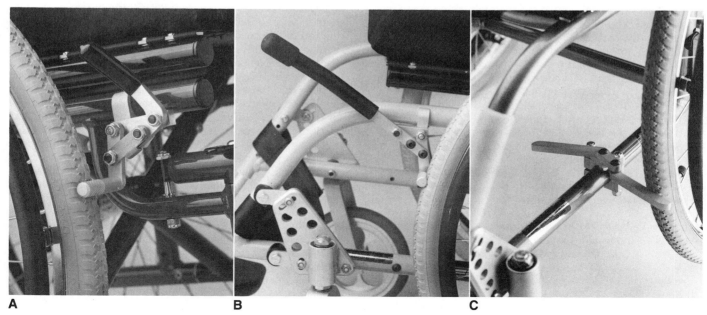

A   B   C

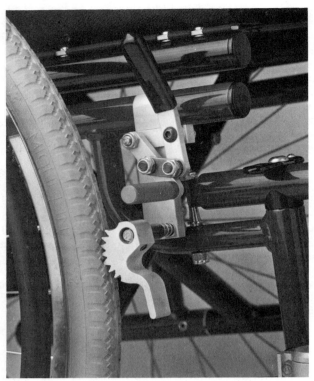

Figure 19-6. Grade aid has spring-loaded teeth which prevent the wheelchair from rolling backward while ascending ramps or inclines.

for types of terrain exist, but are more limited than with manual chairs, though the basic principles remain the same.

POWER AND CONTROL. Power sources consist of batteries, which must be recharged regularly. There are many types of batteries, mounts, casings, and connections, varying with make and model of wheelchair. Two major types of batteries are the fluid acid and gel. The gel batteries do not present problems with acid spills and thus are often transportable on airplanes. They also have less free hydrogen generation, and thus greater presumed safety around open flames, such as in welding.

Motors vary widely in power and durability, and the general rule of thumb is to choose the motor that will perform the task required with the best weight, cost, and energy use characteristics. Speed is a function of the motor and the power linkage. Power linkages are generally of two types: direct drive and belts. Direct drive generally affords a more durable linkage, but puts the motor close to the ground, making repair more involved and costly. Belts allow a greater range of placement, often allow higher speeds, are relatively inexpensive to replace, and provide a margin of protection for the motors. However, they break or slip frequently and are generally the most common source of malfunction.

A feature which can greatly assist the user who has marginal or slowly responsive control of the chair is a braking system which maintains braking when no control input is received. If, for instance, the user lets go of the controls on a grade or ramp, the chair will maintain position until control is regained.

It is desirable to have a control system for a powered wheelchair which is as quick to respond and direct as possible. The *joystick* is the most widely used control system, and can be operated by a hand or arm, the foot, or the chin or tongue. For those unable to use a joystick, *pneumatic switches* operated by "sip and puff" have shown themselves to be a reliable and

functional indirect control system. *Voice-actuated controls* have been around in some form for a considerable period, but have not yet proved widely useful. Significant recent gains in the technology of voice recognition and actuation will probably eventually be incorporated into a highly functional voice-actuated wheelchair control system. Other experimental systems, such as eye position control, ultrasound-mediated head position control, and muscle electrical activity control have shown promise but are still under study.[23] It is often cost-effective to incorporate environmental control and communication functions into wheelchair controls, since the user often has limited functional reach.

An electrically powered, self-reclining wheelchair can indeed be a formidable piece of equipment. It is necessary to remember that the user's expression and interpersonal communication often are centered around the head and face, and so it is imperative that if possible the head and face not be encumbered or surrounded by machinery. The other important aesthetic consideration is the desirability of enclosing wires, tubes, gears, motors, clamps, and any other devices in a rounded, smooth, unobtrusive casing, in order that attention is drawn appropriately to the person in the chair rather than the machinery that surrounds him or her. Another consideration is noise. The quieter the function of the device, the less attention it will draw to itself, and the more effective it will allow the user to be.

SUPPORT. Most often, people who need powered chairs have difficulty maintaining trunk control and stability and so require extra support. The use of thorax pads or shoulder or chest belts, slightly reclining the back, or a combination of these methods can help. It is important to note that by tying a person into the wheelchair, effective weight shifts for pressure relief are made impossible without reclining the chair. Therefore, the user should be confined only enough to maintain acceptable posture and stability.

In patients in whom there is no trunk stability or ability to do independent weight-shifting, a reclining back (paired with elevating footrests and supportive arm- and headrests) is a must (Fig. 19-7). This can be manual or electrically powered. The electrically powered system provides the greatest level of independence; however, these systems require regular maintenance and repair, add significantly to the expense and weight of the unit, and require some control ability on the part of the user.

When prescribing a powered reclining system, there are a number of important considerations. First, seating must be stable and supportive, and provide good pressure relief. The movement of reclining and resuming the upright position, especially when there is spasticity, will often put the user into an uneven posture, which can lead to pressure sores and skeletal deformities unless there is an appropriately supportive seating system. Another important consideration is shear. This is handled in one of three ways: sliding of the seat section, sliding of the back section, or a tilt-back system which maintains the legs and trunk at 90° to each other. Each has its advantages and disadvantages for various patient problems; however, the system using the sliding back is generally applicable to the widest variety of situations.

A third consideration is that all powered recline systems add 1 to 2 inches to the seat height. This increase may be just enough to prevent the user from wheeling up to tables, and as a result may require the basic chair that is ordered from the manufacturer to be lower. Although manual recline systems often require a fair amount of strength and coordination for the attendant to operate, and can be frightening for patient and attendant to use, they may be the best choice if the user needs to recline only occasionally.

Arm and leg support must often be modified to deal with

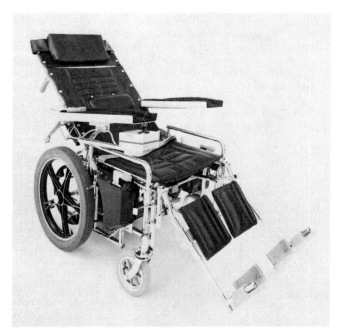

Figure 19-7. A reclining wheelchair is usually necessary for a person who cannot do adequate weight shifts. Armrests and legrests must provide support for the limbs in all positions.

spasticity or lack of body control. Modifications most often used are trough arm or leg rests with appropriate restraints for extremities.

Scooters

There are a number of three-wheeled and four-wheeled devices available to improve mobility. These scooters come in a wide variety of sizes and prices, and are generally most useful for people who are usually ambulatory but who have limited stamina. A major advantage is more portability than with an electric wheelchair. Additionally, the golfcart–like appearance is often more acceptable to the elderly person with little tolerance for disability in himself or others. These devices are seldom adequate for a person who has significant neuromuscular dysfunction and requires a wheelchair for all functions, since transfers and seating stability require fairly good neuromuscular control. Additionally, there are very few modifications available for a person with limited hand function; most scooters were designed for those with normal or near-normal use of their upper extremities.

When considering one of these devices, the physician must be certain that the condition is not progressive so that an actual wheelchair will soon be necessary, and that the patient's perhaps inappropriate fixation on the need for such a device is not a symptom of unhealthy reaction to a significant disability evidenced by unrealistic planning and expectations. However, particularly in elderly patients with stable orthopedic and cardiopulmonary limitations, these devices can greatly improve mobility and self-esteem, and increase general activity level and psychological health.

Special Considerations

WHEELCHAIR CUSHIONS. No wheelchair prescription should be written without consideration for the proper cushion. The two major functions of cushions are to maximize pressure relief over vulnerable areas and to provide a stable seating base, and these are the major considerations in cushion choice.[9] Other considerations include weight, durability, cleanability, cost, temperature, and appearance. In general, the best pressure relief is obtained with a multichambered villous pneumatic cushion.[10] This type of cushion, however, provides very little seating stability and is quite expensive. A firm, contoured foam cushion often provides the best stability with sometimes less-than-optimal pressure relief.[21] A cushion which uses a jelly-filled bladder over a firm, contoured foam base is excellent for some users, but is also costly. Other cushions, including gel, foam, and liquid flotation, all have their adherents and specialized uses; however, all must by judged by the following two absolutes:

1. Is pressure relief adequate for the patient?
2. Does the cushion provide stable, symmetrical seating for the patient?

The cushion to prescribe will be the one that meets both criteria at the lowest cost.

The treatment team can determine the proper cushion after getting to know the user. Some people, especially those who are very active, seldom experience skin breakdown regardless of the type of cushion used[30] These people often prefer a thin foam or simple pneumatic cushion, which serves them very well. Others seem to have skin problems no matter what is done to prevent them and require absolutely the best pressure relief available. In these patients it is often helpful to perform pressure measurements over areas at risk, using one of several available measuring devices.[21] Most wheelchair users fall somewhere between these extremes, and particular uses or needs dictate the type of cushion prescribed. For a person who is active, vigilant about pressure, and has good general health, his or her personal preference is often an important determinant of cushion type.[11]

For children with moderate to severe neuromuscular problems, special or custom seating may be required.[2, 25] This may consist of a modular insert, specifically sized and adjusted to the support needs of the user. The advantage of this system is that it may accommodate for some growth of the user. Another group of systems uses expanded polyethylene spheres, or beads, which form a soft conforming "bean bag" around the user and which hardens in place when a vacuum is applied while the user is seated on it.[26] Then, either the beads themselves form the seat by use of an epoxy-vinyl paint system, or a plaster cast is made and a contoured form seat insert is molded. Though this special seating is expensive, the benefits in positioning the severely spastic or weak child for optimal functioning far outweigh the cost.[27]

UPHOLSTERY. For a person who spends significant time in a wheelchair, color should be another consideration. Patients should be encouraged early on to choose colors and styles, since this is much like a piece of clothing and should be pleasing to the user. Often the act of choosing colors is the first step to reconciliation to use of the chair.[15]

Upholstery which is impervious to body secretions, is easily cleanable and attractive, and does not stretch is optimal. Many of the newer upholstery fabrics are easily removable from the chair and are machine-washable.

STANDING FRAMES AND SUPPORTS. The health benefits of standing for wheelchair-bound individuals may include relief of spasticity, maintenance of range of motion, retardation of bone demineralization, and psychological benefits, although there is little supportive scientific evidence. A wheelchair user may have a vocational need for an upright position, such as for an auto mechanic or a surgeon, and this is often the most important indication for the use of a standing frame. Standing frames may be stationary or mobile, manual or motorized.

Before embarking on a standing program, the patient should have a complete physical examination, concentrating on motion and stability of the trunk, back, and lower extremities. Roentgenograms of the hips, knees, ankles, feet, and long bones should be checked for severe osteoporosis, bone cysts, or joint dislocation. The patient should then undergo a program of mobilization using a tilt table with careful blood pressure monitoring to build tolerance of the upright position. Complications of standing include hypotension and syncope, pressure sores on the feet or knees, lower extremity edema, and fractures. Therefore, a patient starting to use a standing frame should be under close therapist and physician supervision.

A number of different kinds of standing frames are available. The most economical is a rigid, stationary frame into which the user pulls himself or is lifted. This allows standing in one position only; it is used less than mobile frames, which allow the user to change position either passively (wheeled by an attendant) or actively using a manual or electric propulsion system. Getting into a standing frame can be facilitated by a manual or electric lift, which is often necessary for users with poor trunk stability or upper extremity weakness. A feature which may enhance the utility of a standing frame for tasks for which the work surface cannot be moved, such as for an auto mechanic, is the ability to tilt forward. One such device uses retractable legs, which allow a mobile frame to be tipped forward over its front wheels using a forceful shift in body weight. This device requires good trunk stability and excellent upper extremity function.

COMMUNITY MOBILITY

The ability to move about in the community is essential to carry out the important activities associated with independent living, employment, and a productive life-style.

The least expensive means to achieve community mobility is mass transit. Buses, subways, trains, and airplanes, all convey passengers along prescribed routes, according to published time schedules, from station to station. The passenger must arrive at the boarding station, move with the boarding flow, enter the vehicle, pay the fare, take a seat, endure the ride, then reverse the process at his or her destination. For a wheelchair user, anyone of these segments may prove insurmountable. Location of the station, speed of the boarding flow, access, seating space, and fares can be significant deterrents. Accessible bus demonstration programs have been very expensive and grossly underutilized. Mass transit to date is inadequate for the real community mobility needs of wheelchair users.

Taxi transportation is an effective mode for the wheelchair user who can transfer to the passenger seat, if the driver can and will load the wheelchair, and if the passenger can afford the cost. These qualifications effectively eliminate the user of an electric wheelchair because of the problems and hazards related to transfer and loading. Also, persons with communication disabilities are often unable to call and direct the driver. Wheelchair-accessible taxi-vans, available in most large cities, are prohibitive in cost and are often used only when the cost is subsidized by medical insurance.

Vans and minibus transportation systems, the so-called paratransit systems, have been tried in many metropolitan areas. Intended to combine the individualized service of the taxi with the cost savings of shared rides, the paratransit network was instituted specifically for mobility-impaired individuals. These systems have had difficulties remaining fiscally solvent without expensive government support, and are generally successful only in conjunction with independent living complexes, sheltered workshops, and college campuses, where a large number of users share a common origin or destination.

Therefore, the adapted personal vehicle, driven by the disabled person or a family member, remains the only consistently effective means of community mobility for this population. Selecting and configuring a vehicle for its user and training the user in safe and effective operation are specialized functions of most comprehensive rehabilitation centers.

The problems associated with adapting a vehicle to use by a disabled driver are those of access, restraint, and control. First, the user must be enabled to approach the vehicle, open its door, enter, move to and assume a traveling (driving) position, and close the door; and then repeat the process when arriving at the destination. Second, the user must be secured in the traveling (driving) position to facilitate function and ensure safety for both normal vehicle motion and emergency conditions. Third, the user must be interfaced to all vehicle functions over which he or she expects to exercise operational command.

Vehicles and Vehicle Modifications

Passenger Sedan

As a rule of thumb, the sedan is less expensive to purchase, modify, and operate than the van. To qualify for using a sedan, the user must be able to transfer independently to the driver's seat and to load any mobility equipment, especially a wheelchair. To load the wheelchair it is most helpful if the user can at least begin to fold and unfold it. Most experts recommend certain specific types of core and optional equipment. If the user is in a wheelchair, the front door (driver or passenger side) opening should be as wide as possible to permit easier transfer from chair to car. If the chair is to be loaded into the car, a power seat will help provide space behind the seat and a tilting wheel may help achieve space for the driver during loading and transfer.

If at least one arm or leg is nonfunctional, then an automatic transmission should be provided and power steering will be required to assist single-hand or single-foot steering. If driver hand controls will be needed and the car will be driven at highway speeds, a cruise control and power brakes are indicated. If a driver has severe neuromuscular dysfunction, such as a result of spinal cord injury or multiple sclerosis, air conditioning may be necessary to aid in body temperature regulation. Air conditioning is also helpful for many amputees, who experience skin problems and breakdown in extreme heat. Upholstery should be chosen for best breathability and heat dissipation, while being slippery enough to allow easy transfer and positioning.

Posi-traction is useful in areas where there is snow and ice, since the driver will seldom be able to shovel the vehicle out when stuck. Other means of maximizing traction in snowy weather, such as front-wheel or four-wheel drive and studded snow tires, should also be considered. A citizens' band radio is mandatory for those driving alone who are significantly disabled, and power windows, automatic door locks, and delayed-off headlights can maximize personal safety and security.

In general, the passenger sedan is easier to maneuver in traffic, more fuel efficient, and easier to park than the van. The recent popularity of smaller cars has imposed some difficult conflicts on the disabled driver. Although the smaller cars are less expensive to purchase and own, their compact spatial arrangements tend to complicate conversions for hand control and wheelchair loading. The potential driver should carefully evaluate available models before making a purchase. For most people, the full-sized two-door sedan is still the vehicle of choice.

Chair transport for sedans is accomplished in three ways:

with personal assistance, without assistance, and with powered assistance. If relying on personal assistance, the user may choose to have the chair placed inside the passenger compartment, in the trunk (or pickup bed), on an outside rack (roof or bumper), or on a trailer. Obviously, this practice will limit driver independence. Loading the chair without assistance means folding and bringing the chair inside the car, unless the user is ambulatory, in which case the previous options apply. Strong, active paraplegics or lower amputees commonly load the chair behind the front seat (two-door sedans and club cab pickups) or into the bed behind the cab (standard pickup). Four-door sedans are not appropriate because the open rear door blocks movement of the chair. If the user has trouble with the door threshold, he or she can fashion a fold-down ramp and install an overhead hand-cranked rope with which to pull the chair upward. Powered loaders are of two types: inside storing and roof storing. In each case, the user must attach a hook or sling device to the chair before operating the loading motor. Inside storage uses the rear passenger area; outside storage is in a weather-resistant box on the roof.

Driving controls allow the disabled driver to operate the vehicle safely by allowing compensation for disabilities. The least expensive adaptations for driving are levers, knobs, and extensions operated by either the right or left hand. The hand control applies the brake pedal as it is pushed toward the fire wall along the direction of the steering column. Depending on the brand, the throttle pedal is depressed by pulling back (opposite braking), swinging down toward the lap, twisting the level grip (like a motorcycle throttle), or squeezing a lever (like a motorcycle clutch). The dimmer switch (and sometimes the horn) is usually located on the hand control. The turn indicator lever is activated by the fingers of the steering hand.

If the driver has only one functional leg, he or she will operate the throttle and brake pedals either as they are or with a left-side gas pedal. Short legs can often be accommodated with pedal blocks. Short arms may be assisted by a smaller diameter steering wheel. Those with hand dysfunction or upper-extremity prostheses may be aided by steering wheel spinners (knobs, stirrups, or rings). A hearing-impaired driver should be offered extra or large mirrors to help keep track of visual cues.

Vans

For some disabled drivers, the van is the only vehicle that can accommodate their needs. If the user cannot transfer from or to his wheelchair, or does so very slowly or a great energy expense, then a van may be the vehicle of choice, because a van with a lifting device allows the user to enter and exit the vehicle while seated in the wheelchair.

Selection of the type of van and optional equipment will depend on the user, just as with the sedan. If the user is to drive, most of the automatic and power features mentioned for the sedan will be required. It is always advisable to consult the van conversion vendor before purchasing the van to maximize cost-effectiveness. Because most common adaptive modifications add to the vehicle weight, it is usually wise to select a chassis size capable of moderate to heavy load bearing (5/8 ton or greater). Larger V-8 engines are not recommended because they do not produce appreciably greater power and tend to be far more fuel hungry.

Access into a van is most often provided by a wheelchair lift, either folding or swinging. The choice is based on van type and user preference; there is no single best kind. Most lifts may be located in the side cargo opening or the rear cargo opening. Some brands will fit only one or the other. For independent operation, the lift should be fully automatic. Lift operation is

always electric, although the electric power may be applied to mechanical or hydraulic drive trains. Very few wheelchair users can reach and open the van doors to gain access to the lift, so door openers are required for all but the user with an attendant. It is also rare that an unattended user can use a ramp.

When considering van access, it is important to keep in mind two measurements: seated height and wheelchair turning space. Seated height will affect passage into the van and the eye level for driving. It may require that the doorway be extended, the roof raised, or the floor lowered. The turning space will affect location of the lift, seats, and driver station. If possible, the measurement should be taken in a modified van of the brand being considered by the user. The floor of any van will need to be overlaid with a flat plywood surface to eliminate the deep corrugations designed into the floor. Carpeting on the floor should be a close-cut pile or indoor-outdoor type with a strong jute backing. Foam padding should be avoided, and the carpet or mat should be glued to the floor to avoid bunching or twisting under wheelchair tires.

Modifications

Automobile and van seats are designed to provide stability while driving and driver protection for low-speed collisions. Wheelchairs, on the other hand, are inherently unstable, and tend to collapse easily with any significant stress. Therefore, if possible, the user should transfer into the van seat and secure the empty wheelchair. To aid transfer, the seat can be attached to a base that swivels, elevates, or retracts toward the rear of the van (or all of the above). For a person who transfers with difficulty, seat material that is slippery, such as leather or certain smooth fabrics, can be helpful. High-backed, reclining seats with folding armrests can be helpful for effectively shifting weight during stops, relieving fatigue, and promoting torso stability.

If the driver cannot transfer, then the driver's seat must be removed and appropriate alterations performed to accommodate the wheelchair location. The seated height will affect floor treatment. It is very important that the driver's eye level be low enough to allow easy viewing through the windshield and side windows. If it is too high, the floor or the wheelchair seat must be lowered. Lowering the floor in the driver's area is a complicated operation because of the proximity to engine and chassis. Both fixed and movable floor conversions involve radical surgery to the floor and chassis structures and should be ordered only if essential.

The driver and the wheelchair should be restrained separately. Normal vehicle motion and moderate collision impacts should be considered. If the driver needs postural support, a race car–type, double over-the-shoulder belt harness and head restraint should be installed.

The wheelchair-seated driver probably will need alterations to the steering assembly. A column extension will place the steering wheel nearer the operator and a change in column angle will place the wheel nearer the lap. A tilting steering column may aid the angle adjustment and also help in entering or leaving the driving position. Often the wheel is too large in diameter for the range of arm motion. Accessory wheels of smaller diameter may be appropriate.

Many quadriplegics cannot grip the wheel, so a "spinner" device (knob, stirrup, or tri-pin) may be used. The spinner should be located so that the arm is comfortable during straight-ahead driving (neutral position) and can execute a full 360° rotation. The force required to turn the steering wheel, especially when the van is not in motion, may be greater than the capability of the driver. If so, the power steering system can be modified to reduce the required input power force (so-called "reduced effort" or "zero effort" conversions). Since the power steering hydraulic supply pump is driven by the engine, an emergency back-up supply should be added to ensure steering function if the engine dies when the van is in motion.

Throttle and brake controls for sedans and vans are essentially the same. Brake actuating force may be reduced (similar to steering) by a modification to the vacuum booster in the power brake system. Like the modified steering system, the reduced-effort brake should be combined with an emergency back-up vacuum supply.

In many instances the switches and selector levers on the dash panel of the van will be out of reach for the quadriplegic driver. Extended knobs and levers will alleviate some interface problems, but a remote switch console may be required or preferred. Those functions that should be closely examined are ignition, headlights, horn, turn signals, and windshield wiper.

For severely disabled drivers, there are a number of specialized vehicle adaptations available or undergoing development. Most are hydraulically or electrically operated servo systems which put steering, throttle, and braking in a small range and use very low effort. One promising system is the Unistik,[3] in which the vehicle is controlled by a joystick much like that of a wheelchair.

Not all disabled drivers are wheelchair users. For drivers who have no arm function for driving, at least two conversion packages have been developed in add-on devices which allow a person to operate steering and switch function with only the feet.

Candidate Assessment and Driver Training

Most people take driving for granted. It is a relatively simple operation; easily learned by almost everyone. The learning can be acquired from a school, a licensed trainer, or a friend or relative, and can be accomplished with almost any vehicle. Indeed, if a person has a driver's license, it is expected that he or she can drive any car without special training or adjustment. To a person with a physical disability, however, this process becomes much more complex. He or she may need special driver modifications, or if unable to transfer out of a wheelchair, may require a special vehicle. For such special vehicles and vehicle modifications, specialized training will also be required, and must be provided and supported for these drivers.[8]

The right time to begin driver assessment and training is as soon as the driver has attained appropriate physical and cognitive skills to operate a vehicle safely. Often, for a traumatic disability, this assessment and training period will come within the initial rehabilitative hospitalization. For a person with cognitive dysfunction or severe physical disability, driver evaluation and training may be appropriate only after a long rehabilitation period, and will take place after discharge. On the one hand, it is good to introduce driving skill before the disabled person has gotten used to giving up control over his or her community mobility; but on the other hand, it is essential that the driver's chances of success be maximized.

Initially, tests of vision, hearing, reaction time, reach, strength, and range of motion are necessary to determine whether the person can handle the physical task of driving. He or she must be assessed for perception, cognition, and judgment. If there is a history of brain injury (vascular or traumatic), formal neuropsychological evaluation prior to driving may be indicated. Performance on adapted simulators can also be of assistance in screening candidates; however, their use has thus far been limited because of the narrow range of simulator adaptations available.[16] If preliminary evaluation of the candidate shows adequate driving potential, evaluation and training in an appropriately adapted training vehicle can begin. This can be carried out in many rehabilitation centers and also selected private driving schools which feature driver education for individuals with physical disabilities.

Driver's training may range from one session to show the disabled driver how to operate the hand controls, to a complex process of skill training and ongoing vehicle adaptation, depending on the level of disability. Initial training for the disabled driver should take place on a driving range, if possible, where skill in operation of the vehicle may be attained before having to face traffic. In order to undergo driver's training, the disabled driver must have a valid driver's license or a learner's permit. In order to obtain a license, the driver must bring the vehicle that he or she is going to drive to the license examiner and pass a standard road test. At present, there are essentially no limitations or standards regarding vehicle or driver station modification, except that the driver be consistently able to operate it safely and efficiently, and that normal signal and emergency devices work properly. A license obtained with an adapted vehicle will likely bear a code indicating that the driver drives "with hand controls only." Most agencies do not acknowledge a requirement for other modifications.

There are no conclusive data as to the safety record of disabled drivers, although there have been studies that show them to be safer than nondisabled counterparts.[17] Some insurance companies are very supportive of disabled drivers, while others consider them "assigned risks" and charge accordingly for liability insurance.

ENVIRONMENTAL CONTROL SYSTEMS

Patient Assessment

The initial task in solution of environmental control problems is a thorough rehabilitative evaluation of the patient. Physical rehabilitation should make the fullest use of the patient's abilities possible. It is often more functional and economical, for instance, to use the patient's own muscle power and control to perform a task than to try to develop a device which is less direct, slower, and often more difficult to control. For this reason the rehabilitation engineer, physical therapist, occupational therapist, physician, social worker, vocational rehabilitation specialist, and psychologist need to work closely together with the patient as a team in the development of environmental control systems.

The evaluation should consist of the following:

Complete testing and documentation of muscle strength, range of motion, tone, coordination, and control

Evaluation of activities of daily living and vocational abilities and needs

Assessment of the home and work environment

Testing and documentation of intelligence, perception, and motor planning, as indicated

Determination of eligibilities and entitlements for private and public fiscal support for adaptive devices

Determination of emotional stability, acceptance of the system, judgment regarding safety concerns, and psychosocial impact of the proposed system

Team consensus that the proposed goals are realistic and actually those of the patient as well as those of the treatment team

When evaluation is complete, the entire team should meet together with the patient to develop a plan for maximizing function. It is important at the outset to help the patient understand the limitations of the technology offered. It is often tempting for someone with a severe disability to maintain a "bionic man" fantasy, and it is important that such a person not be set up for disappointment and failure.

Adaptive equipment that maximizes independence should be a part of the rehabilitation process as soon as possible after the onset of disability.[22] When a person becomes severely disabled, his or her first role is an extremely dependent one, and if there is no means and encouragement to take control early on, the patient will often quickly become resigned to a dependent life-style, and will be resistant to attempts to provide means to increase independence and control. For example, during the period of intensive care that often follows major trauma, an adequate nurse call system should be set up, if the patient is unable to handle the usual call system. The occupational therapist will be able to provide a switch manageable by the patient, which can be interfaced with the call system in use. Another important early function is adequate communication. If the patient is unable, even temporarily, to speak, the speech pathologist and occupational therapist should be involved as soon as the patient is alert enough to devise an adequate communication system. A telephone system can also be very useful early on to establish control on the patient's part, and as the patient spends more time awake, control of radio, television, and tape player will greatly enhance his or her positive attitude toward independence. It is important to remember that using adaptive devices to perform tasks that were previously done effortlessly requires a change of attitude and a great deal of energy. This necessitates that the perceived payoff be great enough to warrant the energy expenditure, and that the means of accomplishing the task be accompanied by as little frustration as possible.[23]

A Systems Approach to Solving Control Problems

In choosing or developing an adaptive device or system, the following goals should be kept in mind:

Direct control: The more closely related the control function to actual performance of the task, the faster and more precise the control will be, and the less concentration it will take to accomplish it.

Reliability: Even with non-critical tasks, any failure will be very discouraging to the user, who may become frustrated enough to stop using the device. Ensuring reliability often requires development of redundant, or back-up, systems to prevent catastrophic failure of the primary system.

Simplicity: A control function should seem as automatic as possible, so that the results seem to be worth the user's effort.

Economy: Funding for adaptive devices is difficult to obtain. For this reason, it is essential that systems are as low as possible in cost.

Aesthetics: As an extension of the user, an adaptive device should not distance the user from those with whom he or she must relate.

Systems and devices for the disabled consist of four major components: a human interface or switch; one or more actuators which perform the task; a control system which processes messages from the switch to the actuator, often grouping and categorizing series of simple signals for more complex control; and connections that carry messages between components.

The Human Interface and Switch Selection

The proper human interface is essential for the utility of any device. The control site for a device is determined by the user's particular abilities and needs. Control sites may include all extremities, the head, chin and tongue, as well as the eyebrows, the voice, extraocular motion, the muscles (for electromyographic signals from any muscle that can voluntarily contract), and breath control.[1] In selecting the control site, its other uses should be considered. For example, it is difficult to carry on a conversation while using a mouth stick or voice-actuated controls. Appropriate range, power, resolution, and feedback should be factors in choosing a control site that offers the most direct control.[28]

RANGE. *Range* is the functional motion that is possible by an extremity or control site. For example, a C6 quadriplegic can reach functionally in the major part of a hemisphere in front of him, while a person with no upper extremity function or head control will be limited to control in a very small area of motion of, for example, the eyebrow or the tongue. In general, the larger the range of the control site, the more separate control functions can be managed and the greater the power available, and thus the more direct the control.

POWER. The amount of force that can be generated in a given position over time is an important consideration in selecting switches, actuators, and control systems. For instance, if there is very weak motion, an externally powered actuator will be required, whereas if a powerful motion is possible, a simpler, less expensive mechanical device will suffice.

RESOLUTION. Precision of movement, or *resolution,* is a major determinant of how many independent signals or inputs may be used to control a device. The greater the number of signals possible, the more direct the control achievable. More direct control will allow functions to be accomplished faster and more easily, with less attention to the task.

FEEDBACK. The user must have a way of knowing when a control function is accomplished successfully. In one-step direct-control tasks, the visual or auditory feedback of accomplishing the task is often sufficient. However, with a multi-step function, such as using an automatic dialing telephone with only a two-position switch, the user needs a feedback signal for each completed step. This can be auditory, somatosensory, visual, or a combination of these.

SWITCH OPTIONS. Large Alphanumeric Keyboard (Computer Terminal). A large alphanumeric keyboard is a direct-control interface, requiring the greatest degree of range and resolution. It allows the greatest variety of control modalities, from sophisticated communication to environmental control.

Small Alphanumeric Keyboards. If resolution is a problem, size of the individual keys can be expanded and the number of options can be reduced. If range is a problem, a smaller keyboard can be provided. As choices become fewer, control becomes less direct. An expanded keyboard can be either finger-driven or controlled with a mouth stick or head pointer.

Small Numeric Keypad. If choices must be further limited due to poor resolution of movement or a small functional range, a small keypad can afford as many or as few choices as desired.

Switch Arrays. A switch array, such as a joystick or a roller ball, can afford direct control of the motion of an object, such as a wheelchair. The joystick can also be useful for indirect control function in moving a cursor or other indicator on a screen to an appropriate alternative, as is done with direction keys on a computer keyboard. Other switch arrays may include slot switches, arrays of wafer switches, or arrays of toggles.

Single Switch. This is the most easily adaptable interface and can provide direct control of simple functions, such as turning a light on or off, or indirect control of more complex functions, such as telephone dialing. Single switches may have one or more positions, and may be activated in a number of ways. Hundreds of single switches are available for various purposes. Major categories of these are summarized in Table 19-1.

Voice Control. This is a rapidly developing control area, and allows for reliable and direct control of virtually any function by anyone with distinct, reproducible speech. A number of voice input modules for microcomputer control are commercially available and are becoming increasingly economical and reliable.

Actuators

A major consideration in choosing and developing actuators is the power source. Can the device be mechanical, or if electrically powered, can it be plugged into the wall, or are batteries necessary? How are they replaced or recharged? Electrical safety is another consideration. Will the device get wet? As discussed, durability, reliability, size, appearance and noise are other important considerations.

Signal Controllers

A signal controller is required to process commands unrelated to the function actuated, to control a series of functions, or to interpret a series of signals to effect a single function. The most versatile device for signal control is the personal computer, which can be connected to any of the types of switches described above. Because the computer can serve to integrate multiple environmental control and communication functions, it is often the basis for the most economical integrated control systems for people with severe disabilities. However, there are many functions which do not require microcomputer control, and when too many devices are interfaced with a single controller, the incidence of malfunction rises dramatically. Close cooperation of

the occupational therapist, rehabilitation engineer, and vendor becomes essential when deciding how much integration of various devices is optimal.

Component Connections

Most control systems involve sending a message from the interface to the actuator, sometimes with an intermediate stop at the signal controller. These components are often some distance from one another, and may change in their spatial orientation to each other. Signals may travel as electricity in wires, as high-frequency sound waves, or as light (visible or infrared) or radio waves. Each of these has its use as well as limitations. For instance, multiple wires running across the floor can make a room virtually wheelchair-inaccessible. Light and sound waves require essentially line-of-sight transmission, and radio frequencies available for control of devices in the home are quite limited, so that the control device may receive interference from portable telephones, room monitors, remote controlled toys, garage door openers, and such devices frequently found in the homes of people with disabilities.

Information Resources for Assistive Devices

The selection of assistive devices available increases daily, and with the widening availability and decreasing cost of advanced technology, the prescribing team needs to continually update information on available devices. The most complete and timely such resource is the ABLEDATA system, a national computerized data bank which includes references to thousands of commercially available devices. Information available includes common and tradenames of the products, manufacturers, prices, distributors, description of the product, informal evaluations from users, and available results from formal research or testing programs in abstract form.

Additional resources include many other computerized data bases and various publications which are cited in the reference section.

Table 19-1
Major Categories of Control Switches

Type	Requirements	Examples
Position	Sufficient range of extremity to reach switch and to change switch position	Toggle
Pressure	Movement of head or extremity sufficient to reach and to activate switch, and subsequently to release switch	Leaf switch, pressure pad, pillow switch, foam switch, wobble switch
Pneumatic	Lip, tongue, and pharynx control to close around straw and to direct air forward or backward in mouth	Puff-and-sip control
Mercury	Ability to orient head or extremity in space	Mercury head switch
Sound-activated	Ability to produce appropriate activating sound	Whistle switch, Audiolite
Myoelectric	Activation and relaxation of a specific muscle or group of muscles	Limb control switch

Animal Helpers for the Disabled

No discussion of aids to greater independence is complete without some mention of animal helpers for the disabled. Guide dog programs for the blind are well known and accepted as valuable assets for these individuals. The best-developed program for those with other disabilities is Canine Companions for Independence. This program, funded largely by private donations, breeds, trains, and supplies dogs to clients who meet specific qualifications, and then trains the disabled clients at four centers in the United States to control and use the animals to achieve maximum independence. Signal dogs for the hearing impaired, service dogs for the severely physically disabled, and companion dogs for those with emotional disabilities have been used with a high degree of success as a result of the program.

Some work has also been done in the use of primates as assistants to high-level quadriplegics.[18] Because of their superior manipulative skills, primates are able to provide significant assistance in many areas; however, their very high cost, difficult maintenance, and the difficulty of domesticating and training them makes this option presently open only to a very few.

The future of the use of animals to assist the disabled is uncertain, since this is a new area. Data regarding cost-effectiveness and physical and emotional benefits are not widely available, and acceptance of this concept among people with disabilities has not been tested. At this time, however, it does seem likely that appropriately trained animal assistants may significantly enhance the physical and emotional well-being of individuals with various disabilities.

PERSONAL COMPUTERS FOR THE DISABLED

A computer may make the difference between dependence and independence, between productivity and nonproductivity, or between isolation and communication for the disabled. It may also be a recreational facilitator or instructional mediator. For instance, with a personal computer, the blind, using an inexpensive synthesized voice output, may access news, research, correspondence, and a myriad of other information available to the public through data banks and computer bulletin boards.[19] The deaf can call and converse with any other person who has a computer and modem, no longer dependent upon special communication devices, which are usually limited to other deaf people or relatives. People with learning disabilities are able to interact with a teacher who is infinitely patient, nonjudgmental, and always appropriately reinforcing. People with severe physical disabilities are able to communicate and work more effectively than ever before, and are able, with control only of an eyebrow, tongue, or even extraocular motion, to become fully and independently creative with the computer.

Like anyone else, the person with a disability who has no experience with computers must overcome some misconceptions before he or she is able and willing to interact effectively with computers. The most common and disabling of these is the thought of "ruining something" if keys are pushed in the wrong sequence, that the computer will self-destruct if a prompt or question on the screen is not answered immediately and correctly, or that the computer will somehow quickly "learn" how inexperienced the person is and refuse to cooperate.

A second common misconception is that a computer user must be very bright, a scientific and mathematical genius, or at least understand how computers work. There is still a common belief that one must be able to program computers in order to use them. The best way to dispel this idea is to demonstrate to patients that they can effectively use the computer with little or no prior training, knowledge, or related skills.

A rehabilitation department should have one or more personal computers (usually in the occupational therapy section) with the ability to be moved to the bedside, to demonstrate to patients that the computer is made to serve them, has no intelligence of its own, and is quite durable. There are many attractive introductory programs and games which, when presented properly, will break the ice with even the most wary client. It is important to present the computer early in the course of rehabilitation, especially in the case of severe disability. Often, mastery of the computer, even if it is only playing simple games, will give patients their first measure of control over their environment and an opportunity to be more than passive observers of their world.

Computer Hardware

The choice of computer *hardware*—the physical components of a system—will depend upon the user's needs and will be determined by the choice of software that will meet those needs. *Software* consists of specifically structured digital information, which tells the computer what to do with the data it receives and also tells the user how to interact with the computer to achieve the desired result.

Computer hardware has a number of components which must fit together compatibly and be capable of running the software desired. Many hardware options, as part of compatible systems, are fixed. There are, however, a number of choices which can be made in developing a system for the person with a disability.[20]

Memory

Computers must store and retrieve information from a memory. Memory is in two general categories: ROM (read-only memory) and RAM (random-access memory). ROM is a feature which is constant in and particular to each make and model of computer, and this is what determines a computer's compatibility with software and peripherals. RAM is a quantitative feature which determines how much information may be accessed, changed, and compared at one time. Software programs require a certain amount of RAM to run, and in general, more complex functions require more RAM.

Data Entry

Keyboards are either fixed to the main body of the computer or separate from it, attached by a cord. This may be important if placement of the keyboard in a particular way is necessary for accessibility, such as with limited hand and arm function or use of a mouthstick. Another feature which may be important is feedback. Some keyboards produce a physical or audible click when a key is depressed fully, and will therefore signal a user to go on to the next key. A numeric keypad may be useful if there is significant manipulation of numbers. The other keyboard feature which may either assist or interfere with the disabled user is the presence of function keys. The purpose of these is to signal the computer to make a necessary change in mode of operation. They may be useful in making a function more simple by taking the place of a complex entry; however, they could complicate use of the computer for a person with limited hand function or who uses a mouthstick by requiring more than one key to be pressed at once. Adaptations to overcome this problem are discussed later in this section, as are specialized data input systems for the severely disabled user.

Data Display

A monitor is necessary to display data. It should be chosen with the use of the computer in mind. The major choice is whether to install a color or monochrome monitor. Color monitors enhance the enjoyment of games and may also assist in various teaching programs. Their expense is significant, however, and in general, word processing and data management are more easily displayed on a monochrome display, which yields better resolution.

The capability of displaying material in many colors or of displaying a large number of items on one screen will often require special additions to the basic computer ROM.

Data Storage and Retrieval

Several methods have been developed to load software programs into the computer and to save work done on the computer, including magnetic tape and player, mini-floppy disks and one or more disk drives, a fixed or "hard" disk, or a combination of these. The tape recorder is slow, cumbersome, and requires much physical manipulation, and therefore is seldom an option for the disabled user. Mini-floppy disks with one or more disk drives will meet virtually any data storage and access needs; however, they also require some manipulation. A fixed or hard disk is often valuable for the disabled user, since it can accommodate a number of frequently used software programs as well as a large amount of data, which is accessible through keyboard manipulation alone.

Communication

A device which interfaces the computer with a telephone for the purpose of communication is called a *modem*. The reader is referred to basic computer books[20, 24] for a description of the types available. In general, a modem is very valuable for any disabled user who is serious about the computer and who wishes to access the myriad networks available. A modem is a must for the deaf user, as discussed later in this section.

Printers

Most people who use a computer at some time require "hard copy," or a printed form of the output of the computer. A printer may be interfaced with the computer for this purpose. There are two types of printers available for home computers: "dot matrix" and "daisy wheel." The former uses ink jets to form tiny dots on the paper in the shape of characters; the latter prints much like a typewriter, producing high-quality print. The greater speed, versatility, and economy of the dot matrix printer usually makes it the best choice for the disabled user.

Computer Software

Computer software is the most important consideration in setting up a system for the disabled user. Software programs have a number of uses, including the following:

Education: Computer-assisted learning is a valuable asset to the disabled user.

Entertainment: Various games can provide hours of enjoyment and a basis of easy interaction with peers, family, and friends.

Communication: The personal computer can provide both written and synthesized speech, and can also provide communication with other computer users by modem. Besides personal communication and information access, a number of remote transactions such as banking and stock market business, can be performed by modem.

Word processing: Word processing is a very important function for most advanced students and also for most professional employment.

Data base management: This consists of storing, accessing, categorizing, and comparing data and is often necessary in management for program evaluation and in many research areas.

Prediction/spread sheets: This software allows analysis of data in terms of trends and predictions. It is useful in manufacturing and business to track costs and profits, and to evaluate the impact of proposed changes. It may also be used as a tool for personal finance management.

Fine arts applications: Most serious composers now use computers to write and orchestrate compositions, and music synthesizers are seen in nearly every musical genre. In addition, computer graphics are often used to illustrate media productions, and most animation is assisted by a computer. The computer as a fine arts medium is becoming increasingly common and accepted.[19]

The business of matching software, hardware, and user is one which is best done by knowledgeable members of the rehabilitation team. A rule of thumb is to provide the disabled user with as many possibilities as funding will allow. Table 19-2 outlines some major hardware requirements for various uses. It is important to remember, however, that compatibility will be the key, and those components advertised as compatible with specific software or other components may not be truly compatible without manipulations beyond the scope of the average user.

Computer Applications and Adaptations

The Mobility-Impaired User

A person with a disability who has good use of his upper extremities and adequate vision and hearing will require no special adaptation in computer hardware.[20] All necessary elements can be purchased at a computer outlet at low cost. What is purchased will depend upon the uses intended and the software required to achieve the client's goals. These considerations, whether they include professional or educational goals, entertainment, home management, or communication and networking, should be worked out with the help of the occupational therapist, vocational rehabilitation counselor, teachers, and others experienced in computers. Since working with computers seldom requires significant mobility, these people can often compete favorably with nondisabled individuals in computer-based jobs, such as word processing, data entry, or even programming. Again, it is important for clients to understand that one does not need to be a computer programmer to work effectively and make a good living using computers.

The Hearing-Impaired User

Adaptation of the personal computer for the deaf person is not difficult, in that all components can be found in any computer store. The most important advance afforded a deaf person by a computer is the ability to communicate instantly and effectively with a wide population of people—virtually anyone who has a personal computer and a modem, and not just those who are attached to a TDD (Telecommunication Device for the Deaf). It also allows access to the latest news and multiple other on-line information networks, without dependence on a later printed

Table 19-2
Common Hardware Options for Software Applications

Function	Necessary RAM	Data Storage	Modem	Monitor	Printer	Other
Games	8K–64K	Tape or disk	—	Color* Monochrome	—	Joystick, other switch controller
Learning programs	8K–64K	Tape or disk	+ / −	Monochrome Color*	May be useful	—
Word processing	64K–640K (20pp → 200pp)	Disks (floppy or fixed*)	—	Monochrome* Color	Necessary	80-column display
Data base management	256K → 640K	Disks (floppy or fixed*)	+ / −	Monochrome* Color	Necessary	80–160 column display
Communication, networking, remote transactions	64 → 640K	Disks (floppy or fixed*)	necessary	Monochrome* Color	Desirable	modem
Prediction/spread sheet	64–640K	Disks (floppy or fixed*)	—	Monochrome or color	Necessary	80–160 column display
Fine arts applications	128–640K	Disks	+ / −	Monochrome or color	Necessary	Various special components

* Indicates preferable choice

copy of such information or sign-language interpreter. Additionally, there is a growing group of people associated with Deaf-Net, a communication and data bank network especially attuned to the needs of the hearing impaired.[20]

Accessing these networks generally presents no special problems. A person who is born deaf, however, may have had some difficulty acquiring advanced language and abstraction skills, and therefore may require some special instruction and practice in order to converse effectively with hearing people. On the other hand, it is expected that practice with computer-based communication will serve to aid the born-deaf in filling the literacy gap to which they are susceptible.

The most important consideration in selecting a computer for a hearing-impaired person is the same as for any other person—the hardware should fit the desired need and run the desired software. Probably the only uniquely desirable item for the deaf is early acquisition of a modem, and perhaps portability. Since operation of the computer is not dependent upon the ability to hear, computer-related employment is often highly accessible to the hearing impaired.

The Vision-Impaired User

Most educated blind adults know touch typing and can operate a numeric keypad. Therefore, input to the computer usually presents few problems. Getting information out of the computer is, on the other hand, a significant challenge. There are two ways to do this: through speech synthesizers and Braille.[6] Speech synthesizers are available at a reasonable cost, and programs are available to instruct the speech synthesizer to read all or selected parts of the computer screen. They work well with linear or sequential functions, such as word processing or electronic mail; however, they have difficulty with programs such as spread-sheets, in which the entire screen has to be read to find one small piece of data. Another difficulty with the speech synthesizer is that some word processing and data base management programs have control functions (word wrap-around, return, tabs, print commands, and so on) embedded invisibly into

the text, and the synthesizer becomes nonfunctional when faced with these embedded "nonsense" characters. It is important to select programs that will not deactivate the speech synthesizer in this way.

There are now programs that will allow input by standard keyboard, review and editing by speech synthesizer, and printing in Grade II Braille using a standard letter-quality printer (the print-out is done backward by using the period and a soft rubber platen).[20] Before computers were available, there was no easy way of correcting or editing Braille text; once you had written the first draft, you were done, unless you wished to write a complete additional draft. Now, all the joys of word processing are available to the vision impaired at a reasonable cost, and with both Braille and printed output.

The Learning-Disabled User

Teachers of learning-disabled individuals have long known that given the right circumstances, virtually anyone can learn, and that learning can take place beyond the expectations of those who live with these individuals in the normal environment. The attributes of a successful teacher for the leaning disabled include patience, energy, availability, and appropriate reinforcement practices. The computer is exquisitely qualified for this role.[14] Software is becoming increasingly available for teaching basic academic skills, as well as for training in perceptual and cognitive tasks.

In many cases, learning disabilities are accompanied by physical disabilities. The special education teacher and occupational therapist must then work closely to develop appropriate adaptive input systems to make computers accessible to these individuals.

The User With Limited or No Hand Function

Individuals with limited or no hand function may have the most to gain from computer use and are those for whom the most significant input modifications must often be made. These individuals often are highly restricted in their mobility, have limited employment opportunities, and often have accompanying impairments in communication.

The first consideration is how the computer and peripherals will be turned on and programs activated. This will depend upon the user's needs, the availability of an attendant during the time when the computer is being used, and available funds. The computer and peripherals can be easily turned on *en masse* using any environmental control system to turn on power to the surge limiter (a multi-outlet device which plugs into the wall socket and protects the computer from electrical bursts) to which all are connected. Software then may be accessed using one of three means: tape player, disk drive(s), or hard disk (in ascending order of cost, and descending order of difficulty of operation). A tape player is often very difficult to use for a person with limited hand function and will usually by operated by an attendant. Various adaptations are available to make mini-floppy disks easier to handle safely and to make disk drives easier to open and close. Since some drives are easier than others to operate, this should be taken into consideration when selecting hardware for these individuals. Particularly, standing the drives on end (with openings upward) should be considered, so that gravity can be used to gently guide the disks in and out. (It must be remembered that this arrangement will increase the susceptibility of the drives and data to dust and other pollutants.) One or a series of hard disks (permanent storage devices built into a computer) make the access of programs easy, since frequently used programs can be stored internally and accessed at will without any physical manipulation.

If a modem is to be used, the process of dialing the telephone and placing the receiver on the modem needs to be considered. The use of a modem that directly connects to the phone line will eliminate the need to manipulate the telephone handset and dial or keypad.

The next problem to be addressed is that of data input. Anyone who can use a typewriter can usually use a computer keyboard with at least as much facility. The ability to move the cursor to correct mistakes or make changes easily and quickly usually enhances the user's facility in written communication. For those unable to move fingers independently, a cuff with rubber-tipped pointer will allow one key at a time to be struck. If coordination is a problem, a keyguard, an inexpensive plate with holes that fits over the regular keyboard, will aid in directing the finger or pointer to the appropriate key and prevent hitting two keys at once. This device is often useful when a mouthstick is used, since precision of movement often is limited with a mouthstick.[13]

A common problem seen with the use of one hand or a mouthstick is the necessity of pressing two keys at once when performing control functions, such as printing, storage or retrieval of information, or moving among various features of a program. This problem can be addressed in one of a number of ways, depending on the computer used and user preference. Some computers have a feature called Smart-Key, which will allow the user to assign the function of a group or series of keys to a single unused key. The upper case key presents a similar problem, since on most computers the "cap lock" key will not activate the upper case of numbers or other symbols. Some computers allow modification of a shift key to function like a universal "cap lock" key; however, with other computers it is necessary to opt for a mechanical device. There are a number of such devices on the market, which attach to the computer case, and with the use of either a ball bearing or springs hold down the control or shift key to allow the necessary function to occur. One should not attempt to attach the device by drilling into the computer case, since that will nullify the warranty. Other ways of attaching these devices can be frustratingly impermanent.

If resolution of functional range of movement is not adequate to use a regular keyboard, it is possible to interface an expanded keyboard with an expanded numeric keypad, a joystick or other switch array, or a single switch (such as a sip-and-puff or eyebrow switch) to effect data input. Obviously, as the input device becomes more limited, data input becomes slower, and in some cases usable software selection also becomes more limited, requiring specialized programs which prompt the user to choose from a small number of possible responses. An example of one of these highly specialized systems is the Adaptive Firmware Card. This is a hardware/software addition to an inexpensive microcomputer which requires only a single input. This input may be an eye blink, brow twitch, puff of air, or any other single switch input to select an appropriate choice. Alternatives may be indicated by a cursor which moves at a programmable speed among columns and rows of letters, numbers, words, phrases, or any other useful category of choices, or Morse code may also be used. Using this device, it is possible to build sentences and paragraphs at a speed of about five to ten words per minute, as well as play games, draw, or produce synthesized speech. Also available are on/off controls for a number of electrical outlets, which may control a radio, television, tape recorder, or other appliance. This device may also be interfaced with a voice-input module.

For those with distinct and reproducible speech, voice control is an attractive input option. It is much more direct and therefore much faster than a single-switch device, and the reliability of voice-input devices is rapidly improving as the cost decreases. A number of voice input devices are available for most popular computers. Most require purchase of a special card to allow the device to "talk" to the computer in the context of other programs. As these devices continue to improve, their utility as fast, direct input devices will grow.

There are many components and systems to allow disabled individuals to use powerful computer systems for word processing, data base management, and fiscal prediction, and their number is increasing rapidly. The key to successful computer accessibility is the same as with any assistive device: the user should be able to perform the desired function as easily, efficiently, and directly as possible with the minimum of adaptive equipment, and the equipment should serve to enhance interaction and communication between the user and other individuals.

New Frontiers

Until recently, computers have been capable only of exact deduction; that is, any conclusions they were able to draw from a situation or data input had to be based on absolutely identical previous data input for which the computer was programmed. For example, for a digital computer to recognize a picture of an elephant, it must have been shown the exact same picture in the exactly identical position, which generated the exact same digital information from an optical scanner, and which was previously identified as an elephant. In fact, a digital computer is not capable of the concept of elephant-ness without being programmed with a series of descriptive terms, and still cannot match those descriptive terms with input from an optical scanner; it can only recognize proximity to its definition of elephant in the exact descriptive terms with which it was programmed.

An exciting breakthrough in the direction of "artificial intelligence" has come with the development of "neural net" computers. This is the use of a number of linked microprocessors to form an entirely different kind of computer. Though their full capabilities are not yet developed or even known, these devices seem capable of induction from incomplete or approximate data. That is, they would be able to recognize an elephant much as we could from a picture of its trunk, foot, or forehead. The applications of such a device to the problems of the disabled are most promising. They might include a better-than-perfect voice recognition system. Not only would it be able to respond perfectly to its master's voice, or any voice if so programmed; it would also be able to interpret severely and inconsistently spastic or dysarthric speech to perform control functions or to enhance communication. It might be able to maintain a running commentary on a small portable screen for the deaf person, eliminating the need for interpretation, or provide a spoken commentary as desired for the blind person to enhance mobility. One could imagine enhanced wheelchair control for the very spastic individual, responding to general commands, ignoring extraneous movements, and recognizing dangerous situations. These computers may even eventually be able to recognize general signs of distress and call for help when it is needed, even if not specifically asked to do so.

Clearly, available technology is growing exponentially, and ever more sophisticated systems will become widely available at more affordable prices. The ongoing task of rehabilitation professionals will be to develop and adapt this new technology to meet the needs of their disabled clients, and to effect appropriate delivery of new adaptive systems to those who need them.

An interdisciplinary approach will become ever-increasingly necessary to maximize delivery and utilization of technology for the disabled user. Refinement of information systems, development of standards, and earlier interaction between clinical and technical professionals will afford the best opportunity to effect and support system delivery, minimize risks, and promote independence, productivity, and self-esteem for individuals with disabilities.

REFERENCES

1. Barker MR, Cook AM: A systematic approach to evaluating physical ability for control of assistive devices. Proc 4th Annu Rehabil Eng Conf, 1981
2. Bowker J, Reed B: A vacuum formed plastic insert seat for neurologically handicapped wheelchair patients. Inter-clinic Information Bull 12:7–17, July 1973
3. Britell CW, Johnson D, Ciciora J: Unistik vehicle controller: A unique approach to driving for high-level quadriplegics. Arch Phys Med Rehabil 65:466, 1984
4. Brubaker CE: Wheelchair prescription: On analysis of factors that affect mobility and performance. J Rehabil R & D 23:19–26, 1986
5. Congressional Office of Technology Assessment: Technology & Handicapped People. New York, Springer-Verlag, 1983
6. Croft DL: A Beginners' Guide to Personal Computers for the Blind and Visually Impaired. Boston, National Braille Press, 1983
7. DeLisa JA, Greenberg S: Wheelchair prescription guidelines. Am Family Phys 25:145–150, 1982
8. DeLisa JA, Quigley F: Assessing the driving potential of cerebral vascular accident patients. Am J Occup Ther 37:474–478, 1983
9. Ferguson-Pell MW, Wilkie IC, Reswick JB, Barbenel JC: Pressure sore prevention for the wheelchair-bound spinal cord injured patient. Paraplegia 18:42–51, 1983
10. Fisher SV, Patterson R: Long term pressure recordings under the ischial tuberosities of tetraplegics. Paraplegia 21:99–106, 1983
11. Garber SL, Krouskop TA: Body build and its relationship to pressure distribution in the seated wheelchair patient. Arch Phys Med 63:17–20, 1982
12. Golpher LAC, Rau MT, Marshall RC: Aphasic adults and their decisions on driving. An evaluation. Arch Phys Med Rehabil 61:34–40, 1980
13. Graystone P: Computer interfaces for severely disabled person. Proc 5th Annu Conf Rehabil Eng, 1982
14. Hagen D: Microcomputer Resource Book for Special Education. Reston, VA, Council for Exceptional Children, 1984
15. Jebsen RH: Essentials of wheelchair prescription. Northwest Med 67:755–758, 1968
16. Kent H, Sheridan BS, Wasco E, June C: A driver training program for the disabled. Arch Phys Med Rehabil 60:273–276, 1979
17. Lehneis HR: The safety achievements of the disabled driver. Biomed Eng 8:438–439, 1973
18. MacFadyen JT: Educated monkeys help the disabled help themselves. Smithsonian 17:125–132, 1986
19. McGlynn DR: Personal Computing, Home, Professional and Small Business Applications. New York, Willey-Interscience, 1979
20. McWilliams PA: Personal Computers for the Disabled. New York, Quantum Press, 1984
21. Merbitz CT, King RB, Bleiberg J: Continuous direct recording of wheelchair pressure relief behavior. Arch Phys Med Rehab 64(abstr): 1983
22. Norback J: Sourcebook of Aids for the Mentally and Physically Handicapped. New York, Van Nostrand Reinhold, 1983
23. Perkins WJ, et al: High Technology Aids for the Disabled. London, Butterworth, 1982
24. Perry RL: Cavan, NY, Owning Your Home Computer, 1980
25. Pritham CH, Leiper CI: A method for custom seating of the severely disabled. Orthotics Prosthetics 35:19–26, 1981
26. Trefler E: Seating for Children with Cerebral Palsy—A Resource Manual. Washington DC, RESNA Publications Service, 1984
27. Trefler E, Tooms RR, Hobson D: Seating for cerebral-palsied children. Inter-Clinic Information Bull 17:1–8, 1978
28. Williams JR: A Guide to Controls: Selection, Mounting, Applications. Bethesda, MD, RESNA Publications Service, 1982
29. Wilson AB: Wheelchairs: A Prescription Guide. Rehabilitation Press, Charlottesville, VA, 1986
30. Zacharkow D: Wheelchair Posture and Pressure Sores. New York, Charles C Thomas, 1984

Part 3

Major Rehabilitation Problems

20

Rehabilitation of the Pediatric Patient

Bruce M. Gans

The rehabilitation of children with physical impairments both resembles and differs from that established for adults. It is a challenging combination of normal child care and the best of rehabilitation intervention strategies. With the understanding that a child is not merely a miniature adult, and that specific physiological parameters exist that either complicate or allow unique intervention opportunities, successful aid may be offered. It is only, however, through an understanding of the long-term outcomes and consequences of disability in adult life that proper management strategies for the young child may be chosen.

This chapter reviews the scope of disabling disorders that occur in childhood, the specific differences between children and adults that relate to their special needs, and the basic principles of management of disabled children. The specific management of various childhood disorders will be found both within this chapter and within relevant sections of other chapters.

Frequently, a semantic issue comes to the fore in the care of children with physical handicaps: do they require rehabilitation or habilitation? While it is true that the developing child who has not acquired an ability and then lost it may more accurately be described as needing habilitation, the convention used in this text generalizes all needs, strategies, and services under the term rehabilitation.

The various disabling disorders that occur in childhood may be characterized according to several parameters of interest, including time of onset and pattern of the natural history of the disease. Disorders that are present from the time of birth are described as *congenital* if they are not due to known external environmental factors during the birth or post-birth period. Those that occur later are generally considered to be *acquired*. Congenital problems may be further specified by cause as either genetic or influenced by some extrinsic factor, even though the effect was expressed in the prenatal period (for example, fetal alcohol syndrome). Acquired disorders should not be confused with congenital (genetic) disorders that are discovered only after birth (for example, Duchenne muscular dystrophy is usually only diagnosed after age 3, but is a genetic disorder detectable at birth).

The temporal pattern of disabling disorders in children may be static, transient, or progressive. The progressive (or degenerative) disorders of childhood represent a relatively unique class of rehabilitation problems because of the simultaneous occurrence of growth, development, disease progression, and deterioration.

The three commonest disabling disorders of childhood seen in a comprehensive rehabilitation setting are cerebral palsy, myelodysplasia, and muscular dystrophy. These and other diseases are categorized by their onset and temporal patterns in Table 20-1. What is known about etiology and epidemiology is shown in Table 20-2. Information about the prevalence of handicapped children being served by the public school system is shown in Table 20-3. The incidence of most disabling disorders has not changed appreciably in this country in the last ten years. The exceptions are a known decline in the incidence of children being born with spina bifida (due, in part, to prenatal detection and therapeutic abortion) and a change in the characteristics, but not numbers, of children developing cerebral palsy. Perinatal brain damage has become more commonly characterized by severe quadriparesis rather than diplegia or total body–involved athetoid patterns.[41]

THE CHILD AS PATIENT: DIFFERENCES TO CONSIDER

Although children may be thought of as small adults, the reality is that adults are merely large children. Maintaining this perspective is perhaps the most fundamental philosophical difference to be emphasized for health professionals who are going to work with disabled children.

Size, Shape, and Weight

The most striking difference between adults and children is size. Knowledge of the patterns of growth and development is key to understanding, anticipating, and managing the difficulties that disabled children experience. In the early years, head circumference, weight, and height are important parameters to monitor. Standard tables of growth and development may be used to record and compare disabled children to the normal population. The pattern of growth shows anticipated bursts and plateaus that are related to sex, age, and even season. Figure 20-1 shows the pattern of height change as a function of age for boys and girls.

The seasonality of growth is shown in Figure 20-2. In sum-

Table 20-1
Common Disabling Conditions of Childhood

	Temporal Pattern		
	Transient	*Static*	*Progressive*
Congenital	Brachial plexus injury	Cerebral palsy Spina bifida Limb deficiency Retardation	Muscular dystrophy Spinal muscular atrophy Cystic fibrosis
Acquired	Guillain-Barré syndrome	Spinal cord injury Traumatic brain injury Traumatic limb amputation Polio	Juvenile rheumatoid arthritis Collagen vascular disease

Table 20-2
Epidemiology of Common Disabling Disorders (per 100,000)

Diagnosis	Incidence	Prevalence
Cerebral palsy	43	250
Spina bifida	43	40
Muscular dystrophy	1.4	60
Spinal cord injury	5.8	2.7
Traumatic brain injury	600	210
Limb deficiency	38	38
Down's syndrome	65	110
Arthritis	220	220

(Gortmaker SL, Sappenfield W: Chronic childhood disorders: Prevalence and impact. Pediatr Clin North Am 31:3–18, 1984; Human Services Research Institute: Summary of Data on Handicapped Children and Youth. Washington, DC, US Government Printing Office, 1985; Anderson DW, McLaurin RL: Report on the national head and spinal cord injury survey. J Neurosurg 53:S1–S43, 1980)

mer growth is faster than in winter, implying that it is wiser to fit new customized orthotic and prosthetic appliances to growing children in the fall, rather than the spring.[40]

Patterns of various tissue growth vary widely. Knowledge of the growth patterns associated with puberty are important for management and even diagnosis. The specific tissue growth curves shown in Figure 20-3 are useful to remember. This growth may represent a change in contour that, for example, would influence a body jacket design for a pubescent girl.

Physiological Performance

Children vary in accordance with age and size in a number of physiological parameters. Normal heart rate, respiratory rate, heat transfer behavior, and various chemical assessments, all change as a function of age. For example, the serum alkaline phosphatase level may be elevated in an adolescent, not because of the presence of an occult heterotopic ossification, but rather because of normal bone growth.

The question of enhanced "neural plasticity" in youth remains open.[18, 68] Conflicting data appear in the literature to support or reject this concept, but the clinical management implications are generally well accepted: the more treatment that is done earlier and younger, the better the outcome seems to be.

A number of neurologically mediated reflex behaviors are age and development dependent. The asymmetric tonic neck reflex is a normal behavior when elicited at certain ages (2 to 6 months), but may be distinctly abnormal when it is persistent and dominant many months later.

Primitive Reflex Patterns

Because they are commonly observed in physically disabled children, the major primitive reflex patterns that may either interfere with or facilitate skilled motor actions should be well understood. These motor patterns may be thought of as "hardwired" or "firm ware," in that they represent fundamental, neurally mediated preferential relationships between body sensors of the internal and external environment and motor patterns. Many of these patterns appear to have evolutionary advantages to the organism, but it is sufficient for the treating physician simply to know of their existence.

The primitive reflexes should probably be renamed primitive motor behaviors, since they really are stereotypical motor responses and spontaneous patterns of movement. For most of the commonly observed patterns, specific stimuli appear to be associated and may be categorized as to proprioceptive, vestibular, or cutaneous senses.[8] The times of appearance and disappearance in the developmental sequence for these reflexes are summarized in Table 20-4.

Proprioceptive Patterns

The proprioceptive patterns may depend upon trunk, head and neck, and limb positions. The most basic patterns are the flexion and extension synergies of the arms and legs. In the upper extremity, the full flexor pattern shows shoulder adduction, flexion, and internal rotation with elbow flexion, wrist pronation and flexion, and finger and thumb flexion (Fig. 20-4). The thumb is frequently tightly adducted and flexed into the palm. The extensor pattern of the upper extremity shows shoulder extension, relative abduction and external rotation, elbow extension, wrist supination, and finger extension (Fig. 20-5).

Lower extremity patterns are similar. The extension posture of the leg includes hip adduction, extension, and internal rotation, along with knee extension, internal tibial rotation, and equinovarus foot posturing (Fig. 20-6). The flexor pattern consists of hip flexion, abduction and external rotation, knee flexion, external tibial rotation, and calcaneovalgus posturing of the foot (Fig. 20-7).

In both of these postures, the fingers and toes appear to be influential in establishing the dominance of one or the other posture. It is frequently noted that forcing the toes into extension will facilitate a full flexor synergy of the leg. Similarly, placing the flexed thumb in an abducted and extended position will frequently facilitate a full extensor response in the arm.

Lateral rotation of the head on the trunk produces the asymmetric tonic neck reflex (ATNR) (Fig. 20-8). This is the classic fencer's posture of extension in the upper and lower extremities on the nasal side, and flexion of both limbs on the occipital side. The symmetric tonic neck reflex (STNR) (Fig. 20-9) describes midline effects of flexing and extending the head on the body. Flexion of the head facilitates flexion in the upper extremities and extension of the lower extremities. Extension produces the opposite pattern.

Table 20-3
Handicapped Children in School Programs in the United States

Type of Handicap		School Year	
		1982–83	1983–84
All conditions	Number served	4,294,815	4,338,783
	Percent of all served	100	100
	Percent of total enrollment	10.76	10.89
Learning disabled	Number served	1,745,120	1,810,579
	Percent of all served	40.63	41.73
	Percent of total enrollment	4.40	4.57
Speech impaired	Number served	1,133,659	1,130,298
	Percent of all served	26.39	26.05
	Percent of total enrollment	2.86	2.86
Mentally retarded	Number served	778,188	749,205
	Percent of all served	18.11	17.26
	Percent of total enrollment	1.92	1.84
Emotionally disturbed	Number served	353,333	362,003
	Percent of all served	8.22	8.34
	Percent of total enrollment	0.89	0.91
Hard of hearing and deaf	Number served	75,063	74,201
	Percent of all served	1.74	1.71
	Percent of total enrollment	0.18	0.18
Orthopedically impaired	Number served	57,474	56,170
	Percent of all served	13.38	1.29
	Percent of total enrollment	0.14	0.14
Other health impaired	Number served	52,012	54,616
	Percent of all served	1.21	1.78
	Percent of total enrollment	0.13	0.13
Visually handicapped	Number served	31,049	31,554
	Percent of all served	0.72	7.27
	Percent of total enrollment	0.07	0.07
Multi-handicapped	Number served	65,123	67,365
	Percent of all served	1.51	1.55
	Percent of total enrollment	0.07	0.07
Deaf-blind	Number served	2,525	2,492
	Percent of all served	0.05	0.05
	Percent of total enrollment	0.01	0.01

NOTE: Includes children (ages 3–21) served under P.L. 94-142 and children (ages 0–20) served under P.L. 89-113. Percentages of total enrollment are based on the total annual enrollment of U.S. public schools, preprimary through 12th grade. Details may not add to totals because of rounding.
(Human Services Research Institute: Summary of Data on Handicapped Children and Youth. Washington, DC, US Government Printing Office, 1985)

The long spinal reflex posture (Fig. 20-10) relates the reciprocal influence of the upper extremity to the ipsilateral lower extremity. The typical hemiplegic posture of flexion in the arm and extension in the leg is an example of this reflex. On occasion, facilitation of the opposite posture in one limb may be achieved by reversing the pattern in the other limb. For example, a better flexor pattern of the leg during gait may be facilitated in a child by superimposing extension positions on the ipsilateral arm.

The crossed extension reflex describes the influence of the body position across the midline. This pattern promotes symmetry of left and right limbs. Thus, flexion of the left arm will facilitate flexion of the right. One commonly observed result of this reflex is the typical diplegic posture seen in children with cerebral palsy (Fig. 20-11).

Vestibular Patterns

The vestibular system mediates static postures and dynamic postural reactions. These are important movement patterns that facilitate the development of mobility skills.[9]

The most commonly seen static vestibular pattern is the tonic labyrinthine reflex (TLR) (Fig. 20-12). This pattern, facilitated by the supine position of the head, demonstrates lower extremity symmetrical extension with upper extremity shoulder abduction and external rotation. In prone position, shoulder adduction and internal rotation are accompanied by lower extremity flexor posturing.

The dynamic vestibular reflexes are all variations on the body's tendency to weight-shift to a point of postural stability,

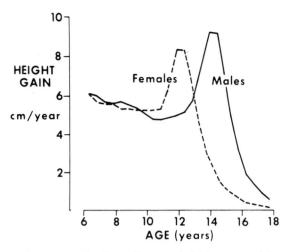

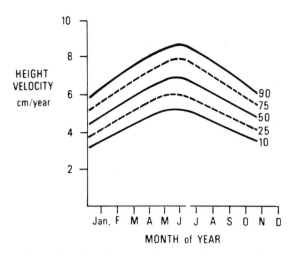

Figure 20-1.   Growth velocity for normal children around the time of puberty. (Tanner JM: Growth at Adolescence. Oxford, England, Blackwell Scientific Publications, 1962)

Figure 20-2.   Growth velocity as a function of the time of year in prepubertal males. (Adapted from Marshall, WA: Arch Dis Child 46:414–420, 1971)

Figure 20-3.   Postnatal growth curves of four major organ systems relative to size attained at age 20. (Tanner JM: Growth at Adolescence. Blackwell Scientific Publications, 1962)

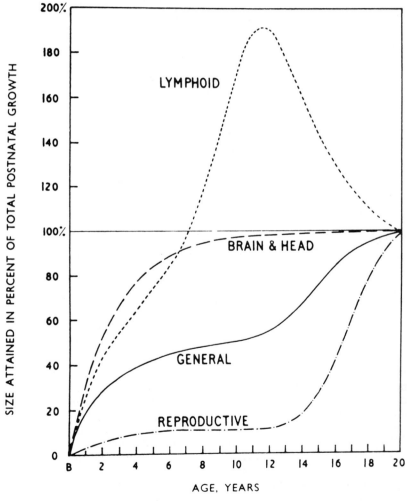

Table 20-4
Normal Acquisition and Regression of Primitive Reflex Behaviors

Reflex	Age of Onset	Age Reflex Disappears
Moro	Birth	6 months
Palmar grasp	Birth	6 months
Plantar grasp	Birth	9–10 months
Adductor spread of patellar reflex	Birth	7 months
Tonic neck	2 months	5 months
Landau	3 months	24 months
Parachute response	8–9 months	Persists

(Swaiman KF, Jacobson RI: Developmental abnormalities of the central nervous system. In Baker AB, Joynt RJ (eds): Clinical Neurology. Philadelphia, Harper & Row, 1984)

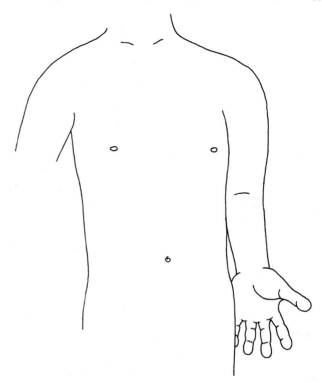

Figure 20-5. The extensor synergy in the upper extremity.

Figure 20-6. The extensor synergy in the lower extremity.

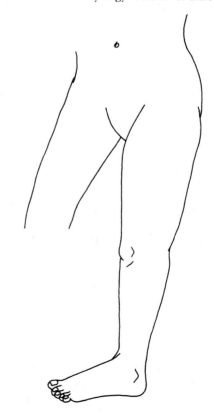

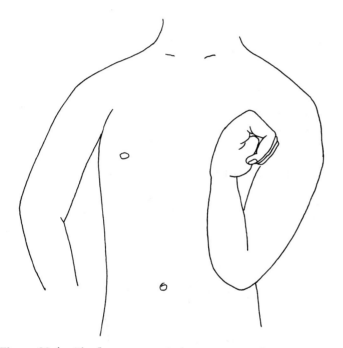

Figure 20-4. The flexor synergy in the upper extremity.

and to extend the upper limbs to oppose the direction of travel in higher velocity movements or more extreme postural deviations.[43] Thus, the protective extension reflexes are seen, in all planes. In the inverted position, this postural reaction is called the *parachute response* (Fig. 20-13), consisting of extension of the upper extremities with downward movement of the head and body.

Cutaneous Mediated Patterns

Cutaneous mediated reflex patterns demonstrate the facilitative relationship between skin tactile receptors and underlying muscle excitation. In general, cutaneous stimulus evokes activation of the muscle groups served by the same sclerotome. In the hand, stroking the palm results in the palmar grasp response. Similarly, in the foot the plantar grasp response occurs with plantar stimulation. Light tactile input to the shin area may evoke

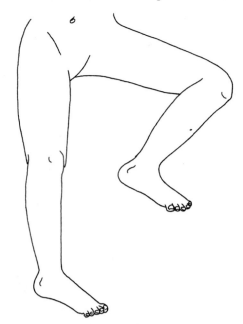

Figure 20-7. The flexor synergy in the lower extremity.

Figure 20-8. The asymmetric tonic neck reflex (ATNR).

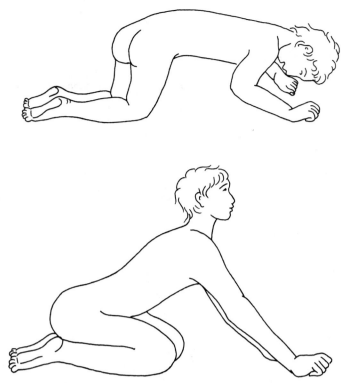

Figure 20-9. The symmetric tonic neck reflex (STNR).

Figure 20-10. The long spinal reflex posture.

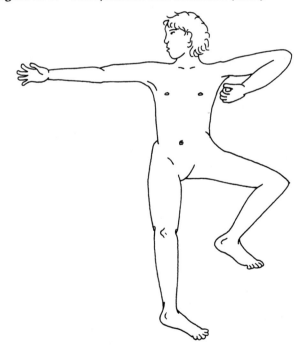

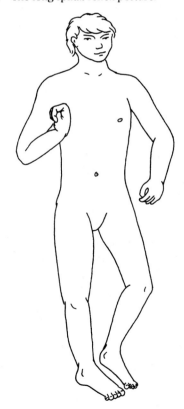

a vigorus full flexor response in children with hyperactive, cutaneously mediated reflex patterns.

Kinesthetic Patterns

The application of vertical load demand to the legs results in several characteristic primitive reflex postures. In young infants, the stepping response will be seen as a result of both loading one limb (by vertical suspension), and also stimulating the dorsum of the opposite foot (presumably a cutaneous influence as well). The positive supporting reaction occurs pathologically in older

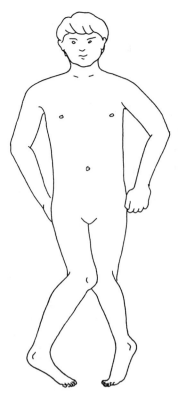

Figure 20-11. Posture in spastic diplegia due, in part, to the dominance of the crossed extension reflex.

Figure 20-12. The tonic labyrinthine reflex (TLR) in the supine position.

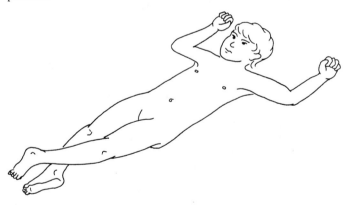

children when a loading of the suspended child's plantar surface results in a symmetric extension pattern of the lower extremities.

Child Development

Physical growth is accompanied by emotional, functional, cognitive, linguistic, and psychosocial development. Many specific methods of quantifying the state of a child's development have been proposed and are used in various settings.[4, 11, 22, 26, 32, 33, 35, 42] What is most important is the recognition of the relative separateness of development along a number of dimensions. For example, there may be next to no correlation between motor development and cognitive skill acquisition. Similarly, language and cognitive functions may be largely independent (for example,

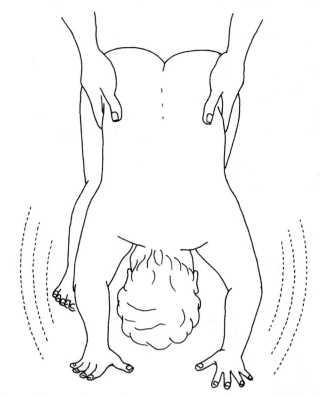

Figure 20-13. The parachute response is a protective response made to downward motion of the head.

the extremely bright but nonspeaking child with athetoid cerebral palsy).[6, 7, 48]

Psychosocial Development

Emotional maturation occurs as a function of experience as well as age.[19, 27] It is frequently easy to misinterpret and misjudge the emotional maturity of disabled children. Frequently, they are infantilized by family and caretakers (the 42-year-old man with severe impairment from cerebral palsy who is still a "Jimmie" instead of a James). They may also be assumed to be more mature than is really the case, particularly if much of their time has been spent in the company of adults in hospital and other health care settings.

Academic achievement must be distinguished from cognitive abilities.[5, 45] Many disabled children experience less than full educational experiences because of a variety of interfering problems, including medical interventions. Formal and standardized testing should be used periodically for disabled children to assess their academic progress.

Adaptation to a child's disability may really be in many cases the parent's adaptation to the child's handicap.[12] Children who grow up with a physical limitation usually do not have a sense of loss of ability. It is usually only later, around adolescence, when social sensitivity and maturity cause adaptation problems to surface. In the early years, it is important to not allow an adult's feelings to be projected upon a child. The most effective strategy appears to be to help the child (and family) identify strengths and abilities the child has, despite the disabilities, in order to build a sense of confidence and self-worth. In many respects this may be similar to the old adage of encouraging the glass to be seen as half full, rather than half empty.

Socially, children are substantially different from adults. They commonly have caretakers available (parents or guardians), and these caretakers are comfortable in that role—indeed, they have emotionally contracted for it. This is in distinction to the spouse who finds him or herself responsible for the care of a newly disabled partner. The emotional commitment in this situation is usually an equal, rather than a strongly dependent, relationship. The result of this fact is that for more seriously handicapped children returning home is generally feasible because of the availability of loving caretakers.[2, 21]

COMMON CONCERNS IN TREATING DISABLED CHILDREN

Medical Problems

Although the disabling disorders of childhood are widely varied, they share a number of common issues and potential as well as active problems. This section will review the common problem areas and appropriate management and treatment strategies for them.

Well Child Care

The most important medical perspective is that of well child care, which concerns itself principally with growth, development, nutrition, and prevention of contagious diseases. These areas of concern are translated into traditional pediatric monitoring strategies, including routine periodic assessment of weight, height, head circumference, and certain specific observations. These may include limb length for a child with an amputation; periodic assessment of developmental status, using either a routine screening instrument such as the Denver Developmental Screening Test[22] or other more sophisticated instruments, depending upon the child's specific problems and developmental level; review of food and liquid intake patterns, bowel and bladder function, and nutritional status as determined by growth and chemical evaluations; and review and preservation of preventive immunization programs.

Immunization deserves special attention in the disabled child. Surprisingly, the more seriously ill child may slip through the cracks of the well child system and be found to be behind in immunizations. The obvious solution is to ensure by routine practice that immunization histories are reviewed regularly. Many children with serious disabilities are at risk for pulmonary infections. Some of these children should also be offered immunization against pneumococcal infections.

Incontinence

The disabled child frequently may be observed to be still in diapers long after it is appropriate from a social developmental perspective. Many times, these children may be converted to classical bowel programs and alternative bladder management strategies with great success. Therefore, they need to be further evaluated to be certain that appropriate medical assessment and intervention have been offered for both of these functions. Investment in these objectives by the parents and consistency of program implementation between home and school personnel are essential for successful control of incontinence in more socially acceptable patterns.

Gastroesophageal Reflux

One of the most common intestinal problems encountered in children with neuromuscular impairment is gastroesophageal (GE) reflux.[20, 31, 38, 53, 56] This may lead to a variety of subtle or dramatic, and occasionally life-threatening, symptoms. In the extreme case, it leads to recurrent aspiration pneumonia, chronic pulmonary disease, and even sudden death. In less severe situations, failure to thrive, difficulty with sleep patterns, and epigastric distress are common. A high index of suspicion should be maintained as to the risk of GE reflux being present, and diagnosis and medical or surgical management pursued when appropriate.

Skin Protection

Small children rarely develop decubitus ulcers. This should not be surprising when one remembers that the principal cause of these lesions is excessive external pressure that exceeds internal capillary filling pressure. Since children are smaller and lighter, they rarely can exceed safe pressure levels for prolonged periods of time. The distribution of subcutaneous fat in children may be a further factor in more evenly distributing forces in a more tolerable manner. A third factor that may contribute is the general activeness of children as a normal aspect of their play and school behaviors.

There are several specific incidences of skin difficulties. The first is pressure irritation from orthoses, splints, and casts. Children will frequently not spontaneously report pain from these appliances, even though they are sensate in the area. Careful inspection and diligence on the part of the parents are essential for the prevention of these problems.

The one common site of pressure damage in children is the occipital protuberance, due to the relatively large mass of the head concentrating pressure over a small bony prominence when the infant or child is supine.

Skin lesions from a variety of other problems that are not specifically related to the disabling disorder also routinely occur in children. Care should be taken to distinguish between skin lesions that are associated with infectious disease, allergy, and other specific diseases (for example, dermatomyositis) and those problems relating to urine contamination, pressure, and shear forces.

Spasticity

Several specific issues regarding spasticity in children deserve mention (see Chapter 22 for a full discussion of spasticity management). Drugs routinely used for spasticity in adults may be used with children, but greater vigilance and monitoring must be given by the managing physician. All of the drugs show more prominent central nervous system side-effects in children, particularly somnolence. In addition, consistent compliance by children and their parents may be difficult to achieve. Although this may not generally be a problem, it can be problematic in several circumstances.

The child with a seizure disorder may be adversely affected by the sudden withdrawal of diazepam, which was being used for spasticity management and not being recognized for its contribution to epilepsy control. In addition, because children may become physiologically addicted to diazepam, slow withdrawal may be necessary.

Baclofen is also a useful drug in certain situations. However, we have observed several incidences of hallucinations in children both on therapeutic levels and with sudden withdrawal. For these reasons careful consideration should be made of the ultimate wisdom of drug management for these problems.

Children tend to be more responsive to physical modalities for spasticity management. The use of positioning, exercise, casting and bracing, and a variety of other modalities has been encouraged. Care should be taken, however, to integrate these management strategies into a child's total daily routine so that normal family, play, and educational experiences continue.

Contractures

Children will develop soft tissue and joint contractures from immobility, inadequate stretching experience, constant muscular contractions, and inflammatory disorders of the joints, soft tissue, or skin. Prevention continues to be the best strategy for management. Whenever possible, protective actions such as tone control, spasticity management, proper positioning, appropriate exercise programs, proper handling techniques, and control of inflammatory disease should be undertaken.

Treatment will depend upon the cause of the contracture. For contractures associated with tonic muscular contraction, serial or inhibitive casting is frequently effective (*e.g.,* in the head-injured child). Surgical intervention may be helpful but needs to be carefully thought through, in terms of the specific indications and procedure as well as in terms of potential deleterious effects. Several examples will illustrate this point. The child with athetoid cerebral palsy may present with a dominant extensor synergy of the lower extremities with concomitant hip adduction posturing. In many cases, if the adductors are surgically released, overwhelmingly dominant flexor tone may result, leading to the rapid development of abduction contractures that may be more disabling than the original adduction posturing.

Children with muscular dystrophy frequently shows the early development of contractures of the heel cords and an associated toe–toe gait. The unknowing surgeon who releases these contractures will likely eliminate the child's ability to walk. The kinesiology of this particular problem frequently reveals that the toe gait and equinus posture are necessary to maintain knee extension stability. After this type of surgery, bracing (at least ankle–foot orthotics) is usually mandatory to resume less functional gait.[39]

Scoliosis

The child with a physical disability is at significant risk for the development of a paralytic scoliosis, due either to weakness or trunk tone asymmetry. In either case, preventive maintenance and routine monitoring are the management strategies of choice. The child with a congenital spinal defect or deformity (such as spina bifida or congenital hemivertebrae) represents a special case for which aggressive treatment with orthotics and surgery must be considered first.

Physical examination of the back for resting posture, dynamic posture, and flexibility should be performed routinely. For children at particularly high risk, routine x-ray evaluation of the spine is appropriate. The ideal x-ray protocol to detect subtle evidence of spinal inflexibility and early curve includes multiple views. In supine, anteroposterior (AP) neutral and maximal left and right bending views are extremely helpful. Sitting AP and lateral views and standing (if possible) AP films will demonstrate the effects of gravity or tight musculature. Views in and out of spinal orthotics are helpful to determine their efficacy. Occasionally, it is useful to take AP sitting views of the patient in a seating device or wheelchair. Assessments made at intervals of 1 to 1½ years during slow growth periods are sufficient. Rapid growth requires closer assessment.

Management of a spinal curve depends on the etiological factors. For flaccid curves, proper positioning and seating, flexibility exercises, and aggressive orthotic management are appropriate. Curves secondary to asymmetric tone and spasticity are dealt with similarly, although tolerance to each of these may be more limited, making tone control more essential. Surgical management of spinal curvatures is becoming increasingly more anticipatory.[44] For example, the boy with muscular dystrophy who can be predicted to develop a serious spinal deformity is better treated by spinal fusion (with intersegmental instrumentation) early on, while he is in good condition from a pulmonary perspective, so that he can tolerate the surgery well and return to active functioning in a short period of time.

In any case, care must be taken that the management of the scoliosis does not interfere greatly with the child's capacity to function. The muscular dystrophy patient is a specific example. It has been commonly observed that the optimal management of a spinal deformity may place the child at a major mechanical disadvantage for the use of his weakened upper extremities. In the extreme, the child may have a straight back at the price of useless upper extremities—a questionable trade-off at best.

Hip Development

The area of the hips and pelvis is a major area for musculoskeletal problems. Children are born with a degree of hip flexion, anteversion, and coxa valga.[16] With normal growth and development, these postures revert to adult norms. Children with any gross motor disorder may show abnormal development in these areas, with either retention or exaggeration of the postures. These can lead to major soft-tissue and bony deformities that ultimately respond best to surgical intervention. Normal developmental aspects of the hip joint range of motion are shown in Figure 20-14 and Table 20-5.

The conservative management of these problems revolves around facilitation of normal positioning, weight-bearing experience, and range-of-motion experiences. The role of hip orthotics is variable, depending upon the specific clinical situation. Objective data confirming or rejecting the benefits of night casts and orthoses of a variety of configurations are limited in the population of children with serious disabilities. Treatment regimes tend to vary more with the regional philosophy than by analysis of objective data.

Asymmetries and obliquities of the pelvis may present profound challenges to the child and care-givers for positioning, seating, and ambulation. Fixed contractures and limitations of pelvic and lower spinal flexibility result in an uneven base for seating and standing. Management is oriented toward identifying the problem, therapy at achieving flexibility, and accommodation at fixing deformities with adapted positioning and seating systems.

Figure 20-14. Femoral anteversion normal findings as a function of age. (Chung SMK: Hip Disorders in Infants and Children. Philadelphia, Lea & Febiger, 1981)

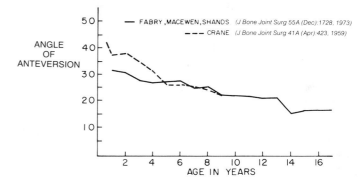

Table 20-5
Normal Passive Range of Hip Motion in Children and Adults

Age	Flexion	Flexion Contracture	Abduction in Extension	Frog-Leg Abduction	Internal Rotation	External Rotation
Newborn	120°–140°	10°–75°, mean 28°		50°–90°, mean 76°	35°–100°*, mean 62°	45°–110°, mean 89°
6 weeks	120°–140°	6°–32°, mean 19°			16°–36°†, mean 24°	26°–73°, mean 48°
3 months	120°–140°	1°–18°, mean 7°			15°–35°†, mean 26°	37°–60°, mean 45°
6 months	120°–140°	−1° to +16°, mean 7°			15°–42°†, mean 21°	34°–61°, mean 46°
3 years	120°–140°	~0°	80°		~30°–45°*	~35°–45°
4 to 10 years	120°–140°	~0°	60°–70°		~30°–45°*	~35°–45°
Adults	135°	0°	45°	65°	45°*	45°
					35°†	45°

* Measured with hips and knees flexed to 90°
† Measured with hips extended and knees flexed to 90°
(Chung SMK: Hip Disorders in Infants and Children p 67. Philadelphia, Lea & Febiger, 1981)

Lower Extremity Development

The major problems of the lower extremities are in unequal leg length and rotational deformities such as internal tibial torsion. A variety of factors may lead to these deformities. These problems must first be recognized; then they can be treated by adapting shoes, orthotics, prosthetics, or seating systems as appropriate.[63] The routine examination of any physically disabled child for these alignment and structural conditions is therefore necessary.

Common Rehabilitation Problems

Just as there are generic medical problems among diagnoses, so are there common functional issues. Specific management strategies vary with the disease, but the determination of goals and objectives is largely independent of the specific disease.

Communication

The desire and ability to communicate is the first conceptual priority in managing a disabled child. Although it is not the first developmental milestone achieved by an infant (at least as perceived by the parents), communication is essential as a "window to the mind." Frequently, the child with serious physical disability is dependent not so much on his or her abilities to physically manipulate the environment, as on the ability to control it through communication.

Early on, it is important to keep in mind the fact that language development does not need to follow motor development. Simply put, a child's inability to move well independently does not preclude an ability to think and to communicate. In fact, in some extremes, there may be complete disparity between motor and communicative development. For example, in severe athetoid cerebral palsy, the child may be totally unintelligible due to the motor deficit, yet if careful testing and assessment through nonvocal communication techniques is performed, normal to superior receptive language and cognitive function is frequently demonstrated.

For children with physical limitations, the use of an augmentative or alternative system or device for communication enhancement may be necessary. These strategies basically convert the available reliable motor abilities of the child into message-sending actions that are understandable by the listener. Specifically this may mean something as sophisticated as a device that responds to eye position by generating computer synthe-sized speech. What is important is not the technology, but the identification of the potential for communication and the development of a system that allows a child to live up to his or her communicative potential.

Mobility

Second to communication in priority is the child's ability to control his or her motion in three-dimensional space. Frequently, children are provided with passive transportation instead of the technical ability to achieve independent mobility. From a developmental perspective, newborns start experiencing self-directed movement in space in their cribs, and a child who is crawling and creeping is acquiring substantial knowledge about the world and navigation within it. It is therefore important to provide not only convenient transportation for parents, but also to give the child his or her own mobility control.

There are a variety of methods which will provide mobility control. For the child with ambulation potential, various adaptive orthoses and upper extremity aids may allow ambulation. Care should be taken, however, to be critical in assessing both the short-term energy expensiveness of ambulation and also the safety and convenience of this form of mobility. In many cases, while movement of arms and legs may be achieved, it may not be a reasonable or practical means of transportation. Furthermore, many children literally outgrow their ability to ambulate in this manner. Spastic diplegic children frequently lose mechanical advantage and coordination with growth, so that marginal childhood ambulation becomes impractical as an adolescent or adult. Similarly many children with high lumbar or thoracic paraplegia (as in spina bifida) will lose their ability to practically ambulate after growth occurs.

Wheeled mobility is possible through the use of many devices. Floor-level devices include the crawling mobile board and caster carts, which provide seated (at floor level) mobility with large drive wheels. Wheelchairs that are appropriately sized for children are available in abundance. Some have frames that accommodate to growth. The ultralight designs appear to offer mechanical advantages for the weaker child who may not be able to propel a regular chair on his own.[24]

For the child who is unable to propel a manual wheelchair, there are powered vehicles. Some commercially available battery-powered toy motorcycles and cars may offer socially acceptable and inexpensive options for the occasional user. For primary mobility means, however, true pediatric, powered wheelchairs should be considered.[23]

Limited research has been performed that agrees with clinical observations of the age at which a child can control the powered wheelchair.[13, 14] By 18 months, the child may be able to acquire the eye–hand coordination necessary to control a wheelchair with a joystick. The environment for a young child's driving needs, of course, must be carefully controlled to maintain safety. Further, the chair itself may need to be controlled so that excessive velocities cannot be achieved.

Seating and Positioning

Positioning and seating a disabled child are early essential issues that need to be addressed. Passive seating is the normal first step for infants, and children with tone problems, deformities, or other structural difficulties frequently need adapted seating and positioning systems to allow them to achieve a number of developmental goals.[51]

General goals for these devices include the achievement of normalization of tone, symmetric posturing, and proper trunk alignment facilitation. These are offered as a means to other ends, such as use of head or upper extremities for communication or other activities, seating to allow mobility, and preservation of good joint alignment.

Side-lying devices may facilitate function and maintain trunk flexibility for floor- and bed-level activities. Adapted seats are useful for spasticity management and the facilitation of upright activities. Standing devices allow vertical alignment, weight-bearing, and experiences in the upright posture. Car seating that is safe both from a postural as well as a crash safety perspective gives secure travel capacity to the child and family.

The particular positioning or seating device chosen will depend upon features, cost, and current market availability. For individuals actively involved in the care of disabled children, the best arrangement is frequently to have a close working relationship with a dealer in durable medical equipment so that tryout and assessment of new products is ongoing.

Self-Care Activities

The acquisition of independent self-care skills is a major component of normal development. Frequently these skills are delayed in the child with a physical disability. Although physical limitations are often the primary cause, secondary reasons are also common. They include a lack of encouragement from the family to achieve independence and unawareness of the potential for independence through the use of alternative techniques and adaptive aids and devices.

On occasion, expectations for independence may be too demanding. Specifically, the child with an upper extremity deficiency who uses a prosthesis may have unrealistic expectations of function. In many amputee clinics, counseling is found to be necessary to prevent the parents of three-year-olds from concluding that a prosthetic deficiency must exist because their child cannot tie shoelaces yet. Reminding families of appropriate age-related developmental milestones is frequently necessary.

Seriously delayed acquisition of independence may be seen in the myelodysplasia population.[60] Studies of this group provide a useful perspective for the analysis of function in disabled children. Few methods for the quantified assessment of functional abilities in children exist.[25]

Education

Whereas vocational rehabilitation is an important consideration for the adult with a disability, special education is important to the disabled child. The laws and services for disabled children vary with state and local school systems, but some common features are present. In general, the goals of special education are to provide "free and appropriate public education" in the least restrictive environment" for a child. Services that may variably be included in this type of educational program include special education, physical therapy, occupational therapy, speech and language therapy, adaptive physical education, psychological and social work services, and nursing services. In each case, these services become school system responsibilities in that they are necessary for the child to participate in an Individualized Education Program (IEP), a specific educational plan with goals, objectives, definition of services, and time frames.

The role of health professionals in the special education system is an advisory and participatory one. Programs developed within a school setting should be consistent with those established out of school, in both the home and other therapy settings. School programs should not let therapeutic goals obscure their educational objectives. Programs that effectively integrate medical rehabilitation needs with those of education are the most effective.[15]

Play

Disabled children frequently need special assistance in achieving the ability to play successfully. Recreational therapy, music therapy, art therapy, play therapy, and other interventions may be helpful in allowing a child to find mechanisms to express him or herself and to experiment with future skills and roles.[66]

Adapted toys and games are useful. Battery adapters that allow external switch control of any electric or electronic device may give the more severely disabled child the option to play with age-appropriate toys while possessing only limited physical skills.

Children may also need special assistance in experiencing group play. Participation in nursery school programs, play groups, and other endeavors will allow the child to experience play both with other disabled and with able-bodied children. Parental counseling and resource identification may be necessary to facilitate these activities.

Social Skills

Children with disabilities are often found to be deficient in adaptive social skills due to a variety of factors, including limited normal childhood experiences and intensive involvement with the health care community. Efforts may need to be taken to assist a child and family to identify specific behavioral issues and find methods to overcome them. The current concept of a child having acquired "learned helplessness" is useful as a perspective in dealing with these issues.

Parenting Skills

Just as normal child parenting is a challenging experience, so is parenting a disabled child. It is further complicated by the challenges of health and social functions experienced by the child and family. Many parents need assistance and guidance in coping with what are really normal parenting issues in their care for their disabled child.

Common problems include difficulty in setting appropriate levels of expectation of responsible behavior, and discipline maintenance. Counseling for the parents on how to distinguish the special limits and expectations that are appropriate for the disability from normal parenting issues, such as control and authority challenging, may be very helpful. Introducing families to parents of other disabled children is also a very positive strategy.

Sexuality

Managing the emerging sexuality of a disabled child requires knowledge, an openness and willingness to discuss, and anticipatory strategies. Many of the early needs of the disabled child are simply for accurate and age-appropriate information about sex and reproduction in general, as well as the child's specific abilities or limitations based upon the disability. Frequently this knowledge is also needed by the parents.

Education and counseling for the adolescent child is often necessary for these issues. Children may express their underlying sexual concerns through other behaviors, including social withdrawal and depression. A high index of suspicion of the need for sexual education and counseling should be maintained by the involved health professional.

Independent Living

A long-term perspective on the child's potential to live independently should be adopted from an early age. Realistic goal setting is the essential first step for any long-term rehabilitation program and for attaining independence. It is frequently possible to distinguish at an early age the child who will need some tupe of supported living situation in the long term. Helping the family and school system to identify these expectations early on will facilitate appropriate school programming and long-term planning.

It is unfortunately all too frequent that we encounter a seriously developmentally disabled adult (age 30 to 40) who lives with parents until they are infirm or they die. Many times, there has been inadequate planning for legal, estate, and practical matters that suddenly become crises. The solution to these types of problems is prevention by ensuring that they are anticipated long before they become a reality.

MANAGEMENT OF CHILDHOOD DISABILITY

The strategies of management of the disabled child are derived from two fundamental knowledge bases. First is the nature of the child's specific physical and functional impairment. Second is a knowledge of normal development, and a belief that appropriate management of a disabled child is to facilitate their passage (as much as possible) through the stages of normal development.

Assessment

Development is studied in a number of specific manners, but a simple overview will be sufficient for the purposes of the following discussion. The most powerful concept is that different skill categories may be identified and assessed on a relatively autonomous basis. The major categories of development commonly considered include gross motor, fine motor, cognitive, personal-social, and language.[22, 26]

Each of these aspects of development may be measured according to a number of formal tests and evaluation tools. Four different types of developmental assessment tools exist: chronologically normalized attainment scales; criterion referenced descriptive tests; physical/performance assessments with quantitative assessments of performance levels; and functional assessment instruments to describe performance of activities.[17]

Developmental Attainment Scales

The most commonly used screening test for developmental attainment assessment is the Denver Developmental Screening Test.[22] This is an easy to learn and use survey and test instrument that allows a quick screening for deviations from normal development. It is intended for analysis of normal and near-normal children and is insensitive to increments of developmental progress that may occur in children with severe disabilities.

A second commonly used test is the Bayley Scales of Infant Development,[4] designed for children from birth to 30 months. This tool is also relatively insensitive to increments of change in severely disabled children.

Descriptive Tests

Examples of descriptive tests include the Koontz Child Development Program[42] and the Brigance[11] assessments. These tests were developed in response to the need for a tool that would define individual components of an IEP.

Performance Analysis

Quantitative analysis of motor performance of children is accomplished by several strategies. First is the measurement of physical parameters, such as range of motion and strength, and physiological parameters, such as heart rate and respiratory rate. Timed trials of specific activities such as the Jebson Taylor Hand Function test[37, 64] may be useful as norm-referenced comparisons or sequential performance reassessments.

Functional Assessment

Quantitative descriptions of the functional activities of disabled children are essential for monitoring and planning rehabilitation programs. The Barthel Index[47] is an example of an adult-oriented instrument, but few pediatric tools are currently available. The two notable exceptions are the analytic tool for children with spina bifida described by Sousa and colleagues,[60] and the Tufts Assessment of Motor Performance (TAMP).[25] The latter provides a method for structured quantitative description of developmentally oriented activities that are commonly engaged in by seriously disabled children. This and other similar tools should be routinely incorporated into the diagnostic and analytic reviews of a disabled child's rehabilitation progress.

Impact of a Disability on Growth and Development

Serious disabling impairments will affect a child's growth and development. Only by knowing the likely impact will the health professional be able to anticipate problems and optimize the child's health and function. Upper motor neuron lesions (especially of the parietal cortex occurring before age 4) will result in mild diminishment of body growth. The child with hemiplegic cerebral palsy, for example, will show signs of hemihypotrophy of the involved body side. This may include limb, trunk, and even facial asymmetries. Growth is usually not seriously disturbed, but the asymmetry may be noticeable. Trunk asymmetries may be mistaken for scoliosis and need careful assessment.

Monitoring of height and weight and head circumference are important routine management strategies. Use of the normative charts for comparison purposes is appropriate. Significant deviations in the curve of growth should be noted and explained. Difficulties in growth may be the result of chronic illness, nutritional deficiency, and chronic gastroesophageal reflux, along with a host of other specific problems.

The presence of a disabling disorder has an obvious impact on the developmental process. In general, the patterns of development may be thought of as mimicking the patterns of adaptation to a disability. Figure 20-15 shows normal development of function along an arbitrary scale of function; Figure 20-16 shows the impact of a congenital disability on that development. Similarly, Figure 20-17 shows the consequences of an acquired disability. In Figure 20-18, the impact of a progressive degenerative disorder is demonstrated. These time patterns of development and progress incorporate both recovery, rehabilitation therapy effects, and normal growth and development.

Prediction of Outcome

One of the major roles played by the health professional is the establishment of medical and functional prognoses for a disabled child. From these estimates of outcome the specific objectives and plans of management can be drawn that will guide the

daily activities of the child and family. It is therefore most important to both accurately predict and be cognizant of the limits of predictability for any individual child.

Certain common milestones that are considered major objectives in life should be considered early on. The first of these is the question, Will my child be able to walk? It must be recognized that *walking* means different things to a medical professional and to a parent. The parent means, Will my child go everywhere he or she wants to, with no assistive devices, no wheelchair, and no help from anyone else? The professional, of course, will be more comfortable in distinguishing between a variety of types of walking (for example, in the house or in the community) and degrees of dependency upon devices and other individuals. Initial clarity of predictions should be sought.

The second major question that may or may not be spoken is, Will my child be able to live independently and earn his or her own living? This is usually closely related to the third question, Will my child be able to marry and have children? Both are major questions that are not easy to answer. It may be useful to guide parents to define what the specific issues related to their child are, and which of them are predictable. By allowing the family to

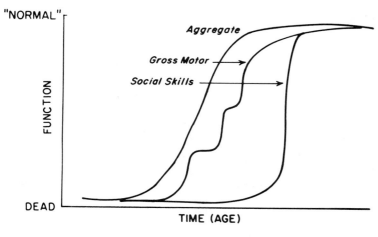

Figure 20-15. Functional development in normal children as a function of age. In the aggregate, development is thought of as a continuous process, but specific individual skills are acquired in a stepwise fashion.

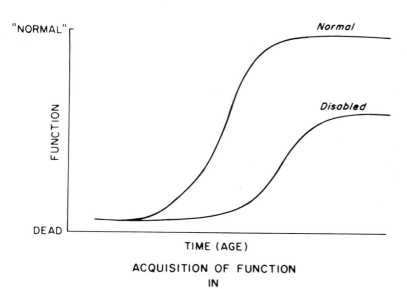

Figure 20-16. Development of function for a child with a congenital or early acquired disability. Note the slower rate of function acquisition and the lower final level of function achieved.

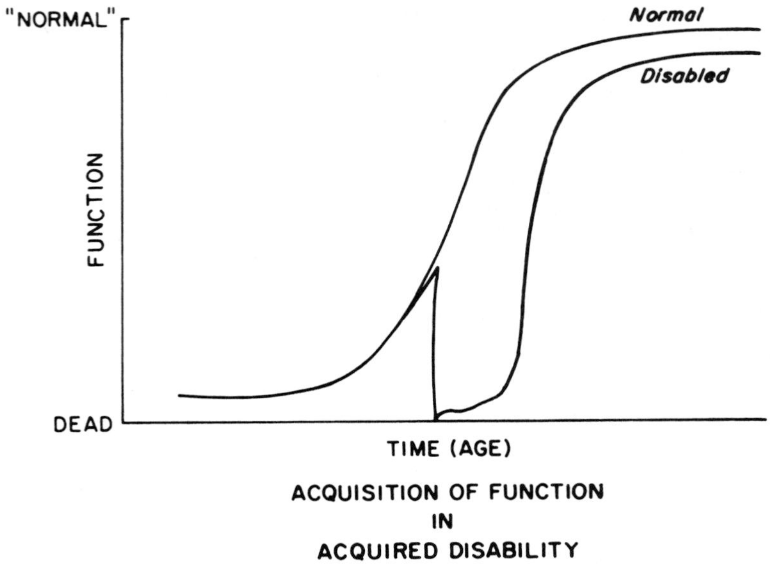

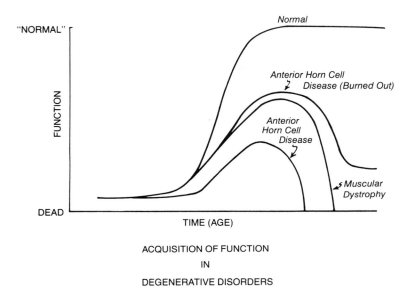

Figure 20-17. Functional development of a child with a late acquired disability. Note the normal pattern that is interrupted by the onset of the new impairment. Relatively rapid early recovery is followed by continuing improvement due to growth and development, as well as possible continuing recovery.

Figure 20-18. Functional development of a child with a progressive degenerative disorder. In some cases, developmental progress (at a lesss than normal rate) may continue while the rate of growth and development exceeds the rate of deterioration from the underlying disease.

participate in the analysis that may lead to answering the questions, greater comfort with the answers may be derived.

In the case of the child with a degenerative disorder, much more serious questions such as How long will my child live? and What will be his or her quality of life? become prominent. The predictions may be obvious, but in our experience, they are frequently difficult and evasive. The greatest harm may be done by providing unnecessarily dogmatic projections in either extreme. For the most pessimistic projection, such as when the child is given only a short time to live, major difficulties come about when the child survives beyond the expected period. The child and family spend the additional lifetime constantly waiting for the end, and more important, frequently nothing is done to allow the child to grow, achieve goals, or face new challenges, because the family adopts a fatalistic, do nothing attitude.

At the other extreme, inappropriately optimistic projections will contribute to unrealistic goal setting and will encourage the child and family to set themselves up for failure to achieve objectives, bringing further frustration and emotional pain.

The right approach is to admit uncertainty when it exists, make cautiously optimistic predictions, and move forward with goals that at least provide for comfort and care for both the child and family, and also give some specific positive objectives.

COMMON CHILDHOOD DISEASES

Cerebral Palsy

Cerebral palsy is the commonest physical disability of childhood seen in practice by rehabilitation professionals. As such, it serves as a useful teaching model for all brain disorders in childhood, including stroke, head injury, tumor, and infections. Cerebral palsy is defined as a motor disorder occurring because of a lesion that is nonprogressive and occurs in the developing brain.[36] This does not preclude other associated problems such as sensory loss, cognitive deficits, language disorders, and so on. Clearly, cerebral palsy is not a specific disease, but rather a collection of disorders with some common features.

The various specific forms of cerebral palsy are generally described along four different parameters that usually are specifically correlated. The four parameters are neuroanatomical lesion; etiology; neurological pattern; and topography of body dysfunction.

The neuroanatomical lesions will either be localized to a physical zone, blood supply distribution, or a distribution that correlates with metabolic sensitivities. Thus, a vascular lesion will lead to a typical stroke pattern, a depressed skull fracture will lead to local cortical findings, and an ischemic or toxic lesion will show more diffuse deficits according to the cells most affected.

The commonest etiologies noted for cerebral palsy include prematurity, ischemia, hypoxemia, hyperbilirubinemia, and trauma (either external or internal).[55, 61]

The neurological pattern of loss shows five major types: spasticity, flaccidity, athetosis, ataxia, and mixed patterns. The distinction between these patterns is not uncommonly difficult, and children frequently evolve from one pattern to another. It is typical, for example, for a flaccid or "floppy" infant to evolve toward spasticity and then, perhaps athetoid patterns, and finally to a mixture of spasticity and athetoid features.

Spasticity in children shows the typical combination of increased resting muscle tone, hyperactive stretch reflexes, clonus, and the spread of reflex responses. *Flaccidity* is usually described in children as low tone or floppiness, and is demonstrated by low resting muscle tone, diminished stretch reflexes, and frequently diminishment of the primitive reflex patterns.

Athetosis is demonstrated in children by several phenomena that are different from those typically thought of as representative of athetosis. First is the observation of markedly variable tone. These children may show major fluctuations in resting tone ranging from flaccidity to opisthotonic rigidity. These changes may or may not be associated with external environmental factors. Associated with the variable tone is the observation of remarkable dominance of primitive reflex patterns throughout the child's motor repertoire. Almost all primitive reflexes are normal findings at certain developmental stages, but their obligatory dominance and preservation over time should never be considered as within normal limits.

Finally, and usually later in development, comes the appearance of the athetoid movement pattern of writhing and flailing motion. Although these motions are described by some as random actions, they typically are not. Rather, they are poorly learned and even more poorly refined efforts at achieving skilled motor control of the limbs. Careful observation of the child with athetosis will show rather consistent and stereotypical patterns of these so-called adventitious movements.

Ataxia is a less common pattern with both trunk and limb involvement. It is commonly associated with cerebellar damage and is seen frequently as a consequence of traumatic brain injury.

The *mixed pattern* may, in fact, be the most common description for cerebral palsy, even though most authors have attempted to minimize this category. The typical child shows features of several patterns. For example, the child with athetoid features, such as poor limb control, variable tone, and dominant primitive reflexes, may also show persistently high tone, even though it varies, and soft tissue contractures. In our experience, the child with pure athetoid patterns will not develop soft tissue contractures; hence, this child shows a mixed spastic-athetoid pattern.

The distribution of the motor deficit over the body is described by the definition of limbs involved. Thus, *monoplegia* implies a single limb is involved; *hemiplegia* suggests the arm and leg on the same side; and *quadriplegia* all four limbs. The term *diplegia* is used when the legs are the major involved limbs, with the arms only subtly affected. The term *paraplegia* is to be avoided, for it implies complete normalcy of the upper limbs. If, in fact, only the lower limbs are involved, the diagnosis of cerebral palsy is most likely incorrect and should be challenged.

Quadriplegia usually also implies that trunk, head and neck control are also deficient. To emphasize this point, the term *total body involved* is sometimes used.

Etiology

The commonest neuroanatomical lesion is damage to the germinal matrix zone in the periventricular region of the premature fetus, usually occurring around 24 to 28 weeks of gestational age.[67] This injury is usually caused by ischemic damage associated with hypoperfusion of the area. This area is susceptible to this type of damage because it is a watershed zone with only marginal blood supply. This lesion tends to be somewhat symmetric, leading to bilateral signs. Further, it occurs in the area of those internal capsular tracts that are more heavily involved in the lower extremities functions. As a consequence, the lesion presents as a spastic diplegia.

Major hypoxic injuries result in diffuse damage to cortical and cerebellar systems, resulting in spastic quadriparesis. There is generally a correlation with the severity of the spasticity and the amount of cognitive dysfunction and likelihood for an associated seizure disorder as well.

More selective damage results from hyperbilirubinemia. This previously common form of damage resulted from Rh incompatibility and resultant erythroblastosis fetalis. As a result of the introduction of Rhogam and fetal transfusions, the consequent damage from kernicterus has been drastically diminished. The pattern of these lesions showed a classical triad of athetosis, sensorineural hearing loss, and paralysis of upward gaze (Parinaud's syndrome). Perhaps more important is the frequently noted major discrepancy between motor dysfunction, speech dysfunction (due to motor difficulties), and the preservation of good cognitive and language function.

More discrete lesions such as cerebral vascular occlusions from emboli or vasculitis result in typical stroke patterns such as hemiplegia. When these occur in infancy and early childhood, their impact on language function is surprisingly minimal. Presumably shifts of cortical dominance occur as compensatory mechanisms to allow relatively good language function to develop.

The typical relationships between these various parameters and the related clinical syndromes are shown in Table 20-6.

Management

The management of the motor deficit of cerebral palsy requires an understanding of the natural history of the disease and the pattern of motor activity available to the child, and a coordinated long-range set of goals for the child.

There are many specific schools of thought about particular therapy programs that may be offered to children. In general, the most effective of these combine knowledge of the reflex behaviors of children with cerebral palsy with knowledge of motor learning.

A variety of specialized therapeutic protocols have been popularized. Little evidence exists, however, to demonstrate the clinical superiority of one over another. Leading systems of care include the traditional orthopedic approach of range of motion, stretch, and strengthening; neurodevelopmental treatment (NDT) for motor learning and tone normalization[10]; sensory integration[3] for a variety of motor and arousal features; and a variety of others.[58] The most commonly used school of therapy in the United States is NDT, as taught by Doctors Berta and Karl Bobath.

Modern therapeutic programs do not rely exclusively on one school of therapy; rather they draw eclectically on a variety of

Table 20-6
Classification and Patterns of Cerebral Palsy

Neurological	Extent	Severity	Other
Hemiplegia			
Flaccid	Right	Mild	Congenital/acquired
Spastic	Left	Moderately severe	Unknown etiology
		Severe	Epilepsy/no epilepsy
Bilateral hemiplegia	—	Mild	Congenital/acquired
		Moderately severe	
		Severe	Epilepsy/no epilepsy
Diplegia			
Hypotonic	Paraplegic	Mild	Congenital:
Dystonic	Triplegic	Moderately severe	Associated with low birthweight
Rigid/spastic	Paraplegic	Severe	Not low birthweight
			Acquired (rare)
			Epilepsy/no epilepsy
Ataxic diplegia	Paraplegic	Mild	Congenital/acquired:
	Triplegic	Moderately severe	With hydrocephalus and/or spina bifida
	Tetraplegic	Severe	No hydrocephalus/spina bifida
			Epilepsy/no epilepsy
Ataxia	Predominantly	Mild	Congenital/acquired:
	Unilateral (rare)	Moderately severe	With hydrocephalus and/or spina bifida
	Bilateral symmetrical	Severe	No hydrocephalus/spina bifida
			Hearing loss/no hearing loss
			Epilepsy/no epilepsy
			Disequilibrium syndrome/no disequilibrium syndrome
Dyskinesia	Monoplegic (rare)	Mild	Congenital:
			Kernicterus/no kernicterus
	Hemiplegic (rare)	Moderately severe	Acquired (rare)
	Triplegic	Severe	
	Tetraplegic		
Other			

(Ingram TTS: Historical review of the definition and classification of the cerebral palsies. In Stanley F, Alberman E (eds): Epidemiology of the Cerebral Palsies, p 8. Philadelphia, JB Lippincott, 1984)

techniques and strategies that will optimize the child's ability to function. Above all, providers of therapeutic services need to be aware of the values and limits, as well as the costs and demands of their interventions, in both financial and human terms. It is important also that they avoid overly burdening the child and family with unlikely or unreasonable therapeutic demands and expectations.

Spinal Dysraphism

One of the commonest congenital defects leading to major physical impairment is spinal dysraphism, variously referred to as myelomeningocele, meningomyelocele, and spina bifida. In general, these disorders represent developmental abnormalities of the spinal axis resulting in spinal cord dysfunction and all the consequences that neurological disruption typically encounters; as in spinal cord–injured patients. Representative patterns of the dysraphic state are shown in Figure 20-19.

Etiology

The cause of spinal dysraphism is believed to be of genetic etiology, with both chromosomal and environmental contributing factors. Major risk factors for the development of a dysraphic

disorder include a family history of dysraphism and increased maternal or paternal age.

Prenatal diagnosis for mothers at risk includes maternal serum alpha fetal protein assessment, amniotic fluid alpha fetal protein elevations, and ultrasound imaging of the fetus for evidence of anomalous development of the spinal axis. Prenatal diagnosis is, of course, indicated principally if consideration is being given to termination of the pregnancy if a defect is identified.[54]

Management

The initial management of a newborn with spinal dysraphism includes decision-making with regard to surgical closure of the lesion and assessment for other associated disorders, especially hydrocephalus. The spinal surgery may range from a simple excision of the empty sack with primary closure, to extensive and meticulous neurosurgical untangling of nerve roots and cord, bony reconstruction, and complex plastic surgical flap rotations.[29]

The management of hydrocephalus (almost a 90% incidence) includes ventricular monitoring (ultrasound while the fontanelle is open, computed tomography or magnetic resonance imaging thereafter), installation of a ventricular shunt (most commonly to the peritoneum), and monitoring of shunt

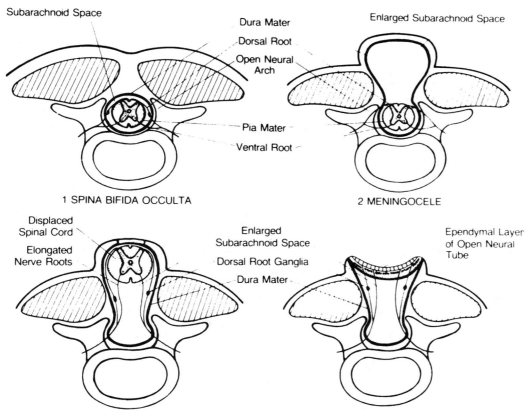

Subarachnoid Space

Dura Mater
Dorsal Root
Open Neural Arch

Pia Mater
Ventral Root

1 SPINA BIFIDA OCCULTA

Enlarged Subarachnoid Space

2 MENINGOCELE

Displaced Spinal Cord
Elongated Nerve Roots

Enlarged Subarachnoid Space
Dorsal Root Ganglia
Dura Mater

Ependymal Layer of Open Neural Tube

3 MYELOMENINGOCELE

4 MYELOCELE

Figure 20-19. Major patterns of spinal dysraphism. The name of the lesion depends on the contents of the abnormal sac. (Menelaus MB: Orthopedic Management of Spina Bifida Cystica, 2nd ed. New York, Churchill Livingstone, 1980)

function (physical examination of the reservoir under the scalp or nuclear scanning of cerebrospinal fluid clearance by the shunt).[57, 65]

The decision to treat or not treat the newborn infant with spinal dysraphism continues to be a complex ethical issue. Objective criteria for determination of indications for not treating (allowing the infant to succumb to central nervous system infection) have been proposed but are still under debate. Increasingly, the clinical tendency is to attempt aggressive surgical intervention in almost all cases.[46, 49, 59]

Early rehabilitation management concerns include bladder and bowel care, prevention of contractures and hip subluxation or dislocation, prevention of spinal deformity, and encouragement of normal mobility (with orthoses and wheelchair use).

Infants with significant bladder detrusor sphincter dyssynergia will benefit from an intermittent catheterization program and appropriate monitoring for urological function (urodynamic studies, renal scan or intravenous pyelogram, recording postvoid residuals, periodic urine cultures). Children developmentally around age 5 may be taught self-catheterization if no perceptual motor problems interfere, although they will continue to require supervision for reliability.

Bowel flow may be managed with traditional bowel program methods. Occasionally, a flaccid anal sphincter without sufficient tone to retain feces is encountered. When it is developmentally appropriate to establish bowel continence (to eliminate the use of diapers), efforts at dietary manipulation to enhance stool consistency may be helpful.

Parents should be taught in the newborn nursery to perform effective range-of-motion exercises for all involved limbs and the trunk. In the early years, range of motion that is performed with each diaper change may result in a compliant institution of this home therapy. Bed positioning should also be reviewed to allow passive stretch of tight hip flexors and spinal restrictions.

Early attention to sitting posture is important. The use of adapted infant and child seats may help to minimize kyphoscoliosis. Frequently a body jacket is effective in controlling spinal alignment against the effects of gravity. Increasingly, early aggressive surgical management (spinal fusion with intersegmental rod instrumentation to avoid prolonged external bracing) is being selected as the management approach of choice.[52] Occasionally, thoracic suspension orthoses for wheelchair positioning are useful.

Early standing using a variety of devices is encouraged. Either a parapodium, standing frame, or knee–ankle–foot orthoses are used. Although few objective substantive studies exist, early standing is believed to enhance hip alignment, bone mineralization, urinary function, and psychosocial functioning. The parapodium, swivel walker, reciprocal orthoses, and traditional orthoses for ambulation training are all advocated by various authors. Moreover, the early institution of good wheelchair skills in parallel with ambulation training offers the needed balance of mobility with ambulation for exercise and function.

Children should be examined for presence of perceptual motor disorders. These are commonly observed, and their presence is likely to be more significant in a child with a history of shunt malfunctions and repeated infections (as is a lower IQ).[50] Frequently, verbal skills may far exceed performance abilities, leading to the "cocktail party personality" behavior. Care should be taken to objectively validate the child's skills and performance of activities, rather than relying on reports by the child.

Later (adolescent) management focuses on ensuring autonomous self-care skills, including personal hygiene and bladder/bowel care, sexual adaptation, and vocational planning. The specific management techniques differ little from those used for the care of spinal cord–injured patients. The complicating factors are the long-standing behavior patterns that have become entrenched, and the frequent presence of mild to moderate cognitive and perceptual deficits. Given that for most children, the long-term survival prognosis is excellent (formerly chronic renal disease was a source of high fatality for long-term survivors), the need for long-range planning and vocational rehabilitation is evident.[30]

REFERENCES

1. Anderson DW, McLaurin RL: Report on the national head and spinal cord injury survey. J Neurosurg 53:S1–S43, 1980
2. Apley J: Care of the Handicapped Child. Philadelphia, JB Lippincott, 1978
3. Ayres AJ: Sensory Integration and Learning Disorders. Los Angeles, Western Psychological Services, 1972
4. Bayley N: The Bayley Scales of Infant Development Manual. New York, Psychological Corporation, 1969
5. Bennett FC: Developmental dysfunction and school failure in the adolescent. In Smith MS (ed): Chronic Disorders in Adolescence. Boston, John Wright, 1983
6. Berninger VW, Gans BM: Language profiles in nonspeaking individuals of normal intelligence with severe cerebral plasy. Augmentative and Alternative Communication 2:45–50, 1986
7. Berninger VW, Gans BM: Assessing word processing capability of the nonvocal, nonwriting. Augmentative and Alternative Communication 2:56–63, 1986
8. Bobath B: Abnormal Postural Reflex Activity Caused by Brain Lesions, 2nd ed. London, Heinemann, 1971
9. Bobath B, Bobath K: Motor Development in the Different Types of Cerebral Palsies. London, Heinemann, 1975
10. Bobath K: A Neurophysiological Basis for the Treatment of Cerebral Palsy. Philadelphia, JB Lippincott, 1980
11. Brigance AH: Brigance Diagnostic Inventory of Early Development. Woburn, MA, Curriculum Associates, 1978
12. Buscaglia L: The Disabled and Their Parents: A Counseling Challenge. Thorofare, NJ, Charles B Slack, 1975
13. Butler C: Effects of powered mobility on self-initiated behaviors of very young children with locomotor disability. Dev Med Child Neurol 28:325–332, 1986
14. Butler C, Okamoto G, McKay T: Motorized wheelchair driving by disabled children. Arch Phys Med Rehabil 65:95–97, 1984
15. Chess S, Fernandez P: The Handicapped Child in School: Behavior and Management. New York, Brunner/Mazel, 1981
16. Chung SMK: Hip Disorders in Infants and Children. Philadelphia, Lea & Febiger, 1981
17. Connolly B, Harris S: Survey of assessment tools. Totline 9:8–11, 1983
18. Cotman CW, Nieto-Sampedro M, Gibbs RB: Enhancing the self-repairing potential of the CNS after injury. Central Nervous System Trauma 1:3–14, 1984
19. Edlin JC, Mitchell JR: Normal adolescent growth and development. In Smith MS (ed): Chronic Disorders in Adolescence. Boston, John Wright, 1983
20. Euler AR, Byrne WJ et al: Recurrent pulmonary disease in children: A complication of gastroesophageal reflux. Pediatrics 63:47–51, 1979
21. Featherstone H: A Difference in the Family: Life with a Disabled Child. New York, Basic Books, 1980
22. Frankenburg WK, Dodds JB: The Denver Developmental Screening Test. Denver, University of Colorado Medical Center, 1966
23. Gans BM, Hallenborg SC: Power wheelchairs: Making the right choices. Rx Homecare, pp 32–41, July 1984
24. Gans BM, Hallenborg SC: Advances in wheelchair design. In Redford JB (ed): Physical Medicine and Rehabilitation: State of the Art Reviews 1:95–109, 1987
25. Gans BM, Mann NR, Hallenborg SC, Haley SC: Tufts assessment of motor performance (TAMP) (abstr). Dev Med Child Neurol 28 (Suppl 53):43, 1986
26. Gesell A, Amatruda GS: Developmental Diagnosis, 2nd ed. London, Harper & Row, 1947
27. Gode RO, Smith MS: Effects of chronic disorders on adolescent development: Self, family, friends, and school. In Smith MS (ed): Chronic Disorders in Adolescence. Boston, John Wright, 1983
28. Gortmaker SL, Sappenfield W: Chronic childhood disorders: Prevalence and impact. Pediatr Clin North Am 31:3–18, 1984
29. Guthkelch AN: Aspects of the surgical management of myelomeningocele: A review. Dev Med Child Neurol 28:525–532, 1986
30. Harrington TF (ed): Handbook of Career Planning for Special Needs Students. Rockville MD, Aspen, 1982
31. Herbst JJ, Book LS, Bray PF: Gastroesophageal reflux in the "near miss" sudden infant death syndrome. J Pediatrics 92:73–75, 1978
32. Herst J, Wolfe S, Jorgensen G, Pallan S: Sewall Early Education Developmental Profiles, 2nd ed. Denver, Sewall Rehabilitation Center, 1976
33. Hoskins TA, Squires JE: Developmental assessment: A test for gross motor and reflex development. Phys Ther 53:117–125, 1973
34. Human Services Research Institute: Summary of Data on Handicapped Children and Youth. Washington, DC, US Government Printing Office, 1985
35. Illingworth RS: Development of the Infant and Young Child: Normal and Abnormal, 7th ed. New York, Churchill Livingstone, 1980
36. Ingram TTS: Historical review of the definition and classification of the cerebral palsies. In Stanley F, Alberman E (eds): Epidemiology of the Cerebral Palsies. Philadelphia, JB Lippincott, 1984
37. Jebson RH, Taylor N et al: An objective and standardized test of hand function. Arch Phys Med Rehabil 50:311–319, 1969
38. Johnson DG, Herbst JJ et al: Evaluation of gastroesophageal reflux surgery in children. Pediatrics 59:62–68, 1977
39. Johnson EW: Pathokinesiology of Duchenne muscular dystrophy: Implications for management. Arch Phys Med Rehabil 58:4–7, 1977
40. Kaplan SL: Normal and abnormal growth. In Rudolph AM, Barnett HL, Einhorn AH: Pediatrics, 16th ed. New York, Appleton-Century Crofts, 1977
41. Kiely J, Paneth N, Stanley F: Monitoring the morbidity outcomes of perinatal health services. In Stanley F, Alberman E (eds): Epidemiology of the Cerebral Palsies. Philadelphia, JB Lippincott, 1984
42. Koontz CW: Koontz Child Development Program: Training Activities for the First 48 Months. Los Angeles, Western Psychological Services, 1974
43. Kottke FJ: Neurophysiologic therapy for stroke. In Licht S (ed): Stroke and Its Rehabilitation. Baltimore, Waverly Press, 1975
44. Lehman M, Hsu AM, Hsu JD: Spinal curvature, hand dominance and prolonged upper extremity use of wheelchair-dependent DMD patients. Dev Med Child Neurol 28:628–632, 1986
45. Lichter P: Educational and vocational aspects of chronic disorders in adolescence. In Smith MS (ed): Chronic Disorders in Adolescence. Boston, John Wright, 1983
46. Lorber J: Results of treatment of myelomeningocele: An analysis of 524 unselected cases with special reference to possible selection for treatment. Dev Med Child Neurol 13:279–303, 1971
47. Mahoney RI, Barthel DW: Functional evaluation: The Barthel index. Maryland State Med J 14:61–65, 1965
48. McCarty SM, St james P, Berninger VW, Gans BM: Assessment of intellectual functioning across the life-span in severe cerebral palsy. Dev Med Child Neurol 28:364–374, 1986
49. McLone DG: Results of treatment of children born with a myelomeningocele. Clin Neurosurg 30:407–412, 1983
50. McLone DG, Czyzewski D et al: Central nervous system infections as a limiting factor in the intelligence of children with myelomeningocele. Pediatrics 70:338–342, 1982
51. Medhat MA, Redford JB, Prescribed seating systems. In Redford JB: Physical Medicine and Rehabilitation: State of the Art Reviews 1:111–136, 1987
52. Menelaus MB: Orthopedic Management of Spina Bifida Cystica, 2nd ed. New York, Churchill Livingstone, 1980
53. Meyers WF, Herbst JJ: Effectiveness of positioning therapy for gastroesophageal reflux. Pediatrics 69:768–772, 1982
54. Milunsky A, Alpert E: The value of alpha-fetoprotein in the prenatal diagnosis of neural tube defects. J Pediatr 84:889–893, 1974
55. Nelson KB, Ellenberg JH: Antecedents of cerebral palsy: Multivariate analysis of risk. N Engl J Med 315:81–86, 1986

56. Orenstein SR, Whitington PF, Orenstein DM: The infant seat as a treatment for gastroesophageal reflux. N Engl J Med 309:760–763, 1983

57. Schmidt K, Gjerris F et al: Antibiotic prophylaxis in cerebrospinal fluid shunting: A prospective randomized trial in 152 hydrocephalic patients. Neurosurg 17:1–5, 1985

58. Scrutton D (ed): Management of the Motor Disorders of Children with Cerebral Palsy. Philadelphia, JB Lippincott, 1984

59. Shurtleff DB, Hayden PW et al: Myelodysplasia: Decision for death or disability. N Engl J Med 291:1005–1011, 1974

60. Sousa JC, Gordon LH, Shurtleff DB: Assessing the development of daily living skills in patients with spina bifida. Dev Med Child Neurol (Supply 37) 18: 134–142, 1976

61. Stanley F, Alberman E: Epidemiology of the Cerebral Palsies. Philadelphia, JB Lippincott, 1984

62. Swaiman KF, Jacobson RI: Developmental abnormalities of the central nervous system. In Baker AB, Joynt RJ (eds): Clinical Neurology. Philadelphia, Harper & Row, 1984

63. Tachdjian MO: Pediatric Orthopedics. Philadelphia, WB Saunders, 1972

64. Taylor N, Sand PL, Jebsen RH: Evaluation of hand function in children. Arch Phys Med Rehabil 54:129–135, 1973

65. Tew B, Evans R et al: Results of a selective surgical policy on the cognitive abilities of children with spina bifida. Dev Med Child Neurol 27:606–614, 1985

66. Tizard B, Harvey D: Biology of Play. Philadelphia, JB Lippincott, 1977

67. Wigglesworth J: Brain development and its modification by adverse influences. In Stanley F, Alberman E (eds): Epidemology of the Cerebral Palsies. Philadelphia, JB Lippincott, 1984

68. Young W: A critical overview of spinal injury research presented at the First International Symposium on CNS Trauma. Central Nervous System Trauma 1:81–88, 1984

21

Rehabilitation of the Geriatric Patient

Gary S. Clark

Patrick K. Murray

GENERAL ASPECTS OF AGING

Aging, in and of itself, is not a disease or disability. Although a significant proportion of elderly develop disabilities, they are secondary to the often multiple chronic diseases that may be associated with aging. Geriatric rehabilitation focuses primarily on two populations: elderly who become disabled and disabled who become elderly. The increasing health care attention and concern shown to these groups is demonstrated by Brotman[14] who writes, "persons aged 65 + are subject to more than twice as much disability, have four times the activity limitation, see physicians 42% more often, and have about twice as many hospital stays that last about 50% longer than persons under 65."

Demography of Aging

At the turn of the century, every 25th American was an *older person* (defined as age 65 or over); now, it is every ninth.[14] By the year 2030, it is projected that every 5th American will be 65 or older.[119] This means that the current 11% of the population age 65 and over (25 million) will more than double to 21% (64 million) within the next 5 decades.[14, 119]

Of even greater importance is the rapidly increasing relative proportion of the 65 and over population who are 75 and over (termed *old-old*). This group includes many of the so-called frail elderly, with a disproportionately high prevalence of disabilities and consumption of health services. While 39% of the elderly were 75 and over in 1980, it is estimated that this figure will be approximately 50% by the year 2000.[119] Even more impressive are estimates that the *oldest-old*, those age 85 and over, will increase from the current 2.3 million to over 16 million by the year 2050.[119]

Currently, approximately 5,200 Americans turn 65 every day, and about 3,600 people age 65 and over die each day, resulting in a net increase of 1,600 older people *every day*.[14] The average life expectancy at age 65 is now more than 16 years.[14]

It is well known that with increasing age there is an increasing incidence of chronic and multiple diseases.[119] Although there are no one-to-one correlations between disease and illness,[131] or disease and disability,[24] a significant proportion of elderly are limited in the amount or kind of usual activity or mobility secondary to chronic impairments. In fact, over 60% of adults with functional impairments due to chronic health problems are age 65 or over.[41] Many of these chronic diseases are not amenable to cure, and may even be progressive. The challenge to health care providers is to prevent or minimize functional impairments resulting from the various chronic and multiple illnesses to which elderly are prone.

Psychosocial Issues in Aging

Myths About Aging

Butler coined the term *ageism* to describe biased perceptions of older people by the younger population in today's youth-oriented culture, as well as perceptions of old age by the elderly themselves.[17] There are a number of prevalent and misleading ageism myths.[58] The myth that most elderly live in institutions is countered by the reality that only about 5% do.[119] The common notion that elderly are not interested in sexual activity is simply not true. Although there is some decline in physiological abilities, the majority of elderly maintain sexual interest and desire.[12] The overwhelming preference of elderly to live alone independently is at odds with the myth that they want to live with their adult children.[118]

Another popular misconception is that people suffer a progressive decline in intelligence as they age. The reality is that although some aspects of fluid intelligence decline with aging, crystal intelligence is preserved. The ability to learn is preserved, albeit at a slower rate.[65]

Ageism perpetuates the myth that all older persons eventually become sick and dependent. Although there is a high incidence and prevalence of disease (and often multiple diseases) with aging, only a relative minority actually become dependent (Fig. 21-1).[41] Even in the 85 and over group, only about 40% require assistance in activities of daily living (ADL) or homemaking. The majority of elderly are cognitively intact, live independently in the community, and are fully independent in ADL.[97]

The patient "looks younger [or older] than stated age" is a common expression of the concept that functional or physiological age is more significant medically than actual chronological age. There is actually little evidence to support this concept.[64] The most significant factors in aging appear to be proximity to genetically determined maximum life span, and presence or

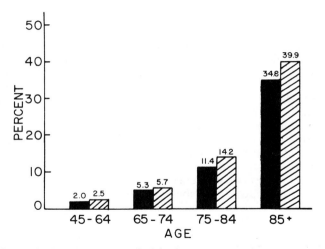

Figure 21-1. Percentages of adults, by age group, who require assistance because of chronic disease in performing basic activities (*solid bar:* walking, bathing, dressing, using the toilet, transferring from bed to chair, eating, and going outside) and in home-management activities (*striped bar:* shopping, chores, meals, and handling money). (Rowe JW: Health care of the elderly. N Engl J Med 312:827–835, 1985. Reprinted, by permission of The New England Journal of Medicine.)

absence of risk factors or disease, especially those affecting more than one organ system.[64]

There is increasing awareness of the critical inter-relationships, particularly for the elderly, of physical health, mental health, and life circumstances. The emotional/life stress associated with major losses is well documented,[44] and elderly are typically progressively exposed to multiple significant losses: health, functional ability, independence, spouse, siblings, friends, income, work role, social roles and status, and self-esteem.[6] The latter losses are particularly stressful. There are few norms or role expectations regarding appropriate behavior in old age.[6]

Alienation of old persons from their families also appears to be a myth.[108] Usually the elderly live near their children and visit frequently; those who do not live nearby maintain telephone contact. Elderly without children tend to maintain closer ties with young relatives or with siblings. It is important to consider family or kin (cousins, in-laws, and others) with regard to support networks, rather than just immediate household members.[108]

Another false myth contends that families "dump" their elderly. In fact, institutionalization of an impaired person is usually the last resort for families, used only when all other efforts fail.[118] Families, rather than the "formal" system of government and agencies, provide the bulk (up to 90%) of personalized long-term care for their disabled elderly relatives.[13] This includes home health and nursing care, personal care, household maintenance, transportation, and shopping.

Support Networks

With advancing age, however, the elderly tend to have increasingly limited and relatively fragile support systems. Dependency in aging parents results in significant physical, emotional, and financial stresses on their family network.[13, 44] An alternative support system may evolve gradually over a period of time, as the elderly person loses family support (through death of spouse and siblings, and children moving away and unable to actively assist). Such a system might include friends and neighbors in an informal network to assist with shopping, cooking, cleaning, and

self-care. With either type of support system, a significant additional insult (*e.g.,* onset of new disease or complication) may overtax an already marginal system. If the elderly person is hospitalized for a prolonged period, the network often dissipates and may be difficult or impossible to reassemble. The critical importance of maintaining the integrity of support networks is illustrated by the observation that for every aged impaired person in a nursing home there are two equally impaired elderly people living in the community.[97] The difference is the role played by the latter's informal support systems, which provide some 80% of their long-term care.

Functional Impact

Physically impaired older people tend to become socially isolated, which can result in exacerbation of medical problems, functional deficits, and mental health problems (particularly depression).[67] Other factors contributing to a vicious cycle of depression, withdrawal, and functional decline may include the stress of multiple losses, malnutrition, chronic ill health, and adverse drug effects.[44] Unfortunately, dependency is too often fostered by the environment. A classic illustration is the acute hospital setting, where the focus is on routinely providing care and assistance, rather than encouraging self-care.[59]

There are additional psychosocial barriers which can interfere with maintaining or improving functional ability in the elderly. Handicapping sequelae of ageism include "devaluation" of elderly disabled (by themselves as well as others), lack of interest among health care professionals in their problems, and limited opportunity for access to appropriate rehabilitation services.[67] Further attitudinal obstacles encountered among disabled elderly include the "right of dependency" (perceived as earned by virtue of longevity) and the "apathy of fatigue" (physical and emotional) associated with multiple illnesses and hospitalizations.[59]

The obvious conclusion, and why rehabilitation plays a key role in restoring function in the disabled elderly, is the importance of awareness and intervention regarding significant psycho-emotional and social factors influencing their health. Many of these can be anticipated and prevented, or at least minimized in terms of their adverse effects. As with any complication, prevention is the best treatment.

Theories of Aging

According to Shock, aging "represents the irreversible progressive changes that take place in the performance of a cell, tissue, organ, or total individual animal with the passage of time. As the probability of an individual's death increases with age, most of the changes associated with aging are apt to represent decrements in performance."[109] Strehler categorizes primary aging changes as *universal* within the species, *intrinsic* to the organism (not due to environmental factors), gradually *progressive* (*e.g.,* excluding stroke and myocardial infarction as normal aging processes), and *deleterious* in nature.[117] From a physiological standpoint, normal aging involves steady erosion of organ system reserves and homeostatic controls.[130]

Despite extensive research, no single definitive theory of aging has gained general acceptance. Despite observational or experimental evidence to support each major hypothesis, a significant question remains: Is the observed change a direct *cause* of aging, or merely the result of changes occurring at a more fundamental level.[56] The multiple theories of aging can be organized by level of proposed action, and have been reviewed in greater detail elsewhere.[18, 56, 103, 117, 122]

Molecular Factors

On a molecular level, oxidation-reduction reactions have been extensively studied.[103] Free radicals, produced as short-lived intermediates during normal metabolic reactions, are molecular subgroups with an unpaired electron, which renders them highly unstable and therefore very potent as oxidizing agents. It is hypothesized that they cause aging changes by combining with and deactivating essential molecules (*e.g.,* DNA, proteins) on a progressive basis. Indeed, antioxidants fed to experimental organisms appear, in some instances, to increase longevity.[56, 103]

Aldehydes, also a product of oxidation, form stable cross-linkages in collagen and other macro-molecules, resulting in the progressive loss of flexibility seen with aging.[117] Since collagen is widespread and plays a critical role in transport and exchange of materials among cells, changes in its physical chemistry may have profound effects on physiological function.

A further consequence of oxidation involves the deposition of insoluble lipofuscin (also known as age pigments) in cell cytoplasm in vital organs. These lipid pigments have been observed to increase with age and may interfere with cellular function.[103]

Cellular Factors

On a cellular level, there has also been considerable interest in environmental and genetic influences on the aging process. Theories of environmental damage hold that there is cumulative and progressive injury from various toxins and radiation, leading to inactivation and mutation of vital genes.[18] Various genetic theories, from differing perspectives, propose intrinsic intracellular mechanisms for the same end result.[56, 117]

The error theory holds that there is an increasing frequency of errors in protein synthesis. The redundant message theory proposes that key genes are selectively repeated as redundant messages, with longer lived species having more back-up key genes. The observed age-related increases in DNA-helix stability, which increase the energy required to separate strands, give rise to the transcription theory: strand separation is a key step in transcription of genetic information into messenger RNA; blocking the process (due to excessive energy requirements) will result in loss of genetic information within the cell.

Since biological development and maturation appear to be controlled by signals originating from information-containing structures (DNA, RNA), it may be reasonable to attribute aging changes to a similar system of programmed genetic signals. The Hayflick phenomenon, demonstrating a finite reproductive capacity of human fibroblast cells *in vitro,* is a landmark study lending credence to this programmed theory.[56] Aging could accordingly be viewed as resulting from an underlying series of orderly programmed genetic events that shut down or slow down key physiological processes in a planned sequence. Hayflick refers to the span of time during which functional decrements finally result in death of the organism as the "mean time to failure."[56] Using an analogy of mechanical systems, he suggests that programmed failure of cell and organ function occurs at predictable times, which are influenced by reliability of synthesis and repair systems. Thus, the mean time to failure may vary among individual cells, tissues, or organs.

Organ System Factors

At the organ system level, a number of immunological theories are based on age-related changes noted in immune system competence.[56, 103] There is decreasing effectiveness with age, resulting in reduced capacity to deal with infection, and a breakdown of immune tolerance with formation of antibodies against one's own cells (*e.g.,* autoimmune diseases). The major criticism of these theories of aging, as well as the intriguing neuroendocrine "pacemaker" (thymus gland or hypothalamus) hypotheses,[18, 122] is that it remains unclear if these observed changes are the underlying basis for aging, or merely expressions of more fundamental processes.[56]

With continuing research it appears that there is probably no single cause of aging. The concept which comes closest to a unifying theory might integrate hypotheses based on passive (random) or active processes of genetic programming, perhaps with superimposed nongenetic mechanisms that could result in varying individual vulnerability.[56] Certainly this would help explain the well-documented phenomenon of *differential aging,* whereby different people appear to age at different rates. Multiple levels of research suggest that rates of aging are affected to varying extents by heredity, life-style, environment, occurrence of disease, and psychological coping abilities.[109, 122]

In view of the apparent multiple mechanisms and levels of aging, it appears unlikely that there will be a single global intervention for life extension. More recent research trends are focusing on potential segmental interventions which may have significant impact on specific components of the aging process.[103] One example is the attempt to arrest or reverse the decline in immunocompetence that occurs with aging, thereby delaying the increased susceptibility to infections, with resulting improved quality and quantity of life. The continuing application of new knowledge and techniques in molecular biology, immunology, nutrition, endocrinology, exercise physiology, and the neurosciences holds promise for future effective segmental interventions.[103]

PHYSIOLOGY OF NORMAL AGING

The normal aging process involves insidious and gradual declines in organ system capabilities and homeostatic controls which are relatively benign in the absence of disease.[130] Although the older individual progressively adapts to these changes without need or desire for outside intervention, the steady erosion of reserves does predispose the elderly to both acute and chronic illness.[19] Characteristics of aging include a decreased reserve capacity of organ systems (only apparent during periods of maximal exertion or stress); decreased internal homeostatic control (*e.g.,* blunting of the thermoregulatory system and decline in baroreceptor sensitivity); decreased ability to adapt in response to different environments (*e.g.,* vulnerability to hypo/hyperthermia with changing temperatures, or orthostatic hypotension with change in position); and decreased capacity to respond to stress (such as exertion, fever, anemia).[19, 109, 130] The end result of these age-related declines is an increased vulnerability to disease and accidents. Older people, in comparison to their younger counterparts, get sick more often, have more chronic diseases, and often have multiple chronic health problems with more and longer hospital stays.[14]

Problems in Study Design

Definition of Normal

A significant concern, in view of the heterogeneity of the aging population, is what is truly normal. There is much variability in rates of aging among healthy elderly, and wide variations in individual performance. Further complicating any analysis is a distorted and spread-out "normal" distribution of skills due to frequency of significantly impaired function from disease.[64] More than 80% of the 65 and over population has at least one chronic disease, and half have two or more disorders.[119] Should the relative minority of elderly who have escaped serious illness be considered normal? This issue has led to criticisms of some studies as characterizing a "supernormal" elderly population.[61, 95] Katzman suggests it is more appropriate to define elderly populations to be studied in terms of either functional abilities or states (working *vs.* retired, athletic *vs.* sedentary), or exclusion of specific impairments or disabilities, rather than considering global normality.[64]

Nonetheless, it is important clinically to be able to differentiate the physiological consequences of aging from those of accompanying disease. Since detection of disease depends on determination that a patient is different from normal, it is critical to define appropriate age-adjusted criteria for clinically relevant variables in the elderly.[95] Some values do not change with age, so that abnormalities should not be inappropriately attributed to old age (*e.g.,* hematocrit and serum electrolyte concentrations).[97] A number of age-related changes may resemble the changes associated with a specific disease. For example, an age-related decline in glucose tolerance is well documented.[1, 80] So dramatic is this change that most people over the age of 60 would be diagnosed as diabetic if standard criteria (based on studies of primarily young patients) were applied.[95] Other changes occurring with aging may actually represent disease, in that they have specific adverse clinical sequelae.[97] Menopause is one example; although an accepted concomitant of aging, it is associated with an increased risk of osteoporosis and atherosclerosis.

Methodology Limitations

There are a number of methodological problems associated with the study of aging. Well recognized are frequent discrepancies in age reporting, with a tendency to upwardly distort.[64] This is coupled with difficulties in verifying reported ages, due in part to lost or nonexistent birth records. Classic examples of this phenomenon include the reports of unusual longevity in the valley of Vilcabamba, Ecuador, and the province of Georgia, USSR. Close analysis of birth dates revealed age exaggeration of up to 46%.[64]

A major problem in the design and evaluation of aging studies is the relative validity of both cross-sectional and longitudinal studies.[64, 95] Cross-sectional studies, although easier and less costly (in time and money) to perform, tend to overemphasize age changes. This is in large part due to significant differences in educational, nutritional, health, and social experiences of persons born in different decades. Contributing further to this distortion is the high proportion of elderly in the United States who were foreign born, with relatively less schooling. This has major implications for studies of psychological and cognitive changes with aging.[64]

A further flaw of cross-sectional studies involves variables related to survival. A *selective mortality* error is encountered for study populations over age 75, since they represent a sample of biologically superior survivors (from a cohort that has experienced at least a 75% mortality).[95] Another variable is the potential survival benefit of the relatively recent fitness movement, as compared to prior less fitness-conscious cultures.[64]

Longitudinal studies tend to underestimate changes due to aging, primarily due to high drop-out rates from death, illness, or relocation. Some studies have experienced as much as 50% drop-out over just a ten-year period.[64] On examination, initial scores of survivors are usually found to be higher than initial scores of those who dropped out. This leads to questions of self-selection for relative preservation of function, and again, the issue of supernormals.[64] Subtle changes in methodology over several years may introduce "laboratory drifts" that are difficult to differentiate from true age-related changes.[95] Another problem whenever serial measurements are made is potential distortion due to learning or stress effects.

A cohort-sequential design has been described, which combines both cross-sectional and longitudinal approaches in a single methodology.[101] By using cohorts of overlapping ages followed longitudinally, it is possible (with sophisticated statistical analysis) to differentiate between cohort effects and age effects.

Mean vs Maximal Performance

Another concern in the characterization of aging is that a focus on averaged or mean changes in various parameters can hide remarkable individual variation, particularly of peak performance.[48] Consider marathon running, which although involving a very select population, does measure maximal performance. A middle-aged male runner with a time of three and one-half hours is in the 99th percentile for his age group, yet not until age 73 would that time set an age group record. Although there is also a slow linear decline in maximal performance with aging (based on world age-group records), this is only on the order of about 1% per year between the ages of 30 and 70.[48]

Effects of Age on Organ System Performance

There are several general principles regarding aging effects on performance of various organ systems[109]:

Wide Individual Differences in Rate of Aging. Variation between healthy individuals of the same age is far greater than the variation due to age, and the range of variability increases with aging.[48] Linear regressions show average changes with aging, but variation between subjects is so great that it is not possible to accurately determine whether age decrements are linear over the entire age span or whether the rate of decline accelerates in later years.[109]

Different Organ Systems Age at Different Rates. There is great variation in the rate of decline for various organ system functions.[130] As depicted in Figure 21-2, there is a 60% decline in maximal breathing capacity with aging, but only a 15% decline in nerve conduction velocity and basal metabolic rate. Another demonstration of this principle is the fact that localized cellular growth, aging, and death occur continually in some tissues and organs (*e.g.,* hematopoietic system, skin, mucosa). Further, longitudinal studies have documented that significant decline in function of one organ system (*e.g.,* kidney) does not entail a similar decline in other organ systems.[109]

Age Changes Greater in Complex Performances. Complex performances will show greater changes with aging because of the need to coordinate and integrate multiple organ system function, as opposed to simple performances involving a single system.[65, 109]

Greatest Age Changes in Adaptive Responses. Adaptive responses (*e.g.,* to temperature change) are most affected by aging, owing to a decline in effectiveness of physiological control mechanisms (sensory/feedback), which is magnified with stress situations (sudden changes in environment, disease).[95, 109, 130]

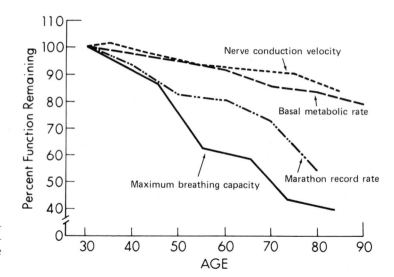

Figure 21-2. Physiological decrements measured in cross-sectional studies approximate a linear decline. (Katzman R: Demography, definitions, and problems. In Katzman R, Terry R [eds]: The Neurology of Aging, pp 1–14. Philadelphia, FA Davis, 1983)

Figure 21-3. The effect of conditioning and increasing age on organ function. The upper curve represents the maximal possible performance of a given organ system, whereas the lower curve is the rate of atrophy when the system is never stressed. Organ function always occurs at some point between the two curves. The slope of the upper curve defines the change in function resulting from aging. (Williams ME: Clinical implications of aging physiology. Am J Med 76: 1049–1054, 1984)

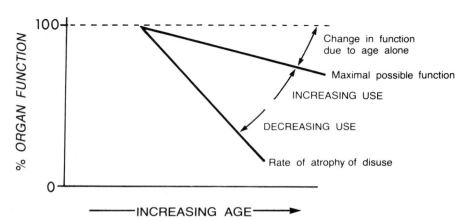

Prevention/Reversability of Physiological Decline

There is little question that biological systems, regardless of direct effects of aging, can be profoundly influenced by environment and life-style.[109, 130] Obvious examples include the effects of smoking, and sedentary vs. active life-styles. Figure 21-3 illustrates this concept, with the implication that the potential for significant decline increases with aging.[32] In further support of this principle, mean hand movement speeds were found to be significantly faster in active 60- to 70-year-olds compared to inactive 20- to 30-year-olds.[112]

The modifiability (or plasticity) of aging is demonstrated by studies in which performance can be bettered despite age, within relatively broad ranges.[48] Physical training in the elderly can lower blood pressure and increase cardiac output.[73, 85] There is also suggestive evidence that exercise may reverse or retard age-related changes in synaptic function and nerve conduction velocity.[120]

Functional Implications of Organ System Aging

The clinician must be aware of specific age-related physiological changes to properly understand disease in the elderly, since they significantly influence not only the presentation of disease, but response to treatment and potential complications that often ensue.[95] Such knowledge is similarly essential to understand underlying mechanisms of functional deterioration secondary to disease, and to formulate effective rehabilitation approaches. The following is a summary of clinically significant physiological changes that occur with aging.

HEMATOLOGICAL SYSTEM. Whether anemia can be considered a normal consequence of aging is controversial, although most authors assert that "anemia of old age" is not an appropriate diagnosis and should always be investigated.[97] In anemia is present in an elderly person, it is usually due to either blood loss (e.g., bowel carcinoma, polyps, or peptic ulcer disease) or decreased production (e.g., iron deficiency).[20, 71] The cause of anemia in otherwise healthy elderly may not be apparent even after investigation; it should still be considered pathological and is most likely due to decreased hematopoiesis.[77] There is no significant difference between healthy elderly and their younger counterparts with regard to hemoglobin, mean corpuscular volume, serum iron, total iron binding capacity, B_{12} or folate levels; however, elderly have significantly higher ferritin values.[77] There is an overall reduction in red cell mass with advancing age (in conjunction with reductions in lean body mass and total body water),[54, 77] but no change in total blood volume or plasma volume.[115]

The functional consequences of anemia can be significant, since there is further reduction of reserve capacity. Symptoms of various disease states may appear earlier than otherwise (e.g., orthostatic blood pressure changes, or change in anginal pattern with lower exercise tolerance). A very anemic patient may present in a confusional state with the potential for misdiagnosis and mistreatment.[100, 130]

There are several physiological changes with aging that can affect drug distribution and pharmacology. Decreased drug binding for highly protein-bound drugs (*e.g.,* warfarin, meperidine, tolbutamide) may result in a higher unbound, or free, drug concentration with correspondingly magnified actions.[22, 54] This effect is even more significant for patients taking multiple drugs (which is common in the elderly) because of competition for fewer binding sites.

Commonly an altered volume of distribution exists, due to reduction in total body water and relative increase in body fat.[22, 54] As a result, water-soluble drugs (*e.g.,* digoxin) tend to have a smaller volume of distribution (with higher plasma concentrations and greater pharmacological effect). Conversely, fat-soluble drugs (*e.g.,* diazepam, phenobarbital) usually have a larger volume of distribution because of relatively greater storage in fatty tissue. Although this may result initially in lower plasma concentrations (with reduced effectiveness relative to dose), the drug effects are markedly prolonged after dosage reduction or discontinuation because of the amount of drug stored in adipose tissue.[54]

GASTROINTESTINAL SYSTEM. The primary changes in the aging intestine involve decreased motility and a relatively hypotonic colon, leading to longer stool transit time, greater stool dehydration, and commonly, constipation.[10] As a result, laxative abuse in the elderly is common, and is the most frequent cause of diarrhea in this age group. More appropriate interventions include increasing diet fiber, using bulk agents or stool softeners, and avoiding routine or frequent use of enemas or laxatives.[19]

Esophageal motility is also often decreased with aging, with decreased peristaltic response, increased nonperistaltic response, delayed transit time, or decreased relaxation of the lower esophageal sphincter.[10] The latter may be associated with achalasia, whereas the other alterations may contribute to dysphagia. Unrecognized, voluntary reduction in caloric intake may result.

A number of age-related changes in the gastrointestinal tract potentially can alter drug absorption. There is less effective surface area available for absorption, decreased motility, and reduced splanchnic blood flow.[54] The overall effect is a less complete, slowed, and less reliable absorption process. Despite evidence of altered absorption of dietary thiamine and calcium, drug absorption in general is probably more significantly affected by concomitant administration of multiple drugs; in particular, antacids and laxatives bind or reduce dissolution of other medications.[54]

HEPATIC SYSTEM. The primary change in the hepatic system with aging is a slowing of hepatic metabolism of drugs (specifically biotransformation), related to decreases in microsomal enzyme activity and hepatic blood flow.[54] This has major implications for circulating concentrations of drugs and their metabolites, the amount of drug reaching effector sites, and on resultant therapeutic outcome. Decreases in hepatic blood flow with aging can be exacerbated by development of congestive heart failure, resulting in even less prompt and incomplete metabolism of those drugs largely inactivated by a single pass through the liver (*e.g.,* lidocaine, meperidine, propranolol, propoxyphene).[54] Inactivation of other drugs (*e.g.,* theophylline, chlorpromazine, diazepam) will be affected more by the reduced hepatic metabolism.[54] By the same token, these drugs will take longer to achieve steady-state concentration, potentially resulting in either delayed therapeutic benefit or unexpectedly delayed onset of toxicity.[22]

RENAL SYSTEM. There are a number of age-related changes in the kidney, including decreases in renal mass, renal plasma flow, and glomerular filtration rate.[96] The latter is associated with a decrease in creatinine clearance (mean decrease of 0.75 ml/min/year),[76] although a corresponding decline in daily urinary creatinine excretion (reflecting decreases in muscle mass) results in no net significant change in serum creatinine level with age.[96] On the other hand, modest rises in blood urea nitrogen may be noted with aging, particularly after age 70.[49] These changes have major implications for drug excretion, with prolonged half-lives of those drugs cleared primarily by glomerular filtration (*e.g.,* aminoglycosides, digoxin, penicillin).[10, 54]

Decreases in tubular function lead to glucose threshold increases, with glycosuria at higher serum glucose levels.[49] This can complicate both the diagnosis and management of diabetes mellitus in older persons.[1]

Related to these changes are significant alterations in fluid and electrolyte control. The aging kidney shows a blunted response to sodium deficiency, as well as impaired ability to concentrate or dilute urine.[115] The resulting salt-losing tendency is a function of both nephron loss (with increased osmotic load per remaining nephron) and mild osmotic diuresis.[96] This difficulty in concentrating urine can result in a hypernatremic state (with attendant mental confusion) if an elderly person is stressed by higher than usual insensible losses (*e.g.,* high or prolonged fever) with poor fluid intake. This is pertinent in a rehabilitation setting, as patients are often engaged in vigorous activities and may relatively easily become overheated or dehydrated. Certainly an acute intercurrent illness with inadequate fluid and salt intake can result in severe extracellular fluid volume depletion, with a vicious cycle of secondarily impaired cardiac, renal, and mental functioning.[96]

Just as older patients are prone to volume depletion when salt-deprived, volume expansion from an acute sodium load (*e.g.,* inappropriate intravenous fluids, dietary indiscretion, intravenous radiographic contrast dye) can be problematic.[96] This complication can occur even in elderly patients without pre-existing myocardial disease. A further potential complication of use of radiocontrast materials in the elderly is the risk of acute renal failure, which is aggravated by the presence of pre-procedure dehydration.[49]

Hyponatremia due to water intoxication may be the most serious electrolyte disorder of geriatric patients.[96] Most frequently complicating an acute illness, the clinical picture includes nonspecific signs of depression, confusion, lethargy, anorexia, and weakness. Serum sodium concentrations below 110 mEq/liter may result in seizures and stupor. The syndrome of inappropriate antidiuretic hormone (ADH) secretion, with water retention and hyponatremia, can be associated with infection (*e.g.,* pneumonia, meningitis), stroke, various drugs (including diuretics), or the stress of anesthesia and surgery.[49, 96]

Renin and aldosterone plasma concentrations are decreased by 30% to 50% in the elderly, with obvious implications regarding control of hypertension.[96] These alterations in the renin-aldosterone system with aging also appear to contribute to the increased susceptibility of elderly to hyperkalemia, particularly in clinical situations leading to acidosis. Potassium-sparing diuretics (*e.g.,* spironolactone, triamterene) should be used with caution in elderly patients.[49, 96]

PULMONARY SYSTEM. If cardiovascular and neuromuscular systems are intact and free of disease the general progressive decline in pulmonary function that occurs with age is primarily a loss of reserve capacity without functional limitations.[66] Changes seen with aging reflect both effects of aging *per se* (pulmonary as well as cardiovascular and neuromuscular systems) and the cumulative effects of inhaled noxious agents (especially cigarette smoke and air pollutants) and infectious processes.[11, 66]

Progressive decline in a number of pulmonary function tests has been documented with aging, including vital capacity, maximum voluntary ventilation (MVV), expiratory flow rate (EFR), and forced expiratory ventilation (FEV_1).[11] All of these tests require maximum forced inspiration and expiration. The declines in values may be due primarily to weakening of intercostal and abdominal muscles, together with small airway narrowing (from decreased elastic function), independent of changes in the lungs.[66] Residual volume and functional residual capacity increase, related to the loss of elastic recoil. Total lung capacity remains unchanged throughout adult life.[11]

Normal gas exchange requires both uniform ventilation of alveoli and adequate blood flow through the pulmonary capillary bed. With increasing age there is a slight increase in lung dead space (well-ventilated but poorly perfused areas), along with less-uniform ventilation, which results in a greater ventilation/perfusion imbalance.[66] Added to this is a mild degree of impaired gas exchange, resulting in a decline in oxygen partial pressure (Po_2) with aging.[11, 66] There is no change in carbon dioxide partial pressure (Pco_2) or pH, and oxygen saturation is normal or only slightly reduced. The reduction in arterial oxygen tension is clinically relevant because it represents a further loss of reserve. Elderly patients are more vulnerable to significant hypoxia from a relatively minor insult (*e.g.,* anemia or respiratory infection), since they are closer to the steep slope of the oxygen-hemoglobin dissociation curve.[66] This vulnerability is further exacerbated by blunting of chemoreceptor responsiveness in the elderly: both hypercapnic and hypoxic ventilatory responses markedly diminish with aging, independent of lung mechanics.[115] Apparently related to this is the significant increase in sleep-related breathing disorders noted with aging.[115]

Regular exercise to improve fitness is critical with aging. Although maximal oxygen consumption (an overall measure of cardiopulmonary function) does decrease with age, it is possible to improve fitness with training at any age.[66, 73, 85] The resultant increase in maximal oxygen consumption and decreased oxygen cost of effort (improved efficiency) lead to improved cardiopulmonary reserves for the elderly, with reduced vulnerability to future stresses (*e.g.,* infections, anemia). The tendency of physicians and society to emphasize decrease in activity among the elderly probably contributes more to poor pulmonary function than aging alone.[66]

Although most attention regarding the high incidence of pneumonia in the elderly is focused on immunological declines, there appear to be contributing factors relating to the lung directly or indirectly. Since most pneumonias result from aspiration of the infecting organism, impaired mucociliary function and decreased chest wall compliance (with impaired ability to clear aspirated material or secretions) probably play a role.[10, 66] Other nonimmunological contributing factors may include dysphagia, disruption of the lower esophageal sphincter, various esophageal disorders, and reduced levels of consciousness.[11]

CARDIOVASCULAR SYSTEM. A number of changes have been documented in the aging cardiovascular system, although recent research is changing traditional concepts. Of major importance regarding activity tolerance are decreases in maximal oxygen consumption and maximal exercise heart rate, resulting in reduced capacity for work.[88] There is no significant change with aging in resting heart rate, although a progressive decline in maximal heart rate in response to exercise (possibly related to decreased chronotropic responsiveness to adrenergic stimuli) is observed.[115] The common clinical formula reflecting this decline indicates the maximal potential heart rate is approximately 220

minus the individual's age, although a more specific formula of $185 - (0.70 \times age)$ has been documented.[92]

Although a number of studies previously have found cardiac output to decrease (along with stroke volume) with age at rest and during exercise, a recent study of subjects rigorously screened to exclude latent coronary artery disease found *no* significant age-related change in cardiac output either at rest or with exercise.[92] Of note was that exercise end-systolic volume was higher and ejection fraction lower in the elderly, but these factors (as well as the age-related decline in maximal heart rate) were offset by age-related increases in end-diastolic volume and stroke volume.[92] Thus, with advancing age there is a shift during exercise from a catecholamine-mediated response (increase in heart rate and reduction in end-systolic volume) to a greater reliance on the Frank-Starling mechanism.[92, 115]

Both cross-sectional and longitudinal studies demonstrate decreases in maximal oxygen consumption with aging, regardless of habitual activity level.[88] However, physically active individuals show significantly smaller decreases in both maximal cardiac output and maximal aerobic capacity with aging than their sedentary counterparts.[73] In fact, trained elderly subjects may have greater maximal oxygen consumption than sedentary subjects who are much younger. Furthermore, endurance training, even when begun in old age, can significantly improve exercise capacity.[88] Of significance is that the energy of walking represents a larger percentage of the total aerobic capacity with advancing age, such that walking becomes a very effective physical conditioning activity.[73]

Aging is associated with progressive, gradual increases in both systolic and diastolic arterial blood pressure, apparently owing more to loss of arterial elasticity than to neurogenic factors (*e.g.,* increases in circulating norepinephrine).[115] This progressive increase in blood pressure with aging was long regarded as a normal consequence of aging (*i.e.,* without clinical significance).[10] However, findings of the Framingham study and more recently of the Hypertension Detection and Follow-Up Program (HDFP) have demonstrated that elevated blood pressure is a significant risk factor for cerebrovascular and cardiovascular diseases, regardless of age.[8, 10] Prevalence of hypertension in the 60- to 69-year-old group in the HDFP was more than 25% for isolated systolic hypertension (systolic blood pressure greater than or equal to 140 mm Hg with diastolic less than 99 mm Hg), and 40% for diastolic hypertension (diastolic blood pressure greater than or equal to 90 mm Hg).[8] Stepped-care treatment reduced the incidence of stroke in these individuals by more than 50%, with minimum side-effects. Based on these findings, hypertension in the elderly cannot be considered either normal or acceptable, and should be treated.[8]

A final age-related physiological change in the cardiovascular system with important clinical applications is decreased baroreceptor sensitivity.[115] This results in a diminished reflex tachycardia upon rising from a recumbent position, and accounts in part (possibly along with blunted plasma renin activity, and reduced angiotensin II and vasopressin levels) for the increased incidence of symptomatic orthostatic hypotension in the elderly, as well as cough and micturition syncope syndromes.[115]

IMMUNOLOGICAL SYSTEM Significant alterations in immune competence occur with aging. The total number of lymphocytes does not appear to change with age, although there are subtle changes in lymphocyte subpopulations and enzyme alterations that resemble immunodeficient states.[129] Associated with these changes is an impaired cell mediated immunity: older humans have less vigorous delayed hypersensitivity reactions, and graft-*versus*-host reactivity is decreased in aging animal models.[43, 129]

Similarly, while there is little change in total concentration of immunoglobulins, distribution of immunoglobulin class is altered (increased IgA and IgG, decreased IgM serum concentrations).[129] The elderly have well-documented impaired humoral immune responses, with significantly reduced specific antibody responses to foreign antigens, and increased levels of autoantibodies.[43, 129]

The increased susceptibility of the elderly to infection is a function of both the above age-related changes in immune function and the frequency of concomitant factors, which further impair host defenses. The latter include diabetes, malignancy, vascular disease, and malnutrition.[43] Resistance to infection is often further compromised by altered local barriers to infection, such as skin breakdown or an indwelling urinary catheter. Common infectious processes in the elderly include pneumonia, urinary tract infection, sepsis, cholecystitis, diverticulitis, and meningitis.[111]

Of particular clinical relevance is the fact that the elderly react differently to infections than their younger counterparts. There is a less active leukocytosis in response to inflammation; the total white blood cell count is often not increased, although there is usually still a shift of the differential count to the left.[111] The older patient may have less pain or other symptomatology, and frequently low-grade or absent fever.[100]

ENDOCRINE SYSTEM. The endocrine system also undergoes major changes with aging. There is a gradual decrease in glucose tolerance with aging, although the fasting blood sugar level remains constant.[80] If criteria developed and applied for young subjects are used, almost half of all elderly could be classified as chemically diabetic following a glucose challenge.[1] The physiology of these changes remains unclear, although there is increasing evidence for an age-related reduction in insulin sensitivity.[10] Fasting insulin levels are lower in the elderly, but post-glucose insulin response and specific insulin binding are comparable in young and elderly subjects.[80]

Of clinical importance is the high frequency of hyperosmolar nonketotic coma in type II (maturity onset) diabetic patients, with high mortality if associated with inciting stress of an infection or cardiovascular event.[10] Administration of certain drugs (*e.g.,* thiazide diuretics, glucocorticoids, furosemide) can result in significant carbohydrate intolerance in elderly patients with previously normal blood sugars.[31] In insulin-dependent diabetics, hypoglycemia can result in a number of complications in the elderly, including pseudostroke syndromes, combative behavior, seizures, or extension of myocardial infarction.[31] Post-hypoglycemic hyperglycemia may further confuse the clinical situation.

There are multiple other endocrine changes associated with aging. Both animal and human studies have shown that the effects of thyroid hormone may be blunted in the elderly, even though circulating levels of thyroxine (T_4), and probably triiodothyronine (T_3), are unchanged.[31] The primary clinical impact of altered thyroid physiology is the need to maintain a high index of suspicion for the unusual presentation of thyroid disease. Common presenting signs and symptoms of the elderly thyrotoxic patient include palpitations, congestive heart failure, angina, atrial fibrillation, major weight loss (associated with anorexia), and diarrhea or constipation).[50] Goiter and serious opthalmopathy are frequently absent.[31] Apathetic hyperthyroidism may not be recognized until late in the course of illness. Patients appear depressed and withdrawn, with clinical clues of muscle weakness, dramatic weight loss and cardiac dysfunction.[50] Signs and symptoms of hypothyroidism are essentially unchanged with aging, but the diagnosis may still be delayed because of the many similarities between the stereotype of senescence and the hypothyroid state (*e.g.,* psychomotor retardation, withdrawal, constipation).[31] The virtual nonoccurrence of myxedema coma under the age of 50 underscores the significance of such delays.

Basal and adrenocorticotropic hormone (ACTH)–stimulated serum cortisol levels are unchanged with aging, and primary adrenocortical disease is uncommon in the elderly.[31] Significant hyponatremia or hyperkalemia, suggestive of adrenocortical insufficiency, is not uncommon in the elderly, but is often iatrogenic secondary to drugs (*e.g.,* thiazide diuretics, chlorpropamide, carbamazepine).[115]

Basal serum calcitonin levels decline progressively with age in both sexes, although serum calcium and phosphate appear to decline only slightly.[31] Elderly patients who become hypercalcemic on thiazide diuretic therapy should be considered hyperparathyroidism suspects and given appropriate diagnostic work-up.[31] Substituting furosemide or ethacrynic acid, both calciuretic, for thiazides may help lower serum calcium to clinically acceptable levels.

Age-related changes in gonadal function are well documented. There is no age-related decline in serum testosterone levels in healthy males, and no indication for routine androgen replacement.[31, 91] The post-menopausal declines in estrogen levels are well documented, with clinical expression variably including vasomotor instability syndrome (hot flashes), atrophic vaginitis, and osteoporosis.[10, 97] Controversy continues regarding prophylaxis and treatment of the latter, particularly with regard to potential benefits of dietary supplements and exercise[97] (see Chapter 44).

THERMOREGULATORY SYSTEM. The elderly have impaired temperature regulation, due in large part to a decline in effectiveness of the autonomic nervous system activity regulating peripheral blood flow.[109] As a result, they have a reduced ability to maintain body temperature with changes in environmental temperature, and are vulnerable to both hypothermia and hyperthermia (heat stroke).[134] Exposure to ambient temperatures of 5° to 15°C for 45 to 120 minutes results in an insignificant change in rectal temperature for younger subjects, but causes a 0.5° to 1°C decrease in elderly subjects.[109] The marked increase of death due to heat stroke among elderly is well documented, reflecting this impairment in regulatory systems. This has major implications for rehabilitation exercise programs, particularly considering the tendency in the elderly for dehydration.[73]

SENSORY SYSTEM. The elderly experience a gradual deterioration of most sensory modalities, including vibratory perception (although only in the lower extremities), touch sensitivity (Von Frey hair perception, index finger touch-pressure threshold), and deep pain perception.[102]

Deterioration of vision is one of the most recognized changes occurring with aging. The most common visual change with increasing age is a gradual loss of the ability of the lens to increase thickness and curvature to focus on near objects (*presbyopia*), and physiological miosis.[19] Cataract formation, with opacification of the lens, occurs to some degree in 95% of the over-65 population.[63] The elderly are also at significantly higher risk for further disease-related visual decrements, such as glaucoma, macular degeneration, and diabetic retinopathy. The result of these various changes is a loss of visual acuity, decrease in lateral fields of vision, decline in dark adaptation ability (and speed of adaptation), and higher minimal threshold of light perception.[93] These changes have obvious implications in relation to the higher incidence of falls in the elderly, particularly at night.[123]

Gradual decline in hearing acuity (*presbycusis*) is also characteristic of aging, although again a number of treatable disorders can cause superimposed damage (*e.g.,* wax occluding the outer canal, cholesteatomas, acoustic neuromas).[98] The elderly most commonly manifest a conductive hearing loss (possibly due to increased stiffness of the basilar membrane) or distortion of perceived sound (with increase in threshold sensitivity, narrow range of audibility, abnormal loudness, and difficulty discriminating complex sounds).[98] Continuing advances in hearing aid technology make remediation of such hearing deficits increasingly feasible. Early recognition and treatment of hearing impairments is particularly critical in the presence of cognitive deficits, to avoid adverse sequelae of social isolation and development of paranoid ideations or frank psychiatric reactions.[98]

NEUROLOGICAL SYSTEM. Numerous changes have been noted in relation to functioning of the neurological system with aging. The three most important areas of dysfunction accompanying normal aging include loss of short-term memory, loss of speed of motor activities (with slowing in the rate of central information processing), and impairment in stature, proprioception, and gait.[65]

The major controversy regarding neurological changes with aging concerns cognitive functioning. In general, there appears to be consensus that *crystallized intelligence* (intellectual performance as measured by tests of verbal abilities in vocabulary, information, and comprehension) is maintained, in the absence of disease, at least until the mid-seventies.[65]

On the other hand, *fluid intelligence* (timed cognitive performance tasks, associative memory, logical reasoning, abstract thinking) appears to decline slowly throughout life.[65] A significant proportion of these changes may be related to a decrease in the rate of central information processing in the elderly. Performance on timed motor or cognitive tasks, including abstraction (*e.g.,* digit symbol substitution test), reaction time tasks, and other tests requiring speed in processing of new information, deteriorates progressively after age 20.[65] Although there are declines with aging in motor and sensory nerve conduction velocities and rate of muscle contraction, they account for only a fraction of these slowed responses.

The primary factor leading to an increased simple reaction time is slowed central processing.[126] Choice reaction time, involving additional time for central decision-making, is increased to a greater degree in the elderly than simple reaction time.[65] In general, it appears that the more complex the mental task, the greater will be the age effect. Further evidence confirming age-related increases in central processing time includes documentation of "backward masking"[126] and increased latency of late components of visual, auditory, and somatosensory evoked potentials in older individuals.[65]

Many aspects of learning and memory remain relatively intact during normal aging, including immediate or primary memory (digit span recall), retrieval from long-term storage, storage and retrieval of overlearned material, and semantic memory.[65] However, age-related impairments have been consistently documented in tasks involving episodic short-term memory and incidental learning. Examples include difficulties with free recall of long (supraspan) lists of digits or words, as well as paired associate and serial rate learning for both visually and verbally presented material.[65] There is good evidence that these latter difficulties with short-term memory and learning experienced by the elderly are related to slowed central processing. What these investigations indicate, as shown in Figure 21-4, is that older adults are capable of new learning, but at a slower rate.[36]

Since much of rehabilitation involves learning, these findings have major implications for rehabilitation programming for the disabled elderly. This is particularly true in the context of

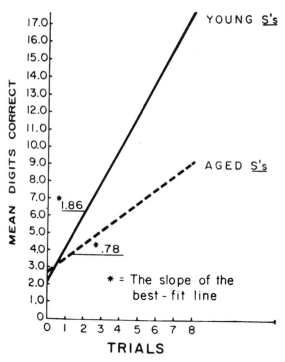

Figure 21-4. Mean learning curves of young and aged subjects (*S's*) asked to recall supraspan digits; plotted by mean slope and *y* intercept. (Drachman DA, Leavitt J: Memory impairment in the aged: Storage versus retrieval deficit. J Exper Psychol 93:302–308, 1973. Copyright 1973 by The American Psychological Association. Reprinted by the permission of the author.)

superimposed cognitive deficits, given that intellectual impairment is an important determinant of effectiveness of a standard geriatric rehabilitation program.[105]

A final area of age-related physiological changes involves stature, proprioception, and gait. In the peripheral nervous system, declines in nerve conduction velocities have already been discussed. This may relate to the decline in speed of motor activities that occurs with aging, although as previously noted, this is influenced to a great extent by relative level of activity.[112] The elderly in general demonstrate progressive declines in coordination and balance, perhaps related in part to impaired proprioception.[65] Another factor that may contribute to these changes is the progressive loss of nigrostriatal neurons with advancing age.[120] The basal ganglia play a major role in control of movement and regulation of muscle tone; in fact, clinically the aging process resembles Parkinson's disease in some respects, since older persons frequently have a fixed posture, muscle rigidity, akinesia, tremor, weak voice, and shuffling gait.[120]

This has significant implications for degree of mobility and stability, although there are a number of common, potentially concomitant, pathological changes that may further contribute to gait problems in the elderly (*e.g.,* vertebral compression fractures with kyphosis, arthritis, degenerative cerebral changes, cerebral infarcts).[65] Table 21-1 summarizes the major physiological changes occurring normally in the aging neurological system between ages 25 and 75.

MUSCULOSKELETAL SYSTEM. The number of motor units decreases with age, as do overall muscle mass, muscle fiber size, number of myofibrils, and concentration of mitochondrial enzymes; these changes occur regardless of level of activity.[102, 120] Muscle strength is relatively preserved through middle age, with

Table 21-1
*Major Physiologic Changes in the Aging Neurological System
Between Ages 25 and 75*

Functions	% Decline
Vocabulary, information Comprehension, digit span recall Touch sensation, two-point discrimination	None
Simple reaction time Hand or foot tapping, finger dexterity	<20%
Rising from chair with support Putting on shirt, cutting with knife Speed of handwriting Digit symbol substitution One leg standing, eyes open	20%–40%
Vibration sense, upper extremities Leg flexion	40%–60%
Vibration sense, lower extremities One leg standing, eyes closed	>60%

(Katzman R, Terry R: Normal aging of the nervous system. In Katzman R, Terry R (eds): The Neurology of Aging, pp 15–50. Philadelphia, FA Davis, 1983)

a 20% to 30% loss between ages 60 and 90.[120] Earlier and greater decrements in maximum power output (work rate) have been observed, with a 45% decline between ages 50 and 80.[120] Muscle endurance appears to increase or remain stable during aging; this may reflect fiber type regrouping with increasing type II fiber preponderance with age.[102]

The high prevalence of osteoporosis and degenerative joint disease (osteoarthritis) in the elderly again raises the question concerning "normal" physiological changes *vs.* ubiquitous pathology.[4, 97] The physiological changes and sequelae associated with osteoporosis are discussed in detail in Chapter 44.

Distinction of the disease of osteoarthritis from the normal aging changes that occur in weight-bearing joints also depends on development of related morbidity.[106] Degenerative joint changes in weight-bearing joints are essentially a universal occurrence in both sexes by age 60. These changes include biochemical alteration of cartilage (especially the proteoglycan component) with reduced ability to bear weight without fissuring, focal fibrillation and ulceration of cartilage, and eventual exposure of subchondral bone.[106] The "wear and tear" hypothesis of osteoarthritis suggests that this process is the result of the cumulative stresses of a lifetime of joint use. Accordingly, primary osteoarthritis results from the stress of repetitive weight-loading (spine, knees) or strain (distal interphalangeals), while secondary osteoarthritis may be related to occupational factors or congenital factors with unusual pattern of stress (congenital hip dysplasia).[4, 106] However, there appear to be other factors operating, including specific hereditary trends. Furthermore, obesity appears not to accelerate joint destruction, but rather increases the probability of experiencing pain symptoms.[106] Osteophytes, or bony spurs, are reactive protrusions of bone and cartilage that occur at margins of involved joints. Fortunately, significant symptoms and disability occur in only a fraction of those with radiographically identifiable degenerative changes; there is often a poor correlation between x-ray findings and the clinical picture.[4]

GENITOURINARY SYSTEM. Benign prostatic hyperplasia is an almost universal occurrence in men over the age of 40, and

develops under hormonal rather than neoplastic influence.[91] Of note is that the median lobe of the prostate, which is not palpable rectally, can cause a ball-valve obstruction during micturition; patients with persisting obstructive symptomatology but minimal prostatic tissue on rectal examination should have a cystoscopy to detect median lobe hypertrophy.[91] In spite of an increasing array of evaluative techniques, it remains difficult to predict which patients will progress to urinary retention or obstructive uropathy.[132] Usual indications for surgical intervention (prostatectomy) include increasing obstructive symptoms, recurrent hematuria, bladder calculi, recurrent infections, and post-void residual volumes greater than 100 ml.[91]

Incontinence in the elderly, although increasingly prevalent with advancing age, should be regarded as a symptom of underlying disease; it does not result from the natural aging process.[90, 91, 132] Normal aging probably results in reductions in bladder capacity, ability to postpone voiding, urethral and bladder compliance, maximal urethral closure pressure, and urinary flow rate.[90] Post-void residual volumes are higher, and uninhibited detrusor contractions occur more commonly. Each of these changes predispose the elderly to incontinence, but none alone precipitates it.[90] A further causative factor for incontinence in women is loss of the normal posterior urethrovesical angle, which can result from reduced pelvic floor muscle tone (from normal aging, multiparity, or surgical manipulation).[132] Other common causes of incontinence can include confusional states, urinary tract infection, atrophic urethritis, a wide variety of drugs (including sedatives, anticholinergics, and calcium channel blockers), limited mobility, and constipation.[97]

The primary clinical significance of these predisposing factors is that the new onset (or exacerbation) of incontinence in an older person is likely due to a precipitating factor outside the urinary tract.[90] Usually remedial intervention can restore continence without necessarily correcting the underlying urological abnormalities.

Contrary to popular belief, the majority of elderly retain sexual interest and desire, and to a variable extent, capability.[12] Males experience decrease in ability to have psychogenic erections and require more intense physical stimulation for erection; erections may be partial, and orgasm with ejaculation may occur without full engorgement.[12, 91] The force of ejaculation is less, along with a less-intense sensation of orgasm.[12] Females experience post-menopausal changes, including increased fragility of the vaginal wall, as well as decreased lubrication.[12] Other factors that may further limit sexual functioning of the elderly include effects of disease (*e.g.,* diabetes) or medication (*e.g.,* methyldopa), as well as psychosocial issues (*e.g.,* anxiety after a period of inactivity, lack of a partner).[12, 91]

VULNERABILITY OF ELDERLY TO FUNCTIONAL DECLINE

Cumulative Effects of Disease

The effects of frequently multiple and chronic illnesses are usually gradual over time (with cumulative erosion of organ reserves), leaving the elderly person reasonably functional with various adaptations, such as walking more slowly or taking more frequent rests.[21] In reality, however, they may well be only marginally functional with little or no reserve capacity, so that even a relatively minor superimposed acute complication or disease process (such as influenza) may result in functional decompensation. Of even greater concern is that the significant functional decompensation may not be reversible even though the intercurrent acute illness is appropriately treated and resolves.[83]

As a group, the elderly are more vulnerable to functional sequelae of diseases for a variety of reasons. They commonly suffer from under-reporting of symptomatology related to illness.[97, 130] Health care providers may subscribe to the myth that elderly are hypochondriacs, and ignore vague and inconsistent symptoms. The elderly themselves often exhibit ageism, thinking that such vague symptoms are a natural result of aging.[97] As a result, the disease process may become quite advanced before care is sought, making treatment much more difficult.[29]

From the older person's viewpoint, the available system of care may seem unresponsive.[130] Physician offices are frequently inconveniently located, with inadequate parking and poor access for the physically impaired. A brief encounter with a physician may not allow for development of rapport and full elaboration of symptoms. Physicians tend to adopt an authoritarian attitude, and may impatiently treat the patient almost as a child; generation and education gaps evolve.[29] Busy office staff may convey an image of disinterested and/or discourteous health care workers.

Other issues may contribute to under-reporting of illness. There may be denial of disease coupled with fear of consequences, especially financial.[97] Depression is common among the elderly and may result in the attitude: "What have I got to gain?"[130] Increasing isolation, with decreasing opportunities for others to observe and react to changes in appearance or behavior, are additional barriers. Finally, the elderly may not recognize significant symptoms or seek medical attention because of cognitive impairments, which not infrequently may be secondary to or aggravated by an underlying and potentially reversible disease process.[97]

There is often an altered response to illness in the elderly, which contributes to delayed or incorrect diagnosis.[100] Many specific diseases present with atypical and nonclassic signs and symptoms. For instance, the presentation of a myocardial infarction in an elderly person is less likely to include classic retrosternal chest pain; more often it will involve nausea, dizziness, syncope, or congestive heart failure with decreased activity tolerance.[100] Furthermore, a wide variety of diseases may present with similar nonspecific symptoms, including confusion, weakness, weight loss, and general "failure to thrive."[97] Accordingly, the differential diagnosis of possible disease processes is much wider in the elderly.

Further confounding accurate elucidation of the underlying illness are the frequent changes in disease patterns and distribution.[130] Abnormalities in one organ system are often accompanied by resultant abnormalities in another. Traditional medical training focuses on disease recognition and treatment in a relatively young population, with emphasis on synthesizing multiple signs and symptoms into a single unifying diagnosis.[131] The elderly more typically have concurrent symptomatology relating to multiple diseases. Although accurate diagnosis is important, the functional impact of each disease (and, in particular, the cumulative and additive impact of multiple diseases) must be determined.[26, 97]

There is an increased frequency of many chronic diseases in this population, including anemia, osteoarthritis, osteoporosis, cardiovascular disease, malignancy, and malnutrition. Palliation and prevention of secondary complications is frequently the more appropriate and realistic goal, rather than cure.[131] However, there are often atypical and potentially confusing behaviors and responses to treatment, secondary to co-existing diseases and decreased functional reserves of multiple organ systems (*e.g.,* altered drug metabolism and distribution).[54]

The elderly are also more prone to a wide variety of concomitant and complicating diseases, which may further cloud diagnosis and treatment decisions. These include thrombophlebitis, dehydration, fluid and electrolyte disturbances, adverse drug interactions or toxicity, decubitus ulcers, pneumonia, and general deleterious effects of deconditioning due to inactivity (occurring earlier and with greater severity in the elderly).[9, 70]

Effects of Acute Hospitalization

There is increasing recognition of the multiple deleterious effects of acute hospitalization on the elderly, separate and distinct from sequelae due primarily to their presenting illness.[29, 53, 127] Disorientation due to the foreign hospital environment and relatively infrequent and brief interactions with unfamiliar health care personnel may contribute to bizarre and inappropriate behavior, including agitation.[127] Contributing to this is the relative sensory and social isolation with few familiar environmental cues or social interactions,[29] especially if confined to a private room or intensive care setting. Moreover, there is an unfamiliar (and often questionable quality) diet and atypical routines and schedules (*e.g.,* bowel and bladder procedures, blood drawing, and vital sign checks at odd hours). This coupled with unusual noises (paging, other patients, machines) often contributes to insomnia. The patient is typically treated with a hypnotic, which may begin a cycle (or cascade) of drug side-effects and interactions which may adversely affect the patient's health.[53, 83]

Increased incidence of medical and iatrogenic complications in the elderly is well documented.[54, 130] Drug side-effects, complications, and toxicity, together with adverse interactions related to polypharmacy, make up a large proportion of such morbidity.[130] There is also a greater frequency of diagnostic and therapeutic misadventures in this age group, related in part to decreased organ reserve with resultant increased vulnerability.[53]

There a variety of emotional sequelae of hospitalization which may affect health and functional status. Anxiety and confusion relating to the underlying illness and prognosis (or just to hospitalization itself) may interfere with cooperation with treatment or therapy programs.[44, 67] Depression from similar origins may result in dependency and poor motivation to cooperate or improve function. Functional dependency frequently is reinforced during acute hospitalizations, both from the elderly who expect hospital staff to assist, and from hospital staff who tend to routinely perform self-care tasks without taking the extra time to supervise the patient performing his or her own self-care.[59] On the other hand, brief hospitalization may actually serve as a respite for the elderly patient, with greater social interaction and attention.[29]

In addition to significant implications for health care in the hospital setting, these sequelae related to acute hospitalization often affect social support systems and discharge disposition.[29] The elderly patient may experience loss of confidence or motivation as a result of multiple insults and complications, coupled with erosion of functional abilities from deconditioning.[70] This in and of itself will put greater stress on often relatively fragile social support systems, making it difficult or impossible for elderly patients to return home to their prior living situation.[13]

Exaggerated Effects of Deconditioning

The debilitating sequelae of inactivity and disuse occur earlier, and with greater severity, in the elderly[9] (see Chapter 23). This is due in large part to the significant erosions in organ reserves with aging, with resultant increased vulnerability. Of even greater concern is that many of these changes are correspondingly more difficult to reverse.[70] For elderly persons who cannot tolerate intensive reconditioning programs, and who have less reserve capacities to begin with, the time required to restore pre-inactivity levels of fitness and function (if indeed possible) will be significantly prolonged.[70]

The obvious implication is that for the elderly in particular, it is critical to mobilize as soon as feasible, and maintain activity at all costs.

MEDICAL MANAGEMENT CONCERNS

Evaluation of Presenting Diagnosis

Among the tasks that confront the physician upon admission of an elderly individual to a rehabilitation program is confirmation of the admitting diagnosis. The specific questions that must be addressed include whether the stated diagnoses are correct, and whether there are additional unrecognized diagnoses. The diagnostic errors encountered can be divided into three types: overdiagnosis, misdiagnosis, and underdiagnosis.

Overdiagnosis occurs most often when a physician fails to appreciate the changes in normal test values in the elderly, or when the physician attempts to treat symptoms when etiology is not clear. Examples of the first problem include a failure to appreciate the high incidence of "pathological" dysrhythmias found on Holter monitoring,[47] the change in arterial Po_2, the altered definition of diabetes, and the incidence of pseudohypertension[82] in the elderly. An example of the latter problem is the effort to treat disabling dizziness in an elderly person without a definite treatable diagnosis. The result of a therapeutic trial without a clear diagnosis is frequently additional dysfunction.

To avoid these problems the physician should be conversant with alterations in test characteristics in the elderly, and carefully review the evidence supporting all diagnoses as well as the rationale for all therapy.

Misdiagnosis, or an error in the primary diagnosis, occurs in less than 5% of all admissions to rehabilitation services,[114] but may cause monumental problems when it occurs. Cancer causing hemiplegia or paraplegia is a common misdiagnosis in the rehabilitation setting, and can dramatically alter the prognosis for both survival and function. Whenever the history is atypical the physiatrist must carefully review the supporting diagnostic data.

Underdiagnosis in the elderly is caused most frequently by ageism. Too often mental status changes, incontinence, unexplained falls, and even pain are attributed to age without even an attempt to look for a cause. These problems frequently have causes that are eminently treatable, and their evaluation and treatment must be familiar to all physicians.[81, 99, 123, 132]

Pessimism about the usefulness of medical therapy in the elderly is also frequently unfounded. There is often too little concern about the potential toxic effects of medications (see the following section) and too much concern about the risk of potentially helpful surgical procedures. It has been well demonstrated that the risk of surgical procedures is far more dependent on the severity of the illness than the age of the surgical candidate. For example, in coronary artery bypass surgery, 95% of those over age 70 had a three-year survival and improvement in symptoms.[68]

A final problem related to underdiagnosis is the failure to treat common problems that are associated with aging. Failure to attend to proper footwear in the elderly with gait problems, failure to refer patients with nonreversible visual problems to low vision centers, and the failure to provide well-designed amplification for the hearing impaired are all too frequent in the elderly referred to a rehabilitation facility. Attending to these relatively common problems will often be rewarded by striking improvements in the patient's overall function.[38, 52, 69, 78]

In the rehabilitation facility, problems of intercurrent or iatrogenic illnesses may develop. The presentation of illness in the elderly is frequently nonspecific.[60] A fall, change in mental status, or decline in functional status may be the only signal of the onset of a major, new illness. Pneumonia, pulmonary emboli, urinary tract infection, exacerbation of heart failure, dehydration, or chronic lung disease may all present with nonspecific symptomatology.[100] When these nonspecific symptoms occur, a thorough examination of the patient is indicated. The use of laboratory examinations should be carefully considered, as diagnostic tests by themselves may cause dysfunction.[39]

Avoiding Adverse Drug Effects

More important than the iatrogenic consequences of diagnostic procedures in the elderly are problems with drug therapy. The incidence of adverse drug reactions approaches 25% in persons over age 80.[130] When one considers that the average hospitalized Medicare patient receives ten prescription drugs it is easy to understand the concern about iatrogenic drug effects in the elderly.[87] The reasons for drug problems in the elderly revolve around five key (and interrelated) areas: polypharmacy, adherence or compliance, increased susceptibility to adverse reactions, and altered pharmacokinetics and receptor sensitivity.

Polypharmacy is frequent in the elderly and often compounded by the frequent use of nonprescription drugs. All medications should be carefully reviewed on admission, and regularly thereafter. The hospital setting is an excellent one in which to discontinue drugs of questionable value, since careful monitoring is possible. Special attention should be paid to digitalis preparations, nonsteroidal anti-inflammatory drugs (NSAID), and psychotropic medications.[54]

A further complication related to polypharmacy is that of potential adverse drug interactions. Reviews of institutionalized patients have shown that up to half of all patients' drug profiles show the potential for clinically important drug interaction.[15]

Adherence or *compliance* with prescribed drug regimens is poor in one-third to one-half of all patients.[57] Patients over 75 years old who live alone are especially likely to have adherence problems.[87] Failure to adhere can cause post-discharge deterioration, and patient education prior to discharge is critical to avoiding such problems. Allowing the patient to self-medicate in the hospital may be a useful way to monitor adherence and reinforce the need for medications.

A second problem that can develop related to adherence is drug toxicity when a nonadherent patient comes into the hospital and begins taking all the drugs that have been prescribed. Such a problem should be suspected when a patient shows a decline in cognitive or functional status 5 to 10 days after admission and other medical work-up is unrevealing.

Adverse drug reactions appear to be more common in the elderly, even when medications are given in proper dosages.[107] This may be related to a relative lack of resiliency in their homeostatic mechanisms.

There are a number of age-related *changes in pharmacokinetics,* previously reviewed. While drug absorption declines for many drugs in the elderly, this is not usually clinically important.[54] Elimination is also slowed for many drugs. The decline in renal excretion parallels the age-related decline in creatinine clearance.[76] Renally excreted drugs must accordingly be given in doses that reflect the patient's creatinine clearance. This is especially true for drugs that have small therapeutic/toxic ratios, such as digoxin and the aminoglycosides.

Age-related alterations in hepatic elimination are a result of slowed oxidative capacity of the microsomal enzyme systems.[54] Nortriptyline, propranolol, and quinidine are common drugs whose elimination will be slowed because of such changes. Changes in hepatic metabolism of drugs cannot be detected by standard hepatic enzyme or other liver functions measures.[87]

With aging, body composition changes: lean body mass declines and total body water declines 10% to 20%, with a proportionate increase in adipose tissue.[22, 54] The distribution of water-soluble drugs (*e.g.,* digoxin) thus declines, with a corresponding increase in serum levels. Fat-soluble drugs (*e.g.,* diazepam) have an increased volume of distribution. Although they have less immediate pharmacological effect per dose, fat-soluble drugs accumulate with delayed effects, which can persist after dosage changes or discontinuation because of adipose tissue storage.[54] Serum albumin declines with aging, and hence drugs that are predominantly protein-bound often compete for fewer available binding sites.[22] Drug interactions related to this phenomena can be very dramatic in the elderly. Warfarin (Coumarin) is particularly problematic in this regard.

Age-related *changes in receptor sensitivity* to drug effects are a final reason for untoward drug effects in the elderly. There is evidence that benzodiazepines and warfarin have greater effect at similar concentrations in the young compared to the elderly.[87] Such changes are difficult to evaluate separately from the pharmacokinetic changes related to aging.

In summary, the common statement "go low, go slow" is sound advice when prescribing drugs for the elderly. Evaluation of response to drug therapy is critical, and elimination of any nonessential medicines mandatory for maximizing function in the elderly. Patient and family education in the use of drugs is particularly important in this population in order to maximize adherence to medical regimens.

Managing Common Complications

Incontinence

An all too common complication, devastating to patient self-esteem and family commitment to patient care, is *urinary incontinence.* (For diagnostic classification and evaluation procedures, see Chapter 26.) Treatment for incontinence in the older patient hinges on proper diagnosis, which is usually possible with a complete history and careful neurological, pelvic, rectal, and mental status examinations. Laboratory studies should include urine analysis and culture, maturation index of the vaginal epithelia, and post-void check of residual volume. A continence chart is often helpful in determining the nature of the problem; cystometrics may also be indicated.[90]

Treatment is directed at the cause of the incontinence. Unfortunately, many of the etiologies have no uniformly successful therapy, and there may even be multiple causes. A timed voiding program is extremely useful in many patients. The nurse offers the patient a toileting opportunity at regular intervals, attempting to keep him or her dry. Initially, the intervals are very short, and increase as indicated.

Surgical procedures are useful in the treatment of prostatic hypertrophy and sphincteric incompetence. Anticholinergics are frequently useful in the management of detrusor instability. Overflow incontinence due to detrusor decompensation may require long-term indwelling catheterization, although intermittent catheterization and cholinergic drugs (to stimulate detrusor contraction) may be helpful.[132]

Bowel incontinence usually implies severe bilateral brain disease or loss of sensory input from the rectal ampulla.[51] Bio-feedback has been shown to be helpful in managing sensory bowel incontinence,[79, 125] but the management of incontinence secondary to diffuse brain disease usually requires a behavioral approach with bowel movements induced by suppositories at regular intervals.

Sleep Disorders

Sleep disorders and daytime fatigue are related problems common in the hospitalized elderly person.[53] The hospital environment alone can disrupt the sleep cycle and is further compounded by the routines of vital signs and medication administration, noises from the ward and neighboring patients, and the depression often associated with the onset of a new major chronic illness. Sleep deprivation at night leads to fatigue during the day. Napping during the day further disrupts nocturnal sleep patterns, and a vicious cycle can ensue.

Hypnotics are generally not the answer. The therapy schedule itself, if filled with enough activity of interest to the patient, will go a long way toward correcting this problem. Disruption of the sleep-wake cycle may be exacerbated by bed rest. It may be better to avoid a post-lunch period of bed rest for the patient having difficulty sleeping at night. If hypnotics are used, they should be of the short acting type to avoid hangover effects.[54] If fatigue persists, a careful review of medications will usually yield a likely cause. Finally, in the patient who remains persistently fatigued without clear organic cause, occult depression should be suspected.[32]

Depression

Depression is a common occurrence in the elderly population, and is very frequent in the setting of the rehabilitation hospital because of the loss of function that necessitates rehabilitation. The physician should maintain a high index of suspicion for the presence of depression in the elderly disabled.

Presenting symptoms in the elderly may be the classic ones of sleep disturbance, loss of appetite, dysphoric mood, impaired memory, poor concentration, fatigue, or thoughts of death or suicide. More commonly, however, there are nonspecific somatic complaints.[72] These can include pain syndromes, ill-characterized dyspnea, or obstipation. Occasionally the depressed elderly patient will appear demented.

In many patients with mild reactive depression the activity and milieu of the rehabilitation unit will alleviate the depression. Progress in therapy and the support of peers and staff are often very therapeutic. When the depression is more profound, antidepressants are frequently very useful. Tricyclic antidepressants should be started at low doses in the elderly, while monitoring for cardiac, orthostatic, and anticholinergic effects.[72] The drugs are frequently tapered after 3 to 6 months of therapy, with careful monitoring for relapse.

Electroconvulsive therapy may also have an important role in treatment of depression in the elderly, and will avoid many of the side-effects of long-term tricyclic use. Resulting memory loss has been minimized with the use of unilateral stimulation.[45]

Agitation

Another problem, common in the newly hospitalized older patient, is agitation. Characterized by nonpurposeful excessive motor activity, agitation has many potential causes and proper diagnosis is important to successful management.[3] Depression, as well as pre-existing psychoses, can present with agitation. The former usually responds to the more sedating tricyclic antidepressants (*e.g.,* doxepin, amitriptyline). Paraphrenia is an example of a psychosis occurring in the elderly which usually presents with agitation.[3] A paranoid psychosis with onset typically late in life, it is characterized by bizarre paranoid delusions in a socially isolated person. Antipsychotics are critical to the management of this problem, coupled with therapeutic alliance with a physician and an attempt to redevelop social contacts for the patient.

History of pre-existing psychiatric disorders should always be sought in the agitated person. Schizophrenia can continue into old age, although exacerbations respond well to antipsychotics.

Anxiety resulting from a change in environment can cause agitation if severe enough.[67] Supportive listening and cautious use of low-dose, short-acting benzodiazepines usually are therapeutic.

Organic mental disorders are the most frequent cause of agitation in the elderly.[110] Delirium, a syndrome characterized by the rapid onset of fluctuating cognitive deficits, can cause sleep disturbances, hallucinations, and agitation. It can coexist with a dementia, making accurate diagnosis very difficult. Any acute medical illness can present in the elderly with delirium without the classic signs of the underlying acute illness.[134] Infections, dehydration, stroke, hypothermia, uremia, heart or liver failure, and pulmonary emboli are the most common examples of this phenomena. Drug toxicity is another frequent cause of delirium in the elderly, with common offenders including digitalis, antidepressants, sedatives, anticholinergics and antihypertensives.[3] Delirium represents a medical emergency, and identifying the cause is critical to its resolution.[134]

Poor Nutrition

Ensuring adequate nutrition is a key component to facilitating optimum progress in an active rehabilitation program. Disabled elderly often present with complex nutritional concerns related to their underlying, often multiple, chronic illnesses together with various potential cognitive or behavioral difficulties.[113] The clinician must consider both the short-term provision of adequate nutrients and long-term therapeutic concerns (see Chapter 28).

Hypotension

Symptomatic orthostatic hypotension occurs in many older patients after even relatively short periods of bed rest.[70] It is accordingly a frequent problem during early mobilization of elderly patients in rehabilitation settings. Symptoms can persist if there are underlying problems with blood pressure maintenance related to drug therapy, salt restriction, or autonomic dysfunction.[115] Orthostatic hypotension is defined as a blood pressure drop of 25 mm Hg systolic and 15 mm Hg diastolic when rising from supine to standing. The patient will also experience symptoms of dizziness or lightheadedness with the position change.[121]

Evaluation of the patient should include a review of medications (particularly antihypertensives, levodopa, phenothiazines, and tricyclic antidepressants), examination for recent fluid loss, and laboratory tests to rule out abnormalities in aldosterone and cortisol levels.[134] Metanephrines should be evaluated when hypotension occurs with episodic hypertension, a hallmark of pheochromocytoma.

Treatment for idiopathic orthostasis potentially includes mechanical measures, plasma expansion, and vasoconstrictor drugs.[134] Mechanical measures, directed at decreasing venous pooling, include use of pressure garments (elastic stockings, abdominal binder) and elevating the head of the bed. High sodium diet and a 9-α-fluorohydrocortisone (an aldosterone analog) are useful for plasma expansion, while ephedrine, vasopressin, and amphetamines are potentially effective vasoconstrictor agents.[121] For severe refractory orthostasis, multiple measures are usually required.

Prescription of Rehabilitation Programs

Appropriate therapeutic prescription is critical to the success of a rehabilitation program. It must be based on a careful analysis of the patient's limitations in terms of aerobic capacity, muscle strength, and range-of-motion, in conjunction with neurological recovery and functional impairments. Social and cultural barriers to certain kinds of exercises or activities must also be taken into account. The patient must comprehend and accept the overall program structure and understand its relevance to his or her own goals. Without a strong therapeutic alliance between all health professional team members and the patient, progress will be slow or nonexistent.

Aerobic conditioning is a critical part of most therapeutic programs because exercise tolerance is almost always a limiting factor in the elderly with disabling conditions.[88] A specific program should be developed to provide 20 to 30 minutes of continuous exercise three or four times per week.[73] The intensity of exercise should be predetermined and constant, and should mildly tax the patient's cardiorespiratory systems. Guidelines to determine safe intensity of exercise usually include establishing a target heart rate between 70% to 85% of age-adjusted maximal heart rate, or alternatively, corresponding to anaerobic threshold.[88] Most elderly patients can tolerate and benefit from such an approach, although a pre-training clinical and ergometric screening evaluation should be performed.[88] This should include history and detailed physical, electrocardiogram (ECG), pulmonary function testing, blood tests (to rule out anemia, thyroid disorders, or electrolyte imbalances), and exercise ECG. An ECG is particularly critical if there is known underlying cardiac disease; however, cardiac disease is certainly not a contraindication to properly structured and supervised aerobic exercise.[73] Motivation for participation in such programs can be enhanced by group work and behavioral contracting.[59]

Formal strengthening programs can present many problems in the elderly. Gains in strength tend to be slower, and motivation to persist with traditional repetitive exercise programs is often poor.[16] If repetitive exercises are used, weights must be increased in very small increments. Brief maximal isometric exercise guided by an individual therapist may be a productive approach to strengthening in the elderly.[75] Formal strengthening programs may not be necessary to reach functional goals; repetitive work on the actual functional goal may provide adequate strengthening.[16]

Functional training approaches are usually well accepted by most older patients because of their obvious relevance and importance. Many therapeutic goals can be achieved by incorporating formal therapy techniques into the context of functional tasks. Examples of this approach include remediating perceptual problems during eating or meal preparation, increasing range of motion with dressing training, strengthening through inclined sanding projects, and aerobic conditioning by adapted competitive sports.

Prescription of the rehabilitation program must be tailored to the individual in order to accommodate limitations imposed by existing multiple medical problems. Guidelines for cardiovascular restrictions should be established with target heart rate ranges and monitoring of blood pressure response to exercise. If oxygen desaturation is a potential problem, the use of supplemental oxygen should be considered. If restrictions on weight-bearing limit therapy, water exercise can be prescribed. Since many elderly disabled patients have low endurance, therapy sessions scheduled in sequential one-hour blocks may not be tolerated. Therapy should be arranged in intervals and sequences designed to suit individual needs. Potential complications of excessive exercise include sudden death, nonfatal myocardial infarction, excessive fatigue, hyperthermia, and significant musculoskeletal problems.[73]

Realistic goal-setting is complex in any rehabilitation setting, but is further complicated in the elderly by at least two unique concerns. First, the elderly frequently have potential care-givers (spouse, siblings, or children) who are also approaching retirement and have medical problems of their own; fitness of the proposed care-giver after discharge must be considered in the initial discharge planning process.[13] The second problem relates to the limited remaining life expectancy of the older disabled patient. For example, diabetic amputees over age 65 have average survivals of little more than a year.[7] With so little time remaining in their lives, prolonged inpatient rehabilitation may not be in their best interests.

SPECIAL CONSIDERATIONS IN REHABILITATION

Dementia

Severe dementia occurs in about 5% of those over age 65 (with mild to moderate forms in another 10%), and in about 20% of those over age 80.[97, 134] It is found in more than half of nursing home residents, and is the most common precipitating cause of admission.[97] Women appear to be affected more frequently than men. Insidious onset of memory loss, loss of abstract reasoning and problem-solving ability, impairment of judgment and orientation, and personality changes (with relatively intact alertness and awareness) are hallmarks of the disease.[134] Often a patient with early dementia, premorbidly not interfering with daily activities, can become severely disoriented during an acute hospitalization. This agitated confusion may resolve without any specific therapy in 1 to 2 weeks. Appreciation of this possibility is important with regard to evaluating and working with this population in rehabilitation settings.

Fifty to sixty percent of dementia patients represent senile dementia of the Alzheimer type (SDAT), and another 20% are multi-infarct in origin.[134] The remaining large number of potentially reversible causes of dementia include subdural hematoma, brain tumor, occult hydrocephalus, syphilis, hypo- or hyperthyroidism, hypercalcemia, vitamin B$_{12}$ deficiency, niacin deficiency, drug toxicity, depression, and cardiac, renal or hepatic failure.[97, 134] Diagnostic evaluation should always be performed to rule out these possible causes. However, even if one of these potentially treatable etiologies is established, reversibility of the dementia may be limited because of permanent damage from the condition.

A standard dementia work-up, in addition to detailed history and physical examination, should include a serological test for syphilis, sedimentation rate, electrolytes, serum calcium, blood urea nitrogen, complete blood count, thyroid evaluation, vitamin B$_{12}$ and folate levels, electroencephalogram, chest x-ray, ECG, and computed tomography (CT) of the brain.[134] A trial off all medications is probably warranted in all patients with new onset of dementia. Many clinicians also routinely give a trial of antidepressants to newly identified dementia patients because an occult depression frequently coexists with mild dementia.[81] Amelioration of the depression may improve overall functioning in this situation.

Patients with moderate or severe dementia usually do not fare well in rehabilitation settings because their ability to form new memory is poor.[105] This limits day-to-day carryover and makes therapeutic gains nearly impossible. Rehabilitation admission may still be justified in such situations when the goal is to train the family in appropriate care of a patient with a new disability.

When evaluating the elderly patient for admission to a rehabilitation program, it is critical to determine the mental status *prior* to onset of the new disability. Too often the mental status that is seen in the acute hospital setting underestimates the patient's cognitive function when healthier and in a supportive and stimulating environment, such as a rehabilitation unit.[5]

Falls and Hip Fractures

Many of the age-related physiological declines in multiple organ systems combine to dramatically increase the incidence of falls in the elderly, including decreased vision and balance, impaired gait, orthostatic hypotension, and vertigo (due to degenerative or vascular changes in the vestibular apparatus).[93] Other factors contribute to the risk of falling, including adverse effects of medications, concomitant disease states (acute or chronic), unfamiliarity with environment, depression, apathy, or confusion.[123, 134] In situations involving rehabilitation of an elderly patient after repair of hip fracture secondary to a fall, it is critical to evaluate and treat the cause of the incident fall. Otherwise, the risks of another subsequent fall are great.

There are a number of controversies involving proper care of the elderly patient post hip fracture. A tendency to conservatively (nonoperatively) treat hip fractures in demented elderly patients is countered by findings of better function with less morbidity and mortality with surgical management.[35] For patients with severe cardiovascular disease which contraindicates general anesthesia, percutaneous pinning with Ender rods under local anesthesia can be performed.[35]

Femoral neck fractures can be treated either by resection of the femoral head with endoprosthesis (with immediate postoperative weight bearing) or internal fixation (with delayed weight-bearing). Earlier reports of higher morbidity and mortality associated with endoprosthesis may have been due to biased patient selection.[135] The benefits of early postoperative mobilization with weight-bearing are well documented.[23]

Although the intertrochanteric fractures are traditionally managed by internal fixation with nail or compression screw with delayed weight-bearing, more recent studies suggest patients can be mobilized much earlier without complication, and with improved morbidity and function.[74]

The urgency of early mobilization after repair of hip fracture is twofold: the vulnerability to many postoperative complications (including pulmonary problems, thromboembolism, and genitourinary sequelae), and the risk of secondary complications from bed rest or relative inactivity.[35]

Arthritis and Joint Replacements

Management of arthritic conditions in the elderly, just as in a younger population, must be individualized with close monitoring of benefits.[4, 34] Treatment principles are comparable, although the balance between rest and activity is much more delicate because of the adverse sequelae of inactivity in the elderly.[34] There is evidence that elderly arthritics may respond better to therapeutic programs and are often more patient and compliant with long-term exercise and activity programs.[4] Treatment goals include relief of fear, fatigue, stiffness, and pain; suppressing the inflammatory process; and prevention or correction of deformity.[133] This is accomplished by a combination of psychological, pharmacological, physical, and surgical measures.[4, 34, 133]

Although the elderly are frequently resistant to use of various assistive devices, provision of a firm chair of appropriate height with arm rests, built-up handle devices, elevated toilet seat with grab bars, or ambulation aids (cane or walker) may help maintain independent community living.

Age should not be a primary factor in considering potential benefits of surgical intervention in the elderly arthritic patient.[55] Significant functional gains may be realized with an appropriately timed procedure (*e.g.,* ligament or tendon repair, osteotomy, arthroplasty, prosthetic joint replacement) to improve stability and range, or to decrease pain.[55, 133] Attention to preoperative and postoperative therapy programs and early mobilization is critical to maximize functional gains and minimize secondary complications from inactivity.[34] (Further details of rehabilitation management, including principles for prescription of medication and therapeutic modalities, can be found in Chapter 39.)

Stroke

Although the cost benefits of stroke rehabilitation in general have been documented,[40] appropriateness of intensive rehabilitation for the elderly stroke patient is still questioned clinically. This ageism appears to be related to assumptions that elderly stroke patients have more severe strokes, or are less likely to recover neurologic function, or have too many complicating diseases to enable them to participate in or benefit from an intensive therapy program. While this may apply to individual stroke patients (at any age), research does not seem to support these factors as holding in general for the elderly.[28, 124] Some studies have suggested that elderly stroke patients may require longer lengths of stay to achieve the same functional gains as their younger counterparts,[124] although others found no significant difference.[28] Certainly an older disabled age group in general tends to have fewer social supports, such as a spouse or siblings. As a result, functional ability is even more critical in their case for discharge to a community independent living setting than for a patient with an available relative to assist or supervise.

The elderly stroke patient may present a number of challenges from a rehabilitation standpoint. Severe cardiovascular disease may limit exercise tolerance; exercise programs to increase strength and endurance may also serve as functional cardiac rehabilitation programs. Certainly patients with borderline anginal or congestive heart failure syndromes may decompensate with intensive therapy programs and must be closely monitored. Diabetics similarly often experience changing insulin needs in the face of increasing activity (to avoid hypoglycemic reactions).

Certainly cognitive deficits, whether premorbid or secondary to the stroke, can interfere with ability to cooperate with the therapist.[51, 105] Emotional and behavioral sequelae of stroke can further interfere with the patient's cooperation and motivation.[51] In particular, depression and the pseudodementia of depression may be problematic.[134] The therapeutic milieu of the rehabilitation program, with emphasis on "small victories," is often sufficient to promote continuing efforts to improve. Antidepressant medications must be used judiciously in view of their multiple side-effects (particularly cardiac). (For further discussion of stroke, see Chapter 29.)

Amputation

As with stroke, there are many ageisms regarding the elderly amputee. A major ageism is that age should be a criteria in the decision as to whether to prescribe a prosthesis; this is inappropriate.[26, 133] Many studies have documented the successful outcomes of rehabilitation programs for older amputees.[26] The knee is even more critical to preserve in elderly amputees than in their younger counterparts, in view of the proprioceptive, neuromuscular control, and energy cost considerations.[26] Energy costs of ambulation with a prosthesis are considerably higher for elderly patients, particularly during their training; there is considerable upper extremity work involved in transfers and ambulation with a walker or crutches.

Similar to stroke rehabilitation, concurrent medical problems may complicate or limit rehabilitation efforts in the elderly amputee. Significant cardiovascular disease may become symptomatic during ambulation; this is particularly true during the training phase.[26]

Prescription of a prosthesis is usually indicated, even in the presence of such major medical problems. The prosthesis in this situation may still be therapeutic and functional, whether from the standpoint of standing, transfers, or just cosmesis.[133] In view of this, and the fact that crutch ambulation (non-weight-bearing on the amputated side) has a higher energy cost than prosthetic ambulation, the old criteria of successful crutch ambulation to justify prosthetic prescription is not justified.[26]

For bilateral amputees, energy costs are significantly higher and ambulation training more difficult, particularly for the elderly patient with simultaneous bilateral amputations. Ambulation may be primarily therapeutic (from both an aerobic exercise and psychological standpoint), or for short distances within the house. In this situation, wheelchair locomotion may be a preferable alternative for longer distance travel at lower energy costs.[37]

Spinal Cord Injury

Spinal cord injury (SCI) is usually considered a disability of the younger population, but it is increasingly occurring in the elderly. Not only is there a significant incidence of SCI among the elderly (5.4% in the 61- to 90-year age group),[116] but also there is increased survival in an aging population injured earlier in their lives.[33] The result is a much greater prevalence of elderly SCI patients, subject to the usual age-related morbidity and mortality. Similarities have been observed between aging morbidity and that of chronic (not old) SCI patients.[86]

Epidemiology of SCI with older age at onset differs from that of younger populations. The etiology of injury is much more likely to be falls (60% in the 75 and over age group), followed by motor vehicle accidents (32% in the 75 and over age group).[116] There is a marked increase in incidence of quadriplegia (QC) and quadriparesis (QI) in the elderly (67% in the 61- to 75-year age group, 88% in those 75 and over), as opposed to the more nearly equal distribution between paraplegia (PC) and paraparesis (PI) and QC/QI in younger age groups.[116] Elderly SCI patients are three times more likely to be QI than QC.

There is a progressive disparity in 10-year survival rates between SCI and non-SCI populations with advancing age at injury.[116] For ages 70 to 98, SCI 10-year survival is 32%, compared to 48% for the non-SCI counterparts. Life expectancies reported for SCI patients differ depending on whether or not patients who die prior to discharge from rehabilitation programs (usually within the first year post-injury) are included in the analysis. If such first-year fatalities are included, life expectancy for SCI patients injured at age 60 is 6.5 years for PI, 5.9 years for PC, 4.2

Table 21-2
Life Expectancies (Years) for Spinal Cord Injury Victims

Age at Hospital Discharge (years)	General Population (Male/Female)	Paraplegia		Quadriplegia	
		Incomplete	Complete	Incomplete	Complete
10	59.09/65.59	57.22/64.09	42.20/50.94	49.88/58.05	28.60/37.81
20	49.65/55.85	47.85/54.41	33.73/41.75	40.88/48.55	21.57/29.56
30	40.61/46.24	38.95/44.82	26.29/32.85	32.57/39.24	16.45/21.83
40	31.53/36.80	29.98/35.47	18.55/24.40	24.13/30.27	10.49/14.77
50	23.08/27.84	21.70/26.64	11.96/17.03	16.61/22.06	5.90/ 9.29
60	15.75/19.50	14.65/18.52	7.08/10.94	10.61/14.86	2.97/ 5.37
70	9.72/11.84	9.00/11.15	3.93/ 6.02	6.29/ 8.68	1.50/ 2.55

(DeVivo MJ, Fine PR, Maetz HM, Stover SL: Prevalence of spinal cord injury: A reestimation employing life table techniques. Arch Neurol 37:707–708, 1980)

years for QI, and 1.9 years for QC (compared to 20 years for the non-SCI population).[116] This contrasts with significantly higher life expectations depicted in Table 21-2 for SCI patients discharged alive from rehabilitation programs.[33]

These significant life expectancies make rehabilitation efforts appropriate even for elderly SCI patients. Good functional outcomes are expected in those with incomplete injuries, but most elderly cord-injured patients with complete injury remain dependent for transfers and self-care despite prolonged therapy, even for injury levels which in younger patients usually allow independent functioning.[84]

SYSTEMS OF CARE FOR DISABLED ELDERLY

Significance of Functional Status

Reference has already been made to the critical nature of functional status with regard to ability to live independently in the community. Elderly people often live alone and must perform their own self-care and other daily activities, including homemaking. Issues of safety in this home environment are frequently raised, particularly after an acute adverse event or illness (such as a fall with hip fracture). A patient who achieves a level of mobility (ambulation or transfers) requiring just close supervision or contact guarding (because of occasional loss of balance) may not be able to safely return home alone. Home-based supervision by an aide, unless paid privately, is typically only available a few hours a day, five days a week, for relatively brief intervals. Return to a community setting may be possible if a relative is available to live with the patient. If not, the patient may not even qualify for a boarding home or intermediate care facility (ICF); most ICF admission criteria include independent safe locomotion. This patient conceivably could be relegated to a skilled nursing facility (SNF) with other patients who are totally dependent for all care. Unfortunately, there is usually no alternative setting to provide a structured environment with available supervision for safety.

Role of the Physiatrist

There is a great deal of overlap between geriatric medicine and rehabilitation medicine.[128] Their history and development show many similar features. Both are concerned with preserving func-

tion in the face of often multiple impairments and preventing secondary complications. Both employ a multidisciplinary team to accomplish holistic goals of maintaining overall health and functioning.[94] Because much of rehabilitation involves elderly disabled, it is necessary for the physiatrist to have a special interest and expertise in care and treatment of older persons. The physiatrist accordingly may fulfill a number of roles relating to geriatrics, including primary care in a rehabilitation inpatient setting[42] or long-term care setting.[104] Other roles include acting as a consultant in various health care settings, such as acute care hospital, SNF, day hospital, or home.[30, 104, 133] In these settings, the physiatrist coordinates and monitors benefits of individualized rehabilitation programs.

Alternative Levels of Rehabilitation Care

In view of the multiple factors relating to severity and reversability of functional deficits in the elderly, it would appear ideal to have access to a system of rehabilitation care at varying levels of intensity and different settings.[27] There is increasing evidence of potential cost benefits of providing structured rehabilitation at levels of intensity less than the acute hospital-level rehabilitation program (*i.e.*, at an SNF level).[2, 25] This seems logical when one considers that insurance provider criteria require a minimum of three hours of therapy daily for hospital-level rehabilitation.[62] Many elderly disabled patients cannot tolerate this intensity of exercise, either because of underlying cardiovascular or other diseases, or because of deconditioning secondary to illness, inactivity, or previous acute care hospitalization. An SNF-level rehabilitation program could provide a less intensive program, as "pre-rehabilitation" to build up endurance to the level of the hospital-level program, or as "post-rehabilitation" to fine-tune self-care and mobility skills prior to discharge home.[25]

Another setting for rehabilitation is the day hospital for relatively intensive and structured therapies to facilitate maintenance of the patient at home with family.[30, 46] Therapy is more intense, with a wider array of equipment and under closer medical supervision than is feasible in a home-based treatment program. With typical lengths of stay of 1 to 2 months, day hospitals allow earlier transition to the more familiar and comfortable home setting, with lower health care costs.[30]

These alternative levels and settings of rehabilitation for the elderly, if combined with more traditional options of home-based care, outpatient therapies, acute hospital (consult) therapy, and comprehensive hospital-level rehabilitation, would provide a spectrum of programming for individually tailored rehabilitation care. It would also facilitate movement between various levels of intensity, as an elderly patient's rehabilitation needs change.

Finally, although a small minority of elderly patients reside in nursing home settings (5%),[119] the potential benefits of formalized rehabilitation input are great.[89, 104] Although only a few may benefit from structured therapy programs to the point of transfer to lower levels of care, benefits can be substantial just in terms of the decreased physical assistance required. Even small gains in function translate to significant improvement in quality of life.

REFERENCES

1. Andres R: Aging and diabetes. Med Clin North Am 55:835–846, 1971
2. Aronow HU, Jenkins JH: Skilled nursing facilities: Can they do it for less? Arch Phys Med Rehabil 63:535, 1982
3. Barnes R, Raskind M: Strategies for diagnosing and treating agitation in the aging. Geriatrics 35:111–119, 1980
4. Baum J: Rehabilitation aspects of arthritis in the elderly. In Williams TF (ed): Rehabilitation in the Aging, pp 177–197. New York, Raven Press, 1984
5. Beck JC, Benson DF, Scheibel AB et al: Dementia in the elderly: The silent epidemic. Ann Intern Med 97:231–241, 1982
6. Bengston VL: The Social Psychology of Aging. Indianapolis, Bobbs Merrill, 1977
7. Bodily KC, Burgess EM: Contralateral limb and patient survival after leg amputation. Am J Surg 146:280–282, 1983
8. Borhani NO: Prevalence and prognostic significance of hypertension in the elderly. J Am Geriatr Soc 34:112–114, 1986
9. Bortz WM II: Disuse and aging. JAMA 248:1203–1208, 1982
10. Boss GR, Seegmiller JE: Age-related physiologic changes and their clinical significance. West J Med 135:434–440, 1981
11. Brandstetter RD, Kazemi H: Aging and the respiratory system. Med Clin North Am 67:419–431, 1983
12. Bray GP: Sexuality in the aging. In Williams TF (ed): Rehabilitation in the Aging, pp 81–95. New York, Raven Press, 1984
13. Brody EM: Informal supports systems in the rehabilitation of the disabled elderly. In Brody SJ, Ruff GE (eds): Aging and Rehabilitation: Advances in the State of the Art, pp 87–103. New York, Springer, 1986
14. Brotman HB: Every ninth American: An analysis for the chairman of the Select Committee on Aging, House of Representatives. Comm. Pub. No. 97-332. Washington, DC, U.S. Government Printing Office, 1982
15. Brown MD, Boosinger JK, Henderson M et al: Drug-drug interactions among residents in homes for the elderly—A pilot study. Nursing Res 26:47–52, 1977
16. Brown M, Rose SJ: The effects of aging and exercise on skeletal muscle: Clinical considerations. Top Geriatr Rehabil 1:20–30, 1985
17. Butler RN: Age-ism: Another form of bigotry. Gerontologist 9:243–246, 1969
18. Cape R: Biologic gerontology. In Cape R: Aging: Its Complex Management, pp 39–62. Hagerstown, MD, Harper & Row, 1978
19. Cape R: Physical aspects of aging. In Cape R: Aging: Its Complex Management, pp 13–38. Hagerstown, MD, Harper & Row, 1978
20. Cape RDT: Nutrition and the elderly. In Cape RDT, Coe RM, Rossman I (eds): Fundamentals of Geriatric Medicine, pp 295–307. New York, Raven Press, 1983
21. Cape RDT: The geriatric patient. In Cape RDT, Coe RM, Rossman I (eds): Fundamentals of Geriatric Medicine, pp 9–15. New York, Raven Press, 1983
22. Carruthers SG: Clinical pharmacology of aging. In Cape RDT, Coe RM, Rossman I (eds): Fundamentals of Geriatric Medicine, pp 187–196. New York, Raven Press, 1983
23. Ceder L, Lindberg L, Odberg E: Differentiated care of hip fracture in the elderly: Mean days and results of rehabilitation. Acta Orthop Scand 51:157–162, 1980
24. Clark GS: Functional assessment in the elderly. In Williams TF (ed): Rehabilitation in the Aging, pp 111–124. New York, Raven Press, 1984
25. Clark GS: Comparison of hospital vs skilled nursing level rehabilitation programs. Arch Phys Med Rehabil 67:624–625, 1986
26. Clark GS, Blue B, Bearer JB: Rehabilitation of the elderly amputee. J Am Geriatr Soc 31:439–448, 1983
27. Clark GS, Bray GP: Development of a rehabilitation plan. In Williams TF (ed): Rehabilitation in the Aging, pp 125–143. New York, Raven Press, 1984
28. Clark GS, Williams ME: Effect of age on stroke rehabilitation. Arch Phys Med Rehabil 64:495, 1983
29. Coni N, Davison W, Webster S: Lecture Notes on Geriatrics. London, Blackwell Scientific Publications, 1971
30. Cummings V, Kerner JF, Arones S, Steinbock C: Day hospital service in rehabilitation medicine: An evaluation. Arch Phys Med Rehabil 66:86–91, 1985
31. Davis PJ, Davis FB: Endocrinology and aging. In Reichle W (ed): Clinical Aspects of Aging, 2nd ed, pp 396–410. Baltimore, Williams & Wilkins, 1983
32. Dement WC, Miles LE, Carskadon MA: "White paper" on sleep and aging. J Am Geriatr Soc 30:25–50, 1982
33. DeVivo MJ, Fine PR, Maetz HM, Stover SL: Prevalence of spinal cord injury: A reestimation employing life table techniques. Arch Neurol 37:707–708, 1980
34. Ditunno J, Ehrlich GE: Care and training of elderly patients with rheumatoid arthritis. Geriatrics 25:164–172, 1970
35. Dorr LD: Treatment of hip fractures in elderly and senile patients. Orthop Clin North Am 12:153–163, 1981
36. Drachman DA, Leavitt J: Memory impairment in the aged: Storage versus retrieval deficit. J Exper Psychol 93:302–308, 1973
37. DuBow LL, Witt PL, Kadaba MP et al: Oxygen consumption of elderly persons with bilateral below knee amputations: Ambulation vs wheelchair propulsion. Arch Phys Med Rehabil 64:255–259, 1983
38. Elwood TW: Older persons' concerns about foot care. J Am Podiatry Assoc 65:490–494, 1975
39. Etienne PE, Dastoor D, Goldapple E et al: Adverse effects of medical and psychiatric workup in six demented geriatric patients. Am J Psychiatry 138:520–521, 1981
40. Feigenson JS: Stroke rehabilitation: Effectiveness, benefits, and cost. Some practical considerations. Stroke 10(1):1–4, 1979
41. Feller BA: Americans needing help to function at home. Public Health Service No. 92. (DHHS Pub. No. 83-1250). Hyattsville, MD: National Center for Health Statistics, Sept 14, 1983
42. Felsenthal G, Cohen BS, Hilton EB et al: The physiatrist as primary physician for patients on an inpatient rehabilitation unit. Arch Phys Med Rehabil 65:375–378, 1984
43. Felser JM, Raff MJ: Infectious diseases and aging: Immunologic perspectives. J Am Geriatr Soc 31:802–807, 1983
44. Filner B, Williams TF: Health promotion for the elderly: Reducing functional dependency. In Somers AR, Fabian DR (eds): The Geriatric Imperative: An Introduction to Gerontology and Clinical Geriatrics, pp 187–204. New York, Appleton-Century-Crofts, 1983
45. Finlayson RE, Martin LM: Recognition and management of depression in the elderly. Mayo Clin Proc 57:115–120, 1982
46. Fisk AA: Comprehensive health care for the elderly. JAMA 249:230–236, 1983
47. Fleg JL, Kennedy HL: Cardiac arrhythmias in a healthy elderly population: Detection by 24-hour ambulatory electrocardiography. Chest 81:302–307, 1982
48. Fries JF: Aging, natural death, and the compression of morbidity. N Engl J Med 303:130–135, 1980
49. Frocht A, Fillit H: Renal disease in the geriatric patient. J Am Geriatr Soc 32:28–43, 1984
50. Gambert SR, Tsitouras PD: Effect of age on thyroid hormone physiology and function. J Am Geriatr Soc 33:360–365, 1985
51. Gibson CJ, Caplan BM: Rehabilitation of the patient with stroke. In Williams TF (ed): Rehabilitation of the Aging, pp 145–159. New York, Raven Press, 1984
52. Gilchrist AK: Common foot problems in the elderly. Geriatrics 34:67–70, 1979
53. Gillick MR, Serrell NA, Gillick LS: Adverse consequences of hospitalization in the elderly. Soc Sci Med 16:1033–1038, 1982

54. Goldberg PB, Roberts J: Pharmacologic basis for developing rational drug regimens for elderly patients. Med Clin North Am 67:315–331, 1983
55. Harris CM: Joint replacement in the elderly. In Williams TF (ed): Rehabilitation in the Aging, pp 81–95. New York, Raven Press, 1984
56. Hayflick L: Theories of aging. In Cape RDT, Coe RM, Rossman I (eds): Fundamentals of Geriatric Medicine, pp 43–50. New York, Raven Press, 1983
57. Haynes RB, Taylor DW, Sackett DL (eds): Compliance in Health Care. Baltimore, MD, The Johns Hopkins University Press, 1979
58. Hess BB: Stereotypes of the aged. J Communication 14:76–85, 1974
59. Hesse KA, Campion EW, Karamouz N: Attitudinal stumbling blocks to geriatric rehabilitation. J Am Geriatr Soc 32:747–750, 1984
60. Hodkinson HM: Non-specific presentation of illness. Br Med J 4:94–96, 1973
61. Horn JL, Donaldson G: On the myth of intellectual decline in adulthood. Am Psychol 31:701–719, 1976
62. Johnston MV, Miller LS: Cost-effectiveness of the Medicare three-hour regulation. Arch Phys Med Rehabil 67:581–585, 1986
63. Kasper RL: Eye problems of the aged. In Reichle W (ed): Clinical Aspects of Aging, 2nd ed, pp 479–488. Baltimore, Williams & Wilkins, 1983
64. Katzman R: Demography, definitions and problems. In Katzman R, Terry R (eds): The Neurology of Aging, pp 1–14. Philadelphia, FA Davis, 1983
65. Katzman R, Terry R: Normal aging of the nervous system. In Katzman R, Terry R (eds): The Neurology of Aging, pp 15–50. Philadelphia, FA Davis, 1983
66. Keltz H: Pulmonary function and disease in the aging. In Williams TF (ed): Rehabilitation in the Aging, pp 13–22. New York, Raven Press, 1984
67. Kemp B: Psychosocial and mental health issues in rehabilitation of older persons. In Brody SJ, Ruff GE (eds): Aging and Rehabilitation: Advances in the State of the Art, pp 122–158. New York, Springer, 1986
68. Knapp WS, Douglas JS Jr, Craver JM et al: Efficacy of coronary artery bypass grafting in elderly patients with coronary artery disease. Am J Cardiol 47:923–930, 1981
69. Kornzweig AL: New ideas for old eyes. J Am Geriatr Soc 28:145–152, 1980
70. Kottke FJ: Deterioration of the bedfast patient: Causes and effects. Public Health Reports 80:437–450, 1965
71. Kravitz SC: Anemia in the elderly. In Reichel W (ed): Clinical Aspects of Aging, pp 443–452. Baltimore, Williams & Wilkins, 1983
72. Lakshmanan M, Mion LC, Frengley JD: Effective low dose tricyclic antidepressant treatment for depressed geriatric rehabilitation patients: A double blind study. J Am Geriatr Soc 34:421–426, 1986
73. Larson EB, Bruce RA: Health benefits of exercise in an aging society. Arch Intern Med 147:353–356, 1987
74. Laskin RS, Gruber MA, Zimmerman AJ: Intertrochanteric fractures of the hip in the elderly: A retrospective analysis of 236 cases. Clin Orthop 141:188–195, 1979
75. Liberson WT: Brief isometric exercises. In Basmajian JV: Therapeutic Exercise, pp 307–326. Baltimore, Williams & Wilkins, 1984
76. Lindeman RD, Tobin J, Shock NW: Longitudinal studies on the rate of decline in renal function with age. J Am Geriatr Soc 33:278–285, 1985
77. Lipschitz DA, Udupa KB, Milton KY, Thompson CO: Effect of age on hematopoiesis in man. Blood 63:502–509, 1984
78. Margolis LM: Hearing disorders. In Libow L (ed): The Core of Geriatric Medicine. St Louis, CV Mosby, 1981
79. Marzuk PM: Biofeedback in gastrointestinal disorders: A review of the literature. Ann Intern Med 103:240–244, 1985
80. McConnell JG, Buchanan KD, Ardill J, Stout RW: Glucose tolerance in the elderly: The role of insulin and its receptor. Euro J Clin Invest 12: 55–61, 1982
81. McKhann G, Drachman D, Folstein M et al: Clinical diagnosis of Alzheimer's disease. Neurology 34:939–944, 1984
82. Messerli FH, Ventura HO, Amodeo C: Osler's maneuver and pseudohypertension. N Engl J Med 312:1548–1551, 1985
83. Mold JW, Stein HF: The cascade effect in the clinical care of patients. N Engl J Med 314:512–514, 1986
84. Murray PK, Muller J, Clark GS: Functional prognosis in the elderly spinal cord injured. Arch Phys Med Rehabil 63:513–514, 1982
85. Naughton J: Physical activity and aging. Primary Care 9:231–238, 1982
86. Ohry A, Shemesh Y, Rozin R: Are chronic spinal cord injured patients (SCIP) prone to premature aging? Medical Hypotheses 11:467–469, 1983
87. Ouslander JG: Drug therapy in the elderly. Ann Int Med 95:711–722, 1981
88. Posner JD, Gorman KM, Klein HS, Woldow A: Exercise capacity in the elderly. Am J Cardiol 57:52C–58C, 1986
89. Reed JW, Gessner JE: Rehabilitation in the extended care facility. J Am Geriatr Soc 27:325–329, 1979
90. Resnick NM, Yalla SV: Management of urinary incontinence in the elderly. N Engl J Med 313:800–805, 1985
91. Riehle RA Jr, Vaughan ED Jr: Genitourinary disease in the elderly. Med Clin North Am 67:445–461, 1983
92. Rodeheffer RJ, Gerstenblith G, Becker LC et al: Exercise cardiac output is maintained with advancing age in healthy subjects: Cardiac dilatation and increased stroke volume compensate for a diminished heart rate. Circulation 69:203–213, 1984
93. Rodstein M: Falls by the aged. In Cape RDT, Coe RM, Rossman I (eds): Fundamentals of Geriatric Medicine, pp 109–116. New York, Raven Press, 1983
94. Rossman I: Physician as geriatrician. In Cape RDT, Coe RM, Rossman I (eds): Fundamentals of Geriatric Medicine, pp 17–23. New York, Raven Press, 1983
95. Rowe JW: Clinical research on aging: Strategies and directions. N Engl J Med 297:1332–1336, 1977
96. Rowe JW: Influence of age on renal function. In Cape RDT, Coe RM, Rossman I (eds): Fundamentals of Geriatric Medicine, pp 69–74. New York, Raven Press, 1983
97. Rowe JW: Health care of the elderly. N Engl J Med 312:827–835, 1985
98. Ruben RJ, Kruger B: Hearing loss in the elderly. In Katzman R, Terry R (eds): The Neurology of Aging, pp 123–147. Philadelphia, FA Davis, 1983
99. Sabin TD: Biologic aspects of falls and mobility limitations in the elderly. J Am Geriatr Soc 30:51–58, 1982
100. Samiy AH: Clinical manifestations of disease in the elderly. Med Clin North Am 67:333–344, 1983
101. Schaie KW, Baltes PB: On sequential strategies in development research: Description or explanation. Hum Dev 18:384–390, 1975
102. Schaumburg HH, Spencer PS, Ochoa J: The aging human peripheral nervous system. In Katzman R, Terry R (eds): The Neurology of Aging, pp 111–122. Philadelphia, FA Davis, 1983
103. Schneider EL, Reed JD Jr: Life extension. N Engl J Med 312:1159–1168, 1985
104. Schuman JE, Beattie EJ, Steed DA et al: Rehabilitative and geriatric teaching programs: Clinical efficacy in a skilled nursing facility. Arch Phys Med Rehabil 61:310–315, 1980
105. Schuman JE, Beattie EJ, Steed DA et al: Geriatric patients with and without intellectual dysfunction: Effectiveness of a standard rehabilitation program. Arch Phys Med Rehabil 62:612–618, 1981
106. Scileppi KP: Bone and joint disease in the elderly. Med Clin North Am 67:517–530, 1983
107. Seidel LG, Thornton GF, Smith JW, Cluff LE: Studies on the epidemiology of adverse drug reactions III: Reactions in patients on a general medical service. Bull Johns Hopkins Hosp 119:299–315, 1966
108. Shanas E: Social myth as hypothesis: The case of the family relations of old people. Gerontologist 19:3–9, 1979
109. Shock NW: Aging of regulatory systems. In Cape RDT, Coe RM, Rossman I (eds): Fundamentals of Geriatric Medicine, pp 51–62. New York, Raven Press, 1983
110. Simon A, Cohen RB: The acute brain syndrome in geriatric patients. Psych Res Rep 16:8–10, 1963
111. Smith IM: Infectious disease problems in the elderly. In Reichle W (ed): Clinical Aspects of Aging. 2nd ed, pp 218–234. Baltimore, Williams & Wilkins, 1983
112. Spirduso WW, Clifford P: Replication of age and physical activity

effects on reaction and movement time. J Gerontology 33:26–30, 1978

113. Steffee WP: Nutrition intervention in hospitalized geriatric patients. Bull NY Acad Med 56:564–574, 1980

114. Steinberg FU: Diagnostic responsibilities of rehabilitation departments—Second look. Arch Phys Med Rehabil 62:509, 1981

115. Stern N, Tuck ML: Geriatric cardiology: Homeostatic fragility in the elderly. Cardiol Clin 4:201–211, 1986

116. Stover SL, Fine PR (eds): Spinal Cord Injury: The Facts and Figures. Birmingham, The University of Alabama at Birmingham, 1986

117. Strehler BL: Time, Cells, and Aging, 2nd ed. New York, Academic Press, 1977

118. Stuart MR, Snope FC: Family structure, family dynamics, and the elderly. In Somers AR, Fabian DR (eds): The Geriatric Imperative: An Introduction to Gerontology and Clinical Geriatrics, pp 137–152. New York, Appleton-Century-Crofts, 1981

119. Taeuber CM: America in Transition: An Aging Society. Current Population Reports, series P-23, No. 128. Washington, DC, Bureau of the Census, 1983

120. Teravainen H, Calne DB: Motor system in normal aging and Parkinson's disease. In Katzman R, Terry R (eds): The Neurology of Aging, pp 85–109. Philadelphia, FA Davis, 1983

121. Thomas JE, Schirger A, Fealey RD, Sheps SG: Orthostatic hypotension. Mayo Clin Proc 56:117–125, 1981

122. Timiras PS, Choy VJ, Hudson DB: Neuroendocrine pacemaker for growth, development and ageing. Age Ageing 11:73–88, 1982

123. Tinetti ME: Performance-oriented assessment of mobility problems in elderly patients. J Am Geriatr Soc 34:119–126, 1986

124. Wade DT, Langton-Hewer R, Wood VA: Stroke: The influence of age upon outcome. Age Ageing 13:357–362, 1984

125. Wald A: Biofeedback therapy for fecal incontinence. Ann Intern Med 95:146–149, 1981

126. Walsh DA: Age differences in central perceptual processing: A dichoptic backward masking investigation. J Gerontol 31:178–185, 1976

127. Warshaw GA, Moore JT, Friedman SW et al: Functional disability in the hospitalized elderly. JAMA 248:847–850, 1982

128. Wedgwood J: The place of rehabilitation in geriatric medicine; An overview. Int Rehabil Med 7:107–108, 1985

129. Weksler ME: Senescence of the immune system. Med Clin North Am 67:263–272, 1983

130. Williams ME: Clinical implications of aging physiology. Am J Med 76:1049–1054, 1984

131. Williams ME, Hadler NM: The illness as the focus of geriatric medicine. N Engl J Med 308:1357–1360, 1983

132. Williams ME, Pannill FC III: Urinary incontinence in the elderly: Physiology, pathopysiology, diagnosis, and treatment. Ann Intern Med 97:895–907, 1982

133. Wolcott LE: Rehabilitation and the aged. In Reichle W (ed): Clinical Aspects of Aging, 2nd ed, pp 182–204. Baltimore, Williams & Wilkins, 1983

134. Wolfson LI, Katzman R: The neurologic consultation at age 80. In Katzman R, Terry RD (eds): The Neurology of Aging, pp 221–244. Philadelphia, FA Davis, 1983

135. Zindrick MR, Daley RJ, Hollyfield RL et al: Femoral neck fractures in the geriatric population: The influence of perioperative health upon the selection of surgical treatment. J Am Geriatr Soc 33:104–108, 1985

22

Spasticity and Associated Abnormalities of Muscle Tone

James W. Little

John L. Merritt

This work was supported in part by the Veterans Administration, Rehabilitation Research and Development Service.

Spasticity comprises a variety of clinical manifestations that accompany upper motoneuron (UMN) disease. Specifically, spasticity is the increased resistance to passive movement that results from the appearance of hyperactive spinal and brain stem reflexes following UMN lesions. Spasticity is often associated with, but is separate from, the deficiency symptoms of UMN disease, that is, weakness and manifestations of that weakness.

Spasticity may be seen after lesions of the cerebral cortex, brain stem, or spinal cord. However, not all increased muscle tone is called spasticity. Pathologic conditions affecting muscle and peripheral nerve, the spinal cord, the basal ganglia, and other areas of the central nervous system (CNS) can result in various kinds of muscle hypertonus that are clinically or electrophysiologically distinguishable from the manifestations of spasticity (Table 22-1).

MANIFESTATIONS OF SPASTICITY

The hyperreflexia of UMN lesions varies with the site and extent of the CNS lesion. Injury to the cerebral cortex yields different manifestations of spasticity than does injury to the brain stem, and these differ from the spasticity of spinal cord injury.[70, 142] Likewise, small lesions of the cerebral cortex or spinal cord yield different manifestations of spasticity than do large lesions.

The manifestations of spasticity depend on the time after injury. Spasticity gradually evolves in the first few months after CNS injury. Spinal and brain stem reflexes are usually depressed acutely, then gradually return in the first few days to weeks and can become hyperactive. Following spinal cord injury, spasticity of flexor muscles is usually noted first, followed by extensor group spasticity. Guttmann and others have suggested that extremity positioning during the appearance of spasticity greatly affects its ultimate manifestations, although this remains to be proven. In infancy, developmental changes in the CNS superimposed on UMN lesions may also affect the patterns of hyperreflexia that develop.[13]

The abruptness of onset of the CNS lesion is another variable affecting the manifestations of spasticity. With slow-onset lesions (*e.g.,* tumors, spinal stenosis, slowly progressive demyelinating disease) there is usually no spinal shock, extensor hypertonus may predominate early, and paresis appears late. The appearance of hyperactive reflexes and spasticity is often the earliest manifestation of a cerebral or spinal pathologic process.

Other transient factors may also affect spasticity. Nociceptive input, whether from a urinary tract infection, a ureteral stone, an acute abdomen, or other source, increases spasticity. In anesthetic patients such as complete quadriplegics, this increase in spinal reflexes may be the earliest sign for both patient and physician that an acute pathologic process is present. Finally, joint and muscle contractures may eventually mask hyperreflexia.[69]

Complete Spinal Cord Injury

Acutely after complete spinal cord injury, spinal reflexes below the lesion are absent or depressed, although priapism or bulbocavernosus reflexes may be present. This initial depression of spinal reflexes has been termed *spinal shock* and is thought to represent loss of normal tonic descending facilitation (see Pathophysiology). Over the next few days to months, various neuronal mechanisms act to increase reflex excitability as these spinal reflexes return and then become hyperexcitable. The full appearance of these hyperactive spinal reflexes requires 6 months or more.[98, 110]

Muscle stretch, whether by passive joint movement, tendon tap, or tendon vibration, can precipitate reflex contractions. These stretch reflexes can be of two varieties: phasic or tonic. Phasic stretch reflexes are elicited by rapid but not by slow movements, and the reflex muscle contraction rapidly extinguishes within several seconds even though the muscle stretch is maintained. In contrast, tonic stretch reflexes result from slow as well as rapid joint movements, and the muscle contraction persists as long as muscle stretch is maintained.

Hyperactive phasic stretch reflexes are manifest in several ways:

1. Low-threshold, large-amplitude tendon jerks that often spread to other joints and to the opposite limb
2. Clonus (repetitive muscle contractions to rapid maintained

Table 22-1
Distinguishing Spasticity from Other Hypertonus

	Velocity Sensitive	Anatomical Distribution	Range of Joint Motion Affected	Associated Pain	EMG	Other Features
Spasticity						
Hyperactive phasic stretch reflexes	Yes	Flexors in upper extremities, extensors in lower extremities	Early range, clasp-knife	Painless	Active	Clonus, extensor spasms, Hoffman's reflex
Hyperactive tonic stretch reflexes	No	Flexors	Last half of range	Painless	Active	Incomplete spinal cord injury
Hyperactive cutaneo-muscular reflexes	No	Flexors	Throughout range	Painless, unless sustained	Active	Spontaneous flexor-spasms, Babinski response, triple flexion
Other Hypertonus						
Myotendinous contracture	No	Any, often two joint muscles	End of range	Painless	Silent	
Decerebrate rigidity	Yes/No	Extensors in all extremities, opisthotonus	Throughout range, clasp-knife	Painless	Active	
Decorticate rigidity	Yes/No	Flexors in upper extremities, extensors in lower extremities	Throughout range, clasp-knife	Painless	Active	
Parkinsonian rigidity	No	Axial and proximal muscles	Throughout range, cog-wheeling	Painless	Active	Bradykinesia, pill-rolling resting tremor, loss of postural reactions, shuffling gait
Cramps	No	Localized	Throughout range	Painful	Active, high-frequency	
Stiff-man syndrome	No	Axial and proximal limb muscles	Throughout range	Painful	Active	
Metabolic contracture (McArdle's)	No	Distal muscles	Throughout range	Painful	Silent	Brought on by exercise/ischemia

stretch), typically observed in ankle plantarflexors, knee extensors, and finger flexors.

3. A velocity-sensitive increase in tone in knee extensors that often manifests a clasp-knife quality such that knee flexion beyond a certain point (*e.g.,* 30° to 60°) results in a sudden giving way of the resistance to this passive movement.

4. Extensor hypertonus in which rapid hip extension elicits a tonic contraction[91] of knee extensors, hip adductors, and ankle plantarflexors for 5 to 15 seconds followed by relaxation.

Another spinal reflex that usually becomes hyperactive after complete spinal cord injury is the cutaneomuscular (flexor withdrawal or spinal withdrawal) reflex. Noxious input to the extremity elicits triple flexion of the hip, knee, and ankle (ankle dorsiflexion). Often these flexor spasms appear spontaneously, without any external stimulus, every several seconds or minutes in an extremity. Uninhibited bladder contractions may elicit some "spontaneous" flexor spasms in the extremities. Spasms of the external urethral sphincter, including detrusor-sphincter dyssynergia, are thought to be another example of hyperactive flexor reflexes.[79] Occasionally the extremities may be in tonic

flexor spasm. This usually occurs in the presence of pressure sores or other sources of continuous noxious input. A vicious cycle of flexor spasms can be caused by a heel pressure sore that can lead to increased noxious stimulation from the skin, with resulting greater flexor spasms and greater skin shear and skin breakdown.[37] Joint contracture is a common end result, which in itself may increase noxious input to the spinal cord.

These manifestations of spasticity have significant functional impacts. Spasticity may interfere with positioning or independent turning in bed, although many patients learn to use their spasms to help position their legs. Spasticity may interfere with sliding board or push-up transfers. However, most paraplegic or quadriplegic patients manage well as long as they anticipate the possibility of a flexor or extensor spasm or clonus and proceed slowly, allowing spasms to subside. Spasms have been implicated in falls from wheelchairs or from patient lifts.

In driving, spontaneous lower extremity flexor spasms or clonus may be distracting or may even cause the driver to involuntarily strike the hand controls. Clonus of wrist or finger flexors can limit the use of hand controls. For most patients with spinal cord injuries, spasticity does not interfere with driving.

Dressing, bathing, and toileting are occasionally limited, although again most patients or caregivers readily learn to proceed slowly, working around the increased tone, flexor, or extensor spasms. Perineal hygiene and catheter care may be complicated by increased hip flexor and adductor tone or spasms producing scissoring of the hips.

Spasticity can cause skin breakdown. Flexor spasms may jerk the legs backward against the heel-loops on a wheelchair or some other sharp object. During a wheelchair-to-car transfer, an extensor spasm may cause the dorsum of the foot to strike the door. Repetitive clonus or flexor spasms can cause skin shear. Ankle malleoli and heels are at greatest risk. Increased hip adductor tone can pull the thighs together, leading to shear and skin breakdown over the medial knees. Difficulty positioning in bed may lead to pressure points over the greater trochanters, scapulae, sacrum, and heels. Frequently, those with spasticity complain that it interferes with sleep. Even those with complete spinal cord injuries may be kept awake at night by the repetitive jarring of the body from recurrent flexor spasms or clonus.

Not all effects of spasticity are adverse. Spasms may be elicited by the patient to help position the legs. Spasticity is also thought to aid lower extremity circulation via the muscle pump action of the spasms, although a convincing study to document this effect remains to be reported. Muscle contractions may in that way reduce the dependent edema or perhaps reduce the risk of deep venous thrombosis, often seen in paralyzed extremities. Spasms certainly help maintain muscle mass by partially reversing disuse atrophy. It has been suggested but not proven that they may also help to maintain bone mineralization in paralyzed extremities. In quadriplegia, forced vital capacity gradually increases over the first 6 months after injury. This in part results from less paradoxical breathing (*e.g.,* less collapse of the chest and collapsing inward at intercostal spaces) because of spasticity in intercostal muscles. Spasticity of thoracic and abdominal muscles may also assist coughing and clearing of bronchial secretions.

Incomplete Spinal Cord Injury

As in complete injuries, spinal reflexes are initially depressed, although often less so. Tendon reflexes, clonus, and hypertonus often return sooner following incomplete (as compared with complete) spinal cord injury and usually accompany the return of voluntary movement. The bulbocavernosus and flexor reflexes may be delayed in their return or may not be as hyperactive. There is a gradient of spasticity that roughly correlates inversely with preservation of voluntary movement. Thus, patients with sparing of strong, well-controlled voluntary movements tend to have less spasticity; those with minimal sparing of voluntary movement tend to have more severe spasticity.

One less well described manifestation of spasticity seems to be peculiar to some patients with incomplete spinal cord injury, not being found in complete injuries. There is a distinctive end of arc tonic stretch reflex activity present in flexor muscles of the hip and knee. The knee can be extended through most of the range with little resistance. Even rapid passive movements can be performed through the first half or two-thirds of the joint range with little resistance. In the latter half of the range, a fixed resistance is felt, indistinguishable from contracture. Electromyographic (EMG) recordings, however, reveal continuous muscle activity, which is present with static stretch but not with the muscle relaxed. This tonic stretch reflex in flexor muscles is often associated with significant hip and knee flexor contractures (Fig. 22-1).[23]

Patients with incomplete spinal cord injury who are ambulatory may experience increased hip adductor tone with scissoring or knee or ankle clonus that interferes. On the other hand, some patients with no or minimal muscle strength may learn to use knee and ankle extensor hypertonus to assist knee extension (Fig. 22-2).

Some who have incomplete cord injuries perceive pain below their injuries; yet flexor and extensor spasms and clonus are not commonly painful. One exception is severe tonic flexor spasms, with continuous muscle activity in flexor muscles. This may be extremely painful, probably because of the associated overuse of muscles.

Demyelinating Disease

Spasticity is common and often severe in multiple sclerosis,[90, 122] but its manifestations are quite varied. It may be manifest as hypertonus, clonus, flexor or extensor spasms, and/or decerebrate or decorticate rigidity, but most commonly parallels that of incomplete paraplegia or quadriplegia. The spasticity may be

Figure 22-1. Tonic stretch reflex. (*A*) Tonic electrical activity from the medial hamstrings elicited by static stretch and associated with knee flexion contracture (*B*) in a patient with incomplete spinal cord injury. EMG activity was recorded with surface electrodes overlying the muscle.

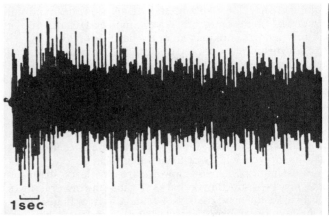

1 sec

A

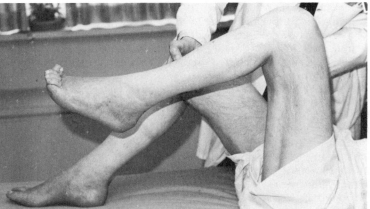

B

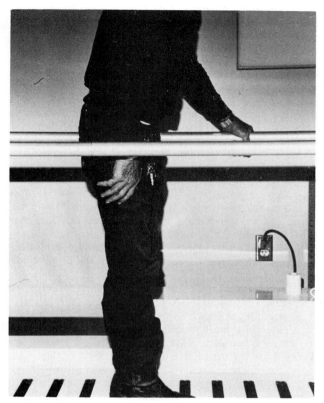

Figure 22-2. Reflex standing. This patient with traumatic spinal cord injury is sensory incomplete but motor complete in his lower extremities, except for slight toe movements bilaterally. He has severe extensor spasms with hip adduction and extension, knee extension, and ankle plantarflexion elicited bilaterally after reclining from sitting and often sustained for more than 5 minutes. He uses these extensor spasms to stand beside his truck while he loads and unloads his wheelchair.

associated with joint contractures, ataxia, weakness, and fatigue.[72]

Stroke

As in spinal cord injury, reflexes and voluntary movement are depressed initially and muscles are flaccid. They begin to return within days to weeks, then become hyperactive over a period of weeks to several months.[166] They become less hyperactive as voluntary strength and control recover. This recovery may become arrested at any point, leaving residual weakness and hyperreflexia.

Spasticity after a stroke typically includes hyperactive phasic stretch reflexes with velocity-sensitive hypertonus, most prominent in the hip adductors, knee extensors, and ankle plantarflexors. Low-threshold, large-amplitude tendon reflexes and clonus appear typically in the ankle plantarflexors, knee extensors, elbow flexors, and wrist and finger flexors. In contrast to spinal cord injury, cutaneomuscular (flexor withdrawal) spasms are not as prominent in stroke spasticity, although a Babinski sign is characteristic. Some hyperactive suprasegmental postural reflexes, such as tonic neck reflexes or symmetrical and asymmetrical tonic labyrinthine reflexes, may be present in hemiplegia, in contrast to quadriplegia and paraplegia. Synergy is characteristic of intermediate recovery of volitional movements. Synergy is the simultaneous mass contraction of synergistic muscles that act on different joints in an extremity. Patients are unable to contract individual muscles in isolation (*i.e.,* "out of synergy").

So-called associated or synkinetic reactions are also common in hemiplegia. These, like the synergistic reactions, are present in normal people[167] but are exaggerated in hemiplegia. Movements in an affected extremity are accompanied by muscle contraction on the opposite side, or in the other extremity on the same side.

Most hemiplegic patients recover some ambulation, although this may be aided by use of a cane and/or ankle-foot orthosis. Ankle or knee clonus and hip adductor hypertonus with scissoring are the most common abnormalities due to the hyperreflexia of a hemiplegic stroke. Additionally, a deficiency of hip, knee, and ankle flexion during the swing phase of gait, often compensated for by hip circumduction, and exaggerated knee and ankle extension during the stance phase are characteristic of hemiplegic stroke (Wernicke-Mann posture).[88, 129] In the hemiplegic upper extremity, flexor tone and voluntary activation predominate over extensor strength and control.

Head Injury

A wide spectrum of hypertonicity may be observed following head injury.[59] Decorticate or decerebrate rigidity are common acutely but tend to decrease in intensity over weeks, when recovery occurs. Over a similar time period, hyperactive phasic stretch reflexes develop, with velocity-sensitive hypertonus, hyperactive tendon reflexes, and clonus being evident. These classic manifestations of spasticity are often superimposed on other hypertonus, such as ataxia and rigidity from cerebellar or basal ganglia involvement. The hypertonus is often enhanced by exaggerated tonic neck and labyrinthine reflexes. This cerebral spasticity interferes with mobility and self-care, in addition to the impairment of voluntary motor function from paresis itself.

Decorticate and Decerebrate Rigidity

Midbrain or bilateral forebrain lesions, whether due to trauma, cerebrovascular accident, tumor, or severe metabolic disorder, commonly result in one of two stereotyped motor responses referred to as decorticate and decerebrate rigidity. Decorticate rigidity is associated with bilateral cortical lesions and is manifest as upper extremity flexion and lower extremity extension bilaterally. In decerebrate rigidity, the lesion involves either the diencephalon bilaterally or the midbrain and is manifest as rigid extension of all extremities, often with neck hypertension (*i.e.,* opisthotonus). These postures appear immediately after injury, in contrast to the spasticity of cerebral hemiplegia or of spinal cord injury, in which there is initial flaccidity. Decorticate or decerebrate rigidity may be present continuously or wax and wane in appearance. A noxious stimulus often exaggerates the abnormal posture, and tonic neck reflexes may appear superimposed on the underlying hypertonus. These abnormal postures are associated with varying degrees of impaired consciousness and tend to resolve as coma lessens. Decorticate rigidity has been associated with a 37% survival rate and decerebrate rigidity with a 10% survival rate.[134] Severe functional impairments are likely in those who do survive.

Cerebral Palsy

Altered muscle tone is often one of the earliest signs of cerebral palsy.[113] An early hypotonia lasting a few weeks or months to as long as 1 year after birth gives way to hypertonicity and abnormal postures, such as scissoring and extension of the lower extremities or persistent flexion and a fisted hand in the upper extremities. Reflex abnormalities accompany the hypertonus. Tendon reflexes are hyperactive and clonus develops. Primitive infantile reflexes persist abnormally and become hyperactive, as do tonic neck, Moro, and palmar and plantar grasp reflexes. The nature of the movement disorder in spastic cerebral palsy is a combination of hypertonus, impaired postural control, persistent primitive reflexes, and associated weakness.[65] These neurological abnormalities eventually lead to muscle shortening and other viscoelastic changes in muscle.[13] Joint capsule tightness and osseous deformities commonly follow and result in further functional deterioration. Common musculoskeletal complications of spastic cerebral palsy include elbow flexion and pronation contractures, wrist and finger flexion deformities, heel cord tightness with equinovarus or occasionally equinovalgus, hip flexion and adduction contractures with femoral anteversion, coxa valga, and hip subluxation or dislocation.

Cerebral palsy is often manifest as spastic hemiplegia, spastic diplegia, or spastic quadriplegia. In the athetoid form, associated with basal ganglia involvement, involuntary writhing or twisting movements of one or all extremities are observed. These slow, sinuous movements of athetosis are distinguished from, but may be seen with, the more rapid, localized movements of chorea or with the sustained, exaggerated postures of dystonia. Purposeful voluntary movements are superimposed on these involuntary movements; co-contraction of antagonists and rigidity are common, but spinal reflexes may or may not be hyperactive.

PATHOPHYSIOLOGY OF SPASTICITY

The pathophysiology of spasticity is complex and controversial.[14, 28, 93, 170] Many different spinal and supraspinal pathways are contributing, and multiple neuronal mechanisms are seemingly responsible for the increases in reflex excitability. Furthermore, the neuronal pathways and neuronal mechanisms responsible for hyperreflexia are still incompletely understood. The following discussion represents one interpretation of the pathophysiology of spasticity.

The Final Common Pathway

Fundamental to comprehending spasticity is understanding Sherrington's concept of the final common pathway. The α-motoneurons in the ventral horn of the spinal cord or in the brain stem are the final common path through which all motor output is conveyed. Each motoneuron receives and summates excitation and inhibition from thousands of spinal and supraspinal inputs. The amount of input and the relative balance of excitation and inhibition determines whether that motoneuron will fire at any given moment and, if so, at what rate. Each discharge of the motoneuron is conducted down the motor axon and results in a contraction of that motor unit. At fast rates of discharge (*e.g.,* 20 to 30 Hz) the muscle contraction becomes tetanic and therefore stronger. Voluntary supraspinal input, reflex spinal or supraspinal input, or a combination of both may discharge motoneurons and cause muscle contractions. Spasticity represents the appearance of hyperexcitable spinal or supraspinal reflexes following degeneration of some or all suprasegmental input.

Initially, following a CNS lesion, the segmental reflexes are often depressed or absent (so-called spinal or cerebral shock). Sherrington, among others, has argued that there has been a loss of tonic descending facilitation that would normally summate with reflex input to allow elicitation of spinal reflexes. After spinal cord injury or stroke, that tonic descending facilitation is lost and spinal reflexes have insufficient excitatory input to depolarize the α-motoneurons voluntarily. Hence, the period of spinal or cerebral shock is observed. Animal studies have shown that a cold block of the spinal cord results in hyperpolarization of motoneurons such that they are more difficult to discharge, which is consistent with Sherrington's postulated loss of tonic descending facilitation.[8]

Within several days, neuronal mechanisms within the spinal cord effect an increase in reflex excitability (Fig. 22-3).[97, 100] One mechanism proposed to explain this increase in reflex excitability is denervation supersensitivity. This mechanism is well known in the peripheral nervous system at muscle and sympathetic ganglia, where denervation causes increased excitability of the end organ within several days. At least in some instances, this denervation supersensitivity results from increased numbers of neurotransmitter receptors on muscle or neuronal membranes. There is some evidence that denervation of neurons, in the spinal cord and other parts of the CNS, results in increased numbers of neurotransmitter receptors and increased sensitivity to neurotransmitter-like substances.[26, 145, 154] Such a mechanism may partially explain the return of and increase in excitability of spinal reflexes several days following a spinal cord or cortical injury.

Another mechanism has been identified in animals that may contribute to later increases in reflex excitability. This mechanism, termed *collateral sprouting* or *reactive synaptogenesis,* involves growth of new synaptic connections by reflex afferents onto the motoneurons and interneurons of the spinal cord, which are partially denervated as a result of the upper motoneuron lesion. The slow growth of new excitatory synaptic terminals by reflex afferents may also explain the gradual appearance of hyperactive spinal reflexes, especially those increases over a period of weeks to months.

Animal and human studies following complete spinal cord injuries have revealed several temporal phases when reflexes become hyperexcitable, consistent with the hypothesis that several mechanisms with differing time courses of appearance develop sequentially to mediate the appearance of hyperreflexia.[97, 98, 100]

TIME COURSE of APPEARANCE

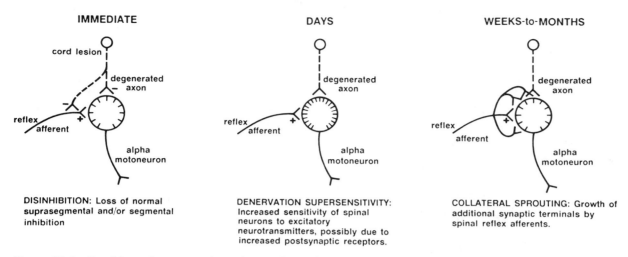

Figure 22-3. Possible mechanisms mediating hyperreflexia. Three mechanisms postulated to mediate the appearance of hyperactive spinal reflexes following upper motoneuron lesions include disinhibition, denervation supersensitivity, and collateral sprouting.

Some have postulated that spasticity results from a relative loss of normal inhibition acting on reflex pathways.[93] Such disinhibition is likely the explanation for decerebrate rigidity, in which there is immediate onset of extensor hypertonus following midbrain lesions. Presumably there is tonic inhibitory control from the cerebral hemispheres to the reticular and vestibular nuclei in the brain stem. Loss of this normal inhibitory input, because of a motor cortex, internal capsule, or midbrain lesion, results in increased excitatory input from vestibulospinal and/or reticulospinal pathways to α- and/or γ-motoneurons in the spinal cord.

Spasticity has been equated with decerebrate rigidity, but the very delayed and gradual onset of spasticity suggests that neuronal mechanisms other than disinhibition likely play a greater role in spasticity. It seems likely that two or more of these neuronal mechanisms, and perhaps others as well, contribute to the appearance of spasticity. Various segmental and suprasegmental pathways that underlie spasticity will now be examined.

Exaggerated Segmental Reflexes

Several sensory receptors that respond to stretch have been identified in muscle; these stretch receptors mediate proprioceptive reflexes from muscle. The dominant receptor is the muscle spindle, which has two types of afferents, group IA and group II. The IA afferents respond primarily to velocity of muscle stretch. They yield a large burst of activity during a rapid stretch but only a small burst during slow stretch. Furthermore, the bursts are brief, subsiding quickly as movement slows, although they do show some tonic firing with maintained stretch. In contrast, the group II afferents respond primarily to muscle length. They discharge at a steady rate that varies with the length of the muscle, and not with the velocity of muscle stretch. Based primarily on animal studies, group IA and II afferents also have different central connections.[17] IA afferents have monosynaptic excitatory connections to α-motoneurons of the same muscle and its synergists (Fig. 22-4). Group II fibers make polysynaptic connections to α-motoneurons that appear to be inhibitory to extensor motoneurons and excitatory to flexor motoneurons

(Fig. 22-5). There are also presynaptic inhibitory terminals on the IA afferents, and the α-motoneurons send recurrent collaterals back to small interneurons in the ventral horn called the Renshaw cells, which inhibit the α-motoneurons.

Efferent γ-motoneurons innervate muscle spindles and maintain tension in the spindle; thus IA and II afferents can respond to changes in muscle length even in a shortened muscle.

When stretch reflexes become hyperactive in spasticity, synaptic excitability from IA afferents to α-motoneurons appears to increase. This may be the result of increased IA synaptic transmission due to sprouting by IA afferents to partially denervated motoneurons or to loss of presynaptic inhibition on the afferent terminals.[9] Another factor could be increased α-motoneuron excitability due to denervation supersensitivity of the motoneuron or loss of postsynaptic inhibition of the motoneuron from Renshaw cells, Ia-inhibitory interneurons,[169] or other sources.

The long-held view that γ-motoneuron activity increases after UMN lesions, resulting in increased muscle spindle sensitivity, appears to be less compatible with current observations.[21] In patients with spasticity, microelectrode recordings from IA afferents by some investigators have failed to demonstrate increased responsiveness to muscle stretch,[64] although others have reported increased discharges.[161] Nerve block does not alter the nerve afferent potential to tendon tap recorded below the block in human subjects.[21] In animal models of spasticity, involving either cerebral or spinal lesions, there has also been a failure to record increased peripheral sensitivity of the muscle spindle, whereas increased central excitability in association with the appearance of hyperactive spinal reflexes has been demonstrated.[3, 56, 96, 108]

Clonus is thought to be a self-sustaining oscillation of phasic stretch reflexes due to recurrent bursts of IA afferent discharge and hyperexcitable IA-motoneuronal synaptic transmission.[44, 135]

Irradiation of tendon reflexes has been examined and is postulated to result in some cases from mechanical spread of the vibration[94, 164] but in other cases from increased central excitability of IA afferent connections to synergistic muscles.[41] The clasp-knife phenomenon, characteristic of knee extensors, has been attributed to group II muscle spindle activity from the

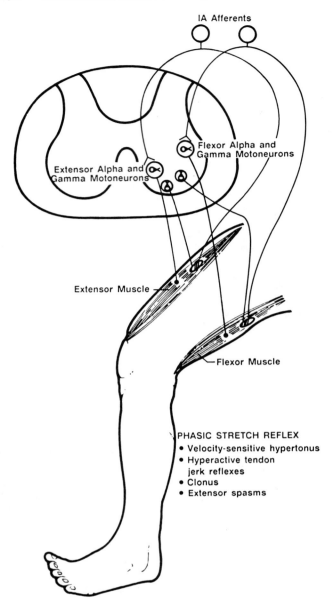

Figure 22-4.   Phasic stretch reflex. This schematic represents reflex pathways that may underlie hyperactive phasic stretch reflexes of spasticity. Possible clinical manifestations are listed.

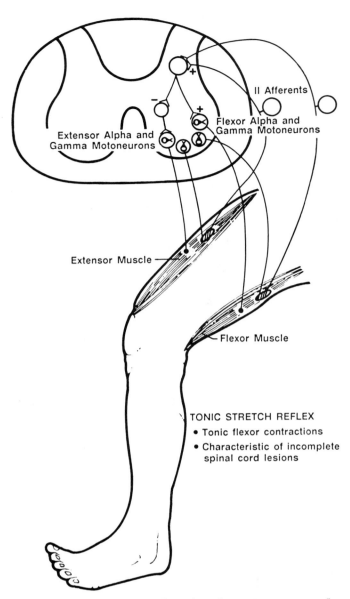

Figure 22-5.   Tonic stretch reflex. This schematic represents reflex pathways that may underlie hyperactive tonic stretch reflexes of spasticity.

quadriceps femoris muscle, which is thought to be centrally inhibitory to extensor motoneurons.[22] Others have suggested that Golgi tendon organs[75] or other free nerve endings in muscle[140] are responsible for the clasp-knife inhibition of the stretch reflex. The shortening reaction has been described in the tibialis anterior and hamstring muscles and may be due to group II muscle spindle discharges from the opposing extensors (*i.e.,* gastrocnemius-soleus and quadriceps femoris, respectively). Group II afferents are postulated to be excitatory to flexor motoneurons. The shortening reaction in the tibialis anterior is seen in subjects with UMN weakness but also in parkinsonian and cerebellar ataxia patients and some normal subjects.[12]

Tonic stretch reflexes imply that tonic stretch of muscle will cause tonic muscle activity (see Fig. 22-5). This seems to be present in some cases after incomplete spinal cord lesions (see Fig. 22-1). It is present in hip flexors and knee flexors[23] and is clinically indistinguishable from contracture except that tonic electrical activity is recorded.[52] It is proposed that group II

muscle spindle afferents from flexor muscles mediate this tonic activity; animal studies have shown that these group II afferents fire tonically and increase their firing rate with muscle stretch, and, centrally, they facilitate flexor and inhibit extensor motoneurons.[77] Some tonic stretch reflex hyperactivity may result from IA afferents since they do maintain some continuous firing with maintained stretch.

Cutaneomuscular (flexor withdrawal or exteroceptive) reflexes (Fig. 22-6) are long-latency polysynaptic, polysegmental reflexes to noxious stimuli, mediated by myelinated (A-delta) and unmyelinated (C) fibers, which spread primarily to flexor and to a lesser extent to extensor muscles.[62, 144] Hyperexcitability of these reflexes presumably results from increases in central excitability with abnormal activation of widespread pathways.[9]

Whether this hyperexcitability occurs at the primary afferent–interneuron synapse or interneuronal afferent–α-motoneuron synapse is unknown. Joint or muscle nociceptive afferents and autonomic afferents (*e.g.,* from the bladder) also

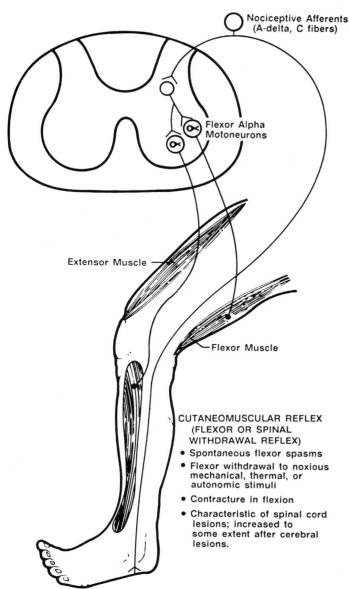

Figure 22-6. Cutaneomuscular (flexor withdrawal) reflex. This schematic represents reflex pathways that may underlie the hyperactive cutaneomuscular reflexes of spasticity.

contribute.[31, 55, 126] Disinhibition,[106] denervation supersensitivity, or collateral sprouting or a combination of these neuronal mechanisms might mediate such hyperexcitability and widespread irradiation. A descending inhibitory pathway, called the dorsal reticulospinal pathway, has been identified in cats.[99] Bilateral section of this pathway results in hyperactive cutaneomuscular (flexor withdrawal) reflexes. This pathway is intact with upper brain stem or cerebral lesions and may explain why hyperactive cutaneomuscular (flexor withdrawal) reflexes and tonic stretch reflexes are more prominent after spinal cord lesions than after more rostral lesions.

Exaggerated Suprasegmental Reflexes

If the UMN lesion is rostral to the brain stem, then suprasegmental reflexes through the upper spinal cord and brain stem may become hyperactive. Thus, tonic neck and labyrinthine reflexes may become hyperactive. They seem to become particularly

prominent after early CNS injury, such as in cerebral palsy, but may also develop in adult-onset cerebral injury, such as after traumatic head injury or after stroke.

Again, the reason for increased reflex excitability may be due to disinhibition, denervation supersensitivity, collateral sprouting, and/or some other unknown factor.

Abnormal Voluntary Control

Paralysis, weakness, and/or impaired voluntary control frequently follow disruption of UMN pathways. This weakness and impaired voluntary control are not spasticity, but they interact with spasticity to produce motor dysfunction. Coactivation of antagonists, common after stroke and incomplete spinal cord injury may, however, result in subsequent reciprocal inhibition of agonists and thus impair voluntary activation.[84] Spasticity and weakness are only mild after pyramidal lesions disrupting the corticospinal tract.[18] Disruption of the extrapyramidal cortical brain stem or brain stem–spinal pathways is presumably of greater significance in producing spasticity.

Normally, in voluntary contraction of muscle, both α- and γ-motoneurons discharge. This allows muscle spindles to remain sensitive and to provide feedback regarding muscle length and movement during the contraction. The effect of UMN lesions and consequent hyperactive group IA– and group II–mediated stretch reflexes on this α-γ coactivation is not currently well understood. UMN lesions usually result in weakness or paralysis. If some voluntary movement is present, it may be limited in strength or range of motion. This impairment of movement is often due to the UMN weakness itself.[95, 142] Spared descending input is not sufficient to allow recruitment of the largest α-motoneurons, while the smallest motoneurons discharge at slow rates to produce weak, unfused (not tetanic) muscle contractions. However, other factors may be contributing:

1. Agonist–antagonist co-contraction due to central coactivation[103] or possibly the result of deficient reciprocal inhibition between agonist and antagonist[33, 170]
2. Agonist–antagonist co-contraction due to hyperactive segmental reflexes, either stretch reflexes, or cutaneomuscular reflexes[87]
3. Changes in the viscoelastic properties of muscle itself[42]

A reduction of antagonist co-contractions, either via nerve block[169] or via antispasticity medication,[85] can enhance the strength of voluntary agonist contractions.

Normally, very strong voluntary contractions of individual muscles are accompanied by simultaneous contraction of synergists on the same and opposite side. Following partial UMN lesions those synergistic and synkinetic contractions are often exaggerated; thus, there is less ability to selectively activate muscles.

Decorticate and Decerebrate Rigidity

The often-observed immediate onset of decerebrate and decorticate rigidity suggests a disinhibition mechanism is involved. The lesion must lie in the pons, midbrain, or diencephalon to cause decerebrate rigidity and involves disinhibition of the lateral vestibular nuclei, which are excitatory to extensor motoneurons, and disinhibition of γ-motoneurons with a resulting increase in muscle spindle discharges. Thus, in contrast to the apparent absence of increased γ-motoneuron activity and muscle spindle discharges in human spasticity, increased γ-motoneuron activity does contribute to the hyperactive stretch reflexes of decerebrate rigidity in the cat.[19] A clasp-knife phenomenon is observed in decerebrate rigidity as well as spasticity.[36, 147, 167]

CLINICAL EVALUATION OF SPASTICITY

Spasticity may be either beneficial or deleterious. Functionally, extensor spasms may help maintain rigidity of the lower extremity in standing and walking, but spasticity can also interfere in those with preserved voluntary control. However, not all compromise of standing and walking following UMN lesions is due to hyperactive stretch reflexes. Deficient descending facilitation, antagonist co-contraction, and altered viscoelastic properties of muscle may interfere as well.[42, 85] Spontaneous flexor spasms can occur during standing or walking and disrupt the gait cycle or throw the patient off balance.

Occasionally, clonus of ankle plantarflexors, quadriceps femoris, or hamstring muscles can also cause loss of balance or impose a slow gait on the patient such that rapid movements do not elicit clonus. Exaggerated hip adduction (i.e., scissoring) is common, resulting in a smaller base of support and difficulty with the swing phase of gait owing to rubbing of thighs. Difficulty clearing the foot during the swing phase of gait often results from deficiency syndromes and muscle imbalance (i.e., ankle plantarflexors and knee extensors are more activated than ankle dorsiflexors and knee flexors) rather than hyperactive stretch reflexes. Extensor spasms may interfere with push-up, sliding board, or hydraulic lift transfers; since these spasms usually subside within 15 to 30 seconds, safe transfers are usually possible by proceeding slowly. Wheelchair positioning may be compromised as well. Flexor spasms, extensor spasms, or clonus may pull the feet off the footrests. Asymmetrical spasms may lead to asymmetrical sitting and scoliosis.

Flexor and extensor spasms can throw the foot against sharp objects, such as the heel-loop bolts on wheelchair footrests or car doors. Hip flexor and adductor spasms often occur together and lead to recurrent shear of the medial knees, with resulting skin breakdown. The presence of severe hip and knee flexor spasms often limits the patient to right or left side-lying, since prone and supine positions are not tolerated or cannot be maintained; this may lead to trochanteric decubiti.

Hip flexors and adductors, knee flexors, ankle plantarflexors, shoulder adductors, elbow flexors, and wrist and finger flexors are at greatest risk for developing contractures after UMN lesions. Tonic reflex activity, such as that occasionally seen in hip and knee flexors after incomplete spinal cord lesions, often results in contracture. Likewise, frequent hip and knee flexor spasms or low threshold ankle clonus may lead to contracture of respective muscles. Knee extensor spasms are usually transient, subsiding within seconds; thus, knee extensor contracture is uncommon.

Patients with spasticity commonly complain of recurring flexor spasms, or less commonly, of clonus, which prevents them from going to sleep or wakes them frequently.

Lower extremity clonus, flexor spasms, or extensor spasms may interfere with driving. Clonus and extensor spasms may be triggered by vibration of the vehicle. The leg may pull up and strike the hand controls or steering wheel or simply cause a distraction. Upper extremity spasms and clonus may directly interfere with using hand controls. Specific vocational tasks may be compromised by spasticity.

Hip adductor and flexor spasms may further interfere with sexual function for both males and females. Pain is an uncommon manifestation of stable spasticity. One exception is that of severe, continuous flexor spasms. Muscles may be constantly painful and tender, and facilitation of muscle activity by cutaneous stimulation or joint movement can further increase pain. Other causes of pain, such as bursitis, tendonitis, or wounds, can be aggravated by spasms.

Routine Evaluation

The functional impact of spasticity cannot be established by physical examination alone. History taking is essential. The physician must determine what manifestations are present, which muscle groups are involved, and whether these manifestations are beneficial or deleterious. Specific questioning is necessary to determine which extremities and muscle groups are most involved. Questions about the frequency of spasms, any diurnal variation present, precipitating factors, and any recent increase or decrease in the level of reflex activity are important. Particularly in patients with spinal cord pathology, in which anesthesia accompanies spasticity, an increase in the frequency and/or intensity of spasms may be the earliest sign of a noxious stimulus such as a bladder infection, skin breakdown, bowel impaction, or acute abdomen.[37, 110] Finally, the functional uses and hindrances of the spasticity need to be explored.

The common feature of all manifestations of spasticity is increased muscle tone. Usually it is a transient increase in tone following rapid passive movements, but occasionally it may be present with slow movements (i.e., independent of movement velocity). The anatomical distribution of the hypertonus should also be described.

Reflex threshold is decreased and amplitude is increased when tendon reflexes are hyperactive. There may be spread or irradiation of the reflex contraction to adjacent or contralateral muscles (e.g., biceps tendon tap may elicit contractions of long finger flexors and thumb adductor as well as the biceps itself; a tap to the medial femoral epicondyle may elicit bilateral adductor contractions). Tendon reflexes can be readily tested in the upper extremity for the biceps brachii, triceps brachii, brachioradialis, pectoralis major, and long finger flexor muscles. In the lower extremity, quadriceps femoris, triceps surae, hip adductor, and medial hamstring muscle reflexes are readily tested.

Tendon tap or rapid stretch will often elicit clonus (repetitive involuntary muscle contractions) in spastic muscles. If resistance is applied, such as resisted ankle plantarflexion after rapid stretch into ankle dorsiflexion, then repetitive synchronous contractions may continue as long as resistance is applied (i.e., sustained clonus) or consist of only several beats. Clonus is also commonly elicited by a sharp downward pull on the patella, or by sudden passive extension of the wrist or fingers.

The examiner should observe for spontaneous flexor spasms and look for Babinski and triple flexion responses to stroking a blunt object along the plantar aspect of the foot. The cutaneomuscular (flexor withdrawal) reflex may have a lower threshold, larger amplitude, longer duration, and/or be more widespread following UMN lesions. Notation is made of the muscles participating (e.g., hip flexors, hamstrings, ankle dorsiflexors, toe dorsiflexors), the intensity of the contraction is graded, and any spread to the opposite extremity is described.

Voluntary muscle strength can be tested and graded on the usual five-point scale. However, motor strength is often much better than motor control. Some patients are able to use their hyperactive spinal stretch reflexes to facilitate static strength and "use their spasticity to stand or walk" (see Fig. 22-2). To assess motor control, the examiner should observe a patient's ability to contract rapidly and relax and to activate selectively individual muscles. Simultaneous contraction of other flexors or extensors in the same leg (i.e., flexor or extensor synergy) or in the oppo-

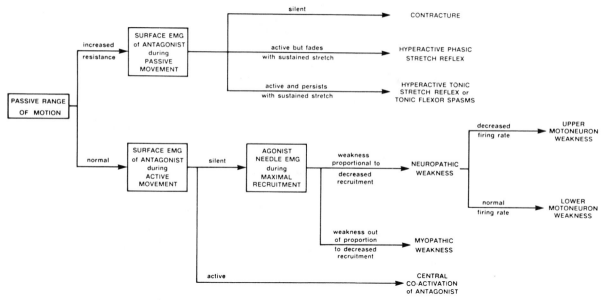

Figure 22-7. Restraint of voluntary movement. Decision tree distinguishing various factors, including hyperactive spinal reflexes, that may restrain voluntary movement.

site leg (*i.e.,* synkinesis) should be described. Any limitation in speed or range of motion (ROM) of voluntary movement should also be noted (Fig. 22-7). If such restraint is present, then the presence or absence of antagonist co-contraction should be noted and can be confirmed by surface EMG recordings. If simultaneous antagonist contraction is not present, then deficient prime mover (agonist) activity is present. This can often be confirmed by needle EMG study.

If both passive and active ROM are significantly limited, then surface EMG recording of the antagonist or anesthetic block of the nerve to the antagonist can be used to distinguish contracture from antagonist muscle reflex activity or co-contraction activity.[23, 33, 52, 84, 112]

Postural effects should also be considered. Does head or body position, (prone vs. supine position or supine vs. sitting or standing) affect tone and voluntary movements? These observations allow one to assess the contributions of tonic neck and labyrinthine reflexes.[155, 156]

Finally, patient function should be examined, focusing on those functions in which the patient describes spasticity interfering. Bed mobility, coming from supine to sitting, coming from sitting to standing, standing, walking, and sliding board transfers, need to be observed along with other self-care skills such as eating, dressing, toileting, and writing. The functional impairments must be correlated with reflex and voluntary movement observations to attempt to identify whether hyperactive reflexes, weakness, contracture, or a combination are primarily limiting function and to identify which muscle groups are most involved.[29, 30, 95, 137]

Other Evaluation Methods

Electrophysiological and mechanical methods are available for evaluating the hyperactive spinal and brain stem reflexes of spasticity. However, for patient management, the history, physical examination and functional examination are of greatest importance. Presently, the quantitative methods are time consuming, require specialized instrumentation not commonly available, often fail to assess the anatomical distribution, and fail to assess

the functional impact of spasticity. These quantitative methods are currently most helpful as a supplement to a thorough clinical and functional examination or in research on specific manifestations of spasticity.

The most available and clinically useful electrophysiological method for evaluating spasticity is dynamic multichannel EMG. Surface electrodes are taped over selected muscles, and the EMG activity is recorded during passive or active movements or in response to cutaneous stimuli.[45, 85] As noted previously, this is particularly useful for distinguishing contracture from antagonist muscle activity in restrained voluntary movements.[32, 52, 70, 104, 112] It may also be useful for identifying which muscle group is primarily contributing to a particular manifestation of spasticity or for following the response to therapy in a semiquantitative way.

Gait analysis is an extension of such multichannel EMG recording, using small radio transmitters or cables to relay EMG signals and force and joint angle information from the lower extremity muscles to recording equipment. The usefulness of gait analysis has been demonstrated in planning tendon lengthening and tendon transfers in spastic cerebral palsy patients.[34, 131, 159] It is a sophisticated way to relate muscle activity to function; and with increasing development of specialized video equipment, miniaturized amplifiers, and microcomputers, it may become a more widely available method for evaluating the functional impact of spasticity. Four-channel EMG equipment is now commonly available, allowing simultaneous recording from four different muscles. Some have even used 16-channel EEG equipment, which does allow widespread sampling of muscle hyperactivity.

H reflexes, first described and named after Hoffmann,[73] are similar to tendon jerks except that they are elicited electrically. Most commonly the tibial nerve is stimulated behind the knee and the response is recorded from the triceps surae muscles. At low intensity stimulation, a reflex potential is recorded at a latency of about 30 msec. This is thought to represent a monosynaptic reflex from IA muscle spindle afferents to α-motoneurons. As stimulus intensity is increased, an M response appears with a latency of about 5 msec. This represents stimulation of motor axons that have a higher threshold than IA afferents and that conduct from the knee to the calf directly. With a further increase in stimulus intensity, the M response reaches a plateau at a maximum amplitude and the H reflex is abolished. Presumably, all motor axons are depolarized at this stimulus intensity and antidromic conduction in these axons collides with the reflex-elicited discharges to abolish the H reflex. Such H reflexes can often also be recorded from the flexor carpi radialis and quadriceps femoris muscles to median and femoral nerve stimulation, respectively.

Tibial H reflexes have been used as a measure of stretch reflex excitability. One parameter that has been used is maximum H reflex amplitude (peak-to-peak) divided by maximum M response amplitude (peak-to-peak).[2, 101] This procedure estimates that proportion of motor units that can be excited reflexly. The H/M ratio tends to be higher in spastic patients with hyperactive tendon jerks. However, there is considerable overlap with the wide range of H/M ratios recorded in normal subjects.[2, 98] The H/M ratio has been most useful in serial studies on spasticity. The effects of cooling, electrical stimulation, and spasmolytic medication on H/M amplitude ratios have been examined. The evolution of spasticity has also been described by recording H/M ratios serially over weeks to months following a UMN lesion.[98] These studies have demonstrated an increase in H/M ratio that accompanies the appearance of hyperactive tendon jerks.

Another parameter of reflex excitability is the ratio of H reflex amplitude during vibration to the amplitude without vibration. Vibration inhibits H reflexes, in part due to presynaptic inhibition by reflex afferents. Subjects with spasticity tend to have less vibratory inhibition of the H reflex than do nonspastic subjects. Curiously, following traumatic spinal cord injury, both the increase in H/M amplitude and the decrease in vibratory inhibition develop some months later, although some manifestations of spasticity are present earlier.[4] Yet another measure of H reflex excitability that has been used in evaluating spasticity is the amount of inhibition that results from a conditioning stimulus given 5 to 500 msec previous to the test H reflex stimulus. This is referred to as the H reflex recovery curve. In spastic patients, inhibition of the H reflex by a conditioning shock is of shorter duration than in normal subjects.[157, 171]

All of these H reflex methods examine only the phasic stretch reflex to one muscle group. They also are quite tedious, particularly the H reflex recovery method. Delwaide[40] has used these various H reflex tests to identify different modes of action of different spasmolytic medications. He suggests that such tests may aid in choosing the optimal muscle relaxant for a given patient with spasticity, which, if confirmed, could be quite helpful clinically.

Electrophysiological methods have also been used to electrically elicit and record cutaneomuscular (flexor withdrawal) reflexes.[107, 165] In spastic patients, various electrophysiological changes of cutaneomuscular reflexes have been described: (1) delayed reflexes,[50, 74] (2) disruption of cutaneomuscular organization,[11, 43, 60] and (3) dishabituation of reflexes.[43] These methods do not as yet have demonstrated clinical usefulness. Pederson[125] has recorded the frequency of flexor spasms at night. This technique allows objective confirmation of sleep disruption by spasticity and allows monitoring of therapeutic effects.

F-waves have also been used to assess excitability of α-motoneurons. Some changes have been described, but they are subtle and the method requires many repetitions of high-intensity stimulation,[48] hampering its usefulness.

The pendulum test (Fig. 22-8), an electrogoniometric recording of knee motion and oscillation after dropping the foot from a position of full knee extension, has been used to quantify spasticity of the quadriceps femoris and hamstring muscles.[7] This test includes the calculation of a "relaxation index," which has

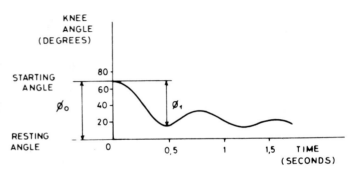

Figure 22-8. Pendulum test. Electrogoniogram of knee angle during a pendulum test showing moderate spasticity of the knee extensors. The relaxation index (R) is calculated as $\theta_1/1.6 \times \theta_0$ where θ_1 is the amplitude of the first swing measured in degrees of joint rotation and θ_0 is the difference between the starting angle and the resting angle. In this subject R is 0.49. In normal subjects, θ_1 is 1.6 times larger or more than θ_0; thus, R is larger than 1.0. (Bajd T, Vodovnik L: Pendulum testing of spasticity. J Biomed Eng 6:9–16, 1984)

been proposed as an index of spasticity. The pendulum test requires relatively inexpensive and readily available equipment, but multiple testing and calculation of average values must be performed. Clinical experience is as yet limited.

Mechanical recording of muscle force has been used to evaluate spasticity, but the need for large, complex, and expensive equipment has limited this to research facilities. More recently, an isokinetic ergometer with peripherally located force sensors has become commercially available. This computer-assisted isokinetic ergometer (Kin-Com) can record, display, and analyze concentric and eccentric torque values. This allows both active and passive velocity-controlled resistances to be evaluated. Active and passive torque curves can be coupled with surface multichannel dynamic EMG recordings for assessment of agonist and antagonist activity at preset velocities. Knutsson reports good repeatability using this combination, and further evaluations are underway.[84, 85]

Anesthetic nerve blocks are sometimes useful in evaluating spasticity. If the block is complete or near complete, and this can be confirmed by nerve stimulation above the block site, then hypertonus can be clearly distinguished from joint capsule tightness or myotendinous contracture. Temporary anesthetic motor point or nerve blocks are often performed prior to long-lasting phenol or alcohol blocks to simulate the effect of the latter. However, the anesthetic blocks are only approximations of the long-lasting blocks in that they usually have a greater effect on the tone and they may also result in loss of sensation that will not be present with motor-point blocks. Nevertheless, local anesthetic blocks are often helpful in assessing the impact on function of contemplated phenol or alcohol blocks before these destructive blocks are performed.

TREATMENT METHODS

Stepped Care

Rarely can all manifestations of spasticity be eliminated. Furthermore, that may not be desirable, since some spasticity is beneficial. The usual goal is to minimize the adverse effects of hyperactive reflexes. Stepped care for spasticity begins with conservative methods that carry the least side-effects and progresses to aggressive treatments with most side-effects (Fig. 22-9).[109]

First and foremost is to identify and eliminate any remediable sources of nociception that may be aggravating spasticity.

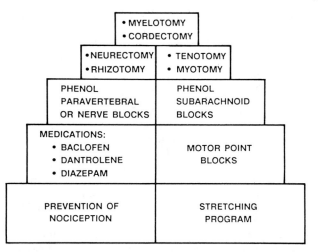

Figure 22-9. Stepped care for spasticity. The initial foundation and subsequent levels of care for spasticity. (Merritt JL: Management of spasticity in spinal cord injury. Mayo Clin Proc 56:614–622, 1981)

This is particularly important in patients with recent aggravation of their hyperreflexia. Urinary tract infection, bowel impaction, pressure sore, fracture, paronychia, and acute abdomen are all examples of nociceptive sources that may increase spasticity.[37, 39, 109]

The acute onset of a UMN lesion is a special case in which one attempts to prevent the development of hyperactive reflexes. Some observations suggest that positioning muscles in a stretched position, minimizing nociceptive input, and using early motor-point and nerve blocks may be helpful in minimizing the ultimate severity of spasticity that develops,[61] but further confirmation of these observations is needed. Further understanding is needed of the mechanisms that mediate the appearance of hyperreflexia and interventions that can prevent that process.

A significant element in treating spasticity is patient education. The benefits and adverse effects of spasticity need to be outlined for the patient, and the patient should be educated regarding the use of slow movements and passive great toe dorsiflexion for minimizing velocity-sensitive hypertonus and clonus. Triggering useful extensor or flexor spasms during transfers or bed mobility can be learned. Patients can be instructed to use foot protection devices and to remove heel-loop bolts from wheelchair footrests if skin breakdown is a risk due to spasms. Waist or chest straps or contact guarding by another person may be needed if spasms are severe to prevent falls from a wheelchair or during transfers. Education will allow patients to minimize the adverse effects of their spasticity and to function despite spasticity.

Physical Modalities

Daily range-of-motion (ROM) exercises are an essential component of spasticity management. The hypertonus and imbalance of muscle activity following UMN lesions predisposes patients to fixed muscle shortening and joint capsule tightening. Daily ROM, whether performed by the patient or an attendant, prevents the development of joint movement limitations. For spasticity, ROM should also include slow, steady end of arc stretching. There is evidence that muscle stretching, particularly daily static stretching, will result in a reduction of stretch reflex hyperactivity that may last for several hours after the exercise.[123] Most therefore recommend ROM and stretching twice daily at a minimum. Some suggest that passive bicycling may help reduce spasticity in some patients.[37]

Standing is another form of static stretch for hip flexors, knee flexors, and ankle plantarflexors. It can reverse early contracture and may reduce stretch reflex excitability. Upright positioning can also help to shift the balance of facilitation toward extensor motoneurons in those with incomplete UMN lesions. This influence comes, at least in part, from tonic labyrinthine reflexes. Other body positions or head positions can be used to minimize facilitation that is contributing to hypertonus and to maximize facilitation to muscles that have reduced voluntary recruitment.[15, 155] Hip adductor scissoring may be marked in infants with cerebral palsy. Parents are taught to hold the infant straddled over their thigh or hip to stretch these hypertonic muscles and prevent contracture. Dynamic stimuli such as tilting while sitting on a large beach ball, spinning in a swing, or tilting on a balance board to elicit phasic labyrinthine reflexes and to counterbalance the maldistribution of muscle tone have been used in children with spasticity. Tendon vibration may also help in facilitating voluntary movement and inhibiting associated spasticity.[14, 63]

Biofeedback, using either EMG or joint position sensors, and providing auditory and/or visual feedback has been described as reducing spasticity in patients with some preservation of voluntary motor control.[10, 20]

Prolonged static stretching of muscles with upper and lower extremity splints,[123] serial casting,[51, 59] or orthotics has also been used. Cutaneous stimulation from the orthosis is in some instances thought to facilitate motoneuron activity, as well as provide static stretching to reduce stretch reflex activity and reverse contracture.[153] In some patients with multiple sclerosis, with excessive ankle plantarflexion tone in standing, and with difficulty initiating the swing phase of walking, rocker shoes have improved the speed and reduced the net energy cost of walking.[130]

Ankle-foot orthoses are used to control spastic equinus deformity at the ankle. Medial or lateral T-straps or anterior flare of a plastic brace can be added to help control varus or valgus. Knee-ankle-foot orthoses or a parapodium may be of use for standing or limited walking in those with marked UMN weakness and hypertonus.

Muscle cooling is of benefit in spasticity, particularly with respect to phasic stretch reflex activity and clonus.[67] Muscle cooling, however, requires prolonged application. The early effect of skin cooling is often to facilitate spasticity. Because cooling is only transient (*i.e.,* lasting 1 to 2 hours) and because it requires prolonged application (*i.e.,* for 15 minutes or more), it is often not practical for day-to-day improvement of function. However, cooling can be used in conjunction with an intense program of physical or occupational therapy, particularly in patients with recent stroke or spinal cord injuries, or in conjunction with static stretch to help overcome hyperactive stretch reflexes predisposing to contracture.[86, 122]

Electrical stimulation at nearly all levels of the nervous system has been reported to be of some benefit in relieving spasticity. Peripheral stimulation of muscle or nerve for 15 minutes reportedly relieves velocity-sensitive hypertonus and clonus for up to several hours after the stimulation is stopped.[76] Even transcutaneous electrical nerve stimulation (TENS) has been reported to decrease spasticity in some patients with spinal cord injury.[6] More recently, Shindo[148] has reported a reduction of spasticity, by clinical evaluation, lasting 8 to 72 hours after each session of a neuromuscular re-education program using agonist–antagonist reciprocating multichannel functional electrical stimulation. Further study of these techniques is warranted.

Medications

There are currently three widely available, effective, and relatively safe medications for the treatment of spasticity: baclofen, diazepam, and dantrolene sodium. Baclofen is thought to act at the level of the spinal cord, possibly on inhibitory synapses that have γ-butyric acid (GABA) as the neurotransmitter, although other sites of action have also been described.[89] It is most useful in treating flexor spasms[144] but also reduces stretch reflex activity in patients with spinal pathology.[86] Benefit in patients with cerebral lesions has been reported but has not been convincingly demonstrated.[59] Patients whose spasticity is notably reduced by muscle cooling (cryotest positive)[86] and those whose voluntary movements are impeded by spasms benefitted most from baclofen.[102] Side-effects are uncommon and generally mild, although rebound spasticity[139] and withdrawal seizures have been reported when the drug is stopped abruptly without tapering gradually and an occasional patient may experience hallucinations, particularly those with brain injury. Experimental studies with continuous intrathecal administration of baclofen have shown that it can eliminate hypertonus and improve function, even when oral therapy with baclofen has failed.[128]

Like baclofen, diazepam is thought to be primarily central acting, possibly facilitating GABA-mediated inhibition within the brain and brain stem, and to a lesser extent in the spinal cord. When given intravenously it can markedly reduce hypertonus, clonus, and flexor spasms. Orally, it can decrease these manifestations of spasticity. CNS side-effects such as sedation and memory impairment are more pronounced with diazepam than baclofen.[139] These limiting CNS effects are often most severe in head injury or severe multiple sclerosis with some symptoms of impaired mentation. Diazepam is also addictive in some patients and can lead to respiratory depression in high doses. However, it may be a useful agent when used in combination with baclofen for flexor spasms and to modulate nociception-induced spasms while definitive treatment is underway.

Dantrolene sodium is a unique drug, acting peripherally on the excitation–contraction coupling mechanism of muscle fibers.[133] It blocks calcium ion release from the sarcoplasmic reticulum and thus inhibits muscle contraction. It seems to selectively reduce stretch reflex hyperactivity and clonus, possibly by preferentially acting on intrafusal over extrafusal muscle fibers. An uncommon but potentially fatal side-effect is hepatotoxicity; this is most common in women, in patients over age 35, and in patients receiving estrogen. Also, weakness may result if a high dose is required as extrafusal muscle fibers are increasingly affected. Rarely, this weakness has been associated with respiratory failure.

Several other medications have reported spasmolytic effects, including clonidine,[118] glycine, chlorpromazine with phenytoin,[30] vincristine, and tizanidine.[68] Epidural morphine and fentanyl suppress flexor and adductor spasms[158] and may prove to be clinically useful. However, none is as yet a widely accepted treatment for spasticity.

Surgery and Chemical Nerve Blocks

Chemical agents can be applied to individual nerves to reduce localized spasticity. Anesthetics can block nerve function for several hours. Phenol (2% to 10% in water, saline, or glycerol) or ethyl alcohol can block spasticity for 6 to 12 months or longer.[49, 168] These neurolytic agents are usually applied to distal motor nerve branches to produce a "motor-point" block or intramuscular phenol neurolysis. Some have performed neurolytic blocks of cutaneous nerves to relieve flexor spasms.[37] If major nerve trunks are injected, containing a significant number of cutaneous nerve fibers, then there is a 10% to 30% risk of the development of painful paresthesias.[16, 82, 132] Some practitioners accept this risk, noting that paresthesias usually disappear gradually over weeks to months, or they can be abolished with repeated phenol injections. The nerves or motor-points are localized percutaneously by electrical stimulation with a hypodermic needle cathode, Teflon-coated except at the tip, through which the neurolytic agent can be injected. A large surface anode is placed near the cathodal needle. Current density is highest at the needle tip. Thus, the motor nerves can be localized at the site where the least current is required to elicit a muscle contraction. Occasionally, an open procedure is performed and phenol is injected intraneurally.[17]

Those manifestations of spasticity that are most amenable to phenol motor-point blocks are clonus and velocity-sensitive tone. Non-velocity-sensitive tone, flexor spasms, and voluntary muscle contractions seem to be less affected by phenol motor-point blocks. This selective action on some aspects of spasticity with relative sparing of voluntary motor control, and ability to titrate the effect during the procedure, make motor-point blocks particularly useful in rehabilitation. Voluntary contractions may also increase in strength following motor-point blocks of antagonists, presumably by eliminating exaggerated reciprocal inhibition.[169] However, those manifestations of spasticity that are least effectively blocked, such as severe flexor spasms, are often most incapacitating. The reason for the selective block of phasic stretch reflexes with sparing of voluntary motor control is not clear. A selective block of γ-efferents has been proposed, but histologic studies in animals have failed to demonstrate selective degeneration of smallest diameter axons.[24, 121]

The most commonly performed motor-point blocks are to triceps surae, tibialis posterior, hamstring, and finger and wrist flexor muscles.[54, 66, 83] Blocks of the obturator (Fig. 22-10), tibial, musculocutaneous, and paravertebral lumbar spinal nerves have been used to relieve hip adductor, ankle plantarflexor, elbow flexor, and hip flexor spasticity.[5, 16, 105, 114, 132]

Intramuscular nonselective infiltration with 45% to 50% ethanol is also of reported benefit.[27, 124, 162] A large area of muscle is infiltrated at multiple sites without attempts to identify the intramuscular motor points or motor nerves. Although this procedure is less painful and time consuming, its efficacy as compared with phenol blocks is not known.

Phenol or alcohol has also been injected epidurally or intrathecally (i.e., subarachnoid) for severe spasticity in the lower extremities, but in those with incomplete UMN lesions, loss of voluntary movement, bowel and bladder control, and sexual function and subsequent muscle atrophy are risks.[25, 81, 119, 146, 160]

Studies suggest that skin desensitization with a topical anesthetic will reduce hypertonus[141] and decrease clonus amplitude.[111] The clinical usefulness of these modalities remains to be explored.

Various peripheral orthopedic procedures are used for spasticity. These can be undertaken for several reasons: (1) to improve function, (2) to prevent or relieve deformity (Fig. 22-11), and/or (3) for cosmesis. The reason(s) need to be clear to the patient. Procedures include section and lengthening or transfer of tendons of involved muscles. Such procedures have been used most successfully in cerebral palsy to improve borderline ambulation.[47, 51, 143] Hamstring tendon section or transfer of insertion has been used for knee flexion contractures.[136] Achilles tendon section or lengthening for equinus deformities, and tibialis posterior tendon section or transfer for varus deformities of the foot have been common procedures in cerebral palsy. Adductor tendon section, with or without obturator neurectomy, may relieve hip adductor spasms. Iliopsoas tendon or muscle

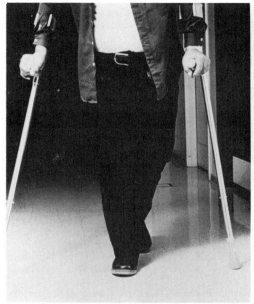
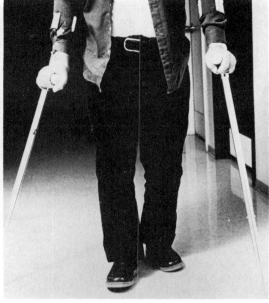

A   **B**

Figure 22-10. Obturator nerve blocks. Patient with spastic quadriparesis secondary to cervical stenosis is shown (*A*) before and (*B*) after phenol block of the obturator nerves bilaterally. Before the block, velocity-sensitive hypertonus and hyperactive tendon jerks were manifest in hip adductor muscles bilaterally, as well as scissoring (*A*) of the lower extremities in adduction during ambulation. Post block, the scissoring, tendon jerks, and hypertonus were abolished (*B*), although some voluntary contraction was preserved. The patient had a wider, more stable stance post block, and this beneficial effect was still present 6 months later.

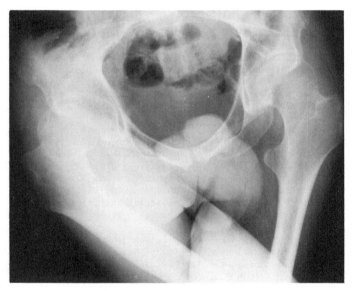

Figure 22-11. Hip flexor/adductor spasms with subluxation. Right hip subluxation due to severe hip flexion and adduction spasms in a patient with motor-incomplete (Frankel grade C) thoracic spinal cord injury.

section has been used for flexor spasms.[1] Subtalar fusion or triple arthrodesis may improve standing balance and gait in the presence of spasticity.[51] When gait is borderline, careful preoperative analysis of gait is necessary, ideally via multichannel dynamic EMG recordings in a gait analysis laboratory, to avoid compromising the current function of the child with cerebral palsy.[159] Early postoperative mobilization is essential to maximize benefits from the operative procedure. These selective procedures reportedly bring about a more generalized reduction of spasticity since the reflexogenic spread of spasticity is decreased. Tenotomies or tendon-lengthening procedures may, however, be followed by a recurrence of the original deformity (*e.g.,* equinus) because of muscle adaptation in which the number of

sarcomeres in the muscle decreases,[163] or the alternate deformity (*e.g.,* calcaneus) may develop.

Tendon lengthening, tendon transfers, and selected joint fusions can also be useful in the upper extremity in the presence of spasticity.[115] Often anesthetic nerve blocks are useful in helping to assess the potential benefit of tendon transfer procedures.

Surgical approaches to spasticity include a variety of operations on the nervous system. Peripheral neurectomy abolishes all muscle tone but is not selective in that any voluntary activity is abolished as well.[47] It is also associated with profound muscular atrophy and with sensory loss. Section of the obturator nerve to relieve hip adductor spasms is the most common application of this procedure. Selective peripheral neurectomies have been performed using microsurgical techniques and intraoperative electrical stimulation.[150] This allows selective section of most but not all nerve fibers to a muscle, thus preserving some voluntary muscle activity and preventing atrophy; cutaneous sensory branches of the nerve are preserved.

Surgery of the CNS has also been used to relieve spasticity. Direct section of the spinal cord in a longitudinal plane, dividing it into anterior and posterior halves from T12 to L5, is one of the most successful approaches. Such a myelotomy divides reflex arcs of the lumbosacral enlargement but may preserve some long-tract motor control and some bladder, bowel, and sexual function.[35, 92, 116] However, for reasons not completely understood, many have a recurrence of spasticity several months after this procedure.

Another commonly used neurosurgical procedure for spasticity is rhizotomy.[9, 53, 120] Section of the posterior roots is easier to perform than section of the anterior roots and does not result in a profound denervation atrophy of muscle that can predispose to pressure sores. Posterior rhizotomy disrupts spinal reflex arcs but will not abolish hypertonus mediated by suprasegmental pathways. The disadvantages of posterior rhizotomy are the sensory loss and associated ataxia and the frequent recurrence of spasticity. Open rhizotomy at multiple levels requires a long laminectomy, which may predispose to spine instability. Percutaneous radiofrequency rhizotomies have been performed with good success, thus avoiding laminectomy,[71, 80] but the long-term results are still to be determined. Selective posterior rhizotomy of the lateral dorsal root entry zone has reduced spasticity and pain in the upper extremities of hemiplegic patients while sparing sensation.[151]

Cordotomy, cordectomy, and cauda equina transection have been performed in extreme cases of spasticity, when other less radical procedures have been unsuccessful.[37, 152] Such procedures are not appropriate when useful voluntary control is preserved or when motor recovery is a possibility. When α-motoneurons or their axons are destroyed, profound muscle atrophy will result with some increased risk of pressure sores over bony prominences.

Epidural electrical stimulation over the dorsal columns has reportedly decreased spasticity in patients with spinal cord injury, multiple sclerosis, and spastic hemiplegia,[78, 117, 138, 149] with a carryover effect reported for hours to days in some patients. More effective control of spasticity has been observed in patients with incomplete than complete spinal cord injuries.[46] However, Gottlieb and co-workers[57] failed to demonstrate objective evidence for a reduction of spasticity following epidural electrical stimulation. Cerebellar stimulation has also reportedly reduced hypertonus in some patients with cerebral palsy.[32, 38, 58, 127] Functional gains are not universal and have not been well-described for CNS stimulators. Stereotactic thalamic and dentate lesions are also performed to control dystonia of cerebral origin.

A large array of physical, pharmaceutical, and surgical techniques are thus available for addressing the various manifestations of spasticity. The selection of the most appropriate method or methods for each patient remains the challenge for the clinician.

REFERENCES

1. Anderson JT, Comfort TH, Strand PJ, Winter RB: Coordinated care for cerebral palsy. Minn Med 61:161–164, 1978
2. Angel RW, Hoffmann WW: The H reflex in normal, spastic and rigid subjects. Arch Neurol 8:591–596, 1963
3. Aoki M, Mori S, Fujimori B: Exaggeration of knee-jerk following spinal hemisection in monkeys. Brain Res 107:471–485, 1976
4. Ashby P, Verrier M, Lightfoot E: Segmental reflex pathways in spinal shock and spinal spasticity in man. J Neurol Neurosurg Psychiatry 37:1352–1360, 1974
5. Awad EA: Phenol block for control of hip flexor and adductor spasticity. Arch Phys Med Rehabil 53:554–557, 1972
6. Bajd T, Gregoric M, Vodovnik L, Benko H: Electrical stimulation in treating spasticity resulting from spinal cord injury. Arch Phys Med Rehabil 66:515–517, 1985
7. Bajd T, Vodovnik L: Pendulum testing of spasticity. J Biomed Eng 6:9–16, 1984
8. Barnes CD, Joynt RJ, Schottelius BA: Motoneuron resting potentials in spinal shock. Am J Physiol 203:1113–1116, 1961
9. Barolat-Romana G, Davis R: Neurophysiological mechanisms in abnormal reflex activities in cerebral palsy and spinal spasticity. J Neurol Neurosurg Psychiatry 43:333–342, 1980
10. Basmajian JV, Kukulka CG, Narayan MG et al: Biofeedback treatment of footdrop after stroke compared with standard rehabilitation technique: Effects on voluntary control and strength. Arch Phys Med Rehabil 56:231–236, 1975
11. Bathien N, Bourdarias H: Lower limb cutaneous reflexes in hemiplegia. Brain 95:447–456, 1972
12. Berardelli A, Hallett M: Shortening reaction of human tibialis anterior. Neurology 34:242–245, 1984
13. Berger W, Quintern J, Dietz V: Pathophysiology of gait in children with cerebral palsy. Electroencephalogr Clin Neurophysiol 53:538–548, 1982
14. Bishop B: Spasticity: Its physiology and management. Phys Ther 57:371–401, 1977
15. Bobath K: A Neurophysiological Basis for the Treatment of Cerebral Palsy. Philadelphia, JB Lippincott, 1980
16. Brattstrom M, Moritz U, Svantesson G: Electromyographic studies of peripheral nerve block with phenol. Scand J Rehabil Med 2:17–22, 1970
17. Braun RM, Hoffer MM, Mooney V et al: Phenol nerve block in the treatment of acquired spastic hemiplegia in the upper limb. J Bone Joint Surg 55:580–585, 1973
18. Brodal A: Neurological Anatomy, 2nd ed. New York, Oxford University Press, 1969
19. Brooks VB: The Neural Basis of Motor Control, pp 151–159. New York, Oxford University Press, 1986
20. Brown DM, DeBacher GA, Basmajian JV: Feedback goniometers for hand rehabilitation. Am J Occup Ther 339:458–463, 1979
21. Burke D: Critical examination of the case for or against fusimotor involvement in disorders of muscle tone. In Desmedt JE (ed): Motor Control Mechanisms in Health and Disease. New York, Raven Press, 1983
22. Burke D, Gillies JD, Lance JW: The quadriceps stretch reflex in human spasticity. J Neurol Neurosurg Psychiatry 33:216–223, 1970
23. Burke D, Gillies JD, Lance JW: Hamstrings stretch reflex in human spasticity. J Neurol Neurosurg Psychiatry 34:231–235, 1971
24. Burkel WE, McPhee M: Effect of phenol injection into peripheral nerve of rat: Electron microscope studies. Arch Phys Med Rehabil 51:391–397, 1970
25. Cain HD: Subarachnoid phenol block in the treatment of pain and spasticity. Paraplegia 3:75–76; 152–160, 1965
26. Cannon WB, Haimovici H: The sensitization of motoneurons by partial "denervation." Am J Physiol 126:731–740, 1939
27. Carpenter EB, Seitz DG: Intramuscular alcohol as an aid in management of spastic cerebral palsy. Dev Med Child Neurol 22:497–501, 1980
28. Chapman CE, Wiesendanger M: The physiological and anatomical basis of spasticity: A review. Physiother Canada 34:125–136, 1982
29. Chyatte SB, Birdsong JH, Bergman BA: The effects of dantrolene sodium on spasticity and motor performance in hemiplegia. South Med J 64:180–185, 1971
30. Cohan SL, Raines A, Panagakos J, Armitage P: Phenytoin and chlorpromazine in the treatment of spasticity. Arch Neurol 37:360–364, 1980
31. Conrad B, Aschoff JC: Effects of voluntary isometric and isotonic activity on late transcortical reflex components in normal subjects and hemiparetic patients. Electroencephalogr Clin Neurophysiol 42:107–116, 1977
32. Cooper IS, Riklan M, Amin I et al: Chronic cerebellar stimulation in cerebral palsy. Neurology (Minneap) 26:744–753, 1976
33. Corcos DM, Gottlieb GL, Penn RD et al: Movement deficits caused by hyperexcitable stretch reflexes in spastic humans. Brain 109:1043–1058, 1986
34. Csongradi J, Bleck E, Ford WF: Gait electromyography in normal and spastic children with special reference to quadriceps femoris and hamstring muscles. Dev Med Child Neurol 21:738–748, 1979
35. Cusick JF, Larson SJ, Sances A: The effect of T-myelotomy on spasticity. Surg Neurol 6:289–292, 1976
36. Davis L: Decerebrate rigidity in man. Arch Neurol Psychiatry 13:569–579, 1925
37. Davis R: Spasticity following spinal cord injury. Clin Orthop 112:66–75, 1975
38. Davis R, Gray E, Ryan T, Schulman J: Bioengineering changes in spastic cerebral palsy groups following cerebellar stimulation. Appl Neurophysiol 48:111–116, 1985
39. DeLisa J, Little JW, Managing spasticity. Am Fam Physician 26:117–122, 1982
40. Delwaide PJ: Electrophysiological analysis of the mode of action of muscle relaxants in spasticity. Ann Neurol 17:90–95, 1985
41. Denny-Brown D, quoted in Feldman RG et al (eds): Spasticity: Disordered Motor Control, p 182. Chicago, Year Book Medical Publishers, 1980
42. Dietz V, Berger W: Normal and impaired regulation of muscle stiffness in gait: A new hypothesis about muscle hypertonia. Exp Neurol 79:680–687, 1983
43. Dimitrijevic M, Nathan P: Studies of spasticity in man: V. Dishabituation of the flexion reflex in spinal man. Brain 94:349–368, 1968
44. Dimitrijevic M, Nathan P, Sherwood AM: Clonus: The role of central mechanisms. J Neurol Neurosurg Psychiatry 43:321–332, 1982

45. Dimitrijevic M, Sherwood A: Spasticity: Medical and surgical treatment. Neurology 30:19–27, 1980

46. Dimitrijevic MM, Dimitrijevic MR, Illis LS et al: Spinal cord stimulation for the control of spasticity in patients with chronic spinal cord injury: I. Clinical observations. Central Nerv System Trauma 3:129–144, 1986

47. Eggers GWN, Evans EB: Surgery in cerebral palsy. J Bone Joint Surg [Am] 45:1275–1305, 1963

48. Eisen A, Odusote K: Amplitude of the F-wave: A potential means of documenting spasticity. Neurology (Minneap) 29:1306–1309, 1979

49. Felsenthal G: Pharmacology of phenol in peripheral nerve blocks: A review. Arch Phys Med Rehabil 55:13–16, 1974

50. Fisher MA, Shahani BT, Young RR: Electrophysiologic analysis of the motor system after stroke: The flexor reflex. Arch Phys Med Rehabil 60:7–11, 1979

51. Fixsen JA: Surgical treatment of the lower limbs in cerebral palsy: A review. J R Soc Med 72:761–765, 1979

52. Foley J: The stiffness of spastic muscle. J Neurol Neurosurg Psychiatry 24:125–131, 1961

53. Fraioli B, Guidetti B: Posterior partial rootlet section in the treatment of spasticity. J Neurosurg 46:618–626, 1977

54. Garland DE, Lilling M, Keenan MA: Percutaneous phenol blocks to motor points of spastic forearm muscles in head-injured adults. Arch Phys Med Rehabil 65:243–245, 1984

55. Garnett R, Stephens JA: The reflex responses of single motor units in human first dorsal interosseous muscle following cutaneous afferent stimulation. J Physiol (Lond) 303:351–364, 1980

56. Gilman S, Lieberman JS, Marco LA: Spinal mechanisms underlying the effects of unilateral ablation of areas 4 and 6 in monkeys. Brain 97:49–64, 1974

57. Gottlieb GL, Myklebust BM, Stefoski D et al: Evaluation of cervical stimulation for chronic treatment of spasticity. Neurology 35:699–704, 1985

58. Grabow JD, Ebersold MJ, Albers JW: Cerebellar stimulation for the control of seizures. Mayo Clin Proc 49:759–774, 1974

59. Griffith ER: Spasticity. In Rosenthal M et al (eds): Rehabilitation of the Head-Injured Adult. Philadelphia, FA Davis, 1983

60. Grimby L: Pathological plantar responses: I. Flexor and extensor components in early and late reflex parts. II. Loss of significance of stimulus site. J Neurol Neurosurg Psychiatry 28:469–481, 1965

61. Guttmann L: Spinal Cord Injuries. Oxford, Blackwell, 1976

62. Hagbarth KE: Spinal withdrawal reflexes in the human lower limbs. J Neurol Neurosurg Psychiatry 23:222–227, 1960

63. Hagbarth KE, Eklund G: The muscle vibrator—a useful tool in neurological therapeutic work. Scand J Rehabil Med 1:26–34, 1969

64. Hagbarth KE, Wallin G, Lofstedt L et al: Muscle spindle activity in alternating tremor of parkinsonism and in clonus. J Neurol Neurosurg Psychiatry 38:636–641, 1975

65. Halpern D: Rehabilitation of children with brain damage. In Kottke FJ et al (eds): Krusen's Handbook of Physical Medicine and Rehabilitation, 3rd ed. Philadelphia, WB Saunders, 1982

66. Halpern D, Meelhuysen FE: Phenol motor point block in the management of muscular hypertonia. Arch Phys Med Rehabil 47:659–664, 1966

67. Hartviksen K: Ice therapy in spasticity. Acta Neurol Scand 38 (suppl 3):79–84, 1962

68. Hassan N, McLennan DL: Double blind comparison of DS103–282, baclofen and placebo for suppression of spasticity. J Neurol Neurosurg Psychiatry 43:1133–1136, 1980

69. Herman R: The myotactic reflex: Clinico-physiological aspects of spasticity and contracture. Brain 93:273–312, 1970

70. Herman R, Freedman W, Meeks SM: Physiological aspects of hemiplegic and paraplegic spasticity. In Desmedt JE (ed): New Developments in Electromyography and Clinical Neurophysiology, vol 3, pp 579–588. Basel, Karger, 1973

71. Herz DA, Parsons K, Pearl L: Percutaneous radiofrequency foraminal rhizotomies. Spine 8:729–732, 1983

72. Hewer RL: Multiple sclerosis: Management and rehabilitation. Int Rehabil Med 2:116–125, 1980

73. Hoffmann P: Über die Beziehungen der Sehnenreflexe zur willkürlichen Bewegung und zum Tonus. Z Biolog 68:351–370, 1918

74. Horstink MWI, Notermans SLM: Local sign in flexor reflexes. Acta Neurol Scand 60 (suppl 73):209, 1979

75. Houk JC, Henneman E: Responses of Golgi tendon organs to active contractions of the soleus muscle of the cat. J Neurophysiol 30:466–481, 1967

76. Hufschmidt H: Die Spastik: Theoretische Überlegungen zu einer neuen Therapie. Nervenarzt 39:2, 1968

77. Hunt CC, Perl ER: Spinal reflex mechanisms concerned with skeletal muscle. Physiol Rev 40:538–579, 1960

78. Illis LS, Sedgwick EM, Tallis RC: Spinal cord stimulation in multiple sclerosis. J Neurol Neurosurg Psychiatry 43:1–14, 1980

79. Jolesz FA, Xu C-T, Ruenzel PW, Henneman E: Flexor reflex control of the external sphincter of the urethra in paraplegia. Science 216:1243–1245, 1982

80. Kasdon DL, Lathi ES: A prospective study of radiofrequency rhizotomy in the treatment of posttraumatic spasticity. Neurosurgery 15:526–529, 1984

81. Kelley RE, Gautier-Smith PC: Intrathecal phenol in the treatment of reflex spasms and spasticity. Lancet 2:1102–1105, 1959

82. Khalili AA, Betts HB: Peripheral nerve block with phenol in the management of spasticity: Indications and complications. JAMA 200:1155–1157, 1967

83. Khalili AA, Harmel MH, Forster S et al: Management of spasticity by selective peripheral nerve block with dilute phenol solutions in clinical rehabilitation. Arch Phys Med Rehabil 45:513–519, 1964

84. Knutsson E: Assessment of motor function in spasticity. Triangle 21:13–20, 1982

85. Knutsson E: Analysis of gait and isokinetic movements for evaluation of antispastic drugs or physical therapies. In Desmedt JS (ed): Motor Control Mechanisms in Health and Disease. New York, Raven Press, 1983

86. Knutsson E, Lindblom U, Martensson A: Differences in effects in gamma and alpha spasticity induced by the GABA derivative baclofen (Lioresal). Brain 96:29–46, 1973

87. Knutsson E, Martensson A: Dynamic motor capacity in spastic paraparesis and its relation to prime mover dysfunction, spastic reflexes and antagonist co-activation. Scand J Rehabil Med 12:93–106, 1980

88. Knutsson E, Richards C: Different types of disturbed motor control in gait of hemiparetic patients. Brain 102:405–430, 1979

89. Koella WP: Baclofen: Its general pharmacology and neuropharmacology. In Feldman RG et al (eds): Spasticity: Disordered Motor Control, pp 383–396. Chicago, Year Book Medical Publishers, 1980

90. Kraft GH, Freal JE, Coryell JK: Disability, disease duration and rehabilitation service needs in multiple sclerosis: Patient perspectives. Arch Phys Med Rehabil 67:164–168, 1986

91. Kuhn R: Functional capacity of the isolated human spinal cord. Brain 73:1–51, 1950

92. Laitinen L, Singounas E: Longitudinal myelotomy in the treatment of spasticity of the legs. J Neurosurg 35:536–540, 1971

93. Lance JW: The control of muscle tone, reflexes and movement: Robert Wartenberg Lecture. Neurology 30:1303–1313, 1980

94. Lance JW, DeGail P, Neilson PD: Tonic and phasic spinal cord mechanisms in man. J Neurol Neurosurg Psychiatry 29:535–544, 1966

95. Landau WM: Spasticity: What is it? What is it not? In Feldman RG et al (eds): Spasticity: Disordered Motor Control, pp 17–24. Chicago, Year Book Medical Publishers, 1980

96. Lieberman JS: Physiological correlates of clinically observed changes in posture and tone following lesions of the central nervous system. Int Rehabil Med 4:195–199, 1982

97. Little JW: Serial recording of reflexes after feline spinal cord transection. Exp Neurol 93:510–521, 1986

98. Little JW, Halar EM: H-reflex changes following spinal cord injury. Arch Phys Med Rehabil 66:19–22, 1985

99. Lundberg A: Control of spinal mechanisms from the brain. In Tower DB (ed): The Nervous System, vol 1. New York, Raven Press, 1975

100. Malmsten J: Time course of segmental reflex changes after chronic spinal cord hemisection in the rat. Acta Physiol Scand 119:435–443, 1983

101. Matthews WB: Ratio of maximum H reflex to maximum M response as a measure of spasticity. J Neurol Neurosurg Psychiatry 29:201–204, 1966

102. McLellan DL: Co-contraction and stretch reflexes in spasticity dur-

ing treatment with baclofen. J Neurol Neurosurg Psychiatry 40:30–38, 1977

103. McLellan DL, Hassan NH: The use of electromyograms to assess impaired voluntary movement associated with increased muscle tone. Electroencephalogr Clin Neurophysiol (Suppl) 36:169–171, 1982

104. McLellan DL, Selwyn M, Cooper IS: Time course of clinical and physiological effects of stimulation of the cerebellar surface in patients with spasticity. J Neurol Neurosurg Psychiatry 41:150–160, 1978

105. Meelhuysen FE, Halpern D, Quast J: Treatment of flexor spasticity of hip by paravertebral lumbar spinal nerve block. Arch Phys Med Rehabil 49:717–722, 1968

106. Meinck HM, Benecke R, Kuster S, Conrad B: Cutaneomuscular (Flexor) reflex organization in normal man and in patients with motor disorders. In Desmedt JE (ed): Motor Control Mechanisms in Health and Disease, pp 787–796. New York, Raven Press, 1983

107. Meinck HM, Kuster S, Benecke R, Conrad B: The flexor reflex—influence of stimulus parameters on the reflex response. Electroencephalogr Clin Neurophysiol 61:287–298, 1985

108. Meltzer GE, Hunt RS, Landau WM: Fusimotor function: III: The spastic monkey. Arch Neurol 9:133–136, 1963

109. Merritt JL: Management of spasticity in spinal cord injury. Mayo Clin Proc 56:614–622, 1981

110. Michaelis LS: Spasticity in spinal cord injuries. In Vinken PJ, Bruyn GW (eds): Handbook of Clinical Neurology, Injuries of the Spine and Cord, vol 26, Part II, pp 477–487. New York, Elsevier, 1976

111. Mills WJ, Pozos RS: A decrease in clonus amplitude by topical anesthesia. Electroencephalogr Clin Neurophysiol 61:509–518, 1985

112. Mizrahi EM, Angel RW: Impairment of voluntary movement by spasticity. Ann Neurol 5:594–595, 1979

113. Molnar GE, Taft LT: Pediatric rehabilitation: I. Cerebral palsy and spinal cord injuries. Curr Probl Pediatr 7:1–55, 1977

114. Moritz U: Phenol block of peripheral nerves. Scand J Rehabil Med 5:160–163, 1973

115. Mowery CA, Gelberman RH, Rhoades CE: Upper extremity tendon transfers in cerebral palsy: Electromyographic and functional analysis. J Pediatr Orthop 5:69–72, 1985

116. Moyes PD: Longitudinal myelotomy for spasticity. J Neurosurg 31:615–619, 1969

117. Nakamura S, Tsubokawa T: Evaluation of spinal cord stimulation for postapoplectic spastic hemiplegia. Neurosurg 17:253–259, 1985

118. Nance PW, Shears AH, Nance DM: Clonidine in spinal cord injury. Can Med Assoc J 133:41–42, 1985

119. Nathan PW: Intrathecal phenol to relieve spasticity in paraplegia. Lancet 2:1099–1102, 1959

120. Nathan PW, Sears TA: Effects of posterior root section on the activity of some muscles in man. J Neurol Neurosurg Psychiatry 23:10–22, 1960

121. Nathan PW, Sears TA, Smith MC: Effects of phenol solutions on the nerve roots of the cat: An electrophysiological and histological study. J Neurol Sci 2:7–29, 1965

122. Nicholas J: Physiotherapy for multiple sclerosis. Physiotherapy 68:144–146, 1982

123. Odeen I: Reduction of muscular hypertonus by long-term muscle stretch. Scand J Rehabil Med 13:93–99, 1981

124. O'Hanlan JT, Galford HR, Bosley J: The use of 45% Alcohol to control spasticity. Va Med Monthly 96:429–436, 1969

125. Pederson E, Klemar B, Torring J: Counting of flexor spasms. Acta Neurol Scand 60:164–169, 1979

126. Pederson E, Petersen T, Schroder HD: Relation between flexor spasms, uninhibited detrusor contractions, and anal sphincter activity. J Neurol Neurosurg Psychiatry 49:273–277, 1986

127. Penn RD, Gottlieb GL, Agarwal GC: Cerebellar stimulation in man: Quantitative changes in spasticity. J Neurosurg 48:779–786, 1978

128. Penn RD, Kroin JS: Continuous intrathecal baclofen for severe spasticity. Lancet 2:125–126, 1985

129. Perry J, Giovan P, Harris LJ, et al: The determinants of muscle action in the hemiparetic lower extremity (and their effect on the examination procedure). Clin Orthop 131:71–89, 1978

130. Perry J, Gronley JK, Lunsford T: Rocker shoe as walking aid in multiple sclerosis. Arch Phys Med Rehabil 62:59–65, 1981

131. Perry J, Hoffer MM: Pre-operative and post-operative dynamic electromyography as an aid in planning tendon transfers in children with cerebral palsy. J Bone Joint Surg [Am] 59:531–537, 1977

132. Petrillo CR, Chu DS, Davis SW: Phenol block of the tibial nerve in the hemiplegic patient. Orthopedics 3:871–874, 1980

133. Pinder RM, Brogden RN, Speight TM, Avery GS: Dantrolene sodium: A review of its pharmacological properties and therapeutic efficacy in spasticity. Drugs 13:3–23, 1977

134. Plum F, Posner JB: The Diagnosis of Stupor and Coma, 3rd ed, p 68. Philadelphia, FA Davis, 1982

135. Rack PMH, Ross HF, Thilmann AF: The ankle stretch reflexes in normal and spastic subjects: The response to sinusoidal movement. Brain 107:637–654, 1984

136. Ray RL, Ehrlich MG: Lateral hamstring transfer and gait movement in the cerebral palsy patient. J Bone Joint Surg [Am] 61:719–723, 1979

137. Read DJ, Matthews WB, Higson RH: The effect of spinal cord stimulation on function in patients with multiple sclerosis. Brain 103:803–833, 1980

138. Richardson RR, Cerullo LJ, McCone DG et al: Percutaneous epidural neurostimulation in modulation of paraplegic spasticity: Six case reports. Acta Neurochir 49:235–243, 1979

139. Roussan M, Terrence C, Fromm G: Baclofen versus diazepam for the treatment of spasticity and long-term follow-up of baclofen therapy. Pharmatherapeutica 4:278–284, 1985

140. Rymer WZ, Houk JC, Crago PE: Mechanisms of the clasp-knife reflex studied in an animal model. Exp Brain Res 37:93–113, 1979

141. Sabbahi MA, DeLuca CJ, Powers WR: Topical anesthesia: A possible treatment method for spasticity. Arch Phys Med Rehabil 62:310–314, 1981

142. Sahrmann SA, Norton BJ, Bomze HA, Eliasson SG: Influence of the site of the lesion and muscle length on spasticity in man. Phys Therapy 54:1290–1296, 1974

143. Samilson RL, Hoffer MM: Problems and complications in orthopaedic management of cerebral palsy. In Samilson RL (ed): Orthopaedic Apects of Cerebral Palsy, Clinics in Developmental Medicine, No 52/53, p 258. Philadelphia, JB Lippincott, 1975

144. Shahani BT, Young RR: The flexor reflex in spasticity. In Feldman RG (ed): Spasticity: Disordered Motor Control, pp 287–297. Chicago, Yearbook Medical Publishers, 1980

145. Sharpless SK: Supersensitivity-like phenomena in the central nervous system. Fed Proc 34:1990–1997, 1975

146. Shelden CH, Bors E: Subarachnoid alcohol block in paraplegia: Its beneficial effect on mass reflexes and bladder dysfunction. J Neurosurg 5:385–391, 1948

147. Sherrington CS: On reciprocal innervation of antagonistic muscles. Proc R Soc Lond 80:552–578, 1908

148. Shindo N: Compensated monophasic low impedance electric treatment used for the reduction of spasticity in spinal patients. Paraplegia (in press); presented at International Medical Society of Paraplegia, Edinburgh, Scotland, September 1985

149. Siegfried J, Krainick JU, Haas H et al: Electrical spinal cord stimulation for spastic movement disorders. Appl Neurophysiol 41:134–141, 1978

150. Sindou M, Abdennebi B, Sharkey P: Microsurgical selective procedures in peripheral nerves and the posterior root-spinal cord junction for spasticity. Appl Neurophysiol 48:97–104, 1985

151. Sindou M, Mifsud JJ, Boisson D, Goutelle A: Selective posterior rhizotomy in the dorsal root entry zone for treatment of hyperspasticity and pain in the hemiplegic upper limb. Neurosurgery 18:587–595, 1986

152. Smolik EA, Nash FP, Machek O: Spinal cordectomy in the management of spastic paraplegia. Am Surg 26:639–645, 1960

153. Snook JH: Spasticity reduction splint. Am J Occup Ther 33:648–651, 1979

154. Stavraky GW: Supersensitivity Following Lesions of the Nervous System. Toronto, University of Toronto Press, 1961

155. Stejskal L: Postural reflexes in man. Am J Phys Med 58:1–25, 1979

156. Stichbury JC: Assessment of disability following severe head injury. Physiotherapy 61:268–272, 1975

157. Strassburg HM, Oepen G, Thoden U: The late facilitation in H-reflex recovery cycles in different pyramidal lesions. Arch Psychiat Nervenkr 228:197–204, 1980

158. Struppler A, Ochs G, Burgmayer B, Pfeiffer HG: The therapeutic use of epidural opioids in flexor reflex spasm. Electroencephalogr Clin Neurophysiol 56:5178, 1983

159. Sutherland DH: Gait analysis in cerebral palsy. Dev Med Child Neurol 20:807–813, 1978

160. Swerdlow M: Intrathecal neurolysis. Anaesthesia 33:733–740, 1978

161. Szumski AJ, Burg D, Struppler A, Velho F: Activity of muscle spindles during muscle twitch and clonus in normal and spastic human subjects. Electroencephalogr Clin Neurophysiol 37:589–597, 1974

162. Tardieu G, Tardieu C, Hariga J: Selective partial denervation by alcohol injections and their results in spasticity. Reconstr Surg Traumat 13:18–36, 1972

163. Tardieu G, Thuilleux G, Tardieu C, Huet de la Tour E: Long-term effects of surgical elongation of the tendon calcaneus in the normal cat. Dev Med Child Neurol 21:83–94, 1979

164. Teasdall RD, Van Den Ende H: The crossed adductor reflex in humans: An EMG study. Can J Neurol Sci 8:81–85, 1981

165. Torring J, Pedersen E, Klemar B: Standardisation of the electrical elicitation of the human flexor reflex. J Neurol Neurosurg Psychiatry 44:129–132, 1981

166. Twitchell T: The restoration of motor function following hemiplegia in man. Brain 74:443–480, 1951

167. Walshe FMR: A case of complete decerebrate rigidity in man. Lancet 2:644–647, 1923

168. Wood KM: The use of phenol as a neurolytic agent: A review. Pain 5:205–229, 1978

169. Yanagisawa N, Tanaka R, Ito Z: Reciprocal Ia inhibition in spastic hemiplegia of man. Brain 99:555–574, 1976

170. Young RR, Shahani BT: Spasticity in spinal cord injured patients. In Bloch RF, Basbaum M (eds): Management of Spinal Cord Injuries. Baltimore, Williams & Wilkins, 1986

171. Zander OP, Diamantopoulos E: Excitability of spinal motor neurons in normal subjects and patients with spasticity, Parkinsonian rigidity, and cerebellar hypotonia. J Neurol Neurosurg Psychiatry 30:325–331, 1967

23

Contracture and Other Deleterious Effects of Immobility

Eugen M. Halar

Kathleen R. Bell

The deleterious effects of prolonged bed rest and immobility have been increasingly recognized during the past four decades. Although bed rest and immobilization have been widely used for over a century in the management of trauma and acute illnesses, the physiological effects have never been fully understood and explained.[13, 78, 100] It has been generally assumed that inactivity fosters healing of the affected part of the body. However, it has not always been appreciated that this same physical inactivity can be harmful to the healthy parts of the body. For example, the immobilization of long bones with a cast has a beneficial effect on bone healing following fractures. However, adverse effects of prolonged immobilization such as joint contracture and muscle and bone atrophy of the healthy parts of the limb may result. Clinical studies on enforced bed rest in normal subjects and on astronauts in space have revealed that, indeed, the adverse effects of immobility may override its therapeutic effects, becoming more problematic than the primary disease (Fig. 23-1).[23, 26, 32, 68, 69, 76, 78] It is therefore, important to anticipate the complications that may result from prolonged immobility. Many are easily prevented and treated if recognized in time, impacting not only on the expense and complexity of medical treatment but also on the functional outcome.[94]

Although these adverse effects of immobility do not spare any age or gender, chronically sick, aged, and disabled populations are particularly susceptible. For instance, a healthy subject placed on total bed rest for one week will develop tightness in the musculature of the back and legs, especially those muscles that are shortened with hip and knee flexion. In similar circumstances, a patient with motor neuron disease and its accompanying limb weakness and spasticity can be expected to develop the same musculoskeletal complications but at a much accelerated rate. The degree to which each of these patients is affected is quite different. The healthy subject may have some degree of stiffness and discomfort; the neurologically impaired subject will likely lose significant independent functions. Therefore, the prevention of such complications should be one of the basic principles of any rehabilitation management plan.

The effects of prolonged bed rest are never confined to only one body system (Fig. 23-2). Immobilization reduces the functional reserve of the musculoskeletal system, resulting in weakness, atrophy, and poor endurance. This, in turn, will place increased demands on a cardiovascular system that has also been negatively impacted as evidenced by reduced cardiac work ca-

pacity and postural hypotension. All of these body system dysfunctions may be grouped together under the general term *deconditioning*. Deconditioning, therefore, may be defined as a reduced functional capacity of all body systems and may be considered a separate disease entity from the original process that led to a curtailment of normal activity.

In this chapter the widespread effects of immobility on the body are described (Table 23-1) and therapeutic and prophylactic approaches to counteract these complications are reviewed.

MUSCULOSKELETAL SYSTEM

The adverse effects of prolonged bed rest and inactivity are most frequently encountered in the musculoskeletal system.[2, 5, 9] Because these complications may not initially cause functional limitations, they are frequently neglected. For the desperately ill patient or multiple trauma victim, considerations such as preserving functional range of motion (ROM) may seem trivial. However, these simple factors are responsible for prolonging hospital stays, increasing utilization of health care systems, and prolonging dependency for mobility and activities of daily living.[84, 117]

Joint Contractures

A general definition of a contracture is the lack of full active or passive ROM due to joint, muscle, or soft tissue limitations. A variety of conditions may initiate limited joint movement. Joint pain, paralysis, or primary muscle damage may all begin the process. However, the single most frequent factor contributing to the occurrence of fixed contractures is the absence of mobility at a joint, that is, the lack of joint mobilization throughout the full allowable range. Any joint *immobilized in a faulty position,* for whatever reason, will develop a contracture. It will be apparent to the astute clinician that the presence of joint contractures will reduce mobility still further in the inactive person, resulting in even higher risks for progressive ROM limitation.

Contractures that are caused by anatomical changes in the joints and muscles can be classified into three groups (Table 23-2): arthrogenic, soft tissue, and myogenic. It is important to remember, however, that all tissues surrounding a joint may

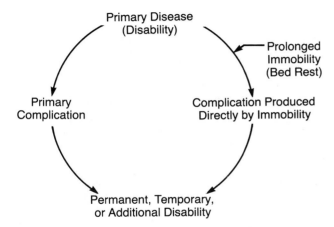

Figure 23-1. Prolonged bed rest and immobility will aggravate primary disease or its complications and will add to the incomplete or total disability.

become secondarily involved in joint contracture regardless of the initiating disease process. All fixed contractures have in common a rearrangement or proliferation of collagen fibers.

Mechanical Properties and Synthesis of Collagen Tissue

Following trauma, inflammation, or degeneration of the muscle or soft tissue, undifferentiated mesenchymal cells start to migrate to the site of injury and gradually change into mature fibroblasts (Fig. 23-3). The fibroblasts tend to travel along fibrin layers, multiply, and develop collagen-producing organelles.[11]

Two main types of polypeptide chains, α_1 and α_2, are produced in the endoplasmic reticulum. Combinations of three α chains, or two α_1 and an α_2 polypeptide in a helix, are connected by special hydrogen bonds or by bonds formed by modification of certain amino acids. The triple helical structures and their intracellular cross-links are responsible for the mechanical properties of collagen. Outside of the fibroblast in the ground substance, the procollagen molecules begin to attach to each other through new intermolecular cross-links. The newly formed fibrils bind among themselves, creating thicker and longer collagen fibers.

The new collagen fibers are usually randomly arranged in a loose connective tissue. The metabolism of collagen is characterized by continuous synthesis and breakdown. If synthesis exceeds breakdown, an excessive fibrosis will result. Thus, the mechanical properties of the newly formed collagen are the

Table 23-1
Deleterious Effects of Prolonged Inactivity and Bed Rest on Body System

System	*Effect*
Musculoskeletal system	Contractures Muscle weakness Disuse atrophy Immobilization osteoporosis
Cardiovascular system	Orthostatic hypotension Reduction of blood plasma volume Reduction of cardiovascular performance Thromboembolic phenoma Cardiovascular deconditioning
Integumentary system	Skin atrophy Pressure sores
Respiratory system	Increased mechanical resistance to breathing Reduced cough and bronchial ciliary activity Reduced tidal and minute volume Hypostatic pneumonia Pulmonary embolism
Genitourinary system	Urinary stasis Urinary stones Urinary tract infections Decreased initiation and emptying of bladder
Disturbance of mineral metabolic balance	Negative nitrogen balance Negative calcium balance Negative sulfur and phosphorus balance Other minerals (magnesium, potassium, sodium)
Hormonal disturbances	Decreased androgen and spermatogenesis Reduced insulin binding sites Growth hormone alteration to glucose Increased parathyroid hormone production
Gastrointestinal system	Constipation Loss of appetite
Nervous system	Sensory deprivation Confusion and disorientation Anxiety and depression Decrease in intellectual capacity Impaired balance and coordination

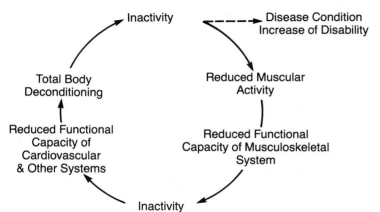

Figure 23-2. The influence of inactivity, immobility, and prolonged bed rest on total body functioning.

Table 23-2
Anatomical Classification of Contractures

I. Arthrogenic Contracture
  A. Cartilage damage, joint incongruency
    (congenital deformities, inflammation, trauma, degenerative joint disease, infection)
  B. Synovial proliferation, effusion
    (inflammation, pannus formation, capsular distention)
  C. Capsular fibrosis
    (trauma, inflammation, immobilization)

II. Soft Tissue Contracture
  A. Soft tissue around the joint
    (trauma, inflammation, immobilization)
  B. Skin, subcutaneous tissue
    (trauma, burns, infection, systemic sclerosis)
  C. Tendon and ligaments
    (tendonitis, bursitis, ligamentous tear)

III. Myogenic Contractures
  A. Intrinsic, structural
    1. Trauma (bleeding, edema, immobilization)
    2. Inflammation (myositis, polymyositis)
    3. Degenerative changes (muscular dystrophy)
    4. Ischemic (diabetes, peripheral vascular disease, immobility)
  B. Extrinsic
    1. Spasticity (strokes, multiple sclerosis, spinal cord injuries upper motor neuron disease, muscle imbalance)
    2. Flaccid paralysis (faulty position, muscle imbalance)
    3. Mechanical (faulty position in bed or chair, immoblization in foreshortened position)
  C. Mixed contracture

result of the amount of collagen produced, its intracellular and intercellular bonds, and the orientation of the collagen fibers in the tissue.

Trauma with bleeding into the soft tissue and muscle, inflammation, degeneration, or ischemia, all could trigger an increased synthesis of collagen. It appears that, owing to immobilization, the collagen fibers become tightly packed, perhaps because of new cross-link formation between collagen molecules (Table 23-3). In some genetically determined diseases of collagen metabolism (*e.g.,* Ehler-Danlos disease), the actual production of collagen and formation of cross-links among the fibers is diminished. On the other hand, collagen degradation is increased in some conditions. In rheumatoid arthritis, for instance, the enzyme collagenase is released from polymorphonuclear leukocytes, causing the direct cleavage and destruction of the collagen in joint cartilage. The balance between synthesis and degradation is also disturbed by physical factors such as prolonged immobilization and inactivity.[40]

The muscle fiber itself contributes very little to the development of contracture. In advanced contractures, the muscle membrane, containing type IV collagen and myofibrils, becomes significantly shortened and contributes to the late stages of myogenic contracture development. Spector and co-workers[98, 99] have shown that the position in which a joint is immobilized also has a significant influence on the number of sarcomeres present in the muscle. Immobilization in a shortened position may cause muscle fibers to lose 40% of their sarcomeres. Hence, the joint should be immobilized in a neutral position to keep opposing muscles at equal length and tension.[99, 100, 103, 104]

Arthrogenic Contracture

Contracture may result directly from pathology involving parts of the joint itself, such as cartilage, synovium, or the joint capsule. Usually, tissue degeneration, acute trauma, inflammation, or infection is present as a precipitating factor. The cartilage loss seen in degenerative joint disease of the elderly and its associated pain may cause involuntary splinting of the joint, leading to a decrease in ROM. Synovial proliferation and fibrosis with associated edema and pain is seen in a variety of the rheumatoid arthropathies and may also result in contracture. That pain and not necessarily the loss of cartilage or synovial fibrosis is implicated in the development of contracture is illustrated by those patients with absent pain and proprioception who sustain severe destruction of cartilage and joint surfaces (Charcot joint) yet have relatively well-preserved ROM or even hypermobility of the involved joint.[34, 36, 37, 40, 89]

The joint capsule can become involved on the basis of inflammatory changes or from collagen fiber shortening secondary to inadequate joint positioning. Initially, collagen fiber shortening occurs, followed by connective tissue proliferation. In most cases, ROM is compromised in all directions of movement, significantly reducing joint function. Certain joints are more commonly involved than others, particularly the shoulder. Initiating factors may include bicipital tendonitis, subdeltoid bursitis, rotator cuff damage, or inflammation. Progression of capsular contractures will result in end-stage frozen shoulder. The posterior knee capsule is another common area for capsular shortening as a consequence of prolonged flexion (*e.g.,* in wheelchair-bound patients).

Soft Tissue Contracture

Soft tissue contracture is also due to collagen fiber shortening and proliferation. However, in contrast to capsular tightness, soft tissue shortening will usually limit movement in only one plane or axis. Burned skin is particularly susceptible to contracture during the healing process; burns across any joint must be positioned in such a way as to oppose this shortening effect.

Topical steroid and vitamin E applications have failed to reduce soft tissue contracture or postoperative scar formation following reconstructive joint surgeries. Vigorous active and passive ROM exercises, placement of the joint in a functional position, and the use of compressive garments are recommended to prevent the development of contracture in burn patients.

Myogenic Contracture

Myogenic contracture is shortening of the muscle itself owing to intrinsic or extrinsic causes. *Intrinsic* changes are structural and may be associated with inflammatory, degenerative, or traumatic processes. *Extrinsic* muscle contracture is secondary, resulting from neurological abnormalities or mechanical factors. The diagnosis of muscle contracture should be made only after careful physical examination, which should include an evaluation of active and passive ROM. An erroneous conclusion of fixed contracture can be made by observing limitation of active ROM only; this could just as likely be due to muscle weakness alone.

A variety of conditions may be responsible for the muscle tissue alterations seen with intrinsic contractures. Inflammation, ischemia, trauma, and associated hemorrhage have all resulted in the restructuring of muscle tissue components. The muscular dystrophies are primary examples of a degenerative process. The most significant histological changes are those of muscle fiber loss, abnormal residual muscle fibers, segmental necrosis

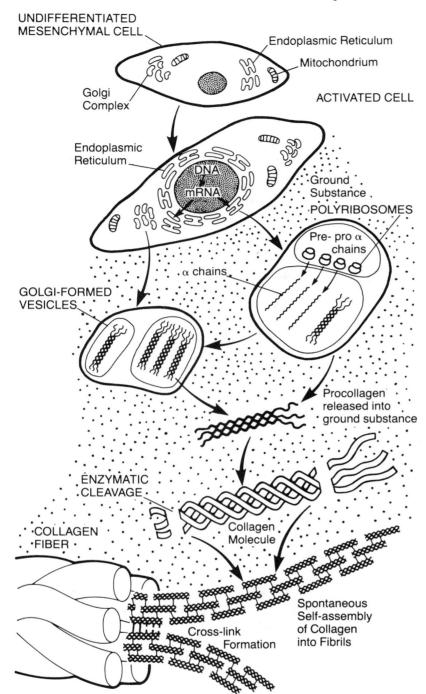

Figure 23-3. Collagen synthesis. Procollagen released by a fibroblast into the extracellular space undergoes enzymatic cleavage of its polar ends by proteases found in ground substance. After removal of the free helical ends, the collagen molecule is formed, which then aggregates into collagen fibrils. The collagen molecule overlaps with its neighbor by a fourth of its length, allowing the development of cross-links between the adjacent molecules. The strength of collagen fiber is, in part, determined by the presence of these intermolecular cross-links. Certain drugs and inherited diseases destroy these cross-links, producing characteristic pathological conditions.

of muscle fibers, and increased amounts of lipocytes and fibrosis. The replacement of functioning muscle fibers with collagen and fatty tissue in concert with chronically shortened positioning results in contracture. Fibrosis is also implicated as a sequela of direct muscle trauma. After hemorrhage into a muscle, fibrin deposition occurs. Within 2 to 3 days, the fibrin fibers are replaced by reticular fibers, which then assemble into a loose connective tissue network. If the muscle is kept immobilized, this rapidly progresses into a dense network that is resistant to stretching. The inflammatory myopathies are a broad category of disease in which muscle fibers are replaced by increasing amounts of collagen and connective tissue in association with lymphocytic infiltration.

Among the processes that may cause intrinsic muscle shortening, heterotopic ossification is the only one that involves deposition of bone rather than of collagen. This ossification is most commonly noted after trauma, joint surgery (especially of the hip), spinal cord injury, or other central nervous system injury, but the actual initiating factor is unknown; a local alteration in metabolism or blood flow may be responsible, in conjunction with the systemic alteration in calcium metabolism that occurs with immobility.[101] Although no truly effective treatment exists, ROM should be aggressively maintained. Surgical resection of the bone may be considered after the bone matures. However, this is often associated with a rebound phenomenon, worsening the extent of bone deposition. Prophylaxis can be accomplished

Table 23-3
Types of Collagen

Type	Distribution	Characteristics*
I	Interstitial tissue, skin, tendon, ligaments, fascia, bone, blood vessels	Most common type; widespread distribution; forms large banded fibrils; contains α_1 and α_2 chains in 2:1 ratio in its helix molecule
II	Cartilage, nucleus pulposus, vitreous	Contains three α_1 chains in helix
III	Distribution same as in type I, but not found in bones	Contains three α_1 chains that are loosely arranged; prominent in distensible and stretchable tissue
IV	Basement membrane (glomerulus, sarcolemma)	Three α_1 chains in helix
V	Vascular tissue, fetal membranes, minimal content in bone and cartilage	Three α_B or two α_B and one α_A chain arrangement

*Each collagen molecule is made up of three polypeptides (α chains), which are arranged in a triple-helix formation. Each α chain contains about 1,000 amino acids and is characteristically twisted a complete turn at every third amino acid. Three chains are also twisted, producing the tight triple helix formation of the basic collagen molecule. There are two types of α chains; α_1 and α_2 and the difference is determined by type and sequence of amino acids. (Types α_A and α_B are subsets of these.)

through the use of disodium etidronate, a diphosphonate compound that prevents the calcification of ground substance.

Extrinsic myogenic contractures are the most common type seen in both healthy and disabled people with prolonged immobilization. It is useful, in planning a therapeutic approach, to identify the cause of an extrinsic contracture as paralytic, spastic, or biomechanical.

Because a paralyzed muscle cannot provide adequate resistance to the opposing muscle across a joint, the antagonist will eventually become shortened. A common example of this is the shortened triceps surae seen in chronic peroneal nerve palsy. Although proper positioning of the ankle will not affect neurogenic paresis, it will enable the effective use of a dorsiflexor assist device. Stretch applied to the normal muscle is essential to prevent contracture in this situation; strengthening of the weak muscle or neuromuscular re-education techniques may be beneficial as well.

In the presence of spasticity, a dynamic imbalance of muscle control exists in the involved extremity. The resting length of spastic muscle is reduced owing to increased muscle tone, which encourages faulty joint positioning (Fig. 23-4). Therefore, it is often difficult to clinically identify the actual onset of structural (intrinsic) changes. If full ROM is unobtainable even after prolonged stretch under adequate tension, then an intrinsic shortening must also be present. Treatment is directed at stretching the abnormal muscle; other antispasticity measures also may be of use, especially local nerve or motor point blocks.

Mechanical factors are the final group to cause extrinsic muscle contracture. Some degree of muscle shortening is present even in the healthy sedentary person, especially in those muscles that cross multiple joints. The hamstrings and back

Figure 23-4. Tension–length diagram of 14 hemiplegic patients with spasticity of the gastrocnemius/soleus muscles. The curve for spastic muscle is shifted to the left; the resting length of muscle belly, but not tendon, is reduced. At 2.5, 5, 10, 20, and 40 pounds of tension, the amount of elongation of spastic and unaffected muscles is not different. This indicates that elongation characteristics are essentially unchanged for spastic muscle although the resting length of muscle is reduced. The gastrocnemius/soleus muscle belly elongates about 1.5 cm during full dorsiflexion.

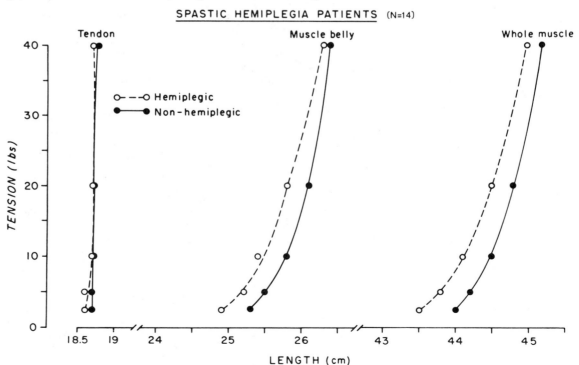

muscles are the most commonly shortened; hip flexors, rectus femoris, gastrocnemius, and tensor fascia lata are the next most likely to shorten. In the upper extremities, the internal rotators of the shoulder are the most frequently contracted. For those on bed rest, the tendency toward tightness in these muscles is accelerated by the typical position of comfort: hips and knees flexed, ankles plantarflexed (Fig. 23-5). Frequent position changes, prone lying, and ankle splints in addition to daily ROM exercises will prevent overall functional loss.

Certain patients have an increased tendency to form mechanically induced contractures. Knee and hip contractures in the lower limb amputee are one such example. The above-knee amputee loses much hip adductor and hamstring influence and will therefore develop contracture in a flexed and abducted position. The below-knee amputee who maintains prolonged hip flexion will develop a significant decrease in knee extension owing to tight hamstrings and soft tissue behind the knee. On the other hand, the below-knee amputee treated with a rigid postoperative dressing in full-knee extension may develop quadriceps muscle tightness preventing full flexion of the knee.

Muscular dystrophy patients are yet another example. In muscular dystrophy, plantarflexion contracture is not only due to intrinsic muscle changes but also to biomechanical forces. Hip extensors are often very weak, forcing the patient into excessive lumbar lordosis; in order to thrust the center of gravity behind the hip joints, the patient tends to walk on his or her toes.[65] Walking on the toes prevents natural stretching of the triceps surae during the stance phase of the gait, encouraging the fibrotic muscle to become even more contracted. If a clinician does not recognize this sequence of events, he or she might assume that weakness and fibrosis are the only reasons for a plantarflexion contracture. A surgical lengthening of the Achilles tendon in such a case may not give the expected improvement. The lengthening of the tendon may shorten the muscle belly, thereby increasing the weakness of the plantarflexors, diminishing the ability of these patients to walk on their toes. Since walking on their toes is the only feasible method of ambulation, the result of an ill-advised tendon lengthening may be a wheelchair-dependent patient.

A muscle held in a foreshortened position for 5 to 7 days will demonstrate initial shortening of the muscle belly. This is due, presumably, to shortening of collagen fibers. Under normal conditions, collagen fibers are coil-shaped and loosely arranged, allowing elongation to occur. However, if the foreshortened position is maintained longer than three weeks, the loose connective tissue in the muscle and around the joint will gradually change into dense connective tissue. This new dense connective tissue is composed primarily of type I collagen rather than the type III fiber commonly found in the endomysial, epimysial, and perimysial layers. The relative proportions of type I and III collagen fibers may also be altered in the soft tissue surrounding a joint, further compounding the problem (see Table 23-3). In situations such as burns, the proliferation of new collagen tissue will cause a more rapid development of multiple joint contractures.

Multiple factors affect the rate of development of contracture such as precipitating causes, duration and degree of immobilization, and preexisting joint restrictions. Edema, ischemia, bleeding, and other alterations to the microenvironment of muscle can hasten the development of fibrosis. Advanced age must also be considered; both muscle fiber loss and a relative increase in the proportion of connective tissue in the body are present in the elderly.[9, 84, 102]

Contractures have their major impact in two areas: (1) in interference with mobility and the ability to perform basic activities of daily living and (2) in the general nursing care of the patient. Lower extremity contractures can significantly alter the gait pattern and, in extreme cases, may eliminate ambulation (Figs. 23-6 and 23-7). Hip flexion contracture, for instance, reduces hip extension, shortens the stride length, and requires the patient to walk on the ball of the foot with an increased lumbar lordosis and subsequent increase in energy consumption. For biomechanical reasons, hip flexion contractures will cause the hamstring muscles to become relatively shorter, which in turn flex the knee. It is not uncommon to see a patient with hip contracture develop knee and ankle joint limitations, especially if the joints are not aggressively mobilized (see Fig. 23-5). Plantarflexion contractures will cause an absence of heel strike and an abnormal push-off, resulting in decreased momentum of forward progression. Hip extension contractures are not frequently encountered. Wheelchair ambulation is impaired in advanced hip and knee extension contractures (see Fig. 23-7). Car transfers may also be difficult with the knee fixed in extension. Limitations in upper extremity ROM may lead to impaired reaching, dressing, grooming, eating, and performance of fine motor tasks.[56]

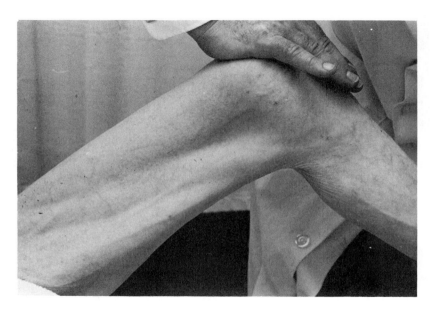

Figure 23-5. A sequence of contracture development from hip to knee in a patient with traumatic hip fracture treated operatively with pins. Owing to hip flexion contracture and immobility, the hamstrings became tight, causing knee flexion contracture with tightness of the posterior capsule and soft tissue. The patient was not able to place his foot on the floor and could not walk independently. Such advanced contractures are best treated with dynamic splinting, casting, or surgery.

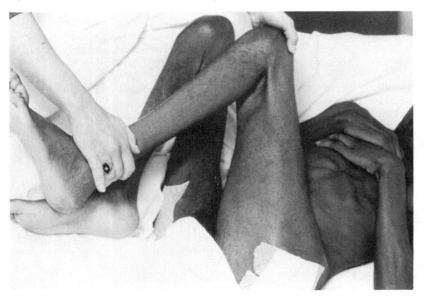

Figure 23-6. A patient with multiple sclerosis, severe spasticity, and pressure sores over the trochanters. Surgery to repair the pressure sores were deferred until the contracture could be reduced. Obturator nerve and nerve root phenol neurolysis may be contemplated to reduce spasticity and permit more effective stretching of the contracted muscles.

Figure 23-7. A patient with multiple joint contractures following hemiplegia due to lack of ROM exercises and mobility. This advanced knee flexion contracture limits his wheelchair mobility, since it prevents him from keeping his leg on the leg rest.

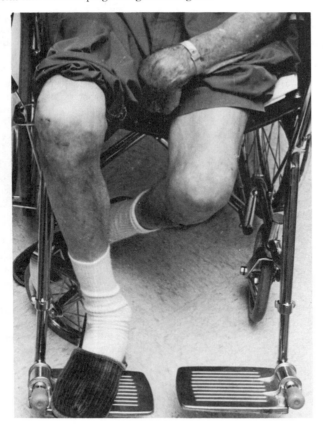

Multiple joint contractures severely interfere with adequate bed positioning and mobility so that perineal hygiene and skin care may be difficult. In addition, joint contractures tend to accentuate areas of increased pressure on skin, leading to skin breakdown that may be impossible to treat (even surgically) without first correcting the contracture (see Fig. 23-6).

Therapeutic Approach and Management

ANALYSIS.   The basis for initiating treatment for contractures is a careful determination of the predisposing factors and a knowledge of what joint component is actually involved. A careful neuromuscular examination emphasizing active and passive ROM is essential. Particular attention should be directed at those muscles crossing two joints. In patients with severe uncontrolled spasticity, it may be necessary to obtain accurate ROM measurements with the use of anesthesia; this is particularly helpful when surgery to repair a decubitus ulcer is contemplated. Of course, the best treatment is prevention and so a careful analysis of positioning and ROM needs should be undertaken with any patient immobilized by disease or by the treatment of disease.

STRETCH (RESTORATION OF LENGTH).   Once a contracture has occurred, the sine qua non for treatment is active and passive ROM combined with a sustained terminal stretch (Table 23-4).[47, 70] For mild contracture, a shorter sustained stretch lasting 20 to 30 minutes twice a day may be effective. Prolonged stretches of 30 minutes or more are necessary for more severe contractures. This is generally more successful when used with heat application to the musculotendinous junction or joint capsule. Ultrasound as a heat source is most popular for large joints; its properties allow therapeutic heating of 40°C to 43°C, which will increase the viscous properties of connective tissue and maximize the effect of stretching.[44]

When applying terminal stretch to a joint, the proximal body part should be well stabilized; in many cases, slight distraction of the joint during stretch will prevent joint compression and possible soft tissue impingement (particularly in the small joints of the hand). The shoulder is commonly a site of contracture, particularly in the adducted and internally rotated position. In this position, the normal downward sliding and rotation of the humeral head on the glenoid fossa does not occur; forced abduction will, therefore, simply cause impingement of the rotator cuff tendon against the acromion, resulting in pain. Stretch applied in forward flexion and external rotation will restore some of this motion and should be attempted prior to abduction.

Sustained stretch of 2 hours or more can be obtained by the use of serial casting or dynamic splinting. Serial casting is the application of plaster or polymer bandages with careful padding over bony prominences. The cast is applied immediately after

Table 23-4
Basic Principles in the Prevention and Treatment of Contractures

---

Prevention*
    Proper positioning
    ROM exercises, active or passive (two-jointed muscle)
    Early mobilization

Treatment
    Passive ROM exercises with terminal stretch
    Prolonged stretch (low passive tension, heat)
    Progressive (dynamic) splinting
    Treatment of spasticity (motor point or nerve blocks)
    Surgical release (tendon lengthening, osteotomies, joint replacement)

---

*Active and passive ROM exercises with early mobilization must be supplemented with proper positioning of an extremity at risk.

heat and manual stretch have been used to obtain maximal ROM. After the initial cast has dried and has been worn for 2 to 3 days, it should be removed and the skin checked for pressure areas. Reapplication of the cast can occur every 2 to 5 days. Serial casting is particularly useful for plantarflexion and knee flexion contractures.

Another method of obtaining repeated stretch is through dynamic splinting. While movement is allowed, a spring or elastic band provides tension in the desired direction. This type of splinting is often used in the hand and arm since it allows a measure of function while providing stretch.

A variation on the use of sustained stretch is the continuous passive mobilization (CPM) device. Its use has become relatively routine for postoperative ROM to the knee, but only recently has become adopted for use on other joints. ROM is provided to the degree chosen, and the device functions at a slow continuous speed. CPM is recommended for the early mobilization of infected joints, synovectomized knees and hips, knee fractures, ligamentous repairs, total knee joint replacement, or any incipient arthrogenic contractures.[6] Early passive mobilization with CPM has been shown to promote the exchange of joint fluid, reduce the need for pain medication after surgery, and prevent contractures. During CPM therapy, muscles around the joint remain relaxed and pain is usually minimal. CPM is typically prescribed for 8 to 12 hours a day for a total of 3 to 5 days postoperatively.

POSITIONING. Prevention and treatment of contracture in a bed-bound patient starts with the selection of an adequate bed and mattress, proper bed positioning, and a mobility training program.

The patient should be moved out of bed as soon as his medical condition allows. The total time allotted to bed rest is gradually reduced to 8 hours. If bed rest is unavoidable, then bed positioning and bed mobility are incorporated into a patient's nursing management program. A firm mattress is in order to prevent sagging, to avoid hip flexion contracture, and to facilitate mobility. The effect of footboards is limited since the foot and ankle are only supported in a supine position. Moving a footboard 4 inches away from the end of the mattress allows the heel or forefoot to be placed between them, providing pressure relief for the feet. To assist a patient in turning side to side or in coming up into a sitting position, partial side-rails should be a standard part of bed equipment. An overhead trapeze is useful for the patient with impaired bed mobility. With the use of the upper extremities and trapeze, a patient should be able to roll side to side, scoot up and down, attain a sitting position, and assist in transferring into and out of bed.

If a patient with paretic or otherwise compromised extremities must be on prolonged bed rest, a variety of assistive devices are used to keep the joints in functional positions. Owing to the recumbent position and weight of the arm, the shoulder tends to assume an adducted and internally rotated position. If this position is maintained through the day, and ROM provided only for a half-hour daily, then shortness of the internal rotators and adductors will result. With the use of pillows, the shoulder can be effectively maintained in abduction and neutral rotation. A palmar roll or hand splint is used to maintain hand, thumb, and finger joints at optimal position. If flexors of the hand and fingers become tighter, then a resting splint in more extension can provide stretch to contracted muscles.

For lower extremity positioning, the trochanter roll is used to counteract excessive external rotation. Plantarflexion contractures are best prevented by the use of a custom-made splint encompassing the foot, ankle and, lower leg with a removable derotation bar. It should be worn at night and for several hours during the day.

While positioning is of most use in the prevention of joint contractures, it can be an important supplement to the treatment of existing joint contractures. Splinting or bracing a joint with a locked adjustable hinge allows maintenance of existing range, which can be increased as other methods of stretching become effective. Serial casts provide excellent position maintenance as well as prolonged stretch.

In order to achieve the best position, it is sometimes necessary to obtain tendon lengthening by surgical means. The benefits and risks of tendon lengthening should be carefully considered. It must be remembered that the muscle belly will remain shortened even though the tendon is longer; therefore, full active ROM may not be restored. Tendon lengthening combined with muscle transfer procedures in spastic or paralytic contractures may give better results since it attempts to restore equilibrium around the joint (particularly effective at the ankle using the tibialis posterior muscle). In other situations, such as hip adductor contractures secondary to spasticity, tenotomy may be combined with neurolysis to obtain optimal results.

FUNCTION. The last major area to be considered in the treatment of contractures is the restoration of function. Encouraging the use of the limb for ambulation or other activities will assist in maintaining the function of uninvolved joints as well as focusing attention on the normal use of the affected joint. Muscle strengthening should be a primary concern to obtain a balance of forces across joints. Electrical stimulation applied to paretic muscles to obtain full muscle contraction will accelerate the strengthening process; its use with electromyographic feedback may also benefit the patient's ability to incorporate the weakened muscle appropriately into normal activities.[24, 48] The elimination of poor habits in ambulation and posture and the use of a strength maintenance and general endurance program are necessary to maintain gains and prevent recurrent joint contractures.

Muscle Weakness and Atrophy

Immobility will directly affect muscle strength and size in addition to the perceived weakness associated with cardiovascular deconditioning (Table 23-5). Although in most patients these effects are easily reversible, for those with preexisting neurological or musculoskeletal disease, the results may be functionally devastating.[10, 33, 52, 53, 91]

With complete bed rest, a muscle will lose 10% to 15% of its strength per week, or about 1% to 3% per day. If at bed rest and

Table 23-5
Effect of Immobilization on Skeletal Muscle

Component	Characteristic Effect*
SDH (succinodehydrogenase, an oxidation enzyme)	Aerobic function decreases
Glycogen	Storage levels are depleted
CP (creatinine phosphokinase, an energy starter enzyme)	Storage levels are depleted
Creatinine (an energy starter)	Storage levels decrease
Type I fiber	Size and area decrease 25%
Type II fiber	Size and area decrease 35%
VO₂ maximum	Consumption is reduced

* Significance of these changes remains unclear.

immobilized for 3 to 5 weeks, a patient will lose half of his muscle strength. The reduction in muscle activity compounded by incomplete muscle contraction may compromise the blood supply, affecting metabolic activity and impairing muscle endurance. Decreased oxidative capacity and lowered tolerance to lactic acid and oxygen debt are at least partly responsible for poor endurance.[2, 35, 60, 88] Certain muscles will atrophy more quickly than others; the quadriceps and back extensor muscles in particular are affected, leading to difficulties walking upstairs and to backaches. Generalized muscle weakness may also result in poor coordination and quality of movement when the patient is eventually remobilized.[39, 98, 99]

Fortunately, disuse weakness is relatively simple to prevent. In addition to encouraging normal activities, muscle strength can be maintained with a program of daily muscle contractions of 20% to 30% of maximal tension for several seconds each day.[88] Alternatively, a more vigorous contraction (50% of maximum) performed for 1 second a day will be effective. Isolated muscle group weakness and atrophy may also be prevented by the use of electrical stimulation.[48] For example, applying local stimulation to the quadriceps while a long leg cast is in place may assist in preserving muscle bulk and strength and may shorten rehabilitation time (a factor that may be particularly important in the athlete). A typical program will consist of three sessions per day for 30 minutes using direct rectangular biphasic pulse stimulation.

Osteoporosis

Maintenance of skeletal mass depends largely on the stresses applied to bone by tendon pull and the force of gravity. Studies performed on normal animals and humans in a weightless state or during enforced immobilization have demonstrated that significant osteopenia can result.[2] Monkeys kept in a semirecumbent position with mobility eliminated demonstrated a loss of both compact and trabecular bone. Histological sections showed an intensification of osteoclastic activity with osteoblastic inhibition. Resumption of normal activity led to the formation of new bone within 2 months; however, trabecular bone was not yet fully restored. Six or more months are required for a return to baseline.[16]

This type of bone loss is accelerated in the presence of a neurogenic paralysis. Patients with spinal cord pathology (*e.g.,* due to trauma or myelodysplasia) usually have enough osteopenia to warrant care in prescribing intensive exercise or ambulation programs to avoid fracture. Another population at increased risk for bone loss during immobilization is those with preexisting osteoporosis of hormonal origin. Particular attention should be paid to continuing activity during illness in these patients.

The biochemical bases for immobilization osteopenia will be further discussed in the section on negative calcium metabolism.

The Effect of Bed Rest on Low Back Pain Syndrome

Clinical observations have provided ample information that prolonged bed rest may cause low back pain, especially after resumption of mobility. This pain is related to several factors, including tightness of the back and hamstring muscles or weakness of the back and abdominal muscles. Any shortening of these muscles will alter spinal alignment and posture. Abdominal and spinal muscle weakness contributes to the increase in spinal curvature and weight-bearing on the small apophyseal lumbar joints. Immobilization osteoporosis of the spine is also a possible contributor to the development of back pain. Abdominal muscle strengthening exercises as well as strengthening and sensible stretching of paraspinal and hamstring muscles with general conditioning may prevent these complications of bed rest.

Acute low back pain, on the other hand, has been treated with bed rest. However, the therapeutic value of prolonged bed rest has been disproven. In a well-controlled and randomized study, Deyo and co-workers[25] have clearly shown that patients with acute and chronic low back pain who were prescribed 2 days of bed rest subsequently had less time lost from work than patients who received 1 week of bed rest. There was no difference, however, between the two groups in respect to functional outcome. This study reinforces the principle that prolonged bed rest should not be considered as a therapeutic tool in the treatment of low back pain syndrome.

CARDIOVASCULAR SYSTEM

Postural Hypotension

One of the most significant effects of prolonged bed rest is the impaired ability of the circulatory system to adjust to the upright position.[14] When a normal person is tilted up from a supine position, redistribution of the blood volume occurs. About 700 ml of blood shifts from the thorax into the legs. As a consequence, the ankle venous pressure increases from 15 cm H₂O in the supine position to 120 cm H₂O in the upright position. A decrease in the stroke volume and the cardiac output results, leading to a transient drop in the systolic blood pressure of an average of 14 mm Hg.

To prevent an excessive drop of blood pressure on standing and quickly restore the normal blood pressure and central blood volume, protective sympathetic reflexes are activated. These adrenergic reflexes, deriving from the great thoracic veins and the right atrium (acting as a low pressure baroreceptor), cause an increase in plasma norepinephrine levels. The adrenergic system influences the release of renin and angiotensin II, which potentiate the sympathetic response. The end result is a transient increase in pulse rate up to 15 beats/min and a more prolonged vasoconstriction of lower extremity vessels and of mesenteric blood supply, thus maintaining normal blood pressure.[78]

However, in postural hypotension due to recumbency, the

circulatory system is unable to maintain a stable extended blood pressure and, for unknown reasons, is unable to mount an adequate sympathetic response. In addition, plasma renin and aldosterone secretion after tilting are not diminished to a normal extent.[122] As a consequence, blood pools in the lower extremities, decreasing the circulating blood volume and venous return. This decrease in venous return along with the rapid heart rate prevents optimal ventricular filling during diastole. Stroke volume, which depends on diastolic filling, may not then be sufficient to maintain adequate cerebral perfusion.[20, 61, 71]

The clinical signs and symptoms of postural hypotension are tingling, burning in the lower extremities, dizziness, lightheadness, fainting, vertigo, increased pulse rate (more than 20 beats/min), decrease in systolic pressure (greater than 20 mm Hg), and decrease in pulse pressure.[5] In patients with coronary artery disease, anginal symptoms may also be prominent since decreased coronary blood flow will accompany inadequate diastolic filling.[38]

In normal people, adaptability to the upright position may be completely lost following 3 weeks of complete bed rest. A significant increase of heart rate and drop in systolic pressure may occur after only several days of recumbency in those who have associated problems of sepsis, major trauma, major medical illness, or advanced age. Older people are also slower to reestablish normal blood pressure and heart rate levels during remobilization. The process of restoring normal postural cardiovascular responses can vary from 20 to 72 days.[7, 20, 61]

As a group, quadriplegic patients are quite susceptible to orthostatic hypotension. When these patients are tilted up, they show a significant decrease in mean arterial pressure, an increase in heart rate, and an increase in both sympathetic and plasma renin activities as measured by serum dopamine-β-hydroxylase and plasma renin radioimmunoassay. Two possible mechanisms may account for orthostatic hypotension in patients with spinal cord injury. First, the normal increase in plasma norepinephrine that occurs on tilting is delayed in quadriplegic patients. Second, the efficacious use of antigravity suits in treating quadriplegics with postural hypotension indicates that venous pooling may play an important role in the occurrence of orthostatic hypotension.

Early mobilization is the most effective way of countering orthostatic hypotension and should include ROM, strengthening exercises, ambulation, and calisthenics, as tolerated by the patient. Abdominal strengthening and isotonic/isometric exercises involving the legs are optimal for reversing venous stasis and pooling. Elevating leg rests and reclining backs may be used to assist during the reconditioning process. Occasionally a tilt table may be necessary with the goal of tolerating 20 minutes at 75° of tilt. Supportive garments such as Ace bandage wraps, full-length elastic stockings, and a variety of abdominal binders are regularly used.[5, 96, 118, 121] Ephedrine and phenylephrine are sympathomimetic agents that help to maintain blood pressure; fludrocortisone (Florinef), a mineralocorticoid, is the next choice of drug to be used. Maintaining an adequate salt and fluid intake will prevent any worsening of hypotension secondary to blood volume contraction.

Impaired Cardiovascular Performance

During periods of bed rest, the resting pulse rate increases 1 beat per minute per 2 days, indicating decreased cardiac efficiency. After 3 weeks of bed rest, the pulse rate after 30 minutes of walking at 3.5 miles per hour up a 10% grade increases an average of 35 to 45 beats above normal and requires 26 to 72 days of continued activity to return to pre–bed rest level. This is calculated to be a 25% decrease in cardiovascular performance. In addition to this, there is a gradual elevation of the systolic blood pressure in response to increased peripheral vascular resistance. The absolute systolic ejection time is shortened, and the length of diastole is reduced, resulting in stroke volume reduction. Work capacity, which is a derivative of the left ventricular pressure and force of ventricular contraction, is also reduced. Overall declines in cardiac output, stroke volume, and left ventricular function may be observed, with prolonged immobility.[17, 61, 108–111]

Redistribution of Body Fluids

Normally, 20% of total blood volume is contained within the arterial system, 5% in the capillaries and 75% in the venous system. On lying down, 700 ml of blood shifts to the thorax with a consequent decrease in heart rate and an increase of cardiac output of 24%; cardiac work is calculated to increase approximately 30%. During lengthy periods of bed rest, there is a progressive decrease in blood volume over 30 days with the maximum reduction on the sixth day. This reduction of blood volume is due mainly to a reduced hydrostatic blood pressure. A reduction of plasma volume rather than the red cell mass occurs, leading to increased blood viscosity and, possibly, to thromboembolic phenomena. By the fourth day of recumbency, the loss of plasma volume can reach 12% of the pre–bed rest level. The extracellular fluid volume remains unchanged, however, for the longer periods of bedrest the decrease in the extracellular fluid is noted.[62, 66, 87, 108, 112, 115, 119]

For normal subjects on bed rest, the reduction of plasma volume can be diminished by exercise. Therapeutically, isotonic exercises are almost twice as effective as isometric exercises in preventing plasma volume reduction.[49–51]

The studies have shown a significant reduction of plasma volume and plasma protein after prolonged bed rest. The loss of plasma proteins during recumbency can be reduced by exercising. Although short periods of intensive exercise produce a small loss of plasma proteins, sustained submaximal exercise actually induces a net gain in plasma protein, which contributes to the stabilization of plasma volumes.[104, 105] The combination of hypovolemia and stasis of the circulation due to bed rest are important precipitating factors in thrombogenesis.

Thromboembolic Events

Immobilization exposes the patient to two factors that are contained in Virchow's triad (factors contributing to clot formation): stasis and increased blood coagulability. The third factor, injury to the vessel wall, is all that is required to increase the patient's risk of thromboembolism.[32, 46]

Stasis of blood flow occurs in the lower extremities owing to decreased pumping activity of the muscles. Other factors that can contribute to stasis are surgery, age, obesity, prior deep venous thrombosis (leading to abnormal blood flow mechanics), malignancy, and congestive heart failure. A hypercoagulable state is then produced via dehydration and increased blood viscosity. A direct relationship between the frequency of deep venous thrombosis and the length of bed rest has been observed.[83]

Clinical detection of deep venous thrombosis begins with the observation of signs and symptoms including edema, tenderness, hyperemia, venous distention, and Homans's sign. When deep venous thrombosis is suspected on clinical grounds, further diagnostic studies include the following:

1. *Doppler ultrasound study.* This study may be 95% accurate depending on the skill of the examiner. However, this method cannot be used to detect thrombi above the level of the femoral vein.[12]
2. *Impedance plethysmography.* Impedance plethysmography is a fairly sensitive method that is useful for detecting thrombi located in the thigh.[113]
3. *^{125}I fibrinogen scanning.* Radioisotope fibrinogen scanning can detect an actively forming thrombus. However, it is not useful for very proximal locations or after heparinization has been instituted.[113]
4. *Radionuclide venography.* Radionuclide venograms are both sensitive and specific for thrombi above the knee but cannot detect calf thrombi or distinguish between old and new disease (unless, of course, the patient has a previous study available for comparison).[81]
5. *Contrast venography.* Dye venography remains the "gold standard" for diagnosis. It is, however, invasive, time consuming, painful, and irritating to the venous lining.[12]

Pulmonary emboli are manifested by a sudden onset of dyspnea, tachypnea, tachycardia, or a cardiac murmur and are often associated with a preexisting deep venous thrombosis. Diagnosis rests on arterial blood gases, ventilation–perfusion scans, and pulmonary angiography.

The most common means of prevention of thromboembolic complications is the use of low-dose subcutaneous injections of heparin (5,000 units twice a day). Other preventive methods include external intermittent leg compression, elastic leg wrappings, active exercise, and early mobilization.

METABOLIC SYSTEM

Negative Nitrogen Balance

Although energy sources at rest are derived from carbohydrates and fat, daily nitrogen loss is increased during prolonged bed rest (Fig. 23-8). Restriction of muscular activity accelerates the breakdown of protein and reduces protein synthesis leading to hypoproteinemia. This protein deficit is exacerbated via gastrointestinal mechanisms such as loss of appetite, reduced intestinal absorption, and constipation (Fig. 23-9).

The daily loss of nitrogen for an immobilized healthy person is about 2 g. This compares with 12 g/day during starvation, and 8 g/day during the first few days after long bone fractures. Increased nitrogen loss usually begins on the fifth or sixth day of recumbency, with a peak loss in the second week.[47, 79] It takes 1 week to restore nitrogen balance if the person has been on bed rest for 3 weeks. However, 7 weeks of bed rest will require 7 weeks of activity to restore a positive nitrogen balance.

Urinary excretion of creatine is minimal under normal conditions except during pregnancy or in infants. The excretion of creatine is greater during certain pathological conditions, such as starvation, diabetes, muscular dystrophy, hyperthyroidism, fever, rheumatoid arthritis, and prolonged inactivity.[29] Prolonged bed rest or weightlessness causes a significant increase in both creatine and creatinine excretion. The increased excretion in urine during immobilization is not well understood.[58]

Negative Calcium Balance

Despite a normal serum calcium level, immobilized patients are markedly hypercalciuric. Urinary calcium excretion increases above normal levels on the second and third days of recumbency.

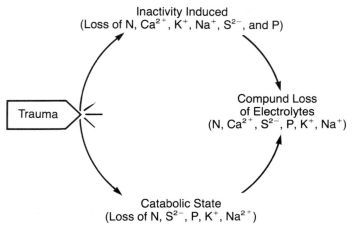

Figure 23-8. Negative metabolic balance induced by trauma can be aggravated by negative metabolic balance produced by prolonged bed rest and immobility.

Figure 23-9. Negative nitrogen balance during prolonged bed rest results from a decrease in nitrogen synthesis and an increase in nitrogen breakdown, and leads to hypoproteinemia.

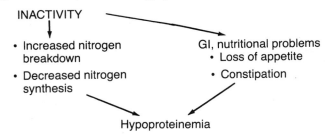

Maximum loss occurs during the fourth or fifth week when the urinary calcium excretion doubles above the level of the first week; on the average, calcium loss is 1.5 g/wk. This decrease in total calcium continues even after resumption of physical activity. At 3 weeks after resumed physical activity, calcium losses of up to 4.0 g have been measured. This negative calcium balance can last for months and even years.[29]

Calcium loss is primarily attributed to reduced activity of the muscular system. Skeletal mass depends in large part on the stresses applied to bone over tendons and to gravitational forces. Osteopenia due to immobilization is characterized by the loss of calcium and hydroxyproline from the cancellous bone of long bone epiphyses and metaphyses. This probably occurs through the suppression of the parathormone (PTH)–1,25-dihydroxyvitamin D axis. Increased resorption of bone is the primary process responsible for disuse osteoporosis, although the precise nature of this resorption is unknown.[86, 116] Disuse osteoporosis can be prevented by the regular use of isometric or isotonic exercises. Ambulation or at least standing on a tilt table may retard the loss of calcium. Calcium loss is restored much less quickly than nitrogen balance.[95]

Another consequence related to disordered calcium metabolism is the syndrome of immobilization hypercalcemia seen particularly in adolescent boys after acute spinal cord injury. Symptoms include anorexia, abdominal pain, nausea, vomiting, constipation, confusion, and ultimately coma.[27, 31, 59, 63, 72, 93]

Treatment relies on achieving adequate calcium excretion through hydration with normal and half-normal saline and diuresis with furosemide.

Negative calcium balance can be induced by decreased physical activity alone without actual confinement to bed. The sedentary person tends to progressively lose calcium from bone. Several well-controlled studies have shown that normal subjects on a year-long program of exercises will increase their bone mass in contrast to those who are sedentary.[116] Protracted negative balance can lead to secondary complications such as hip and vertebral bone fractures after minimal trauma or ectopic calcification around the large joints.[45, 55, 57]

Negative Balance of Phosphorus, Sulfur, Sodium, and Potassium

Both immobility and trauma will negatively affect the metabolic balance of sodium, sulfur, phosphorus, and potassium, compounding their individual effects. A decrease in total body sodium occurs in tandem with the diuresis seen early during bed rest. Serum sodium levels do not correlate well with the severity of orthostatic hypotension. Hyponatremia will be manifested especially in the elderly by lethargy, confusion and disorientation, anorexia, and seizures. Potassium levels progressively decrease during the early weeks of bed rest as well. Although immobility alone will rarely cause a serious metabolic disturbance (except for calcium), patients with multiple medical illnesses may be affected by even slight abnormalities (see Fig. 23-8).

GENITOURINARY SYSTEM

Many compromises in the metabolic and physical function of the urinary tract occur in response to prolonged bed rest; the end result of these alterations is an increased incidence of bladder and/or renal stones and urinary tract infections. Hypercalciuria is a frequent finding in the immobilized patient.[18] This, combined with the altered ratio of citric acid to calcium and the increased urinary excretion of phosphorus, is one important factor. The other is urinary stagnation. In the supine position, urine must flow uphill from the renal collecting systems to be drained via the ureters. Often, patients simply find it difficult to initiate voiding while supine, a situation not ameliorated by reduced intra-abdominal pressure secondary to muscle weakness and deconditioning. Incomplete bladder emptying results in an ideal situation for stone formation. The most common types of stones are struvate and carbonate apatite found in 15% to 30% of immobilized patients. Bladder stones allow bacterial growth and cause decreased efficacy of standard antimicrobial treatment.[57, 74, 95] Irritation and trauma to the bladder mucosa by stones can encourage bacterial overgrowth and infection. Urea-splitting bacteria will then increase the urine pH and ammonium concentration, leading to further precipitation of calcium and magnesium. These complications are aggravated by the presence of neurological disease affecting bladder function such as spinal cord injury or diabetes mellitus.

Treatment of these problems lies first in prevention, which includes adequate fluid intake, use of the upright position for voiding, and scrupulous avoidance of bladder contamination during instrumentation. Other therapeutic approaches might include acidification of the urine through the use of vitamin C, urinary antiseptics, and, in those populations at highest risk of stone-forming, an urease inhibitor. Treatment of stones after they have formed may require surgical removal or the use of newer techniques of ultrasonic lithotripsy.[18] Appropriate antibiotic selection based on urine cultures and sensitivity trials is required to eliminate urinary tract infection.

RESPIRATORY SYSTEM

The respiratory complications of immobility are better recognized than most because of the life-threatening nature of the resulting illnesses. Tidal volume, minute volumes, and maximal breathing capacity are diminished. Vital capacity and functional reserve capacity may also be reduced 25% to 50%. Mechanisms for this may include diminished diaphragmatic movement in the supine position and decreased chest excursion (in part due to a progressive decrease in the ROM allowed at the costovertebral and costochondral joints). For the same reasons breathing tends to be shallower with subsequent increases in respiratory rate.[106]

This decreased movement of the diaphragm and the intercostal muscles will eventually lead to a loss of their strength as with any other muscle, adversely affecting overall endurance. Clearance of secretions is more difficult. The bronchi are not covered evenly with secretions. The dependent (usually posterior) walls accumulate more secretion, whereas the upper parts (anterior) become dry, rendering the ciliary lining ineffective in clearing secretions while supine. This allows pooling of secretions in the lower bronchial tree. Coughing is impaired because of ciliary malfunction and abdominal muscle weakness. Regional changes in the ventilation–perfusion ratio occur as dependent areas become poorly ventilated and overperfused. This may lead to significant arteriovenous shunting with lowered arterial oxygenation. Atelectasis and hypostatic pneumonia may be the ultimate result. Treatment and/or prevention rests with early mobilization, frequent respiratory toilet (deep breathing, coughing, and suctioning, if necessary), and frequent position changes. Percussion and postural drainage may be indicated in more advanced cases of obstruction.[88]

GASTROINTESTINAL SYSTEM

Gastrointestinal changes are due to inactivity and immobility. The loss of appetite, atrophy of the intestinal mucosa and glands, slower rate of absorption, and distaste for protein-rich food all lead to nutritional hypoproteinemia. Constipation results from the interaction of multiple factors. Immobilization causes increased adrenergic stimulation, which inhibits peristalsis and causes sphincter contraction. The loss of plasma volume and dehydration aggravates constipation. In addition, the use of a bedpan for fecal elimination places the patient in an unphysiological position, and the desire to defecate is reduced owing to a social embarrassment when using the bedpan in bed. The end point of this process is fecal impaction requiring enemas, manual removal, or in extreme cases, surgical intervention.

Prevention of constipation requires an adequate intake of an appealing fiber-rich diet including raw fruits and vegetables and of liberal amounts of fluids. Stool softeners and bulk-forming agents are helpful in maintaining bowel function. The use of narcotic agents should be limited since they produce slowed peristalsis as well. The limited use of glycerin or peristaltic-stimulating suppositories in combination with a regularly timed bowel program will further assist in the prevention of impaction.[64]

ENDOCRINE SYSTEM

A lack of physical activity can cause altered responsiveness of hormones and enzymes, which may be clinically undetected early during immobilization. However, numerous changes have been demonstrated to occur in the endocrine system. Significant carbohydrate intolerance has been noted after 8 weeks of immobility. The duration of immobility is positively correlated to the degree of carbohydrate intolerance.[15, 77, 92, 107, 120] This glucose intolerance induced by bed rest can be improved by isotonic but not isometric exercises of the large muscle groups in the legs.[28] It appears that inactivity causes a reduction in insulin-binding sites on the muscle membrane, as well as a qualitative reduction of insulin action.[8] A second major hormonal effect is seen with the increase in serum parathyroid hormone.[3, 75] This may be related to hypercalcemia of immobility, although the precise mechanism of this disorder is still unknown. In addition, alterations are seen in androgen levels and spermatogenesis,[21] in the growth hormone response to hypoglycemia, in adrenocorticotropic hormone, and in catecholamine secretion from the sympathomedullary system. Exercise has been shown to increase hydrocortisone levels and decrease plasma norepinephrine levels.[67, 73, 82, 90]

NERVOUS SYSTEM

Sensory deprivation is a silent hazard of prolonged bed rest. Normal subjects placed on strict bed confinement for 3 hours and required to wear gloves, cuffs, goggles, and earplugs to reduce sensory input experienced hallucinations and disorientation. One might predict that significant changes in mental concentration, orientation to space and time, and other intellectual skills occur after several days.[4] Restlessness, anxiety, decreased pain tolerance, irritability, hostility, insomnia, and depression may occur. Such behavioral effects will result in a lack of motivation and will drastically affect the ability of the patient to effect optimal healing and restoration of function.[22, 30, 97]

Balance and coordination are also impaired following immobilization. This impairment of balance appears not to be due to muscle weakness, but rather to unknown factors of neural control.[19, 54, 94, 97, 114]

CONCLUSIONS

In 1862, John Hilton, and English surgeon advocated that bed rest was a basic physiological approach in the treatment of human illnesses. Since that time, bed rest has been indiscriminately used in the treatment of acute and chronic illnesses. However, the complications of prolonged bed rest have been increasingly recognized and reported since the mid 1940s. After World War II, clinical investigators, particularly Deitrick and co-workers[23] in 1948, have revealed that prolonged bed rest causes multiple adverse effects in many organs and body systems. In the 1960s, studies on astronauts have greatly advanced knowledge of the deleterious effect of bed rest and weightlessness. Clinicians are now more aware of possible deleterious effects of prolonged bed rest.

The new era of advocating exercises and cardiovascular conditioning has begun. Studies have indicated that prolonged bed rest and inactive sedentary life-styles have negative effects on human body functioning. The principles advocated by rehabilitation medicine have significantly contributed to the current philosophy on the use and misuse of immobility.

REFERENCES

1. Altman DF, Baker SD, McCally M, Peimme TE: Carbohydrate and lipid metabolism in man during prolonged bed rest. Clin Res 17:543, 1969
2. Arnold JS, Bartley MH: Skeletal changes in aging and disease. Clin Orthop 49:17–38, 1966
3. Balsam A, Leppo LE: Assessment of the degradation of thyroid hormones in man during bed rest. J Appl Physiol 38:216–219, 1975
4. Banks R, Cappon D: Effects of reduced sensory input on time perception. Percept Motor Skills 14:74, 1962
5. Bassey EJ, Fentem PH: Extent of deterioration physical condition during postoperative bed rest and its reversal by rehabilitation. Br Med J 4:196–196, 1974
6. Bentham JS, Brereton WDS, Eng P et al: Continuous passive motion device for hand rehabilitation. Arch Phys Med Rehab 68:248–250, 1987
7. Birkhead NC, Maupt GJ, Myers RN, Daly JW: Circulatory and metabolic effects of prolonged bed rest in healthy subjects. Fed Proc 22:520, 1963
8. Blotner H: Effect of prolonged physical inactivity in tolerance of sugar. Arch Intern Med 75:39–44, 1945
9. Bonner CD: Rehabilitation instead of bed rest? Geriatrics 24:109–118, 1969
10. Booth FW, Gollnick PD: Effects of disuse on the structure and function of skeletal muscle. Med Sci Sports Exerc 15:415–420, 1983
11. Bornstein P, Byers PH: Collagen Metabolism, Current Concepts (pamphlet). Kalamazoo, MI, Upjohn, 1980
12. Browse NL: Diagnoses of deep vein thrombosis. Br Med Bull 34:163, 1978
13. Browse NL: The Physiology and Pathology of Bed Rest. Springfield, IL, Charles C Thomas, 1965
14. Browse NL: Effect of bed rest on resting calf blood flow of healthy adult males. Br Med J 1:1721, 1962
15. Buhr PH: On the influence of prolonged bodily inactivity in the blood sugar curves after oral glucose loading. Helv Med Acta 30:156–175, 1963
16. Cann CE, Genant HK, Young DR: Comparison of vertebral and peripheral mineral losses in disuse osteoporosis in monkey. Radiology 134:525–559, 1980
17. Cardus D, Vallbona C, Spencer WA: The effect of bed rest on various parameters of physiological function: VI. The effect of the performance of periodic Flack maneuvers on preventing cardiovascular deconditioning of bed rest, publication No. NASA CR-176. US National Aeronautics and Space Administration, Washington, DC, April 1965
18. Carlson HE, Ockerblad NF: Stones of recumbency. South Med J 33:582, 1940
19. Chase GA, Grave D, Rowell LB: Independence of changes in functional and performance capacities attending prolonged bed rest. Aerospace Med 37:1232–1238, 1966
20. Chobanian AV, Lillie RD, Tercyak A, Blevins P: The metabolic and hemodynamic effects of prolonged bed rest in normal subjects. Circulation 49:551–559, 1974
21. Cockett AT, Elbadawi A, Zemjanis R: The effects of immobilization on spermatogenesis in subhuman primates. Fertil Steril 21:610–614, 1970
22. Corrodi H, Fuxe K, Kokfelt T: The effect of immobilization stress on the activity of the central monoamine neuron. Life Sci 7:107–112, 1968
23. Deitrick JE, Whedon GD, Shorr E: Effects of immobilization upon various metabolic and physiologic functions of normal men. Am J Med 4:3–32, 1948
24. Demida BF, Machinski I: Use of rehbilitation measures for restoration human physical work capacity after the prolonged limitation of motor activity. Kosm Biol Avialkosm Med 12:74–75, 1979
25. Deyo RA, Diehl AK, Rosenthal M: How many days of bed rest for acute low back pain? N Engl J Med 315:1064–1092, 1986
26. Dock W: Evil sequelae of complete bed rest. JAMA 125:1083–1085, 1944
27. Dodd K, Graubarth H, Rapport S: Hypercalcemia and encephalopathy following immobilization. Pediatrics 6:124, 1950
28. Dolkas CB, Greenleaf JE: Insulin and glucose responses during bed rest with isotonic and isometric exercise. J Appl Physiol 43:1033–1038, 1977
29. Donaldson CL, Hulley SB, Vogel JM et al: Effect of prolonged bed rest on bone mineral. Metabolism 19:1071–1084, 1970

30. Downs FS: Bed rest and sensory disturbances. Am J Nurs 74:434–438, 1974

31. Drivas G, Ward M, Kerr D: Immobilization hypercalcemia in patients on regular haemodialysis. Br Med J 3:468, 1975

32. Eastman NJ: The abuse of rest in obstetrics. JAMA 125:1077–1079, 1944

33. Eichelberger L, Roma M, Moulder PV: Effects of immobilization on the histochemical characterization of skeletal muscle. J Appl Physiol 12:42, 1958

34. Eichler J: Proceedings: Pre-arthrosis due to immobilization. Z Orthop 112:571–573, 1974

35. Eldrige L, Liebhold M, Steinback JH: Alterations in cat skeletal neuromuscular junctions following prolonged inactivity. J Physiol 313:529–545, 1981

36. Enneking WF, Horowitz M: The intra-articular effects of immobilization on the human knee. J Bone Joint Surg [Am] 54:973, 1972

37. Evans EB, Eggers GWN, Butler JK, Blumel J: Experimental immobilization and remobilization of rat knee joints. J Bone Joint Surg [Am] 42:737, 1960

38. Fareeduddin K, Abelmann WH: Impaired orthostatic tolerance after bed rest in patients with myocardial infarction. N Engl J Med 280:345–350, 1969

39. Ferguson AB, Vaughn L, Ward L: A study of disuse atrophy of skeletal muscle in the rabbit. J Bone Joint Surg [Am] 39:583–596, 1987

40. Finsterbush A, Friedman B: Early changes in immobilized rabbit's knee joint. Clin Orthop 131:279, 1972

41. Fournier M, Roy R, Perham H et al: Is limb immobilization a model of muscle disuse? Exp Neurol 80:147–156, 1983

42. Fuller JH, Bernauer EM, Adams WC: Renal function, water and electrolyte exchange during bed rest with daily exercise. Aerosp Med 41:60–72, 1970

43. Garcia-Bunuel L, Garcia-Bunel VM: Connective tissue metabolism in normal and atrophic skeletal muscle. J Neurol Sci 47:69-77, 1980

44. Gersten JW: Effect of ultrasound on tendon extensibility. Am J Phys Med 34:360–362, 1955

45. Giannetta CL, Castleberry HB: Influence of bed rest and hypercapnia upon urinary mineral excretion in man. Aerosp Med 45:750–754, 1974

46. Gibbs NM: Venous thrombosis of the lower limbs with particular reference to bed rest. Br J Surg 191:209–235, 1957

47. Goldspink DF: The influence of immobilization and stretch on protein turnover in rat skeletal muscle. J Physiol 264:267–282, 1977

48. Gould N, Donnermeyer D, Pope M, Ashikaga T: Transcutaneous muscle stimulation as a method to retard disuse atrophy. Clin Orthop 164:215–220, 1982

49. Greenleaf JE, Bernauer EM, Young HL et al: Fluid and electrolyte shifts during bed rest with isometric and isotonic exercise. J Appl Physiol 42:59–66, 1977

50. Greenleaf JE, Bernauer EM, Morse JT et al: +Gz tolerance in man after 14-day bed rest periods with isometric and isotonic exercise conditioning. Aviat Space Environ Med 46:671–678, 1975

51. Greenleaf JE, Young HL, Bernauer EM et al: Effects on Isometric and Isotonic Exercise on Body Water Compartments during 14 Days' Bed Rest. Aerospace Medical Association Preprints, Washington, DC, 1973

52. Haggmark T: A study of morphologic and enzymatic properties of skeletal muscles after injuries and immobilization in man, thesis. Stockholm, Sweden, Karolinska Institute, 1978

53. Haggmark T, Jansson E, Eriksson E: Fiber types area and metabolic potential of the thigh muscle in man after knee surgery and immobilization. Int J Sports Med 2:12–17, 1981

54. Haines RF: Effect of bed rest and exercise on body balance. J Appl Physiol 36:323–327, 1974

55. Halvorsen S: Osteoporosis, hypercalcemia and nephropathy following immobilization of children. Acta Med Scand 149:401, 1954

56. Hamrin E: Anatomical and functional changes in joints and muscles during long-term bed rest. Nord Med 85:293–298, 1970

57. Heath HJ III, Earll JM, Schaaf M et al: Serum ionized calcium during bed rest in fracture patients and normal men. Metabolism 21:633–640, 1972

58. Heilskov NCS, Schonheyder F: Creatinuria due to immobilization in bed. Acta Med Scand 151:51–56, 1955

59. Henke JA, Thompson NW, Kaufer H: Immobilization hypercalcemia crisis. Arch Surg 110:321–323, 1975

60. Henriksson R, Reitman JS: Time course of changes in human skeletal muscle succinate dehydrogenase and cytochrome oxidase activities and maximal uptake with physical activity and inactivity. Acta Physiol Scand 99:91–97, 1977

61. Holmgren A, Mossfeldt F, Sjostrand T, Strom G: Effect of training on work capacity, total hemoglobin, blood volume, heart volume and pulse rate in recumbent and upright positions. Acta Physiol Scand 50:73–83, 1960

62. Hyatt KH, Kamenetsky LG, Smith WM: Extravascular dehydration as an etiologic factor in post-recumbency orthostatism. Aerosp Med 40:644–650, 1969

63. Hyman LR, Boner G, Thomas JC, Segar WC: Immobilization hypercalcemia. Am J Dis Child 124:723–727, 1972

64. Ivy AC, Grossman MI: Gastrointestinal function in convalescence. In symposium on physiological aspects of convalescence and rehabilitation. Fed Proc 3:236–239, 1944

65. Johnson EW: Pathokinesiology of Duchenne muscular dystrophy: Implications for management. Arch Phys Med Rehab 54:4–7, 1977

66. Johnson PC, Briscoll TB, Carpentier WR: Vascular and extravascular fluid changes during 6 days of bed rest. Aerosp Med 42:875–878, 1971

67. Katz FH, Romfh P, Smith JA: Episodic secretion of aldosterone in supine man: Relationship to cortisol. J Clin Endocrinol Metab 35:178–181, 1972

68. Kottke FJ: Deterioration of the bedfast patient. Public Health Rep 80:437–447, 1965

69. Kottke FJ: The effects of limitation of activity upon the human body. JAMA 196:117–122, 1966

70. Kottke FJ, Pauley DL, Ptka RA: The rationale for prolonged stretching for correction for shortening of connective tissue. Arch Phys Med Rehabil 47:345–352, 1966

71. Lamb LE, Stevens PM, Johnson RL: Hypokinesia secondary to chair rest from 4 to 10 days. Aerosp Med 36:755-763, 1965

72. Lawrence GD, Loeffler RG, Martin IG, Conner TB: Immobilization hypercalcemia. J Bone Joint Surg [Am] 55:87, 1973

73. Leach CS, Hulley SB, Rambaut PC, Dietlein LF: The effect of bed rest on adrenal function. Space Life Sci 4:415–423, 1973

74. Leadbetter WF, Engster HE: Problems of renal lithiasis in convalescent patients. J Urol 53:269, 1957

75. Lerman S, Canterbury JM, Reiss E: Parathyroid hormone and the hypercalcemia of immobilization. J Clin Endocrinol Metab 45:425–488, 1977

76. Lieberson S, Mendes DG: Walking in bed. Phys Ther 59:1112, 1979

77. Lipman RL, Schnure JJ, Bradley EM, Lecocq FR: Impairment of peripheral glucose utilization in normal subjects by prolonged bed rest. J Lab Clin Med 76:221–230, 1970

78. Long CL, Bonilla LE: Metabolic effects of inactivity and injury. In Downey JA (ed): Physiological Basis of Rehabilitation Medicine. Philadelphia, WB Saunders, 1971

79. Lynch TN, Jensen RL, Stevens PM et al: Metabolic effects of prolonged bed rest: Their modification by simulated altitude. Aerosp Med 38:10–20, 1967

80. Mack PB, Montgomery KB: Study of nitrogen balance and creatine and creatinine excretion during recumbency and ambulation of five young adult human males. Aerosp Med 44:739–746, 1973

81. McDonald G: Radionuclide venography. J Nucl Med 14:528, 1973

82. Melada GA, Goldman RH, Luestscher JA, Zager PG: Hemodynamics, renal function, plasma renin, and aldosterone in man after 5 to 14 days of bed rest. Aviat Space Environ Men 46:1049–1055, 1975

83. Micheli LJ: Thromboembolic complications of cast immobilization for injuries of the lower extremities. Clin Orthop 108:191–195, 1975

84. Miller MG: Iatrogenic and neurogenic effects of prolonged immobilization of the ill aged. J Am Geriatr Soc 23:360–369, 1975

85. Miller PB, Johnson RL, Lamb LE: Effects of four weeks of absolute bed rest on circulatory functions in man. Aerosp Med 1194–1200, 1964

86. Moore Ede MC, Burr RG: Circadian rhythm of urinary calcium excretion during immobilization. Aerosp Med 44:495–498, 1973

87. Morse JT, Staley RW, Juhos LT, Van Beaumont W: Fluid and electro-

lyte shifts during bed rest without isometric and isotonic exercises. J Appl Physiol 42:59–66, 1977

88. Muller EA: Influence of training and of inactivity on muscle strength. Arch Phys Rehabil Med 449–462, 1970

89. Partridge REH, Duthie TTR: Controlled trial of the effect of complete immobilization of the joints in RA. Ann Rheum Dis 22:91, 1963

90. Pawlson LG, Field JB, McCally M et al: Effect of Two Weeks of Bed Rest on Glucose, Insulin and Human Growth Hormone Levels in Response to Glucose and Arginine Stimulation. Aerospace Medical Association Preprints, Washington, DC, 1968

91. Pestronk A, Drachman B, Griffin JW: Effect of muscle disuse on acetylcholine receptors. Nature 260:352–353, 1976

92. Piemme TE: Effects of two weeks of bed rest on carbohydrate metabolism, hypogravity and hypodynamic environments, NASA Special Publication No. 269. US National Aeronautics and Space Administration, Washington, DC, 1971

93. Rosen FJ, Woolin DA, Finberg L: Immobilization hypercalcemia after single limb fracture in children and adolescents. Am J Dis Child 132:560–564, 1978

94. Ryback RS, Lewis OF, Lessard CS: Psychobiologic effects of prolonged bed rest (weightlessness) in young healthy volunteers (study II). Aerosp Med 42:529–535, 1971

95. Sekutz B Jr, Blizzard JJ, Birkhead NC, Rodahl K: Effect of prolonged bed rest on urinary calcium output. J Appl Physiol 21:1013–1020, 1966

96. Sieker HO, Burnum JF, Hickman JB, Penrod KE: Treatment of postural hypotension with a counterpressure garment. JAMA 161:132–135, 1956

97. Smith MJ: Changes in judgment of duration with different patterns of auditory information for individuals confined to bed. Nurs Res 24:93-98, 1975

98. Spector SA: Effects of elimination of activity on contractile and histochemical properties of rat soleus muscle. J Neurosci 5:2177–2188, 1985

99. Spector SA, Simard CP, Fournier SM et al: Architectural alterations of rat hind limb skeletal muscle immobilized at different lengths. Exp Neurol 76:94–110, 1982

100. Spencer WA, Vallbona C, Carter RE: Physiologic concepts of immobilization. Arch Phys Med Rehabil 46:89–100, 1965

101. Spielman G, Gennarelli TA, Rogers CR: Disodium etidronate: Its role in preventing heterotopic ossification in severe head injury. Arch Phys Med Rehabil 64:539–542, 1983

102. Steinberg FU: The Immobilized Patient: Functional Pathology and Management. New York, Plenum Press, 1980

103. Stolov WC, Fry LR, Riddel WM, Weilepp TG Jr: Adhesive forces between muscle fibers and connective tissue in normal and denervated rat skeletal muscle. Arch Phy Med Rehabil 154:208–213, 1974

104. Stremel RW, Convertino VA, Greenleaf JE, Bernauer EM: Response to maximal exercise after bed rest. Fed Proc 33:327, 1974

105. Stremel RW, Convetino VA, Bernauer EM, Greenleaf JE: Cardio-respiratory deconditioning with static and dynamic leg exercise during bed rest. J Appl Physiol 41:905–909, 1976

106. Svanberg L: Influence of posture on the lung volumes ventilation and circulation in normals. Scand J Clin Lab Invest 9:25, 1957

107. Takayama H, Tomiyama M, Managawa A et al: The effect of physical exercise and prolonged bed rest on carbohydrate, lipid and amino acid metabolism. Jpn J Clin Pathol 22(suppl):126–136, 1974

108. Taylor HL: The effects of rest in bed and of exercise on cardiovascular function. Circulation 38:1016–1017, 1968

109. Taylor HL, Erickson L, Henschel A: The effect of bed rest in the blood volume of normal young men. Am J Physiol 144:227–232, 1945

110. Taylor HL, Henschel A, Porozek J, Keys A: Effects of bed rest on cardiovascular function and work performance. J Appl Psych 2:223–229, 1949

111. Taylor HL, Henschel A, Bozek J, Keys A: Effects of bed rest on cardiovascular function and work performance. J Appl Physiol 2:223, 1949

112. Thompson WO, Thompson PK, Dailey ME: The effect of posture on the composition and volume of the blood in man. J Clin Invest 5:573–604

113. Todd J: Deep venous thrombosis in acute spinal cord injury: A comparison of 1251 fibrinogen ligament scanning, impedance plethysmyography and venography. Paraplegia 14:50, 1976

114. Trimble RW, Lessard CS: Performance Decrement as a Function of Seven Days of Bed Rest. USAF School of Aerospace Medicine Technical Report 70–56, 1970

115. Turner AH: The circulatory minute volume of healthy young women in reclining, sitting, and standing positions. Am J Physiol 80:601–630, 1927

116. Uhthoff HK, Jaworski ZFG: Bone loss in response to long-term immobilization. J Bone Joint Surg [Br] 60:420–429, 1978

117. Vallbona C: Bodily responses to immobilization. In Kottke FJ, Stilwell GK, Lehmann JF (eds): Krusen's Handbook of Physical Medicine & Rehabilitation, pp. 963–976. Philadelphia, WB Saunders, 1982

118. Vallbona C, Spencer WA, Cardus D, Dale JW: Control of orthostatic hypotension in quadriplegic patients with the use of a pressure suit. Arch Phys Med Rehabil 44:7–18, 1963

119. Van Beaumont W, Greenleaf JE, Juhos L: Disproportional changes in hematocrit, plasma volume, and proteins during exercise and bed rest. J Appl Physiol 33:55–61, 1972

120. Varnikos-Danellis J, Winget CM, Leach CS: Circadian endocrine and metabolic effects of prolonged bed rest: Two 56-day bed rest studies. NASA Technical Bulletin, No. Tm V-3051. US National Aeronautic and Space Administration, 1974

121. Vogt FB: Effect of intermittent leg cuff inflation and intermittent exercise on the tilt table response after ten days' bed recumbency. Aerosp Med 37:943–947, 1966

24

Movement Disorders, Including Tremors

Steven G. Scott

Involuntary movements are due to dysfunction or diseases involving the extrapyramidal system, principally the basal ganglia and the related brain stem structures. Lesions in the central nervous system can also produce abnormalities of movement, such as the production of involuntary movements. Involuntary movement disorders can be easily categorized as having too much or too little movement: hyperkinetic or hypokinetic movement disorders.

Hypokinetic movement disorders are characteristic of parkinsonian syndrome (PS) and supranuclear palsy, whereas tremors, chorea, athetosis, myoclonus, and dystonias are hyperkinetic movement disorders (Table 24-1). Most movement disorders are thought to occur because of an imbalance of neurotransmitters and may be idiopathic or induced by injury or drugs. The basic involuntary hypokinetic and hyperkinetic movement disorders and their treatment are described here.

HYPOKINETIC MOVEMENT DISORDERS

Parkinsonian Syndrome

Parkinsonian syndrome (PS) is a degenerative brain disorder that affects 200,000 people in the United States. Approximately 1% of those more than 50 years of age have PS.[30] The disorder accounts for half of the people who suffer from involuntary movement disorders. It occurs equally in men and women, most frequently from the sixth to the eighth decade of life. Parkinsonian syndrome was first described by James Parkinson in 1817. However, it was recognized in ancient medical writings. The most common clinical symptom of PS is tremor. Victims also develop bradykinesia, muscular rigidity, gait disturbances, postural changes, dementia, slow ocular movements with visual changes, and speech that is often slurred, slow, and monotonous.

A common clinical feature of PS is bradykinesia or slowness in movement. This can be easily misinterpreted as a primary depression or withdrawal behavior. There is slowness in performing motor tasks owing to deficient motor planning. Bradykinesia can be disabling and is most pronounced when initiating movements; at times the patient has a tendency to "freeze." PS decreases facial expression (masked faces) and the frequency of eye blinking. Often the patient appears to have a reptilian stare when he or she looks straight ahead without blinking. The voice also tends to be monotonal, slurred, and decreased in amplitude. Arm swing is decreased when the patient walks, and synergistic movements are lost. Activities of daily living, such as buttoning clothing and feeding, are usually slower and more difficult to perform. There is usually a loss of spontaneity in conversation and interaction with the family. Spontaneous movements, such as crossing the legs, readjusting posture when sitting in a chair, and gesturing with the hands and arms during speech, may be diminished or lost.

Tremors of PS are regular and rhythmic and are most pronounced at rest. The frequency of tremors is from three to five cycles per second, and they usually involve the distal muscles. The face, tongue, and lips may also be involved, with alternate contractions of flexion and extension. The tremor is aggravated by emotional tension, and it disappears during sleep. Tremors are usually the least disabling aspect of PS. An anatomical basis for the tremors is unknown, although improvement usually follows treatment with anticholinergic drugs, indicating a possible cholinergic and dopaminergic chemical imbalance as the cause. The tremors often begin in the upper extremities (usually the hands), and they are frequently unilateral. They vary in amplitude and frequency and fluctuate throughout the day. They are usually made worse by emotional stress, and they decrease with relaxation. Physical and emotional distraction often decrease the tremors.

Rigidity is probably the most disabling clinical feature of PS. Rigidity increases resistance to passive movement and is a disorder of reciprocal inhibition. As tremors are superimposed on the rigidity, cogwheeling, or a ratchet-like rigidity, develops. Cogwheeling can lead to further disability because it may limit the range of motion of the joint. It usually appears first in the proximal muscles of the arms and legs. The person can feel stiffness of the neck and develop back and neck pain. Often the wrists are extended; the hand is slightly flexed at the metacarpals and extended at the proximal and distal interphalangeals. The fingers can become adducted and the great toe can become extended.

Another clinical feature of PS is gait dysfunction. The person usually develops a shuffling gait with postural instability. It can consist of retropulsion, in which the patient falls backward, or lateral pulsion, in which the patient falls sideward. Postural problems include the person assuming a flexed, stooped posture with the arms in internal rotation. Also, the person has a de-

Table 24-1
Involuntary Movement Disorders

Hypokinetic
Parkinsonian syndrome
Progressive supranuclear palsy

Hyperkinetic
Tremors
Tics
Gilles de la Tourette syndrome
Myokymia
Dystonias
Hemifacial spasm
Athetosis
Tardive dyskinesia
Chorea
Myoclonus
Asterixis
Hemiballismus

creased arm swing and difficulty turning and taking small steps and initiating gait movements. Often these patients develop a propulsive style in which the steps become faster as the person loses his or her balance.

Dementia is also an important clinical characteristic of PS, occurring in more than half the patients.[13] It occurs 10 times more frequently in people with PS than in the normal population. These patients can develop perceptual abnormalities and have difficulty with block design and object assembly.

Patients often develop postural disturbances in the musculoskeletal system, with abnormal reflexes and loss of normal postural reflexes. Grasp, snout, and palmomental reflexes can be present and indicate diffuse cerebral dysfunction. The classic PS posture is head flexed, thorax in a kyphotic position, and shoulders protracted in abduction with the trunk flexed. The patient often develops weakness and becomes easily fatigued. Muscle pain may also occur and may be severe; flexion contractures and decreased range of motion can develop with this posture.

Patients also develop hypokinetic dysarthria, with decreased mobility, restricted range of motion, and a decreased rate of repetitive movements of the muscles involving speech. The muscles of respiration, phonation, and articulation are all limited in excursion. Loudness level is decreased, variability in pitch and loudness are decreased, and the patient learns to produce shorter, hurried units of speech.

The loss of autonomic reflexes is another disturbing problem. The patient with PS often has hypertension, cardiovascular disease, bladder and bowel dysfunction, and hypomotility of the gastrointestinal tract. The patient chews and swallows slowly and has prolonged esophageal and bowel transit times. Often the patient is constipated and also develops excess amounts of perspiration or oily skin. Drooling is a problem as a result of the inability to hold the head erect and the loss of the swallowing response, which results in accumulation of saliva in the mouth. Other clinical symptoms include sialorrhea, seborrhea, tearing, micrographia, and limitation of eye movements, especially upward gaze and convergence.

The prognosis and natural history of PS are unpredictable. If the disorder is mainly a disease of tremor, it usually has a favorable prognosis.[41] The more severe the tremor, the slower is the progression of the disease. However, if there is akinesia, which is an extreme form of bradykinesia, this may indicate a rapidly developing disease.[38] When treated, the disease usually progresses slowly and the patient eventually becomes immobilized. The rate of deterioration varies widely. Elliott[7] stated that within 5 years, 25% of untreated patients are severely disabled; by 10 years, this increases to 66%.

The pathogenesis of PS may be cellular loss throughout the basal ganglia and cerebral cortex. This is characterized by alteration, depigmentation, and neuronal loss within the substantia nigra. A reduction in the dopamine content of the substantia nigra and neostriatum has been demonstrated. Homovanillic acid and dopa decarboxylase levels have also been found to be reduced. Many syndromes with presumed degenerative origin have parkinsonian features. The most consistent finding in PS is degeneration of the melanin-containing neurons in the zona compacta of the substantia nigra. The cause of this selective cell loss is unknown. The cells of the zona compacta of the substantia nigra give rise to the dopaminergic neurons that terminate in the striatum, and the manifestation of the disease is proportionate to the deficiency in dopamine activity as a consequence of the cell loss. Often PS appears spontaneously, with no known cause. It can also occur as a result of inflammation from postencephalitic syndrome, a consequence of an epidemic of the early 1920s. The disorder is also seen in arteriosclerosis of the brain, in episodes of repeated head trauma in boxers, and with manganese intoxication.

Parkinsonian syndrome takes several different forms. Idiopathic PS involves abnormal neurological functions such as drowsiness, stiffness, gait disturbance, abnormal speech, and ocular signs. The second type is the Shy-Drager syndrome, which includes degeneration of the intermediolateral cells of the spinal cord with resultant central nervous system symptoms, autonomic irregularity, and, often, cerebellar ataxia. A third classification is secondary symptomatic PS due to dopamine-depleting or dopamine-blocking drugs. Butyrophenones (*e.g.,* haloperidol), phenothiazines, reserpine, and tetrabenazine are drugs that have been known to cause secondary or symptomatic PS. The disorder can occur when an antipsychotic drug is given and effectively blocks the dopamine systems in the cortex. However, the drug also blocks the striatal dopamine system and produces parkinsonian symptoms that are indistinguishable from idopathic PS.

A fourth type of PS is the postencephalitic or postinfection type, which is distinguished by oculogyric crisis. This type occurred after an epidemic of encephalitis in 1918 to 1926. In addition to the typical PS, these patients also had tics, abnormal walking behavior, oculogyric crisis, sudden dystonia, and rolling of the eyes. An unusual gait, consisting of a hop up and down and then a normal walk, also developed. Parkinsonian syndrome can also occur secondary to exposure to toxic metals (manganese), strokes, neoplasm, or metabolic abnormalities such as Wilson's disease.

Treatment

Treatment options for PS include rehabilitation, medication, and operation. Rehabilitation of a parkinsonian patient is by a team approach involving a physiatrist, physical therapist, occupational therapist, psychologist, and speech therapist.

PHYSICAL THERAPY. Therapy should concentrate on the goal of restoration of normal body alignment. It is important to stimulate balance reactions to give the patient a sense of how to regain balance to regulate these movements. Therefore, activities that encourage weight transfer with the correct head and trunk movements lead to improvement in the patient's ability to regain balance when there is a change in the center of gravity.

The use in therapy of a wobbleboard or tiltboard may be of some benefit.

Physical therapy should also improve the ability to initiate movements and increase the excursion of all movements, particularly those of rotation and extension, which are often decreased. This is because patients often lose range of motion owing to tremors, bradykinesia, and rigidity. For tremors, there is no specific treatment except to ensure that the patient understands the importance of relaxation and freedom from anxiety, effort, and stress, which all tend to increase tremors. At times, weight-bearing on a tremorous lower extremity can cause a temporary reduction of tremor. Exercises for range of motion can include passive stretching, active assistance, and proprioceptive neuromuscular facilitation exercises.

Specific therapy can include shoulder-girdle exercises with a broomstick handle to stretch the upper extremities and trunk. The arms and shoulders can also be exercised with a pulley to improve range of motion. Back flexion and extension exercises can be helpful in addition to exercises to improve balance when sitting and standing. Frankel exercises for coordination (repeated movements of the feet in adjacent squares on the floor) are helpful. Training in this type of exercise enhances the patient's ability for accurate foot placement during the gait cycle. Quadriceps and hip extensor isometric strengthening exercises can improve the ability to climb stairs or get out of a chair. Facial exercises can also be prescribed to maintain flexibility of the facial muscles for expression. Thoracic breathing exercises are also helpful to maintain thoracic mobility.

Good posture focuses on maintaining good head control and proper balance when sitting and standing. In PS, there is a tendency for a general flexion to occur involving the trunk, head, and limbs. When sitting, the patient may compensate for extreme flexion by leaning backward at the hips, which gives the impression that the patient is falling forward. Physical thereapy should emphasize extension of the hips when standing and flexion of the hips when sitting, which will enable more trunk extension, Pelvic-tilt exercises for the low back, stretching the pectoralis muscles, and sitting back-extension exercises will also be helpful in maintaining normal postural alignment.

It is important to emphasize proper posture and to encourage postural exercises, perhaps done in front of a mirror. Extension exercises should be emphasized to decrease any flexion contractures of the trunk. Again, balance and equilibrium exercises on a tiltboard or wobbleboard may be of help.

Mobility is a problem for patients with PS. In walking, the patient should be taught to take large steps, raising the toes as he or she steps forward. Proper heel strike, in which the heel touches the ground first, should be emphasized. The feet should be kept at least 12 to 15 inches apart and the back straight. The patient should be taught to rock side-to-side and raise his or her legs from below, never crossing the legs when turning. Arm swinging is emphasized because it will help take the body's weight off the legs, lessen fatigue, and loosen the arms and shoulders. Walking should be practiced sideways, backwards, and in circles. Turning should be practiced several times per day. The patient should relax back on his or her heels and lift the toes if he or she feels frozen to the floor; this will help eliminate muscle spasms and fear of falling. This can be facilitated by raising the arms from the sides with sudden movements. Also, freezing may be decreased by not walking in narrow spaces.

Normal walking movements need to be reciprocal and bilateral. In PS, these reciprocal movements are often diminished. Therefore, a stationary bicycle or arm ergometer may help to train reciprocal movements, providing increased freedom of movement. Normal arm swing and trunk rotation should be emphasized by the therapist. Using a cane or stick, the therapist can actively assist the arm swing and trunk rotation while the patient walks. The initial passive movements in the arm encourage some rotation of the trunk and, consequently, larger steps. Markings on the floor can aid in visual stimulation and encourage longer steps, and walking over obstacles will encourage weight-bearing on one foot, more purposeful steps, and confidence in walking. Occasionally, music can also be used to help regain rhythmic movement.

The parkinsonian patient frequently has problems getting in and out of chairs and, therefore, should be instructed in helpful techniques while receiving physical therapy. The patient should be taught to back into the chair, getting as close to it as possible. Then he or she should be instructed to sit down by bending sharply forward and moving slowly downward. To get out of the chair, the patient should be instructed to place both feet under the chair, bend forward, and push up vigorously. Raising the back legs of the chair with 2- to 5-inch blocks can also be helpful.

Speech therapy is an important aspect of the rehabilitation of a patient with PS. The movements characteristic of PS, such as bradykinesia, rigidity, and tremor, usually cause these patients to have hypokinetic dysarthria. Therapeutic efforts are designed to improve respiration by teaching the patient diaphragmatic breathing exercises to increase thoracic and abdominal movements when speaking. The patient can be taught to put pressure over the abdomen and to encourage exhalation. Also, general physical therapy exercises to improve posture and flexibility can improve vital capacity. By learning to take deep breaths before speaking, the volume of the sound and the number of words spoken per breath can increase.

General cardiovascular fitness exercises should also be prescribed for aerobic conditioning. Exercises such as swimming, walking, and the use of a stationary bicycle should be encouraged. Conditioning exercises will improve general mobility, pulmonary and cardiac functional capacity, and sense of well-being.

The lack of movement with general increased muscle tone and rigidity can be improved by having the patient sing or read aloud with forceful movements of the lip and tongue. Also, practicing speech in front of a mirror and emphasizing exaggerated facial movements during recitation of the alphabet or counting numbers may be helpful.

Occupational therapists can assist parkinsonian patients with problems of swallowing and difficulties in activities of daily living. They can also provide proper environmental aids. Parkinsonian patients often have difficulty in swallowing because of the tremors and rigidity. There is variability in the prevalence and type of swallowing disorders of the parkinsonian patient. The patient may have poor bolus formation, misdirected swallow, abnormal pharyngeal mobility and pharyngeal status, and abnormal cricopharyngeal function. Also, there is slow esophageal transient time. Tongue and mandibular excursions are limited, and formation of the posterior bolus is difficult. It is usually assumed that the patient has difficulty in oral bolus formation, with a loss of coordination between the oral and pharyngeal phases of swallowing.

The patient should be taught to eat smaller portions more frequently, especially in feeding times that are restricted. Usually, the patient does well with general, not special, diets. Timing of medications should coincide with mealtime so that their effects can facilitate oral and pharyngeal movements.

There are various swallowing and stimulation techniques: use of ice, upward stroking under the chin, manual vibration of the laryngopharyngeal musculature, and tilting the head forward as the patient prepares to swallow. Position should be emphasized; the head should be positioned slightly forward to avoid neck extension. Food texture, taste, and temperature are also important. General stimulation techniques to improve the patient's mental status, such as a well-lighted room, proper upright sitting position, and a favorable time of day, should be initiated.

Increased muscle tone can be relaxed with facilitating techniques such as digital compression, muscle stretching, light touching over the skin or muscle areas, or high-frequency vibration. Facilitation techniques can also improve muscle tone, strengthen desired muscles, and redistribute the balance of muscle power. If the muscles are weak, then oral and facial weakness can be improved with various exercises. Exercises such as broadly smiling and tight frowning of lips can be used for the lips and buccal and jaw muscles. Lip pursing and retraction as well as resistant lip exercises can also be done to strengthen muscles. Other exercises, such as blowing on a match, straw, or whistle, are often practiced. These exercises can be done in front of a mirror to improve facial symmetry.

Tongue movements are important, and exercises to strengthen the tongue can be initiated to aid retraction, protraction, lateralization, elevation, and depression. General exercises can include pronouncing certain sounds or pushing the tongue against the depressor. Also the patient can count with the tongue and push the tongue against the side of the cheek, the roof of the mouth, and against the lower lip with isometric contractions.

Adaptive equipment can be used to assist in eating. If the patient is uncoordinated, large-rimmed dishes or plate guards help to keep food from sliding off the plate. Plates can also be weighted on the table to prevent easy displacement from hand tremors. Also, cups can have weighted or large handles to help patients with a poor grip to hold onto the cup. Swivel utensils that make it easier to glide food into the mouth are also available for patients with limited range of motion.

There are various environmental aids that may be helpful to the person with parkinsonian disease. These include zippers or Velcro closures in garments instead of buttons. Also, kitchen and eating utensils with large comfortable handles and appliances that have large handles and knobs may be helpful. Grab-rails are also helpful for the bathtub, toilet, and bedside. The bed and chair should not be too low, and the use of raised toilet seats may help mobility. Stairways should have strong handrails on both sides. Environmental control aids, such as electronic scanning devices and typewriters, are available. In addition, if the patient needs an electrically powered wheelchair, there are control joysticks that can be helpful for independent mobility.

Depression is common in PS patients; some degree of dementia may be present. Therefore, early psychological counseling, involving the entire family, is important in the rehabilitation process.

Bladder dysfunction, with urinary incontinence or retention, has been reported in 45% to 90% of patients.[3, 39] This may be due to the abnormalities in the basal ganglia, medications, preexisting prostatic hypertrophy, or dementia. Bradykinesia, tremors, and rigidity of the extremities can often cause failed attempts at bladder retraining or make the independent use of self-intermittent catheterizations impractical. Levodopa and other antiparkinsonian drugs can cause urinary retention. Proper management of this problem should first include urodynamic testing and cystoscopy. Most patients have hyperreflexive detrusors (bladder); a few have areflexia, and infrequently there is detrusor-sphincter dyssynergia.[39] Anticholinergics, such as propantheline or oxybutynin (Ditropan), are often used for hyperreflexic detrusors. Straining, Credé's maneuver, or catheterizations can be attempted for management of areflexic detrusors. It is important to eliminate urinary tract infections and have the person on a schedule for voiding (e.g., every 3 to 4 hours) and fluid intake.

Parkinsonian patients frequently have bowel problems with chronic constipation as a result of eating poorly, drinking little water, or a general slowing of the muscular action of the bowels.

Patients should make an effort to drink more water and eat foods with high fiber content. Often bulk laxatives, such as Metamucil, are helpful. A fecal softener, dioctyl sodium sulfosuccinate, is another useful laxative. If these approaches are inadequate, a laxative that stimulates the bowel directly may be required, such as bisacodyl (Dulcolax).

Sexual dysfunction also occurs in parkinsonian patients for various reasons from the limitations of body movements to side-effects of several medications. Discussions concerning sexuality and the treatment approach should be individualized to meet the needs of the patient and spouse.

Parkinsonian patients may need to irrigate the eyes with artificial tears because of the discomfort resulting from reduced frequency of blinking. Also seborrhea can usually be controlled with good hygiene.

MEDICATIONS. Pharmacologic therapy for PS is based on the theory that there is a dopamine depletion in the striatum and that the restoration of dopamine toward normal levels will improve symptoms. Multiple medications can be used, such as anticholinergic, antihistaminergic, and dopaminergic drugs. Anticholinergics and antihistaminergics act to improve tremor and some degree of rigidity. They block the unopposed striatal cholinergic system. Side effects are common: early symptoms include dry mouth and later features are vomiting, mental confusion, and hallucinations. They also have atropine-like side effects and can cause urinary retention, dry mouth, poor vision, and constipation.

Dopamine replacement therapy is based on the findings of decreased dopamine content in the substantia nigra and recovery of the patient when normal levels are restored. The pharmacological strategy is an attempt to replace the decreased neurotransmitter. Dopamine is used as the treatment of choice for bradykinesia and rigidity of PS. Incidence of nausea and vomiting and other peripheral side effects can be reduced by combining levodopa with a peripheral decarboxylase inhibitor (Sinemet).

Another drug treatment for PS involves dopamine agonists. The dopamine agonist directly stimulates the dopamine receptors by bypassing the metabolic pathways with synthesized dopamine. Bromocriptine is the most widely studied dopamine agonist, and its clinical efficacy is comparable to that of levodopa.[17] Generally, dopamine agonists are relegated to the role of adjunct therapy, and they are usually used with levodopa or Sinemet.

Peripheral side effects of medical therapy can include psychosis, confusion, memory impairment, hallucinations, and delirium, probably owing to overstimulation of the dopamine receptors in the limbic system. Some patients have sleep disruptions, night tremors, visual hallucinations, and nightmares.

The second problem associated with medical therapy is dyskinesia, or abnormal voluntary movements such as chorea or dystonia. These can be serious and are usually due to excessive dopamine receptor stimulation in which the dopamine receptors may be denervated and highly sensitive.

A serious limitation of chronic dopamine therapy is the "off-and-on" phenomenon in which sudden and dramatic fluctuations in parkinsonian symptoms occur. Increased mobility can suddenly alternate with periods of severe akinesia. The "on" episodes are usually accompanied by a dyskinesia of varying intensity. These stages may last from minutes to hours and can occur at any time and in an unpredictable fashion. It is estimated that 50% of these patients are affected if the treatment lasts longer than 5 years. The mechanism of this "off-and-on" phenomenon may be an increased dosage of medications, increased frequency of drug ingestion, decreased dietary intake, or the use of dopamine adrenergic medication. Reducing the dosage of dopamine and taking drug-free holidays may be helpful in improving the "off-and-on" phenomenon.

In summary, medical therapies for parkinsonian disease use a symptomatic approach. They probably do not prevent the progression of this disorder. Only improved understanding of the different causes of PS will lead to improved treatment.

SURGERY. Surgical options are increasing for patients with parkinsonian disease. Stereotaxic thalamotomy may be useful in patients who have tremors as their primary disabling symptom.[43] The operation improves tremors and partially relieves rigidity but has no effect on bradykinesia, which is often the most disabling aspect of the disease. If bilateral tremors are present, the operation has to be performed bilaterally, and this may result in dysarthria and hemiparesis; death may occur as a complication of the surgery.

Supranuclear Palsy

Progressive supranuclear palsy (PSP) was first described by W. C. Posey in 1904.[42] Only a small percentage of patients with parkinsonian symptoms develop clinical signs consistent with progressive PSP. The onset of this movement problem is in the fifth and sixth decades and there is a slight male predominance. The symptoms of onset are often vague, with disequilibrium occurring in the majority of these patients and mental changes or disturbed vision occurring in a large percentage. Often there are associated symptoms such as dementia, cerebellar abnormalities, dysphasia, and marked dysarthria. Progressive supranuclear palsy is usually more progressive than parkinsonian symptoms and the majority of these patients die within the first decade after onset.[29] The most distinguishing feature of supranuclear palsy is supranuclear ophthalmoparesis.[29] The initial complaints are difficulty in walking and frequent falling. Tremor is lacking in PSP. However, PSP is similar to PS in that both include bradykinesia, rigidity, and postural instability. In PSP, the rigidity predominantly affects the axial musculature, resulting in hypertonicity of the neck extensors, whereas it is more diffuse in idiopathic PS. Gait is often stiff and broad based, and the facial expression of a person with PSP is one of worry and anguish.

Patients with PSP develop pseudobulbar palsy, with hypokinetic dysarthria, dysphagia, sialorrhea, explosive cough, hyperactive gag reflex, and emotional lability. The main clinical feature is vertical gaze palsy. It can lag behind diagnosis of other features by months or years. In addition, 25% to 31% of these patients complain of difficulty with downward gaze during the early stages of the disease.[25] Also, many complain of poor vision, dry or tearing eyes, photophobia, diplopia, and eyelids that close involuntarily. The vertical gaze palsy is easily overcome early in the disease process by oculocephalic maneuvers, confirming the supranuclear origin of the ophthalmoparesis. Initially, downward gaze is impaired, but later the upper lateral gaze and conversion become involved and impaired. Later in the disease process oculocephalic or even caloric stimulation may not be sufficient to overcome the oculomotor palsy, indicating extensive brain stem involvement.

Neurobehavorial features, including forgetfulness, irritability, withdrawal, depression, sleep disturbances, spatial disorientation, and apraxia, may be present. There is often subcortical dementia or degeneration within the brain stem or in the basal ganglia. Most of these patients do poorly on psychological tests because of the visuomotor and visual scanning problems and dysarthria. When the disorder involves the cerebellum,

there are associated symptoms of a broad-based gait and motor incoordination of the hands and feet.

The laboratory features include a normal blood cell count and a negative brain scan. The electroencephalogram is often abnormal and the computed tomographic scan may show atrophy.[25] Pathologically there is a mild-to-moderate atrophy, particularly in the brain stem and cerebellum, with dilation of the third and fourth ventricles. Histological examination reveals neuron loss, gliosis, granulovacuolar degeneration, and neurofibrillary tangles. Histological abnormalities are also found broadly in the brain stem and basal ganglia regions.

Patients usually have marked functional abnormalities in eating, reading, writing, and dressing, and they have difficulty in ambulation and deficiencies in vision. A small percentage may have bladder and bowel dysfunction, whereas others have difficulty with swallowing.

Rehabilitation usually involves a team approach with a neurologist and physiatrist, a psychologist, and physical, occupational, and speech therapists. The therapeutic goals and approaches are similar to those mentioned in the treatment of PS, except that adaptive aids (prism glasses) and environmental aids (mirrors) are needed to compensate for the visual gaze palsy. In addition, because of the rapid downhill course of the disease, closer supervision and more frequent follow-up are needed.

The pharmacological management includes antiparkinsonian drugs. In the early stages of the disorder, anticholinergics or carbidopa-levodopa may be helpful.[1] Dopamine agonists (*e.g.,* bromocriptine) may also have some benefit. Unfortunately, medication does not slow the progression of the disorder.

HYPERKINETIC MOVEMENT DISORDERS

Tremors

Tremors are the most common form of involuntary movement disorder. They tend to be repetitive, stereotyped movements that are irregular and are produced by involuntary contraction of the reciprocally innervated antagonistic muscles.[26] The antagonist and agonist muscles may be contracting alternately or in synchrony, and the movements may be continuous or intermittent. During normal muscle action, motor units are constantly discharged independently to maintain posture, and this regulates movement of the limb. When the motor unit discharges become synchronized or arrhythmic to the degree that they impair normal activity, tremors become noticeable and a functional problem can develop.

Tremors can be classified as physiological, resting, action, and intentional tremors. Physiological tremors are usually peripheral and are normal. They are caused by circulating catecholamines landing on different receptors, causing a motor unit to fire in a synchronized rhythmic fashion.[36] These tremors often increase with any emotional stress, especially anxiety, fright, nervousness, or anger. They also are aggravated by fatigue, hypoglycemia, thyrotoxicosis, pheochromocytoma, exercise, alcohol, and fever, and they can be drug induced. Usually they are not of any clinical significance, and they can be blocked with β-blockers such as propranolol. Usually the patient needs to avoid the aggravating activities and be assured that there is nothing seriously wrong.

Resting tremors are pathognomonic of parkinsonian disease and are most commonly seen in this disorder. They are also characteristic of essential tremors and anxiety and can be seen in patients who have thyrotoxicosis or are taking lithium treatments. In these tremors, the antagonistic muscles alternately contract at a rate of approximately three per second.[44] They usually do not limit functional activities, are present at rest, and decrease on action. These tremors can easily be treated with anticholinergic drugs such as trihexyphenidyl and benztropine.

Action tremors are common and usually occur during motor tasks. This tremor has a synchronous quality; the agonist and antagonist muscles contract together at a rapid rate of approximately nine per second.[26] A person whose voice shakes when he or she gives a talk in public has a type of action tremor. An essential tremor is classified as an action tremor but has no known cause. It is usually a benign and familial disorder that is more pronounced on intention and is aggravated by anxiety and disappears during sleep. Titubation of the head and tremors of the voice are frequent features of these tremors. The symptoms often progress with age. People with this type of tremor often seek some relief because it interferes with their normal daily activities. Often they cannot work because the tremor becomes embarrassing. Prevalence of essential tremors or action tremors is approximately 4.2 per 1,000 in the United States, or approximately 500,000 people.[26] They usually develop in adolescence or in adulthood and may be progressive. Often the person is not aware of it until someone points it out. If they involve the upper extremities, the tremors are usually asymmetrical and absent at rest. When the arms maintain any static postural position, the tremor is usually produced. Often there are abduction-adduction movements of the fingers with flexion-extension movements of the hand that are seen when patients hold their hands straight in front of them. These movements often interfere with normal daily activities such as writing, drinking, or eating. Head and voice tremors can also occur. When they occur in the trunk or leg, they can interfere with lower extremity coordination. The pathology of these tremors is unknown. Unlike resting tremors, they tend to progress more into the proximal muscles, and they have an increased frequency of approximately 7 to 11 contractions per second. Also, unlike resting tremors, they are exacerbated by intensive voluntary control and by emotional and physical stress.

Action tremors can also be treated with β-blockers such as propranolol and benzodiazepines such as diazepam (Valium) or chlordiazepoxide (Librium). Measures to reduce or alleviate anxiety are often helpful for these patients. Occupational therapy can help these patients. They can be taught to use straws when drinking if their facial tremors are marked and to press hard with a felt-tipped pen and limit the size of script so as to prevent a sudden jerking when writing. The use of weights on the extremities to decrease tremors may improve the patient's ability to do fine motor activities.

Another type of tremor is the intentional tremor, which is often seen in cerebellar disorders. It is both a postural and a kinetic tremor and appears on initiation of movement or during the movement. The tremor is often coarse and has a side-to-side component. The amplitude of the tremor increases as the arm is extended or as it reaches toward the target. It is often due to lesions of the lateral cerebellar nuclei. Tremor frequency is generally three to five contractions per second.[1] Oscillating movements become wider as the arm approaches its target and when reaching for different objects. Titubation of the head is often involved: the head nods by alternating contraction of the flexor and extensor muscles of the neck. Treatment is usually unsatisfactory, but the tremor can be improved by weighting the affected limb.[23]

The various types of tremors mentioned can affect speech when they involve the extrinsic and intrinsic muscles of the larynx and result in dysphonia. The voice becomes quivery, with rhythmic alterations in pitch and loudness. Speech therapy may be beneficial for patients who require clarity of speech.

Tics

Tics are sustained nonrhythmic muscle contractions[18] that are stereotyped, purposeless, and rapid. They usually occur in the same extremity or body part. Often the person is able to suppress the tics voluntarily, but it requires great effort and is often difficult to sustain. Usually, the tic occurs in moments of tension or psychological stress. Most often, the muscles of the face and neck are involved, and movements are usually of a rotational type away from the midline of the body. Most patients have a single type of tic, such as eye-blinking or involuntary rotary movements of the head. The shoulder is also commonly affected, followed by the trunk, limb girdle, and distal extremities. The symptoms occur mainly in males. Twelve to 24% of normal children have a tic, which occurs between the ages of 5 and 10 years.[46] They can often be seen in children who have no abnormalities of personality or intelligence, and they usually disappear by the end of adolescence. Tics have not been noted to cause any physical impairment in function; however, a tic may make the person withdraw from social contacts because of the embarrassment of the tic movements. Often, an increase of anxiety increases tic movements, followed by even more anxiety. The exact etiology is unknown, although it is thought that it may represent either repressed desires or conflicts, subtle brain damage, or transient maturational changes that occur in the central nervous system.

Treatment has been largely unsuccessful, since neither psychosocial therapies nor medication has more to offer than spontaneous remission. Prognosis is usually good because most tics disappear spontaneously, and only a small percentage of patients carry these movements into adult life. If the tics become multiple, Gilles de la Tourette syndrome should be considered. Rehabilitation is directed toward measures to decrease anxiety and provide relaxation. The use of biofeedback to decrease tics has not been evaluated.

Gilles de la Tourette Syndrome

Gilles de la Tourette syndrome is an involuntary movement disorder characterized by onset in childhood of multiple tics and unusual vocalizations. The disorder is named after George Gilles de la Tourette who, in 1885, described nine patients with multiple tics, strange cries, echolalia, and coprolalia.[15] This syndrome occurs mainly in males, and its typical onset is between 4 and 12 years of age, with a median age of 7 years. It has been estimated that approximately 100,000 Americans may have this disorder.[8, 31] In one study, the prevalence was 4.6 per million per year.[10, 33] The primary symptoms of this disorder are multiple facial motor tics accompanied by vocal tics. It can begin as a simple tic involving the eye or facial grimacing, which is often replaced by a second tic symptom. It can appear quite suddenly with movements of the head and neck, shoulders, trunk, or legs. The severity of the tics varies greatly, and there are transient complete remissions.

The vocal tics occur along with motor tics, and the disorder may first manifest itself as a nervous cough or snorting sound. This occurs because of spontaneous contractions of the respiratory and phonation muscles. At times, explosive vocalizations occur with jerking of the head and with loud cries and yips. The person often develops restlessness and appears hyperactive with a short attention span owing to the motor and vocal tics. This often leads to poor school performance.

Patients have different tic sensations at different times in their lives. Sometimes the patient has few symptoms whereas at other times he or she is socially incapacitated. Tic movements usually increase with stress, especially when the person is in public, but the movements disappear with sleep.

Coprolalia, the involuntary use of obscenities, is present in 60% of these patients and is the most socially disabling aspect of Gilles de la Tourette syndrome. It can be the initial symptom in young adolescents and must be distinguished from voluntary cursing. Often patients conceal the curse by verbalizing only the first syllable or altering a letter.

Other features of this syndrome include copropraxia, in which the patient uses obscene gestures, and echolalia. Some echo whole sentences, where as others only echo a few words. Echopraxia, the imitation of other people's mannerisms, also occurs.

Emotional problems are common in children who have Gilles de la Tourette syndrome. Attention-deficit disorders and learning problems are also common in these children.[8] Self-destructive behavior, aggressive outbursts, antisocial behavior, and delinquent behavior have been reported. Many of these patients may have behavior difficulties in adult life.

Owing to the multiple manifestations of Gilles de la Tourette syndrome, it has been confused with many other conditions. Usually, it is confused with transient tics of childhood, which are common in youngsters. These benign and transient tics usually occur in one or two muscle groups and most frequently involve eye movements.

There is no cure for Gilles de la Tourette syndrome and, therefore, treatment is usually symptomatic. Haloperidol is widely used and is generally effective.[45] Benzodiazepines and clonazepam help by reducing anxiety; however, they can produce addiction and withdrawal effects. Psychotherapy is indicated in patients having behavioral problems. Early identification and special education of children with learning disorders are needed. Relaxation exercises and biofeedback reduce anxiety and may also have some benefit. Surgery, such as stereotaxic surgery, is not recommended, except in incapacitating cases.

Myokymia

Myokymia is characterized by continuous, fine, rhythmic, undulating, wavelike fascicular twitchings of muscles. It can involve facial muscles, or it can be generalized, as in peripheral neuropathy, thyrotoxicosis, and after physical exertion. A localized form has been associated with multiple sclerosis, brainstem tumor, and Guillain-Barré syndrome. In multiple sclerosis, myokymia may disappear spontaneously in approximately 6 weeks. In brain stem tumors, myokymia is often the initial symptom and may be the only symptom for years, gradually giving way to paralysis. In either condition, contractions often persist during sleep and disappear after nerve blockage. In Guillain-Barré syndrome, myokymia usually occurs in clinically weak muscles and is often bilateral and transient.

It is believed that in brainstem tumors, myokymia is caused by disordered activation of the facial nucleus by the tumor. In myokymia associated with multiple sclerosis, it may result from the release of the inhibitory influence of the reticular formation secondary to demyelination. Treatment is usually of the underlying disease, because the movement disorder causes no functional limitations.

Dystonia

Dystonia is probably the least understood of the movement disorders. It consists of slow, sustained torsional movements of the somatic musculature. These movements can occur anywhere on the body but most often on the trunk, neck, and proximal limb muscles. The movement disorder may be generalized, segmental, or focal, and it is usually not progressive. Dystonia resembles athetosis, but the movement is a more sustained isometric muscle contraction. Dystonia can be an isolated disorder or may be associated with other neurological symptoms. It has been defined by Herz as slow, long-sustained turning movements of the head and trunk and rotation of the upper and lower extremities.[22] The rapid movements are usually continuous and repetitive. Dystonia usually increases with anxiety, pain, emotional or physical stress, or fatigue, and it ceases with sleep. Quality and severity of movement vary throughout the day. It can be absent in the morning and more pronounced in the evening. Dystonia can have characteristics of any one of a wide range of movement disorders. When it involves slow movements, it often overlaps with athetoid movements. When the movements become more rapid, it can be labeled as chorea.

Frequently, patients develop methods to decrease the dystonic movements. Change in posture and touching of the affected body part can stop or decrease abnormal movements. The use of sensory stimulation can also help in diagnosis. It has been commonly misdiagnosed in the past as being a hysterical voluntary-movement problem.

The anatomical and pharmacological bases of dystonia are unknown. It can be seen in association with other movement disorders. It also can be a feature of Wilson's disease, encephalitis, and hyperparathyroidism. Reversible dystonias may occur as a side-effect of neuroleptic or levodopa therapy. Ofter there is a dopamine-acetylcholine imbalance that appears to be important in dystonia, as shown by the worsening of dystonia with physostigmine therapy and by the more consistent improvement with anticholinergic therapy than with dopaminergic agents.[9]

Dystonias can be either primary or secondary.[9] The primary dystonias have no other neurological abnormalities, whereas the secondary dystonias have other neurological findings. The primary dystonias are characterized by a slow, progressive course that can plateau at any time. Primary dystonia usually begins as an action dystonia and dystonic postures rarely develop. In contrast, the secondary dystonias begin with dystonia at rest and dystonic posture is sustained. Secondary dystonias that involve a metabolic disease, such as Wilson's disease, tend to have a rapid progressive course. However, the secondary dystonias, that are due to environmental causes, such as head exposure to toxins, tend to have a clinical course that stabilizes and does not progress.

Dystonias have been classified into four different types: focal, segmental, multifocal, and generalized (Table 24-2).[10, 37] Focal dystonia refers to the presence of dystonic movements in a single body part, such as the neck (torticollis), periorbital region

Table 24-2
Types of Dystonia

Focal
Torticollis (neck)
Blepharospasm (periorbital)
Oromandibular (mouth or jaw)
Writer's or occupational cramp (arm or leg)

Segmental
Cranial
Brachial
Crural

Multifocal
Generalized
Dystonia musculorum deformans

(blepharospasm), mouth and jaw (oromandibular dystonia), and limbs (writer's or occupational cramps or leg dystonia). Segmental dystonias are dystonic movements that start in one body part and spread to other regions. The dystonia spreads in a contiguous fashion such as leg to trunk to neck to arm, arm to neck to trunk, or face to jaw to neck to larynx to arm.[37] Such movement disorders are described as cranial dystonia, brachial dystonia (arm with and without trunk), and crural dystonia (leg with and without trunk). The third type of dystonia is the multifocal type, which occurs in more than one focal area but is not generalized. Generalized dystonia usually involves the trunk, at least one leg, and an additional body part and frequently affects walking. Generalized dystonias, such as dystonia musculorum deformans, usually have their onset in childhood.

Speech can also be affected in dystonia because of unusual postures of the speech musculature. Slurred speech often occurs along with a hyperkinetic dysarthria, marked irregularities in precision of articulation, and inconsistent control of loudness. Speech is often slow, with prolongation of certain intervals between syllables and with the insertion of inappropriate silent periods.

There is no effective medical therapy for dystonia. Symptomatic therapy usually consists of trials of sedatives, phenothiazines, muscle relaxants, and antiparkinsonian drugs. They rarely have any significant benefit. Levodopa has both improved and aggravated the dystonic condition. Drug-induced dystonia requires elimination of the offending drug. It is important to rule out certain disease states, such as Wilson's disease, which often responds well to D-penicillamine.

Physical therapy is given to maintain range of motion, strength, and mobility. Often these patients develop tension myalgia; therefore, heat modalities and sedative massage are helpful. The use of electric therapy and biofeedback for patients with dystonia needs further investigation.[2] Relaxation exercises and steroid injections at painful trigger points are usually of some benefit. Occupational therapy is also needed for many patients to instruct them in the use of adaptive aids, energy-saving techniques, swallowing methods, and chair and bed positioning. Orthoses help to stabilize abnormal posture if the dystonic movements are quick and the orthosis is used at intervals.

There are surgical options such as stereotaxic surgery, but the side-effects (e.g., pseudobulbar palsy) can be serious.

Oromandibular Dystonia

Oromandibular dystonia involves muscles of the jaw, pharynx, and tongue. The mentalis and platysma muscles may also be involved. The jaw or mandible is pulled down or up during this movement disorder. The movements are repetitive, with occasional retraction. The jaw can be retracted and at times is deviated to the side. In lingual dystonia, the tongue has abnormal movements when the patient begins to speak or is tempted to bring food to the back of the pharynx during deglutition. When this dystonia is present during speaking, the tongue tends to protrude between the teeth, producing a marked lisping. When this dystonia is present during eating, the tongue tends to force the food forward out of the mouth instead of backward toward the pharynx. Occupational and speech therapy can help to improve swallowing and speech problems. Techniques such as the ones reviewed for patients with PS can be used.

Meige's Syndrome

Meige's syndrome was described by Jankovic and Ford[27] as a combination of blepharospasm and orofacial-cervical dystonia. It was first described by Henri Meige in 1910 and consists of sustained forceful closure of the eyelids or grimacing, platysma contractions, and sustained neck flexion. Women are usually affected more than men. The mean age at onset is usually in the sixth decade of life. It is a rare movement disorder and is frequently misdiagnosed. This movement disorder has been studied neuropathologically in only a few cases. One case was normal, and another showed patchy neuronal loss, with severe gliosis of the dorsal striatum. Usually the person has central tremors and other movement disorders such as dystonia of the neck, trunk or extremities. Patients are often treated with pharmocotherapies that include anticholinergics, baclofen, benzodiazepines, haloperidol, monoamine oxidase inhibitors, phenothiazines, and tetrabenazine. Therapeutic exercises to improve or maintain posture, relaxation, and range-of-motion exercises can be prescribed.

Blepharospasm

Blepharospasm usually begins with increased blinking of the eyelids. Some patients may complain of eye irritability or the feeling of sand in the eyes. With progression, there is more sustained closure of the lids; with further progression there is forceful closure of the lids. Episodes are usually brief or can be prolonged and vary throughout the day. Sunlight and driving tend to make the blepharospasm more pronounced. Transient remissions occur while talking, humming, and singing. Recently, botulism toxin injections have been used with temporary success.[12]

Writer's or Occupational Cramp

Writer's cramp is a focal dystonia involving the dominant hand and wrist. It appears as an uncontrollably tense grip of a pen or a pencil, accompanied by flexion of the wrist and marked pressure of the point against the paper. It may be associated with jerking or sustained movements. Usually, other coordinated movements of the hand are normal. It is an action dystonia in which a specific activity such as writing, or other occupational activity, brings on involuntary movement. Other specific dystonias have also been reported and are usually related to the person's occupation, especially those in which the arm maintains a specific posture; those dystonias include musician's cramp in pianists, violinists, and harpists and telegrapher's cramp. Often the movement varies with the posture of the trunk and shoulder girdle. Patients may be able to write while standing at a blackboard but have difficulty when writing at a desk. A history of always having gripped a pen or pencil tightly and always having found prolonged writing to be difficult is usually noted in these patients.

Physical therapy is directed at maintenance of a normal range of motion and re-education for movement patterns related to the dystonic posture. Relaxation exercises are helpful. In addition, occupational therapy can be of help in teaching the patient to use the opposite hand to write, in improving posture, or in making splints that can prevent the dystonic posture. Biofeedback from the involved muscles has been used, but the results appear to be short term.

Spasmodic Torticollis

Spasmodic torticollis is an involuntary movement disorder characterized by variable-rate, hyperkinetic, usually asymmetrical contractions of the muscles about the cervical spine. These contractions result in a variable degree of repetitive semiarrhythmic movements of the head. The condition is presumed to be of central nervous system origin, although the site and mechanism of the pathophysiology are unknown.[5]

The patients are usually female, and onset of this movement

disorder is usually in the fourth or fifth decade of life. The muscles most involved in the dystonic (hypertonic) process are the sternocleidomastoid, trapezius, and posterior neck muscles. The movement can be tonic, dystonic, or choreic and the head can be in an antecolic (forward) or retrocolic (backward) position. Patients usually have restricted cervical spine motion, facial dyskinesia, horizontal and vertical head tremors, and reduction of the ipsilateral arm swing with walking. A smaller number have associated speech dysfunction (hyperkinetic dyskinesia) and static hand tremors. Abnormal structural finding on roentgenograms can include thoracolumbar scoliosis and upper cervical scoliosis.

Historically, different activities have a marked effect on the severity of torticollis symptoms. Improvement or disappearance of symptoms occurs with sleeping, in the first several minutes of awakening, with relaxation, and with distraction. Activities that aggravate the symptoms include emotional stress, walking, increased muscular activity, sitting for longer than 30 minutes, and being in a cool and humid climate. Usually the patient's posture influences the severity of symptoms. Improvement of symptoms occurs with the use of antagonistic gestures of either hand to various head or facial sites. Lying supine and dangling the head also improve symptoms. Symptoms are frequently aggravated by prolonged standing or walking and direct ocular gazing contralateral to the direction of the face and chin rotation.

Spontaneous remission can occur in a small percentage of patients, and the rate of remission is highest in younger females.[11] However, recurrence after remission is possible.

Many patients have a family history of other movement disorders, and some have close relatives who have spasmodic torticollis. An association with thyroid disease has been reported.

All patients have limitations of their functional capabilities beginning within 6 to 12 hours of the onset of torticollis symptoms. Most experience limitations at work, and some are forced to quit or retire early owing to their torticollis. The type of work that is limited ranges from secretarial work to the practice of law. The increased muscular activity, pain, and restrictive postures and the need to reduce stress are usually the reasons cited for the limited ability to work.

Patients are also limited in their ability to participate in sports and hobbies. Sports commonly limited are golf and bowling, which involve standing, looking down, and swinging of the upper extremity. Hobbies that involve looking down and using the hands, such as knitting, are also limited.

Driving is difficult for most patients because of the abnormal posture of the head, limiting vision; prolonged sitting; and emotional stress. Many patients limit the distances driven and use high-backed seats and cervical collars for bi-occipital support. Many patients feel restricted in their social life. They often feel embarrassed, lack confidence, and state, "everywhere I go people stare at me."

Rehabilitation of spasmodic torticollis involves a team approach with neurology, physiatry, occupational and physical therapy, and other therapies. The objective of physical therapy is to minimize any abnormal proprioceptive input to the central nervous system by prescribing exercises and physical modalities to relieve painful stimuli, reduce muscle spasms, and correct postural malalignment.

Heat modalities and sometimes cryokinetics, as well as deep sedative massage, are used over painful areas. In addition, trigger-point steroid injections have been helpful. Cervical range-of-motion exercises, usually with the head supported, dangling, or while the patient is supine, can maintain symmetrical range of motion around the neck. Shoulder girdle exercises, consisting of shoulder shrugs and pectoralis stretching, are prescribed for

patients who have a marked degree of trapezius involvement of a shoulder. Isometric exercises to strengthen the contralateral noninvolved sternocleidomastoid and reciprocal relaxation to the involved sternocleidomastoid muscle are helpful for decreasing discomfort. Relaxation exercise with biofeedback over involved muscles and regular biofeedback exercises to decrease muscle tone can be used. Use of a mirror for postural alignment may also be helpful. Although Brudny and co-workers[4] reported a 50% improvement with biofeedback, it is not often helpful because multiple muscles are involved. Electrical stimulation to decrease the spasticity of the torticollis, thus far, has not been proven to be of benefit.

Several medications can be used to treat spasmodic torticollis. Patients are usually started on perphenazine/amitriptyline (Triavil) therapy, and, if needed, benztropine is added later to potentiate its action. If this therapy is unsuccessful, or if the movement disorder was retrocollis, then haloperidol, with benztropine and amitriptyline to minimize its side effects, has been of benefit. Other medications, such as lithium and trihexyphenidyl, have been tried and are successful. If the patient has associated tremors, various benzodiazepine derivatives and propranolol are used.

Various surgical procedures have been attempted to correct spasmodic torticollis. These have included myotomy of the sternocleidomastoid, neurectomy of the spinal accessory nerves unilaterally or bilaterally, and stereotaxic, multiple cervical rhizotomies.[20] Numerous complications occurred, including dysarthria, tremors, and ataxia with combined spinal accessory nerve section. Cervical fusion has no benefit and may be complicated by breaking of the fusion postoperatively.

Treatment of spasmodic torticollis was also reported by suppression of labyrinthine mechanisms.[6] Dorsal cord stimulation has also been used, with electrodes inserted at the C1-C2 levels and extending down to the C5-C6 level.[14]

In summary, spasmodic torticollis can be a disabling disorder in which cervical motion is restricted and dystonic muscular contractions lead to significant disfigurement and discomfort. Almost every aspect of daily living can be affected. Activities, particularly those involving the use of the upper extremities and cervical muscles, cold or humid climate, and unsupported upright posture, frequently exacerbate the symptoms of torticollis. This leads to difficulties in work, driving, and recreational activities. Associated neurological findings also lead to difficulties in eating and communication. Psychosocial problems frequently encountered are usually related to poor self-concept generated by the torticollis or associated neurological phenomena (facial dyskinesia, dysarthria, tremor). Therefore, recommendations for treatment involve a full rehabilitation program, including medical, physical, speech, and occupational therapy and social, psychological, and vocational counseling.

Dystonia Musculorum Deformans

Dystonia musculorum deformans is a specific entity that is a rare hereditary disease that occurs most frequently in families of Russian-Jewish descent. The onset of symptoms begins between age 5 and 15 years, and they consist of sustained movements with torsional spasms initially involving the lower extremity and pelvis, resulting in a gait disturbance. The muscles of the upper extremity, neck, and face may be involved later in the course of the disease. Symptoms consist of dysarthria, facial grimacing, and torticollis. Involuntary movements and spasm often increase with volitional movements or anxiety and disappear with sleep. The disease often is confused with hysterical and other psychological disturbances, and it usually progresses to death within 5 to 10 years in the more severe forms.

Pathological changes in the basal thalamus have been observed, but no specific lesion has been found. Treatment often involves the use of anticholinergic drugs, with a slowly increased dose to produce the optimal effect without any unacceptable side-effects. These medications can consist of trihexyphenidyl and clonazepam. In addition, diazepam and baclofen have been tried.

Physical therapy includes the start of range-of-motion exercises, positioning in a chair or bed, mat activities, and mobility training. Occupational therapy is used for activities of daily living, environmental aids, adaptive equipment, energy-saving techniques, and communication aids.

Hemifacial Spasm

Hemifacial spasm is the most frequent form of facial hyperkinesia. It is uncommon and has an insidious onset of paroxysmal involuntary hyperkinetic facial movements. It is usually twice as frequent in women, usually in middle life, and rarely occurs beyond the fifth and sixth decades.[32] It can cause physical limitations by interfering with vision. In addition, it can cause a great amount of social and psychological discomfort. Often it is aggravated by emotional stress, fatigue, and involuntary facial movements. Spontaneous remission is rare and hemifacial spasms can easily increase in frequency over time. Occasionally, there is a tonic contraction in which sustained involuntary contraction can occur, with eye closure and with elevation of the corner of the mouth. The spasms are usually tonic, beginning in the orbicularis oculi muscle and later involving other muscles innervated by the seventh cranial nerve. Rarely is the frontalis muscle involved. The exact etiology of hemifacial spasm is unknown, but it may involve the cerebral cortex, facial nucleus, or the peripheral end of the facial nerve. The current controversy about the pathogenesis centers around the hypothesis that vascular compression of the facial nerve in the posterior fossa may be responsible for the hemifacial spasm.[32]

The diagnosis of hemifacial spasm is made from the history and clinical examination. It is important that other causes are ruled out and, therefore, computed tomographic scans, roentgenograms, angiograms, electromyograms, and electronystagmograms should be obtained. These will rule out any serious problem.

Numerous medical treatments for hemifacial spasm have been tried and include vasodilators, anticholinergics, local anesthetics, and antipsychotic agents. Also, biofeedback has been attempted.[34] Thus far, none of these measures have been successful. Usually carbamazepine (Tegretol) is the initial treatment of choice. However, control studies of its benefits are lacking.[47] Overall, hemifacial spasm has proven refractory to medical management in the vast majority of cases.

Surgical methods have included injection of alcohol or local analgesics, acupuncture, neurotomy, needle insertion, and decompression within the temporal bone and other variants of this operation. Newer surgical techniques include percutaneous thermolysis, radiofrequency coagulation, and microsurgical decompression.[1] Recent success has involved a retromastoid craniotomy to relieve pressure on the facial nerve. However, complications such as dysfunction of the seventh and eighth cranial nerves have occurred.[32] Microvascular decompression completely relieved symptoms in 81% of 44 patients. However, 15% had permanent hearing loss.[1]

Physical therapy can be given to these patients and includes facial exercises, relaxation exercises, and counseling to help minimize the social and psychological stress of this problem.

The effectiveness of electric therapy, such as transcutaneous nerve stimulation, has not been adequately researched.

Athetosis

Athetosis was first described by Hammond[19] in 1871 as involuntary, irregular, slow, writhing, and repeated movements. It consists of cramplike spasmodic movements that are slower than choreiform movements and less sustained than dystonia. Its movement characteristics are between the extremes of chorea and dystonia. Athetoid movements may be separate from or in combination with either of these two other movement disorders. It is usually a result of relatively sustained, unequal contractions of the agonist and antagonist muscle groups. It often leads to a bizarre but characteristic disturbance of posture. These abnormal movements and postures are often exacerbated by voluntary movements or mental effort and are relieved by relaxation or sleep.

Any body part may be affected, but the face and distal upper extremities are more often involved and athetosis may be accompanied by hemiplegia. Various types of athetosis have been reported. One is a generalized idiopathic form, but most often athetosis is a secondary or acquired disorder that follows cerebral infarction, hemorrhage, tumor, central nervous system storage diseases, Wilson's disease, and Hallervorden-Spatz disease.

Treatment is usually symptomatic and not particularly effective. Hemiathetosis has been helped by stereotaxic thalamotomy, but the outcome of the procedure is variable and difficult to predict. It should only be carried out by someone experienced in the procedure. Physical therapy is directed toward maintaining normal range of motion and strength, correcting postural abnormalities, and maintaining the patient's independent mobility. Occupational therapy is directed at using adaptive aids to help open cans and doors and to handle keys. In addition, weighting the limbs with 1- to 3-pound weights can be of help.

Tardive Dyskinesia

Tardive dyskinesia is an abnormal, involuntary movement of the tongue, lips, and facial muscles that is sometimes described as choreiform movement or dystonic movement. These involuntary movements are sometimes called buccal-lingual-masticatory dyskinesia. Tardive dyskinesia can also involve mouthing, chewing, sucking, and licking movements of the tongue, as well as puckering, smacking, and other lip movements. It is more common in females and in the elderly and is often seen after prolonged use of antipsychotic drugs, such as phenothiazines and butyrophenones. The prevalence of tardive dyskinesia can be as high as 56% in patients being treated with neuroleptics for prolonged intervals.[10, 28] The pathogenesis of this movement disorder has been related to chronic dopamine receptor-site blockage and the resultant receptor-site hypersensitivity. The neuroleptics probably alter the central dopaminergic balance and cause this overactivity of the dopaminergic system.

The prognosis is often not good, since symptoms frequently become worse. However, if drug induced, the disorder can often be reversed after withdrawal of the neuroleptic drug. Usually, the earlier the symptoms are recognized, the more effective drug withdrawal is in improving the prognosis for recovery. Most often, symptoms disappear in 1 to 2 months after withdrawal, and patients can continue to improve for up to 2 years.[1] Usually, the more mildly affected patients are more likely to experience complete remission.

Medications that have been used to decrease tardive dyskinesia include reserpine, which is used to deplete the brain of dopamine (usually administered in a low dose that is gradually increased) and medications to increase the cholinergic effect, in an attempt to effect a dopaminergic and cholinergic chemical balance.

Prevention of tardive dyskinesia is the best treatment. This can be done by decreasing the dose and by the use of neuroleptic medications. "Drug vacations or holidays" may prevent the disorder. Even more important, early detection of tardive dyskinesia and rapid withdrawal of medication are an optimal approach.

Once tardive dyskinesia occurs, proper posture of the head, neck, and shoulders can make it easier to function and should be taught to the patient. Patients should have adequate dental care, especially if dentures are ill fitting. The patient's movements are usually more apparent when they are relaxed. Therefore, it may be of some value for patients to increase their general activity with walking, swimming, or stationary bicycling. Some patients attempt to control the movements voluntarily and may chew gum. Oral-lingual and facial exercises can be done along with biofeedback, but their effectiveness in tardive dyskinesia is not known.

Chorea

Chorea is a movement disorder characterized by involuntary nonstereotyped, unpredictable, and jerky movements that interfere with coordinated movements.[16] The movements are often rapid and erratic, complex, and often purposeless and can involve any or all body parts. Chorea usually involves the lips, mouth, and tongue. The distal muscles seem to be more affected than the proximal muscles, but generally the movements are diffuse. Often the movements increase with stress and disappear with sleep. A mild form of chorea may be mistaken for restlessness or nervousness. When it is confined to a single limb or joint, it can be mistaken for a tic, which is usually a more stereotyped movement disorder. When it becomes severe, there is prominent facial grimacing, darting movements of the tongue, and twitching or turning of the head, neck, limbs, and trunk. When chorea involves larger muscles, it disrupts voluntary movements and produces an uncoordinated jerking appearance. At times, the person may be able to briefly suppress the abnormal movements but will be unable to maintain the posture of the involved limb. The classic sign of chorea is the "milkmaid's grip." This occurs when the patient is asked to maintain a firm grip on the examiner's hand; the patient's hand begins to alternately contract and relax.

Chorea can be classified as an acute or chronic movement disorder. It may occur acutely in almost any disease of the central nervous system, because it is observed in vasculitis and encephalitis. The use of drugs, including levodopa, is probably the most common cause of acute chorea in many patients being treated for parkinsonian disease. Also, drugs such as amphetamine, opium, and phenytoin have been associated with chorea. Chorea is often associated with other diseases, such as Sydenham's chorea, thyrotoxicosis, systemic lupus erythematosus, and cirrhosis. Structural damage to the subthalamic nucleus from infarction and from stereotaxic thalamotomy have also been known to cause chorea-type movements. Its most familar generalized form is Huntington's chorea, which will be described as a separate movement disorder.

In chorea, the vocal cords occasionally tighten and raise the vocal pitch. Chorea interferes with the normal movements of respiration and articulation. This leads to "jerky" speech, various levels of loudness, breathlessness, hoarseness, and hypernasality.

The drugs used to treat chorea either decrease dopamine availability or increase anticholinergic activity. The major side-effect of this approach is reversible parkinsonian-like symptoms due to dopamine deficiency. Usually the drugs modify the symptoms of chorea but do not affect the underlying disease. Drugs such as phenothiazines and butyrophenones block dopamine as well as the membrane pump, which is necessary for reuptake of dopamine. The main disadvantage of this is that it may damage the dopamine receptors and lead to tardive dyskinesia. The second group of drugs used includes reserpine and tetrabenazine, which block the uptake of dopamine into the presynaptic granules and deplete the brain of dopamine. A third group is represented by α-methyl-*p*-tyrosine, which inhibits tyrosine hydroxylase and prevents the synthesis of dopamine and norepinephrine. Cholinergic stimulators, such as choline and lecithin, have been used to inhibit the release of dopamine.

Rehabilitation can include exercise to maintain range of motion and strength. In addition, adaptive equipment or orthoses that help to stabilize the proximal muscles and trunk are helpful. Weighted cuffs on the hands and feet seem to help some patients coordinate the distal extremities. Stereotaxic thalamotomy has been used, but the outcome of the procedure is not predictable.

Huntington's Chorea

Huntington's chorea is a terminal, involuntary movement disorder. It is a hereditary disorder that is transmitted through autosomal dominant genes. It was first described by George Huntington in 1872 and its prevalence is 4 to 6 persons per 100,000 population.[21, 24] More than 1,000 cases in the United States have been traced to two brothers who migrated from Europe to Long Island. The onset of symptoms can begin anytime from childhood to the seventh and eighth decades. Only a small percent of patients have symptoms that begin in childhood and adolescence, but these patients usually have the more severe course. Usually the choreic movements occur first in the fingers, toes, and facial regions. The early stages of the disorder include choreic movements of the face and extremities that are abrupt and purposeless. Often dysarthria, facial grimacing, and grinding of the teeth are observed. The choreic movements often develop in association with progressive dementia and emotional disturbance.

As this disease progresses, parkinsonian features, dystonia, and restricted eye movements replace chorea as the primary motor problems. Progressive incoordination, immobility, unsteadiness of gait, and dysarthria are also present. The course is often rapid; within a few years there can be constant movements of the extremities, face, and trunk, with almost no purposeful movement. Intellectual impairment begins early and progresses rapidly. Eventually, dementia becomes the most disabling problem. Alcoholism, psychosis, and even violence may occur and lead to suicide.

The psychosis of Huntington's chorea is quite severe. Many of these patients are depressed, become violent, and have schizophrenic symptoms or personality disorders. Ultimately, the patient is institutionalized because of the psychosis. Many of these patients get divorces, have morbid sexual jealousy, and engage in indecent exposure, incest, voyeurism, assault on females, and promiscuity. There is a high incidence of neglect of children and child abuse. The suicide rate is 2,000 times greater than the national average.

The pathology and etiology of Huntington's chorea include deterioration in the basal ganglia, particularly the caudate nucleus. Victims of Huntington's chorea often deteriorate in various stages. At first, occupational skills erode owing to progressive dementia and personality changes. Later, self-care skills deteriorate and are eventually lost. Finally, in the terminal stages of Huntington's chorea, the patient requires constant skilled nursing care. Death usually results from aspiration pneumonia. Symptoms progress over a 10- to 25-year period. Medical therapies have had little beneficial effect on the progression of the disease.[48]

The currently available pharmacotherapy for Huntington's chorea remains limited to symptomatic relief of the movement disorder, depression, and the psychotic manifestations of the disease. In general, these therapies provide only transient benefits and are associated with potentially disabling side-effects. Therapy for the choreic movements often causes unwanted sedation, lethargy, and depression. Treatment with haloperidol or phenothiazines may cause tardive dyskinesia. If patients are receiving these medications, frequent drug-free holidays are encouraged to prevent side-effects. In patients who have disabling parkinsonian features, particularly those with the juvenile onset, antiparkinsonian agents may be beneficial and will help restore mobility and functional capability. If the patient has an affective disorder, various antidepressant therapies may be attempted. Psychotic problems are often not helped by antipsychotic medications. Generally, the patient needs good supportive measures and proper genetic counseling.

Decline in function is usually steady, without any period of remission or exacerbation. The decline varies a great deal and cannot be predicted, especially early in the disorder when work performance initially becomes unsatisfactory. Usually it is necessary at this early stage to have someone else begin financial and estate planning to prepare the person and the family for the further decline in function. The family should be evaluated fully by a social worker during this time.

With progression of the disease, domestic skills begin to wane and additional support is needed at home. The patient will need help to perform normal household duties, such as cleaning, laundering, and preparing meals. The family bears the direct burden during this time because of the loss of domestic skills. Outside help, such as organized community health resources and volunteer agencies, can be useful during this time. Occupational therapy can also be prescribed to help maintain independence at home with adaptive and environmental aids. Physical therapy to maintain mobility should be initiated as the patient becomes more disabled. However, independence in ambulation and daily functioning will eventually be lost, requiring further medical support to assist the patient with speech, swallowing, bladder and bowel function, and general physical care. Later, the patient will need chronic care outside the home because of the large degree of psychological disturbances. Psychotherapy should also involve the family members.

Myoclonus

In 1861 Reynolds first described chronic spasms of epileptics. The term *myoclonus* was first used by Friedreich, as he described the syndrome of paramyoclonus multiplex.[35] Myoclonus means quick movement of muscle. Myoclonic involuntary movement arises from the central nervous system in well-defined short bursts of jerky movements that may be stereotyped. It can occur as polymyoclonus, involving a group of muscles, or it may appear as a repetitive contraction of one muscle. The rapid muscle contractions usually cause joint movement and are quite

similar to the muscle contractions produced by electric shock to a peripheral motor nerve. The movements can be either rhythmic or arrhythmic. In addition, myoclonus can be stimulus linked or occur spontaneously.

Myoclonus can occur in normal people when they are falling asleep. It is also seen in diffuse central nervous system dysfunctions such as acute intoxications, Alzheimer's disease, myoencephalitis, and Jakob-Creutzfeldt disease. Patients may have an overlap between myoclonus and various other dystonic movements. This is called myoclonus dystonia. Unlike tremors that have a sinusoidal movement pattern, the arrhythmic contraction of myoclonus is more like a square wave with a rest interval between each movement.[35]

Myoclonus classification is based on etiology: physiological, essential, epileptic, or symptomatic.[1] Physiological myoclonus occurs in normal people when they are falling asleep, while walking, or when they become anxious. Such things as sleep jerks, anxiety or exercise jerks, and hiccups can be classified as physiological myoclonus. Essential myoclonus occurs when there is no neurological deficit noted in these patients. The pathology is unknown, and the myoclonic jerks often increase with activity. They often produce a disability and are usually aggravated by emotional stress.[35]

The third type of myoclonus is epileptic. The patient usually has no other evidence of cerebral disease. The seizure disorder often dominates the symptomatology. There is no encephalopathy noted with this particular type of myoclonus.

The fourth type is symptomatic myoclonus, which is part of a more widespread encephalopathy and can be either progressive or static. The patient may or may not have epilepsy with this particular type of myoclonus. Symptomatic myoclonus is usually due to an underlying disorder. Myoclonus may occur secondary to the central nervous system storage diseases, spinocerebellar degeneration, dementias, metabolic encephalopathies, and focal central nervous system damage, such as that seen after strokes.[35]

Treatment for myoclonus can include the use of drugs, which has been proven effective for some patients. These drugs include diazepam (Valium), 5-hydroxytryptophan, and clonazepam (Clonopin). Transcutaneous nerve stimulation also has been used with a degree of success.[49]

Asterixis

Asterixis, or absence of a fixed posture, is a sudden and irregular movement disorder characterized by a brief lapse of muscle tone or posture followed by a jerking and rapid movement of the extremities, similar to a bat's wings flapping.[26] Electrophysiologically, it may be a form of "negative myoclonus" produced by an inhibition of the neuron system that controls tonic extension of a limb.[44] Asterixis has been observed in the wrists of patients with Wilson's disease. It usually occurs in the diffuse encephalopathy that follows liver or renal failure. It can also occur in cerebral infarction, in malabsorption syndromes, and with phenytoin (Dilantin) therapy.[40] Treatment is directed at the underlying disorder.

Hemiballismus

Hemiballismus is a rare movement disorder consisting of extremely violent flinging movements of the arms and legs, usually on one side of the body. It is thought to be due to partial destruction of the contralateral subthalamic nucleus, which results in loss of inhibitory influences on the output of the globus pallidus. The lesion could be due to hemorrhage or infarction but may also occur as a result of tumor, abscess, or thalamic injury. If these movements are left unchecked, they can result in exhaustion and, ultimately, death. Neuroleptic agents have been tried in the past with some success. Placing weights on the extremities to slow down the flinging movements may be of some benefit.

REFERENCES

1. Auger RG, Piepgras DG, Laws ER Jr: Hemifacial spasm: Results of microvascular decompression of the facial nerve in 54 patients. Mayo Clin Proc 61:640–644, 1986
2. Bird BL, Cataldo MF: Experimental analysis of EMG feedback in treating dystonia. Ann Neurol 3:310–315, 1978
3. Bradley WE: Neurological disorders affecting the urinary bladder. In Krane RJ, Siroky MD (eds): Clinical Neuro-Urology, pp 245–255. Boston, Little, Brown & Co., 1979
4. Brudny J, Grynbaum BB, Korein J: Spasmodic torticollis: Treatment by feedback display of the EMG. Arch Phys Med Rehabil 55:403–408,1974
5. Duane DD: Torticollis-dystonia-tics. Paper presented at ACP course "Neurology for the Internist," March 7, 1979
6. Duane DD, Svien HJ: Preliminary evaluation of labyrinthine suppression in the treatment of spasmodic torticollis (abstract). Neurology 22:399, 1972
7. Elliott FA, cited in Davis JC: Team management of Parkinson's disease. Am J Occup Ther 31:300–308, 1977
8. Erenberg G, Cruse RP, Rothner AD: Tourette syndrome: An analysis of 200 pediatric and adolescent cases. Cleve Clin Q 53:127–131, 1986
9. Fahn S: The varied clinical expressions of dystonia. Neurol Clin 2:541–554, 1984
10. Fahn S, Jankovic J: Practical management of dystonia. Neurol Clin 2:555–569, 1984
11. Friedman A, Fahn S: Spontaneous remissions in spasmodic torticollis. Neurology 36:398–400, 1986
12. Frueh BR, Felt DP, Wojno TH, Musch DC: Treatment of blepharospasm with botulinum toxin: A preliminary report. Arch Ophthalmol 102:1464–1468, 1984
13. Gaspar P, Gray F: Dementia in idiopathic Parkinson's disease: A neuropathological study of 32 cases. Acta Neuropathol 64:43–52, 1984
14. Gildenberg PL: Comprehensive management of spasmodic torticollis. Appl Neurophysiol 44:233–243, 1981
15. Gilles de la Tourette G: Étude sur une affection nerveuse caractérisée par de l'incoordination motrice accompagnée d'écholalie et de coprolalie. Arch Neurol 9:19–42; 158–200, 1885
16. Godwin-Austen RB: The treatment of the choreas and athetotic dystonias. J R Coll Physicians Lond 13:35–38, 1979
17. Godwin-Austen RB, Smith NJ: Companion of the effects of bromocriptine and levodopa in Parkinson's disease. J Neurol Neurosurg Psychiatry 40:479–482, 1977
18. Golden GS: Tics and Tourette's: A continuum of symptoms? Ann Neurol 4:145–148, 1978
19. Hammond WA: A Treatise on Diseases of the Nervous System. New York, D Appleton, 1871
20. Hassler R, Dieckmann G: Stereotactic treatment of different kinds of spasmodic torticollis. Confin Neurol 32:135–143, 1970
21. Hayden MR: Huntington's Chorea. New York, Springer-Verlag, 1981
22. Herz E: Dystonia: I. Historical review; analysis of dystonic symptoms and physiologic mechanisms involved. Arch Neurol Psychiatry 51:305–318, 1944
23. Hewer RL, Cooper R, Morgan MH: An investigation into the value of treating intention tremor by weighting the affected limb. Brain 95:579–590, 1972
24. Huntington G: On chorea. Med Surg Reporter 26:317–321, 1872
25. Jankovic J: Progressive supranuclear palsy: Clinical and pharmacologic update. Neurol Clin 2:473–486, 1984
26. Jankovic J, Fahn S: Physiologic and pathologic tremors: Diagnosis, mechanism, and management. Ann Intern Med 93:460–465, 1980
27. Jankovic J, Ford J: Blepharospasm and orofacial-cervical dystonia: Clinical and pharmacological findings in 100 patients. Ann Neurol 13:402–411, 1983
28. Klawans HL, Goetz CG, Perlik S: Tardive dyskinesia: Review and update. Am J Psychiatry 137:900–908, 1980
29. Kristensen, MØ: Progressive supranuclear palsy—20 years later. Acta Neurol Scand 71:177–189, 1985
30. Kurland LT: Epidemiology: Incidence, geographic distribution and genetic considerations. In Fields WS (ed): Pathogenesis and Treatment of Parkinsonism, pp 5–43. Springfield, IL, Charles C Thomas, 1958
31. Lees AJ: Tics and Related Disorders, pp 22–56. New York, Churchill Livingstone, 1985
32. Loeser JD, Chen J: Hemifacial spasm: Treatment by microsurgical facial nerve decompression. Neurosurgery 13: 141–145, 1983
33. Lucas AR, Beard CM, Rajput AH, Kurland LT: Tourette syndrome in Rochester, Minnesota, 1968–1979. Adv Neurol 35:267–269, 1982
34. Maroon JC: Hemifacial spasm: A vascular cause. Arch Neurol 35:481–483, 1978
35. Marsden CD, Fahn S: Movement Disorders. Boston, Butterworth Scientific, 1982
36. Marsden CD, Foley TH, Owen DAL, McAllister RG: Peripheral β-adrenergic receptors concerned with tremor. Clin Sci 33:53–65, 1967
37. Marsden CD, Harrison MJG, Bundey S: Natural history of idiopathic torsion dystonia. Adv Neurol 14:177–186, 1976
38. Marttila RJ, Rinne UK: Disability and progression in Parkinson's disease. Acta Neurol Scand 56:159–169, 1977.
39. Murnaghan GF: Neurogenic disorders of the bladder in parkinsonism. Br J Urol 33:403–409, 1961
40. Murphy MJ, Goldstein MN: Diphenylhydantoin-induced asterixis: A clinical study. JAMA 229:538–540, 1974
41. Pollock M, Hornabrook RW: The prevalence, natural history and dementia of Parkinson's disease. Brain 89:429–448, 1966
42. Posey WC, cited in Jankovic J: Progressive supranuclear palsy: Clinical and pharmacologic update. Neurol Clin 2:473–486, 1984
43. Selby G: Stereotactic surgery for the relief of Parkinson's disease: II. An analysis of the results in a series of 303 patients. J Neurol Sci 5:343–375, 1967
44. Shahani BT, Young RR: Asterixis: A disorder of the neural mechanisms underlying sustained muscle contraction. In Shahani M (ed): The Motor System: Neurophysiology and Muscle Mechanisms, pp 301–306. Amsterdam, Elsevier Scientific, 1976.
45. Shapiro AK, Shapiro E, Wayne H: Treatment of Tourette's syndrome: With haloperidol, review of 34 cases. Arch Gen Psychiatry 28:92–97, 1973
46. Shapiro E, Shapiro AK: Tic disorders. JAMA 245:1583–1585, 1981
47. Shaywitz BA: Hemifacial spasm in childhood treated with carbamazepine. Arch Neurol 31:63, 1974
48. Shoulson I: Huntington disease: Functional capacities in patients treated with neuroleptic and antidepressant drugs. Neurology 31:1333–1335, 1981
49. Toglia JU, Izzo K: Treatment of myoclonic dystonia with transcutaneous electrical nerve stimulation. Ital J Neurol Sci 6:75–78, 1985

25

Pressure Ulcers

William H. Donovan

Susan L. Garber

Steven M. Hamilton

Thomas A. Krouskop

Gladys P. Rodriguez

Samuel Stal

Decubitus ulcers, bed sores, pressure sores, and pressure ulcers are simply different names for a pervasive and persistent medical complication affecting people with restricted mobility. Pressure ulcers are "localized areas of cellular necrosis"[49] that derive their various names from the perceived principal causative factor: increased pressure on a small area of soft tissue due to lying or sitting in one position for too long.

The largest group at risk for the development of pressure ulcers are patients with spinal cord injury. However, anyone with an acute or chronic loss of mobility may develop them. Persons with quadriplegia and paraplegia are equally at risk of developing pressure ulcers,[94] with incomplete injuries having a smaller incidence than complete injuries.[75, 95] Other studies[1, 19] have given conflicting results as to the incidence and location of pressure ulcers, but the report by Young and Burns[94, 95] has the largest, most complete and current data on this aspect of the problem and revealed a nearly equal occurrence between paraplegia and quadriplegia.

Besides patients with spinal cord injuries, many other patients with impaired sensation and/or mobility are susceptible to develop pressure ulcers. If, in addition, there is urinary and/or fecal incontinence, and perhaps a modicum of mental confusion, the risk increases.[65] Elderly and hemiplegic patients and those with multiple sclerosis or hip replacement often develop pressure ulcers.[3, 13] In acute care hospitals, the incidence of pressure ulcers might be as low as 3%, but in chronic care hospitals it could be as high as 45%.[19]

The mental and emotional cost of a pressure ulcer is hard to quantitate, but the financial cost, which is considerable, is not quite as difficult to assess. Spinal cord-injured patients who develop no sores during their initial hospitalization have a mean injury-to-home period of 4 months. Patients who developed severe pressure ulcers had a mean hospitalization period of 8 months. Those who developed more superficial ulcers were hospitalized for approximately 6 months.[94] Assuming an average daily hospital cost of $500 (a conservative estimate),[88] each additional month in the hospital would mean $15,000 additional rehabilitation cost. In the years following the injury, the difference in mean hospital costs between patients who had no pressure ulcers and those who had severe ulcers has been approximately $19,000 (in 1980 dollars).[95]

Even if one disregards the mental and emotional costs and considers the economic costs, the prevention and cure of pressure ulcers is a very pressing matter indeed. The magnitude of the problem is further emphasized when an analysis similar to those done by Robinson in Canada,[76] Noble in Australia,[62] and Motloch in California[59] is performed on the problem in the United States. Using the assumptions and data from these analyses, the medical costs associated with curing pressure sores in the United States are estimated to exceed $2 billion per year. The most commonly cited causes of pressure sores include the following:

1. Prolonged sitting during daily activities, particularly during travel and in recreational activities, such as card playing and video games
2. Use of old, deteriorated wheelchair cushions
3. Activities that involve sitting on uncushioned areas such as a bathtub or a floor to play with young members of the family
4. Falls while transferring from a wheelchair or bed
5. Sitting too soon after a surgical procedure to correct a vertebral defect, or even during the comprehensive rehabilitation process
6. Excessive sweating or irregular attention to one's skin condition.[5]
7. Wearing clothing that has exaggerated seamlines such as jeans, which cause pressure to concentrate on areas that would normally not carry significant loads

BIOMECHANICAL FACTORS

Pressure ulcers are characterized by an open wound where tissue necrosis has developed in response to externally applied loads. The normal structure of skin and the physiological processes involved in maintaining healthy tissue are fairly well understood, but in contrast the exact causes and mechanisms of soft tissue breakdown resulting in pressure sores are not as certain. During normal activities such as sitting, lying, and leaning against another surface, relatively small volumes of flesh are compressed between the internal bony skeleton and the external surface. Since most of the body weight is carried by the skeleton, extremely high tissue stresses can be generated. Classically, decubitus ulcers are assumed to be caused by pressure-induced vascular ischemia, resulting in tissues being deprived of oxygen and nutrients. The nonrigid walls of blood and lymph vessels collapse under pressures that are higher than that of the fluids inside. Also mechanical deformations of the flesh due to high levels of sustained load or more moderate, repetitive forces are of importance in producing tissue damage. During the past 25 years, a number of scientific studies have advanced our knowledge of the factors involved in the formation of pressure sores and have provided a basis for improving preventive techniques.[2, 17, 26, 36, 48, 51, 55, 63, 64, 83, 93] A number of investigators have studied blood flow and tissue mechanics in attempts to quantify the relationship between externally applied loads and the internal stresses that result in cessation of blood flow.[11, 12, 22, 27, 43, 44, 51, 52, 61, 73, 85, 86] In Kosiak's classic study, the variables governing soft tissue breakdown were extended to include "time at pressure."[48] Although Kosiak's relationship between "time at pressure" and breakdown has considerable variance associated with it, the clinical significance was shown by Rogers in the early 1970s.[81] As these early studies became well publicized, investigators began to appreciate that tissue breakdown was probably a multifactorial process. The variables identified included such factors as pressure, shear loading, general metabolic condition of the person, local tissue integrity and viability, age, edema, repeated pressure, altered sensation, neurotrophic effects, and psychological factors.[21, 93] Unfortunately, most studies have isolated for examination only one or two of the variables, leaving the other variables uncontrolled or assumed to be constant, even though other investigators have identified them as significant contributing factors. For example, the age, metabolic condition, and levels of general neuroendocrine stress in subjects (human and animal) have not been controlled in most studies. The shape of the experimental load applicator has only recently been structured so as to control the shearing load that is applied. Consequently, it is difficult and often impossible to compare the results obtained in one laboratory directly with the results from another. General trends may be noted to agree, but specific values are often found to be incompatible.

Many studies have been designed with animal models. Typically, the animals have been subjected to various externally applied pressure loads using indentors having very different geometries. As a result, substantial data have been collected indicating that pressures ranging from 20 mm Hg upward are necessary to produce tissue breakdown.[25, 48] Several studies have been conducted to elucidate the relationship between externally applied pressure and cessation of blood flow in a region. One of the most widely used models is based on the Krough cylinder. These studies have produced useful information for determining where, when, and how long blood flow will cease after an area has been loaded with externally applied pressure. Unfortunately, the magnitude of the pressure and load duration times typically derived from these studies are inconsistent with conditions existing in a hospital or nursing home setting. The animal studies indicate that "healthy" tissue can withstand pressure of 300 mm Hg[17] for periods up to 18 hours with reversible damage. Consequently, investigators have started to look for additional factors causing blood reduced circulation and/or tissue damage.

Bennet and co-workers[8] and Reichel[74] have researched the role of shear stress. Bennett and co-workers theorized that in addition to shear forces produced by friction, the shear resulting from large variation in compressive forces will produce severe mechanical stress in the soft tissues.[5–7, 60] They concluded that shear force plays a significant part in the occlusion of blood vessels but large compressive forces must already be applied in order for suitable shear conditions to develop. This work indicates that the pressure level capable of disrupting blood flow can be reduced by one-half by the presence of significant shear forces.

Brand[10] has contributed most to our knowledge about the effects of repetitive stress on soft tissue breakdown. Repetitive subcritical loads were applied to the foot pads of rats over a period of 3 weeks in different patterns,[10, 54] creating necrotic areas in the soft tissue that had characteristics similar to those of pressure sores. Of particular importance was the finding that introduction of rest intervals followed by re-stressing caused the soft tissue region to hypertrophy and become capable of bearing much greater external loads than before. Based on Brand's work, design criteria have been developed and used in the fabrication of shoes for people with insensitive or severely deformed feet, as found in leprosy, peripheral neuropathies, and peripheral vascular disorders associated with diabetes.

Analytical and experimental studies have also been conducted to investigate the effects of altered lymphatic drainage and the role of interstitial fluid on the formation of pressure sores.[73] The results have been used to provide a basis for understanding the "time at pressure" phenomenon noted in the earlier work done by Kosiak[48] and Rogers.[81]

Moisture also predisposes to tissue necrosis. As early as 1852 Brown-Séquard demonstrated that soiling and moisture greatly increased the effects of pressure on the skin of guinea pigs.[19, 65] Incontinence is well known to be associated with decubitus ulcers. In the Greater Glasgow Health Board Survey[47] it was found that while 3.7% of fully continent patients had significant pressure sores, the incidence rose to 15.5% and 39.7% among those with urinary and fecal incontinence, respectively. The observation must be attributed in part to the susceptibility of moist skin to maceration through direct trauma or exposure to pressure. Wet skin is also most likely to adhere to clothing and bed linen, thus enhancing the generation of substantial shearing forces. An additional factor in the case of fecal incontinence is mechanical attrition of the epidermis combined with the introduction of infection into any breach of the body defense.

Poor nutrition, resulting in loss of weight and reduced padding of bony prominences, is another important factor.[56, 57] The body's normal tissue integrity is dependent on a correct nitrogen balance and vitamin intake. Hypoproteinemia leading to edema causes the skin to become less elastic and more susceptible to inflammation as the rate of oxygen transfer from the capillaries to the tissue is reduced, thus compromising the skin's vitality.

The role of skin temperature and perspiration in the process of soft tissue breakdown has recently become an active area of research.[31, 53, 91] Slight changes in tissue temperature, particularly temperature increases, produce dramatic effects by increasing the metabolic demands of the cells in the local region. A rise of 2°F to 3°F can change the metabolic demands of a region, and the use of temperature as a predictive tool has been explored in several laboratories. In a number of studies, infrared thermography has been employed to study thermal changes in the skin related to the effects of repetitive stresses and to monitor the rate of healing of established pressure sores.[54]

BIOCHEMICAL FACTORS

Kosiak[49] stated that there was no increased susceptibility to pressure ulcers in the skin of the paraplegic rats. But, two facts were not considered. Rats are loose-skinned animals that do not have the same skin structure and vascularity as humans; and the experimental rats had been paraplegic only for a few hours, not long enough to have developed the metabolic changes brought on by spinal cord injury. Experiments done on swine, animals whose skin structure closely resembles that of humans, showed that animals that had been rendered paraplegic approximately 4 weeks before had a reduced pressure-duration threshold for the production of pressure ulcers.[23] This effect could be accounted for, at least partly, by the wasting of the lower limbs of the paraplegic pigs so the soft tissue covering over the bony prominences was greatly reduced.

The muscle to fat ratio of patients with spinal cord injuries is significantly lower than normal (predictively lowering skin tolerance to pressure).[39] Yet in one study quadriplegics unable to do weight shifts were reported ulcer free in spite of excessive times between pushups.[30] The great variability in the individual response to pressure underscores the multifactorial nature of the ulcer development process mentioned earlier.

Other indirect effects of spinal cord injury may be implicated in the heightened sensitivity to pressure in these patients. Guttman[38] explained that the loss of vasomotor control would make it easier to interrupt blood flow in spinal cord-injured patients and produce ischemia. The density of α-adrenergic receptors in the skin of spinal cord–injured patients decreases as length of time since injury increases, and the decrease is more pronounced in patients injured above the T6 level.[80] Skin blood flow in the buttocks of adult sitting paraplegics has been measured as being approximately equal to that of geriatric subjects but only one-third that of normal subjects of similar age.[8] Blood circulation below the level of injury in spinal cord–injured patients is impaired,[45] and that may account for the finding that there was a fivefold increase in the incidence of wound healing complications in wounds occurring below the level of injury in patients with spinal cord injury.[4] The impaired circulation could affect nutrient delivery to the cells, interfere with cell biosynthesis of collagen, and might account for the variations in collagen content in the skin of spinal cord–injured patients. The

concentration of hydroxyproline, a collagen-specific amino acid, in the skin below the injury of patients injured longer than 3 years is lower than in skin below the injury of patients injured less than 3 years. Electron microscopy studies revealed epithelial thinning, thickening of the basal lamina, a decreased number of fibrils in the papillary dermis, a transformation from a compact heterogeneous population of fibrils in collagen bundles in the reticular dermis to dispersed collagen fibrils of a small diameter, and a decrease in the longitudinal banding pattern (Figs. 25-1 and 25-2).[15] The skin of spinal cord-injured patients below the level of injury has a much lower concentration of proline, hydroxyproline, lysine, and hydroxylysine than above the level of injury, and the degree of hydroxylation of proline is much less.[77] This has implications for the tensile strength of the skin and its ability to withstand pressure since the hydroxyl groups of hydroxyproline stabilize the collagen helix by forming water bridges within the molecule. In addition, studies of a small number of patients have shown that while the activity of the enzyme lysyl hydroxylase in skin above the level of injury is approximately the same as that in skin from normal controls, the activity of the enzyme in skin below the level of injury is well below control values.[77]

Increases in the urinary excretion of a collagen metabolite associated with the preferential degradation of skin collagen, glucosyl galactosyl hyroxylysine, can be detected approximately 1 month before clinical signs of an incipient pressure ulcer can be detected (Fig. 25-3).[78, 79] Evidence for abnormal skin collagen synthesis in spinal cord injury is accumulating. The existence of a defective collagen matrix in the skin of spinal cord-injured pa-

Figure 25-1. Transmission electron micrographs *A* and *C* are of skin biopsy specimens of a patient with a C7 spinal cord lesion at 2 years after injury. Micrographs *B* and *D* are of skin biopsy specimens of a patient with a T12 spinal cord lesion 12 years after injury. Micrographs *A* and *B* (×9,200) show the thickening of the basal lamina (*arrow*) secreted by the stratum basale (*SB*). At 2 years after injury, the basal lamina is 600 A (*A*); at 12 years after injury, the basal lamina is 1250 A (*B*). Note the decrease in the number of collagen fibrils within the papillary dermis (*PD*). Micrographs *C* and *D* (×13,200) show the decrease in the density of collagen fibrils within the papillary dermis as a function of years after spinal cord injury. (Courtesy of Frank Kretzer, Ph.D., Baylor College of Medicine)

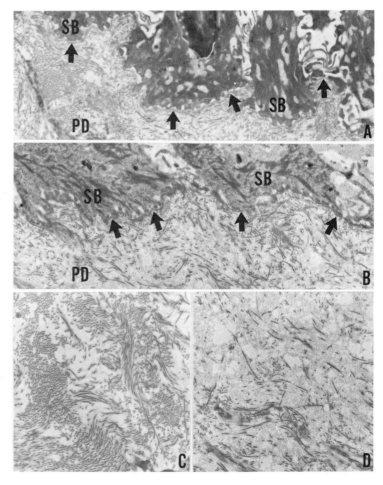

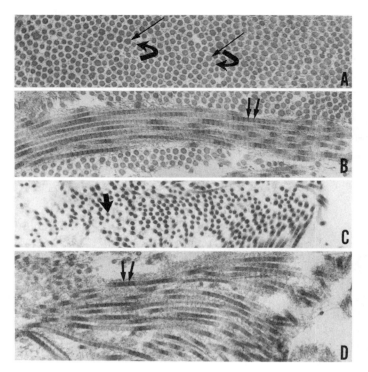

Figure 25-2. Transmission electron micrographs *A* and *B* are of skin biopsy specimens of a patient with a C7 spinal cord lesion 2 years after injury. Micrographs *C* and *D* are of skin biopsy specimens of a patient with a T12 spinal cord lesion 12 years after injury. These micrographs (×26,000) demonstrate the change in the nature of the collagen bundles within the reticular dermis as a function of years after injury. At 2 years after injury (*A*), the collagen bundles are a compact, heterogeneous population of 600 A (*curved arrows*) and 1000 A (*diagonal arrows*) diameter fibrils with a longitudinal periodicity (*B*) of 680 A (*small arrow*). In contrast, at 12 years after injury (*C*), the collagen bundles are composed of a dispersed population of 500 A (*wide arrow*) diameter fibrils with a longitudinal periodicity (*D*) of 620 A (*small arrows*). (Courtesy of Frank Kretzer, Ph.D., Baylor College of Medicine)

work of collagen and elastin fibers that characterize the gross mechanical properties of the tissue, working together as parallel springs transmitting loads between the external surface of the tissue and the underlying skeletal surface. Collagen breakdown and synthesis is very sensitive to many physiological factors, including the concentration of oxygen and trace elements such as copper within the tissue. When suitable biochemical conditions are not present, a collagen trihelix forms that is not stable at body temperature and is water soluble.

It may be hypothesized that the capacity of soft tissue to support mechanical forces without inflammatory or necrotic changes is fundamentally related to its inherent elastic properties, which determine the extent to which force applied externally to the skin will be distributed within subdermal tissue layers. In conditions that affect the elastic properties of soft tissue it is further hypothesized that collagen within the soft tissue is progressively broken down and washed out of the subdermal matrix, leaving an increasing proportion of the load distributing function of the tissue to the elastin fibers. As more and more collagen is lost from the tissue, the increasing stress placed on the vascular and lymphatic elements causes a reduction in the availability of nutrients essential for all metabolism in association with impeded performance of the lymphatic system in removing waste products. An additional effect of removal of collagen from the soft tissue is reduction of tissue resistance due to the displacement of interstitial fluid and ground substance that normally perform the function of separating cells and maintaining a localized hydrostatic state of stress. When a sufficient volume of interstitial fluid and ground substance has been removed from a region under pressure, the cushioning effect is lost and cell-to-cell contact may occur. Contact stresses under these conditions may then become high enough to cause distortion and rupture of the cell membranes.[70, 72] If damage does occur and the lymphatic system is unable to cleanse the region of toxic intracellular materials, the remaining cells in the region may be poisoned causing a larger necrotic area to develop.

MEDICAL FACTORS

The level of injury, completeness of lesion (both motor and sensory), etiology, race, employment status, level of education, and familiarity with spinal cord injury care needs have been named as eight factors identifying a person at risk for developing pressure ulcers.[87] In addition, satisfaction with the activities of life and degree of responsibility shown for their own skin care have been shown to be significantly associated with the incidence of pressure ulcers in quadriplegics.[1]

Maintenance of health, both physical and emotional, and the receipt of comprehensive rehabilitation are therefore important in the prevention of pressure ulcers[62] since there are certain pathophysiological factors that can be identified that if allowed to develop can predispose to skin breakdown. They include malnutrition, anemia, infection, severe spasticity, contractures, edema, and psychological disturbance, particularly depression.

Malnutrition among hospitalized patients is well documented.[9] Patients with spinal cord injury require a balanced intake of nutrients. Their nutritional requirements will, of course, vary depending on the length of time since their injury.[32, 66] Patients seen in the acute trauma center, immediately after injury may require 3500 to 4000 kcal/day.[84] This requirement will be increased if pressure sores are allowed to develop during this period because of the loss of body protein through the ulcers and the metabolic demands posed by the combating of

tients, if proven, would certainly be a powerful predisposing factor for ulcer formation.

Correlations with other factors associated with spinal cord injury have also been found. In 131 patients studied, a high correlation was found between the presence of heterotopic ossification and the incidence of pressure ulcers.[40] Anemia, especially if there was low serum iron and low serum iron binding capacity, was associated with the development of large, deep ulcers while nonanemic patients developed small, superficial sores.[67]

Research into the prevention of pressure ulcers by biochemical means is limited. Vitamins A, E, and C as well as zinc have been suggested as possible factors to enhance the skin's ability to withstand pressure.[19]

Several investigators[14, 18, 69] have studied changes in collagen metabolism following spinal cord injury and the possible interrelation of these changes with susceptibility to soft tissue breakdown. At this time studies in this area remain speculative, and yet the qualitative information provided to date serves as a useful framework for the development of a model of pressure sore etiology. One such model has been proposed by Krouskop and associates[50] and is based on the following information:

Soft tissue may be represented as a matrix composed of cells, vascular networks, and interstitial fluid supported by a net-

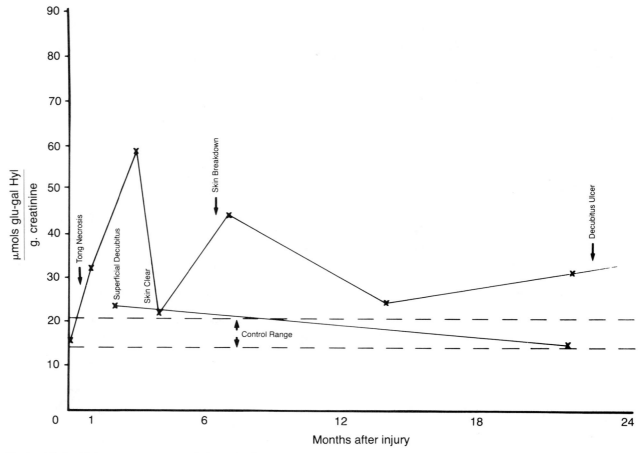

Figure 25-3. Urinary concentration of glucosyl galactosyl hydroxylysine (glu-gal Hyl) in micromols per gram of creatinine versus time since injury. Solid lines are values of two patients, one of which had several episodes of skin-related problems in contrast to the other patient who had an uneventful recovery. Dashes represent mean control value ± standard deviation.

infection and healing at the ulcer site. Patients who develop pressure ulcers at some time well past their original injuries may require fewer calories depending on their nutritional status and the size of the wound.[84]

Anemia decreases the oxygen-carrying capacity of the blood and thus impairs the ability of the body to heal and to react to the ischemic effects of pressure.[67] Ischemia itself, when chronic, decreases one's healing capacity and has been shown in rats with femoral artery ligation to decrease tolerance for pressure by one half as compared with normal rats.[46] A hemoglobin value below 10 g/dl needs to be corrected. The means of correction depends on the urgency of the situation. Patients getting ready for surgery should be transfused prior to the surgical procedure up to a level of 12 g/dl. However, the anemia usually seen in patients with pressure ulcers that have been present for an extended period of time and who are undernourished is often the "anemia of chronic disease." One frequently sees not only a low serum iron value but also a low iron-binding capacity along with an elevated serum ferritin value in this condition. If the iron level is low, it should be corrected; however, the larger problem is the body's failure to use the existing iron stores in the bone marrow and to create new erythrocytes. The underlying "chronic disease" needs to be corrected, otherwise the anemia will remain constant and transfused blood cells after they have expired will not be replaced by the patient's own marrow. Therefore, every effort must be taken to correct the nutritional deficiencies and to treat any chronic infection that may be present either in the decubitus

(soft tissue or underlying bone) or in places other than the decubitus such as the urinary bladder.

Chronic infection as mentioned will likely impair the patients' general health even in the absence of systemic reactions. Examples include an afebrile urinary tract infection and a chronic pressure ulcer. The latter may worsen spasticity and thereby create problems with posturing, leading to increased pressure over selected bony prominences. If, however, a febrile systemic response is present, more frequent turning or position changing should be done every 2 hours since this has been observed to decrease skin tolerance.[53] During such bouts of systemic illness, patients often do not eat and the nutritional intake suffers.

Spasticity is common in spinal cord-injured and other neurologically impaired patients and, as mentioned, may interfere with turning and body positioning and can lead to contractures of joints, particularly the hips and knees. This will remove the prone and supine position as options for lying in bed and force increased time on the trochanteric areas. Spasticity is an issue that must be assessed and corrected as much as possible prior to surgical repair of pressure ulcers.[20, 28]

If a pharmacological regime is unsuccessful in controlling spasticity, then careful attention should be given to other means, particularly if the risk of separation of a surgically repaired wound by a sudden spasm is very high. This risk is particularly high in flaps intended to cover ischial and sacral pressure sores.

Contractures especially of the hip and knee, if present, will also interfere with positioning during the postoperative period. If contractures of the hip are so severe that they preclude posturing the patient in the prone position, correction of the contractures should be accomplished first, prior to repairing the pressure sore. In some instances, it may be possible to perform the surgical procedure and place the patient in the supine position using an "air fluidized" (*e.g.,* Clinitron or Mediscus) bed. Such beds allow the positioning of a patient so that weight can be borne through the surgical flap. There have been anecdotal reports of successful healing of a flap even when the patient is allowed to lie on it (something that is not possible in any other bed regardless of the mattress chosen). This is not recommended however unless it is absolutely necessary. Even if the pressure on the newly designed flap does not exceed the critical capillary closing pressure, venous drainage is impeded when the patient is lying with the flap in the dependent position.

Edema decreases the diffusion of oxygen and nutrients in proportion with the distance it places between the capillary and the cell membrane. This can be a significant problem in the extremities and therefore affects the tolerance of the skin over the malleoli, the heels, and other bony prominences of the feet. Elevation of the lower extremities at night and the use of elastic hose during the day while the legs are dependent in the wheelchair will help to decrease this predeposition to skin breakdown.

Several investigators have noted the influence of psychosocial factors on the incidence of decubiti; namely, the patient's acceptance of responsibility for skin care, satisfaction with activities of daily living, and sense of self-esteem correlate well with the risk of skin ulceration.[43, 94] A person's understanding of the causes and risks of skin breakdown, combined with a positive attitude toward health and independent living, is also expected to heavily influence the effects of potentially dangerous mechanical factors encountered during everyday life. There are many emotional burdens that the spinal cord-injured patient must endure. As difficult as it is, an adjustment must be made wherein the patient accepts the reality of the situation and adopts the necessary attitudes and behaviors that are required to maintain intact skin. The amount of psychological support required will vary widely among individuals. However, if they are placed in a supportive environment where they are cared for by staff whom they can trust, in facilities that they know are adequate, and among other patients with similar problems from whom they can learn and share, this will do much to allay anxiety and fears (which fuel anger and depression) and create a learning attitude. Some patients will require psychiatric intervention on a continuous basis, and many will likely profit from antidepressant medication, particularly amitriptyline.

MANAGEMENT

Definition and Classification

Despite the multitude of contributing factors that can be associated with the development of pressure sores, pressure remains the central biomechanical and pathophysiological agent related to creation and evolution of pressure ulcers. Clinically, pressure sores range from superficial inflammation and excoriation to large infected cavities, which occasionally involve underlying bone. The most widely accepted classification is as follows.

Grade 1—Skin area with erythema or induration overlying a bony prominence (*i.e.,* an incipient sore)

Grade 2—A superficial ulceration that extends into the dermis

Grade 3—An ulcer that extends into the subcutaneous tissue but not into muscle

Grade 4—Deep ulceration that extends through muscular tissue down to the underlying bony prominence

Grade 5—An extensive ulcer with widespread extension along bursae into joints or body cavities (*e.g.,* rectum, intestine, vagina, bladder)

A clear classification of these ulcers is important since definitive local treatment of the wound will be determined by its grade, or more specifically, its depth and tissue involvement (Fig. 25-4).[24]

Treatment

The treatment of pressure sores falls into two broad categories: systemic and local wound therapy. Systemic treatment consists of correction of the factors discussed previously that contribute to the patient's impaired ability to resist pressure injury or fight infection.

Patients should be evaluated according to the local wound characteristics described in the previous grading system and separated into conservative (topical therapy with closure by secondary intention alone) and surgical treatment groups. Those candidates for surgical treatment require equally aggressive topical therapy preoperatively in order to promote wound contraction, decrease tissue infection, and remove necrotic debris. The wound grading system provides a convenient reference point to predict successful therapy of a pressure injury. For instance, patients with grade 1 ulcers will usually require reevaluation and treatment of the intrinsic and extrinsic factors that contribute to pressure injury. In particular, the patient requires alteration of padding and frequent turning, and the general state of health of the patient needs to be carefully reevaluated and appropriate therapy instituted. Frequently, these early pressure sores can be completely resolved with these simple measures. Grade 2 ulcers, with superficial ulceration into the dermis, require similar evaluation and aggressive topical therapy to promote wound healing by secondary intention. Such conservative methods promote wound contraction and eventual reepithelialization. As in topical therapy of deeper wounds, the immediate goal of local therapy is a conservative débridement of necrotic tissue, suppression of infection, and frequent dressing changes. The list of recommended topical agents published for treatment of these shallow ulcers is extensive and includes enzymes, topical antibiotics, elements and simple compounds, tannic acid, honey, sugar, and povidone-iodine. However, there remains a lack of objective evidence that any of these agents are superior to normal saline wet-to-dry gauze dressings. Therefore, following conservative débridement of any superficial necrotic debris, wet-to-dry dressings changed every 6 to 8 hours appear to help promote healing by secondary intention while providing adequate mechanical débridement of any accumulated debris. Appropriate wet-to-dry dressings involve placement of gauze material moistened with normal saline, with care taken to remove sufficient saline from the gauze to allow for adequate evaporation and drying and secondary adherence to the walls of the ulcer cavity in order to better promote mechanical débridement with the next dressing change. This form of dressing can also be used with a dilute hypochlorite (Dakins) solution or povidone-iodine (Betadine) in those wounds that continue to show signs of superficial infection with anaerobic or microaerophilic organisms such as *Bacteroids* or *Peptococcus.*

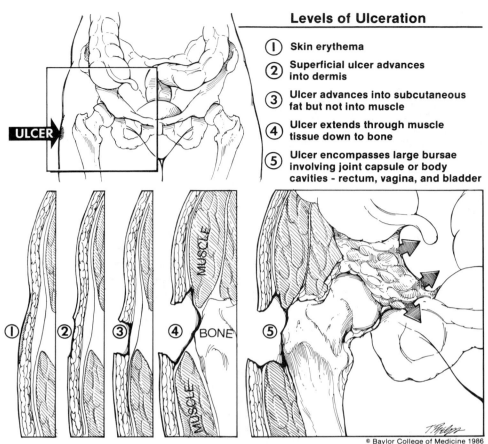

Levels of Ulceration

(1) **Skin erythema**

(2) **Superficial ulcer advances into dermis**

(3) **Ulcer advances into subcutaneous fat but not into muscle**

(4) **Ulcer extends through muscle tissue down to bone**

(5) **Ulcer encompasses large bursae involving joint capsule or body cavities - rectum, vagina, and bladder**

© Baylor College of Medicine 1986

Figure 25-4. The depth of tissue involvement for each grade of pressure ulcer is shown.

General Principals of Surgical Therapy for Wound Closure

Ulcers of grades 3 to 5 will generally require a surgical procedure. Before discussing specific methods of wound coverage and closure it is important to address the initial management of necrotic and infected ulcers. In many cases, it is necessary to perform surgical débridement first and then close the wound as a second stage after adequate cleansing has been accomplished, and after results of cultures taken from the surrounding tissue and bone (if bone is involved, or suspected of being involved) have been obtained.

If bone is involved, and osteomyelitis is present, antibiotics should be continued for 6 weeks. If only soft tissue is involved, then 2 weeks of antibiotic therapy is all that is necessary. The diagnosis of osteomyelitis is difficult and should be made on the basis of positive cultures and characteristic appearance on histological study.[89] Results of bone scans and gallium scans are often misleading.

Although sinography, ultrasonography, and computed tomography have been found useful in some instances to further define and delineate the extent of tissue involvement and the presence of sinus tracts or abscesses, one can only be sure of the presence of osteomyelitis by the combined histological and bacteriological studies mentioned.[41] Before definitive closure of a deep ulcer, the wound should appear absolutely clean, deep swabs should reveal no growth of microorganisms, and all devitalized tissue must have been removed. As long as these conditions are met, a wound with osteomyelitis may be closed before the 6 weeks of specific antibiotic treatment have elapsed.

Certain general principles of surgery apply to all types of plastic procedures used on patients with decubitus ulcers, namely, proper handling of tissues, closure of all dead space, evacuation of fluid by judicious use of drains, use of healthy tissues to pad bony prominences, meticulous suture for strength, and prevention of infection.[37, 42]

An important aspect of planning for surgery is the evaluation of previous surgical procedures with the intent to preserve tissue that may be used for flaps in the future.

Surgical Procedures

Skin grafts, skin flaps, muscle flaps, musculocutaneous flaps, neurovascular flaps, and free flaps can all be used to provide wound closure after excision of pressure sores. A brief description of each, and their appropriate use, follows.

SKIN GRAFTS. Skin grafts consist of either split-thickness or full-thickness skin. In general, intermediate or split-thickness skin grafts are usually applied to surgical closure of small, superficial wounds. Ordinarily, split-thickness skin grafts are meshed 1½ to 1 and applied unexpanded. Applied in this manner, these grafts will conform to irregular wounds and concavities in a superior fashion and present fewer problems with subgraft collection of blood or purulent material. In flat, easily accessible areas, sheet grafts can be applied with small incisions made in the graft to allow for drainage. In chronic, highly contaminated wounds, smaller "postage stamp" grafts can also be successfully used. In the postoperative period, it is important that the grafts remain covered and constantly moist for at least 2 to 3 days. Occasionally, rolling the graft with cotton-tipped swabs aids in the removal of fluid collecting beneath the graft. The donor site, treated as a superficial burn, heals in 10 to 14 days by reepithelialization from epidermal elements from deeper adnexal structures. After appropriate healing of donor and recipient areas, care must be given to lubricate these regions since sweat gland function is often impaired.

The clinical application of skin grafts to pressure ulcer management falls into two distinct categories: (1) the superficial full-thickness ulcer that is small, relatively clean, and impractical for the patient to treat by lengthy topical therapy and closure by secondary intention and (2) massive ulceration that is not immediately amenable to more definitive flap closure. In the latter case, skin grafts can be applied to those ulcers after appropriate topical therapy to convert a dirty wound into a relatively clean one. Since frequently this category of patient tolerates surgery poorly, stamp grafts applied sequentially over the extensive denuded areas of the body would allow for progressive epithelial closure of these wounds, decrease protein and fluid losses, and ultimately stabilize the patient for possible further definitive care.

SKIN FLAPS. Skin flaps are cutaneous territories elevated surgically and hinged on their blood supply. The blood supply to these flaps may consist of distinct cutaneous vessels, supplying a specific skin territory (called an axial or arterialized flap), such as the deltopectoral flap supplied by the secondary intercostal branch of the internal mammary artery and the groin flap supplied by the superficial circumflex iliac artery.

Skin flaps may also receive their blood supply from perforating musculocutaneous vessels at the base of the flap. It is important to note that the distal portion of these territories (called random flaps) is then nourished from small vessels within the subdermal layer. These subdermal extensions place a limit on the size of the flap that can be nourished from these perforating branches. Therefore, the surgeon will generally design a random flap so the length will not exceed the base by one and one-half times in size.

Skin flaps can be raised with or without the underlying muscle fascia; however, elevation with the underlying fascia generally ensures incorporation of additional perforating muscle blood supply. Skin flaps are generally designed for transposition over areas of previous ulceration after en bloc débridement of the ulcer and underlying bony prominence. In general, skin flaps alone are reserved for ulcers without a significant underlying dead space; otherwise, muscle tissue accompanying the skin flap, or elevated separately, is required to treat more extensive ulcers, such as those found in grades 4 or 5. In general, grade 3 ulcers are most amenable to skin flap closure alone.

MUSCLE FLAPS. It can be demonstrated that most muscles have their major neurovascular bundle entering at the proximal end of the muscle belly. Therefore, minor distal neurovascular pedicles can be divided and the origin and insertion of these muscles can be detached. The muscle can then be used for transposition into areas of significant deep tissue loss to fill the cavity and provide padding. Examples of muscles used for this purpose are the biceps femoris muscle, vastus lateralis, gluteus maximus, and gracilis.

MUSCULOCUTANEOUS FLAPS. Growing awareness that blood supply from skin is derived from perforating musculocutaneous vessels has led to the design of larger and more reliable composite flaps for complete reconstruction of extensive pressure ulcers. As in muscle flaps, these flaps are carefully designed and carried out to preserve the proximal perforating vessels of the muscle with care to avoid perforating vessels that are present in the areolar tissue between the muscular fascia and overlying cutaneous territory. The tensor fascia lata flap, the posterior hamstring advancement flap, and the gluteal myocutaneous flap, all fall into this category of often-used composite flaps or musculocutaneous flaps.

NEUROVASCULAR SKIN FLAPS. Neurovascular flaps consist of arterialized flaps that contain a sensory nerve supply in the cutaneous territory elevated along with the flap. In general, these flaps are designed off intercostal vessels and nerves and are transposed to regions in the sacrum in order to provide protective sensation. This especially shows promise in patients with more distal lumbar lesions.

FREE FLAPS. Free flaps consist of a skin flap or more typically a musculocutaneous flap, that is harvested from a remote or distant portion of the body, such as the latissimus dorsi or tensor fascia latta, and transplanted by microvascular anastomosis to the site of ulcer resection. Technically, it is also possible to restore arterial, venous, and possible nerve function by direct anastomosis or a nerve interposition graft. This technique is reserved for the "end stage," extremely large pressure sore where local tissue is not sufficient for adequate coverage.

Specific Ulcers

In review of the literature of surgical treatment for pressure ulcer management in quadriplegics and paraplegics, three ulcers stand out in prevalence and also in number of related surgical procedures: sacral, trochanteric, and ischial ulcers. Discussion will be limited to these ulcers, but the same principles apply to the surgical reconstruction of all other pressure sores. In evaluation of these patients, the decision for appropriate flap coverage involves precise preoperative planning, allowing for occasional flap failures or, more frequently, recurrences. Thorough preoperative planning for appropriate soft tissue manipulation and eventual closure of these ulcers includes appropriate radiographic studies, bone scans, wound cultures, and, when necessary, sinograms and CT scans to appreciate the extent of ulcer involvement.

SACRAL ULCERS. Local and distant tissue is available for appropriate soft tissue coverage of sacral ulcers. Skin grafts should not be used in quadriplegia in the sacral region since significant padding is required in that area; however, they could be considered for higher sacral lesions in paraplegia with shallow defects and especially in those who maintain some sensibility. Owing to the generally even topography of the underlying sacral bony structure, ulcers in this region appear to have less extensive dead space to fill, and flaps in this region tend to demonstrate a higher success rate, perhaps owing to more diffuse pressure characteristics. As a result, local flaps are usually sufficient for reconstruction in this region.

ISCHIAL ULCERS. Ischial ulcers present more demanding reconstructive requirements. The recurrence rate is high in this group, perhaps owing to documented higher pressures over the ischiae when sitting than other areas of the body. Ischial ulcers are also frequently associated with large underlying dead space; therefore, they require more significant soft tissue augmentation with local or distant muscle tissue. The significant soft tissue loss associated with ischial ulceration is complicated by the muscle atrophy in the paralyzed patient, especially in patients with spina bifida and those with cauda equina injury. This may result in insufficient bulk of appropriate muscle tissue to successfully reconstruct extensive ischial ulceration. It is particularly important in the care of ischial ulcers to aggressively address any bone involvement. Frequent bone involvement with histological evidence of osteomyelitis is associated with persistent drainage; therefore, appropriate ischiectomy and perioperative antibiotic therapy is considered a standard of treatment in significant ischial wounds. Choice of reconstructive measures for closure of ischial ulcers is made relatively simple by lack of many alternatives for successful reconstruction. Skin grafts usually are not sufficient coverage for ischial sores owing to an obvious lack of padding and deep tissue. Local flaps, such as biceps femoris or gluteal musculocutaneous flaps, should be carried out in an appropriate order with care to preserve alternate local tissues for possible salvage procedures should the flap fail or recur. Furthermore, use of local tissue and design of incisions should be planned in initial reconstructive schemes to preserve blood supply of more distant tissue that may possibly be needed for advancement into this region for salvage procedures. Free flaps are also considered in this region after exhaustion of other local and regional tissue.

TROCHANTERIC ULCERS.   Clinically, the extent of trochanteric ulcers can be misleading owing to an often-extensive underlying bursa with occasional extension into the articular space of the hip. These ulcers are rarely treated with skin graft unless they are extremely superficial. Local flaps, especially the tensor fascia lata, are the method of choice for closure of this category of ulcer. When joint involvement is encountered, reconstruction of the dead space, following appropriate débridement by disarticulation of the hip joint and ostectomy, is accomplished with use of the vastus lateralis muscle flap with skin graft coverage. Distant flaps for trochanteric ulcer reconstruction include the gluteal thigh flap, and of course a free flap remains an option in this case as well.[92]

COMBINED ULCERS.   Combined ulcers consist of a combination of any of the previously discussed ulcers unilaterally or bilaterally. These patients frequently present after multiple episodes of breakdown and usually have had one or more surgical closures in the past. The large soft tissue defects, as well as extensive bone involvement, present a difficult challenge. As mentioned previously, conservative topical therapy is frequently the treatment of choice in this difficult population while systemic factors are corrected. Skin grafting can be considered a temporizing measure until the patient's condition stabilizes and he or she is able to maintain a positive nitrogen balance. Extensive assessment by the rehabilitation team is important to determine if this patient is a candidate for surgery, not only physically but also psychologically. Social service must also be involved to help ensure compliance after the patient goes home.

Reconstruction of these multiple defects has become possible with the development of more aggressive procedures using one of the lower extremities as a single musculocutaneous composite flap after fillet amputation. Successful examples exist of reconstruction of more than five ulcers with a lower extremity used as an extensive musculocutaneous flap. These flaps are tremendous undertakings and should be considered only in those patients deemed capable of tolerating a lengthy and stressful operation; they require care and experience on the part of the surgical team. These procedures are carried out by disarticulation of the skeletal structure of the lower extremity and its subsequent removal from the soft tissue. The leg is opened up in an anterior or posterior direction to allow for appropriate rotation and transposition in either direction. With deepithelialization, the lower extremity can be transposed and tunneled into multiple sites, both ipsilaterally and contralaterally, to close multiple regions of soft tissue defects due to chronic pressure ulcers.

Postoperative Care

The postoperative care in many ways reflects the same concerns addressed in the preoperative care of the patient. Positioning is of primary importance postoperatively to avoid pressure on the flap that could compromise the blood supply; therefore, patients with reconstructive procedures, especially in the three areas discussed previously, require positioning in the prone position for approximately 4 weeks while allowing for adequate healing and stabilization of the flap (Fig. 25-5). Antibiotics are chosen on the basis of documented surface cultures, as well as results of deep tissue and bone biopsies. Therapy with these agents is maintained for 24 to 48 hours for clean-appearing wounds showing minimal bacterial growth. Wounds that had previously appeared grossly infected should be treated with antibiotics for at least 10 to 14 days, and wounds that had shown histopathologically confirmed osteomyelitis are treated for a full 6 weeks for definitive treatment of deep osseous infection. Drains are left in for approximately 2 weeks to allow for removal of fluid that may accumulate beneath the flap, and special care is given to stripping of the drains in the immediate postoperative period to avoid clotting of the drains and subsequent hematoma formation. Spasticity must be maximally suppressed during the postoperative period to avoid excess movement leading to bleeding and hematoma formation. With the patient in the prone position, appropriate padding is necessary to avoid secondary iatrogenic pressure injury due to immobilization in this position for 4 weeks. Care must be taken for appropriate perineal padding and support to avoid scrotal and penile edema, and indwelling cathe-

Figure 25-5.   The postoperative positioning with the appropriate padding and arrangement of surgical drains and indwelling catheter is shown.

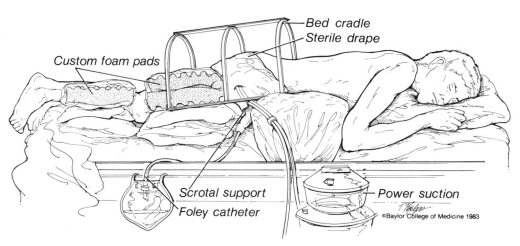

Bed cradle
Sterile drape
Custom foam pads
Scrotal support
Foley catheter
Power suction
©Baylor College of Medicine 1983

ters are required to prevent unnecessary turning from side to side in the initial postoperative period. Gastrointestinal management frequently includes constipating regimens preoperatively and postoperatively; however, the use of incontinence bags, applied similarly to colostomy dressings, has obviated the need for these extended periods of constipation and clear liquid diets, thus allowing continued adequate nutrition of these patients during their reconstructive phase. Some patients will not tolerate the prone position for 4 weeks, especially patients with low pulmonary reserve, in particular, the high quadriplegic or obese population. Therefore, an air-fluidized bed is recommended so that these patients may be maintained in the supine position without undue force placed over the flap site. In patients requiring more than one flap procedure, these fluidized support systems are ideal to protect multiple sites from pressure injury during recovery from a single flap reconstruction, while protecting other injured areas awaiting appropriate reconstructive measures. There is, however, no substitute for consistent nursing evaluation and monitoring of the patient's skin.[90]

Complications

Flap necrosis secondary to hematomas or seromas or disruption of the blood supply and infection remain the most common complications. After successful recovery from the initial reconstructive procedure, some studies list a recurrence rate of up to 44% within 4 years of surgery. A high recurrence rate can be linked to similar contributory factors that give rise to the initial ulcer; however, persistent osteomyelitis, residual sinus tracts, inadequate ostectomy, and overlying scar, all may play a role in the high recurrence rate seen in this patient population. Apart from the reconstruction procedure, follow-up care must include patient education, routine postoperative visits, and appropriate pressure analysis and padding.

PREVENTION

Prevention is clearly the easiest, least expensive, and most successful mode of therapy. The essential elements of an effective prevention program include an integrated team management approach emphasizing good medical and nursing care, proper training and education of patients, encouragement of patient compliance with these recommendations, and the proper prescription of pressure relief devices.

The prevention of pressure sores begins during the acute phase of hospitalization and continues through the rehabilitation process. Initially, careful positioning on proper support surfaces is the key factor in reducing the risk of tissue breakdown. Therefore, early medical management must include consideration of the patient's pressure relief requirements since patients left in one position for even short periods of time may develop severe tissue breakdown. If allowed to develop, pressure ulcers will greatly interfere with the rehabilitation process and the person's active participation in programs that are intended to help achieve maximal functional potential.

Turning and Positioning

The turning and positioning of patients and the proper use of special pressure-relief devices, such as therapeutic mattress surfaces, are essential if pressure sores are to be prevented. Turning regimens usually consist of 2 hours on one side, 2 hours on the back, and 2 hours on the opposite side.[29, 68] As a person builds up skin tolerance, the length of time between turns may be in-

creased in 30-minute increments. All turns are performed with extreme care to avoid shearing and friction of the skin against the bed surface. Patients are lifted or gently rolled into place and never dragged across the bed surface.

In the supine position, the anatomical areas most vulnerable to breakdown are the heels and the sacrum, the latter particularly if the head of the bed is elevated. Shear forces create friction between the skin and the supporting surfaces, causing tissue damage on the skin surface, particularly in the sacral region, when the head of the head is raised and lowered. Sores form as the skin and underlying tissue are eroded away by the constant movement of the skin against the other surface.[58, 81] When the patient is supine, his or her legs should be elevated 15° with the calves resting on a pillow to improve venous drainage and prevent heel pressure (Fig. 25-6A). For patients who must endure long periods of time on their side, the trochanter is the area most vulnerable to breakdown. A side-lying position in which the inferior leg is flexed 20° at the hip and knee and the superior leg is extended at the hip and flexed 35° at the knee so that the foot of that leg is well behind the midline of the body (Fig. 25-6B) has been identified as being optimum for decreasing trochanteric pressure.[35] This position significantly lowers the trochanteric pressure and allows the person to tolerate longer periods of time on that side. It does not, however, eliminate the need for turning.

The prone position is frequently used following surgery to repair pressure sores of the ischium, sacrum, or trochanters. The knees are the most vulnerable to breakdown in this position,

Figure 25-6. (A) In the supine position, the calves are elevated to remove pressure from the heels. (B) In the side-lying position pressure on the trocanter is lessened when the legs are positioned as shown. (C) In the prone position, the iliac crests and knees are relieved of pressure by the arrangement of pillows or foam as shown.

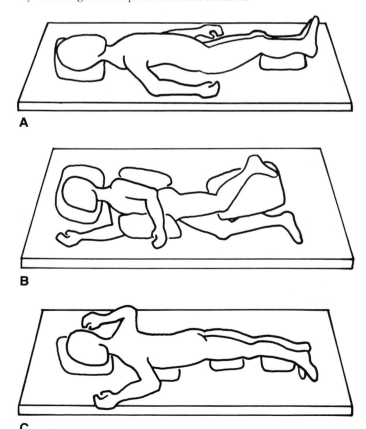

A

B

C

although the anterior iliac crests, shins, dorsa of the feet, and toes are also at risk. Proper prone positioning to prevent tissue breakdown can be accomplished with soft pillows, a static air mattress, or specially constructed foam devices that use a "bridging" technique that not only relieves pressure from vulnerable areas but allows adequate drainage of catheters and colostomy devices (Fig. 25-6C).

Under some circumstances it may be necessary to employ one of the pressure-relief devices designed for beds. These devices are categorized as either therapeutic mattress surfaces, mattress overlays, or pressure relief beds. A therapeutic mattress surface is defined as a device that is placed directly on top of the hospital bed mattress. Its effectiveness in relieving pressure depends on either its design or the material of which it is fabricated. The different types of therapeutic mattress surfaces include polyurethane foams (solid or convoluted), air-filled static mattresses, alternating air-pressure mattresses, gel pad inserts, and water-filled inserts.[50] (Gel and water inserts may also be used in conjunction with polyurethane foam mattress surfaces. The foam is cut out in the desired location, such as under the pelvis, and the insert is placed within the cut out.)

Special Beds

In addition to therapeutic mattress surface, there are several pressure-relief beds that are designed specifically to reduce pressure and the risk of ulceration. Examples of these include the air-fluidized bed, the alternating air-pressure bed, and the kinetic therapeutic bed. These highly specialized beds as noted earlier are usually used while the person is still in the hospital, especially if he or she has just had multiple episodes of severe pressure sores or surgery to correct pressure sores. These beds are also available on a rental basis for home use. It is suggested that a physician, therapist, or nurse familiar with these types of devices be consulted prior to ordering one for use at home.

Frequent turning and the use of appropriate pressure-relief devices are essential to minimize the risk of pressure sores for those confined to bed. Most patients with physical disabilities develop good skin tolerance on the standard hospital mattress when there are conscientious turning regimens during the early phases of rehabilitation. The special mattresses and beds should be reserved for difficult cases (*e.g.,* multiple ulcers, severe contractures, or inability to tolerate the prone position).

Wheelchair Mobility

The transition from confinement in bed to the use of the wheelchair is an important milestone for patients undergoing rehabilitation. An accurately measured and fitting wheelchair and one that is properly maintained contributes to optimum functional positioning, balance, stability, and weight distribution. Critical factors that must be considered when prescribing a wheelchair include seat width and depth, back height, seat to floor height, leg rests or foot pedals, arm rests, cushion compatibility, the patient's weight, and the anticipated use of the chair.

Because there are now many different styles of wheelchairs and because there are many options to be considered when ordering a chair, it is recommended that this equipment be ordered only after one is thoroughly familiar with all current options and how they affect pressure distribution and function.

A wheelchair can last 5 or 6 years, if properly maintained. The seat and back vinyl upholstery probably will have to be replaced periodically because it becomes stretched out, ultimately affecting positioning and pressure distribution. The frame requires attention to prevent or correct bending that will also interfere with balance, pressure relief, and mobility.

Weight Shifts

For the patient with a spinal cord injury or other neurological or musculoskeletal disability the achievement of vertical tolerance to 90° in the wheelchair enables him or her to participate in many functional tasks and engage in educational, social, and recreational activities. When 90° is reached, the sitting time may also be gradually increased. During this time, the risk of developing pressure sores is greatly increased. Those areas at risk include the ischial tuberosities, coccyx, and trochanters.

The performance of weight shifts by the patient allows for the periodic and routine relief of pressure while sitting. This is especially important for the patient with a spinal cord injury who has absent or diminished sensation below the level of the injury and is not aware of the pressure overload that may result in tissue breakdown. Weight shifts are performed either independently or with varying degrees of assistance depending on any limits in range of motion or strength.

Studies on blood flow and the lymphatic system[71] as well as clinical observation of spinal cord-injured subjects have formed the basis of recommending weight shifts every 30 minutes for a duration of 15 seconds. For those patients who require assistance to perform a weight shift the recommended time frame is every hour for 30 seconds.

Wheelchair Seating and Pressure-Relief Devices

Wheelchair cushions or pressure-relief devices are frequently prescribed to reduce the risk of pressure sores in patients with physical disabilities. The primary functions of the wheelchair cushion are to

- Relieve pressure in the anatomical areas vulnerable to breakdown by providing an additional protective layer between the seating surface and the body
- Distribute the body's weight away from bony prominences
- Stabilize the body for balance and functional positioning

In general, wheelchair seating is classified by function: seats or devices designed for postural control and seats or devices designed to relieve pressure and prevent tissue breakdown. It is the latter that will be addressed here. Seating surfaces for pressure relief are categorized further as either dynamic or static devices. Dynamic wheelchair cushions (and their mattress counterparts) are designed to produce alternating high and low pressures at any point on the sitting and lying surface of the body. Dynamic cushions are dependent on an external power source such as a battery or wall socket. This factor limits mobility and may interfere with a person's functional independence. Static wheelchair cushions are those devices that are placed on the wheelchair seat, and their ability to relieve or reduce pressure is determined by either their material and by their design. The three major categories of wheelchair cushions are air-filled, flotation, or foam.[33] Each category has distinct advantages and disadvantages as described in Table 25-1.

Over the past 10 years, the choices for the prescription of wheelchair cushions have increased dramatically. This has occurred for the following reasons:(1) the development of new and improved materials; (2) the advances in design technology; and (3) the availability of knowledge and information on pressure sore formation, treatment, and prevention. Furthermore, the

Table 25-1
Characteristics of Static Wheelchair Cushions

Category	Definition	Advantages	Disadvantages
Air-filled	An inflatable membrane appropriately filled with air	Lightweight Easy to clean	Subject to puncture Not easily repaired Requires monitoring of air pressure
Flotation-filled	Chemically treated water or other liquid within plastic or rubber membrane	Adjusts to body's movement Easy to clean	Heavy May leak if punctured Difficult to transfer
Flotation-gel	Plastic-like material simulates body fat tissue. Ideally, compression of one area of flotation cushions allows liquid or gel to flow into other noncompressed areas.	Adjusts to body's movement Acts as a shock absorber	Same as flotation-filled
Polyurethane foam	Solid blocks or layers of foam Compression of one area has little effect on other areas. Pressure distribution depends on design and firmness.	Readily available Lightweight Can be cut into any size, shape, or thickness Easy to transfer Provides stability and good balance	Wears out quickly (average 6 months) Cannot be washed or cleaned Subject to changes in temperature Should not be exposed to direct sunlight

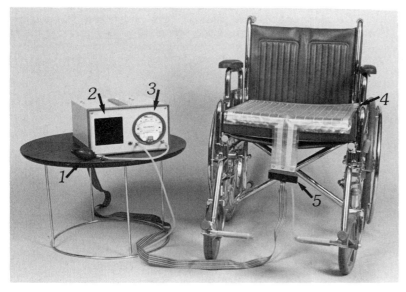

Figure 25-7. A device for measuring pressure under every part of the patient's sitting surface called a Texas Interface Pressure Evaluator (TIPE). (*1,* pump; *2,* readout display; *3,* gauge; *4,* sensing pad; *5,* connector)

cushion prescribed during a first admission for rehabilitation may not be satisfactory once a patient returns to his or her home, family, job, school, and social activities. Whereas one type of cushion initially may promote good balance and posture, increased sitting tolerance, and pressure relief, it may not be practical on a long-term basis. Therefore, other cushions should be considered when the person returns for a progress assessment 6 months to 1 year following discharge from the rehabilitation hospital. These devices may be selected following pressure evaluation, a technique for assessing the amount of pressure between the body and another surface (*i.e.,* a bed or a wheelchair). It is used to individualize the prescription of a wheelchair cushion for patients with physical disabilities (Fig. 25-7).

Pressure evaluation is indicated for the following situations:

1. The development of tissue breakdown on the current cushion
2. During recovery from surgery undertaken for the correction of pressure sores, once the patient has at least 1½ hours of sitting tolerance
3. In a person at high risk to develop pressure sores (very thin and bony)
4. When there is a change in level or type of activities at home, work, or school that requires a change in the cushion.

Pressure evaluators are currently commercially available.* However, despite the controversy that continues to surround such instrumentation, it is clear that the pressure itself is not the only factor in determining a wheelchair pressure-relief device. Since the mid 1970s, researchers have documented other factors that must be considered when selecting effective devices.[16, 34, 50] These are listed in Table 25-2.

---

*For example, the Texas Interface Pressure Elevator (TIPE) and the Scimedics Pressure Evaluator Pad.

Table 25-2
Factors That Determine the Effective Selection of Wheelchair Cushions

1. Diagnosis
2. Number of hours spent daily in the wheelchair
3. Types of activities performed from the wheelchair
    a. Self-care/independent living skills
    b. Vocational
    c. Educational
    d. Recreational/social
    e. Homemaking
4. Posture and trunk stability
5. Usage environment
    a. Climate, temperature, humidity
    b. Pollution
    c. Terrain
    d. Continence
6. Living arrangements
    a. Independent
    b. Assisted by family, friends, attendants, or nurses
7. Tissue history
    a. Pressure sores
    b. Surgery to correct pressure sores
    c. Decreased sitting tolerance secondary to specific medical or social factors
8. Body build based on height, weight, age, and sex
9. Wheelchair style and size
10. Pressure
    a. Magnitude
    b. Distribution

It is important to remember that there is no single cushion on the market today that is effective for all patients. Therefore, consumers of these products are encouraged to communicate with their physicians and therapists in order to select the best device for their individual needs and life-styles. Patients who rely on this type of equipment are cautioned against purchasing a cushion based on the recommendations of another person with a physical disability, even one in the same diagnostic category. This might result in a needless expense as well as the risk of pressure sores if the device proves inappropriate or ineffective.

Regardless of the accuracy of the pressure-relief device prescription, long-term outcomes depend on proper use of these devices by the patient. This, in turn, depends on adequate patient compliance and education.

A Philosophy for Tissue Pressure Management

Because pressure sore formation is a constant threat to patients with spinal cord injuries or other neurological or musculoskeletal impairment, education concerning pressure sore prevention should begin early in the rehabilitation program. The patient must be brought into the educational process as an active participant. While they perform routine activities such as bed positioning, turning, and range of motion, nurses and therapists should first introduce to the patient and the family the concept of pressure sore prevention. The importance of these activities as early interventions must be emphasized. As the patient progresses in the rehabilitation program, all the disciplines should incorporate specific pressure sore prevention information during the various therapies and instruction. In this regard consideration must be given to skin hygiene, nutrition, equipment, and communication.

Skin Care

The principles of skin care begin with good personal hygiene. The skin must be kept clean and dry. Moisture and bacteria from perspiration or incontinence may irritate the skin already stressed over bony prominences in the sitting or lying position. In addition, absent or diminished sensation and reduced circulation contribute to the formation of pressure sores in patients with disabling conditions. The skin should be cleansed using a mild, nonallergenic soap in order to avoid rashes or the loss of natural moisture from the superficial layers of the skin. If the skin becomes dry, flaky, or cracked, a lotion should be applied to the affected areas. Exposure to the sun should be limited to very short periods of time initially. Tolerance may be slowly increased over time. In very hot climates, the skin should be protected from the sun by using sunscreens or other effective sunburn protective ointments. Any alteration of the skin such as a rash caused by allergy or irritation from drugs, alcohol, or medication should be treated as though it were a pressure sore. If it arises on a weight-bearing surface, pressure should be kept off it until it is healed. An infection that results in the elevation of body temperature changes the general body metabolism. Therefore, sitting times and activity levels should be reduced and turning schedules modified. Spasms may also result in tissue breakdown either from shearing forces or by shifting the body out of the ideal alignment in the chair. Poorly fitting or tight shoes and clothing or appliances such as braces, orthoses, corsets, and leg-bag attachments can erode soft tissue and must be checked regularly. Proper fit and careful observation are essential to preventing tissue breakdown.

Skin Assessment

Routine skin assessment, performed twice each day by the patient independently or by a caregiver, identifies the following early signs of impending tissue breakdown:

1. Changes in color of the skin
2. Blisters
3. Burns
4. Rashes
5. Swelling
6. Pimples and ingrown hairs
7. Bruises
8. Breaks in the surface of the skin

Assessment of the skin in the morning determines whether positioning during the night, wrinkles in sheets and pajamas, or possibly a foreign object (*e.g.,* food, utensils) caused pressure that resulted in a change in the color or the texture of the skin. A night assessment, after the person transfers from the wheelchair to the bed before retiring, provides information on whether the daily sitting time and schedule, transfers, or traumas created any skin problems. Mirrors are helpful when checking areas difficult to see such as the backs of the legs, buttocks, hips, and back. If areas of unusual redness or discoloration remain visible on the skin surface for more than 30 minutes, these areas must be considered potentially dangerous and should be relieved of pressure until they return to their normal color.

Communication

The success of any pressure sore prevention program is also dependent on the cooperative interaction between patients vulnerable to the effects of pressure and the rehabilitation health care professionals. One of the most effective and beneficial means of promoting pressure sore prevention is by establishing small group sessions in which therapists or nursing staff present tissue pressure management and pressure sore prevention techniques to patients and their family members. Short lectures or more in-depth seminars accompanied by visuals, handouts, and interactive discussion maximize retention of pertinent information.

It is the responsibility of all health care professionals to keep informed about current practices in pressure sore prevention. Experimental and new commercially available products and devices appear on the market and require clinical evaluation. Related research findings and the clinical experiences of other practitioners are frequently presented at professional meetings and published in professional journals.

Although the main thrust of promoting pressure sore prevention and awareness occurs during hospitalization, the education process must continue after the patient's discharge from the hospital environment. A constant, daily vigil must be kept against the effects of pressure. Routine follow-up visits to the hospital and physicians where a person received rehabilitation are often scheduled at intervals of 1, 3, 6 and 12 months following discharge to identify changes or problems in medical management including urinary, respiratory, circulatory, skin, and psychosocial issues. These visits provide an extended series of scheduled follow-up contacts essential for continuity of care. Patients are encouraged to call for an earlier appointment should any problems, such as tissue breakdown, develop prior to the scheduled visit.

Tissue pressure management clinics have been established in the United States and other countries to provide and maintain individualized pressure sore prevention programs. Tissue problems are assessed by a team of professionals, including the patient's main physician, a plastic surgeon, nurse, therapist, and social worker. It is during such a clinic visit that the person's individual program can be assessed and modified. Recommendations may include the following:

1. Conservative medical management
2. Reduction of sitting time
3. Replacement of wheelchair cushion
4. Evaluation for a new wheelchair cushion
5. Repair of the wheelchair
6. Curtailment of activity
7. For grade 3 ulcers: instruction in dressing application
8. For grade 4 and 5 ulcers: admission to hospital for culture, débridement and antibiotics if indicated and evaluation for surgical repair.

CONCLUSIONS

Pressure sores interfere with every aspect of the physically disabled patient's life from active participation in a rehabilitation program to returning to the community as a productive and creative person. Although the cost for the surgical repair of pressure sores may now exceed $25,000, this is only a fraction of the total burden on society. Other aspects of this burden derive from the loss of productive employment with its concomitant economic impact on the patient and the family, the reduced educational opportunities with their long-term impact on vocational potential, the separation from the family unit with its impact on psychological and social development, and, finally, a loss of general personal independence and productivity that contributes to a severe bereavement of self-esteem.

Many factors alone or in combination are responsible for tissue breakdown. Therefore, the importance of a comprehensive, multidisciplinary approach to tissue pressure management for patients with physically disabling conditions cannot be overemphasized. This approach must have at its core a treatment component and an extensive educational component in which many pressure sore prevention methods and techniques are presented to patients and family members. These methods include personal hygiene and skin assessment, weight shifts, nutrition awareness, prescription and care of wheelchairs, and the proper selection and use of pressure-relief devices. Furthermore, it has been demonstrated that comprehensive tissue management programs do in fact reduce the recurrence rate of pressure sores.[50]

The success of the educational component depends not only on the family and the health care team but on the individual patient's willingness to be an active participant in the prevention process. Only in combination will the prevention activities result in healthy skin, free of the tissue erosion that reduces productivity and independence. And, only by reducing or ameliorating the threat of tissue breakdown, and incorporating practical tissue management into the rehabilitation program, can a patient with a physical disability achieve his or her highest potential.

REFERENCES

1. Anderson TP, Andberg MM: Psychosocial factors associated with pressure sores. Arch Phys Med Rehabil 60:341–346, 1979
2. Artigue RS, Hyman WA: The effect of myoglobin on the oxygen concentration in skeletal muscle subjected to ischemia. Ann Biomed Eng 4:128–137, 1976
3. Barton A, Barton M: The Management and Prevention of Pressure Sores. London, Faber & Faber, 1981
4. Basson MD, Burney RE: Defective wound healing in paraplegic patients. Surg Forum 32:78–80, 1981
5. Bennett L: Transferring load to flesh: VIII. Stasis and stress. Bull Prosthet Res 10(Spring):202–210, 1975
6. Bennett L: Transferring load to flesh: V. Experimental work. Bull Prosthet Res 10(Fall):88–103, 1973
7. Bennett L: Transferring load to flesh: II. Analysis of compressive stress. Bull Prosthet Res 10(Fall): 45–63, 1971
8. Bennett L, Kavner D, Lee BY et al: Skin stress and blood flow in sitting paraplegic patients. Arch Phys Med Rehabil 65:186–190, 1984
9. Blackburn GL, Bistrian BR, Maini BS et al: Nutritional and metabolic assessment of the hospitalized patient. J Parenter Enteral Nut 1:11–12, 1977
10. Brand PW: Pressure sores. In Kenedi RM, Cowden JM, Scales JT (eds): Bed Sore Biomechanics, pp 19–25. London, Macmillan Press, 1976
11. Branmark PI: Microvascular function reduces flow rates. In Kenedi RM, Cowden JM, Scales JT (eds): Bedsore Biomechanics. London, Macmillan Press, 1976
12. Cherry GW, Ryan TJ: The effects of ischemia and reperfusion of tissue survival. Maj Probl Dermatol 7:93, 1976
13. Clark MO, Barbenel JC, Jordan MM, Nicol SM: Pressure sores. Nurs Times 74:363–366, 1978
14. Claus-Walker J, DiFerrante N, Halstead LS, Tavella D: Connective tissue turnover in quadriplegia. Am J Phys Med 61:130–140, 1982
15. Claus-Walker J, Kretzer FL: Insensitive skin properties of spinal cord injured patients. Arch Phys Med Rehabil 62:521, 1981
16. Cochran GVB, Palmieri V: Development of test methods for evaluation of wheelchair cushions. Bull Prosthet Res 17(Spring):9–30, 1980
17. Cochran GVB: The Pig as a Model for Soft Tissue Experiments. Presented at the Workshop on the Effects of Mechanical Stress on Soft Tissue, Dallas, Texas, November 5–7, 1980
18. Cohen K: Biochemistry of Collagen. Presented at the Workshop on the Effects of Mechanical Stress on Soft Tissues, Dallas, Texas, November 5–7, 1980
19. Constantian MB: Pressure Ulcers: Principles and Techniques of Management. Boston, Little, Brown & Co, 1980
20. Cousins MJ, Mather LE: Intrathecal and epidural administration of opioids. Anesthesiology 61:276–310, 1984

21. Cull JB, Smith OH: A preliminary note on demographic and personality correlates of decubitus ulcer incidence. J Psychol 85:225–227, 1973

22. Daly CH, Chimosky JE, Holloway GA, Kennedy D: The effects of pressure loading on the blood flow rate in human skin. In Kenedi RM, Cowden JM, Scales JT (eds): Bedsore Biomechanics, pp 69–78. London, Macmillan Press, 1976

23. Daniel RK, Priest DL, Wheatley DC: Etiologic factors in pressure sores: An experimental model. Arch Phys Med Rehabil 62:492–498, 1981

24. Daniel RK, Hall EJ, MacLeod M: Pressure sores: a reappraisal. Ann Plastic Surg 1:53–63, 1979

25. Daniels R: Skin. Presented at the Workshop on the Effects of Mechanical Stress on Soft Tissues. Dallas, Texas November 5–7, 1980

26. Dinsdale SM: Decubitus ulcers: Role of pressure and friction in causation. Arch Phys Med Rehabil 55:147–152, 1974

27. Dinsdale SM: Decubitus ulcers in swine: Light and electron microscopy study of pathogenesis. Arch Phys Med Rehab 54:51–56, 1973

28. Donovan WH: Effect of Clonidine on Spasticity: A Clinical Trial. Presented at the 12th Annual Scientific Meeting, American Spinal Injury Association, San Franscisco, CA, 1986

29. Dowling AS: Pressure sores: Their cause, prevention and treatment. MD State Med J 6:131–134, 1970

30. Fisher SV, Patterson P: Long-term pressure recordings under the ischial tuberosities of tetraplegics. Paraplegia 21:99–106, 1983

31. Fisher SV, Szymke TE, Apte SY, Kosiak M: Wheelchair cushion effect on skin temperature. Arch Phys Med Rehabil 59:68–71, 1978

32. Fleck A: Protein metabolism after surgery. Proc Nutr Soc 39:125–132, 1980

33. Garber SL: A classification of wheelchair seating. Am J Occup Ther 10:652–654, 1979

34. Garber SL: Wheelchair cushions for spinal cord injured individuals. Am J Occup Ther 39:722–725, 1985

35. Garber SL, Campion LJ, Krouskop TA: Trochanteric pressure in spinal cord injury. Arch Phys Med Rehabil 63:549–552. 1982

36. Garber SL, Krouskop TA, Carter RE: System for clinically evaluating wheelchair pressure-relief cushions. Am J Occup Ther 32:565–570, 1978

37. Griffiths BH: Advances in treatment of decubitus ulcers. Surg Clin North Am 43:245–260, 1963

38. Guttman L: Spinal Cord Injuries: Comprehensive Management and Research, pp 512–515. Oxford, Blackwell Scientific, 1973

39. Hancock DA, Reed GW, Atkinson PJ et al: Bone and soft tissue changes in paraplegic patients. Paraplegia 17:267–271, 1979

40. Hassard GH: heterotopic bone formation about the hip and unilateral decubitus ulcers in spinal cord injury. Arch Phys Med Rehabil 56:355–358, 1975

41. Hendricks RW, Calenoff L, Lederman RB, Neiman HL: Radiology of pressure sores. Radiology 138:351–356, 1981

42. Herzog SJ, Harding RL: Surgical treatment of pressure ulcers. Arch Phys Med Rehabil 59:193–200, 1978

43. Hickman KE, London O, Reswick JB, Scalan RH: Deformation and flow in compressed skin tissues. Proceedings of the symposium on Biomechanics and Fluid Mechanics, American Society of Mechanical Engineers, April 25–27, 1966

44. Holloway GA, Daly C, Kennedy D, Chimosky J: Effects of external pressure loading on human skin blood flow measured by xenon clearance. J Appl Physiol 40:597–600, 1976

45. Hunt RK, Connally WB, Aronson SB, Goldstein P: Anaerobic metabolism and wound healing: An hypothesis for the initiation and cessation of collagen synthesis in wounds. Am J Surg 135:328, 1978

46. Hussain T: Experimental study of some pressure effects on tissues with reference to the bed sore problem. J Pathol Bacteriol 66:347–358, 1953

47. Jordan MM, Clark MO: Report of Incidence of Pressure Sore in the Patient Community of the Greater Glasgow Health Board Area. University of Strathclyde, January 21, 1977

48. Kosiak M: Etiology and pathology of ischemic ulcers. Arch Phys Med Rehab 40:62–69, 1959

49. Kosiak M: Etiology of decubitus ulcers. Arch Phys Med Rehabil 42:19–29, 1961

50. Krouskop TA, Noble P, Garber SL, Spencer WA: The effectiveness of preventive management in reducing the occurrence of pressure sores. J Rehabil RD 20:73–83, 1983

51. Larsen JB, Holstein P, Lassen NA: Pathogenesis of bed sores—Skin: Blood flow cessation by external pressure on the back. Scand J Plast Surg, 13:347–350, 1979

52. Lindan O: Etiology of decubitus ulcers: An experimental study. Arch Phys Med Rehabil 42:774–783, 1961

53. Mahanty SD, Roemer RB: Thermal response of skin to application of localized pressure. Arch Phys Med Rehab 50:584–590, 1979

54. Manley MT, Darby T: Repetitive mechanical stress and denervation in plantar ulcer pathogenesis in rats. Arch Phys Med Rehab 61:171–177, 1980

55. Manley MT: Incidence of contributing factors and costs of pressure sores. S Afr Med J 53:217–222, 1978

56. Moolten SE: Bed sores in the chronically ill patient. Arch Phys Med Rehabil 53:430–438, 1972

57. Moolten SE: Suggestions on the prevention and management of bed sores. Med Times 101:52–56, 1973

58. Morley MH: Decubitus ulcer management: A team approach. Canad Nurse 10:41–43, 1973

59. Motloch WM: Analysis of Medical Costs Associated with Healing of Pressure Sores in Adolescent Paraplegics. Unpublished report, University of San Francisco, 1978

60. Murphy E: Transferring load to flesh: I. Concept. Bull Prosthet Res 10(Fall):38–44, 1971

61. Newell PH Jr, Thornburgh JD, Fleming WC: The management of pressure and other external factors in the prevention of ischemic ulcers. ASME Trans J Basic Eng 93:590–596, 1970

62. Noble PC: The Prevention of Pressure Sores in Persons with Spinal Cord Injuries. World Rehabilitation Fund. International Exchange of Information in Rehabilitation, Monograph No. 11, 1981

63. Nola GT, Vistnes LM: Differential response of skin and muscle in the experimental production of pressure sores. Plast Res Surg 66:728–733, 1980

64. Palmieri VR, Haelen G, Cockran GVB: A comparison of interface pressure measurements on seat cushions between air cell transducers and miniature diaphragm pressure transducers. Bull Prosthet Res 17(Spring):5–8, 1980

65. Parish LC, Witkowski JA, Crissey JT: The Decubitus Ulcer. New York, Masson Publishing, 1983

66. Peiffer SCI, Blust P, Llysom JFJ: Nutritional assessment of the SCI patient. J Am Dietetic Assoc 78:501–507, 1981

67. Perkash A, Brown M: Anaemia in patients with traumatic spinal cord injury. Paraplegia 20:235–236, 1982

68. Pinel C: Pressure sores. Nurs Times 2:172–174, 1976

69. Prockop DJ, Kivirikko KI: Hydroxyproline and the metabolism of collagen. In Gould BS (ed): Treatise on Collagen, vol 2, pp 215–246. New York, Academic Press, 1968

70. Reddy NP: A Discrete Model of the Lymphatic System, dissertation. Texas A&M University, College Station, Texas, 1974

71. Reddy NP, Cockran GVB, Krouskop TA: Interstitial flow as a factor in decubitus ulcer formation. J Biol 14:879–881, 1981

72. Reddy NP, Cochran GVB: Phenomenological theory underlying pressure-time relationship in decubitus ulcer formation. Fed Proc 38:1153, 1979

73. Reddy NP, Krouskop TA, Newell PH Jr: Biomechanics of a lymphatic vessel. Blood Vessels 12:261–278, 1975

74. Reichel SM: Shear force as a factor in decubitus ulcers in paraplegics. JAMA 166:762–763, 1958

75. Richardson RR, Meyer PR: Prevalence and incidence of pressure sores in acute spinal cord injuries. Paraplegia 19:235–247, 1981

76. Robinson CE, Coghlan JK, Jackson G: Decubitus ulcers in paraplegics: Financial implications. Canad J Public Health 69:199, 1978

77. Rodriguez GP: Lysyl hydroxylase activity: Relationship to skin collagen metabolism in spinal cord injury patients. Final report, Mary Switzer Fellowship, NIHR, August 1985

78. Rodriguez GP, Claus-Walker J: Measurement of hydroxylysine glycosides in urine and its application to spinal cord injury. J Chromat 308:65–73, 1984

79. Rodriguez GP, Claus-Walker J, Kent MC, Carter RE: Urinary collagen metabolite concentration as a predictor of complications in spinal cord injury. ASIA Abstracts Digest. 11th Annual Scientific Meeting, April 15–17, 1985

80. Rodriguez GP, Claus-Walker, Kent MC, Stal S: Adrenergic receptors in insensitive skin of spinal cord injury patients. Arch Phys Med Rehabil 67:177–180, 1986

81. Rogers JE: Annual Report of the Rehabilitation Engineering Center. Rancho Los Amigos Hospital, Downey, California, 1973

82. Romanus M: Microcirculatory reactions to local pressure induced ischemia. Acta Chir Scand 143:5–30, 1977

83. Romanus ME: Microcirculatory reactions to controlled tissue ischemia and temperature: A vital microscopic study on the hampster's cheek pouch. In Kenedi RM, Cowden JM, Scales JT (eds): Bedsore Biomechanics, pp 79–82. London, Macmillan Press, 1976

84. Ruberg RL: The role of nutrition in plastic surgical practice: A review. Plast Reconstr Surg 65:363–375, 1980

85. Ryan TJ: Blood supply and decubitus ulcers. Int J Dermatol 18:123–134, 1979

86. Seiler WO, Stahelin HB: Skin oxygen tension as a function of imposed skin pressure: Implication for decubitus ulcer formation. J Am Geriatr Soc 27:298–301, 1979

87. Shea JD, Sepulveda JA: Pressure sore profile. Presented at ASIA Meeting, Atlanta, April 15–17, 1985

88. Smith CR: Pressure sores. Rehabil Rept 1:2–3, 1985

89. Sugarman B: Osteomyelitis beneath pressure sores. Arch Intern Med 143:683–688, 1983

90. Stal S, Serure A, Donovan W, Spira M: The perioperative management: The patient with pressure sores. Ann Plast Surg 11:347–356, 1983

91. Van der Leun JE, Lowe LB, Beerens EGJ: The influence of skin temperature on dermal-epidermal adherence: evidence compatible with a highly viscous bond. J Invest Dermatol 62:42–46, 1974

92. Vasconez LO, Schneider WJ, Jurkiewicz MJ: Pressure Sores. In Ravitch M (ed): Current Problems in Surgery. Chicago, Year Book Medical Publishers, 1977

93. Williams A: A study of factors contributing to skin breakdown. Nurs Res 21:238–243, 1972

94. Young JS, Burns PE: Pressure sores and the spinal cord injured: I. SCI Digest 3(Fall):9–16, 1981

95. Young JS, Burns PE: Pressure sores and the spinal cord injured: II. SCI Digest 3(Winter):11–19, 1981

26

Neurogenic Bladder and Bowel

Joachim L. Opitz

Gudni Thorsteinsson

Ann H. Schutt

David M. Barrett

Patricia K. Olson

With the advent of antibiotics, intermittent catheterization, and the increasing ability to explore, define, and measure urodynamically the various neurogenic dysfunctions of the lower urinary tract, members of the rehabilitation team are now able to assist the patient in satisfactory, regular emptying of the bladder, prevention of marked bladder hypertrophy, maintenance of urinary continence, and avoidance of potentially life-threatening urological complications. A similar evolution has occurred in regard to the management of neurogenic bowel dysfunction. The purpose of this chapter is to assist the interested health care professional of the rehabilitation team in the diagnosis and management of neurogenic bladder and bowel dysfunctions.

NEUROGENIC BLADDER DYSFUNCTION

Anatomical and Physiological Considerations for the Urinary Tract

The Kidneys

The kidneys are capable of producing a concentrated solution of metabolic waste products. They are highly vascular, demanding just under 25% of cardiac output. Each day, 180 liters of primary urine are filtered through the glomeruli, from which an average daily urine volume of approximately 1 liter is produced. A fluid intake of approximately 1800 ml/day produces a urine volume of approximately 1400 ml without undue renal metabolic work and a reasonably low urine concentration.

The Ureters

The ureters channel the urine by peristalsis from the renal pelvices to the bladder over a distance of 25 to 30 cm. The vesicoureteral junction prevents vesicoureteral reflux of urine. The one-way valve mechanism can remain competent only as long as the oblique course of the ureters within the bladder wall is maintained. The vesicoureteral junction becomes incompetent, permitting vesicoureteral reflux, when bladder hypertrophy causes the course of the distal ureter to become progressively perpendicular to the inner surface of the bladder (Fig. 26-1). Once ureteral reflux occurs, the ureter dilates markedly

and hydronephrosis results. Reflux is often further complicated by acute or chronic pyelonephritis with progressive renal failure. Therefore, maintenance or reestablishment of a competent vesicoureteral junction should be a basic goal in the management of neurogenic bladder dysfunction. Maintenance of normal voiding pressures of the bladder detrusor appears to be the key issue.

The Bladder

The bladder has the abilities of low-pressure storage of urine, complete emptying, protecting the kidneys from reflux, and maintaining the urinary tract free of infections. The capacity of the normal bladder is 400 to 500 ml. During progressive filling, the low transmural pressure of the bladder is maintained until near capacity is reached. The muscle bundles of the bladder detrusor extend into the wall of the proximal urethra, forming the internal urethral sphincter mechanism at its base.[56]

During emptying, the detrusor contracts to a normal voiding pressure of up to 60 cm H_2O. The contraction of the detrusor shortens the bladder neck and pulls it open. The bladder neck then assumes the shape of a funnel.[56] The bladder empties to a residual urine volume of 0 ml. The flow rate of urine during emptying (micturition) should be at least 10 ml/sec peak or mean flow. It may reach 30 to 40 ml/sec.

The Urethra

The urethra consists of involuntary smooth muscle proximally and of voluntary skeletal muscle distally. The male urethra is considerably longer (18 cm) than the female urethra (4.5 cm). The urethra has two sphincters: (1) the involuntary internal sphincter mechanism of the bladder neck and (2) the voluntary external urethral sphincter muscle.

The course of the male urethra is S-shaped. The posterior portion of the proximal urethra in men (between the base of the bladder and the external urethral sphincter) is surrounded by the prostate. The channels for the transport of semen extend through the prostate and enter the urethra proximally to the external urethral sphincter at the verumontanum (colliculus seminalis).

The course of the female urethra is straight. It runs adjacent

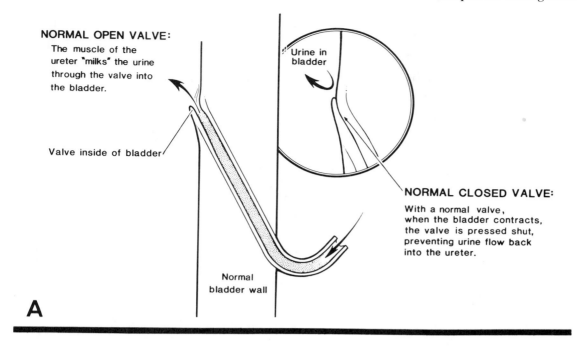

NORMAL OPEN VALVE:
The muscle of the ureter "milks" the urine through the valve into the bladder.

Valve inside of bladder

Urine in bladder

NORMAL CLOSED VALVE:
With a normal valve, when the bladder contracts, the valve is pressed shut, preventing urine flow back into the ureter.

Normal bladder wall

A

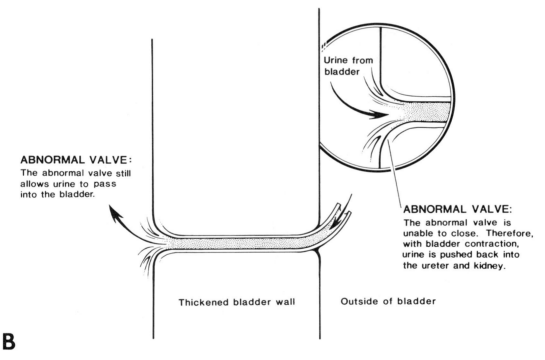

ABNORMAL VALVE:
The abnormal valve still allows urine to pass into the bladder.

Urine from bladder

ABNORMAL VALVE:
The abnormal valve is unable to close. Therefore, with bladder contraction, urine is pushed back into the ureter and kidney.

Thickened bladder wall   Outside of bladder

B

Figure 26-1. Vesicoureteral junction. (*A*) One-way valve mechanism is created by oblique course of ureter within wall of bladder. (*B*) Decompensated vesicoureteral junction due to bladder hypertrophy. Note straight course of ureter, perpendicular to inner surface of bladder, and obliteration of valve leaflet.

to the anterior wall of the vagina. The short, straight course favors incontinence and ascension of bacteria from the perineum (anus) into the bladder, especially when voiding is irregular and incomplete.[1]

In men, infected urine may be pressed into the seminal pathways in cases of voiding dysfunctions associated with co-contraction of the external urethral sphincter and high-pressure voiding. This event may lead to prostatitis and epididymitis.

Innervation of the Lower Urinary Tract

The bladder and proximal urethra receive their efferent and afferent nerve supply through the parasympathetic (pelvic nerves) and the sympathetic (hypogastric nerves) nerve systems. The striated, voluntary pelvic floor muscles, including the external urethral sphincter, receive their efferent and afferent nerve supply somatically via the pudendal nerves.[19, 71]

The *parasympathetic nerve system* provides the main motor innervation to the detrusor muscle. It originates in the intermediolateral sacral gray matter from S2–S4 (detrusor nucleus) and runs via the pelvic nerves to synapse in the extramural and intramural detrusor ganglia. Because most of the parasympathetic cell bodies are located within the detrusor muscle itself, destruction of the pelvic nerves leads to decentralization rather than to true denervation of the bladder. The postsynaptic fibers travel to the motor endings of the myosyncytium of the detrusor. Liberation of acetylcholine leads to membrane depolarization. The wave of depolarization spreads throughout the detrusor muscle via delicate cytoplasmic connections (nexus) between the fibers of the myosyncytium.[27, 28, 62, 81]

Sensory impulses, predominantly from the stretch receptors within the bladder wall, travel proximally in the pelvic nerves to the sacral micturition center (S2–S4).

The *sympathetic nerve system* provides innervation to the bladder and the proximal urethra.[41] The sympathetic nerve supply originates in the intermediolateral gray matter of the thoracolumbar cord (T11–L2). Sympathetic nerve impulses then travel via the ventral roots, the trunk ganglia, and the inferior mesenteric and hypogastric plexus to the hypogastric nerves and then to the entire bladder and proximal urethra. Norepinephrine is liberated at the sympathetic nerve endings. The bladder neck and the proximal urethra, which possess predominantly α-adrenergic receptors, respond to the appearance of norepinephrine with contraction. In contrast, the fundus of the bladder possesses predominantly β-adrenergic receptors[27] and responds with relaxation to the liberation of norepinephrine. Figure 26-2 illustrates the distribution of autonomic receptors in the bladder and proximal urethra. Sensory afferent fibers are also carried in the hypogastric nerves proximally. They originate predominantly from the submucosal layers of the bladder and proximal urethra.[41]

Sympathetic stimulation is also responsible for contraction of the ejaculatory ducts of the prostate and seminal vesicles, causing emission of semen. The co-contraction of the bladder neck and proximal urethra prevents retrograde ejaculation into the bladder.

The *somatic nerve supply via the pudendal nerves* provides innervation to the skeletal muscles of the proximal urethra, the urogenital diaphragm, and the external urethral sphincter. It arises from the anterior horn cells of the second to the fourth sacral cord segments and is under voluntary control. Afferent fibers are also carried in the pudendal nerves to the sacral micturition center from muscle spindles, stretch receptors, and other peripheral sensory organs of the pelvic floor, including those from the external anal sphincter, the perineum, the clitoris and labia of the female, and the scrotum, penis, and ischial and bulbocavernosus muscles of the male.

Central Regulation of Normal Micturition

Agreement exists about the common final pathways of micturition and storage of urine, as mediated through the thoracolumbar cord (sympathetic) and sacral cord (parasympathetic and somatic). In humans, the spinal cord centers of micturition by themselves lack the ability to effect well-coordinated storage of urine and micturition. Considerable disagreement exists about the specific location and functional interrelationships of supraspinal micturition centers.[5,19,71]

The following is a simplified description of the normal regulation of urine storage and micturition (Fig. 26-3). The actual coordinating center for reflexes affecting normal micturition and storage of urine seems to be located in the pons with ascending (dorsal and lateral funiculi) and descending (ventral reticulospinal and pyramidal tracts) spinal cord pathways connecting the pontine with the spinal micturition centers. Superimposed on the pontine micturition center are complex, modifying cortical (frontal, singulate gyrus), and subcortical areas (genu of corpus callosum, cerebellum, and midbrain). They exert learned, powerful, conscious inhibitory and, perhaps, less powerful facilitory influences on the pontine micturition center.[19, 71]

Normal Urodynamics of Filling and Emptying of the Bladder

Besides protecting the kidneys from hydrostatic pressure, the bladder has two dynamic functions, the progressive filling (storage) and the active, complete expulsion of urine at a time when it is socially acceptable.

During the *filling phase,* the pressure inside the bladder (transmural pressure) rises very slowly, mostly owing to the loose viscoelastic properties of the bladder wall (Fig. 26-4). When the stretch receptors within the bladder wall finally become stimulated, their increased nerve impulses are carried directly via pelvic nerves and the posterolateral funiculi to the pontine micturition center and to sensory-relating cortical areas, which then inhibit the pontine micturition center. The inhibited micturition center sends impulses probably via the ventral reticulospinal tracts to the thoracolumbar cord and to the sacral cord.[5, 19, 71] At the thoracolumbar cord, the sympathetic impulses via the hypogastric nerves effect contraction of the internal urethral sphincter mechanism (α-sympathetic receptors) and relaxation of the fundus of the bladder (β-sympathetic receptors). At the sacral cord, somatic impulses via the pudendal nerves cause increasing contraction of the external urethral sphincter and pelvic floor muscles. The normal bladder capacity is 400 to 500 ml.

The *emptying phase* is normally initiated by the consciously perceived sensation of fullness and urgency. The cortical and subcortical centers of micturition are capable of strong voluntary inhibition of the pontine micturition center until the right time and place for urination have been reached.[5, 19, 71] At that time, cortical facilitation of the pontine micturition center causes impulses to reach the thoracolumbar cord and the sacral micturi-

Figure 26-2. Distribution of autonomic receptors of bladder and proximal urethra. (Khanna OP: Nonsurgical therapeutic modalities. In Krane RJ, Siroky MB [eds]: Clinical Neuro-Urology, pp 159–196. Boston, Little, Brown Co, 1979. By permission of the publisher.)

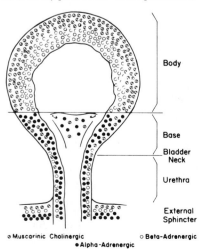

Body

Base

Bladder
Neck

Urethra

External
Sphincter

⊘ Muscarinic Cholinergic   ○ Beta-Adrenergic
● Alpha-Adrenergic

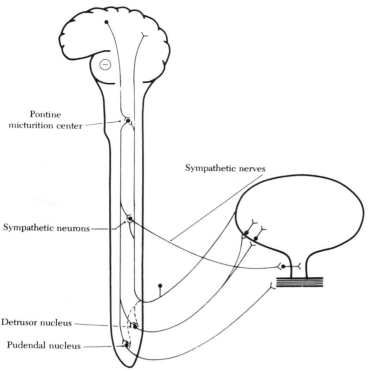

Figure 26-3. Spinal and supraspinal micturition centers. (Krane RJ, Siroky MB: Classification of neuro-urologic disorders. In Krane RJ, Siroky MB [eds]: Clinical Neuro-Urology, pp 143–158. Boston, Little, Brown Co, 1979. By permission of the publisher.)

Figure 26-4. Normal cystometrogram/pelvic floor electromyogram shows (*1*) bulbocavernosus reflex, (*2*) progressively increasing electrical activity (contraction) of pelvic floor muscles during later phase of filling, (*3*) functional bladder capacity, (*4*) detrusor contraction during voiding, (*5*) abrupt electrical silence during voiding, and (*6*) electrical activity of pelvic floor muscles during voluntary inhibition.

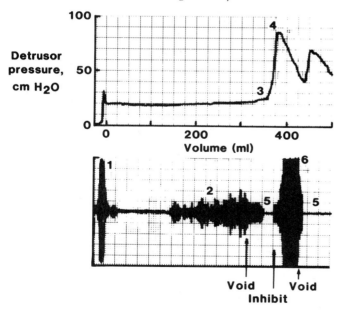

Mechanisms

Uninhibited neurogenic bladder dysfunction is caused by neurological lesions between the cortical or subcortical micturition areas of the brain and the pontine micturition center. The patient with uninhibited neurogenic bladder dysfunction does not become sufficiently aware of a full bladder, insufficiently suppresses the activity of the pontine micturition center, and voids prematurely.

Urodynamically, the micturition dysfunction is minimal (reduced capacity) because the pontine micturition center functions normally (Fig. 26-5).

Upper motor neuron bladder dysfunction is caused by neurologic lesions between the pontine and sacral micturition centers. The spinal micturition centers are rendered hyperreflexic and incoordinated (spastic). Urodynamically, the external urethral sphincter co-contracts with the detrusor muscle (detrusor/external urethral sphincter dyssynergia). The more spastic the cord is or the stronger the detrusor stretch reflex is acting, the more pronounced are the co-contractions (Fig. 26-6).

Upper motor neuron bladder dysfunctions are characterized by a hyperactive bulbocavernosus reflex, a reduced bladder capacity (usually less than 300 ml), and detrusor/external urethral sphincter dyssyrgia (Fig. 26-6). The resulting high voiding pressure leads to progressive detrusor hypertrophy with potential vesicoureteral reflux.

Spinal lesions above T10 tend to result in additional increases in sympathetic discharges from T11–L2, with an increase in tension of the internal sphincter mechanism resulting in detrusor–internal sphincter dyssynergia and probably some reduction of the detrusor–detrusor reflex.

Complications of upper motor neuron bladder dysfunction are primarily related to the high outflow resistance, owing to detrusor–sphincter dyssynergia. A vicious cycle starts to build when the spastic detrusor is allowed to work against high outflow resistance with elevated voiding pressures of more than 80 to 90 cm H_2O. The consequences are progressive detrusor hypertro-

tion center. From the thoracolumbar cord, the sympathetic impulses cease, which causes the internal sphincter mechanism to relax and the detrusor to be uninhibited. From the sacral cord, parasympathetic impulses cause a strong detrusor contraction, and the somatic impulses to the external urethral sphincter cease, which causes its relaxation. Voiding then commences (Fig. 26-4).

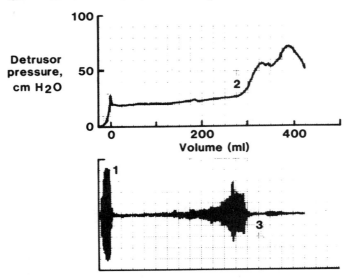

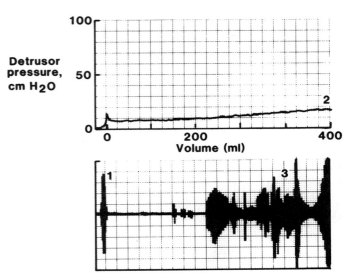

Figure 26-5. Cystometrogram/electromyogram in a patient with complete, uninhibited neurogenic bladder dysfunction shows (*1*) brisk bulbocavernosus reflex, (*2*) spontaneous detrusor contraction at reduced bladder capacity, and (*3*) associated silence of pelvic floor muscles (external urethral sphincter).

Figure 26-6. Cystometrogram/electromyogram in a patient with complete upper motor neuron bladder dysfunction shows (*1*) brisk bulbocavernosus reflex, (*2*) reduced bladder capacity, (*3*) high intravesical pressure during detrusor contraction, and (*4*) marked electrical activity of pelvic floor muscles during detrusor contraction (detrusor/external urethral sphincter dyssynergia).

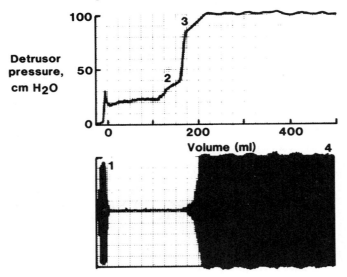

phy and an increase in residual urine volumes of more than 100 ml, causing recurrent urinary tract infections.[87] Both the increased pressure work of the detrusor and the frequently coexisting cystitis promote higher levels of cord spasticity and dyssynergia. The development of ureteral hypertrophy with dilatation, pseudodiverticula formation of the bladder, and vesicoureteral reflux with progressive destruction of the upper tracts are sequelae.[10, 89]

Mixed type A neurogenic bladder dysfunction is caused by neurological lesions in the sacral micturition center, which destroy the detrusor nucleus and render the nucleus of the pelvic floor muscles (external urethral sphincter) hyperreflexic.

Figure 26-7. Cystometrogram/electromyogram in a patient with complete mixed type A neurogenic bladder dysfunction shows (*1*) brisk bulbocavernosus reflex, (*2*) marked increase of bladder capacity with absent detrusor contractions (detrusor areflexia), and (*3*) hyperactive pelvic floor muscle activity (external urethral sphincter).

Urodynamically, mixed type A neurogenic bladder dysfunction is characterized by an absent or markedly hypoactive detrusor in the presence of a hyperactive internal or external urethral sphincter (Fig. 26-7). Therefore, the patient is unable to void in the presence of a markedly increased bladder capacity.

Type A neurogenic bladder dysfunction may also be caused by the development of myogenic bladder insufficiency[29, 81] (as a result of chronic overfilling of the bladder) or possibly by a marked spasticity of the thoracolumbar (sympathetic) micturition center in spinal cord injury above T10. Mixed type A neurogenic bladder dysfunction is the more common of the two mixed neurogenic bladder dysfunctions.

Complications are abdominal pain from overstretching of the bladder and urinary tract infections with overflow voiding (constant dribbling). Vesicoureteral reflux is rare.

Mixed type B neurogenic bladder dysfunction is postulated as a neurological lesion just above the sacral micturition center, affecting the pelvic floor nucleus but leaving the detrusor nucleus spastic. The result is detrusor hyperreflexia associated with flaccid paralysis of the pelvic floor.

Urodynamically, mixed type B neurogenic bladder dysfunction is characterized by a marked hyperreflexic detrusor with decreased bladder capacity and a hypoactive, flaccid external urethral sphincter (Fig. 26-8). The patient has a low bladder capacity with uncontrollable, frequent urinary incontinence.

Complications may consist of bladder hypertrophy, marked incontinence, and, rarely, vesicoureteral reflux with its associated consequences.

Lower motor neuron bladder dysfunction is caused by neurological lesions destroying the sacral micturition center or the relating nerve supply to the lower urinary tract. Urodynamically, it is characterized by flaccid paralysis of the detrusor and pelvic floor muscles (including the external urethral sphincter) with increased bladder capacity (Fig. 26-9). The bladder neck (internal sphincter mechanism), however, may have increased tension leading to some increase in outflow resistance in the presence of an intact thoracolumbar (sympathetic) micturition center. Patients harbor large volumes of infected urine and void only by constant dribbling when the bladder cannot expand any farther (overflow voiding).

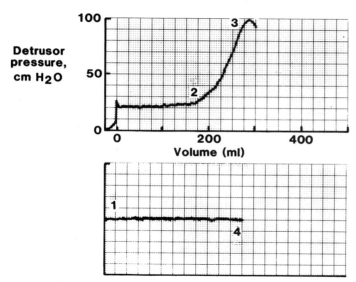

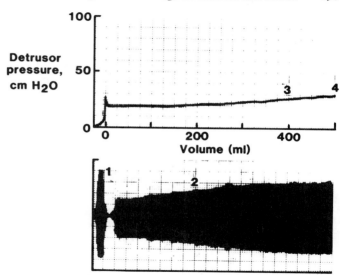

Figure 26-8. Cystometrogram/electromyogram in a patient with complete mixed type B neurogenic bladder dysfunction shows (*1*) no bulbocavernosus reflex, (*2*) decreased functional bladder capacity, (*3*) spontaneous detrusor contraction to abnormally high voiding pressure, and (*4*) no electrical activity of pelvic floor muscles (external urethral sphincter).

Figure 26-9. Cystometrogram/electromyogram in a patient with complete lower motor neuron bladder dysfunction shows (*1*) absent bulbocavernosus reflex, (*2*) absence of major detrusor contractions, (*3*) no pelvic floor muscle activity (external urethral sphincter), and (*4*) large bladder capacity.

Figure 26-10. Cystometrogram/electromyogram in a patient with complete myogenic detrusor insufficiency shows (*1*) brisk bulbocavernosus reflex, (*2*) habit voluntary contraction of pelvic floor muscles (external urethral sphincter), (*3*) no detrusor contraction, and (*4*) large bladder capacity.

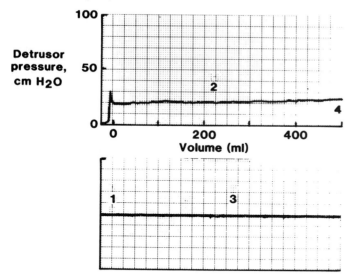

Complications are abdominal pain from overstretching of the bladder, frequent infections of the lower urinary tract, and skin complications with urinary incontinence. Vesicoureteral reflux is rare.

Myogenic detrusor insufficiency may be caused by cellular separation, intercellular fibrosis, and disruption of intercellular cytoplasmic processes (nexus) as sequelae of acute or recurring bladder overdistentions.[29, 81] Myogenic detrusor insufficiency may be present before or may be acquired during earlier stages of neurogenic bladder dysfunction.

Urodynamically, myogenic detrusor insufficiency is characterized by the presence of a bulbocavernosus reflex, voluntary control of the pelvic floor muscles including the external urethral sphincter, a noncontracting or poorly contracting detrusor muscle, and increased bladder capacity (Fig. 26-10). The bethanechol test is negative. The patient, therefore, has large retention of usually infected urine and overflow voiding, as described previously for lower motor neuron bladder dysfunction.

Micturition dysfunction is the main abnormality of myogenic detrusor insufficiency because of the missing expulsive force of the bladder. Micturition dysfunction may be further enhanced by a contracted bladder neck, which has become stiff because of little opening over prolonged periods as a result of existing overflow voiding or the use of intermittent catheterization. Habit contraction of the pelvic floor muscles at the time of attempted voiding may also further complicate and enhance the micturition dysfunction.[63, 74]

Classifications

Several classifications have been developed.[70] A classification should help members of the rehabilitation team arrive at a proper understanding and categorization based on the urodynamic characteristics of a particular dysfunction.

The classification presented in Table 26-1 is a modification of the classification of Perkash.[102] Issues of complete versus incomplete and of isolated sensory versus motor paralysis have been left out of the classification intentionally because they seem to be of less importance in practice. Neurological diseases that produce unstable or multiple lesions of the central nervous system, such as multiple sclerosis and polyradiculitis, are not included.

Early Management

Acute, Medically Unstable Phase

Neurogenic bladder dysfunction during the acute stage, while the medical status is either unstable or being evaluated, is by indwelling urethral catheter.[101] During this stage the patient

Table 26-1

Coordination of Clinical Disorders, the Resulting Neurological Lesions, the Related Urodynamic Abnormalities, and the Terminology of Neurogenic Bladder Dysfunctions

Clinical Disorder	Level of Neurological Lesion	Urodynamic Abnormalities
I. Delayed central nervous system maturation (childhood) Brain injury Brain neoplasms Stroke Cerebral arteriosclerosis (old age)	Between cerebral cortex and pontine micturition centers	Detrusor hyperreflexia with coordinated detrusor–sphincter interaction (uninhibited bladder dysfunction)
II. Traumatic spinal cord injury Syringomyelia Arteriovenous malformation Transverse myelitis Herniated intervertebral disk Spinal cord neoplasms (primary and secondary)	Between pontine and sacral micturition centers	Detrusor hyperreflexia with incoordinated, dyssynergic detrusor–sphincter interaction (upper motor neuron bladder dysfunction) Detrusor hyporeflexia or areflexia with external urethral sphincter hyperreflexia (mixed type A bladder dysfunction)
III. Traumatic spinal cord injury Syringomyelia Arteriovenous malformation Transverse myelitis Herniated intervertebral disk Myelodysplasia Poliomyelitis Spinal cord neoplasms (primary and secondary)	Lesion involving sacral micturition center	Detrusor hyporeflexia with external urethral sphincter hyperreflexia (mixed type A bladder dysfunction) Detrusor hyperreflexia with external urethral sphincter hyporeflexia or areflexia (mixed type B bladder dysfunction) Detrusor and external urethral sphincter hyporeflexia or areflexia (lower motor neuron bladder dysfunction) Detrusor and external urethral sphincter hyporeflexia or areflexia
Traumatic injury of pelvic and/or pudendal nerves Iatrogenic injuries of pelvic and/or pudendal nerves Peripheral neuropathies	Peripheral nerves between sacral micturition center and lower urinary tract	
IV. Acute or chronic bladder overdistention for organic and/or dysfunctional psychogenic reasons	Intramural disruption of nexus	Weak or absent detrusor contractions with normal external sphincter functions or dysfunctional (habit) co-contraction of external urethral sphincter and pelvic floor muscles during attempted micturition (myogenic detrusor insufficiency)

needs parenteral fluids and close monitoring of multiple organ systems. For the rare incidences of injury to the genitourinary system, as may be associated with pelvic fractures, cystocatheterization may be indicated. The following factors should be routinely monitored: temperature, fluid intake and output, complete blood cell count, and serum creatinine and urea. Urinalysis should also be performed regularly, and urine culture and sensitivity tests should be performed every other day. Frequent culturing of urine is essential during the acute phase.

Acute, Medically Stable Phase

When organ systems have become stable and parenteral treatment has been discontinued, a decision should be made about whether the bladder is to be drained by indwelling urethral catheter or by intermittent catheterization. Depending on the choice, fluid intake, prophylaxis for infections of the urinary tract, and treatment of urinary tract infections vary. Intermittent catheterization is the preferred method because it is associated with fewer complications.[6,46] If indwelling urethral drainage is selected, the fluid intake should be about 3000 ml/day, asymptomatic bacteriuria should not be treated, and antimicrobial prophylaxis of the urinary tract is not recommended.

However, cleanliness and changing of the indwelling catheter every 2 weeks are mandatory.

Before discontinuation of indwelling catheterization, the results of a recent urine culture and sensitivity tests should be available, specific antimicrobial therapy should be started, and the daily fluid intake should be decreased from 3000 to 1800 ml/day. Intermittent catheterization may be started once the daily urine output has decreased to 1400 ml and the results of a Gram stain are negative.

Intermittent catheterization should then be done with sterile technique every 6 hours, or more frequently if necessary, in order to keep the retention volumes less than 400 ml. Once the urine has become sterile (by culture), the patient should receive urinary tract antimicrobial prophylaxis. The management of significant infection is discussed below. In cases of symptomatic urinary tract infection, intermittent catheterization needs to be discontinued and continuous drainage started. In cases of asymptomatic urinary tract infection, intermittent catheterization may be continued if specific antimicrobial therapy can be started promptly. Otherwise, continuous drainage may be safer until specific antimicrobial treatment can be initiated.

During hospitalization and intermittent catheterization, urine should be cultured weekly or as needed if any symptoms develop that suggest urinary tract infections (see discussion below on urinary tract infections). External collection devices can be used for male patients if they are incontinent between intermittent catheterizations, unless one prefers to suppress the spontaneous detrusor contractions with anticholinergic medications.

Evaluation of Patients[86, 102]

History

The history of the present illness should be clearly identified, as should the other systems involved by injury or disease or as a sequela. These can significantly affect a patient's ability to comprehend or participate in a complex bladder management program that demands learning skills, some manual skills, transfers, and a change of living habits. A detailed past medical, sexual, and psychosocial history is needed to determine whether comprehension, motivation, learning skills, fitness, manual skills, transfers, or family support have been affected. Histories of past genitourinary tract disease or operations are also important because they can significantly influence goals and management.

Physical Examination

A neurological examination will determine mental status, motor and sensory level, and the presence of spinal shock. Determining the level of the spinal cord lesion allows predictions about future management and independence. During the rectal examination, anal sensation and tone, presence of the bulbocavernosus reflex, and any voluntary sphincter control are evaluated. During the abdominal examination, the status of the gastrointestinal tract, the kidneys, the bladder, and the abdominal wall is evaluated. The genitalia need to be examined both externally and internally. Fertile female patients need to be tested for pregnancy. Genital sensations should be determined, and a history about erections should be obtained.

Laboratory Examinations

Excretory urography should be done when the patient is medically stable, or earlier if indicated, but before definitive management by bladder retraining or intermittent catheterization. The excretory urogram gives information about structural changes of the kidneys, renal pelvis, ureters, and bladder and evidence of differences in the excretion of the radiopaque dye between the two sides or of significant delay in excretion. Overview roentgenography of the abdomen should be done to exclude the presence of visible stones.[86]

A renal scan may be indicated to determine renal size, shape, and position and to study renal function, urinary outflow tract obstruction, space-occupying lesions, changes in renal size, and major deformities of the upper urinary tracts. Renal scans may be useful for evaluating the upper urinary tracts in cases of allergy to radiopaque dye.[129]

Serum creatinine and urea values give baseline information about kidney function. Various renal clearance tests can be used to evaluate this, including creatinine clearance and several isotope studies, one of which is the short renal clearance test (of glomerular filtration rate) using ^{125}I-iothalamate.[129] Urinalysis is needed to determine the urine pH and osmolality and to study microscopically the urine sediment to determine the presence of bacteria,[60] leukocytes, and other elements.[86] A positive Gram stain of the urine correlates well with bacterial colony counts of more than 10^5 colonies/ml.[86] A positive leukocyte esterase dipstick test indicates pyuria. In cases of bacteriuria without significant tissue invasion, the leukocyte esterase dipstick test may be falsely negative.[72]

Urine cultures and sensitivity tests are needed at regular intervals, once per week to every other week, until the goal of permanent bladder management has been reached.

Residual urine volumes or retention volumes should always be checked when indwelling catheterization is discontinued and either intermittent catheterization or bladder retraining is instituted. For intermittent catheterization, retention volumes need to be checked in order to avoid bladder overdistention and to determine the frequency of catheterization. For bladder retraining, residual urine volumes need to be determined regularly in order to evaluate the efficiency of voiding. Elevated residual urine volumes are associated with a higher frequency of urinary tract infection.[87]

Cystoscopy should be performed before starting bladder retraining for catheter-free voiding, and before intermittent catheterization as definitive management. Voiding cystourethrography (video urodynamic test) may be indicated if findings on excretory urography or cystoscopy indicate lower tract abnormalities. More often, cystourethrography is used in combination with video urodynamic tests to delineate the location of urethral obstruction in patients who encounter difficulties during bladder retraining (Figs. 26-11 and 26-12.)

Urodynamic Testing

Before the bladder retraining program is started, diagnostic urodynamic studies should be done. A urologist should be consulted at that time to become acquainted with the patient and to rule out relative or actual contraindications to bladder retraining.[97, 102] Diagnostic urodynamic testing should be performed just before instituting bladder retraining. The lower urinary tract should be free of irritants such as infection, stones, or indwelling catheters. This study is usually done in the operating room and is followed by cystoscopy. Cystoscopy done before the urodynamic study usually irritates the genitourinary tract and distorts the findings.

Subsequent urodynamic studies can be done in the urodynamic laboratory. They are indicated when there is lack of progress in bladder retraining and are used to determine the optimal voiding techniques or the effect of neuro-urologic medications.

The cystometrogram provides information about volume–pressure relationships inside the bladder and about detrusor activity during the gradual filling of the bladder. Simultaneously, the activity of the external sphincter is determined with electromyography.[7, 12, 26, 68, 135] Techniques used for increasing bladder pressure (suprapubic tapping, straining, and the Credé maneuver) are evaluated, and the effects on bladder pressure and external sphincter activity are noted. The therapeutic urodynamic study is done with the patient on a bedside commode to simulate the conditions under which the bladder training is actually done.

Before the bladder is filled, the presence or absence of the bulbocavernosus reflex and any voluntary sphincter control is established. Cystometrography records the intravesical pressure as produced by detrusor activity. This gives information about the detrusor with regard to spasticity or flaccidity, spontaneous activity, ability to inhibit, and maximal pressure produced by bladder stimulation, straining, or the Credé maneuver.[12, 26, 68, 135] The maximal filling is usually limited to 500 ml, but it may be necessary to fill to 600 ml if no detrusor contraction can be elicited.

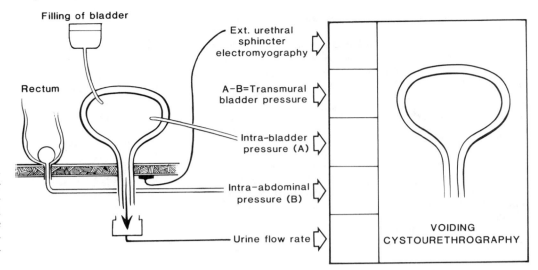

Figure 26-11. Urodynamic factors tested: external (ext.) sphincter electromyographic activity, intravesicular pressure, intra-abdominal pressure, and urine flow rate. (The actual access to the bladder for filling and measurement of intra-bladder pressure is transurethral.)

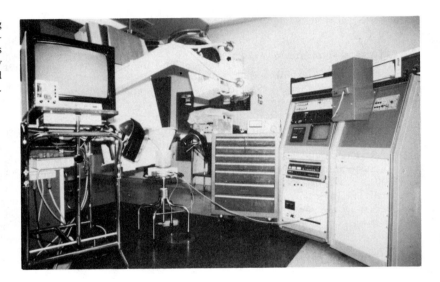

Figure 26-12. Urodynamic laboratory in an operating room. *Left to right:* monitor to follow fluoroscopy, cystometrography/electromyography, and fluorometry tracings during video urodynamic studies; adjustable fluoroscopy table; fluoroscope; urine flowmeter; video recorder; and cystometrograph/electromyograph fluorometry recorder.

Simultaneous electromyography of the external sphincter gives information about the coordinated or incoordinated (dyssynergic) activity between the detrusor and the external urethral sphincter.[7] If there is evidence of dyssynergia, the effects of anal sphincter stretching on relaxation of the external sphincter may be evaluated.[100]

The urethral pressure profile is a measure of the outflow resistance within the urethra. Several techniques have been described. The usefulness of the urethral pressure profile is not clear at this time, and therefore urethrocystography is often needed.[4, 13, 84, 122, 127]

The bethanechol (Urecholine) test should be done in patients with areflexic detrusors.[14] The test helps to determine the presence of bladder denervation (as indicated by a positive test). The bethanecol test is based on the fact that the denervated detrusor, unlike the innervated detrusor, shows increased tension in the presence of bethanechol. The test has several contraindications. It should not be performed on patients with the following conditions: hypertension, peptic ulcer disease, vagotonia, bronchial asthma, any heart disease (including coronary artery disease, sinus bradycardia, or heart block), seizure disorder, Parkinson's disease, chronic obstructive pulmonary disease, hypotension (symptomatic), and intestinal obstruction.

Test results should be interpreted in conjunction with the clinical status of the patient because false-positive results are possible.[14]

Transrectal ultrasonography seems to be promising for studying otherwise unexplained urethral outflow obstructions.[103]

Considerations in the Evaluation of Children

The evaluation of children with neurogenic voiding dysfunctions is much the same as that of adults but with special considerations for the size of the lower urinary tract and the cooperation of the patient.

Imaging studies of the kidney that are used are excretory urography or renal sonography. If possible, awake, voiding cystograms are important to determine the urological anatomy. In the presence of abnormal structures, further studies are indicated. Endoscopic procedures are rarely needed.

Residual urine volumes are difficult to determine in very young children. Bladder size and kidney size can be determined by real-time ultrasonography[52] and by computed tomography if needed. Urodynamic studies can be helpful for the selection of therapy and the understanding of reflux.[9, 15, 85, 114] They can be done in newborns[11, 114] to identify children at risk for upper or lower urinary tract deterioration. Outflow obstruction in the form of detrusor–sphincter dyssynergia is an ominous finding and leads to impairment of urinary tract drainage in infants. All newborns with myelodysplasia should be evaluated urodynamically as soon as possible after the neurosurgical conditions are stabilized.[114] Thus, newborns at risk can be identified early, followed closely, and treated aggressively at the first sign of urinary tract deterioration.[11, 114] Cystometrography-electromyography may also be helpful.

Definitive Management

Bladder management may be accomplished through various methods, depending on the patient's level of function, motivation, and cognitive ability to follow a particular program of bladder care. Regardless of the method of bladder management, an interdisciplinary team approach improves patient care and leads to a more coordinated and efficient program.

A well-organized team should include representatives from various specialties. The patient is, of course, an integral part of any team because it is the patient's responsibility to carry through and apply the program of bladder care. The principal coordinator of the management program is the physiatrist, who is responsible for establishing the proper diagnosis on the basis of the urodynamic findings and coordinating the various team interventions related to management.

The urologist is a necessary team member. He or she participates in the diagnostic workup before initiation of bladder management, performs surgical procedures when indicated, and sees the patient in consultation during follow-up.

The physical therapist, or an equally trained rehabilitation nurse, is responsible for patient education and teaches the necessary motor skills for catheter-free voiding (bladder retraining), including biofeedback of the pelvic floor muscles when indicated. The physical therapist or nurse also provides specific information about the status of a patient's ability to transfer independently and perform the necessary activities of daily living required for independent catheter-free voiding. The physical therapist or nurse, therefore, assists the physician in assessing the practicality of catheter-free voiding versus other methods of bladder management that may be preferable in certain patients.

In association with the physical therapist, the occupational therapist assists with evaluation of the activities of daily living and modifies clothing, when indicated, to improve the efficiency of donning and doffing for voiding. The occupational therapist also assesses hand function and dexterity needed for intermittent self-catheterization and for application and use of external urinary collection devices.

The primary rehabilitation nurse reinforces drinking/voiding or catheterization schedules and assists the patient in applying newly acquired knowledge and skills to the home environment.

Urotechnicians assist the physicians with diagnostic urodynamic testing and the patients by teaching intermittent self-catheterization techniques. They also perform intermittent catheterization for hospitalized patients. Internists in nephrology and infectious disease are essential for assisting with the management of specific problems. Data about the results of diagnostic tests, urological complications, and the success or failure of the bladder management program provide the basis for follow-up and program evaluation.

As indicated, bladder management can be accomplished through various methods, including catheter-free voiding (blad-der retraining), voiding with an external collection device, long-term intermittent self-catheterization, indwelling urethral catheterization, suprapubic cystostomy, and urinary diversion by an ileal conduit. Before a specific type of bladder management is chosen, all patients with a neurogenic bladder dysfunction should have a complete urological workup to identify indications and contraindications and to delineate the optimal method of management.

Bladder Retraining for Catheter-Free Voiding

Bladder retraining is the method used to develop catheter-free voiding. Catheter-free voiding requires low residual urine volumes, normal voiding pressures, and regular drinking–voiding schedules. It is indicated for patients who have the proper motivation, hand dexterity, and cognitive ability to adhere to a drinking–voiding schedule and perform the required psychomotor skills. It is appropriate only after the patient is out of spinal shock and has a sterile urinary tract, as verified by urine culture. It is contraindicated for patients with vesicoureteral reflux, hydronephrosis, pyelonephritis, or advanced renal failure. Urinary tract infection and bladder or kidney stones are relative contraindications that need to be resolved before bladder retraining can proceed. Likewise, the patient should be free of general medical problems, such as uncontrolled hypertension, severe diabetes mellitus, autonomic hyperreflexia, deep venous thrombosis, or severe coronary artery disease, that may interfere with the methods of catheter-free voiding. Finally, the patient needs to have the endurance necessary for toilet transfers and regular voiding attempts and the functional capacity required for donning and doffing clothing.

The goals of bladder retraining are to

- Preserve the function of the vesicoureteral valve in order to protect kidney function
- Maintain regular (every 3 hours) and complete (less than 100 ml residual urine volume) emptying of the bladder in order to preserve abacteriuria
- Maintain continence
- Assist the patient in learning methods of solving problems related to the urinary system and thus enhance acceptability and independence in the community setting

Adherence to drinking–voiding–catheterization schedules is essential to an organized program of bladder retraining.[98] The drinking schedule is set up to provide an adequate volume of fluid for renal function but not so much as to overfill the bladder. A typical drinking schedule is to drink 400 ml with major meals (breakfast, lunch, and supper) and to drink 200 ml at 10 AM, 2 PM, and 4 PM to a total of 1800 ml/24 hr. Usually no fluids are taken after 6 PM. All drinking is done at the scheduled hours. Foods with a high water content, such as ice cream, soup, gelatin, and fruit, are counted as fluids.

The voiding schedule is structured in relation to the drinking schedule so that voiding is attempted at regular intervals when the bladder is optimally filled. In this fashion, overfilling of the bladder is prevented and the incidence of urinary tract infections is decreased.

The usual voiding schedule is every 2 to 3 hours depending on the bladder dysfunction. Regular and complete emptying on a voiding schedule also assists in maintaining continence. Once catheter-free voiding is accomplished, the voiding schedule may need to be modified to correspond to the patient's daily home drinking schedule. Usually the following guidelines are used after dismissal:

1. Void on awakening
2. Void 1 to 1½ hours after the main fluid intakes (breakfast, lunch, and supper)
3. Void every 2 to 3 hours
4. Void before going to bed at night and, if needed, once during the night

The catheterization schedule during bladder retraining provides for catheterizations every 6 hours; patients attempt to void just before the catheterizations to determine residual urine volumes. If the residual urine volumes are consistently more than 500 ml, fluid intake may need to be restricted initially. Fluids should not be restricted, however, to less than 1200 ml/day. If the residual urine volumes continue to be more than 500 ml with decreased fluids, the catheterization schedule may have to be increased to every 4 hours temporarily.[98]

Patient education is another essential component at the onset of bladder retraining. The relating health professionals, such as the physical therapist and the primary rehabilitation nurse, may be responsible for the education related to the urinary system and the patient's bladder dysfunction. They teach the anatomy of the urinary system and basic information about normal micturition and the patient's individual bladder dysfunction based on the diagnostic cystometrogram-electromyogram. They instruct the patient in the correct drinking–voiding–catheterization schedules and how to record these values on the intake–output bladder sheets and graphs (Figs. 26-13 and 26-14).[98] They also provide information about the signs and symptoms of urinary tract infection.

Three basic voiding techniques are taught (Fig. 26-15). The specific technique used for a patient is based on the detrusor and external urethral sphincter responses during diagnostic or therapeutic cystometrography-electromyography. The optimal voiding technique is the one that produces the greatest increase in intravesical pressure with the least amount of external urethral sphincter activity.

Light suprapubic tapping (used for patients with upper motor neuron bladder dysfunction) relies on the response of the stretch reflex of the detrusor via the sacral micturition center to cause a detrusor contraction. The patient taps lightly with the fingertips over the suprapubic area of the abdominal wall (Fig. 26-15A). Quadriplegic patients may need to use the side of the hand to produce an effective tapping force. The goal of light tapping is to cause an effective contraction of the bladder muscle without a strong co-contraction of the external urethral sphincter. Hard tapping may produce greater intravesical pressures owing to a stronger detrusor response, but usually at the expense of increased dyssynergia. As dyssynergia increases, it leads to progressive detrusor hypertrophy and eventual vesicoureteral reflux.

Straining (Valsalva maneuver) provides an external force (intra-abdominal pressure) to compress the bladder and to open the bladder neck (Fig. 26-15B). The patient begins the straining procedure by placing one arm over the abdomen to support it. The patient then leans forward with the elbow resting on top of the thigh. Before starting to strain, the patient takes three "quick" breaths in order to be able to hold the breath for a longer time and thus produce a more effective strain. Then the patient takes a deep breath, holds it, and bears down firmly, such as when having a bowel movement, while pushing the abdomen out against the support of the arm, further increasing the intra-abdominal pressure. The strain should be held as long and as hard as is possible without causing lightheadedness or a headache. Straining needs to be repeated, interrupted by rest periods, until no more urine can be expressed.

The Credé maneuver (like straining) compresses the bladder and opens the bladder neck (Fig. 26-15C). Deep massage of the bladder with the fingertips may increase bladder tone and make the Credé maneuver more effective. Next, a fist is made with the dominant hand, placing it about an inch below the navel. Without holding one's breath, the patient pushes the fist into the abdomen toward the tailbone. Then, the patient leans forward slowly and directs the push downward onto the bladder. The patient continues performing the Credé maneuver until the stream stops and repeats it until voiding ceases completely.

Sometimes catheter-free voiding is achieved by using a combination of voiding techniques.

GUIDELINES FOR SPECIFIC BLADDER DYSFUNCTIONS. In *uninhibited bladder dysfunction*, the detrusor contracts spontaneously, and the result is urinary incontinence because the patient lacks adequate awareness of a full bladder. The voiding dynamics are normally undisturbed, the capacity is moderately decreased, and emptying is usually complete. Measures for bladder retraining are aimed at causing the patient to become adequately aware of bladder fullness in order to check voiding and prevent incontinence. Therefore, the patient is offered a urinal or commode frequently, usually 1 hour after meals and every 2 hours, even if there is no definite sensation of a need to void. The patient is instructed to spend 10 minutes trying to void. The verbal cues given the patient are to relax, to feel for the sensation of fullness, and to concentrate on voiding. The noise of running water or light suprapubic tapping may facilitate voiding.

Incontinence due to reflex voiding may improve as the patient improves neurologically, becomes more mobile, is better able to communicate his or her needs to the nursing staff, and follows an intake–voiding schedule. However, if incontinence does not resolve, anticholinergic medications may be added to relax the detrusor and decrease incontinence and increase bladder capacity. In some cases, the patient may require the use of protective clothing containing high-absorption pads or an indwelling catheter to manage refractory incontinence, especially if there is significant ongoing cognitive impairment.

In *upper motor neuron bladder dysfunction*, the detrusor and the external urethral sphincter are hyperreflexic. Often, there is significant detrusor–external sphincter dyssynergia. The goal, therefore, is to trigger an effective detrusor contraction with minimal external sphincter co-contraction. The preferable technique to accomplish this goal is light suprapubic tapping.

α-Sympathetic blockers for the bladder neck and/or antispasticity medications for the external urethral sphincter may be helpful for decreasing bladder outlet resistance. Limited external sphincterotomy may be needed in men with significant detrusor–external sphincter dyssynergia to decrease sufficiently the outflow resistance for efficient catheter-free voiding.

However, if bladder pressures continue to be excessively

Figure 26-13. Daily record sheet on which patients receiving bladder retraining record time and volumes of fluid intake, intentional and unintentional voidings, and residual urine volumes. (Opitz JL: Treatment of voiding dysfunction in spinal-cord-injured patients: Bladder retraining. In Barrett DM Wein AJ [eds]: Controversies in Neuro-Urology, pp 437–451. New York, Churchill Livingstone, 1984. By permission of the publisher.)

Record Of Bladder Retraining

Date _____   Name _____   MC No. _____

Time	Fluid Intake — All beverages, also include soup, ice cream, jello	Intentional — Volitional (*NOT* triggered, strained or manually expressed)	Intentional — Triggered, Strained or Manually Expressed	Unintentional — Incontinence or Spontaneous voidings	Catheterization — Residual Checks or Retentions — Self	Catheterization — Residual Checks or Retentions — Team
1:00 AM						
2:00						
3:00						
4:00						
5:00						
6:00						
7:00						
8:00						
9:00						
10:00						
11:00						
12:00 N						
1:00 PM						
2:00						
3:00						
4:00						
5:00						
6:00						
7:00						
8:00						
9:00						
10:00						
11:00						
12:00 MN						
SUBTOTAL						

TOTAL IN: _____   TOTAL OUT: _____

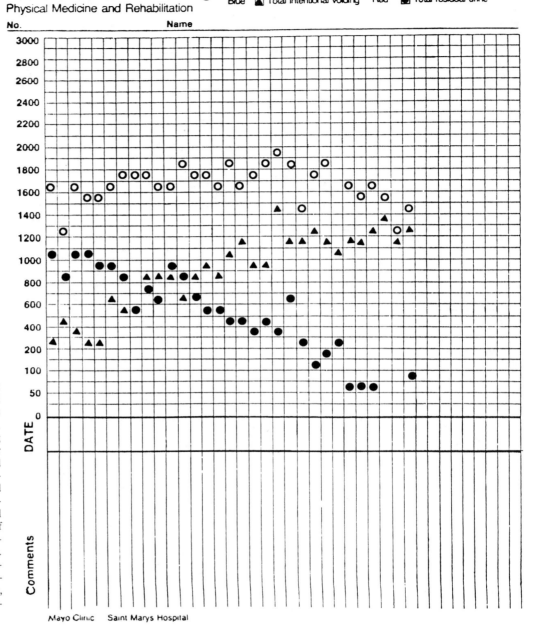

Record of Bladder Training
Physical Medicine and Rehabilitation

Black ▣ Total intake   Green △ Total unintentional voiding
Blue ▲ Total intentional voiding   Red ◙ Total residual urine

No. _____   Name _____

Figure 26-14. Data from woman with complete, flaccid detrusor and external urethral sphincter paralysis after disk compression of sacral cord. The patient recorded (by filling in appropriate squares and color coding) her 24-hour volumes of fluid intake, intentional voidings, and residual urine volumes, as determined of 6 hourly intermittent catheterizations. She had no unintentional voidings. (Optiz JL: Treatment of voiding dysfunction in spinal-cord-injured patients: Bladder retraining. In Barrett DM, Wein AJ [eds]: Controversies in Neuro-Urology, pp 437–451. New York, Churchill Livingstone, 1984. By permission of the publisher.)

high, it may be necessary to suppress the detrusor with anticholinergic medications. The patient then needs to manage the bladder by intermittent catheterization or an indwelling urethral catheter, depending on the residual functional capacity of the patient. Occasionally, especially in women, if urinary incontinence due to detrusor hyperreflexia cannot be controlled with anticholinergic medications, chemical rhizotomy of S2–S5 by intrathecal phenol in glycerin is helpful. It transforms the hyperreflexic detrusor and external sphincter to a flaccid (lower motor neuron) state allowing for management by catheter-free voiding, intermittent catheterization, or indwelling catheter, again depending on the patient's residual function.

In *lower motor neuron bladder dysfunction,* the detrusor and external urethral sphincter are flaccid. The key to voiding in this type of dysfunction is to apply an external force to compress the bladder and open the bladder neck so that voiding can occur.

The external force can be applied by either straining or the Credé maneuver. Often, it is necessary to add α-sympathetic blockers or cholinergic medications before voiding becomes efficient.

In *mixed type A neurogenic bladder dysfunction,* the bladder is flaccid and the external urethral sphincter is hyperreflexic. As in lower motor neuron bladder dysfunction, straining or the Credé maneuver is the voiding technique of choice. Unfortunately, because the external sphincter is hyperreflexic, it tends to contract, obstructing the flow of urine during attempted voiding. Various methods, such as biofeedback from the pelvic floor muscles, rectal stretch, and antispasticity medications, are used to decrease or minimize the inappropriate contraction of the external sphincter. By slowly increasing the intra-abdominal pressure during straining, the patient may be able to minimize the co-contraction of the pelvic floor muscles. A cystometro-

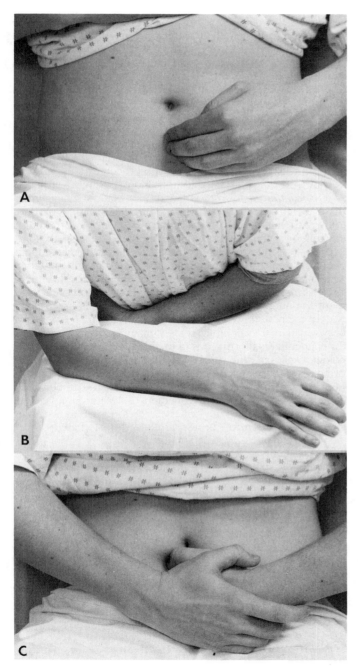

Figure 26-15. Techniques of catheter-free voiding. (*A*) Light suprapubic tapping (spastic detrusor). (*B*) Straining with forearm supporting abdominal wall (flaccid detrusor). (*C*) Credé maneuver (flaccid detrusor). (Opitz JL, Mitros MM: Bladder retraining. In Sinaki M [ed]: Basic Clinical Rehabilitation Medicine, pp 194–206. Burlington, Ontario, BC Decker, 1987. By permission of the Mayo Foundation.)

when combined with straining, leads to improved voiding with decreased bladder outlet resistance. Finally, antispasticity medications or a limited external sphincterotomy in men may assist in decreasing the force of co-contraction of the external sphincter adequately for voiding to occur.

In *mixed type B bladder dysfunction,* the detrusor is hyperreflexic and the external urethral sphincter is flaccid. The key to successful bladder retraining is a combination of a regular, frequent voiding schedule and light tapping to trigger a detrusor contraction before the detrusor contracts spontaneously.

If significant incontinence continues between voiding attempts, anticholinergic medications may be helpful to decrease incontinence by increasing bladder capacity. At times, it may be difficult to suppress the detrusor adequately to allow for continence. In that case, the detrusor may have to be partly denervated by selective sacral rhizotomy.

In *myogenic bladder dysfunction,* the detrusor is flaccid and unable to contract because of prolonged overstretching by overfilling of the bladder. The pelvic floor muscles are under voluntary control and usually are in a pattern of habit contraction during voiding. Because the bladder is flaccid, straining or the Credé maneuver is the appropriate voiding technique. However, emptying the bladder cannot be accomplished efficiently using these techniques unless the pelvic floor muscles are relaxed during voiding. Biofeedback is helpful to re-educate the patient for relaxation of pelvic floor muscles. Neuromuscular re-education then progresses from lying on the side, to sitting, and eventually to voiding with the pelvic floor muscles relaxed. In addition to biofeedback techniques for the pelvic floor muslces, *a*-sympathetic blockers or cholinergic medications may be necessary to assist in complete emptying of the bladder.[98]

Finally, once voiding occurs regularly (every 2 to 3 hours) and completely (less than 100 ml), the catheterizations may be discontinued when the patient feels self-assured about being able to empty the bladder regularly and completely. The patient is dismissed on a drinking–voiding schedule that is compatible with the home situation.

Scheduled rechecks are set up at 3 months, 6 months, 1 year, and then yearly for 5 years. Thereafter, if the patient remains stable, rechecks are scheduled every 2 years. During rechecks, team members assess the status of the urinary system and the patient's performance. They address, with the patient, any problem that is identified. Occasionally, a few sessions as an outpatient may be necessary to reinforce previously learned bladder retraining skills.

Voiding with the use of an *external urinary collection device* is another method of bladder management for men. It is used in association with catheter-free voiding. Often, a condom-type "external" provides independence in voiding for quadriplegic men with upper motor neuron bladder dysfunction who lack the hand dexterity, strength, and sitting balance to don or doff pants independently and place a urinal for voiding. However, it is essential that a person using an "external" for independent voiding adhere to a regular drinking–voiding schedule, as previously described, and not just allow the bladder to overflow or trigger spontaneously into the "external."[94]

An "external" may also be used to maintain continence if spontaneous voiding cannot be prevented between scheduled voiding attempts. Unfortunately, although several external collection systems are available for women, none have so far proved to be totally effective for keeping them dry because the devices become dislodged easily with transfers.[67]

The disadvantages to wearing an "external" are associated with skin breakdown of the penis and urinary tract infections. Good skin inspections and hygiene are essential to prevent penile skin ulcerations. The patient also needs to avoid the use of

graphy–electromyography machine may be used as a biofeedback device to monitor the intravesical pressure produced by straining and/or the electromyographic activity produced by the pelvic floor muscles during straining. Such therapeutic use of cystometrography-electromyography may be of substantial assistance in achieving an effective straining method with minimal or no co-contraction of the pelvic floor muscles. Manual stretching of the anal sphincter, called rectal stretch, will usually improve voiding in mixed type A bladder dysfunction.[100] Rectal stretch inhibits the contraction of the external urethral sphincter and,

a posey (which causes compression of the urethra during erections), any twisting of the condom or the "external" at the site of the drainage tube attachment, or any bending of the tubing itself, all of which may lead to urethral obstruction. The obstructed urethra then interrupts the flow of urine, which causes reflux of infected urine into the bladder and incomplete emptying.[67, 94]

Long-term intermittent self-catheterization is an effective method of management in a person whose bladder is flaccid or overstretched and who, even with medications to increase detrusor contractility and decrease bladder outlet resistance, is unable to empty the bladder completely.[33, 80, 93] Intermittent catheterization is also beneficial for patients who are not motivated to achieve catheter-free voiding and, therefore, elect to manage the bladder with intermittent self-catheterization. It may also be an alternative method of management in patients with prostatic outlet obstruction when operation is contraindicated.[67]

If the detrusor can be suppressed with anticholinergic medications in patients with upper motor neuron bladder dysfunction, intermittent catheterization is an effective method of bladder management as long as high intravesical pressure can be avoided. Depending on the patient's residual level, the patient, an attendant, or a family member can perform the catheterization every 6 hours. All patients managed by intermittent catheterization should continue to follow an 1800-ml fluid schedule and keep all retention volumes less than 500 ml.[98]

It is important that the patient be careful in either sterile or clean intermittent self-catheterization techniques in order to decrease the incidence of urinary tract infections. For most patients, a clean technique with use of individual sterile catheters will be sufficient to maintain abacteriuria.[67] However, there are reports of bladder calculi forming around the nidus of pubic hairs introduced during self-catheterization.[3, 116]

Indwelling urethral catheterization is a reasonable method of bladder management for various medical conditions. It is indicated in patients with severe cognitive impairment after stroke or closed-head injury and in seriously ill or debilitated patients with either total retention or incontinence refractory to medications who are unable to follow a program of intermittent catheterization. An indwelling urethral catheter may also be necessary for quadriplegic women who are unable to transfer to a commode for voiding and lack the hand dexterity to do intermittent self-catheterization and for quadriplegic men who, even after limited external sphincterotomy to relieve bladder outlet resistance, do not have the muscle strength and endurance needed for a regular tapping schedule and complete emptying.[67] If other caregivers are not available to do intermittent catheterization, an indwelling catheter used in combination with anticholinergic medications to decrease detrusor hyperreflexia, if present, is a reasonable alternative form of bladder management. Anticholinergic medications decrease the likelihood of ulceration of the bladder wall against the catheter tip.

Complications can, however, arise with the use of an indwelling catheter. Probably the most common of these are severe cystitis due to chronic urinary tract infection, injury of the bladder by the catheter tip, and bladder stone formation. Drinking at least 3000 ml/day may assist in decreasing symptomatic urinary tract infections by a constant "washing out" effect. The indwelling catheter should be changed every 2 weeks because encrustations of calcium salts on the catheter tip may chip off and form the beginning of bladder stones, especially in a chronically infected bladder. Care in maintaining the urinary bag below the level of the bladder to prevent the retrograde flow of urine back into the bladder and the use of a closed drainage system may also limit infection.

Complications such as penoscrotal fistulas can be prevented by taping the catheter to the abdominal wall. In women, the catheter is taped to the inner aspect of the thigh. Taping the catheter also prevents accidental traction on the catheter, which may lead to hematuria. In quadriplegics, it is important to prevent catheter blockage and overfilling of the urinary bag, which can lead to urinary retention and autonomic hyperreflexia.[67]

With proper care and close monitoring, an indwelling catheter is an effective and reasonable choice of bladder management when indicated. Patients with long-term use of a urethral or suprapubic catheter should have a yearly urinalysis, urine culture, cytologic examination of the urine, and cystoscopy to examine the bladder mucosa carefully and for removal of bladder stones or debris, if present. Follow-up procedures also address quickly and efficiently any complications that have occurred.

Suprapubic cystostomy is a method of bladder management that is useful for patients who have neurogenic bladder dysfunction in association with urethral injury or sepsis, severe urethral strictures, or other urethral complications. Problems with suprapubic cystostomy are well recognized, including deterioration in renal function.[32, 49] The management of a suprapubic catheter is similar to the management of an indwelling urethral catheter.

Urinary diversion by ileal conduit is a method of management for neurogenic bladder dysfunction that is not used as widely today as previously because of the high incidence of upper urinary tract complications. It may, however, be of benefit for congenital malformations of the bladder, for pelvic or gynecologic cancer in which the bladder itself or other portions of the urinary structures must be removed, and for persistent hydronephrosis with progressive deterioration of the upper tracts refractory to conservative management.[48, 53] Many complications have been associated with urinary diversion, such as acute and chronic pyelonephritis, ureteral reflux, stomal changes, renal calculi, ureteroileal obstruction, and acidosis.[53, 54, 111]

For patients treated with urinary diversion, good skin care is mandatory to maintain skin integrity. Aggressive cleaning of the peristomal skin, aggressive removal of the adhesive, or improperly applied appliances may cause irritation or damage to the peristomal skin.[123]

The urinary appliance is part of a closed drainage system with a leg bag. Frequent checks of the tubing and appliance connections are necessary to prevent any obstruction of the free flow of urine from the conduit. A high-fluid intake (2500 to 3000 ml/day) is recommended for its beneficial "washing out" effect on infection of the ileal pouch.

Pediatric Considerations

Normal Development of Urine Storage and Voiding

During the first months of infancy, bladder evacuation normally occurs through an unconscious brain stem reflex. The detrusor responds to stretching by forceful, uninhibited contractions. Synergy of detrusor and sphincter is coordinated, and bladder emptying is completed with normal pressure.[9] There is a transition from the reflex voiding of infancy to controlled voiding as the child matures.[9] With time, experience, and conditioning, the response of the bladder to stretching becomes increasingly under voluntary control. The child learns to label the sensation of a full or contracting detrusor and can consciously retard micturition. The age (from 12 to 36 months) at which this occurs depends on neurological and musculature maturity, locomotion, vocabulary, and social reinforcement, as well as voluntary control of the contraction and relaxation of the sphincter when the detrusor is contracting. Often, the perception of bladder sensation and central voluntary control of the detrusor mechanism do not develop as early as the ability to contract the sphincter. This can lead to enuresis.[9] In these cases, the child has only a last-minute warning that a detrusor contraction is in progress.

With maturation, voluntary control of the bladder improves and episodes of uncontrolled detrusor contraction lessen. Development of more accurate perception of bladder sensation and unconscious as well as voluntary detrusor control allow controlled voiding of normal bladder volumes at normal frequency.

During the developmental period these new skills are often unreliable and fragile. Incontinence may be precipitated by any condition that increases the sensibility of the bladder (cystitis) or reduces central inhibition (sleep, preoccupation with play, or stress). Normal children can be expected to exhibit certain elements of dysfunctional voiding for brief periods.[9, 95]

If these dysfunctional mechanisms persist or there is a neurological cause for the dysfunction, special methods of voiding training may be necessary. These are determined by the level of the neurological lesions or the cause of the dysfunction. The ability to ambulate and to transfer on and off the toilet, the intellect of the child and of the parent, growth, maturation, stress, genetics, experience, and motivation are all factors that have an impact on the ability for bladder training. Other factors that help bladder training in children with or without neurologic problems are responsibility, reinforcement, and a regular drinking–voiding schedule during the day. With this drinking schedule, adjusted for the age and size of the child, the child has three larger amounts of fluids at meals and regular amounts of fluids at mid-morning and mid- and late-afternoon. Only small amounts of fluids are given after the evening meal. In children, limiting fluids is not recommended but regularly scheduled drinking and voiding are important. Regular, frequent (every 2 hours) voiding times with attempts at postponement of voiding when it is not time to void help to condition the bladder to empty and fill. Practicing of stopping and starting urination and conditioning by timed voiding as well as an alarm device at night, all work to some extent and lead to improved attention to and perception of bladder stimulation or bladder emptying. With these methods, more consistent detrusor voluntary control is possible. Adherence to drinking and voiding schedules is needed with the use of intermittent catheterization.

Recurrent cystitis in girls, usually between the ages of 3 and 8 years, is a common, often transient, and usually benign form of neurogenic bladder dysfunction.[9, 61, 95] They usually develop regular voiding habits in infancy, but episodes of dysuria, frequency, urgency, small volume incontinence, and nocturia occur. Cross-legged posture, facial grimaces, curtsying, squatting on the floor, sitting up on the heels, or holding the genitalia are often clues to this problem. Suppressive antibiotics, time, and maturation usually take care of this problem.[9] Urethral dilation does not change the pattern of infection. Meticulous skin cleaning and wiping techniques from front to back can be helpful.

Urodynamic studies in recurrent cystitis have demonstrated an obstruction that is not fixed but is dysfunctional. It produces voluntary, dyssynergic co-contractions of the external sphincter with the detrusor.

Management of Dysfunctions

Possible clinical signs of neurogenic bladder dysfunction are the inability to empty the bladder, urinary infections, incontinence, reflux of urine into the kidneys, and upper tract deterioration. The management of children with a neurogenic bladder dysfunction has changed profoundly during the past 10 years.[11]

An indwelling urethral catheter, external sphincterotomy, and urinary diversion have become undesirable methods of management.[2, 39, 77] Cass and colleagues[20–22] reported on the use of clean, intermittent catheterization for the management of children. They found that 49% of the children managed with clean, intermittent catheterization were totally continent and 17% were slightly damp. Preexisting ureteral reflux deterioration was present in 25% of their 84 children, which, with clean, intermittent catheterization, cleared in 35% of the patients and was unchanged in 40%; preexisting upper tract deterioration improved in 12.5% and was unchanged in 87.5%. With clean, intermittent catheterization and antibiotic medication, 90% of the children had sterile urine and only 7.5% had 10^6 colonies/ml or more on urine cultures.[20–22]

The complications were minor: only 20 episodes of difficulty passing the catheter, 21 episodes of a sore urethra or swelling of the penis, 9 episodes of urethral bleeding, 1 case of urethral discharge, 1 case with a stone on a hair in the bladder, and 2 cases of incorrect techniques or scheduling.[20–22]

Neuro-urologic medications, such as oxybutynin and propantheline, increase bladder capacity and decrease reflex bladder activity. Ephedrine increases urethral resistance at the internal sphincter mechanism. These medications are used in children.[20–22]

Methods of clean, intermittent catheterization, antibiotic medications, when used with bacteria-suppressing antibiotic medications, and anticholinergic medications in cases of detrusor hyperreflexia have proved to be effective for achieving continence and allowing children, even when reflux is present, to grow and resolve the anatomical abnormalities.[16, 20–22, 65, 104]

When an antireflux operation is necessary, the success rate of management with intermittent catheterization improves dramatically.[9] The acceptance of intermittent catheterization by parents, patients, and school personnel depends on factors such as careful teaching, kind supervision, psychodynamics, self-image, and sexuality.[15, 121] Appropriate counseling, training, and supervision are vital for the success of intermittent catheterization. The earlier intermittent catheterization and proper parental training are instituted, the less likely are complications of the upper urinary tract. The development of independence in bladder management depends on the level of the lesion. This independence can be achieved at ages 4 to 7 years in lower lesions but not until the age of 10 to 11 years in higher lesions. Independence may not be achieved until 17 to 18 years of age in the most handicapped patients.[121]

In the newborn who cannot be catheterized because of size or parental acceptance, cutaneous vesicostomy can be an excellent temporary form of diversion.[11] Location of the stoma should allow for draining into a diaper. The bladder neck and the external sphincter mechanisms are not altered so continence can be obtained by intermittent catheterization after closure. The major complications of permanent diversion such as refluxing of the ureteroileal conduit, risk of subsequent operations, and major kidney infections are avoided.[2, 39, 77] The temporary diversions allow the bladder to be rehabilitated after closure of the diversion.

Implantation of an artificial urinary sphincter has gained considerable popularity.[91] The artificial sphincter device is not suitable for everyone. Better results are accomplished with careful selection of patients and consideration of the appropriateness for the child's age (after 10 years is recommended), allowing for maturation.

Neuro-urological Medications

Neuropharmacological management can assist the lower urinary tract to store and to empty urine (Table 26-2). Because both storage and emptying dysfunctions relate to the detrusor function and the function of the urethral sphincters, both the de-

Table 26-2
Neuro-urological Medications Used for the Management of Neurogenic Bladder Dysfunctions

Neuro-urologic Medication	Upper Motor Neuron	Lower Motor Neuron	Mixed Type A	Mixed Type B
Anticholinergic	+ or ++	−	−	++
Cholinergic	− −	(+)	(+)	− −
α-Sympathetic blocker	+	+	+	− −
Sympathomimetic	− −	(+)	−	(+)
Antispasmatic	++	−	++	−

*The medication: (+), may be tried; +, is indicated; ++, is strongly indicated; −, is contraindicated; − −, is strongly contraindicated.

trusor and the sphincters need to be considered when using neuro-urological medications.[51]

Treatment of Storage Dysfunctions

Storage dysfunctions may be caused by either hyperreflexia of the detrusor or insufficient function of the urethral sphincters. Both dysfunctions may lead to low bladder capacity and urinary incontinence.

Hyperreflexia of the detrusor may be decreased with the use of anticholinergic medications, such as propantheline bromide (Pro-Banthine) (7.5 to 15 mg three or four times daily). Oxybutynin chloride (Ditropan) (5 mg three or four times daily) is also effective, acting on the bladder muscle itself. Use of β-adrenergic stimulation is less effective and usually has marked side effects.

Ineffective closure of the internal urethral sphincter mechanism may be improved with α-sympathetic stimulating medications, such as phenylephrine, ephedrine, or imipramine. Long-term use, however, may have undesirable cardiovascular consequences.

Ineffective closure of the voluntary external sphincter may respond to neuromuscular re-education and strengthening or surgical procedures rather than to any neuro-urological medication.

Treatment of Emptying Dysfunctions

Emptying dysfunctions may be caused by insufficient contraction of the detrusor (weak expulsive force) or by hyperactivity of the internal or external urethral sphincter. Video urodynamic testing allows diagnosis of urethral obstruction by the internal or external urethral sphincter.

Weak expulsive force of the detrusor may be improved with cholinergic medications, such as bethanechol (Urecholine) (25 to 50 mg orally, three to four times daily, 30 minutes before voiding). Bethanechol is not used often anymore because the expulsive force of the bladder can be improved more effectively with straining. However, bethanechol may improve detrusor tone and thus make the Credé maneuver more effective. Bethanechol is contraindicated in patients with elevated detrusor pressures.

The tension of a *hyperactive internal sphincter mechanism* may be reduced with the use of α-adrenergic blockers, such as phenoxybenzamine (Dibenzyline) (10 mg three or four times

daily). Phenoxybenzamine is a long-acting medication and may have cumulative effects if used too aggressively. Some questions exist regarding the possible mutagenic effects of phenoxybenzamine during long-term use. It may be of particular help early during bladder retraining after prolonged periods of intermittent catheterization or drainage by an indwelling catheter. It is especially helpful during the early phase of bladder retraining in women with lower motor neuron bladder dysfunction.

Unfortunately, the tension of a *hyperactive external urethral sphincter* cannot be reduced effectively with antispasmodic medications, such as baclofen, diazepam, and dantrolene sodium. However, any measure that leads to a lowering of the level of spasticity of the spinal cord, especially meticulous prevention of any complications of spinal cord injury, is likely to lower the degree of detrusor–external sphincter dyssynergia. Antispasmodic medications are completely ineffective in neurologically normal patients with emptying dysfunction due to habit contraction of the pelvic floor muscles during attempts at voiding. Neuromuscular re-education of the pelvic floor muscles is then the treatment of choice.[74]

Surgical Treatment

The goal of treatment of neurogenic bladder dysfunction is to reinstate the normal functions of the lower urinary tract. Treatment should provide low-pressure collection and storage of urine, continence with adequate emptying, effective control of infection, and preservation of the upper urinary tract. Treatment planning must consider several factors, including the underlying disease, the ability of the patient to move around and reach the bathroom quickly, and the reliability of the patient's family.

Surgical therapy is directed at correcting incontinence, improving voiding, and preventing complications. Careful preoperative evaluation and counseling are necessary to avoid the unhappiness that stems from a failure to achieve the high expectations that most patients with neurogenic bladder dysfunction have before undergoing operation. Preoperatively, the patient must understand that further operative procedures, intermittent catheterization, or prolonged pharmacological management may continue to be necessary.

Operation to Promote Bladder Emptying

Patients may be unable to empty their bladders efficiently because of problems with the bladder outlet or problems with decreased detrusor contractility or both. Most often, operation to enhance bladder emptying is directed at the bladder outlet. It is at this level that the sphincteric mechanisms are composed of both skeletal and smooth muscle. Urodynamic study generally allows for adequate definition of bladder outlet obstruction due to the types of detrusor–sphincter dyssynergia.

Transurethral Sphincterotomy

Sphincterotomy as a means of decreasing outlet resistance due to dyssynergia is most commonly considered in the male patient; in the female patient, it generally leads to unacceptable incontinence. Sphincterotomy is performed to decrease high intravesical pressures mediated by bladder contraction against the dyssynergically contracted distal or proximal sphincter and also thereby to improve bladder emptying. Although external sphincterotomy improves bladder emptying in 70% to 90% of cases,[69, 110] a second or even third sphincterotomy may be required to provide for a successful outcome.

Different techniques have been used for transurethral external sphincterotomy, including incisions at the 5 and 7 o'clock positions, the 3 and 9 o'clock positions, or the so-called limited external sphincterotomy at the 12 o'clock position. The one that has gained the most popularity is the 12 o'clock sphincterotomy. This "limited" procedure involves considerably less bleeding and a minimal risk of inducing erectile dysfunction because the line of incision is well away from the cavernous nerves. The sphincterotomy can be performed with a coagulation current, a cutting current with a Collings knife, or a true transurethral resection of sphincteric tissue with the loop. The area of excision or incision in this procedure should be no longer than 2 to 3 cm at the level of the external sphincter. Perforation of the spongy tissue of the bulbous urethra must be avoided because it may result in profuse bleeding.

When a combination of internal and external sphincteric dyssynergia is identified, the sphincterotomy is extended to include the smooth muscle of the bladder neck and proximal urethra. In older male patients, this may involve a partial resection of prostatic tissue if it has become hypertrophic and obstructive. The prostate itself can be obstructive. It must be considered when designing the operation in conjunction with various degrees of sphincteric dyssynergia.

Postoperatively, the use of a nonreactive silicone urethral catheter ranging from No. 20 to 24 F is recommended. The catheter should remain indwelling for at least 6 days postoperatively, at which time the patient's ability to empty the bladder can be efficiently monitored with intermittent catheterization. The complications of sphincterotomy include bleeding, bladder neck or bladder perforation, extravasation of urine, and urosepsis. Urethral stricture rarely occurs after sphincterotomy in patients with neurogenic vesical dysfunction, but it may appear as a late complication with longer periods of follow-up.[107]

Pudendal Nerve Block and Neurectomy

The pudendal nerve block outlet regulates external sphincter activity. Blocking the function of the external sphincter unilaterally or bilaterally can improve bladder emptying. A pudendal block can be produced by injecting lidocaine (Xylocaine) 1% into the area medial to the ischial tuberosity. The efficacy of the block can be assessed by urethral pressure profilometry before and after the injection, by studying the voiding pattern under fluoroscopy before and after injection, and by sphincter electromyography, which becomes silent after bilateral pudendal block.[108, 109] Although permanent pudendal block can be achieved by injection of phenol or alcohol, it may produce necrosis of normal tissues and impotence owing to total inactivation of the nerve. Pudendal block may, however, be used diagnostically to assess the potential effect of external sphincterotomy. If the external sphincter pressure can be reduced and the urinary flow improved by pudendal block, external sphincterotomy should improve a patient's condition.

Unilateral pudendal neurectomy is recommended over bilateral pudendal neurectomy because the latter is associated with higher incidences of impotence and fecal incontinence.[30] The acceptance of transurethral external sphincterotomy has practically eliminated the use of pudendal neurectomy as a means of reducing bladder outlet resistance.

Procedures to Promote Urine Storage

In patients with neurogenic bladder dysfunction who have urinary incontinence, certain surgical procedures can be undertaken to either decrease detrusor contractility and thereby promote urinary continence or enhance outlet resistance by a procedure at the bladder neck or proximal urethra.

Denervation Procedures to Decrease Detrusor Contractility

CENTRAL DENERVATION. In subarachnoid blocks (or "spinal" anesthesia), the sacral reflexes, somatic pudendal nerve, and parasympathetic nerves are affected, and an areflexic bladder and lax external sphincter are produced. However, even when a hyperbaric solution is used, the procedure is not as selective as a root block and may occasionally affect unintended levels. Impotence is common, and perianal anesthesia or paraparesis of the legs may also develop. Even with injection of phenol, the effect may wear off after a year or more.

SACRAL RHIZOTOMY. Sacral rhizotomy may include sectioning of the anterior, posterior, or entire root. This form of treatment, although effective for a functionally low-capacity bladder secondary to hyperreflexia, may not improve bladder capacity in patients with diminished compliance. The third sacral root predominates in bladder motor function. Although sectioning of the entire root is more effective than sectioning of the anterior portion only,[90] the former is associated with a higher rate of impotence.[79, 90]

PERIVESICAL DENERVATION. Perivesical denervation can be achieved transvaginally[55, 58] or abdominally.[73, 78, 92, 126, 133] With the transvaginal approach, both inferior vesical pedicles are exposed and divided, and success rates are as high as 60% to 80%.[55] A more promising and conservative approach to perivesical denervation may be transvesical or transvaginal injection of phenol into the bladder base in an attempt to eradicate the autonomic innervation in this area.[92]

Perivesical denervation by a transabdominal approach may be achieved by detrusor myotomy,[78] bladder transection,[126] or cystolysis.[73, 92, 133] For all practical purposes, cystolysis is the only procedure that has gained some popularity for total bladder denervation at the local level. Cystolysis was first reported by Worth and Turner-Warwick[133] for the treatment of interstitial cystitis. Leach and co-workers[73] used a similar technique in patients with detrusor hyperreflexia and a bladder capacity of more than 150 ml during anesthesia. When the bladder capacity is smaller, this technique is used in combination with augmentation cystoplasty. Results are good in most patients, at least initially. In the male patient, the risk of losing erectile function is of concern because total mobilization of the bladder and prostate will also impair the cavernous nerves, which regulate erectile function.

Enterocystoplasty

Augmentation cystoplasty is the most major of the surgical procedures designed to treat the functionally and anatomically contracted bladder. However, it may well be the most uniformly efficient way of increasing vesical functional capacity and decreasing intravesical pressure during urine storage. The wider acceptance of intermittent catheterization and the improved results with the newer models of the artificial urinary sphincter most likely will lead to increased use of this approach.[8, 36, 38, 64, 75, 76, 106, 115, 131]

Cystourethropexy

In the female patient with a relatively incompetent outlet and manageable detrusor contractility, cystourethropexy can be considered as a means of increasing outlet resistance and thereby enhancing urinary control. This procedure, because of its obstructive nature, is contraindicated in patients with marked detrusor hyperreflexia or decreased bladder compliance. If the patient already has an areflexic detrusor, it is reasonable to assume that some additional therapy to augment bladder emptying will be required after the vesicourethropexy. This generally is in the form of intermittent self-catheterization. The method for this type of suspension can be the Stamey needle technique, a Marshall-Marchetti-Krantz operation, or a pubovaginal sling procedure.[50, 83, 118]

Bladder Neck Tubularization

Bladder neck tubularization is designed to modify the bladder neck and proximal urethra through surgical molding of the tissues to enhance outlet resistance. The Young-Dees procedure, the Tanagho procedure, and the Leadbetter modification of the Young-Dees procedure have all been used with some degree of success in patients with sphincteric urinary incontinence. Again, these are obstructive, and intermittent catheterization may be required to assist in complete vesical emptying. These procedures, like all that create a dynamic outlet obstruction, are contraindicated in patients with high-pressure detrusor hyperreflexia.

Artificial Urinary Sphincter

The use of totally implantable, externally controlled devices for the treatment of urinary incontinence has achieved widespread clinical acceptance during the past decade. Major advances in the mechanical aspects of the artificial sphincter device have led to the currently used AS 800 model (manufactured by American Medical Systems; Fig. 26-16). Although ideally suited for pure sphincteric incontinence and normal detrusor function, numerous categories of patients with neurogenic bladder dysfunction may qualify as candidates for implantation of the artificial urinary sphincter. It may be implanted around the bladder neck or bulbous urethra in male patients and around the bladder neck in female patients. In general, patients who have high-pressure detrusor hyperreflexia are not good candidates for implantation of the sphincter unless their detrusor function can be modified through pharmacological manipulation, neurologi-

Figure 26-16. Artificial urinary sphincter, AS 800 device.

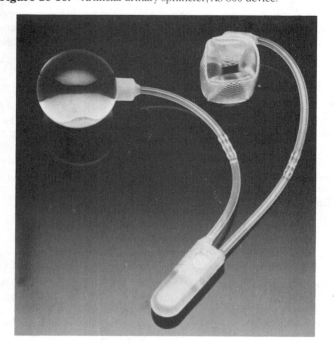

cal blockade, or augmentation cystoplasty. As in other procedures that modify the outlet, bladder emptying may require augmentation with intermittent self-catheterization.

Electrical Stimulation

In patients with hypotonic, areflexic bladders that result in decreased contractility, electrical stimulation directly to the bladder[17, 18] or by way of the spinal cord[44, 45] has been attempted. The results have been poor. Problems usually stem from stimulus of the urogenital diaphragm, which causes functional outlet obstruction during voiding, and additional procedures, such as sphincterotomy and neural blockade, may be required to decrease outflow resistance. Pain, the worst problem with bladder stimulation, occurs in at least 20% of patients and arises from electrical current migration. The application of these techniques has met with little enthusiasm and only partial success. Research, however, continues, and it is hoped that selective neural stimulation of the detrusor and the bladder outlet will meet with more success in the next decade.

Urinary Diversion, Continent Pouches, and Reservoirs

Urinary diversion can be achieved by any of several ways, including an indwelling urethral catheter, cystostomy (tube or tubeless), ureterostomies, nephrostomies, ileal conduit, colonic conduit, and various forms of continent pouches. In general, this means of managing the lower urinary tract is reserved as a last resort in patients with neurogenic vesical dysfunction.

Management of Urinary Tract Infection and Urinary Calculi

Urinary Tract Infection

Every effort should be made to protect the genitourinary tract from the damage of infection. Three-fourths, if not more, of patients with neurogenic bladder dysfunction will have infection at one time or another. The high degree of susceptibility to infection, however, should not mean that infection should be allowed to develop.[119] The benefit of aggressive management of urinary tract infection is evident by the decreasing incidence of renal failure as a major cause of death in patients with spinal cord injury.[128, 134]

Mechanical washout is considered to be the most effective barrier to infection.[86] This mechanism is often defective in neurogenic bladder dysfunction. High residual urine volumes, which are favorable for bacterial growth, also affect the antibacterial activity of the bladder wall. Other host defenses are the urine pH and osmolality and the function of the vesicoureteral valve mechanism.

The consequences of urinary tract infection are structural damages and dysfunctions of the genitourinary tract. The danger of urinary tract infection is that it may leave permanent damage (especially to the kidneys), promote recurrence and spread of infection, and eventually interfere with successful treatment. Examples of structural damages are prostatitis, epididymitis, trabeculation and thickening of the bladder wall, bladder stone formation, ureteritis, and the development of incompetence of the vesicoureteral junction. Recurrent upper urinary tract infections may lead to irreversible kidney damage and renal failure.

Asymptomatic infections of the lower urinary tract may lead to incontinence (because of increased bladder irritation), increased detrusor–sphincter dyssynergia with increased residual urine volumes, and further increased colony counts.

Systemic dysfunctions secondary to urinary tract infections consist of increased spasticity, autonomic hyperreflexia, and potentially life-threatening urosepsis.

Prevention of urinary tract infections is, therefore, important. Infections of the lower urinary tract are often asymptomatic in patients with neurogenic bladder dysfunction.[86] Therefore, early recognition of asymptomatic bacteriuria and prompt and specific antimicrobial therapy prevent it from becoming symptomatic.

The usual symptoms of lower urinary tract infection such as urinary frequency, urgency, nocturia, and dysuria are unreliable in neurogenic bladder dysfunction. More reliable clinical evidence includes increased spontaneous voiding, a change in residual urine volumes, cloudy urine, abnormal smell of urine, increased spasticity, and autonomic hyperreflexia.

When symptoms of urinary tract infection develop in patients with neurogenic bladder dysfunction, they may remain rather nonspecific, such as fever, chills, sweating, and abdominal discomfort. With the occurrence of such symptoms, one should suspect significant tissue invasion by the infection, such as pyelonephritis, epididymitis, prostatitis, or severe cystitis.

A urine culture is the most reliable method to determine the significance of bacteriuria and the type of bacteria present. However, the reliability of a urine culture depends on the type of urine sample (clean voided or catheter) and the time elapsed between obtaining the sample and culturing because the growth of bacteria may be rapid, especially if the specimen is kept unrefrigerated. Because of the risk of causing infection by performing a catheterization (the estimated infection rate is 2% per catheterization), midstream urine samples should be used whenever possible. Midstream urine samples with significant colony counts on the first sample have been shown to correlate to 80% with significant bacteriuria from catheter specimens. Repeat cultures of midstream urine samples often are helpful for confirming the presence or absence of lower tract infection. Bacterial colony counts of 10^4 to 10^5/ml in midstream urine specimens demand repeat culture without starting treatment. Colony counts of more than 10^5/ml in catheter or suprapubic specimens are considered indicative of the presence of an infection and call for treatment. Colony counts of 10^4 to 10^5/ml on catheter specimens should be considered significant, especially when gram-negative organisms are present. Under these circumstances, one should repeat the culture and probably start specific antimicrobial therapy. Bacteria counts of less than 10^3/ml are not diagnostic of infection. However, culture should be repeated while treatment is being withheld. If a patient is symptomatic in the presence of low colony counts, a repeat urine culture showing similar colony counts should be obtained before the institution of treatment.

Several other laboratory studies help supplement the information about urinary tract infection, but by themselves they are not sufficiently reliable for the diagnosis of lower urinary tract infection. These include urinalysis,[60] a spun sediment urine Gram stain, the leukocyte esterase dipstick test, blood chemistry studies, excretory urogram, or renal scans. The washout test of Farley and the test for urinary antibody-coated bacteria have been used in attempts to differentiate upper from lower urinary tract infections. These tests are cumbersome and not sufficiently sensitive to be useful by themselves.[86]

In patients with indwelling catheters, the incidence rate of infection is 90% at any one time. Patients on intermittent catheterization are reported to have variable infection rates. The frequency of positive urine cultures per week for patients on intermittent self-catheterization has been reported to range from 0% to 20%. During the course of bladder retraining for inpatients, 77% have infection at least once.[119] For patients on long-term

intermittent catheterization, the reported incidence of infection ranges from 13% to 18%.[124] The infection rates for outpatients receiving antimicrobial prophylaxis (methenamine salts or co-trimoxazole) have been reported to range from 0% to 20% in those managed with intermittent self-catheterization and in those managed with catheter-free voiding after bladder retraining.[88]

No single bacterium is most common in recurrent urinary tract infection associated with neurogenic bladder dysfunction. Patients on intermittent self-catheterization tend to develop *Escherichia coli* infections, followed in decreasing order of frequency by *Streptococcus* coagulase-negative, *Klebsiella pneumoniae, Pseudomonas aeruginosa,* and *Streptococcus* infections.[125] The most frequent bacteria observed in inpatients on team intermittent catheterization are *Streptococcus* coagulase-negative, *Klebsiella pneumoniae, Pseudomonas aeruginosa,* and *Escherichia coli.*[125]

The type of antimicrobial prophylaxis seems selective for certain bacteria when lower urinary tract infections recur. Patients receiving methenamine hippurate (Hiprex), with or without ascorbic acid, tend to become infected with *Escherichia coli;* those receiving trimethoprim-sulfamethoxazole tend to become infected by resistant *Klebsiella pneumoniae;* and patients who are not receiving prophylaxis tend to become infected with gentamicin-sensitive *Pseudomonas aeruginosa.*[125]

When treating asymptomatic urinary tract infections, one has to determine whether the patient is going to be managed by continuous drainage (indwelling urinary catheter) for an extended time, by intermittent catheterization, or by catheter-free voiding. Patients with indwelling catheters should not be treated with antimicrobial agents unless the urinary tract infection becomes symptomatic. High fluid intake, careful avoidance of any obstruction of the drainage system, changing the catheter every 2 weeks, and avoiding pressure of the catheter within the urethra is the basic treatment for patients with indwelling catheters. While the patient is hospitalized, urine should be cultured regularly to detect infection with resistant organisms.

For patients managed by intermittent catheterization or catheter-free voiding, significant asymptomatic bacteriuria should be treated according to sensitivities. Any foreign bodies (stones or catheters) within the genitourinary tract should be removed. Reculture should always be done after the patient has been receiving specific antimicrobial treatment for 48 hours to ascertain treatment effectiveness. The duration of treatment depends on the degree of structural changes or tissue infiltration present in the genitourinary tract and especially on whether the upper tracts are involved. The usual duration of treatment is 7 to 14 days. The urine should be recultured 48 hours after discontinuing treatment to ascertain the effectiveness of the therapy. Subsequent urine culturing should be performed weekly.

In the presence of drug-resistant organisms (gram-negative bacteria resistant to gentamicin and to two other antibiotics or *Staphylococcus aureus* resistant to oxacillin), isolation of the patient is mandatory. One may consider "rehabilitation" isolation, which involves extra precaution in handling the genitourinary tract, the catheter, clothing, the toilet, and the wheelchair. Such precautions allow the patient to have an open drainage system (otherwise, a closed drainage system is used consistently) and to participate in the rehabilitation program outside the room. All handling of the genitourinary tract occurs in the patient's room. A soiled wheelchair or clothes are not allowed outside the room.

An important factor in prophylaxis is cleanliness. Sterile intermittent catheterization is preferred over clean intermittent catheterization when the patient is on intermittent self-catheterization in the hospital, because this will further protect the patient from acquiring hospital-based resistant organisms. Once the patient is home, clean, intermittent catheterization is the technique of choice.

The basic principle of antimicrobial prophylaxis is to extend the time of freedom from infection. Methenamine hippurate, trimethoprim-sulfamethoxazole, and methenamine mandelate seem to be equally effective; the incidence of negative weekly urine cultures is 90%, and that in patients who are not receiving prophylaxis is 75%.[124] The use of ascorbic acid does not seem to add to the protection against infection;[124] however, acidification with ammonium chloride (1 g every 6 hours) is effective when used with methenamine mandelate.[66]

Urinary Tract Calculi

The most common cause of urinary tract calculi in patients with neurogenic bladder dysfunction is infection, especially infection with urea-splitting bacteria. Urea tends to precipitate on foreign bodies within the urinary tract, such as cellular debris, catheters, or hairs, especially when there is stagnation.[43]

Stones should be suspected when a patient exhibits recurrent urinary tract infection (*Escherichia coli, Pseudomonas,* or multiple organisms) despite what seems to be adequate treatment. The presence of urinary calculi is definitively diagnosed by roentgenography or cystoscopy. Urea stones are not visualized roentgenographically.

Most commonly, urinary stones are localized to the bladder in patients with neurogenic bladder dysfunction and are frequently a complication of indwelling catheters.

The treatment of stones is removal. This can be accomplished through the cystoscope when dealing with bladder stones. Upper tract stones can be removed in various ways. A recently added method is extracorporeal shock wave lithotripsy, which may be applied in about 65% of cases. The indication depends on the size of the stone, the presence or absence of infection, and the size of the patient. Percutaneous removal of upper urinary tract stones by nephroscopy is accomplished in about 30% of cases and is the treatment of choice in stones that are infected.[112, 113] The prophylaxis of urinary calculi is related to proper management of the genitourinary tract.[43]

Follow-Up

After initiation of long-term management, patients with neurogenic bladder dysfunction should be examined regularly, regardless of what method of management is being used. With intermittent self-catheterization and catheter-free voiding, the function of the urinary tract is usually rechecked at 3 months and 6 months and annually thereafter, and the urine is cultured monthly and later every 3 months if no infection occurs. Asymptomatic bladder infections, once suspected and identified, should be treated promptly and specifically. In cases of catheter-free voiding, the goals of regular follow-up visits are to ensure that the patient can

- Maintain acceptable voiding pressures of not more than 90 cm H_2O, to safeguard against excessive bladder hypertrophy, vesicoureteral reflux, and upper tract deterioration
- Void to residual volumes of less than 100 ml (preferably less than 50 ml), to safeguard against recurrent urinary tract infections
- Maintain a sterile urinary tract
- Maintain urinary continence by appropriately adhering to drinking–voiding schedules

- Maintain normal function and normal structure of the upper urinary tracts
- Make commonsense decisions in the day-to-day management of bladder dysfunction

During the follow-up visit, history-taking relates to the frequency and duration of voiding, changes in characteristics of the urinary stream, duration of voiding, incidence of recurrent, asymptomatic (or symptomatic) urinary tract infections, effectiveness of antibiotic therapy, use of bacteriostatic medications, and a review of systems.

The physical examination consists of an examination of vital signs, the abdomen, the flanks, and, in men, the external genitalia and of a neurological examination in regard to spinal cord functions. The rectal examination includes determining the presence or absence of sensation, voluntary control of the anal sphincter, the bulbocavernosus reflex, and anal sphincter tone; the response of the sphincter to gentle, prolonged stretching (in hyperreflexic sphincters) is noted; and the rectum and prostate are examined.

Laboratory examinations that are performed are urinalysis, urine culture and sensitivity tests, and routine blood chemistry profiles. Hemoglobin concentration, leukocyte count, erythrocyte sedimentation rate, and residual urine volume are determined. Presence or absence of stones is assessed from a roentgenogram of the kidneys, ureter, and bladder. The structure of the upper urinary tracts is evaluated by an excretory urogram consisting of a 20-minute postinjection film. An isotope renal scan may give information about gross structural changes of the urinary system and about renal function.[129] It is less cumbersome for the patient because it does not require special preparations for the patient and requires much less time.

Especially important is the urodynamic study in patients with hyperreflexic detrusors. Cystometrography-electromyography may be directed by the physiatrist. The urologist then examines the patient in association with the physiatrist, and they both determine the best action for the patient. Explanations are given freely about the findings and optimal management. A review of the roentgenograms and the urodynamic tracing with the patient may have motivating results regarding the firm establishment of new preventive living habits. Possible further implications of beginning complications need to be discussed in detail. If defects in knowledge, skills, and attitudes are detected, remedial interactions between the patient and members of the rehabilitation team are advised and arranged if agreed to by the patient, either during the same visit or, if necessary, later in the form of a "refresher course."

Follow-up examinations of patients on intermittent self-catheterization need not take issue with voiding characteristics but instead relate to the technique and use of intermittent self-catheterization, the function of the urinary tract (especially of detrusor pressure if the detrusor is hyperreflexic), and the presence or absence of infection and of bladder stones.[3] Because of the relative frequency of stone formation, cystoscopy should be done regularly in these patients.

Long-Term Results of Management

The morbidity and mortality of patients with spinal cord injury have improved considerably over the past decades, especially since the advent of antibiotics, intermittent catheterization, and bladder retraining.[34, 47, 96] Initially, the methods of choice after World War II were indwelling urethral or suprapubic catheters. These methods have now been largely replaced with intermittent self-catheterization and with bladder retraining for catheter-free voiding. Long-term results with indwelling catheters indicate maintenance of renal function[105] and substantial numbers of patients with stone formation, cystitis, and infection.[59] Reports of long-term management with intermittent self-catheterization[3, 101, 120] show satisfactory maintenance, as do reports of management with bladder retraining and continued catheter-free voiding.[31, 37, 86, 88, 97, 98, 117, 128]

Overall, either method may give satisfactory results. However, all methods require some change of living habits by the patient and regular follow-up examinations for an indefinite time so that changes in urodynamics, renal function, stone formation, and infection are detected early and thus the actual clinical complications of neurogenic bladder dysfunction are avoided.

NEUROGENIC BOWEL DYSFUNCTION

Anatomical and Physiological Considerations for the Colon, Rectum, and Anus

The Colon

The main function of the colon is the absorption of water, sodium, other minerals, and vitamins. The colon converts the 1000 to 2000 ml of isotonic chyme that enters through the ileocolic valve (one-way valve) each day from the ileum to about 150 g of semisolid feces. Colonic motility includes segmentation contractions for mixing, peristaltic waves for propulsion, and mass action contractions for expulsion (defecation) of content. The colon is innervated through the superior hypogastric plexus (ascending and transverse) and the inferior hypogastric plexus (descending colon and sigmoid). In contrast to the bladder, with denervation, the colon continues to function independently with near-normal motility, because of the intramural myenteric plexus along its entire length. Ingested food reaches the cecum in about 4 hours, the hepatic flexure in about 8 hours, and the pelvic colon in about 12 hours.

The Rectum

The rectum is 10 to 15 cm long. It is angulated distally above the anus at nearly 90° posteriorly, follows the concavity of the sacrum, and borders to the sigmoid in a transverse fold. Both the proximal transverse fold and the distal angulation have quasi-valvelike function, especially when the rectum is empty and the intra-abdominal pressure is elevated. Distally, the rectum is pulled forward by the levator ani. The rectum is innervated from sacral cord segments S2–S4 via the pelvic nerves.

The Anus

The *anal canal* is surrounded by the internal anal sphincter proximally. It consists of smooth muscle. It is sympathetically innervated, similar to the internal urethral sphincter mechanism from the thoracolumbar cord (T11–L2). The *external anal sphincter* encircles the internal anal sphincter in part and extends around the distal part of the anal canal. It consists of skeletal muscle and is innervated, like the external urethral sphincter, from the sacral spinal cord (S2–S4) via the pudendal nerves.

Central Regulation of Normal Defecation

Relatively little is known about the organization and interaction of the centers of defecation. Some evidence, however, supports the hypothesis that the reflexes of storage and of emptying in the rectum and anus are integrated in the central nervous system in a fashion similar to that of the lower urinary tract, with the spinal defecation center located at S2–S4 and T11–L2, interacting with a supraspinal defecation center at the pons[130] and multiple cortical-relating areas.

Normal Rectal Sphincter Dynamics

Storage

Electromyographic studies have shown ongoing electrical activities in both anal sphincters when the rectum is not distended. These reflexes are important for the maintenance of rectal continence. With filling of the rectum, the rectum contracts and the internal anal sphincter relaxes in response to stretch sensors in the rectal mucosa.[35] With relaxation of the internal anal sphincter, the anal mucosa is exposed to the rectal content. The anal mucosa is richly supplied with sensory endings with which the cerebral cortex may distinguish solid, liquid, and gaseous matter. As soon as the anal sensations are perceived and rapidly interpreted by cortical sensory areas, the pontine defecation center is then either inhibited or facilitated as a conscious, learned process. If the pontine center is inhibited by the cortex, the external anal sphincter increases in tone, and the motor action spreads progressively to other muscles of the pelvic floor, especially the levator ani, all maintaining anal continence.

Defecation

In response to rectal distention, the cortex facilitates the pontine defecation center when defecation is socially acceptable and the external anal sphincter relaxes, permitting defecation to take place. Straining occurs, and the colonic mass action comes into play. It is facilitated and maintained by stimulation from the anal mucosa via the myenteric plexus and by central actions of the pontine defecation center.

Mechanical or chemical stimulation of the proximal anorectal mucosa digitally or by suppositories also initiates reflex activities that lead to stimulation of the myenteric plexus, mass action contraction of the colon, and defecation.

Filling of the stomach with food tends to initiate contractions of the rectum, which often are associated with a desire to defecate. This response is called the gastrocolic reflex, even though there is some evidence that it is not neurally mediated but is due to the action of gastrin on the colon.

Abnormal Rectal Sphincter Dynamics

Uninhibited bowel dysfunction is caused by neurologic lesions interfering with the cortical interrelationships with the pontine defecation center. In patients with stroke, brain injury, or other such neurological lesions, when stimulated by anorectal filling, the pontine defecation center may not become sufficiently suppressed to prevent fecal incontinence.

Upper motor bowel dysfunction occurs with neurological lesions interrupting the pontine from the spinal defecation centers in patients with spinal cord injury above the sacral cord. There is evidence that with rectal filling not only the internal but also, by spinal reflex, the external anal sphincter relaxes.[35, 130] Defecation then occurs through mass action contraction, as mediated through the stimulated myenteric plexus of the colon. Clinical experience indicates that a similar process is initiated with mechanical or chemical stimulation of the rectal mucosa, probably using the same spinal and myenteric activities.

Lower motor neuron bowel dysfunction is caused by neurological lesions destroying either the sacral defecation center or the relating nerve supply to the rectum and anus. Electromyographic evidence shows that the external anal sphincter is denervated and that the internal anal sphincter relaxes with filling of the rectum, as it does in people with normal control.[35] Defecation, indeed, is possible through stimulation of the myenteric plexus of the colon and rectum, which occurs with distention of the colon and filling of the rectum, leading to mass action peristalsis and internal sphincter relaxation. The same process may be initiated by mechanical or chemical stimulation of the anal mucosa.

Classification and Management

Acute Phase

Adynamic ileus is the most frequent gastrointestinal complication in the acute stage of neurogenic bowel dysfunction, occurring in about 63% of patients with spinal cord injury.[40] Management of this condition is important because it may last from days to more than a week.

Management of adynamic ileus is nasogastric suction in order to prevent further gastrointestinal dilatation and respiratory compromise. Close monitoring of fluid balance with a central intravenous line is indicated, and intravenous therapy needs to be instituted. Peristalsis of the gut may be stimulated by abdominal massage or transcutaneous electrical stimulation.[40, 57]

As soon as bowel sounds reappear, a clear liquid diet may be introduced and, at the same time, a regular bowel emptying program is instituted. This is done with suppositories (bisacodyl) or manual extraction.

Long-Term Management

Bowel evacuation in patients with neurogenic bowel dysfunction is done on a bedside commode as soon as sitting balance allows because sitting facilitates emptying. Regular, adequate fluid intake (1500 to 2000 ml) is important and needs to be correlated with the management of the urinary tract.

During the reparative phase after spinal cord injury, the diet should be high in protein, high in calories, and high in fiber.

Several types of medications assist in bowel regulation.[24] Bulk cathartics promote intestinal evacuation by retaining a considerable amount of water while in the colon. The most commonly used medications of this type are the hydrophilic colloids, such as psyllium hydrophilic mucilloid (Metamucil, Fiberall). Another commonly used bulk cathartic is milk of magnesia, usually taken 8 hours before planned bowel care.

Irritant cathartics, such as castor oil or bisacodyl (Ducolax) tablets, are usually avoided because they may cause unpredictable degrees of stool softness and promote mucus production and fecal incontinence. Bisacodyl suppositories, however, are commonly used to stimulate evacuation. Furthermore, surface active agents or fecal softeners are popular, such as docusate sodium (dioctyl sodium sulfosuccinate or Colace). Peri-Colace may or may not be helpful; it is a combination of docusate sodium and the mild stimulant laxative casanthranol. It may cause cramping discomfort and irregular bowel action.

In bowel retraining, the regulation and regularity of bowel movement are the most important issues. Goals of bowel retraining are to make the patient continent and socially acceptable and to lead to consistently regular and normal bowel evacuations. The frequency of regular bowel movements is variable. It may be daily, every other day, or every third day. Problems with incontinence, constipation, and impaction usually develop if patients delay bowel actions beyond every 3 days. Patients with lower motor neuron bowel dysfunction may have much more frequent bowel movements because they need to strain or use the Credé maneuver for bladder emptying. Men with lower motor neuron bowel dysfunction who rely on straining of Credé maneuvers to empty the bladder may have to sit down for bladder emptying because of frequent, associated bowel movements.

Surgical bowel diversion procedures may have to be done when fecal incontinence continues to be a problem interfering with the rehabilitation program and reentry into the community. However, the need for surgical intervention is extremely rare in patients with neurogenic bowel dysfunction. Surgical procedures used to treat fecal incontinence secondary to conditions other than neurogenic bowel dysfunction include muscle loop procedures. They are dependent on sensory feedback or muscle being available for transposition.[23, 25]

To initiate a regular bowel movement, one usually has to use either bisacodyl (Dulcolax) or glycerin suppositories. Patients have to be encouraged to have bowel action at the same time each day. Use of gastrocolic reflex is often helpful when bowel care is done approximately 1 hour after breakfast or supper. Maintenance of regular mealtimes is also important. If medications are needed, bulk cathartics are the first to be added to the program and then surface active agents, and, finally, more stimulating medications are used only until a satisfactory program is established. With long-term management, one attempts to achieve freedom from all medications and suppositories. Often, digital stimulation is sufficient to encourage bowel evacuation when done regularly. Digital extraction may be necessary, especially in cases of lower motor neuron bowel dysfunction.

Enemas should be used only when bowel movement has not been accomplished by any of the above-described measures and impaction may be imminent. Patient and family education is of vital importance in a program of bowel retraining.

Marked spasticity of the external anal sphincter may significantly interfere with successful bowel care. It may lead to cramping abdominal pain and marked bloating. Intramuscular neurolysis of the anal sphincter may be tried to accomplish better bowel evacuation.[99]

Biofeedback may also be tried, especially in patients with lower motor neuron bowel dysfunction in whom incontinence rather than constipation is the problem. Biofeedback has been reported to be successful in the treatment of fecal incontinence in children with spina bifida.[132]

Complications

Complications of neurogenic bowel dysfunction are well described.[40] Some of these have already been mentioned, such as ileus, peptic ulcer (common during physical stress), and fecal impaction. These conditions account for 45% of complications. Superior mesenteric artery syndrome is rare because halo vests instead of halo casts are now being used for immobilization of the cervical spine. Other complications are hiatal hernia, gastroesophageal reflux, and diverticulosis.

Fecal incontinence *per se* can cause complications and may necessitate more aggressive means of control. These complications are skin irritation with skin breakdown and ulcerations. Also, soiling of the genitalia may cause recurrent urinary tract infections. Autonomic hyperreflexia can be precipitated by fecal impaction and necessitates close monitoring of vital signs and blood pressure during release of the impaction. Liberal use of lidocaine (Xylocaine) jelly during digital extraction can be helpful. Patients with neurogenic bowel dysfunction can develop irritable bowel syndrome. This necessitates the same treatment used for patients without neurogenic bowel dysfunction (that is, diet and sedatives). Patients with neurogenic bowel dysfunction are often sensitive to spicy food. They should be warned of this to avoid embarassment in public places after dining out.

Anticholinergic medications, used for the management of neurogenic bladder dysfunction, can significantly interfere with bowel management. They may cause severe constipation or even adynamic ileus. Also, antidepressant medications with significant anticholinergic side-effects may interfere with bowel management.

Proctalgia is one of the pain syndromes that may develop as a sequela of spinal cord injury. It may be central in origin or a neuralgia as part of a cauda equina syndrome. It may be annoying and difficult to manage. Antidepressant medication may be of help for controlling the pain. Furthermore, transcutaneous electrical nerve stimulation should be tried, especially in cases associated with neuralgia from a cauda equina syndrome.

Pediatric Considerations

The evaluation of anal tone may influence bowel training. However, Sullivan-Bolyai and associates[121] found no detectable difference in learning bowel care between children with spastic anal sphincters and a strong anal wink and those with an absent or weak anal tone.

Several factors need to be taken into consideration in training for bowel continence. There must be a regular time for evacuation.[42] This regular evacuation should be 30 to 45 minutes after a meal in order to use the gastrocolic reflex. The child should have a diet with adequate fiber content—at least eight fiber-rich foods per day.[42, 82]

Adequate intake of fluid is important not only for bladder training but also for proper consistency of the feces. Insertion of pediatric bisacodyl or glycerin suppositories next to the bowel wall is helpful. When the suppository is inserted into the bowel, the rectal sphincters and rectal sigmoid junction should be stretched in order to stimulate the relating reflexes. In an infant, the fifth finger can be used to insert the suppository. A stool softener such as docusate sodium (Colace) or bulk expanders such as psyllium hydrophilic mucilloid (Metamucil) have been suggested but are not often necessary if the diet has adequate fiber.[42, 82, 132] A small expansion enema has been used after failure with other methods of bowel care.[42, 132] Milk of magnesia or mineral oil is not suggested.

Biofeedback and behavior modification techniques were described by Whitehead and colleagues[132] for the management of incontinence. These techniques of providing visual feedback and rewards for successful strong sphincter contractions in the training sessions and the use of 50 sphincter contractions daily proved helpful for bladder and bowel continence. In combination with behavior modifications involving attempts to defecate immediately, attempts to have a bowel movement after an evening meal each day, receiving rewards for bowel movements on the toilet without an enema and suppository, and the use of enemas only if unsuccessful for 2 consecutive days resulted in a reduction in the frequency of incontinence of more than 50% in 64% of their patients.[132] These techniques seem to result in maintenance of continence at 1-year follow-up.[132]

Chronic constipation and delayed bowel movements for longer than 2 days can lead to chronic impactions and overstretching of the bowel. Associated findings are further destruction of nervous control of the bowel wall, enlargement of the bowel, and even urinary obstruction. In some reports, urinary infections have resulted from impactions.[42, 121, 132]

Some reasons for failure or delayed toileting are mental retardation, family disruption, physical difficulties such as kyphoscoliosis, braces, inability to sit on a toilet, arthrogryposis, irritable bowels, abnormalities of the anus, and renal complications.[42, 132] Factors that interfere with the success of toilet training are failure of the family to comply, emotional disturbances, and failure of the school to cooperate.[42, 132] A few children react idiosyncratically to certain foods or medications, such as anticholinergic medications, and develop loose stools.[121, 132] For handicapped children, active involvement of a school nurse and nursing consultants in writing informed individual education plans should help to ensure inclusion of toilet training and toileting maintenance needs. A private place for bowel and bladder procedures; verbal reminders from parents, teachers, nurses, therapists, and physicians; praises for even small gains; and assistance in toileting programs allow for optimal success in bowel training for children.[121]

REFERENCES

1. Adatto K, Doebele KG, Galland L et al: Behavioral factors and urinary tract infection. JAMA 241:2525–2526, 1979
2. Ahmed S, Carney A: Urinary undiversion in myelomeningocele patients with an ileal conduit diversion. J Urol 125:847–852, 1981
3. Amendola MA, Sonda LP, Diokno AC et al: Bladder calculi complicating intermittent clean catheterization. Am J Roentgenol 141:751–753, 1983
4. Awad SA: Urethral pressure profile: Clinical value of liquid profilometry. In Barrett DM, Wein AJ (eds): Controversies in Neuro-Urology, pp 47–53. New York, Churchill Livingstone, 1984
5. Bagley NA, O'Shaughnessy EJ: Urodynamic evaluation of voluntary detrusor response in healthy subjects. Arch Phys Med Rehabil 66:160–163, 1985
6. Barkin M, Dolfin D, Herschorn S et al: The urologic care of the spinal cord injury patient. J Urol 129:335–339, 1983
7. Barrett DM: Electromyography: The practical approach. In Barrett DM, Wein AJ (eds): Controversies in Neuro-Urology, pp 85–92. New York, Churchill Livingstone, 1984
8. Barrett DM, Furlow WL: Incontinence, intermittent self-catheterization and the artificial genitourinary sphincter. J Urol 132:268–269, 1984
9. Bartholomew TH: Neurogenic voiding: Function and dysfunction. Urol Clin North Am 12:67–73, 1985
10. Barton CH, Vaziri ND, Gordon S et al: Renal pathology in end-stage renal disease associated with paraplegia. Paraplegia 22:31–41, 1984
11. Bauer SB: Editorial: Management of neurogenic bladder dysfunction in children. J Urol 132:544–545, 1984
12. Bhatia NN, Bradley WE: Cystometry: Gas. In Barrett DM, Wein AJ (eds): Controversies in Neuro-Urology, pp 1–8. New York, Churchill Livingstone, 1984
13. Bhatia NN, Bradley WE: Urethral pressure profile. Gas. In Barrett DM, Wein AJ (eds): Controversies in Neuro-Urology, pp 39–46. New York, Churchill Livingstone, 1984
14. Blaivas JG: A critical appraisal of specific diagnostic techniques. In Krane RJ, Siroky MB (eds): Clinical Neuro-Urology, pp 69–109. Boston, Little, Brown & Co, 1979
15. Borzyskowski M: Management of neuropathic bladder in childhood. Dev Med Child Neurol 26:401–404, 1984
16. Borzyskowski M, Mundy AR, Neville BGR et al: Neuropathic vesicourethral dysfunction in children: A trial comparing clean intermittent catheterization with manual expression combined with drug treatment. Br J Urol 54:641–644, 1982
17. Boyce WH, Lathem JE, Hunt LD: Research related to the development of an artificial electrical stimulator for the paralyzed human bladder: A review. J Urol 91:41–51, 1964
18. Bradley WE, Chou SN, French LA: Further experience with the radio transmitter receiver unit for the neurogenic bladder. J Neurosurg 20:953–960, 1963
19. Bradley WE, Timm GW, Scott FB: Innervation of the detrusor muscle and urethra. Urol Clin North Am 1:3–27, 1974
20. Cass AS, Luxemberg M, Gleich P et al: A 22-year followup of ileal

conduits in children with a neurogenic bladder. J Urol 132:529–531, 1984

21. Cass AS, Luxemberg M, Gleich P et al: Clean intermittent catheterization in the management of the neurogenic bladder in children. J Urol 132:526–528, 1984

22. Cass AS, Luxenberg M, Johnson CF et al: Management of the neurogenic bladder in 413 children. J Urol 132:521–525, 1984

23. Cohen M, Rosen L, Khubchandani I et al: Rationale for medical or surgical therapy in anal incontinence. Dis Colon Rectum 29:120–122, 1986

24. Comarr AE: Bowel regulation for patients with spinal cord injury. JAMA 167:18–21, 1958

25. Corman ML: Follow-up evaluation of gracilis muscle transposition for fecal incontinence. Dis Colon Rectum 23:552–555, 1980

26. Cytometry: editorial comment. In Barrett DM, Wein AJ (eds): Controversies in Neuro-Urology, p 37. New York, Churchill Livingstone, 1984

27. De Groat WC: Nervous control of the urinary bladder of the cat. Brain Res 87:201–211, 1975

28. DeLaere KPJ, Debruyne FMJ, Michiels HGE et al: Prolonged bladder distention in the management of the unstable bladder. J Urol 124:334–337, 1980

29. Dewey MM: The anatomical basis for propagation in smooth muscle. Gastroenterology 49:395–402, 1965

30. Engel RME, Schirmer HKA: Pudendal neurectomy in neurogenic bladder. J Urol 112:57–59, 1974

31. Erickson RP, Merritt JL, Opitz JL et al: Bacteriuria during follow-up in patients with spinal cord injury: I. Rates of bacteriuria in various bladder-emptying methods. Arch Phys Med Rehabil 63:409–412, 1982

32. Faure JJ, Retief PJM, Key AG: Urological management of the patient with spinal cord injury. S Afr Med J 58:682–686, 1980

33. Frankel HL: Intermittent catheterization. Urol Clin North Am 1:115–124, 1974

34. Freed MM, Bakst HJ, Barrie DL: Life expectancy, survival rates, and causes of death in civilian patients with spinal cord trauma. Arch Phys Med Rehabil 47:457–463, 1966

35. Frenckner B: Function of the anal sphincters in spinal man. Gut 16:638–644, 1975

36. Furlow WL, Barrett DM: The artificial urinary sphincter: Experience with the AS 800 pump-control assembly for single-stage primary deactivation and activation—a preliminary report. Mayo Clin Proc 60:255–258, 1985

37. Gjone RN, Ween E: Results of bladder training 1966–1974. Paraplegia 15:47–54, 1977–1978

38. Goldwasser B, Webster GD: Augmentation and substitution enterocystoplasty. J Urol 135:215–224, 1986

39. Gonzalez R, Sidi AA: Preoperative prediction of continence after enterocystoplasty of undiversion in children with neurogenic bladder. J Urol 134:705–707, 1985

40. Gore RM, Mintzer RA, Calenoff L: Gastrointestinal complications of spinal cord injury. Spine 6:538–544, 1981

41. Gosling JA, Dixon JS: The structure and innervation of smooth muscle in the wall of the bladder neck and proximal urethra. Br J Urol 47:549–558, 1975

42. Greecher CP, Cohen IT, Ballantine TVN: Survey of nutritional problems encountered in children with neuromotor disorders. J Parenter Enteral Nutr 4:490–493, 1980

43. Griffith DP: Infection-induced stones. In Coe FL (ed): Nephrolithiasis: Pathogenesis and Treatment, pp 203–228. Chicago, Year Book Medical Publishers, 1978

44. Grimes JH, Nashold BS, Anderson EE: Clinical application of electronic bladder stimulation in paraplegics. J Urol 113:338–340, 1975

45. Grimes JH, Nashold BS, Currie DP: Chronic electrical stimulation of the paraplegic bladder. J Urol 109:242–245, 1973

46. Guttmann L, Frankel H: The value of intermittent catheterisation in the early management of traumatic paraplegia and tetraplegia. Paraplegia 4:63–84, 1966–1967

47. Hackler RH: A 25-year prospective mortality study in spinal cord injured patient: Comparison with long-term living paraplegic. J Urol 117:486–488, 1977

48. Hackler RH: When is an ileal conduit indicated in the spinal cord injured patient? Paraplegia 16:257–262, 1978–1979

49. Hackler RH: Long-term suprapubic cystostomy drainage in spinal cord injury patients. Br J Urol 54:120–121, 1982

50. Hadley HR, Zimmern PE, Staskin DR et al: Transvaginal needle bladder neck suspension. Urol Clin North Am 12:291–303, 1985

51. Halstead LS, Claus-Walker J: Neuroactive Drugs of Choice in Spinal Cord Injury: A Guide for Using Neurologically Active Medications in Spinal Injured Patients. The Institute of Rehabilitation and Research. Houston, TX, Baylor College of Medicine, 1980

52. Hederström E, Forsberg L: Accuracy of ultrasonography compared with urography in detection of intrarenal dilatation in children. Acta Radiol [Diag] 26:201–207, 1985

53. Hendry WF: Urinary stomas: I. Surgical procedures and complications. Clin Gastroenterol 11:303–317, 1982

54. Hensle TW, Nagler HM, Goldstein HR: Long-term functional results of urinary tract reconstruction in childhood. J Urol 128:1262–1269, 1982

55. Hodgkinson CP, Drukker BH: Infravesical nerve resection for detrusor dyssynergia: The Ingelman-Sundberg operation. Acta Obstet Gynecol Scand 56:401–408, 1977

56. Hutch JA: Anatomy and Physiology of the Bladder, Trigone, and Urethra. New York, Appleton-Century-Crofts, 1972

57. Hymes AC, Raab DE, Yonehiro EG et al: Acute pain control by electrostimulation: A preliminary report. Adv Neurol 4:761–767, 1974

58. Ingelman-Sundberg A: Partial denervation of the bladder: A new operation for the treatment of urge incontinence and similar conditions in women. Acta Obstet Gynecol Scand 38:487–502, 1959

59. Jacobs SC, Kaufman JM: Complications of permanent bladder catheter drainage in spinal cord injury patients. J Urol 119:740–741, 1978

60. Jenkins RD, Fenn JP, Matsen JM: Review of urine microscopy for bacteriuria. JAMA 255:3397–3403, 1986

61. Jones KV, Asscher W, Jones RV et al: Renal functional changes in schoolgirls with covert asymptomatic bacteriuria. Contrib Nephrol 39:152–163, 1984

62. Jørgensen L, Mortensen SO, Colstrup H et al: Bladder distention in the management of detrusor instability. Scand J Urol Nephrol 19:101–104, 1985

63. Kaplan WE, Firlit CF, Schoenberg HW: The female urethral syndrome: External sphincter spasm as etiology. J Urol 124:48–49, 1980

64. Kass EJ, Koff SA: Bladder augmentation in the pediatric neuropathic bladder. J Urol 129:552–555, 1983

65. Kass EJ, Koff SA, Diokno AC et al: The significance of bacilluria in children on long-term intermittent catheterization. J Urol 126:223–225, 1981

66. Kevorkian CG, Merritt JL, Ilstrup DM: Methenamine mandelate with acidification: An effective urinary antiseptic in patients with neurogenic bladder. Mayo Clin Proc 59:523–529, 1984

67. Khanna OP: Nonsurgical therapeutic modalities. In Krane RJ, Siroky ME (eds): Clinical Neuro-Urology, pp 159–196. Boston, Little, Brown & Co, 1979

68. Khanna OP: Cystometry: Water. In Barrett DM, Wein AJ (eds): Controversies in Neuro-Urology, pp 9–29. New York, Churchill Livingstone, 1984

69. Koontz WW Jr, Smith MJV, Currie RJ: External sphincterotomy in boys with meningomyelocele. J Urol 108:649–651, 1972

70. Krane RJ, Siroky MB: Classification of voiding dysfunction: Value of classification systems. In Barrett DM, Wein AJ (eds): Controversies in Neuro-Urology, pp 233–251. New York, Churchill Livingstone, 1984

71. Kuru M: Nervous control of micturition. Physiol Rev 45:425–494, 1965

72. Kusumi RK, Grover PJ, Kunin CM: Rapid detection of pyuria by leukocyte esterase activity. JAMA 245:1653–1655, 1981

73. Leach GE, Goldman D, Raz S: Surgical treatment of detrusor hyperreflexia. In Raz S (ed): Female Urology, pp 326–334. Philadelphia, WB Saunders, 1983

74. Libo LM, Arnold GE, Woodside JR et al: EMG biofeedback for functional bladder-sphincter dyssynergia: A case study. Biofeedback Self Regul 8:243–253, 1983

75. Light JK, Engelmann UH: Reconstruction of the lower urinary tract:

Observations on bowel dynamics and the artificial urinary sphincter. J Urol 133:594–597, 1985

76. Linder A, Leach GE, Raz S: Augmentation cystoplasty in the treatment of neurogenic bladder dysfunction. J Urol 129:491–493, 1983
77. MacGregor PS, Kay R, Straffon RA: Cutaneous ureterostomy in children—long-term followup. J Urol 134:518–520, 1985
78. Mahony DT, Laferte RO: Studies of enuresis: IV. Multiple detrusor myotomy: A new operation for the rehabilitation of severe detrusor hypertrophy and hypercontractility. J Urol 107:1064–1067, 1972
79. Manfredi RA, Leal JF: Selective sacral rhizotomy for the spastic bladder syndrome in patients with spinal cord injuries. J Urol 100:17–20, 1968
80. Maynard FM, Diokno AC: Clean intermittent catheterization for spinal cord injury patients. J Urol 128:477–480, 1982
81. Mayo ME, Lloyd-Davies RW, Shuttleworth KED et al: The damaged human detrusor: Functional and electron microscopic changes in disease. Br J Urol 45:116–125, 1973
82. McCallum G, Ballinger BR, Presly AS: A trial of bran and bran biscuits for constipation in mentally handicapped and psychogeriatric patients. J Hum Nutr 32:369–372, 1978
83. McGuire E: Retropubic operative procedures for stress urinary incontinence. In Raz S (ed): Female Urology, pp 241–251. Philadelphia, WB Saunders, 1983
84. McGuire EJ: Urethral pressure profile: Technique and application. In Barrett DM, Wein AJ (eds): Controversies in Neuro-Urology, pp 67–81. New York, Churchill Livingstone, 1984
85. McGuire EJ, Savastano JA: Urodynamic studies in enuresis and the nonneurogenic neurogenic bladder. J Urol 132:299–302, 1984
86. Merritt JL: Urinary tract infections, causes and management, with particular reference to patient with spinal cord injury: A review. Arch Phys Med Rehabil 57:365–373, 1976
87. Merritt JL: Residual urine volumes: Correlate of urinary tract infection in patients with spinal cord injury. Arch Phys Med Rehabil 62:558–561, 1981
88. Merritt JL, Erickson RP, Opitz JL: Bacteriuria during follow-up in patients with spinal cord injury: II. Efficacy of antimicrobial suppressants. Arch Phys Med Rehabil 63:413–415, 1982
89. Mirahmadi MK, Vaziri ND, Ghobadi M et al: Survival on maintenance dialysis in patients with chronic renal failure associated with paraplegia and quadriplegia. Paraplegia 20:43–47, 1982
90. Misak SJ, Bunts RC, Ulmer JL et al: Nerve interruption procedures in the urologic management of paraplegic patients. J Urol 88:392–401, 1962
91. Mitchell ME, Rink RC: Experience with the artificial urinary sphincter in children and young adults. J Pediatr Surg 18:700–705, 1983
92. Mundy AR, Stephenson TP: The urge syndrome. In Mundy AR, Stephenson TP, Wein AJ (eds): Urodynamics: Principles, Practice and Application, pp 212–228. Edinburgh, Churchill Livingstone, 1984
93. Nanninga JB, Wu Y, Hamilton B: Long-term intermittent catheterization in the spinal cord injury patient. J Urol 128:760–763, 1982
94. Newman E, Price M: External catheters: Hazards and benefits of their use by men with spinal cord lesions. Arch Phys Med Rehabil 66:310–313, 1985
95. Nielsen JB, Nørgaard JP, Djurhuus JC: Enuresis as protective factor in vesicoureteral reflux. Urology 26:468–473, 1985
96. Nyquist RH, Bors E: Mortality and survival in traumatic myelopathy during nineteen years, from 1946 to 1965. Paraplegia 5:22–48, 1967
97. Opitz JL: Bladder retraining: An organized program. Mayo Clin Proc 51:367–372, 1976
98. Opitz JL: Treatment of voiding dysfunction in spinal-cord-injured patients: Bladder retraining. In Barrett DM, Wein AJ (eds): Controversies in Neuro-Urology, pp 437–451. New York, Churchill Livingstone, 1984
99. Opitz JL, Lutness MP: Anal motor point blocks in the treatment of symptomatic anorectal dyssynergia in paraplegic male (abstr). Arch Phys Med Rehabil 66:559–560, 1985
100. O'Shaughnessy EJ, Clowers DE, Brooks G: Detrusor reflex contraction inhibited by anal stretch. Arch Phys Med Rehabil 62:128–130, 1981
101. Pearman JW, England EJ: The Urological Management of the Patient Following Spinal Cord Injury. Springfield, IL, Charles C Thomas, 1973
102. Perkash I: Management of neurogenic dysfunction of bladder and bowel. In Kottke FJ, Stillwell GK, Lehmann JF (eds): Krusen's Handbook of Physical Medicine and Rehabilitation, 3rd ed, pp 724–745. Philadelphia, WB Saunders, 1982
103. Perkash I, Friedland GW: Real-time gray-scale transrectal linear array ultrasonography in urodynamic evaluation. Semin Urol 3:49–59, 1985
104. Plunkett JM, Braren V: Five-year experience with clean intermittent catheterization in children. Urology 20:128–130, 1982
105. Price M, Kottke FJ, Olson ME: Renal function in patients with spinal cord injury: The eighth year of a ten-year continuing study. Arch Phys Med Rehabil 56:76–79, 1975
106. Raezer DM, Evans RJ, Shrom SH: Augmentation ileocystoplasty in neuropathic bladder. Urology 25:26–30, 1985
107. Raz S, Bradley WE: Neuromuscular dysfunction of the lower urinary tract. In Harrison JH, Gittes RF, Perlmutter AD et al (eds): Campbell's Urology, 4th ed, vol 2, pp 1215–1270. Philadelphia, WB Saunders, 1979
108. Raz S, Bruskewitz R: Surgical treatment of the neurogenic bladder. Am Urol Assoc Update Series, vol 1, lesson 35, 1982
109. Raz S, Magora F, Caine M: The evaluation of pudendal nerve block by measurements of urethral pressure. Surg Gynecol Obstet 133:453–457, 1971
110. Schellhammer PF, Hackler RH, Bunts RC: External sphincterotomy: An evaluation of 150 patients with neurogenic bladder. J Urol 110:199–202, 1973
111. Schmidt JD, Hawtrey CE, Flocks RH et al: Complications, results, and problems of ileal conduit diversions. J Urol 109:210–216, 1973
112. Segura JW: Endourology. J Urol 132:1079–1084, 1984
113. Segura JW, Patterson DE, LeRoy AJ et al: Percutaneous removal of kidney stones: A review of 1,000 cases. J Urol 134:1077–1081, 1985
114. Sidi AA, Dykstra DD, Gonzalez R: The value of urodynamic testing in the management of neonates with myelodysplasia: A prospective study. J Urol 135:90–93, 1986
115. Smith RB: Use of ileocystoplasty in the hypertonic neurogenic bladder. J Urol 113:125–127, 1975
116. Solomon MH, Koff SA, Diokno AC: Bladder calculi complicating intermittent catheterization. J Urol 124:140–141, 1980
117. Sperling KB: Intermittent catheterization to obtain catheter-free bladder function in spinal cord injury. Arch Phys Med Rehabil 59:4–8, 1978
118. Stamey TA: Endoscopic suspension of the vesical neck for urinary incontinence. Surg Gynecol Obstet 136:547–554, 1973
119. Stover SL, Fleming WC: Recurrent bacteriuria in complete spinal cord injury patients and external condom drainage. Arch Phys Med Rehabil 61:178–181, 1980
120. Stover SL, Lloyd LK, Nepomuceno CS et al: Intermittent catheterisation: Follow-up studies. Paraplegia 15:38–46, 1977–1978
121. Sullivan-Bolyai S, Swanson M, Shurtleff DB: Toilet training the child with neurogenic impairment of bowel and bladder function. Compr Pediatr Nurs 7:33–43, 1984
122. Tanagho EA: Urethral pressure profile: Membrane catheter. In Barrett DM, Wein AJ (eds): Controversies in Neuro-Urology, pp 55–65. New York, Churchill Livingstone, 1984
123. Thielman D: Patient teaching guidelines. J Enterostomal Ther 10:166–168, 1983
124. Thorsteinsson G, Keys T: The frequency and type of urinary tract infections in patients on intermittent catheterization and by catheterization team (abstr). Arch Phys Med Rehabil 64:519, 1983
125. Thorsteinsson G, Keys TF: The influence of urinary tract prophylaxis on the type of urinary tract infections in patients on intermittent catheterization: Preliminary report (abstr). Arch Phys Med Rehabil 64:520, 1983
126. Turner-Warwick RT, Ashken MH: The functional results of partial, subtotal and total cystoplasty with special reference to ureterocaecocystoplasty, selective sphincterotomy and cystocystoplasty. Br J Urol 39:3–12, 1967
127. Urethral pressure profile: editorial comment. In Barrett DM, Wein AJ (eds): Controversies in Neuro-Urology, pp 83–84. New York, Churchill Livingstone, 1984
128. Viera A, Merritt JL, Erickson RP: Renal function in spinal cord injury: A preliminary report. Arch Phys Med Rehabil 67:257–259, 1986
129. Wahner HW: Radioisotopes in medical diagnoses. In Spittell JA Jr

(ed): Clinical Medicine, vol 1, chap 37. Philadelphia, Harper & Row, 1985

130. Weber J, Denis P, Mihout B et al: Effect of brain-stem lesion on colonic and anorectal motility: Study of three patients. Dig Dis Sci 30:419–425, 1985

131. Webster GD, Goldwasser B: Management of the contracted bladder. In Krane RJ, Siroky MB (eds): Clinical Neuro-Urology, 2nd ed. Boston, Little, Brown & Co (in press)

132. Whitehead WE, Parker L, Bosmajian L et al: Treatment of fecal incontinence in children with spina bifida: Comparison of biofeedback and behavior modifications. Arch Phys Med Rehabil 67:218–224, 1986

133. Worth PHL, Turner-Warwick R: The treatment of interstitial cystitis by cystolysis with observations on cystoplasty. Br J Urol 45:65–71, 1973

134. Young JS, Burns PE, Bowen AM et al: Spinal cord injury statistics: Experience of the regional spinal cord injury systems. Phoenix, AZ, Good Samaritan Medical Center, 1982

135. Zinner NR, Sterling AM, Ritter RC: Cystometry: A word of advice. In Barrett DM, Wein AJ (eds): Controversies in Neuro-Urology, pp 30–36. New York, Churchill Livingstone, 1984

27

Sexual Functioning: Medical and Psychological Aspects

Stanley Ducharme

Kathleen Gill

Susan Biener-Bergman

Louisa Fertitta

Over the past decade there has been an increasing awareness that the field of rehabilitation medicine must address concerns of sexuality. This need has demanded a better understanding of how disability affects sexual functioning on both physiological and psychological levels. Although funding for such research has been noticeably poor, clear progress has been made and service delivery programs have been established at major rehabilitation facilities.[103] Today, sexual health is an integrated component of most rehabilitation programs and the importance of this information to patients and families has been clinically documented.

In order to clarify issues discussed in this chapter it is important to first define sexuality. *Sexuality* is the integration of physical, emotional, intellectual, and social aspects of an individual's personality that express maleness or femaleness. Sexuality is an expression of the total personality evident in everything done by a person. Interactions with others, personal hygiene, dress, speech, and expressions of affection are all an important part of sexuality. Given the broad scope of sexuality it is therefore safe to state that a person's sexuality is not determined by physical characteristics or abilities. It is also understood that given the total integration of sexuality into an individual's personality, no one is too disabled to be sexual. Disabled people are therefore not asexual and do not lose their sexuality after the onset of a traumatic disability. These negative stereotypes are a function of our society.

The sexual issues of people with disabilities are not so different than the issues of the able-bodied population. Nevertheless, there is a tendency to emphasize the differences rather than the similarities that exist between able and disabled people. Obviously, this tendency goes much deeper than issues of sexuality and is a function of society's discomfort with people who have disabilities. The sexual rights and responsibilities of disabled people are identical to those of all people. Humans have the right to information about sexuality. Everyone has the right to sexual expression and the right to develop the fullest potential in all aspects of life.

THE PHYSIOLOGY OF HUMAN SEXUALITY

In the early 1960s, Masters and Johnson introduced the four stages of human sexual response. These stages were defined as excitement, plateau, orgasm, and resolution[66] and were ob-served in extensive laboratory investigations and are seen in both men and women. However, demarcation between stages is somewhat arbitrary and may differ between individuals and circumstances. Although a complete discussion of the anatomy, physiology, and endocrinology of human sexuality is beyond the scope of this chapter, several points bear reviewing.

Excitement Stage

Excitement occurs in response to sexual stimulation either due to touch (reflexogenic) or imagination (psychogenic) in both men and women. This stage is governed mainly by the parasympathetic nervous system through S2, S3, and S4 via the cauda equina. The sympathetic nervous system (T11–L1) is also involved, but to a lesser extent.[31]

In men, the excitement stage is characterized by penile erection as a result of vasocongestion in the spongy tissue. The scrotum contracts and the testes are brought close to the body. In some men, nipple erection occurs as well.

In women, the excitement stage is characterized by vaginal lubrication, with vasocongestion leading to a transudate of fluid.[56] Other changes include expansion of the inner two-thirds of the vagina and elevation of the uterine body, cervix, and labia majora. The clitoris enlarges as well. Nipples become erect, and the breasts may swell.

Plateau Stage

The plateau stage consists of the high levels of sexual arousal that precede the threshold levels required to trigger orgasm. The duration of the plateau stage varies considerably.

In men, vasocongestion continues; the penis enlarges farther and can deepen in color. The testes elevate and rotate anteriorly, coming to rest against the perineum.

In women, the processes of vaginal expansion and clitoral and nipple engorgement continue. A "sex flush" may spread over the abdomen, breast and chest wall.

Extragenital features of this stage seen in men and women include tachypnea, tachycardia, elevated blood pressure, and generalized myotonia.

Orgasm

Masters and Johnson theorize that orgasm is triggered by a neural reflex arc once the orgasmic threshold is reached.

In the male, accessory sex organ contraction concentrates seminal fluid (consisting of live sperm and prostatic seminal vesicle and vas deferens secretions). The man first feels a sensation of "ejaculatory inevitability." The internal sphincter of the bladder closes to ensure the forward propulsion of seminal fluid. Orgasm is felt as rhythmic contractions of the pelvic muscles, prostate, and penile shaft.

In the female, orgasm is also felt as rhythmic muscular contractions. These include the uterus, the anal sphincter, and the outer third of the vagina, although women who have had a hysterectomy or clitoridectomy may still experience orgasm. More diffuse responses are noted as well, including peripheral muscular contractions and changes in electroencephalographic activity.

This stage is under sympathetic control in both sexes.

Resolution

Males undergo a refractory period immediately after ejaculation. Further ejaculation cannot occur, although an erection can. The length of this period varies and tends to increase with age.

Women do not experience a refractory period and have the potential to experience several successive orgasms.

During this stage, vasocongestion and the changes that have occurred during the previous phases reverse.

THE PHYSICAL EXAMINATION

The physical examination of the person with a disability can provide a challenge and a reward for both the patient and the health care provider. Optimal care demands good communication. Although communication may be difficult when discussing sexuality, it is essential if a trusting relationship is to develop.

A detailed history should be taken by the examiner. A more extensive history is appropriate when referral for sexual counseling is undertaken. The sexual history should include data from several categories. The congenitally disabled person should be asked to briefly describe the adolescent experience. Personal and parental attitudes regarding puberty, dating, sexual activity, and childbearing are significant factors in the development of the adult role and need to be discussed at this time.

Those with acquired disability should be asked about premorbid and post-traumatic changes in terms of their desire for sexual activity, what they do, who they do it with, and their own gratification. It is appropriate to ask questions about the patient's sexual partner. It would be ideal to offer the patient an opportunity to invite the partner to be present for any part of the evaluation. All history-taking should be completed with the open-ended question, "Is there anything else I haven't asked about or you think I should know about you?"

The examiner should use this opportunity of the physical evaluation to check the patient's knowledge of sexually transmitted diseases (STD). All patients who are sexually active in nonexclusive relationships without STD precautions (condoms used consistently) should be screened for infection. Most patients, female and male, are not aware of the signs or symptoms of STDs, nor are they aware of the fact that a significant portion of the infected population is without signs or symptoms.

Attitude of the Examiner

A gentle, empathic, and organized approach is the most useful. Gentle, respectful physical diagnosis skills yield the best results. An empathic attitude requires careful thought about the desired quality of care provided. The examiner must realize that the person with the disability will often require more time in pre-examination preparation (*e.g.,* emptying the urinary bag), history-taking, setting up on an examining table, conducting an examination, and providing postexamination care (*e.g.,* after genital-rectal examination). The examiner should have a plastic apron available for the occasional accident. Sufficient equipment and lines should be handy. Professional and ancillary staff should be knowledgeable and able in both attitude and skills most helpful to the patient. The examiner should know what he or she wishes to accomplish, what these tasks require, and what possible problems can occur, such as bladder and bowel accidents.

Pre-examination Preparation

Bladder and bowel care should be completed before the examination. Just prior to the examination, the bladder should be emptied. The day before the examination, the patient should be assessed for bowel status. Necessary steps should be taken to empty the lower bowel. Anatomical assessment can be inaccurate or inadequate secondary to a bowel distended with stool. The female is at special risk because a speculum inserted into a vagina with posterior wall distention due to stool can cause discomfort, embarrassment, trauma, and/or bleeding. Diaphragm size can be incorrect if the stool distends the vagina and alters the examiner's perception of distance from the symphysis to the posterior fornix.

Positioning on the Examining Table

The patient should be positioned on the examining table in such a way as to ensure a sense of stability. This may require safety belts, ancillary staff on both sides of the table, and a resourceful approach to the situation. Small pillows may be helpful for positioning.

Knowledge and use of good body mechanics are essential in the examination of the person with a disability. An ancillary person on each side and the examiner at the foot of the table during the genital-rectal examination allows the examiner to conduct the examination with good control over safety and to maximize this opportunity for evaluation.

Conducting the Physical Examination

The Female Patient

Breast examination is essential. Breast self-examination (BSE) should be taught or arrangements made for every female patient to have her breasts examined at least every 3 months. Patients at high risk for breast cancer need monthly BSE. If the patient is not able to conduct BSE without assistance, a friend, relative, home health care aide, personal care attendant (PCA), or visiting nurse can be recruited.

Women with disabilities can have special concerns about their breasts. Congenitally disabled women may have concerns about whether their breasts are too large or too small. This may carry over to a sense of inadequacy in childbearing and parenting ability. The patient should be given ample opportunity to discuss this if the examiner believes that there is concern.

Women whose disabilities are acquired suffer a sense of loss about body changes, and this includes the breasts. Prior to illness or injury, the breasts were perhaps not only different in appearance but also a symbol of femininity. After injury, the breast size can suddenly seem "too large" if one has difficulty sitting upright without support. Large or pendulous breasts can be subject to excoriation beneath the breast if proper support and cushioning are not provided. Finally, breast palpation should include neck, supraclavicular, and axillary nodes and nipple evaluation for discharge.

THE PELVIC EXAMINATION. Flaccid buttocks may need cushioning on the examination table. A protective plastic-coated pad under the buttocks is useful for unexpected bladder/bowel accidents. Two layers of such pads are helpful if the patient is difficult to move. The examination table should conceal a basin at the foot of the table. The placement of legs and feet in stirrups must be arranged for each patient with an individual approach. Sensitive skin may require swaddling with a soft towel so as to avoid skin-to-skin pressure areas. Feet can be secured in stirrups with Velcro or Kerlix. It is important to note that the labia minora and majora of women in wheelchairs can appear more atrophic than age would suggest. This is usually due to muscle atrophy from injury.

Speculum insertion must be conducted gently and carefully. Metal specula continue to be the instruments of choice because of their maneuverability and reliability. There is a wide range of sizes available (pediatric through adult). Pediatric sizes can be especially appropriate for the congenitally disabled female. Care should be taken to test the temperature of the instrument before insertion. Too cold an instrument can trigger autonomic dysreflexia. Too warm an instrument can damage vaginal mucosa sufficient to cause fistula formation.

Several more points should be noted. A mirror should be available to demonstrate findings to the patient. Observation and inspection of the skin of the lower back, the buttocks, and the genitals should be conducted at the time of examination. Inspection of the clitoris by retraction of the clitoral hood should be performed by employing gentle contact. Bimanual examination, including occult blood testing, should be performed on each patient. Finally, in obtaining Papanicolaou smears, samples from the endocervix and the exocervix should be gathered before any STD samples are taken. This ensures that any abnormal cells are retrieved for cytological evaluation and not lost to the microbiology laboratory analysis.

The Male Patient

The classic male genitalia examination should be conducted. Special care and attention should be paid to the skin of the penis and scrotum. As in female patients, body image concerns may be important and merit evaluation.

Postexamination Care

Skin should be carefully and gently washed after genital-rectal examination. Plain water will dissolve water-soluble jelly. A cloth or suitable disposable towel can be used to pat dry. Cornstarch or talc can be used to absorb moisture.

Female patients may require a sanitary napkin or a tampon to absorb any lubricating jelly from the vagina.

Assistance with dressing should be provided as needed. All fabric edges or ridges and zippers should be checked to avoid skin injury.

Evaluation

Evaluation of sexual difficulties, like any other medical evaluation, depends on a thorough history and physical examination (Table 27-1). In addition to sexual history-taking described previously, the sexual assessment must include a knowledge of any drugs a person is taking, both prescription and nonprescription (Table 27-2).

PSYCHOSOCIAL ASSESSMENT

A number of authors[28, 51, 59] have emphasized the increasing awareness of physicians of the importance of including a sexual history as a part of the standard data base. One reason the sexual history is relevant is the high incidence of sexual dysfunctions in a medical patient population, including those with chronic physical disabilities. Another is that, by requesting such information, the physician gains a valuable perspective in understanding the patient's life context, quality of relationships, values, psychological adjustment, and health-maintaining behaviors. In addition, comprehensive treatment of a patient may include referral for psychotherapy to address individual, marital, or sexual adjustment problems that are revealed through the sexual history. Taking a sexual history also provides an invitation for the patient to ask questions regarding special considerations around sexual adjustment for his or her unique physical abilities, such as the concerns a cardiac patient may have about the risks of repeated heart attack from intercourse, the management of an indwelling catheter or of dysreflexia for a spinal cord-injured patient, and so on.

There are several excellent sources that provide an in-depth sexual history of the type used for developing treatment plans for patients with specifically sexual problems.[49, 50, 54, 63] These are comprehensive assessments, requiring at least 2 to 3 hours of interview time, which include questions regarding early childhood learning about affection, trust, and the nature of interpersonal relationships; the emotional climate in which one was raised; religious values and attitudes; sexual learning history; dating behavior; adjustment in prior relationships; extramarital relationships; development and quality of the present relationship; communication; life-style issues; children; definition of the presenting complaints; current sexual repertoire; attempts at solving the problem; traumatic sexual experiences; goals for treatment; and resistance to change. Clearly, this level of evalua-

Table 27-1
Sexual Aspects of the Physical Examination

System	Observation
General	Demeanor, posture, cognitive status
Skin	Scars, rashes, open wounds, skin lesions
HEENT	Visual and hearing disorders, dysphagia
Lungs	Cough, consolidation, signs of chronic obstructive pulmonary disease
Cardiac	Arrhythmias, heaves, rubs, murmurs
Abdomen	Presence of ostomy equipment
Genital	Normal genital anatomy, open lesions, urinary collection devices
Rectal	Open lesions
Neurological	Paralysis, sensory deficits: presence and distribution
Musculoskeletal	Contractures, presence of painful, inflamed joints, restricted range of motion

Table 27-2
Drugs Affecting Sexual Functioning

	Effect
Anticholinergics	These drugs include probanthine and similar agents used to treat detrusor hyperacitvity. These agents inhibit the parasympathetic nervous system and thus interfere with vasocongestion, penile and clitoral erection, and vaginal lubrication of the excitement and plateau stages.[56]
Histamine Antagonists	Cimetidine has been cited as a cause of both impotence and gynecomastia.[106]
Tricyclic Antidepressants	These drugs include: amitriptyline and imipramine. Sexual effects of such drugs may be related to anticholinergic side-effects, although these agents can also interfere with ejaculation.[7]
Antispasmodics	The effects of this class of drugs on sexual function can be beneficial to the extent that anxiety (in the case of the benzodiazepines) or spasticity inhibits sexual expression. Impairment of erection can occur with high doses of diazepam. The benzodiazepines may be associated with menstrual irregularities,[107] but this is controversial.[37] Teratogenic effects of benzodiazepines are also possible.[70] The teratogenic effects of baclofen are unknown.
Antihypertensives	Drugs that function by sympathetic blockade (especially α-blockers) can result in inability to ejaculate. Drugs such as methyldopa can impair libido and arousal,[77] possibly secondary to fatigue and depression. Methyldopa can also increase circulating prolactin and thus cause gynecomastia or galactorrhea.[95] Clonidine, an antihypertensive that can also be used to treat spasticity, acts by a central mecahnism to lower sympathetic outflow; 10% to 20% of male users report impotence or decreased libido.[75]
Corticosteroids	Effects on sexuality are dose related. Dosages greater than the equivalent of 20 mg cortisol will suppress the hypothalamic-pituitary-adrenal axis; higher doses can lead to impaired glucose tolerance and increased susceptibility to infections. Even higher doses can depress spermatogenesis.[65]
Anticonvulsants	Both barbiturates and phenytoin are believed to be teratogenic. Barbiturates can lower circulating levels of both testosterone and estrogen via the induction of the liver enzymes that metabolize them. The actual effect on people who use low-dose barbiturates on a therapeutic basis is unclear.[56]

tion is too detailed for use with every physically disabled client, many of whom are functioning sexually to their satisfaction.

Sexual adjustment is defined here as intimate communication, involving a mutually pleasurable and practical repertoire of behavior (which may or may not emphasize genital behavior). The patient and his or her partner define whether their current sexual adjustment is adequate for them. A simplified history, which is feasible for standard inclusion in the data base, can assess this. One model for use in determining whether referral for sexual counseling is needed is provided in Table 27-3.

Training of health care professionals to deliver sexual information and assessment services stresses the importance of the practitioner's attitudes toward both sexuality and disability.[17, 28] A nonjudgmental stance, which respects the values and the preferences of the patient, is necessary to maintain rapport, to foster the patient's autonomy, and to promote candor. Most training programs include specific opportunities for the practitioner to understand and evaluate his or her own values so as not to impose them on the patient. Open-ended questions, such as those modeled in the sample interview format, promote this nonevaluative atmosphere. This lack of judgmentalism must necessarily stop short of sanctioning attitudes or practices that are psychologically or physically harmful to the patient or his or her sexual partners (*e.g.,* sadomasochistic activity, sexual relations with children, or autoerotic asphyxia).

The language of the interview should be neither too technical nor too casual. In practice, many clients present with some anxiety about sexual topics and language used by the interviewer can help reflect an atmosphere of permission to discuss the topic as well as to be explicit about sexual matters. Examples of terms that carry a pejorative connotation are *frigidity* and *impotence.* Although these terms may accurately reflect true feelings, the terms *nonorgasmic* and *erection problems* are more accurate

and carry less stigmatizing meanings. *Intercourse* is preferable to the more vague *doing it* or even *lovemaking.* Regarding the changes in sexual functioning that may be the sequels of physical disability, the terms *handicaps* or *impairments* should be avoided; *disabilities* is a term in common usage, although it has been suggested that *differently abled*[24] connotes a healthier attitude toward the process of coping with illness or injury. The interviewer models a sensitive and matter-of-fact attitude while listening carefully to the attitudes expressed by the patient's language. It can be helpful to the interview process to comment on the patient's apparent discomfort, if it occurs, with a statement such as, "Not many people find it easy to discuss such private matters with a relative stranger. Are you feeling embarrassed by this?" Gentle humor, or a pause to take a deep breath and relax, generally allows the interview to proceed more openly. More difficult topics are reserved for later in the interview when greater rapport and trust are better established. Finally, open-ended questions are another way of conveying permission for the patient to be candid in answering. Contrast the more open-ended, "When did you first experience sexual feelings?" to the less universalized, "Did you play doctor or masturbate as a child?" which has the impact of requiring a confession from the patient.

In order to understand the patient's sexual adjustment, it is essential to get a clear picture of the relationship context in which this adjustment occurs. The impact of disabling medical conditions on patients' and their family members' psychological status is part of that context. When a referral is made to treat clients with sexual problems, the therapist needs to assess the couple's readiness for sex therapy based on whether the relationship itself is stable and whether they are readily able to negotiate and resolve disputes. Only then can the sensitive issues of sexual intimacy be addressed. If there are more basic issues that need to

Table 27-3
Sample Interview Format

Category	Question/Statement
Introduction	I'd like to discuss with you your present sexual functioning. (Assurance of confidentiality)
Curent sexual functioning (general)	Are you sexually active at present?
	Have you ever been sexually active?
	Are you satisfied with your current sexual relationship(s)? or with your current sexual adjustment?
	How has your illness or injury affected your enjoyment of or ability to engage in sexual relations? (Frequency, quality, course of adjustment)
	What is your sexual repertoire? Or what type of sexual and affectionate behavior do you engage in?
	Is self-stimulation (or masturbation) one of the options that you choose?
	Do you have any concerns or questions about your sexual functioning? (Stop if no questions or concerns)
Current sexual functioning (specific)	(Men) Are you able to have and maintain an erection sufficient for intercourse? Is this a problem to you or your partner? Under what circumstances do you have difficulty?
	(Women) Are you able to reach orgasm? From intercourse, or by means of other stimulation? In what situations do you have difficulty?
	Are you able to have sexual relations without pain or discomfort? Are you sufficiently lubricating? Under what circumstances?
Partner satisfaction/ relationship history	Are you able to stimulate and satisfy your partner? Does your partner know what pleases you?
	Are you able to communicate effectively about sex? About other aspects of the relationship?
	How long have you been in your present relationship? Have you been able to work out a compatible adjustment? What difficulties have you encountered, and how did you resolve them successfully?
	How has having children/not having children affected your relationship?
Other effects on the relationship	How stable is your health at present? Future?
	Do you take any prescription medication?
	What method of contraception do you use? Are you satisfied with it?
	Do you use alcohol or other drugs? How often? How does this effect your relationship? Your sexual relationship?
	Have you had any negative or traumatic sexual experiences?
Follow-up	Would you be interested in speaking with a specialist in sexual functioning about the questions or problems that you've raised in this interview?

be resolved, sex therapy is postponed. One major example of a more basic problem is alcohol or drug abuse. Kaplan[51] categorically states that this is a contraindication for sex therapy, and most practitioners will refuse to treat a couple with an active substance abuse problem. The reasoning is not only because of the impact of drugs on psychological functioning but also because of the pathological interpersonal and family relationships that are present in substance-abusing clients. A referral for family treatment of these problems is a prerequisite to formal work on sexual issues if any long-lasting progress is to be achieved.

Opinions vary regarding when to address sexual adjustment. It was earlier suggested that a sexual history routinely accompany the physical examination. The initial sexual history might be conducted as soon as the patient's medical condition has stabilized to the point of ensuring survival. At the other extreme, the topic is reserved until close to the time of discharge from the rehabilitation setting. Those who say "wait until the patient brings it up" may find that the topic is never addressed owing to patients' concerns that the subject is taboo. A useful rule of thumb, then, is to integrate this topic into the total rehabilitation program, raising it along with other aspects of patient education and allowing patients to decline detailed inquiry if they so desire. Some patients will not be ready to address their own sexual adjustment in depth until years after the onset of the disabling condition, but the permission to discuss the issue that is conveyed by sexual history questions can be extremely valuable in promoting later adjustment.

PSYCHOSOCIAL ASPECTS OF SEXUAL FUNCTIONING

Sexual functioning involves both the ability to sustain intimacy and a prescribed series of genital behaviors.[33] Similarly, when studying the impact of disability on patient adjustment, the health care professional must consider the patient's entire life-style including his or her health, diagnosis, status, relationships, vocation, role, self-esteem, body image, independence, as well as intellectual capacity and ability to communicate. If a patient's status, appearance, or mobility is not "standard" according to cultural prescriptions, the patient may suffer and conclude that he or she is not only disabled but also handicapped. Health care practitioners can combat societal stereotypes and discrimination by focusing on the abilities that the patient retains after illness or injury.[17] In sexual rehabilitation the emphasis that succeeds is on the remaining strengths; in this way patients may learn to value themselves again.

Several basic premises guide the practitioner who delivers health care services to a disabled population. There is not one "right" way to express sexuality. Everyone who acts in a responsible way has a right to make choices about sexual expression. Everyone has both abilities and disabilities. Everyone is sexual where "sexual" is defined as a "health entity,"[17] that is, something that implies self-love and respect, aliveness, and vitality and something that contributes to the entire well-being of the person, apart from considerations of whether that person is sexually active.

In this section the psychosocial sequelae of physical disability that affect sexual functioning will be addressed.

Psychological Adjustment to Congenital Disability

A survey of the literature reveals that the task of adaptation to disability differs for those who are disabled from infancy and for those who acquire their disability through later illness or injury. Although societal stigma of asexuality may impinge on both groups, the congenitally disabled are frequently overprotected and isolated, causing a decreased opportunity to socialize and learn appropriate interpersonal skills. The practical necessity of being dependent on one's caretakers to survive often brings with it shyness and passivity, neither of which enhances the ability to form balanced, mature relationships in which sex could thrive. In traumatic disability, the person may have had the opportunity for normal socialization but is faced with loss of previous expectations and of familiar behavior. Frequently a period of adjustment, which resembles mourning, is a normal feature in the traumatically disabled patient's rehabilitation process. Anything that generates anxiety, depression, relationship conflict, or fatigue decreases the probability of satisfying sexual experiences, and all of these are common occurrences for people in rehabilitation settings. Physical disabilites can influence such sexual feelings as desire, pleasure, comfort, and competence even though most do not directly affect sexuality through loss of genital functioning.[16] Family and relationships, self-esteem, and body image are constantly impacted by the disability that touches all aspects of one's life throughout all the critical developmental stages. The relationship between the subjective impact of the disability and the social impact is circular: how you perceive yourself influences how you act and therefore what you draw from other people; and how they perceive you, in turn, influences how you perceive yourself.

The birth of a disabled child or an early illness produces a profound trauma for the parents, which may include deep sadness, depression, guilt, anger, embarrassment, rejection, or a feeling of failure.[4] In addition, the sick or disabled child requires even more parental caretaking than the normal child, which may tax and fatigue the parents beyond their ability to cope. All this is undoubtedly communicated to the offspring in direct and indirect ways, accounting for the higher risk of a negative self-image and passivity and shyness, or aggravation and demanding behavior, in social situations. In addition, the amount of attention that must be paid to survival or maintenance functions decreases the amount of concern and investment available to be given to the child's intellectual, personal, social, and sexual development. Impairments of mobility, cognition, perception, and communication severely handicap the child's ability to acquire normal developmental experiences and learnings. Common errors of parenting disabled children (*e.g.,* placing less responsibility on the child or tolerating more deviant behavior) exacerbate the problem. Again, the problems are magnified if the child is placed in an institution. Even if the parents and siblings are able to deal successfully with their emotional reactions and the child is able to learn personal and social skills vicariously (rather than through interaction with and manipulation of the environment), there is still a potentially hostile societal reaction to be confronted.

The peer group is the other major impact on the child's socialization process. Potential rejection and practical limitations on the child's ability to interact with able-bodied peers present another dilemma. There is controversy over the placement of a child in a school environment that exposes him or her only to other disabled youngsters versus children of the majority "culture." The advantages of the segregated placement are protection from abuse, specialized attention, and exposure to role models who have successfully adapted to disability; the advantage of mainstreaming is the opportunity to learn to interact successfully with the nondisabled so as to acquire a sense of equal worth. Both opportunities would appear to be valuable and desirable.[4] Pervasive discriminatory attitudes will inevitably touch the disabled child, but genuine attachment and caring from family members, teachers, health care professionals, and age-mates can compensate for the negative experiences by providing rewarding social opportunities, which in turn promote a healthy self-concept.

Adolescence, which is normally a time of developing sexual awareness and social experimentation, can be especially frustrating for a disabled young person since the immature values of adolescence (appearance, conformity, popularity) may weigh heavily on those who are seen as different and therefore less "marketable" on the dating scene. As in all aspects of sexual growth, replacement of superficial values with more mature human values is an asset. Young people who learn to value themselves as people complete with strengths and weaknesses, who communicate feelings, and who learn to give as well as receive have a good chance of establishing loving, meaningful sexual relationships regardless of disability. In all of these areas there is more than one way to achieve the goal; if the person is limited in his or her ability to communicate verbally, for example, nonverbal methods can be used (such as a caring touch or smile). Some people may discover these alternatives through trial and error. A more effective and facilitative method involves sex education, which, unfortunately, is lacking on a widespread and high-quality basis. Among the components of an effective sex education curriculum are basic anatomy and physiology, social skills training, assertiveness, values clarification, self-esteem, making choices, birth control, genetic counseling, identifying and communicating feelings, handling sexual feelings, and masturbation.[8, 20, 29, 35, 87] This information should be presented in a way that takes into account the limitations of the audience since disabled youngsters have less opportunity of learning from books and socialization and in some cases have more difficulty with social judgment and impulse control.

For example, patients with cerebral palsy frequently have speech problems, visual and hearing impairments, and sometimes mental retardation. In order to effect sexual relations, they may require assistance in positioning because of muscle spasm, paralysis, muscle and bone deformity, weakness, and impaired balance. Athetoid movements may increase in states of emotional excitement, including during sexual activity. Diaphragms and condoms may be difficult to apply. Even undressing can be difficult. Body image problems may result from the severe disfiguration and need for prosthetic devices (such as a wheelchair). Overprotection and architectural barriers limit social contacts. Even the opportunity to be touched may be deprived from patients with cerebral palsy owing to ingrained attitudes toward attractiveness and beauty held both by able-bodied and disabled people.[87]

Simply handing a person with this condition a book on sexuality would hardly constitute sexual education. A more comprehensive approach would be to teach parents to sanction the independence and desirability of their growing offspring and to reassure their apprehensions. The educational material for the client would have to be presented visually (through pictures or sign language) instead of through printed material, auditorily or in a tactile way, depending on the remaining sensory channels available. Practice (such as through role playing) of social approaches would have to be provided. Practical issues of positioning and dealing with personal care attendants would need to be included. Exposure to people with disabilities who have successfully adjusted would be both validating and instructional.[67]

In the case of mentally retarded or brain-injured children, social skills, awareness of appropriate social behavior, education concerning inhibiting impulses, and understanding the motivations implied by social cues are absolutely basic to their sexual functioning. It is not the case that these people are childlike as adults, although reference to "mental age" in reporting IQ levels may mislead the public into thinking this way. Many people, including parents and professionals, would insist that withholding sexual information from people in these categories protects them from exploitation, unwanted pregnancy, or sexual acting out. The opposite is true; lack of information does not deter sexual activity and promotes fearfulness, lack of responsible choice, inappropriate behavior, and confusion.[87] A model program for traumatically head-injured adolescents[96] teaches the basic information and skills necessary to promote healthy sexual functioning by "starting at where the client is." Young people who have had a head injury frequently lack social judgment, have difficulties in communication, are impulsive, have impaired memory, show reduced speed of processing information, and have low frustration tolerance. The remediation program teaches them how to identify whether a potential date is interested; what to say; how to slow the conversation down; how to compensate for memory problems; and, in a step-by-step way, how to identify an accepting social network in the community. The teachers set limits on impulsive behavior in a consistent fashion, so that the social gains can be gradually generalized to life outside the structured program. The sexual adjustment counseling they provide promotes patient awareness by reviewing what things were previously important to patients in the social sphere and then helps them identify their current values, strengths, and weaknesses. When they are ready to take action, a detailed plan is established that identifies their strengths and equips them to overcome their deficits in the practical areas of hygiene and appearance, transportation, social skills (including anxiety reduction), assertiveness (initiating social contact, handling rejection), and getting in contact with social and religious groups where they can meet people. A realistic timetable is set up and practice is given. This program has achieved marked success from the clients' perspective, and many professionals, aware of the difficulties faced by their patients in this area, also endorse its comprehensive structure and practicality.

Marriage and childbearing, although major responsibilities, should not be considered beyond the scope of options for mentally retarded and brain-injured patients. However, support services will probably be necessary to help them successfully achieve these goals.

Psychological Adjustment to Traumatic Disability

Turning to discussion of the task of adjustment in traumatic injury or illness, successful coping, or what might be referred to as psychological rehabilitation, is a process, a gradual course in learning to live with what is lost when a disabling illness or injury occurs, a resolution of the feeling of loss through grieving, and the development of coping strategies and improved attitudes that validate the meaningfulness of the "new" postinjury life. Some period of upset is normal and expected, but a full-blown depression is not a necessity. The changes produced by the illness or injury create a crisis in which growth can occur. Most people have little motivation to examine their sexual attitudes or self-worth, especially if things are going along tolerably well; when all their previous expectations are forced to change they can enter a period of sexual growth. Successful adjustment depends

on the recognition that choice is still available. Focusing on the tragedy immobilizes the patient; selecting from among the many options that are still available promotes adaptation.

Certainly, the process of coping varies from person to person and depends on a great number of factors, including previous psychological adjustment, quality of the support system, age at onset, gender, physical health, patient's belief system, and type of illness or injury.

Because of this diversity of adjustment tasks, a standard pattern of grieving losses and mourning the past cannot be given. What may be observed as a normal reaction to illness and injury are fear and anxiety, shock or denial, anger and blame, refusal to participate actively in rehabilitation, impatience and demanding behavior, bargaining, sadness, and eventually acceptance. Depression, defined as a constellation of sad affect, sleeping disturbance, eating disturbance, anhedonia, and loss of energy, is not normal but can be activated by the illness and should be evaluated and treated with medication and psychotherapy. Mourning is a healing process in which the patient recognizes that changes in behavior, goals, and relationships have occurred, grieves the former circumstances, and relinquishes them. What follows is a series of adjustments that restores the person to effective functioning.

Feelings are best dealt with by acknowledging and expressing them; then they are able to be worked through instead of stored (leading to what is called a "protracted grief reaction"). This is not to say that the patient needs to be constantly immersed in his or her feelings of loss. The defense mechanism of denial can take on both healthy and unhealthy forms. Healthy denial, which aids survival and rehabilitation, is adaptive and should be encouraged. Unhealthy denial interferes with rehabilitation and needs to be gradually replaced with acceptance of the disability through reality-based feedback if progress is to occur.

The changes in the patient create a crisis that affects not only the patient but also the members of the family system, who may feel angry and guilty about their anger. Their anger may be expressed toward the patient, or toward the staff, as a projection of their feelings of helplessness or as a result of actual insensitivity of the staff to the family's distress. Family members may intrude, avoid contact, become overly solicitous, fall apart emotionally, or express conflict within the family. Adult children may experience some setbacks in achieving autonomy from the family, much as in the case of congenital illness. Although there is limited research addressing the question, one report found the divorce rate in the population with spinal cord injury no higher than the national average.[25] Previous problems in the relationship may be exacerbated by an illness or injury causing the dissolution of the marriage, but in previously stable relationships the crisis can be negotiated successfully. Staying in the relationship out of obligation may occur but is not the most common reason for sustaining the marriage. Good family adjustment can improve rehabilitation success by providing warm, loving, consistent, autonomy-generating support to the patient. The implication is to include the family in the rehabilitation process through meetings with the rehabilitation team and through family support groups. The role of staff toward patients and family members is ideally one of empathy, alliance with their health-engendering behavior, and sufficient perspective regarding their health-endangering behavior so as to confront it without attacking or alienating them.

Rehabilitation is a difficult job for staff as well, and ideally opportunities for preventing or dealing with burnout need to be available. Finally, although compliance with hospital structure may be appreciated by staff, it may not be associated with maximum patient and family adjustment since a more successful transition to independent living requires active, assertive, autonomous behavior rather than passivity and dependence.[55] A focus on empowering the patient, by engaging him or her as a decision-making member of the rehabilitation team, facilitates long-term adjustment. An educational model that emphasizes relearning coping skills, rewards gradual progress, and focuses on gains conveys this message of empowerment.

Despite the best efforts of staff, families, and friends, there is an increased rate of suicide and of alcohol and drug abuse among the severely disabled. These may also be seen as coping mechanisms, albeit dysfunctional ones. All represent ways to withdraw from and avoid the pains of adjustment and are frequently associated with a lifelong, learned pattern of handling difficulty through avoidance. Two high-risk periods of suicidality have been identified: (1) the diagnostic phase, in which the illness and its prognosis are uncertain and the patient questions whether he or she will ever be himself or herself again, and (2) the postdischarge phase (with the highest death rate occurring at 1 to 2 years after injury), in which the patient is faced with a new level of understanding of the ramifications of the illness or injury. Psychotherapeutic treatment of suicidal depression and of substance abuse (including participation in Alcoholics Anonymous and similar organizations with proven records of effectiveness) is essential.[23]

A common fear expressed by disabled people is increased vulnerability to physical and sexual assault. Conditions that result in cognitive impairment, weakness, and balance or mobility problems increase the risk of being vulnerable. Preventive programs of self-defense and programs to assist victims have been instituted.[1, 97] Psychotherapy and prevention may assist patients in planning ways to reduce vulnerability and in feeling and acting competent and powerful.

Sexual Adjustment

Turning now to consideration of sexual adjustment following traumatic injury or illness, the same principles apply as are true for adjustment in general. The losses need to be mourned so that the remaining strengths can be developed and nurtured. Everyone has some ability to function sexually—some repertoire of behavior that can communicate sexual feelings. Frequently, however, patients go through a period of reduced sexual drive or performance. Choosing celibacy is not always a sign of giving up but must also be considered a viable option if it is agreeable to the patient and his or her partner. However, substantial numbers of patients fail to resume an active sex life owing to fear, misinformation, or problems of adjustment. Others go through a period of sexual acting out, presumably to validate their survival.

Those who do resume sexual relations are advised to keep separate the roles of caretaker and partner in order to preserve intimacy, which is diluted when one spouse is perceived as needy and helpless compared with the other. The process of sexual adjustment, and the balancing of the roles, can be facilitated by providing information and counseling.

It has been said that sexuality, broadly defined, is the most important part of rehabilitation because of its relationship to self-esteem, body image, interpersonal attachment, and motivation.[88] Although this may be an overstatement, traditional definitions of mental health also highlight its importance. Freud, for example, defined mental health as the ability to love and to work. To the extent that the disabled person can learn to value his or her new sexual abilities (as opposed to trying to regain the same sexual life as before) and establish some method of communication, he or she will achieve a satisfying sexual adjustment. Disabled patients who achieve success in sexual functioning do so because of increased communication and a willingness to experiment with

developing romance and intimacy, as well as technique. They are secure enough to realize not every experiment will work, and they value nongenital erogenous zones. Their partners feel that their present lovemaking with the disabled partner is far more satisfactory than previous relationships with nondisabled partners. They would not want to give up these patterns of making love even if genital function returned.[33] Especially important is the development of skills in communication and intimacy. The need for specific and immediate communication between sexually involved partners is essential for a satisfactory relationship among the disabled, as well as the able-bodied.[81] These, in fact, are the same principles used in sexual enhancement programs for the able bodied; everyone who will sexually grow has to work at it. Although especially important to the disabled, everyone can benefit from the debunking of myths about the importance of sexual performance, or about achieving orgasms as the only goal of a sexual encounter, or about needing to have "the body beautiful" in order to enjoy the experience. Spontaneity is reduced if extra self-care is required for sex, but "letting nature take its course" is largely a romantic idealization anyway. Also, it is harder to meet partners after disability, but it can be argued that a mate who will appreciate the strengths and uniquely positive qualities of a disabled person rather than responding to the packaging is probably a better choice anyway.

PHYSICAL EFFECTS OF DISABILITY ON FUNCTIONING

Although psychological considerations need to be addressed in all discussions regarding sexuality, basic physical information is equally important. Often an open, sensitive discussion regarding topics such as sensation, birth control, lubrication, and erections can be very supportive. Such topics are usually on the minds of most patients, but their anxiety prevents a thorough discussion with appropriate health care professionals. Physical changes in sexuality after spinal cord injury are summarized in Table 27-4.

Erections and Lubrication

The capacity of psychogenic erections in men and lubrication in women is either partially or completely lost in most disabilities that involve damage to the central nervous system. These may include traumatic events, such as spinal cord injury and stroke, or progressive disabilities, such as multiple sclerosis. As expected, the capabilities for sexual response vary according to the level of injury in the spinal cord as well as the completeness of the lesion. For purposes of this discussion, upper motor neuron lesions refer to spinal cord lesions that preserve the sacral cord. Such patients will have external anal sphincter tone and a bulbocavernosus reflex. Such lesions are generally T12 or higher. Lower motor neuron lesions imply disruption of the sacral cord. Patients with these lesions will have a lax anal sphincter and the absence of a bulbocavernosus reflex. As a rule, the incidence of erections and lubrication is greater in patients with incomplete upper motor neuron lesions.[87]

When the sacral area of the spinal cord has been left intact, it is common for patients to experience a reflexogenic erection. Although such erections may not be sustained for intercourse, they can be achieved by manual stimulation of the genital area. Frequently, touching, a full bladder, or rubbing the penis on clothing or bed linen will be sufficient for a male patient to achieve at least a partial reflexogenic erection. However, once stimulation has been removed, the erection may no longer be sustained.[87]

Table 27-4
Sex and Spinal Cord Injury

	Men	Women
Sexual Desire	Remains intact, although psychological factors may reduce libido during periods of adjustment.	Same
Genital Response	*Erection:* Depends on level and completeness of injury. Higher lesions are associated with a greater chance of achieving and maintaining erection. The chance is also greater with incomplete lesions. Psychogenic erections are found in incomplete, lower lesions; reflexogenic erections are characteristic of complete, higher lesions. Erectile capacity may gradually return during the first year of recovery. The majority of men are able to achieve erection of some type.	Sensations in the genital area are lost in complete lesions, as they are with males; sensations above the level of injury, however, may be enhanced and become erotically responsive producing para-orgasm. Movement of the pelvic area is limited. Lubrication is more probable in incomplete, lower lesions.
	Ejaculation: Most men are unable to ejaculate. Those who do are likely to have incomplete, lower lesions. Retrograde ejaculation is common. Orgasm does not invariably accompany ejaculation, although para-orgasm is possible (a sensation of pleasurable release). Spasticity may increase at the point of ejaculation.	Alternatives to intercourse such as kissing, oral-genital contact, manual erotic pleasuring of genital and non-genital areas, and use of vibrators are widely used and can provide sexual satisfaction among both male and female patients.
Intercourse	The ability to complete intercourse varies widely; if sufficient erections are not available, "stuffing" the non-erect penis into the vagina is an alternative, as well as penile implant surgery and papavarine injections to supply erection.	Intercourse is generally possible despite absent or altered sensation and movement. Vaginal lubrication can be used if natural lubrication is insufficent.

Since lubrication may also be altered in a variety of disabilities, it is common for many disabled women to experience painful sensations during intercourse. Although this may be resolved with lubricating jelly, there are also psychological ramifications of this physiological change. Women frequently question their attractiveness and their femininity. Fear of rejection, affecting their relationships or potential relationships, can emerge.

Sensation

The most severe sensory problem is lack of sensation, as in spinal cord injury. Classically, patients with spinal cord injury are insensate below the level of their lesion. Afferent sensory impulses are interrupted on their way to the cortex at the level of the lesion. These patients sometimes report heightened erotic sensation at their cutoff sensory level.[31] This is especially common at the T4 or T5 level. The mechanism of this is unclear.

Other entities in which sensory disturbances are common include peripheral neuropathy and stroke. Peripheral neuropathy can be due to diabetes, renal failure, toxic exposure, or entrapment. Diabetes frequently causes impotence on the basis of interference with both the nerve and the vascular supply to the genitals. Diabetic women have difficulty with lubrication and orgasm.[27, 74, 108]

Stroke can have a profound effect on sexual activity in both sexes. Sensory impairment rather than paresis is cited as a cause of decreased libido, decreased frequency of intercourse, and erectile and orgasmic difficulty.[92] Fear of sustaining another stroke is also seen as a reason for decreased sexual activity in stroke patients.[71]

Pain

The presence of pain, whether acute or chronic, can severely limit enjoyment of sexual activity, especially in positions where weight is borne by the painful area or where the painful area is subjected to undue movement. Entities in which pain plays a role include all types of arthritis, chronic low back or neck pain, ischemic ulcers, and amputations (including phantom pains).

Motor Deficits

Numerous disabilities involve motor deficits, including paralysis, weakness, absence of a body part (amputations, mastectomy, or other ablative surgery for cancer or in congenital limb deficiency), contractures (arthritis, cerebral palsy, spastic conditions), and decreased endurance (cardiac patients). Some of these entities limit positioning during sexual activity. Others affect the person's self-concept and body image.

Urinary Incontinence

The fear of involuntary urination and subsequent rejection are major issues to be confronted across disabilities. Bladder accidents can result as a medical complication of multiple sclerosis, spinal cord injury, diabetes, and a variety of other disabilities. Urinary tract infection may also cause chronic urgency and loss of bladder control during sexual intercourse. Thus, in many disabilities there is a reality that a bladder accident may occur at any time throughout courtship or overt sexual activity.

This fear, perhaps one of the greatest for many people, creates undue anxiety and is often regarded as a major reason for social isolation or the termination of relationships. Social stereotypes make communication especially difficult and associate incontinence with embarassment and humiliation. When the possibility of a bladder accident is not discussed prior to sexual activity, it can be a devastating experience for the disabled person. When it has been discussed and prepared for, it can be incorporated into the lovemaking and treated as a temporary inconvenience.

Failure to empty the bladder prior to sexual activity is the most common cause for such problems. For those familiar with intermittent catheterization, this should be performed prior to sex. Indwelling catheters can be taped on the side of the penis with a condom placed over the catheter. Females can engage in sexual intercourse despite the presence of a catheter by taping the catheter to the abdomen. For either sex, fluids should be limited during the hours preceding sexual activity, with towels being available should problems arise.

Fertility

People with many types of disabilities retain their ability to conceive and bear children. Such disabilities include the arthritides, cerebral palsy, amputations, multiple sclerosis, chronic pain, and many other entities. However, some disabilities can destroy fertility. Spinal cord injury remains the most extensively studied and best understood of the neurogenic sexual dysfunctions.

Male Fertility

Many studies exist detailing the male sexual potential after spinal cord injury.[10, 38, 101] Erections occur in 54% to 87% of male patients with spinal cord injuries. Men with incomplete upper motor neuron lesions (99%) are more likely to achieve erections than those with complete lower motor neuron lesions (7%). In men with upper motor neuron lesions, erections are usually reflexogenic and may not always be sustained. Men with lower motor neuron lesions tend to have psychogenic erections, especially those with incomplete lesions. Most of these men experience return of their erections within the first year after injury. In addition to the effects of the injury itself on sexual function, it is important to realize that sphincterotomy can diminish or abolish erectile function in up to 56% of patients.[102] Erections obtained after spinal cord injury are sufficient for coitus in 80% of those with incomplete lower motor neuron lesions, 63% of those with incomplete upper motor neuron lesions, 53% of those with complete upper motor neuron lesions, and 23% of those with complete lower motor neuron lesions, or about 50% overall.[10]

Ejaculation occurs much less often than erection. Only 1% of men with complete upper motor neuron lesions report ejaculation, while up to 70% of men with incomplete lower motor neuron lesions report it. A distinction is made between seminal emission (seminal fluid entering the urethra) and actual ejaculation (expulsion of fluid from the urethra to the outside).[38] When ejaculation occurs, it is often dribbling or retrograde into the bladder (because of failure of closure of the internal sphincter).

Orgasm is reported even less frequently; it is least frequent in men with complete upper motor neuron lesions. The sensation of orgasm is attributed to afferent feedback associated with adnexal smooth muscle contractions of emission and with the striated muscle contractions of the second phase of ejaculation.[38] Orgasm is variably described as a sudden increase in spasticity followed by generalized muscle relaxation, pleasurable sensations in the lower abdomen, pelvis, or thighs (complete lower motor neuron lesions), and occasionally as painful sensations (incomplete upper motor neuron lesions). Orgasm may also be felt at the cutoff sensory level, genitals, or other erogenous zones (*e.g.,* neck, ears).

The ability to sire a child correlates with frequency of ejaculation and seminal emission.[38] Successful pregnancy rates of sex partners range from 0% to 5%. Men with incomplete lesions are more likely to become fathers than those with complete lesions; those with incomplete lower motor neuron lesions are more likely to be fertile than those with incomplete upper motor neuron lesions. Possible mechanisms for male infertility in this setting include retrograde ejaculation, repeated urinary tract infections, and altered testicular temperature.[14] Testosterone and gonadotropin levels are usually found to be in the normal range.[21, 42, 54] Testicular biopsy specimens frequently show decreased spermatogenesis and interstitial sclerosis. The reasons for this remain unclear.[60]

Female Fertility

Following spinal cord injury, a woman's menses may continue without interruption or they may temporarily cease, returning to normal within about 6 months. Once her menstrual periods return, fertility returns to preinjury levels and the woman needs reliable birth control.

Choosing appropriate birth control for women with spinal cord injury is difficult because of the risk of thromboembolic disease with oral contraceptives and the need for adequate hand function or a cooperative partner to insert a diaphragm or contraceptive sponge. Foam and condoms represent a safe and effective method but also depend on a cooperative partner. Intrauterine devices are contraindicated.[85]

In women, vaginal lubrication and clitoral engorgement are analogous to male penile erection. Little formal data are available on the physiological changes in women with spinal cord injury during sexual activity. However, based on their observations of a woman who participated in studies of the sexual response cycle prior to her injury and who was re-studied after sustaining a complete lower motor neuron lesion, Masters and Johnson state that pelvic vasocongestion is impaired and that the orgasmic platform does not form.[56] In this woman breast changes occurred, as did changes in the lips and mouth analogous to changes in the outer portion of the vagina. Her case "apparently illustrates not only the ability to transfer erotic zones from one region of the body to another (a phenomenon already observed by several authors in relation to the spinal cord injured) but also the transfer of a physiologic erotic reflex from its ordinary location (in this case, the non-innervated vagina) to a remote but physiologically similar location.[56] This transfer of erotic feelings has been corroborated by other surveys.[24]

As in men, some women with spinal cord injury experience orgasm as a sudden increase in spasticity followed by sudden muscular relaxation.[39]

In both men and women, libido, especially if considered in the broader psychosexual sense, does not change after spinal cord injury.[31, 100]

Pregnancy

The decision to become a parent is a difficult one since parenting skills do not come naturally but must be learned.[83] Parents with disabilities must cope with the same doubts and fears as everyone else, and then some. However, the essential component of parenting—love—is no less represented in a physically disabled population.[104] Well-chosen adaptive equipment and helpful partners and families can make parenthood much easier for disabled parents.

People with nontraumatic disabilities must also consider whether the condition will be inherited. There has been much progress in screening, preventing, and diagnosing certain inherited disabling conditions. Individualized answers can be obtained by consulting a specially trained genetic counselor.[83] The question of pregnancy termination is one that is highly personal and involves many considerations.

Once a disabled woman becomes pregnant, pregnancy, labor, and delivery can progress with surprisingly little difficulty. Disabled women should receive regular prenatal care with a gynecologist who is knowledgeable about disabled women. The physiatrist can play a role here in educating both patients and other physicians. Possible problems (and solutions) include urinary tract infections (acidification and hydration can help with management); anemia (the hematocrit should be monitored and transfusion or iron therapy considered); constipation (this can be managed with suppositories and stool softeners); and altered balance secondary to the expanding uterus (this can be dealt with by modification of the seating system; if the patient is ambulatory, she may need assistive devices to prevent falls and possible fractures.)

Labor takes place normally since the uterus retains its ability to contract despite denervation.[82] Because of a lack of sensation, the mother with a spinal cord injury may not be able to feel the onset of labor. To prevent a precipitous, unsupervised birth, it is prudent to admit such a mother to the maternity ward about 10 days in advance of her estimated date of confinement. Spinal cord injury *per se* is not an indication for cesarean section; a cesarean section may be needed for purely obstetrical reasons.

In a woman with lesion about T6 (the origin of the sympathetic outflow), autonomic dysreflexia may occur during labor.[85] It is vital for the obstetrician to be familiar with this phenomenon and not to confuse it with preeclampsia or eclampsia. It can be managed with epidural anesthesia to diminish the noxious stimulus, antihypertensives, or immediate delivery if the blood pressure cannot be controlled by any other means.[82]

There may be an increased incidence of small-for-date and premature infants after spinal cord injury, but no increase in number of spontaneous abortions has been noted. An increase in congenital disabilities and cerebral palsy has also been reported for mothers who are pregnant when injured.[34]

Disabled mothers can successfully breast feed their infants. As in all nursing mothers, medications should be carefully reviewed. Any agent that is not absolutely necessary for the mother's health should be discontinued.

Medical Interventions

For men whose self-esteem depends heavily on being able to achieve erection and penetration, surgical implantation of a penile prosthesis may be helpful. Indications for a penile prosthesis include impotence from vascular or neurological disorders, trauma, or various types of surgery (*e.g.,* sphincterotomy, prostatectomy, cystectomy, or aneurysm repair).[56]

Types of prostheses include the fixed rod and the inflatable. Fixed rod prostheses (such as the Small-Carrion type made of two partially foam-filled silicone rods) are relatively easy to implant but result in a state of permanent semierection.[93] The inflatable type is technically more difficult to implant but is more physiological. It consists of two inflatable cylinders implanted adjacent to the corpora cavernosa, connected to a pump placed in the scrotum. A fluid reservoir is placed in the prevesical space, which the wearer can activate by compressing a bulb in the scrotum. Fluid moves from the reservoir to the cylinders, resulting in penile erection. Erection is released by activating the bulb again, causing fluid to move back into the reservoir.[56]

Complications of penile prostheses include infection (especially in diabetic or already infected patients) and erosion of the corpus cavernosus with migration of the Small-Carrion prosthesis into the urethra. Preventive management strategies include ensuring a sterile urine, careful preoperative skin preparation with povidone-iodine, and therapy with systemic antibiotics. Selecting appropriately sized prostheses intraoperatively can prevent migration of a too-large prosthesis into the urethra.[57]

A technique that shows a great deal of promise is autoinjection of phentolamine (Regitine) into the corpora cavernosa.[111] Patients and/or their spouses can learn this technique on an outpatient basis. It results in an erection that lasts between 2 and 4 hours and carries minimal risk of infection.[52]

Male infertility after spinal cord injury is much more difficult to treat, although research continues in this area.[30] Intrathecal injections of neostigmine (Prostigmin) have been employed to obtain semen that can be used for artificial insemination.[15] Electrical stimulation using a vibrator applied to the glans penis has also been used to induce ejaculation.[12, 13] Autonomic dysreflexia is the major risk of these techniques in patients with spinal cord lesions above T6; hypertension in this setting can be severe. Infusions of prostaglandin E_2 have been used to control the hypertension without interfering with ejaculation. Still, the technique must be used with caution.[76]

The idea of sperm banking is tantalizing, especially since sperm obtained in the first few days after injury tends to be normal. More research in this area is needed.

SPECIAL MEDICAL CONDITIONS

Stroke

In general, the hazards that may face the stroke patient and his or her partner include decreased libido (due to personality changes), decreased enjoyment (due to personality changes, changes in sensation, or psychological factors), decreased excitement (due to the interference of fear or pain), decreased mobility affecting sexual performance (due to paralysis), and decreased ability to perceive and exchange sexual cues and affectionate expressions with the partner (due to aphasia, or impaired processing of nonverbal communications, such as facial expression and "body language").

The reduced rates of sexual activity among stroke patients and their increased incidence of sexual problems are probably due to psychological factors, although further research is needed.[45, 71, 80, 109] Depending on the extent of cerebral damage, the following are unusual, but possible, results of organic pathology: partial or absent erection, retarded ejaculation, retrograde ejaculation, and decreased vaginal lubrication (with resultant pain).[9, 22, 80] Sensation may be reduced or distorted on the affected side of the body, including in the genital area. Visual field disturbances and unilateral neglect can also reduce sexual stimulation. Motor changes can decrease coordination and balance and produce weakness and spasm, thereby affecting sexual positioning, and can result in wetting and soiling. Facial paralysis may affect kissing and swallowing (which can lead to drooling). The ability to touch and be touched is impaired, resulting in decreased sexual satisfaction. Fatigue is more likely.

There are well-documented personality syndromes described in the clinical literature on stroke.[46] The patient with right hemisphere damage may be impulsive and overtalkative, demonstrating exaggerated self-confidence and denying any need to adjust since no impairment is acknowledged or recognized. The patient with left hemisphere damage may be cautious and hesitant, disorganized and emotionally labile, or depressed in response to his or her awareness of physical changes; thus, these patients may demonstrate a greater loss of libido than those with right hemisphere damage, at least initially. These personality changes, when present, undoubtedly require changes in the patient's spouse and other relationships and contribute stress.

Even in the absence of the stroke-related personality changes, normal psychological reactions occur that can impair sexual functioning. Grief and depression can decrease sexual desire. Anxiety (particularly the commonly reported fear of sexual activity causing another stroke or the fear of the sensations of orgasm that may appear to the patient to resemble stroke sensations) decreases sexual excitement and can lead to disturbances of erection or orgasm. Stroke patients may be concerned about their appearance, their masculinity or feminity, and their desirability as a sexual partner. They may be feeling rejected by a spouse who also may have a negative response to the changes in the patient. They may be upset by role changes in the relationship or in regard to their vocation. Most patients acknowledge sexual problems as a sequel to stroke.[109]

The best adjustment is achieved by patients with good premorbid sexual adjustment who are sensitive to the emotional changes in themselves and their partners. These patients and their partners are able to respond supportively to necessary role changes and are able to develop a positive body image. Counseling around sexual issues is important in this population, since it is related to better success in rehabilitation in general and because communication breakdowns in couples facing adjustment to stroke frequently occur even when no aphasia is present.[19, 69, 73] Physicians should reassure their patients about the medical risks of resuming sexual activity, advise them about the effects of antihypertensive or other medicines on sexual functioning, suggest ways of positioning to reduce problems with paralysis, and sanction continued communication about sexual topics and all aspects of adjustment between the partners.

Traumatic Brain Injury

The cognitive and emotional changes that can result from head injury are again the major contributors to sexual dysfunction;

organic factors have not been clearly identified in sexual changes, except those associated with limbic system or brain stem structures and epilepsy.[9] Contrary to popular belief, hypersexuality is not common, but a high incidence of impulsivity or inappropriate sexual remarks may be seen in disinhibited patients with frontal lobe injury.[22]

Emotional lability (crying, laughing excessively and unpredictably), social withdrawal or overtalkativeness, concreteness, and impaired judgment have a great deal of impact on the ability to form and maintain a sexual relationship without any impairment in the physical ability to perform sexual acts. In addition, the psychological adjustment reaction common to all disability may reduce sexual drive or impair performance, at least initially.[53, 78] The more severe the cerebral damage, the more serious the impairments in personal, social, and sexual functioning. Head-injured adults may need basic re-education in social skills as described previously for head-injured adolescents; counseling spouses will assist them in the difficult decisions about the future of their relationships and in the mechanics of living with a brain-injured partner as well as how to restore a satisfactory (although altered) sexual life once they complete a recovery process of coming to terms with the effects of the injury.[6, 22, 61, 105]

Alzheimer's and Huntington's Diseases

The severe cognitive and emotional changes resulting from the irreversible degenerative organic brain syndromes of Alzheimer's and Huntington's diseases interfere with sexual functioning. In addition to the psychological adjustment reaction to recognizing that one is deteriorating, which is common to both disorders, in Huntington's disease the patient's anxieties about passing the disease on to offspring are an additional stress that can impair sexual functioning. Counseling focuses on the spouse's loss of their familiar partner, preparation for the dying process, and facilitating the couple's decision regarding the place that sex and affection hold in their relationship as the disease progresses.

Renal Disease

Patients with chronic renal disease, who are treated with dialysis or are facing renal transplantation, frequently withdraw from their usual sexual activity owing to side-effects of their illness and treatment.[58, 90] Fatigue, lethargy, and despondence are commonly reported reactions. Uremia also decreases sexual functioning (frequency of contact and level of desire and of satisfaction) both by exacerbating the fatigue and threatening the patient with a worsening of his or her condition. Among women patients, menstruation may cease or become irregular, fertility may decrease, orgasm may become less intense, and vaginal lubrication and breast tissue mass may be reduced, all as a result of chronic renal insufficiency.[11] Dialysis itself often produces excessive or even painful menstruation.[11] Counseling involves the larger context of the place of the disease in the patients' lives, and the quality of their life and of their relationships as well as specific sexual advice. Kidney dialysis is a very confining procedure that can elicit feelings of dependency and that produces frequent adjustment problems. The suicide rate is high in this population. On the other hand, successful transplant surgery is sometimes followed by improvement in sexual functioning because it allows patients greater automony, better health, and hope; it can also restore fertility.

Chronic Obstructive Pulmonary Disease

Chronic shortness of breath may lead to anxiety about participation in any physical activity. The increases in blood pressure, heart, and respiration rates are reasonably low during sex so the reluctance may represent an irrational fear (such as suffocation) or reflect other concerns, which counseling should address. Coughing and physical changes (pectus or emphysematous chest) may be a source of embarassment; fatigue may be a factor.[53] A comprehensive rehabilitation program, including preventive elements (smoking cessation, active exercise, and counseling), may eliminate many of the barriers to sexual functioning in this population.

Spinal Cord Injury

Sexual sequelae of spinal cord injury have been extensively studied[25, 39, 40, 41, 72, 79, 84, 87, 91] (see Table 27-4); the physical impairments of erection, ejaculation, orgasm, male fertility, and vaginal lubrication have been well documented, although more investigation is needed into the sexual responsivity of the vagina and uterus in spinal cord–injured women.[87] Psychosocial factors in sexual adjustment to spinal cord injury are better understood than in other disability categories. During the previous decade much of this education has come about because of the availability of sexual attitude reassessment seminars for professionals and clients.[17]

Multiple Sclerosis

With its onset in young adulthood and the unpredictably progressive course of the disorder, multiple sclerosis (MS) represents a difficult psychological and sexual adjustment problem. MS affects sensory and motor neurons, impairing both sensation and movement. In men, erectile dysfunction may occur sporadically or there may be a failure to maintain erection at all. Ejaculation may also be impaired. Fatigue, weakness, irritability or euphoria, and other personality changes can affect both genders. Women patients may suffer from thigh spasms making intercourse impossible, decreased vaginal lubrication, numbness, and reduced frequency of orgasm. Libido, however, is not impaired in either male or female patients. Pregnancy is possible but may exacerbate a woman's symptoms of MS; another concern about offspring is the increased incidence of MS in children of MS patients. Bladder and bowel problems have to be managed, as in spinal cord injury. The constant adjustments that need to be faced as the disorder progresses add stress, and the loss of mobility and altered appearance can also create psychological barriers to sexual functioning. Cognitive deficits, speech problems, social withdrawal, increased dependency, and partners' reactions are all part of the adjustment picture that faces MS patients and that may be worked through in counseling or in support groups for MS families.[3, 53, 67, 90]

Amyotrophic Lateral Sclerosis

Amyotrophic lateral sclerosis (ALS) is characterized by a degeneration of the motor neurons in spinal cord and brain stem. It affects people unpredictably, with onset in middle age. It can cause decreased sexual functioning (ejaculation, erection, lubrication). However, it has been reported that some patients retain their sexual ability even at the terminal stages of this illness.[18] While libido and sensation areas are intact, movement of upper and lower extremities and speech and respiratory musculature are impaired.[48]

Diabetes

Sexual drive remains intact in the diabetic population, but sexual functioning frequently declines with age.[26, 27, 74, 81, 99, 108, 110] The majority of diabetic men over age 60 are unable to achieve or maintain an erection compared with a minority of diabetic men under age 30. Surveys report that for women, as well as men, there is a loss of sensation with aging, but problems with vasocongestion usually develop first with a progressive onset, later becoming chronic. Ejaculation in men may be retrograde, reducing fertility. Orgasm may occur with or without ejaculation since this function is physiologically distinct and is apparently not affected by diabetic peripheral neuropathy. In women, pain may contribute to reduced orgasmic capacity resulting from decreased vasocongestion and decreased lubrication. It is possible for a diabetic woman to achieve orgasm, provided vaginal lubricants are used to enhance pleasure so the sexual response cycle may proceed to resolution. As in men, orgasm may occur without first-stage sexual response. The mechanism underlying these effects appears to be neuropathy affecting the pelvic parasympathetic nerves, which control erection in men and clitoral and labial enlargement in women as well as lubrication. Hormonal changes do not appear to be involved. Complicating the sexual adjustment of diabetics are associated illnesses, such as circulatory problems, that may impair other stages of the process.

Treatment involves good medical management of the diabetes with diet and medication. Alternatives to intercourse and feelings about the changes may be explored in sexual rehabilitation counseling. When erectile dysfunction is neurogenic, penile implant surgery or papaverine injections may be recommended, provided that the marital relationship is stable and, characterized by good previous sexual adjustment and that the couple realizes that the procedures only correct the absence of erection, not sensation, orgasm, or relationship problems. Older or more traditional couples may respond more favorably to restoration of previously familiar sexual behavior rather than to learning new repertoires.

Alcoholic Neuropathy

Long-term alcohol abuse can also cause persistent peripheral neuropathy as well as hormonal changes that impair erection, ejaculation, and female arousal and orgasm.[51, 90] Erectile dysfunction, which initially is reversible but later becomes permanent, is increased as a result of decreased sensory and motor function in the peripheral nerves and hypothalamic-pituitary suppression resulting from chronic liver disease. This also causes feminization, characterized by gynecomastia, decreased beard, reduced prostate size, testicular atrophy, and sterility. In addition, libido is decreased for both male and female alcoholics. Women patients appear to suffer decrements in all stages of the sexual response cycle as well.

Cardiac Illness

In many cases of arteriosclerotic heart disease and postmyocardial infarction, patients have recovered well enough to be able to safely manage the work load on the heart caused by sexual intercourse, but estimates are that only 25% resume sexual activity.[94] The reported reduction in libido and ability to function sexually are not physically mediated. Certainly there are cases of coronary artery disease that can reduce circulation enough to physically impair sexual performance; some antihypertensive medication can impair sexual functioning; and unstabilized congestive heart failure patients and patients with arrhythmias should be advised not to resume sexual or other activity until the condition is managed.[43] The estimate above refers to cases in which sexual activity is physically possible.

By far the most common reason for abstaining is fear of death or a repeat heart attack, even in cases in which patients have been counseled about the safety of resuming intercourse. Depression following heart attack is common and is also incompatible with active sexual functioning. Other contributing factors are misinformation, partner's fears, anginal pain, fatigue, anger, and a stressful life-style.[32]

There is no increased mortality associated with a gradual but full return to premorbid levels of activity, including sexual activity.[36, 44] A comprehensive cardiac rehabilitation program is encouraged that emphasizes education, nutrition, smoking cessation, caffeine reduction, vocational counseling, psychological and sexual counseling, exercise programs, stress reduction, social service support, and medical treatment. If electrocardiographic and stress tolerance are in normal limits by the 8- to 12-week follow-up, there is no reason to advise against resuming sexual relations, provided the patient is rested, not under stress (such as after drinking or a heavy meal), and does not experience shortness of breath or angina. Nitroglycerin may be taken before sexual activity to prevent angina. Exercise has definitely been shown to increase the cardiac work load, and relaxation training methods can actually improve cardiac functioning and resistance to stress. Although sexual capacity is not the main reason for pursuing exercise and relaxation, it is certainly enhanced by these procedures.

The most common psychogenic sexual problems in male cardiac patients are decreased desire and erectile dysfunction; in female patients it is decreased desire. When sexual dysfunction is due to medication that cannot be changed, and other medical treatments (*i.e.,* bypass surgery) are not feasible, the patient may face a dilemma involving his or her health or sex life. In these cases, counseling can suggest alternative ways of communication of affection short of intercourse and assist the patient in coping with the changes and losses resulting from the illness.

Arthritis/Pain Syndromes

Pain, fatigue, and lack of mobility can interfere with sexual functioning and are common for arthritics and patients with back pain.[2, 11] Managing pain is exhausting, reducing desire and responsiveness. Corticosteroid treatment may also increase libido. In rheumatoid arthritis, sexual activity has been reported to be therapeutic, increasing the level of natural cortisone by stimulating the adrenal cortex.[19] Sexual activity has an analgesic effect while sexual frustration and stress can exacerbate arthritis pain. A variety of methods of reducing pain, including self-hypnosis, hot baths, massage, and medication, can be employed to enhance the ability to enjoy sexual stimulation. Planning sexual activity for times when the pain is minimal helps, as does experimenting with positioning. Abstinence from sexual activity is recommended in conditions in which bones are brittle (as in severe osteoporosis following the use of corticosteroids) and for several weeks after hip replacement surgery until healing is well established. In cases of chronic pain, psychological evaluation and treatment is recommended to provide support and to identify and reduce any health-risk behavior that may be exacerbating the condition or interfering with medical treatment.

Amputation

Except for cases in which associated illnesses (diabetes, circulatory problems) physically prevent sexual functioning, pain and psychological adjustment problems are the main deterrents to sexual functioning among amputees. Phantom pain can be persistent and severe, limiting sexual activities. Reducing pain permits greater openness to sexual experience.[19]

The adjustment reaction to amputation may initially decrease sexual desire and frequency. Body image concerns are common, as are feelings of dependency and frustration over lack of mobility. In successful cases, once the prosthesis has been fitted and its use mastered, mood improves and adjustment proceeds. At the other extreme, the denial that is mobilized by patients in an unhealthy way to cope with the trauma of the amputation can exacerbate the underlying condition further by interfering with compliance with medical regimens, rehabilitation progress, and healthy life-style. A period of mourning is normal, and sexual activity may temporarily be suspended; the more pervasive adjustment problems may be associated with long-standing personality problems and/or sexual difficulties, and these patients may be candidates for psychotherapy.

Simple reassurance of continued attractiveness and independence and advice on pain management and positioning are recommended for all amputee patients.

Cancer

Although the psychological impact of a cancer diagnosis may itself reduce sexual functioning, cancers of the breast and genital organs are frequently accompanied by either psychogenic or organic sexual dysfunction.[11, 58, 67] Prostate cancer, treated by prostatectomy, frequently results in erectile dysfunction due to damage of the nerve supply to the penis by the surgery. (When prostate surgery is performed for prostatitis, the rate of organic erectile dysfunction is lower but retrograde ejaculation is common. In an older population in whom fertility is not a major issue, this represents a minor inconvenience. Without physician reassurance, however, patients' worries may cause psychogenic sexual problems.) Testicular cancer is treated by surgery or irradiation, which can result in organic erectile dysfunction or infertility. Guilt over sexual practices that are erroneously blamed for the illness, or false beliefs about the decrease of masculinity due to testicular removal, can produce a psychogenic erectile dysfunction even in the absence of organic impairment.

Breast cancer may result in a similar false belief about the loss of femininity and produce psychogenic sexual dysfunction in women unless staff and spouse support are provided. Cervical cancer may result in dyspareunia if scarring follows from surgery or irradiation. Cancer of the uterus, treated by hysterectomy, generally does not impair physical sexual functioning. It can cause reduced sexual responsiveness if it is seen as compromising femininity or if vaginal dryness or hormone effects are not compensated for. Cancers that result in ostomy may also impair sexual functioning owing to body image concerns about stoma or appliances. Preventive measures involve instruction in self-care and counseling regarding feelings of attractiveness.

Aging

Although certainly not synonymous with disability, many patients are aging and cultural stereotypes have prevented the elderly from receiving information on sexual functioning. Information can serve to promote full sexual expression by reducing fear and correcting myths.

For both men and women, there is a reduction in hormone secretion and a decrease in sensory and motor functioning. Women may experience decreased elasticity and muscle tone in the vaginal wall and decreased lubrication, leading to pain if lubricants or hormone treatments are not applied. Men may have reduced frequency of orgasm, no longer experiencing it with each intercourse; the refractory period may lengthen; and there may be a loss of awareness of impending orgasm. Men may also require more direct stimulation to produce arousal and erection. Counseling should validate the elders' attractiveness and the appropriateness of their sexual interest. Sexual adjustment (activity, interest, and pleasure) that is established early in life is correlated with maintaining sexual adjustment in older age.[98]

PSYCHOLOGICAL INTERVENTIONS

Individual Counseling

A distinction between sexual rehabilitation counseling and sex therapy should be made. The principles are similar, but sex therapy assumes that sex is the highest priority issue to be dealt with at the time of treatment. Usually, sex therapy deals with sexual problems caused by stress or other psychological variables (*i.e.,* psychogenic sexual dysfunction), including conflict in the family or couple system. Sexual rehabilitation counseling assumes the presence of a physical disability and further assumes that sexual adjustments are only one of a constellation of changes that are being dealt with by the client. Focusing specifically on enhancing intercourse or alternatives to intercourse may be appropriate in a simple sex therapy procedure but is too narrow for sexual rehabilitation counseling when there may be organic or even interpersonal skill deficits that serve as barriers to psychological and sexual adjustment.[89]

However important it is to view the client as part of a social context encompassing partner, family, friends, co-workers, neighbors, and even the hospital milieu, there are a number of psychotherapeutic issues that need to be addressed by the person in order to promote psychosocial and sexual functioning. The issues of identity, dependency, self-esteem, and values are among the major concerns the patient needs to face in the course of his or her adjustment to disability.[55] Identity refers to questions of who one is, and was, and can become in the face of altered physical capacities—of who one is as a sexual person. Dependency involves not only the issue of increased reliance on others for help subsequent to disability but also much broader emotional issues about personal power and locus of control. In the sexual context, lack of resolution of this issue contributes to serious relationship conflict and inability to take responsibility for one's own sexual needs and behavior. Self-esteem, referring to body image as well as an accurate but compassionate evaluation of oneself, is seriously challenged by disability. It is necessary for optimum sexual functioning and is more a matter of attitude than of attributes. The issue of values includes ethical principles of behavior, the meaning of life and of the disability, and deeper spiritual considerations. Sexual values guide behavior, and an awareness of one's value promotes healthier and more honest choices.

Because of the personal nature of these issues, an individual therapy format is recommended; this may precede or accompany couple therapy if indicated. It is also the treatment of choice for single parents (who have a right to sexual information and counseling) of those in relationships in which the partner is unwilling to participate in the therapy.

Marital Therapy

The initial stage of therapy with couples around sexual rehabilitation concerns involves the establishment of therapeutic rapport. The couple must come to understand that the therapist will not take sides but is the agent of change for the relationship. In the first session, the couple begins to trust the therapist, to receive validation of their feelings and permission to be open about their sexual issues. The next stage of the process is a thorough assessment of their physical, psychological, interpersonal, and sexual strengths and weaknesses. This information is gathered from interview, psychological and medical testing, a review of the records, and input from other team members who work with the patient and the partner. The process of the interview requires a nonjudgmental stance and open-ended questions in order to put the clients at ease and to promote the most accurate and open reporting. The content of the assessment has been described previously.

The next stage of therapy is to integrate these data into an individualized treatment plan. It is very helpful to provide feedback to the couple on how the therapist conceptualizes the problem and how the course of treatment will be responsive to the problems they have reported and to the clients' goals. The central issues are addressed first, and it is important to build in early success so as to motivate the clients to continue to work in a step-by-step, gradual way toward change. Engaging the clients actively in the planning and review of the treatment empowers them and fits the interventions to their unique needs. An example of this is to dispense with the usual couple format (in which both partners are present in the therapy meetings) in a case in which one partner has a severe memory deficit. Teaching the able-bodied partner to be an effective sexual partner and then relying on that person to guide the patient to be an effective partner in return is less frustrating for the patient and more practical.

The next phase of the therapy is to provide education and information relative to the sexual changes encountered, ways of coping with altered body image, alternatives to the previous repertoire, and emotional communication skills. Many therapists include a course of systematic relaxation training that eliminates any contribution of anxiety to the sexual dysfunction and that is compatible with learning increased awareness and consciousness of feelings and sensations. The couple is instructed to experiment at home with new behavior and new attitudes, again in a gradual, nonthreatening way, thereby increasing the effectiveness of their sexual technique and building a "team-ness" between the couple to replace the common pretreatment adversarial stance between the partners.

A common progression is to begin with attitude exercises whose results are shared in the session and then some "sensate focus" or massage exchange, first of nongenital areas, then of genital regions. Often partners are asked to experiment with self-stimulation in order to access information about their sexual responses, needs, and preferences. Later this information is shared with the partner, and the improvements in sexual stimulation are generalized to the couple. Communication throughout this process is absolutely vital since it is assumed that the couple has mutual responsibility for the solution of sexual dilemmas (as opposed to mutual blame, or individual blame, which does not assist behavior change). Frequently, the solution of the sex problem involves a broader change, away from destructive interaction patterns, life-styles, or sex roles.[62, 64]

In brief, the principles of sexual adjustment counseling are the same for able-bodied and disabled clients: relax/go slow, get information/experiment, and communicate. A case example will illustrate the above principles:

> A couple, the young husband of which had suffered a stroke with resultant aphasia, presented to therapy in conflict. The husband was able to perform sexually with the wife; he was, however, subject to spontaneous erections when there was no opportunity to act on sexual feelings. Interview revealed that the wife's need for reassurance and reconnection with the husband was being expressed as pressure to perform sexually. Communication had broken down because of the language impairment but more saliently because the wife was "afraid to put pressure on him" by speaking about her concerns. The husband was initially depressed, owing to necessary life-style changes, as well. Six months post stroke, both of them were frustrated and willing to ask for therapeutic assistance. Gradual opening of communication and nonpressured practice restored their previously satisfying sexual adjustment and the balance of power in their relationship.

Family Therapy

Sexual growth for a disabled child will frequently involve a family format in which the parents' ability to separate from their offspring in a mature way is fostered. The child's individuation from the family on whom he or she has been emotionally and physically dependent can be a lengthy and difficult process. Individual work for the patient can supplement the family treatment and explicitly address the sexual topics that are private between the generations.

Another indication for family therapy is the case of sexual or physical abuse of the children, which requires the support of social service agencies to ensure the safety of the victims.

In addition, family therapy can assist adjustment in families in which the disabled member is a parent and there may be role changes that threaten the family homeostasis and in chronic illnesses in which maladaptive patterns and chronic stress disrupt adequate family functioning.

> The parents of a head-injured young man were upset when the patient expressed his intention to resume his residence with a male roommate after discharge from the rehabilitation center. The roommate had been a devoted supporter of the patient throughout his inpatient stay, visiting daily. A family meeting was called to discuss discharge plans, and the roommate was included, since he was directly involved in the outcome. During the session, the therapist described the level of responsibility and commitment that would be involved for the roommate if the patient returned to their home. The roommate acknowledged his willingness to assume the responsibility and further disclosed that he and the patient were homosexual lovers, which was new information to the parents. During follow-up therapy, the parents' reactions were processed and they came to appreciate the high quality of the relationship between the two men, while disagreeing with the nature of their liaison based on their own value system. The male couple was able to work on the imbalance of the relationship roles that the injury had produced and made a commitment to a long-term partnership.

Group Therapy

Traditional group therapy assumes that there will be sufficient duration of stable and somewhat homogeneous group membership to allow the development of group cohesiveness, which is the matrix for change in the group setting. This may take up to 6 months to establish before significant work can begin. These characteristics of group therapy are impractical in most inpatient settings, and even if outpatient follow-up is provided, group membership is often variable.

Despite deviations from the ideal group structure, groups with disabled persons have several advantages. It is cost effective to see clients in groups, especially educationally oriented ones rather than to try to provide preventive health principles to each patient individually. Also, the presence of other disabled group members provides perspective, reassurance, and a sense of shared burden as opposed to the notion that one is "in it alone." A common criticism of able-bodied therapists by disabled clients is, "What do you know about it? You haven't experienced it." In individual work, the client is asked to say how it is; in group work, there are others there who have experienced it. The members of the group, the consumers of the therapy services, are able to look at the problems with many points of view and generate solutions that are realistic from their perspective. There have been reports of success at conveying information around sexual issues in a short-term structured group format.[5]

Therapy groups can also include the topic of sexuality among the many other issues that such groups deal with. The advantage of including sex as an ongoing topic in the group, or even of focusing specifically on the topic for the short periods in the context of a continuing group, is that there is much more opportunity for members to express their feelings and concerns (as opposed to being recipients of sexual information as in the educational groups). Group members set the agenda rather than having it detailed to them. Guidelines for establishing and maintaining sex counseling groups include gradually more personal exploration of sexual topics; the role of the group leader in keeping the discussion on topic, in giving permission to discuss the subject, and in creating a warm, nonthreatening atmosphere; the confidential nature of the material discussed; the possibility of relationships forming within the group and how to deal with them; and the types of topics that patients have found valuable.[68]

Finally, a third type of group format is the self-help group.[47] This type of group is formed by and for patients, or in some cases by patients' families, to provide peer support, assist in problem solving, and fill a need that is frequently unfilled by health care providers. The main advantage of this format is that responsibility for behavior change is placed directly in the hands of the consumers instead of the person "being helped" with its connotation of helplessness. The success of these types of organizations is well documented. Although not focused specifically on sexual topics, interpersonal issues are clearly a large component of the issues covered by self-help groups.

REFERENCES

1. Aiello D, Capkin L, Catania H: Strategies and techniques for serving the disabled assault victim: A pilot training program for providers and consumers. Sexuality Disability 6:135–144, 1983
2. Arthritis Information Clearing House: Sexuality and the Rheumatic Diseases: An Annotated Bibliography 1970–1982. Arlington, VA, 1982
3. Barrett M: Sexuality and Multiple Sclerosis. Toronto, MS Society of Canada, 1977
4. Battle CU: Disruptions in the socialization of a young, severely

handicapped child. In Marinelli RP, Dell Orto AE (eds): The Psychological and Social Impact of Physical Disability. New York, Springer, 1984

5. Berkman AH, Macaluso E: A sex counseling program in groups in a hospital setting. AASECT/SSS Combined Annual Meeting. Boston, June 6–10, 1984

6. Blackerby W: Disruption of sexuality following a head injury. Natl Head Injury Found News 7(1): 2; 8, 1987

7. Blackwell B, Stefopoulos A, Enders P, Adolphe A: Anticholinergic activity of two tricyclic antidepressants. Am J Psychiatry 135:722–724, 1978

8. Blum G, Blum B: Feeling Good About Yourself. Mill Valley, CA, Feeling Good Associates, 1983

9. Boller F, Frank E: Sexual Dysfunction in Neurological Disorders. New York, Raven Press, 1982

10. Bors E, Comar AE: Neurological disturbances of sexual function with special reference to 529 patients with spinal cord injury. Urol Surv 10:191–222, 1960

11. Boston Women's Health Book Collective: The New Our Bodies, Ourselves. New York, Simon & Schuster, 1984

12. Brindley GS: Electroejaculation: Its technique, neurological implications, and uses. J Neurol Neurosurg Psychiatry 44:9–18, 1981

13. Brindley GS: Reflex ejaculation under vibratory stimulation in paraplegic men. Paraplegia 19:299–302, 1981

14. Brindley GS: The fertility of men with spinal injuries. Paraplegia 22:337–338, 1984

15. Chapelle PA, Jonet M, Durand J, Grossiord A: Pregnancy of the wife of a complete paraplegic by homologous insemination after an intrathecal injection of neostigmine. Paraplegia 14:173–177, 1977

16. Cole TM: Sexuality and the physically handicapped. In Green R (ed): Human Sexuality: A Health Practitioner's Text. Baltimore, Williams & Wilkins, 1975

17. Cole TM, Cole SS: The handicapped and sexual health. SIECUS Rep 4(5):1–2; 9–10, 1976

18. Comfort A: Sex counseling of the disabled in medical practice. In Comfort A (ed): Sexual Consequences of Disability, pp 5–9. Philadelphia, George F Stickley Co, 1978

19. Conine TA, Evans JH: Sexual reaction of chronically ill and disabled adults. J Allied Health pp 261–270, November, 1982

20. Cook R: Sex education program service model for the multihandicapped adult. Rehabil Lit 35:264–267; 271, 1974

21. David A, Ohry A, Rozin R: Spinal cord injuries: Male infertility aspects. Paraplegia 15:11–14, 1977–1978

22. Ducharme S: Sexuality and physical disability. In Caplan B (ed): Rehabilitation Psychology Desk Reference, pp 419–435. Rockville, MD, Aspen Publishers, 1987

23. Ducharme S: Working with the suicidal client. Paper presented at Current Issues in Rehabilitation Psychology, University Hospital, Boston, November 15, 1985

24. Duffy Y: All Things Are Possible. Ann Arbor, MI, A.J. Garvin & Associates, 1981

25. Eisenberg MG, Rustad LC: Sex and the Spinal Cord Injured: Some Questions and Answers. Washington, DC, U.S. Government Printing Office, 1974

26. Ellenberg M: Impotence in diabetes: The neurologic factor. In LoPiccolo J, LoPiccolo L (eds): Handbook of Sex Therapy. New York, Plenum Press, 1978

27. Ellenberg M: Diabetes and female sexuality. Women's Health 9:75–70, 1984

28. Ende J, Rockwell S, Glasgow M: The sexual history in general medicine practice. Arch Intern Med 144:558–561, 1984

29. FitzGerald D, FitzGerald M: Sexual implications of deafness. Sexuality Disability 1:57–69, 1978

30. Francois N, Maury M, Jouannet D et al: Electroejaculation of a complete paraplegic followed by pregnancy. Paraplegia 16:248–251, 1978

31. Freed MM: Traumatic and congenital lesions of the spinal cord. In Kottke FJ, Stillwell KG, Lehmann JF: Krusen's Handbook of Physical Medicine and Rehabilitation. Philadelphia, WB Saunders, 1982

32. Friedman JM: Sexual adjustment of the postcoronary male. In LoPiccolo J, LoPiccolo L (eds): Handbook of Sex Therapy. New York, Plenum Press, 1978

33. Glass DD, Padrone FJ: Sexual adjustment in the handicapped. J Rehabil 44:43–47, 1978

34. Goller H, Paeslack V: Pregnancy damage and birth: Complications in the children of paraplegic women. Paraplegia 10:213–217, 1972

35. Gordon S: Missing in special education: Sex. J Special Ed 5:351–354, 1971

36. Green AW: Sexual activity and the postmyocardial infarction patient. Am Heart J 89:246–252, 1975

37. Greenblatt DJ, Shader RI: Benzodiazepines in Clinical Practice. New York, Raven Press, 1974

38. Griffith ER, Tomko MA, Timms RJ: Sexual function in spinal cord injured patients: A review. Arch Phys Med Rehabil 54:539–543, 1973

39. Griffith ER, Trieschmann RB: Sexual functioning in women with spinal cord injury. Arch Phys Med Rehabil 56:18–21, 1975

40. Griffith ER, Trieschmann RB: Sexual training of the spinal cord injured male and his partner. In Ami Sha'ked (ed): Human Sexuality and Rehabilitation Medicine: Sexual Functioning Following Spinal Cord Injury. Baltimore, Williams & Wilkins, 1981

41. Griffith E, Trieschmann RB, Hohmann GW et al: Sexual dysfunctions associated with physical disabilities. Arch Phys Med Rehabil 56:8–13, 1975

42. Guttman L, Walsh JJ: Prostigmin assessment test of fertility in spinal man. Paraplegia 9:39–51, 1971

43. Hellerstein HK, Friedman EH: Sexual activity and the post-coronary patient. Med Aspects Hum Sexuality, pp 70–96, 1969

44. Hellerstein HK, Friedman EH: Sexual activity and the post myocardial infarction patient. Arch Intern Med 125:987–999, 1970

45. Humphrey M, Kinsella G: Sexual life after stroke. Sexuality Disability 3:150–153, 1980

46. Imes C: Interventions with stroke patients. Cognitive Rehabil 2(5):4–17, 1984

47. Jaques ME, Patterson KM: The self-help group model: A review. In Marinelli RP, Dell Orto AE (eds): The Psychological and Social Impact of Physical Disability. New York, Springer, 1974

48. Janiszewski D, Caroscio J, Wisham L: Amyotrophic lateral sclerosis: A comprehensive rehabilitation approach. Arch Phys Med Rehabil 64:304–307, 1983

49. Kaplan HS: The New Sex Therapy: Active Treatment of Sexual Dysfunctions. New York, Brunner/Mazel, 1974

50. Kaplan HS: The New Sex Therapy: Volume II: Disorders of Sexual Desire. New York, Brunner/Mazel, 1979

51. Kaplan HS: The Evaluation of Sexual Disorders: Psychological and Medical Aspects. New York, Brunner/Mazel, 1983

52. Katz HT, Sarkarati M, Fam B: Autoinjection of vasoactive medications: A new effective treatment of impotence in spinal cord injured males (abstr). Arch Phys Med Rehabil 66:548, 1985

53. Keller S, Buchanan DC: Sexuality and disability: An overview. Rehabil Dig 15:3–7, 1984

54. Kikuchi TA, Skowsky WR, El-Torai I, Swerdolff R: The Pituitary-gonadal axis in spinal cord injury. Fertil Steril 27:1142–1145, 1976

55. Kir-Stimon W: Counseling with the severely handicapped: Encounter and commitment. Psychother Res Pract 7:70–74, 1970

56. Kolodny RC, Masters WH, Johnson VE: Textbook of Sexual Medicine. Boston, Little, Brown, & Co, 1979

57. Kramer SA, Anderson EE, Bredall J, Paulson DF: Complications of Small-Carrion penile prosthesis. Urology 13:49–51, 1979

58. Labby D: Sexual concomitants of disease and illness. Postgrad Med 58:103–111, 1975

59. Leiblum SR, Rosen RC: Guidelines for taking a sexual history. Unpublished manuscript, Sexual Counseling Service, Rutgers Medical School

60. Lerich A, Berard E, Vauzelle JL et al: Histological and hormonal testicular changes in spinal cord patients. Paraplegia 14:274–279, 1976

61. Lezak M: Living with the characterologically altered brain-injured patient. J Clin Psychiatry 39:592–598, 1978

62. LoPiccolo L: Techniques for Resolution of Sexual Problems. Workshop, Boston, June 14–15, 1985

63. LoPiccolo L, Heiman J Jr: Sexual assessment and history interview. In LoPiccolo J, LoPiccolo L (eds): Handbook of Sex Therapy. New York, Plenum Press, 1978

64. LoPiccolo J, LoPiccolo L (eds): Handbook of Sex Therapy. New York, Plenum Press, 1978

65. Mancini RE, Lavieri JC, Juller F et al: Effect of prednisone upon normal and pathologic human spermatogenesis. Fertil Steril 17:500–513, 1966

66. Masters WH, Johnson VE: Human Sexual Response. Boston, Little, Brown, & Co, 1966

67. Masters W, Johnson V, Kolodny R: Masters and Johnson on Sex and Human Loving. Boston, Little, Brown, & Co, 1986

68. Mayers KS: Sexual and social concerns of the disabled: A group counseling approach. Sexuality Disability 1:100–111, 1978

69. McIntyre K, Elesha-Adams M: Sexual limitations caused by stroke. J Sex Ed Ther 10:57–59, 1984

70. Milkovich L, VanDenBearg BJ: Effects of prenatal meprobamate and chlordiazepoxide hydrochloride on human embryonic and fetal development. N Eng J Med 291:1268–1271, 1974

71. Monga T, Lawson JS, Inglis J: Sexual dysfunction in stroke patients. Arch Phys Med Rehabil 67:19–22, 1986

72. Mooney T, Cole TM, Chilgren R: Sexual Options for Paraplegics and Quadriplegics. Boston, Little, Brown, & Co, 1975

73. Muckleroy RN: Sex counseling after stroke. Med Aspects Hum Sexuality, pp 115–116, December, 1977

74. Newman A, Bertelson A: Sexual dysfunction in diabetic women. J Behav Med 9:261–270, 1986

75. Nickerson M, Ruedy J: Antihypertensive agents and the drug therapy of hypertension. In Goodman LS, Gilman A (eds): The Pharmacologic Basis of Therapeutics, 5th ed. New York, Macmillan, 1975

76. Nininger JE: Inhibition of ejaculation by amitriptyline. Am J Psychiatry 135:750–751, 1978

77. Page LB: Advising hypertensive patients about sex. Med Aspects Hum Sexuality 9:103–104, 1975

78. Price JR: Promoting sexual wellness in head-injured patients. Rehabil Nurs pp 12–13, Nov–Dec, 1985

79. Rabin BJ: The Sensuous Wheeler: Sexual Adjustment for the Spinal Cord Injured. Santa Ana, CA, Joyce Publications, 1974

80. Renshaw DS: Sexual problems in stroke patients. Med Aspects Hum Sexuality 9:68–74, 1975

81. Renshaw DC: Impotence in diabetics. In LoPiccolo J, LoPiccolo L (eds): Handbook of Sex Therapy. New York, Plenum Press, 1978

82. Robertson DNS: Pregnancy and labour in the paraplegic. Paraplegia 10:100–212, 1972

83. Robmault IP: Sex, Society, and the Disabled. New York, Harper & Row, 1978

84. Romano M: Counseling the spinal cord injured female. In Sha'ked A (ed): Human Sexuality and Rehabilitation Medicine: Sexual Functioning Following Spinal Cord Injury. Baltimore, Williams & Wilkins, 1981

85. Rossier A, Ruffieus M, Ziegler WH: Pregnancy and labour in high traumatic spinal cord lesions. Paraplegia 19:210–215, 1981

86. Saxton M: Born and unborn. In Raditti A et al (eds): Test Tube Women. London, Pandora Press, 1984

87. Sex and Disability Project. Who Cares? A Handbook on Sex Education and Counseling Services for Disabled People. Washington, DC, George Washington University, 1979

88. Sha'ked A: Human Sexuality in Physical and Mental Illnesses and Disabilities: An Annotated Bibliography. Bloomington, IN, Indiana University Press, 1978

89. Shrey DE, Diefer JS, Anthony WA: Sexual adjustment counseling for persons with severe disabilities: A skill-based approach for rehabilitation professionals. J Rehabil, pp 18–33, April–June, 1979

90. Sidman JM: Sexual functioning and the physically disabled adult. Am J Occup Ther 31:81–85, 1977

91. Singh SP, Magner T: Sex and self: The spinal cord injured. Rehabil Lit 36:2–10, 1975

92. Sjogren K, Fugl-Meyer A: Adjustment to life after stroke with special reference to sexual intercourse and leisure. J Psychosom Res 26:409–417, 1982

93. Small MP: The Small-Carrion penil prosthesis: Surgical implant for the management of impotence. Sexuality Disability 1:272–281, 1978

94. Stein RA: Sexual counseling and coronary heart disease. In Leiblum SR, Pervin LA (eds): Principles and Practice of Sex Therapy. New York, Guilford Press, 1980

95. Steiner J, Cassar J, Mashiter K et al: Effects of methyldopa on prolactin and growth hormone. Br Med J 1:1186–1188, 1976

96. Strauss D: Sexuality: Treatment interventions for professionals working with head injured. Paper presented at Braintree Hospital Traumatic Head Injury Conference, Braintree, MA, October 23–25, 1985

97. Stuart CK, Stuart VW: Sexual assault: Disabled perspective. Sexuality Disability 4:246–253, 1981

98. Sviland MAP: Helping elderly couples become sexually liberated: Psychosocial issues. In LoPiccolo J, LoPiccolo L (eds): Handbook of Sex Therapy. New York, Plenum Press, 1978

99. Symposium on Sex and Diabetes. Diabetes Care 2:4–30, 1979

100. Talbot HS: Psychosocial aspects of sexuality in spinal cord injured patients. Paraplegia 9:37–39, 1971

101. Talbot HS: The sexual function in paraplegia. J Urol 73:90–101, 1955

102. Thomas DG: The effect of transurethral surgery on penile erections in spinal cord injured patients. Paraplegia 12:286–289, 1976

103. Trieschmann RB: Psychological, Social and Vocational Adjustment in Spinal Cord Injury: A Strategy for Further Research. New York, Pergamon Press, 1980

104. Turk R, Turk M, Assejev V: The female paraplegic and mother–child relations. Paraplegia 21:191–196, 1983

105. Valentich M, Gripton J: Facilitating the sexual integration of the head-injured person in the community. Sexuality Disability 7:28–42, 1984

106. Van Thiel DH, Gavalen JS, Smith WI Jr, Paul G: Hypothalamic pituitary gonadal dysfunction in men using cimetidine. N Engl J Med 300:1012–1015, 1979

107. Whitelaw MJ: Menstrual irregularities associated with use of Methaminodiazepoxide. Journal of Sex Education and Therapy 175:400–401, 1961

108. Whitley MP, Berke PA: Sexual response in diabetic women. J Sex Ed Ther 9:51–56, 1983

109. Wiig, E: Counseling the adult aphasic for sexual readjustment. Rehabil Counseling Bull, pp 111–119, December, 1973

110. Woods F: Sexuality and chronic illness: Diabetes and heart disease. In Human Sexuality in Health and Illness. St. Louis, CV Mosby, 1979

111. Zorgniotti AW, Lefleur RS: Autoinjection of the corpus cavernosum with a vasoactive drug combination for vasculogenic impotence. J Urol 133:39–40, 1985

28

Nutrition

Donna L. Frankel

Nutrition is the study of foods, the nutrients that foods contain, and the way in which nutrients support health and life. Good nutrition is essential to the promotion of optimal health, growth, and physical and mental function. Nutritional status as a significant factor in both the outcome of acute illness and the course of chronic disease is now accepted as fact.[16, 21, 43, 44, 72, 96, 103, 105, 171, 177] Additionally, the capacity for collection and use of historical, clinical, and laboratory data to assess nutritional status and monitor the effect of nutritional intervention is continually expanding.[23, 45, 59, 69, 72, 73, 103, 105, 108, 116, 121, 155] This is coupled with advances in nutritional support for patients for whom the normal oral route of feeding is impossible.[39, 47, 79, 94, 109, 110, 114, 136, 138, 146–148, 150, 169, 178] In the presence of disability, whether temporary or permanent, the relationship of nutritional status to health and function persists.

An overview of the basic information necessary for the application of the principles of good nutrition to the care of the disabled person, in both the acute and the chronic situation, is presented in this chapter. The study of nutritional assessment and nutritional intervention in this population group is in an early stage of development. The present challenge is twofold: (1) to apply the present knowledge base with a critical and open mind, recognizing the potential for variation in physiological function in patients who have congenital or acquired disability and (2) to pursue basic and applied research that will allow further identification of the special nutritional needs of the disabled.

BALANCED NUTRITION

Food is made up of chemical substances. Those substances that must be consumed by living organisms to sustain life are known as nutrients. Other substances, which may also affect health and function, are present in some food. An adequate diet is achieved by balancing the substances in food in amounts appropriate for a given person.

Nutrients

Nutrients include six major categories of chemical compounds: water, protein, carbohydrates, fats, vitamins, and minerals. The specific categories of nutrients are based on their chemical composition. Water is the most basic compound essential for life, comprising more than 50% of total body mass, and is an integral part of cell structures and the basic medium for body fluids. Protein, carbohydrates, and fats share the function of sources of energy. Additionally, they each have a unique chemical composition and serve unique functions in areas of body composition, cell structure, and metabolic activity. Vitamins are divided into two categories, based on their solubility in fat or water (Table 28-1). Vitamins function primarily as cofactors for enzymatic reactions to support metabolic needs of the body. Their daily requirements vary with the size and activity of the person. The fat-soluble and some of the water-soluble vitamins are stored in the body to some extent, so that not all vitamins must be obtained daily to maintain balanced nutrition. Minerals include inorganic elements, classified according to the relative quantities in the diet (Table 28-2).

Although all nutrients are considered essential to life, the amounts of some nutrients necessary for health are variable with the overall diet composition because functions overlap. An example of this variability is the proportion of protein, fat, and carbohydrates needed for health. Because all share the function of providing energy to the body, for this purpose alone the proportions of these three nutrients in the diet can vary. However, there are also some very unique roles for these nutrients, especially protein and fat. Because of the inability of the body to make some of the basic components of protein (specific essential amino acids) and of fats (specific essential fatty acids) there is a basic essential requirement for these substances in the diet not reflected in the energy requirements. The specific amino acids and fatty acids that are essential vary with the age and health of the person.[86, 100] There is also evidence that excessive amounts of any of these three classes of nutrients in the diet may have detrimental effects on the body. Therefore, there appear to be limits to both the absolute amounts and the specific proportions of these nutrients that are healthy. An example of this is that when amino acids, the basic components of protein, are used for the body for energy they must be modified chemically in the liver to remove the nitrogen. The ability to remove nitrogen and excrete it has finite limits, which if exceeded may lead to increased ammonia in the body. Additionally, the metabolic activity necessary for this chemical transformation increases overall caloric requirements. Therefore, protein as the sole source of energy is potentially

Table 28-1
Vitamins

Water-soluble
  B-complex
    Energy releasing
      Thiamine (vitamin B_1, anti-beriberi factor)
      Niacin (niacinamide, nicotinic acid, nicotinamide)
      Riboflavin (vitamin B_2, lactoflavin)
      Pantothenic acid (anti-gray hair factor, vitamin B_3)
      Biotin (anti-egg white factor)
    Hematopoetic
      Folacin (folic acid, pteroylglutamic acid, PGA)
      Cyanocobalamin (vitamin B_{12}, cobalamin, anti-pernicious anemia
        factor)
    Other
      Pyridoxine (vitamin B_6)
      Choline*
      Inositol* (myoinositol)
      p-Aminobenzoic acid*
      Coenzyme Q*
      Lipoic acid*
  Non–B-Complex
    L-Ascorbic acid (vitamin C)

Fat-soluble
  Vitamin A (retinol, retinal, retinoic acid)
  Vitamin D (1,25-dihydroxycholecalciferol; cholecalciferol, D_3;
    ergocalciferol, D_2; antirachitic factor)†
  Vitamin E (the trocopherols)
  Vitamin K (the naphthoquinones)

---

* Dietary substances that are sometimes considered to be vitamins, but a specific requirement for such status has not yet been identified.

† Vitamin D can be manufactured to a limited extent in the body, thus its classification as a vitamin or a hormone is subject to debate.

(Adapted from Anderson CE: Vitamins. In Schneider HA, Anderson CE, Coursin DB [eds]: Nutritional Support of Medical Practice, 2nd ed, p 24. Philadelphia, J. B. Lippincott, 1983)

Table 28-2
Minerals

Macronutrients
  Required in amounts of 100 mg/day or greater
    Calcium
    Phosphorous
    Sodium
    Potassium
    Chlorine
    Magnesium
    Sulfur

Micronutrients
  Required in amounts of less than 20 mg/day
    Iron
    Cobalt
    Manganese
    Molybdenum
    Fluorine
    Copper
    Zinc
    Iodine
    Selenium
    Chromium
  Present in trace amounts in food, but specific requirements not
    established
    Nickel
    Tin
    Silicon
    Vanadium

Trace Contaminants
  Lead
  Mercury
  Barium
  Boron
  Lithium
  Rubidium
  Antimony
  Cadmium
  Arsenic
  Strontium
  Aluminum
  Beryllium
  Silver

(Adapted from Anderson CE: Minerals. In Schneider HA, Anderson CE [eds]: Nutritional Support of Medical Practice, 2nd ed, pp 54–55. Philadelphia, JB Lippincott, 1983)

harmful. Thus, there are optimal ratios of these three substances that one should try to achieve in developing a balanced diet.

Another major factor affecting the requirements of various nutrients is the ability of the body to store them. Fats are stored as adipose tissue, which is the storage form of all excessive energy whether derived from protein, carbohydrate, or fat in the diet. Minimal quantities of carbohydrates are stored in the form of glycogen; otherwise it must be produced from absorbed food substances or from fat stores as needed. There is no particular storage form of protein. When protein in the diet is limited, the protein of skeletal muscle will be broken down to meet the metabolic requirements for life-sustaining functions.

Other Components of the Diet

Fiber

Fiber refers to carbohydrates and related substances in the diet that are not digestible; therefore, it is not classified as a nutrient. However, fiber does perform several physiological functions in the gastrointestinal system.[166] The primary properties of fiber in the gut seem to be its hydrophilic capacity, which increases stool bulk and decreases transit time, and its ability to bind other dietary substances, such that changes in the fiber content of the diet will alter absorption and bioavailability of both nutrients and toxins. These functions may sound quite

simple, but the overall impact of fiber in the diet is quite diverse and varies with the type of fiber consumed. The physiological consequences have been shown to have an effect on the control of diabetes mellitus, disorders of lipid metabolism, and obesity. Additionally, the fiber content of the diet is implicated to be associated with the incidence of some types of cancer.

Cholesterol

Cholesterol is a member of the sterol group of organic compounds. It is derived from fats and can be manufactured in the body in sufficient quantities for metabolic demand. It is an integral part of cell structures and also a precursor of some hormones and vitamin D. Cholesterol is also present in some foods and absorbed during the process of digestion. Dietary sources of cholesterol have been shown to be important in the development of atherosclerosis in some people.[51, 118] The effect of dietary cholesterol on the development of atherosclerosis in disabled patients has not been evaluated.

Food Additives

Food additives are a diverse group of chemical substances that are added to foods during processing to improve shelf life and enhance appearance or flavor. Their role in the development and continuation of some clinical abnormalities remains controversial. Some additives are substances that are found naturally in the diet, and others are compounds that have been synthesized specifically for use in foods. There is no question that our food supply is more diverse and more consistently available because of the use of additives. However, the long-term effects of many of these substances on health are unknown or questionable.[122, 172]

Adequate Diet

The purpose of dietary recommendations is to translate the information about nutrients required for health and the nutrient composition of food into amounts of food that should be consumed for meeting nutritional needs. Several schemata have been developed to serve this purpose. One of the most widely used methods for general nutrition education purposes is to classify foods into the basic four food groups: milk and dairy products; meats, fish, and eggs; fruits and vegetables; and breads and cereals. There are guidelines for serving sizes and numbers of recommended servings for children of various ages, teenagers, adult men and women, and pregnant and lactating women. The caloric content of the diet will vary primarily by the specific food choices within a group and food preparation techniques.[159, 161] With the recent recognition of the role of excessive amounts of some substances in the diets of people living in developed countries, the basic four food groups have been adapted to reflect the need to control the intake of salt, fat, sugars, and alcohol in the general diet.[24, 126] This basic scheme, with the associated modifications, continues to work well for many purposes.

For therapeutic diets, a flexible approach has been to develop "exchange" lists, which are lists of foods categorized by similarities of nutrient content with specific serving sizes for each food within a group. The registered dietitian works with the patient to develop a diet plan based on the requirements of the diet prescription and the food habits, interests, and economic status of the patient. This is translated into numbers of servings per day of food from each of the exchange lists.[159, 172] This approach allows a reasonable amount of flexibility, with minimum effort on the part of the patient on a day-to-day basis.

Getting adequate amounts of eight of ten specific nutrients in a diet that includes a variety of foods will ensure that all the required nutrients are consumed. These eight to ten nutrients have been identified as *indicator nutrients* and are the basis on which the information on nutritional labels of food products has been developed. The labels give the percentage of an average daily requirement of each of ten nutrients in any specific food. If the total adds up to 100% of each, then the diet is probably adequate to protect against deficiencies.[161] The use of indicator nutrients has not been adapted to protect against excesses in the diet.

Another concept is to identify a method of rating the nutritional content of each food, in a numerical way so that its nutritional value can be compared with other foods. This method includes consideration of nutrient content of the food; content of salt, fat (+ / − cholesterol), and sugar; and the "nutrient density,"

which expresses the proportion of nutrients relative to calories in the food. This is best applied as a teaching and information tool to illustrate the relative nutritional value of various foods rather than the basis of a diet plan alone.[48, 160]

MALNUTRITION

Malnutrition exists when a person is not taking in nutrients in the optimal amounts for health maintenance, tissue repair, and/or tissue growth. Historically, malnutrition has been considered to exist primarily because of a lack of one or more nutrients in the diet. However, the problems of excessive and imbalanced nutrient intake have also become evident as life expectancy increases, food supplies in the developed nations of the world have stabilized at abundant levels, and the metabolic basis of chronic disease states has been identified. Thus, any one of three conditions can result in suboptimal function secondary to malnutrition:

1. Nutrient deficiency. This condition develops when insufficient amounts of one or more nutrients are taken in to meet metabolic needs.
2. Nutrient excess. This condition is the result of an excessive intake of one or more nutrients.
3. Nutrient imbalance. This condition develops when a person consumes a diet that is not balanced in nutrients. Therefore, some nutrients might be consumed in excessive amounts and others in insufficient amounts.

The development of malnutrition follows a continuum that initially develops as body stores of a nutrient are changed from a balanced state to one of imbalance, involving depletion and/or excess of one or more nutrients. Further imbalance of nutrient intake then leads to alterations of metabolism at the biochemical level. If the imbalance continues, overt disease will result. Specific function may be altered at any point along this continuum, which is illustrated in Figure 28-1.

When considering the problem of malnutrition, there is a tendency to focus on the specifics of food intake alone. The development of malnutrition is truly multifactorial, and its solution requires recognition of the potential for contribution from any one of these factors (Fig. 28-2). People are at risk of going from the well-nourished state to one of malnutrition when any one of these factors is altered.

By understanding the multifactorial etiologies of the clinical problem of malnutrition, it is possible to develop realistic approaches to recognizing and solving the problem. It is quite obvious that the acutely injured person who has a sudden onset of physiological trauma that will result in disability is by definition at risk for malnutrition because of the combination of increased demands for nutrients by the metabolic response to injury and the decreased regularity of oral feedings as a result of gastrointestinal malfunction, surgery, or diagnostic tests.[15, 33, 41, 52, 75, 87, 92, 95, 96, 140, 162, 163, 171] Likewise, there is increased recognition of the need for specific attention to nutritional status and nutritional support in patients admitted to rehabilitation units.[5, 6, 13, 35, 37, 64, 76, 119, 120, 125] However, there continues to be insufficient awareness of the fact that malnutrition can develop without physiological trauma because of the effects of nonphysiological factors on food intake.

Of additional importance is the recognition of the need for a team approach to the solution of the problem of malnutrition. Many factors are totally out of the control of the physician and other members of the health care team (*e.g.,* the general level of food supply in a given community or the income of a family).

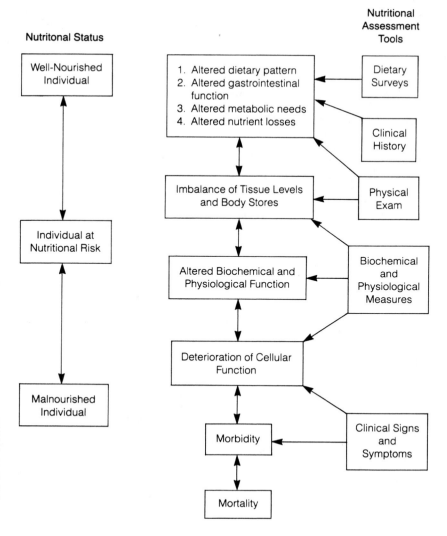

Figure 28-1. Individual variability of nutritional status. (Adapted from Wellman NS: The evaluation of nutritional status. In Howard RB, Herbold NH [eds]: Nutrition in Clinical Care, 2nd ed, p 382. New York, McGraw-Hill, 1982, and Young VR: Nutrition. In Steinberg FU [ed]: Care of the Geriatric Patient in the Tradition of E.V. Cowdry, 6th ed, p 221. St Louis, CV Mosby, 1983)

Figure 28-2. Multifactorial etiology of malnutrition.

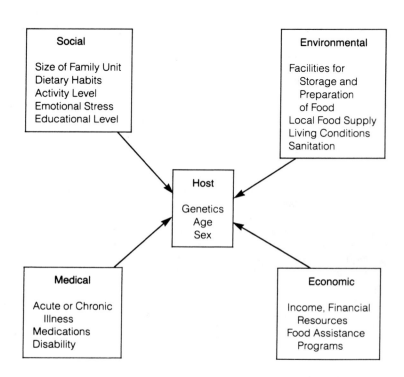

Causative factors may respond to social intervention or the reduction of architectural barriers in the community resulting in increased independence for the disabled person, thus increasing the person's level of responsibility for food intake. It might be necessary to educate the patient's caregiver in the principles of nutrition or in the principles of budgeting. Thus, it is only through open-minded assessment and use of the talents of a diverse team that malnutrition will be fully recognized and successfully combatted.

NONPHYSIOLOGICAL FACTORS AFFECTING FOOD INTAKE

Nonphysiological factors can be instrumental in the development of malnutrition and are impacted by the presence of disability. It is because of these factors that malnutrition can persist even when the ideal diet for a given person can be defined. Although the primary physiological reason for eating is to meet the metabolic needs of the body, the consumption of food has many meanings and fulfills multiple psychological needs as well. The availability of food and selection of specific types of foods includes many social and economic factors, in addition to consideration of a person's health.

Economic Status

Food must be obtained before it can be eaten. In developed countries, most people are dependent on food purchases for the majority of their diet. Thus, one factor influencing the amount and type of food available to a person is his or her financial resources. The sudden onset of disability is often accompanied by a loss of earning power and an increase in medical expenses. Therefore, less money may be available for food purchases and the quality of the diet may decline. The very real correlation between the quality of the diet and the economic level of the family unit has been documented in one study of food intake in disabled children.[19] Limited financial resources could also limit the mobility of patients because of the cost of transportation, either private or public, resulting in less opportunity for shopping. When there is insufficient income for maintaining utility payments, food preparation may become the limiting factor. Therefore, the impact of a disability on economic status can have a significant effect on one or several factors related to the adequacy of the diet.

Environment

The place of residence is an important contributing factor to adequacy of food intake. When a person lives in private housing, factors such as the proximity to stores, access to transportation for shopping, facilities for food storage, preparation, and clean up within the home have major importance. When a person lives in an institutional setting, factors such as the facilities for dining and the congeniality of residents and staff may become the major environmental factors contributing to adequacy of food intake. Adequacy of the diet is also dependent on provision of nutritionally sound food choices for the residents of institutions.[8]

Social Factors

The most obvious social factor involved in influencing food intake is the pervasive presence of foods and beverages at social gatherings. Choices are generally based on taste, convenience, and cost, resulting in a relative abundance of foods high in fat, salt, and sugar. Frequently there is a pervasive presence of alcoholic beverages as well. Thus, an active social life often promotes poor nutritional habits. Conversely, because of the association of eating with socialization, people who are isolated and lonely are also at increased risk of inadequate or imbalanced food intake.

The second pervasive social factor involved in food intake is the presence of massive advertising campaigns for food products, especially manufactured ones, many of which have questionable nutritional value. Some foods become status symbols and are consumed because they are the "in" thing, not because of nutritional content.

Food may be used as a reward for good behavior, or it may be seen as a punishment for people with significant feeding disorders. Once these values are attached to food, changing the behavior will not necessarily change the meaning of the food. The meaning of food, specific or general, will then have significant impact on food consumption.

NUTRITIONAL ASSESSMENT

Nutritional assessment is the evaluation of nutritional status, providing the means to determine the presence of any form of malnutrition. Additionally, it provides a data base from which the effect of nutritional intervention can be monitored over time. The assessment process may be applied to individuals or groups. The information critical to successful comprehensive nutritional assessment includes direct measurement or estimation of food and nutrient intake and the use of subjective and objective measures of clinical, anthropometric, biochemical, and physiological status as a reflection of the person's nutritional status.[4, 16, 69, 103, 105, 151, 167] The appropriate assessment techniques vary depending on the goals to be achieved by the assessment.[165]

Accurate nutritional assessment is the key to successful, appropriate nutritional support. In applying the principles of nutritional assessment to the disabled population, three questions, adapted from the work of Bowman and Rosenberger,[17] must be kept in mind:

1. Are the standards established in able-bodied people applicable to the evaluation and monitoring of nutritional status in those with disability?
2. Does the physiological adaptation to disability result in changes of body composition and/or biochemical function as a result of the natural history of the process causing the disability or as a result of the development of malnutrition?
3. When altered nutritional status is observed in a disabled person, does it represent an imbalance of diet or a change in digestion, absorption, metabolism, or excretion related to the disability or management of the disability?

Evaluation of Food/Nutrient Intake

A record of food intake is necessary to determine the nutrient content of the food consumed. Ideally, the level of nutrient intake is compared with standards so that the adequacy of the diet can be determined. Various methods exist for obtaining this information, all of which have advantages and limitations.[153, 175, 176]

Methods of Collection of Food Intake Information

Several of the more common dietary survey methods will be reviewed here, with the intention of concentrating on both their strengths and weaknesses. Information of this type is crucial to selecting the type of data collection needed to meet the needs of any given patient care situation.[176]

24-HOUR FOOD RECALL. The registered dietitian or trained technician interviews the patient to determine what foods and fluids have been consumed in the previous 24 hours. Through the use of food models and/or measuring utensils and tableware, there is also an attempt to estimate the quantity of each item consumed. The type of preparation is also determined. If pre-packaged or pre-prepared foods are consumed, the specific brand is identified. Questions about snacks, condiments, and additives are included in the interview.

MULTIPLE DAY FOOD INTAKE RECORD. Recording the food and fluid consumed over several days (usually 3 to 7) can be done. Because food habits vary, especially between weekdays and weekends, it is important to know what specific days have been included. Records for outpatients are kept by each patient or by the patient's caregiver. Accuracy is increased if portions are measured or weighed as prepared and waste is subtracted. For institutionalized patients, the record may be kept by the patient or by nursing or dietetic personnel.

FOOD FREQUENCY RECORD. The frequency with which major groups of foods are consumed (daily, weekly, monthly, sporadic, or never) can also be surveyed. A standard portion size provides the base against which the number of portions for a given time interval are determined. Information is obtained through a questionnaire or interview.

Obviously, the most accurate methods record food intake as it is eaten. The alternative is to use standard measures of portion size and then estimate the percentage of portions consumed. A major disadvantage to such methods is the time and attention required to obtain these data. Additionally, there is the risk of introducing bias from the close observation of eating habits.

There is less bias on actual food intake behavior when a recall method of survey is used. However, this type of survey is subject to the problems inherent in historical recall. It requires that the subject being interviewed have an intact functional memory. Inaccuracies may be introduced by poor recall of actual foods eaten, poor estimates of portion size, or filtering of the information based on the subject's idea of what the interviewer wants to hear, rather than what was actually consumed.

Methods that sample only one day's food intake do not reflect total food intake accurately. People may vary their food intake according to the day of the week, their activity level, their emotional status, the temporal relationship with a paycheck or support payment, special sales items in stores, and many other factors. Thus, significant misconceptions about dietary adequacy can result from surveys because of time limits.

It is important to obtain information on ethanol consumption and use of nutritional supplements as part of the survey. It is also helpful to have information about minerals in the water supply. Sodium content of the diet may be highly variable, even within communities, depending on the presence of in-house water conditioning systems. If supplements are consumed, it is important to get information on their nutrient content directly from packaging material because combinations and amounts of ingredients vary among brands.

Common sense would dictate that the reliability of any of the methods will increase with repetition. Through the use of a combination of food intake survey methods, one can also achieve increased reliability.[90] By combining a food intake survey with the measurement of related biochemical parameters it is possible to build in some ability to validate the accuracy of the dietary

intake information. This concept has been successfully applied to the study of dietary protein intake.[14]

Methods of Determining Adequacy of Nutrient Intake

The dietary information collected by methods such as those reviewed previously must be translated into information about nutrient composition. Methods that assess frequency of food or food group intakes are usually evaluated for nutrient content by comparing the diet pattern of the patient with standard intake patterns, such as the basic four food groups. If a significant imbalance is evident, there is indication of a possibility of malnutrition on the basis of poor dietary habits.

When actual food intake is recorded or recalled, it may be compared against patterns of food intake with food surveys, or specific nutrient/energy content may be calculated by information available from food composition tables.[2, 127, 168] Historically, this was a very tedious task; however, with the advent of the widespread availability of computer software to transform food intake data into nutrient intake, this is now a trivial task. Such reports are produced with a degree of precision that is deceptive. The specific nutrient content of any food depends on where it was produced, the conditions and length of storage, and the type of preparation. The information in food composition tables is based on average data from small samples at a remote time. Caution in interpretation of nutrient intake data must be urged. Even though information may be reported to the nearest milligram, it must be recognized as an approximation. For metabolic balance studies it is necessary to perform nutrient analysis on samples of the food being consumed by the subjects of the study to achieve a sufficiently high level of validity for investigative purposes.

Standard of Adequacy of Nutrient Intake

The need for establishing reference standards of specific nutrient intake became apparent as individual vitamin deficiencies were recognized to be the cause of unique disease states. Since 1941, the recommended dietary allowances (RDAs) have served this purpose for the population of the United States. There are equivalent governmental and international standards that have been developed and applied in other parts of the world. To date, the philosophical basis on which the RDAs were developed has been to provide an estimation of nutrient allowances, based on available (often limited) scientific evidence, which if met in population groups would be adequate to prevent the development of deficiency states in the majority of healthy Americans.[55]

Historically, the RDAs have been revised approximately every 5 years, without a change in the philosophical basis on which they were established. However, the science of nutrition is entering a new era. The dietary problems in the more developed parts of the world include disease states secondary to excessive amounts of nutrients and nutrient imbalances. Individual variations in nutrient requirements and response to specific dietary components contribute to morbidity and mortality. Nutritional support techniques have been developed that bypass significant parts of or the entire gastrointestinal tract. This has resulted in a recognition of the need to reformulate the basic assumptions underlying the RDAs to expand the concept from one of defining adequate levels to prevent deficiency to that of safe ranges of intake to optimize health.[56] Thus, despite 5 years of effort, the 1985 revision of the RDAs was not published.

The RDAs presently in use by nutritionists continue to be the ninth edition, published in 1980. The information base from which these recommendations have been derived is discussed in the report itself.[55] Additional critical comments about their application and limitations can be found in review articles.[7, 23, 56, 115, 116] The RDAs have been applied to nutritional assessment and management of individuals as well as groups, but for such application to be successful, the assumptions underlying their development and the limitations of their value as a result of these assumptions must be clearly understood. This is an especially important concept to work with in evaluating the adequacy of nutrient intake of disabled people. Disability results from physiological alterations of the physical and/or mental capacity of the patient. These changes must be understood before appropriate modifications of the RDAs can be made for application to the needs of the disabled. Additionally, it is necessary to recognize that the spectrum of causes and effects of disability is vast, and thus it is impossible to categorize nutritional requirements solely on the presence of a specific disability. Each person must be considered individually. Major factors known to affect the nutrient requirements of specific individuals are listed in Table 28-3. These factors will be discussed to a greater extent in the following sections on specific components of nutritional assessment.

Methods for Screening for Nutritional Risk Related to Inadequate Food Intake

In daily clinical practice it is necessary to be able to identify subjects at risk for malnutrition because of poor dietary habits or poor food intake. For patients in an institutional setting a tray monitor is quite helpful. This involves recording the food left over on a patient's tray after eating. The nutrient value of the institutional diet is based on standards so that it is assumed to have a known nutritional content that is adequate for the needs of most patients on that particular diet, general or therapeutic, if consumed in its entirety. Thus, estimates of calories and other nutrients consumed can be made easily from monitoring the food consumed. This is only valid if the person has no other sources of food. Thus, tray monitors require the cooperation of the patient being monitored, family and/or friends, and staff for accuracy.

For people who are followed as outpatients there is a need to use simple screening tools to first identify those with alterations in any of the multiple factors that can affect nutritional status (Fig. 28-3).

When patients are identified as being at nutritional risk, simple screening tools that can be completed quickly and scored by people with training in use of the specific instrument can be

---

Table 28-3
Factors for Which It Is Necessary to Adjust the Recommended Dietary Allowances

1. Age
2. Sex
3. Body size
4. Activity
   Physical
   Metabolic
5. Environmental Extremities
6. Acute or chronic illness/injury
7. Medical use

(National Research Council, Committee on Dietary Allowances: Recommended Dietary Allowances, 9th ed. Washington, DC, National Academy of Sciences, 1980)

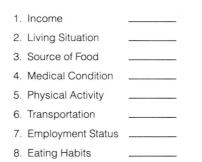

Has there been a change in any of the following?

1. Income   _____
2. Living Situation _____
3. Source of Food   _____
4. Medical Condition _____
5. Physical Activity _____
6. Transportation   _____
7. Employment Status _____
8. Eating Habits   _____

If there is a change in any of these since last evaluated, there is a new risk of malnutrition and further screening of nutritional status should be undertaken.

Figure 28-3. Screening for risk of malnutrition.

---

used. The identification of a variance from the standard score is an indication for referral of the patient to the registered dietitian, freeing this professional to devote time to the patients at highest risk and most likely to benefit from such intervention.[6, 26, 70, 83, 90, 105, 157]

Food/Nutrient Intake in the Disabled

There is a rapidly expanding base of information about food and nutrient intake in disabled patients. The major message that comes through in a review of the literature is a confirmation of the diversity of these patients.

Evaluation of nutrient intake is important for several reasons:

1. Patients with chronic disease and disability are the target of "quacks" who sell nutritional "cures." This can result in waste of precious economic resources for unproven, potentially harmful substances or combinations of nutrients.[9]
2. Food may be used as part of a behavioral modification program, leading to imbalances in the diet unperceived by the patient or caregiver unless based on sound nutritional principles.
3. Patients with disability are by definition at risk for nutritional problems.
4. Nutrient intake must be quantified if dietary recommendations are to be considered for modification as part of a therapeutic regimen.

In reviewing the literature on studies of food intake in the disabled, it is important to keep in mind that the standards with which they are compared are taken primarily from the RDAs or some equivalent, thus being subject to the concerns discussed previously.

The food/nutrient intake of children with disabilities has been studied extensively. Although the methods of study have varied, the information seems to be valid because of similarities in the findings among studies. Of major importance is the finding that food/nutrient intake varies widely. Some children appear to have adequate diets; others appear to have poor diets. The reason for the poor diets is sometimes due to the disability or to associated feeding difficulties.[19, 67] However, factors such as family income,[19] the level of education of parents,[67] and the quality of the food offered to children residing in institutions[9] are also quite significant in determining the adequacy of food/nutrient intake. Other factors that have been shown to affect diet quality include the level of supplements in the diet[18,67] and the level of salty, high fat, and sweet foods consumed.[18] Thus, it seems that besides the effect of mechanical feeding problems, the factors associated with poor dietary habits are no different than those in able-bodied children.[90]

Dietary surveys of adults with disability have demonstrated wide individual variations in both calorie and nutrient intake.[5,80,120,125] There are reports of a relative decrease in caloric intake in people with physically disabling chronic illness[77,152] and increased caloric intake in adults with mental retardation.[70] In patients with amyotrophic lateral sclerosis, it has been shown that the adequacy of the diet was poorer in those with more severe swallowing problems.[152] Litchford and Wakefield[101] identified a strong correlation between the nutrition knowledge of caregivers and the adequacy of the diet of adults disabled by mental retardation. Dysgeusia has also been shown to be a critical factor in the adequacy of diets.[106]

The results of multiple dietary surveys of the elderly are summarized by Bowman and Rosenberg.[17] Average energy intakes are below two-thirds of the RDAs, but less than 10% have intakes of calcium, iron, vitamin A, and water-soluble vitamins below two-thirds of the RDAs. In a study of elderly veterans, it was shown that dietary adequacy was correlated with the self-perception of chewing problems to a greater extent than with clinically determined dental status or the degree of social isolation.[66]

Historical dietary information shows a wide variation of nutrient intake in the groups studied. Factors such as food supply, financial resources, and nutritional knowledge of caregivers have a significant impact on nutrient intake. Thus, the presence of a physical/mental disability alone does not result in poor dietary habits. Multiple factors beyond a person's physical/mental ability affect the consumption of food and thus his or her nutritional status.

Clinical Evaluation of Nutritional Status

The value of the clinical history and examination in identifying people with malnutrition should not be overlooked. Baker and co-workers[4] clearly demonstrated this fact in their study of 59 general surgical patients, finding both a high level of agreement on classification of nutritional status between two examiners and a high correlation of the results of clinical assessment with more objective measures. Because of the lack of standards for objective measures in much of the disabled population, it seems that careful clinical evaluation for indicators of malnutrition is certainly a reasonable and necessary place to focus our attention. Certainly clinical evaluation should be a part of all nutritional assessment and monitoring because of the ease of gathering such information and the fact that no particular equipment is required for its successful application.

Historical Information

Much information about nutritional status can be gained from questions included in the general medical history. Of particular concern is information about a change in body weight (especially if this was not the result of specific dietary intervention), change in appetite or eating habits, change in activity level, change in gastrointestinal function, presence of acute or chronic medical-surgical problems, specific feeding or swallowing problems, and regular medication/supplement usage. A sample of such questions is presented in Figure 28-4. There are several examples of historical surveys in the literature, which either stand by themselves or are used in conjunction with objective data.[26,83,90,144] It is important to define the significance of several of these historical factors further in this section.

ACUTE OR CHRONIC ILLNESS. Acute and chronic illness may affect the nutritional status of patients, whether able bodied or

Figure 28-4. Historical information suggesting nutritional risk.

Check if answer to question is yes. Nutrition risk increases as the number of checks increases.

1. Are you on a special diet? _____
2. Have you had a change in your eating habits? _____
3. Has your weight changed? _____
4. Do you have any cravings or desires for specific food, liquid, or other substances to eat or drink? _____
5. Has your appetite changed? _____
6. Do you eat most of your food away from home? _____
7. Are you experiencing any of the following?
   a. Difficulty seeing at night? _____
   b. Dry skin or rashes? _____
   c. Nausea or vomiting? _____
   d. Constipation or diarrhea? _____
   e. Swelling of legs? _____
   f. Change in hair color, texture, or thickness (other than chemically or mechanically induced by hair care)? _____
   g. Yellow skin or eyes? _____
   h. Easy bruising? _____
   i. Swollen, tender joints? _____
   j. Poor healing of minor cuts or scratches? _____
8. Have you been ill or had surgery? _____
9. Are you taking any medicines or supplements? _____
10. Do you avoid any foods, liquids, or additives because of allergies or bad reactions? _____

disabled, by altering the metabolic activity of the body, changing the bioavailability of nutrients, changing body composition, and changing the activity level.[43, 55, 177]

There are some conditions that are seen more frequently in disabled people. When decubitus ulcers develop there is an increased loss of nutrients through the dead tissue and seepage of body fluids. There is no direct way of measuring the loss in the clinical setting, but common sense would dictate an increase in nutritional needs of healing. When edema is present, there is a relative increase in the extracellular water compartment of the body. This can affect electrolyte balance and the distribution of pharmaceutical agents. Respiratory tract and urinary tract infections are seen with a greater frequency. Energy requirements are increased as body temperature rises. The impact of infection on nutritional requirements is outlined in Table 28-4.

ENVIRONMENT. Climatic conditions, especially temperature extremes, can affect energy and fluid electrolyte balance.[55, 143] The potential of effects of new equipment and treatments on environmental factors cannot be overlooked. An example is the widely recognized increase in fluid requirements of patients on air-fluidized mattresses because of the drying effect of the equipment when in operation.

INTERMITTENT OR CONTINUOUS MEDICATION USAGE. Food intake, nutritional status, and efficacy of pharmaceutical agents are all intimately interrelated. The effects of food/nutrient intake on drug therapy result from alterations in absorption, metabolism, and/or excretion of drugs. Additionally, drugs can affect nutritional status by their effect on appetite, gastrointestinal function, psychological state, and renal and/or hepatic metabolism.[3, 135] It is important to keep this intimate interrelationship in mind when working with the disabled patient, regardless of the state of nutrition.

The effect of any drug on appetite or nutrient absorption may mean the difference between adequate nutrition and malnutrition in the person who has marginal nutritional status. Therefore, it is important to be familiar with the drug–nutrient interactions and use this information in planning therapy for disabled patients with the intention of optimizing, not jeopardizing, nutritional status. (When is is possible to choose between two drugs, consider using the one with the least adverse effect on nutritional status whenever this information is available.) If there are known drug–nutrient interactions, this information can be obtained most easily from the pharmacist or registered dietitian. The other easily accessible sources of information are the various forms of drug literature, such as the *Physicians' Desk Reference* or

---

Table 28-4
Effects of Infection on Nutrient Requirements

1. Nutrient losses: Most nutrients, especially intracellular minerals and nitrogen. Exception is retention of water and salt, after initial losses.
2. Increased metabolic rate from fever
3. Decreased food intake secondary to anorexia
4. Functional nutrient loss, secondary to overuse, diversion, and sequestration of nutrients
5. Hypermetabolism and accelerated use of cellular energy with phagocytosis

(Beisel WR: Infectious diseases. In Schneider HA, Anderson CE, Coursin DB [eds]: Nutritional Support of Medical Practice, 2nd ed, pp 443–457. Philadelphia, JB Lippincott, 1983)

---

information sheets that accompany the drugs at the point of distribution. Additionally, information can be obtained from reference texts and journal articles. The astute clinician will always keep the possibility of drug–nutrient interactions in mind in day-to-day management of patients so that new or unrecognized interactions may be identified and reported. Information available on some drugs commonly used in the management of people with disability is presented in Table 28-5.

Physical Examination

Although one rarely encounters specific physical changes from isolated nutrient deficiencies in developed countries, there are abnormalities on the physical examination that should alert the physician to the potential for malnutrition. The physical consequences of specific nutrient deficiencies are most frequently seen in patients on long-term nutritional support with manufactured nutritional supplements or elemental formulations,[94] and the physiological manifestations of specific nutrient excesses have been identified in people who take large amounts of nutritional supplements.[142] Thus, an awareness of specific findings is important. These physical findings should be familiar to all members of the rehabilitation health care team. Some of these specific findings are given in Table 28-6.

Physical findings can reflect three different stages of the development of malnutrition. The integrity of body tissues with a rapid turnover, such as skin and mucous membranes, reflects the adequacy of recent nutritional support. The condition of body tissues that have developed over time, such as hair and nails, may reflect changes in nutritional status during variable growth periods. The proportions of body tissues that serve as reservoirs of nutrients, such as skeletal muscle and adipose tissue, reflect chronic nutritional status. Additionally, with severe malnutrition, one may find changes in the size and/or function of specific organ systems that can be observed on clinical examination and reflect malnutrition.

Determination of Energy Balance

Energy is necessary for all activities of life, including the internal work of metabolic processes for maintenance and repair of bodily tissues and external work done by the person on the environment. The optimal state of nutrition regarding energy in the stable person is one of equilibrium: the amount of energy ingested is equal to the amount of energy expended. In the person who is growing, either as part of the natural life cycle or as recovery from the loss of or injury to body tissue, energy balance must be positive: the amount of energy ingested is greater than the amount of energy expended. If insufficient energy is taken in to meet the internal demand of metabolic activity or the external demands for interaction with the environment there will be an energy deficit, and body tissues will be metabolized for transformation into energy. Conversely, with the consumption of excessive amounts of energy, beyond that needed for normal maintenance and/or growth, the substrate will be converted into extra body tissue, primarily adipose tissue.

The major sources of energy in the diet are carbohydrates, protein, and fat (Table 28-7). Ethanol is also a source of energy and may provide a substantial amount of calories in the diets of some people. The traditional unit for expression of energy content of foods and energy requirements is the kilocalorie. This is the amount of heat necessary to raise the temperature of 1 kg of water from 15°C to 16°C. The energy content of foods and nutrients has been determined through calorimetric techniques

Table 28-5
Examples of Potential Drug–Nutrient Interactions in the Disabled

Medication	Potential Effect on Nutritional Status	Potential Effect of Nutrition on Medication
Antispasticity Medications		
Diazepam	Weight gain	Increased sedation with ethanol
Baclofen	Nausea, constipation	Increased sedation with ethanol
	Transient increase in blood glucose	
Dantrolene sodium	Diarrhea, constipation, dysphagia, abdominal cramps, gastric irritation	
Anticonvulsant Medications		
Phenytoin	Decreased bone density	Increased rate of metabolism with ethanol, with folate supplement
	Decreased serum folate, vitamin B_{12}, pyridoxine, vitamin D, calcium	
	Increased serum copper	
	Associated with megaloblastic anemia and peripheral neuropathy	
Phenobarbital	Decreased serum folate, vitamin B_{12}, pyridoxine, vitamin D, calcium	Increased rate of metabolism with ethanol
	Decreased bone density	Food decreased effectiveness of absorption
	Decreased red blood cell folate	
Tricyclic Antidepressants	Alters appetite, taste, diarrhea, epigastric distress, dry mouth, weight change	
Didronel	Decreased serum phosphate, diarrhea, nausea	Food decreases absorption; should not be taken within 2 hours of a meal
Bisacodyl		Tablets should not be taken within 1 hour of consuming antacids or milk.
Metamucil		Taken with plenty of liquid
Docusate sodium	Bitter taste of liquid may irritate throat or cause nausea	
Coumadin		Vitamin K supplements may decrease effectiveness of given dose.

(Data from references 3, 74, 104, 135, and individual product information)

Table 28-6
Physical Findings Indicative of Malnutrition

Body System	Clinical Findings	Possible Nutritional Causes
Hair	Lack of natural shine; dull dry, sparse, loss of curl, dyspigmentation, easily plucked	Protein–calorie Malnutrition; often multiple nutrient deficiencies
Face	Malar and supraorbital increased pigment; nasolabial seborrhea	Low calories, B-complex vitamin deficiencies, especially niacin, riboflavin, and pyridoxine
	Edema	Protein deficiency
	Pallor	Iron deficiency, general undernutrition
Eyes	Pale conjunctivae	Iron deficiency
	Bitot's spots, conjunctival and corneal xerosis, keratomalacia, exophthalmus	Vitamin A deficiency
	Angular palpebritis	Niacin, riboflavin, and/or pyridoxine deficiency
	Blepharitis	B-complex vitamin deficiency
	Ophthalmophlegia	Thiamine deficiency
Lips	Redness and swelling	Niacin or riboflavin deficiency
	Angular fissures and scars	B-complex or protein deficiency
Tongue	Red, raw and fissured, swollen (glossitis)	Folic acid, niacin, vitamin B_{12} or iron deficiency
	Magenta coloration	Riboflavin deficiency

(Continued)

Table 28-6 *(Continued)*

Body System	Clinical Findings	Possible Nutritional Causes
Tongue	Pale, atrophic	Iron deficiency
	Filiform papillary atrophy	Niacin folic acid, vitamin B_{12}, or iron deficiency
	Fungiform papillary hypertrophy	General undernutrition
Teeth	Carious or missing	Excess sugar
	Mottled enamel	Excess fluoride
Gums	Spongy, bleeding	Vitamin C deficiency
Glands	Thyroid enlargement	Iodine deficiency
	Parotid enlargement	General undernutrition, especially protein
Skin	Follicular hyperkeratosis	Vitamin A deficiency
	Xerosis with flaking	Vitamin A deficiency or excess, fatty acid deficiency
	Hyperpigmentation	Vitamin B_{12}, folic acid, or niacin deficiency
	Yellow coloration	Excess carotene
	Petechiae	Vitamin C deficiency
	Pellagrous dermatitis	Niacin or tryptophan deficiency
	Scrotal or vulval dermatosis	Riboflavin deficiency
Nails	Spoon nails (koilonychia)	Iron deficiency
	Brittle nails	Iron deficiency, excess vitamin A
Musculoskeletal	Muscle wasting	Protein–calorie malnutrition
	Epiphyseal swelling; soft, thin infant skull, persistently open anterior fontanelle, knock knees or bowed legs	Vitamin D deficiency
	Beading of ribs	Vitamin D and calcium deficiency
	Subperiosteal bleeding	Vitamin C deficiency
Gastrointestinal	Hepatomegaly	Chronic malnutrition
	Hard small cirrhotic liver	Hemochromatosis
Nervous	Mental confusion and irritability	Chronic undernutrition, thiamine or niacin deficiency
	Sensory loss, loss of lower extremity deep tendon reflexes	Thiamine or vitamin B_{12} deficiency
	Ataxia	Vitamin B_{12} deficiency, pyridoxine excess
	Weakness, paresthesias of legs	Thiamine, pyridoxine, vitamin B_{12}, pantothenic acid deficiency
Cardiovascular	Cardiomegaly	Thiamine deficiency
	Congestive heart failure	Thiamine deficiency, hemo-chromatosis

(Adapted from Wellman NS: The evaluation of nutritional status. In Howard RB, Herbold NH [eds]: Nutrition in Clinical Care, 2nd ed, pp 387–388. New York: McGraw-Hill, 1982, and Butterworth CE Jr, Weinsier RL: Malnutrition in hospitalized patients: Assessment and treatment. In Goodhard RS, Shils ME [eds]: Modern Nutrition in Health and Disease, 6th ed, pp 667–684. Philadelphia, Lea & Febiger, 1980)

and is available for use in determining the energy value of the food consumed.[2, 127, 168]

Measures of Energy Expenditure

It is necessary to be able to have at least a reasonable estimate of the energy requirements of a given person in order to provide optimal energy sources in the diet and prevent the complications of insufficient or excessive energy intake. With the advent of successful methods of nutritional support and the recognition of the potential for deleterious effects from either overfeeding or underfeeding, the need for accuracy in determin-

ing energy requirements has been recognized. The level of accuracy required, however, is quite dependent on the clinical situation.

In a steady state, energy requirements can be determined by observing the change in body weight over time with the energy calculated to be present in the food consumed during that same period of time. If the person is losing weight, the energy intake (a known quantity calculated from food composition information) is less than that required to maintain weight. If there is weight gain during that time, the energy intake exceeds expenditure; and if weight is stable, energy requirement is known and equal to the energy in the food consumed. This approach is rather crude

Table 28-7
Sources of Energy in the Diet

	kcal/g (average)
Carbohydrates	
Monosaccharides	3.8
Polysaccharides	4.2
Protein	4.0
Fat	9.0
Ethanol	7.1

(Adapted from Silberman H, Eisenberg D: Evaluation of nutritional status. In Silberman H, Eisenberg D [eds]: Parenteral and Enteral Nutrition for the Hospitalized Patient, p 37. Norwalk, CT, Appleton-Century-Crofts, 1982)

but can be quite appropriate in establishing long-term dietary goals for a person who desires to maintain weight in the face of a sudden change in diet or the person who needs to change dietary habits to produce a change in body weight.

The above approach does not allow for the determination of significant day-to-day fluctuations in energy expenditure, which have been recognized to occur in patients during the immediate post-traumatic period.[140] Additionally, there is a failure to account for the fact that body weight can be altered significantly by variations in the state of hydration.

Direct calorimetry is the standard method for directly measuring heat loss from the body, thus determining energy expenditure. It requires that the patient be in an insulated chamber. The amount of heat given off directly is determined by temperature measures. Additionally, the heat removed by vaporization of water from the body surfaces is calculated from information obtained by measuring the amount of moisture added to the air in the chamber. This method is cumbersome and time consuming and thus is applicable only to laboratory research.[130, 150]

Techniques of indirect calorimetry allow the calculation of energy expenditure through the estimation of heat production from measures of gaseous exchange (oxygen consumed and/or carbon dioxide produced) during normal respiration.[130, 143] With the development of portable equipment for gaseous sampling and analysis, it is now possible to apply this technique clinically, as an aid to direct determination of energy expenditure in both the acutely ill patient and the patient with chronic disability, during rest and activity.[33, 41, 111, 140, 162]

Techniques for Estimation of Energy Requirements

It is also possible to estimate the energy requirement of an individual. Very crude estimates can be made from standards such as those of the Joint FAO/WHO/UNU Expert Consultation.[89] The value of estimates such as these is primarily in working with patients who are in a steady-state condition.

For care of the acutely ill patient, more specific formulae, such as the Harris-Benedict equation, have been used to attempt to provide an accurate estimation of resting energy expenditure, with specific adjustments included to account for increased metabolic needs.[137, 150]

Formulae have been widely used as the basis for estimating the energy needs of disabled people, both acutely after injury[52, 92] and at later stages in recovery.[5, 13, 120, 125] Critical assessments of these formulae have demonstrated a significant variation from actual energy expenditure, as determined by direct measures.[38, 150] Studies have demonstrated the errors in the calcula-

tion of energy requirements using such formulae in the acute stages of conditions such as spinal cord injury,[93] head injury,[33, 41] and burns.[140, 163] Cox and colleagues[35] have demonstrated the inaccuracy of the use of several formulae for estimating the energy expenditure in stable patients with remote spinal cord injury.

Thus, it seems appropriate to recommend the use of indirect calorimetry measures in the acute stages of disorders associated with disability whenever this technique is available. Because of expense and time considerations, it would be impractical to recommend the application of indirect calorimetry to the routine care of patients in the chronic stages of disability. Estimations based on calculations from specific formulae, however, must be recognized as giving only rough estimates of caloric requirements. When nutritional assessment or nutrition support recommendations are based on such information, subjects need close observation, with adjustments as indicated by both subjective and objective clinical parameters. For research purposes, the use of indirect calorimetry is necessary for accuracy in determinations of energy expenditures in the more stable chronic stages of disability as well as the acute stages.

For the assessment of energy needs in stable disabled children, it is important to consider requirements for normal growth, in addition to all other requirements. Energy requirements to support growth have been found to be related to both height and mobility status, more than the presence or absence of motor dysfunction *per se.*[36]

Alterations in Energy Expenditure With Disability

Energy expenditure varies with the effects of multiple factors, including body size, body composition, activity level, environmental conditions, presence of illness or injury, and medication usage, on metabolic activity and with body temperature and amount of specific types of body tissues.[55, 143]

One frequently sees a reference to amount of energy per kilogram of body mass or per centimeter of height. With the onset of disability, there may be a sudden, dramatic change in body size, such as in the traumatic amputee, or a slower, more insidious alteration in body composition, such as the alterations seen after spinal cord injury. There are theoretically two stages during which the effect of altered body size must be factored into the estimation of energy requirements in the disabled: (1) the time period during which the body is undergoing physiological adaptation to the disabling condition and thus overall body size is undergoing change and (2) the time period after physiological adaptation when body size is theoretically stabilized. In disabled children the nutritional needs for normal growth must also be factored in during both of the above two periods.

The onset of disability changes the level of activity of the body, metabolically and physically. After acute trauma, either from intrinsic causes (*e.g.,* intracranial hemorrhage from a ruptured aneurysm or gangrene of the leg from a clot in the popliteal artery) or from extrinsic causes (*e.g.,* head injury from a fall or gunshot or traumatic amputation from an accident with a power saw), there is an increase in metabolic requirements from a stress reaction of the body. This is a time of catabolism, which may not be entirely reversible even with the best nutritional support.[23, 41, 75, 95, 96, 162, 174] Thus, it may be impossible to achieve a condition of energy balance.

After the stage of acute injury has passed there is a period of adaptation during which there may be further adjustments of energy consumption and metabolic rate; this adaptation is followed by a period of relative stability when the steady-state of body composition and activity has been achieved.[9, 35, 71, 78, 124]

Disabled persons, as well as their healthy cohorts, have variable levels of activity. Even persons with the same disability, such as a high level of cervical injury resulting in complete quadriplegia, and total dependence on extrinsic assistance for all activities of daily living, mechanical or physical, will have a variable level of activity depending on whether spasticity exists and is controlled. In children with cerebral palsy the presence of spasticity will inhibit purposeful activity and therefore produce a relative decrease in activity, whereas the athetoid forms result in higher activity levels.[11, 36, 50]

A paraplegic who is able to walk with crutches and/or orthoses will have a far different level of activity than one who depends entirely on a wheelchair for mobility. The energy expenditure with a given activity may even vary with the type of orthosis used.[111]

Evaluation of Body Composition

Knowledge of body composition is important both as a measure of nutritional status (is it optimal or not?) and as a basis on which to estimate nutrient and caloric needs (energy and nutrient requirements to maintain lean body mass are greater per kilogram of tissue than are the requirements to maintain adipose tissue mass). Major divisions of the body include lean body mass, intracellular fluid, extracellular fluid, and body fat. Body composition at the chemical level is also of interest but related to the relative proportions of major body divisions.

Anthropometric Measures

Measures of body size, weight, and proportions are all anthropometric techniques that are useful in assessing and following nutritional status. The most widely recognized measures are those of height and weight. (The need for routine measuring and recording of this information must be stressed.) Other anthropometric techniques include skinfold thickness measures, from which one can calculate estimates of total body fat stores; bony measures, such as elbow breadth to estimate "frame size" and skeletal mass; and limb circumference, which can be combined in a formula with skinfold thickness to yield an estimate of muscle mass. These techniques allow caregivers to obtain objective measures with relatively simple, low-risk, noninvasive techniques. However, because of the deceptive simplicity of these measures, there is real potential for erroneous data collection. Well-trained examiners, who pay meticulous attention to anatomical detail and use the same equipment for repetitive data collection, are necessary for the collection of reliable, valid information.[45, 133, 172]

The information gained from anthropometric measures can be used in the nutritional management of patients in two ways:

1. It can provide the basis for comparison of a person with a group normal standard, classifying a person as to his or her relative position within a group. (Patient A weighs less than the average adult of the same sex and height.)
2. It can provide baseline information from which to monitor change over time, and thus the effectiveness of nutritional intervention or nutritional maintenance. (Patient A has gained 2 pounds in the past month.)

When these data are used as a measure reflecting nutritional status at a given time, it is important that the measured values are compared with norms derived from an equivalent population group.[58, 130, 170] There is a dearth of normative data for people with disability, resulting in the primary difficulty in estimating nutritional status of a given disabled person from anthropometric information obtained at a single time. If these data are used alone, only gross departures from the norm are of any meaning, and these levels of variation are usually quite apparent by clinical observation alone.[4, 130, 170] Anthropometric measures will fluctuate on a daily basis relative to hydration status as much or more so than as a reflection of general nutritional status or total amount of body tissue, lean or adipose. Height, when measured in a standing person, varies with posture and hydration status of the intervertebral disk spaces. For many disabled people, it is necessary to determine height in the supine position. In the case of a person with lower extremity amputations, height cannot be accurately determined. Other standards, which have not yet been developed, must be used for this group of people.

With the use of anthropometric measures, it is theoretically possible to estimate the size of specific body compartments, such as skeletal muscle mass and subcutaneous fat tissue. However, the formulae for extrapolation are less than perfect and have been derived from information gained from studies of physiologically normal people.[45, 88] Thus, present information is insufficient to extrapolate this type of information to body compartment size in many people with disability. The most useful current application of anthropometric data gathered at one time is to provide a basis for a rough estimation of caloric and nutrient needs from height and weight data.

The value of anthropometric studies in providing quantitative data for longitudinal follow-up of patients and a monitor of the effectiveness of nutritional intervention is much greater. However, until normative data are collected, the nutritional significance of such changes in disabled patients will not be known. Additionally, one must recognize potential sources of error when interpreting this information. This can best be accomplished by understanding the factors that affect anthropometric measures. Changes in body weight with time will reflect hydration status and/or total body tissue mass. Edema secondary to venous stasis and/or hypoalbuminemia can result in falsely increased skinfold thickness and limb girth measures. Conversely, relative dehydration may falsely decrease these values. If myositis ossificans has developed, there may be changes in the anthropometric measures as well. If these variables can be controlled, repetitive measures can be of value in assessing changes in subcutaneous fatty tissue and skeletal muscle mass.

Another variable to consider is the physiological response to neurological damage. One would expect decreased muscle mass in a paralyzed flaccid limb. One would also expect the muscle mass to increase in normal limbs that are compensating for the loss of function in a damaged limb. There is a need for serial studies in the disabled population to establish normative data to see if these expectations during successful recovery are correct. This would provide the baseline information necessary for successful application of the use of anthropometric techniques in nutritional assessment and management of the disabled.

Alterations in Anthropometric Measures in the Disabled

It is apparent that, in general, children with severe developmental disabilities are of a shorter stature than their able-bodied counterparts.[18, 36, 67] However, there are significant proportions of disabled children at both extremes of the weight-for-height norms.

Although there is usually an initial weight loss in adults after spinal cord injury, patients stabilize at a variety of weights, some over and some under predicted weights from normative data.[5, 35, 71, 112, 125] Pierce and Nickel[129] suggest that the guidelines for recommended weight be 10 to 15 pounds below ideal body weight for paraplegics and 15 to 20 pounds below ideal body weight for quadriplegics when compared with the 1959 Metropolitan Life Tables. Others have recommended that spinal cord–injured patients who weigh less than 10% below the mean of ideal body weight be considered at risk for undernutrition.[112, 125] Reduced weight below these suggested levels has not been related to changes in functional outcome. Thus, the specific recommended levels of weight for height for patients after spinal cord injury for optimal nutritional status have yet to be established.

Relative weights have been reported in other studies of disabled adults as well. Green and McIntosh[70] found 48% of mentally retarded adults in a small survey (21 subjects) to be overweight. Five of 20 outpatients with amyotropic lateral sclerosis were found to have lost more than 10% of usual body weight and therefore were considered to be underweight.[152]

When growth is the goal, increased height can reflect this. For the assessment of growth in disabled children, it is recommended that the goal be to maintain growth within the percentile that the child falls into initially, if initial nutritional status is judged to be adequate.[149] This information can be recorded graphically, allowing for easy monitoring of goal attainment.

Anthropometric data are basically of no value in patients with large burns, and other measures must be chosen.[140]

Thus, the value of anthropometry in assessing and monitoring nutritional status of disabled patient is quite limited at the present time. It is anticipated that the clinical value will increase through the collection of normative data.

Other Methods for Determination of Body Composition

Through the use of standard and innovative techniques to determine body composition, the general effects of some chronic illnesses on body composition are being elucidated. There are some excellent examples of this work in the areas of oncology and nephrology.[78, 124, 148]

Standard laboratory techniques for estimation of body composition include measures of body density by underwater weighing, estimates of specific body compartment sizes by multiple isotope dilution techniques, radiographic estimates of fatty tissue layers and bony sizes, creatinine–height index, and whole-body liquid scintillation counting to determine total body potassium content.[15, 57, 68, 130, 158] Newer techniques for the study of body composition include the use of ultrasound and computed tomographic scanners to determine sizes of specific body tissue layers and organs.[78] Other techniques being assessed at present include infrared interactance[34] and dual-photon absorptiometry.[108]

The optimal body composition for the disabled person has not yet been defined. Specific information will be quite elusive because of the multitude of disabling conditions seen today and the extreme variability in the way a specific disability will affect any one person. However, standard techniques, such as those mentioned previously, have been applied to a limited extent in the evaluation of disabled children[10] and adults with spinal cord injury.[25, 27, 71, 97] These studies have shown the following:

1. There is generally a depletion in lean body mass.
2. There is a tendency toward an increased proportion of body fat.
3. There is an increase in total body fluid.
4. There is a high degree of intersubject variability.

To summarize, the physiological adaptation to disability includes an alteration in the proportion of body tissue compartments from that known to exist in able-bodied people. The need for further study to clarify the effects of disability on body compartment size is great.

Initially, the time course of normal physiological adaptation to disability and its impact on body composition must be determined. It is necessary to identify both the extent of body composition changes and the time course for moving from the changing adaptive state to a steady-state of chronic physiological adaptation. This would allow for more precise application of nutrition support. It would also allow for a more intense focus of nutritional assessment and nutritional support needs on the patients with continually changing requirements during the time of physiological adaptation to the disability.

Additionally, the effect of altered body composition on the significance of biochemical measures of organ function must be recognized. The most obvious, yet frequently overlooked, example is the mistaken impression that the serum creatinine value reflects renal function in a patient with greatly decreased skeletal muscle mass, such as the patient who has a high-level flaccid quadriplegia or who has sustained bilateral high above-knee amputations. When muscle mass is decreased below a relative level there is insufficient creatinine produced to raise the serum creatinine value in levels proportional to the impairment of renal function. Creatinine clearance measures are necessary to assess renal function in patients with greatly reduced skeletal muscle mass.

It is also important to recognize the potential for altered physiological activity of pharmaceutical agents with changes in body composition. Some drugs are distributed throughout the total body water space; others are stored in fatty tissue. Both the half-life of the drug and the effective serum levels may be affected by changes in body composition. Thus, in some instances, it may be necessary to monitor serum drug levels more closely and adjust dosage according to clinically observed effects or signs of toxicity in the patient with disability.

Objective Biochemical and Physiological Measures of Nutritional Status

Biochemical and physiological measures of nutritional status can provide two types of information, static or functional.[156] The most widely accepted diagnostic tools are in the category of static measures, which quantify the amount of a given nutrient, metabolite of the nutrient, or nutrient-specific carrier protein in body fluids or tissues. There are many limitations to the successful application of this information to nutritional status evaluation of a person, whether able bodied or disabled (Table 28-8).

Recognition of such limitations has resulted in a growing interest in developing functional measures of nutritional status, which are tests of performance (biochemical, physiological, or behavioral) that can be objectively measured and vary with alterations of nutritional status. Since optimal biological function is the goal of the application of the principles of nutrition to the care and management of patients, functional measures of nutritional status appear to provide the most logical solution to the problems encountered in assessing nutritional status and monitoring the outcome of nutritional intervention.[154, 155, 165] The major advantage of the functional approach to nutritional assessment is the fact that the patient can serve as his or her own control. The measure of adequacy of nutritional status is a plateau of function, rather than a specific value. Therefore, whereas the adequacy of static indices depends on whether the values fall into a given "normal" range (usually average $+/-$ 2 SD), the function of a patient will tend to plateau when nutritional status is optimal and drop off in the face of either deficient or excessive amounts of any given nutrient that affects that function.

Table 28-8
*Pitfalls and Limitations of Static Indices in the Assessment
of Nutritional Status*

1. Samples may be subject to exogenous contamination.
2. Circulating nutrient levels may be homeostatically regulated and protected so that stores are depleted before circulating concentrations decline.
3. Circulating nutrient levels may be independently affected by infections, diseases, hormonal status, drugs, and other deficiency states.
4. Binding capacity for a nutrient (available binding sites on transport proteins) may determine circulating levels.
5. The index may reflect only recent intake of nutrient or precursor and not reflect stores.
6. Convenient biopsy material such as hair or blood cells may only represent active (target) tissue, while storage pools may be inaccessible for biopsy.
7. Interpretation can be obscured by "shotgun" therapy with the nutrient.

(Solomons NW: Assessment of nutritional status: Functional indicators of pediatric nutriture. Pediatr Clin North Am 32:319–334, 1985)

The remainder of this section will provide a brief discussion of some of the more widely used indices of nutritional status, both static and functional. There will also be a brief discussion of one of the newer functional measures being studied currently. There are some excellent reviews that can be used for gaining more information.[65, 128, 141, 154, 155, 165]

Static Measures

SERUM HEMOGLOBIN AND HEMATOCRIT. Serum hemoglobin and hematocrit values are routinely obtained for most patients, and normative standards are available. The presence of anemia may reflect a deficiency of iron, vitamin B_{12} or folic acid. Additionally, anemia may reflect a generalized state of protein–calorie malnutrition. Polycythemia may be the result of dehydration. However, nonnutritional factors that may cause abnormalities must be considered in assessing the nutritional significance of this information. Nonnutritional factors that may lead to anemia include blood loss, hemolysis, or bone marrow failure. All of these abnormalities may occur acutely or chronically. Polycythemia may be present as a result of the need for increased oxygen-carrying capacity, usually from chronic pulmonary disease or as the result of adaptation to reduced atmospheric oxygen pressure at high altitudes, or from hyperprolific disorders of the bone marrow.

PLASMA PROTEINS. Albumin. Albumin is the major protein in the plasma, functioning as a carrier of small molecules and as the major molecular agent of colloidal osmotic pressure. Low serum albumin has been recognized as an indicator of depleted visceral protein stores. However, the serum albumin value can also be altered by liver disorders, because it is manufactured in the liver, and by renal disease, because it can be wasted through urinary excretion in some types of renal disease. In the absence of liver or kidney disease, albumin has served best as an indicator of long-term nutritional status because its rate of turnover is low. Thus, it has not been of value in following nutritional support when weekly reassessments of nutritional status are necessary.

Other Plasma Proteins. There are other plasma proteins that reflect nutritional status changes more acutely because of rapid turnover, including transferrin, thyroxine-binding prealbumin, and retinol-binding protein. These levels are, however,

subject to fluctuation from metabolic changes in liver function as well. These proteins are sensitive to nutritional factors other than just protein status. Endocrine abnormalities may also affect the level of thyroxine-binding prealbumin.

TOTAL LYMPHOCYTE COUNT. The total lymphocyte count has been found to be correlated with nutritional status, with lower values reflecting poor nutrition. It can also be decreased in response to bone marrow failure from any reason.

SERUM LIPIDS. Measures of serum lipids, including cholesterol, triglycerides, and lipoproteins, are not usually included in the screening tests of acutely chronically ill patients for malnutrition. However, these factors should be assessed in any evaluation of nutritional status because abnormalities are associated with morbidity and mortality and dietary factors have been shown to be correlated with excessive levels in many cases. This information would be most useful at this point in helping the registered dietitian determine what proportions of calories in the diet should be provided by protein, carbohydrates, and fats and the types of fats and carbohydrates to include in the diet. Abnormalities may also be helpful in deciding how aggressively to pursue treatment of obesity in some patients.

Functional Measures of Nutritional Status

DELAYED HYPERSENSITIVITY. Testing for delayed hypersensitivity involves the ability of the immune system to mount an antigenic response to common antigens. Impairment has been shown to be associated with poor nutritional status, including protein–calorie malnutrition and trace mineral deficiencies.

PROTHROMBIN TIME. The prothrombin time is sensitive to vitamin K intake.

OTHER FUNCTIONAL TESTS. Numerous other biochemical and physiological tests have been used or are being considered for use in assessment and follow-up of nutritional status in situations of specific intervention (Table 28-9).

One type of physiological functional assessment technique that seems of particular interest is the application of measures of skeletal muscle function to the assessment of nutritional status. Both the force of contraction with rapid repetitive stimuli and the maximal relaxation rate of the abductor pollicis brevis were studied for this functional test. Suboptimal performance was found in malnourished patients with chronic renal failure.[12] In a small group of obese patients, skeletal muscle function became abnormal during a 2-week period of a very low calorie diet (400 kcal/day), persisting during an additional 2 weeks of fasting. Function returned to normal after a 2-week period of refeeding. Standard parameters of nutritional status including serum albumin and transferrin values, creatinine height index, anthropometric measures, and total body nitrogen and potassium levels did not change during this study.[139] Grip strength has been shown to be a more sensitive indicator of nutritional status in surgical patients than standard anthropometric measures or serum albumin.[84] These studies are good examples of the innovative thought going into solution of the problem of finding more useful objective indicators of nutritional status.

Nutrient Balance

The final concept or review in the discussion of nutritional assessment is that of balance. The theoretical basis of this con-

Table 28-9
Functional Tests That May Reflect Nutritional Status

System	Nutrients
Strucural integrity	
Erythrocyte fragility	Vitamin E, selenium
Capillary fragility	Vitamin C
Tensile strength of skin	Copper
Experimental wound healing	Zinc
Collagen accumulation in implant sponge	Zinc
Lipoprotein peroxidation	Vitamin E, selenium
Host Defense	
Leukocyte chemotaxis	Protein/Energy, zinc
Leukocyte phagocytic activity	Protein/Energy, iron
Leukocyte bacteriocidal capacity	Protein/Energy, iron, selenium
Leukocyte metabolism	Protein/Energy
Serum opsonic activity	Protein/Energy
White cell interferon production	Protein/Energy
Lymphocyte (T-cell) blastogenesis	Protein/Energy, zinc
Delayed cutaneous hypersensitivity	Protein/Energy, zinc
Rebuck skin window	Protein/Energy
Transport	
Intestinal absorption	
Iron	Iron
Cobalt	Iron
Plasma/tissue transport	
^{65}Zn uptake by erythrocyte	Zinc
^{75}Se uptake by erythrocyte	Selenium
Retinol relative-dose-response	Vitamin A
Post–glucose plasma chromium response	Chromium
Post–glucose urine chromium response	Chromium
Thyroid radioiodine uptake	Iodine
Hemostasis	
Prothrombin time	Vitamin K
Platelet aggregation	Vitamin E, zinc
Reproduction	
Sperm count	Energy, zinc
Nerve function	
Dark adaptation	Vitamin A, zinc
Color discrimination	Vitamin A
Central scotoma	Vitamin A
Olfactory acuity	Vitamins A and B_{12}, zinc
Taste acuity	Vitamin A, zinc
Nerve conduction	Protein/Energy, vitamins B_1, B_6, and B_{12}
Skin conductivity	Protein/Energy
Abducens nerve function	Vitamin B_1
Electroencephalography	Protein/Energy
Sleep pattern	Protein/Energy
Work capacity/hemodynamics	
Task performance/endurance	Protein/Energy, vitamins B_1, B_2, B_6, and iron
VO$_2$ max	Protein/Energy, iron
VO$_2$ submax	Protein/Energy, iron
Heart rate (cumulative)	Protein/Energy, iron
Vasopressor response	Vitamin C
Unclassified	
d-Uridine suppression test	Vitamin B_{12}, folic acid

(Solomons NW, Allen LH: The functional assessment of nutritional status: Principles, practice and potential. Nutr Rev 41:33–50, 1983)

cept is the assumption that the optimally nourished person is in a state of equilibrium, with the amount of nutrients used or lost in daily metabolic activity being replaced by nutrients in the diet. When a person is in a physiological stage of growth or tissue repair, it is necessary for the balance to become positive, with a greater amount of nutrients in than out. For healthy weight loss, it is necessary for energy balance to become negative (more energy used than consumed), but without loss of lean body mass, so other nutrients, such as protein, should remain in balance. Balance for any given nutrient fluctuates with time, but over a given time period, such as a day or week, one can assess the overall direction of balance for most nutrients, if desired.

Nitrogen Balance

Nitrogen balance reflects the equilibrium of the body as regards protein status and therefore provides useful information for monitoring the adequacy of nutritional support, especially in patients with high rates of metabolic activity and those requiring supplemental feedings. Without nutritional support, significant negative nitrogen balance will develop rapidly in the face of acute illness or trauma. It has generally been assumed that nitrogen balance must be positive for successful healing in the face of trauma.[95] However, the inability to totally reverse the catabolic response to massive trauma, even with aggressive nutritional support, is now recognized.[33, 96, 103, 177] Nutritional support, even if positive nitrogen balance is not achieved acutely, has been shown to improve outcome after severe trauma.[87] There is a need for further research in this area, because excessive amounts of protein (or amino acids) in the diet increase the metabolic work of digestion, since these compounds are metabolized in the liver. Patients, already in a hypermetabolic state from severe trauma, do not need this additional metabolic burden of protein or amino acid intake greater than necessary to protein specific functions.

The determination of nitrogen balance is theoretically simple. One measures the nitrogen content of the diet and any supplements, the nitrogen content of any material lost from the body (*e.g.,* via urine and feces), and determines the difference between intake and output. Measures of nitrogen intake can be accurately determined in the hospital setting for patients on total enteral or parenteral feedings because the amount of substrate administered and its protein or nitrogen content are known. However, if one recalls all the factors affecting the accuracy of dietary surveys, the difficulty in obtaining accurate quantities of dietary nitrogen for patients eating regular meals becomes apparent. Accurate determination of nitrogen losses is a much more difficult problem. The most easily measured, largest source of nitrogen loss is that excreted in the urine. Thus, nitrogen balance studies require accurate, complete 24-hour urine collections. The urinary urea nitrogen value is generally measured and a correction factor applied for non–urea nitrogen. Clifton and co-workers[33] have demonstrated that use of a standard correction factor may underestimate total urinary nitrogen excretion when a major catabolic insult (*e.g.,* severe head injury) has occurred; therefore, accuracy in such cases requires the determination of non–urea nitrogen in the urine also. Additional estimates are generally used for approximation of the non–urea nitrogen losses in feces and skin. However, in the patient with a protein-losing enteropathy, use of such formulae will greatly underestimate the total protein lost. In patients with burns, decubitus ulcers or abscesses there is no accurate way to measure the protein and nitrogen loss secondary to fluid exudate or necrotic tissue sloughs. Therefore, the application of accurate nitrogen balance studies to routine nutritional monitoring is still limited.

Fluid Balance

Fluid balance is generally monitored in the acute hospital setting by measuring fluid intake and urine output. The need to adjust intake to exceed urine output at greater amounts is usually recognized in the presence of diarrhea, vomiting, or fever.

There has been little study of the effect of disability on the insensible water loss (the water lost through perspiration and evaporation from the skin). Kuhlemeier and colleagues[97] reported that the insensible water loss in paraplegics was within the range of that for normal adults but that quadriplegics had a significantly lower amount of insensible water loss than normal adults. Although this study involved only 24 subjects, it demonstrates the need for further investigation of this topic.

Electrolyte Balance

There is an excellent series of articles by Claus-Walker and Halstead in which they review the information in the literature on metabolic response to spinal cord injury, including electrolyte balance.[27–31] Some of the findings include a negative fluid balance in the initial 3 to 4 weeks after injury and a relative depletion of exchangeable potassium ions and relative excess of exchangeable sodium ions. Urine sodium losses are decreased in quadriplegics, and in the acute stages of injury the response of urine sodium and potassium excretion to a low sodium intake or thiazide diuretics is blunted. There is an increase of skin and bone collagen metabolism, accompanied by increased urinary losses of bone minerals during the acute period after spinal cord injury, accompanied by hyperphosphatemia and hypermagnesemia, but only rarely is hypercalcemia seen. Calcium balance is negative in the acute period of spinal cord injury. Obviously there is a need for further information of this nature in the spinal cord–injured patient and those with other disabilities.

MANAGEMENT OF FEEDING PROBLEMS

To achieve and maintain optimal nutritional status in the disabled person it is necessary to address the multiple factors related to the act of food consumption, as well as the previously discussed issues of nutrient requirements and nutritional status assessment.

Factors Influencing Successful Oral Feeding

When a person with a disability loses previous independence in selecting and preparing food, there is a loss of control over a significant factor in daily living. Part of the rehabilitation process involves working toward achieving the maximal level of independence in those living skills that the person is capable of through the application of available physical, emotional, and economic support. This level is dependent on many factors, which vary considerably with each patient. Through the availability of adapted transportation and accessible shopping facilities, adaptations of the kitchen and utensils, and careful selection of prepared and/or packaged foods to simplify preparation, it can be possible for disabled people to recover independence in these activities to some extent. However, a significant percentage of disabled people remain dependent on others for these functions, whether living independently or in an institution.

The loss of food choices may adversely affect the appetite or may lead to the development of food as an object of a power struggle, rather than a basic need for health. The development of problems such as these that interfere with optimal nutrition can be discouraged by allowing the disabled person to have a choice in food selection or preparation whenever possible. If an attendant will be required after discharge from an institution, it is important that the caregiver, as well as the disabled person, be included in discharge planning and discharge education. The support staff responsible for feeding patients in institutions need to understand basic principles of nutrition to maintain optimal nutrient intake in disabled patients. The correlation of nutritional status of dependent subjects with the nutrition knowledge and resources of the family has been documented.[19, 67] Likewise, the nutritional status of disabled patients living in institutions has been shown to be dependent to some extent on the nutrition knowledge of the staff.[101]

The loss of the ability to feed oneself is frequently a critical determinant in the potential for a semi-independent or independent existence. Thus, when loss of physical capacity of the upper extremities develops, it is important to look carefully at the deficit and determine whether an assistive device can reestablish independence for that patient. An analysis of motions of the upper extremity necessary for self-feeding is provided in Table 28-10. It also includes a list of adaptive devices to be considered in overcoming any particular problem. Through the advances of environmental control systems, high technology electronics can also be used to solve individual feeding problems for the severely handicapped.

Proper oral function for successful feeding is a truly complex process that requires integrity of anatomical structures and appropriate control of oral musculature. Attention to positioning and posture of the entire body may be necessary to control or use uninhibited reflex posturing to improve oral function or swallowing. Therefore, the assessment of oral functions in the disabled patient requires a comprehensive evaluation of body position, presence of primitive reflexes, consistency of dietary substances, and length of feeding time. It is very difficult to integrate all this information into an objective scale of oral function, but this has been done quite nicely by Stratton.[156] Her instrument allows for a quantifiable objective assessment of the multiple factors for contributing to successful oral feeding and allows for the collection of measurable data over time to assess the effect of alterations in any one of these factors on oral function.

There are multiple sources of additional information on this topic.[60, 82, 102, 172] For successful application of this information to the feeding of a disabled patient, it is crucial to keep three basic facts in mind:

1. Feeding management systems are only as successful as their acceptance by those who must use them on a day-to-day basis: the disabled person and, when involved, family members, the personal care attendant, or institution staff. The perception of a feeding problem by these key individuals is a crucial factor to developing a workable solution.[66]
2. The economic, social, and psychological status of the disabled person must be given equal consideration to the physical or cognitive disabilities present. An expensive, high-tech, electronic feeding device may be essential to giving a disabled person the independence necessary to return to work and may be affordable because of the potential earnings of that person. However, for a disabled person who lives alone without outside activities, personal assistance at meal times may provide an opportunity for socialization that is essential to maintenance of optimal psychological health.
3. Solutions should optimize the use of existing resources.

Table 28-10
Motions of the Upper Extremity Necessary for Self-Feeding

Body Part	Motion	Purpose	Substitution	Loss	Device Used to Compensate
Hand	Pick up: palmar prehension	Pick up and	1. Lacing spoon between fingers	Minimal	1. Utensil interlaced in fingers (some shaping may be necessary)
			2. Adduction of fingers		2. Moleskin or tape over handle to prevent slipping
	Holding: lateral prehension to middle finger (modified lateral pinch)	hold utensil	3. Hook grasp	Moderate	3. Built-up handle (wood, sponge, or other material)
					4. Grip-shaped handles
					5. Handle with horizontal and vertical dowels (pegged handle)
					6. Handle with finger rings
				Severe	7. Warm Springs type short opponens with C-bar and utensil attachment
					8. Plastic and metal holder
				Complete	9. ADL (universal) cuff
					10. Prehension orthosis
					• Manually operated
					• Power operated
Wrist	Stabilization (slight flexion and extension of radial and ulnar deviation normally used depending on whether grasp is hook or pinch)	Positioning of hand for optimal function (to prevent wrist flexion)	1. Use of finger or thumb extensors	Partial stability	1. ADL wrist support, dorsal (leather with spring steel insert)
					2. Flexible, adjustable nylon wrist support or Klenzac joints
				Complete	3. Tubular spring-clip (ADL) orthosis
					4. Cock-up splint, rigid palmar
					5. Warm Springs type long opponens
Forearm	Pronation	Pick up food on utensil	1. Shoulder abduction and internal rotation	Partial or complete	1. Swivel spoon
			2. Raise forearm to vertical position and then rotate		2. Bent fork or spoon
	Supination	Keep utensil level while putting food in mouth to avoid spill	3. Shoulder adduction and exernal rotation		1. Swivel spoon
					2. Placing fork or spoon over thumb, use thumb extensors
Elbow	Flexion of forearm	Raising hand to mouth	1. Use of knee	Partial or complete	1. Balanced forearm orthosis (ball bearing feeder)
			2. Shoulder abduction		2. Overhead sling with "feeder" attachment
			3. Trunk flexion		3. Overhead sling with built-up lapboard
	Extension	Lowering hand to plate	4. Rock forearm on edge of table		4. Long-handled utensil
					5. Functional arm orthosis
Shoulder	Stabilization against hyperextension and internal rotation in position of • Slight flexion • Slight abduction plus slight active active flexion and extension	Provides positioning and assists in raising hand to level of mouth	1. Trunk flexion	Partial or complete	1. Pillow behind upper arm
			2. Prop elbow on table		2. Overhead sling
					3. Balanced forearm orthosis
					4. Functional arm orthosis hyperextension stop

(Zimmerman ME: Activities of daily living. In Willard HS, Spackman GS [eds]: Occupational Therapy, 4th ed, p 228. Philadelphia, JB Lippincott, 1971)

Alternate Feeding Routes

Patients who are unable to take sufficient nutrition by oral feeding require nutritional support by an alternative route, either enteral or parenteral, or a combination of both.[150, 159] The reasons are generally physiological, but psychological factors may be contributory to the decision to use an alternative feeding route. The major purposes for the delivery of nutrients through alternate feeding routes include supplementation, which provides part of nutritional requirements via the alternate route; alimentation, which provides the entire basic requirement of nutrients via the alternate route; and hyperalimentation, which provides nutrients in excess of usual demands via the alternate route. Alternate feeding routes may be used to prevent the development of malnutrition in a patient with a severe feeding disturbance or with a massive increase in nutritional requirements or to restore the person to a state of balanced nutrition.

There are several reports of the benefits of using alternate feeding routes in patients who are acutely disabled as the result of burns or trauma.[33, 46, 52, 96, 132, 162, 164] There are only sporadic reports of the effectiveness of alternate feeding routes in promoting optimal nutritional status in patients who have entered the chronic or recovery stage of disabling injury.[13, 119]

There are risks as well as benefits from the use of alternate feeding routes. Foremost, one must realize that the use of an alternative feeding route, enteral or parenteral, bypasses the homeostatic control mechanisms of the body that regulate food and fluid intake. Therefore, objective monitors must be used routinely to assess the adequacy of nutritional support because of the high risk of overfeeding or underfeeding.[103] This monitoring should include gross observations, such as daily records of intake and output, frequent checking of weight, and monitoring of vital signs. Additionally, nitrogen balance, serum electrolyte and glucose levels, and liver and kidney function may need to be evaluated regularly.

The decision for use of, and specific types of, alternate feeding routes is multifactorial, including the needs of the patient and the capacity of the health care delivery system. The value of an in-house nutrition support team, as well as nutrition support manuals, cannot be stressed too strongly. These resources allow for the implementation of specific guidelines and protocols for the provision and maintenance of nutrition support through alternative feeding methods, based on the strengths and resources of the particular institution. Many communities now have access to nutritional support teams for patients who require the use of alternate feeding routes after hospital discharge. These resources should be used and if not present should be developed if alternate feeding routes are used at all in hospital or at home. The team approach greatly enhances the success of utilization of this technology, while decreasing the complications. Further information on this topic can be found elsewhere.[39, 94–96, 103, 110, 114, 136, 138, 150, 159, 169, 178]

Enteral Feeding

Enteral feeding uses the gastrointestinal tract for site of food intake but bypasses any proximal obstacles to feeding that might exist and delivers blenderized food, liquid nutritional supplements, or elemental nutrient solution to either the stomach or the small intestine. Enteral routes include nasogastric, nasoenteric, esophagogastric, gastrostomy, and jejunostomy. Enteral feeding is indicated when there is sufficient gastrointestinal function for safe administration and absorption of dietary substances but oral feeding is impossible or when there is an inability to move food through proximal structures of the gastrointestinal tract despite normal oral function.[114, 136, 145, 167] In general, enteral feeding is the least expensive alternate feeding route, has lower risks of complications from access or induced metabolic abnormalities, and provides the most physiological alternate feeding route.

The primary unique risk for tube feedings that deliver substrate to the stomach is aspiration. When there is a depressed gag reflex and/or impaired swallowing, there is no natural protective mechanism to prevent aspiration pneumonia if there is gastroesophageal reflux or misplacement of the tube such that it lies more proximal than intended (*i.e.,* in the esophagus or pharynx).

The direct gastrostomy or jejunostomy routes are considered most desirable when it is anticipated that tube feedings will continue for several weeks or more. These routes are also more cosmetically acceptable than routes with nasal access. Because of the slight risk from sedation or anesthesia in their placement, techniques have been developed for percutaneous placement of small-bore tubes.[62, 110, 173] The advantages of this type of insertion include the ability to start feeding less than 24 hours after surgery and avoidance of the risk of general anesthesia. Large-bore tubes placed surgically, with the creation of a permanent stoma, have the advantage of being easily inserted and removed so that the tube only needs to be in place during meal time, such as the Janeway gastrostomy and the esophagogastrostomy procedures.[109, 110] Placement of the tube via jejunostomy minimizes the risk of aspiration. The disadvantages of more distal placement of the feeding tubes are related to the decreased absorptive capacity of the remaining gut, including less tolerance of high osmolar loads and altered absorption of some pharmaceutical agents and nutrients.

The rate of administration may be intermittent bolus or continuous drip and should be established based on consideration of the needs and tolerance of the patient and the staffing and equipment support available. Administration of tube feedings by continuous drip requires a mechanical pump to control flow rate. This apparatus may interfere with therapeutic activities of the patient in a rehabilitation setting. Activity tolerance may be limited by the physiological response to a full stomach. Bolus feedings can be problematic because of limited gastric capacity and delayed gastric emptying. When possible, continuous drip feeding, limited to the late evening and night, provides a means of minimizing complications while maximizing patient freedom. Patients receiving gastric feedings while in bed must be maintained in a position with the head elevated. This may, in some situations, compromise skin care, illustrating once again the need to consider the patient holistically for determination of optimum means of nutritional support.

Parenteral Feeding

Parenteral feeding uses the venous system for direct delivery of elemental forms of nutrients to the body. This is generally done through a central venous access line, which allows for the administration of the entire day's nutrient requirements. However, peripheral venous access may also be used in limited circumstances. Total parenteral feeding is indicated when the gut is nonfunctional or must be kept free of food for extended periods of time. Parenteral supplementation is indicated when gastrointestinal function is temporarily interrupted or in the presence of hypermetabolic states that require nutrients in excess of the absorptive capacity of the gut.

The proper administration of parenteral nutrition requires recognition that this is a nonphysiological means of delivering nutrients. Nutrients are delivered in elemental forms. Initial estimates of nutrient requirements were extrapolated from the RDAs, which were established based on administration of food through the gut. Some nutrients are manufactured in the gut by intestinal bacteria, and essentially all nutrients are absorbed into the portal venous system, thus passing through the liver for metabolism prior to general distribution through the body. Therefore, patients dependent on parenteral feeding require close observation and frequent monitoring of nutritional status. Complications from both nutrient deficiency and nutrient excess have been identified in patients receiving parenteral feeding. The optimal elemental composition of parenteral solutions varies widely, and recommendations are being modified on a regular basis as research and experience with parenteral nutrition continues.[39, 63, 94, 138, 178]

There are very real risks with the delivery of parenteral alimentation through a central line. The initial risk is associated with the insertion of the central venous catheter, especially for pneumothorax. The risk of infection of the catheter during use is ever present, as is the risk of contaminated substrate. Fluid and electrolyte balance must be closely monitored. The optimal ratio of carbohydrate and protein must be achieved so that nitrogen retention is optimized, without placing excessive metabolic demands on the liver and kidneys for amino acid metabolism and elimination of nitrogen waste products. The requirement of sufficient lipid to supply essential fatty acids has been recognized for several years, but the value of lipids in relatively significant quantities is still a subject of research.[63] The ratio of the basic nutrients that provide energy affects the amount of substrate and fluid required because lipids are a more concentrated source of calories than carbohydrates or protein. Carbohydrate metabolism is associated with greater carbon dioxide production than lipid metabolism, a factor that is now recognized to contribute significantly to carbon dioxide levels and thus affect respiratory drive in patients with respiratory compromise.[59, 85, 121]

It is impossible to achieve the delivery of a full day's nutrient requirements through a peripheral line, because the high osmolar concentration of the substrate results in chemical phlebitis. Peripheral venous supplementation is beneficial, however, as a source of fat or carbohydrate when oral feeding must be held for less than a week or as a source of fluids and extra nutrients in the patient who is unable to eat sufficient amounts of food to meet nutrient requirements and a small supplement is indicated.[169]

The psychosocial impact of long-term use of alternate feeding route has been reviewed.[123] It seems that enteral feeding routes are less problematic than parenteral feeding routes. The psychosocial problems associated with enteral feeding include gustatory deprivation, dry mouth, and tube-related discomforts. With parenteral feeding, there were problems identified owing to the loss of normal eating ability and associated body image changes, as well as depression and decreased sexual activity. Additionally, there was note of stress associated with fear of the apparatus, its maintenance, and its function. There is a great need for more information on this aspect of nutritional support, encompassing patients with a variety of disabilities.

CONCLUSIONS

The preceding discussion has included a large amount of information about nutrients, diet, nutritional requirements, nutritional assessment, and feeding problems with the identification of specific information and/or gaps in knowledge for application of basic nutritional principles to the care of the disabled person. Each disabled individual is nutritionally unique. The need for extensive research on the application of nutritional assessment techniques to the disabled to allow them the full benefit of nutritional support should be obvious at this point. Recently, the focus of nutritional evaluation and management has been on

institutionalized patients, especially those in the acute and subacute stages of disability. A report by Gaffney[61] illustrates the need to look at nutritional care of the homebound as well. The entire rehabilitation team may be involved in the solution of nutritional problems and support of good nutrition in the disabled person.

Despite the multiple questions that remain, it is possible to apply the information that is available to the clinical management of some specific problems that are frequently encountered in the practice of rehabilitation medicine and make some basic recommendations about general dietary practices for the person with remote disability that is now stabilized.

Specific Clinical Problems with Nutritional Implications

Urinary Tract Stones

The increased incidence of urinary tract stones in patients with a neurogenic bladder is of concern. The increased rate of calcium loss from bone with spinal cord injury and immobilization is well known and difficult to control.[32, 91, 107, 117] The causes of urinary tract stones are multifactorial.[1, 42, 134] Diet may be critical in some instances. Recommendations for dietary modification in an attempt to control the production of stones have included a low calcium diet (400 to 500 mg/day), a low sodium diet, and combination of thiazides and a low calcium diet.[1, 99] There is a report that the use of a high protein diet, as is now being done more frequently in the acute stages of post-trauma management to help control the adverse effects of nitrogen depletion, may increase calcium excretion in the urine.[53] However, there is no conclusive evidence that control of hypercalciuria will actually decrease the incidence of stone formation.

There has been concern about the potential for oxalate stone formation in the urinary tract of patients on large (several grams) intakes of vitamin C, a dietary supplement commonly used by patients with a neurogenic bladder.[98] Work by Fituri and associates[54] has shown that the purported increase in urinary oxalate excretion associated with high vitamin C intake was actually an artifact induced by the laboratory assay used in the earlier studies. This subject is succinctly reviewed in a letter by Hoffer.[81]

A general recommendation for adequate fluid intake can be made. Sufficient fluid intake to support adequate urine volume (at least 2 to 2.5 liters/day) will keep the urine more dilute and therefore decrease the tendency of substances to crystallize out because of high concentration.[131, 159] This fluid output is, however, difficult to maintain in patients are are managed with an intermittent catheterization program. Thus, the tendency to form stones can only be one factor in deciding optimal fluid intake for the patient with a neurogenic bladder.

The pH of the urine can also be manipulated to reduce the tendency to form any particular type of stones. The urinary pH is best controlled through medication. Although one still encounters recommendations for altering urinary pH through the use of acid and alkaline ash diets, it is difficult to implement consistent changes in urine pH through dietary methods.[49]

Decubitus Ulcers

The problem of skin breakdown continues to be a significant cause of morbidity, as well as a very expensive complication of disability. Despite numerous studies of this problem, prevention has not been achieved to a full extent. Thus, health care practitioners must continue to face this complication and strive to achieve healing as rapidly and inexpensively as possible.

Although the immediate cause of decubitus ulcers is pressure that has not been controlled, if one looks at the effect of pressure at the microscopic level, it becomes apparent that the cells break down because of inability to sustain metabolism, secondary to poor delivery of nutrients and poor exit of waste products. Thus, local cellular nutrition imbalance is at the crux of the problem.

When a decubitus ulcer is present there is an increase in nutritional needs. However, the extent of the increase has yet to be defined objectively. Obviously, fluid that contains proteins, vitamins, and minerals is lost continuously through the open surface of the wound. There is also the need for sufficient nutrition to support tissue repair. Therefore, the nutritional status of patients with decubitus ulcers should be evaluated closely and followed carefully with frequent adjustments in diet as indicated by results of the follow-up.

Moolton[113] reports an association of low albumin levels with the incidence of decubitus ulcers. Additionally, obesity may be a factor contributing to the development of decubitus ulcers because there will be greater tissue compression in any position if there is more weight pressing down and frequent position changes are more difficult for the obese person with disability, whether or not that person is dependent on others for turning.

Edema

The presence of decreased muscle activity in dependent limbs will result in edema from venous pooling. If not controlled, the edema will have adverse effects on the tissues involved. When this problem exists, it is important to be certain that venous pooling is the only cause of the edema. Therefore, the serum albumin value should be checked, since a low serum albumin level may cause edema because of decreased plasma oncotic pressure.

The treatment of edema usually involves elevation of the dependent extremities and/or compression with elastic stockings. However, the practice of giving diuretics to decrease total body fluid and/or decrease sodium intake through low sodium diets also continues. There are two major concerns with these practices:

1. The patient with neuromuscular disability and flaccid paralysis has a decreased lean body mass and therefore decreased total body potassium. Thus, there is a greater risk of dangerous levels of potassium depletion with the use of potassium-wasting diuretics in disabled patients than in able-bodied subjects. It is important to monitor the serum potassium value closely when diuretics are instituted.
2. Decreased plasma volume as a result of low sodium diet and/or diuretics will aggravate the tendency toward orthostatic hypotension in disabled patients, unless the reason for venous pooling is changed.

Constipation

There is a consensus that the standard bowel programs used on most rehabilitation units are excellent for control of the problems accompanying neurogenic bowel syndromes. One important aspect of the bowel program is a regular source of fiber in the diet or as a supplement (*e.g.,* psyllium). Quantities of fiber up to 25 to 30 g/day may be required to control constipation in some disabled patients, especially if there is a combination of immobility and previous laxative abuse.[20] Successful alteration of fiber intake in the diet will generally require individual dietary instruction, which should include consideration of the means to achieve increased fiber intake and the potential for this increased intake to affect the balance of other nutrients in the diet.[166]

Sometimes there is the patient for whom the bowel program has been tried but failed. Frequently, the failure is the result of inadequate fluid intake (which is probably being rigidly controlled because of problems with bladder management), and relief of constipation will result from increasing fluid intake to a minimum of 2 or more liters per day.

Obesity

Obesity is encountered frequently among the disabled, especially those with a significant decrease in activity level and as a result of head injury with associated cognitive impairment. Management is optimal if there can be a way to increase activity level as well as decrease caloric intake. Successful nutritional intervention may require application of behavioral techniques to control food intake, along with general nutrition information.

Recommendations

By reviewing the factors associated with malnutrition, it should be obvious that all patients admitted to a rehabilitation unit for therapy are at nutritional risk. Therefore, nutritional assessment should be part of the initial evaluation and nutritional status should be monitored at a regular interval during the admission. If dietary modifications are indicated, the registered dietitian should work with the nursing staff on dietary instruction throughout the period of the hospital stay. For patients with feeding problems, combined efforts of all members of the rehabilitation team will be required to establish a successful solution.

The ideal monitors of nutritional status for the disabled person have yet to be established. There are some reports of present activities in rehabilitation units for nutritional assessment and monitoring.[5, 37, 64, 76, 90, 120, 125] There is a need to collect baseline information and follow complications closely on large numbers of rehabilitation unit patients so that standards for monitoring can be developed. This will require a multicenter effort. One example of the type of data collection that would provide a valuable information base, with minimal cost, is presented in Table 28-11.

For the healthy disabled person, who is presumably in a steady-state, routine screening for new risk factors of malnutrition (see Fig. 28-4) should be included in regular care. If new risk factors are identified, further assessment of nutritional status is needed, with dietary modification and follow-up as indicated by

---

Table 28-11
Suggested Basic Data Collection for Nutritional Status Monitoring of Patients in Rehabilitation Units

Parameter	Frequency of Evaluation
Height	Twice annually
Weight	Twice weekly
Serum albumin	Monthly
Hemoglobin/hematocrit	Monthly
Total lymphocyte count	Monthly
Presence of infections or skin breakdown	Daily
Medication record reviewed	Weekly
Mobility level	Weekly
Level of independence/dependence in feeding	Weekly
24-Hour protein and calorie intake	Monthly
Clinical signs or symptoms of malnutrition	Monthly

the results of the assessment. Daniel and Gorman[40] have provided an excellent review of the application of presently known nutritional principles to the dietary needs of the disabled athlete.

REFERENCES

1. Abraham PA, Smith CL: Medical evaluation and management of calcium nephrolithiasis. Med Clin North Am 68:281–299, 1984
2. Adams CF: Nutritive Value of American Foods in Common Units. Agriculture Handbook No. 456, US Department of Agriculture. Washington, DC, US Government Printing Office, 1975
3. Awad AG: Diet and drug interactions in the treatment of mental illness—a review. Can J Psychiatry 29:609–613, 1984
4. Baker JP, Detsky AS, Wesson DE et al: Nutritional assessment: A comparison of clinical judgement and objective measurements. N Engl J Med 306:969–972, 1982
5. Barboriak JJ, Rooney CB, El Ghatit AZ et al: Nutrition in spinal cord injury patients. Am J Paraplegia 6:32–36, 1983
6. Baugh E: Actions to improve nutrition care on a general rehabilitation unit. J Am Diet Assoc 85:1632–1634, 1985
7. Beaton GH: Uses and limits of the use of the Recommended Dietary Allowances for evaluating dietary intake data. Am J Clin Nutr 41:155–164, 1985
8. Berg K: Effect of physical activation and of improved nutrition on the body composition of school children with cerebral palsy. Acta Paediatr Scand 204(suppl):53–69, 1971
9. Berg K: Somatic adaptation in cerebral palsy—summary and general discussion. Acta Paediatr Scand 204(suppl):81–93, 1971
10. Berg K, Isaksson B: Body composition and nutrition of school children with cerebral palsy. Acta Paediatr Scand 204 (suppl):41–52, 1971
11. Berg K, Olsson T: Energy requirements of school children with cerebral palsy as determined from indirect calorimetry. Acta Paediatr Scand 204(suppl):71–80, 1971
12. Berkelhammer CH, Leiter LA, Jeejeebhoy KN et al: Skeletal muscle function in chronic renal failure: An index of nutritional status. Am J Clin Nutr 42:845–854, 1985
13. Bildsten C, Lamid S: Nutritional management of a patient with brain damage and spinal cord injury. Arch Phys Med Rehabil 64:382–383, 1983
14. Bingham SA, Cummings JH: Urine nitrogen as an independent validatory measure of dietary intake: A study of nitrogen balance in individuals consuming their normal diet. Am J Clin Nutr 42:1276–1289, 1985
15. Bistrian BR, Blackburn GL, Sherman M, Scrimshaw NS: Therapeutic index of nutritional depletion in hospitalized patients. Surg Gynecol Obstet 141:512–516, 1975
16. Blackburn GL, Thornton PA: Nutritional assessment of the hospitalized patient. Med Clin North Am 63:1103–1115, 1979
17. Bowman BB, Rosenberg IH: Assessment of the nutritional status of the elderly. Am J Clin Nutr 35:1142–1151, 1982
18. Brown JE, Davis E, Flemming PL: Nutritional assessment of children with handicapping conditions. Ment Retard 17:129–132, 1979
19. Bryan AH, Anderson EL: Dietary and nutritional problems of crippled children in five rural countries of North Carolina. Am J Pub Health 55:1545–1554, 1965
20. Burr M, Alton M: Constipation in immobile patients. Med J Aust 1:446–447, 1984
21. Burton BT, Foster WR: Health implications of obesity: An NIH consensus development conference. J Am Diet Assoc 85:1117–1121, 1985
22. Butterworth CE Jr, Weinsier RL: Malnutrition in hospitalized patients: Assessment and treatment. In Goodhard RS, Shils ME (eds): Modern Nutrition in Health and Disease, 6th ed, pp 667–684. Philadelphia, Lea & Febiger, 1980
23. Caldwell MD, Kennedy-Caldwell C: Normal nutritional requirements. Surg Clin North Am 61:489–507, 1981
24. New American Eating Guide. Center for Science in the Public Interest, NA, 1755 S Street, NW, Washington, DC, 20009
25. Chantraine A, Delwaide PA: Hydroelectrolytic determination in paraplegics. Paraplegia 14:138–145, 1976
26. Christensen KS, Gstundtner KM: Hospital-wide screening improves basis for nutrition intervention. J Am Diet Assoc 85:704–706, 1985
27. Claus-Walker J, Halstead JL: Metabolic and endocrine changes in spinal cord injury: I. The nervous system before and after transection of the spinal cord. Arch Phys Med Rehabil 62:595–601, 1981
28. Claus-Walker J, Halstead LS: Metabolic and endocrine changes in spinal cord injury: II (section 1). Consequences of partial decentralization of the autonomic nervous system. Arch Phys Med Rehabil 63:569–575, 1982
29. Claus-Walker J, Halstead LS: Metabolic and endocrine changes in spinal cord injury: II (section 2). Partial decentralization of the autonomic nervous system. Arch Phys Med Rehabil 63:576–580, 1982
30. Claus-Walker J, Halstead LS: Metabolic and endocrine changes in spinal cord injury: III. Less quanta of sensory input plus bedrest and illness. Arch Phys Med Rehabil 63:628–631, 1982
31. Claus-Walker J, Halstead LS: Metabolic and endocrine changes in spinal cord injury: IV. Compounded neurologic dysfunctions. Arch Phys Med Rehabil 63:632–638, 1982
32. Claus-Walker J, Spencer WA, Carter RE et al: Bone metabolism in quadriplegia: Dissociation between calciuria and hydroxyprolinuria. Arch Phys Med Rehabil 56:327–332, 1975
33. Clifton GL, Robertson CS, Contant CF: Enteral hyperalimentation in head injury. J Neurosurg 62:186–193, 1985
34. Conway JM, Norris KH, Bodwell CE: A new approach for the estimation of body composition: Infrared interactance. Am J Clin Nutr 40:1123–1130, 1984
35. Cox SAR, Weiss SM, Posuniak EA et al: Energy expenditure after spinal cord injury: An evaluation of stable rehabilitating patients. J Trauma 25:419–423, 1985
36. Culley WJ, Middleton TO: Caloric requirements of mentally retarded children with and without motor dysfunction. J Pediatrics 75:380–384, 1969
37. Curtin HC, Harvey RF, Jellinek HM: Role of the clinical nutritionist as a member of a rehabilitation team. Nutr Supp Serv 2:25–31, 1982
38. Daly JM, Heymsfield SB, Head CA et al: Human energy requirements: Overestimation by widely used prediction equation. Am J Clin Nutr 42:1170–1174, 1985
39. Daly JM, Long JM III: Intravenous hyperalimentation: Techniques and potential complications. Surg Clin North Am 61:583–592, 1981
40. Daniel M, Gorman D: Nutritional considerations for the wheelchair athlete. Sports 'n Spokes (Sept-Oct):8–13, 1983
41. Dempsey DT, Guenter P, Mullen JL et al: Energy expenditure in acute trauma to the head with and without barbiturate therapy. Surg Gynecol Obstet 160:128–134, 1985
42. DeVivo MJ, Fine PR, Cutter GR, Maetz HM: The risk of renal calculi in spinal cord injury patients. J Urol 131:857–860, 1984
43. Dickerson JWT: Vitamin requirements in different clinical conditions. Bibl Nutr Dieta 35:44–52, 1985
44. Dickhaut SC, DeLee JC, Page CP: Nutritional status: Importance in predicting wound-healing after amputation. J Bone Joint Surg [Am] 66:71–75, 1984
45. Dixon JK: Validity and utility of anthropometric measurements: A survey of cancer outpatients. J Am Diet Assoc 85:439–444, 1985
46. Dominioni L, Trocki O, Fang CH et al: Enteral feeding in burn hypermetabolism: Nutritional and metabolic effects of different levels of calorie and protein intake. J Parenter Enter Nutr 9:269–279, 1985
47. Dudrick SJ, Rhoads JE: Metabolism in surgical patients. In Sabiston DC (ed): Davis-Christopher Textbook of Surgery, 12th ed, pp 144–171. Philadelphia, WB Saunders, 1981
48. Duyff RL: The adequate diet—the prudent diet. In Howard RB, Herbold NH (eds): Nutrition in Clinical Care, 2nd ed, pp 13–39. New York, McGraw-Hill, 1982
49. Dwyer J, Foulkes E, Evans M, Ausman L: Acid-alkaline ash diets: Time for assessment and change. J Am Diet Assoc 85:841–845, 1985
50. Eddy TP, Nicholson AH, Wheeler EF: Energy expenditures and dietary intake in cerebral palsy. Dev Med Neurol 7:377–386, 1965
51. Ernst ND: NIH consensus development conference on lowering blood cholesterol to prevent heart disease: Implications for dietitians. J Am Diet Assoc 85:586–588, 1985

52. Fabiani C, Candy S: Oral hyperalimentation in the nutritional management of burned patients. S Afr Med J 67:768–770, 1985
53. Fellstrom B, Danielson BG, Karlstrom B et al: Urinary composition and supersaturation on a high protein diet. Contrib Nephrol 37:27–30, 1984
54. Fituri N, Allawi N, Bentley M, Costello J: Urinary and plasma oxalate during ingestion of pure ascorbic acid: A reevaluation. Eur Urol 9:312–315, 1983
55. Food and Nutrition Board: Recommended Dietary Allowances, 9th ed. Washington DC, National Research Council, National Academy of Sciences, 1980
56. Food and Nutrition Board: Recommended dietary allowances: Scientific issues and process for the future. J Nutr Ed 18:82–87, 1986
57. Forbes GB, Bruining GJ: Urinary creatinine excretion and lean body mass. Am J Clin Nutr 29:1359–1366, 1976
58. Frisancho AR: New standards of weight and body composition by frame size and height for assessment of nutritional status of adults and the elderly. Am J Clin Nutr 40:808–819, 1984
59. Fuel mixtures for critically ill patients given total parenteral nutrition. Nutr Rev 43:17–20, 1985
60. Furse A, Levine E: Food, nutrition and the disabled: An annotated bibliography. Toronto, Nutrition Information Service, Ryerson Polytechnical Institute Library, 1981
61. Gaffney JT, Singer GR: Diet needs of patients referred to home health. J Am Diet Assoc 85:198–202, 1985
62. Gallo S, Ramirex A, Elizondo J et al: Endoscopic placement of enteral feeding tubes. J Parenter Enter Nutr 9:747–749, 1985
63. Gilder H: Parenteral nourishment of patients undergoing surgical or traumatic stress. J Parenter Enter Nutr 10:88–99, 1986
64. Glenn MB, Carfi J, Belle SE et al: Serum albumin as a predictor of course and outcome on a rehabilitation service. Arch Phys Med Rehabil 66:294–297, 1985
65. Goodhart RS, Shils ME: Modern Nutrition in Health and Disease, 6th ed. Philadelphia, Lea & Febiger, 1980
66. Gordon SR, Kelley SL, Sybyl JR et al: Relationship in very elderly veterans of nutritional status, self-perceived chewing ability, dental status, and social isolation. J Am Geriatr Soc 33:334–339, 1985
67. Gouge AL, Ekvall SW: Diets of handicapped children: Physical psychological, and socioeconomic correlations. Am J Mental Defic 80:149–157, 1975
68. Grande F, Keys A: Body weight, body composition and calorie status. In Goodhart RS, Shils ME (eds): Modern Nutrition in Health and Disease, 6th ed, pp 3–34. Philadelphia, Lea & Febiger, 1980
69. Grant JP, Custer PB, Thurlow J: Current techniques of nutritional assessment. Surg Clin North Am 61:437–463, 1981
70. Green EM, McIntosh EN: Food and nutrition skills of mentally retarded adults: Assessment and needs. J Am Diet Assoc 85:611–613, 1985
71. Greenway RM, Houser HB, Lindan O, Weir DR: Long-term changes in gross body composition of paraplegic and quadriplegic patients. Paraplegia 7:301–318, 1969
72. Haider M, Haider SQ: Assessment of protein–calorie malnutrition. Clin Chem 30:1286–1299, 1984
73. Hannaman KN, Penner SF: A nutrition assessment tool that includes diagnosis. J Am Diet Assoc 85:607–609, 1985
74. Hansten PD: Drug Interactions, 5th ed. Philadelphia, Lea & Febiger, 1985
75. Hausmann D, Mosebach KO, Rommelsheim K: Combined enteral-parenteral nutrition versus total parenteral nutrition in brain-injured patients: A comparative study. Intensive Care Med 11:80–84, 1985
76. Hecht JS, Grabois M, Kunioki S, Hart WD: Nutritional assessment of newly spinal cord injured patients (abstr). Arch Phys Med Rehabil 62:527, 1981
77. Hewson DC, Phillips MA, Simpson KE et al: Food intake in multiple sclerosis. Hum Nutr Appl Nutr 38A:355–367, 1984
78. Heymsfield SB, McManus CB: Tissue components of weight loss in cancer patients: A new method of study and preliminary observations. Cancer 55:238–249, 1985
79. Hinsdale JG, Lipkowitz GS, Pollock TW et al: Prolonged enteral nutrition in malnourished patients with nonelemental feeding: Reappraisal of surgical technique, safety, and costs. Am J Surg 149:334–338, 1985
80. Hodges P, Sauriol D, Man SFP et al: Nutrient intake of patients with cystic fibrosis. J Am Diet Assoc 84:664–669, 1984
81. Hoffer A: Letter: Ascorbic acid and kidney stones. Can Med Assoc J 132:320, 1985
82. Howard RB, Fetters L, MacDonald DM: Nutrition in neurological disorders and in the care of the disabled. In Howard RB, Herbold NH (eds): Nutrition in Clinical Care, 2nd ed, pp 594–628. New York, McGraw-Hill, 1982
83. Hunt DR, Maslovitz A, Rowlands BJ, Brooks B: A simple nutrition screening procedure for hospital patients. J Am Diet Assoc 85:332–335, 1985
84. Hunt DR, Rowlands BJ, Johnston D: Hand grip strength: A simple prognostic indicator in surgical patients. J Parenter Enter Nutr 9:701–704, 1985
85. Irwin MM, Openbrier DR: A delicate balance: Strategies for feeding ventilated COPD patients. Am J Nurs (March):274–280, 1985
86. Jackson AA: Aminoacids: Essential and non-essential? Lancet 1:1034–1037, 1983
87. Jensen TG, Long JM III, Dudrick SJ, Johnston DA: Nutritional assessment indications of postburn complications. J Am Diet Assoc 85:68–72, 1985
88. Johnston FE: Relationships between body composition and anthropometry. Human Biol 54:221–245, 1982
89. Joint FAO/WHO/UNU Expert Consultation: Energy and protein requirements. WHO Tech Rep Ser 724, 1985
90. Kalisz K, Ekvall S: A nutritional interview for clients with developmental disorders. Ment Retard 22:279–288, 1984
91. Kaplan PE, Gandhavadi B, Richards L, Goldschmidt J: Calcium balance in paraplegic patients: Influence of injury duration and ambulation. Arch Phys Med Rehabil 59:447–450, 1978
92. Kaufman HH, Rowlands BJ, Stein DK et al: General metabolism in patients with acute paraplegia and quadriplegia. Neurosurgery 16:309–313, 1985
93. Kearns PJ, Pipp TL, Quirk M, Campolo M: Nutritional requirements in quadriplegics (abstr). J Parenteral Enter Nutr 6:577, 1982
94. Klein GL, Rivera D: Adverse metabolic consequences of total parenteral nutrition. Cancer 55:305–308, 1985
95. Kudsk KA, Stone JM, Sheldon GF: Nutrition in trauma. Surg Clin North Am 61:671–679, 1981
96. Kudsk KA, Stone JM, Sheldon GF: Nutrition in trauma and burns. Surg Clin North Am 62:183–192, 1982
97. Kuhlemeier KV, Miller JM III, Nepomuceno CS: Insensible weight loss in patients with spinal cord transection. Paraplegia 14:195–201, 1976
98. Lamden MP, Chrystowski GA: Urinary oxalate excretion by man following ascorbic acid ingestion. Proc Soc Exp Biol North Am 85:190–192, 1954
99. Lamid S, El Ghatit AZ, Melvin JL: Relationship of hypercalciuria to diet and bladder stone formation in spinal cord injury patients. Am J Phys Med 63:182–187, 1984
100. Lands WEM: Renewed questions about polyunsaturated fatty acids. Nutr Rev 44:189–195, 1986
101. Litchford MD, Wakefield LM: Nutrient intake of institutionalized developmentally disabled individuals: Impact of the nutrition knowledge of paraprofessionals. J Am Diet Assoc 85:690–692, 1985
102. Loosen BM: Self-help aids. In Redford JB (ed): Orthotics Etcetera, 2nd ed, pp 650–681. Baltimore, Williams & Wilkins, 1980
103. MacBurney M, Wilmore DW: Rational decision making in nutritional care. Surg Clin North Am 61:571–582, 1981
104. March DC: Handbook: Interaction of Selected Drugs with Nutritional Status in Man. Chicago, American Dietetic Association, 1978
105. Margen S: Evaluation of nutritional status in the outpatient setting. Med Clin North Am 63:1095–1101, 1979
106. Mattes-Kulig DA, Henkin RI: Energy and nutrient consumption of patients with dysgeusia. J Am Diet Assoc 85:822–826, 1985
107. Maynard FM, Imai K: Immobilization hypercalcemia in spinal cord injury. Arch Phys Med Rehabil 58:16–24, 1977
108. Mazess RB, Peppler WW, Gibbons M: Total body composition by dual-photon (153Gd) absorptiometry. Am J Clin Nutr 40:834–839, 1984
109. McGovern B: Janeway gastrostomy in children with cerebral palsy. J Pediatr Surg 19:800–802, 1984

110. Meguid MM, Eldar S, Wahba A: The delivery of nutritional support: A potpourri of new devices and methods. Cancer 55:279–289, 1985

111. Merkel KD, Miller NE, Merritt JL: Energy expenditure in patients with low-, mid-, high-thoracic paraplegia using Scott-Craig knee-ankle-foot orthoses. Mayo Clin Proc 60:165–168, 1985

112. Mirahmadi MK, Barton CH, Vaziri ND et al: Nutritional evaluation of hemodialysis patients with and without spinal cord injury. Am J Paraplegia 6:36–40, 1983

113. Moolton SE: Bedsores in the chronically ill patient. Arch Phys Med Rehabil 53:430–438, 1972

114. Moore MC, Greene HL: Tube feeding of infants and children. Pediatr Clin North Am 32:401–417, 1985

115. Munro HN: Major gaps in nutrient allowances. J Am Diet Assoc 76:137–141, 1980

116. Munro HN: Evolving scientific bases for the Recommended Dietary Allowances—a critical look at methodologies. Am J Clin Nutr 41:149–154, 1985

117. Naftchi NE, Viau AT, Sell GH, Lowman EW: Mineral metabolism in spinal cord injury. Arch Phys Med Rehabil 61:139–142, 1980

118. NIH Consensus Development Conference Statement: Lowering blood cholesterol to prevent heart disease. Arteriosclerosis 5:404–412, 1985

119. Newmark SR, Simpson S, Daniel P et al: Nutritional support in an inpatient rehabilitation unit. Arch Phys Med Rehabil 62:634–637, 1981

120. Newmark SR, Sublett D, Black J, Geller R: Nutritional assessment in a rehabilitation unit. Arch Phys Med Rehabil 62:279–282, 1981

121. Orme JF: Nutrition and ventilator-dependent patients. West J Med 144:351–352, 1986

122. Oser BL: Chemical additives in foods. In Goodhart RS, Shils ME: Modern Nutrition in Health and Disease, 6th ed, pp 506–519. Philadelphia, Lea & Febiger, 1980

123. Padilla GV, Grant MM: Psychosocial aspects of artificial feeding. Cancer 55:301–304, 1985

124. Panzetta G, Guerra U, D'Angelo A et al: Body composition and nutritional status in patients on continuous ambulatory peritoneal dialysis (CAPD). Clin Nephrol 23:18–25, 1985

125. Peiffer SC, Bluse P, Leyson JFJ: Nutritional assessment of the spinal cord injured patient. J Am Diet Assoc 78:501–505, 1981

126. Pennington JAT: Considerations for a new food guide. J Nutr Ed 13:53–55, 1981

127. Pennington JAT, Church HN: Bowes and Church's Food Values of Portions Commonly Used, 14th ed. Philadelphia, JB Lippincott, 1985

128. Pi-Sunyer FX, Woo R: Laboratory assessment of nutritional status. In Simko MD, Cowell C, Gilbride JA (eds): Nutrition Assessment: A Comprehensive Guide for Planning Intervention, pp 139–174. Rockville, MD, Aspen Systems, 1984

129. Pierce DS, Nickel VH: The Total Care of Spinal Cord Injuries. Boston, Little, Brown & Co, 1977

130. Pike RL, Brown ML: Nutrition: An Integrated Approach, 2nd ed. New York, John Wiley & Sons, 1975

131. Power C, Barker DJP, Nelson M, Winter PD: Diet and renal stones: A case-control study. Br J Urol 56:456–459, 1984

132. Rapp RP, Young B, Twyman D et al: The favorable effect of early parenteral feeding on survival in head-injured patients. J Neurosurg 58:906–912, 1983

133. Robbins GE, Trowbridge FL: Anthropometric techniques and their application. In Simko MD, Cowell C, Gilbride JA (eds): Nutrition Assessment: A Comprehensive Guide for Planning Intervention, pp 69–92, Rockville MD, Aspen Systems, 1984

134. Robertson WG, Peacock M: Metabolic and biochemical risk factors in renal stone disease. Contrib Nephrol 37:1–4, 1984

135. Roe DA: Interactions between drugs and nutrients. Med Clin North Am 63:985–1007, 1979

136. Rombeau HL, Barot LR: Enteral nutritional therapy. Surg Clin North Am 61:605–620, 1981

137. Roza AM, Shizgal HM: The Harris Benedict equation reevaluated: Resting energy requirements and the body cell mass. Am J Clin Nutr 40:168–182, 1984

138. Rudman D, Williams PJ: Nutrient deficiencies during total parenteral nutrition. Nutr Rev 43:1–13, 1985

139. Russell DMcR, Leiter LA, Whitwell J et al: Skeletal muscle function during hypocaloric diets and fasting: A comparison with standard nutritional assessment parameters. Am J Clin Nutr 37:133–138, 1983

140. Saffle JR, Medina E, Raymond J et al: Use of indirect calorimetry in the nutritional management of burned patients. J Trauma 25:32–39, 1985

141. Sauberlich HE, Skala JH, Dowdy RP: Laboratory Tests for the Assessment of Nutritional Status. Cleveland, CRC Press, 1974

142. Schaumberg H, Kaplan J, Windebank A et al: Sensory neuropathy from pyridoxine abuse: A new megavitamin syndrome. N Engl J Med 309:445–448, 1983

143. Shils ME: Food and nutrition relating to work, exercise and environmental stress. In Goodhart RS, Shils ME (eds): Modern Nutrition in Health and Disease, 6th ed, pp 814–851. Philadelphia, Lea & Febiger, 1980

144. Shils ME: Nutrition assessment in support of the malnourished patient. In Simko MD, Cowell C, Gilbride JA (eds): Nutrition Assessment: A Comprehensive Guide for Planning Intervention, pp 237–252. Rockville, MD, Aspen Systems, 1984

145. Shils ME, Randall HT: Diet and nutrition in the care of the surgical patient. In Goodhart RS, Shils ME (eds): Modern Nutrition in Health and Disease, 6th ed, pp 1082–1124. Philadelphia, Lea & Febiger, 1980

146. Shires GT, Cornezin PC, Lowry SF: Fluid, electrolyte, and nutritional management of the surgical patient. In Schwartz SI, Shires GT, Spencer FC, Stover EH: Principles of Surgery, 4th ed, pp 45–80. New York, McGraw-Hill, 1984

147. Shizgal HM: Body composition and nutritional support. Surg Clin North Am 61:729–741, 1981

148. Shizgal HM: Body composition of patients with malnutrition and cancer: Summary of methods of assessment. Cancer 55:250–253, 1985

149. Siddall CNM: The nutritional care of the multiply handicapped person. J Can Diet Assoc 42:317–320, 1981

150. Silberman H, Eisenberg D: Parenteral and Enteral Nutrition for the Hospitalized Patient. Norwalk, CT, Appleton-Century-Crofts, 1982

151. Simko MD, Cowell C, Gilbride JA: Nutrition Assessment: A Comprehensive Guide for Planning Intervention. Rockville, MD, Aspen Systems, 1984

152. Slowie LA, Paige MS, Antel JP: Nutritional considerations in the management of patients with amyotrophic lateral sclerosis (ALS). J Am Diet Assoc 83:44–47, 1983

153. Smiciklas-Wright H, Guthrie HA: Dietary methodologies: Their uses, analyses, interpretations, and implications. In Simko MD, Cowel C, Gilbride JA (eds): Nutrition Assessment: A Comprehensive Guide for Planning Intervention, pp 119–138. Rockville, MD, Aspen Systems, 1984

154. Solomons NW: Assessment of nutritional status: Functional indicators of pediatric nutriture. Pediatr Clin North Am 32:319–334, 1985

155. Solomons NW, Allen LH: The functional assessment of nutritional status: Principles, practice and potential. Nutr Rev 41:33–50, 1983

156. Stratton M: Behavioral assessment scale of oral functions in feeding. Am J Occup Ther 35:719–721, 1981

157. Strohmeyer SL, Massey LK, Davison MA: A rapid dietary screening device for clinics. J Am Diet Assoc 84:428–432, 1984

158. Szeluga DJ, Stuart RK, Utermohlen V, Santos GW: Nutritional assessment by isotope dilution analysis of body composition. Am J Clin Nutr 40:847–854, 1980

159. Taylor KB, Anthony LE: Clinical Nutrition. New York, McGraw-Hill, 1983

160. Tseng RYL, Sullivan MA, Downes NJ: A proposed method for the nutritional rating of foods. J Nutr Ed 18:67–74, 1986

161. Tuckerman MM, Turco SJ: Human Nutrition. Philadelphia, Lea & Febiger, 1983

162. Turner WW: Nutritional considerations in the patient with disabling brain disease. Neurosurgery 16:707–713, 1985

163. Turner WW, Ireton CS, Hunt JL, Baxter CR: Predicting energy expenditures in burned patients. J Trauma 25:11–16, 1985

164. Twyman D, Young AB, Ott L et al: High protein enteral feedings: A means of achieving positive nitrogen balance in head injured patients. J Parenteral Enter Nutr 9:679–684, 1985

165. Underwood BA: Evaluating the nutritional status of individuals: A critique of approaches. Nutr Rev (suppl)44:213–224, 1986

166. Vahouny GV: Conclusions and recommendations of the symposium on Dietary Fibers in Health and Disease, Washington, DC, 1981. Am J Clin Nutr 35:152–156, 1982

167. VanLandingham SB, Key JC, Symmonds RE: Nutritional support of the surgical patient. Surg Clin North Am 62:321–331, 1982

168. Watt BK, Merrill AL: Composition of Foods: Raw, Processed, Prepared. Agriculture Handbook No. 8, US Department of Agriculture. Washington, DC, US Government Printing Office, 1963

169. Watters JM, Freeman JB: Parenteral nutrition by peripheral vein. Surg Clin North Am 61:593–603, 1981

170. Weigley ES: Average? Ideal? Desirable? A brief overview of height–weight tables in the United States. J Am Diet Assoc 84:417–423, 1984

171. Weinsier RL, Hunker EM, Krumdieck CL, Butterworth CE Jr: Hospital malnutrition: A prospective evaluation of general medical patients during the course of hospitalization. Am J Clin Nutr 32:418–426, 1979

172. Williams SR: Nutrition and Diet Therapy, 4th ed. St. Louis, CV Mosby, 1981

173. Wills JS, Oglesby JT, Burke WA: Percutaneous gastrostomy: A safe, cost-effective alternative to surgical gastrostomy and intravascular hyperalimentation. Nutr Supp Ser 6:10–15, 1986

174. Wolfe BM, Chock E: Energy sources, stores, and hormonal controls. Surg Clin North Am 61:509–518, 1981

175. Wotecki CE: Improving estimates of food and nutrient intake: Applications to individuals and groups. J Am Diet Assoc 85:295–296, 1985

176. Wotecki CE: Dietary survey data: Sources and limits to interpretation. Nutr Rev (suppl)44:204–213, 1986

177. Wretlind A: Nutrient requirements in various clinical conditions. Bibl Nutr Dieta 35:31–43, 1985

178. Zlotkin SH, Stallings VA, Pencharz PB: Total parenteral nutrition in children. Pediatr Clin North Am 32:381–400, 1985

Part 4

Rehabilitation of Specific Disorders

29

Rehabilitation of the Stroke Patient

Susan J. Garrison

Loren A. Rolak

Robert R. Dodaro

Anthony J. O'Callaghan

DEFINITION

A cerebrovascular accident (CVA) can be defined as infarction of the brain, causing disruption of brain function due to ischemia or hemorrhage. *Stroke* is actually a term for any sudden-onset focal neurological deficit. A CVA is the most common cause, but other underlying lesions can cause acute focal neurological deficits. For this chapter, the terms *stroke* and *CVA* are used synonymously.

Hemiparesis is the most common manifestitation of stroke. In describing hemiparesis, confusion can arise if care is not taken to distinguish the anatomy of the brain lesion from the clinical signs and symptoms it causes. The description "left-sided stroke" does not convey whether the patient has weakness of the left side of the body or a left hemisphere lesion. The use of a precise description such as "left hemisphere stroke with right hemiparesis" avoids confusion.

DIFFERENTIAL DIAGNOSIS

The physician should not assume that any neurological symptom that appears suddenly must be due to vascular disease. Many common features of a CVA are seldom due to vascular disease when they occur alone, unaccompanied by other evidence of neurological damage (Table 29-1). The lists of differential diagnoses for a patient with acute-onset vertigo, dysarthria, headache, or diplopia alone are long, with vascular disease less common than many other causes. It is also particularly important that changes in mental status not be attributed to cerebrovascular disease until other more likely metabolic, toxic, and infectious etiologies have been excluded: confusion, delirium, amnesic memory loss, and coma are rarely caused by stroke.[91]

Epilepsy mimics CVA more often than any other condition. In one large study of 821 consecutive patients admitted to a CVA unit, 13% had a disease other than CVA.[86] Almost 40% of these misdiagnosed patients had seizures. The next largest group of mistaken diagnoses involved patients with confusion from drugs, alcohol, or metabolic abnormalities. Mass lesions such as cerebral tumor or subdural hematoma may present as stroke. Occasionally labyrinthitis, encephalitis, multiple sclerosis, brain abscess, hypoglycemia, migraine, and hysterical or psychogenic symptoms may be erroneously diagnosed as CVA (Table 29-2).[86] However, a well-trained physician can usually differentiate cerebrovascular disease from other processes on the basis of clinical features alone at least 80% of the time.[84, 117]

EPIDEMIOLOGY

CVA is the most common serious neurological problem in the world, and in the United States it is second only to head trauma as the leading cause of neurological disability. Half of all patients hospitalized for acute neurological disease have a CVA.[128] It is the third most common cause of death in the Western World, behind heart disease and cancer.[51] Nearly half a million new CVAs occur in the United States annually, about 200,000 of which are fatal. The survivors, added to previous cases, comprise about 1.7 million disabled victims. The estimated financial impact on society related to stroke exceeds 7 billion dollars per year.[66, 122] The human costs are immeasurable.

The incidence of CVA rises with increasing age. There is a doubling of incidence rate in each successive decade above age 55.[128] The prevalence rate is 66 per 100,000 below age 45, 998 per 100,000 for ages 45 to 64, and 5,063 per 100,000 for age over 65. Both the incidence and mortality are declining in the United States. Despite an increasingly aging population, the total number of deaths has fallen, and stroke rates are declining more rapidly than other complications of atherosclerosis such as cardiac disease. It appears that the rate has declined at about 1% per year since the 1940s, with an acceleration in the past decade dropping the rate at nearly 5% per year.[69] This decline is real and not simply a result of changes in death certificates or inaccuracies in diagnosis.[128] It is not possible to determine how much of the decline in mortality is due to the drop in the incidence rate and how much is from better treatment that has lowered the fatality of CVAs.

Much of the decline in incidence is attributed to better management of hypertension, but mortality was clearly declining for several years before effective antihypertensive therapy became available, so other variables must be involved in this trend. Modern emphasis on weight loss, reduction of salt in the diet, decrease in cigarette smoking, exercise, and promotion of healthy life-styles may also contribute. The ubiquitous use of

Table 29-1
Symptoms Seldom Due to Cerebrovascular Disease

Vertigo alone	Confusion
Dysarthria alone	Memory loss
Dysphagia alone	Delirium
Diplopia alone	Coma
Headache	Syncope
Tremor	Incontinence
Tonic/clonic motor activity	Tinnitus

Table 29-2
Conditions Most Frequently Mistaken for Stroke

Seizures	Peripheral neuropathy
Metabolic encephalopathy	Multiple sclerosis
Cerebral tumor	Hypoglycemia
Subdural hematoma	Encephalitis
Cerebral abscess	Migraine
Vertigo, Ménière's disease	Psychogenic

antiplatelet agents may also play a role, and there has been a decrease in other cardiac diseases responsible for CVA, including myocardial infarction, atrial fibrillation, mitral stenosis, and rheumatic heart disease.[49, 50, 123]

RISK FACTORS

Age is one of the main risk factors for stroke (Table 29-3). In most age groups, CVA is as common in women as in men. CVA is the only major complication of atherosclerosis in which men are not at greater risk.

Hypertension is the greatest treatable risk factor for ischemic as well as hemorrhagic CVAs. The risk is related to the level of blood pressure throughout its range: the incidence of stroke rises as the pressure rises.[60] Systolic pressure, even isolated systolic hypertension, is most closely linked to risk of CVA.[128]

Data consistently show higher incidence and death rates among blacks than whites, at least in the United States. Race is thus a risk factor most likely as a reflection of the propensity to hypertension in blacks. Cardiac impairment ranks third, following age and hypertension, as a risk factor. This is especially true of ischemic coronary artery disease, but nonatherosclerotic heart disease is also an important cause of CVA.[5, 50] Coronary artery disease is the major cause of death among stroke survivors, just as it is in patients with transient ischemic attacks (TIAs) or carotid bruits.[112] The coexistence of coronary artery disease is also a factor that may influence stroke rehabilitation by limiting the patient's level of participation. The risk is more than doubled in both men and women with coronary heart disease, and the presence of congestive heart failure adds an even greater increase in risk.

The heart can serve as a source of emboli that subsequently travel to the brain, so the presence of thrombogenic heart diseases other than myocardial infarction is also a risk factor. Most important is atrial fibrillation, which even in the absence of rheumatic heart disease or other valvular problems, is a frequent precursor. Even in patients with chronic stable atrial fibrillation, the risk of CVA is five times normal. Other arrhythmias such as

Table 29-3
Major Risk Factors for Stroke

Age
Hypertension
Cardiac disease
Diabetes
Previous stroke or transient ischemic attack (TIA)

sick sinus syndrome are also important, although ventricular arrhythmias seem to be less significant.[43, 59, 126]

A CVA is itself a risk factor for another CVA. Patients with prior stroke, TIAs and even asymptomatic carotid bruits are more likely to suffer further cerebrovascular disease. In the case of the asymptomatic carotid bruit, the increased risk of CVA is not necessarily ipsilateral to the diseased vessel.[127] From 10% to 50% of all CVAs are preceded by TIAs. A patient with a TIA has approximately a 5% chance per year of having a CVA at some time.[9, 12, 18, 38, 107] TIAs, thus, are also a risk factor for stroke. Diabetics also develop stroke at an increased rate, about twice the risk of nondiabetics.[128]

Some risk factors for atherosclerosis in other vessels, such as the coronary arteries, are only mild risk factors for stroke. The relationship between stroke and elevated cholesterol, including high-density lipoprotein subfractions, is very weak. There is no relationship between level of triglycerides and risk of stroke. Obesity by itself is not a risk for stroke, except in as much as it is associated with hypertension or diabetes. Similarly, cigarette smoking, coffee drinking, sedentary life-style, or behavioral factors (type A personality) provide minimal, if any increased risk for stroke.[128]

ANATOMY AND ETIOLOGY

One of the most important clinical determinations in the evaluation of the patient with cerebrovascular disease is whether the symptoms arise from the anterior circulation (the carotid artery and its main branches, the anterior and middle cerebral arteries) or the posterior circulation (vertebral, basilar, and posterior cerebral arteries). The pathogenesis, diagnostic workup, therapy, and prognosis of stroke in these two vascular regions are usually different.

Anterior Circulation

Unfortunately, few signs or symptoms allow a reliable distinction between anterior and posterior ischemia, and interconnections between the systems (especially through the circle of Willis) permit shunting of blood that can obscure the anatomy of the lesion. Eighty percent of strokes happen in the carotid distribution, with a hemiparesis, ranging from mild weakness to complete paralysis of the limbs on one side of the body, typically involving the face, arm, or leg in any combination. There is often some degree of numbness or sensory loss in a similar distribution as the weakness. Aphasia, dysarthria, headache, and visual field cuts may also occur (Table 29-4). However, the corticospinal tracts and spinothalamic tracts that mediate weakness and numbness extend from the cerebral cortex through the brain stem, so a syndrome of weakness and numbness on one side of the body could be caused by interruption anywhere along their length, including the brain stem. Thus, hemiparesis or hemi-

Table 29-4
Most Common Symptoms of Carotid Circulation Ischemia

Symptom	Frequency
Hemiparesis	65%
Hemisensory loss	60%
Monocular blindness	35%
Facial numbness	30%
Lower facial weakness	25%
Aphasia	20%
Headache	20%
Dysarthria	15%
Visual field loss	15%

Table 29-5
Most Common Symptoms of Vertebrobasilar Circulation Ischemia

Symptom	Frequency
Ataxia	50%
Crossed or hemisensory loss	30%
Vertigo	30%
Crossed or hemiparesis	25%
Dysarthria/dysphagia	25%
Syncope or lightheadedness	25%
Headache	20%
Deafness or tinnitus	10%
Diplopia	10%

anesthesia does not reliably differentiate posterior circulation from anterior circulation ischemia.

The two symptoms that most accurately indicate carotid circulation involvement are aphasia and monocular blindness. The capacity for language resides in the dominant (usually left) hemisphere, within the territory of the carotid artery. A stroke causing aphasia must therefore be in the carotid distribution. Similarly, the blood supply of the eye is largely via the ophthalmic artery, a direct branch from the carotid artery. Therefore, monocular ischemia implicates the carotid artery circulation.

Posterior Circulation

Because the brain stem contains more compactly arranged neurological structures than the cerebral hemispheres, clinical syndromes in the posterior circulation are usually more complex than those in the cerebral hemispheres.[21, 85, 124] In brain stem stroke, bilateral signs are frequently present and cranial nerve and cerebellar abnormalities are usually prominent (Table 29-5). The most reliable indication of brain stem disease is cranial nerve dysfunction such as dysarthria, dysphagia, diplopia, or dizziness in conjunction with hemiparesis and hemisensory loss, which may be crossed. Deviation of the eyes may also help in the localization of stroke. In hemispheric lesions (carotid circulation) damage to the frontal lobe gaze centers will cause the patient to look away from the hemiparetic side of the body, whereas patients with a brain stem stroke (posterior circulation) with damage to the pontine gaze centers, will look toward the hemiparetic side. Facial weakness may also be a valuable sign, since weakness of the lower part of the face alone suggests damage in the cerebral hemispheres, whereas a stroke affecting the brain stem and damaging the facial nerve nucleus itself will paralyze the entire side of the face. Dysarthria and dysphagia most frequently arise from brain stem lesions, but may occur with facial and tongue weakness owing to hemispheric damage and therefore are unreliable localizing signs.

Few clues exist that absolutely differentiate carotid from vertebrobasilar ischemia. Doubt is usually resolved in favor of carotid disease, since it probably accounts for 80% of all strokes. This anatomical distinction has practical importance for the patient and physician. The middle cerebral and internal carotid arteries are the major points of attack for atherosclerosis in the cerebrovascular system, and strokes in the carotid distribution are due to atherosclerotic stenosis and thrombosis of these vessels. Most emboli from the carotid artery or the heart travel to the middle cerebral artery. In contrast, artherosclerosis is less

prominent in the posterior circulation and emboli seldom travel through the vertebral arteries. Brain stem strokes are thus generally due to small, penetrating arterioles emerging directly from the vertebrobasilar arteries becoming thrombosed and occluded. Evaluation of a patient with carotid ischemia will therefore usually focus on atherosclerotic disease of the neck, sometimes with a view toward carotid endarterectomy, and on cardiac sources of emboli.

Extensive workup of brain stem ischemia is seldom indicated, since surgical repair is usually not feasible, cardiac emboli to this region are rare, and therapeutic options are more limited. The most important aspect of management of the patient with symptomatic vertebrobasilar disease is to determine and correct the mechanisms that trigger the attacks, since correction of the underlying disease is seldom feasible. However, prognosis may be better for posterior circulation strokes. Although the brain stem is a vital region in which damage may have catastrophic effects, the blood supply is largely through multiple tiny vessels. Therefore, brain stem strokes are often small and patients have an excellent prognosis for recovery. Large strokes are often fatal; but most people who survive brain stem strokes recover well, with little functional impairment. The prognosis for recovery from carotid strokes is highly variable and depends on many factors, but in general it is less complete than in brain stem strokes.[50]

STROKE PATHOGENESIS

Vascular disease of the brain takes four major forms: thrombotic, embolic, lacunar, and hemorrhagic. Each has a different etiology, a different emphasis in its diagnostic workup, a different therapy, and a different prognosis (Table 29-6).

Thrombotic Stroke

Thrombotic strokes are the most common kind of stroke, accounting for about 40% of all ischemic cerebrovascular disease.[78] Thrombotic strokes are usually due to the atherosclerotic stenosis or occlusion of a large blood vessel, especially the carotid or middle cerebral artery. The clinical effects of internal carotid stenosis, internal carotid occlusion, and middle cerebral artery stenosis may be quite similar depending on the richness of collaterals, the speed of occlusion, and the individual vascular anatomy. Because thrombotic occlusion of a vessel commonly occurs as a gradual process, the deficit it produces often has a

Table 29-6
Pathogenesis of Stroke

Type	% of All Strokes	Onset	Preceding TIAs	Seizure at Onset	Headache at Onset	Coma	Atrial Fibrillation	Known Coronary Artery Disease	Angiography or Noninvasive Tests	CT Scan	Other Features
Thrombotic	40%	Stuttering, gradual	50%	1%	20%	5%	10%	50%	Large vessel stenosis or occlusion	Ischemic infarction	Carotid bruit, stroke during sleep
Embolic	30%	Sudden	10%	10%	10%	1%	35%	35%	May have stenosis or ulceration	Superficial (cortical) infarction	Underlying heart disease, peripheral emboli or strokes in different vascular territories
Lacunar	20%	Gradual or sudden	30%	0%	5%	0%	5%	35%	Normal	Normal, or small, deep infarction	Pure motor or pure sensory stroke
Hemorrhagic	10%	Sudden	5%	10%	35%	25%	5%	10%	Normal, mass effect intracranially	Hyperdense mass	Nausea and vomiting, decreased mental status

TIA, transient ischemic attack.

slower onset than other kinds of strokes. It may present as an evolving deficit or a stuttering or stepwise progression of symptoms over hours or even days. Warning signs may precede the stroke, and as many as half of patients with thrombotic strokes report previous TIAs.[78]

Thrombosis commonly occurs at night; therefore, the patient who awakens in the morning with a new deficit has probably had a thrombotic stroke. Because atherosclerosis generally involves large vessels, the ischemia produced by thrombotic strokes tends to be extensive and the patients are often severely impaired.[24]

Embolic Stroke

Emboli cause perhaps 30% of all strokes. Their relative importance may be increasing as antihypertensive drugs and better control of atherosclerotic risk factors begin to lower the incidence of thrombotic stroke.[22, 78] Embolic strokes arise from platelets, cholesterol, fibrin, or other bits of hematogenous material breaking off from an arterial wall or from the heart. Most strokes occurring in the setting of myocardial infarction are the result of cardiac emboli. Embolic strokes have a very abrupt onset since the embolic material travels up the arterial tree to lodge suddenly in a smaller caliber blood vessel. Because emboli float in the circulation until encountering a vessel with a sufficiently small diameter to stop them, they usually occlude distal, small cortical vessels. For this reason, cortical deficits are the hallmark of embolic strokes, including seizures, aphasia (dominant hemisphere), and neglect (nondominant hemisphere). Although the region of infarcted brain may be superficial and small, the effect on the patient's daily activities may be great because of the importance of cortical functions affected. Although emboli may be scattered among multiple vessels, they occasionally cause repeated strokes in the same vascular territory.

Lacunar Stroke

Lacunar strokes comprise approximately 20% of all strokes.[40, 77, 80] These are very small infarctions, by most definitions less than one cubic centimeter in size, that occur only where small perforating arterioles branch directly off large vessels. This distinctive vascular anatomy occurs in the depths of the brain in the region of the basal ganglia, internal capsule, and brain stem. Therefore, these are the regions where lacunes develop. Because these very small perforating arterioles are exposed to the same constant high pressures and flows of the large arteries from which they branch, they become damaged over the years, particularly if hypertension is present. They become thickened, hyalinized, and thrombosed, resulting in small infarcts in the discrete territory supplied by the arteriole. This chronic process may produce symptoms resembling thrombosis, including a gradual onset and preceding TIAs. Since they occur in distinctive subcortical regions of the brain, lacunes produce characteristic clinical features and they do not cause aphasia, neglect, seizures, or other cortical symptoms. In fact, they are recognized by the discrete and specific subcortical deficits they produce, by far the most common being the pure motor stroke, or hemiparesis without any sensory loss.[39] Similarly, a pure sensory stroke that produces numbness but no motor deficits may also occur.[41] Although these deficits may be severe, infarctions are small and the prognosis is generally excellent, with about 85% of patients experiencing a very good recovery.[79]

Hemorrhagic Stroke

Intracerebral hemorrhage accounts for only 10% of all strokes, making it the rarest but the most catastrophic type of CVA. Typically, the onset is very sudden, although bleeding may continue over minutes or hours. The clinical key to recognition of hemorrhagic stroke is the presence of increased intracranial pressure resulting from the sudden outpouring of blood into the brain, causing headache, nausea and vomiting, and a decreased level of consciousness.[78] The stroke patient who is lethargic or comatose probably has bled.[91] Hemorrhages tend to occur in exactly the same location as lacunes, namely, deep within the brain in the region of the basal ganglia, internal capsule, and brain stem.[53, 65] Here, hypertension can rupture the penetrating arterioles and cause subsequent hemorrhage. Subcortical deficits are thus most common, although generally much more extensive than those seen with lacunes because of the large mass of blood. Hemiplegia, hemisensory loss, and visual field defects are common, in addition to altered mental status. The prognosis for hemorrhagic stroke is very poor, with an initial mortality of 50% to 70%. If the patient does recover, the blood may be reabsorbed, leaving only mild deficits.

INTERVENTION

Medical Intervention

Following a completed stroke, care of the patient should emphasize supportive measures. Patients are generally admitted to the hospital following the acute event. Of course, supportive treatment of vital functions is necessary if the patient is comatose or unstable. There is some controversy regarding how long patients should be at bed rest to avoid postural hypotension and conditions that may aggravate their stroke versus whether they should be allowed to ambulate early for active rehabilitation and prevention of deep venous thrombosis, pulmonary embolism, and other complications. Most clinicians favor early ambulation. Stroke patients who are either bedridden or have lost mobility in their limbs are at high risk for deep venous thrombosis, and pulmonary embolism is one of the leading causes of morbidity and mortality following a stroke.[118] Prophylaxis for pulmonary embolism is a controversial subject, but a case can be made for low-dose heparin therapy, such as 5000 units given subcutaneously twice daily.[74]

It is usually preferable to err on the side of hypertension in patients with ischemic stroke since lowering the blood pressure too quickly may further enlarge the area of ischemia.[87] Most patients have a transient blood pressure elevation after their stroke, and this can usually be monitored without intervention. Other support includes maintenance of hydration and normal glycemia as well as proper electrolyte balance. Another leading cause of morbidity after stroke is aspiration pneumonia, so patients should have their oral intake restricted until it is clear their swallowing mechanism is adequate. Fever and other evidence of infection after a stroke should prompt a search for pneumonia.

Aside from supportive measures, little can be done to alter the outcome of a completed infarction. If there is an edematous swelling of the brain, as may occur after hemorrhage or massive ischemic infarction, the use of hyperosmolar agents such as intravenous mannitol, urea, or glycerol can osmotically remove water from the brain and hence shrink its size. Thus more room is available for the blood or swollen brain within the tight confines of the cranium. Diuretics such as furosemide (Lasix) may also help reduce the water content of the brain. Corticosteroids, which are often employed for this purpose, probably have little benefit.[62]

Many other agents have been used in attempts to preserve remaining function in the damaged, but not destroyed, brain

tissue in the region of a stroke; others have been employed to aid in recovery of already lost functions. The list (Table 29-7) includes vasodilators such as papaverine, dilutional or hypoviscosity agents such as dextran, agents to prevent neuronal damage such as calcium channel blockers, and a variety of other drugs including steroids, naloxone, barbiturates, β-adrenergic blockers, and antioxidants. There are various opinions concerning the usefulness of these agents, but no adequate study has demonstrated the effectiveness of any of them.

Most stroke therapy has thus shifted to the prevention of strokes, especially after TIAs. Unfortunately, again, the evidence supporting either medical or surgical treatment as effective in preventing subsequent stroke is meager.

Anticoagulation, either with heparin or warfarin compounds, is sometimes recommended for patients who have had a TIA. A review of the many past studies of anticoagulation following a TIA again reveals a mix of both optimistic and pessimistic results, but the overall information available does not prove its efficacy.[15] Nevertheless, many clinicians continue to use these drugs, often for 3 to 12 months following a TIA, during which time the risk of stroke is highest. Patients with a cardiac source of TIA or those having multiple TIAs, or those with a tight stenosis of a major vessel (*e.g.,* the internal carotid artery, middle cerebral artery, or basilar artery) are often chosen as candidates for anticoagulation. After several months to a year, the risks of chronic anticoagulation therapy probably exceed the benefits in stroke reduction, so such treatment is seldom prolonged beyond this time. Uncontrolled hypertension, peptic ulcer disease, and other bleeding diatheses are, of course, contraindications to this type of therapy.

Antiplatelet agents have become the mainstay of stroke therapy. Aspirin is the primary drug used. Several large-scale, prospective, randomized, double-blind, multicenter, long-term studies of aspirin for the prevention of stroke in patients with previous stroke or TIA have been conducted.[9, 12, 18, 19, 38, 95, 107] There are some differences in design and methodology among these studies, making results difficult to compare reliably. Some studies have suggested that aspirin can reduce the number of strokes in such patients,[9, 18] but most studies have failed to show such benefit (Table 29-8).[12, 19, 38, 107] However, because some of the data suggest a possible benefit from aspirin, and since it is a relatively benign drug with few complications or risks to the patient, it is almost universally employed in patients with cerebrovascular disease. Large studies have cited dosages of 1 g or more of aspirin per day. However, some clinicians, based on theoretical reasons rather than clinical data, prefer a lower dose, such as one aspirin per day. Treatment is usually continued indefinitely.

Other antiplatelet agents such as sulfinpyrazone (Anturane) and dipyridamole (Persantine) are also occasionally used. The evidence that they are of benefit is even weaker than for aspirin, and it is likely that these drugs have no real usefulness in prevent-

---

Table 29-7
Some Agents That Have Been Used to Treat Strokes

Steroids	Barbiturates
Dextran	Antioxidants
Hyperventilation	Calcium channel blockers
Vasodilators	β-Adrenergic blockers
Naloxone	

Table 29-8
Prospective, Randomized, Double-Blind, Controlled Trials of Aspirin for the Prevention of Stroke

Study	No. of Patients	Follow-up	Daily Aspirin Dose	Stroke		Myocardial Infarction		All Deaths		Comments
				On Aspirin	Not on Aspirin	On Aspirin	Not on Aspirin	On Aspirin	Not on Aspirin	
American Fields et al[38]	178	24 mo	1300 mg	11/88 (12%)	14/90 (15%)	2 Fatal	3 Fatal	3	7	No benefit for aspirin. Some trends favored aspirin.
German Reuther et al[95]	58	24 mo	1500 mg	0/29	4/29	Not studied	Not studied	0	0	No benefit for aspirin (numbers too small), but trend favored aspirin.
Canadian Barnett et al[18]	585	26 mo	1300 mg	36/390 (12%)	48/295 (16%)	Not studied	Not studied	17	25	Claimed benefit for aspirin (only in men without heart disease), but controversial statistical manipulations.
Italian Candelise et al[19]	124	11 mo	1000 mg	2/63 (4%)	2/61 (4%)	0	1	0	1	No benefit for aspirin; no trend.
French Bousser et al[9]	604	36 mo	1000 mg	35/400 (11%)	31/204 (18%)	7	11	18	7	Claimed benefit for aspirin in men and women.
Danish Sorenson et al[107]	203	25 mo	1000 mg	17/101 (17%)	11/102 (11%)	6	14	7	7	No benefit for aspirin; trend favored placebo.
Swedish Britton et al[12]	505	24 mo	1500 mg	12/253 (5%)	13/252 (5%)	8(?)	6(?)	13	13	No benefit for aspirin; no trend.

ing strokes.[1,9,18] There is hope that research on new antiplatelet agents, such as ticlopidine, will produce more effective drugs.

Surgical Intervention

The value of carotid endarterectomy in preventing strokes remains controversial and poorly documented.[31] Surgical procedures are seldom subjected to the rigorous testing of efficacy that is required of drugs, and no adequate prospective controlled trial has shown carotid endarterectomy to be superior to drug management or even placebo for the prevention of strokes. Nevertheless, surgical therapy is the standard practice in most communities in the United States; carotid endarterectomy is one of the most frequent operations performed. If such an approach is considered, patients who have TIAs or very mild or recovered strokes in a carotid artery distribution, when medically stable, will undergo cerebral angiography. If a significant stenosis of 50% to 70% or more is discovered in the carotid artery, or ulcerated plaques are found, carotid endarterectomy will usually

be performed. There is much debate regarding the true morbidity and mortality of this surgery, either in the hands of experienced surgeons or in the community at large, as well as the actual reduction in risk that successful surgery imparts. A prospective randomized study underway in the United Kingdom comparing carotid endarterectomy with antiplatelet therapy may help answer these questions.

Some patients with TIAs or minor strokes have a completely occluded internal carotid artery or a vessel with stenosis or ulceration in a surgically inaccessible site. For this reason, a surgical bypass of the lesion was once advocated, using an anastomosis between an extracranial blood vessel, usually the superficial temporal artery, and an intracranial blood vessel, such as the middle cerebral artery or one of its branches. A careful prospective, randomized, controlled trial of extracranial to intracranial artery bypass patients who had TIAs failed to demonstrate any benefit from surgery, either in general or in any specific subgroups of patients.[32] There is no longer any clear indication for this procedure for the prevention of stroke.

Surgical bypass or endarterectomy involving the posterior

circulation is being performed with increasing frequency. Although there are reports of successes, these procedures remain largely experimental.

Conclusions

It seems certain that a great potential for recovery after stroke exists, since many neurons affected by stroke are merely damaged rather than destroyed. Therapy to salvage these reversibly damaged cells could have a major impact on improving stroke outcome. Similarly, our basic scientific knowledge of atherosclerosis, platelet function, microcirculation, and biochemical mechanisms of hypoxia in cell injury, as well as pharmacology of drugs that affect these processes, has expanded enormously in recent years. The nihilistic view that stroke will remain forever an untreatable condition is thus not warranted.

Unfortunately, these advances have not yet been translated into clinical benefits, and the situation today is one in which a wide variety of medical and surgical treatments are applied to stroke victims, often aggressively and dogmatically, despite the flimsiest of evidence that any of these treatments are effective. In fact, despite the vast increase in our understanding of cerebrovascular disease, the clinician today has little more to offer than did physicians of a generation ago. There is no treatment, medical or surgical, that has been proven to alter the natural history of TIAs or strokes.

CONTROL OF RISK FACTORS

Until more effective medical and surgical therapy for stroke is available, the best hope for ameliorating the enormous public health impact of stroke is by reduction of risk factors. Preventive medicine is much more effective in this setting than therapy after the fact. Since excellent control of high blood pressure can be achieved with available antihypertensive agents, this is probably the single most important intervention a physician can make to minimize the risk of stroke. Although there is debate regarding the effectiveness of tight glucose control in diabetics to prevent complications such as stroke, it seems reasonable to control glucose as well as possible. Life-style changes, including the cessation of smoking and dietary restrictions on lipids, while altering only minor risk factors for stroke, also seem sensible. Attention to the heart, with good management of coronary artery disease, congestive heart failure, and arrhythmias, also minimizes the possibility of stroke.

STROKE REHABILITATION CONTROVERSY

Stroke survivors are often left with severe mental and physical disabilities, which create a major economic and social impact. An idea of the magnitude of the public health problem of stroke can be seen in statistics showing that 71% of stroke survivors have impaired vocational capacity, 16% remain institutionalized, 31% need assistance in self-care, and 20% require assistance in ambulation. With increasing numbers of elderly persons in the population, stroke and its prevention are a matter of great concern to society.[128]

The value of rehabilitation following a stroke remains hotly debated. Some authorities believe "many studies have demonstrated that stroke rehabilitation is effective and that it can significantly improve functional ability even in patients who are elderly, medically ill, and who have severe neurological and functional deficits."[37]

Other authorities believe "experts in stroke rehabilitation abound, but none of them has ever proved anything about rehabilitation to the satisfaction of anyone else."[56] Proof of efficacy of a treatment, whether a drug or rehabilitation therapy, requires prospective, randomized, blinded controlled trials, usually with large numbers of people followed for a long period of time. No such studies acceptable by modern standards have been performed evaluating rehabilitation therapy after a stroke. Indeed, such evaluations may be impossible because so many variables may influence the results.[29] Stroke outcome is related to the cause of the stroke, its severity, and its location. The age of the patient, his or her motivation, the family and socioeconomic system, and the specific neurological deficits all affect the outcome of rehabilitation. Different aspects of physical therapy of importance include the timing (how soon after the stroke?) type (activities of daily living, speech therapy, occupational therapy, interdisciplinary team approach versus individual therapy), duration, and intensity. It is not even clear how best to evaluate the results of rehabilitation—whether to use mortality, length of hospitalization, performance of activities of daily living, or standardized disability scales.

Although many studies have addressed the value of rehabilitation after stroke, there are many differences among them that make comparisons and generalizations impossible. They arrive at disparate conclusions, some supporting rehabilitation[2, 36, 68, 104, 130] and some finding no benefit,[44, 70, 89, 121, 125] but all have sufficient flaws to make their results suspect. Rehabilitation therapy is an expensive and limited resource, but the factors that determine which patients would most benefit from it remain uncertain. Nevertheless, most patients and families desire rehabilitation, and most physicians request it for all but the most severely involved cases.

STROKE REHABILITATION

Accurate data regarding stroke incidence and prevalence is lacking since there is no national stroke registry. However, from various local studies it has been observed that of the patients who survive longer than 1 month after stroke, 10% experience an almost complete spontaneous recovery. Another 10% do not benefit from any form of treatment owing to the severity of disability. It is the remaining 80%, with significant neurological deficits, who may benefit from rehabilitation.[108] Again, statistics vary, but this represents from 150,000 to 200,000 people per year. The estimated prevalence of stroke in the United States is around 1 million.

Candidates for Rehabilitation

There are some general considerations that may be helpful in selection of candidates for rehabilitation. Patients whose physical condition prevents them from engaging in therapies should be excluded. Because learning is an integral aspect of rehabilitation, patients who demonstrate inability to follow verbal or gestural instructions or who evidence severe memory problems will not be able to compensate for physical deficits through rehabilitation. Some authors have suggested that certain demented patients actually regress with traditional rehabilitation techniques.[103] Although it is difficult to characterize the best candidate for rehabilitation, statements can be made regarding patients who have little chance of benefitting.[34, 35, 111] In a review of 33 studies of prediction of function after stroke, it was found that poor prognostic indicators include previous stroke, older age, urinary and bowel incontinence, and visuospatial deficits. There was no correlation found between functional outcome and sex or hemisphere affected.[58]

"Stroke rehabilitation" is not well defined; it ranges from specialized stroke units, where all patients are medically managed and therapies are primarily nursing responsibilities, to general acute care settings, where physical therapy is ordered, to comprehensive stroke rehabilitation offered by rehabilitation teams. These teams include physicians who have had special training or experience in rehabilitation, physical therapists, occupational therapists, speech pathologists, rehabilitation nurses, neuropsychologists, and other professionals whose main interest and experience is in stroke management. Perhaps these differences of treatment setting account for some of the variability in outcome studies. For example, in one randomized controlled study of elderly acute stroke patients, independence in self-care activities was achieved more quickly by patients on the stroke unit than by those on medical units.[105] Although it is unrealistic to assume that all patients can be rehabilitated in specialized programs, it is appropriate to expect that some type of stroke rehabilitation should be made available to each patient who may have a chance of improved quality of life and greater independence in activities of daily living.[3] This concept becomes increasingly important in an aging population by decreasing the dependence on nursing services. The challenge remains to better define the group who might benefit from rehabilitation. In practice, this selection process often takes the form of a 1- to 2-week trial of rehabilitation.

Typical Deficits

There are well-recognized patterns of deficits secondary to the localization of ischemic strokes. Lesions that involve the anterior cerebral artery usually result in paralysis and cortical hypesthesia of the contralateral lower limb. There may be mild involvement of the contralateral arm. This may be accompanied by mental changes of impaired judgment and insight. There may be apraxia of gait, a sucking reflex and grasping reflexes of the contralateral side, as well as incontinence of bowel and bladder.

The more commonly seen middle cerebral artery infarction results in a contralateral hemiplegia. Usually the arm is more affected than the leg; however, there may be paralysis of the face alone, one limb alone, or even part of one limb. Impairment of sensation occurs in the same areas as motor loss (cortical sensory deficit or cortical hypesthesia). There may be blindness in one half of the visual field (hemianopsia), difficulty in speaking or in understanding language (dysphasia), or inability to recognize people and things (visual agnosia). Deficits will be present depending on hemispheric laterality.

Posterior cerebral artery lesions result in inability to recognize or comprehend written words (alexia), mental change with memory impairment, and an inability to recognize people and things (visual agnosia), which is often temporary. There may be paralysis or palsy of the third cranial nerve. Visual deficits include hemianopsia or cortical blindness (unawareness by the patient that he or she cannot see).

Each patient therefore presents a unique challenge for the rehabilitation team based on the localization of the lesion and resultant neurological deficits, and management should be as individualized as possible.

Patterns of Recovery

In typical classic stroke, the affected limbs are totally paralyzed. When accompanied by absence of tendon reflexes, the affected extremity is said to be flaccid. Deep tendon reflexes usually return within 48 hours.[115] Characteristically, there is a gradual continuous progression from flaccidity to spasticity to normal muscle tone, while complete motor paralysis resolves through synergy patterns to voluntary segmental movements. Synergy patterns are mass, composite motor movements; for example, a patient who attempts to flex his or her elbow will have movement at the shoulder, wrist, and possibly the fingers.

In the upper extremity, flexor activity predominates, so that the posture assumed is that of scapular retraction and depression, internal rotation and adduction of the shoulder, pronation of the forearm, and flexion of the elbow, wrist, and fingers. In the lower extremity, overactivity of the extensors typically results in an anatomical retraction and elevation of the pelvis; extension, adduction, and internal rotation of the hip; extension of the knee; and plantarflexion of the ankle and inversion of the foot. Strengthening of the muscle groups in the affected extremity that are not predominantly affected may improve function. Typically, proximal function returns prior to distal function.

The process of recovery may be halted at any phase; an upper extremity may remain flaccid or synergy patterns may never yield to voluntary isolated movement. Poor prognosis for functional recovery is related to prolonged flaccid period, late onset of motion (2 to 4 weeks), absence of voluntary hand movement (4 to 6 weeks), severe proximal spasticity, and late return of reflexes.[115]

Along with return of motor function, another important area for consideration is sensory function. Impairment of proprioception and tactile senses may prohibit the patient with good motor ability from using the limb functionally. This is especially relevant to tasks involving manual dexterity and affects ambulation when the patient lacks proprioceptive feedback of foot placement.

The stroke patient should undergo frequent comprehensive neurological assessment so that functional neurological recovery can be documented. Rather than focusing solely on neurological deficits, other factors, such as age-related disorders, intellectual impairment, and medication effect should be taken into consideration when neurological status is assessed for prognostic reasons.[114]

Stroke Rehabilitation Techniques

Conventional Therapies

Conventional methods of stroke rehabilitation include various combinations of range of motion and muscle strengthening exercises, mobilization activities, and compensatory techniques. There is debate regarding which type of traditional exercise program is more advantageous. One study showed that a program of selective stretching, training in activities of daily living, and progressive resistive exercise was more effective in aiding patients to achieve functional independence in 1 month than a program of training in activities of daily living alone, or in combination with active exercise.[55]

Neurophysiological Therapies

More controversial are the neurophysiological/developmental based methods, in which the therapeutic exercise program incorporates neuromuscular re-education techniques. These include the techniques popularized by Brunnstrom, Rood, Bobath, and Kabat, Knott, and Voss. Brunnstrom's approach attempts to enhance specific synergies through the use of cutaneous and proprioceptive stimuli as well as central facilitation, following Twitchell's stages of recovery. Rood advocates modifications of muscle tone and voluntary motor activity through use of cutaneous sensory stimulation. Bobath emphasizes the use of specific postures appropriate for task, while suppressing synergies with sensory input and motor feedback. Kabat, Knott, and Voss use reflexes and a patterning technique for proprioceptive neuromuscular facilitation (PNF).[42]

In a study by Stern, patients who were treated with conventional therapy did just as well as patients treated with PNF and Brunnstrom techniques in areas of self-care, mobility, and strength.[110] Dickstein compared conventional treatment, PNF, and Bobath techniques and also found no difference in outcome.[28] Despite these findings, some aspects of these more controversial techniques are usually combined with traditional therapies for most patients, since a specific technique may be beneficial in an individual case.

Biofeedback

Biofeedback attempts to modify autonomic functions, pain, and motor disturbances through acquired volitional control by way of auditory, visual, and sensory clues. In applying biofeedback to patients with neurological disorders, several factors require consideration. One is "acquired volitional control"; the patient must be able to understand what is required of him or her. Speech, language, and cognition must be intact and functioning at near normal levels. The patient must also have enough control of voluntary functions so that abnormal myoneural firing can be inhibited.[4] Proprioceptive impairment is also a negative influence.[129] Electrode placement sites may be over primary mover or antagonist muscle groups, or both, and may be used for facilitation or inhibition of muscle contraction. The success of biofeedback is dependent on the cognitive function and the ability to acquire volitional control. This is often compromised by the amount of central nervous system deficit making other treatment techniques more effective in the initial recovery rehabilitation period.

In the upper extremity, biofeedback has been employed in attempts to control shoulder subluxation and to improve hand function.[6, 17] Wolf found that biofeedback was more successful in restoration of function in the lower than in the upper extremity.[129]

Functional Electrical Stimulation

Functional electrical stimulation (FES) is commonly employed in both upper and lower extremities to improve strength, encourage and augment early active range of motion, assist in the management of dependent peripheral edema through forceful isotonic muscle contraction, and establish early proprioceptive joint sense in the sensory-compromised patient.[64, 75, 131] It has also proven effective in aiding the reduction of antagonistic muscle spasticity and reduction of joint contractures.[131] FES is used for improving gait and for wrist and finger muscle activity. It is not useful for completely paralyzed muscles. FES and positional feedback has been advocated as a treatment modality for facilitating wrist extension.[10]

Typical Problems

In addition to absent or weak muscular strength after stroke, typical functional problems include joint contractures, incoordination, and abnormalities of muscle tone, particularly hypertonicity. The main treatment of contractures is prevention, through range of motion exercises. When muscle tone over-

comes the ability to move the joint through full range of motion, antispasticity medications should be considered. Incoordination may be a result of weakness, poor proprioception, or neglect and may respond to specific training techniques.

Antispasticity medications are typically used when spasticity interferes with mobility or activities of daily living or is a significant source of pain. These medications include dantrolene sodium (Dantrium), diazepam (Valium), and baclofen (Lioresal). Stroke patients rarely benefit from diazepam or baclofen since they may alter reflexes but not affect synergy patterns. Diazepam should not be used in the depressed patient. Both of these agents act as central nervous system depressants, although baclofen's main site of action is the spinal cord. Dantrolene, working directly at the skeletal muscle level, may help in the bedridden patient for nursing care of positioning and hygiene. Doses of these medications should be adjusted so that loss of spasticity does not interfere with ambulation, since the spasticity may provide support to weak muscles. Abrupt withdrawal of any of these medications should be avoided. Currently, there is no medication effective in treating the abnormally increased tone of the stroke patient.[132] Muscle relaxants are not antispasticity medications and should not be used in the stroke patient, since they may impair cognition.

Ideally, spasticity treatment should affect only targeted muscle fibers and be long lasting. This has been attempted through the use of peripheral nerve blocks with phenol.[90] These are most often used in the tibial nerve, to diminish spasticity of foot plantarflexion and ankle clonus. Complications have included development of painful paresthesias in a few patients.[90] Since the nerve may be destroyed, there should be no clinical evidence of neurological improvement, motor or sensory, for several months prior to the procedure. Other nerves may also be blocked.

Surgical management of spasticity in the stroke patient consists of tendon releases and/or transfers.[113, 119] Bone or joint procedures are not usually necessary. Generally, surgical procedures have proven more successful on the lower extremity than the upper, although this may be due to patient selection. Although improvement may be anticipated, no patient will be made "normal" by a surgical procedure.[113]

Specific Age Groups Affected by Stroke

As the population ages, more and more elderly patients are affected by a stroke. A significant number of these patients will have already sustained a previous stroke. The impact on the patient's potential as a rehabilitation candidate have already been discussed.

Infrequently, children are affected by stroke. There is a paucity of literature on this subject. One major review of 86 children with acute hemiplegia evaluated prognosis for future seizures, residual hemiparesis, intellectual capacity, and behavior disorders. The etiology of the stroke was classified as unknown in 41 of these children. Seizures as a presenting symptom were present in a majority of children under 2 years of age; this was related to increased mortality, motor deficits, intellectual problems, and further seizures. Older children usually had no seizures at the onset. Approximately 50% of the 41 children had mild to moderate residual motor deficit but normal intellect and behavior without seizures.[106]

In many ways the rehabilitation of children is similar to that of adults. However, it is important that allowances be made for physical growth in equipment prescriptions. Nonfunctional extremities may be neglected, and the child may become very adept at one-handed techniques. Fortunately, most affected children remain ambulatory.

Complications in upper and lower extremity management are similar. Movement disorders (tremor, dysdiadochokinesis) affecting the previously hemiplegic upper extremity may severely impede functions; anticholinergic medications have not been of benefit. Biofeedback techniques may be helpful.[92]

Cognitive Aspects of Stroke

To successfully participate in a comprehensive rehabilitation program, a patient must be capable of following commands and learning. This is one of the areas in which the difference between right hemiplegia and left hemiplegia is readily apparent. The patient's mental status will influence these abilities: a person who is not oriented may have great difficulty in learning new skills (new information) while someone who may not be able to relate the date can show progress in ambulation, a previously mastered skill. The amount of functional disability to be overcome also plays a role: someone who is severely disabled will need more awareness and ability to learn new methods of function to become independent.

In a study of outcomes of patients with dual disability of hemiplegia and lower extremity amputation, it was found that patients who underwent amputation prior to stroke had a better functional outcome. Patients with left hemiplegia who later had amputations demonstrated the poorest outcomes. This was attributed to perceptual problems and difficulty in learning prosthetic ambulation with preexisting neurological weakness.[116]

A frequent reason for exclusion from rehabilitation is poor motivation, particularly in the geriatric population. This may be attributed to such factors as response to disability, interference from medical and psychiatric conditions, or lack of understanding of rehabilitation goals.[52] The rehabilitation team should identify and investigate these potential problems, rather than attributing lack of progress to "poor motivation." If solutions are available, the patient may then be given a rehabilitation trial.

Some patients benefit from neuropsychological testing to define specific areas of involvement and outline methods of treatment. Occupational therapists, speech pathologists, and psychologists may all be involved with aspects of cognitive retraining. The approaches used should be reinforced in as similar a fashion as possible by the rehabilitation nursing staff and other rehabilitation team members, as well as the patient's family. The team's approach should include a stimulation program to enhance memory skills, specific methods for the presentation of new materials to be used by all team members, and consideration for safety factors on discharge. Cognitive retraining or communicative retraining may be used to address orientation, mental alertness, attention span, short- and long-term memory, sequencing, abstract reasoning, categorization, and basic problem solving.

Many types of activities are employed to help improve the cognitive status of the patient. Patients often respond well to computer training owing to the flexibility, diversity, and multiple visual and auditory feedback mechanisms built into these programs. Cognitive retraining can also be accomplished through use of pictures of family members, reference to clocks or calendars, and attendance at special activity groups. Memory books containing an ongoing log of the patient's activities, written by the patient, are particularly useful, as are prominently posted schedules of the day's activities.

Patients with cognitive deficits often require 24-hour supervision after discharge; this recommendation should be thoroughly discussed with the patient and family well before discharge and documented in the medical record. The neuropsychologist may help make decisions regarding legal competence and return to education and vocational situations and provide outpatient follow-up of the cognitively impaired patient. As the neuropsychologist works with the patient and the family throughout rehabilitation, it can be reinforced that the patient's behaviors are a result of brain damage, not psychiatric disturbance.[20] However, accommodations must be made for the patient's anticipated behaviors after discharge. "Lifeline" type telephone services may be necessary for patients who are left unattended. In addition, Medic Alert tags and readily available lists of current medications may help in emergency situations when the patient is incapable of relating a medical history.

Left Hemiplegia Versus Right Hemiplegia

There are significant differences between the cognitive abilities of patients with left hemiplegia (right hemisphere injured) and right hemiplegia (left hemisphere injured). These so influence the way the patient perceives and learns that the rehabilitation professionals must use different approaches depending on the laterality of the lesion.

The left hemiplegic patient often demonstrates visuomotor perceptual impairment, loss of visual memory, and left-sided neglect. However, this patient may retain verbal fluency, so that the deficits may not be readily apparent. In fact, only with a high degree of suspicion and specialized testing, such as cognitive evaluation by speech therapist, occupational therapist, or neuropsychologist, may problems be documented. The patient may clinically appear impulsive or unorganized in performing activities of daily living. Furthermore, he or she lacks insight into these problems; he or she may become a safety problem on the rehabilitation unit with many falls, or may smoke cigarettes unsupervised when told repeatedly to do so only with someone else present. This lack of insight and judgment and inability to follow through is inconsistent with typical rehabilitation goals of independence and self-reliance. The patient "cannot be trusted." He or she does not learn from mistakes or from observing others. This must be stressed over and over again to families who are misled by the patient's verbal abilities. Neglect is more common in the left hemiplegic than the right hemiplegic. Not only affecting vision, it also is present in touch, proprioception, and hearing. Some patients deny the involved extremity, even attributing it to another person. Rehabilitation in such severe cases is difficult or impossible. Learning is impaired. The patient's performance may not improve despite repeated practice. If one task does improve, it cannot be assumed that the achievement will generalize to improve other activities.[27]

Perceptual remediation techniques should be attempted. Gordon and associates integrated basic visual scanning, somatosensory awareness and size estimation training, and complex visuoperceptual organization into a sequentially administered remediation program for right hemisphere–damaged stroke patients. At discharge, the study group demonstrated greater gains in all three areas than the control group; however, the control group continued to show improvement while the study group reached a plateau 4 months after discharge.[47]

The left hemiplegic patient frequently becomes engaged in battles with staff to be discharged (prematurely) from inpatient rehabilitation, seemingly on a whim. Lacking insight into the problem, he or she may demand discharge while literally walking into a wall. Even in mild cases of neglect, patients should be strongly discouraged from driving or operating hazardous machinery, including lawn mowers, golf carts, and power tools. Families must prevent such behavior.

The right hemiplegic patient is unable to communicate effectively. Both vocabulary and auditory retention span are reduced. However, intact right hemisphere functions such as visuomotor perception and visuomotor memory provide ways in which learning may proceed. Behaviors to be learned should be visually demonstrated step-by-step, encouraging imitation. Limiting or eliminating words is the best approach. Family members and unknowledgeable staff often incorrectly assume the patient comprehends much more than he or she does, for he or she will pick up ideas of conversations through body language, tone of voice, expression, and even the speaker.[27] This can be demonstrated by relating a known humorous story with inappropriate emotions and gestures, such as sadness or anger. The patient will take cues and react as the story teller. If the listeners react appropriately, the patient may become confused, indicating lack of verbal comprehension. This socially autonomous behavior may fool the casual observer. When the patient fails to follow a direction or respond appropriately to a question, he or she may have difficulty benefitting from rehabilitation. In contrast to the person with left hemiplegia, one with the right hemiplegia will learn from mistakes, is able to synthesize parts of a task, and will learn from observing others in the therapy department.

Post-Stroke Depression

Post-stroke mood disorders have been attributed to a simple psychological reaction to physical or cognitive impairment. In fact, brain lesions may alter signs and symptoms of depression. Communication impairment may restrict the verbal psychiatric history, while depression in those who speak but who have flattened affect from right frontal lesions may not be fully appreciated by the team. Denial of illness may prevent the patient from giving accurate emotional reports, while euphoric behaviors may hide depression.[101]

Robinson, through a series of studies on post-stroke depression, has found that 26% of a group of 103 stroke patients had symptoms of major depression; another 20% had symptoms of minor depression. He cites a third mood disorder associated with stroke that is characterized by an indifferent, apathetic mental state associated with inappropriate cheerfulness.[96] The prospective study of acute stroke patients over the first 2 years post stroke suggests that "post-stroke depressions are long-term disorders which are not simply a reflection of the clinical course of stroke rehabilitation."[98]

There is evidence that depression is more common in patients with left hemisphere than right hemisphere injury and that severity of the depression correlates with the proximity of the lesion to the frontal pole.[99] Diagnosable depression may occur in up to 70% of patients with left frontal injury, while only 15% of right hemisphere–injured patients have diagnosable depression in the acute post-stroke period.[96] In addition, patients between 6 months and 2 years after stroke have an increased prevalence of depression.[97] It is hypothesized that biological depression following stroke could be related to catecholamine-containing neurons, which may be partially damaged by focal brain injury. There may be differences that depend on hemispheric involvement as well.[96]

Signs of depression may include slowed or inconsistent recovery, poor cooperation, management problems, or clinical deterioration from a previously stable neurological deficit. The family as well as the patient should be interviewed regarding depression; the patient may deny it. A patient who does not have pseudobulbar palsy but displays inappropriate laughing or crying is probably depressed. The patient's behaviors may be very different from his or her statements about depression.[100]

The dexamethasone suppression test (DST) has been used as a biological marker to document the existence of depression. In one study, this test was abnormal in almost 50% of patients 7 weeks after stroke. Differences between left and right hemi-

plegia were not significant, and the results of the DST did not correlate with rehabilitation outcome.[93]

Psychological/psychiatric support or antidepressants, or both, are indicated for post-stroke depression. Nortriptyline (Pamelor) has been shown to be an efficacious treatment. Care must be taken to observe for side-effects of such drugs, such as bladder distention, particularly in the elderly population. All patients who demonstrate depression after stroke should be evaluated and given a trial of antidepressant medication.[71]

Communication Rehabilitation

There is controversy over when rehabilitation of communication impairment following stroke should begin and for how long treatment should last. The first 6 weeks to 2 months following a stroke has traditionally been known as a period when spontaneous recovery takes place. Some specialists believe that this recovery will take place regardless of intervention by the speech pathologist. However, early intervention by the speech pathologist has a number of advantages. Early diagnosis of the communication impairment will aid in recovery by identifying the patient's specific communication problems. Often the patient is thought to be able to understand what is heard when he or she does not. Aphasic patients will often respond to questions with head nods and appropriate eye contact with the speaker. Any patient has a 50% chance of answering a question correctly if it requires a yes or no response.

Assessment of communicative deficits is necessary so that the patient's family and the rehabilitation team can understand the nature and extent of the communication impairment and provide the best possible treatment. The patient with aphasia suddenly becomes unable to understand, read, speak, or write. He or she is unable to communicate the simplest of needs and becomes frustrated and angry as attempts to communicate fail. (See Chapter 6 for a discussion of the evaluation and treatment of communication impairment.)

Acute Rehabilitative Intervention

Immediately after the patient sustains a stroke, problems may occur due to immobility. The person who lives alone, and therefore may not be discovered for several hours or even days following an event, is particularly prone to dehydration and the development of pressure sores. Even during the hospital evaluation, similar problems may develop. Positioning is a primary concern. Lying on the affected side may lead to edema and/or early contractures of the paralyzed arm and leg. Elevating the head of the bed may cause shear forces, leading to sacral sores.

The bed should be left flat to prevent hip and knee contractures and pressure sores. An egg-crate mattress will provide extra pressure relief. A second egg-crate mattress should be used for the patient who will be transported on stretchers for diagnostic testing. When the patient is positioned, care should be taken to prevent placement of undue stress on the paralyzed extremities by tugging or pulling. Family members should also be educated with regard to this precaution. Positions of side lying should be changed approximately every 2 hours. The prone position, although not always accepted by adults, decreases the risk of hip and knee contractures. Footboards are of questionable use in preventing footdrop because of constant repositioning needs and potential increase in spasticity; however, they may function to prevent tight, heavy bed sheets from causing injury to the affected lower extremity. A space of 10 to 15 cm between the mattress and the footboard can be used for free clearance of the heels. Another method of prevention of heel ulcers is the use of heel protector boots. The use of boots with large external plastic foot positioners is unsafe because the device may injure the affected extremity when worn bilaterally.

The patient's bed should be situated so that the majority of activities occur on the patient's unaffected side, minimizing problems secondary to visual neglect. Later, as compensatory training progresses, the telephone, bedside table, and other items may be placed on the affected side.

At approximately 48 hours after stroke, if the patient appears medically stable, bedside physical therapy, occupational therapy, and speech therapy, if indicated, should be started. The patient will receive passive range of motion to the involved extremities as well as active assistive or active range of motion to the unaffected extremities by both physical therapy and occupational therapy. The type of motion employed depends on the level of consciousness of the patient and the patient's ability to follow simple commands. Active resistive exercise can be used when the patient's awareness level improves. Occupational therapists will perform early bedside evaluation of activities of daily living. Physical therapy will pursue progressive mobilization including assessment and treatment of sitting balance, head and trunk control, and bed mobility. The impaired patient can usually learn to use the bed rails for assistance early in treatment. The overhead trapeze bar is not usually functionally appropriate for this patient. As the patient's tolerance to sitting improves, bedside therapy should be replaced by therapy in the departments.

Family members should be given as much information as possible regarding potential stroke outcomes by the rehabilitation team. They can be involved in assisting with feeding and employ passive range of motion activities, as taught by therapists, but should not assume the patient's responsibility for participating in rehabilitation. Often one family member appears to function as the family "nurse" to the exclusion of others. However, it may be another family member who must assume care at home. The team should be aware of this to better help the family cope with the situation.

During the acute phase, there should be a stable neurological status, normal blood pressure, appropriate glucose levels, and maintenance of adequate nutritional status. Advancing the diet too rapidly may increase the risk of aspiration. Food pocketing on the affected side of the mouth, poor cough, choking on liquids, or refusal to eat are some of the warning signs. Absence or presence of a gag reflex does not correlate well with swallowing. Assessments should be made early by the speech pathologist and the diet modified as needed. Dysphagia will be discussed more fully later.

Intravenous lines should not be placed in the affected extremity, particularly if the limb is sensory impaired or severely neglected. Such placement interferes with passive range of motion activities, increasing chances of contracture, as well as predisposing to phlebitis. Foley catheters should be removed as soon as there is no need to closely monitor urinary output. Often voiding can be managed by offering the urinal or bed pan every 2 hours. Constipation should be avoided from the outset through hydration, diet, and resumption of the patient's usual methods of bowel management. Bedside commodes, rather than bedpans, should be used as soon as the patient's sitting balance and transfer abilities allow. Use of adult diapers should be avoided, except for the patient who otherwise cannot attend therapy because of bladder or bowel incontinence.

Other acute interventions include use of methylcellulose eye drops and taping of eyelids when necessary; use of lotions for dry skin, and application of antiembolic hose. Appropriate oral hygiene is a must. All of the patient's personal devices such as glasses, dentures, and hearing aid, if used, should be readily available and worn daily.

The patient's and family's participation in early therapy will give some indication of the patient's suitability as a rehabilitation candidate.

Lower Extremity Management

Although ambulation is an indicator of independence following stroke, it must be remembered that the majority of patients have arm involvement that is greater than lower extremity involvement. Most patients eventually ambulate with assistive devices and training but still may be dependent in care activities because of upper extremity involvement.

The physical therapist uses a variety of progressive activities aimed toward independent mobility and ambulation. A well-equipped, well-lighted physical therapy gymnasium with mats, parallel bars, mirrors, and appropriate space for maneuvering wheelchairs and ambulating with assistive devices is essential. Initial evaluation should include documentation of a manual muscle test and notation of sensory disturbances, problems of tone, spasticity, and synergies. The program first emphasizes sitting and standing balance activities at the bedside and later on the mat and at the parallel bars.

Good sitting and standing balance are prerequisites for functional transfers and ambulation. Therapists use feedback mechanisms to correct the patient's tendency to lean toward the affected side. Dynamic sitting balance is achieved through trunk exercises, use of mirrors, and verbal feedback regarding position.

Ambulation

Potential ambulatory ability should be assessed by standing the patient in the parallel bars. At times, a patient who cannot move his or her leg in bed will have enough antigravity muscle activity to support weight on the affected leg in a functional position and later ambulate. Far too often, well-meaning attendants report a patient to be "ambulating" when actually the patient is being dragged by the trunk by two attendants while unable to advance the affected extremity. This is not ambulation and usually gives false hope to the patient and family regarding prognosis.

The patient should be taught bed-to-chair transfer activities as soon as sitting balance and weight shifting activities allow. Nurses and family members should employ these transfer techniques consistently, with the patient functioning as independently as possible. These activities are just as important for patients in whom full ambulation is predicted as well as those who appear to be wheelchair bound. The hemiplegic patient is taught to do lateral transfers toward the unaffected side. For the patient who is able to come to standing and shift some weight to the affected extremity, a standing pivot transfer is preferred.

If gait belts are used, it is best if the patient is issued a belt to be used both in therapy and by nursing staff and family members when they assist the patient in transfers or ambulation. It is generally most helpful to walk on the patient's unaffected side. For safety reasons, the patient will often practice ambulation with a more advanced gait-assistive device in the physical therapy department but continue to use previously mastered equipment on the rehabilitation unit and during home visits.

The hemiplegic patient who lacks independent ambulation should be assigned a "hemiplegic" wheelchair early in the rehabilitation process. In this chair the seat is lower than a conventional wheelchair, which allows for the nonambulatory or minimally ambulatory patient to propel the chair independently using the unaffected arm on the rim and the foot on the floor for propulsion and steering. A typical chair for a patient who is severely limited in ambulation might be a hemiplegic chair with removable desk arms and swing-away, detachable footrests. The "sportie" lightweight models may be more desirable, particularly when family members cannot perform heavy lifting. The patient should have access to an appropriate chair, preferably his or her own, throughout the inpatient rehabilitation stay. Families should be discouraged from purchasing wheelchairs or borrowing from others without specific input from the rehabilitation team. If the patient already has a chair, it should be assessed for appropriateness and modified if necessary. Important equipment may include a seat belt, an arm trough, overhead sling,[81] foam cushion, or a lapboard, depending on upper extremity involvement and ambulatory status.

A patient whose hip flexors and extensors remain too weak will not ambulate independently, since there is yet no satisfactory hip bracing available. If knee extensors are weak, the knee can be maintained in extension by adequate hip extensors. Such a patient is at risk for hyperextension of the knee (genu recurvatum). Hyperextension can cause knee pain and damage; it should be addressed and eliminated whenever possible. It can be decreased in some patients using an ankle–foot orthosis (AFO) with some dorsiflexion. The characteristic spastic gait of the hemiplegic patient is typified by pelvic rotation, circumduction of the leg, equinovarus of the foot, and short stride on the affected extremity.

The ankle dorsiflexors and evertors are typically the last to show improvement in function. Usually, appropriate substitution can be made by the use of a plastic AFO. This may be prescribed as a relatively inexpensive, off-the-shelf prefabricated device, as a custom-fitted orthosis with a trim line posterior to the malleoli, or as a total contact orthosis trimmed anterior to the malleoli for more mediolateral stability. Use of a plastic AFO usually necessitates a larger size shoe on the affected foot. Whereas braces are usually covered by third party payers, shoes often are not. The most carefully fabricated AFO will not function correctly in an inappropriate shoe.

Plastic AFOs may be more cosmetic, but their rigidity may be a drawback. A double upright metal AFO may be more appropriate for the patient who experiences increasing tone after stroke. If severe spasticity causes the foot to plantarflex, a fixed plantarflexion stop is indicated.[67] Other modifications, such as the placement of a T-strap to control excessive inversion or eversion at the ankle, can be used.

Corcoran[23] found that a patient walking with a metal brace did not expend more energy than with a plastic brace. Ambulation with either type of brace significantly decreased oxygen consumption. Regardless of the type of orthosis used, the goal is to approximate normal gait patterns.[67] In a study covering a 10-year period, Ofir[88] found that there was a definite change from the use of metal to plastic bracing. Also, the total number of ambulatory patients who were braced decreased. The number of patients who achieved functional ambulation was constant, regardless of the type of bracing or even the presence of bracing. As mentioned, the hemiplegic patient rarely requires or benefits from a long leg brace, since functioning hip extensors with an appropriate ankle brace will prevent knee flexion.[108]

As lower extremity function improves, ambulation activities may be upgraded with the use of assistive devices. Because of upper extremity involvement, stroke patients can rarely use devices that require two-handed use. Devices such as hemiwalkers, wide-based or narrow-based quad canes or straight canes, for the most advanced patients, may be employed. All such devices should be adjusted for proper height and steadiness; rubber tips should be replaced as often as necessary to allow for firm contact with the floor.

Over time, endurance and speed of ambulation should be addressed. Patients should be guided through crowded halls and taken on uneven surfaces and through tight spaces. Patients with visual field deficits must be taught to compensate. Climbing stairs should be practiced, using both double and single bannisters. Safety is of prime importance; the therapy should continue until the patient demonstrates confidence and competence in these areas. A good gait pattern should be the goal. However, a therapist should not continually nag the patient about problems but reinforce appropriate movements.[14]

Lower Extremity Complications

In addition to contractures, spasticity, incoordination, and sensory impairment, the affected lower extremity is prone to complications as a result of motor weakness. Deep venous thrombosis is discussed in the section on general medical complications, as are musculoskeletal problems, including hip fracture and amputation. It must be remembered that the unaffected extremity will be subject to additional stress and potential trauma as the patient uses it more, so that careful observation of both lower extremities is essential.

Upper Extremity Management

Lack of movement, often accompanied by lack of sensation, is frightening and frustrating for a stroke patient. When the dominant hand is affected, the patient may be so overwhelmed that use of compensatory coping skills may be ignored. Therefore, he or she may be more dependent in feeding, bathing, and dressing activities than necessary. Evaluations made by the occupational therapist address all of these activities that compromise the post-stroke patient's independence in self-care activities. Formal evaluation procedures are performed in all areas of self-care, such as bathroom skills, oral and personal hygiene, dressing, feeding, kitchen activities, cleaning, personal hobbies, and child care skills, if appropriate, and are repeated at intervals and before discharge from occupational therapy services. One-handed skills are most successfully learned when the nondominant hand is affected and there are few, if any, cognitive visuoperceptual problems. The occupational therapist also employs and teaches passive range of motion exercises for the affected upper extremity. The patient and family should be taught to carry out range of motion exercises at least daily. Nurses should employ passive range of motion while assisting the patient with bathing.

As motor function improves, the therapist adds active range of motion, coordination, strengthening, and dexterity exercises to the program. Muscle re-education, including proprioceptive neuromuscular facilitation techniques, biofeedback, and functional electrical stimulation may be employed. Once the patient can tolerate sitting for long enough periods to be transported to the occupational therapy department, therapy sessions should occur there twice daily except for some morning training in activities of daily living that may be performed more appropriately in the patient's room. This is not to be considered a situation in which the occupational therapist is bathing and dressing the patient but a learning situation for the practice of skills.

Devices to assist in activities of daily living include reachers and specially adapted eating utensils, plates and cups, can openers, chopping boards, key holders, pens, and many other items. In prescribing such equipment, it must be remembered not to overload the patient with many gadgets that will not be used. Such equipment should not be delivered the day of discharge; the patient should be given the opportunity to use the devices as needed as an inpatient for a full evaluation and training period.

The occupational therapist may provide a custom-fitted

wrist–hand orthosis (WHO), if indicated. WHOs are used to prevent joint contractures secondary to abnormal posturing or to help minimize increased tone in the spastic hand. WHOs are not indicated in patients who have significant active movement or in the flaccid hand. The occupational therapist's involvement in the training with AFOs is related to ambulation evaluation and training during functional activities such as housework, cooking, and bathroom and dressing activities, including donning and doffing the AFO. The occupational therapist and the physical therapist assist in prescribing the wheelchair and training the patient in its use. Areas evaluated include the recommendation and use of the appropriate type and size of pressure-relief cushion and considerations for the use of solid seats and solid backrests, lapboards, forearm troughs, and slings. Other equipment routinely used includes protective boots, elbow pads, neurodevelopmental treatment approach positioners, prefabricated and custom-made splints, and various types of work-simplification utensils and equipment.

The occupational therapist may modify undergarments and shoes to facilitate independent dressing activities. The therapist also counsels the patient on types of clothing that may be easier to use. The nonambulatory patient may be taught to dress himself or herself in bed, using the assistance of gravity.

Shoulder Subluxation

Shoulder subluxation, a common problem, is often documented but not adequately treated. The diagnosis is clinical; there is a palpable gap between the acromion and the humeral head on the affected side more apparent than that on the unaffected. There is as yet no standard criteria for the diagnosis of shoulder subluxation, clinically or radiologically. The exact cause of subluxation remains unknown; any change in the mechanical maintenance of glenohumeral joint stability may result in shoulder subluxation. These may include the angle of the glenoid fossa, support of the scapula on the rib cage, the effect of the supraspinatus muscle on the seating of the head of the humerus, support from the superior portion of the joint capsule, and contraction of the deltoid and rotator cuff muscles when the humerus is slightly abducted.[17] In the patient with increasing upper extremity tone, shoulder subluxation may lead to problems with tone and contractures. Some patients, over time, will develop enough upper extremity tone that the head of the humerus will be pulled into the glenoid fossa when the patient stands and ambulates, although subluxation may be present when sitting. These patients may not need slings.

The use of slings to treat shoulder subluxation is controversial.[17, 54] There are many types of slings, with no clear advantage to any type. A sling that does not fit properly, or cannot be easily donned by the patient, even with assistance, will be of little benefit. Slings often do not mechanically reposition the head of the humerus into the glenoid fossa and may contribute to flexion synergies by the position in which the affected upper extremity is maintained. This may ultimately lead to contractures. Most sources agree that a flaccid upper extremity should be in a sling when the patient is ambulating, if simply to protect it, but others believe it impedes balance and standing activities.[17] A sling worn for shoulder subluxation is only necessary when the arm cannot be supported by other means, such as the armrest of a wheelchair. The sling should not be worn when the patient is in bed. The patient and family should be educated in appropriate times for use of the sling. If recovery progresses, the sling may eventually be discarded.

Another alternative is a forearm trough. Attached to the armrest of the wheelchair, the patient's arm is positioned in slight elbow flexion, the forearm pronated with the wrist and fingers extended and the thumb abducted. The elbow may require a protective pad. The forearm trough is useful for the patient who has poor upper extremity recovery, whose shoulder subluxation is minimal, and who may ambulate only short distances and therefore be primarily a wheelchair user.

Patients who are not ambulatory may use an overhead sling, attached to the wheelchair, for the prevention of hand edema as well as treatment for shoulder subluxation. An alternative for this type of patient is the use of a lapboard. Preferably clear acrylic, to diminish chances of further impairment of body image, and to allow the patient to see the floor, the lapboard should have rounded edges and be securely attached to the wheelchair. The affected arm should be placed in partial extension at the elbow, using an elbow protector. The wrist should not be allowed to dangle over the forward edge of the board.

Brachial Plexus Injury

If an atypical progression of upper extremity recovery is observed, a diagnosis of brachial plexus injury should be investigated. Clinical findings may include flaccidity and atrophy of the supraspinatous, infraspinatus, deltoid, and biceps muscles, with increased muscle tone or movement in the distal musculature of the affected extremity. Electromyography, documenting lower motor neuron involvement in a pattern consistent with a brachial plexus lesion that is not normally present in hemiplegia, will confirm the diagnosis. These injuries may represent traction injury to the affected upper extremity from improper positioning and transfer techniques. Such a problem may impede rehabilitation progress. Treatment should be directed toward education of families, nurses, and transport personnel regarding proper handling of the affected upper extremity.[17, 61, 82]

Other Peripheral Nerve Injuries

In addition to brachial plexus injury, other nerve problems may occur. These are usually secondary to improper positioning of an insensate, motor-impaired extremity.[82] The radial, ulnar, and median nerves are all at risk from pressure neuropathies, particularly in patients confined to wheelchairs. Slings, lapboards, and arm troughs may be causative agents in the affected upper extremity. Canes and other gait-assistive devices may cause compression neuropathies in the hand of the unaffected extremity.

Shoulder–Hand Syndrome

Shoulder–hand syndrome (SHS), or reflex sympathetic dystrophy of the upper extremity, is a well recognized post-stroke phenomenon. Clinical symptoms typically include painful active and passive range of motion, particularly abduction, flexion, and external rotation at the shoulder with localized tenderness; severe pain on wrist extension accompanied by edema over carpals and tenderness to deep palpation; mild edema over metacarpals without tenderness; and moderate fusiform edema of digits with severe pain on passive flexion of metacarpophalangeal and proximal interphalangeal joints.[25] Most stroke patients develop SHS between the second and forth months after stroke.[25] Thus, owing to shorter length of stay in hospital, the patient may develop problems as an outpatient, delaying diagnosis and treatment. Early recognition of SHS is paramount to appropriate resolution of this problem. There may be painful rapid loss of range of motion in affected joints. However, symptoms may occur only in the hand of the affected extremity. There should be daily observation of the hand to evaluate for edema. When such edema occurs, immediate application of a compression glove with increased range of motion exercises may be effective. The stroke patient who is transferred out of the rehabilitation unit for intensive medical or surgical therapy and is no longer treated daily by rehabilitation professionals is at risk.

Treatment objectives are to decrease pain so that passive stretching may be accomplished. This should result in diminished pain and swelling in less than 1 week. In patients with severe SHS, a short course of oral steroids (prednisone, 30 mg/day) has been shown to be helpful combined with application of superficial heat or cold prior to passive stretching of the affected joints to increase pain tolerance. Slings or resting splints may be necessary. Use of overhead slings as well as pneumatic compression units may be helpful in reducing massive hand edema.[17, 25, 81] The affected painful shoulder may awaken the patient at night; low dosages of amitriptyline (Elavil) may be helpful for sleep. Patients may benefit from oral analgesics such as aspirin, but narcotics should be avoided. A transcutaneous electrical nerve stimulation (TENS) unit may aid in pain management. Local injections of analgesics or corticosteroids have been used. Sympathetic block of the stellate ganglion or upper thoracic ganglion with an average of seven blocks required for control of symptoms has been reported. It is believed that if a series of three to four blocks or a continuous block for several days does not result in improvement, this treatment should be discontinued.[81, 109]

Patients should receive explanations of reassurance that the pain will diminish over time but that immobility will only increase the pain. They should also continue in the full rehabilitation program. If the problem recurs, the patient should undergo a second course of treatment.

Heterotopic Ossification

Heterotopic ossification is seen infrequently but may affect the elbow or the shoulder.[81] It is characterized in early stages by pain, moderate swelling, local warmth, tenderness, and decreasing passive range of motion. In the elbow, flexion is limited and there is usually no history of trauma. Radiological examination in the early stage may reveal no abnormalities, but after several months it may show calcification about the olecranon process. The calcification only occurs on the extensor surface of the elbow; therefore, a fixed extension contracture may occur but there is no limitation of forearm pronation or supination, since the proximal radioulnar joint is not involved.[83] Treatment should be directed toward continued efforts at mobilization and modalities for local pain relief. Etidronate disodium (Didronel) may be helpful in preventing further ossification.

Other Upper Extremity Problems

Thrombophlebitis may also occur.[81] The affected extremity should not be used for intravenous lines in order to prevent thrombophlebitis. If thrombophlebitis occurs, the extremity should be elevated and warm compresses applied. When evaluating shoulder complaints, rotator cuff tears and adhesive capsulitis should be ruled out.

Upper Extremity Surgery

Surgery in the affected upper extremity may be performed to diminish pain or correct flexion deformities caused by increased tone. In the functional hand, surgery can improve extension of the wrist, thumb, or fingers when hand function is impaired by increased tone. Preoperatively, local median or ulnar nerve blocks can aid in the differentiation of spasticity from contracture. Careful preoperative evaluation of motor and sensory function is essential in the selection of appropriate candidates. In the nonfunctional upper extremity, surgery can correct flexion deformities of the hand, elbow, or shoulder causing pain or preventing hygiene.[120] One study showed that in patients with localized shoulder pain and spasticity of the internal rotator mechanism, surgical release and immediate postoperative exercise program diminished pain and increased range of motion.[11]

General Medical Complications

It is rare for a stroke to occur as a single illness in a previously healthy person. Any patient who is generally deconditioned secondary to chronic medical illness and prolonged bed rest due to complications from stroke will be slower to rehabilitate and is at higher risk of developing the problems relating to immobility noted previously.

Deep Venous Thrombosis and Pulmonary Embolism

Deep venous thrombosis (DVT) in the legs and the accompanying risk of pulmonary embolism is a well-recognized complication of immobility. Phlebothrombosis occurs in approximately 30% of patients with stroke. Not surprisingly, the incidence is greater in the affected leg. Many cases are not diagnosed on a clinical basis alone. In one study using 125 fibrinogen technique, 53% of the patients were found to have developed DVT in the paralyzed leg.[118] Clinically, the lower extremities must be examined daily for edema, discoloration, or pain on movement. Well-fitting antiembolic stockings, early ambulation, and protection of the affected extremity, including proper positioning, should aid in prevention. Mini-dose heparin is advocated by many. Patients in whom DVT is clinically suspected should undergo full heparinization prior to either invasive or noninvasive diagnostic testing. The risk of pulmonary embolism following stroke is approximately 10% with DVT.[118] After diagnosis, the patient should be placed at bed rest with the affected extremity elevated with warm compresses. All therapy to the extremity should be discontinued. After full heparinization, the patient should be converted to oral anticoagulation prior to a return to full activities.

Seizures

Seizures occur in 10% to 15% of stroke patients, with half of these appearing in the acute period.[81] Seizures are more common following embolic than thrombotic strokes.[16] Patients should not be treated prophylactically for seizures. If seizures do occur, phenytoin sodium (Dilantin) is the drug of choice. The patient who is overmedicated may become lethargic. Therapeutic levels should be maintained. When seizures leave behind a temporary increase in neurological deficit (Todd's paralysis), or when they occur frequently or are not observed, the event may be misdiagnosed as another stroke.

Stroke

A patient who has sustained a stroke is at greater risk for having another. Medical management and surgical intervention in selected cases can be offered. Any neurological changes experienced by the patient should be accurately documented and carefully assessed.

Medication

Evaluation of medications, on at least a weekly basis, may be helpful in decreasing chances of drug interactions and dependency on pain medication. Hypotension, extrapyramidal symptoms, delirium, and lethargy may all result from medication effects. Patients whose caloric intake is poor will need adjustment of hypoglycemic agents. Timing of medications also plays a role. The patient who is incontinent of urine in the morning therapy session may be experiencing bladder overflow caused by a diuretic. In addition, dehydration may be a problem in patients who are oversedated.[81] Adequate fluid should be available and offered in therapy. Also common is a day/night reversal of the sleep cycle. Medication effect must be considered for all of these problems. The use of sleeping medications such as flurazepam (Dalmane), which may accumulate, should be avoided. Psychotropic medications should be monitored closely, particularly in the elderly.[46]

Nutrition

Many patients are malnourished when they reach rehabilitation owing to chronic medical illness, dietary interruption for testing, and prolonged NPO status. Factors such as visual neglect, communication impairment, cranial nerve dysfunction, and upper extremity paralysis may result in poor caloric intake. Calorie counts should be obtained and supplements added if needed. Obvious problems that may result from poor nutrition in these patients include general weakness and, therefore, the inability to fully participate in the rehabilitation program. There may also be increased risk of the development of pressure sores.

Dysphagia

In addition to disrupting speech processes, a stroke may affect the functioning of the oral and pharyngeal musculature for chewing and swallowing. This is called dysphagia. Swallowing problems have been reported in patients who have suffered brain stem lesions[30] and unilateral cerebral lesions.[76] Logemann reports that the most prevalent swallowing problem in brain stem or anterior unilateral stroke is the absence or severe delay in the swallowing reflex.[72] With an absent or delayed swallowing relfex, material will fall over the base of the tongue into the vallecula until the vallecula fills. Material will then fall into the open airway. Patients with hemiparesis of the oral and pharyngeal musculature (lips, tongue, cheeks, jaw, and vocal cords) will experience a reduction in oral and pharyngeal transit time, an increase in saliva control, pocketing of material on the side of the hemiparesis, and reduced laryngeal airway protection. The warning signs of swallowing difficulty secondary to neurological impairments include the following: confused mental state, dysarthria, complaint of obstruction, nasal regurgitation, mouth odor, aspiration, gastroesophageal reflux, speech and voice abnormality, pain, weight loss, pneumonia, previous medical history, and medications.[48, 72, 73]

Once the dysphagia evaluation is completed, some considerations should be made prior to initiation of swallowing training. These include the risk of aspiration, level of patient alertness, and extent of oral impairment that might interfere with swallowing function. Treatment should begin immediately to improve the strength, precision, and range of motion of the lips and tongue for improved oral motor control of the bolus, stimulation of the swallowing reflex to decrease its delay when the swallow is initiated, and exercises to increase adduction of the vocal cords to improve airway protection.[7, 30] Modification of food consistency may also be recommended. Patients who aspirate may tolerate a pureed diet better than a full liquid diet. Patients with severe oral motility problems may benefit from a pureed diet rather than from a full solid or mechanical soft diet. Thermal stimulation exercises may be employed with an iced oral mirror to facilitate recovery. These exercises may be taught to nurses and family members.

For the patient who is unable to swallow without significant risk of aspiration, nasogastric feeding is recommended. Many of these patients are at risk for aspiration and development of pneumonia. If long-term tube feeding is indicated due to prolonged absence of swallowing, jejunostomy with constant drip is preferred over gastrostomy feeding. Particularly with bolus feeding, a patient fed through a gastrostomy tube is likely to aspirate if the stomach becomes overextended.

Cardiac Problems

Cardiac problems are frequent in stroke patients and may dictate the pace of rehabilitation. Records of electrocardiograms should be available and electrocardiography repeated whenever clinically indicated.[81] Cardiac medications can quickly cause adverse effects in elderly patients, particularly hypotensive episodes. In these patients all exercise should be undertaken with cardiac precautions. The patient on the rehabilitation unit who vomits prior to breakfast may be exhibiting digitalis toxicity.

Urinary and Fecal Incontinence

Urinary incontinence is common, but usually transient, following stroke. Some believe that incontinence is related more to motor deficit, lack of mobility, and mental impairment than to involvement of neurological pathways; however, this view has been challenged.[8, 13, 63] Fecal incontinence relates to immobility and may result from constipation.[13] It may also indicate bilateral hemispheric involvement. Bladder and bowel training should be employed. Urological evaluation should be obtained in patients in whom urinary incontinence cannot be overcome by voiding management techniques.[26]

Sexual Concerns

Following a stroke, sexual functioning is rarely addressed by the patient, spouse, or the health care professional. In general, the more sexually active a person has been, the more active he or she remains, even into later life. There are little scientific data on post-stroke sexual functioning. Most patients' post-stroke sexual problems are related to emotional causes, such as fear, anxiety, or guilt regarding the stroke itself. Medications may have some effect. Routine sexual counseling and professional "permission" to engage in sexual activities should be given. Specific positioning and potential bowel or bladder incontinence are usually areas of patient concern.[94]

Falls

Falls are a significant cause of complications. Drug problems, alcohol abuse, lack of judgment (as in left hemiplegic patients), and visual problems all have a role. Orthostatic hypotension should be ruled out, particularly in the elderly. The stroke patient usually falls toward the paretic side. As noted, gait belts should be used at all times. Use of bedside commodes will decrease the length of bathroom trips at night. As part of the general rehabilitation program, the patient should be taught to rise from the floor. An ambulatory stroke patient who sustains a hip fracture should undergo aggressive orthopedic operative intervention and weight bearing as soon as is feasible. These patients should not be immobilized for any length of time, since morbidity and mortality rates are high.[81]

Musculoskeletal Injuries

Old musculoskeletal injuries may jeopardize the patient's ability to achieve independence, particularly those involving the unaffected extremities. For example, a patient with frozen shoulder of the unaffected extremity will have greater difficulty in performing activities of daily living. Because of atherosclerosis, many patients who have sustained strokes have experienced dysvascular limb loss or may be expected to undergo amputation in the future. One study showed that the affected extremity is more likely to be amputated than the unaffected after a stroke. Patients with diabetes mellitus were at greater risk for earlier amputation. Suggested causes include unobserved trauma due to decreased sensation, or alteration in muscle fiber usage.[45]

Endurance

Many patients need adequate periods for rest spaced throughout the day. Endurance and tolerance for activity improve gradually over time. Therapy sessions should be scheduled so that there is enough time for meals, rest, and transport to and from the therapy departments.

Psychosocial Aspects

The psychosocial aspect of stroke recovery should receive significant attention in the rehabilitation setting. It is important for the team to recognize the patient as a person with hopes, dreams, and desires that are now altered by a disability. "Motivation" becomes an issue. Fears of aging and loss of independence may be overwhelming. The patient's self-esteem and self-worth are important in rehabilitation assessment and outcome. Physical appearance plays a role. Although mirrors are employed frequently for feedback in position sense and ADL training, some patients demonstrate aversion to viewing themselves, as they perceive, disheveled and unkempt. Most rehabilitation units require patients to dress in comfortable street clothes rather than hospital gowns or personal pajamas and robes. Women are encouraged to wear makeup if desired; men are to shave as needed. Hairstyling may be encouraged. Although this is a part of rehabilitative training in activities of daily living, it also serves to reinforce a "wellness" concept. Attention to physical appearance often signals a time when the patient is ready to put forth more effort in rehabilitation.

The role of the rehabilitation social worker is crucial in providing psychosocial evaluation and follow-up during rehabilitation. He or she should be involved from the onset of the acute event, as a resource and support person for the patient and family. The social worker should be adept at interpreting insurance coverage, Medicare, Supplemental Security Income (SSI), disability, and other types of medical and financial payment systems. Aware of local agencies such as "Meals on Wheels," senior citizens groups, and stroke club support systems, the social worker serves a vital link in enabling the patient to reintegrate into the community. The social worker may also make inquiries into physical layout of the house, family members living at home, and availability of local assistance. A primary role is in making referral to extended care facilities or nursing homes and documenting other domestic details that have significant impact. In large established rehabilitation areas, social workers may facilitate regularly scheduled family–patient discussion groups, focusing on adjustment to perceived disability. The social worker can work closely with the neuropsychologist on particular cases and the home care coordinator in all cases.

There are many psychosocial problems facing stroke patients and families, including those related to psychological, social, familial, and economic stressors.[33] It is important to remember that these problems may not emerge until after discharge, rather than during the acute rehabilitative phase. Although there are community services available, without assistance from health care professionals with knowledge about such services, the patient's needs often go unmet after discharge. Particularly affected may be the patient's socialization; Schmidt found that only 33% of patients functioned at their prior social level, while physical abilities were at 76% of the premorbid level.[102] This may impede stroke recovery and adjustment.

Vocational Aspects

Stroke outcome studies vary on the reports of successful return to work. This may represent social and cultural influences of the "sick role." Vocational impairment affects 70% of stroke victims.[46] Simply because a patient is physically capable of returning to work following a stroke, it cannot be assumed that he or she is mentally capable. Neuropsychological assessment and appropriate cognitive treatment, when indicated, is imperative. If the patient lacks insight into the problem, the family must be recruited and encouraged first to recognize the problem and then to reinforce appropriate behaviors. Lack of driving skills and inability to operate other hazardous machinery in the workplace may also prevent return to work.

Discharge Planning

Discharge planning of the stroke patient should begin prior to admission to the rehabilitation unit. Typically this involves the social worker and the home care coordinator. Issues of house accessibility, need for supervision at home, and potential date of discharge must be discussed with the patient and family. A home evaluation should be conducted if necessary to assess the need for architectural modifications. Forms for handicapped parking permits and transportation should be completed by the physician. Information regarding the operation of motor vehicles should be made available, since licensing requirements and restrictions vary from state to state.

Equipment needs at home must be assessed. Generally, the use of a hospital bed at home is discouraged for the stroke patient. It is not necessary for mobility, may be too high for appropriate transfers, causes crowding of furniture (thereby becoming a safety hazard), and reinforces the "sick role." Other equipment needs include possible installation of ramps, bathroom grab bars, or raised toilet seats.

Plans for homebound or outpatient physical, occupational, and speech therapies or nursing follow-up, as needed, should be made several days prior to discharge. Appropriate prescriptions for therapies should be generated and be readily retrievable in case of question. The team as a whole can discuss these issues with the family at a discharge planning conference. Any further teaching that the patient or family requires for care at home should be carried out by nurses and/or therapists.

Functional outcome of stroke rehabilitation does not always predict placement after discharge from the rehabilitation facility. Often, family members will take home dependent patients who require significant nursing care and will manage rather well. Other patients who may be more independent but demonstrate slow recovery sometimes must be referred to extended-care facilities for further, slower-paced, physical, occupational, or speech therapy if they live in remote areas without family support or access to homebound or outpatient therapy.

Follow-up

Ideally, follow-up care of the stroke patient is provided by the physician who managed the inpatient program in order to ensure continuity. Patients with severe general medical complications should retain their internists for general care and medication renewal. Multiple medications from various physicians should be discouraged. Communication among specialists is the key to outpatient follow-up. The stroke patient typically returns to the rehabilitation physician as an outpatient 1 month after discharge and at monthly to quarterly intervals thereafter as dictated by progress or complications. Blood pressure and weight should be obtained, and medications reviewed. The patient's report of activities and progress should be validated by an accompanying family member. Reports from home care or outpatient therapists should be reviewed and discrepancies noted. The patient should demonstrate the ability to perform the home program. Direct inquiry regarding psychosocial issues at home, known through previous inpatient contact, should be made. The patient and family should be encouraged to bring a list of questions to the office visit, with ample time allowed for discussion.

A neurological examination should be documented, focusing on function, such as the ability to rise from a chair and ambulate. Gait should be assessed with appropriate assistive devices. All of the patient's equipment should be checked. Wheelchairs should be inspected for hammock effect of the seat, indicating a need for replacement of the upholstery, adequate brakes, and maneuverability. All orthotic devices should be checked for stability and appropriate fit. Shoes should be checked for fit and pattern of wear on the sole. Slings should be checked for appropriate application.

All of the above should occur prior to renewing any home care or outpatient therapy. Physicians should not order therapy without reexamination of the patient. Particularly when upgrading the use of an assistive device, the patient should not be discharged too quickly from physical therapy. Unfortunately, reducing or discontinuing therapy often gives the unintended message to the patient and family that the situation is "hopeless." It must be explained that natural recovery may be slow and that a well-practiced home program will be beneficial. If there is little or no improvement in occupational and speech therapy as time progresses, recommendations must be made about decreasing or discontinuing therapy. The patient and family are often adamant about continuing therapy. This requires patience and continued teaching and support from the entire team regarding the individual pattern of stroke recovery.

CONCLUSIONS

Comprehensive rehabilitation of the stroke patient is an exciting challenge. Although there are general principles of stroke recovery, no two patients share the same experience. Thus, the rehabilitation professional must employ basic knowledge as well as that gained through clinical experience in tailoring each program to meet individual needs. Trends that are already having an impact on providers of stroke rehabilitation include the decreasing incidence of stroke, balanced by the general aging trend in the population. Governmental regulations regarding delivery of rehabilitative care, such as the 3-hour therapy rule, have already changed the way in which rehabilitation is practiced.[57] Other factors that will affect rehabilitation include the decreasing inpatient length of stay, with a shift toward outpatient and homebound therapies. Funding limitations in these areas also affect care. The influences on outcomes require further investigation. Although there will continue to be controversy over the justification of stroke rehabilitation, the importance of the achievement of independent function following rehabilitation cannot be denied.

REFERENCES

1. American-Canadian Cooperative Study Group. Persantine aspirin trial in cerebral ischemia: II. End point results. Stroke 16:406, 1985
2. Anderson TP, Baldridge M, Ettinger MG: Quality of care for completed stroke without rehabilitation: Evaluating by assessing patient outcomes. Arch Phys Med Rehabil 60:103–107, 1979
3. Anderson TP, Kottke FJ: Stroke rehabilitation: A reconsideration of some common attitudes. Arch Phys Med Rehabil 59:175–181, 1978
4. Baker M, Regenos E, Wolf S, Basmajian J: Developing strategies for biofeedback: Applications in neurologically handicapped patients. Phys Ther 57:402–408, 1977
5. Barnett HJM: Heart in ischemic stroke: A changing emphasis. Neurol Clin 1:291–316, 1983
6. Basmajian JV, Gowland C, Brandstater ME et al: EMG feedback treatment of upper limb in hemiplegic stroke patients: Pilot study. Arch Phys Med Rehabil 63:613–616, 1982
7. Beukelman DR, Yorkston KM: A communication system for the severely dysarthric speaker with an intact language system. J Speech Hear Disord 42:265–270, 1977
8. Borrie MJ, Campbell AJ, Caradoc-Davie TH, Spears GF: Urinary incontinence after stroke: A prospective study. Age Ageing 15:177–181, 1986
9. Bousser MG, Eschwege E, Haguenau M et al: "AICLA" controlled trial of aspirin and dipyridamole in the secondary prevention of atherothrombotic cerebral ischemia. Stroke 14:5–14, 1983
10. Bowman BR, Baker LL, Waters RL: Positional feedback and electrical stimulation, automated treatment for hemiplegic wrist. Arch Phys Med Rehabil 60:497–502, 1979
11. Braun RM, West F, Mooney V et al: Surgical treatment of the painful shoulder contracture in the stroke patient. J Bone Joint Surg 53:1307–1312, 1971
12. Britton M, Helmers C, Samuelsson K: High dose acetylsalicylic acid after cerebral infarction. Stroke 17:132, 1986
13. Brocklehurst JC, Andrews K, Richards B, Laycock PJ: Incidence and correlates of incontinence in stroke patients. J Am Geriatr Soc 33:540–542, 1985
14. Brunnstrom S: Walking preparation for adult patients with hemiplegia. J Am Phys Ther Assoc 45:17–29, 1965
15. Brust JCM: Transient ischemic attacks: Natural history and anticoagulation. Neurology 27:701–707, 1977
16. Buonanno F, Toole JF: Management of patients with established ("completed") cerebral infarction. Stroke 12:7–16, 1981
17. Calliet R: The Shoulder in Hemiplegia. Philadelphia, FA Davis, 1980
18. Canadian Cooperative Study Group: A randomized trial of aspirin and sulfinpyrazone in threatened stroke. N Engl J Med 299:53–59, 1978
19. Candelise L, Landi G, Perrone et al: A randomized trial of aspirin and sulfinpyrazone in patients with TIA. Stroke 13:175–179, 1982
20. Caplan B: Neuropsychology in rehabilitation: Its role in evaluation and intervention. Arch Phys Med Rehabil 63:362–366, 1982
21. Caplan LR: Vertebrobasilar disease: Time for a new strategy. Stroke 12:111–114, 1981
22. Cerebral Embolism Task Force: Cardiogenic brain embolism. Arch Neurol 43:71–84, 1986
23. Corcoran PJ, Jebsen RH, Brengelmann GL, Simons BC: Effects of plastic and metal leg braces on speed and energy cost of hemiparetic ambulation. Arch Phys Med Rehabil 51:69–77, 1970
24. Corston RN, Kendall BE, Marshall J: Prognosis in middle cerebral artery stenosis. Stroke 15:237–241, 1984

25. Davis SW, Petrillo CR, Eichberg RD, Chu DS: Shoulder–hand syndrome in a hemiplegic population: A 5-year retrospective study. Arch Phys Med Rehabil 58:353–356, 1977

26. DeLisa JA, Mikulic MA, Melnick RR, Miller RM: Stroke rehabilitation: II. Recovery and complications. Am Fam Physician 26(6):143–151, 1982

27. DeLisa JA, Miller RM, Melnick RR, Mikulic MA: Stroke rehabilitation: I. Cognitive deficits and prediction of outcome. Am Fam Physician 26(5):207–214, 1982

28. Dickstein R, Hocherman S, Pillar T, Shaham R: Stroke rehabilitation: Three exercise therapy approaches. Phys Ther 8:1233–1238, 1986

29. Dombovy ML, Sandok BA, Basford JR: Rehabilitation for stroke: A review. Stroke 17:363–369, 1986

30. Donner MW: Swallowing mechanism and neuromuscular disorders. Semin Roentgenol 9:273–282, 1974

31. Dyken ML: Carotid endarterectomy studies: A glimmering of science. Stroke 17:355–358, 1986

32. EC-IC Bypass Study Group: Failure of extracranial-intracranial arterial bypass to reduce the risk of ischemic stroke: Results of an international randomized trial. N Engl J Med 315:1191–1200, 1985

33. Feibel JH, Berk S, Joynt RJ: The unmet needs of stroke survivors. Neurology 29:592, 1979

34. Feigenson JS, McCarthy ML, Greenberg SD, Feigenson WD: Factors influencing outcome and length of stay in a stroke rehabilitation unit: II. Stroke 8:657–662, 1977

35. Feigenson JS, McCarthy ML, Greenberg SD et al: Factors influencing outcome and length of stay in a stroke rehabilitation unit: I. Stroke 8:651–656, 1977

36. Feigenson JS, McCarthy ML, Moose PD et al: Stroke rehabilitation: Factors predicting outcome and length of stay. NY State J Med 77:1426–1430, 1977

37. Feigenson JS: Stroke rehabilitation: Effectiveness, benefit and cost: Some practical considerations. Stroke 10:1–3, 1979

38. Fields WS, Lemak NA, Frankowski RF, Hardy RJ: Controlled trial of aspirin in cerebral ischemia. Stroke 8:301–314, 1977

39. Fisher CM, Curry HB: Pure motor hemiplegia of vascular origin. Arch Neurol 13:30–44, 1965

40. Fisher CM: Lacunar strokes and infarcts: A review. Neurology 32:871–876, 1982

41. Fisher CM: Pure sensory stroke involving face, arm, and leg. Neurology 15:76–80, 1965

42. Flanagan EM: Methods of facilitation and inhibition of motor activity. Am J Phys Med 46:1006–1011, 1967

43. Friedman GD, Loveland DB, Ehrlich SP Jr: Relationship of stroke to other cardiovascular disease. Circulation 38:533–541, 1968

44. Fudman DJ, Lee PR, Unterecker J et al: Comparison of functionally oriented medical care and formal rehabilitation in management of patients with hemiplegia due to cerebrovascular disease. J Chronic Dis 15:297–310, 1962

45. Garrison JH, Shankara B, Mueller MJ: Stroke hemiplegia and subsequent lower extremity amputation: Which side is at risk? Arch Phys Med Rehabil 67:187–189, 1986

46. Goodstein RK: Overview: Cerebrovascular accident and the hospitalized elderly—a multidimensional clinical problem. Am J Psychiatry 140:2:141–147, 1983

47. Gordon WA, Hibbard MR, Egelko S et al: Perceptual remediation in patients with right brain damage: Comprehensive program. Arch Phys Med Rehabil 66:353–359, 1985

48. Groher M: Dysphagia: Diagnosis and Management. Boston, Butterworths, 1984

49. Hachinski V: Decreased incidence of mortality of stroke. Stroke 15:376–378, 1984

50. Hachinski V, Norris J: The Acute Stroke. Philadelphia, FA Davis, 1985

51. Hertyke JF: Epidemiology of cerebrovascular disease. In Siekert RG (ed): Cerebrovascular Survey Report, p 135. Bethesda, MD, National Institute of Neurologic and Communicative Disorders and Stroke, 1980

52. Hesse KA, Campion EW: Motivating the geriatric patient for rehabilitation. J Am Geriatr Soc 31:586–589, 1983

53. Hier DB, Davis KR, Richarson EP, Mohr JP: Hypertensive putaminal hemorrhage. Ann Neurol 1:152–159, 1977

54. Hurd MM, Farrell KH, Waylonis GW: Shoulder sling for hemiplegia: Friend or foe? Arch Phys Med Rehabil 55:519–522, 1974

55. Inaba M, Edberg E, Montgomery J, Gillis M: Effectiveness of functional training, active exercise and resistive exercise for patients with hemiplegia. Phys Ther 53:28–35, 1973

56. Isaacs B: Problems and solutions in rehabilitation of stroke patients. Geriatrics 33(7):87–91, 1978

57. Johnston MV, Miller LS: Cost-effectiveness of the Medicare three-hour regulation. Arch Phys Med Rehabil 67:581–585, 1986

58. Jongblood L: Prediction of function after stroke: A critical review. Stroke 17:765–776, 1986

59. Kannel WB, Abbott RD, Savage DD et al: Epidemiologic features of chronic atrial fibrillation: The Framingham study. N Engl J Med 306:1018–1022, 1982

60. Kanner WB, Wolf PA, Vortor J et al: Epidemiologic assessment of the role of blood pressure in stroke: The Framingham study. JAMA 714:301, 1970

61. Kaplan PE, Meredith J, Taft G, Betts H: Stroke and brachial plexus injury: A difficult problem. Arch Phys Med Rehabil 58:415–418, 1977

62. Katzman R: Treatment of cerebral edema in brain infarction. In Price TR, Nelson E (eds): Cerebrovascular Disorders, pp 199–207. New York, Raven Press, 1979

63. Khan Z, Hertanu J, Yang W et al: Predictive correlation of urodynamic dysfunction and brain injury after cerebrovascular accident. J Urol 128:86–88, 1981

64. Kralj A, Vodovnik L: Functional electrical stimulation of extremities: I. J Med Eng Technol, No. 1, Part II, No. 2, 1977

65. Kushner MJ, Bressman SB: The clinical manifestations of pontine hemorrhage. Neurology 35:637–643, 1985

66. Lambo TA: Stroke: A worldwide health problem. In Goldstein M et al (eds): Advances in Neurology, vol 25. New York, Raven Press, 1979

67. Lehmann JF: Biomechanics of ankle–foot orthoses: Prescription and design. Arch Phys Med Rehabil 60:200–207, 1979

68. Lehmann JF, DeLateur BJ, Fowler RS et al: Stroke: Does rehabilitation affect outcome? Arch Phys Med Rehabil 56:375–382, 1975

69. Levy RI: Stroke decline: Implications and prospectives. N Engl J Med 300:490–491, 1979

70. Lind K: Synthesis of studies on stroke rehabilitation. J Chronic Dis 35:133–149, 1982

71. Lipsey JR, Pearlson GD, Price TR et al: Nortriptyline treatment of post-stroke depression: A double blind study. Lancet 1:297–300, 1984

72. Logemann J: Evaluation and Treatment of Swallowing Disorders. San Diego CA, College-Hill Press, 1983

73. Logemann J: Manual for the Videofluoroscopic Examination of Swallowing. San Diego, College-Hill Press, 1986

74. McCarthy ST et al: Low dose heparin as a prophylaxis against deep-vein thrombosis after acute stroke. Lancet 2:800, 1977

75. McNeal D, Reswick J: Control of skeletal muscle by electrical stimulation. In Advances in Biomedical Engineering, vol 6. New York, Academic Press, 1976

76. Meadows J: Dysphagia in unilateral cerebral lesions. J Neurol Neurosurg Psychiatry 36:853–860, 1973

77. Miller VT: Lacunar stroke: A reassessment. Arch Neurol 40:129–134, 1983

78. Mohr JP, Caplan LR, Melski JW et al: The Harvard cooperative stroke registry. Neurology 28:754–762, 1978

79. Mohr JP, Kase CS, Wolf PA et al: Lacunes in the NINCDS pilot stroke data bank. Ann Neurol 12:84, 1982

80. Mohr JP: Lacunes. Stroke 13:3–11, 1982

81. Moskowitz E: Complications in the rehabilitation of hemiplegic patients. Med Clin North Am 53:541–558, 1969

82. Moskowitz E, Porter JI: Peripheral nerve lesions in the upper extremity in hemiplegic patients. N Engl J Med 269:776–778, 1963

83. Moskowitz E, Steinman R: Heterotopic calcification in the hemiplegic upper extremity. NY State J Med 432–435, 1964

84. Murray V, Britton M: Diagnosis in suspected stroke. Stroke 17:141, 1986

85. Naritomi H, Sakai F, Meyer JS: Pathogenesis of transient ischemic attacks within the vertebrobasilar arterial system. Arch Neurol 36:121–128, 1979

86. Norris JW, Hachinski VC: Misdiagnosis of stroke. Lancet 1:328–331, 1982
87. Olesen J: Cerebral blood flow: Methods for measurement, regulation, effects of drugs and changes in disease. Acta Neurol Scand 50(suppl 57):1, 1974
88. Ofir R, Heiner S: Orthoses and ambulation in hemiplegia: Ten year retrospective study. Arch Phys Med Rehabil 61:216–220, 1980
89. Peacock PB, Riley CP, Lampton TD et al: Birmingham stroke, epidemiology and rehabilitation study. In Stewart GT (ed): Trends in Epidemiology, pp 231–345. Springfield, IL, Charles C Thomas, 1972
90. Petrillo CR, Chu DS, Davis SW: Phenol block of the tibial nerve in the hemiplegic patient. Orthopedics 3:871–874, 1980
91. Plum F, Posner JB: The Diagnosis of Stupor and Coma, 3rd ed. Philadelphia, FA Davis, 1980
92. Quaglieri CE, Chun RWM, Cleeland C: Movement disorders as a complication of acute hemiplegia of childhood. Am J Dis Child 131:1009–1010, 1977
93. Reding M, Orto L, Willensky P et al: The dexamethasone suppression test: An indicator of depression in stroke but not a predictor of rehabilitation outcome. Arch Neurol 42:209–212, 1985
94. Renshaw DC: Stroke and sex. In Comfort A (ed): Sexual Consequences of Disability, pp 121–132. Philadelphia, George F. Stickley, 1978
95. Reuther JR, Dorndorf W: Aspirin in patients with cerebral ischemia and normal angiograms or nonsurgical lesions. In Breddin K, Dorndorf W, Loew D, Marx R (eds): Acetylsalicylic Acid in Cerebral Ischemia and Coronary Heart Disease, pp 97–106. Stuttgart, FK Shattauer Verlag, 1978
96. Robinson RG, Kubos KL, Starr LB et al: Mood disorders in stroke patients: Importance of location of lesion. Brain 107:81–93, 1984
97. Robinson RG, Price TR: Post-stroke depressive disorders: A follow-up study of 103 patients. Stroke 13:635–641, 1982
98. Robinson RG, Starr LB, Kubos KL et al: A two year longitudinal study of post-stroke mood disorders: Findings during the initial evaluation. Stroke 14:736–741, 1983
99. Robinson RG, Szetela B: Mood change following left hemispheric brain injury. Ann Neurol 9:447–453, 1981
100. Ross ED: Right hemisphere's role in language, affective behavior and emotion. Trends Neurosci 7:342–346, 1984
101. Ross ED: The aprosodias: Functional-anatomical organization of the affective components of language in the right hemisphere. Arch Neurol 38:561–569, 1981
102. Schmidt SM, Herman LM, Koenig P et al: Status of stroke patients: Community assessment. Arch Phys Med Rehabil 67:99–102, 1986
103. Schuman JE, Beattie E, Steed DA et al: Geriatric patients with and without intellectual dysfunction: Effectiveness of a standard rehabilitation program. Arch Phys Med Rehabil 62:612–618, 1981
104. Sivenius J, Pyorala K, Heinonen OP et al: The significance of intensity of rehabilitation of stroke trial. Stroke 16:928–931, 1985
105. Smith ME, Garraway WM, Smith DL, Akhtar AJ: Therapy impact on functional outcome in a controlled trial of stroke rehabilitation. Arch Phys Med Rehabil 63:21–24, 1982
106. Solomon GE, Hilal SK, Gold AP, Carter S: Natural history of acute hemiplegia of childhood. Brain 93:107–120, 1970
107. Sorenson PS, Pedersen H, Marguardsen J et al: Acetylsalicylic acid in the prevention of stroke in patients with reversible cerebral ischemic attacks: A Danish cooperative study. Stroke 14:15–22, 1983
108. Steinberg FU: Rehabilitating the older stroke patient: What's possible? Geriatrics 41:3:85–97, 1986
109. Steinbrocker O: The shoulder–hand syndrome: Present perspective. Arch Phys Med Rehabil 49:388–395, 1968
110. Stern PH, McDowell F, Miller JM, Robinson M: Effects of facilitation exercise techniques in stroke rehabilitation. Arch Phys Med Rehabil 51:526–531, 1970
111. Stern PH, McDowell F, Miller JM, Robinson M: Factors influencing stroke rehabilitation. Stroke 2:213–218, 1971
112. Toole JF, Janbuay R, Choi K et al: Transient ischemic attacks due to atherosclerosis: A prospective study of 160 patients. Arch Neurol 32:5, 1975
113. Treanor WJ: Improvement of function in hemiplegia after orthopaedic surgery. Scand J Rehab Med 13:123–135, 1981
114. Turney TM, Garraway WM, Sinaki M: Neurologic examination in stroke rehabilitation: Adequacy of its description in clinical textbooks. Arch Phys Med Rehabil 65:92–94, 1984
115. Twitchell TE: The restoration of motor function following hemiplegia. Brain 74:443–480, 1951
116. Varghese G, Hinterbuchner C, Mondall P, Sakuma J: Rehabilitation outcome of patients with dual disability of hemiplegia and amputation. Arch Phys Med Rehabil 59:121–123, 1978
117. Von Arbin M, Britton M, DeFaire U et al: Accuracy of bedside diagnosis in stroke. Stroke 12:288–293, 1981
118. Warlow C, Ogston D, Douglas AS: Deep venous thrombosis of the legs after strokes. Br Med J 1:1178–1183, 1976
119. Waters RL, Perry J, Garland D: Surgical correction of gait abnormalities following stroke. Clin Orthop 131:54–63, 1978
120. Waters RL: Upper extremity surgery in stroke patients. Clin Orthop 131:30–37, 1978
121. Waylonis GW, Keith MW, Aseff JN: Stroke rehabilitation in a western country. Arch Phys Med Rehabil 54:151–155, 1974
122. Weinfeld FD (ed): The national survey of stroke. Stroke 12(suppl 1):1–71, 1981
123. Whisnant JP: The decline of stroke. Stroke 15:160–167, 1984
124. Williams D, Wilson TG: The diagnosis of the major and minor syndromes of basilar insufficiency. Brain 85:741–774, 1962
125. Wolcott LE, Wheeler PC, Pallard P et al: Home care vs institutional rehabilitation of stroke: A comparative study. Mo Med 63:722–724, 1966
126. Wolf PA, Dawber TR, Thomas HE Jr et al: Epidemiologic assessment of chronic atrial fibrillation and risk of stroke. Neurology 28:973–977, 1978
127. Wolf PA, Kannel WB, Sorlie P: Asymptomatic carotid bruit and risk of stroke: The Framingham study. JAMA 245:1442–1445, 1981
128. Wolf PA, Kannez WB, Verter J: Current status of risk factors for stroke. Neurol Clin 1:317–343, 1983
129. Wolf SL, Baker MP, Kelly JL: EMG biofeedback in stroke: Effect of patient characteristics. Arch Phys Med Rehabil 60:96–102, 1979
130. Wylie CM: Value of early rehabilitation in stroke. Geriatrics 31:107–113, 1970
131. Ylvisaker CJ, Fields RW: A Clinical Assessment of PIRD-Y: A New Therapy for Rehabilitation of Stroke and Other Neurological Deficits. Portland, OR, Pird-Y Stroke Rehabilitation, 1985
132. Young RR, Delwaide PJ: Drug Therapy Spasticity: I and II. N Engl J Med 304:28–33; 96–99, 1981

30

Rehabilitation of the Patient With Head Injury

John Whyte

Mitchell Rosenthal

NATURE OF THE PROBLEM

Head injury has been identified as a major health problem in the United States and other countries where vehicular accidents, sporting accidents, and interpersonal violence are commonplace. The systematic study of the residual effects of head injury can be traced to World War II and the work of Alexander Luria,[111] Kurt Goldstein,[64] and others. In this early work, much was learned about the deficits following penetrating injuries to the brain in soldiers with gunshot wounds. The pattern of residual dysfunction often corresponded to a focal lesion caused by the bullet passing through the brain. These focal deficits resulting from penetrating head injuries were similar to focal deficits observed in cerebrovascular accidents.

The vast majority of peacetime head injuries seen in hospitals are classified as "closed" head injuries, where the skull is not actually penetrated. The nature of injury sustained in vehicular accidents (blunt impact, acceleration-deceleration) often results in multifocal lesions and diffuse brain damage with a variety of physical and neurobehavioral impairments that are unique to each patient and pose a great challenge for the rehabilitation team.

The Range of Outcomes: Death to Complete Recovery

The pattern and severity of injury and resultant outcome are also highly variable. In some injuries, commonly referred to as "mild or minor," the patient may suffer no loss of consciousness or only a very brief period of altered consciousness. In these cases, the patient may be seen in a hospital emergency department, held for observation, and released several hours later. In the absence of any further medical complications, the patient may return to normal activities within a few days. In other "minor" injuries, a post-traumatic syndrome consisting of headaches, vertigo, fatigability, memory disturbance, and emotional irritability may follow and cause a disruption of vocational activity up to 3 months after injury.[146] In a small percentage of cases, physical and psychosocial symptomatology may be reported for months and years after injury.[153] Minor head injuries constitute the vast majority of head injuries within the United States—approximately 290,000 per year.[118]

Most rehabilitation efforts are focused on those patients with severe closed head injuries (*i.e.,* unconsciousness for 6 hours or longer). There are 50,000 to 75,000 people per year in the United States who suffer severe head injuries.[57] Within this broad category, a variety of outcomes may be observed. In most studies, approximately 50% of patients with severe head injuries die.[89] Of the survivors, global outcome is usually defined by the following categories taken from the *Glasgow Outcome Scale*[86]: vegetative state, severe disability, moderate disability, and good recovery. The percentages of survivors in these categories at various time periods after injury are shown in Table 30-1. However, even those who achieve a "good recovery" status according to the *Glasgow Outcome Scale* may have significant psychosocial impairments that preclude a return to premorbid level of function.

Measures of Injury Severity

Duration of coma has been commonly considered to be an index of the severity of traumatic brain injury. A severe brain injury is often defined as coma lasting 6 hours or longer. Longer periods of coma are typically associated with poorer outcomes. Although this may have validity in certain populations (*e.g.,* children[23]), duration of coma is no longer considered to be the best measure of injury severity. With the advent of the *Glasgow Coma Scale,*[166] a more precise, objective definition of coma and the *depth of unconsciousness* can be obtained, as shown in Table 30-2. Coma is defined as (1) not opening the eyes, (2) not obeying commands, and (3) not uttering understandable words. A *Glasgow Coma Scale* score of 8 or less is operationally defined as a comatose state.[20]

Russell[154] was the first to describe *post-traumatic amnesia* as a measure of severity. The duration of post-traumatic amnesia is determined by the duration of time from the point of injury until the patient has continuous memory of ongoing events. A scale of severity and its relationship to post-traumatic amnesia is shown in Table 30-3.

Researchers have used post-traumatic amnesia as an index of injury severity and an important predictor of outcome.[102] Unfortunately, post-traumatic amnesia is often measured retrospectively through inspection of medical records and only a rough approximation of the duration of the amnesia can be achieved. The use of the *Galveston Orientation and Amnesia Test (GOAT)*

Table 30-1
Outcome in Survivors of Severe Head Injury

Outcome	3 Months (n = 534)	6 Months (n = 515)	12 Months (n = 376)
Vegetative state	7%	5%	3%
Severe disabiilty	29%	19%	16%
Moderate disability	33%	34%	31%
Good recovery	31%	42%	50%
Moderate-good (combined)	64%	76%	81%

(Jennett B, Teasdale G: Management of Head Injuries, p 309. Philadelphia, FA Davis, 1981)

Table 30-3
Relationship Between Post-traumatic Amnesia and Severity of Injury

Length of Amnesia	Severity of Injury
Less than 5 minutes	Very mild
5 to 60 minutes	Mild
1 to 24 hours	Moderate
1 to 7 days	Severe
1 to 4 weeks	Very severe
More than 4 weeks	Extremely severe

(Jennett B, Teasdale G: Management of Head Injuries, p 90. Philadelphia, FA Davis, 1981)

Table 30-2
Glasgow Coma Scale

	Examiner's Test	Patient's Response	Assigned Score
Eye Opening	Spontaneous	Opens eyes on own	4
	Speech	Opens eyes when asked in a loud voice	3
	Pain	Opens eyes when pinched	2
	Pain	Does not open eyes	1
Best Motor Response	Commands	Follow simple commands	6
	Pain	Pulls examiner's hands away when pinched	5
	Pain	Pulls a part of the body away when pinched	4
	Pain	Flexes body inappropriately when pinched (decorticate posturing)	3
	Pain	Body becomes rigid in an extended position when pinched (decerebrate posturing)	2
	Pain	Has no motor response to pinch	1
Verbal Response (Talking)	Speech	Carries on a conversation correctly and tells examiner where he or she is, who he or she is, month and year	5
	Speech	Seems confused or disoriented	4
	Speech	Talks so examiner can understand victim but makes no sense	3
	Speech	Makes sounds that examiner cannot understand	2
	Speech	Makes no noise	1

(Teasdale G, Jennett B: Assessment of coma and impaired consciousness. Lancet 2:81, 1974)

developed by Levin and co-workers provides a more objective, reliable way of measuring post-traumatic amnesia.[104]

EPIDEMIOLOGY OF HEAD INJURY

The incidence of head injury requiring hospitalization is generally estimated to be 200 to 225 per 100,000 population in the United States.[57] In all, approximately 500,000 new cases of head injury occur annually in the United States.[55] Precise measures of prevalence within the population are unknown; however, within the past 10 years epidemiological studies have shown a great uniformity in the yearly incidence of head injuries. Approximately 44,000 people per year survive severe head injury with moderate to severe physical or neurobehavioral sequelae.[100]

The age distribution of head injury is bimodal, with young adults (aged 15 to 24, 200 to 225 / 100,000) and the elderly (aged 65 to 75, 200 / 100,000) showing the highest incidence. The elderly population has the highest level of mortality.[5] Elderly

patients have a much slower and more uncertain recovery process, compared with the young adult population.

In all studies of head injury, males outnumber females by at least 2 : 1. Furthermore, male head injury mortalities are three to four times greater than in the female population.[57] Concerning racial background, several studies have noted that head injury tends to occur with slightly greater frequency among minority groups.[184]

About half of all head injuries are caused by transportation-related accidents. The other half are the result of falls, assaults, and other causes.[57] There are some age and socioeconomic factors that affect patterns of causation. In the Olmstead County study, the peak mortality group was aged 65 to 75, with suicide attempts and falls as predominant causes of head injuries.[5] Studies in the Bronx, New York, and in Harris County, Texas, show a 40% to 44% incidence of gunshot wounds as a cause of head injury.[34, 56] Of those who survive the initial injury, 49% of those in persistent vegetative state die within the first year after injury.[87] There are no long-term studies that document life expectancy of patients with moderate to severe disability, but there is no reason to expect a great shortening of life span.

A variety of risk factors have been identified as influential in determining who is likely to sustain a head injury. The most common factor cited is alcohol intake prior to the head injury.[102] Other factors have been noted, such as preinjury personality disturbance, family discord, or antisocial behavior, but little systematic research has been done to relate these factors to risk of injury.[25, 170]

The economic and social impact of head injury is considered enormous, but has not been carefully studied. In the Head and Spinal Cord Injury Survey of the National Institute of Neurological and Communicative Disorders and Stroke (NINCDS), costs attributable to head injury in 1974 were estimated to be 4 billion dollars, exclusive of lost wages or extended rehabilitation costs in institutional settings or from home health care agencies.[93] Estimates of return to work vary greatly, from 15% to 100%.[17] Head injury causes marital strain, affects role relationships, fosters economic hardship, and creates a great burden on the family.[113] These issues will be discussed further later in this chapter.

OUTCOME AFTER HEAD INJURY

Types of Deficits

The majority of survivors of severe head injury emerge from coma and achieve remarkable progress toward regaining their preinjury functional abilities. However, in most cases, the patient is left with a combination of physical, cognitive, and integrative deficits that may persist for many months or years after the injury. For a given patient, the specific pattern of deficits is a consequence of the severity of the injury, nature of brain damage, and medical complications. Thus, the pattern of deficits varies greatly from one head-injured patient to the next. In this section, a cursory description of the major deficits following head injury is presented. These problem areas are described in greater detail later in this chapter.

In the *physical* sphere, a variety of movement disorders may be observed, including paresis, abnormal muscle tone, contractures, ataxia, tremors, and apraxia. Even a head-injured person with many of these deficits may ambulate functionally within a few months after injury. The normal physical appearance of most head-injured patients after several months may be quite deceiving. Although gross movement may appear generally intact, smoother, fine movements, which require greater coordination and speed, are usually impaired. For example, a head-injured adult may be able to walk ten blocks but cannot run, hop on one foot, or perform rapid alternating movements. Even with a residual upper extremity paresis, most head-injured adults can use their arms and hands for dressing and personal hygiene but often have difficulty with handwriting, cutting meat, or picking up small items. Sensory deficits frequently observed include visual field cuts, impaired sense of smell, visuoperceptual problems, diplopia, hearing disorders, and vestibular dysfunction. Disorders of taste and somatic sensation are less frequently observed but can present great subjective discomfort for the affected person.[71]

Cognitive deficits are almost always present after a severe head injury. These impairments vary in magnitude but tend to greatly alter the capacity of the patient to acquire, store, and retrieve new information and exercise good judgment. A listing of some of these deficits appears in Table 30-4. Initially, the patient has a decreased level of alertness and arousal and is observed to fluctuate in the ability to concentrate. Although

Table 30-4
Common Cognitive Disabilities

Disorders of consciousness
Disorientation
Memory deficits
Decreased abstraction
Decreased learning abilities
Language/communication deficits
General intellectual deficits
Deficits in processing/sequencing information
Illogical thoughts
Poor judgment
Poor quality control
Inability to make decisions
Poor initiative
Verbal, motor perseveration
Confabulation
Difficulty in generalization
Difficulty in sustaining attention
Distractability
Fatigability
Perplexity
Dyscalculia
Reduced motor speed
Reduced eye–hand coordination
Poor depth perception
Spatial disorientation
Poor figure–ground perception
Auditory perceptual deficits
Anosognosia
Autotopagnosia
Tactile, auditory, visual neglect
Apraxias

(Rosenthal M, Griffith ER, Bond MR et al: Rehabilitation of the Head Injured Adult, p 29. Philadelphia, FA Davis, 1983)

alertness and arousal level stabilize, attentional deficits are still pronounced but take the form of reduced speed of information processing or of difficulty in sustaining attention or shifting attention from one task to another. Difficulties in remembering may take several forms. As described earlier, post-traumatic amnesia typically follows emergence from coma. In addition to this loss of functional memory for everyday events, retrograde amnesia, for a period of minutes to hours preceding the injury, usually occurs. Despite this loss, remote memory of personal events and social history is usually well preserved.

Head injuries can produce a variety of impairments in executive functions, manifested by perseveration, impulsivity, concreteness, poor problem solving, and slowness in the rate and complexity of information processing. Speech and language disabilities are commonly found, although not typically in the form of a classic aphasic syndrome. The most frequent language problems include anomia, tangentiality, and circumlocution.[140, 155] Other disorders include dysphasia, dysarthria, dyslexia, and dysprosody. Perceptuomotor and constructional disorders are also commonly observed after head injury. Loss of spatial perception and visual field awareness and motor sequencing difficulties are common and have great impact on the injured person's capacity to learn and perform routine skills needed in activities of daily living.

The third major sphere of dysfunction can be termed *integrative deficits*. This refers to the ability to perform complex, multifaceted tasks that require the *integrated* operation of numerous perceptual, motor, cognitive, and regulatory processes.

Table 30-5
Common Changes in Behavior and Personality

Apathy
Impulsivity
Irritability
Aggressiveness
Anxiety
Depression
Emotional lability
Silliness
Lack of goal-directed behavior
Lack of initiation
Poor self-image, reduced self-worth
Denial of disability and its consequences
Aggressive behavior
Childlike behavior
Bizarre, psychotic ideation and behavior
Loss of sensitivity and concern for others: selfishness
Dependency, passivity
Indecision
Indifference
Slovenliness
Sexual disturbances
Drug, alcohol abuse

(Rosenthal M, Griffith ER, Bond MR et al: Rehabilitation of the Head-Injured Adult, p 29. Philadelphia, FA Davis, 1983)

Complex activities of daily living, appropriate social functioning, and vocational success may be considered integrative functions.

Changes in behavior and personality after head injury have been documented by many investigators and are considered by many clinicians to be among the most difficult problems to manage effectively (Table 30-5).[19, 105, 107] Behavior problems range from minor irritability and passivity to disinhibited and psychotic behavior. Many behavioral changes can be traced to the presence of specific patterns of neurological damage.[3] The severely head-injured patient often appears similar to an egocentric child and requires a highly structured, consistent, positive-reinforcing environment. Problems in mood, often in the form of depression, are also difficult to treat. In some cases, behavioral management strategies and psychotropic medications can be helpful in reducing the frequency of maladaptive behavior. The result of cognitive and behavioral dysfunction is usually a loss of social relationships and the occurrence of family distress. The severely head-injured person usually cannot return successfully to premorbid educational or vocational pursuits. In turn, this lack of vocational activity can lead to economic losses that place an even greater stress on the patient's and family's adaptive abilities.

Outcome Measurement

The process of outcome measurement has recently received increased attention. As neurosurgeons have developed more sophisticated intervention techniques that have reduced mortality and increased survival, questions about outcome and quality of life have been posed. In the past, large group, multicenter studies have investigated a host of epidemiological, demographical, medical, and other variables to determine how they correlate with outcome.[88] These studies, by definition, can provide guidelines for prediction of the "average" head injury case but only provide rough guidelines for predicting outcome in individual cases. Because the outcome categories used in these studies are

Table 30-6
Glasgow Outcome Scale

Score/Category	Definition
1. Death	As a direct result of brain trauma Patient regained consciousness and died thereafter from secondary complications or other causes.
2. Persistent vegetative state	Patient remains unresponsive and speechless for an extended period of time. Patient may open the eyes and show sleep/wake cycles but an absence of function in the cerebral cortex as judged behaviorally.
3. Severe disability (conscious but disabled)	Dependent for daily support by reason of mental or physical disability, usually a combination of both. Severe mental disability may occasionally justify this classification in a patient with little or no physical disability.
4. Moderate disability (disabled but independent)	Can travel by public transport and work in a sheltered environment and can therefore be independent as far as daily life is concerned. The disabilities found include varying degrees of dysphasia, hemiparesis, or ataxia, as well as intellectual and memory deficits and personality change. Independence is greater than simple ability to maintain self-care within the patient's home.
5. Good recovery	Resumption of normal life even though there may be minor neurological and pathological deficits

(Jennett B, Bond MR: Assessment of outcome in severe brain damage: A practical scale. Lancet I:480–484, 1975)

global, it is rare that a true picture of a person's level of functional skills can be obtained. In contrast, the process of extensive, detailed serial investigation of a single case can allow one to predict more precisely that person's outcome but does not enable one to generalize to the larger population.

The major outcome scale that has been used in virtually all studies of head injury is the *Glasgow Outcome Scale* (Table 30-6). The *Glasgow Outcome Scale* consists of five global categories, ranging from good recovery to death. It has been shown to have a high degree of interrater reliability in large, multicenter, international studies,[88] and it has been used to correlate early injury severity measures and outcome at 6 months after injury. Several major weaknesses in the use of the scale for rehabilitation purposes have been identified: (1) the categories are so broad that it is not a sensitive measure of progress during rehabilitation; (2) the global categories do not provide a real indication of functional abilities; and (3) cognitive and behavioral dysfunctions are not really addressed in the outcome categories. Despite these limitations, it continues to have widespread use for its intended purpose—to provide a quantitative, general way of describing outcome.

To address the shortcomings in the *Glasgow Outcome Scale,* Rappaport and colleagues devised an instrument known as the *Disability Rating Scale.*[142] This scale produces a quantitative

Table 30-7
Rancho Los Amigos Levels of Cognitive Function Scale

I. No response
II. Generalized response to stimulation
III. Localized response to stimuli
IV. Confused and agitated behavior
V. Confused with inappropriate behavior (nonagitated)
VI. Confused but appropriate behavior
VII. Automatic and appropriate behavior
VIII. Purposeful and appropriate behavior

(Hagen C, Malkmus D, Durham P: Levels of cognitive functions. In Rehabilitation of the Head-Injured Adult: Comprehensive Physical Management. Downey, CA, Professional Staff Association, Rancho Los Amigos Hospital, 1979)

index of disability across ten levels of severity: none, mild, partial, moderate, moderately severe, severe, extremely severe, vegetative state, extreme vegetative state, and death. Interrater reliability has been reported to be quite high—.97 to .98.[75] In the study reported by Hall and co-workers, the usefulness of the *Glasgow Outcome Scale* and the *Disability Rating Scale* were compared by evaluating a series of head-injured patients at 2, 4, 6, 12, and 24 months after injury. They found that 71% of patients showed a change in categories on the *Disability Rating Scale,* as compared with 33% on the *Glasgow Outcome Scale* during their hospital rehabilitation. Their conclusion was that the *Disability Rating Scale* was a more sensitive index of change of status during rehabilitation.[75]

Yet a third scale has been commonly used to describe outcome—the *Rancho Los Amigos Levels of Cognitive Functioning Scale* (Table 30-7).[74] In this scale, each level of cognitive functioning is accompanied by a lengthy description of behavior that meets the criteria for placement at that level. A comparison of this scale with the *Disability Rating Scale* revealed that it has lower validity and reliability.[67] It is used primarily as a descriptive tool for charting the patient's level of awareness and capacity to interact appropriately and effectively with the environment. In addition, the scale has been used extensively as a basis for planning specific therapeutic, educational, and vocational interventions as well as a means of categorizing groups of head-injured patients within large facilities for the treatment of head injury.

Prediction of Outcome

The *Glasgow Coma Scale* is the most widely used measure of injury severity and is a primary basis for most predictions of outcome. The total coma score when taken at 2 to 3 or 4 to 7 days after injury is highly predictive of outcome at 6 months, as measured by the *Glasgow Outcome Scale.*[89] Scores less than 8 are usually predictive of poor outcome. Duration of post-traumatic amnesia is also highly correlated with ultimate outcome, with amnesia for more than 14 days associated with a greater likelihood of moderate and severe disability.[89]

Multimodality evoked potentials have also been used as an early means of assessing neurological status and predicting outcome, and it appears that they improve the prognostic value of the *Glasgow Coma Scale* and correlate with outcome measures such as the *Disability Rating Scale.*[141] Greenberg and co-workers found that maximal recovery occurs in approximately 3 months with minimal evoked potential abnormalities.[68] However, the presence of severe evoked potential abnormalities suggests that maximal recovery may extend to 12 months, if rehabilitation occurs during that time period.

Reactive pupils are associated with better outcomes than nonreactive pupils: 50% of those with reactive pupils achieve the moderate disability or good recovery range, while only 4% with nonreactive pupils progress to these outcome categories.[90] The oculovestibular response, elicited by injecting ice water into the ear of a comatose patient, has also been used to predict outcome. If no movement of the eyes is obtained, there is indication of severe brain stem dysfunction and poorer outcome.[126] The presence of an intracranial hematoma appears to increase the chance of a poor outcome when the patient is under 20 years of age.[89]

In most studies reporting correlations between age and outcome, children and young adults appear to have a generally more positive prognosis than older adults. Children, in general, appear to have less physical and neurobehavioral sequelae after deep or prolonged coma. They seem to have accelerated recovery of physical and cognitive functions as compared with the adult population. However, very young children (under age 5) and older adults (above age 65) have the greatest mortality.[55]

The research from Glasgow and other major head injury centers strongly suggests that the vast majority of neurological recovery from acute brain injury occurs within the first 6 months after injury. The *maximal* duration of recovery is somewhat more controversial. Some researchers affirm that neurological recovery is virtually complete by 1 year, while others assert that recovery can extend at least until 2 years or more after injury.[128] It is clear, however, that certain areas of dysfunction recover more quickly than others. For example, recovery of physical abilities and functional skills such as mobility occurs rapidly, often within 3 months after injury.[78] The same is generally true for recovery of speech and language functions. Verbal abilities as measured by IQ scores recover rapidly and reach a plateau by 6 months after injury, whereas perceptuomotor skills, as assessed by performance IQ, do not reach a plateau until 12 months after injury.[116] This, however, may be a function of the differential nature of task demands on verbal versus performance subtests (untimed versus timed) and the nature and complexity of the tasks (verbal—old learning; performance—novel tasks), rather than neurological recovery itself. Neuropsychologists generally recognize that "formal IQ" does not provide a true indication of the presence of residual cognitive deficits.

Preinjury medical and psychological factors may also affect the recovery process. For example, a head injury or neurological deficit prior to the injury is likely to slow the recovery process. Also, if cognitive or behavioral abnormalities existed prior to the injury, there is a greater likelihood of a slower and less complete recovery. The presence of brain damage is thought to exacerbate preexisting behavior disorders.[21]

PATHOPHYSIOLOGY OF HEAD INJURY

The pathophysiology of head trauma includes both immediate, impact-related (primary injury) and delayed brain injury (secondary injury). The ultimate morbidity and mortality relates to the sum of these pathophysiological processes. It is mainly in secondary injury where therapeutic advances can be expected. Some useful generalizations can be made from data on pathophysiology of traumatic brain injury derived from animal simulations and human autopsy.

Primary Injury

Diffuse axonal injury (DAI) is the distinguishing feature of traumatic brain injury. Acceleration/deceleration and rotational forces that commonly result from motor vehicle accidents produce diffuse axonal disruption. DAI is most severe in the upper brain stem and corpus callosum[7] and is primarily responsible for the initial loss of consciousness (Fig. 30-1).[44] The precise mechanism of axonal damage remains controversial but includes microscopic hemorrhage and "retraction balls" of extruded axoplasm in white matter.[120] This pathology, in a subtle form, is seen even after minor head injury and may be a risk factor for later dementia.[127, 139]

Cerebral contusions are another form of primary injury. These cortical "bruises" occur at the crests of the gyri and extend to variable depths depending on severity. Contusions occur primarily on the undersurface of the frontal lobes and at the temporal tips regardless of the site of impact (Fig. 30-2).[120] The lesions are usually bilateral but may be asymmetrical.[31] Cerebral contusions may produce focal cognitive and sensorimotor deficits and are risk factors for seizure disorders but are not directly responsible for loss of consciousness.[120] In contrast to DAI, cerebral contusions may result from relatively low velocity impact such as

blows and falls.[7] A given patient's pattern of functional deficits may be more focal (from contusions) or diffuse (from DAI) or may include features of both.[7]

Secondary Injury

The initial injury may set in motion a variety of pathological processes that result in more severe and widespread brain damage. Any factor that leads to increased intracranial pressure (ICP) can decrease cerebral perfusion pressure and cause ischemic damage. Expanding hematomas or acute hydrocephalus lead to dramatic pressure changes.[120] Vasogenic edema related to disruption of the blood–brain barrier can occur in tissue near areas of contusion.[171] Increases in cerebral blood volume and hence ICP may accompany hypoxia, hypercapnia, or venous obstruction. Once increased ICP compromises perfusion, further cytotoxic edema creates a self-perpetuating cycle.[120] Indeed, inter-

Figure 30-1. Brain regions particularly involved by diffuse axonal injury (DAI), including corpus callosum and parasagittal white matter, as well as dorsolateral quadrants of the midbrain. (Auerbach SH: Neuroanatomical correlates of attention and memory disorders in traumatic brain injury: An application of behavioral subtypes. J Head Trauma Rehabil 1:1–12, 1986. Reprinted with the permission of Aspen Publishers, Inc., © 1986)

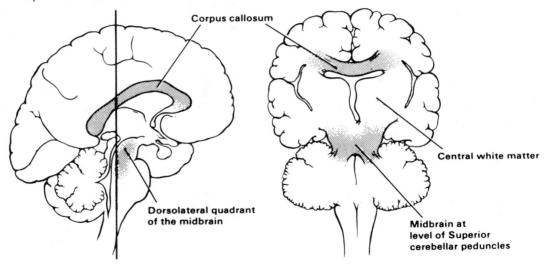

Figure 30-2. Areas predominantly affected by cortical contusions. Darker shading represents more frequently involved areas. Anterotemporal and orbitofrontal regions are particularly involved. Note relative sparing of dorsolateral frontal lobe and medial temporal lobe. (Adapted with permission from Courville. Mythology of the Central Nervous System. Mountain View, CA, Pacific Press Publishing, 1937.)

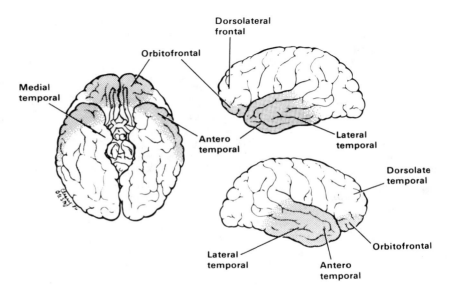

mittent peaks in ICP during the first 24 hours are a risk factor for sustained increases in ICP.[96]

ICP is now routinely monitored in severe head injury and managed with hyperventilation, hyperosmotic diuresis, steroids, muscle paralysis, and barbiturate coma.[125, 126] These treatment modalities act on different components of the pressure equation (cerebral blood flow, interstitial edema, and metabolic activity) and are not all equally well validated.[85, 179] Intractable increases in ICP can lead to diffuse ischemic injury, focal vascular occlusion, and tentorial herniation.[126]

Systemic factors such as blood loss and hypotension, pulmonary injury, and cardiac or respiratory arrest may also contribute to secondary brain injury. Brain infection may occur from open skull fractures or cerebrospinal fluid rhinorrhea or iatrogenously from ICP monitoring.[96, 120] Protracted seizures can also lead to deterioration via increased metabolic requirements, disruption of spontaneous respirations, and aspiration.

POSSIBLE MECHANISMS OF FUNCTIONAL RECOVERY

Recovery from head injury is often incomplete. Reports have identified mild but persistent deficits after even minor head injury.[10, 114] Yet many head-injured patients make tremendous gains from coma to the reemergence of a variety of complex skills. This recovery is believed to occur at multiple levels, from alterations in biochemical processes to alterations in family structure.[186] The precise mechanisms of these same recovery processes are not entirely clear. Even less clear are the relative contributions of various types of recovery throughout the postinjury period. Some of the potential contributions to recovery are identified below.

Resolution of Temporary Factors

On impact, some brain tissue is irreparably damaged by gray matter contusion or axonal disruption. A variety of secondary processes, however, may magnify the extent of functional impairment. Brain edema may depress metabolic activity of intact neurons and cause ischemia to intact neural structures. Associated pulmonary and cardiac problems may contribute to hypoxia and ischemia.[59, 164] Administration of anticonvulsants may depress marginal neural activity.[77] These and many other processes may impair the activity of relatively spared neural structures. In extreme cases, further brain tissue is lost to these secondary processes. Brain tissue that is functionally impaired but not destroyed, however, may gradually resume functioning as medical status stabilizes and edema resolves. This type of recovery mechanism would be expected to operate in the first days to weeks after injury.

Neuronal Regeneration

There is increasing evidence that central nervous system neurons are capable of dendritic and axonal sprouting following an injury in a variety of animal species.[51, 117] This represents a potential mechanism for reestablishment of neural connections over time that could contribute to functional recovery. At present, however, the importance of fiber growth to the recovery process is unclear for several reasons:

- Research on fiber sprouting has been performed primarily in relatively simple species and may be more prevalent in non-mammalian species.[52]

- Fiber sprouting may be age dependent, occurring more readily in infancy during normal neural development.[110]
- Fiber sprouting is likely to occur to different degrees in different brain systems. Phylogenetically, old unmyelinated fibers show more sprouting than newer myelinated systems.[165]
- The "purposefulness" of fiber sprouting is unclear. Fibers may sprout in response to specific chemical signals that allow functional reconnection.[161] Alternatively, fibers may sprout in a random way that, only by chance, allows useful function.[183]
- Fiber sprouting is more easily demonstrated over short distances.[173] Reconnection of distant structures is more questionable and may be inhibited by intervening glial proliferation.[76]

Clearly, more research on fiber sprouting in adult higher animals is necessary. If this process plays a role in functional recovery, however, it is likely that it does so over relatively longer periods of time (weeks to months). It is possible that there is a role for experience and functional training in promoting fiber sprouting or in selecting and perpetuating new "useful" connections. This possibility is suggested by evidence that enriched environments increase synaptic connections and dendritic spines in normal infant rats[70] and provide some behavioral protection against brain damage.[159]

Synaptic Alterations

Central nervous system neurons depend on a variety of inputs for their ongoing activity. Sudden loss of stimulating inputs can lead to marked depression of undamaged structures (diaschisis).[40] For example, cerebral blood flow on the *uninvolved* side is markedly diminished following cerebrovascular accident for as long as 1 month.[124] Robinson and colleagues have shown that widespread changes in catecholamine neurotransmitter concentrations persist for several weeks after localized lesions in rats.[147] It appears that a lesion of the central nervous system, therefore, can potentially disrupt not only functions served by that region but also those served by a variety of regions to which it projects.

Alterations can occur in receptor sensitivity to remaining neurotransmitters. This process is analogous to denervation supersensitivity or tachyphylaxis occurring in the periphery. There is potential for partially disrupted neural connections to reexert normal levels of function if neurotransmitter receptor regulation leads to increased sensitivity to residual transmitter levels. There is considerable evidence in several animal species and some in humans that certain receptor agonists can hasten functional recovery while doses of antagonists cause regression.[49]

The ability to apply this concept in rehabilitation of patients with head injury is limited at present. Our knowledge of the many neurotransmitter systems and their interconnections is primitive, and the multifocal nature of traumatic brain injury limits the ability to apply existing knowledge of neurotransmitter localization. Furthermore, alterations in receptor sensitivity could also lead to disproportionate importance of particular neural inputs, producing dysfunctional results.

Functional Substitution

A patient with a particular deficit may have difficulty accomplishing a task in the usual way. In theory, however, such a patient may discover another strategy for accomplishing the task that relies on neural systems that remain intact.[162] It has been difficult to systematically study the role of functional substitution in human recovery because the alternate strategy can only be inferred from observing the outcome. The more successful the alternate strategy is in achieving the outcome, the more invisible the strategy becomes. However, some possible examples of functional substitution strategies have been proposed:

- Reliance on a different sensory modality to guide behaviors formerly guided by another sensory/perceptual system that is damaged[52]
- Recoding verbal material into visual images or nonverbal material into verbal statements to maximize reliance on relatively spared cognitive systems[92]
- Discovery of existing motor synergy and reflex patterns that can be called on for certain movement goals[26]

The ability to develop broadly applicable alternate strategies is likely to vary with the neural system damaged. A highly specialized system may be less capable of functional replacement. Damage to multiple systems would be expected to complicate the development of alternate strategies by limiting the availability of systems capable of substituting function. Finally, the degree to which compensatory strategies can become generally applicable, spontaneous, and relatively automatic is unclear.

Learning of Specific Skills

Patients with more severe deficits may find it difficult to learn general alternate strategies applicable to a broad range of circumstances. This need not, however, indicate an inability to learn specific useful skills. For example, a patient with an acquired reading disorder may not be able to reacquire the ability to sound out unfamiliar words but may be able to acquire a list of specific sight words useful in daily tasks. Similarly, a patient with a significant verbal memory deficit may not be able to develop any general strategies for improving memory performance but may, through repetition, learn the names of caregivers and the locations of therapy activities. In order to maximize the usefulness of this recovery strategy, training must obviously be concretely tailored to the patient's anticipated environment and functional tasks. In contrast to the biological mechanisms previously discussed, this type of recovery need not be time limited because preserved learning capacities may be applied to specific tasks at any time.

In summary, numerous avenues to functional recovery are theoretically possible after traumatic brain injury. Much more research is needed to clarify the roles of these mechanisms in clinically important improvement. Furthermore, our ability to intervene is limited mainly to the more psychological and behavioral levels at present. With time, however, systematic encouragement of neuronal reconnection and neurotransmitter function may be added to the rehabilitation armamentarium.

THE ASSESSMENT AND TREATMENT PLANNING PROCESS

Time Frame of Intervention: Potentially Life-Long

The rehabilitation needs of the survivor of severe head injury often begin at the roadside (or site of emergency care) but are not likely to end for many years after the injury. As described earlier, a variety of physical, cognitive, and integrative deficits persist after a traumatic brain injury. Despite the interindividual differences in residual dysfunctions, the research of Bond,[21] Brooks,[24] Levin and co-workers[102] and Thomsen[169] has documented that long-term psychosocial deficits are routinely found and require prolonged intervention. Although many medical conditions and physical deficits stabilize within 1 year after injury, the presence of long-term psychosocial disorders often necessitates a variety of interventions, including behavioral management and cognitive rehabilitation.

Variety of Treatment and Support Options

In considering the scope of medical and rehabilitative interventions necessary to prolong, sustain, and achieve a reasonable quality of life, one must consider a broad spectrum of services that may be provided in hospital, community-based, or home settings, depending on the severity of injury and residual sequelae.

Initial medical management takes the form of early, aggressive neurosurgical intervention designed to evacuate hematomas, reduce brain edema, treat hydrocephalus, and monitor ICP. When the patient's condition stabilizes, the physiatrist may be called in as a consultant even when the patient is still in the intensive care unit. The role of the physiatrist is to assist the acute care team in preventing complications such as contractures, decubitus ulcers, and bowel and bladder problems that may impede later rehabilitation. Such complications, if not prevented acutely, may consume resources that would otherwise be directed to functional training.[158] In addition, the physiatrist may assist in choosing medications that minimize sedation of recovering patients. Following neurosurgical intensive care, a tremendous variety of treatment programs may be appropriate for a given patient at various points in the recovery process.[36] Some of these are briefly described below.

In the acute rehabilitation phase, the patient typically is medically stable and emerging from coma. Such patients may have multiple medical/physical problems and display confusion, agitation, and post-traumatic amnesia. Comprehensive rehabilitation services are provided in an inpatient hospital setting and include medical management; physical, occupational, and speech therapy; neuropsychological assessment; cognitive rehabilitation; behavior management; nursing care; family counseling; and discharge planning. During this period, patients often regain a measure of physical mobility, capacity to perform routine activities of daily living, a better recall of day-to-day events, improved communication skills, and increased awareness of their condition and the surrounding environment. This phase often lasts several months but is variable based on rate of recovery and presence of medical complications.

When the patient is ready to be discharged, several options are available for the post-acute rehabilitation phase. These options are dependent on the expressed and perceived needs of the patient and family. If comprehensive daily rehabilitation is still required, but a slow rate of progress is expected, the patient may be referred to an extended-care facility. These facilities often have categorical head injury programs and can provide rehabilitation services for many months or years (depending on reimbursement). In other cases, when a patient can be managed at home but continues to display a variety of physical or neurobehavioral problems, a day treatment program may be recommended. This type of treatment, a recently developed modality, is often conducted in a rehabilitation center and provides extensive cognitive rehabilitation, behavior management, training in daily life skills, community activities, and prevocational activities. These services are usually delivered 4 to 5 days/wk for 4 to 6 hours/day.[16, 140] Professional services usually include neuropsychology, speech therapy, occupational therapy, special education, social services, and recreational therapy.

Some head-injured patients display disinhibited, aggressive, self-abusive, or otherwise inappropriate behavior that cannot be managed effectively within the home. For this reason, residential, behavioral management programs have been developed. In such programs, a primary objective is the modification of inappropriate behaviors and the teaching of more effective means of communication and social interaction. Often, these programs use a contingency management approach, frequently a token economy, along with other techniques.[46] Other restorative and therapeutic services are also provided at these facilities.

When a head-injured person has regained the ability to learn, remember, exercise good judgment, and interact appropriately with others, community-based treatment alternatives may be considered. In the transitional living model, the head-injured person lives in a supervised group home setting and is given instruction and progressively increasing responsibility in skills needed to live independently (*e.g.,* cooking, cleaning, money management, community mobility, job seeking). After a 6- to 12-month period, head-injured adults may be ready to "graduate" into their own apartment or into an unsupervised apartment with a roommate.

A final step in community reintegration is return to work. There are a number of vocational rehabilitation facilities within the United States that have programs designed for the head injured. These programs provide intensive vocational assessment, work adjustment training, vocational training, and placement into a job in the community or a sheltered work setting. Participation in these programs is often under the sponsorship of the state vocational rehabilitation agency. Unfortunately, many state vocational rehabilitation agencies have only recently recognized the unique needs of head-injured patients and do not yet have programs specifically designed to address their needs. However, the vocational rehabilitation agency can provide a variety of vocational services and assistance in financial planning that can be valuable for many head-injured clients.

Varying Role of Medical Versus Social Support Services

In the early stages of recovery from head injury, medical needs predominate and affect the types of services rendered. As the patient's condition becomes stable and reaches maximal physical function, the emphasis switches to psychosocial needs and programming. The involvement of the physician, however, does not cease on discharge from the hospital. Because of the risk of seizures, physiatrists, neurologists, or neurosurgeons provide follow-up for several years to provide and monitor antiseizure medication. Physicians may also provide medical management for other medical problems (*e.g.,* contractures, spasticity, sensory deficits). Physiatrists perform a variety of roles. They plan rehabilitation treatment and prescribe therapies. After discharge, the physiatrist is often asked to provide routine medical management for several years after injury and is requested to provide recommendations on driving, disability determination, fitness for employment, and medicolegal matters.

A critical social support role is that of *case manager.* This person coordinates the provision of services for many years after the injury. This role is often filled by a rehabilitation nurse, vocational counselor, social worker, or insurance rehabilitation specialist. The case manager serves as a liaison between the patient, family, and service providers and gathers medical records, arranges for medical visits, screens programs and facilities, and helps coordinate admission and discharge. The case manager often assists with financial and insurance matters, which are of critical importance in long-term planning.

Patient Assessment and Treatment Planning

Rehabilitation services are traditionally organized on a team model to promote coordination and information sharing across disciplines. There is perhaps no disability group in which this interdisciplinary process is more critical than the head injured. The cognitive deficits are highly varied and unique to each patient. A specific cognitive deficit may interfere with the performance and retention of a mobility, language, or activity of daily living task. Disruptive behaviors and lack of initiation cut across all therapy domains. Each of these problems requires the development of a unified team view of the patient's deficits and needs and the development of a unified treatment plan.

When a patient enters a rehabilitation service, an initial assessment is needed to guide treatment planning. Typically, a member of each discipline conducts an individual assessment in his or her area of expertise. The goals of this assessment will vary with time since injury. A recently injured patient has the potential for considerable recovery. Therefore, assessment is usually aimed at defining broad functional areas in need of treatment (*e.g.,* impaired mobility, memory deficits). As the pace of recovery slows and discharge to home or another facility approaches, assessment must shift to identification of the specific skills and behaviors that will be prerequisites in the new environment (*e.g.,* toilet transfers, learning a daily schedule). Assessment also depends on injury severity. It will be focused more on physical function and basic sensory processing in the severely impaired, and on cognitive, social, and vocational function in the mildly impaired.

Discipline-specific assessments must be melded into a patient-oriented assessment for treatment planning purposes (see Chap. 8). The different theoretical and clinical backgrounds of various disciplines may present an obstacle. For example, a patient's inability to retain treatment instructions may be identified as a memory deficit by an occupational therapist, an attentional deficit by a neuropsychologist, and a language comprehension deficit by a speech pathologist unless group definitions have been developed. The development of a unified problem code with shared problem definitions can foster team communication.

Typically, severely injured patients have a large number of medical, physical, cognitive, and behavioral problems. Therefore the team must develop priorities for treatment, based on such factors as estimated length of stay, functional importance of each deficit, and prognosis for improvement. Treatment priorities are also affected by the patient's degree of cooperation and treatment tolerance.

At present, data on the recovery potential of various deficits are sparse. As such data are accumulated, treatment strategies will be modified. For example, there is now considerable evidence that true memory function cannot be generally improved through repeated memory exercises.[63] Therefore, memory remediation *per se* should be of low priority. However, teaching the patient to remember certain key environmentally relevant facts either through repeated drill or by using a journal or microcomputer as a memory aid may be critical.

Another key factor in planning treatment is the age at the time of injury, particularly in the case of children and adolescents. This area has not been well studied, but some general guidelines may be established. Children under the age of 5 who sustain a severe head injury may be especially prone to developmental delays or arrested development in physical, neurobehavioral, or integrative functions. This is attributable to the immaturity of the central nervous system. In such cases, very close medical, therapeutic, and neuropsychological follow-up is desirable to evaluate the effects of brain injury. Often, a special preschool educational setting is desirable to provide the required intensive therapy and education.

Older children, between early childhood and preadolescence, are in the midst of developing a sense of personal and social identity and may suffer a great loss of self-esteem and capacity to establish effective peer relationships. This is also a period in which many basic academic skills, such as reading, writing, and mathematics, are taught. Cognitive and communication impairments may limit the head-injured child's capacity to learn and retain important skills. Educational programs should be developed for the head-injured child and preadolescent that take into consideration the child's residual strengths and weaknesses as well as the need for the development of age-appropriate peer relationships.

Adolescents who sustain a head injury are often in the process of completing their education and planning their vocational future. The injury greatly disturbs this normal developmental process. Often, preestablished goals for higher education and vocation need to be modified. For a head-injured student in high school, the process of completing the necessary coursework to receive a diploma may be greatly prolonged. Special tutoring, modified class subjects and schedules, and remedial work are often required. Early contact with the appropriate vocational agencies is often advisable, owing to the inability of many head-injured students to continue with graduate studies.

Identified treatment priorities should be framed in terms of long- and short-term goals (see Chap. 8). Certainly this is important for accountability, but it is also very useful for clarifying the team's thinking. For example, the goal "Patient will demonstrate improved memory" has quite different implications from "Patient will remember where his room is with the help of a map." As time passes, the goals are likely to become more specific and functionally oriented such that "Patient will have increased ROM in all joints" becomes "Patient will have adequate hip flexion for erect sitting throughout the day." Identification of the patient's physical and cognitive strengths can be very helpful in determining the best way to circumvent a specific deficit.

Some treatment goals (e.g., improved ambulation) may be discipline specific while others (e.g., decreased aggression) may be common to many or all team members. In general, once the problem and goal are identified, appropriate team members accept responsibility for carrying out each intervention. Complete division of labor, however, defeats the interdisciplinary purpose. A communication strategy designed by a speech pathologist, for example, should be carried out by nurses and other therapists to promote generalization of the skill.

The neuropsychological assessment is important in clarifying cognitive mechanisms responsible for various behavior and skill deficits. In the severely impaired patient, formal testing may be impossible. However, the neuropsychologist's informal observation of the patient may still be helpful. Higher level patients should receive formal testing of such core cognitive areas as attention, learning, and remembering; language comprehension and production; visual perception; and planning, reasoning, and organization.[33] Such testing is useful in clarifying strengths and weaknesses but should not be the end of the neuropsychologist's involvement. Of particular importance is the periodic problem-oriented assessment by the neuropsychologist in response to clinical questions raised by other team members. In some post-acute programs the neuropsychologist is the primary coordinator of treatment planning.

Patient reassessment by the team should be conducted continuously on an informal basis and periodically in a more structured fashion. Such reassessment has several functions. It allows objective documentation of changes in status that should prompt re-discussion of treatment goals and plans. It provides program evaluation data with which to judge the success of a program's various treatment objectives. In addition, reassessment may lead to more appropriate distribution of resources to areas amenable to change or redesign of interventions to more adequately treat difficult problems.

MEDICAL PROBLEMS AFTER HEAD INJURY

Head injury most often occurs in situations that predispose to multiple trauma. Therefore, management of the head-injured patient frequently requires management of multiple-system dysfunction. Some associated problems, such as fractures, may be viewed as independent injuries that will have functional consequences, while others, such as pulmonary injuries, may play a direct role in the severity of brain injury.

Medical problems associated with head injury may persist well beyond the period of initial stabilization. The physiatrist will manage some of these problems directly. In other cases, he or she will coordinate the services of consultants while keeping in mind the functional goals of treatment.

Neurodiagnostic Techniques

A variety of imaging and neurophysiological technologies are available to assist in management of head injury. In the acute postinjury period, CT scanning can detect intracranial hematomas, brain swelling, hydrocephalus, and infarction.[31, 95] However, it is not sensitive in identifying small contusions and white matter injury.[167] In the post-acute phase, CT scanning is useful in evaluating the progress of hydrocephalus and cortical atrophy.

Magnetic resonance imaging (MRI), a newer anatomical imaging modality, has advantages over CT scanning, including lack of x-ray exposure, greater resolution in the brain stem, better identification of isodense collections of blood, and detection of small white matter lesions.[103]

Brain scintigraphy has been largely replaced by the above modalities. Its current use includes primarily cerebrospinal fluid flow assessment in normal pressure hydrocephalus and cerebrospinal fluid leakage (cisternography) and assessment of cerebral perfusion in confirmation of brain death.[157]

Positron emission tomography (PET) is a modality that can provide information about brain function as well as anatomy. Labeled metabolic substrates such as 2-deoxyglucose or labeled blood components are taken up by brain tissue in proportion to metabolic demand or blood flow. Thus metabolically hypoactive but anatomically normal tissue may be identified. This method is very limited in availability. However, it is the only imaging method that has the potential to correlate directly with neuropsychological performance by demonstrating metabolic hypoactivity in regions subserving specific cognitive functions in the absence of gross structural change.[54]

The standard electroencephalogram can provide gross information about the severity, location, and extent of brain damage. In addition, epileptiform activity may suggest seizure risk. However, interictal electroencephalograms have low sensitivity for seizure disorders especially in areas distant from the cortical convexities (e.g., medial temporal lobes).[145] Sensitivity can be increased by sleep deprivation or prolonged monitoring with behavioral correlation.[145] Electroencephalographic measures may at times be misleading, as in the case of improvement of a patient with an isoelectric electroencephalogram.[6]

Much research has been done on evoked potentials in head trauma (see Chap. 12). In group studies, it has been shown that multimodality evoked potentials (MEPs) add to the prognostic accuracy of the *Glasgow Coma Score*.[22, 143, 144] The ability to make accurate prognostication about individual patients remains more limited. Rappaport reports the use of MEPs to allocate rehabilitation resources to patients with a potential to benefit.[144] It remains to be demonstrated that this decision strategy is superior to allocation on clinical grounds.

The clinical utility of MEPs for individual patients is clear in at least three situations. They may document organic pathology in patients with minor head injury who might otherwise be viewed as neurotic.[152] MEPs may help localize the site of neurological deficit.[69] Finally, in patients who are unconscious or uncooperative, MEPs provide a way of diagnosing somatosensory, hearing, or visual deficits that might interfere with rehabilitation treatments and allow the selection of optimal modalities for communication and environmental stimulation.[144]

Seizures

Post-traumatic epilepsy is common after significant head injury. The risk of ongoing seizures is related to injury severity, specifically depressed skull fracture, intracranial hematoma, early seizure, and prolonged disturbance of consciousness.[89] The risk of seizure development is greatest in the first 2 years after injury and gradually declines. Spontaneous resolution of a seizure disorder also occurs, indicating the need for periodic reevaluation.

Most seizures are diagnosed clinically on the basis of focal or generalized motor activity. Patients with muscle spasms or tremors may present diagnostic dilemmas. In such cases, routine or sleeping electroencephalography may reveal epileptiform activity. More definitive is a 24-hour electroencephalogram that is correlated with observations of the suspicious activity. Seizures in limbic areas may lead only to altered behavior or states of consciousness, presenting further diagnostic challenges.[21]

Seizure prophylaxis remains controversial. Several studies of prophylactic use of phenytoin or phenobarbital have failed to show reduction of seizure incidence.[134, 192, 193] However, none of these has succeeded in maintaining therapeutic serum concentrations for the duration of the study. In many acute care centers, patients at high risk are begun on parenteral anticonvulsants in the intensive care unit. Unfortunately, phenytoin and phenobarbitol have been shown to impair cognitive performance in epileptic patients. Therefore, it is prudent to substitute more cognitively benign drugs such as carbamazepine and valproic acid when use of oral medication becomes feasible.[168, 172, 188]

There are no standard recommendations on duration of treatment. However, most clinicians withdraw anticonvulsants after 1 to 5 seizure-free years. In view of the expense and potential toxicity of anticonvulsants it would seem appropriate to withdraw medications cautiously after that time in most seizure-free patients.

Hydrocephalus

Ventricular dilation occurs in up to 40% of patients with severe head injury and usually begins to appear within 2 weeks of injury.[95] However, in most instances ventriculomegaly is due to diffuse atrophy or focal infarction of brain tissue (hydrocephalus ex vacuo). Flattening of the cortical sulci and periventricular lucency tend to support the diagnosis of clinically important hydrocephalus.[9]

Hydrocephalus in head injury is most often of the communicating or normal pressure type.[9] Unfortunately, the classic triad of incontinence, gait disorder, and dementia is of little help in severely disabled patients.[188] Failure to improve or deterioration in cognitive and behavioral realms should prompt assessment with a CT scan. If the results of the scan are equivocal, cisternography may resolve the ambiguity. Patients with ventricular shunts may experience shunt failure. Thus, a deterioration in such patients should also prompt a follow-up CT scan and a shunt flow study or pressure measurements.

Frequently the patient's therapists and nurses are the best judges of subtle cognitive improvements and deteriorations. Hydrocephalus and shunt failure may not be identified through the standard neurological examination, especially in a patient with abnormal baseline findings on the initial examination. Thus, it is critical that consulting neurologists and neurosurgeons incorporate the entire team's assessments of cognitive and behavioral fluctuations into their evaluation.

Hypertension

Hypertension is common in the acute postinjury period for the severely injured and is believed to be due to the intense sympathetic outflow associated with brain injury and increased ICP.[72, 188] Therefore, β-blockers represent the most specific intervention in this patient group and will control associated tachycardia as well. Propranolol and methyldopa cause cognitive impairments in hypertensive patients.[160] Consequently, use of highly polar β-blockers such as atenolol may be preferable. Atenolol crosses the blood−brain barrier very little in normals,[39] but this has not been studied in diffuse brain injury in which the blood−brain barrier may be disrupted.

Sustained hypertension is infrequent after head injury unless there was preexisting hypertension. When hypertension does exist, diuretics and polar β-blockers are least likely to cause cognitive impairment.[38, 160] If medication with central nervous system side-effects must be used, it is wise to inform therapy staff so that subtle cognitive deterioration is noted and reported to the physiatrist.

Cardiopulmonary Disorders

Head trauma may have a number of acute effects on cardiopulmonary function. Severe injury can produce cardiorespiratory arrest or dysrhythmias.[59] Such disturbances of respiratory control are both indications of severe brain injury and causes of further hypoxic injury. Cardiac injury occurs as a result of blunt trauma to the right ventricle against the sternum. This results in early elevations of cardiac enzymes, cardiac wall motion abnormalities, and decreased cardiac output.[164] Central sympathetic hyperactivity can lead to ongoing myocardial necrosis over the next few days.[72] Although these injuries may result in lasting electrocardiographic changes (Q waves and ST segment alterations), their relevance to long-term cardiovascular health of survivors is unknown.

Multiple trauma often causes pneumothorax, pulmonary contusions, and lacerations. In addition, intense α-adrenergic outflow is believed to cause noncardiogenic pulmonary edema.[8, 59] These and other problems can further compromise cerebral oxygenation.

Many head-injured patients will require tracheostomies for ventilation and suctioning in the acute period. In some instances tracheal stenosis will prevent decannulation and will require dilatation or surgical management. Patients who require long-term tracheostomies but have begun to vocalize may benefit from one of the varieties of tubes that permit vocalization. Pneumonia in patients with tracheostomies is common, but attempts to use antibiotics prophylactically are unwarranted.[66]

Long-term survivors of severe head injuries have been reported to show decreased lung capacity, vital capacity, and forced expiratory volume. The etiology of these abnormalities is not entirely clear but there appears to be a combination of muscle weakness and incoordination, decreased compliance, and deconditioning.[12] The role of cardiopulmonary conditioning in head injury has not been systematically assessed.

Hypothalamic and Endocrine Dysfunction

An autopsy study of 100 head-injured patients revealed a 62% incidence of pituitary injury.[98] Hypothalamic injuries coexisted in some patients. Less is known about endocrine status in survivors of head injury. Case reports document a variety of endocrine dysfunctions, but no study has evaluated prevalence in a population with varying severity of injury or prevalence longitudinally during recovery. Potentially, head injury may directly injure the pituitary or may impair hypothalamic excitatory or inhibitory control.

Head injury may result either in diabetes insipidus or in the syndrome of inappropriate secretion of antidiuretic hormone (SIADH). Antidiuretic hormone is secreted from neuroendocrine cells in the posterior pituitary. The mechanism of traumatic SIADH is unknown, but it may relate to the loss of cortical or limbic inhibition of the hypothalamus.[42] Diabetes insipidus occurs as a result of impairment or necrosis of the posterior pituitary. It may appear as late as 1 month after injury perhaps because dying tissue can release stored antidiuretic hormone for that period.[73] Both disorders can be managed acutely by controlling fluid and electrolyte intake and monitoring serum electrolytes and osmolality. Persistent or late appearance of diabetes insipidus is usually permanent and may be managed with a synthetic antidiuretic hormone analog.

Anterior pituitary damage may range from panhypopituitarism to selective loss of gonadal stimulating hormones, thyrotropin, or adrenocorticotropic hormone.[53,97] Clinical signs may be subtle and confounded with other causes of cognitive, behavioral, and physiological abnormalities. Hypotention or hypothermia or cognitive decline may be indicators of endocrine dysfunction. Secondary amenorrhea in female patients is common and may predispose to osteoporosis.

During the acute postinjury period, elevated serum cortisol is common. It is related to increased ICP but only in the presence of an intact brain stem.[50] The mechanism is unknown since it is not associated with elevated secretion of adrenocorticotropic hormone.[50]

Gynecomastia and galactorrhea occur from elevations in prolactin. In normals, prolactin secretion is controlled by tonic hypothalamic inhibition. Therefore, brain injury frequently disrupts these inhibitory influences.[43] Chest trauma and a number of medications may also result in galactorrhea.

Sexual dysfunction in head-injured males is more common than can be accounted for on the basis of endocrine dysfunction but is related to other indices of injury severity.[99] Although it is suggested that this represents hypothalamic dysfunction, it is difficult to rule out more psychosocial etiologies.

In summary, it appears that endocrine dysfunction is common at least in the severely injured and may remit with neurological recovery.[53] Clinical evaluation may be difficult because of confounding deficits, so the clinician should have a high index of suspicion. Uncorrected endocrine disorders may limit cognitive and behavioral recovery and lead to serious physical sequelae.

PHYSICAL DEFICITS

Cranial Nerve Dysfunction

Olfactory nerve injuries commonly accompany significant head trauma owing to the delicate anatomy of the fibers exiting the cribriform plate; they are particularly likely in association with cerebrospinal fluid rhinorrhea.[89] The diagnosis may be missed owing to incomplete sensory testing. Serial testing may reveal some degree of recovery. Olfactory deficits may play a role in altered feeding behavior.

Visual impairment may occur as spotty scotomata that differ in the two eyes, as homonymous hemianopsia, or as complete blindness. Optic nerve pathology must be distinguished from hemi-inattention, cortical blindness, and visual agnosia. Early assessment can be done in gross terms through fundoscopic examination, visual evoked response studies, and pupillary reflex assessment. Therapists may make behavioral assessments of visual fixation and tracking in response to novel objects at various locations. Crude measurement of visual acuity can be performed with an optokinetic drum.[18] When cooperation allows, more precise visual field and acuity testing should be performed. Neuropsychological assessment may clarify visuospacial perceptual disorders. Information about field cuts and acuity should be shared with all team members to ensure that therapeutic stimuli are of appropriate size and placement.

Extraocular movements may be affected by damage to cranial nerves or their brain stem nuclei or by impairment of coordinative structures in the midbrain and cerebellum.[27] In addition, orbital fractures or damage to the extraocular muscles may produce disconjugate gaze.[18] Neuro-ophthalmologic examination may help clarify the pathophysiology of the deficit. Alternating or unilateral eye patching can eliminate diplopia. Use of prisms and strabismus surgery require that the patient be capable of ocular fusion in order to achieve binocular vision, but surgery may sometimes be appropriate solely for cosmetic purposes. Many medications can exacerbate diplopia.[101]

Temporal bone fractures may disrupt facial nerve function temporarily or permanently.[18] This must be differentiated from cortical or subcortical central facial weakness. Early nerve conduction and electromyographic studies may clarify the prognosis for facial nerve recovery.[65] Facial weakness, when combined with corneal insensitivity due to trigeminal pathology, can lead to corneal ulceration. Corneal lubricants or tarsorrhaphy may be indicated.

Skull fractures may also disrupt the auditory or vestibular pathways. Ossicular dislocation can lead to conductive hearing loss.[18] Brainstem auditory evoked responses (BAERs) can be helpful in assessment of auditory function in comatose or uncooperative patients. However, if no response is seen at normal intensity, the hearing threshold should be evaluated with increasing intensities. Caloric and oculovestibular testing can provide information about vestibular function. Later, standard audiologic evaluation including speech perception should be performed. Hearing aids or ossicular repair can be helpful in selected patients. The patient's auditory capabilities should be shared with the entire treatment team so that care can be taken to communicate in the environment and style that optimizes comprehension.

Movements of the tongue, pharynx, and larynx are often impaired by severe head injury at various levels in the central nervous system. Evaluation of oral motor function, cough and gag reflexes, and indirect laryngoscopy may help clarify the location and extent of the pathology. Such disturbances will be relevant for safe oral feeding as well as vocal communication.

Sensory Deficits

Traumatic brain injury can produce disturbances of any of the sensory modalities. Depending on the location and severity of the damage, these may be disturbances of basic sensation (*e.g.,* decreased visual acuity) or of perceptual processing of that sensation (*e.g.,* impaired visual spatial perception). Both forms of disturbance can be disabling.

Cranial nerve sensory deficits were discussed previously. Disorders of somesthetic sensation can result from damage to a variety of brain structures and may distort touch, pain, temperature, and positional information. Pain syndromes may result from central injury to the thalamus or other cerebral structures.[71]

Basic sensation can be assessed in each modality as soon as the patient is able to cooperate. Visual, auditory, and somesthetic sensation can be grossly assessed earlier with evoked potential studies. However, the presence of normal basic sensation does not ensure that the patient can form the complex perceptions needed to recognize a visually presented object through tactile exploration or identify a letter through stereognosis.

When patients fail at a task for which basic sensory input is intact, other causes of inability to perform can be explored. A patient recovering from cortical blindness, for example, may have full visual fields and functional acuity but may be unable to name visually presented objects. Neuropsychological assessment can help to differentiate among object-naming disorders, visual agnosias, scanning disorders, and disorders of complex visual perception.

There is no uniform strategy for coping with sensory deficits. Rather, treatment is planned around the severity of the deficit, strength of remaining sensory capabilities, and cognitive status of the patient. All team members should be involved in this planning since the patient's sensory, motor, and cognitive capacities are all relevant to the process.

Heterotopic Ossification

Heterotopic ossification occurs in 11% to 76% of severely injured patients, primarily in proximal joints of the upper and lower extremities.[62] The etiology of heterotopic ossification in brain injury (as in spinal cord injury and hip replacement) is unknown. Risk factors include prolonged coma and increased muscle tone in the involved extremity.[163]

A study using historical controls suggests that diphosphonates may have a role in prevention of heterotopic ossification after head trauma.[163] However, Garland has reported that patients who remain severely cognitively and physically impaired have a high rate of recurrent bone formation after surgical treatment.[60] This may imply an ongoing stimulus for heterotopic ossification in such patients, raising questions about the efficiency of time-limited prophylaxis. More research is needed on the role of prophylaxis in various subgroups of head-injured patients.

Heterotopic ossification may present as pain, warmth, swelling, and contracture formation, but it may be occult. Earliest diagnosis is possible with a bone scan, but subsequently ossification is visible on plain roentgenograms.[58] The role of diphosphonates in treatment of established heterotopic ossification is controversial. Range of motion exercises are indicated to prevent ankylosis. If ankylosis seems inevitable despite exercises, it should be encouraged to occur in the most functional position.

Surgery for removal of ectopic bone should be undertaken only for clear functional goals, such as improved standing posture or ambulation or independent dressing and feeding. In general, surgery is not undertaken earlier than 18 months after injury.[60] More functional patients with normal alkaline phosphatase levels are less likely to experience recurrence.[60] Diphosphonate prophylaxis should be done perioperatively and range of motion exercises continued.

Increased Muscle Tone and Contractures

Increased muscle tone following head trauma may include true spasticity (increased phasic stretch reflexes). Other disorders of tone such as dystonia, posturing in response to head position and cutaneous stimulation, and extrapyramidal syndromes are also common. The mere existence of abnormal tone is not an indication for treatment. Treatment should be based on functional considerations, such as those listed in Table 30-8.

Physical modalities such as heat, cold, stretch, and inhibitory postures can be helpful in mild to moderate tone but are unlikely to provide lasting control or control of severe tone. Medications such as dantrolene sodium, baclofen, or diazepam may be used. It has been claimed that only dantrolene is effective in spasticity of cerebral origin,[195] although this remains controversial.[94, 136] Dystonia, a severe functional problem, rarely responds dramatically to antispasticity drugs. Furthermore, all three agents produce sedation often enough to raise concerns about their effects on marginal cognitive function.[188, 195, 196] Little research has been done on any of these medications specifically in head injury. It is not clear that drug effects assessed in patients with cerebrovascular accident or spinal cord injury predict response in head injury given the high prevalence of brain stem and midbrain pathologic processes in the latter diagnosis.

Phenol nerve and motor point blocks are an effective strategy in severe disorders of tone. Although their efficacy is best documented in true spasticity,[47] they have been found to be effective to varying degrees in spasms, posturing, and dystonia. Multiple muscle groups may need to be blocked and blocks repeated periodically. The advantage, however, is the effectiveness in severely increased tone and the lack of cognitive side-effects.[61]

Contractures following head trauma usually result from increased tone or heterotopic ossification. Ideally, contractures should be prevented through range of motion exercises, splinting, and treatment of tone. The functional prognosis of patients cannot be accurately predicted early after injury. Therefore, at this point, attempts should be made to treat all contractures by nonsurgical means such as ultrasound, traction, and serial casting. Contractures in patients with head injuries in the more distant past should be treated only for clear functional goals such as improved hygiene, positioning, or active movement. Surgical treatment of contractures should be undertaken only for clear functional goals after conservative measures have failed.

Table 30-8
Indications for Treatment of Increased Muscle Tone

Interference with active movement
Contracture formation or progression in a posturing limb
Interference with appropriate positioning or hygiene
Self-inflicted trauma during muscle spasms
Excessive pain on range of motion or during muscle spasms
Excessive therapy time devoted to contracture prevention rather than
  functional activities

Motor Disturbances

A variety of motor disturbances result from significant head injury. The diffuse and multifocal nature of the neuropathologic processes often challenges a precise neurophysiological diagnosis. Disorders of muscle tone have been previously discussed. Additional deficits include paralysis or paresis involving isolated muscle groups, combinations of limbs, or the whole body. Weakness, especially in combination with disorders of tone can have profound effects on mobility, status of activities of daily living, and employment.

Disorders of balance and coordination may result from cerebellar or other injuries. Patients with good muscle strength may be unable to ambulate or even sit independently owing to profound ataxia. Similarly, limb ataxia may preclude self-feeding, writing, and independent activities of daily living. Tremors, bradykinesia, and parkinsonism may accompany basal ganglia and substantia nigra lesions.[131]

The patient's movement abilities should be assessed by the physiatrist, physical therapist, and occupational therapist. Weakness can be addressed through active assistive range of motion and progressive resistive exercises. Distal weakness accompanied by atrophy should raise the question of peripheral nerve injury and should prompt nerve conduction and electromyographic studies.

Ataxia is notoriously difficult to treat. A weighted walker, wrist cuffs, and propranolol may be of modest benefit. Other drug interventions are under investigation. If ataxia varies markedly from proximal to distal joints, selective splinting or strategies to stabilize the extremity may be useful.

An attempt should be made to specifically diagnose tremors with reference to their frequency, amplitude, and occurrence during action, rest, and sleep. Levodopa and propranolol have both been used in movement disorders such as tremors and ataxia, but functional tests should be performed on and off medication to assess efficacy in individual patients.[48] Orthotics and adaptive devices may assist weak or ataxic patients in performing functional tasks. Dexterity exercises may be used to increase manual speed and coordination.

Slowed motor responses are among the most common deficits associated with head injury and may significantly limit self-care and employment productivity. However, it appears that much of this motor slowness can be attributed to central processing delays rather than a motor deficit *per se*.[175] There is, as yet, no consensus on how to treat this generalized slowness.

Nutrition and Feeding

Head injury can produce dramatic increases in basal metabolism, with catabolism, weight loss, and low serum albumin levels. These metabolic responses occur independent of steroid treatment.[194] Thus, the acutely injured patient must have increased caloric and protein intake. However, the degree to which aggressive enteral or parenteral feeding can improve recovery as opposed to aggravating metabolic derangement is not clear.

The obtunded patient can usually be fed via a nasogastric tube relatively soon after injury. There is no consensus regarding how soon to consider gastrostomy or jejunostomy in patients who remain obtunded or lack oral motor capability, but tube placement improves cosmesis and lowers the risk of aspiration.[174] Tube feeding may be performed via bolus or continuous methods and during the day, night, or over 24 hours. Although nocturnal feedings are conveniently scheduled and ensure an empty stomach during therapy times, it is difficult to keep patients positioned with their heads elevated during sleep, and the effects of nocturnal feeding on diurnal rhythm are unknown.

Gastroesophageal reflux is common following brain injury even in those without nasogastric tubes.[176] It may lead to aspiration and esophagitis. Antacids and acid suppressants may improve esophagitis. Metoclopramide increases gastroesophageal sphincter tone, but it can cause sedation and extrapyramidal side-effects.[123] Head elevation may reduce aspiration.

Obstacles to oral feeding following head trauma include both cognitive and oral motor deficits.[189] Attempts at oral feeding generally begin with assessment of the reflexive and voluntary components of oral motor function by a speech, occupational, or physical therapist experienced in dysphagia treatment. This is followed, if necessary, by an oral motor facilitation treatment program to decrease the latency of the swallowing reflex and improve oral motor strength and coordination.

When appropriate, small quantities of pureed foods are introduced and increased in amount to build endurance. As performance improves the variety of thickness and texture is increased until liquids can be safely handled. Failure to become a functional feeder is associated with persistently poor intraoral manipulation or cognitive levels below V on the Rancho Los Amigos Scale.[189]

Patients who appear to be candidates for oral feeding but who have frequent coughing or an episode of clinical aspiration may benefit from video fluoroscopy performed collaboratively by an experienced feeding therapist and radiologist (see Chap. 6).[109] By using different food textures and placements it may be possible to determine a strategy to normalize swallowing.

When the patient has made maximal progress in terms of food quantity and texture, the family and nursing staff should be trained in the optimal oral feeding methods.

Bowel and Bladder Dysfunction

Pathologic conditions affecting the frontal lobe, so common in head injury, can impair inhibitory control over bowel and bladder evacuation, leading to urgency and incontinence.[4] Clinically, post-void residuals are rarely elevated in incontinent head-injured patients, suggesting that if neurogenic bladder exists, it is of the uninhibited detrusor type. However, detrusor–sphincter dyssynergia can occur, particularly with significant brain stem involvement below the pontine micturition center.[135] Slowed mobility, poor communication, and impaired initiation also contribute indirectly to incontinence.

The presence of a neurogenic bladder can be assessed by noting the frequency and volume of individual voids and measuring the post-void residual. Normal residuals with frequent small voids suggest an uninhibited detrusor reflex. The patient can be managed with frequent toileting. If the needed frequency is not feasible, anticholinergic medications may increase bladder capacity.[181] However, one must be aware of potential urinary retention and sedation.

Once a feasible voiding pattern is established, a behavioral toileting program designed around the patient's high probability voiding times is instituted. When the patient is successful on this program, attempts should be made to teach initiation of toileting.

If a toileting program is unsuccessful, a CMG/electromyogram may help clarify the patient's degree of sensation and voluntary control. If continence is not a feasible goal a condom catheter is an option for males. Condom catheters carry an increased risk of urinary tract infection when used in agitated patients who manipulate or kink the tubing.[84] Absorbent pads for females are less ideal but have a lower risk of infection than indwelling catheters.

Bowel management is similar to other neurological disabilities. Regulation of stool consistency and induction of a regularly timed bowel movement will help the majority of patients remain continent.

COGNITIVE DEFICITS AFTER HEAD INJURY

Head injury is by nature a diffuse and multifocal brain insult. For this reason, there is great variability in the patterns of cognitive deficits that such patients display. These deficits depend on the pattern and severity of focal gray matter lesions as well as white matter disruption. Neuropsychological investigation of individual patients can be highly informative. Questions and hypotheses generated by therapy staff may be clarified by such investigations.

Despite the variability in cognitive deficits, certain common patterns exist. This is most likely related to the common areas of gray matter injury (frontal and temporal poles) and white matter damage (midbrain and corpus callosum). Even mildly injured patients may complain of difficulty with alertness, memory, and concentration.[153] These same deficits appear in more severe forms in seriously injured patients who may have, in addition, significant disorders of perception, communication, and interpersonal behavior.

The rehabilitation of cognitive deficits is in its infancy. Cognitive retraining, cognitive remediation, or cognitive rehabilitation are names used interchangeably to refer to a variety of treatment techniques intended to improve cognitive function and minimize psychological deficits. There is no formal definition for this area of work, and the approaches vary in terms of how much they make use of computer technology versus traditional therapy tasks, how much they focus on isolated components of cognition versus the cognitive aspects embedded in functional tasks, and how much they seek to directly improve impaired cognitive processes versus encourage compensatory strategies. Thus, it is important to critically assess the content of cognitive remediation programs on an individual basis when making clinical referrals. For those engaged in this pursuit, it will be important to continually integrate advances in the neurosciences into the clinical treatment approach.

Disorders of Arousal and Attention

Deficits in arousal and attention are among the most widespread in head injury and affect the entire spectrum of severity.[175] The comatose patient suffers from profoundly impaired arousal, and many of the cognitive and emotional complaints in minor head injury are hypothesized to be attentional.[175]

Arousal may be defined as the general state of responsiveness to environmental stimuli. Normally, arousal undergoes slow fluctuations in relation to diurnal rhythm, temperature, and activity level (tonic arousal). Arousal can also be modulated over brief intervals by demands in the environment (phasic arousal).[138] The reticular activating system (RAS) has a primary role in control of arousal, exerting its influence over diffuse cortical regions and receiving cortical inputs in return.[137] Damage to the RAS plays a critical part in coma onset.[44, 52]

A deficit in tonic arousal can lead to generalized impairments in responsiveness and profound slowing of information processing. Impaired phasic arousal may interfere with the ability to modify arousal to cope with cognitively demanding situations.

Attention may be considered to be the selective channeling of arousal. Awareness is directed to a particular set of internal or external stimuli out of the infinite set of possible targets of awareness. Attention is not a unitary phenomenon either in psychological or neurophysiological terms,[132] and there is no precise agreement about how to divide up its component processes. One can at least distinguish the following phenomena:

- *Selection:* the ability to focus on a particular stimulus
- *Concentration:* the ability to inhibit attention to competing stimuli over a period of time
- *Spatial attention:* the ability to attend to both sides of space
- *Capacity:* the quantity of information that can be held in mind at one time (sometimes referred to as immediate or working memory and measured by digit span)
- *Divided attention:* The ability to concurrently perform two or more activities requiring attention

Numerous brain regions appear to play a role in attentional processes. Research has particularly highlighted the roles of the right hemisphere and prefrontal regions in attentional function.[41, 122] Disorders of attention may impair learning and performance. Affected patients may have difficulty focusing on any task, may be easily distracted, or may show hemispatial neglect. Decreased attentional capacity can lead to secondary decreases in language comprehension or visuospatial processing because the patient's information processing is limited to such small units. Inability to divide attention might be manifested, for example, in the inability to attend simultaneously to task instructions and monitor one's own performance. It has been suggested that posttraumatic amnesia is most appropriately considered a confusional state related to attention deficit rather than a true memory disturbance.[7] Similarly, frontal lobe disorders such as impulsivity and perseveration may be interpreted in attentional terms. These disorders may reflect a loss of goal-directed control over attention such that attention is easily pulled or dysfunctionally fixed on irrelevant aspects of a task.[41]

Arousal and attention are best assessed by a combination of formal neuropsychological tests such as line bisection,[81] letter cancellation,[121] digit span,[180] and behavioral observation by all disciplines. It is critical to arrive at more precise diagnoses than "impaired attention," since impairments of different components of attention have different therapeutic implications. In general, treatment of these disorders can be grouped in terms of pharmacological, behavioral, and compensatory strategies (Table 30-9). Teaching strategies and the environment can always be modified to help accommodate attentional deficits (compensatory strategies). The roles of medications and behavioral treatments in specific disorders are still under investigation but have shown promise in certain instances. For example, stimulant medications have been used clinically to increase alertness and decrease distractibility.[35] Behavioral approaches have been used to improve hemispatial attention and attention to task.[191]

Many medications used for other purposes have negative effects on arousal, attention, and general cognitive function. Anticonvulsants such as phenytoin and phenobarbital, antihypertensives such as methyldopa and propranolol, and antispasticity drugs such as diazepam, baclofen, and dantrolene may all impair cognitive performance.[160, 168, 195, 196] Therefore, attempts should be made to withdraw such medications or replace them with less sedating alternatives (*e.g.,* carbamazepine, hydrochlorothiazide, atenolol, phenol nerve blocks).[61, 188]

The interdisciplinary team should reach consensus regarding the nature of a patient's attentional deficits and agree on consistent approaches in terms of behavioral and compensatory treatments. Medication trials and behavioral treatments can then be monitored in terms of their effects on objective variables such as on-task behavior, amount of cueing needed to overcome neglect, and so on.

Table 30-9
Treatment of Disorders of Arousal and Attention

Deficit in:	Pharmacological	Behavioral	Compensatory
Arousal	Avoid sedating drugs. Psychostimulants*	Reinforce "alert behaviors" (*e.g.*, eyes open).	Provide environmental stimulation and work when most alert.
Selection	Avoid sedating drugs. Psychostimulants*	Reinforce "focusing."	Use highly salient stimuli.
Concentration (distractability)	Avoid sedating drugs. Psychostimulants*	Reinforce "on-task behavior."	Work in nondistracting environment, take breaks, and change tasks.
Spatial attention		Training in spatial attention	Present material on "good side."
Capacity			Present information in small amounts and provide breaks to allow processing.
Divided attention			Avoid tasks that require divided attention.

* Investigational status.

In normal people, extensive practice of virtually any task leads to the ability to perform it with minimal attention (*i.e.* "automatically").[185] This phenomenon has received little study in brain-damaged patients. However, it would seem possible to deal with some attentional impairments by practicing the activities to such a degree that they no longer place much demand on the disordered attentional processes.

One of the concerns in treatment is to ensure that strategies learned in a therapy environment are carried over into a variety of functional activities. Therefore, if a team member is training spatial attention in, for example, reading, interdisciplinary plans should be made to transfer the same protocol to other settings such as ambulation and activities of daily living.

Disorders of Learning and Remembering

Memory can be grouped into the component processes of encoding (analyzing and restructuring information into storable forms), storage (the actual maintenance of stored memories), and retrieval (the locating and returning to awareness of stored information). Head injury frequently results in a combination of retrograde and anterograde memory deficits.[112] Retrograde amnesia is defined as the inability to recall events preceding the injury. The time period affected by retrograde amnesia varies with severity of injury but typically shrinks over time, leaving an episode of minutes unaccounted for.[132] Usually more remote memories are intact. Although this may be subjectively disturbing to patients, it is not of great functional significance.

Anterograde memory disturbance (difficulty in acquiring new information) is the most widespread cognitive complaint of patients and families. One must distinguish between a core memory deficit or amnesia and other deficits that secondarily limit ability to remember in everyday life. Damage to the medial temporal lobes and hippocampus or to portions of the thalamus can lead to profound anterograde amnesia with relative preservation of other cognitive capacities.[7] Such patients perform normally on immediate tests of cognitive performance but moments later are unable to recall that they have even taken these tests. Unilateral damage to the above structures produces material-specific impairments in memory for verbal (if left sided) or nonverbal (if right sided) material.[132]

Profound damage to these neuroanatomical structures is relatively uncommon in head injury.[7] Therefore, it appears likely that a portion of the memory deficits reported in such patients is due to secondary effects of other deficits. In general, material to be remembered must be attended to, and the deeper and more elaborately it is processed, the better it will be remembered. Given the prevalence of attentional deficits in head injury, it appears that much "memory impairment" can be attributed to defective processing of information at the time of presentation.[112, 132] Similarly, disorders of planning and organization may lead to a disorganized pattern of information storage and a disorganized mental search at the time of retrieval.[112]

Regardless of the precise etiology, functional disorders of memory are of profound significance. They limit the ability of patients to learn new tasks during the rehabilitation process. Even familiar or routine tasks may be disrupted by the patients' inability to regain their place if they become distracted or their inability to recall minor changes required from day to day.

Assessment of memory dysfunction should include formal neuropsychological testing aimed at the following questions:

1. Does the patient have a disorder of functional memory, and, if so, is it global or material specific?
2. To what extent can the disorder be attributed to attention deficits?
3. To what extent can the disorder be attributed to organizational deficits?

The most widely used test of memory, the *Wechsler Memory Scale,* is an inadequate assessment tool for this purpose, but alternatives have been reviewed.[112] In addition, the interdisciplinary team and the family should identify the environmental situations in which the disorder disrupts function.

Treatment of core memory deficits has had limited success. Medications that may impair memory, such as diazepam, should be avoided or, if used, should be accompanied by memory assessment before and after initiation of therapy.[148] Memory-augmenting drugs are under study and may provide therapeutic alternatives in the future.[35]

There is no convincing evidence that exercise of the "memory muscle" will produce generalized improvement in memory function.[63] Thus, the plethora of computer-driven memory exercise and game drills appear to lack therapeutic value in core memory disorders. The ability to use nonverbal memory to compensate for verbal memory deficits or vice versa has shown some promise in laboratory settings, but it has not been demonstrated that patients use the strategy spontaneously, perhaps because it requires considerable conscious effort.[63] Various prosthetic devices have also been tried, such as diaries, computer entries, and alarms. These approaches, however, are complicated by the patients' lack of awareness of what they will need to record and by failure to refer to the recorded information. Such prostheses represent incomplete but potentially useful compensations. The ability of profoundly amnestic patients to acquire some habits and skills (procedural memory) is well documented.[32, 37] Some investigators are exploring ways to make use of this phenomenon in rehabilitation.[63]

In theory, disorders of functional memory attributable to attentional or organizational deficits can be ameliorated by treating the contributing deficits. However, this approach has yet to be clinically validated. It remains difficult to specify the mechanism by which various organization deficits impair memory, and it remains unclear how effectively such deficits can be treated.

Clearly, effective remediation of memory disorders is at a primitive stage with many potential options under investigation. At present, however, certain strategies seem justified:

- Drills can be effective in teaching particular pieces of functionally important information. These might include important facts such as locations, schedules, or names, or important strategies such as "there's a calendar on my wall." They should not be expected to improve memory for other material.
- Prosthetic devices such as diaries and alarms are likely to have benefit only to the degree that the patient can be taught when to use them and what information to record.
- The functional goals of any experimental memory remediation strategy should be articulated and regular team discussions held regarding the degree of functionally important changes seen.

Disorders of Communication

Communication disorders following traumatic brain injury may take many forms depending on the site and extent of the lesion(s). Unlike the stroke patient, classic aphasic syndromes are not prominent following brain injury, unless there is a focal left frontotemporal lobe lesion. Sarno reported that 30% of her head-injured patients were clinically aphasic at 1 year after injury.[155, 156] In many cases aphasia that presents in an early stage tends to resolve within the first 6 months.[86] Dysarthria is sometimes noted after brain injury and may be the result of either peripheral or central nervous system damage affecting motor control of the speech mechanism. It has been found to occur in patients with focal mass lesions of the left hemisphere[169] and in cases of diffuse injury.[155] Anomia, commonly referred to as a word finding or object naming disturbance, is perhaps the most common language disorder seen in traumatic brain injury. Levin and co-workers reported that anomic aphasia usually takes the form of semantic errors, circumlocution, and concretism.[102] The neuroanatomical locus is considered to be the dominant parietal area. Anomia is often accompanied by signs of dysgraphia, dyslexia, and dyscalculia, as reported by Heilman and colleagues.[80] Verbal fluency may be affected more generally by left frontal or bifrontal lesions.[14]

A variety of nonaphasic language disturbances may also manifest after traumatic brain injury. The problem of talkativeness has been described by Prigatano, who found this problem in 16% of 48 consecutive head-injured patients who were seen at least 16 months after injury.[140] He noted that relatives of head-injured patients reported that this problem was accompanied by other difficulties, such as belligerence, negativism, anxiety and depression. Levin and co-workers noted that the tangential expression of ideas, reflective of fragmented thought processes, was also characteristic of many head-injured patients.[104] Peculiar phraseology, as shown when patients speak of themselves in the third person, is another interesting language phenomenon. Dysprosodia, which is an impairment of the melody, affective coloring, and cadence of speech, may be seen with right hemisphere lesions.[28] Alexia, most often accompanied by agraphia, which involves severe reading and writing deficits, is associated with a lesion in the posterior margin of the angular gyrus of the temporoparietal lobes.[30]

In everyday life, it is often difficult to separate communication disorders from the cognitive impairments that may appear concomitantly. For example, a patient with anomia may have significant attentional, memory, and visuospacial perceptual problems, all of which may contribute to an inability to recall items from a shopping list. Another patient may respond inappropriately to questions asked by a person in a crowded, noisy room owing to problems in auditory comprehension, complex information processing, or dividing attention. In a job situation, a head-injured person who is employed in telephone sales may perform poorly owing to circumlocutory speech, as well as a difficulty with the rate of information processing. For the majority of head-injured patients, basic functional communication skills will recover in 6 months after injury so that the head-injured person may appear functionally normal to the casual observer. However, in a more challenging environment such as school or work, communication difficulties become more easily identified and pose major problems to successful reentry.

The treatment of communication disabilities is often delegated to the speech-language pathologist on the rehabilitation team. In the case of aphasia, techniques such as visual-auditory cueing, use of gestures, and object-naming exercises are often employed. The dysarthric patient receives oral motor strengthening and coordination exercises to improve articulation, a palatal lift for nasality, and breath support training to improve sustained volume. Pragmatic disorders of communication, such as tangentiality, circumlocution, and aprosodia are often treated within "communication groups" in which audiotape, videotape, and listener feedback are immediately provided. In addition, other group members and leaders attempt to model good communication skills. For the severely impaired patient who has limited expressive communication skills but relatively intact comprehension, augmentative communication devices may be provided (see Chap. 6).

It is important to ensure that the strategies that optimize communication are shared among all disciplines so that consistent communication demands are placed on the patient in all environments. Another critical part of treatment involves the education and counseling of family members. Speech pathologists, as well as other team members, provide specific information to families about the nature of communication disorders, their relationship to the brain injury, prognosis for recovery, and ways in which family members can facilitate recovery of communication skills or compensatory techniques to circumvent fixed deficits. The role of the family in facilitating communication is very important because a primary frustration for head-injured patients is often their inability to communicate their needs to family members.

Disorders of Visuospatial Perception and Construction

Visuospatial disorders are less commonly observed than other neurobehavioral disorders after head injury, perhaps because the posterior areas of the brain are less often damaged than the frontal and temporal areas. A head-injured patient may perform poorly on visually mediated activities owing to deficits in attention, problem solving, poor manual dexterity, or ataxia rather than visuospatial deficits *per se.*

Nevertheless, several types of visuospatial perception disorders can be identified. Prosopagnosia, the inability to recognize familiar faces, is an unusual disorder that has been studied extensively by Benton.[13] This disorder has been correlated with lesions of the right inferior occipitotemporal region.[13, 119] Other visuospatial deficits include disturbances in body schema, problems in motor planning, and impaired perception of form, spatial relations, color, and figure–ground relationships.[178]

A variety of assessment procedures can be used to determine the presence of visuospatial dysfunctions and to differentiate visuospatial from visuoconstructive disorders. Assessment of visual neglect has been described previously. Disturbances in body schema are often evidenced by completion of drawing tasks, such as the *Draw-a-Person.* Tests such as the *Frostig, Rey-Osterreith Complex Figure, Block Design,* or *Picture Completion* subtests can reveal difficulties in the visuospatial domains. The *Motor Free Visual Perception Test* is often used to ascertain whether a gross visuospatial problem exists independent of constructional abilities.

A variety of constructional disorders (with or without perceptual deficits) may arise from lesions to the posterior association cortex, particularly in the parietal area. A defective spatial orientation is seen in cases of dyscalculia, in which the patient has difficulty in manipulating numbers in spatial relationships even though mathematical reasoning skills may be intact. Brain-injured patients may also show impairment on tasks that require the copying of designs or construction of two- and three-dimensional figures. In performing such tasks, a patient with a right hemisphere lesion may take a fragmented approach and miss the total configuration while accurately producing internal details. This type of performance is frequently manifested on the *Block Design* subtest of the *Wechsler Adult Intelligence Scale.* In contrast, left hemisphere lesions will cause a patient to reproduce accurately the entire figure but not internal details. Patients with right hemisphere lesions will tend to display greater impairment in perceptual and constructional functions than those with left hemisphere lesions.[106]

Visuospatial disorders have functional consequences in many areas of daily life skills such as dressing, grooming, preparation of meals and eating, driving a vehicle, ambulating, writing, and performing manual assembly tasks.[11]

In the rehabilitation setting, the occupational therapist is most often the team member who treats visuospatial disorders, although the neuropsychologist may have performed the initial assessment to identify the presence of these dysfunctions. A variety of treatment techniques may be used to attempt to remediate or compensate for these problems. Visual scanning exercises may be used to treat visual field deficits or visual neglect. Completing human figure puzzles or using a mirror to provide visual feedback while dressing may be used to treat disturbances of body schema. Extensive verbal or written cues instead of gestures may help in treating patients with more generalized visuospatial problems when working on functional activities such as ambulation, transfers, or dressing.

Disorders of Cognitive and Behavioral Regulation

The mark of intelligent performance is the ability to adapt to change, solve problems, and cope with novel situations, not the ability to perform a particular task well. This capacity requires such abilities as cognitive flexibility, self-monitoring, generation of multiple alternatives, and anticipation of consequences. These abilities, in turn, are highly dependent on prefrontal cortical function.[41] It is perhaps not surprising, then, that head injury (which often involves damage to the frontal poles) commonly leads to disorders of reasoning, planning, and problem solving and to impulsivity or perseveration. These deficits may also manifest themselves in aberrant personal and social behaviors, such as inappropriate sexual gestures or bizarre speech.

In normal people the focus of attention is sometimes externally controlled. For example, one attends to a loud noise or bright object. However, normal people also modulate their attention in the service of higher-level goals. For example, if one's goal is to get to an appointment as rapidly as possible, one will be more likely to attend to street signs and less likely to attend to store windows. For such modulation to occur, emotional and motivational states must be linked to the control of attention and action and frontolimbic structures coordinated with perceptual and motor structures.

It has been argued that many of the disorders of cognitive and behavioral regulation experienced by head-injured patients can be attributed to loss of goal-directed modulation of attention and action.[81] Thus, the head-injured patient who behaves in a sexually inappropriate manner may be controlled more by the salience of the stimuli (*e.g.,* "My therapist is attractive") than by an internal goal (*e.g.,* "I don't want to offend my therapist").

These deficits are among the most difficult to address for several reasons. They are the least understood in terms of their neuropsychological and neurophysiological underpinnings. By their nature, they are least obvious in highly structured and routine environments. Finally, because these disorders relate to ability to deal with novelty and change, they cannot be seen within specific tasks but must be looked for in changing tasks.

Attempts to treat disorders of cognitive and behavioral regulation have been based on two perspectives. At one extreme, one may conclude that the basic deficits are unremediable and, hence, one would seek to train patients how to solve *specific* problems of functional importance and display *specific* socially acceptable behaviors. To the extent that clinicians can predict situations a patient is likely to face, this will be of some value, but one would not predict a general improvement in self-regulation.

At the other extreme, one may seek to remediate the essential processes of cognitive flexibility, self-monitoring, and so on, in the hope of improving the ability to face a broad range of unanticipated circumstances. To the extent that the patient's deficit is dependent on a particular problem such as impulsivity, adoption of a single strategy such as "stop and think" may be of broad benefit. However, many patients' difficulties with problem solving are due to a collection of interacting deficits. To remediate the complex interactions of all these deficits would amount to training the patient to increase general intelligence. The ability to train intelligence in other populations has not been demonstrated.

The disorders of cognitive and behavioral regulation are of profound functional significance for severely head-injured patients and are major obstacles to independent living and employment. More research is needed on the efficacy of various treatment strategies. Until such information is available however, it would seem prudent not to focus exclusively on retraining abstract capacities, but to include the particular functional problems such as planning a meal or organizing transportation.

All team members are likely to be involved in addressing these problems. The neuropsychologist may be able to suggest treatment strategies applicable to all disciplines. In addition, each therapist can assist the patient to solve the specific problems faced within that discipline. For example, the physical therapist helps the patient plan how to navigate around obstacles and the occupational therapist helps the patient learn strategies for organizing a menu.

Anosognosia

The failure of head-injured patients to acknowledge the presence of a neurological deficit, particularly manifested by the denial that a paretic extremity belongs to them, is termed *anosognosia*.[81, 140] This phenomenon has been closely associated with nondominant (particularly right hemisphere) lesions, occurs most frequently in the acute stages after brain injury, and frequently dissipates over the following weeks. Anosognosia is often equated with psychological denial, which involves the refusal to acknowledge the severity of a brain injury or its long-term implications. Frequently, it is difficult to clinically distinguish between the two phenomena. However, in the case of anosognosia, there is often a generalized reduction in emotional responsivity and a decreased capacity for self-awareness.

Whether primarily neurologically or psychologically mediated, failure to appreciate deficits creates a significant obstacle to progress in the rehabilitation process. Patients with anosognosia may be unmotivated to practice tasks that they see no need for and may be unwilling to consider employment retraining or changes in educational plans. In extreme cases, they may see no purpose in the entire rehabilitation effort. This problem is often dealt with in the rehabilitation setting by retraining patients to attend to their affected side and by confronting their unrealistic appraisal of their deficits in a group psychotherapy format.[81, 82, 140]

DISORDERS OF INTEGRATIVE FUNCTION

Integrative function can be thought of as those high-level adaptive functions whose performance is dependent on the integration of numerous component physical and cognitive processes. Deficits in integrative function may result from disorders in one or more component processes. Hence, they may be treated both through treatment of component deficits and directly at the level of retraining of the particular integrative function.

Impairments in Mobility

Mobility may be impaired for a variety of reasons (Table 30-10), ranging from the purely physical to the purely cognitive. Many patients will have multiple physical and cognitive deficits contributing to impairments in mobility. A physical assessment by the physiatrist, physical therapist, and occupational therapist will identify contractures and motor disturbances that limit mobility. Aggressive attempts should be made in the early months after injury to improve these deficits. Purchase of permanent assistive devices should be postponed until the patient's ultimate level of physical function is relatively certain.

Before purchasing an electric or one-arm-drive wheelchair for a patient with limited physical function, it is wise to assess the patient's spatial attention and motor planning abilities. Testing of visuospatial perception may contribute to this assessment, but a trial of the equipment with assessment by the relevant therapists will provide more definite information about the patient's ability to learn the chair's operation and navigate the environment.

Patients who can safely navigate on foot or in a wheelchair may nevertheless get lost or confused. In most cases this should be handled in some other way than by mobility restriction. The ability to be mobile, even aimlessly, in response to environmental stimuli may contribute to quality of life.

Table 30-10
Some Component Processes Relevant to Mobility

Component	Role in Mobility
Range of motion	Must allow for required movements
Strength	Necessary for ambulation, wheelchair propulsion, or switch operation
Balance/postural reflexes	Necessary for safe ambulation and transfer and adjustment to sudden perturbations
Muscle tone	Must allow for effective use of strength
Visuospatial perception	Necessary for environmental navigation
Spatial attention	Necessary for awareness of both sides of space
Concentration	Necessary for maintenance of locomotion in presence of distractions
Memory	Necessary for using previous experience of routes and locations
Planning/organization and reasoning skills	Necessary for mobility in unfamiliar environments and using public transportation
Initiation	Necessary for turning plans into action

Less disabled patients may have all the physical prerequisites for mobility yet have difficulty learning routes and mastering bus schedules and mobility services. Such patients may benefit from maps, written sequences of instructions, training in reading of schedules, and use of the telephone to arrange mobility services, depending on their particular patterns of strengths and weaknesses. Many patients may have difficulty transferring these strategies to a new environment. Therefore, it appears most useful to teach community mobility skills in the community where the patient will reside.

Impairment in Activities of Daily Living Skills

As with mobility, independence in activities of daily living may be limited by a complex combination of physical and cognitive impairments. A similar process of interdisciplinary physical and cognitive assessment may lead to identification of particular component processes that are especially significant (see Chap. 5).

Basic skills such as dressing, bathing, and feeding may be improved with a treatment program aimed at three components:

1. Attempts to improve salient physical or cognitive deficits such as serial casting for contractures or graded constructional exercises for visuospatial constructional deficits.
2. Attempts to compensate for salient physical or cognitive deficits such as provision of assistive devices for physical deficits or written or pictorial cue cards for cognitive deficits.
3. Attempts to provide retraining in a task at the level of integrative function without specific regard for the contributing deficits using behavioral training methods (breaking down into small steps, backwards chaining, reinforcement).

Patients who master basic skills in daily living may progress to home management skills such as cooking, shopping, budgeting, and cleaning. Similar treatment principles are involved, but these tasks place greater emphasis on the cognitive components in that they are less routine and require more planning and organization.

Skills needed for activities of daily living may suffer when the patient returns to an environment in which the stimuli are different and demands placed by family members differ from those experienced in the rehabilitation setting. This problem should be anticipated and training should be provided to family members. Ideally, the patient should be phased into the home environment gradually and communication with the therapy staff maintained to assist in the transition. This can be accomplished through the use of periodic home passes with follow-up communication between the family and team, by systematic home visits by team members, or by a transition from inpatient to full-time outpatient to part-time outpatient status.

Disruptive, Combative, and Disinhibited Behavior

Behaviors such as screaming, striking out, and sexual fondling or public masturbation are not tolerated in the social or vocational environment and may preclude the reintegration of severely injured patients. Such behaviors are typical of a generally agitated state as patients emerge from coma and will often resolve spontaneously. This may be because increasing alertness eventually allows coherent processing of the environment in place of confusion. This agitated behavior has been termed *hypomania*. A number of factors may contribute to the persistent occurrence of such behaviors.

Patients with premorbid histories of aggressive, impulsive, and disinhibited behavior may be at risk for head injury (see Chap. 3). Premorbid patterns may persist or intensify after injury at a time when other effective strategies for getting needs met have been lost. A premorbid personality history derived from family, school, or employer is useful in setting realistic treatment goals.

The frontolimbic structures so frequently damaged by head injury are believed to play an important role in inhibition of impulsive and inappropriate behaviors.[21] Thus, in head-injured patients a minimal provocation can lead to a dramatic outburst of noise or aggression. It has been suggested that such outbursts reflect limbic seizure activity or temporal lobe epilepsy.[190] Alternatively, impaired impulse control may accompany damage to frontolimbic structures independent of seizure activity.[190] This suddenly aggressive behavior pattern in "normal" people has been referred to as the episodic dyscontrol syndrome and is associated with an increased incidence of subtle neurological signs such as nonlocalizing electroencephalographic abnormalities.[115]

Impairments of other cognitive processes such as concentration and language comprehension or expression may contribute to behavior problems indirectly. Such deficits may foster confusion, misunderstanding, and frustration, which, in someone with limited options, may predispose to agitated, aggressive behavior. With specific reference to sexually inappropriate behaviors, lack of availability of receptive partners, lack of private places to masturbate, and perhaps loss of preinjury sexual relationships may predispose to inappropriate sexual behavior.

Medications may have unwanted effects on behavior. Benzodiazepines and other sedatives can produce paradoxical agitation[77] perhaps by making the patient less able to coherently process the environment's events and by further impairing inhibitory mechanisms. Psychostimulants given to improve alertness and attention may lead to excessive stimulation and agitation.[182]

Patients who are aware of their deficits may have difficulty in adjusting to their disability. This can lead to anger, hostility, and depression. Depression as a direct result of brain damage has been noted in other neurological populations.[79] These mood and adjustment issues can also contribute to maladaptive behavior.

Patients who have been institutionalized for some time may have been unintentionally taught their maladaptive behaviors. They may, for example, have discovered that screaming or striking out receives the prompt attention of staff members.

Treatment of maladaptive behavior may include behavior modification, other forms of psychotherapy, and psychoactive medications. The optimal combination of these elements has not been precisely identified nor are there agreed-on guidelines for matching patients and treatments. A possible stepwise behavior management protocol is, however, outlined below:

1. *Watchful waiting.* Recently injured patients may rapidly move through stages of combative and agitated behavior. In such instances, the best strategy may be to provide intensive staffing, remove dangerous objects, and wait for the patient to calm spontaneously. Inadvertent reinforcement of maladaptive behavior should be avoided.
2. *Baseline data.* Patients who persist in their maladaptive behaviors require more active intervention. Sedatives and other behaviorally active medications should be withdrawn whenever possible to allow accurate assessment of the relevant "natural" behaviors. Staff members must be prepared for exacerbation but will be surprised by how often the behaviors improve or at least remain stable when sedatives are withdrawn.

   Baseline data should be collected by all disciplines using an agreed-on operational definition of the behavior (*i.e.,* "screaming," "pounding fist," rather than "agitation"). Data should document frequency, duration, or intensity of the behavior; possible environmental factors that may have contributed to it (*e.g.,* a difficult task, a late-arriving meal); and the consequences that followed it (*e.g.,* a need was met, the patient was scolded).
3. *Treatment planning.* The entire rehabilitation team should meet to share and analyze data for patterns. A mood disturbance may be revealed by occurrence of a behavior at times of family contact, by episodes of crying, or by vegetative signs. Other cognitive deficits that contribute may be identified if the behavior occurs primarily when working on one content area, or when frustrated by attempts at communication. Plans should be made to compensate for these deficits by altering the difficulty of tasks or the method of giving instructions.

   Too often, planning revolves around what to do once a maladaptive behavior occurs. The emphasis should be shifted to positive reinforcement of appropriate behaviors. This might include training patients in appropriate ways to notify therapists of increasing frustration, to express anger, or to ask to have needs met. The reinforcements used to strengthen these alternative behaviors include food, tokens, and rewards with special significance to the patient, such as looking in the mirror or going outside (see Chap. 3). Environmental restructuring may also be undertaken. If aggression occurs primarily in large group activities, the patient can be treated only in small groups and gradually introduced to larger groups as behavior improves.

   Consequences for the maladaptive behavior can range from simple nonreinforcement to time out, loss of privileges, or restitution. It is critical for these consequences to be planned by the team at a dispassionate moment, not invoked by angry staff members concerned with making the "punishment fit the crime."
4. *Reassessment.* It is crucial for the whole team to adopt a

uniform treatment approach until reassessment takes place. Continued data collection may reveal dramatic improvement, partial response, or no improvement. Reanalysis may clarify the reasons and allow for modification of the treatment plan. Subjective assessment of change is notoriously unreliable and must be avoided.[187] If behavioral analysis reveals partial response or no response, adjunctive medication may prove useful.

5. *Medication trial.* Few guidelines exist to assist in choosing behaviorally active medications. Medication efficacy is assessed through the same behavioral data collection as described previously. However, it should be noted that there is no medication effective specifically against, for example, "screaming." Therefore, a drug that decreases screaming may also decrease numerous other, more adaptive behaviors. Therapists should note unwanted changes. Deteriorating performance may also be revealed by repeated neuropsychological tests.

Medications useful in control of aggression and agitation have been adopted from the psychiatric and mental retardation literature. However, one must be careful in extrapolation from these populations in the absence of data specifically on head injury. Superficially similar symptoms may have different mechanisms and drug responses, and head-injured patients are likely to be especially sensitive to the cognitive effects of medications.

Several medications have been reported to decrease agitated or aggressive behavior in selected patients (Table 30-11). The selection of an appropriate medication for an individual patient remains a challenge. Patients with prominent disorders of arousal and attention may benefit from psychostimulants or tricyclic antidepressants, in a manner analogous to children with attention deficit disorder. Drugs effective in acute mania (lithium carbonate, carbamazepine) have been of use in agitated and aggressive patients. In many patients, neuroleptics have a nonspecific depressant effect on behavior. Thus, they are used relatively infrequently in crisis situations when sedation is the overt treatment goal and less toxic drugs have proved inadequate. Occasional patients may benefit from low doses of neuroleptics used chronically and experience minimal sedation, but this should be assessed on an individual basis, usually after other agents have failed. All psychoactive medications should be reassessed periodically by attempted tapering to determine their continued usefulness and lowest effective dose. Double-blind placebo-controlled trials with behavioral ratings have been of great clinical value in determining drug efficacy for individual patients.[187]

When acceptable behavior has been achieved in the controlled clinical environment, it should be generalized into home and community settings. Family members should be taught relevant interventions and told to expect some "testing" by the patient in new environments. When family and staff pass these tests, they promote generalization of the adaptive behaviors to various settings. Explicit attention to generalization of appropriate behavior has been shown to allow transition to less restrictive environments in severely impaired patients.[46]

Impaired Initiation

Some head-injured patients simply fail to act without extensive cueing or imposed structure. In extreme cases, patients may be able to verbally describe a course of action but simply do not do it. This type of deficit may accompany particular patterns of neurological damage that disrupt the linkage between limbic motivational inputs and cognitive and motor activities.[130]

Impaired initiation appears to be a fairly specific frontally mediated deficit. However, it may, at times, be difficult to differentiate from depression or impaired arousal. This may be a problem of differential diagnosis. Alternatively, it may be a reflection of some common underlying neurophysiological mechanisms subserving mood, arousal, and initiation such that these are not independent phenomena. One of us (J.W.) has treated some patients who demonstrated striking increases in initiation in response to psychostimulants or "activating" tricyclics such as protriptyline in the absence of overt signs of depression or lethargy.

Commonly used behavioral approaches to impaired initiation include physical, verbal, written, or pictorial cues for the steps involved in a task, with behavioral reinforcement for proceeding from one step to the next rather than for completion of the previous step. Structured time frames for task completion may also be of help.

Difficulty is often encountered in generalizing to varied tasks. That is, the patient learns to initiate a morning sequence of daily living activities but shows no improvement in working on homework independently. Development of prompting strategies that can be used across tasks may be of help. For example, if a patient learns to use a sequence of flash cards to prompt a dressing sequence, it may be possible to use a sequence of cards for many other tasks with minimal new learning required. Obviously, this requires interdisciplinary treatment planning.

Disorders of initiation can have profound effects on independent living. Whereas patients with severe physical disabilities can often have the help of personal care attendants, little appreciation is given to the need for "cueing" or "prompting attendants." In some instances, patients might be able to live semi-independently with the assistance of someone to periodically check their progress and prompt completion of necessary tasks.

Depression

Depression may accompany head injury of all levels of severity.[107] Depressive psychoses are found more commonly than hypomanic states after traumatic brain injury, yet still comprise a rather small percentage of overall cases.[2] Affective disorders are often transient and may be accompanied by a confusional state, paranoid ideation, and aggressive outbursts. A variety of factors have been postulated to contribute to the manifestation of these conditions, including the direct effect of brain injury; the influence of a preexisting personality disposition; the effect of trauma as a nonspecific stress that precipitates the condition, aside from the brain damage itself[108]; and a secondary emotional reaction to the primary mental or physical deficits.[21]

Depressive reactions after head injury may manifest in various forms and levels of severity. Intensity of depression does not appear to be well correlated with lateralization of lesion, level of neuropsychological impairment, or severity of brain damage.[140]

Table 30-11
Psychoactive Medications for Behavioral Management

Psychostimulants (methylphenidate, dextroamphetamine, pemoline)
Tricyclic Antidepressants
Carbamazepine
Lithium Carbonate
Beta blockers
Benzodiazepines*
Neuroleptics*

---

*Less frequently used.

In most follow-up studies of head-injured patients, depressed mood is reported by both patient and family for years after the injury. Prigatano defined depression secondary to head injury as a constellation of symptoms including "feelings of worthlessness, helplessness, loss of interest in work and family activities and decreased libido."[140] Reactive depression appears to be the most common form of depression after head injury. It may occur weeks, months, or years after the initial neurological insult but often signals the patient's fuller recognition of the deficits or life changes caused by the injury. As in other cases of reactive depression, the best treatment is often active involvement in therapeutic work or social activities that can induce increased self-esteem and reduce feelings of worthlessness. In some cases psychotherapy or psychostimulant or tricyclic antidepressant medication may prove useful. However, tricyclics should be used with caution owing to their effects on seizure threshold.[91]

Severe depression can lead to suicidal ideation and suicide attempts. Hilbom studied 3,552 war veterans and found that 37 (1.4%) of the total sample had committed suicide.[83] Similarly, Vauhkonen followed 3,700 brain-injured soldiers and found 1% had committed suicide by 1957.[177] Achte and Anttinen noted that the frequency of suicide tended to rise after 15 to 19 years after injury and that over one-half of their suicidal cases had been psychotic at some point since the injury.[1] The subjects in each of these studies were head-injured veterans, predominantly male, and likely suffering penetrating, rather than closed, head injury.

Social Function

Many severely head-injured adults appear "childlike" in their behavior, show a lack of regard for conventional social norms, and have great difficulty maintaining preinjury relationships or establishing new ones. Much of this behavior may be attributable to the frequency of frontal lesions that can destroy the "sense of self." Head-injured patients seem to lack an "observing ego" (i.e., the ability to monitor and ascertain the correctness of their social behavior). Other difficulties in interpersonal relationships may be related to subtle language problems, such as tangential discourse, circumlocution, excessive talkativeness, and peculiar phraseology.[140] Group psychotherapy conducted by a psychologist or conjointly with a social worker, speech pathologist, or other team member may prove helpful.[29, 82, 140]

Only a few investigators have examined the effects of head injury on leisure and recreational activities. Bond found that work and leisure activities were the most disrupted of all daily activities after head injury.[19] Oddy and co-workers found that the most severely head-injured in their sample of 50 young head-injured adults did not return to all of their leisure activities at 12 months after injury.[133] Clinicians working in rehabilitation settings have recognized that residual physical and neurobehavioral sequelae prevent many head-injured patients from returning to their premorbid recreational pursuits. Since many do not return to work either, loss of leisure activity may be psychologically devastating. In recent years, as specialized head injury units have been developed, the recreational therapist has become an integral team member, performing leisure skills assessments and developing individualized and group treatments to teach new ways of occupying leisure time or adaptive methods for performing favorite premorbid activities (see Chap. 1).

In recent years, the effects of head injury on the family have been systematically studied by a number of investigators. Bond studied 56 severely injured patients within 2 years after injury and found that family cohesion was primarily affected by mental, as opposed to physical, disability.[19] Rosenbaum and Najenson examined marital relationships 1 year after injury in Israeli brain-injured veterans.[149] They found increased interpersonal tension within the family; feelings of loneliness, depression, and isolation in the wives; lack of sexual contact with husbands due to loss of feelings of attractiveness and personality changes; and role changes within the family. They also found that many of the difficulties in marital relationships were associated with the wives' depressed mood.

McKinlay and associates attempted to identify the major sources of psychosocial burden on 55 relatives of the brain-injured patients within 1 year after injury.[113] They identified three types of burdens: objective burden type 1—changes in family routine, family health, housing conditions, financial status, and leisure activities; objective burden type 2—post-traumatic symptoms and changes in patient's behavior; and subjective burden—stress felt by the caregiver resulting from presence of objective burden. Their results focused primarily on objective burden type 2. The most frequent symptoms reported by relatives at 12 months after injury were irritability, impatience, tiredness, and poor memory.

Inclusion of the family into the rehabilitation program has become a standard practice within the past 10 years. Previous studies have indicated that families often feel disappointed and upset about the lack of detailed information received from health care providers. Perhaps in response to this, a great emphasis has been placed on individualized or group family education.[45] Other types of treatments for family include family counseling, family therapy, and family support groups.[151] Most commonly, the rehabilitation psychologist, neuropsychologist, and social worker are the members of the team who deliver these services to the family.

Disturbances in sexual function have been often noted by clinicians but have not been well studied. Sexual dysfunctions may include hypersexuality, hyposexuality, impotence, loss of feelings of attractiveness, inability to find appropriate partners, and incapacity to engage in intimate interpersonal relationships requiring the interpretation and expression of complex emotions. Staff members and relatives are often dismayed by the sexual dysfunctions after head injury and have difficulty in effectively managing these problems. More recently, rehabilitation facilities have developed sexual re-education programs for head-injured patients, in which specific information is provided about sexual function and basic social skills regarding interpersonal intimacy are taught. Sexual behavior is most often perceived by staff as a problem when the patient engages in overtly inappropriate behavior (e.g., public masturbation or continual advances toward rejecting partners). In these cases, team members such as the psychologist or social worker are often asked to intervene to help re-educate and redirect the patients toward more appropriate expression of their sexual drives.

Inadequate sexual function is too often neglected since it creates fewer problems for family and staff. Patients may have hormonal or neurological disorders that interfere with sexual function and may lack the relevant psychosocial skills for forming intimate relationships. As in other patient groups, such information is rarely elicited unless solicited. Furthermore, patients with memory impairments or lack of awareness of their disabilities may be unable to accurately report presence of erections, lubrication, orgasm, and so on.

Educational, Prevocational, and Vocational Function

The presence of disabling motor impairments, such as paralysis, weakness, and incoordination, and of cognitive deficits, such as poor memory, decreased attention, and deficient planning and organization, adversely affect the patient's capacity to reenter the educational system, whether at an elementary, secondary, or postsecondary level. Although Public Law 94-142 "guarantees" educational opportunities for head-injured children up to age 21 (as well as other disability groups), the implementation of special accommodations for head-injured children varies greatly, depending on the local school district's educational philosophy, available resources, and understanding of the nature of the problem. For the elementary and secondary school child, transition back into school can be traumatic. For this reason, it is advisable for school personnel, rehabilitation team members (particularly psychologists, occupational therapists, and speech therapists), and the family to help the school develop an individualized education plan (IEP). A variety of broad options need to be considered: tutoring at home or school; regular class placement; regular class placement with a variety of support services (*e.g.,* speech therapy, physical therapy, counseling, adaptive physical education); resource room services; self-contained classroom; and full-time, 12-month residential program.[129]

For the postsecondary school adolescent or adult, further educational and vocational services may be required. There are a growing number of community colleges and universities that offer educational programs tailored to the head-injured person. At these schools, remedial courses in basic skill areas such as reading or mathematics are provided. In other cases, supplemental tutoring may be made available. To assist with daily living needs, a group living situation with assistance from a residential counselor is sometimes available. These modifications allow a head-injured person to progress at a slower pace, with a great deal of support and a far greater likelihood of academic success than in a typical college environment.

Vocational goals are important to many head-injured patients once they complete their acute rehabilitation. The major problem is that vocational goals may be based on their premorbid abilities or vocation and may be unrealistic. Some comprehensive rehabilitation programs include prevocational assessment and vocational training.[15] After the patient completes a period of extensive cognitive rehabilitation, a vocational counselor in the program designs a vocational program that usually involves "work trials" within the rehabilitation setting. If this proves successful, the patient may be placed into a transitional employment placement. In this setting, a "job coach" can provide on-the-job instruction and guidance to the client and advise the employer as to potential job modifications needed to maximize the patient's performance.

Every state has a Department of Vocational Rehabilitation. Head-injured patients are routinely referred to the state vocational rehabilitation agency by the rehabilitation team members, often the social worker or psychologist. The vocational counselor meets with the client and family to determine what a feasible vocational goal might be and develops an individualized written rehabilitation plan. This plan may include any of a wide variety of services, including prevocational assessment, vocational assessment, work adjustment training, sheltered workshop training, or a "supported work" program (a program in which the head-injured client is taught specific job skills and then gradually integrated into an actual competitive work situation with assistance provided by an on-site "job-coach"). Vocational assessment, which is accomplished through the administration of standardized work samples, tests of ability and vocational interest, physical endurance, and work habits, forms the basis for much of the vocational planning. The neuropsychological assessment is usually requested by vocational counselors as an essential component on which to base the vocational plan.

FINANCIAL AND MEDICOLEGAL ISSUES

A head injury not only taxes the adaptive resources of the family but also the financial resources. Programs have been developed that provide extended rehabilitation services for months and years after the injury, but these programs are costly. Cost is not a problem for a few patients who have gained large settlements from personal injury litigation, have worker's compensation, or benefit from living in a no-fault insurance state. For the vast majority of survivors of severe head injury, third party reimbursement and personal finances become exhausted within the first few months or year after injury. Federal and state programs, such as Medicare and Medicaid, do not generally support long-term residential programs, day treatment, transitional living, or behavioral management. To achieve financial as well as psychosocial survival, many patients and their families must gain access to public welfare funds or Social Security disability or engage in private fund-raising efforts.

A variety of medicolegal issues can complicate the rehabilitation process. There is often the need to determine the competency of the head-injured person to manage financial affairs, make important decisions, engage in vocational pursuits, or manage medical needs. If the court deems a head-injured person to be incompetent, a conservator may need to be appointed to manage financial affairs or a guardian named to make decisions for the person. Another issue for many is personal injury litigation, which often results from accident cases. In this circumstance, the head-injured person tries to recoup financially for past medical expenses, pain and suffering, and past and future lost wages. Although a large settlement can be very beneficial for the patient, it often takes 5 years or longer for a case to be settled in the courts. This produces a severe stress on the patient and the family. Furthermore, head-injured patients can be their own worst witnesses because of their memory impairments and "normal" physical appearance and many achieve minimal financial gain.[150]

A variety of professionals can assist head-injured patients and their families to deal with these complex financial and medicolegal problems. The social worker or case manager is often relied on to assist in financial planning, in obtaining governmental benefits, and in locating needed home health services after discharge from the hospital. A lawyer is frequently hired to represent the head-injured person in various types of litigation. Unfortunately, most attorneys are not knowledgeable about head injury and must be educated by health care professionals. All of the members of the rehabilitation team may be asked to assist in medicolegal cases, although typically the physician specialists (neurologist, neurosurgeon, and physiatrist) and psychologist (neuropsychologist or rehabilitation psychologist) are those who are asked to provide detailed records and provide testimony in court.

CONCLUSIONS

Increased interest has been focused on head injury in recent years as more patients survive severe injury and as the long-term sequelae of all grades of injury become clearer. During this time, head injury rehabilitation has emerged as a subspecialty of interest to physiatrists, nurses, psychologists, and therapists.

The focused interest in head injury has led to a number of important advances in knowledge. The epidemiology, pathophysiology, and course of recovery have been substantially defined. Our ability to estimate prognosis has improved. The medical, physical, cognitive, and behavioral sequelae of head injury have been more clearly identified and classified.

Treatment advances have also occurred. The acute management of patients with head injury has benefited from the advances in neurosurgical intensive care. Medical management of the complications of head injury has also improved. The physical sequelae of head injury such as paralysis, contractures, and heterotopic ossification have been lessened by the same treatments used in the rehabilitation of other physical and neurological disabilities. Yet the cognitive and behavioral deficits of many head-injured patients represent their most significant obstacles to community reintegration. It is in these cognitive and behavioral realms that the ability to improve function is least clearly defined.

Much research is in progress to refine the classification of cognitive and behavioral deficits, to clarify the extent to which they are remediable, and to identify the most effective remediation strategies. However, because each head-injured patient's pattern of deficits is unique, it will always remain a challenge to apply the knowledge gathered from group studies to the management of the individual patient. For this reason, a thoughtful interdisciplinary treatment planning process that considers the complex interactions of the many physical, cognitive, and behavioral deficits is essential.

REFERENCES

1. Achte KA, Anttinen EE: Suizide bei Hirngeschadigten des Krieges in Finland. Fortschritte der Neurologic, Psychiatrie 31:645–667, 1963
2. Achte KA, Hilbom E, Aalberg V: Post-traumatic Psychoses Following War Injuries, vol 1. Helsinki, Rehabilitation Institute for Brain Injured Veterans in Finland, 1967
3. Alexander MP: Traumatic brain injury. In Benson DF, Blumer D (eds): Psychiatric Aspects of Neurologic Diseases, vol 2. New York, Grune & Stratton, 1982
4. Andrew J, Nathan PW: Lesions of the anterior frontal lobes and disturbances of micturition and defaecation. Brain 87:233–262, 1964
5. Annegers JF, Grabow JD, Kurland LT: The incidence, causes and secular trends of head trauma in Olmstead County, Minnesota. Neurology 30:912–919, 1980
6. Askenazy JJ, Sazbon L, Hackett P et al: The value of electroencephalography in prolonged coma: A comparative EEG–computed axial tomography study of two patients one year after trauma. Resuscitation 81:181–194, 1980
7. Auerbach SH: Neuroanatomical correlates of attention and memory disorders in traumatic brain injury: An application of behavioral subtypes. J Head Trauma Rehabil 1(3):1–12, 1986
8. Baigelman W, O'Brien JC: Pulmonary effects of head trauma. Neurosurgery 9:729–740, 1981
9. Bakay L, Glasauer FE: Post-traumatic hydrocephalus. In Head Injury. Boston, Little, Brown & Co, 1980
10. Barth J, Macciocchi S, Giordani B et al: Neuropsychological sequelae after minor head injury. Neurosurgery 13:529–533, 1983
11. Baum B, Hall KM: Relationship between constructional praxis and dressing in the head injured adult. Am J Occup Ther 35:438–442, 1981
12. Becker E, Bar-Or O, Mendelson L et al: Pulmonary functions and responses to exercise of patients following craniocerebral injury. Scand J Rehab Med 10:47–50, 1978
13. Benton AL: Behavioral consequences of closed head injury. In Odom GL (ed): Central Nervous System Trauma Research Status Report, pp 220–231. Bethesda, MD, National Institute of Neurological and Communicative Disorders and Stroke, 1979
14. Benton AL: Differential behavioral effects of frontal lobe disease. Neuropsychologia 6:53–60, 1968
15. Ben-Yishay Y et al: Neuropsychological rehabilitation: Quest for a holistic approach. Semin Neurol 5:252–259, 1985
16. Ben-Yishay Y, Diller L: Cognitive remediation. In Rosenthal M, Griffith ER, Bond MR, Miller JD (eds): Rehabilitation of the Head Injured Adult. Philadelphia, FA Davis, 1983
17. Ben-Yishay Y, Silver S, Piasetsky E et al: Relationship between employability and vocational outcome after intensive holistic cognitive rehabilitation. J Head Trauma Rehabil 2(1):35–48, 1987
18. Berrol S: Medical assessment. In Rosenthal M, Griffith ER, Bond MR et al (eds): Rehabilitation of the Head Injured Adult. Philadelphia, FA Davis, 1983
19. Bond MR: Assessment of the psychosocial outcome of severe head injury. Acta Neurochir 34:57–70, 1976
20. Bond MR: Standardized methods of assessing and predicting outcome. In Rosenthal M, Griffith ER, Bond MR, Miller JD: Rehabilitation of the Head Injured Adult pp 97–113. Philadelphia, FA Davis, 1983
21. Bond MR: The psychiatry of closed head injury. In Brooks N (ed): Closed Head Injury: Psychological, Social and Family Consequences. Oxford, Oxford University Press, 1984
22. Born JD, Albert A, Hans P et al: Relative prognostic value of best motor response and brain stem reflexes in patients with severe head injury. Neurosurgery 16:595–600, 1985
23. Brink JD et al: Recovery of motor and intellectual function in children sustaining severe head injuries. Dev Med Child Neurol 12:565–571, 1970
24. Brooks N (ed): Closed Head Injury: Psychological, Social and Family Consequences. Oxford, Oxford University Press, 1984
25. Brown G, Chadwick O, Shaffer D et al: A prospective study of children with head injuries: III. Psychiatric sequelae. Psychol Med 11:63–78, 1981
26. Brunnstrom S: Movement Therapy in Hemiplegia. Hagerstown, MD, Harper & Row, 1970
27. Burde RM, Savino PJ, Trobe JD: Clinical Decisions in Neuro-Ophthalmology. St. Louis, CV Mosby, 1985
28. Burns MS, Halper AS, Mogil SI: Clinical Management of Right Hemisphere Dysfunction. Rockville, MD, Aspen, 1986
29. Carper M, Rosenthal M: The value of group psychotherapy with the brain injured. Presented at the Annual Meeting of the American Psychological Association, Washington, DC, August 1986
30. Charness A: Stroke/Head Injury: A Guide to Functional Outcomes. Rockville, MD, Aspen, 1986
31. Clifton GL, Grossman RG, Makela ME et al: Neurological course and correlated computerized tomography findings after severe closed head injury. J Neurosurg 52:611–624, 1980
32. Cohen NJ, Squire LR: Preserved learning and retention of a pattern analyzing skill in amnesia: Dissociation of knowing how and knowing that. Science 210:207–209, 1980
33. Cohen RF: Hypothesis testing approach to neuropsychological assessment for treatment planning. Paper presented at the conference on Neurological Syndrome: Pathophysiology, Neuropsychological Assessment, and Treatment, Boston, November 1985
34. Cooper KD, Tabbador K, Hauser WA: The epidemiology of head injury in the Bronx. Neuroepidemiology 2:70–88, 1983
35. Cope DN: The pharmacology of attention and memory. J Head Trauma Rehabil 1(3):34–42, 1986
36. Cope N: Traumatic closed head injury: Status of rehabilitation treatment. Semin Neurol 5:212–220, 1985
37. Corkin S: Acquisition of a motor skill after bilateral medial temporal lobe excision. Neuropsychologia 6:255–265, 1968
38. Cove-Smith JR, Kirk CA: CNS-related side effects with metoprolol and atenolol. Eur J Clin Pharmacol 28(suppl):69–72, 1985
39. Cruikshank JM, Neil-Dwyer G: Beta-blocker brain concentrations in man. Eur J Clin Pharmacol 28(suppl):21–23, 1985
40. Dail WG, Feeney DM, Murray HM et al: Responses to cortical injury: II. Widespread depression of the activity of an enzyme in cortex remote from a focal injury. Brain Res 211:79–89, 1981
41. Damasio AR: The frontal lobes. In Heilman KM, Valenstein E (eds): Clinical Neuropsychology, 2nd ed. New York, Oxford University Press, 1985
42. Davis BP, Matukas, VJ: Inappropriate secretion of antidiuretic hormone after cerebral injury. J Oral Surg 34:609–615, 1976
43. de Leo R, Petruk KC, Crockford P: Galactorrhea after prolonged traumatic coma: A case report. Neurosurgery 9:177–178, 1981
44. Denny-Brown D, Russell WR: Experimental cerebral concussion. Brain 64:93–164, 1941
45. Diehl L: Patient-family education. In Rosenthal M, Griffith E, Bond MR, Miller JD (eds): Rehabilitation of the Head Injured Adult. Philadelphia, FA Davis, 1983

46. Eames P, Wood R: Rehabilitation after severe brain injury: A follow-up study of a behaviour modification approach. J Neurol Neurosurg Psychiatry 48:613–619, 1985
47. Easton JKM, Ozel T, Halpern D: Intramuscular neurolysis for spasticity in children. Arch Phys Med Rehabil 60:155–158, 1979
48. Ellison PA: Propranolol for severe head injury action tremor. Neurology 28:197–199, 1978
49. Feeney DM, Gonzalez A, Law WA et al: Amphetamine, haloperidol, and experience interact to affect the rate of recovery after motor cortex injury. Science 217:855–857, 1982
50. Feibel J, Kelly M, Lee L et al: Loss of adrenocortical suppression after acute brain injury: Role of increased intracranial pressure and brain stem function. J Clin Endocrinol Metab 57:1245–1250, 1983
51. Field PM, Colman DE, Raisman G: Synapse formation after injury in the adult rat brain: Preferential reinnervation of denervated sites by axons of the contralateral fimbria. Brain Res 189:103–113, 1980
52. Finger S, Stein DG: Brain Damage and Recovery. New York, Academic Press, 1982
53. Fleischer AS, Rudman DR, Payne NS et al: Hypothalamic hypothyroidism and hypogonadism in prolonged traumatic coma. J Neurosurg 49:650–657, 1978
54. Foster NL, Chase TN, Fedio P et al: Alzheimer's disease: Focal cortical changes shown by positron emission tomography. Neurology 33:961–965, 1983
55. Frankowski RF, Annegers JF, Whitman S: The descriptive epidemiology of head trauma in the United States. In Becker DP, Povlishock JT (eds): Central Nervous System Research Status Report, pp 33–43. Bethesda, MD, National Institute of Neurological and Communicative Disorders and Stroke, 1985
56. Frankowski RF, Klauber MR, Tabbador K: Head injury mortality: A comparison of three metropolitan counties. Bethesda, MD, National Institute of Neurological and Communicative Disorders and Stroke, 1980
57. Frankowski RF: The demography of head injury in the United States. In Miner M, Wagner KA (eds): Neurotrauma, vol 1, pp 1–17. Boston, Butterworths, 1986
58. Freed MM: Traumatic and congenital lesions of the spinal cord. In Kottke FJ, Stillwell GK, Lehmann JF (eds): Krusen's Handbook of Physical Medicine and Rehabilitation, 3rd ed. Philadelphia, WB Saunders, 1982
59. Frost EA: Respiratory problems associated with head trauma. Neurosurgery 1:300–306, 1977
60. Garland DE, Hanscom DA, Keenan MA et al: Resection of heterotopic ossification in the adult with head trauma. J Bone Joint Surg [Am] 67:1261–1269, 1985
61. Glenn MB: Update on pharmacology: Nerve blocks in the treatment of spasticity. J Head Trauma Rehabil 1(3):72–74, 1986
62. Glenn M, Rosenthal M: Rehabilitation following severe traumatic brain injury. Semin Neurol 5:233–246, 1985
63. Glisky EL, Schacter DL: Remediation of organic memory disorders: Current status and future prospects. J Head Trauma Rehabil 1(3):54–63, 1986
64. Goldstein K: Aftereffects of Brain Injury in War. New York, Grune & Stratton, 1942
65. Goodgold J, Eberstein A: Electrodiagnosis of Neuromuscular Diseases, 3rd ed. Baltimore, Williams & Wilkins, 1983
66. Goodpasture HC, Romig DA, Voth DW et al: A prospective study of tracheobronchial bacterial flora in acutely brain-injured patients with and without antibiotic prophylaxis. J Neurosurg 47:228–235, 1977
67. Gouvier WD, Blanton PD, LaPorte KK et al: Reliability and validity of the Disability Rating Scale and the Levels of Cognitive Functioning Scale in monitoring recovery from severe head injury. Arch Phys Med Rehabil 68:94–97, 1987
68. Greenberg RP, Becker DP, Miller JD, Mayer DJ: Evaluation of brain function in severe head trauma with multimodality evoked potentials. II. Localization of brain dysfunction and correlation with post-traumatic neurological conditions. J Neurosurg 47:163–177, 1977
69. Greenberg RP, Stablein DM, Becker DP: Noninvasive localization of brain-stem lesions in the cat with multimodality evoked potentials: Correlation with human head-injury data. J Neurosurg 54:740–750, 1981
70. Greenough WT: Experiential modification of the developing brain. Am Scientist 63:37–46, 1975
71. Griffith ER: Types of disability. In Rosenthal M, Griffith ER, Bond MR et al (eds): Rehabilitation of the Head Injured Adult. Philadelphia, FA Davis, 1983
72. Hackenberry LE, Miner ME, Rea GL et al: Biochemical evidence of myocardial injury after severe head trauma. Crit Care Med 10:641–644, 1982
73. Hadani M, Findler G, Shaked I et al: Unusual delayed onset of diabetes insipidus following closed head trauma. J Neurosurg 63:456–458, 1985
74. Hagen C, Malkmus D, Durham P: Levels of cognitive functioning. Downey, CA, Rancho Los Amigos Hospital, 1972
75. Hall K, Cope DN, Rappaport M: Glasgow Outcome Scale and Disability Rating Scale: Comparative usefulness in following recovery in traumatic brain injury. Arch Phys Med Rehabil 66:35–37, 1985
76. Harvey J, Strebnik H: Locomotor activity and axon regeneration following spinal cord compression in rats treated with L-thyroxin. J Neuropath Exp Neurol 26:666–668, 1967
77. Harvey SC: Hypnotics and sedatives. In Gilman AG, Goodman LS, Gilman A (eds): The Pharmacological Basis of Therapeutics, 6th ed. New York, Macmillan, 1980
78. Head Injury Rehabilitation Project: Final Report: Severe Head Trauma—Comprehensive Medical Approach, project 13-P-591569. San Jose, CA, Santa Clara Valley Medical Center, 1982
79. Heilman KM, Bowers D, Valenstein E: Emotional disorders associated with neurological diseases. In Heilman KM, Valenstein E (eds): Clinical Neuropsychology, 2nd ed. New York, Oxford University Press, 1985
80. Heilman KM, Safran A, Geschwind N: Closed head trauma and aphasia. J Neurol Neurosurg Psychiatry 34:265–269, 1971
81. Heilman KM, Watson RT, Valenstein E: Neglect and related disorders. In Heilman KM, Valenstein E (eds): Clinical Neuropsychology, 2nd ed. New York, Oxford University Press, 1985
82. Helffenstein D, Wechsler F: The use of interpersonal process recall in the remediation of interpersonal and communication skill deficits in the newly brain injured. Clin Neuropsychol 4:139–142, 1982
83. Hilbom E: Aftereffects of brain injuries. Acta Psychiatr Neurol Scand 142(suppl. 60):36–47, 1960
84. Hirsh DD, Fainstein V, Musher DM: Do condom catheters cause urinary tract infections? JAMA 242:340–341, 1979
85. Hoff JT: Cerebral protection. J Neurosurg 65:579–591, 1986
86. Jennett B, Bond MR: Assessment of outcome after severe brain damage: A practical scale. Lancet 1:480–484, 1975
87. Jennett B, Pitts L, Teasdale G et al: Fate of vegetative and severely disabled patients after severe head injury. Unpublished report, 1984
88. Jennett B, Snoek J, Bond MR, Brooks DN: Disability after severe head injury: Observations on the use of the Glasgow Outcome Scale. J Neurol Neurosurg Psychiatry 44:285–293, 1981
89. Jennett B, Teasdale G: Management of Head Injuries, pp 317–332. Philadelphia, FA Davis, 1981
90. Jennett B, Teasdale G, Braakman R et al: Prognosis in series of patients with severe head injury. Neurosurgery 4:283, 1979
91. Jick H, Dinan BJ, Hunter JR et al: Tricyclic antidepressants and convulsions. J Clin Psychopharm 3(3):182–185, 1983
92. Jones MK: Imagery as a mnemonic aid after left temporal lobectomy: Contrast between material-specific and generalized memory disorders. Neuropsychologia 12:21–30, 1974
93. Kalsbeek WD et al: The national head and spinal cord injury survey: Major findings. J Neurosurg 53:519, 1980
94. Kendall PH: The use of diazepam in hemiplegia. Ann Phys Med 7(6):225–228, 1964
95. Kishore PR, Lipper MH, Girevendulis AK et al: Post-traumatic hydrocephalus in patients with severe head injury. Neuroradiology 16:261–265, 1978
96. Klauber MR, Toutant SM, Marshall LF: A model for predicting delayed intracranial hypertension following severe head injury. J Neurosurg 61:695–699, 1984
97. Klingbell GE, Cline P: Anterior hypopituitarism: A consequence of head injury. Arch Phys Med Rehabil 66:44–46, 1985
98. Kornblum RN, Fisher RS: Pituitary lesions in craniocerebral injuries. Arch Pathol 88:242–248, 1969

99. Kosteljanetz M, Jensen TS, Norgard B et al: Sexual and hypothalamic dysfunction in postconcussional syndrome. Acta Neurol Scand 63:169–180, 1981

100. Kraus JF, Black MA, Hessol N et al: The incidence of acute brain injury and serious impairment in a defined population. Am J Epidemiol 119:186–201, 1984

101. Leigh RJ, Zee DS: The Neurology of Eye Movements. Philadelphia, FA Davis, 1983

102. Levin HS, Benton AL, Grossman RG: Neurobehavioral Consequences of Closed Head Injury. New York, Oxford University Press, 1982

103. Levin HS, Kalisky Z, Handel JF et al: Magnetic resonance imaging in relation to the sequelae and rehabilitation of diffuse closed head injury: Preliminary findings. Semin Neurol 5:221–232, 1985

104. Levin HS, O'Donnell VM, Grossman RG: The Galveston orientation and amnesia test: A practical scale to assess cognition after head injury. J Nerv Ment Dis 167:675–684, 1979

105. Lezak MD: Living with the characterologically altered brain injured patient. J Clin Psychiatry 39:592–598, 1978

106. Lezak M: Neuropsychological Assessment, 2nd ed. New York, Oxford University Press, 1983

107. Lishman WA: Brain damage in relation to psychiatric disability after head injury. Br J Psychol 114:373, 1968

108. Lishman WA: Organic Psychiatry. pp 191–261. Oxford, Blackwell Scientific Publications, 1978

109. Logemann J: Evaluation and Treatment of Swallowing Disorders. San Diego, College Hill Press, 1983

110. Lund RD, Cunningham TJ, Lund JS: Modified optic projections after unilateral eye removal in young rats. Brain Behav Evol 8:51–72, 1973

111. Luria AR: Higher Cortical Functions in Man. New York, Basic Books, 1966

112. Mack JL: Clinical assessment of disorders of attention and memory. J Head Trauma Rehabil 1(3):22–33, 1986

113. McKinlay WW, Brooks DN, Bond MR et al: The short-term outcome of severe blunt head injury as reported by relatives of the injured persons. J Neurol Neurosurg Psychiatry 44:527–533, 1981

114. McLean A, Temkin N, Dikmen S et al: The behavior sequelae of head injury. J Clin Neuropsychol 5:361–376, 1983

115. Maletzky BM: The episodic dyscontrol syndrome. Dis Nerv Syst 34:178–185, 1973

116. Mandleberg IA: Cognitive recovery after severe brain injury: III. WAIS verbal and performance IQs as a function of post-traumatic amnesia duration and time from injury. J Neurol Neurosurg Psychiatry 39:1001–1007, 1975

117. Marshall JF: Neural plasticity and recovery of function after brain injury. Int Rev Neurobiol 26:201–247, 1985

118. Marshall L, Marshall S: Current clinical head injury research in the U.S. In Becker DP, Povlishock JT (eds): Central Nervous System Research Status Report, pp 45–52. Bethesda, MD, National Institute of Neurological and Communicative Disorders and Stroke, 1985

119. Meadows JC: The anatomical basis of prosopagnosia. J Neurol Neurosurg Psychiatry 37:439–450, 1974

120. Mendelow AD, Teasdale GM: Pathophysiology of head injuries. Br J Surg 70:641–650, 1983

121. Mesulam MM: Attention, confusional states, and neglect. In Mesulam MM: Principles of Behavioral Neurology. Philadelphia, FA Davis, 1985

122. Mesulam MM et al: Acute confusional states with right middle cerebral artery infarctions. J Neurol Neurosurg Psychiatry 39:84–89, 1976

123. Metoclopramide (Reglan) for gastroesophageal reflux. Med Lett Drugs Ther 27:21–22, 1985

124. Meyer JS, Shinohara M, Kanda T et al: Diaschisis resulting from acute unilateral cerebral infarction. Arch Neurol 23:241–247, 1970

125. Miller JD: Barbiturates and raised intracranial pressure. Ann Neurol 6:189, 1979

126. Miller JD: Early evaluation and management. In Rosenthal M, Griffith ER, Bond MR, Miller JD (eds): Rehabilitation of the Head Injured Adult. Philadelphia, FA Davis, 1981

127. Mortimer JA, Pirozzolo FJ: Remote effects of head trauma. Dev Neuropsychol 1:215–229, 1985

128. Najenson T, Mendelson L, Schechter I et al: Rehabilitation after severe head injury. Scand J Rehabil Med 6:5–14, 1974

129. National Head Injury Foundation: An Educator's Manual. Framingham, MA, NHIF, 1985

130. Naute WJH: Some thoughts about thought and movement: An essay based on Hughlings Jackson's notions. In Frontiers of Neuroscience, Symposium in honor of WJH Naute, Massachusetts Institute of Technology, Cambridge, May 28, 1986

131. Nayernouri T: Post-traumatic parkinsonism. Surg Neurol 24:263–264, 1985

132. Nissen, MJ: Neuropsychology of attention and memory. J Head Trauma Rehabil 1(3):13–21, 1986

133. Oddy M, Humphrey M, Uttley D: Subjective impairment and social recovery after closed head injury. J Neurol Neurosurg Psychiatry 41:611–616, 1978

134. Penry JK, White BG, Brackett CE: A controlled study of pharmacologic prophylaxis of post-traumatic epilepsy. Neurology 29:600–601, 1979

135. Perkash I: Management of neurogenic dysfunction of the bladder and bowel. In Kottke FJ, Stillwell GK, Lehmann JF (eds): Krusen's Handbook of Physical Medicine and Rehabilitation, 3rd ed. Philadelphia, WB Saunders, 1982

136. Pinto OdeS, Polikar M, Debong G: Results of international clinical trials with Lioresal. Postgrad Med J October supplement:18–23, 1972

137. Plum F, Posner JB: The Diagnosis of Stupor and Coma, 2nd ed. Philadelphia, FA Davis, 1972

138. Posner MI, Rafal RD: Cognitive theories of attention and the rehabilitation of attentional deficits. In Meier RJ, Diller L, Benton AL (eds): Neuropsychological Rehabilitation. Guilford Press, NY, 1987

139. Povlishock JT, Becker DP, Cheng CLY et al: Axonal change in minor head injury. J Neuropath Exp Neurol 42:225–242, 1983

140. Prigatano GP: Neuropsychological Rehabilitation after Brain Injury. Baltimore, Johns Hopkins Press, 1986

141. Rappaport, M: Evoked potential and head injury in a rehabilitation setting. In Miner M, Wagner K (eds): Neurotrauma: Treatment, Rehabilitation and Related Issues, pp 189–194. Boston, Butterworths, 1986

142. Rappaport M, Hall KM, Hopkins K, Belleza T: Disability rating scale for severe head trauma: Coma to community. Arch Phys Med Rehabil 63:118–123, 1982

143. Rappaport M, Hall K, Hopkins HK et al: Evoked potentials and head injury: I. Rating of evoked potential abnormality. Clin Electroencephalogr 12:154–166, 1981

144. Rappaport M, Hopkins HK, Hall K et al: Evoked potentials after head injury: II. Clinical applications. Clin Electroencephalogr. 12:167–176, 1981

145. Riley TI: Electroencephalography in the management of epilepsy. In Browne TR, Feldman RG (eds): Epilepsy: Diagnosis and Management. Boston, Little, Brown & Co, 1983

146. Rimel RW, Giordini B, Barth JT et al: Disability caused by minor head injury. Neurosurgery 9:222–235, 1981

147. Robinson RG, Bloom FE, Battenberg ELF: A fluorescent histochemical study of changes in noradrenergic neurons following experimental cerebral infarction in the rat. Brain Res 132:259–272, 1977

148. Romney DM, Angus WR: A brief review of the effects of diazepam on memory. Psychopharm Bull 20:313–316, 1984

149. Rosenbaum M, Najenson T: Changes in life patterns and symptoms of low mood as reported by wives of severely brain injured soldiers. J Consult Clin Psychol 44:681–688, 1976

150. Rosenthal M, Kolpan K: Head injury rehabilitation: Psycholegal issues and roles for the rehabilitation psychologist. Rehabil Psychol 31:37–46, 1986

151. Rosenthal M: Strategies for family intervention. In Edelstein B, Couture E (eds): Behavioral Approaches to the Traumatically Brain Damaged. New York, Plenum Press, 1984

152. Rowe MJ III, Carlson C: Brain stem auditory evoked potentials in postconcussion dizziness. Arch Neurol 37:679–683, 1980

153. Ruff RM, Levin HS, Marshall L: Neurobehavioral methods of assessment and the study of outcome in minor head injury. J Head Trauma Rehabil 1(2):43–52, 1986

154. Russell WR: Cerebral involvement in head injury. Brain 35:549–603, 1932

155. Sarno MT: The nature of verbal impairment after closed head trauma. J Nerv Ment Dis 168:685–692, 1980

156. Sarno MT: Verbal impairment after head injury: Report of a replication study. J Nerv Ment Dis 172:475–479, 1984

157. Silberstein EB: Brain scintigraphy in the diagnosis of the sequelae of head trauma. Semin Nucl Med 13:153–167, 1983

158. Singer W, Giebler K, Feldman P et al: The cost of rehabilitating contractures. Poster presented at the third annual Houston Conference on Neurotrauma, Houston, February 25–27, 1987

159. Smith CJ: Mass action and early environment. J Comp Physiol Psychol 52:154–156, 1959

160. Solomon S, Hotchkiss E, Saravay SM et al: Impairment of memory function by antihypertensive medication. Arch Gen Psychiatry 40:1109–1112, 1983

161. Sperry RW: Chemoaffinity in the orderly growth of nerve fiber patterns and connections. Proc Natl Acad Sci 50:703–719, 1963

162. Sperry RW: Effect of crossing nerves to antagonistic limb muscles in the monkey. Arch Neurol Psychiatry 58:452–473, 1947

163. Spielman G, Gennarelli TA, Rogers CR: Disodium etidronate: Its role in preventing heterotopic ossification in severe head injury. Arch Phys Med Rehabil 64:539–542, 1983

164. Sutherland GR, Amacher AL, Sibbald WJ et al: Heart injury in head-injured adolescents. Childs Nerv Syst 1:219–222, 1985

165. Svengaardt NA, Bjorklund A, Stenevi U: Regeneration of central cholinergic neurons in the adult rat brain. Brain Res 102:1–22, 1976

166. Teasdale G, Jennett B: Assessment of coma and impaired consciousness. Lancet 2:81, 1974

167. Teasdale G, Mendelow D: Pathophysiology of head injuries. In Brooks N (ed): Closed Head Injury: Psychological, Social, and Family Consequences. Oxford, Oxford University Press, 1984

168. Thompson PJ, Trimble MR: Anticonvulsant drugs and cognitive functions. Epilepsia 23:531–544, 1982

169. Thomsen IV: Evaluation and outcome of aphasia in patients with severe closed head trauma. J Neurol Neurosurg Psychiatry 38:713–718, 1975

170. Tobis J, Pure K, Sheridan J: Rehabilitation of the severely brain injured patient. Presented at the American Congress of Rehabilitation Medicine, San Diego, California, November 1976

171. Tornheim PA, Prioleau GR, McLaurin RL: Acute response to experimental blunt head trauma: Topography of cerebral cortical edema. J Neurosurg 60:473–480, 1984

172. Trimble MR, Thompson PJ: Sodium valproate and cognitive function. Epilepsia 25(suppl 1):60–64, 1984

173. Tsukahara N: Synaptic plasticity in the red nucleus. In Cotman C (ed): Neuronal Plasticity. New York, Raven Press, 1978

174. Twomey PL, St. John JN: The neurological patient. In Rombeau JL, Caldwell MD (eds): Clinical Nutrition, vol 1, Enteral and Tube Feeding. Philadelphia, WB Saunders, 1984

175. van Zomeran AH, Brower WH, Deelman BG: Attention deficits: The riddles of selectivity, speed, and alertness. In Brooks N (ed): Closed Head Injury: Psychological, Social, and Family Consequences. Oxford, Oxford University Press, 1984

176. Vane DW, Shiffler M, Grosfeld JL et al: Reduced lower esophageal sphincter (LES) pressure after acute and chronic brain injury. J Pediatr Surg 17:960–964, 1982

177. Vauhkonen V: Suicide among the male disabled with war injuries to the brain. Acta Psychiatr Neurol Scand [Suppl] 137:90–91, 1959

178. Wahlstrom PE: Occupational therapy evaluation. In Rosenthal M, Griffith ER, Bond MR, Miller JD (eds): Rehabilitation of the Head Injured Adult. Philadelphia, FA Davis, 1983

179. Ward JD, Becker DP, Miller JD et al: Failure of prophylactic barbiturate coma in the treatment of severe head injury. J Neurosurg 62:383–388, 1985

180. Wechsler D: A standardized memory scale for clinical use. J Psychol 19:87–95, 1945

181. Weiner N: Atropine, scopolamine, and related antimuscarinic drugs. In Gilman AG, Goodman LS, Gilman A (eds): The Pharmacological Basis of Therapeutics, 6th ed. New York, Macmillan, 1980

182. Weiner N: Norepinephrine, epinephrine, and the sympathomimetic amines. In Gilman AG, Goodman LS, Gilman A (eds): The Pharmacological Basis of Therapeutics, 6th ed. New York, Macmillan, 1980

183. Weiss P, Taylor AC: Further experimental evidence against "neurotropism" in nerve regeneration. J Exp Zool 95:233–257, 1944

184. Whitman S, Coonley-Hoyanson R, Desai BT: Comparative head trauma experiences in two socioeconomically different Chicago-area communities: A population study. Am J Epidemiol 119:186–201, 1984

185. Whyte J: Automatization of a motor skill: Practice makes perfect, dissertation. University of Pennsylvania, August 1981

186. Whyte J: Mechanisms of recovery of function in the central nervous system. In Griffith ER, Rosenthal M, Bond MR et al (eds): Rehabilitation of the Child and Adult with Traumatic Brain Injury, 2nd ed. Philadelphia, FA Davis, (in press)

187. Whyte J, Wroblewski B, Tankle R et al: Clinical drug evaluation: The use of the single case double-blind placebo controlled study. Paper presented at the annual convention of the American Academy of Physical Medicine and Rehabilitation/American Congress of Rehabilitation Medicine, Orlando, FL, October 19, 1987

188. Whyte J, Glenn MB: The care and rehabilitation of the patient in a persistent vegetative state. J Head Trauma Rehabil 1(1)39–53, 1986

189. Winstein CJ: Neurogenic dysphagia: Frequency, progression, and outcome in adults following head injury. Phys Ther 63:1992–1997, 1983

190. Wood Ll: Rehabilitation of patients with disorders of attention. J Head Trauma Rehabil 1(3):43–53, 1986

191. Wood R: Behavior disorders following severe brain injury: Their presentation and psychological management. In Brooks N (ed): Closed Head Injury: Psychological, Social, and Family Consequences. Oxford, Oxford University Press, 1984

192. Young B, Rapp RP, Norton JA et al: Failure of prophylactically administered phenytoin to prevent early post-traumatic seizures. J Neurosurg 58:231–235, 1983

193. Young B, Rapp RP, Norton JA et al: Failure of prophylactically administered phenytoin to prevent late post-traumatic seizures. J Neurosurg 58:236–241, 1983

194. Young B, Ott L, Norton J et al: Metabolic and nutritional sequelae in the non-steroid treated head injury patient. Neurosurgery 17:784–791, 1985

195. Young RR, Delwaide PJ: Drug therapy: spasticity: I. N Engl J Med 304:28–33, 1981

196. Young RR, Delwaide PJ: Drug therapy: spasticity: II. N Engl J Med 304:96–99, 1981

31

Rehabilitation of the Patient With Multiple Sclerosis

Nancy D. Cobble

Carolyn Wangaard

George H. Kraft

Jack S. Burks

In multiple sclerosis (MS), discrete demyelinating lesions scattered throughout the central nervous system (CNS) cause variable combinations of motor, sensory, and coordination impairments. The course of MS, the most commonly diagnosed neurological disorder of young to middle-aged adults, ranges unpredictably from occasional mild relapses over an entire lifetime to total disability within a few months.[63, 84, 113] The uncertain course requires patients and families to make ongoing physical, emotional, social, and vocational readjustments, over a usually normal life span.

MS is the third leading cause of significant disability (after trauma and arthritis) in the 20- to 50-year age range—the period of life with greatest expectations and responsibilities. In the United States there is an incidence of at least 8,000 new cases per year. The prevalence is approximately twice that of spinal cord injury.[84, 121] In spite of the continuing or fluctuating disabilities and the uncertain future course, patients with MS can create productive, satisfying lives.[15, 96, 112] Fragmented or inaccessible medical care and psychosocial support increase the difficulties brought by the disease.[27, 170] Comprehensive rehabilitation using the team approach best provides the training, tools, and strategies to cope with the demands and changes caused by MS.[24, 158, 170]

MULTIPLE SCLEROSIS: PATHOLOGY, ETIOLOGY, AND NATURAL HISTORY

Understanding the nature, etiology, and risks of MS is fundamental for the clinician to recommend interventions, evaluate treatment effectiveness, estimate future course, and answer patients' questions.

Pathology

MS is characterized by focal inflammatory lesions scattered throughout white matter tracts of the CNS. Lesions (plaques) recur or enlarge, and new inflammatory plaques develop alongside old gliotic plaques.[73, 99]

Initial discrete points of white matter perivenular inflammation enlarge by outward extension and coalescence.[99, 185] The typical distribution and the size of plaques are shown in Figure 31-1. In active lesions, massive edema, due to blood–brain barrier damage, accompanies a marked inflammatory response. Immunocompetent lymphocytes presumably leave the circulation and enter the CNS in response to antigenic stimulation. Myelin lamellae are sequentially stripped from axons and ingested by activated macrophages. Ultimately axons are left bare, but they characteristically remain relatively well preserved even in chronic lesions.[40, 106, 168, 185, 190]

Older plaques are progressively less inflammatory, as oligodendrocytes are destroyed and astrocytes proliferate. Astrocytes lay down glial fibers and bare axons become invested by astrocytic processes. The plaque assumes a firm "sclerotic" texture.[99, 106, 147, 168, 185, 190]

Neurological dysfunction results from partial, complete, or intermittent block of nerve conduction through demyelinated areas. A nerve impulse reaching a demyelinated area is unable to continue by either saltatory or sequential conduction. Current leaks through the demyelinated segments, preventing the buildup of electrical potential sufficient to cause depolarization at the adjacent internode. The demyelinated region also cannot conduct current sequentially because the internode axon membrane lacks necessary sodium–potassium channels. Additional symptoms due to demyelination may relate to increased nerve excitability (sustained paresthesias), the inability to sustain high-frequency transmission (muscle weakness and fatigability), or ephatic cross-activation (paroxysmal symptoms).[2, 79, 102, 117, 147]

The role of neuroelectrical blocking factors remains undefined. Such factors are postulated since nerve transmission in early lesions appears to be suppressed before myelin destruction occurs. Possible factors include pressure from edema, changes in extracellular ionic composition, destructive enzymes released by inflammation, or serum neuroblocking agents entering the CNS through the damaged blood–brain barrier.[102, 117]

Recovery of function (remission) may be due to resolution of inflammation or edema pressure, removal of humeral factors, reattachment of paranodal myelin, partial remyelination, or rerouting of nerve transmission through alternative pathways. Factors that allow clinical remission seem to operate more frequently and completely in the early lesions.[40, 79, 100, 101, 102,]

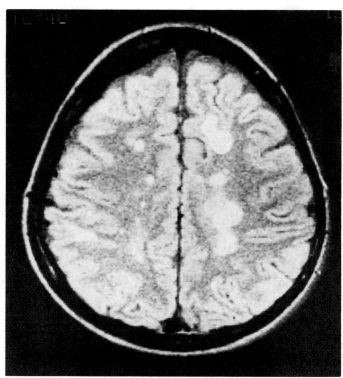

Figure 31-1. Typical pattern of multiple sclerosis lesions on cerebral magnetic resonance imaging.

Table 31-1
Characteristics of People at Risk to Develop Multiple Sclerosis

Residence before age 15 years: Temperate climate
Socioeconomic level: Higher > lower
Age: Onset 20 to 40
Racial background: White > black > Asian
Family history of MS: Siblings > parents > others
Sex: Female > male 2 : 1

(Data from Ellison GW, Visscher BR, Graves MC, Fahey JL: Multiple sclerosis. Ann Intern Med 101:514–526, 1984; Multiple sclerosis: A national survey, NIH Publication No. 84-2479. Bethesda, MD, US Department of Health and Human Services, Public Health Service, National Institutes of Health, 1984; Paty DW, Power C: Clinical symptoms and signs of multiple sclerosis: In Power CM, Paty DW, Scheinberg L et al [eds]: The Diagnosis of Multiple Sclerosis, pp 27–43. New York, Thieme-Stratton, 1984)

[117, 147, 168] In addition, some form of conduction is restored in the demyelinated CNS nerve, but the nature of conduction and the factors influencing its restoration remain unknown. Sodium–potassium channels may spread from nodal to internodal areas to allow sequential conduction, similar to unmyelinated fibers. Astrocyte proliferation and axon ensheathment may act as replacement insulation.[79, 102, 117, 147, 168]

Restored conduction is not normal. Velocities are slow (2.5% to 5% of normal), high-frequency impulse transmission cannot be maintained, and an estimated 50 to 200 times more energy is required for nerve transmission.[79, 102, 117, 147] As myelin thins, the safety factor decreases that normally enables conduction despite potentially adverse conditions. When conduction can barely occur, the smallest additional environmental insult produces a block. Environmental factors that can temporarily block a marginally functioning nerve and cause a brief aggravation of neurological symptoms include edema, relatively minor elevation of core body temperature, emotional stress, hypocalcemia, or certain chemicals.[2, 114, 117, 126, 138, 147]

Etiology

The etiology of MS is unknown, but characteristics of people at higher risk for MS have been identified (Table 31-1).[40, 121, 132] Best evidence for etiology suggests a multifactorial cascade of events; exposure to a common environmental agent triggers a dysregulated immune response in a genetically susceptible person.[6, 40, 106, 148]

An unequally distributed environmental agent is suggested by the distinct predilection of MS for temperate climates and economically developed countries.[40, 52, 106, 132] Exposure appar-

ently occurs during childhood or early adolescence since geographical risk is based on childhood residence, not on residence at the time symptoms appear. Epidemics in isolated populations are compatible with the introduction and spread of an infectious etiological agent.[35, 40, 52, 89, 106, 186]

The specific environmental agent has not yet been identified, but a viral agent is most suspected. A virus theoretically could directly alter cell functions and persist in the CNS, with intermittent reactivation, or induce a dysregulated autoimmune response and then disappear.[6, 40, 101, 106, 168] Attempts to confirm the identification or isolation of a specific virus, or to consistently transmit MS by direct inoculation techniques, have not yet succeeded.[40, 106, 148, 168, 185]

Susceptibility to MS seems to be under multigenic control. Family risk is around 10 times the general population, and increased risk is also associated with certain HLA antigens and racial backgrounds.[6, 26, 101, 106, 132, 186] However, the disease itself is not inherited since even monozygotic twins show much less than a 100% concordance rate for developing MS. It appears that environmental exposure must be coupled with genetic predisposition for MS to develop. Thus, one who is predisposed but never meets the hypothetical agent will not develop the disease, and vice versa.[6, 26, 52]

As understanding of immunity improves, evidence increasingly supports the view that MS is a virally induced, immunopathologically mediated disease, even though a specific white matter antigen has not yet been conclusively identified.[2, 6, 32, 40, 106, 148, 185, 186] Both humoral and cell-mediated immunity may be involved. In MS, a large amount of central nervous system IgG is produced by plasma cells within MS plaques. The immunological process may involve nonspecific, mitogenic stimulation of CNS plasma cells rather than response to a specific infection, since studies have demonstrated antibodies to one or more viruses, as well as many unidentified antibodies, in the cerebrospinal fluid (CSF) of MS patients. Cell-mediated immunity may also be important. T lymphocytes and macrophages within plaques appear to be involved in the primary disease process. Changes in levels of peripheral and CNS T-cell subpopulations have been tentatively correlated with acute episodes of MS. Low levels of interferon leading to poor natural killer cell function against virus-infected cells have also been demonstrated.[2, 40, 148] Finally, immunosuppressive therapies have had beneficial effects, consistent with the premise that immune mechanisms contribute to MS lesions. The true nature of the proposed immune dysregulation is controversial, but once triggered the immune response may not be appropriately regulated.[2, 6, 40, 106, 148, 185]

Natural History

Signs and Symptoms

Signs and symptoms depend on the size, intensity, and location of lesions. Individual symptoms and signs are similar to any localized CNS lesion, but the characteristic pattern of multiple, remitting/recurring, fairly symmetrical dysfunction identifies MS.[100, 139] Plaques do not follow specific nerve tracts. A few involve gray matter, but most show predilection for certain CNS white matter regions, resulting in typical impairments[99, 101, 106, 137, 168]:

- Optic nerves—optic neuritis
- Cerebrum (especially periventricular areas, frontal lobes)—cognitive, behavioral changes
- Spinal cord (especially cervical)—weakness, spasticity, numbness, bowel, bladder, and sexual dysfunctions
- Brain stem—vertigo, nystagmus, internuclear ophthalmoplegia, dysarthria, dysphagia
- Cerebellum/basal ganglia—ataxia, tremor

Common MS signs and symptoms are listed in Table 31-2. Trigeminal neuralgia of young adults and Lhermitte's sign (a transient, electric-like sensation radiating down the spine following neck flexion) are classic, but not pathognomonic, for MS.

Infrequent impairments include epilepsy, aphasia, paroxysmal attacks (brief, repetitive, stereotyped sensorimotor patterns), movement disorders, autonomic disturbance (sweating, cardiovascular),[177] and impaired hearing or taste.[100, 101, 115] In addition, some patients may embellish or exaggerate true symptoms and signs.[55, 115, 139] Detailed reviews of the neurological examination are presented elsewhere.[2, 38, 46, 76, 100, 101, 115, 121, 123, 132, 156, 163]

Course and Prognosis

MS typically follows either a relapsing-remitting or a progressive course, with several variations (Fig. 31-2).[63, 84, 101, 106, 113, 154, 155] Underlying pathological features are common to all forms of MS despite variable presentations, implying that the disease is a single pathophysiological entity.[106]

Table 31-2
Common Signs and Symptoms in Multiple Sclerosis

Motor/Cerebellar	Sexual
Weakness	Impaired erections
Spasticity	Impaired genital sensation
Incoordination	Decreased libido
Ataxia	Decreased vaginal lubrication
Dysarthria	
Dysphagia	*Visual*
	Nystagmus
Sensory	Decreased activity
Numbness/paresthesias	Extraocular muscle impairments
Pain	
Lhermitte's sign	*Cognitive/Affective*
Trigeminal neuralgia	Memory
	Attention
Bladder	Concentration
Urgency	Sequencing
Frequency	Problem solving
Incontinence	Depression
Hesitancy/retention	Emotional lability, euphoria
Bowel	*Fatigability*
Constipation	
	Heat Intolerance

The initial course for 85% of patients is relapsing-remitting. Relapses or exacerbations are new and significant recurrent neurological dysfunctions lasting more than 24 to 48 hours that reflect a disturbance of CNS white matter. Onset usually evolves over several days with progression of severity and type of symptoms. Duration lasts several weeks.[2, 17, 33, 121] During an exacerbation multiple new CNS lesions develop and existing lesions expand, but only some are clinically detectable.[73, 77, 169, 185] Remissions, with partial and sometimes complete resolution of symptoms by definition last more than 24 to 48 hours and may persist months or years. The likelihood of recovery is inversely proportional to the duration of symptoms, so that by 12 months only 10% of remissions are complete.[8, 17, 84, 113, 158, 159] The cumulative effect of exacerbating disease depends on relapse rate, severity, and degree of recovery.[17]

Progression from onset is more common in older patients. Also, most people with a remitting pattern eventually develop progressive disease as later relapses last longer and resolve less completely.[39, 102] With progression, cumulative impairment depends on type and rate of deterioration.[84, 113]

Specific prognostication for any given patient is impossible, but a poor prognosis is more accurately predicted than a favorable one.[17, 76, 84, 101, 132, 155] Guidelines indicating a probable poor or favorable course are listed in Table 31-3. Once the disease is established (3 to 5 years from diagnosis, or 10 years from symptom onset), the most recent course roughly predicts the immediate future course. Careful documentation of symptom onset and subsequent course rate gives a rough estimate of disease activity (*i.e.,* severity of impairments given the duration of disease).[84, 101, 113]

The difficulty in accurate prognostication is due in part to the lack of an independent marker of disease activity and to the discrepancy between underlying disease activity and the clinical expression of that activity.[102] Prolonged clinical inactivity is not synonymous with cure or disease "burnout" since silent lesions may be developing during times of apparent clinical remission.[32, 33, 77, 102, 106, 113, 185] In addition, acute clinical exacerbation does not always represent a new lesion. An old lesion may reach sufficient size to create new symptoms, or nerve transmission through a previously silent but marginally functioning lesion may be lost.[102]

Health care professional are usually biased by seeing only the more severely involved patients,[27, 128] but in spite of the tendency to progression MS carries a much better overall prognosis for life and activity than is generally believed.[27, 84, 106, 113, 121, 134, 157, 159]

Morbidity and Mortality

Life expectancy from onset is normal for 85% of MS patients but ranges from a few weeks to over 60 years.[17, 84, 134, 159, 171] Deaths are primarily from complications of pneumonia, renal involvement, decubiti, septicemia, or depression. Only rarely is death due directly to MS plaque causing such events as respiratory failure or intractable seizures.[113, 180]

Morbidity and hospitalizations result from complications, medication side-effects, need for special problem management, failure of long-term care resources, and neurological exacerbation/progression. No other illnesses have been shown to be specifically associated with MS.[17, 27, 113, 114, 140]

Risk Factors

Factors associated with an increased risk of onset or exacerbation of MS are controversial. Emotional stress, physical overexertion, vaccination, trauma, surgery, lumbar puncture, anesthe-

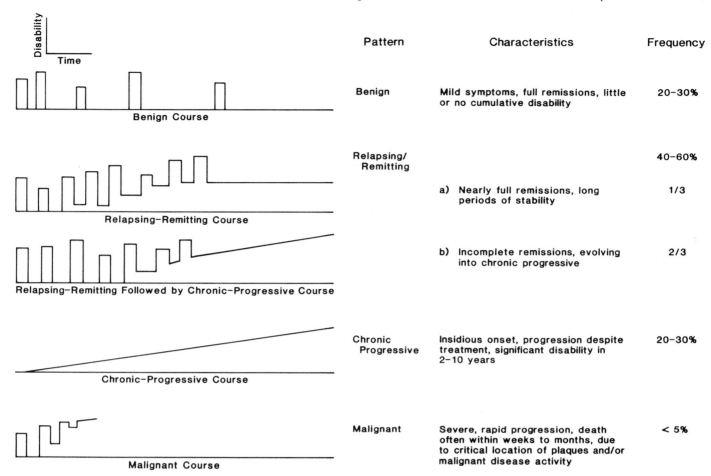

Figure 31-2. Patterns of multiple sclerosis. (Modified from Burks JS, Thompson DS: Multiple sclerosis. In Earnest M [ed]: Neurologic Emergencies, p 362. New York, Churchill Livingstone, 1983; Kraft GH, Freal JE, Coryell JK et al: Multiple sclerosis: Early prognostic guidelines. Arch Phys Med Rehabil 62:55, 1981; McAlpine D: Symptoms and signs. In McAlpine D, Lumsden CE, Acheson ED [eds]: Multiple sclerosis: A reappraisal , p 214. Edinburgh, ES Livingstone, 1972)

Table 31-3
Guidelines for Prognosis in Multiple Sclerosis

	Favorable	*Unfavorable*
Early MS		
Age at onset	Younger (<35)	Older (>35)
Symptom(s)	Monosymptomatic	Polysymptomatic
Symptom type	Optic neuritis/sensory	Early motor, cerebellar
Pattern	Sudden onset, good recovery, long remissions	Progression or frequent exacerbations
Established MS*		
Symptom type	Sensory brain stem, visual	Motor, cerebellar
Disability	Mild to moderate, ambulatory	Moderate to severe, nonambulatory

* 10 to 20 years after onset or 5 to 10 years after diagnosis
(Data from Kraft GH, Freal JE, Coryell JK et al: Multiple sclerosis: Early prognostic guidelines. Arch Phys Med Rehabil 62:54–58, 1981; McAlpine D: Multiple sclerosis: A review. Br Med J 2:292–295, 1973; Paty DW, Power C: Clinical symptoms and signs of multiple sclerosis. In Poser CM, Paty DW, Scheinberg L et al [eds]: The Diagnosis of Multiple Sclerosis, pp 27–43. New York: Thieme-Stratton, 1984)

sia, intercurrent infection, and pregnancy are some of the factors that have been investigated.[76, 114, 126, 138, 140, 166, 179, 180, 187] Retrospective studies and anecdotal reports implicate all these factors, but inherent weaknesses in study design make it difficult to draw definite conclusions. More recent prospective or controlled studies have generally demonstrated no associations between suspected risk factors and MS activity, with the possible exceptions of negative emotional stress,[48] spinal anesthesia,[51, 180, 187] the postpartum period of pregnancy,[51, 76, 141, 180] and electrical injury.[166] Also, although trauma and surgery themselves may not increase disease activity, subsequent bed rest often delays or prevents recovery to preinjury functional levels, especially in those already significantly disabled. Therefore, most authors traditionally advise caution with regard to possible risks.

The physician may be asked to provide legal expert opinion on the connection between risk factors and onset, exacerbation, or progression of MS. The apparent temporal connection between a symptom and a risk factor can be explained in several ways. Symptoms of insidious onset may remain unrecognized until after an injury or stressful event. Similarly, after a flare, people search for circumstances that might explain their relapse. Finally, as discussed previously, MS symptoms and signs are often not synonymous with new lesions but represent loss of nerve transmission through marginally functional preexisting lesions. Lacking full knowledge of the cause of MS, most authors agree that there is no evidence on which to base an opinion supporting or negating a relation between a given injury and any subsequent alteration in disability or disease course. Definite opinions must await further studies.[114, 126, 138]

STRATEGIES FOR REHABILITATION

Of the five treatment approaches to MS (Table 31-4), rehabilitation is the most effective. To develop strategies for rehabilitation, the team must appreciate both the nature of CNS damage and the impact of the special psychosocial aspects of this disease.

Special Aspects of Multiple Sclerosis Affecting Rehabilitation

Physical

In multiple sclerosis, CNS dysfunction reflects the cumulative effect of variable, incomplete, multilevel lesions causing both impaired neural output and distorted sensory input.[19, 33, 110] MS uniquely combines disorders of strength, sensation, and coordination, and no two people have exactly the same problems and course. Stability of disease is often more important for successful rehabilitation than degree of disability,[157] that is, long remissions with severe relapses may be easier to adapt to than mild relapses with short remissions.

Interacting or interdependent impairments compound the total level of disability and increase the complexity of rehabilitation. For example, minimal gait problems may arise from either mild ataxia or mild proprioceptive loss but the combination produces far greater gait difficulty. Similarly, mild urinary frequency may be fairly easily tolerated but combined with poor transfer skills it often leads to incontinence.[25, 34] Interventions helpful for one impairment may be detrimental to another. For example, resistive exercise helps disuse weakness but aggravates fatigue and spasticity, and weighting ataxic limbs dampens tremor but limits function when weakness is also present.

Functions controlled or integrated by diverse parts of the CNS such as cardiovascular autonomic regulation, cognition,

Table 31-4
Treatment Approaches to Multiple Sclerosis

Approach	Goal	Effectiveness
Prophylactic	Prevent initial shock	– –
Curative	Arrest progress	+ –
	Prevent future attacks	– –
	Shorten attacks	+ –
Restorative	Repair damaged tissue	– –
	Restore normal function	– –
Symptomatic	Prevent/relieve symptoms	+
Rehabilitative	Help patient/family adjust to disability, achieve maximal function	+ +

(From Liversedge LA: Treatment and management of multiple sclerosis. Br Med Bull 33:78–83, 1977; Scheinberg L, Holland NJ, Kirschenbaum M et al: Comprehensive long-term care of patients with multiple sclerosis. Neurology 31:1121–1123, 1981)

bladder function, speech, or swallowing are impaired by different mechanisms in different patients, depending on plaque location.[11, 34, 137, 152, 177] Therefore, unlike conditions for which functional goals can be specified once the diagnosis is established (*i.e.*, below-knee amputee, C6 spinal cord injury), outcome is less predictable for MS. Goals must be based on careful assessment and the patient's response to treatment.[24, 27, 109]

Finally, the characteristic disease fluctuation and progression require that the team provide ongoing, goal-oriented involvement of varying intensity, rather than a one-time program.[25]

Psychosocial

Certain experiences are common to MS and influence how a patient approaches treatment. MS most often develops during the productive years of life in people who are highly educated, goal directed, and otherwise generally health.[27, 78, 114, 166] A person who has been accustomed to a well-planned life suffers major disruptions and unpredictabilities.

Patients with MS differ from acutely ill or injured patients in their experience with the medical system. The diagnostic process is often prolonged (average 2 years), and stress-induced symptoms may compound disease symptoms.[27, 78, 111, 178] Patients may initially receive incorrect diagnoses or hear the message that "nothing can be done." The team must therefore help patients with anger, despair, or inappropriate expectations that have already developed.

Disease variability and unpredictability complicate adaptation. Adjustment to a clearly defined loss is usually not possible, and people often live a "borderline" existence—well at times, disabled at times, but never able to clearly identify with either.[18, 45, 60] Beyond the potential for exacerbations and remissions, patients with MS must deal with daily, or even hourly, fluctuations in function and sense of well-being due to variation in nerve transmission through completely or partially demyelinated plaques. Finally, many symptoms such as fatigability, sensory impairment, or emotional pain are invisible, resulting in inappropriate expectations and loss of credibility, from others and from themselves.[18, 45, 78, 178]

Overreaction may occur in one of two extremes. With "anticipation of disability," patients function below capacity. Conversely, they may also feel driven to attempt activities beyond true abilities. Either extreme precludes successful function. A realistic, structured rehabilitation program encourages healthier adaptation.[65, 111]

At some point, often when disabilities begin to accumulate, many patients and families are tempted to deplete health and financial resources on fad "cures." Flamboyant claims seem to provide an answer, while sober counsel to improve health practices, to await scientific proof, and to carefully weigh the risks of currently available treatments may fail to adequately touch a patient's inner desperation.[2, 97, 106, 171] A person who pursued recent unsubstantiated claims could choose, among many other options, removal of all dental fillings ("mercury burden"), potentially toxic megadoses of vitamins, or venom treatments at a serpentarium. Trust in a well-informed, easily accessible, empathetic medical team helps patients withstand the pressure to pursue unsubstantiated treatments.

Points of Intervention

Specific points of intervention can be identified for each clinical situation (Table 31-5). Every patient should receive a baseline evaluation and begin work with a comprehensive care team as early as possible. Recently diagnosed patients usually seek comprehensive care resources,[85, 111] and these should be made available, even where no major impairments exist. Early intervention sets a pattern for later successes.

In established disease any threatened or recent loss of function should be evaluated carefully for reversible components. Apparent progression may reverse with treatment of such problems as occult infection, symptoms responsive to medication, general discouragement, or loss of home support.[110]

Table 31-5
Rehabilitation Interventions for Various Clinical Situations in Multiple Sclerosis

MS	Goals
Benign	Wellness Adjustment Long-term retraining
Acute relapse	Support recovery with medical/physical interventions Follow closely during recovery phase Facilitate adjustment to new residual impairment/disability
Static residual disability	Symptomatic treatment Rehabilitate to maximal function Emphasize home programs for maintenance
Progressive disability	Rehabilitate to less than current maximal function so that function gained can be sustained over a period of time Manage reversible components that contribute to progression
Fluctuating disability	Train for best performance in a variety of situations

(From Colville PL: Rehabilitation. In Hallpike JF, Adams DWM, Tourtellotte WW [eds]: Multiple Sclerosis: Pathology, Diagnosis and Management, pp 631–654. Baltimore, Williams & Wilkins, 1983; Kraft GH, Freal JE, Coryell JK et al: Multiple sclerosis: Early prognostic guidelines. Arch Phys Med Rehabil 62:54–58, 1981; Maloney FP: Rehabilitation of the patient with multiple sclerosis. In Maloney FP, Burks JS, Ringel SP [eds]: Interdisciplinary Rehabilitation of Multiple Sclerosis and Neuromuscular Disorders, pp 75–83. Philadelphia, JB Lippincott, 1985)

Settings

Hospitalization allows intensive team treatment but is costly and relatively short term, and skills learned must be transferred to the home. The difficulties of travel, fatigue, and brief contacts generally outweigh benefits for long-term outpatient treatment,[118] but outpatient care effectively updates home programs. Homebound therapy often lacks coordinated goal setting and supervision, but new skills are learned in the setting in which they will be used.[45]

Functional Assessment

Management must be based on realistic goals determined by careful assessment of each patient's impairments and the environmental factors in his or her life that determine disabilities and handicaps. Functional assessment also provides an estimate of assistance required from family or outside resources. Reassessment evaluates intervention effectiveness and identifies new problems.[25, 54, 120]

A thorough understanding of each patient requires evaluation in each of the following areas[25, 70, 110, 120, 155]:

- Impairments (neurological examination): loss or abnormality of psychological, physiological, or anatomical function or structure
- Disability (activities of daily living): any restriction or lack (resulting from an impairment) of ability to perform an activity in the manner or range considered normal for a human
- Handicap (vocation, social, health care needs): a disadvantage for a given person resulting from an impairment or disability that limits or prevents the fulfillment of a role that is normal depending on age, sex, social, and cultural factors for that person

When assessing treatment effectiveness, the examination should account for factors that may cause symptom fluctuation: fatigue, heat, anxiety, and time of day. When assessing to plan for treatment or recommend assistance, the entire range of function for a given patient should be evaluated in various situations.[46, 118]

Many scales have been developed to evaluate specific problems or rate overall status.[8, 25, 42, 84, 110, 169] Two scales developed specifically for MS have been widely used in clinical settings. The *Kurtzke Expanded Disability Scale* rates eight separate neurological systems (pyramidal, cerebellar, brain stem, sensory, bowel and bladder, visual, mental) from normal to severely impaired. These ratings then define a single overall disability score, often used in MS literature as a quick summary of impairment. For example, Kurtzke 1 = minimal signs but no disability; 4 = severe disability but able to work full time; 6 = assisted walking; and so on. The Kurtzke scale is complicated, weighted heavily on pyramidal functions, and rather insensitive since significant clinical changes can occur without changes in ratings. Even so, the scale has been widely used since it was shown to accurately summarize other impairment evaluations in the first large multicenter treatment trial in MS.[88, 120, 150]

The *Minimal Record of Disability,* developed by the International Federation of Multiple Sclerosis Societies, is designed as a minimum but comprehensive data set that can be used in any medical setting for any culture. On this instrument impairments are rated by the Kurtzke scale. Disabilities are rated on the *Incapacity Status* (a survey based on the *Pulses Profile, Barthel Index,* and *Granger's ESCROW rating system*).[54, 120] The *Environmental Status Scale* assesses social handicaps resulting from chronic illness.[120]

For rapid screening, a simple *7-Point Mobility Scale* has been developed.[83, 84]

General Guidelines for Comprehensive Care

All areas in which patients might have problems are evaluated, including a complete review of systems and functional examination. Treating only the patient's chief complaint is insufficient. Patients rarely volunteer all information, because they believe their symptoms are not worth mentioning or cannot be treated. However, some areas that patients are least likely to mention, such as bladder problems, fatigue, or sexual dysfunction, may be most amenable to treatment.

The past course, disease activity, and current functional levels are determined to provide guidelines to initial goal selection. The clinician can help the patient prioritize what is most disruptive to life-style, what is most likely to cause future complications, and how various problems interact. Issues can then be addressed in order of importance.

A long-term relationship is based on clear, concise, honest communication in order to facilitate long-term management and patient and family adjustment. Health care professionals inform, ask, listen, share what is known and unknown, and reflect feelings as well as facts.[18, 53, 142, 155, 159, 160, 180]

Specific return appointments are scheduled for counseling, education, early detection of new problems, and becoming familiar with the patient as well as the disease course.[18, 53] Phone consultations are important to answer questions and screen new problems.

Patients are encouraged to pursue good general health practices and develop a wellness life-style. Diet should be well balanced and low in fat to maintain optimal weight and nutrition. No specific diet has been shown to affect the course of MS.[7, 118, 140, 159, 180] Exercise and rest should be balanced to avoid the complications of either inactivity or exhaustion. Exposure to colds, to flu, and to factors causing uncomfortable temporary aggravation of symptoms should be avoided. Unhealthy practices, such as smoking, should be discontinued.[33, 45, 46, 86, 180]

People with MS should be helped to become managers of their own health care. Patients are encouraged to learn about MS, to evaluate critically any proposed treatments and fads, to develop a variety of care resources, to become effective health care consumers, and to take control of their professional and personal lives.

MANAGEMENT

Medical Care

Diagnosis

Diagnosis should be reconfirmed for every patient referred to a comprehensive care setting, based on review of history, supportive laboratory evidence, and current neurological examination in order to ensure appropriate treatment and realistic planning.[27, 100, 103, 139]

Multiple sclerosis is not the only illness that can present as multiple, relapsing, or progressive symptoms. The differential diagnosis includes CNS primary or metastatic neoplasms, vascular disorders, connective tissue diseases, chronic infections, and cervical spondylopathy.[17, 76, 125, 139]

The diagnosis of MS requires the demonstration that white matter damage has occurred in multiple areas on more than one occasion (dissemination in time and space).[46, 103] No single symptom, sign, or laboratory abnormality is specific for MS. Thus, a number of schemes to define diagnostic categories have been formulated.[41, 71, 76, 103, 116, 139, 164, 167] Until recently, criteria have been based exclusively on clinical signs documenting the presence of lesions (Schumacher Committee, 1965).[164] More recently, the Poser Committee has established criteria for the inclusion of historical and laboratory evidence for patients in research studies.[71, 103, 116, 139] "Laboratory supported" evidence demonstrates CSF immunological abnormalities; "paraclinical" evidence identifies multiple sites of CNS damage.[103] Various tests useful in diagnosing MS are listed in Table 31-6.

Laboratory-supported evidence includes increased CNS IgG production and CSF oligoclonal bands in the absence of serum bands.[17] "Oligoclonal" refers to the fact that several (oligo) clones of B cells produce antibodies, each of which migrates as a discrete band on electrophoresis. CSF oligoclonal bands are present in 90% to 98% of patients with clinically definite MS but are also found in other neurological diseases of immunological or viral origin.[103, 106, 148] Other CSF findings in MS include elevated myelin basic protein representing active but nonspecific demyelination during exacerbations. Mildly increased protein or cells may also be detected, but these findings can be seen in any CNS inflammatory process.

Paraclinical evidence documenting multiple lesions is useful when only one area of the CNS shows clinical abnormalities in early, mild, or spinal cord progressive forms of MS. However, laboratory abnormalities indicate only the presence of lesions not the etiology.[106, 116] Visual, auditory, and somatosensory evoked potentials detect slow nerve conduction in various sensory axons. More than 80% of clinically definite MS patients will show slowed conduction on one or more evoked potentials.[17, 103, 106, 116, 139, 172] The blink reflex is less sensitive than evoked potentials but can be performed more quickly and economically. When positive, the blink reflex localizes lesions in the brain stem more precisely than the brain stem auditory evoked response.[75] The hot bath test uses the known heat sensitivity of many MS patients to uncover new signs and symptoms.[32] The test is cumbersome, nonstandardized, uncomfortable, possibly dangerous, and not generally recommended for diagnosis.[149]

CNS imaging also provides evidence of multiple, but nonspecific, lesions.[72, 73, 131] Computed tomography (CT scanning), especially high-volume delayed (HVD) contrast enhancement, discriminates acute lesions from old lesions. Acute enhancement probably results from blood–brain barrier breakdown during an exacerbation.[131] Magnetic resonance imaging (MRI) is approximately ten times more sensitive than CT scanning at detecting numbers of lesions. It is being evaluated as an objective marker of disease activity and response to treatment.[72, 73, 77] However, in early or mild MS, when additional evidence is most needed, MRI is frequently negative.[72, 73]

All laboratory-demonstrated abnormalities are nonspecific and must therefore be interpreted only within the appropriate clinical context[103]:

- Age: 10 to 59
- Attacks: Two separate occurrences 6 months apart or progression longer than 6 months of neurological dysfunction with clinical demonstration or past documentation by a competent examiner
- Separate lesions: Symptoms cannot be explainable on the basis of a single lesion.
- Features typical of MS: Features that derive from the known sites of white matter tract predilection
- No better explanation for the signs and symptoms

Table 31-6
Diagnostic Testing in Multiple Sclerosis

Test	Purpose	Findings
Cerebrospinal fluid analysis	Evidence of immune activation Evidence of inflammation Evidence of myelin breakdown during acute exacerbation	Increased proteins, cells Relative increase in IgG, oligoclonal bands* Myelin basic protein

Electrodiagnostic tests
  Visual evoked potential*
  Brain stem auditory evoked response
  Somatosensory evoked potential
  Blink reflex
	Demonstrate presence of clinically silent neurological lesions	Prolonged latency

Imaging
  Magnetic resonance imaging*—spinal cord or cerebral
  Computed tomography with contrast
	Demonstrate multiple lesions
	Most sensitive to variations in quantity and size of lesions in established (>3 years) MS
	Differentiates acute lesions with blood–brain barrier breakdown
		Multiple lesions
		Multiple lesions
		
		Enhancing lesions

Other tests Myelography, electroencephalography, electromyography, blood tests	Rule out other disease states	Examples include cerebrospinal fluid obstruction, peripheral nerve compression, tumor, toxins

* Greatest sensitivity.

In summary, to establish or confirm a diagnosis, the clinician should first evaluate current and documented clinical evidence, then cautiously include laboratory evidence.[59, 103, 139]

General Health

Since multiple problems occur in MS, there is a natural tendency to ascribe all new problems to MS.[7, 17] New symptoms and signs require careful evaluation to rule out other treatable general health problems such as infection, diabetes, arthritis, or peripheral nerve compression.

Acute MS Exacerbations

Not all new symptoms result from new MS lesions. Temporary aggravation of symptoms in old and previously silent lesions may be caused by fever, heat, stress, fatigue, or other medical problems, especially pulmonary or urinary tract infection, dehydration, or medication side-effects.[113, 160] Aggravating factors and other medical problems must either be identified and treated or ruled out.

Any flare of neurological symptoms, regardless of cause, can acutely decrease function and require treatment with any of the following measures in addition to medications:

1. Relative rest—defer stressful activities and resistive training programs, continue flexibility exercises, and defer emotionally stressful situations if possible.
2. Bladder drainage—use intermittent catheterization or temporary indwelling catheter if bladder is acutely flaccid or distended.
3. Bowel evacuation—use bowel program if patient is constipated or bowel is impacted.
4. Sensorimotor assistance and protection—provide passive range of motion, positioning, and skin protection.
5. Dysphagia protection—evaluate swallowing, prevent aspiration, and ensure nutrition, including temporary alternate feeding routes if necessary.
6. Vertigo and nausea from a brain stem lesion—provide bed rest, rehydration, and antiemetics.

MS Course

The goals for medical intervention in the course of MS are to improve neurological function of stable disease; decrease frequency and severity of relapses; improve recovery and shorten duration of morbidity after an acute exacerbation; and stabilize, halt, or reverse progression.[16, 118] Some research attempts to enhance conduction through demyelinated areas (goal 1),[147, 175] but most focuses on altering disease activity (goals 2 through 4).

Patients and their physicians must carefully weigh expected benefits with side-effects and costs of any proposed treatment.[3, 105, 119, 140] In 1986 dollars, a year's worth of plasmapheresis costs $11,000 and a 2-week course of cyclophosphamide costs $10,000. Progression seems to resume whether treatment is continued, and long-term risks are unknown.[39, 118, 119, 176, 180, 188, 189] For some patients and their physicians, the risks of steroids are worth the chance of shortening the duration of a relapse, even though the degree of eventual disability is unchanged. Similarly, for some, the risks of immunosuppression are worth the possibility of slowing or halting progression, even for only a few weeks or months. For others, the risks are too high and the benefits are insufficient. Given accurate information, people base their choices on personal values.

Steroids in short bursts at high doses are used for their antiinflammatory and antiedema properties to shorten the duration of acute relapses.[2, 106, 118, 155, 181] Protocols vary among physicians and have never been specifically compared in controlled studies. Intrathecal administration of steroids is specifically contraindicated because of the risk of arachnoiditis.[127] ACTH or prednisone, either alone or in combination, may be used. An example of an appropriate course would be prednisone, 100 mg/day, in a single dose for 4 days and tapered off within 2 weeks. The drug has fewer side-effects when given in the morning with elimination of table salt, replacement of potassium, and administration of antacids, if necessary.

The expected benefits of steroids are to shorten the duration of morbidity. However, residual disability is unchanged. Side-effects and risks include mood swings, fluid retention, electrolyte imbalance, gastrointestinal disturbance, insomnia, acne, or steroid dependence. Optic neuritis, brain stem, motor, and some acute pain problems, and bowel and bladder symptoms are more responsive than sensory or cerebellar dysfunction.[17, 118] Long-term use is not beneficial since risks for hypertension, osteoporosis, diabetes, or cataracts increase and disease activity resumes despite continued treatment.[40] Recently a short course of high-dose intravenous methylprednisolone (1000 mg/day with taper) has been studied experimentally for immunosuppressive effects that may more reliably stabilize disease and further shorten morbidity.[37, 40, 144]

Patients with chronic progression of gravely disabling symptoms, who are intolerant or unresponsive to steroids, may be candidates for immunosuppressive therapy under a formal experimental protocol.[51, 118, 155, 183, 188] Altering the immune system involves several risks. Since the nature of the immune dysfunction in MS is not understood, experimental treatments (γ-interferon, transfer factor, and levamisole) have sometimes aggravated signs and symptoms by causing other immune system–related problems or possibly by "turning off" the "wrong set" of lymphocytes.[104, 105, 118] In addition to acute risks (infection, nausea, liver dysfunction, gonadal suppression, or alopecia), late lymphoma, leukemia, or other malignancies may develop after years.[93] A final risk is the patient's increased psychological vulnerability. No matter how well prepared, patients always harbor some hope of miraculous cure when they submit to an extraordinary treatment.[189]

Cyclophosphamide has been used for progressive MS with short duration of severe disability. In one major study, 75% of chronic progressive patients responded to cyclophosphamide within 3 to 5 weeks and stabilized for 12 months,[61] but longer term follow-up showed that progression resumed in 1 to 3 years for most patients.[188] Booster protocols with intermittent dosing are being evaluated to determine if stabilization can be maintained.

Azathioprine for chronic or relapsing-chronic progression is under study. The major effect is expected within 2 to 4 months.

Past studies have been conflicting as to effectiveness, and malignancy is also a late risk.[2, 39, 40, 51, 118, 119, 156, 180, 183] Total lymphoid irradiation is also being evaluated as a means of immunosuppression.[28] Some recent experimental approaches to alter the course of MS are listed in Table 31-7.

In the search for a cure, researchers are trying to find the following:

1. The specific mechanism of myelin destruction.[186]
2. A valid marker of disease activity. Such a marker would identify what treatments are effective and who is at risk for aggressive disease. Clinical changes, evoked potentials, and CSF findings do not represent actual disease activity.[1, 72, 116] Magnetic resonance imaging shows promise as an anatomical marker, but a marker of immunological activity is being sought.[72, 73]
3. More specific agents or combinations of agents with lower toxicity
4. The best protocol for drug treatment.[2, 40]

In summary, current drugs and investigations point the way to new research but are not yet safe or effective cures of multiple sclerosis. Current treatment will continue to be based on "the exercise of clinical judgment when faced with a disease that can be devastating."[183]

Symptom Management

Symptoms that may be managed by medication are listed in Table 31-8. Since most symptoms respond best to interdisciplinary management of interrelated factors, detailed discussion is presented later in the chapter. As symptoms fluctuate, doses of drugs need to be readjusted. Under medical supervision, patients often learn to titrate drugs themselves for symptom control.

Rehabilitation Management

Impairments

WEAKNESS. Lower extremities are usually involved earlier and more severely than upper extremities; mobility is usually more affected than activities of daily living. Spasticity, ataxia,

---

Table 31-7
Experimental Approaches to Altering the Course of Multiple Sclerosis

Theoretical Cause	Proposed Intervention	Treatments Under Investigation
Disordered immune regulation		
Autoimmunity	Antigen block	Copolymer I
	Immune suppression	Cyclohosphamide
		Azathioprine
		Cyclosporin A
		Monoclonal antibodies
		Total lymphoid irradiation
Immune complex or demyelinating serum factors	Remove agents	Plasmapheresis
Persistent virus (causing direct damage or eliciting immune dysregulation)	Antiviral, Stimulation of natural killer cell function	Selected interferons

Table 31-8
Medications Used in Symptomatic Therapy for Multiple Sclerosis

Symptom	Drug	Usual Dosage Range	Potential Adverse Effects	Expected Benefit
Spasticity	Baclofen*	5–20 mg tid or qid	Weakness, sedation, confusion	Decrease hypertonus, improve movement
	Diazepam	2–10 mg tid or qid	Weakness, sedation, confusion	Decrease hypertonus, improve movement
	Dantolene	25–50 mg tid or qid	Weakness, liver dysfunction	Decrease hypertonus, improve movement
	Clonazepam	0.5–1 mg tid	Sedation	Decrease hypertonus, improve movement
Cerebellar incoordination	Isoniazid and pyridoxine	300 mg bid or tid 100 mg qd	Liver dysfunction	Decrease tremor amplitude Improve truncal stability
	Propranolol	10–20 mg tid or qid	Hypotension, bradycardia	Decrease tremor amplitude Improve truncal stability
Painful sensory disturbance	Carbamazepine*	200–300 mg bid to qid	Weakness, sedation, bone marrow suppression	Decrease pain
	Tricyclic anti-depressants*	25 mg bid or tid	Dry mouth, constipation, urinary hesitancy	Decrease pain
	Baclofen	5–20 mg tid or qid	Weakness, sedation, confusion	Decrease pain
	Phenytoin	300 mg qd	Sedation, confusion, gait impairment, nystagmus	Decrease pain
Paroxysmal symptoms	Carbamazepine*	200 mg bid or tid	Weakness, sedation, bone marow suppression	Suppress paroxysms
Psudobulbar palsy (paroxysmal involuntary facial expressions)	Amitriptyline*	25 mg bid or tid	Sedation, dry mouth, constipation, urinary hesitancy	Suppress expression of emotional lability
Depression	Tricyclic anti-depressants*	25–50 mg bid or tid	Sedation, dry mouth, constipation, urinary hesitancy	Improve mood Decrease insomnia
Bladder hyperactivity	Propantheline*	7.5–15 mg bid or tid	Urinary heistancy, constipation, dry mouth	Decrease bladder urgency and frequency
	Oxybutynin*	5 mg bid or tid	Urinary heistancy, constipation, dry mouth	Decrease bladder urgency and frequency
	Imipramine	100 mg qd	Urinary heistancy, constipation, dry mouth	Decrease bladder urgency and frequency
Fatigue	Amantadine*	100 mg bid	Confusion, increased spasticity	Decrease fatigue
Vertigo and nausea	Scopolamine skin patches*	1 patch q 3 days	Confusion, drowsiness, dry mouth	Suppress dizziness
	Meclizine	12.5–25 mg tid	Confusion, drowsiness, dry mouth	Suppress dizziness

* Medication of choice at Center for Neurological Diseases/Rocky Mountain Multiple Sclerosis Center, University of Colorado Health Sciences Center.
(Modified from Franklin GM, Burks JS: Diagnosis and medical management of multiple sclerosis. In Maloney FP, Burks JS, Ringel SP [eds]: Interdisciplinary Rehabilitation of Multiple Sclerosis and Neuromuscular Disorders, p 44. Philadelphia, JB Lippincott, 1985)

fatigability, and disuse deconditioning compound the problems caused by weakness. Evaluation includes repetitive functional activities, because mild weakness may only become apparent during sustained effort. For example, patients with normal strength ankle dorsiflexors on standard manual muscle testing may develop functionally limiting footdrop while walking down a long hall.

Exercise maintains general conditioning and prevents or reverses disuse atrophy but has not been proven to directly affect weakness due to the upper motor neuron lesions[33, 86, 180] since limited nerve transmission through MS lesions may not be able to generate or sustain sufficient muscle tension to produce muscle fiber hypertrophy.[2, 147] Nevertheless, exercise programs to reverse deconditioning and disuse weakness are beneficial for stable and mild to moderately impaired patients, including those with normal findings on neurological examination. A home program of resistive, aerobic, and endurance training should be specifically prescribed in terms of intensity, type, frequency, duration, and time of day so that training occurs without compromising the patient's ability to perform daily activities.[13, 45, 86] Exercise may be limited by fatigability or heat sensitivity. However, within a supervised program, patients can exercise maximally for training effect if allowed 1- to 5-minute rest intervals during the training session.[13, 25] Physical activity may be limited to cooler environments to minimize elevation of core body temperature. Exercise to the point of fatigue is not harmful, but physical activity to exhaustion can require a prolonged recovery period and may temporarily aggravate old symptoms.

Range-of-motion and functional activities should be encouraged for all patients, even those with severe disabilities. Hydrotherapy in cool water (29°C) provides the advantages of buoyancy, variable resistance, and a temperature-controlled environment.[33, 180] When weakness is severe or rapidly progressive, patients need bracing and splinting to protect weakened muscles and joints and to assist function.

Occasionally, muscle atrophy is present, suggesting lower motor neuron involvement, which presumably results from lesions of myelin extending from the cord around spinal nerve roots. Other reasons for lower motor neuron lesions, such as peripheral nerve compression, need to be ruled out.[115] Hand intrinsics and extensors may show such atrophy, and the flexor spasticity commonly combined with weakness further compromises hand function. Prolonged flexor stretching often should be added to the hand strengthening program.[192]

SPASTICITY. Spasticity ranges from a mild "catch" in passively stretched muscle to severe rigidity and can also present as painful mass spasms. Even mild spasticity can be detrimental to automatic reciprocal motion.[45] Greater degrees directly interfere with other function and aggravate fatigue since the patient moves against constant resistance. Upper extremity flexors and lower extremity extensors are preferentially affected. New or fluctuating spasticity may signal the presence of skin irritations, bladder distention, infections, fractures, fecal impaction, fatigue, or anxiety.[45, 165]

Treatment includes medication, physical interventions, and the elimination of noxious sensory input. Response to treatment varies from patient to patient and must be evaluated by functional measures. Spasticity from spinal cord lesions is more responsive to treatment than spasticity from cerebral lesions. Also, underlying weakness may be revealed if spasticity is reduced, resulting in less, not more, function.[118, 165, 173]

Baclofen, the drug of choice for both hypertonia and flexor spasms in MS, acts at the spinal cord level. Treatment should begin with small doses (5 mg daily to twice daily), with gradual increases until reaching a beneficial effect or limiting side-effect. Dosage usually ranges from 40 to 80 mg/day, although at least one center reports using much higher doses if needed.[158, 159] Limiting side-effects, especially sedation, confusion, and a feeling of weakness, are possibly related to drug action on coexisting cerebral lesions.[25, 33, 118, 165, 173] Initial sedation usually abates within a few days. The feeling of weakness may resolve if the dose can be reduced slightly. The dosage of baclofen must be tapered when discontinued since hallucinations, seizures, and rebound spasticity have been reported after sudden withdrawal.[33, 159, 173] Diazepam is usually less well tolerated, since antispastic effects are more directly proportional to sedative effects, depression may be aggravated in MS patients, or drug dependence may result. However, diazepam is sometimes useful as an adjunct to baclofen, or in patients who cannot tolerate baclofen. Dantrolene is not often recommended because of the risk of hepatotoxicity.[118, 173]

Physical measures to manage spasticity are discussed in Chapter 22. Daily stretching exercises may be sufficient treatment for minimal to moderate spasticity.[14]

More aggressive interventions can be considered when hypertonicity compromises range of motion and function. Peripheral phenol motor point nerve blocks may provide localized relief for several months.[19, 25, 33] Rarely, patients with severe, painful spasticity who have permanently lost lower extremity sensation, strength, and sphincter control, may benefit in dressing, positioning, or hygiene from intraspinal injection of alcohol or phenol, or neurosurgical interruption of the reflex arc.[33, 118, 158, 165, 173]

INCOORDINATION, ATAXIA, TREMOR, DYSMETRIA. Lesions in the cerebellum, cerebellar connections, and dorsal columns can cause or contribute to ataxic gait, head or trunk titubation, intention tremor of limbs, ataxic breathing, dysarthria, and dysphagia. Mild incoordination may be barely detectable as slight uncertainty or a minimally widened stance. Extremes of incoordination can prevent ambulation, standing, unsupported sitting, or self-care.[33, 118]

No intervention is consistently effective. Isoniazid, with monitoring of liver function, or propranolol, with monitoring of pulse and blood pressure, may be worth trials to reduce tremor amplitude. If a response occurs, it will be noticeable within 3 to 5 days; treatment should not be continued unless function improves.[8, 56, 65, 118]

Physical interventions emphasize stabilization, balance, coordination retraining, and relaxation. Weighted cuffs and mobility equipment increase stability by dampening the tremor, but use may be limited by weakness or fatigability.[13, 81, 97, 118, 192] Since the tension and effort involved in stabilization can increase tremor, techniques such as strengthening of proximal musculature or stabilizing limbs against something solid may be more effective if combined with biofeedback relaxation training. Coordination and balance retraining require precise, prolonged efforts for generally subtle gains.

SENSORY DISTURBANCE AND PAIN SYNDROMES. Sensory disturbance falls into four categories: impaired sensation, dysesthesias, chronic pain syndromes, and general musculoskeletal complaints.

Numbness in the MS patient is often difficult to document on neurological testing. Vibratory losses, although common, are usually unimportant, but proprioceptive losses can seriously limit function. With significant sensory loss, patients use visual compensation and precautionary measures to prevent injury.[2, 23, 132, 139]

Pain has long been assumed to be rare in MS but, in fact, is a not uncommon consequence of MS lesions resulting in dysesthesias, chronic pain, or mass spasms. Pain may also develop from a variety of secondary musculoskeletal complaints.[2, 23, 140]

Dysesthesias, which include numbness, tingling, itching, and hot or cold spots, range from mildly annoying to profoundly distressing. Carbamazepine, although effective, is recommended only for disabling discomfort because of risks of bone marrow suppression and side-effects of sedation or weakness. Tricyclic antidepressants, baclofen, and phenytoin are also helpful, sometimes in low doses. Corticosteroids may alleviate a variety of increased pain problems associated with acute MS exacerbation. As with other sensory symptoms, dysesthesias often resolve within several weeks or months so that often medication can be discontinued.[23, 118, 140]

Chronic diffuse pain, which fortunately is rare, is more difficult to eradicate. Chronic pain management strategies should be used along with the medications discussed above, especially tricyclic antidepressants.[23]

Musculoskeletal mechanical discomfort arises from abnormal use and positioning of weak or spastic muscles and joints and from stress-induced chronic muscle tension.[23, 173] Physiatric management improves posture and activity patterns, reduces muscle spasticity, alleviates trigger points, and suppresses pain and inflammation. Painful mass flexor spasms respond to baclofen.

VISUAL IMPAIRMENT. The blurriness, dimness, and ocular pain of acute optic neuritis respond to steroids. Visual acuity usually recovers to a large degree, but residuals of optic neuritis can include photophobia, scotoma, pain, and decreased contrast sensitivity, acuity, and color vision.[46] In addition, patients with MS often find that acuity tends to fluctuate rapidly with heat and fatigue.

Vision may also be impaired by brain stem lesions causing abnormal extraocular muscle movements. Blurred vision, disconjugate gaze, diplopia, or nystagmus results. Internuclear ophthalmoplegia (paralysis of the adducting eye at midline and nystagmus of the abducting eye) is especially common in MS and causes difficulties in focusing quickly, tracking from line to line, or blurred peripheral vision, which compromises safe driving.[123]

Visual impairments are frequently troublesome, even if mild.[15, 25] Patching one eye eliminates double vision, but depth perception is altered. Prism lenses help only when the degree of extraocular muscle weakness is stable. Reading may be easier by moving a guide from line to line. With severe visual impairment, coexisting sensorimotor impairments complicate adaptation.

BLADDER DYSFUNCTION. Bladder dysfunction results in both morbidity from urinary tract infection, fever, or upper tract damage and in significant social disability.[4, 11, 22, 66] Bladder dysfunction develops in nearly all patients and may occur at any point during the course of MS, even as a presenting symptom.[66] Patients especially at risk have other spinal cord involvement, recurrent urinary tract infections, and a greater degree of overall disability.[5, 11] However, all patients need to be specifically questioned about their bladder symptoms, toileting habits, and fluid restriction to control bladder symptoms.

Either the detrusor or sphincter may be overactive or underactive. In addition, bladder and sphincter activity may be incoordinated (bladder–sphincter dyssynergia), which usually takes the form of simultaneous sphincter–detrusor contraction. Bladder–sphincter dyssynergia may be an end-stage pattern.[4, 11, 191]

The patient may experience one of several problems:

- "Failure to store" occurs with an overactive bladder or an underactive sphincter. The symptoms are "irritative" with frequency, urgency, nocturia, and incontinence.
- "Failure to empty" occurs with an underactive bladder or an overactive sphincter. The symptoms are either "obstructive" with hesitancy, retention, and infections, or "irritative" with frequent spillover of residual urine.
- A combination of problems occurs with bladder–sphincter dyssynergia. Uninhibited bladder contractions cause frequency and urgency, but incoordinated sphincter activity prevents complete bladder emptying. Patients are most at risk for complications because of large amounts of residual urine or high pressure voiding of infected residual urine against a closed sphincter.[4, 5, 11, 66, 191]

Treatment should be based on the mechanism of dysfunction not just on the symptoms. Evaluation of bladder dysfunction is similar to other conditions (see Chap. 26).[4, 5, 11, 66] In settings where urodynamic testing is not readily available or when patients are reluctant to undergo such testing successful management is often possible using the following schema[4, 11, 64, 66, 67]:

1. Initial treatment of nonneurogenic factors. Urinary tract infection should always be adequately treated before any other testing. Constipation may cause reflex spinal cord activity to overflow to the bladder. Severe fluid restriction increases bladder wall irritability. Many medications have side-effects on bladder function. A toileting disability may lead to incontinence, even with very mild bladder dysfunction.
2. Careful history of symptoms and storage problems
3. Calculation of bladder capacity in a well-hydrated patient by measurement of residual and voided urine
4. Selection of initial bladder management directed toward the probable mechanism of dysfunction based on the above assessment
5. Evaluation of initial management. Persistent problems require formal urodynamic study.

Treatment strategies are outlined in Table 31-9 (see Chap. 26 for details).

Since bladder function is likely to change over time and may even revert to normal, each patient should be followed regularly with monitoring for residual urine, infection, and change in bladder function that may warrant a change in treatment program. Patients should learn how to recognize new symptoms and when to seek treatment.[34, 65, 66, 159, 191] Changes may also occur if overmedication with anticholinergics causes iatrogenic flaccidity or if regular intermittent catheterization relieves a chronically overdistended detrusor so that it can contract with greater force.[64] Cystoscopy is indicated for persistent urinary debris or

---

Table 31-9
Bladder Dysfunction in Multiple Sclerosis: Initial Evaluation and Management

Symptoms	Residual	Patient's Problem	Most Common Mechanism	Intervention	Follow-up
Irritative	Low	Failure to store	Overactive bladder	Anticholinergics Timed voids	Check for residual urine.
Obstructive	High	Failure to empty	Underactive (overstretched) bladder	Intermittent catherization Ascorbic acid and mandelamine	Monitor for urinary tract infection.
Mixed	High	Mixed	Bladder/sphincter dyssynergia	Anticholinergics Intermittent catheterization	Check for residual urine. Monitor for urinary tract infection.

(Data from Blaivas JG, Holland NJ, Giesser B et al: Multiple sclerosis bladder: Studies and care. Ann NY Acad Sci 436:328–346, 1984; Holland NJ, Wiesel-Levison P, Schwedelson ES: Survey of neurogenic bladder in multiple sclerosis. J Neurosurg Nurs 13:337–343, 1981)

hematuria. In dyssynergia or recurrent infections, the upper urinary tract should be evaluated regularly.[4, 11, 66, 67]

In general, an indwelling catheter is used only temporarily, with anticholinergic medication to prevent bladder spasm and hypertrophy. Indications include severe bladder overdistention, absence of a caregiver who can perform intermittent catheterization or help with toileting, presence of a decubitus ulcer, or recent surgery.[67] Surgical procedures such as urinary diversion, sphincterotomy, or destruction of bladder nerve supply are not generally needed.[11, 158]

BOWEL DYSFUNCTION. Spinal cord MS lesions cause decreased gastrointestinal motility and constipation with hard stool and incomplete evacuation. Significant contributing factors include poor dietary habits, relative physical inactivity, medication side-effects, depression, weakness of abdominal muscles, postponement of defecation due to immobility, and fluid restriction to control bladder symptoms.[94]

Essential elements of a program to promote good bowel function are sufficient dietary fiber and fluid to add bulk and consistency so that stools are more easily moved by peristalsis; bladder management to allow adequate fluid intake yet prevent overdistention bladder pressure; a habitual time of day to evacuate; and evacuation 20 to 30 minutes after a meal to make use of the gastrocolic reflex. Specific measures to overcome constipation include specifically prescribed and limited use of suppositories, laxatives, digital stimulation, or bulk supplements.[21, 34, 94, 140, 155] Each new step in a bowel program involves gradual modification of peristaltic and digestive patterns over at least 2 to 4 weeks.[34]

Patients must be encouraged to establish regular bowel habits early in MS to prevent impaction, incontinence, or laxative dependence, which are much more difficult to correct.

Diarrhea and incontinence are uncommon and are likely to be caused by gastrointestinal disease, change in diet, or drugs. Rarely MS causes hyperactive bowel function or diminished rectal sensation and tone. Persistent neurogenic incontinence can sometimes be managed by establishing regular evacuation that keeps the bowels relatively empty.[94]

SEXUAL DYSFUNCTION. Changes in sexual function, transitory or permanent, are common and can occur at any point in MS. A specific history of sexual function and satisfaction should be included at every stage of MS.[58, 182]

Sexual, bowel, and bladder dysfunctions are often associated. Men most frequently report problems in achieving or sustaining an erection or ejaculation, impaired genital sensation, fatigue, or altered desire or experience of orgasm. Women report fatigue, impaired genital sensation, changes in orgasm or desire for sex, and decreased vaginal lubrication.[51, 140, 153, 182]

Most sexual dysfunction in MS results from a combination of specific lesions affecting sexual function, general sensorimotor problems interfering with the ability to be sexually active, and psychological adjustment issues. Medications also frequently have side-effects affecting sexual desire and performance. Contributing factors include general fatigue, motor weakness, numbness, spasticity, pain, contractures, decubiti, bowel or bladder dysfunction, and cognitive impairment. Psychological responses include altered self-image, decreased sense of self-worth, increased anxiety, increased stress, and depression.[58, 78, 115, 153, 182] Evaluation of sexual function assesses the relative contributions of these components. Part of the physical examination includes an evaluation of genital sensation, sacral reflexes, pelvic muscle strength, and general autonomic functions (bowel and bladder and the ability to sweat).[58]

A simple therapeutic approach for patients with sexual dysfunction is the P-LI-SS-IT model.[58] Intervention begins when health care professionals give patients and partners permission to explore the problem and possible alternatives (P = permission), and accurate information about sexual function and satisfying options (LI = limited information). Once good communication between partners has been established so that the focus is on intimacy rather than performance, various positions and techniques can be explored (SS = specific suggestions). Associated problems are managed such as establishing good bowel and bladder programs, diminishing spasticity, or mastering new transfer skills. A water-soluble vaginal lubricant may be helpful. Some men with permanent erectile dysfunction may use a penile prosthesis. Also, sexual activity can be planned for times when fatigue is minimal.[58, 60, 111, 173] Finally, patients who do not respond to the above strategies may be referred to a sex therapist (IT = intensive therapy).[58]

A related issue is reproductive counseling. Families are concerned about the inheritance of MS, the risks of MS on pregnancy, and the risks of pregnancy on the woman with MS. Since only the susceptibility to MS is inherited, not the disease itself, the lifetime risk of developing MS is only slightly increased when a parent has MS (around 1% compared with a 0.1% risk in the general population).[153]

Multiple sclerosis does not increase the risk of congenital malformations or miscarriage. However, some medications used in MS, such as diazepam or azathioprine, do increase risk and need to be discontinued during pregnancy.[51, 153, 179] Aspects of pregnancy that may pose temporary problems are increased fatigue, incontinence, and difficulty ambulating because of a shifted center of gravity. Pregnancy has no long-term effect on disability or prognosis, but there is an increased tendency to exacerbation in the postpartum period.[51, 76, 153, 179] Families need to plan for back-up care of the infant and mother if such a postpartum flare should occur. Long-term options in case of severe progression during the child-raising years should also be considered.[53, 65, 153]

Given this information, the decision to have children is based on personal values. The presence of MS does not automatically exclude having a family.[51, 153]

DYSARTHRIA. Weakness, spasticity, ataxia, and fatigability of oral pharyngeal, laryngeal, and respiratory musculature contribute to dysarthric speech. Problems include slurred, imprecise, dysmetric, or scanning articulation; low volume; hypernasal or harsh resonance; and strained voice with inappropriate stress patterns.[34, 152] These problems occur in 20% to 25% of MS patients, but unintelligible speech occurs in only 4%.[10, 25] However, even mild impairments may cause disability in social communication. Severe speech difficulties usually occur in patients who are generally more disabled.

During exacerbation, acutely dysarthric patients should conserve energy in communicating.[34] When stable, patients can sometimes improve breath control, oral musculature strength, voice quality, and articulation with speech therapy. Articulation improves by slowing rate and emphasizing key words.[152] A palatal lift may improve voice resonance, and portable voice amplifiers help when low volume limits intelligibility.[34]

With chronic or progressive speech impairment, treatment focuses on preserving effective forms of communication. Communication aids requiring hand or head control are often limited in their effectiveness because of coexisting upper extremity or truncal/head ataxia. However, patients can learn to use short phrases, to overarticulate, and to train their listeners in active listening skills.[34, 152]

DYSPHAGIA. Dysphagia occurs in 3% to 20% of MS patients, often associated with other disabilities. Swallowing disorders are secondary to impairments of cranial nerves V, VII, IX, X, and XII, which cause spasticity, ataxia, muscle weakness, and difficulty with the timing and sequencing of oral manipulation and swallow. Spasticity and weakness of the neck flexors and respiratory and laryngeal muscles also contribute. Because lesions may affect multiple cranial nerves, various types and combinations of swallowing disorders occur. Reduction in pharyngeal peristalsis, delayed swallowing reflexes, and decreased oral, pharyngeal, or laryngeal sensitivity are most common, while reduction in lingual function and laryngeal adduction are associated with more advanced stages of MS.[34, 98, 152, 173] The evaluation and treatment of these disorders are discussed in Chapter 6. In multiple sclerosis, eating and swallowing may cause fatigue during a meal or later in the day, which can be compensated for by taking small bites, eating the largest meal early in the day, or eating several small meals throughout the day.[34, 152]

COGNITIVE/AFFECTIVE IMPAIRMENTS. Cognitive/affective and behavioral changes cause some of the most difficult problems for patients, families, and rehabilitation teams. Contrary to the historical view that mental deterioration is absent in MS, studies using neuropsychological tests detect cognitive changes in most patients with MS who have significant numbers of cerebral plaques.[55, 62, 136, 137] These findings are generally mild and isolated in relapsing-remitting MS but more frequent and significant in chronic-progressive MS.[62] Since MS can produce lesions anywhere in the cerebrum, there is no single pattern of deficit.[137] Only a small subgroup of patients (5% to 20%) show severe impairment.[27, 85, 115, 184] However, even minor changes in cognition or affect can be distressing.

In the individual patient, it is not always possible to clearly identify whether cognitive/affective changes result from organic damage or from an emotional reaction to the experience of the disease.[84, 107, 112, 137] If organicity is detected, then cognitive strengths can be used and patient, family, and team expectations for behavior, treatment, and vocation outcome can be readjusted. Behavior that is understood as organically based, not stubborn or unmotivated, is more easily tolerated. In fact, patients who have been experiencing problems often express relief at knowing that some cognitive impairment may be a possibility and that they are not "going crazy."

Impairments in cognition or affective control are due to white matter lesions in the frontal lobe cerebral association tracts resulting in "disconnection syndromes." The degree of cognitive impairment is correlated with extent and location of cerebral MS.[47] Occasionally, cognitive/affective changes can present in isolation and may progress independently from physical disability. Conversely, some patients with severe physical impairments due to spinal cord/brain stem plaques may have little, if any, cognitive loss.[62, 136, 137] Advanced frontal lobe disease manifests as apraxic gait, primitive release reflexes, pseudobulbar affect, and other typical frontal lobe signs. However, since verbal skills are relatively well preserved, significant involvement is often not immediately apparent. Family and team may note what seems to be a lack of initiative in problem solving, or the patient may report difficulties at work.

The bedside mental status examination, developed primarily for detection of gray matter lesions, is inadequate in predicting the cognitive status of MS patients.[62, 136, 137] Formal neuropsychiatric screening or full testing for subcortical cognitive dysfunction should be obtained, unless obvious cognitive impairment precludes valid testing.[49, 129] If testing services or other types of psychological evaluation are unavailable, special atten-

tion should be paid during the neurological examination to abstraction, attention, short-term memory, language, and spatial skills.[137]

Automatic, long-standing, and overlearned verbal skills are highly preserved. The functions that are most vulnerable to loss, often affecting new learning and rehabilitation efforts, occur in the following[49, 55, 62, 136, 137, 145, 146]:

- Short-term memory, especially verbal or visuomotor learning
- Abstract conceptualizations: planning, organizing, problem solving, concentration, judgment, focusing, flexibility, using feedback to modify a plan of action
- Psychomotor tasks: speed and accuracy (affected only in part by motor/sensory impairment)

Behavioral changes that may have some organic basis include impaired insight and judgment, perseverative behavior, adynamia, insensitivity to the needs and viewpoints of others, impulsiveness, and difficulty adapting to new situations.[55, 184] Affective disorders (substantial and relatively persistent disturbances of mood) include depression, irritability, emotional lability,[162] and euphoria or eutonia (inappropriate cheerfulness or sense of physical well-being out of keeping with the physical-social circumstances). Rarely, MS may cause or reveal an underlying psychosis.

Depression, possibly due to lesions involving the limbic system, is especially common and further complicates the patient's problem solving, initiative, and coping. The depression responds to tricyclics and psychotherapy.[55, 160] Studies implicate an organic rather than only a reactive basis for the depression because patients with MS have a significantly higher rate of affective disorders, including depression, than similarly disabled patients who have diseases that do not affect the cerebrum.[55, 91, 161]

Intervention for cognitive dysfunction focuses on compensatory techniques: teaching patients to use associations, rehearsal, imagery, lists, preplanning, and cuing. When impairments are severe, new stimuli and expectations are introduced in small increments. A single method is taught with extensive repetition, instead of showing the patient a variety of ways to accomplish a task. Families are helped to structure a stable environment and regular routines that allow patients to use cognitive strengths.[137, 184]

Disabilities

ADJUSTMENT. Every patient needs to deal with the fact that he or she has an incurable, potentially incapacitating disorder. Fear, anxiety, anger, and stress can be more disabling than physical impairments and can interfere with memory, problem solving, building relationships, and the ability to use help.[18, 42, 74, 85, 92, 111, 178] Healthy adjustment plays a crucial role in managing the effects of MS.

The way in which a person reacts to MS does not necessarily relate to the severity of the disease.[18] Adjustment is influenced by the disease but also by psychosocial factors: the person's internal coping skills, self-esteem, social support system, degree of other life stressors, and knowledge and attitudes about MS.[15, 30, 78, 92, 107, 111, 112] As in other chronic diseases, psychological recovery is possible even when physical recovery is not.

Adjustment to MS is a dynamic process. Patients usually attribute early symptoms to some nonserious cause and do not see themselves as sick. This perception gradually changes as symptoms return or get worse, often leading into a stressful interval of sustained apprehension and changing self-identity.

The patient may feel that something is seriously wrong, but this suspicion is not easily verified, since many of the early MS symptoms are invisible (fatigue, tingling) and physicians are often reluctant to make a tenuous early diagnosis for such a serious disease. Diagnosis is a critical point in the adjustment process, bringing relief from the unknown but introducing the stress of having an incurable, progressive disease.[60, 178] Early emotional reactions include shock, denial, anger, fear, loss of self-esteem, and some element of guilt.[15, 31, 45, 78, 92, 111] The denial phase helps patients "get used to" having MS, but, if unchallenged, leaves patients clinging to denial for years, or pinning all hope on cure so that available help is refused.

Later, in a healthy adjustment process, patients are able to acknowledge the reality of having MS, both privately and publicly, and are able to grieve over losses, express appropriate anger, and deal with anticipatory anxiety over potential disability and with the fear of being rejected or abandoned. Rehabilitation and "doing something about MS" are actively pursued. Patients rebuild self-esteem on reordered priorities and values.[15, 78, 111, 112]

Finally, successful adaptation for many patients involves the integration of MS as only a part of their lives, allowing them to move on to new personal satisfactions.[15, 112] The adjustment process can take 2 to 3 years or longer,[132] and the process recycles with subsequent exacerbations or progression.[74, 78, 107] Patients often report unmet needs in dealing with their initial reactions to the disease, but early attention to adjustment prepares for later successes.[29, 84, 85, 111]

Intervention begins with permitting and encouraging patients and families to explore the feeling and meaning side of their experiences.[65, 111, 112, 142] A realistic approach by the team assures the patient and family that the best care will be provided to keep a person functioning and to mobilize resources. Psychological help should be offered as a tool to increase coping skills not as a sign of yet one more area of dysfunction.[74] Health care knowledge is increased, and the patient is encouraged to assume personal responsibility for those aspects of wellness he or she can control. Many patients benefit from specific training in stress management techniques.[111] Antidepressants may be helpful when indicated or in combination with counseling.

Individual and group counseling helps patients and families deal with current and reactivated stresses, with excessive grief reactions, and with the development of stronger communication and coping skills. Groups especially designed for MS patients and families offer education, support, problem solving, accountability, and the benefits of shared experience. They are most effective when organized around common experiences (e.g., minimally handicapped, progressive, young families).[31, 60, 74, 91, 92, 111, 133]

By enhancing healthy adjustment, patients gain control over their responses to, and the meaning of, an otherwise largely controllable disease.[30, 31, 60, 78, 92, 111] Those who are emotionally able to deal with MS make better use of health care resources and see more options. They feel better and stay healthier.[15, 29, 74, 84, 133]

FATIGABILITY/HEAT INTOLERANCE. Fatigue in MS is distinctly different from that experienced by normal healthy adults and is probably related to the increased energy required for nerves to transmit through or around demyelinated areas.[2, 17, 50, 87] Patients with MS may experience fatigue in one or more of four ways: (1) tiredness related to time of day (usually afternoon and evening); (2) a sense of tiredness after minimal activity; (3) a sense of continuous exhaustion; and (4) fatigue (loss) of function with sustained effort, for example, footdrop after walking one block or blurry vision after reading a few minutes.[15, 50, 87, 124]

Disabling fatigue may present at any point, often prior to onset or exacerbations, and frequently limits physical function, meeting daily responsibilities, and ability to engage in intensive rehabilitation. It is a common cause of social and vocational handicaps that is easily misinterpreted by others. Return or aggravation of old symptoms may be associated with generalized fatigue.[25, 33, 50, 87, 124]

Many CNS stimulants such as pemoline, methylphenidate, amantadine, or caffeine have been tried, but none has proven to be uniformly helpful.[33, 50, 124, 158] Although the connection between fatigue and depression is unconfirmed, some clinicians report that small doses of antidepressants may help.[87, 155]

Other interventions include moderate conditioning exercise, "real" rest periods (15 to 30 minutes prior to or at the onset of fatigue), adequate regular sleep patterns, energy conservation and work simplification techniques, including handicapped parking. During a rehabilitation program, patients better tolerate several short therapy sessions with regularly scheduled rest intervals rather than a single uninterrupted 30- to 60-minute session. Patients learn to organize their time and use periods when energy is most reliably available, such as mornings or after rest periods.[13, 25, 50, 192]

Although aggravating and potentially disabling, fatigue is not in itself harmful. Total exhaustion should be avoided, since recovery can be prolonged, and there have been anecdotal reports linking exhaustion to exacerbations.[15, 33, 50, 180, 192]

Heat intolerance manifests as fatigue and transiently aggravated neurological symptoms. A patient may lose significant function during a fever, by exposure to a hot environment, or with sustained general physical activity that increases core body temperature. Air conditioning is a legitimate medical expense for these patients.[25, 86] Activity patterns need to be relocated to cooler environments with frequent breaks to avoid overheating. Pools, baths, and showers should be around 29°C, too cool for comfort for many people.[33, 86]

Both fatigability and heat intolerance have recently been acknowledged by Social Security as a cause of disability. Objective documentation is required for each patient.[151]

MOBILITY. About 70% of patients have mobility dysfunction ranging from decreased endurance of fairly normal walking to complete dependence, even for bed mobility. Weakness, spasticity, and ataxia impair mobility, complicated by fatigability, vertigo, sensory impairment, and upper extremity involvement that limits use of walking aids. Mobility problems increase in frequency and severity with patient age and duration of MS.[9, 13, 25, 34, 88, 135]

Treatment aims to improve safety, decrease energy cost, and increase endurance and rate. Gait training focuses on appropriate aids, balance, upper extremity control of assistive devices, and visual training to compensate for sensory loss.[13, 45, 135]

The subject of assistive devices for mobility is closely tied to complicated emotional issues. Sometimes a person who walks unsteadily may use a cane in order to identify himself or herself as disabled instead of as drunk. More commonly, gaiting aids are resisted as symbols of disability/dependence. Patients need help to separate emotional responses from realistic needs. The potential to improve safety, cosmesis, energy conservation, and range of activity should be emphasized.[25, 33, 45, 51]

Up to two-thirds of patients with MS continue to walk with no more than a single cane for decades after diagnosis.[121, 134] Lightweight double forearm crutches often sustain walking ability with moderate weakness and ataxia; walkers provide even more stability. Lightweight plastic bracing stabilizes paretic or mildly spastic ankles and improves toe clearance and knee control. A metal brace, although heavier, is more adjustable for controlling knee and ankle stability as changes occur over time.[13, 33] Rocker shoes occasionally help patients with a very specific combination of deficits.[135] A significant number of patients with MS depend on the assistance of another person, walls, or furniture for stability, instead of walking independently by means of aids and braces.[9] A standard wheelchair or motorized three-wheeled power scooter may be used on a part-time basis, even when the patient is still ambulatory, to expand long distance mobility and conserve energy.[13, 45, 192]

If the disease progresses, intervention shifts to trunk/sitting balance, transfers, and wheelchair mobility.[13] Special training for safety is needed at this stage since most falls occur during transfers.[25] Patients need to identify when they are capable of safe transfer (usually mornings or well rested) and when they must ask for assistance. Walking as an exercise is encouraged as long as possible, even when it is no longer functional.

Proper wheelchair prescription is essential for optimal wheelchair mobility. Special adaptations compensate for such problems as poor trunk control or lower extremity spasms.[12, 192] Light-weight sports chairs may be useful if back support is added. Power chairs are indicated for independent mobility outside the home or for very disabled patients at home who will be left alone part of the day. Cerebellar and cognitive deficits may limit the independent use of power chairs, although special controls to dampen ataxic movements can be tried.

ACTIVITIES OF DAILY LIVING. Self-care skills are usually maintained longer than general mobility but may come to consume inordinate amounts of time and energy. In evaluating activities of daily living, actual accomplishments should be verified, since patients may not be aware of full capacities and underreport or they may deny problems and overreport.[45, 95] Direct observation and home visits allow an understanding of how patients strategize and problem solve.

Rehabilitation training with appropriate techniques and equipment helps patients conserve energy and improve function, efficiency, and safety. Patients benefit from a reordering of schedules and priorities so that top-priority items are given prime time. Activities of less importance can either be deferred or delegated.[192]

Driving can present special difficulties because of problems with vision, coordination, spasticity, weakness, loss of proprioception, and changes in motor planning or perceptual skills. Adaptive equipment and training may help, but the team may have to advise against driving in some situations.

Handicaps

VOCATION. Employment usually becomes modified to fewer hours or a less strenuous position and too often is lost entirely owing to the disabilities and fears caused by MS.[8, 20, 68, 85, 111, 121, 157] Primary factors interfering with full vocation are mobility problems, incoordination of the upper extremities, bladder dysfunction, fatigue, visual losses, communication disorders, transportation difficulty, depression, anticipation of disability, and employer fears.[8, 10, 68, 82, 157]

Vocational issues need to be addressed early, since it is much easier to maintain than to resume employment.[68, 82, 85] The Vocational Rehabilitation Act has been specifically applicable to patients with multiple sclerosis since 1977.[20, 111, 157] However, vocational counselors often have little experience with MS patients and they benefit from information about both the individual patient and the disease. Patients with benign MS qualify for long-term retraining. Those with progressive disease can at least engage in short-term retraining. Patients with relapses will have some job absence and may need adjustments to residual disability on recovery.[82, 84, 96]

The team helps determine the person's ability to continue working in his or her own field or helps plan for a transfer to another occupation. The team can also help employers understand the capabilities of patients with MS and the special modifications that will make "reasonable accommodation" in accordance with federal requirements. Jobs should be accessible, task-oriented rather than time-oriented, and low stress, with flexibly scheduled rest and demand periods. The physical environment should be cool and physical demands light. Corresponding to these recommendations, most patients who remain in their original vocation are in managerial or professional positions[68, 86, 157, 192] Seventy to 75% of people with MS in the United States are unemployed; yet a significant proportion of these patients have good employability characteristics: strong educational backgrounds, normal life span, minimal cognitive involvement or pain, and generally good prognosis (60%) for only mild to moderate disability.[82, 84, 111, 140, 157]

RECREATION/FINANCES/PERSONAL RESIDENCE/PERSONAL ASSISTANCE/FAMILY ROLES. To pursue recreational activities, patients with MS should slowly build up endurance, plan for the effects of time of day and temperature, and develop awareness of their physical responses that indicate that maximum tolerable activity has been reached. Given these qualifications, most recreational endeavors, including extensive travel, are adaptable. Impairments do not have to limit interests.[7, 174]

MS is costly to patients and to society, and costs increase with degree of disability.[69, 111, 121] In one center, 36% of patients received Social Security benefits, 12% received Supplemental Security Income or welfare, and 47% were supported in whole or part by their families.[25] Early expenses center around diagnosis. Later expenses deal with medical and rehabilitative care, attendant/assistance costs, housing modifications, and lost wages.[27, 42, 69] A nationwide survey estimated that nearly half the total income for an average MS patient was lost to the disease.[121] Many are uninsured because they are unemployed. Private insurance, Medicare, and Medicaid, even when available, do not adequately meet needs for life-long chronic care.[25, 44, 69]

Not only the patient's current needs for architectural changes or equipment to improve accessibility and safety but also his or her projected future needs must be evaluated, especially when financial resources are limited.

The amount of assistance is determined so that patients and families have realistic expectations of one another. The team helps the family understand exactly what kind of help they can provide and what help may need to be supplied by resources outside the family.

Family and other strong support systems are among the most important factors for overall success, and they must also be treated and nourished.[21, 44, 45, 78, 90, 107, 111, 142, 143] The person with MS often faces a change in his or her role associated with changes in ability to work, fulfill home responsibilities, and physically "do for" others. Families feel the loss of the patient's role, while at the same time they are faced with corresponding new responsibilities and roles.[18, 44, 74, 111, 153] Even the anticipation of such changes is stressful. The family may become socially isolated by choice or necessity. Mutual activities can be lost and finances drained. In the face of chronic stress and despite good intentions, unhealthy family responses can range from smothering overprotection to neglect, abandonment, or outright cruelty.[92, 118, 143]

Intervention helps family members identify changes and new options. Children especially need help understanding the effect of MS on a parent. They need to be relieved of assumed guilt and assured of the continued presence of parental limits and love. Adolescents may have a particularly difficult time of separation.[142, 143, 180] Finally, patients need to be reminded that who they are is much more important than what they do. The ability to love, listen, and guide does not change, even when physical impairments increase. Each patient's special gift to his or her family can be to illustrate how to face adversity with hope, courage, and dignity.

Complications

Many complications are a direct result of inactivity[34, 173] compounded by spasticity, sensory loss, and weakness. The risk of decubitus ulcers, contractures, respiratory compromise, deep venous thrombosis, osteoporosis, and fracture decreases when patients follow a structured activity prescription.

Respiratory problems may develop because of weakness, spasticity, or ataxia of the respiratory muscles, with shallow or irregular breathing and ineffective cough. Rarely CNS lesions may directly impair respiratory control. Function is enhanced by reducing spasticity, deep diaphragmatic breathing, strengthening or supporting abdominal muscles, improving posture, paying attention to pulmonary hygiene, increasing fluids to keep secretions thin, and minimizing exposure to upper respiratory tract infection.[13, 152]

Adequate nutrition may be compromised by dysphagia, depression, fatigue, and impaired ability to prepare meals. Between 10% and 25% of patients lose weight, sometimes for no discernible reason. About 10% become overweight from decreased activity and increased intake of snacks and sweets.[25]

Sleep patterns are sometimes disturbed. Reversible factors include spasms, nocturia, and depression. Antidepressants may correct sleep disturbance within a few days, even in the absence of depression.

Contractures should be managed by positioning, deep heat and stretching, or surgical releases.[13, 25, 34, 86, 118, 159, 165] Lower extremity edema responds to leg elevation and small doses of mild diuretics.

COST BENEFITS

The cost of team care must be weighed against the cost of maintenance medical care without rehabilitation. Since the cost of MS increases with degree of disability,[69] measures that decrease disability and increase personal independence should decrease cost. Available studies indicate that aggressive comprehensive rehabilitation leads to improved functional skills and decreased care requirements, which can be maintained for significant periods of time. Organized comprehensive care requires only a few additional personnel when compared with standard health care and more effectively prevents complications and minimizes disabilities.[42, 43, 158] Consequently, patients and families require less home health care hours and less equipment. Even home modifications, although costly, are only about a third the cost of life-time institutionalization.[25, 27, 69] Ultimately, good comprehensive care should help patients better maintain vocation and family support.

THERAPEUTIC GOALS

Goals for patient quality of life and goals for team operations should be addressed. In addition, for effective use of time and resources, those problems likely to respond to rehabilitation must be identified. Finally, quality research should be a goal for each professional involved in treating MS, since many more answers are needed for effective care.

Patient Care

General therapeutic goals for the person with MS are enhanced function, wellness life-style, and successful adjustment characterized by a balanced use of intellectual, physical, social, and spiritual resources. The degree of impairment sets upper limits on functional improvement but not on wellness and adjustment.

Team Goals

Patient/Family Education

Patients with MS who understand their disease do better and feel more positive about themselves and their medical care.[30, 92] The educational component of comprehensive care addresses personal concerns, medical information and technical skills, adjustment skills, and life planning issues. Common patient questions are listed in Table 31-10 that can be answered by health care team, both directly and by guiding patients to references written for patients and families.[154, 156]

Most importantly, patients need to learn that having MS does not preclude a reasonably normal life. Most disabilities are either temporary or mild to moderate in severity, and all MS problems are, to some degree, manageable.[159]

Long-Term Management

Part of long-term management includes regularly scheduled rechecks for treating new symptoms, preventing predictable complications, and updating treatment programs. Follow-up

---

Table 31-10
Aspects of an Education Program for People with MS

Personal Concerns
What can I expect?
Is my life in danger?
How did I get this disease?
Can I give it to anyone else (contagious, genetics)?
Why do I have so many different symptoms?
Are there parts of me I can trust?

Medical Information
What can I do to stay healthy?
How do I evaluate treatments—established and claimed?
What medical resources can I take advantage of?
What are the benefits of an active life-style?
What are the rationales and side-effects of symptomatic treatments?
What new physical skills do I need?
When do I call my health care providers for help?

Adjustment Skills
What makes me worthwhile if I cannot do what I used to do?
How do I ask for help without becoming dependent?
How do I communicate my feelings and concerns to others?
Why should I work so hard when I may get worse anyway?
How do I cope with this disease over the next 50 years?

Realistic Life Planning
What community resources are available to me?
What kind of work can I do?
Should I have any more children?
What will I do if I become bedridden?
What will I do if I become wheelchair bound?
What will I do if I become unable to walk very far?
What will I do if I become unable to jog?
What will I do if I become nothing different than I am now?

visits allow the opportunity for checking the accuracy of the patient's past learning of both facts and skills. Regular contact builds motivation and provides both accountability and regular encouragement.[24, 25, 65]

The team also helps patients and families prepare for future options by developing the knowledge and skills necessary to assume responsibility for long-term health management. Rehabilitation then becomes one of many resources the patient has learned to use.

Disposition

The primary disposition goal for the person with MS is to continue living well in his or her usual environment. Patients with families overall achieve better adaptation and have less disabilities than those without.[142] However, some patients do live alone, while some use independent living resources.[44, 156]

Even with severe disabilities, families can keep patients within the home, given adequate physical, financial, and emotional resources. Much of the real or anticipated burden on families is relieved when patients maximize their own personal care and coping skills, when family adjustment is supported, and when financial and community resources are secured. Respite care needs to be planned and day care programs used when available. Families then function better over longer periods of time.[25, 44, 57]

Nursing home placement is more often related to family breakdown or decrease in patient cognitive function than to the degree or type of physical impairment. Three to 15% of comprehensive care setting patients enter nursing homes where special programs need to be developed for this younger-than-usual age group.[25, 27, 44, 157]

Conserving and Developing Resources

Since MS is a life-long problem with great financial impact, team members must carefully balance the cost and expected benefits of their recommendations. This is especially true if the MS has entered a phase of progressive disability, when patients and families may feel pressured to seek cure or relief at any price. Team members can help conserve and develop new resources.

Special resources for people and families with MS are listed below:

- The National Multiple Sclerosis Society. Over 150 local chapters provide various services, including educational materials, equipment, groups, and peer support (headquarters: 205 E. 42nd Street, New York, NY 10017).[20]
- State vocational rehabilitation services[82, 85, 96, 111]
- Social Security disability programs[96]
- Veterans Administration. Veterans with documented onset of symptoms within 7 years of discharge are currently eligible to be evaluated for service-connected benefits. Assistance groups, such as the Paralyzed Veterans of America, can help veterans establish a claim.

Cautious Use of Irreversible Procedures

Early in the course of MS, irreversible procedures are not appropriate because of the possibility of remission, even with severe impairment. By the time surgery can be considered for permanent impairment, patients often have multiple significant disabilities and are not good surgical candidates. The most common surgical procedures involve bladder modifications and surgical release of contractures. Other procedures that have been applied to MS problems include neurosurgical interventions for control of pain, spasticity, and tremor.[11, 118, 159, 165]

Effective Team Functioning

Part of the necessary work of the interdisciplinary team includes dealing with difficult emotional issues about the disease itself and about particular patients. In caring for patients who have MS, health care professionals set themselves against an incurable, uncertain, fluctuating, potentially devastating disease. Patients with MS are often peers of team members (i.e., young adults, well-educated, goal-oriented). Feelings of personal discomfort, frustration, inadequacy or resentment if progression continues inevitably arise.[18, 36]

Such difficult responses create stress in team members and can lead to suboptimum care unless these feelings are openly addressed. Team members often conclude that such feelings are inappropriate and mistakenly attempt to ignore the stress or adopt a common style that conceals feelings toward MS patients and families. These strategies only lead to more problems, since ignored stress does not resolve and "concealed" feelings still manifest themselves. Problems can include reduced therapeutic objectivity, unrealistic expectations for team members and for patients, making mistakes, or agreeing with inappropriate patient and family plans. In addition, patients are often aware of a "cover-up" and may feel an increased sense of isolation.

Careful attention to the issue of team response leads to better understanding of, and care for, patients. Team members sometimes mirror patients' experience in working through necessary but difficult phases of adjustment. Attending to these feelings can provide important information about a patient. For example, if a patient feels hopeless, he or she can reproduce that hopelessness in a team member by asking for help or advice, then refusing each counsel offered with a "yes, but . . ." If team members find themselves set against one another, they should be careful to evaluate the possibility that a patient with strongly ambivalent feelings (hostility but dependency) has split the team into "good guys" and "bad guys." Open, professional communication with patients provides a strong model of good adaptive skills,[36] helps patients and families acquire realistic expectations for the rehabilitation program (intervention, not cure),[42] and ensures more objective treatment by team members.

Dealing with difficult feelings requires open intrateam communication and support with a strong team leader to facilitate the process. Each team member learns to pace himself or herself, ask for support, take time to grieve when needed, and use stress management strategies.[24, 36] The team must also develop clear, realistic goals with each patient in order to identify and enjoy the successes patients do achieve.

Problems Responsive to Rehabilitation

Although the underlying mechanism for CNS damage is as yet untreatable, neurological impairments are often managed symptomatically. In addition, contributing factors that compound an impairment are frequently reversible (e.g., noxious stimuli that aggravate spasticity can be removed).

Disabilities are usually directly responsive to rehabilitation, especially general conditioning, balance, toileting, activities of daily living, transfers, wheelchair skills, and training for improved gait in those who still ambulate. Problems that should be evaluated but that have an unreliable or poor outcome include coordination, cognition/perception, and training nonambulators to become ambulatory.[24, 25, 42]

Handicaps also have great potential for improvement, but patients often report unmet needs in these areas,[85, 111] and the results of rehabilitation at this time are only described as "fair."[24, 26, 42, 157]

Rehabilitation Research Relating to MS

Research needs to determine more clearly the pathophysiology and treatment of symptoms deriving from a damaged nervous system. Rehabilitation research can also document comprehensive care effectiveness and outcome in terms of function, coping behaviors, cost-effectiveness, and treatment influence on overall disease course.[14, 42, 43, 101, 108, 111]

Trials to establish effectiveness of any treatment are extraordinarily complex[16, 105, 122] because of the unpredictability of MS and the lack of a true marker of disease activity. In addition, past studies have demonstrated a large placebo response—70% with acute relapse and 50% with chronic progressive.[150, 183]

Good research can be accomplished with strict adherence to the following guidelines.[16, 118, 122, 130] Studies on multiple sclerosis must be controlled (random, double-blind, matched for variables); occur over sufficient time to take into account the naturally occurring wide variation in course between and within patients; have adequate functional measures; and use appropriate statistics. Physiatrists and other rehabilitation specialists have the special opportunity of applying their expertise in evaluating

function to a multitude of unanswered questions about the effect of MS on people and the effect of treatment on disease.

CONCLUSIONS

Effective intervention helps patients with MS gain or sustain function, deal positively with emotional reactions, stay active, plan satisfactory life goals and options, nourish personal resources, and sustain the process of healthy adjustment despite the presence of disease or disability. The principles and benefits or rehabilitation in MS also serve as a model for rehabilitation in other neurological and chronic progressive disorders. Achievable quality of life goals for a person with MS (based on Kottke's schema for quality of life[80]) are listed in Table 31-11. The comprehensive care provided by an interdisciplinary team facilitates these achievements.

REFERENCES

1. Aminoff MJ, Davis SL, Panitch HS: Serial evoked potential studies in patients with definite multiple sclerosis. Arch Neurol 41:1197–1202, 1984
2. Arnason BG: Multiple sclerosis: Current concepts and management. Hosp Pract 17:81–89, 1982
3. Aronson SM (ed): Therapeutic Claims in Multiple Sclerosis. New York, International Federation of Multiple Sclerosis Societies, 1982
4. Augspurger RR: Bladder dysfunction in multiple sclerosis. In Maloney FP, Burks JS, Ringle SP (eds): Interdisciplinary Rehabilitation of Multiple Sclerosis and Neuromuscular Disorders, pp 48–61. Philadelphia, JB Lippincott, 1985
5. Awad SA, Gajewski JB, Sogbein SK et al: Relationship between neurological and urological status in patients with multiple sclerosis. J Urol 132:499–502, 1984
6. Batchelor JR: Immunological and genetic aspects of multiple sclerosis. In Matthews WB (ed): McAlpine's Multiple Sclerosis, pp 281–300. Edinburgh, Churchill Livingstone, 1985
7. Bauer H: A Manual on Multiple Sclerosis. Vienna, International Federation of Multiple Sclerosis Societies, 1977
8. Bauer HJ: Problems of symptomatic therapy in multiple sclerosis. Neurology 28:8–20, 1978
9. Baum HM, Rothschild BB: Multiple sclerosis and mobility restriction. Arch Phys Med Rehabil 64:591–596, 1983
10. Beukelman DR, Kraft GH, Freal J: Expressive communication disorders in persons with multiple sclerosis: A survey. Arch Phys Med Rehabil 66:675–677, 1985
11. Blaivas JG, Holland NJ, Giesser B et al: Multiple sclerosis bladder: Studies and care. Ann NY Acad Sci 436:328–346, 1984
12. Brammell CA, Maloney FP: Wheelchair prescriptions. In Maloney FP, Burks JS, Ringel SP (eds): Interdisciplinary Rehabilitation of Multiple Sclerosis and Neuromuscular Disorders, pp 364–391. Philadelphia, JB Lippincott, 1985
13. Brar SP, Wangaard C: Physical therapy for patients with multiple sclerosis. In Maloney FP, Burks JB, Ringel SP (eds): Interdisciplinary Rehabilitation of Multiple Sclerosis and Neuromuscular Disorders, pp 83–102. Philadelphia, JB Lippincott, 1985
14. Brar S, Cobble N, Smith MB et al: Evaluation of treatment protocols on minimal to moderate spasticity in multiple sclerosis. (submitted)
15. Brooks NA, Matson RR: Social-psychological adjustment to multiple sclerosis: A longitudinal study. Soc Sci Med 16:2129–2138, 1982
16. Brown JR: Problems in evaluating new treatments for multiple sclerosis. Neurology 30:8–11, 1980
17. Burks JS, Thompson DS: Multiple sclerosis. In Earnest M (ed): Neurologic Emergencies, pp 361–385. New York, Churchill Livingstone, 1983
18. Burnfield A: Doctor–patient dilemmas in multiple sclerosis. J Med Ethics 1:21–26, 1984
19. Caillet R: Exercise in multiple sclerosis. In Basmajian JV (ed): Therapeutic Exercise, pp 375–388. Baltimore, Williams & Wilkins, 1978

Table 31-11
Goals for Improved Quality of Life

Psychophysiological Equilibrium
Understanding of the disease, the symptoms, and how to manage them
Understanding of limitations and strengths; functioning up to but respecting limits
Maintenance of function with minimum effort and maximum safety (balancing rest and activity appropriately)
Functional improvement in spite of persistent neurological signs
Return to pre-exacerbation physical status
Altering environment to support independence, diminish disability
Wellness life-style
Mastery over potential uncertainty and loss of control

Interrelatedness
Realistic expectations for patient and family
Preservation of family unit
Learning new ways to fulfill family/friendship roles
Knowing and practicing how to be realistically independent (not being a burden) but also being able to communicate when and how help is needed
Avoiding social isolation
Knowing and appropriately using community resources

Productivity
Developing alternative plans to already establised vocational goals (job, education, other training)
Establishing a productive life (paid or volunteer)

Creativity
Developing problem-solving skills
Developing avocational interests
Reaching important life goals; focusing on remaining possibilities
Developing an enjoyable, personally meaningful life (MS not being the focus of one's life)

(Modified from Cobble ND, Burks JS: The team approach to the management of multiple sclerosis. In Maloney FP et al [eds]: Interdisciplinary Rehabilitation of Multiple Sclerosis and Neuromuscular Disorders. Philadelphia, JB Lippincott, 1985)

20. Campbell NO: The social service worker and the neuromuscular disease patient: A partnership in problem solving. In Maloney FP, Burks JS, Ringel SP (eds): Interdisciplinary Rehabilitation of Multiple Sclerosis and Neuromuscular Disorders, pp 392–401. Philadelphia, JB Lippincott, 1985

21. Catanzaro M: MS, nursing care of the person with MS. Am J Nurs 2:286–291, 1980

22. Catanzaro M, O'Shaughnessy EJ, Clowers FC, Brooks G: Urinary bladder dysfunction as a remedial disability in multiple sclerosis: A sociologic perspective. Arch Phys Med Rehabil 63:472–474, 1982

23. Clifford DB, Trotter JL: Pain in multiple sclerosis. Arch Neurol 41:1270–1272, 1984

24. Cobble ND, Burks JS: The team approach to the management of multiple sclerosis. In Maloney FP, Burks JS, Ringel SP (eds): Interdisciplinary Rehabilitation of Multiple Sclerosis and Neuromuscular Disorders, pp 11–31. Philadelphia, JB Lippincott, 1985

25. Colville PL: Rehabilitation. In Hallpike JF, Adams DWM, Tourtellotte WW (eds): Multiple Sclerosis: Pathology, Diagnosis and Management, pp 631–654. Baltimore, Williams & Wilkins, 1983

26. Compston A: Genetic factors in the aetiology of multiple sclerosis. In McDonald WI, Silberberg DH (eds): Multiple Sclerosis, pp 56–73. London, Butterworths, 1986

27. Conomy JP, Bhasin C, Fisher J et al: The experience of the Mellen Center for Multiple Sclerosis Treatment and Research at the Cleveland Clinic Foundation. Multiple Sclerosis Symposium: Scientific Advances and Interdisciplinary Care, March 1986

28. Cook S, Devereux C, Troiano R et al: Effect of total lymphoid irradiation in chronic progressive multiple sclerosis. Lancet 1:1405–1409, 1986

29. Coryell JK, Barash N, Kraft GH: Psychosocial intervention with recently diagnosed multiple sclerosis patients (abstr). Arch Phys Med Rehabil 62:532, 1981

30. Counte MA, Bieliauakas LA, Pavlou M: Stress and personal attitudes in chronic illness. Arch Phys Med Rehabil 64:272–275, 1983

31. Crawford JD, McIvor GP: Group psychotherapy: Benefits in multiple sclerosis. Arch Phys Med Rehabil 66:810–813, 1985

32. Davis FA: The hot bath test in multiple sclerosis. IN Poser CM, Paty DW, Scheinberg L et al: The Diagnosis of Multiple Sclerosis, pp 44–48. New York, Thieme-Stratton, 1984

33. Delisa JA, Miller RM, Mikulic MA, Hammond MC: Multiple sclerosis: Common physical disabilities and rehabilitation. Am Fam Physician 32(4):157–163, 1985

34. Delisa JA, Miller RM, Mikulic MA, Hammond MC: Multiple sclerosis: II. Common functional problems and rehabilitation. Am Fam Physician 32(5):127–132, 1985

35. Detles R, Visscher BR, Haile RW et al: Multiple sclerosis and age at migration. Am J Epidemiol 108:386–393, 1978

36. Dubovsky SL: Therapist–patient relationship in chronic care of the disabled patient. In Maloney FP, Burks JS, Ringel SP (eds): Interdisciplinary Rehabilitation of Multiple Sclerosis and Neuromuscular Disorders, pp 355–363. Philadelphia, JB Lippincott, 1985

37. Durelli L, Cocito D, Riccio A et al: High-dose intravenous methylprednisolone in the treatment of multiple sclerosis: Clinical-immunologic correlations. Neurology 36:238–243, 1986

38. Ellenberger C (Jr), Daroff RB: Neuro-ophthalmic aspects of multiple sclerosis. In Poser CM, Paty DW, Scheinberg L et al (eds): The Diagnosis of Multiple Sclerosis, pp 49–63. New York, Thieme-Stratton, 1984

39. Ellison GW: Treatment aimed at modifying the course of multiple sclerosis. In McDonald WI, Silberberg DH (eds): Multiple Sclerosis, pp 153–165. London, Butterworths, 1986

40. Ellison GW, Visscher BR, Graves MC, Fahey JL: Multiple sclerosis. Ann Intern Med 101:514–526, 1984

41. Farlow MR, Marhand ON, Edwards MK et al: Multiple sclerosis: Magnetic resonance imaging, evoked responses, and spinal fluid electrophoresis. Neurology 36:828–831, 1986

42. Feigenson JS, Scheinberg L, Catalano M et al: The cost-effectiveness of multiple sclerosis rehabilitation: A model. Neurology 31:1316–1322, 1981

43. Francabandera F, Reding M, LaRocca N et al: Rehabilitation options in multiple sclerosis (abstr). Neurology 36:187, 1986

44. Frankel D: Long-term care issues in multiple sclerosis. Rehabil Lit 45:282–285, 1984

45. Frankel D: Multiple sclerosis. In Umphred DA (ed): Neurological Rehabilitation, vol 3, pp 398–415. St. Louis, CV Mosby, 1985

46. Franklin GM, Burks JS: Diagnosis and medical management of multiple Sclerosis. In Maloney FP, Burks JS, Ringel SP (eds): Interdisciplinary Rehabilitation of Multiple Sclerosis and Neuromuscular Disorders, pp 32–47. Philadelphia, JB Lippincott, 1985

47. Franklin GM, Heaton RK, Filley CM et al: Correlation of neuropsychological and magnetic resonance imaging (MRI) findings in chronic/progressive multiple sclerosis (abstr). Neurology 36:185, 1986

48. Franklin GM, Nelson LM, Heaton RK et al: Stress and its relationship to acute exacerbation in multiple sclerosis (MS). (accepted for publication in the Journal of Neurorehabilitation)

49. Franklin GM, Nelson LM, Filley CM, Heaton RK: Early subcortical dementia in multiple sclerosis—case reports and application of a neuropsychological screening battery. (in preparation)

50. Freal JE, Kraft GH, Coryell JK: Symptomatic fatigue in multiple sclerosis. Arch Phys Med Rehabil 65:135–138, 1984

51. Giesser BS, Holland NJ, Scheinberg LC: Multiple sclerosis. Female Patient 8:4–18, 1983

52. Gonzales-Scarano F, Spielman RS, Nathanson N: Epidemiology. In McDonald WI, Silberberg DH (eds): Multiple Sclerosis, pp 37–55. London, Butterworths, 1986

53. Gorman E, Rudd A, Ebers G: Giving the diagnosis of multiple sclerosis. In Poser CM, Paty DW, Scheinberg L et al: The Diagnosis of Multiple Sclerosis, pp 216–222. New York, Thieme-Stratton, 1984

54. Granger CV: Health accounting—functional assessment of the long-term patient. In Kottke FJ, Stillwell GK, Lehman JF (eds): Krusen's Handbook of Physical Medicine and Rehabilitation, 3rd ed, pp 253–274. Philadelphia, WB Saunders, 1982

55. Grant I: Neuropsychological and psychiatric disturbances in multiple sclerosis. In McDonald WI, Silberberg DH (eds): Multiple Sclerosis, pp 134–152. London, Butterworths, 1986

56. Hallet M, Lindsey JW, Adelstein BD, Riley PO: Controlled trial of isoniazid therapy for severe postural cerebellar tremor in multiple sclerosis. Neurology 35:1374–1377, 1985

57. Halper J, Ressler N, Zdinak A: Respite care and multiple sclerosis. MS Q Rep 5:36–37, 1986

58. Halstead LS: Sexuality and disability. In Halstead LS, Grabois M, Howland LA (eds): Medical Rehabilitation, pp 325–333. New York, Raven Press, 1985

59. Hart RG, Sherman DG: The diagnosis of multiple sclerosis. JAMA 247:498–503, 1982

60. Hartings MF, Pavlou MM, Davis FA: Group counseling of MS patients in a program of comprehensive care. J Chronic Dis 29:65–73, 1976

61. Hauser SL, Dawson DM, Lehrich JR et al: Intensive immunosuppression in progressive multiple sclerosis. N Engl J Med 308:173–180, 1983

62. Heaton RK, Nelson LM, Thompsom DS et al: Neuropsychological findings in relapsing-remitting and chronic-progressive multiple sclerosis. J Consult Clin Psychol 53:103–110, 1985

63. Herndon RM, Rudick RA: Multiple sclerosis, the spectrum of severity. Arch Neurol 40:531–532, 1983

64. Holland N: Intermittent catheterization—application in multiple sclerosis. J Am Urol Assoc Allied 2:5–8, 1982

65. Holland NJ, McDonnell M, Wiesel-Levison P: Overview of multiple sclerosis and nursing care of the MS patient. J Neurosurg Nurs 13:28–33, 1982

66. Holland NJ, Wiesel-Levison P, Schwedelson ES: Survey of neurogenic bladder in multiple sclerosis. J Neurosurg Nurs 13:337–343, 1981

67. Holland NJ, Abransom AS: Bladder and bowel management. In Scheinberg LC (ed): Multiple Sclerosis, A Guide for Patients and Their Families, pp 129–153. New York, Raven Press, 1983

68. Holland NJ, Sprinzeles L, Kaplan SR: Vocational issues. In Scheinberg L (ed): Multiple Sclerosis, Guide for Patients and Their Families, pp 209–216. New York, Raven Press, 1983

69. Inman RP: Disability indices, the economic costs of illness, and social insurance: The case of multiple sclerosis. Acta Neurol Scand 101:46–55, 1984

70. International Classification of Impairments, Disabilities, and Handicaps. Geneva, World Health Organization, 1980

71. Izquerdo G, Hauw J, Lyon-Caen O et al: Value of multiple sclerosis

diagnostic criteria: 70 autopsy confirmed cases. Arch Neurol 42:848–850, 1985

72. Jacobs L, Kinkel WR, Polachini I, Kinkel RP: Correlations of nuclear magnetic resonance imaging, computerized tomography, and clinical profiles in multiple sclerosis. Neurology 36:27–34, 1986

73. Johnson MA, Li DKB, Bryant DJ, Payne JA: Magnetic resonance imaging: Serial observation in multiple sclerosis. AJNR 5:495–499, 1984

74. Kalb R: Psychological counseling and the MS person. MS Q Rep 3:29–31, 1984

75. Kayamori R, Dickens S, Yamada T, Kimura J: Brainstem auditory evoked potential and blink reflex in multiple sclerosis. Neurology 34:1318–1323, 1984

76. Kelly R: Clinical aspects of multiple sclerosis. In Vinken PJ, Bruyn GW, Klawans HL, Koetsier JC (eds): Handbook of Clinical Neurology, vol 47, Demyelinating Diseases, pp 49–78. Amsterdam, Elsevier Science Publishers, 1985

77. Kirschner HS, Tsai SI, Runge M, Price AC: Magnetic resonance imaging and other techniques in the diagnosis of multiple sclerosis. Arch Neurol 42:859–863, 1985

78. Knutson LL: Understanding and managing the psychosocial aspects of multiple sclerosis. In Maloney FP, Burks JS, Ringel SP (eds): Interdisciplinary Rehabilitation of Multiple Sclerosis and Neuromuscular Disorders, pp 157–167. Philadelphia, JB Lippincott, 1985

79. Kocsis JD, Waxman SG: Demyelination: Causes and mechanisms of clinical abnormality and functional recovery. In Vinken PJ, Bruyn GW, Klawans HL, Koetsier JC (eds): Handbook of Clinical Neurology, vol 47, Demyelinating Diseases, pp 29–47. Amsterdam, Elsevier Science Publishers, 1985

80. Kottke FJ: Philosophic considerations of quality of life for the disabled. Arch Phys Med Rehabil 63:60–62, 1982

81. Kraft GH: Movement disorders. In Basmajian JV, Kirby L (eds): Medical Rehabilitation, pp 19–33. Baltimore, Williams & Wilkins, 1984

82. Kraft GH, Coryell JK, Freal JE et al: Multiple Sclerosis: A Handbook for Rehabilitation Counselors with Emphasis on Prognostic Guidelines. Seattle, University of Washington, 1979

83. Kraft GH, Freal JE: Disability ratings in development of prognostic indicators. Acta Neurol Scand 64:80–81, 1981

84. Kraft GH, Freal JE, Coryell JK et al: Multiple sclerosis: Early prognostic guidelines. Arch Phys Med Rehabil 62:54–58, 1981

85. Kraft GH, Freal JE, Coryell JK: Disability, disease duration, and rehabilitation service needs in multiple sclerosis: Patient perspectives. Arch Phys Med Rehabil 67:164–168, 1986

86. Krebs MA: Degenerative disorders of the central nervous system. In Halsted LS, Grabois M, Howland CA (eds): Medical Rehabilitation, pp 251–263. New York, Raven Press, 1985

87. Krupp LB, Alvarez LA, LaRocca NG, Scheinberg LC: Clinical characteristics of fatigue in multiple sclerosis (abstr). Neurology 36:200, 1986

88. Kurtzke JF: Rating neurologic impairment in multiple sclerosis: An expanded disability status scale (EDSS). Neurology 33:1444–1452, 1983

89. Kurtzke JF: Epidemiology of multiple sclerosis. In Vinken PJ, Bruyn GW, Klawans HL, Koetsier JC (eds): Handbook of Clinical Neurology, vol 47, Demyelinating Diseases, pp 259–288. Amsterdam, Elsevier Science Publishers, 1985

90. Lambert G: Patients with progressive neurological disease. In Power PW, Del Orto AE (eds): Role of the Family in the Rehabilitation of the Physically Disabled, pp 264–271. Baltimore, University Park Press, 1980

91. Larcombe NA, Wilson PH: An evaluation of cognitive-behavior therapy for depression in patients with multiple sclerosis. Br J Psychiatry 145:366–371, 1984

92. LaRocca NG: Psychosocial factors in multiple sclerosis and the role of stress. Ann NY Acad Sci 436:435–442, 1984

93. Lhermitte F, Marteau R, Roullet E: Letter: Not so benign long-term immunosuppression in multiple sclerosis? Lancet 1:276–277, 1984

94. Levine JS: Bowel dysfunction in multiple sclerosis. In Maloney FP, Burks JS, Ringel SP (eds): Interdisciplinary Rehabilitation of Multiple Sclerosis and Neuromuscular Disorders, pp 62–74. Philadelphia, JB Lippincott, 1985

95. Lincoln NB: Discrepancies between capabilities and performance of activities of daily living in multiple sclerosis patients. Int Rehab Med 3:84–88, 1981

96. Litvin ME: Vocational rehabilitation and social security disability programs. In Maloney FP, Burks JS, Ringel SP (eds): Interdisciplinary Rehabilitation of Multiple Sclerosis and Neuromuscular Disorders, pp 413–425. Philadelphia, JB Lippincott, 1985

97. Liversedge LA: Treatment and management of multiple sclerosis. Br Med Bull 33:78–83, 1977

98. Logemann J: Evaluation and Treatment of Swallowing Disorders. San Diego, College-Hill Press, 1983

99. Lumsden CE: The neuropathology of multiple sclerosis. In Vinken PJ, Bruyn GW (eds): Handbook of Clinical Neurology, vol 9, Multiple Sclerosis and Other Demyelinating Diseases, pp 132–189. Amsterdam, North-Holland Publishing, 1970

100. McAlpine D: Symptoms and signs. In McAlpine D, Lumsden CE, Acheson ED (eds): Multiple sclerosis: A reappraisal, pp 132–189. Edinburgh, ES Livingstone, 1972

101 McAlpine D: Multiple sclerosis: A review. Br Med J 2:292–295, 1973

102. McDonald WI: The pathophysiology of multiple sclerosis. In McDonald WI, Silberberg DH (eds): Multiple Sclerosis; pp 112–133. London, Butterworths, 1986

103 McDonald WI, Silberberg DH: The diagnosis of multiple sclerosis. In McDonald WI, Silberberg DH (eds): Multiple Sclerosis, pp 1–10. London, Butterworths, 1986

104. McFarlin DE: Use of interferon in multiple sclerosis. Ann Neurol 18:432–433, 1985

105. McFarlin DE: Treatment of multiple sclerosis. N Engl J Med 308:215–217, 1983

106. McFarlin DE, McFarland HF: Multiple sclerosis. N Engl J Med 307:1183–1188, 1246–1251, 1982

107. McIvor GP, Riklan M, Reznikoff M: Depression in multiple sclerosis as a function of length and severity of illness, age, remission, and perceived social support. J Clin Psychol 40:1028–1033, 1984

108. Madonna MG, Holland NJ, Wiesel-Levison P: The value of physical therapy in improving gait in multiple sclerosis: A research design. Rehabil Nurs 10(5):32–34, 1985

109. Maloney FP: Rehabilitation of patients with progressive and remitting disorders. In Maloney FP, Burks JS, Ringel SP (eds): Interdisciplinary Rehabilitation of Multiple Sclerosis and Neuromuscular Disorders, pp 3–8. Philadelphia, JB Lippincott, 1985

110. Maloney FP: Rehabilitation of the patient with multiple sclerosis. In Maloney FP, Burks JS, Ringel SP (eds): Interdisciplinary Rehabilitation of Multiple Sclerosis and Neuromuscular Disorders, pp 75–83. Philadelphia, JB Lippincott, 1985

111. Marsh GG, Ellison GW, Strite C: Psychosocial and vocational rehabilitation approaches to multiple sclerosis. In Pan EL, Bacher TE, Vash CL (eds): Annual Review of Rehabilitation, vol 3, pp 242–267. New York, Springer, 1983

112. Matson RR, Brooks NA: Adjusting to multiple sclerosis: An exploratory study. Soc Sci Med 11:245–250, 1977

113. Matthews WB: Course and prognosis. In Matthews WB (ed): McAlpine's Multiple Sclerosis, pp 49–72. Edinburgh, Churchill Livingstone, 1985

114. Matthews WB: Some aspects of the natural history. In Matthews WB (ed): McAlpine's Multiple Sclerosis, pp 73–95. Edinburgh, Churchill Livingstone, 1985

115. Matthews WB: Symptoms and signs. In Matthews WB (ed): McAlpine's Multiple Sclerosis, pp 96–145. Edinburgh, Churchill Livingstone, 1985

116. Matthews WB: Laboratory diagnosis. In Matthews WB (ed): McAlpine's Multiple Sclerosis, pp 167–209. Edinburgh, Churchill Livingstone, 1985

117. Matthews WB: Patholphysiology. In Matthews WB (ed): McAlpine's Multiple Sclerosis, pp 210–232. Edinburgh, Churchill Livingstone, 1985

118. Matthews WB: Treatment. In Matthews WB (ed): McAlpine's Multiple Sclerosis, pp 233–278. Edinburgh, Churchill Livingstone, 1985

119. Mertin J: Drug treatment of patients with multiple sclerosis. In Vinken PJ, Bruyn GW, Klawans HL, Koetsier JC (eds): Handbook of Clinical Neurology, vol 47, Demyelinating Diseases, pp 187–212. Amsterdam, Elsevier Science Publishers, 1985

120. M.R.D.: Minimal record of disability for multiple sclerosis. New York, National Multiple Sclerosis Society, 1985

121. Multiple Sclerosis: A National Survey, NIH publication No. 84-2479. Bethesda, MD, US Department of Health and Human Services, Public Health Service, National Institutes of Health. 1984

122. Multiple sclerosis—special issue: Proceedings of the international conference on therapeutic trials in multiple sclerosis. Arch Neurol 40(11), 1983

123. Muri RM, Meienberg O: Clinical spectrum of internuclear ophthalmoplegia in multiple sclerosis. Arch Neurol 42:851–855, 1985

124. Murray TJ: Amantadine therapy for fatigue in multiple sclerosis. Can J Neurol Sci 12:251–254, 1985

125. Murray TJ, Murray SJ: Characteristics of patients found not to have multiple sclerosis. Can Med Assoc J 131:336–337, 1984

126. Namerow NS: A discussion concerning physical trauma in multiple sclerosis. Trauma 4:42–50, 1963

127. Nelson D: Arachnoiditis from intrathecally given corticosteroids in the treatment of multiple sclerosis. Arch Neurol 33:373, 1976

128. Nelson LM, Franklin GM, Hamman RF et al: Referral bias in multiple sclerosis research. (submitted)

129. Nelson LM, Franklin GM, Heaton RK: Neuropsychological screening battery. (In preparation)

130. Noseworthy JH, Seland TP, Evers GC: Therapeutic trials in multiple sclerosis. Can J Neurol Sci 11:355–362, 1984

131. Ormerod IE, duBoulay GH, McDonald WI: Imaging of multiple sclerosis. In McDonald WI, Silberberg DH (eds): Multiple Sclerosis, pp 11–36. London, Butterworths, 1986

132. Paty DW, Power C: Clinical symptoms and signs of multiple sclerosis. In Poser CM, Paty DW, Scheinberg L et al: The Diagnosis of Multiple Sclerosis, pp 27–43. New York, Thieme-Stratton, 1984

133. Pavlou M, Hartings M, Davis FA: Discussion groups for medical patients, a vehicle for improved coping. Psychother Psychosom 30:105–115, 1978

134. Percy AK, Nobrega FT, Okazaki H et al: MS in Rochester, Minn.: A 60-year reappraisal. Arch Neurol 25:105–111, 1971

135. Perry J, Gronley JK, Lunsford T: Rocker shoe as walking aid in multiple sclerosis. Arch Phys Med Rehabil 62:59–65, 1981

136. Peyser JM, Edwards KR, Poser CM, Filskor SB: Cognitive function in patients with multiple sclerosis. Arch Neurol 37:577–579, 1980

137. Peyser JM, Becker B: Neuropsychological evaluation in patients with multiple sclerosis. In Poser CM, Paty DW, Scheinberg L, et al (eds): The Diagnosis of Multiple Sclerosis, pp 143–158. New York, Thieme-Stratton, 1984

138. Poser CM: Trauma, stress, and multiple sclerosis. Bull Am Acad Psychiatry Law 7:209–218, 1979

139. Poser CM: The diagnostic process in multiple sclerosis. In Power CM, Papty DW, Scheinberg L, et al (eds): The Diagnosis of Multiple Sclerosis, pp 3–13. New York, Thieme–Stratton, 1984

140. Poser S: Management of patients with multiple sclerosis. In Vinken PJ, Bruyn GW, Klawans HL, Koetsier JC (eds): Handbook of Clinical Neurology, vol 47, Demyelinating Diseases, pp 147–186. Amsterdam, Elsevier Science Publishers, 1985

141. Poser S, Poser W: Letter: MS and postpartum stress. Neurology 34:704–705, 1984

142. Power PW, Sax DS: The communication of information to the neurological patient: Some implications for family coping. J Chronic Dis 34:57–65, 1978

143. Price G: The challenge to the family. Am J Nurs 80:282–285, 1980

144. Pryse-Phillips WEM, Chandra RK, Rose B: Anaphylactoid reaction to methylprednisolone pulsed therapy for multiple sclerosis. Neurology 34:1119–1121, 1984

145. Rao SM, Hammeke TA: Hypothesis in patients with chronic progressive multiple sclerosis. Brain Cognition 3:94–104, 1984

146. Rao SM, Hammeke TA, McQuillen MP et al: Memory disturbance in chronic progressive multiple sclerosis. Arch Neurol 4:625–631, 1984

147. Rasminsky M: Pathophysiology of demyelination. Ann NY Acad Sci 436:68–85, 1984

148. Reder AT, Arnason BGW: Immunology of multiple sclerosis. In Vinken PJ, Bruyn GW, Klawans HL, Koetsier JS (eds): Handbook of Clinical Neurology, vol 47, Demyelinating Diseases, pp 337–395. Amsterdam, Elsevier Science Publishers, 1985

149. Rolak LA, Ashizawa T: The hot bath test in multiple sclerosis: Comparison with visual evoked responses and oligoclonal bands. Acta Neurol Scand 72:65–67, 1985

150. Rose AS, Kuzma JW, Kurtzke JF et al: Cooperative study in the evaluation of therapy in multiple sclerosis: ACTH vs. placebo, final report. Neurology 20:1–59, 1970

151. Rules and regulations. Red Reg 50:50099–60000, 1985

152. Ruttenberg N: Assessment and treatment of speech and swallowing problems in patients with multiple sclerosis. In Maloney FP, Burks JS, Ringel SP (eds): Interdisciplinary Rehabilitation of Multiple Sclerosis and Neuromuscular Disorders, pp 129–142. Philadelphia, JB Lippincott, 1985

153. Sadovnick AD, Baird PA: Reproductive counseling for multiple sclerosis patients. Am J Med Genet 20:349–354, 1985

154. Schapiro RT: Symptom Management in Multiple Sclerosis. New York, Demos Publications, 1987

155. Schapiro RT, van den Noort S, Scheinberg L: The current management of multiple sclerosis. Ann NY Acad Sci 436:425–434, 1984

156. Scheinberg L: Signs, symptoms, and course of the disease. In Scheinberg LS (ed): Multiple Sclerosis: A Guide for Patients and Their Families, pp 35–55. New York, Raven Press, 1983

157. Scheinberg L, Holland N, LaRocca N et al: Multiple sclerosis, earning a living. NY State J Med 80:1395–1400, 1980

158. Scheinberg L, Holland NJ, Kirschenbaum M et al: Comprehensive long-term care of patients with multiple sclerosis. Neurology 31:1121–1123, 1981

159. Scheinberg LC, Giesser BS, Slater RJ: Management of the chronic MS patient. Neurology and Neurosurgery Update Series. 4(21):2–8, 1983

160. Scheinberg LC, Kalb RC, LaRocca NG et al: The doctor–patient relationship in multiple sclerosis. In Poser CM (ed): The Diagnosis of Multiple Sclerosis, pp 205–215. New York, Thieme-Stratton, 1984

161. Schiffer RB, Babigian HM: Behavioral disorders in multiple sclerosis, temporal lobe epilepsy and amyotrophic lateral sclerosis: An epidemiologic study. Arch Neurol 41:1067–1069, 1984

162. Schiffer RB, Herndon RM, Rudick RA: Treatment of pathologic laughing and weeping with anitriptyline. N Engl J Med 312:1480–1482, 1985

163. Schneitzer L: Rehabilitation of patients with multiple sclerosis. Arch Phys Med Rehabil 59:430–437, 1978

164. Schumacher GA, Beebe G, Kebler RF et al: Problems of experimental trials of therapy in multiple sclerosis. Ann NY Acad Sci 122:552–568, 1965

165. Sharkey PC: Spasticity. In Halsted LS, Grabois M, Howland CA (eds): Medical Rehabilitation, pp 307–315. New York, Raven Press, 1985

166. Sibley WA, Bamford CB, Clark K: Triggering factors in multiple sclerosis. In Posner CM, Paty DW, Scheinberg L et al (eds): The Diagnosis of Multiple Sclerosis, pp 14–24. New York, Thieme-Stratton, 1984

167. Sibley WA, Sears ES: Multiple sclerosis: A comparison of diagnostic criteria. In Poser CM, Paty DW, Scheinberg L et al (eds): The Diagnosis of Multiple Sclerosis, pp 230–233. New York, Thieme-Stratton, 1984

168. Silberberg DH: Pathogenesis of demyelination. In McDonald WI, Silberberg DH (eds): Multiple Sclerosis, pp 99–111. London, Butterworths, 1986

169. Slater RJ: Scoring techniques and problems in the evaluation of change in patients. Arch Neurol 40:675–677, 1983

170. Slater RJ: A model of care: Matching human services to patient's needs. Neurology 30:39–43, 1980

171. Slater RJ, Yearwood AC: MS facts, faith, and hope. Am J Nurs 80:276–281, 1980

172. Slimp J, Kraft G, Alvord E: Evoked potentials to arm and leg stimulation in MS patients and EAN monkeys. Electroencephalogr Clin Neurophysiol 56:374, 1983

173. Smith CR, Aisen ML, Scheinberg L: Symptomatic management of multiple sclerosis. In McDonald WI, Silberberg DH (eds): Multiple Sclerosis, pp 166–183. London, Butterworths, 1986

174. Smith MB, Wolf BG: Therapeutic recreation. In Maloney FP, Burks JS, Ringel SP (eds): Interdisciplinary Rehabilitation of Multiple Sclerosis and Neuromuscular Disorders, pp 402–413. Philadelphia, JB Lippincott, 1985

175. Stefoski D, Davis FA, Tyszka MF, Schauf CL: 4-Aminopyridine improves clinical signs (abstr). Ann Neurol 18:131, 1985

176. Steinberg AD: Editorial: Cyclophosphamide, should it be used daily, monthly, or never? N Engl J Med 310:458, 1984

177. Sterman AB, Coyle PK, Panasci DJ, Grimson R: Disseminated abnormalities of cardiovascular autonomic functions in multiple sclerosis. Neurology 35:1665–1668, 1985

178. Stewart DC, Sullivan TJ: Illness behavior and the sick role in chronic disease, the case of multiple sclerosis. Soc Sci Med 16:1397–1404, 1982

179. Thompson DS, Nelson LM, Burks JS, Franklin GM: The effects of pregnancy in multiple sclerosis (MS): A retrospective study. Neurology 36:1097–1099, 1986

180. Tourtellotte WW, Baumhefner RW, Potvin JH et al: Comprehensive management of multiple sclerosis. In Hallpike JF, Adams CWM, Tourtellotte WW (eds): Multiple Sclerosis—Pathology, Diagnosis, and Management, pp 513–578. Baltimore, Williams & Wilkins, 1983

181. Troiano RA, Hafstein MP, Zito G et al: The effect of oral corticosteroid dosage on CT enhancing multiple sclerosis plaques. J Neurol Sci 70:67–72, 1985

182. Valleroy ML, Kraft GH: Sexual dysfunction in multiple sclerosis. Arch Phys Med Rehabil 65:125–128, 1984

183. van den Noort S: Immunosuppressant treatment in multiple sclerosis. Clin Neuropharmacol 8:58–63, 1985

184. Vowels LM, Gates GR: Neuropsychological findings. In Simons AF (ed): Multiple Sclerosis—Psychological and Social Aspects, pp 82–89. London, William Heinemann Medical Books, 1984

185. Waksman BH: Current trends in multiple sclerosis research. Immunol Today 2:87–93, 1981

186. Waksman BH: Mechanisms in multiple sclerosis. Nature 218:104–105, 1985

187. Warren TM: Lumbar epidural anesthesia in a patient with multiple sclerosis. Anesth Analg 61:1022–1023, 1982

188. Weiner HL: An assessment of plasma exchange in progressive multiple sclerosis. Neurology 35:320–322, 1985

189. Weiner HL, Hauser SL, Hafler DA et al: The use of cyclophosphamide in the treatment of multiple sclerosis. Ann NY Acad Sci 436:373–381, 1984

190. Weller O: Pathology of multiple sclerosis. In Matthews SB (ed): McAlpine's Multiple Sclerosis, pp 301–343. Edinburgh, Churchill Livingstone, 1985

191. Wheeler JS, Siroky MB, Pavlakis AJ et al: The changing neurourologic pattern of multiple sclerosis. J Urol 130:1123–1126, 1983

192. Wolf BG: Occupational therapy for patients with multiple sclerosis. In Maloney FP, Burks JS, Ringel SP (eds): Interdisciplinary Rehabilitation of Multiple Sclerosis and Neuromuscular Disorders, pp 103–218. Philadelphia, JB Lippincott, 1985

32

Rehabilitation of the Spinal Cord-Injured Patient

William E. Staas, Jr.

Christopher S. Formal

Arthur M. Gershkoff

Maureen Freda

Judith F. Hirschwald

Gail D. Miller

Leonard Forrest

Beth A. Burkhard

Spinal cord injury (SCI) is a traumatic insult to the spinal cord that can result in alterations of normal motor, sensory, and autonomic function. Optimal management of SCI requires a multidisciplinary team. The team members must be competent as individuals and must work within a system that promotes effective interaction. Each team member should be familiar with the problems and treatment approaches of other team members.

The rehabilitation principles presented here also apply to nontraumatic spinal cord disorders. The reader is referred elsewhere for specific information about these disorders. Pediatric SCI is discussed in Chapter 20, Rehabilitation of the Pediatric Patient. Management of the ventilator-dependent patient is discussed in Chapter 35, Rehabilitation of the Patient with Pulmonary Disease.

CHARACTERISTICS OF SPINAL CORD INJURY

Epidemiology

Quadriplegia accounts for 53% of SCI, and paraplegia accounts for the remaining 47%. Forty-eight percent of quadriplegias are complete, and 60% of paraplegias are complete. Twenty-three percent of quadriplegics have functional preserved motor function at the time of admission, as do 18% of paraplegics. Thirty-one percent of quadriplegics have functional preserved motor function at the end of the initial medical rehabilitation, as do 25% of paraplegics. Six percent of patients admitted with complete quadriplegia have incomplete quadriplegia at the end of the initial medical/rehabilitation period, and 1% have functional preserved function; the figures for patients admitted with complete paraplegia are 4% and 1%, respectively.[215]

SCI occurs primarily in young adults. It is rare in children under age 14, but almost half of all injuries occur in people between the ages of 15 and 24. Eighty-two percent of patients are men. Male patients have a slightly higher percentage of quadriplegias and of complete injuries than do female patients. Seventy-five percent of patients are white, which is below the percentage of whites in the general population. Blacks, Hispanics, and American Indians have a disproportionately high incidence of SCI. Thirty-two percent of patients are married at the time of injury, 60% are employed, and 21% are students.[215] SCI occurs most commonly in July; the incidence then decreases until February before increasing. More injuries occur on Saturday than any other day.[215]

The incidence of traumatic SCI is approximately 55 per million person-years overall, with 35 per million person-years for those who survive to be hospitalized. The prevalence is estimated to be 500 to 900 per million person-years. Thus, the national incidence varies between 7,000 and 10,000 cases each year, with a prevalence of 150,000 to 200,000 cases.[47]

The epidemiology of nontraumatic spinal cord disease is not as well examined. One study found the incidence of nontraumatic disease to be more than twice that of traumatic injury.[137] Cancer alone was a more common cause of cord disease than traumatic injury. Spondylosis was also a common cause. Age had a dramatic effect on cause. Traumatic injury was more than twice as common as nontraumatic disease in patients under age 40. In patients over age 40, cord disease due to cancer was four times as common as traumatic injury.

Etiology

In the United States, the leading cause of SCI is auto accidents (46%), followed by falls (16%), gunshot and stab wounds (12%), and diving accidents (10%).[81]

Outcomes

Approximately 37% of SCI patients die prior to hospitalization. Most deaths occur within 2 hours of injury and are associated with multiple and massive trauma. The reported fatality for patients who survive to be hospitalized ranges from 8.5% to 16.7%. The mortality after hospital admission tends to be higher for complete lesions, higher-level lesions, and the elderly.[59, 81, 87] The leading causes of in-hospital death are pulmonary infections and pulmonary embolus. Mortality is higher among male patients by a 3-to-1 ratio. Life expectancy for SCI is shown for male and female patients, respectively, in Tables 32-1 and 32-2. A 30.2-year mean life expectancy has been estimated.[81] Late deaths are due to cardiovascular diseases, pulmonary disease, suicide, and genitourinary tract disease.[28]

Mechanisms of Injury

Fractures, dislocations, and fracture-dislocations of the occiput C1 and C2 vertebrae are either fatal, owing to the high level of cord involvement above the innervation to the diaphragm, or without neurological consequences. The Jefferson fracture, a burst fracture of the ring of the atlas, resulting from axial compression, is typically without neurological deficit because the fracture itself decompresses the canal.[98] The hangman fracture of the neural arch of the axis is caused by flexion and/or extension and axial compression. An abrasion on the forehead or chin may be present and implies this mechanism of injury. Typically, an SCI is not present with this fracture.[170] Fractures of the odontoid are poorly understood, although a shearing force is a component.[136]

Only 5% of these fractures have associated neurological deficits, owing to the abundance of room to accommodate the spinal cord at this level.[91, 177]

From C3 to C7, there is a relationship between the mechanism of injury, the type of fracture, and the likelihood of neurological deficit. With pure flexion or extension injuries, there is usually no accompanying neurological deficit and the spine is stable.[94] In a flexion injury, the energy is dissipated by producing a compression fracture of the anterior portion of a vertebral body. The ligaments remain intact, and the spinal cord is not compromised. With a pure extension mechanism, the anterior longitudinal ligament is disrupted and there may be an avulsion fracture of the anterosuperior portion of the vertebral body. However, the posterior ligamentous complex remains intact and the spinal cord is typically not disturbed.[158]

When rotation is combined with flexion, the damage to the vertebral column is more severe because the rotational component disrupts the posterior ligamentous complex or produces fractures of the posterior vertebral elements.[94, 158] The flexion component, thus unrestrained, causes a forward dislocation of one or both facet joints or a "teardrop" fracture, with displacement of the remainder of the vertebral body into the spinal canal, causing damage to the cord.[169]

Compression "burst" fractures due to axial loading (such as

Table 32-1
Life Expectancies for Male Spinal Cord Injury Victims by Age at Time of Injury and Impairment Category

| Age at Hospital Discharge (yr) | General Population | Life Expectancy (yr) | | | |
| | | Paraplegia | | Quadriplegia | |
		Incomplete	Complete	Incomplete	Complete
10	59.09	57.22	42.20	49.88	28.60
20	49.65	47.85	33.73	40.88	21.57
30	40.61	38.95	26.29	32.57	16.45
40	31.53	29.98	18.55	24.13	10.49
50	23.08	21.70	11.96	16.61	5.90
60	15.75	14.65	7.08	10.61	2.97
70	9.72	9.00	3.93	6.29	1.50

(DeVivo MJ, Fine PR, Maetz HM, Stover SL: Prevalence of spinal cord injury: A reestimation of employing life table techniques. Arch Neurol 37:707, 1980. Copyright © 1980, American Medical Association)

Table 32-2
Life Expectancy for Female Spinal Cord Injury Victims by Age at Time of Injury and Impairment Category

| Age at Hospital Discharge (yr) | General Population | Life Expectancy (yr) | | | |
| | | Paraplegia | | Quadriplegia | |
		Incomplete	Complete	Incomplete	Complete
10	65.59	64.09	50.94	58.05	37.81
20	55.85	54.41	41.75	48.55	29.56
30	46.24	44.82	32.85	39.24	21.83
40	36.80	35.47	24.40	30.27	14.77
50	27.84	26.64	17.03	22.06	9.29
60	19.50	18.52	10.94	14.86	5.37
70	11.84	11.15	6.02	8.68	2.55

(DeVivo MJ, Fine PR, Maetz HM, Stover SL: Prevalence of spinal cord injury: A reestimation of employing life table techniques. Arch Neurol 37:708, 1980. Copyright © 1980, American Medical Association)

that seen in diving accidents) also frequently result in SCI because the burst fragments are pushed into the canal.[94] Depending on the exact mechanism of injury in a particular case, there may be an additional component of flexion, extension, or rotation.

Fractures and dislocations of the thoracolumbar spine are similar in most respects, with regard to mechanism, stability, and likelihood for neurological deficit, to those of the cervical spine. The following mechanisms are relatively unique to the thoracolumbar spine, however.

The Chance fracture results from a pure distraction force, causing a fracture that extends through the vertebral body, pedicles, and posterior elements.[26] It is most commonly seen in automobile accidents in victims wearing only lap seat belts. Sudden flexion of the upper body over the restraining seat belt is causative. This injury is typically incurred without resultant neurological deficit and is stable secondary to osseous interdigitation.[91]

The second type is the significantly displaced Chance fracture. That is, distraction is coupled with forward translation, shifting the upper portion of the vertebral body forward relative to the lower portion. This is unstable and frequently is accompanied by neurological deficit.

The third mechanism is the shear or translational injury, which results in ligamentous disruption, allowing translation of one vertebra on another. Due to the ligamentous disruption, this injury is unstable and is also commonly associated with neurological injury.[63]

Additional factors contributing to SCI include underlying instability (*e.g.,* rheumatoid involvement of the cervical spine), a congenitally narrow canal, and the presence of osteophytes.

Overall, 10% to 14% of spinal fractures and dislocations result in injury to the spinal cord.[157] Injuries of the cervical spine produce neurological damage in 40% of cases. The incidence is reported to be 10% for the thoracic spine and 4% at the thoracolumbar junction.[160] It is rare that the spinal column trauma actually lacerates or physically transects the cord. Rather, the physical force incites a process within the spinal cord. The direction and force of the insult to the cord in each case will dictate the specific pathological events. However, the basic process has been studied and is as follows: experimentally, there is progressive decrease of the microperfusion at the site of injury, beginning in the central gray matter.[61] Histologically, studies have shown microzones of hemorrhage in the central gray matter within 15 minutes following injury. (By 4 hours, focal coalescence with associated parenchymal and vascular wall necrosis is noted centrally.) Over the next 4 hours, there is the development of the central hematoma and advancing edema.[212] Biochemically, norepinephrine and other bioamines are believed to cause or be contributory to the vasospasm and parenchymal destruction.[145, 211]

Additional mechanisms include gunshot wounds, arterial compromise, and tumors. The central cord syndrome deserves special mention. It is characterized by disproportionately greater motor impairment of the upper extremities than of the lower extremities. It is most commonly seen in older patients with vertebral osteophytes. The mechanism of injury is hyperextension of the neck. By this means, the cord is impinged between the ligamentum flavum posteriorly and the hypertrophic spurs anteriorly.[168] Typically, no fracture or dislocation of the spine is present. The result is hematomyelia, which is confined to the central portion of the cord, with a surrounding "brim" of edema.[126] Since the white matter of the corticospinal tract is laminated with the fibers to the upper extremities closest to the center, it follows that they would be more profoundly involved.

The degree of ultimate recovery is proportional to the resolution of the edema versus cord destruction.[5]

Initial Emergency Management

Usually, the initial person to find an SCI victim will be inexperienced in first aid management. Unless the victim's life is in danger, he or she should not be moved. A conscious victim should be encouraged not to move until experienced personnel can be found. Thus, the team approach begins at the accident site and continues for the patient's lifetime. Guttman[85] has provided specific information concerning initial management of a patient with SCI.

Although each SCI patient presents with unique problems and challenges, the following guidelines for first aid should be considered:

1. All activities should be carried out with the possibility of an SCI kept in mind by securing and continuously monitoring the stability of the spine.
2. The airway/breathing and circulation should be assessed, including monitoring of the patient's vital capacity and blood pressure.
3. The neurological status should be determined. This includes evaluation of the level of consciousness, cranial nerves, sensory and motor deficits, and reflexes.
4. A Foley catheter should be inserted.
5. Associated injuries should be considered, including head, chest, abdomen, and long bones.
6. Plain roentgenograms of the spine, including the lateral view of the cervical spine down to and including C7, should be taken.
7. The team members should by now have identified all of the patient's injuries and are now ready to transfer the patient safely from the backboard to the Stryker frame, or other appropriate bed. Usually five team members, all standing on the same side, move the patient in unison, with one person counting and lifting the patient's head.
8. Tongs may then be applied and appropriate traction instituted.
9. Additional roentgenograms, including a computed tomographic (CT) scan, can be obtained.

Surgical Procedures

The initial surgical management of an SCI involves decompression, stabilization, or both. An unstable spine can be simply defined as one in which there is a possibility of the shift of bone fragments or vertebral relationships. Denis[46] and McAfee and co-workers[120] redefined previous approaches of evaluating for spinal instability with the introduction of a three-column spine concept, in which the anterior column consists of the anterior vertebral body, anterior annulus fibrosus, and anterior longitudinal ligament. The middle column consists of the posterior longitudinal ligament, the posterior annulus fibrosus, and the posterior vertebral body. The posterior column consists of the posterior bony complex and posterior ligaments.

In the case of the unstable spine, the vertebrae involved should be reduced to approximate the premorbid alignment. This can be accomplished by closed means via traction or by open manipulation at the time of surgery. Spinal stabilization procedures at any level can be done posteriorly, anteriorly, or posteriorly and anteriorly, depending on the pathology.

Ultimately, stability is achieved by bony union of the involved vertebrae. In some fractures, this will occur without the addition of bone graft. Usually, however, bone grafting is done and provides the framework for the bony union. Fusion is usually complete in 3 months.

If there is a significant fracture of the vertebral body, reduction of the spinal fracture or dislocation may not completely relieve the problem of impingement of the spinal cord. Decompression of the spinal cord or nerve roots may be necessary. Since the insulting fragments are typically from the vertebral body (and, therefore, anterior to the spinal cord), an anterior approach to the spine is typically made. The vertebral body is removed, including the offending fragments. The adjacent disks are removed, and the space is filled with a strut graft. Following decompression, stability must be assessed.[13, 53, 106] The issue of decompressing the spinal cord months or years following injury is controversial. However, Bohlman[14, 15] has reported some success.

A different approach has been taken by investigators attempting to address the progression of the spinal cord lesion itself. Methods attempting to halt progression of this process include myelotomy, hypothermia, and pharmacological measures. These treatments have been employed experimentally in animal studies, as well as on a limited scale in humans. This topic is discussed in reviews by Hansebout[88] and Northrup and Alderman[142]

Technology is also advancing the assessment of the spinal cord following injury. In this regard, magnetic resonance imaging (MRI) is proving to be of value, particularly with the diagnosis of disk pathology and post-traumatic syrinx.[77] Spinal evoked potentials may also prove useful as a predictor of recovery, as well as for monitoring at the time of surgery.[114]

External Spinal Stabilization

Traction can be used for reduction of the cervical spine as well as for temporary maintenance of spinal stability. Crutchfield,[43] in 1933, introduced skeletal traction with tongs inserted into the skull. Closed reduction is best accomplished by this means.

The halo-plaster body jacket was introduced in 1959 by Perry and Nickel.[149] During the 1970s, a thermoplastic prefabricated vest replaced the plaster jacket for most situations. Today, multiple styles are available, but the principle remains the same. A metal ring is secured by four, heavy, threaded pins placed with the patient under local anesthesia into the outer table of the skull. The ring is, in turn, secured to the vest by two or four upright posts. The advent of the halo-vest was probably the most significant impetus for early rehabilitation of the cervical SCI patient. It stabilizes the cervical spine, allowing easy access to neck incisions, trachostomy sites, and so on, while at the same time allowing the patient to be mobilized and begin a rehabilitation program.

Persistent instability or nonunion, while the patient is in the halo-vest, is reported to be 10% to 15%.[39, 52, 193] Follow-up roentgenograms should be done at regular intervals, particularly during the first month, when most redislocations are noted. A report of neck pain or difficulty in swallowing, sudden increase in spasticity, or any deterioration of strength or sensation requires anteroposterior and lateral cervical spine roentgenograms and perhaps further radiological study.

Other cervical orthoses may be indicated. The Philadelphia collar may be used as primary treatment following stable injuries or may be used for 4 to 6 weeks following removal of the halo-vest. This continues to provide a moderate amount of stability while allowing a limited range of motion. Typically, during the final 2 to 3 weeks of wearing the collar, the patient can be started

on isometric neck exercises and weaned gradually from the collar, as neck strength improves.

For thoracic and lumbar spine trauma, the thermoplastic, custom-molded TLSO is most commonly used. The brace provides total contact and a stable three-point fixation.[204] It may be used as the sole method of treatment or to supplement internal fixation, depending on the stability of the fracture. Following fracture healing or graft fusion, it is best to wean the patient from the TLSO over 1 to 2 weeks to avoid undue strain on the stress-shielded muscles and ligaments.

Other conventional thoracolumbar orthoses such as the Knight-Taylor brace or the Jewett hyperextension orthosis occasionally are used in the SCI patient but their use is more typical following relatively minor spine trauma without neurological injury.

Contractures

In the upper extremity, the most common contractures are adduction/internal rotation of the shoulder, elbow flexion, forearm pronation or supination, and finger/wrist contractures, in positions that are inadequate for using the "tenodesis effect." In the lower extremity, hip flexion/adduction (with compensatory increased lumbar lordosis), knee flexion or extension, and foot–ankle equinovarus are most often encountered. Contractures of muscles or joints under voluntary control can neutralize their usefulness, resulting in the patient functionally "losing" one or more spinal cord levels. Contractures can also contribute to the major complications of fractures and pressure sores. Contractures are covered in detail in Chapter 23.

Lower Extremity Fractures

Lower extremity fractures occurring at the time of the acute injury are best treated according to the usual principles of fracture management. The trend is toward open reduction–internal fixation, which provides early stabilization and is generally associated with fewer complications.[76, 113, 147] The fractures most likely to be diagnosed by the rehabilitation physician, on the other hand, are lower extremity fractures occurring months to years following SCI.

The reported incidence of lower extremity fractures occurring after SCI is 1.5% to 6%.[154] This is despite osteoporosis in lower extremity bones, patient participation in vigorous physical therapy programs, and the ever-present risk of falls and other trauma to the paralyzed limbs. The true incidence, however, is probably somewhat higher than reported since relatively minor fractures of the ankle and foot may go undetected.[154]

The femur is most commonly fractured, while fractures of the ankle and foot are rare.[58, 71, 73, 154] In a retrospective study, fractures occurred two and one-half times as often in paraplegics as quadriplegics and ten times more frequently following complete versus incomplete injuries. A fall during a transfer is the most common cause. A fracture should be ruled out by clinical examination and roentgenograms, if necessary, in all cases of extremity swelling.

For most of these fractures, a pillow splint (or a well-padded splint) is the best management.[58, 73, 154] Generally, the patient may be out of bed and in a wheelchair within several days after the fracture. Traction is rarely indicated, and use of plaster casts or splints should be avoided since inadequate padding can cause pressure sores.[71]

Bone union typically occurs more rapidly in the paralyzed than in the neurologically intact patient.[58] On the other hand, the incidence of heterotopic ossification occurring secondary to the fracture or during the phase of rapid healing is not reported to be increased.[154] The most problematic fractures for healing are the femoral neck and subtrochanteric fractures. The femoral neck fracture will typically develop a nonunion. However, this does not usually cause a problem and may, therefore, be acceptable.[71] Subtrochanteric fractures often develop marked angulation, which may be cosmetically or functionally unacceptable. Open reduction and internal fixation should, therefore, be considered.[71, 124, 143]

Autonomic Hyperreflexia (Dysreflexia)

Autonomic hyperreflexia is characterized by sudden onset of headache and hypertension in a patient with a lesion above the T6 level. There may be associated bradycardia, sweating, dilated pupils, blurred vision, nasal stuffiness, flushing, or piloerection. It usually occurs several months after injury and has an incidence as high as 85% in quadriplegia. Frequently, it subsides within 3 years of injury, but it can recur at any time. Distention of bowel and bladder are common causes. Association has been observed with fecal impactions, rectal stimulation, bladder stones, decubitus ulcers, and ingrown toenails, and in some patients the cause remains unclear. Hypertension is the major concern because of associated seizures and cerebral hemorrhage.

Noxious stimuli initiate afferent impulses, which enter the posterior horn of the spinal cord. Segmental reflexes may be initiated and impulses ascend and synapse with neurons in the intermediolateral columns of the thoracic cord. Vasoconstriction, particularly in the splanchnic bed, is the result. The sympathetic trunks of the thoracolumbar cord are stimulated, resulting in sweating, vasoconstriction, and piloerection. Hyperhidrosis above and below the level of injury may occur. Vasoconstriction results in hypertension, which causes headache and flushing above the level of injury, with pallor below the level of spinal injury.

In non–spinal cord–injured humans, inhibitory impulses from higher brain stem centers cause vasodilatation and prevent sustained hypertension. In those with SCI, however, this cannot happen because the injury level is above the splanchnic bed. Bradycardia results from baroreceptors in the carotid sinus and is mediated by the aortic arch through medullary vasomotor centers.

Because autonomic hyperreflexia is a potentially life-threatening problem, the SCI patient who complains of headache or sweating should have blood pressure and pulse recorded. If the patient is hypertensive, necessary measures should be taken to eliminate the noxious stimuli. The most common causes are bladder distention and bowel distention. Drug management includes short-acting agents such as nitroglycerin and amyl nitrite or longer-acting agents such as guanethidine, mecamylamine, diazoxide, and hydralazine. For a life-threatening episode, intravenous agents or spinal anesthesia may be required.[174]

COMPLICATIONS OF SPINAL CORD INJURY

Pulmonary Complications

There are four major muscle groups involved in respiration: the accessory neck muscles, the diaphragm, the muscles of the chest wall, and the abdominal muscles. Observation of the breathing of a quadriplegic patient reveals elevation of the abdomen during inspiration, as the diaphragm descends. This is accompanied by retraction of the chest wall, which is a passive response to the negative intrathoracic pressure caused by descent of the diaphragm. The retraction is counterproductive because it negates in part the inspiratory force developed by the diaphragm, and it is normally opposed by the muscles of the chest wall. The quadriplegic with a paralyzed chest wall cannot oppose the retraction. If the patient is instructed to breathe out forcefully, or to cough, little force is observed owing to the paralyzed chest wall and abdominal muscles.

Respiratory failure is generally divided into problems of ventilation and problems of oxygenation. The most immediate problem after SCI is ventilatory failure due to muscular paralysis, although preexisting pulmonary disease and complications such as pneumonia and atelectasis can add components of oxygenation failure. The accessory muscles of respiration may be able to provide adequate ventilation in the chronically injured patient but are inadequate in the acutely injured patient.[97] If diaphragmatic function is completely spared, adequate ventilation is usually achieved.

All acutely injured patients should be screened for developing ventilatory failure. Arterial blood gases should be evaluated and vital capacity should be measured. A Pco_2 above 40 mm Hg or vital capacity below 1000 ml suggests that artificial ventilation may be required. A chest roentgenogram should be taken to rule out associated injury to the chest wall. Intubation of a patient with a fracture of the cervical spine is best carried out electively. Acute management should emphasize mobilization of secretions, prevention of atelectasis, and strengthening of muscles of respiration. If applied regularly, these measures will significantly decrease morbidity and mortality.[125]

The pulmonary status of the chronically SCI patient should be constantly self-monitored. Problems should be reported immediately to the managing physician so that early treatment can be instituted. Those with quadriplegia should be encouraged to obtain influenza vaccination each year and pneumoccocal vaccination every 5 years.

Communication and Swallowing Problems

A primary goal during the initial evaluation of the SCI patient is to ascertain the most effective means of communication. Most SCI patients who have undergone tracheostomies, and/or are ventilator dependent, communicate by using an exaggerated mouthing of words/sentences, which the staff and family members then decipher by lip reading. The patient also may be trained to communicate via an established yes/no response.[123] Eye blinks for yes and no are typically not effective unless they are exaggerated, since this is a reflexive response that may be misinterpreted. It is important to refrain from using head nodding/shaking to indicate yes/no, especially if the patient's spine has not been sufficiently stabilized. Tongue clicking may be used as a signal for assistance.

Additional options for communication might include use of a communication board.[9, 10, 123, 167, 202] One form of communication board is organized into quadrants. The patient looks to the specific quadrant on a board, which has a variety of basic needs listed. The listener reads aloud those needs in the designated quadrant until the patient responds affirmatively. With another type of communication board, the patient mouths the number corresponding to the need. Examples of these boards are illustrated in Figure 32-1.

Other communication aids include speaking tracheostomy tubes, the Venti-Voice, and artificial larynxes (Figs. 32-2 through 32-4; see Appendix 32-1 for suppliers). With speaking tracheostomy tubes, oxygen or compressed air is deflected past the vocal cords, resulting in phonation.[105] Examples of these tubes are Pitt, Portex, and Communitrach I.[164] For the Venti-Voice, the sound source is a one-way reed valve that vibrates as the compressed air/oxygen passes its surface.[7,12] A nasal or oral catheter is inserted through which the generated sound travels into the oropharynx. Battery-operated artificial larynxes are produced in two forms: one has a vibrating diaphragm placed against the neck (*e.g.,* Servox, Aurex, and Western Electric), and the second type directs sound into the oral cavity via a tube (*e.g.,* Cooper Rand).[121, 165, 189] As the SCI patient begins the weaning process and the tracheostomy tube is changed to a fenestrated tracheos-

ABC	GHI
DEF	JKL
MNO	TUVW
PQRS	XYZ

SUCTION	HUNGRY
TURN ME	THIRSTY
Tired	Cold
Not	Scared
T.V.	Sleepy

1. Suction
2. Thirsty
3. Pain
4. Family
5. T.V.
6. Turn Me

Figure 32-1. Examples of communication boards.

Figure 32-2. Olympic Trach-Talk. (Courtesy of Olympic Medical)

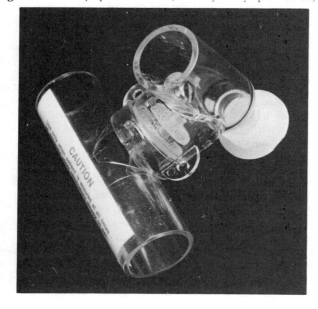

Figure 32-3. Artificial larynx.

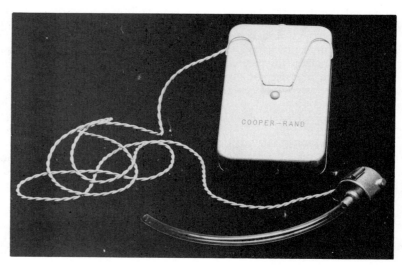

tomy tube, the patient can communicate by having the listener place a finger over the stoma or by using an Olympic Trach-Talk. The Olympic Trach-Talk functions as a one-way valve by opening on inhalation and closing during exhalation to produce phonation. Both of these techniques serve to redirect the air through the fenestration, thus vibrating the vocal cords.[115]

Swallowing ability of the ventilator-dependent patient must be assessed. Swallowing of food or liquid should not be initiated if the patient has an endotracheal tube, since the adduction of the vocal cords against the tube during swallowing may result in trauma to the vocal cords. Stabilization devices may also affect swallowing. For example, if the patient's neck is hyperextended, risk of aspiration is increased owing to an increase in the airway opening. For the swallowing evaluation, various consistencies, amounts, and techniques are attempted. If aspiration is suspected, the patient is kept NPO. Barium videofluoroscopic swallowing and/or gastrointestinal evaluations may be recommended to determine the cause of the aspiration.[30, 82, 115]

Patients can be trained in glossopharyngeal breathing (GPB). The purposes of GPB are to increase chest compliance and to provide respiratory support for survival in case of ventilatory system failure.[31, 38]

Cardiac Complications

SCI can alter cardiac physiology. When an SCI patient exercises there is an increase in heart rate and oxygen uptake, as in normal subjects. However, the levels reached are lower than in normal people, and quadriplegics have lower levels than high-level paraplegics, who have lower levels than low-level paraplegics.[40] This may be due to less functioning muscle mass, poorer venous return, and poorer ventilatory dynamics. Quadriplegics and high-level paraplegics have lost sympathetic connections between brain stem and heart and may have relatively low maximal heart rates. Quadriplegics may demonstrate increased capacities for work if exercised prone in water, owing to improved venous return and ventilatory function.[48] Decreased exercise capacity after spinal cord injury may contribute to lowering the level of high density lipoprotein (HDL) cholesterol, thus increasing the risk of cardiovascular disease.[18]

Orthostatic hypotension is associated with a sudden decrease in systolic and diastolic blood pressures and an elevation of heart rate. It is commonly seen in higher-level SCI patients, generally those with injuries above T6. Patient complaints include dizziness, lightheadedness, or sudden loss of conscious-

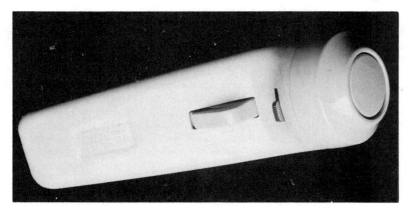

Figure 32-4. Artificial larynx.

ness. Dramatic alteration in pulse and blood pressure can occur in SCI patients with high-level injury and may not produce symptoms. Blood pressures on the order of 100/60 mm Hg are common, especially in younger patients with quadriplegia. Among activities associated with symptomatic hypotension are postural changes, transfer activities, eating, and drinking.

The problem seems to be the result of blood pooling in dependent lower extremities and ineffective vasoconstriction, due to injury to the sympathetic nervous system. Tachycardia results from the vagolytic response from the carotid bodies.

Conservative treatment suffices for almost all cases. Care is taken to slowly elevate the head of the bed in the morning before the patient is moved to a sitting position. Elastic garments are used for the legs and abdomen. Elevating leg rests are used. Liberal salt and fluid intake is encouraged. Supplementary sodium chloride tablets can be given. Sleeping with the head of the bed elevated may be helpful. Progressive elevation in a reclining-back wheelchair or on a tilt-table is begun. The patient is instructed to try to exercise if he or she recognizes the symptoms. Biofeedback, combined with mental imagery (particularly sexual imagery), may be useful. If conservative management proves inadequate, ephedrine, which will act as an α-agonist, can be administered. A mineralocorticoid can be given to promote volume expansion. If all else fails, a trial of a monoamine oxidase inhibitor concomitant with administration of tyramine may be warranted.[214] Orthostatic hypotension can be exacerbated by α-adrenergic blockers such as phenoxybenzamine, which is often used in management of bladder dysfunction. Orthostatic hypotension has been reported to be a consequence of a post-traumatic cyst of the cervical spinal cord.[119] Presumably the cyst could interfere with descending sympathetic tracts.

Severe bradyarrhythmias progressing to cardiac arrest have been reported.[68, 117] The arrest often occurs following tracheal suction. The mechanism is presumed to involve increased vagal tone, induced by the suctioning, with subsequent suppression of the sinus node. This is unopposed by the usual sympathetic response, owing to separation of supraspinal from spinal sympathetic centers, and also owing to absent sympathetic outflow from a spinal cord that is in spinal shock. Hypoxia seems to be a predisposing factor. Treatment involves atropine to oppose the vagal tone. If this fails, a pacemaker may be necessary.[102] It is not usual to observe asymptomatic bradycardia in a quadriplegic patient.

Patients with SCI can develop hyperkalemia and cardiac arrest in response to administration of succinylcholine.[20, 196] Administration of the drug can drive serum potassium levels to over 13 mEq/liter within 2 minutes. Normally succinylcholine acts by strongly binding acetylcholine receptors in the motor end-plate section of muscle fibers. In denervated muscle fibers, and perhaps in muscle fibers whose anterior horn cells have lost

supraspinal innervation, the muscle cell membranes become extremely sensitive to acetylcholine. A drug such as succinylcholine can then cause widespread depolarization and egress of potassium from the large intracellular pool. Patients with SCI should not be administered the drug. Other agents are available.

Deep Venous Thrombosis and Pulmonary Embolism

Deep venous thrombosis is a major cause of early morbidity and mortality after SCI. The published incidence figures are dependent on the criteria used for diagnosis.[16, 64, 197] Contrast venography is generally considered the most accurate test. The period of greatest risk seems to be during the several months after injury, but thrombosis can appear within days of the injury. The cause of this high incidence is unclear. The immobility accompanying flaccid paralysis, as in the recently injured patient in spinal shock, may be pathogenetic. Bors and associates[16] found a lesser incidence when spasticity was present. He also found a greater incidence on the left compared with the right, perhaps reflecting impaired venous return from the left lower extremity. Spinal cord injury may be accompanied by alterations of Factor VIII and platelet function, predisposing to thrombosis.[161]

Diagnosis by physical examination is difficult. Regular physical examination of the legs should nevertheless be performed in all SCI patients. Calf and thigh circumference should be measured bilaterally, at a fixed distance from an anatomical landmark, such as the medial tibial plateau. A difference between sides of 1 cm or more is suggestive.

The high incidence of disease and the low sensitivity of physical examination suggest that supplementary laboratory examination should be carried out. Regular examination by radionuclide scanning and by impedance plethysmography may be employed. The former test is sensitive for clot in the calf, and the latter is sensitive for clot in the thigh. In the event that one of these screening studies is positive, the study may be repeated, or venography may be performed. The presence of persistent unexplained fever may justify venography.

The physical findings of deep venous thrombosis can be produced by other problems common to this patient population. Lower extremity fracture, lower extremity hemorrhage, heterotopic ossification, dependent edema, and postphlebitic edema can all be confused with acute deep venous thrombosis.[29, 144] The presence of one entity from this group does not rule out another.

The high incidence of disease has stimulated a search for effective prophylaxis. Compressive stockings are frequently used. Low doses of heparin are also recommended. Green and co-workers[80] have demonstrated a prophylactic effect for external pneumatic calf compression. The effect was increased by concomitant administration of aspirin and dipyridamole. If deep venous thrombosis is demonstrated by venography, bed rest is begun and lower extremity range of motion is stopped. The lower extremities are elevated. If no contraindication to anticoagulation exists, a bolus of intravenous heparin is given, followed by an infusion. After 3 to 5 days, warfarin is begun, with the goal of achieving a prothrombin time 1.3 to 1.5 times control.

If a contraindication to anticoagulation exists, it can be deferred while surgical consultation is obtained for placement of a vena caval filter. If the clot appears particularly dangerous by venography (such as a large, free-floating clot in a proximal vessel), anticoagulation can be started while a surgeon is consulted.

Anticoagulation is normally carried out for 3 months following deep venous thrombosis. The patient may be mobilized after 7 days, but lower extremity range of motion is usually deferred for another week. When range of motion is restarted, the therapist should not be forceful, owing to the risk of lower extremity hemorrhage in patients taking warfarin.[29]

SCI patients are at risk for pulmonary embolus, particularly during the first several months after injury.[140] This is a significant cause of early mortality. The presentation may be subtle, such as a decline in an already ventilator-dependent patient or the development of referred shoulder or scapular pain in a quadriplegic. Diagnosis usually involves ventilation and perfusion scanning of the lung or pulmonary angiography. Treatment proceeds as outlined for deep venous thrombosis, except that warfarin is continued for at least 6 months. In addition, circulatory and ventilatory support may be needed. A critically ill patient may require thrombolytic therapy or embolectomy by suction or by surgery. If the pulmonary embolus occurs in a patient who is already fully anticoagulated, surgical consultation for placement of a vena caval filter should be considered.

Fever

Fever is a common problem in SCI patients. More than one-half of patients hospitalized will develop fever at some point.[188] Determination of the cause of the fever is necessary for appropriate management.

Evaluation of the febrile SCI patient is similar to evaluation of other febrile patients. Urinary tract infection is a frequent complication as a result of abnormal bladder function and the need for instrumentation of the urinary tract. Typical symptoms of urinary tract infection may be lacking, owing to the spinal cord injury. There may have been a recent episode of bladder distention, and the color of the urine may change or the urine may become cloudy. Urinalysis will reveal pyuria and bacteriuria. Pneumonia is a frequent complication, caused by impairment of the coughing mechanism. Cough may be absent. Physical examination and roentgenograms provide the diagnosis. Intra-abdominal disease may be present with no localizing symptoms or signs. Physical examination may reveal increased spasticity and reflex guarding of the abdomen. Pancreatitis should always be considered, especially in the recently injured patient. Injuries to the extremities, such as a long bone fracture or hemorrhage into a muscle, may cause no symptoms other than fever and may only be noted on close physical examination. Deep venous thrombosis is a common complication and may cause no symptoms or signs. Studies to rule out thrombophlebitis should always be considered in the evaluation of the febrile patient. Occasionally, an unexplained fever develops before the discovery of heterotopic ossification. Areas of pressure ulceration can become infected, causing osteomyelitis and fever.[185-187] Osteomyelitis may

be present in over 10% of patients. It can cause fever, leukocytosis, and an elevated erythrocyte sedimentation rate, although none of these findings may be present. Osteomyelitis can underlie a pressure sore that does not appear infected clinically and can cause nonhealing of a sore. Diagnosis may require aggressive workup, including a bone biopsy. Fever can sometimes be caused by high ambient temperatures, owing to poikilothermia.[50] It is possible that some patients may develop a fever that is caused primarily, in some way, by SCI, but this is not a frequent occurrence, and the diagnosis is one of exclusion. Finally, a high percentage of SCI patients have also suffered a brain injury, which can cause an elevation of body temperature.

Urological Problems

Urological problems as a result of neurogenic bladder dysfunction are common among SCI patients and are discussed in Chapter 26, Neurogenic Bladder and Bowel. With current management, death from renal failure is uncommon, decline in renal function over time can be prevented, and a satisfactory method of long-term bladder drainage can be achieved by most patients.

Gastrointestinal Complications

SCI has been found to affect the physiology of virtually all segments of the gastrointestinal tract. Gastric emptying may be delayed in quadriplegics owing to alterations in autonomic function.[62] Gastric acid secretion may be altered because of changes in autonomic function. Colonic myoelectric activity is abnormal.[1] Baseline activity is increased. This corresponds to a disturbance of colonic functioning, with decreased compliance.[78,130] During the acute phase, when abdominal emergencies are most likely to occur, spinal shock may be present. This can prevent rigidity or guarding from developing when acute disease is present. Conversely, it can result in absent bowel sounds when there is no disease. Abdominal tone may be variable from patient to patient, and it is thus advisable for the physician to be familiar with the patient's baseline abdominal tone so that any changes may be detected. Often the most notable sign associated with abdominal disease is either an increase in spasticity or autonomic dysreflexia.[99]

The SCI patient is at high risk for gastric atony and ileus, which may cause vomiting and aspiration. All acutely injured patients should undergo stomach decompression by placement of a nasogastric tube. If ileus is prolonged, it may respond to metaclopramide.[131] Abdominal emergencies developing within 24 hours of injury are usually due to trauma. Peritoneal lavage may be required to establish the presence of bleeding.

Gastrointestinal bleeding is a common early complication.[8,103] It is usually due to stress ulceration. The risk is greater in patients with complete injuries above the T5 level.[8] During spinal shock, these patients may lack sympathetic input to the stomach, leaving vagal parasympathetic input unopposed, thus increasing acid secretion. Gastrointestinal bleeding is rare in patients with lesions below the T5 level.[112] Artificial ventilation increases the risk.[8] Full heparinization may also increase the risk.[60] The stool should be routinely tested for occult blood. It is common to administer cimetidine or ranitidine prophylactically for 3 months after injury. Administration of antacids may be equally effective.

Pancreatitis is also occasionally noted after SCI and can be lethal.[25] It must be suspected in cases of recurrent nausea and vomiting or of unexplained fever. The classic pain may be absent. It may be due to trauma or to unopposed parasympathetic stimulation of the sphincter of Oddi. Amylase determinations are helpful. The risk may be increased by administration of corticosteroids.[8] Presumably hypercalcemia can also contribute to pathogenesis.

The superior mesenteric artery syndrome has been reported as a cause of recurrent vomiting in quadriplegia.[155] The syndrome results from occlusion of the third part of the duodenum by compression between the underlying aorta and the overlying superior mesenteric artery. Predisposing factors include prolonged supine posture and acute loss of retroperitoneal fat, both of which may be operative after SCI. Occlusion of the duodenum causes vomiting 1 to 2 hours after eating. The syndrome is usually worse in the supine position and can be relieved by lying in the left lateral decubitus position or by sitting upright with forced upward displacement of the abdominal contents. An upper gastrointestinal series will show a cutoff across the third portion of the duodenum, which can be influenced by positioning.

Dependable management of neurogenic bowel dysfunction is important and is covered in Chapter 26.

Changes in Body Composition and Regulation

SCI causes changes in body composition and regulatory processes that can lead to significant clinical problems. Shortly after SCI, body weight decreases as a result of a water diuresis and breakdown of soft tissue and bone.[23, 33] Diuresis can occur for a month or more after injury and is most pronounced at night. Patients on an intermittent catheterization program are thus at greatest risk for overdistention at night. A redistribution of body water occurs, so that extracellular water volume becomes relatively expanded.

Collagen is a major component of soft tissues, such as skin, and of the matrix of bone. It is a protein and includes a large proportion of the amino acid hydroxyproline. Hydroxyprolinuria nearly doubles shortly after SCI, reflecting resorption of soft tissue and bone.[34] This disorder seems to be made worse by inactivity, and thus early mobilization may decrease tissue loss.

Alterations of body composition may contribute to altered drug kinetics, such as the increased clearance of gentamicin.[172] In addition, basal metabolic rate and energy expenditure are decreased after SCI.[135] This may account in part for the fact that, although weight loss is almost always seen soon after SCI, weight can increase later and obesity can develop, which can increase problems of mobility and self-care. Standard formulas for predicting caloric needs overestimate the requirements for SCI.[41] During the acute phase, however, patients may be undernourished.[101]

Hypercalciuria develops soon after SCI and can persist for months.[34, 178] Calcium can be excreted at three times the normal rate. The calcium is derived from bone, principally located in the paralyzed portion of the body. Despite the resorption of calcium, hypercalcemia generally does not develop, since the increased load is excreted by the kidneys. The increased load of calcium causes a decrease in parathyroid hormone and 1,25-dihydroxyvitamin D. These changes limit calcium absorption from the gastrointestinal tract, which implies that restriction of dietary calcium will have little effect on hypercalciuria. The cause of the calcium resorption is ultimately not known but is believed to result from immobilization, since hypercalciuria occurs in immobilized patients who do not have SCI. Conversely, mobilization limits hypercalciuria in SCI.[37, 100]

The increased calcium resorption contributes to the problems of urinary tract calculi and osteoporosis and may contribute to the problem of heterotopic ossification. A fourth problem generated by increased calcium resorption is that of hypercalcemia. As mentioned earlier, hypercalcemia is an unusual problem in the SCI population in general, but it is more common in young, recently injured male patients. The clinical manifestations of hypercalcemia are protean and can include such central nervous system manifestions as lethargy, headache, irritability, or confusion, followed by convulsions and coma. Polyuria and polydipsia can be noted. Gastrointestinal symptoms such as nausea and vomiting can also occur. The manifestations are sufficiently varied that the clinician does well to include hypercalcemia in the differential diagnosis of virtually any otherwise unexplained problem in the recently injured young man. Indeed, such patients should have screening serum calcium levels drawn even if they are asymptomatic.

The pathogenesis is uncertain.[118] Certainly the problem begins with the increased resorption of body calcium, which may overwhelm the excretory capacities of the body. In some patients, hypercalcemia may cause nausea and vomiting, and these may lead to dehydration, decreased renal clearance, and ultimately worsening of the hypercalcemia. It has also been found that hypercalcemic SCI patients do not have depressed parathyroid hormone levels as much as would be expected, based on serum calcium levels.

The treatment of hypercalcemia in these patients has several aspects.[36, 118] The patient should be mobilized in a wheelchair and on a tilt-table as tolerated. Measures to decrease calcium absorption from the gastrointestinal tract may be employed, including oral phosphates, oral steroids, and reduced oral calcium intake. Vitamin D intake may be reduced by eliminating milk from the diet, as well as any multivitamins containing vitamin D. Gastrointestinal calcium absorption is usually minimal, so these measures may not significantly affect the hypercalcemia. A diuresis should be established to increase calcium excretion and also to maintain a dilute urine to minimize the likelihood of precipitation. This is achieved through concomitant administration of saline and furosemide. Calcitonin has also been employed to decrease hypercalcemia[24] and is administered by daily intramuscular injection in a dose of 1 to 2 units/kg. This will have at least a temporary effect. Disodium etidronate, which is typically used to prevent and treat heterotopic calcification, has also been used to treat hypercalcemia.[129] Its mode of action involves modification of calcium crystallization, and can also block dissolution of preformed crystal.[55] Etidronate is administered as a daily oral dose of 10 mg/kg, well spaced between meals. Mithramycin has been suggested for use in emergency situations.

The secretion of several of the nine pituitary-derived hormones is altered after SCI. Secretion of adrenocorticotrophic hormone (ACTH) from the pituitary is normal in response to blood-borne stimuli but may not be appropriate in response to neural-mediated stimuli.[35] The response to stresses such as surgery or pressure ulceration may be deficient. The adrenal cortex remains capable of responding to stimulation by ACTH. Levels of thyroid-stimulating hormone are normal, but levels of thyroxine show a small, transient decrease. Levels of growth hormone may show unusual bursts. The data involving hormones of the pituitary-gonadal axis are inconsistent. Levels of follicle stimulating hormone (FSH) drop transiently.[138] Luteinizing hormone (LH) levels drop transiently in paraplegia but more permanently in quadriplegia. Testosterone levels drop transiently. These hormonal changes may be relevant to the testicular atrophy, sterility, and gynecomastia often observed after SCI. The patterns mentioned may not hold true for patients with damage to the sacral spinal cord segments.[139] These patients may demonstrate chronically elevated FSH levels. In contrast to other SCI patients, they may demonstrate an abnormal response to a challenge with luteinizing hormone releasing hormone (LHRH), with abnormally high FSH and LH levels.

Glucose intolerance may be observed in patients not previously diabetic.[51] This appears to be due to insensitivity to insulin rather than to a deficient insulin response.

Transient anemia usually develops. This is accompanied by a rise in erythropoietin levels, which is sustained in paraplegics but transient in quadriplegics.[32]

Heterotopic Ossification

Heterotopic ossification has been reported to occur in 16% to 53% of patients following SCI.[205] Most commonly the hip is involved, followed by the knee. Less frequently the shoulder and elbow are affected.[180] Heterotopic ossification has only been reported within the area of neurological deficit unless another causative factor, such as extensive burns, is present.[180, 210] The process may occur in patients with spastic or flaccid paralysis and complete or incomplete injuries. Typically, the heterotopic ossification is noted 1 to 4 months following injury, but it has been reported to occur as early as 19 days and as late as several years following injury.[89]

The etiology is poorly understood. Decreased tissue oxygenation or some unknown factor is believed to induce a metaplasia of multipotential connective tissue cells to chondroblasts and osteoblasts.[27, 146] The new bone forms in planes between connective tissue layers.[74] Trauma to the involved area is attractive in theory as a cause; however, this has not been borne out clinically.[181]

The natural history of heterotopic ossification is to progress to mature bone. Depending on the extent of the ossification and its relationship to a joint, restriction of joint motion will occur. In a study reviewing heterotopic ossification prior to modern concepts for treatment, approximately 20% of patients developed complete ankylosis of one or more joints. Overall, ankylosis occurred in slightly more than 10% of affected joints.[210] Restriction of joint range of motion of even a modest degree may impair function or interfere with hygiene. In addition, a pressure sore may occur as a secondary complication. This may occur indirectly from altered positioning related to heterotopic ossification of the hip with increased pressure, particularly beneath the contralateral ischial tuberosity.[90] Heterotopic ossification overlying a bony prominence (e.g., trochanter or ischial tuberosity) will directly predispose to a pressure sore.[44, 66]

The early clinical findings are swelling and heat. Fever may also be present. In the lower extremity, this may be mistaken for deep vein thrombosis.[205] Hematoma, infection, and tumor are other considerations. Over several days, the swelling becomes more firm and localized. Alternately, this inflammatory phase may be subdued and go undetected. In these cases, it is often the physical therapist who calls attention to the decreasing range of motion of a particular joint.

Roentgenograms will reveal the process only after sufficient ossification has taken place. The third, or bone, phase of the bone scan does correlate well and usually precedes roentgenographic findings by at least 7 to 10 days. During the active phase, an elevated alkaline phosphatase level may also be present.[69]

The outcome is best when the condition is diagnosed early and an aggressive passive range of motion program is begun. Disodium etidronate has been shown to be effective in limiting the extent of the ossification, particularly if therapy is started early.[69, 180] The optimum length of treatment with this medication is not yet known. Some recommend continuation for 6 months if the process, when discovered, is of mild to molderate intensity;

continuation for 1 year is advised if the process seems more severe.[179] Studies on the prophylactic use of disodium etidronate are continuing.

When an established heterotopic ossification is causing severely limited range of motion or frank ankylosis that is impairing function, surgery is indicated. A wedge resection of the heterotopic bone is usually performed. However, maturity of the bone must be ensured to prevent massive recurrence. On serial bone scans, isotope uptake that is approaching that of normal bone is the best measure of maturity.[69, 182] The length of time from the onset, a stable clinical examination, a stable roentgenographic appearance, and an alkaline phosphatase level that has returned to normal are not reliable to make this judgment, but they do provide supportive evidence. Disodium etidronate has proven to be effective in preventing recurrence of heterotopic ossification following surgery for as long as the medication is being given. Recurrence following discontinuation of the drug is variable but seems to be inversely proportional to the length of therapy and the size of the initial bone mass.[182]

Pain

Varying types of pain are found in SCI patients. Damage to the spine and soft tissue may cause throbbing or aching in the region of the injury. Nerve root pain is sharp or lancinating or may have an electric shock quality. It may radiate into involved dermatomes and be associated with distal paresthesias. Phantom body pain or spinal cord pain results from damage to the spinal cord and is described by patients as being sharp or burning. It may have an electric shock–like quality or feeling of expanding or exploding tissue. Most often it occurs in the perineal region and the lower extremities and less commonly in the abdominal region or upper extremities. Its incidence varies between 5% and 100%, with severe pain occurring in 5% to 30% of patients. Most commonly, it appears within 6 months of injury, although late onset years after injury has been observed and reported. It more often is seen in cauda equina lesions and less commonly in cervical lesions.

Melzack and Loeser[128] have suggested the source of spinal pain within the spinal cord and brain stem. The loss of sensory input is thought to influence the phantom pain. Neuronal pools at multiple levels within the spinal cord and brain are thought to initiate impulses that project to the brain, are localized, and are perceived as painful.

Treatment includes patient education, emphasizing the normality of this experience in SCI patients. Transcutaneous electrical nerve stimulation (TENS) may be of value. Psychotrophic drugs, including tricyclic antidepressants and phenothiazines, are beneficial to many patients. They seem to increase pain tolerance and may affect the endorphin and enkephalin systems. Relaxation techniques, with biofeedback, may be helpful by reducing pain behaviors. Narcotic analgesics are almost never appropriate or indicated for this problem.[174]

Syringomyelia

The incidence of post-traumatic syringomyelia in SCI patients is between 0.3% and 3%. It is important because of the functional changes that can occur in the patient. Because syringomyelia is progressive, if unrecognized it can result in increased disability. Its occurrence is most frequent in incomplete lesions of the thoracic and lumbar cord. Initial symptoms can appear as early as 8 months to many years following injury. Frequently, pain is the presenting symptom, followed by numbness. Pain may be exacerbated by laughing, coughing, sneezing, or strain. Sensory loss above the site of original injury is often observed. Dissociated sensory loss (*i.e.,* loss of sensation to pain and temperature and loss of proprioception), with retention of touch, may occur in association with numbness. Loss of deep tendon reflexes may also be evident. Spontaneous and excessive sweating may occur and can extend to body segments below the level of spinal injury. Motor weakness and muscle atrophy may be later manifestations.

The pathogenesis of syringomyelia is uncertain. Initial cavitation may occur with liquefaction of intracordal hematoma at the time of original injury. Following this, the syrinx may extend anteroposterior, as well as cephalad to caudad. Following trauma, the spinal cord becomes inflexible and tethered as a result of arachnoid adhesions. It can be affected by sudden changes in venous pressure, such as occurs during straining and Valsalva maneuvers. Increased intrathoracic or intra-abdominal pressure distends eipdural veins and transmits pulsatile waves to cerebrospinal fluid. This can result in damage to weakened sites, such as the gray matter between the dorsal horn and posterior columns, owing to fragile supporting connective tissue.

Diagnosis is based on a high index of suspicion in patients presenting with compatible symptomatology. The confirmation may be established with metrizamide myelography and CT scanning or a magnetic resonance image of the spinal cord and spinal canal. Management is dependent on the clinical status of the patient. Conservative management may include pain control, since numbness, sensory loss, and reflex changes may not change while motor weakness may improve spontaneously. Serial electromyography may be of value for monitoring of denervation. Intractable pain, rapidly progressive weakness with functional decline, and neuropathic joints are considered indications for surgical intervention. Surgical management involves removal of cerebrospinal fluid and prevention of its reaccumulation. Shunting procedures have been used frequently. Results of surgical care have been variable, depending on timing of surgery and the procedure used.[54]

Sexual Dysfunction

Sexual dysfunction is discussed in Chapter 27.

Neurological Impairment

Appropriate classification of the level of injury facilitates communication among professionals and helps to predict functional outcomes. Confusion has resulted from the existence of multiple classifications systems. The American Spinal Injury Association (ASIA) system defines the level as the lowest intact segment where the key muscle grade is "fair" (grade 3 or better). This designation is satisfactory if the patient's injury is "complete." The *Frankel Scale* (Table 32-3) distinguishes between complete and incomplete lesions and qualitatively describes the degree of incompleteness. More recently, the motor score has been developed to quantitatively define the extent of a patient's motor activity.[175]

FUNCTIONAL ASPECTS OF REHABILITATION

The expected functional outcomes for patients with complete SCI are listed in Table 32-4. The achievement of the given level of function is dependent on strengthening of available muscles and substitution of a working muscle to perform an action of which it is capable but would not do under ordinary circumstances. Examples include the following:

Table 32-3
Frankel Scale

1. Complete (A). The lesion is found to be complete both motor and sensory below the segmental level marked. If there is an alteration of level, but the lesion remains complete below the new level, then the arrow would point up or down the complete column.
2. Sensory only (B). There is some sensation present below the level of the lesion but the motor paralysis is complete below that level. This column does not apply when there is a slight discrepancy between the motor and sensory level but does apply to sacral sparing.
3. Motor Useless (C). There is some motor power present below the lesion but it is of no practical use to the patient.
4. Motor Useful (D). There is useful motor power below the level of the lesion. Patients in this group can move the lower limbs and many can walk, with or without aids.
5. Recovery (E). The patient is free of neurological symptoms (*i.e.,* no weakness, no sensory loss, no sphincter disturbance). Abnormal reflexes may be present.

(Frankel HL, Hancock DO, Hyslop G et al: Value of postural reduction in the initial management of closed injuries of the spine with paraplegia and tetraplegia. Paraplegia 7:179–192, 1969)

CLOSED KINETIC CHAIN

- Elbow extension via biceps and shoulder external rotators
- Sitting push-ups via reverse action of the latissimus dorsi bilaterally

OPEN KINETIC CHAIN

- Shoulder abduction to produce elbow flexion
- Shoulder adduction and external rotation producing forearm supination[21]

The maximum functional level that any patient can achieve will be modified by a variety of factors, both medical and nonmedical. In addition to strength, the physical factors that modify or lower maximum levels are age, body proportions and weight distribution, immobilization devices (spinal and extremity), spasms (controllable and triggered *vs.* uncontrolled), joint range limitations, and individual variation in segmental innervation.

Persistent medical complications such as heterotopic ossification and associated soft tissue and head injuries will considerably alter physical outcomes. Not to be ignored are the psychosocial and vocational issues: patient motivation/attitude and goals, family/significant other support system, living arrangements, prior life-style, prior vocation, and educational level. Financial support may be the major determinant in achievement of function. High-tech equipment, as well as most of the basic equipment, is expensive. What equipment and future services (*i.e.,* home modifications, attendants) will be funded are determined by the primary and secondary insurers. In C4 quadriplegia, a power chair with an environmental control unit, purchased by the insurer or from personal resources, will significantly change the functional independence and quality of life achieved.

Acute Interventions

In the acute stage, prevention of pressure sores, contractures, and upper respiratory tract problems is of primary importance. Additionally, the educational process of patient and family re-
(*Text continues on p. 648*)

Table 32-4
Functional Outcomes for Patients with Complete Spinal Cord Injuries

Level of Injury	Pulmonary Hygiene	AM Care	Feeding	Grooming	Dressing	Bathing	Bowel & Bladder Routine
C3 C4	Totally assisted cough	Total dependence	May be unable to feed self. Use of BFOs with universal cuff and adapted utensils indicated; drinks with long straw after set up.	Total dependence	Total dependence	Total dependence	Total dependence
C5	Assisted cough	Independent with specially adapted devices with set up	Independent with specially adapted equipment for feeding after set up	Independent with specially adapted equipment for grooming after set up	Assist with upper extremity dressing; dependent for lower extremity dressing	Total dependence	Total dependence
C6	Some assistance required in supine position; independent in sitting position	Independent with equipment	Independent with equipment; drinks from glass	Independent with equipment	Independent with upper extremity dressing; assistance needed for lower extremity dressing	Independent in upper and lower extremity bathing with equipment	Independent for bowel routine; assistance needed with bladder routine
C7	As above	Independent	Independent	Independent with equipment	Potential for independence in upper and lower extremity dressing with equipment	Independent with equipment	Independent
C8 T1	As above	Independent	Independent	Independent	Independent	Independent	Independent
T2–T10	T2–6 as above T6–10 independent	Independent	Independent	Independent	Independent	Independent	Independent
T11–L2	Not applicable	Independent	Independent	Independent	Independent	Independent	Independent
L3–S3	Not applicable	Independent	Independent	Independent	Independent	Independent	Independent

Table 32-4
Functional Outcomes for Patients with Complete Spinal Cord Injuries

Bed Mobility	Pressure Relief	Wheelchair Transfers	Wheelchair Propulsion	Ambulation	Orthotic Devices	Transportation	Communications
Total dependence	Independent in powered recliner wheelchair; dependent in bed or manual wheelchair	Total dependence	Independent in pneumatic or chin control–driven power wheelchair with powered reclining feature	Not applicable	Upper extremity: external powered orthosis, dorsal cockup splint, BFOs	Dependent on others in accessible van with lift; unable to drive	Read with special adapted equipment; specially adapted phone; unable to write; types with special adaptions
Assisted by other and by equipment	Most require assistance	Assistance of one person with or without transfer board	Independent in powered chair indoors and outdoors; short distances in manual wheelchair with lugs indoors	Not applicable	As above	As above	As above
Independent with equipment	Independent	Potentially independent with transfer board	Independent manual wheelchair with plastic rims or lugs indoors; assistance needed outdoors and with elevators	Not applicable	Wrist-driven orthosis	Independent driving specially adapted van	Independent with phone; writes with equipment; types with equipment; independent in turning pages
Independent	Independent	Independent with or without transfer board including car except to/from floor with assistance	Independent manual wheelchair indoors and outdoors, except curbs, stairs	Not applicable	None	Independent driving car with hand controls or specially adapted van; independent wheelchair into car placement	Independent with equipment for phone, typing, and writing; independent in turning pages
Independent	Independent	Independent including to/from floor and car	Independent manual wheelchair indoors and outdoors; curbs, escalators	Not applicable	None	As above	Independent
Independent	Independent	Independent	Independent	Exercise only (not functional with orthoses); requires physical assist or guarding.	Knee/ankle/foot orthoses with forearm crutches or walker	As above	Independent
Independent	Independent	Independent	Independent	Potential for independent functional ambulation indoors with orthoses; some have potential for stairs using railing	Knee/ankle/foot orthoses on ankle/foot orthoses with forearm crutches	As above	Independent
Independent	Independent	Independent	Independent	Community ambulation: independent indoors and outdoors with orthoses	Ankle/foot orthoses with forearm crutches or canes	As above	Independent

garding the future therapy program must begin. Monitoring for changes in the neurological (sensorimotor) level is a part of daily routine. Changes in neurological status are documented.

Respiratory Care

Techniques that will assist in increasing vital capacity (deep breathing or use of incentive spirometry) and in maintaining good pulmonary hygiene must be used. Vibration, percussion, intermittent positive-pressure breathing (IPPB), and assisted cough techniques are used if appropriate. Because of the paralysis of the abdominals and the intercostal musculature in quadriplegia and high-level paraplegia, attention to respiratory capacity and maintaining a clear chest are paramount.

Prevention of Contractures

Proper positioning of the trunk and extremities will help prevent joint contractures and pressure sores. Use of rotating beds that have positioning troughs for the arms and legs are an aid for the quadriplegic patient. (See Chapter 23 for other details about positioning and range of motion exercises.) Shoulder positioning at 90° has been advised to decrease the later onset of shoulder pain.[171]

Training in Activities of Daily Living

Simple activity of daily living (ADL) tasks should be started while still in bed. Equipment such as touch pad call bells, prism glasses, page turners, and incline table trays may be helpful in quadriplegia to increase the patient's ability to read and/or watch television. Basic ADL devices might be recommended at this time to allow some self-care (e.g., Universal cuffs for eating, wash mitts for bathing). Suspension slings may be adapted to the overhead bar of the bed to support weakened arms to maximize the functional ability of the upper extremities.

Rehabilitation Phase

Progression to the upright position is usually managed by combination of elevating the head of bed and use of a reclining wheelchair with elevating leg rests. Once the upright position has been achieved, active programming begins with a thorough physical assessment, including evaluation of functional abilities, to identify areas on which intensive therapeutic interventions must be concentrated.

Goals based on the level of injury can be assumed until all factors altering the maximum goals are identified at team conference. A treatment plan is established with short-term goals set week to week to ensure that the discharge goals are appropriately met.

Essential early activities that should be addressed are provision of an appropriate wheelchair; establishment of a stable seating base for optimal reduction of pressure and spinal stability and proper total body alignment;[216] teaching of some wheelchair propulsion and selected management skills that will give the patient a sense of independence and control over his or her environment; and static thermoplastic splints to maintain and/or increase range, prevent deformity, protect and stabilize weakened joints, or maintain the proper musculoskeletal alignment. Splints regularly used include volar resting hand splint, dorsal wrist supports with web space straps, wrist cock-up splints, and long/short opponens. These splints may incorporate C-bars (to maintain the web space), and metacarpophalangeal extension stops when needed.

Treatment programming will depend on whether the injury is complete or incomplete, the extent to which the injury is incomplete, and whether stabilization devices interfere with performance of exercises or temporarily mandate the nonperformance of certain functional activities. Standard therapeutic approaches are used for the achievement of strength, range of motion, and endurance.

Biofeedback

Biofeedback involves the use of artificial sensors to provide an individual with information about motor or autonomic function (see Chap. 13). The greatest role of biofeedback in the management of SCI patients is as an adjunct to motor retraining.[79] Biofeedback may also be useful in the management of autonomic problems associated with SCI, such as orthostatic hypotension or uninhibited sweating.

Functional Electrical Stimulation

Electrical stimulation of muscle, either through nerve or through the muscle itself, can be used for therapeutic purposes (see Chap. 15). In SCI patients, it has two general uses: first as a means of avoiding some of the complications of muscle inactivity and second as a means of producing extremity motion for functional activities.

SCI predisposes to the development of deep venous thrombosis. Functional electrical stimulation of lower extremity muscle groups may be useful in lowering the risk. Osteoporosis develops, perhaps due in part to decreased stress from muscle contraction. This technique may be useful in producing muscle contraction. Maximal exercise capacity is lowered after SCI,[40] which results in cardiovascular deconditioning. Functional electrical stimulation can be used to provide a cardiovascular conditioning program.[151] The bulk of muscle, and its strength and endurance in response to the stimulation, can be increased by the stimulation.[67] This can be applied to totally paralyzed muscle after a complete injury or to weakened muscle after an incomplete injury.

Electrical stimulation can be used to produce extremity motion for functional activities, including ambulation. The best results are obtained in patients with incomplete lesions. The technique can then be used on a limited number of muscles where the patient may be deficient.[199] Ambulation by electrical stimulation in patients with complete thoracic level paraplegia is more problematic. If the electrical stimulation is to produce functional ambulation in such patients, it will be through the use of a computerized control system. Use of this treatment modality may improve ambulation in patients using a reciprocating gait orthosis.[56, 148]

Management of Overworked Upper Extremity Syndrome

Upper extremity complications occurring as a result of the excessive work performed by the arms of quadriplegic and paraplegic patients is a problem. An incidence of 51.4% of shoulder pain was reported in SCI patients surveyed by the Spinal Injuries Association of Great Britain.[141] In 42.6%, the pain was severe enough to interfere with sleep.

The magnitude of the problem may range from a mild, tolerable discomfort to a significant impairment of function. Often, there is a delay in the rehabilitation program or a refocusing of therapy time to address the problem.

Included in this overworked upper extremity syndrome is tendonitis, medial and lateral epicondylitis, bursitis, myofascial pain, compression neuropathies, and degenerative joint changes. With the exception of the latter two, these problems typically present during the initial rehabilitation admission.

Long-term upper extremity complications are also beginning to be recognized. Compression neuropathies have been noted to increase with the length of time from injury. In one study, there was a 27% incidence of carpal tunnel syndrome in a group of paraplegic patients who were seen 1 to 10 years after SCI; 54% in those 11 to 30 years after SCI; and 90% in those who were seen 31 or more years after SCI.[4] One report suggests, however, that these compression neuropathies may be present subclinically in a significant number of patients in the early postinjury rehabilitation phase as well.[208] Another study on long-term effects, reviewing the use of wheelchair and/or crutches in patients disabled for more than 5 years, revealed an incidence of hand and wrist pain of 48%, elbow pain of 32%, and shoulder pain of 38%.[11]

The treatment for these various maladies does not differ markedly from the treatment of similar problems in the neurologically intact patient. This includes therapeutic modalities, anti-inflammatory medication, and steroid injections.[22, 166] However, for most treatment protocols, rest of the extremity is an important feature. In the SCI population, this would typically mean a significant, if not total, decline in functional capacity. "Relative rest," therefore, becomes an important concept. By reducing the level of stress on the extremity, nonpainful function can be continued. At the same time, the condition is not being aggravated and is able to resolve.

Tendon Transfer

The opportunity to extend the quadriplegic patient's control over an additional joint, or to create active pinch and hand grasp, offers an array of functional possibilities. This is the goal of tendon transfers. It is important, however, to understand not only what can be achieved but also the requirements for the surgery, as well as the consequences and potential risks.

When considering a patient for tendon transfer, knowledge of the functional cord level alone is insufficient. A detailed examination to determine the specific motor strength of each upper extremity muscle is required. Additionally, the sensation of the hand with regard to two-point discrimination must be evaluated.[134] The classification presented in Table 32-5 is useful as a guideline for understanding and predicting the function that can be gained by a tendon transfer.[72]

Elbow extension can be effected by posterior deltoid transfer to the triceps using the tibialis anterior tendon or brachialis fascia graft, according to the procedure described by Moberg.[132] It is noteworthy that antigravity triceps gained via muscle transfer does not necessarily imply that the patient will be able to perform wheelchair pushups or body transfers independently. These activities require shoulder stabilization, which is provided by the trapezius, costal portion of the pectoralis major, and latissimus dorsi.[133] There typically is, however, an improvement in existing transfers, as well as improvement in one or more of the following: use of a wheelchair, bed mobility, feeding, and grooming.[45, 72, 132, 133, 153]

Wrist extension is obtained by transfer of the brachioradialis

Table 32-5
Prediction of Function After Tendon Transfer

Muscles Active	Function to Be Gained
Deltoid grade 4–5 Biceps 3+ or better	Elbow extension
Above, plus brachioradialis +/− weak wrist extensors	Elbow extension Wrist extension

Above muscles are good to
    normal +/− pronator teres
    grade 4 or better
	Elbow extension
	Lateral thumb pinch
	Active finger flexion

Above, plus triceps, P.T.
    flex or carpi radialis plus
    weak finger flexors/extensors
	Lateral thumb pinch
	    increases strength of
	    finger flexion

All intact except intrinsics	Lateral thumb pinch

(Adapted from Freehafer AA, Kelly CM, Pechham PH: Tendon transfer for the restoration of upper limb function after a cervical spinal cord injury. J Hand Surg [Am] 9:887–893, 1984)

to the wrist extensor. Later a thumb pinch can be gained by transferring an available muscle (*e.g.,* brachioradialis, pronator teres, or extensor carpi radialis longus to the flexor digitorum superficialis and rerouting this tendon through a tunnel at the distal edge of the flexor retinaculum to the abductor pollicis brevis.[195] Alternatively, the brachioradialis can be transferred directly to the flexor pollicis longus. Waters reported results using the brachioradialis to flexor pollicis longus transfer.[206]

Finger flexion is gained or augmented by transfer of an available forearm muscle (brachioradialis, pronator teres, or extensor carpi radialis longus) to the flexor digitorum profundus. This procedure is typically coupled with an opponensplasty to improve overall grasp. If the finger extensors are not strong enough, hand opening is accomplished by wrist flexion and extension tenodesis effect. Although quantification of the results of this procedure is not easily done, improvement in functioning ability of the hand is reported.[70, 72, 132, 133]

Other procedures for the upper extremity in the quadriplegic population include tenodeses and arthrodeses. Tenodesis of the flexor pollicis longus to the radius can help achieve a lateral thumb pinch in the absence of an active muscle available for transfer in a patient with satisfactory wrist extension.[133] Arthrodeses of the thumb interphalangeal and metacarpophalangeal joints will provide stability for an effective lateral pinch and prevent a collapse deformity in a patient with very supple joints.

If the patient does not have adequate sensation on the thumb pulp (1 to 1.2 cm on 2-point discrimination), then only one hand can be controlled visually at a time and, therefore, only one hand is considered for reconstructive surgery.[133]

The following are generally accepted as the requirements of the patient for successful tendon transfer surgery: waiting until at least 1 year after injury; stable neurological status; essentially full passive range of motion of the joints of the upper extremities; no severe spasticity involving that extremity; patient motivation; and clear understanding by the patient of the potential gains, consequences, and potential risks.

Typically only one extremity is done at a time—usually the dominant extremity; if both elbow extension and wrist–hand function are to be addressed, the elbow function is addressed first. Then, following healing and return to function of the elbow, the wrist–hand function is addressed. Typically, the return to function of the extremity is 3 months following each procedure (total is therefore a minimum of 6 months per extremity); if the brachioradialis is used for a transfer, the elbow must be stabilized by the triceps (if functioning), a splint, or posterior deltoid-to-triceps transfer (if needed, this procedure should be done first). The cost of the procedures and postoperative rehabilitation is another factor to be considered. In general, the benefits gained from the surgical procedure are small but can be significant to the patient. The great majority of patients who have had the tendon transfers performed report that they would go through the procedures again for the same benefits.[45, 133]

Range of Motion

For the paraplegic and quadriplegic there are specific joints at which having greater than normal or less than normal range is a distinct advantage. This is often referred to as selected stretch or selected tightness.

Selected stretch is necessary for straight leg range, which in the normal person is 80° to 90°. The range needed by these patients is 120°, to allow activities such as donning trousers, socks, shoes, and knee–ankle–foot orthoses, without producing overstretch and instability of the low back, which in turn results in sitting instabilities. When stretching the hamstrings, the low back should be in the locked position and the leg brought up either with the knee straight or with the hip flexed to 90° and above, and then the knee is extended.

Selected tightness is allowed to develop so that compensations for paralyzed musculature can be accomplished. At the C6 level with wrist extensor, tightness is allowed to develop in the long finger flexors, producing finger flexion (grasp) on wrist extension and finger opening with passive wrist flexion (tenodesis). In quadriplegia and high-level paraplegia, spinal tightening in the erect sitting position should be allowed to occur. Should the trunk musculature and ligament structures become lax, three negative effects could occur: (1) late kyphosis and/or scoliosis with resultant decrease in vital capacity; (2) sitting instability with possible compromise of upper extremity functioning or development of pressure sores; and (3) transfer problems due to the passive lengthening of the spinal column during the push-up phase of the transfer.[216] One caution in allowing back musculature tightness is to repeatedly assess and maintain rib cage flexibility so that vital capacity is not compromised.

Respiratory Function

Improvement of vital capacity and respiratory endurance is continued throughout the program. Once the patient is able to push the wheelchair, gym or hall laps or use of a commercially available wheelchair treadmill (see Appendix 32-1) are excellent ways to improve endurance and upper extremity strength. Because it is so difficult to cough and move secretions out of the lungs, assisted coughing techniques are taught.[3] Included are placing a pillow in the lap, folding arms across the lower rib cage and falling forward; wrapping a towel around the lower rib cage and pulling (sitting or supine—requires good grasp); compression of lower rib cage/epigastric region while supine by folding arms and sharply pressing inward. Family members or caregivers must also be trained in manual coughing techniques.

Hand Function

Maintenance of adequate range of motion is vital to increased hand function. Particular attention is given to the metacarpophalangeal joints, the proximal interphalangeal joints, and the web space. Care is taken to allow the finger flexors to develop the tightness needed for a functional tenodesis grasp.

In quadriplegia, much treatment time will be spent in maximizing hand function. An important factor is the presence of tenodesis action. Patients without active wrist extension may be taught how to use a manually operated ratchet wrist orthosis in order to achieve pinch. Powered prehension orthoses may also be considered.

Patients with active wrist extension are taught how to use tenodesis pinch and gravity-assisted active wrist flexion for release during functional tasks. Some of these patients use a wrist-driven orthosis that mechanically transfers the power of the wrist extensors to the fingers to achieve varying degrees of pinch.

These orthotic devices can be made using thermoplastic materials for temporary training purposes. The patient can practice using the specific device in various graded grasp-release activities. The patient's level of motivation and acceptance can be assessed. A permanent orthosis can then be fabricated from metal or a high temperature plastic.[95, 213]

There are several other devices that can be used in order to compensate for decreased hand function:

- Universal cuff: a leather or webbing cuff has a palm pouch that holds eating utensils, toothbrushes, razors, typing sticks, and so on.
- There are several commercially available writing devices that attach to the hand to stabilize a pen or pencil
- Built-up handles or cuff-type handles can be adapted to many hygiene, grooming, and household items.

In high-level quadriplegia, additional adaptive equipment is needed to aid in upper extremity functional mobility, particularly for prepositioning the weak shoulder musculature in preparation for functional use of the hand. Overhead suspension slings, counterbalance slings, and mobile arm supports are the most commonly used devices. Each device supports the upper extremity in a more functional position. The overhead sling and the counterbalance sling eliminate the force of gravity; the mobile arm supports allow gravity to assist the weakest muscles to move in one direction while the patient exerts his or her own muscle power to move to the opposite direction.[95, 194, 213]

Functional Mobility Training

Training for functional mobility activities (bed mobility, wheelchair propulsion and transfers) is carried out concomitantly with the general exercise program.[19, 65] Selection of which activities will be done independently, with supervision, or with assistance or which will be dependent is made in accordance with physical capacity projections. Some activity training may have to be postponed until the spinal stabilization device can be removed. Acquisition of these activities is accomplished via some basic principles:

1. Sequence the skill from simple to difficult.
2. Break the whole down into accomplishable units and then recombine units into the whole.
3. Use momentum, head motions, and muscle substitutions to augment weakened or absent muscles. For example, use swinging arms side to side to achieve rolling from supine to side-lying as a substitute for absent thoracic and abdominal musculature.
4. When possible, use the body weight as the resistance during exercise. Exercises will need to be done supine, side-lying, long-sitting, short-sitting, semi-reclining, and in the wheelchair.

5. Muscle groups should be exercised in the position in which they are used functionally.

If the patient will not be independent, training is given on two levels: (1) to the patient, who must be competent to instruct another person in the safe accomplishment of that particular activity, and (2) to the significant other, family members, or attendant who must offer assistance on a daily basis. Family involvement occurs as early in the rehabilitation phase as both patient and family are ready emotionally and physically.

A person with paraplegia can perform most grooming and hygiene tasks independently—in bed at first, then from the wheelchair. These independent tasks include hair brushing/combing, shaving, applying makeup, oral hygiene, nail care, and applying deodorant. Bathing is done from the bed initially, with assistance for the back, perineum, and lower extremities. The patient progresses to use of shower chairs and tub benches.

The patient becomes more independent in dressing skills as balance improves. Early on, lower extremity dressing may need to be performed with the use of adaptive equipment. The most frequently used equipment includes reachers, dressing sticks, adapted shoe laces or alternate closure system, and leg-lifting straps.

The issues of activities of daily living and adaptive equipment are especially significant when treating the quadriplegic patient owing to the varying degrees of involvement in the upper extremities and the resulting functional deficits. Mobility limitations are compensated for through the use of assistive devices.[95, 109, 147, 159, 162, 209]

The following are examples of various pieces of adaptive equipment:

FEEDING

- Universal cuffs
- Built-up utensil handles
- Long, flexible straws
- Angled utensils
- Scoop dishes

DRESSING

- Quad handle dressing sticks
- Loops on socks
- Zipper loops
- Button hooks with Universal cuff
- Velcro closures
- Leg ranging straps

GROOMING AND HYGIENE

- Cuff handles on razors and brushes
- Dispensers for toothpaste and deodorant
- Long self-inspection mirrors

BATHING

- Wash mitts
- Soap on rope
- Tub benches
- Hand-held shower
- Shower chairs
- Long-handled sponges

MOUTHSTICKS[75, 111, 183, 200]

- Static, with wooden or other lightweight shaft
- Dynamic, including tongue-activated pincer type

Homemaking and Community Skills

The ability to function independently in household and homemaking tasks is addressed near discharge. This may involve a combination of individual and group sessions. Areas discussed and practiced are meal preparation, food purchase, cooking, serving, laundry, house cleaning (*i.e.,* dusting, vacuuming), and making beds. At this time, other functional tasks such as use of the telephone and operating light switches, stereo, door locks, tape recorder, and similar items are practiced and adapted as needed. The need for any adaptions will be greater in the quadriplegic population because of the decreased upper extremity function.

In order to prepare the patient more adequately for reintegration into the community, many institutions have begun community skills groups. Typical outings include use of public transportation, accessing and using a shopping mall, going to movies, grocery shopping, banking and using automatic teller machines, going to health spas, and eating in restaurants.

Use of Wheelchair

Wheelchair prescription is a complex task. Whoever assumes this responsibility must have current knowledge of the models and brands available and the advantages and disadvantages of each. Each available model has different accessories that are either standard or optional. In prescribing the wheelchair, the input of the entire team is needed, including the patient and the insurance carrier. Some of the factors to be identified are how heavily it will be used; where it will be used; whether the insurance provider places an upper limit on money to be spent; whether the weight of the chair is a factor in propulsion/endurance; and whether the patient needs a special size, cushion, seating system, or propulsion system.

Once this information is gathered, selection of the chair by manufacturer, model, and accessories (frame, weight, upholstery, size specifications, arm rests, foot rest/leg rest assembly, wheels, tires, and rims) may be completed.[163] Proper prescription of a chair is critical not only to the patient's independence but also because of cost. In 1985, the average cost of a light metal alloy standard frame chair was $1,500, and the cost of an "ultra light" frame chair was $2,000. The cushion selected must be compatible with the type of chair and its dimensions.[3, 216]

For the person with high-level quadriplegia, powered wheelchairs may be the only functional mode of mobility. The type of control (hand control, sip 'n' puff, tongue control, mouthstick, head control) that is most easily accessed and comfortable for the patient must be selected. Usually, the patient will have an evaluation period with the recommended chair(s) before a final decision is reached.[122, 150]

Ambulation

Patients with complete SCI want to walk again. Many become so focused on walking that assumption of functional skills or resumption of life-style, vocation, or education in the community is deferred. There is controversy over whether and when a patient should be afforded the opportunity to be braced and attempt ambulation. One opinion is to try ambulation during the initial phase. Another is to complete initial rehabilitation at the wheelchair level, returning after several months of adjusting to life in the community when the patient will have a more realistic perspective. In any case, a trial training program with defined performance and a mutually agreed on level of ambulation may have advantages.

The trial ambulation program defines specific levels of ambulation; has defined graded performance criteria that need to be achieved before orthotic prescription is completed and is designed so that the patient has the opportunity to attempt performance of each sequentially; allows the therapist and physician to assess the effect of such factors as spasms, limitations in range of motion, spinal hypermobility, upper extremity strength, and general endurance; affords the patient the opportunity to exhibit that he or she has the motivation and perseverence to succeed in the activity; and allows the patient to assess the advantages and drawbacks of everyday brace donning and use.[3]

In most centers specializing in spinal cord management four levels of "ambulation" are identified:

1. Standing only (passive standing)
2. Therapeutic ambulation (walks for short distances with the assistance of another for any or all of the following: donning/removal of orthoses, sit-to-stand transfers, balance assist while ambulating, assistance from floor to chair, or standing after a fall). Patient uses ambulation for exercise only.
3. Indoor/functional ambulation. Patient walks full time in orthoses within the home, has the ability to don and remove orthoses and to transfer from sitting to standing from floor to chair or to stand independently, does not use wheelchair inside the home or at work or school, and uses wheelchair outdoors for extremely long distance mobility.
4. Community ambulation. Patient is completely independent at the ambulatory level and does not use the wheelchair at any time.[3]

These guidelines should be viewed as flexible. Orthotic prescription should be considered when there is a specific need or barrier in the environment, and the use of orthoses and ambulatory aids will resolve the problem. Orthoses have been successfully used for many patients who use a chair at all times except when access to an otherwise inaccessible part of the home, school, or office or a particular work/homemaking activity requires just standing or minimal ambulation.

Options for standing only include stand-up wheelchairs (Poirier, Vertecalibre, Levostand), power standing frames (Motostand, Standaid), and stationary frames (see Appendix 32-1). Options for knee–ankle–foot orthoses include the metal or metal/plastic conventional orthoses, Scott Craig metal orthoses, or the LSU reciprocal braces.[49] There have been no studies that prove that the reciprocal braces are more energy efficient than the Scott Craig. All bilateral knee–ankle–foot orthoses require about four times normal energy consumption.

Home Visits/Environmental Accessibility

Part of a comprehensive rehabilitation program involves the assessment of a newly injured person's home environment and the ability of the patient to function within that environment. Home visits are designed to check for accessibility, recommend modifications, assist patient and family in recognizing potential problems, gather specific information regarding home situation (*e.g.*, measurements), and test for functional skills within the home environment.

In making recommendations, the home visit team takes four basic areas into consideration: (1) patient's needs, (2) family's needs, (3) architectural needs/limitations, and (4) financial abilities (*e.g.*, insurance coverage). The process of solving identified problems is usually handled by discussion between family members, staff, the patient, and the insurance representative. The goal is to present both short- and long-term solutions

so as not to overwhelm or complicate the situation. Additionally, the team will try to make the recommendations as simple as possible.

Architectural adaptations that minimize barriers and improve access range from the simple to the complex and from the economical to the expensive. Simple adaptations include ramps and door widening, while the complex or expensive include wheelchair elevators, stairglides, remodeling of the bathroom to include a roll-in shower, or construction of an entirely accessible home.[201]

Adaptations should not be confined solely to the home environment. Adaptations to the school or work setting permit the resumption of a productive life-style.

Returning some measure of control over one's environment is a priority for the high-level quadriplegic patient. One way to restore control is through the use of an environmental control system (ECS). An ECS is a system of electronic components that remotely controls lights, telephones, sound equipment, television, radios, appliances, intercoms, doors, and other items that are powered electrically in a home and office. The systems available today vary greatly in cost and complexity.

The selection of the proper ECS depends on a number of factors, such as the physical abilities or specific limitations in strength and motion of the upper extremities and the head and neck; the physical as well as psychological needs of the patient; the environment to be controlled; the adaptability of the equipment; and their cost and the financial ability of the patient.

Switches for controlling the system include hand controls with specific modifications, mouthsticks, tongue switches, pneumatic switches and brow switches, and a rocking lever that can be operated with the head, hand, or foot.

Choices need to be made regarding the complexity of the system. Some patients require only a remote control unit, which is portable and operates without special wiring. This is most appropriate for patients needing only to control light switches and appliances. Other patients will need to operate special built-in telephones, electrical beds, televisions, window drapes, and doors. These units require complex electrical connections and are more costly and used on a more permanent basis.[57, 96, 104, 173, 203]

Driving Program

Both driving and being a passenger in an appropriate vehicle can be a major problem. There are driver education programs for the disabled. There is also the Association of Driver Educators for the Disabled, which conducts conferences for professionals.

Driving programs may be staffed by occupational or physical therapists. Ideally, a complete program consists of three parts. The pre-driving screening includes assessment of visual acuity, reaction response, field of vision, depth perception, color perception, visual accommodations, judgment, attention, problem solving, sequencing, memory, recognition of signs and symbols, number recognition, upper and lower extremity mobility skills, hand function, and transfer skills. The results of the evaluation will provide the basis for determining the patient's capabilities and specific needs for driving. A driving simulator can be used for parts of the evaluation.

Once the patient is deemed eligible, the next step is the selection of the appropriate vehicle with the necessary modifications or adaptive equipment. There is wide variety of such equipment commercially available, ranging from steering wheel attachments, power seats, console controls, and hand controls for gas and brake to completely converted vans with hydraulic lifts. In making these decisions, the professional takes into consideration the patient's goals and life-style, safety, and insurance coverage.

The final step is the behind-the-wheel training. This requires that the patient have a valid license or learner's permit.

Patients who are not yet ready to drive may receive an abbreviated evaluation aimed at determining the appropriate vehicle or equipment needed to be a passenger.[84, 93, 116, 156, 190]

Recreation/Leisure

Recreation and the constructive use of leisure time enhance one's quality of life. Each patient has both a need and a right to involvement in leisure activities as an integral part of a healthy life-style.

The use of leisure time is often perceived by the newly injured patient as a problem. The patient may see the mobility limitations as obstacles for returning to premorbid leisure activities. Thus, the overall program should include use of community recreational resources; learning of new leisure skills; adaptations for previous leisure skills and interest; and the refinement of functional abilities related to specific leisure activities. Community skills groups feature both discussions and reentry trips to develop the skills necessary to take an active role in recreational opportunities.

One area that has been receiving publicity is wheelchair sports for both recreational and competitive purposes. Wheelchair sports allow the SCI patient to increase his or her activity level, improve strength and endurance, and promote good health. Wheelchair sports also afford the opportunity to aggressively compete with people at the same functional level and provide an arena for excellence with athletic and physical achievement as well as the camaraderie and sportsmanship available to the able-bodied community. Examples of sports activities successfully participated in by SCI men and women include archery, boating, football, camping, hunting, flying, golf, scuba diving, swimming, basketball, table tennis, weight lifting, tennis, horseback riding, distance racing, track and field events, and sit skiing. Many sports and recreational activities that a person participated in before injury can be adapted for participation after injury. In some instances, the disabled can participate in and compete with their able-bodied counterparts. In addition to sports activities, some health spas and fitness centers have incorporated the needs of the disabled into their programs.

The participation in sports and a general fitness program is viewed by many as an expression of well-being and a step toward improved general health. Secondary gains include a more positive self-image, often resulting in better interpersonal relationships.

The learning of appropriate leisure skills and the incorporation of these activities into the individual's life-style will have long-lasting effects. A person who can use leisure time constructively and meaningfully is less likely to become depressed. As in all aspects of rehabilitation, the "choice" belongs to the patient. The SCI patient must take an active role in deciding what direction to take. The discovery and development of "quality" in his or her life-style has its beginning in the discovery that many sources of self-satisfaction and reintegration into society remain open.[2, 83]

Role of Computers

The technological advances in today's microcomputers, coupled with their availability, have a potential impact on the level of independent activity achievable by the quadriplegic population. Computers can be used for money management, word processing, leisure, and vocational activities. Many tasks previously difficult or impossible are made possible.

Most patients will be able to access the keyboard using handheld sticks or mouthsticks. Many of the higher-level quadriplegics will not be able to access the computer in the traditional manner through the keyboard. There are several adaptive interface systems to supply input, including scanning, Morse code, and direct selection.

The computer can be used as an adjunct to an environmental control system, thus increasing independence. It can also be used for working from the home or otherwise increasing a patient's vocational potential.[109, 127, 152]

PSYCHOSOCIAL AND VOCATIONAL ISSUES

Scientific and technological advances within the past 2 decades have significantly improved the survival rate and life expectancy for the SCI patient. However, attention to quality of life issues has lagged behind advances in quantity of life. The impact of this catastrophic injury will influence the patient and the family for a lifetime and be experienced in every aspect of the patient's life. The patient, family, and rehabilitation professionals share the responsibility for rebuilding a different life. This new life will obviously retain many aspects of the preinjury life, but new skills and new coping strategies must be incorporated.

Within the scope of this chapter, only a few of the key issues in this process of adaptation will be addressed: individual adjustment and family issues, independent living issues, and vocational issues. A behavioral analysis of the adjustment to disability, a discussion of the coping skills model of adjustment to disability, a critical analysis of the concept of stages of adjustment following disability, and more details about vocational rehabilitation are provided in Chapters 3 and 4.

Individual and Family Adjustment

A common misconception among lay persons and some rehabilitation professionals is that there exists a "second moment in time," when the patient "accepts" or "adjusts" to the disability. In fact, learning to live with a disability is a lifelong process.[129] Rehabilitation professionals are only beginning to explore the added impact of disability on the "normal" stages of adult development.[110, 184]

Although each person will respond according to his or her unique personality and life process, there are some common issues that confront the patient and family within the first years following injury. Perhaps one of the most significant early issues relates to loss of control and feelings of helplessness. The experience of hospitalization causes universal feelings of loss of control. The loss of control and helplessness extends to all areas of physical functioning, including bowel and bladder functions, tasks that we normally master at an early age. Strategies to minimize loss of control and the issues of denial and motivation are discussed in Chapter 3.

In evaluating the adjustment issues, consideration must also be given to the family and the patient's broader support system. In many respects, the entire family structure must adjust to the disability.[110] The impact on the family is not only emotional but also often physical and economical. The roles and responsibilities assumed by the person with the disability must be temporarily or permanently assumed by other family members. In addition, other responsibilities for the physical care of the disabled person may be assumed by family members. The family must be an integral part of any treatment program, not only to assist them to cope with the disability and their response to the disabled person but also to help them to deal with their own issues, increased responsibilities, and pressures.

Rehabilitation is primarily a learning process, for both the patient and the family. This learning process involves not only the physical skills but also the psychosocial skills that will enable the person to redefine a satisfying life-style and reintegrate into the home and community. The basic physical skills may be learned within the first several years following injury. The learning of psychosocial skills will continue throughout a lifetime.[198]

Independent Living

Although the patient must make certain adaptations and accommodations, these changes lose meaning unless society affords certain opportunities for reintegration into community life. The independent living movement, which gained momentum in the 1970s, started from the premise that the person with a disability should have the same life choices as the nondisabled person. The goal of this consumer movement is to expand choices in such basic areas as where to live, how to live, how to travel, and what recreational or social activities to pursue.[42]

The political activism of the disabled population, as well as a more enlightened attitude among some legislators, has brought about changes. The 1973 Rehabilitation Act and the subsequent 1978 amendments are examples. Debates in many major cities regarding the provision of accessible mass transportation is another. Some breakthroughs have occurred in the provision of affordable, accessible housing and in attendant care. Independent living centers are emerging and receiving some federal, state, and local funding. However, until attitudinal and architectural barriers are eliminated, the disabled person will continue to confront obstacles in the struggle to reintegrate into the community. Thus, the person with a disability must also master skills in system management and advocacy in order to reach the goal of independent living.

Vocational Issues

For many, the attainment of self-sufficiency and independence means a return to work or to training or education leading to return to work. The vocational process should begin early following injury, with the introduction of the work expectation and opportunity for return to work, when this is an appropriate goal.[6]

The vocational process must incorporate two parallel processes: one takes place with the person with the disability, while the second occurs within the business community. For the patient, the process needs to be multifaceted and flexible, allowing the person to enter at the point of need. The basic elements of that program process are as follows:

- Psychological testing, including interest and achievement
- Establishment of an initial vocational plan
- Vocational counseling
- Work evaluation, including standardized work samples
- Occupational and physical therapy assessment, including definition of functional skills and assessment of architectural barriers in the home environment
- Driver education and vehicle modification
- Educational remediation including general educational development (GED) and work-related academic skills
- Communication with state vocational rehabilitation agencies, insurance companies, and other sponsors
- Job analysis and job modification
- Job seeking skills
- Referral to specific training programs or educational institutions
- Involvement of a business advisory group
- Referral to job placement, including employer contacts
- Follow-up.[92]

Obviously, everyone does not require all components of service. However, owing to the severity of SCI and the average age at onset, many patients are faced with the need to both define and redefine vocational options and opportunities. Even an experienced worker with a salable, realistic job skill may need to learn new skills in résumé writing and interviewing to accommodate for the limitations imposed by the disability.

Education of and technical assistance to employers can be a powerful tool in enhancing vocational opportunities for people with disabilities. Many employers are unaware of the person's capabilities or are afraid and unsure of their ability to accommodate a disabled employee. Businesses are unsure of what adaptations may be needed to their physical plant and envision expensive and disruptive modifications. Other employers are reluctant to raise concerns about the physical capabilities and ability to perform certain job tasks. Supervisors may have difficulty in coping with disability-related issues and believe that they need to change standards to accommodate a disabled employee. Specific information may need to be transmitted, technical assistance offered, and myths and prejudices dispelled before an employer is comfortable with hiring a person with a disability. Business advisory groups and federally funded programs, such as Projects With Industry, have helped in opening dialogue between rehabilitation professioinals, disabled employees, and the business community. These efforts have greatly enhanced employment opportunities for the disabled.

THE OLDER SCI PATIENT

Some elderly patients in relatively good health at the time of their SCI have no more medical or psychological complications than previously healthy younger patients and can return to productive independent living. However, declining organ system function and preexisting disease make other patients susceptible to severe medical complications and prolongation of their rehabilitation course.[107]

Early mortality following SCI has been noted to be extremely high in the elderly. When compared with younger populations, elderly patients suffer a large proportion of cervical cord injuries, usually as a result of falls at home. High cervical cord injuries in the setting of declining cardiovascular and pulmonary reserve, atherosclerosis, or chronic obstructive or restrictive pulmonary disease may contribute to mortality. Elderly patients with severe chronic obstructive or restrictive pulmonary disease are also at high risk of prolonged ventilator dependence, poor pulmonary toilet, and pneumonia. Nutritional depletion is almost universal in the elderly, with the serum albumin level falling to low normal levels or below. If this depletion is untreated, delayed wound healing and impaired resistance to infection can result. Diverticulosis predisposes to lower gastrointestinal tract bleeding, while upper gastrointestinal tract bleeding from gastritis or ulcers occurs frequently. Chronic anemia tends to accompany severe pulmonary infection, gastrointestinal bleeding, and severe nutritional depletion and occurs frequently in this population.

Early rehabilitation of the elderly SCI patient can be impeded by many factors. Neurogenic bladder management can be affected by diseases common in the elderly such as diabetic neuropathy, chronic urinary tract infections, prostatic hypertrophy, pelvic floor laxity, and Parkinson's disease. Indwelling Foley catheterization may be favored over intermittent catheterization in patients with severe prostatic hypertrophy, until this can be surgically corrected.[191] Bowel training can be difficult with preexisting laxative abuse. Poor cardiorespiratory reserve will slow and limit endurance training and conditioning programs. Underlying depression and organic brain syndrome may make psychological adjustment to the disability difficult and may prevent attainment of full independence.

Preexisting health problems will complicate the long-term management of the superimposed SCI. Impaired sensation may alter symptoms of cardiac, gastrointestinal, neurological, and endocrine disease, making it more difficult for the patient, family, and health care providers to monitor medical problems. Dietary restrictions, medication regimens (including insulin injections), and other treatments for medical problems common in the elderly may add sufficiently to the complexity of care that the patient and family may be overwhelmed. The spouse and children may have medical problems that limit their physical ability to render care. Close medical and nursing follow-up after discharge is crucial to ensure that all problems are dealt with properly. For the patient who wishes to live alone, yet who needs substantial assistance, finding and training a primary caregiver is a major challenge. This needs to be initiated well before discharge from the rehabilitation facility. Similarly, it is desirable to locate a primary care physician in the patient's locality who is willing to assume responsibility for the day-to-day management of medical problems.

Community resources will often enable patients to return home. Attendant care, transportation, and homemaker services may be needed for the patient to remain at home. As with younger patients following discharge from rehabilitation, close follow-up by a visiting nurse will increase the likelihood of proper bowel, bladder, and skin care, as well as medication intake and patient and family adjustment to the disability. For patients requiring assistance or supervision who lack sufficient family or community support, nursing home placement may be inevitable, but this occurs surprisingly infrequently at the time of discharge from rehabilitation. If family members subsequently become physically ill or emotionally overwhelmed, or if community resources become unavailable, a crisis may occur that places the patient at serious risk for medical complications and may necessitate rehospitalization and nursing home placement.[108, 160, 192, 207]

DISCHARGE PLANNING

Discharge planning should begin at the time of entrance into the acute care system and continue through the in-hospital rehabilitation phase. The focus should be on providing for educational and adjustment needs of the patient and family unit. The educational elements include management of medical and functional needs, becoming expert in performing or directing needed care, recognizing when to seek medical attention, developing knowledge of equipment needs, and recognizing when to seek support for identified needs.

The first meeting with the patient and family may occur in the emergency department or a neurointensive care unit. Sufficient information should be obtained to permit the physician to initiate a discharge plan. The strengths and weaknesses of the family unit must be recognized. Throughout the acute care and rehabilitation phase, many discussions will be necessary to refine the discharge plan. Discharge to home represents only one component of discharge planning.

On initial examination, a diagnosis and medical and functional prognosis should be determined. Thorough knowledge and understanding of the functional significance of the level of spinal injury is necessary in order to estimate an expected outcome. Knowledge of spinal stability and anticipated orthopedic or neurosurgical interventions facilitates the planning for a rehabilitation program and aids in estimating the expected length of hospital stay. Medical needs should be estimated, as should the functional retraining and adaptive equipment needs. Prognosis for further neurological improvement can usually be estimated. A neurologically complete traumatic spinal injury, without motor or sensory improvement within 24 hours, is usually indicative of no further neurological change. Incomplete injuries may improve neurologically and functionally. The longer the time from injury, the less the likelihood for significant improvement.[17, 176] When the discharge date is determined, support systems should be identified and procured, including durable equipment, home modifications, patient/family teaching, transportation, and the family physician. The family physician and community agencies, such as nursing services, must be apprised of the patient's status and needs. Follow-up appointments should be a part of discharge planning.

SYSTEM OF CARE

SCI centers should provide a continuum of care from retrieval through lifetime follow-up. The SCI patient may require continuous monitoring and on-call medical services 24 hours per day. One model system sees patients 1 month after discharge, and then at 3 months, 6 months, and 12 months after discharge. Yearly visits are arranged thereafter.[174] The patient and family physician have access to the model system at all times for problems or questions. If the required intervention exceeds the resources of the family physician, the patient is readmitted into the model system to be returned home and to the care of the family physician when the acute problems are resolved.

Each follow-up visit should include evaluations by the physiatrist, nurse, and social workers. When indicated, the patient should also be seen by a physical therapist, occupational therapist, psychologist, rehabilitation counselor, vocational evaluator, or recreational therapist. In view of the medical problems and the medications that these patients require, periodic laboratory studies, in addition to a complete history and physical examination, should be performed. A complete blood count, urinalysis, urine culture and sensitivity, routine serum chemistries, creatinine clearance, cystogram, renal scan, cystometrogram, and cystoscopy may be needed periodically. The timing for the various studies will depend on patient status and clinical judgment. Occasionally, patients will require brief readmission to the hospital for reassessment of their medical and functional status and to update their management program. Scheduled follow-up visits serve primarily for problem identification. Problem solving frequently occurs during the interim between scheduled visits or on hospitalization.

Devices and Suppliers

Communitrach
Implant Technologies, Inc.
7900 West 78 Street
Minneapolis, Minnesota 55435

Levo Stand Up
American Stair Glide Corporation
4001 E. 138th Street
Grandview, Missouri 64030

Moto-Stand
Advanced Technology Corporation
P.O. Box 19142
Kansas City, Missouri 64141

Olympic Trach-Talk
Olympic Medical
4400 Seventh South
Seattle, Washington 98108

Portex, Inc.
42 Industrial Way
Wilmington, Massachusetts 01887

Stand Aid Power Lift
Aciveaid Distributors
501 E. Tin Street
Redwood Falls, Minnesota 56283

Venti-Voice
Bear Medical Systems, Inc.,
2085 Rustin Avenue
Riverside, California 92507

Verticalibre
Poirier S A
Usene des Roches—Fondettes
37230 Luynes, France

American Wheelchair Rollers
State Aluminum
P.O. Box 987
Paramount, California 90723

REFERENCES

1. Aaronson MJ, Freed MM, Burakoff R: Colonic myoelectric activity in persons with spinal cord injury. Dig Dis Sci 30:295–300, 1985
2. Adams RC, Daniel AN, Rullman L: Games, Sports, and Exercises for the Physically Handicapped. Philadelphia, Lea & Febiger, 1980
3. Adkins HV: Spinal Cord Injury. New York, Churchill Livingstone, 1985
4. Aljure J, Eltorai I, Bradley WE et al: Carpal tunnel syndrome in paraplegic patients. Paraplegia 23:182–186, 1985
5. Allen A: Surgery of experimental lesions of the spinal cord equivalent to crunch injury of fracture dislocation of the spinal column. JAMA 57:878–880, 1911
6. Athelstan GT: Vocational assessment and management. In Kottke FJ, Stillwell GK, Lehman JF (eds): Handbook of Physical Medicine and Rehabilitation, vol 8, pp 163–189. Philadelphia, WB Saunders, 1982
7. Baker BM: Communications Aids for the Ventilator Dependent Patient. Ear, Nose, Throat Journal 64(3–4) entire issue, 1985
8. Berlly MH, Wilmot CB: Acute abdominal emergencies during the first four weeks after spinal cord injury. Arch Phys Med Rehabil 65:687–690, 1984
9. Beukelman DR, Yorkston K: Communication options for patients with brain stem lesions. Arch Phys Med Rehabil 59:337–340, 1978
10. Beukelman DR, Yorkston K: Nonvocal communication performance evaluation. Arch Phys Med Rehabil 61:6, 1980
11. Blankstein A, Shmueli R, Weingarten I et al: Hand problems due to prolonged use of crutches and wheelchairs. Orthop Rev 14:735–740, 1985
12. Blom ED, Singer MI, Harkleroad BA: Self-activated pneumatic voicing system for ventilator dependent patients. Presented at the American Association for Respiratory Therapy Annual Convention and American Speech-Language Hearing Association Annual Convention, 1982
13. Bohlman HH: Surgical management of cervical spine fractures and dislocations. Instr Course Lect 34:163–187, 1985
14. Bohlman H: Indications for late anterior decompression and fusion for cervical spinal cord injuries. In Tator C (ed): Early Management of Acute Spinal Cord Injury, vol 27, pp 315–333. New York, Raven Press, 1982
15. Bohlman H: Late anterior decompression for spinal cord injury: Review of 131 patients with long-term results of neurologic recovery. Am Spinal Injury Assoc Abstr Dig, 205–208, 1986
16. Bors E, Conrad CA, Massell TB: Venous occlusion of lower extremities in paraplegic patients. Surg Gynecol Obstet 99:451–454, 1954
17. Bosch A, Stauffer ES, Nickel VL: Incomplete traumatic quadriplegia: A ten-year review. JAMA 216:473–478, 1971
18. Brenes F, LaPorte R, Shapera R, Landau P: Cardiovascular risk factors in spinal cord injury: Serum magnesium and lipoprotein cholesterol. Am Spinal Injury Assoc Abstr Dig, 1983
19. Bromley I: Tetraplegia and Paraplegia: A Guide for Physiotherapists, 2nd ed. Edinburgh, Churchill Livingstone, 1981
20. Brooke MM, Donovon WH, Stolov WC: Paraplegia: Succinylcholine-induced hyperkalemia and cardiac arrest. Arch Phys Med Rehabil 59:306–309, 1978
21. Brunnstrom's Clinical Kinesiology, 4th ed, rev. Lehmkuhl LD, Smith LK (eds). Philadelphia, FA Davis, 1983
22. Cailliet R: Soft tissue pain and disability. Philadelphia, FA Davis, 1977
23. Cardus D, McTaggart WG: Total body water and its distribution in men with spinal cord injury. Arch Phys Med Rehabil 65:509–512, 1984
24. Carey DE, Raisz LG: Calcitonin therapy in prolonged immobilization hypercalcemia. Arch Phys Med Rehabil 66:640–644, 1985
25. Carey ME, Nance FC, Kirgis HD et al: Pancreatitis following spinal cord injury. J Neurosurg 47:917–922, 1977
26. Chance G: Note on type of flexion fracture of the spine. Br J Radiol 21:452, 1948
27. Chantraine A, Minaire P: Para-osteo arthropathies. Scand J Rehabil Med 13:31–37, 1981
28. Chap TL, Price M: Survival from spinal cord injury. J Chronic Dis 35:487–492, 1982
29. Chen YT, Gershkoff AM: Lower extremity hemorrhage in spinal cord injured patients receiving therapeutic anticoagulation. Arch Phys Med Rehabil 65:263–266, 1984
30. Cherney LR, Cantieri CA, Pannell JJ: Clinical Evaluation of Dysphagia. Rockville, MD, Aspen, 1986
31. Cherney LR, Cantieri CA, Pannell JJ: GPB for high level quads. Rehabil Gazette 19:61–63, 1976
32. Claus-Walker J, Dunn CDR: Spinal cord injury and serum erythropoietin. Arch Phys Med Rehabil 65:370–374, 402, 1984
33. Claus-Walker J, Halstead LS: Metabolic and endocrine changes in spinal cord injury: The nervous system before and after transsection of the spinal cord. Arch Phys Med Rehabil 62:595–601, 1981
34. Claus-Walker J, Halstead LS: Metabolic and endocrine changes in spinal cord injury: Compounded neurologic dysfunctions. Arch Phys Med Rehabil 63:632–638, 1982
35. Claus-Walker J, Halstead LS: Metabolic and endocrine changes in spinal cord injury: Less quanta of sensory input plus bedrest and illness. Arch Phys Med Rehabil 63:628–631, 1982
36. Claus-Walker J, Halstead LS, Rodriquez GP, Henry YK: Spinal cord injury hypercalcemia: Therapeutic profile. Arch Phys Med Rehabil 63:108–115, 1982
37. Claus-Walker J, Spencer WA, Carter RE et al: Bone metabolism in quadriplegia: Dislocation between calciuria and hydroxy-prolinemia. Arch Phys Med Rehabil 56:327–332, 1975
38. Clough P: Glossopharyngeal breathing: Its application with a traumatic quadriplegic patient. Arch Phys Med Rehabil 64:384–385, 1983
39. Cooper P, Maravilla K, Sklar F et al: Halo immobilization of cervical spine fractures—indications and results. J Neurosurg 50:603–610, 1979
40. Coutts KD, Rhodes EC, McKenzie DC: Maximal exercise responses of tetraplegics and paraplegics. J Applied Physiol 55:479–482, 1983
41. Cox SAR, Weiss SM, Posuniak EA et al: Energy expenditure after spinal cord injury: An evaluation of stable rehabilitating patients. J Trauma 25:419–423, 1985

42. Crewe NM, Zola IK: Independent Living for Physically Disabled People. San Francisco, Jossey-Bass, 1983

43. Crutchfield W: Skeletal traction for dislocations of the cervical spine: Report of a case. South Surgeon 2:156–159, 1933

44. Damanski J: Heterotopic ossification in paraplegia. J Bone Joint Surg [Br] 43:286–299, 1961

45. DeBenedetti M: Restoration of elbow extension power in the tetraplegic patient using the Moberg techniques. J Hand Surg [Am] 4:86–89, 1979

46. Denis F: Spinal instability as defined by the three column spine concept in acute spinal trauma. Clin Orthop 189:65–76, 1984

47. DeVivo MJ, Fine PR, Maetz HM, Stover SL: Prevalence of spinal cord injury: A reestimation employing life table techniques. Arch Neurol 37:707–708, 1980

48. DiRocco P, Hashimoto A, Daskalovic I, Langbein E: Cardiopulmonary responses during arm work on land and in a water environment of nonambulatory spinal cord impaired individuals. Paraplegia 23:90–99, 1985

49. Douglas R, Larsens P, D'Ambrosia R, McCall R: LSU reciprocation – gait orthosis. Orthopedics 6/7: 834–839, 1983

50. Downey JA, Darling RC: Physiological Basis of Rehabilitation Medicine. Philadelphia, WB Saunders, 1971

51. Duckworth WC, Jallelpalli P, Solomon SS: Glucose intolerance in spinal cord injury. Arch Phys Med Rehabil 64:107–110, 1983

52. Dunn E, LeClair WE: How to reduce complications in treatment of cervical spine trauma. Instr Course Lect 34:155–162, 1985

53. Dunn H: Anterior stabilization of thoracolumbar injuries. Clin Orthop 189:116–124, 1984

54. Dworkin GE, Staas WE Jr: Post-traumatic syringomyelia. Arch Phys Med Rehabil 66:329–331, 1985

55. Editorial: Diphosphonates: Aimed in a chemical sense. Lancet 2: 1326–1328, 1981

56. Editorial: Paraplegic walking. Lancet 2: 1341, 1342, 1985

57. Efthimiou J, Gordon WA, Sell GH, Stratford C: Electronic assistive devices: Their impact on the quality of life of high level quadriplegic patients. Arch Phys Med Rehabil 62:131–134, 1981

58. Eichenholz S: Management of long bone fractures in paraplegic patients. J Bone Joint Surg [Am] 45:299–310, 1963

59. Eisenberg MG, Tierney DO: Changing demographic profile of the spinal cord injury population: Implications for health care support systems. Paraplegia 23:335–343, 1985

60. Epstein N, Hood DC, Ransohoff J: Gastrointestinal bleeding in patients with spinal cord trauma. J Neurosurg 54:16–20, 1981

61. Fairholm D, Turnbull I: Microangiographic study of experimental spinal cord injuries. J Neurosurg 36:277, 1971

62. Fealey RD, Szurszewski JH, Merritt JL, DiMagno EP: Effect of traumatic spinal cord transection on human upper gastrointestinal motility and gastric emptying. Gastroenterology 87:69–75, 1984

63. Ferguson R, Allen BL Jr: A mechanistic classification of thoracolumbar spine fractures. Clin Orthop 189:77–78, 1984

64. Flinn WR, Peterson LK, Harris JP et al: Recognition and prevention of deep venous thrombosis in acute spinal cord injured patients. Am Spinal Injury Assoc Abstr Dig, 61–62, 1981

65. Ford JR, Duckworth B: Physical Management for the Quadriplegic Patient. Philadelphia, FA Davis, 1974

66. Forrest L, Cohen P, Staas W: Recurrent ischial decubitus ulceration and underlying heterotopic ossification as a late complication of spinal cord injury (abstr). Arch Phys Med Rehabil 66:536, 1985

67. Fournier A, Goldberg M, Green B et al: A medical evaluation of the effects of computer assisted muscle stimulation in paraplegic patients. Orthopedics 7:1129–1133, 1984

68. Frankel HL, Mathia CJ, Spalding JMK: Mechanisms of reflex cardiac arrest in tetraplegic patients. Lancet 2:1183–1185, 1975

69. Freed JH, Hahn H, Menter R, Dillon T: The use of the three-phase bone scan in the early diagnosis of heterotopic ossification and in the evaluation of Didronel therapy. Paraplegia 20:208–216, 1982

70. Freehafer AA: Tendon transfers to improve grasp in patients with cervical spinal cord injury. Paraplegia 13:15–21, 1975

71. Freehafer AA, Hazel CM, Becker CL: Lower extremity fractures in patients with spinal cord injury. Paraplegia 19:367–372, 1981

72. Freehafer AA, Kelly CM, Pechham PH: Tendon transfer for the restoration of upper limb function after a cervical spinal cord injury. J Hand Surg [Am] 9:887–893, 1984

73. Freehafer AA, Mast W: Lower extremity fractures in patients with spinal cord injury. J Bone Joint Surg [Am] 47:683–694, 1965

74. Freehafer AA, Yurish R, Mast WA: Para-articular ossification in spinal cord injury. Med Serv J Can 22:471–478, 1966

75. Garcia S, Greenfield J: Dynamic protractible mouthstick. Am J Occup Ther 35:529–530, 1981

76. Garland DE, Rieser TV, Singer DI: Treatment of femoral shaft fractures associated with acute spinal cord injuries. Clin Orthop 197:191–195, 1985

77. Gelman A, Betz R, DeFilipp G, Mesgarzadek M: Magnetic resonance imaging in evaluation of spinal cord injured children. Am Spinal Injury Assoc Abstr Dig, 45–58, 1986

78. Glick ME, Meshkinpour H, Haldeman S et al: Colonic dysfunction in patients with thoracic spinal cord injury. Gastroenterology 86:287–294, 1984

79. Goldsmith MF: Computerized biofeedback training aids in spinal injury rehabilitation. JAMA 253:1097–1099, 1985

80. Green D, Rossi EC, Yao JS et al: Deep vein thrombosis in spinal cord injury: Effect of prophylaxis with calf compression, aspirin, and dipyridamole. Paraplegia 20:227–234, 1982

81. Griffin MR, Opitz JL, Kurland LT et al: Traumatic spinal cord injury in Minnesota, 1935–1981. Am J Epidemiol 121:884–895, 1985

82. Groher ME: Dysphagia: Diagnosis and Management. New York, Butterworth, 1984

83. Gunn SL, Peterson CA: Therapeutic Recreation Program Design, Principles, and Procedures, Englewood Cliffs, NJ, Prentice-Hall, 1981

84. Gurgold GD, Harden DH: Assessing the driving potential of the handicapped. Am J Occup Ther 32:41–46, 1978

85. Guttman L: Spinal Cord Injuries—Comprehensive Management and Research, 2nd ed, pp 137–141. Boston, Blackwell Scientific Publications, 1976

86. Guttman L: Spinal Cord Injuries—Comprehensive Management and Research, 2nd ed, pp 565–571. Boston, Blackwell Scientific Publications, 1976

87. Hackler RH: A 25-year prospective mortality study in the spinal cord injured patient: Comparison with the long-term living paraplegic. Urology 117:486–488, 1977

88. Hansebout R: A comprehensive review of methods of improving cord recovery after acute spinal cord injury. In Tator C (ed): Seminars in Neurological Surgery—Early Management of Acute Spinal Cord Injury, pp 181–196. New York, Raven Press, 1982

89. Hardy S, Dickson J: Pathologic ossification in traumatic paraplegia. J Bone Joint Surg [Br] 45:76–87, 1963

90. Hassard GH: Heterotopic bone formation about the hip and unilateral decubitus ulcers in spinal cord injury. Arch Phys Med Rehabil 56:355–358, 1975

91. Heppenstall R: Fractures and dislocations of the cervical spine. In Heppenstall R (ed): Fracture Treatment and Healing, Chap 13, pp 292^330. Philadelphia, WB Saunders, 1980

92. Hirschwald JF, Sullivan DC, Ditunno JF: The vocational process—one center's approach. Spinal Cord Injury Digest, 3(1):3–10, 1981

93. Hogan HA: A simulator for objectively evaluating prospective drivers of the Scott Van. Bull Prosthet Res 10-37:19–27, 1982

94. Holdsworth F: Fractures, dislocations, and fracture-dislocations of the spine. J Bone Joint Surg [Am] 52:1534–1551, 1970

95. Hopkins H, Smith HD: Willard & Spackman's Occupational Therapy, 6th ed, pp 407–425. Philadelphia, JB Lippincott, 1983

96. Institute of Rehabilitation Medicine, NY University Medical Center: Environmental Control Systems and Vocational Aids for Persons with High Level Quadriplegia, rehabilitation monograph #55. New York, 1979

97. James WS, Minh VD, Minteer MA, Moser KM: Cervical accessory respiratory muscle function in a patient with a high cervical cord lesion. Chest 71:59–64, 1977

98. Jefferson G: Fracture of the atlas vertebra: Report of four cases and a review of those previously reported. Br J Surg 20:407–422, 1920

99. Juler GL, Eltorai IM: The acute abdomen in spinal cord injury patients. Paraplegia 23:118–123, 1985

100. Kaplan PE, Roden W, Gilbert E et al: Reduction of hypercalciuria in tetraplegia after weight-bearing and strengthening exercises. Paraplegia 19:289–293, 1981

101. Kaufman HH, Rowlands BJ, Stein DK et al: General metabolism in

patients with acute paraplegia and quadriplegia. Neurosurgery 16:309–313, 1985

102. Kay MM, Kranz JM: External transcutaneous pacemaker for profound bradycardia associated with spinal cord trauma. Surg Neurol 22:344–346, 1984

103. Kewalramani LS: Neurogenic gastroduodenal ulceration and bleeding associated with spinal cord injuries. J Trauma 19:259–265, 1979

104. Klause G: Telephone set and environmental control center: VITAL aids disabled people at home and in medical centers. Int J Rehabil Res 3:205–214, 1980

105. Kluin KJ, Maynard F, Bogdasarian RS: The patient requiring mechanical ventilatory support: Use of the cuffed tracheostomy "talk" tube to establish phonotron. Otolaryingol Head Neck Surg 96:625–627, 1984

106. Kostuik J: Anterior fixation for fractures of the thoracic and lumbar spine with or without neurologic involvement. Clin Orthop 109:103–115, 1984

107. Kraus JF, Franti CE, Borhani NO, Riggins RS: Survival with an acute spinal cord injury. J Chronic Dis 32:269–283, 1979

108. Kurtzke JF: Epidemiology of spinal cord injury. Exp Neurol 48:163–236, 1975

109. Lathem PA, Gregorio TL, Garber SL: High level quadriplegia: An occupational therapy challenge. Am J Occup Ther 39:705–714, 1985

110. LeBarron S, Currie D, Zeltzer L: Coping with spinal cord injury in adolescents. In Blum RW (ed): Chronic Illness and Disabilities in Childhood and Adolescents, pp 277–297. New York, Grune & Stratton, 1984

111. Lee KL, Price TL: The mouthstick: An extra-oral attachment for tetraplegic patients. Dent Tech 38:14–16, 18, 1985

112. Leramo OB, Tator CH, Hudson AR: Massive gastroduodenal hemorrhage and perforation in acute spinal cord injury. Surg Neurol 17:186–190, 1982

113. Levine AM, Krebs M, Santos-Mendoza N: External fixation in quadriplegia. Clin Orthop 184:169–172, 1984

114. Levy W, York D: Motor evoked potentials in the evaluation of spinal cord injury. Am Spinal Injury Assoc Abstr Dig, 175–177, 1986

115. Logemann J: Evaluation and Treatment of Swallowing Disorders. San Diego, College Hall Press, 1983

116. Long C: The handicapped driver—a national symposium. J Rehabil 40:34–39, 1974

117. Mathias CJ: Bradycardia and cardiac arrest during tracheal suction: Mechanisms in tetraplegic patients. Eur J Intensive Care Med 2:147–156, 1976

118. Maynard FM: Immobilization hypercalcemia following spinal cord injury. Arch Phys Med Rehabil 67:41–44, 1986

119. Maynard FM: Post-traumatic cystic myelopathy in motor incomplete quadriplegia presenting as progressive orthostasis. Arch Phys Med Rehabil 65:30–32, 1984

120. McAfee PC, Yuan HA, Fredrickson BE, Lubicky JP: The value of computed tomography in thoracolumbar fractures. J Bone Joint Surg [Am] 65:461–473, 1983

121. McCormick G: Modifying the Aurex Neovox Electrolarynx for use by paralyzed/voiceless patients. J Pa Speech Lang Hearing Assoc 17:6–8, 1984

122. McCoy G, Hollings EM, Nichols PJR: Problems of Living on Wheels in Wheelchairs and Outdoor Transport. Wilshere ER et al (eds). London, National Fund for Crippling Diseases, 1971

123. McDonald ET, Schultz AR: Communication boards for cerebral palsied children. J Speech Hear Disord 38:73–88, 1973

124. McMaster W, Stauffer E: The management of long bone fracture in the spinal cord injury patient. Clin Orthop 112:44–52, 1975

125. McMichan JC, Michel L, Westbrook PR: Pulmonary dysfunction following traumatic quadriplegia. JAMA 243:528–531, 1980

126. McVeigh J: Experimental cord crushes with special reference to the mechanical factors involved and subsequent changes in the areas of the cord affected. Arch Surg 7:573–600, 1923

127. McWilliams P: Computers for the Disablaed. Los Angeles, Prelude Press, 1984

128. Melzack R, Loeser JD: Phantom body pain in paraplegics: Evidence for a central "pattern generating mechanism" for pain. Pain 4:195–210, 1978

129. Merli GJ, McElwain GE, Adler AG et al: Immobilization hypercalcemia in acute spinal cord injury treated with etidronate. Arch Intern Med 144:1286–1288, 1984

130. Meshkinpour H, Nowroozi F, Glick ME: Colonic compliance in patients with spinal cord injury. Arch Phys Med Rehabil 64:111–112, 1983

131. Miller F, Fenzi TC: Prolonged ileus with acute spinal cord injury responding to metaclopramide. Paraplegia 19:43–45, 1981

132. Moberg E: Surgical treatment for absent single-hand grip and elbow extension in quadriplegia: Principles and preliminary experience. J Bone Joint Surg [Am] 57:196–206, 1975

133. Moberg E: The Upper Limb in Tetraplegia. New York, Thieme Stratton, 1978

134. Moberg E, Freehafer A, Lamb D et al: International Federation of Societies for Surgery of the Hand: A report from the Committee on Spinal Cord Injuries 1980. Scand Rehabil Med 14:3–5, 1982

135. Mollinger LA, Spurr GB, el Ghatit AZ et al: Daily energy expenditure and basal metabolic rates of patients with spinal cord injury. Arch Phys Med Rehabil 66:420–426, 1985

136. Mouradian WH, Fietti VG Jr, Cochran GV et al: Fractures of the odontoid: A laboratory and clinical study of mechanisms. Orthop Clin North Am 9:985–1001, 1978

137. Murray PK, Kusior MF: Epidemiology of nontraumatic and traumatic spinal cord injury. Arch Phys Med Rehabil 65:634, 1984

138. Naftchi NE, Viau AT, Sell GH, Lowman EW: Pituitary-testicular axis dysfunction in spinal cord injury. Arch Phys Med Rehabil 61:402–405, 1980

139. Nance PW, Shears AH, Givner ML, Nance DM: Gonadal regulation in men with flaccid paraplegia. Arch Phys Med Rehabil 66:757–759, 1985

140. Naso F: Pulmonary embolism in acute spinal cord injury. Arch Phys Med Rehabil 55:275–278, 1974

141. Nicholas P, Norman P, Ennis J: Wheelchair users' shoulder. Scand J Rehabil Med 11:29–32, 1979

142. Northrup B, Alderman J: Non-surgical treatment. In The Cervical Spine, pp 298–305. Philadelphia, JB Lippincott, 1983

143. Nottage W: A review of long bone fractures in patients with spinal cord injuries. Clin Orthop 155:65–70, 1981

144. Orzel JA, Rudd TG, Nelp WB: Heterotopic bone formation (myositis ossificans) and lower extremity swelling mimicking deep venous disease. J Nucl Med 25:1105–1107, 1984

145. Osterholm JL, Matthews GJ: Altered norepinephrine metabolism following experimental spinal cord injury: I. Relationship to hemorrhagic necrosis and post-wounding neurological deficits. J Neurosurg 36:386–394, 1972

146. Ostrowski K, Wlodanski K: Induction of heterotopic bone formation. In Bourne G (ed): Biochemistry and Physiology of Bone, vol III, p 299. New York, Academic Press, 1971

147. O'Sullivan SB, Culler KE, Schmitz TZ: Physical Rehabilitation: Evaluation and Treatment Procedures. Philadelphia, FA Davis, 1981

148. Patrick JH, McClelland MR: Low energy cost reciprocal walking for the adult paraplegic. Paraplegia 23:113–117, 1985

149. Perry J, Nickel V: Total cervical spine fusion for neck paralysis. J Bone Joint Surg [Am] 41:37–60, 1959

150. Pezenik D, Bennethum E, Butler C: Power Wheelchairs: When, How, Why. Camarillo, CA, Everest & Jennings, 1984

151. Phillips CA, Petrofsky JS, Hendershot DM, Stafford D: Functional electrical exercise. Orthopedics 7:1112–1123, 1984

152. Platt H (ed): Equipment for the Disabled: Communication. Horsham, England, National Fund for Research into Crippling Diseases, 1972

153. Raczka R: Posterior deltoid to triceps transfer: A review of the experience at Rancho Los Amigos Hospital. Paraplegia 22:45–54, 1984

154. Ragnarsson KT, Sell GH: Lower extremity fractures after spinal cord injury: A retrospective study. Arch Phys Med Rehabil 62:418–423, 1981

155. Ramos M: Recurrent superior mesenteric artery syndrome in a quadriplegic patient. Arch Phys Med Rehabil 56:86–88, 1975

156. Reger SI, McGloin AT, Law DF et al: Aid for training and evaluation of handicapped drivers. Bull Prosthet Res 10-36:35–39, 1981

157. Riggins RS, Kraus JF: The risk of neurologic damage with fractures of the vertebrae. J Trauma 17:126–133, 1977

158. Roaf R: A study of the mechanics of spinal injuries. J Bone Joint Surg [Br] 42:810–823, 1960

159. Rogers JC, Figone JJ: Traumatic quadriplegia: Follow-up study of self-care skills. Arch Phys Med Rehabil 61:316–321, 1961

160. Rogers L: Radiology of skeletal trauma. In Rothman RH (ed): The Spine, p 273. Philadelphia, WB Saunders Co, 1982

161. Rossi EC, Green D, Rosen JS et al: Sequential changes in factor VIII and platelets preceding deep vein thrombosis in patients with spinal cord injury. Br J Haematol 45:143–151, 1980

162. Runge M: Self-dressing techniques for patients with spinal cord injury. Am J Occup Ther 21:367–375, 1967

163. Ditunno JF: Current therapy in physiatry. In Ruskin AP (ed): Physical Medicine and Rehabilitation. Philadelphia, WB Saunders, 1984

164. Safer P, Grenvik A: Speaking cuffed tracheostomy tube. Crit Care Med 3:23–26, 1975

165. Salmon SJ, Goldstein LP: The Artificial Larynx Handbook. New York, Grune & Stratton, 1978

166. Scheon R, Moskowitz R, Goldberg V: Soft Tissue Rheumatic Pain: Recognition, Management, Prevention. Philadelphia, Lea & Febiger, 1982

167. Schiefelbusch RL: Non Speech Language and Communications: Analysis and Intervention. Austin, TX, Pro Ed, 1980

168. Schneider R, Cherry G, Pantek H: The syndrome of acute central cervical spinal cord injury. Neurosurgery 11:546–577, 1954

169. Schneider R, Kahn E: Chronic neurologic sequelae of acute trauma to the spine and spinal cord: I. The significance of acute flexion or "tear-drop" fracture: Dislocation of the cervical spine. J Bone Joint Surg [Am] 38:985–997, 1956

170. Schneider R, Livingston K, Cave A, Hamilton G: Hangman's fracture of the cervical spine. Neurosurgery 22:141–154, 1965

171. Scott JA, Donovan WH: The prevention of shoulder pain and contracture in the acute tetraplegic patient. Paraplegia 19:313–319, 1981

172. Segal JL, Gray DR, Gordon SK et al: Gentamicin disposition kinetics in humans with spinal cord injury. Paraplegia 23:47–55, 1985

173. Sell GH, Stratford CD, Zimmerman ME et al: Environmental systems for high level quadriplegic patients: Evaluation and prescription. Arch Phys Med Rehabil 60:246–252, 1979

174. Staas WE, Section V: Spinal cord. In Ruskin AP (ed): Current Therapy in Physiatry, pp 378–456. Philadelphia, WB Saunders, 1983

175. Ditunno JF, Roberts JD, Jacobs SR, Naso F et al: Standards for Neurological Classification of Spinal Injury Patients. Chicago, American Spinal Injury Association, 1982

176. Stauffer ES: Diagnosis and prognosis of acute cervical spinal cord injury. Clin Orthop 112:9–15, 1975

177. Steel H: Anatomical and mechanical considerations of the atlantoaxial articulation. Proceedings of the American Orthopedic Association. J Bone Joint Surg [Am] 50:1481–1482, 1968

178. Stewart AF, Adler M, Byers CM et al: Calcium homeostasis in immobilization: An example of resorptive hypercalciuria. N Engl J Med 306:1136–1140, 1982

179. Stover S: Personal communication, 1985

180. Stover SL, Hahn HR, Miller JM III: Disodium etidronate in the prevention of heterotopic ossification following spinal cord injury (preliminary report). Paraplegia 14:146–156, 1976

181. Stover SL, Hataway CJ, Zerger HE: Heterotopic ossification in spinal cord impaired patients. Arch Phys Med Rehabil 56:199–204, 1975

182. Stover SL, Neimann KM, Miller JM III: Disodium etidronate in the prevention of post-operative recurrence of heterotopic ossification in spinal cord injury patients. J Bone Joint Surg [Am] 58:683–688, 1976

183. Stow RW: Grasping mouthstick. Arch Phys Med Rehabil 47:31–33, 1966

184. Strax TE, Wolfson SD: Life cycle crisis of the disabled adolescent and young adult: Implications for public policy. In Blum RW (ed): Chronic Illness and Disabilities in Childhood and Adolescence, pp 47–57. New York, Grune & Stratton, 1984

185. Sugarman B: Fever in recently injured quadriplegic persons. Arch Phys Med Rehabil 63:639–640, 1982

186. Sugarman B: Osteomyelitis in spinal cord injury. Arch Phys Med Rehabil 65:132–134, 1984

187. Sugarman B: Infection and pressure sores. Arch Phys Med Rehabil 66:177–179, 1985

188. Sugarman B, Brown D, Musher D: Fever and infection in spinal cord injury patients. JAMA 248:66–70, 1982

189. Summers J: The use of the electrolarynx in patients with temporary tracheostomies. J Speech Hear Discord 38:335–338, 1973

190. Szeto AY, Hogan HA, Pierce S: Handicapped drivers evaluation and training. Am Rehabil 7:18–25, 1982

191. Tarabulcy E: Neurogenic diseases of the bladder in the geriatric population. Geriatrics 29:123–138, 1974

192. Tator CH, Edmonds VE: Acute spinal cord injury: Analysis of epidemiologic factors. Can J Surg 22:575–578, 1979

193. Tator C, Ekong C, Rowed D et al: Halo devices for the treatment of acute cervical spinal cord injury. In Tator C (ed): Early Management of Acute Spinal Cord Injury. New York, Raven Press, 1982

194. Thenn JE: Mobile Arm Supports. Northern Calif OT Association, 1975

195. Thompson T: Modified operation for opponens paralysis: J Bone Joint Surg [Am] 24:632–640, 1942

196. Tobey RE: Paraplegia, succinylcholine, and cardiac arrest. Anesthesiology 32:359–364, 1970

197. Todd JW, Frisbie JH, Rossier AB et al: Deep venous thrombosis in acute spinal cord injury: A comparison of ^{125}I fibrinogen leg scanning, impedance plethysmography and venography. Paraplegia 14:50–57, 1976

198. Trieschmann RB: The Psychological, Social, and Vocational Adjustment to Spinal Cord Injury: A Strategy for Future Research. Washington, DC, Rehabilitation Administration Publication, 1978

199. Turk R, Obreza P: Functional electrical stimulation as an orthotic means for the rehabilitation of paraplegic patients. Paraplegia 23:344–348, 1985

200. Turner C, Bennett CG: A simple mouthstick prosthesis for a quadriplegic patient. Spec Care Dentist 5:178–179, 1985

201. Uniform Federal Accessibility Standards: Federal Register: General Services Administration, Department of Housing and Urban Development, 1984

202. Vanderheiden GC, Grilley K: Non-vocal Communication Techniques and Aids for the Severely Physically Handicapped. Baltimore, University Park Press, 1976

203. Vanderheiden GC, Thompson CJ (eds): Rehabilitation Aids Resource Book. Ft. Collins, CO, Basic Telecommunications Corp, 1981

204. Van Hanswyk E, Yuan H, Eckhardt W: Orthotic management of thoracolumbar spine fractures with a total contact TLSO. Orthot Prosthet 33:10–19, 1979

205. Venier LH, Ditunno JF Jr: Heterotopic ossification in the paraplegic patient. Arch Phys Med Rehabil 52:475–479, 1971

206. Waters R, Moore KR, Graboff SR, Paris K: Brachioradialis to flexor pollicis longus tendon transfer for active lateral pinch in the tetraplegic. J Hand Surg [Am] 10:385–391, 1985

207. Watson N: Pattern of spinal cord injury in the elderly. Paraplegia 14:36–40, 1976

208. Weiss M: Subclinical median and ulnar nerve compression neuropathy in acute paraplegia. Am Spinal Injury Assoc Abstr Dig, 316, 1983

209. Welch RD, Lobley SJ, O'Sullivan SB, Freed MM: Functional independence in quadriplegia: Critical levels. Arch Phys Med Rehabil 67:235–240, 1986

210. Wharton GW, Morgan TH: Ankylosis in the paralyzed patient. J Bone Joint Surg [Am] 52:105–112, 1970

211. White R: Pathology of spinal cord injury in experimental lesions. Clin Orthop 112:16–26, 1975

212. White R, Albin M, Harris LS, Yashon D: Spinal cord injury: Sequential morphology and hypothermic stabilization. Surg Forum 20:432–434, 1969

213. Wilson DJ, McKenzie MW, Barber LM, Watson KL: Spinal cord injury: A treatment guide for occupational therapist, rev ed. Thorofare, NJ, Slack, 1984

214. Wood CA, Riddle J, Reed R, Paul C: Letter: Quadriplegia, orthostatic hypotension, and phenelzine with tyramine. Ann Intern Med 103:803–804, 1985

215. Young JS, Burns PE, Bowen AM, McCutchen R: Spinal cord injury statistics: Experience of the Regional Spinal Cord Injury Systems. Phoenix, AZ, Good Samaritan Medical Center, 1982

216. Zacharkow D: Wheelchair Posture and Pressure Sores. Springfield, IL, Charles C Thomas, 1984

33

Rehabilitation of the Cancer Patient

David Hirsh

Martin Grabois

Norman Decker

No one who is practicing medicine needs to be reminded of the significant incidence of cancer, the increasing remission and cure rate, or the functional and psychosocial problems seen in patients with cancer. The estimated incidence of cancer is 315 per 100,000 population, or 675,000 people a year in the United States, with an estimated survival rate of at least 34%, or 229,000.[25, 37, 39, 45] There are one million people in the United States currently under active treatment for cancer and approximately 1.5 million considered cured.[77] In all of these patients, the cancer and its necessary therapeutic intervention often produce significant long-term or permanent functional loss, requiring rehabilitation to return the individual to functional independence and improve his or her quality of life.

As in other areas of physical medicine and rehabilitation, the goal in treating cancer patients is to reach their fullest physical, psychological, social, vocational, avocational, and educational potential.[25] These goals must be realistic and consistent with physiological and environmental limitations. Due consideration needs to be given to the affected anatomical site, histology, stage of cancer, treatment used, possible metastases, patient age, and treatment in establishing goals.[25] Because of the large number of problems in patients with cancer, an interdisciplinary comprehensive approach with the health care professionals, using both their technical and psychological skills, is necessary in order to achieve optimal results.[48] Preventive as well as definitive rehabilitation therapy is necessary to reduce the degree of disability and the time needed to reach optimal functional goals.[26]

Dietz notes that therapeutic goals need to be established as early as possible and suggests three categories: restorative, supportive, and palliative.[26] The restorative category envisions a patient returning to premorbid status without remarkable residual handicap. Supportive implies the patient can expect to eliminate as much disability as possible by proper training and treatment, and palliative envisions a patient with increasing disability from progressive disease and an associated decrease in functional capacity, but who will, with appropriate provision of treatment, eliminate or reduce some of the potential complications.

CANCER REHABILITATION PROGRAMS

The development of cancer rehabilitation programs has been very slow. In 1965 the United States Congress passed the Regional Medical Program, which emphasized heart disease, can-

cer, and stroke.[37] Although significant activities were noted in the vocational rehabilitation of heart disease and stroke, few patients with cancer benefited.[37] The National Cancer Act of 1971 placed additional emphasis on cancer rehabilitation with funds to be used in the development of training, demonstration, and research projects in rehabilitation.[37] Despite this increased legislative emphasis and despite the demonstrated need for and benefit from programs in cancer rehabilitation, they still have not reached their optimum in quality and quantity. However, John Healey noted recent success in terms of the increased number of cancer rehabilitation programs.[38]

R. Lee Clark in 1967 noted that formidable barriers would need to be broken down to implement a rehabilitation program for patients with cancer.[16] He identified the primary barrier as an ingrained defeatist or negative attitude on the part of physicians and public alike toward resolving this problem. He suggested a mass education program in the meaning of and potential for cancer patient rehabilitation. Lehmann noted in 1978 that a significant number of rehabilitation problems in cancer patients could be improved with rehabilitation care,[45] but the primary barriers to the delivery of this care were lack of identification of patient problems and lack of appropriate referral by physicians unfamiliar with the concept of rehabilitation. Harvey in 1982 noted that the success of rehabilitation efforts in patients with cancer is likely to depend on referral patterns, team communication, and effective rehabilitation treatment processes.[37] He found a failure to apply comprehensive rehabilitation efforts in the area of cancer, possibly related to a reluctance on the part of rehabilitation personnel to receive the cancer patient referral or to a lack of data showing benefit of cancer rehabilitation programs. Villanueva noted that cancer rehabilitation can give good results only when it is properly executed.[70]

Dietz in 1969 developed and demonstrated a cancer program in two cooperating hospitals, one an acute hospital and one a rehabilitation hospital.[26] He found it essential to establish early recognition of the patient's disability and rehabilitation potential and to stimulate prompt referral for rehabilitation care.

In another model of cancer rehabilitation care, the gaps and barriers to rehabilitation service delivery were closed[45] by using the physiatrist as the link between the clinical oncology team and comprehensive rehabilitation team. Both teams were appropriately trained by formal lectures, demonstrations, and in-service training programs, which presented rehabilitation concepts to the oncology team and advances in cancer care to the rehabili-

Table 33-1
A Typical Cancer Rehabilitation Program

Program Direction
  Rehabilitation medicine physician   33%
  Oncology physician   25%
  Allied health   19%
Team Composition (based on inclusion in more than 50% of the program surveyed)
  Oncology and/or rehabilitation medicine physician
  Social worker
  Psychologist
  Physical therapist
  Oncology nurse
  Occupational therapist
Method of Initiation of Care
  Individual consultation to team members
  Consultation to physician directors/coordinator
  Consultation to team
Delivery of Services
  Individual consultation followed by care
  Team conference with problem-oriented process and/or goal-oriented process
Program Content
  Patient education
  Family involvement
  Protocols for specific sites
  Pain control methods
Expected Patient Characteristics
  Mixed disease status
  Inpatient, 64%; outpatient, 30%; home care, 6%
  Site emphasis (in descending order): breast, gastrointestinal tract, lung, head and neck
Funding Resource
  Fee for service with some grant support
Location (based on perceived success and potential)
  Community hospital   94%
  Cancer center   74%
  University hospital   66%

(Harvey RF, Jellinek HM, Habeck RV: Cancer rehabilitation: An analysis of 36 program approaches. JAMA, 247:2127–2131, 1982)

Table 33-2
Karnofsky Performance Status Index

General Category	Index	Specific Criteria
Able to carry on normal activity, no special care needed	100	Normal, no complaints, no evidence of disease
	90	Able to carry on normal activity, minor signs or symptoms of disease
	80	Normal activity with effort, some signs or symptoms of disease
Unable to work, able to live at home and care for most personal needs, varying amount of assistance needed	70	Cares for self, unable to carry on normal activity or to do work
	60	Requires occasional assistance from others, but able to care for most needs
	50	Requires considerable assistance from others and frequent medical care
Unable to care for self, requires institutional or hospital care or equivalent, disease may be rapidly progressing	40	Disabled, requires special care and assistance
	30	Severely disabled, hospitalization indicated; death not imminent
	20	Very sick, hospitalization necessary; active supportive treatment necessary
	10	Moribund
	0	Dead

(Mor V, Laliberle L, Morris JN, Wiemann M: The Karnofsky Performance Status Scale: An examination of its reliability and validity in a research setting. Cancer 53:2002–2007, 1984)

tation team. All cancer patients treated by the oncology team were screened for potential rehabilitation problems by a rehabilitation nurse coordinator, and those patients that seemed likely to have problems were presented to the physiatrist for consultation and appropriate recommendations.

Harvey in 1982 surveyed 36 out of a known 95 cancer rehabilitation programs and developed a typical cancer rehabilitation program (Table 33-1).[37] This summary can serve as a model for the development and implementation of a cancer rehabilitation program that will meet the comprehensive needs of a patient with cancer.

Rehabilitative Approaches in the Patient With Cancer

The rehabilitation problems encountered in the cancer patient are multifactorial and complicated by the often relentless course of the underlying disease and its treatment. As an example, general weakness, the second most common rehabilitation problem identified in the Lehmann study,[45] could occur as a result of multiple factors, including the following: mechanical effects caused by the primary tumor or its metastases in the central or peripheral nervous system; "remote effects" of malignancy produced at a distance from the primary tumor or its metastases, generally referred to as the paraneoplastic syndrome; the effect of treatment including radiation, chemotherapy, and surgery; the nutritional problems associated with cancer; the complications of immobilization; and the psychological problems associated with cancer. Therefore, the physiatrist needs to establish an accurate diagnosis, have a knowledge of the natural history of the disease and expected complications of treatment, and be able to work closely with other physicians as part of the rehabilitation team.

Oncologists have identified that the functional status of the patient can be correlated with the outcome of the underlying disease.[50] The *Karnofsky Performance Status Scale* has been the most widely used measure of the functional status of cancer patients (Table 33-2). The *Karnofsky Scale* has been found to be reliable and strongly related to other measures of patient functioning, including the *Katz ADL Index*.[52] It is not known if treatment directed specifically at the patient's ability to function will result in an increased survival from cancer.

SYSTEM-SPECIFIC DIAGNOSES

In the following sections the most frequent causes of rehabilitation problems are discussed by the organ system affected. Treatment techniques are emphasized when they differ from techniques used to treat nonmalignant problems of a similar etiology.

Central Nervous System

The central nervous system (CNS) can be affected by an almost bewildering variety of complications associated with cancer, and many patients will have more than one cause of CNS dysfunction. CNS problems are the most common cause of referral to cancer rehabilitation services.

Primary Tumors

Primary CNS tumors are not as common as secondary or metastatic lesions; almost 14,000 new cases occur in the United States each year. Patients with primary CNS tumors are often referred to a physiatrist because their functional problems and rehabilitation treatment are similar to those of patients with cerebrovascular disease.

Primary tumors arise from a variety of cell types, but 60% arise from glial cells. Because the great majority of these tumors arise from astrocytes, astrocytomas can be discussed as a model for other CNS tumors. Astrocytes can give rise to a number of different tumor types from benign to malignant, and are graded according to their histological features. The *Kernohan System* grades astrocytomas from I to IV, with grades I and II considered the most benign and grades III and IV the most malignant.

Headache is the most frequent initial symptom as well as the most frequent symptom at the time of diagnosis.[51] Seizures, characteristically grand mal or focal, occur in one-third to over half of patients sometime before diagnosis. Other common symptoms include focal neurological findings such as hemiparesis, speech difficulties, personality changes, and impaired consciousness. Impaired consciousness is correlated with increasing intracranial pressure and is an unfavorable prognostic sign when present at the time of diagnosis.[32] The computed tomography (CT) scan is currently the most accurate method of diagnosis, but other techniques such as brain scan and angiography have also proved useful.

The cornerstone of treatment for astrocytomas and other brain tumors is surgery and radiation therapy; chemotherapy has a less important role. Surgery can range from biopsy, partial resection, and complete removal to lobectomy. Complete removal of an astrocytoma is considered possible only in low-grade (I and II) tumors and when the tumor is surgically accessible. When the removal is incomplete or the histological grade is more advanced, radiation therapy may also be used. In low-grade astrocytomas routine postoperative irradiation does not exceed 6000 rads and is given to limited fields. The daily dose usually does not exceed 200 rads with four to five treatments per week. High-grade astrocytomas are usually treated with high-dose 6000-rad megavoltage treatment, which lasts from 7 to 7½ weeks.[46, 59] Radiation oncologists attempt to limit the field as much as possible with high-dose megavoltage treatment because of the developments of side-effects in survivors, including intellectual deficits. Corticosteroids, usually in the form of dexamethasone, are often given to control intracerebral edema. Survival is related to the histological grade of the tumor as well as its location.[71] In low-grade malignancies, the patients with complete removal of the tumor at initial operation will have a 5-year survival of greater than 90%. After an incomplete tumor resection and radiotherapy, these patients have a 5-year survival of 40% to 50%. High-grade lesions have a much poorer survival record, ranging from a 40% 1-year and a 20% 5-year survival for grade III astrocytomas, down to no better than a 25% 1-year survival in patients with a grade IV tumor.

The rehabilitation treatment of patients with primary brain tumors is similar to that of patients with similar deficits resulting from cerebrovascular disease. If the functional deficits warrant it, there is no reason that a patient with a low-grade astrocytoma and good prognosis for prolonged survival should not be treated in an intensive inpatient rehabilitation setting. Patients with a higher grade lesion and a more dismal prognosis are often best mobilized to return home as soon as possible. It is difficult to accurately assess a patient's rehabilitation potential immediately after surgery or while the patient is still undergoing postoperative radiation therapy. These patients can be extremely lethargic and unable to participate in an intensive therapy program. Shortly after the completion of radiation therapy, patients can make a very rapid functional recovery and their rehabilitation program will need to be modified to reflect their increasing capabilities. Patients with a primary brain tumor, even with an unfavorable prognosis, will often have many months of relatively symptom-free survival. When the tumor does recur, patients can have an equally rapid and dramatic decline in functional ability from which they do not recover. In selected cases, secondary operations for malignant astrocytomas can be of benefit in patients whose preoperative functional status was good.[75]

Metastatic Brain Tumors

Metastatic brain disease is a serious and common problem in rehabilitation. Autopsy series show that up to 25% to 30% of patients with cancer are found to have cerebral metastasis.[58] The most common sites of tumors that metastasize to the brain are lung, breast, gastrointestinal, cancer from unknown primaries, and malignant melanoma. Metastases to the brain usually involve the cerebrum, with the frontal lobe being the most common site followed by the temporoparietal and occipital regions. Metastases to the cerebellum and the brain stem are much less frequent.

The common symptoms of metastatic disease to the brain include headache, loss of motor function, impaired cognition, seizures, and sensory loss.[67] The CT scan has been very important in increasing the timeliness and accuracy of diagnosis. Patients with lung cancer have a very high incidence of CNS metastases and vague symptoms should be evaluated by a CT scan. The cornerstone of treatment in patients with metastatic brain disease is radiation therapy and large dosages of corticosteroids, with initial dosages as high as 8 to 10 mg of dexamethasone every 8 hours. For longer term maintenance, a lesser dose is required. In some series,[2] 10% to 20% of patients developed a steroid myopathy causing significant weakness.

Radiation therapy is effective in relieving symptoms and increasing survival. The typical radiation technique recommended for most patients is 3000 rads to the whole brain over a 2-week period. Several large studies carried out by the Radiation Therapy Oncology Group have shown that relief of symptoms can be quite dramatic.[7] Over 30% of patients with motor loss, impaired mentation, sensory loss, and lethargy experienced a complete response to radiation therapy with an overall response greater than 70%. Similar improvements were seen in the *Karnofsky Performance Scale* status. Improvements were much greater in ambulatory patients who had the brain as the only site of metastasis. Chemotherapy is less effective in treating CNS metastases because many of these agents cannot penetrate the blood–brain barrier.

The overall median survival in these and other studies is in the range of 15 to 18 weeks, but certain groups do better. Ambulatory patients survive longer than nonambulatory patients, and patients with breast cancer survive longer than lung cancer patients. Ambulatory patients with adenocarcinoma of the lung were found to have a 1-year survival of about 50% and a 2-year survival of approximately 30%.[74] The physiatrist needs to individually evaluate each patient, consulting closely with the oncologist, neurosurgeon, and radiation therapist to establish the optimal rehabilitation program. As with patients with primary brain tumors, these patients will often show a remarkable improvement in function following the completion of radiation therapy, a relatively symptom-free period, and then a final precipitous decline.

Cerebrovascular Complications

In a large survey of patients with cancer, cerebrovascular disease was found in 14.6% of patients.[35] Approximately half of these patients had significant clinical symptoms related to the cerebrovascular disease. The patients were equally divided between those with a cerebral hemorrhage and infarction. The most common cause of intracerebral hemorrhage was from intratumoral hemorrhage, especially in patients with malignant melanoma, and hemorrhage secondary to coagulopathy, frequently in patients with leukemia. The most common etiology of cerebral infarction was atherosclerosis, but this represented only 15% of symptomatic patients. A majority of symptomatic patients with infarction were found to have intravascular coagulation or nonbacterial thrombotic endocarditis. Septic embolus was also a common cause of cerebral infarction.

The clinical presentation of cerebrovascular disease in patients with cancer is more often a diffuse encephalopathy, sometimes without localizing signs, rather than the usual acute onset focal deficit seen in atherosclerotic or hemorrhagic cerebrovascular disease. The rehabilitation techniques used in these patients are similar to those used with patients with cerebrovascular disease without cancer. The patient's survival and the success of the program are related to the course of the underlying cancer. In our experience, patients with cerebrovascular disease and cancer can be successfully treated in an intensive inpatient rehabilitation setting.

Paraneoplastic Syndromes

There are a wide variety of paraneoplastic syndromes that can affect the CNS. Reported syndromes have included subacute cerebellar degeneration, limbic encephalitis, and dementia.[9, 27] All of these, with the exception of dementia, are uncommon. The cerebellar degeneration is a subacute to chronic progressive disorder often with associated dementia. This syndrome is associated with a wide variety of neoplasms including lung, prostate, gastrointestinal, and ovarian. The course is usually progressive, even though there are some reports of improvement with treatment of the underlying malignancy. A mild dementia has often been reported in association with lung cancer, and it is unclear how much this syndrome affects patient function in these very sick individuals with limited survival.

Endocrine and metabolic paraneoplastic syndromes are much more common.[60] Ectopic adrenocorticotropic hormone (ACTH) production is a rare complication usually arising from small-cell lung tumors. Patients may present with severe mental status changes and proximal muscle weakness rather than an overt Cushing's syndrome. Ectopic production of antidiuretic hormone leads to the development of the syndrome of inappropriate secretion of antidiuretic hormone (SIADH). Like many paraneoplastic syndromes, the SIADH syndrome most often presents as a complication of small-cell tumor of the lung.

Hypercalcemia is found in up to 10% of cancer patients in many series.[54] The most common neurological manifestations of hypercalcemia are those of a metabolic encephalopathy. Other rare paraneoplastic syndromes causing metabolic encephalopathy include hypocalcemia, hyponatremia, and hypoglycemia. Although not paraneoplastic syndromes, renal and hepatic failure cause a metabolic encephalopathy that can result in significant functional problems in the cancer patient.

Treatment-Related Encephalopathy

Radiation encephalopathy is a relatively rare effect of CNS radiation therapy in adults.[61] Although mild CNS effects of radiation therapy are often noted, patients with significant deficits are rarely appreciated. When these cases do appear the clinical picture is much like that of a primary CNS tumor with focal deficits. Toxic encephalopathies are rare, but can be seen secondary to chemotherapeutic agents. Drugs which have been implicated include L-Asparaginase, procarbazine, vincristine, methotrexate, and 5-fluorouracil.[1, 42] Drugs widely prescribed to patients with cancer such as corticosteroids, opiates, antidepressants, and anticonvulsants will cause metabolic encephalopathy just as they do in the general population.

Metastatic Cancer to the Spinal Cord

Spinal cord metastases are a significant problem in the rehabilitation of patients with cancer. Most spinal cord injury is due to extradural compression from adjacent metastatic deposits in the vertebral bodies. The common primary sites are lung, breast, lymphomas, and prostate.[33] The most frequent initial symptom is radicular pain, which usually precedes the onset of motor weakness, sensory disturbance, or bowel or bladder dysfunction. In one recent series from a general hospital, almost 50% of the patients were not known to be suffering from malignant disease when they presented with symptoms of spinal metastasis.[64] Physiatrists who are referred patients with back pain, especially those with a known malignancy, must be alert to this possibility. In many cases, the pain will precede neurological symptoms by up to an average of 6 months. Patients with spinal metastatic disease will also have spinal tenderness. Patients with spinal cord metastasis often present later in the course of their disease, and are significantly deconditioned and debilitated. Most of the patients have a clinical picture compatible with a transverse myelopathy, with Brown-Séquard syndrome rarely seen.

As many as 20% of patients with symptoms from spinal metastasis have no findings on plain x-ray films of the spine.[64] Myelography is the method of choice to establish a diagnosis. In patients with breast and renal cancer, complete myelography is necessary because blocks can occur at multiple levels.[8]

Many factors have been identified which affect the outcome. As is the case in many patients with malignancy, the best predictor of outcome is the site of the primary tumor; patients with hematological malignancy, or prostate or breast cancer will do better than patients with lung cancer. Patients who present with an acute onset usually respond less well to treatment than those whose condition is chronically progressive. Patients whose presentation is initially less severe will also be more likely to respond well to treatment and rehabilitation.

Treatment consists of surgery and radiation therapy.[4, 33, 64] Patients with hematological malignancies respond well to radiation therapy alone and surgery is usually not necessary unless it is to establish a diagnosis. Patients with nonhematological malignancies often require surgery to confirm the diagnosis, as a significant number of patients present with spinal metastasis as their initial manifestation of malignancy. Corticosteroids are commonly prescribed, but their efficacy in nonhematological malignancies is controversial.

The techniques of management of patients with spinal metastasis are similar to those with spinal cord injury from traumatic causes; however, one must keep the underlying prognosis in mind. The range of survival in all patients with spinal metastatic disease is quite poor, ranging from 6 to 12 months in most studies. There is a large amount of variation in survival depending on the tumor type, and prognosis is most favorable in patients with hematological malignancies, and breast and prostate cancer. Survival can be prolonged long enough to justify treatment in an intensive inpatient rehabilitation setting.[41, 53]

Peripheral Nervous System

Peripheral nerves can be involved by compression, direct invasion, diffuse infiltration, remotely as one of the manifestations of a paraneoplastic syndrome, and as a side-effect of treatment. Diffuse infiltration of peripheral nerves is usually seen only in the leukemias, lymphomas, and multiple myeloma. This type of involvement is quite rare compared to other forms of involvement of the peripheral nerves.

Tumor in the Paravertebral Spaces, Brachial Plexus, and Lumbosacral Plexus

A syndrome caused by tumors arising in the apex of the lung that grow outward and posteriorly to involve the extraspinal nerve roots and the sympathetic nerves is known as Pancoast's syndrome.[57] The tumor can also involve the substance of the ribs and the corresponding vertebral bodies. The lower cervical and upper thoracic vertebrae are characteristically involved. The clinical picture includes sensory loss and motor weakness in a C8 to T1 distribution, and Horner's syndrome. Local pain and tenderness are often present. When identified early, these tumors can respond to aggressive surgical treatment with radiation therapy. The resulting motor and sensory deficits and pain syndromes are treated as with any other nerve injury.

A tumor can also involve the brachial plexus. Kori, Foley, and Posner[44] reviewed 78 cases of cancer involving the brachial plexus. They found most of these cases due to cancer of the lung, breast, or a lymphoma. The clinical presentation is very similar to Pancoast's syndrome, except the incidence of Horner's syndrome is less.

The main differential diagnosis is usually between tumor involvement and the effects of radiation therapy. In their study, Kori, Foley, and Posner found that pain at presentation, Horner's syndrome, and involvement of the lower trunk of the brachial plexus were more characteristic of metastatic involvement and lymphedema, whereas involvement of the upper trunk was more characteristic of a radiation-induced plexopathy.[44] In addition, electromyography (EMG) can reveal myokymic EMG discharges from patients with radiation plexopathy.

Studies have shown that the risk of developing a radiation plexopathy is related to the dose received, but with modern methods of radiotherapy the incidence has been very low. This differential diagnosis is important because radiotherapy is the treatment of choice for paliation of tumor involvement to the brachial plexus. Rehabilitation treatment of these conditions is similar to that of brachial plexus injury.

The peripheral neuropathies are the most common of the paraneoplastic syndromes. According to Croft and Wilkinson, who studied neuromyopathies in 1,476 patients with cancer, they are usually divided into two syndromes: a sensory neuropathy and a sensory motor neuropathy.[20, 21] The sensory neuropathy, also referred to as a dorsal root ganglionitis, is very rare. It presents with a subacute or chronic onset of sensory loss including proprioception and associated loss of deep-tendon reflexes. However, the muscle strength is often preserved and nerve conduction velocities are within normal limits. In the far more common sensory motor peripheral neuropathy, the symptoms include a symmetrical distal weakness with wasting and sensory loss with areflexia.[19] This syndrome can occur in from 5% of all patients with cancer to over 50% of patients in certain series with lung cancers. Involvement is often subclinical and demonstrated only by nerve conduction studies. As with many paraneoplastic syndromes, these are most common in lung cancers. Recovery from paraneoplastic peripheral neuropathies is very rare, even when the underlying tumor is removed.

Peripheral neuropathies are a common and often a serious symptom in multiple myeloma and associated paraproteinemias. Many different clinical syndromes have been described, but the most usual is a distal, symmetric, progressive sensory motor polyneuropathy in a stocking-glove distribution.[43] Severe sensory symptoms, muscle weakness with atrophy, and loss of deep-tendon reflexes are found. The EMG is consistent with an axonal type of polyneuropathy. Clinical signs of polyneuropathy are reported in approximately 10% to 15% of myeloma patients. Electrodiagnositc or biopsy abnormalities are found in 40% to 65% of patients. The usual peripheral neuropathy with multiple myeloma responds poorly to treatment and progresses with the underlying disease.

Treatment-Related Neuropathy

Many anticancer drugs have been associated with peripheral neuropathy. Vinca alkaloids, especially vincristine, cause a peripheral neuropathy that is dose-related, and in some treatment protocols all the patients will show at least some symptoms of peripheral neuropathy.[14] The initial symptoms are usually sensory and include paresthesias as well as the loss of distal deep-tendon reflexes. More severe cases develop a distal weakness with muscle wasting. These peripheral neuropathies often persist after the sensation of drug therapy. As in all toxic peripheral neuropathies, the clinical syndromes can be much more severe in patients with a pre-existing peripheral neuropathy. Electrodiagnostic studies usually show mild abnormalities in sensory and motor nerve conduction consistent with an axonal neuropathic process. Peripheral neuropathies are less common with other antineoplastic drugs, but peripheral neuropathies have been reported with procarbazine, 5-azacitidine, cisplatin, VP-16-213, and alpha interferon.[15, 42, 73, 76]

The peripheral nervous system is also affected by surgical disruption. Spinal accessory nerve injury can occur as a complication of radical neck dissection.[68, 69] The resulting paralysis of the trapezius can have a very deleterious effect on shoulder alignment and function. Goals of a physical rehabilitation program in accessory nerve injury include avoidance of contracture of the pectoralis muscles, avoidance of neck pain and excess stretching of the trapezius muscle, and strengthening of the compensatory muscles, especially the levator scapulae, rhomboids, and serratus anterior. A number of comprehensive rehabilitation programs have been described, but the results after complete nerve injury are unsatisfactory and shoulder problems are common.[28]

Another frequent cause of peripheral nerve injury in cancer patients is compression due to improper body positioning. Cancer patients have multiple risk factors for the development of this complication, including pre-existing nerve disease such as diabetes mellitus, drug-induced peripheral neuropathies, extreme weight loss, and prolonged immobilization. In our experience, the most common sites of compression are the ulnar and peroneal nerves. Prevention, by means of proper positioning, judicious use of padding and orthotics, and patient education, is much more effective than treatment after the injury has occurred. Once again, treatment techniques are similar to those used in patients with compression neuropathies without cancer.

Skeletal System

Primary Tumors

Metastatic cancer to the skeletal system is a much more common problem than primary bone tumors. Approximately 2,000 cases of primary malignant tumors of the bone are expected in the United States each year, which is less than 0.5% of all cancers.

Bone tumors can arise from any of the tissue types that comprise bone. The most common primary malignant tumors of bone are osteosarcomas.[22] These tumors usually occur in adolescence. The most common sites of involvement are the knee joint and proximal humerus, and these tumors metastasize almost exclusively through the blood. Before the development of adjuvant chemotherapy and limb-sparing procedures, amputation was the usual treatment. The amputation was usually performed one joint above the tumor-bearing bone. Since the development of effective adjuvant chemotherapy, total joint replacement technology, and accurate radiological imaging, limb salvage techniques have been developed.

Not all patients with osteosarcomas are candidates for limb-sparing surgery. Contraindications incude major peripheral nerve and vascular involvement, pathological fractures, infection, extensive muscle involvement, and limited expectations of survival.[62] The procedures themselves consist of tumor resection, skeletal reconstruction, and soft tissue and muscle transfers. These limb-salvage procedures are best carried out in tertiary cancer treatment centers where these patients are often referred. As a result, the physiatrist in general practice will have limited involvement in their rehabilitation.

In reconstruction of osteogenic sarcomas involving the proximal humerus, adequate resection requires removing 15 cm to 20 cm of the humerus and the shoulder joint.[49] Some effort is usually made to preserve the musculocutaneous nerve. A successful operation will result in minimal shoulder motion with effective elbow, wrist, and hand function. Postoperatively it is important to control edema by range-of-motion exercises and the use of elastic sleeves.

Limb-sparing procedures of the lower extremity include resection and reconstruction of the distal femur and proximal fibula.[62] Depending on which muscles or nerves need to be excised, the patient may require an orthosis or cane, or both, for adequate ambulation. If a knee arthrodesis has to be performed, the patients will use a long-leg brace postoperatively and will be nonweight-bearing for 4 to 6 weeks. The functional outcome depends on the level of reconstruction and the amount of corresponding muscle and nerve damage. It is not clear if there are functional advantages to an endoprosthetic limb salvage procedure with a knee arthrodesis as opposed to an above-knee amputation, but the cosmetic and psychological advantages are obvious.[56]

Patients with amputation for the treatment of cancer can usually be fitted with a conventional prosthesis. Complications commonly seen in the cancer patient include weight fluctuations and skin healing problems related to radiation therapy and chemotherapy. Each patient needs to be carefully evaluated and decisions made individually. In addition to the effects of surgery, patients with osteogenic sarcoma will receive chemotherapy or radiation therapy with their associated side-effects.

Metastatic Bone Cancer

The development of bone metastasis is a common and serious problem. More than 50% of all patients with breast, lung, or prostate cancer will eventually develop bony metastasis. These cancers represent more than 75% of the patients with metastatic bone disease. Metastatic bone disease causes pain, pathological fractures, neurological impairment, and associated functional problems. Skeletal management of patients with multiple myeloma, a tumor primary to bone, may also be considered with this group because they represent from 10% to 25% of all patients presenting with pathological fractures.

Pain is the most consistent symptom of metastatic bone disease. This pain is often more severe at night and can often be elicited by percussion tenderness at the site of involvement. Pain is produced by stretching of the periosteum, fractures, or nerve entrapment. Skeletal metastases are rarely solitary. The axial skeleton is involved in over 70% of the cases. When the appendicular skeleton is affected, involvement of the hands, forearms, feet, and distal legs is unusual. The evaluation of metastatic bone disease should include both a radiograph and bone scan. Up to one-third of the patients with positive bone scans will show no x-ray changes on plain films.[3] Less commonly, bone scans will not reveal lesions seen on plain films, especially in multiple myeloma. Plain films are essential to select patients for prophylactic surgery, but lesions less than one cm often go undetected on plain films.

Bony metastases require treatment with multiple modalities to relieve pain and prevent fractures. Radiation therapy is highly effective and offers significant relief in over 75% of the patients treated.[40] Chemotherapy in the form of hormonal manipulation is used to relieve or reduce pain in metastases from breast or prostate cancer. Chemotherapy is often equally effective in treating multiple myeloma or metastases from hematological malignancies.

Immobilization is useful in relieving pain and forestalling the developoment of a pathological fracture. The upper extremity can be immobilized using slings or binders. Cervical spine lesions are usually immobilized with a halo and body jacket or a skull occiput mandibular immobilization (SOMI) brace. Cervical collars will usually not relieve pain and do not provide effective immobilization of the cervical spine. Thoracic spine lesions are best treated by plastic molded body jackets. In our experience, patients do not well tolerate other types of orthoses to stabilize this region. Lumbar lesions can often be effectively stabilized and the pain reduced by a corset.

When pain cannot be relieved by conventional means or a pathological fracture is impending or has occurred, surgical treatment is necessary. The first surgical procedure usually has the best prognosis, and as much diseased bone as possible should be replaced. Many procedures use methylmethacrylate, which allows for rapid mobilization and does not interfere with radiation therapy.

The majority of symptomatic metastases in the upper extremity are from breast cancer, followed by multiple myeloma and renal cancer. More than 90% of the lesions involve the humerus. Surgery using a rod and cement is necessary when 50% of the cortex is destroyed, lesions are greater than 3 cm in diameter, or the patient has intractable pain.[63] The patient should not remain immobilized for more than 3 or 4 days after the operation and should have full use of the extremity in 7 to 10 days.

The most common types of metastases involving the hip joint include breast cancer, lymphoma, lung, and prostate cancer. Unlike long bones, the hip cannot be treated with prophylactic procedures. However, fractures or intractable pain on weight-bearing are an indication for surgery. The surgical treatment usually involves total hip replacement. Rehabilitation techniques are similar to those involved with total hip replacement in patients without cancer. In most series, patients who were ambulatory before surgery were ambulatory postoperatively.[47]

The frequent tumor types involving the femur are breast

and kidney cancer, multiple myeloma, lung, and prostate cancer. Surgery should be considered prophylactically in any patient with lesions greater than 2.5 cm in diameter, when 30% to 50% of the cortex is destroyed, or when intractable pain is present with weight-bearing.[36] All surgical procedures in the femur make use of methylmethacrylate. After surgery, the techniques of rehabilitation are similar to those of nonmetastatic disease, and the prescription of weight-bearing must be decided individually. The combined results of several studies show that pain relief is obtained with surgery in 90% to 97% of the patients. Over 90% of the patients ambulatory prior to the operation will continue to walk. However, those patients that were not ambulatory prior to the operation will only be ambulatory in 25% of the cases.[36] Median survival in patients treated by surgery for metastatic bone disease ranges from 6 months to over 1 year depending on the primary tumor type.

Neuromuscular System

Primary tumors of muscle are very rare, and there are only scattered case reports of metastatic cancer to muscle that does not arise from the growth of a contiguous nonmuscle metastasis. This section will discuss the remote effects of cancer that primarily affect muscle and neuromuscular junction.

Cachexia and Asthenia

Cachexia and asthenia are characteristic symptoms of cancer. *Asthenia* is a syndrome that includes as its major manifestations fatigue and lethargy, which coexist with normal muscle strength; there is no other demonstrable cause for these symptoms.[66] There is no satisfactory explanation of its etiology. Treatment, aside from therapy for the primary tumor, is supportive. *Cachexia* is generalized weight loss with muscle weakness.[18] There are a variety of contributing factors to the cachexia of malignancy, which include but are not limited to anorexia, alterations of the sensation of smell and taste, oropharyngeal and esophageal lesions and infections associated with radiation and chemotherapy, problems with the digestion and absorption of food, and preferential nutrient utilization by the tumor. Many studies have demonstrated that these patients have an unusually high caloric and protein need similar to patients with burns or major trauma. It is not known to what extent such factors as immobilization contribute to the clinical picture seen in these patients. As is the case with asthenia, treatment is directed toward the primary tumor and establishing adequate nutrition. Enteral and intravenous hyperalimentation has been used to treat this disorder with mixed results.[10] The rehabilitation approach to these patients makes use of proper positioning, avoidance of immobilization, maintenance of normal range of motion, and exercises designed to increase endurance. Experiments have not yet been performed to determine the appropriateness or success of this approach in increasing function in these patients.

There are conflicting descriptions in the literature of syndromes that are termed *carcinomatous neuromyopathies*.[13, 19, 20] The most common description includes muscle weakness and wasting, often greater proximally, with depressed distal deep-tendon reflexes. The most characteristic electrodiagnostic findings include myopathic EMG abnormalities with fibrillations and fasciculations and variable nerve conduction velocity abnormalities.[13] This syndrome is not uncommon and is associated with mild to moderate functional difficulties. Treatment of the underlying tumor usually does not improve the weakness, depressed deep-tendon reflexes, or EMG abnormalities. In our experience these patients can benefit from a program similar to that described above for patients with cachexia.

Dermatomyositis and polymyositis occur with a higher frequency in patients with cancer than in the general population. The rehabilitation treatment of these disorders is like that for those in patients without cancer.

Disorders of Neuromuscular Transmission

Most cases of the Eaton-Lambert syndrome are associated with a small-cell cancer of the lung. Symptoms include muscle weakness and fatigue, especially in those tasks associated with the proximal muscles. A corresponding autonomic peripheral neuropathy and sensory peripheral neuropathy with paresthesias is not uncommon. As expected, the neurological examination demonstrates proximal muscle weakness, which is improved with effort. Electrodiagnostic testing is definitive and reveals facilitation of the response to 3 Hz supermaximal stimulation after exercise or high-frequency stimulation (10–50 Hz). The defect in Eaton-Lambert syndrome is felt to be an incomplete calcium-mediated release of acetylcholine from the nerve terminals. Guanidine hydrochloride, an anticholinesterase drug, is often prescribed alone or in combination with pyridostigmine. This treatment is often not completely effective and these drugs have numerous side-effects that can preclude their use.[55] A small number of cases will show improvement with removal of the primary tumor, and some have reported benefit from plasmapheresis in combination with immunosuppressive therapy.[23] Patients are usually not seriously disabled from the effects of the Eaton-Lambert syndrome, but suffer more problems from the underlying malignancy.

Breast Cancer

The treatment of local and regional disease in breast cancer has undergone a number of changes in the past decade, which has greatly decreased the incidence of tumor-related problems of the shoulder and upper extremity. In the early 1970s, approximately 50% of patients treated for primary breast cancer had a radical procedure. With the much increased use of lesser surgical procedures, problems of restricted shoulder mobility and edema following primary surgery for breast cancer are now infrequent. Nonetheless, the basic goals of rehabilitation of the post-mastectomy patient have not changed. These include pain-free, edema-free use of the upper extremity with a normal range of motion, as well as those components of rehabilitation common to all cancer patients, that is, return to full psychological health, restoration of physical appearance by prosthesis or breast reconstruction, and occupational and vocational rehabilitation.[12]

Even with lesser surgical procedures, a careful focus on preventive measures will lessen the complications. Postoperatively, the arm should be positioned at 90° abduction with the elbow free rather than pinned to the chest wall.[24, 25] Three to five days after mastectomy, the patient can begin active range of motion to the elbow, wrist, and fingers of the operated extremity and to the nonaffected upper extremity. After the drains are out, active range-of-motion exercises of the affected extremity can start in the supine position; isometric exercises of the biceps, triceps, and more distal muscle groups can also begin. When the sutures are removed, the program can proceed with exercises prescribed in the erect position. The goal of these exercises should be a full range of motion at the time of discharge. The patient should be given a home program with clear instructions on range-of-motion exercises two or three times daily for at least 6 months to a year after the operation.

When the shoulder musculature and lymphatics have been disrupted by surgery, the affected extremity should be compressed by elastic wrap to prevent the development of edema. This wrap may have to be continued, or a custom-fitted gradient pressure garment prescribed, if the edema persists.

There is a wide variation in the reported frequency of lymphedema after radical and modified radical mastectomies, varying from 7% to 63%.[11] Severe edema occurs in a much smaller percentage of these patients. No single factor or combination of factors such as radiation therapy, infection, or recurrent tumor has been adequate to exlain or predict who will develop significant lymphedema after mastectomy and its treatment. As previously mentioned, positioning, maintaining a full range of motion, and isometric exercises are an important part of the treatment of post-mastectomy lymphedema. If these measures are not successful, then pneumatic intermittent compression can be tried.[34] Depending on the manufacturer, units are available with a cuff that inflates and deflates alternately or one that inflates sequentially distal to proximal rather than all at once. We have encountered patients that responded only to the sequentially inflating machine, but no well-controlled comparison studies have been performed.[65] Treatment may vary from 2 to 12 hours a day, and when the treatment must be continued for long periods of time, home units are available. In between compression, the arm needs to be maintained in a custom-fitted gradient pressure garment, which should not be prescribed until the size of the limb has stabilized. Diuretic therapy as well as salt restriction has been tried, but with much less success than mechanical methods of treatment. The patient suffering from lymphedema needs to be educated to protect the arm from potential injury or constriction. Most physicians recommend prompt antibiotic therapy at the first sign of infection.

PAIN MANAGEMENT

Pain is a significant morbidity problem in patients with cancer, becoming increasingly prevalent with the progression of the disease. The incidence of moderate to severe pain ranges from 40% in patients with intermediate-stage cancer to 60% to 80% in patients with advanced cancer.[5, 6, 72] Thus, pain represents a justified fear and has a significant impact on the quality of life and functional abilities of the patient with cancer.

Seventy-five percent of pain seen in the patient with cancer is estimated to be directly related to the cancer either from primary or metastatic invasion of normal tissue.[31, 72] Approximately 20% is associated with cancer therapy in the form of surgery, radiation, and chemotherapy.[31, 72] Pain unrelated to cancer is experienced by only 5% of patients with cancer, ranging from indirect complications of the cancer to coincidental pain due to non-cancer-related etiologies.[31, 72] Foley[31] has classified patients with pain into acute and chronic with further subdivision into the following five groups:

I. Patients with acute related pain associated with diagnosis of cancer or associated with therapy
II. Patients with chronic cancer-related pain associated with cancer progression or therapy
III. Patients with pre-existing chronic pain and cancer-related pain
IV. Patients with history of drug addiction and cancer-related pain
V. Patients dying with cancer-related pain

It is obvious that cancer patients with different etiologies and types of pain will respond differently to therapy. Therefore, adequate evaluation, including history, physical examination, and appropriate diagnostic studies, is necessary in accurately diagnosing the etiology and extent of the pain as well as its psychosocial components. Foley notes that, like other medical problems seen in patients with cancer, chronic pain is treated most effectively with a multidisciplinary approach that includes adequate analgesic drug therapy, neurosurgical and anesthetic procedures, behavioral methods, and supportive therapy.[31]

Analgesic Drug Therapy

The management of cancer pain primarily relies on medications; physical modalities, neurosurgical and anesthetic techniques, and behavior approaches are used secondarily or in combination with drug therapy. Non-narcotic analgesia is the first choice of medication for mild to moderate pain. For severe pain, these drugs are still useful in the potentiation of the effects of narcotic analgesic agents and may have a unique role in the management of certain kinds of pain from bone metastases.[31]

Narcotic agents are the preliminary form of therapy for moderate to severe pain.[30] Often the concern for physical dependency and addiction results in the inadequate use of this type of medication. However, it has been demonstrated in patients with cancer that although tolerance and physical dependence occur, psychological dependency or addiction is rare.[31]

Table 33-3 serves as a good guideline for narcotic analgesic use in cancer pain management.[31] There is no best narcotic analgesic agent, but instead a series of agents with similar properties but different equivalent dosages, durations, methods of administration and possible side-effects. Most have a mechanism that is central and are metabolized by the liver. Narcotic elixirs seem to show no increased beneficial effect over a single narcotic in patients with cancer pain and generally are not indicated.[72] Medication should be administered orally if possible and on a regular basis, with the dosage based on the patient's need and the duration of the analgesic effect. Continuous dosage of narcotic as well as epidural and intrathecal administration can be used as an alternative to oral administration, especially in the terminal patient. Many times an increase in the normal dosage of drugs is safe and can continue to produce additional analgesia in patients with cancer pain because the calculated maximal dosage of narcotic drugs is related mainly to postoperative single-dose studies. Side-effects of the medication should be prevented or treated. When tolerance to a medication finally develops, alternative narcotics, addition of non-narcotic agents, adjuvant analgesic agents, or other types of treatment are indicated. Adjuvant analgesic agents, such as phenothiazines, antidepressants, and anticonvulsant agents, can serve to increase the effectiveness of narcotic agents by acting on the mood or producing analgesia by methods not clearly established.[72]

Physical Modalities

Multiple physical modalities have been suggested to relieve cancer pain. We found them to be an adjuvant treatment, rather than the primary or sole treatment modality. Vibration, transcutaneous electrical stimulation, massage, and thermal modalities are the most frequently suggested and used.[72]

Anesthetic Neurosurgical and Behavioral Approaches

Anesthetic approaches to pain management in the form of nerve blocks and local freezing are most useful in patients with localized, well-defined pain secondary to tumor infiltration. Neu-

Table 33-3
Guidelines for the Use of Narcotic Analgesics in Pain Management

1. Start with a specific drug for a specific type of pain.
2. Know the pharmacology of the drug prescribed:
   - Duration of the analgesic effect
   - Pharmacokinetic properties
   - Equianalgesic doses and route of administration
3. Adjust the route of administration to the patient's need.
4. Administer the analgesic on a regular basis after initial titration of the dosage.
5. Use drug combinations to provide additive analgesia and reduce side-effects (*e.g.,* nonsteroidal anti-inflammatory drugs, antihistamine [hydroxyzine], amphetamine [Dexedrine]).
6. Avoid drug combinations that increase sedation without enhancing analgesia (*e.g.,* benzodiazepine [diazepam] and phenothiazine [chlorpromazine]).
7. Anticipate and treat side-effects:
   - Sedation
   - Respiratory depression
   - Nausea and vomiting
   - Constipation
8. Watch for the development of tolerance:
   - Switch to an alternative narcotic analgesic.
   - Start with one-half the equianalgesic dose and titrate the dose for pain relief.
9. Prevent acute withdrawal:
   - Taper drugs slowly.
   - Use diluted doses of naloxone (0.4 mg in 10 ml of saline) to reverse respiratory depression in the physically dependent patient, and administer cautiously.
10. Do not use placebos to assess the nature of pain.
11. Anticipate and manage complications:
    - Overdose
    - Multifocal myoclonus
    - Seizures

(Foley KM: The treatment of pain in the patient with cancer. CA-A Cancer Clinicians 36(4):194–215, 1986)

rosurgical approaches in the form of neurectomy, rhizotomy, and cordotomy, as well as most central destructive procedures are the most common surgical procedures to relieve pain in the patient not responsive to other means of pain control. Behavioral modification and behavior approaches are used as an adjuvant method of pain control in addiction to appropriate medications.[17, 31, 72] Their mechanism of action is mainly secondary to their ability to modulate the affective response to painful stimuli.[31] Relaxation training, distraction, guided imagery, hypnosis, and cognitive and behavioral training help by increasing the patient's sense of control, by calming the patient and diverting attention, and by breaking the pain–anxiety–tension cycle.[17, 31, 72]

Supportive Therapy

Supportive therapy includes the appropriate use of facilities such as the hospital, hospice, and home environment and the early and continuous involvement of the rehabilitation team specialists, especially in the social and psychological aspects.[72] Availability of a supportive physician with an excellent knowledge of pain control approaches and methods who responds appropriately to the patient's need is vitally important.

PSYCHOSOCIAL PROBLEMS

Matthew P., a 47-year-old concert violinist watched his world unravel after an intra-abdominal lymphoma was diagnosed. He felt too ill to perform and had to cancel a concert tour and a scheduled recording session. Although he, his wife, and two children lived well, they had lived to the extent of his earnings and had little economic reserve. Medical costs that were not covered by insurance benefits rapidly eroded his reserve, and he had to borrow money from family and friends. The combination of illness and deleterious effects of chemotherapy led to major weight loss, baldness, an appearance of physical frailty, and premature aging, all culminating in Matthew losing pride and confidence in his body. Several attempts to play the violin were catastrophic. Matthew did not have the endurance to play for more than a few minutes, and he felt clumsy and unable to play well. He developed a mild encephalopathy caused by chemotherapy and discovered that he had forgotten music he had known for years.

His wife, Dorothy, had not worked for years, since the birth of their first child. She returned to work as a secretary, but found that much of her earnings went into child care. She could also work only sporadically, since Matthew needed her assistance much of the time. His self-esteem was eroded by the role reversal and the necessity of his wife returning to work. He received another blow when Dominick, his 15-year-old, son began to fail at school and was caught smoking marijuana in the school bathroom. He and Dominick did not talk much about his illness.

Matthew became severely depressed and considered suicide, but never followed through with his ideation. Treatment was successful and his lymphoma went into remission. Improvement of his depression and loss of self-esteem took longer. It was 2 years before he was able to seriously return to the violin, and he never regained his former success. His relationship with Dorothy ended in divorce. Dominick did attempt suicide and required lengthy psychiatric care.

This case history demonstrates some common features of the emotional and adaptational disruptive effects on patients and their families as a result of cancer. These effects are similar to those occurring in other persons with serious physical illness or disability (see in Chapter 3, "Psychological Adjustment to Disability"). As with other conditions, psychosocial impairment may persist after the underlying physical problem has resolved or improved. Because the stress extends to the entire family, successful treatment must include the family as well as the patient. Denial may occur. Depression is not universal, but when it does occur, it requires specific treatment. If grieving occurs, the patient and family should be guided toward an adaptive adjustment, if possible.

Although these problems and their management are similar to those that occur with other disabling conditions, there are some problems more specific to cancer patients and their families. Pain, and the fear of pain, occurs much more frequently in cancer than in most other disabling conditions. Both the disease and its treatment may be painful, and patients must be assured and reassured that the pain can be controlled. The discomfort and nausea that can occur with chemotherapy can sometimes be alleviated by shaping, relaxation, or hypnosis techniques. These techniques may also be applicable for a stress reaction that occurs after emotionally traumatic episodes, such as especially painful treatments or seeing oneself in a mirror for the first time after disfiguring surgery.

When the illness progresses, the patient must be helped to adapt to multiple stepwise losses and uncertainty over the future. Preparatory mourning can occur as family members begin to emotionally detach from the patient while he or she is still alive and functional, and even when cure is still a realistic possibility. Empathetic confrontation of the family, including exploration of why the detachment is occurring, and help in planning supportive strategy can guide the family members to become more supportive while the patient is alive. If the patient dies, the family is then more likely to detach and grieve adaptively and to suffer less guilt and disruption of self-esteem later.

Bereavement is also specific to cancer and other disabling conditions that progress to death of the victim. The bereaved are at risk for physical and psychosocial illness. Follow-up care of the family can help the bereaved to adapt to their loss in constructive rather than destructive ways.

Cancer sometimes has a paradoxical salutary effect on both patient and family members. Sometimes the successful facing of the specters of mortality and finiteness leads to a readjustment of life values, which the patient and family perceive as an improvement over pre-cancer existence. Everyday existence may be viewed as vivid and rich, and the patient may see his remaining time as an opportunity to deepen relationships and contribute to society. This reaction may occur both in patients who achieve a cure and in those with a terminal prognosis. Although this phenomenon has received little study, it may be possible for the rehabilitation team to lead the patient in this direction.

REFERENCES

1. Abelson HT: Methotrexate and central nervous system toxicity. Cancer Treat Rep 62:1999–2001, 1978
2. Afifi AK, Bergman RA, Harvey MC: Steroid myopathy: Clinical, histologic, and cytologic observations. Johns Hopkins Med J 123:158–173, 1968
3. Blair RJ, McAfee JG: Radiological detection of skeletal metastases: Radiographs versus scans. Int J Radiat Oncol Phys 1:1201–1202, 1976
4. Boland PJ, Lane JM, Sundareson N: Metastatic disease of the spine. Clin Orthop 169:95–102, 1982
5. Bond MR: Cancer Pain: Psychological substrates and therapy. Clin J Pain 1:99–104, 1985
6. Bonica JJ: Treatment of cancer pain: Current status and future needs. Adv Pain Res Ther 9:589–616, 1985
7. Borgelt B, Gelber R, Kramer S et al: The palliation of brain metastases: Final results of the first two studies by the radiation therapy oncology group. Int J Radiat Oncol Bioll Phys 6:1–9, 1980
8. Bowers TA, Murray JA, Charnsangavej C et al: Bone metastases from renal carcinoma. J Bone Joint Surg 64A:749–754, 1982
9. Brain NR, Wilkinson M: Subacute cerebellar degeneration associated with neoplasms. Brain 88:465–482, 1965
10. Brennan MF: Total parenteral nutrition in the cancer patient. N Engl J Med 305:375–382, 1982
11. Britton RC, Nelson PA: Causes and treatment of post mastectomy lymphedema of the arm: Report of 114 cases. JAMA 180:95–102, 1962
12. Burdick D: Rehabilitation of the breast cancer patient. Cancer 36:645–648, 1975
13. Campbell MJ, Paty DW: Carcinomatous neuromyopathy. J Neurol Neurosurg Psychiatry 37:131–141, 1974
14. Casey EB, Jellife AM, LeQuesne PM et al: Vincristine neuropathy: Clinical and electrophysiological observations. Brain 96:69–86, 1973
15. Clark AW, Parhad IM, Griffin JW et al: Neurotoxicity of cis-platinum: Pathology of the central and peripheral nervous systems. Neurology 30:429, 1980
16. Clark RL, Moreton RD, Healey JE, MacDonald EJ: Rehabilitation of the Cancer patient. Cancer 20:839–845, 1976
17. Cleeland CS: The impact of pain on the patient with cancer. Cancer 54:2635–2641, 1984
18. Costa G: Cachexia of neoplastic diseases. Career Res 37:2317–2325, 1977
19. Croft P, Urich H, Wilkinson M: Peripheral neuropathy of the sensorimotor type associated with malignant disease. Brain 90:31–66, 1967
20. Croft P, Wilkinson M: The incidence of carcinomatous neuromyopathy in patients with various types of cancer. Brain 88:427–434, 1965
21. Croft PB, Wilkinson MSP: The course and prognosis in some types of carcinamatous neuromyopathy. Brain 92:1–8, 1969
22. Dahlin DC: Bone Tumors: General Aspects and Data on 6,221 Cases, 3rd ed. Springfield, IL, Charles C Thomas, 1978
23. Dau PC, Denzs EH: Plasmapheresis and immunosuppressive drug therapy in the Eaton-Lambert syndrome. Ann Neurol 11:570–575, 1982
24. Degenshein GA: Mobility of the arm following radical mastectomy. Surg Gynecol Obstet 145:77, 1977
25. DeLisa JA, Miller RA, Melnick RR et al: Rehabilitation of the cancer patient. In Devita V, Hellman S, Rosenberg S, (eds): Principles and Practices of Oncology, 2nd ed, pp 2155–2188. Philadelphia, JB Lippincott, 1985
26. Dietz JH: Rehabilitation of the cancer patient. Med Clin North Am 53:607–624, 1969
27. Dorfman LH, Forno LS: Paraneoplastic encephalomyelitis. Acta Neurol Scand 48:556–572, 1972
28. Dudgeon BJ, DeLisa JA, Miller RM: Head and neck cancer: A rehabilitation approach. Am J Occup Ther 34:243–251, 1980
29. Elmquist D, Lambert EH: Detailed analysis of neuromuscular transmission in a patient with the myasthenic syndrome sometimes associated with bronchogenic carcinoma. Mayo Clin Proc 43:689–713, 1968
30. Foley KM: Pharmacologic approaches to cancer pain management. Adv Pain Res 9:629–653, 1985
31. Foley KM: The treatment of pain in the patient with cancer. CA-A Cancer J Clinicians 36(4):194–215, 1986
32. Gehan EA, Walker MD: Prognostic factors for patients with brain tumors. Natl Cancer Inst Monogr 46:189–195, 1977
33. Gilbert RW, Kim JH, Posner JR: Epidural spinal cord compression from metastatic tumor: Diagnosis and treatment. Ann Neurol 3:40–51, 1979
34. Grabois M: Rehabilitation of the postmastectomy patient with lymphedema. Cancer 26:75–79, 1976
35. Grauss F, Rodgers LR, Posner JB: Cerebrovascular complications in patients with cancer. Medicine 64:16–35, 1985
36. Haberman ET, Sachs R, Stern RE et al: The pathology and treatment of metastatic disease of the femur. Clin Orthop 169:70–82, 1982
37. Harvey RF, Hellinek HM, Habeck RV: Cancer rehabilitation: An analysis of 36 program approaches. JAMA 247:2127–2131, 1982
38. Healey JE: The quality of success in the treatment of cancer. Oklahoma State Med Assoc J 65:147–151, 1972
39. Healey JE, Zislis J: Cancers. In Stolov WC, Clowers MR (eds): Handbook of Severe Disability. Washington, DC, US Government Printing Office, 1981
40. Hendrickson FR, Sheinkop MB: Management of osseous metastasis. Semin Oncol 2:399–415, 1975
41. Jameson RM: Prolonged survival in paraplegia due to metastatic spinal tumor. Lancet 8:1209–1211, 1974
42. Kaplan RS, Wiernik PH: Neurotoxicity of antineoplastic drugs. Semin Oncol 9:103–128, 1982
43. Kelly JJ, Kyle RA, Miles JM et al: The spectrum of peripheral neuropathy in myeloma. Neurology 31:24–31, 1981
44. Kori SH, Foley KM, Posner JB: Brachial plexus lesions in patients with cancer: 100 cases. Neurology 31:45–50, 1981
45. Lehmann JF, DeLisa JA, Warrne G et al: Cancer rehabilitation: Assessment of need, development, and evaluation of a model of care. Arch Phys Med Rehabil 59:410–419, 1978
46. Leibel SA, Sheline GE, Wara WM et al: The role of radiation therapy in the treatment of astrocytomas. Cancer 35:1551–1557, 1975
47. Ley RN, Sherry HS, Siffert RS: Surgical management of metastatic disease of bone at the hip. Clin Orthop 169:162–169, 1982
48. Lynch PD, Schaefer S, Eckert D: Cancer rehabilitation issues for occupational and physical therapists: A conference report. Progress in Cancer Control IV: Research in the Cancer Center 443–453, 1983
49. Marcove RC, Lewis MM, Huvos AG: En bloc upper humeralinterscapular resection: The Tikhoff-Linbergg Procedure. Clin Orthop 124:219–228, 1977
50. Maurer IH, Pajak H: Prognostic factors in small cell carcinoma of the lung: A cancer and leukemia group B study. Cancer Treat Rep 65:767–774, 1981

51. McKeron RO, Thomas DGT: The clinical study of gliomas. In Thomas DGT, Graham DI (eds): Brain Tumors: Scientific Basis, Clinical Investigation, and Current Therapy, p 202. London, Butterworth, 1980

52. Mor V, Laliberle L, Morris JN, Wiemann M: The Karnofsky Performance Status Scale: An examination of its reliability and validity in a research setting. Cancer 53:2002–2007, 1984

53. Murray PK: Functional outcome and survival in spinal cord injury secondary to neoplasia. Cancer 55:197–201, 1985

54. Myers WPL: Differential diagnosis of hypercalcemia and cancer. Cancer 27:258–272, 1977

55. Norris FH, Eaton JM, Milke CH: Depression of bone marrow by guanidine. Arch Neurol 30:184–185, 1974

56. Otis JC, Lane J, Hillyer CD: Energy consumption in postoperative osteogenic sarcoma patients. In Chao Eys, Innis JC (eds): Design and Application of Turner Prosthesis for Bone and Joint Reconstruction, pp 385–396. New York, Thieme Straton, 1983

57. Paulson DL: Carcinomas in the superior pulmonary sulcus. Ann Thorac Surg 28:3–4, 1979

58. Posner JB, Cheonik M: Intracranial metastases from systemic cancer. Adv Neurol 19:579–592, 1978

59. Scanlon PW, Taylor WF: Radiotherapy of intracranial astrocytomas: Analysis of 417 cases treated from 1960 through 1969. Neurosurg 5:307–308, 1979

60. Schneider BS, Manalo A: Paraneoplastic syndromes: Unusual manifestations of malignant disease. Disease-A-Month 2:1–60, 1979

61. Sheline GE, Wara WM, Smith V: Therapeutic irradiation and brain injury. Int J Radiat Oncol Biol Phys 6:1215–1228, 1980

62. Sim FH, Bowman UUE, Chao EYS: Limb salvage surgery and reconstructive techniques. In Sim FH, Thorofare NJ, Stock CB (eds): Diagnosis and Treatment of Bone Tumors: A Team Approach, pp 75–105. Thorofare, NJ, Slack, Inc, 1983

63. Sim FH, Pritchard DJ: Metastatic disease in the upper extremity. Clin Orthop 169:83–94, 1982

64. Stark RJ, Henson RA, Evans SJW: Spinal metastases: A retrospective survey from a general hospital. Brain 105:189–213, 1982

65. Stillwell GK: Treatment of postmastectomy lymphedema. Mod Treatm 6:396–412, 1969

66. Theologides A: Asthenia in cancer. Am J Med 73:1–3, 1982

67. Vieth RG, Odorn GL: Intracranial metastases and their neurosurgical treatment. J Neurosurg 23:375–383, 1965

68. Villanueva R: Orthosis to correct shoulder pain and deformity after trapezius palsy. Arch Phys Med Rehabil 58:30–34, 1977

69. Villanueva R, Chandra A: The role of rehabilitation medicine in physical restoration of patients with head and neck cancer. Cancer Bull, 29:46–54, 1977

70. Villanueva R, Drane JB, Gunn AE et al: Rehabilitation of the cancer patient. In Cancer Patient Care at M.D. Anderson Hospital and Tumor Institute, pp 671–691. Houston, TX, 1976

71. Walker MD: Chemotherapy: Adjuvant to surgery and radiation therapy. Semin Oncol 2:69–72, 1975

72. Walsh NE: Pain management for cancer patients. Cancer Rehabilitation Symposium, 48th Annual Assembly of the American Academy of Physical Medicine and Rehabilitation, Baltimore, October 1986

73. Weiss HD, Walker MD, Wiernik PH: Neurotoxicity of commonly used antineoplastic agents. N Engl J Med 291:75–81, 127–133, 1974

74. West J, Maor M: Intracranial metastases: Behavioral patterns related to primary size and results of treatment by whole brain irradiation. Int J Radiat Oncol Biol Phys 6:11–15, 1980

75. Young B, Oldfield EH, Morkesbery WR et al: Reoperation for glioblastoma. J Neurosurg 55(b):917–921, 1981

76. Young DF, Posner JB: Nervous system toxicity of chemotherapeutic agents. In Vinken PJ, Bruyn (eds): Handbook of Neurology, chapter 4, pp 92–129. Amsterdam, Elsevier, 1979

77. Zislis JM: Rehabilitation of the cancer patient. Geriatrics 25:150–158, 1970

34

Rehabilitation of the Cardiac Patient

H. L. Brammel

Diseases of the heart and blood vessels remain among the major medical problems of the civilized world. In the United States, these conditions affect over 60 million persons, are responsible for almost 1 million deaths, and result in costs of more than $85 billion each year.[48] Systemic hypertension affects the greatest numbers—roughly 20% of the adult population—but atherosclerotic coronary artery disease accounts for the majority of the cardiovascular deaths and the major portion of the financial burden.[59] There are approximately 1.5 million heart attacks each year in the United States, and 4.7 million persons are known to have coronary artery disease.

Although the total number of persons with coronary disease has not decreased substantially, the mortality rate from cardiovascular disease has fallen significantly—about 25%—in the past 20 to 25 years.[113] The implication for cardiac rehabilitation programs is clear: more persons are surviving acute cardiac events, thereby increasing the number of those who might be served by rehabilitation.

Despite the apparent increase in candidates for cardiac rehabilitation programs, use of program services remains fairly low. The *Directory of Cardiac Rehabilitation Units—1981*, compiled by the American Heart Association identifies over 700 programs in the United States.[25] Of the estimated 540,000 survivors of myocardial infarction and over 100,000 survivors of coronary artery bypass graft surgery, only 30,000 are enrolled each year in formal cardiac rehabilitation programs.[23]

This chapter is a review of the concepts, programs, practice, and outcome of cardiac rehabilitation. The basic model for discussion is coronary artery disease. Most patients who require cardiac rehabilitation will have coronary disease, usually acute myocardial infarction, coronary bypass graft surgery, percutaneous coronary angioplasty, or angina pectoris.

CARDIAC REHABILITATION

Cardiac rehabilitation may be defined as the process of restoring a person with heart disease to, and maintaining that person at, his or her optimal physiological, psychosocial, vocational, and educational status. As with all rehabilitation programs, the practitioner's obligation is to identify those areas or aspects of the patient's life that are adversely affected by the disabling condition, and areas that may, if uncorrected, lead to further disability. The program is made up of activities which minimize current disability, and which attempt to prevent additional subsequent disability.

Cardiac rehabilitation, and rehabilitation in general, when properly practiced, could be described as a wellness program, since the goal is not only to treat and remove signs and symptoms, but also to help the patient to achieve the highest level of wellness consistent with the existing disability. Most cardiovascular diseases are diseases of life-style whose natural history is directly related to how one lives, which means that much of the cardiac rehabilitation/wellness program must deal with the identification and modification of unhealthful life-style practices.

General Features

There are several features of the cardiac rehabilitation program which help determine its content and direction.

The program is longitudinal. Most persons with cardiovascular disease have a condition that is long-standing, unlikely to be reversed, and with a high potential for progression. Although certain phases of the program will have well-defined end points, the practices and activities of the program are continued indefinitely.

The program must be participatory in nature. Contemporary medicine demands that patients take an active role in their own care. To do so requires a strong sense of self-responsibility on the part of the patient. The patient must assume responsibility for his or her health outcomes and the outcomes to be realized from the rehabilitation program. The concept of self-responsibility must be continually fostered and nurtured by the program staff. If the patient is unwilling to assume an active role in achieving meaningful life-style change, no substantial or sustained benefit from the program can be anticipated.

The program is preventive in nature. Most patients on entry will have experienced one or more cardiac events: angina pectoris, myocardial infarction, angioplasty, or coronary artery bypass graft surgery. The program activities must be designed toward preventing additional clinical events or complications—that is, secondary prevention. It is the responsibility of the program managers to stay abreast of research in this area and to make timely program modifications as new information becomes available.

To some extent the program may be personalized. Although broad conceptual and programmatic generalizations can be made, each patient served by the program will have a unique profile: risk factors, physiological sequelae, vocational concerns, personal circumstances, and emotional response to the illness. The program and the staff which administers it must work to identify the unique features and specific needs of each patient which may affect the rehabilitation outcome.

Components

There are four major components of the cardiac rehabilitation program: physiological, psychosocial, vocational, and educational. Failure to optimize the patient's status in each area may impede or prevent full rehabilitation. In addition, other areas may need to be recognized which, if not addressed, may affect the outcome for a particular patient. For example, cultural or ethnic issues may be crucial for some.

Physiological Component

Physiological activities, which are designed to enhance body functions of the participant, include medical and surgical management, activity counseling, and nutrition.

MEDICAL AND SURGICAL MANAGEMENT. The highest quality traditional medical and surgical care is necessary for an optimal rehabilitation outcome. Physiological sources of disability must be identified, treated, and, if possible, prevented. The most common sources of physiological disability in patients with heart disease are symptoms of pump failure, chest pain, and symptoms associated with cardiac dysrhythmias. In addition, the management of other medical conditions such as hypertension or diabetes should be optimized. Cardiac rehabilitation program staff must be trained to recognize those symptoms which indicate a change in a patient's clinical status. Communication with, and referral to, the primary care or referring physician should result in prompt treatment and maintenance of optimal medical care. The efforts of the family practitioner, cardiologist, physiatrist, internist, and cardiac surgeon should be directed toward maintaining the best possible medical/surgical outcome.

As a word of caution, the management of medical problems resides with the patient's primary care physician, not the medical director of the cardiac rehabilitation program. Any medical problem uncovered during participation in the rehabilitation program must be referred to the primary physician for disposition.

ACTIVITY COUNSELING. For the person with heart disease, activity must be prescribed much like medications. The patient's response to activity must be observed, usually during an exercise stress evaluation, and an individualized activity prescription written for work, recreation, and exercise conditioning. The motor-driven treadmill is usually used for the exercise evaluation, but a bicycle ergometer or other methods such as telemetry or Holter monitored modeling of job activities may be useful as well.

A detailed job task assessment is often helpful as a supplement to the treadmill evaluation in writing the exercise training prescription. It allows job-specific exercises to be included in the training program, thereby increasing the likelihood of a successful return to the pre-event job.

NUTRITION. Specific nutritional prescriptions are often required for persons with heart disease to help manage body weight, hyperlipidemias, hypertension, heart failure, or glucose intolerance. Nutritional counseling and monitoring should usually be delegated to an experienced nutritional consultant, since physicians may not have either the time or the expertise necessary for this component of the program.

Psychosocial Component

Psychosocial issues may have a significant effect on the rehabilitation outcome. Some degree of assessment of key psychosocial variables should be made of patients who are enrolled in the cardiac rehabilitation program. Often, this assessment is quite informal, performed by conversation or interview between program staff and the patient and family. Some clinics will conduct a more intensive, systematic evaluation, which may include psychometric testing and interviews by an experienced psychologist, psychiatrist, or medical social worker. Whatever approach is used, it should include assessment of the patient's personality; the number, nature, and severity of stressors in the patient's life; the amount of distress caused by anxiety, depression, or hostility; and any significant financial or marital problems. In addition, unhealthful behaviors such as cigarette smoking, which may require behavior modification interventions, should be identified.

The most common emotional responses to heart attack are anxiety and depression.[13, 41] For most, these reactions are transient and do not interfere with a successful return to normal living. The presence of good coping skills prior to a heart attack is associated with less sense of disability and a greater likelihood of returning to full normal vocational and avocational activities after convalescence. In addition, denial has been shown to be a valuable psychological mechanism for coping with anxiety and depression. Patients who use denial successfully tend to have lower hospital mortality and an improved vocational outcome.[107]

The most common psychosocial intervention in cardiac rehabilitation programs is stress management. Other activities may include individual and group counseling, formal behavior modification programs, time management training, and financial planning. It is, of course, not practical for most of these latter programs to be provided by the rehabilitation team. An appropriate referral is made for those patients with a specific need.

Vocational Component

For the younger cardiac patient, a return to work often defines a successful rehabilitation outcome. Indeed, for the patient who was working at the time of the acute cardiac event, a return to work, usually to the pre-event job, is expected. Seventy percent to 80% of postinfarction patients will return to work,[75] although percentages as low as 31% of men in a lower socioeconomic population have been reported.[37]

The vocational assessment should include a review of the patient's education and training, a detailed work history, and an in-depth evaluation of the patient's current position. This assessment is particularly important for patients who have physically demanding jobs or who may have to make a job change because of anticipated residual physical impairment.

Vocational interventions may include contact with the patient's supervisor, a visit to the job site when the working environment or job tasks are unclear, job-specific exercises built into the exercise conditioning program, work hardening, and the prescription for return to work.

Educational Component

To a significant degree, a successful cardiac rehabilitation requires a long-term commitment to a life-style change. Most patients are unable or unwilling to make and maintain the necessary changes without understanding why they should be made, the potential benefits resulting from the changes, and how to go about effecting the changes. The education program is designed to provide the information necessary to increase each person's acceptance of the need for change and the personal responsibility required to achieve maximal benefits from the program.

The educational program typically provides up-to-date information on how the heart functions in health and disease, on exercise, nutrition, blood pressure control, smoking cessation, stress management, cardiovascular warning symptoms, and medications. The education sessions should be comprehensive yet clearly understandable by the layman. Open discussion should be encouraged, and spouses should be made welcome.

If the patient does not reach an optimal status in any component of the cardiac rehabilitation program, then a degree of residual disability exists. Achieving a high functional capacity through exercise conditioning is not enough. If the patient continues to be significantly stressed and is unemployed, then psychosocial and vocational disability remains. The rehabilitation team members must remind themselves of the comprehensive nature of the cardiac rehabilitation program and must ensure that the assessments are thorough and on-going, that the interventions are appropriate to the individual, and that they are designed to meet specific, identified goals.

Phases of Cardiac Rehabilitation

Cardiac rehabilitation programs are generally considered to have three phases: phase I, in-hospital; phase II, early post-hospitalization; and phase III, maintenance.

Activities of the in-hospital portion (phase I) of the program typically include progressive ambulation, low-level exercise, patient and family education, initial vocational and psychosocial assessment, and other necessary interventions.

The early post-hospitalization program (phase II) is usually based in an institution and is highly supervised by medical personnel. This phase generally begins within 2 weeks after the patient leaves the hospital and is the most intensive of the three phases. Exercise sessions are often monitored by telemetry, and a physician is present in the immediate exercise area. Phase II is also the most expensive segment of the program, currently costing between $1500 and $2500 for a 12-week program. Eighty percent of these costs are generally reimbursed by major medical insurors and Medicare. By the time phase II is completed, the patient should be close to optimal status in the major component areas and should have the basic information and skills which will permit continuation of the life-style change activities learned in the program.

The maintenance rehabilitation program (phase III) is designed to complete the key life-style changes begun in phase II, and to provide the resources to help the patient sustain those changes as long as possible. This program is usually conducted outside of the hospital or clinic and does not require close medical supervision or monitoring. It can function concurrently with an adult fitness primary prevention program. The apparently well participants of such a program are often surprised at the energy, stamina, and functional capacity of those who have completed the phase II program.

Candidates for Rehabilitation

Most participants in the cardiac rehabilitation program will have some form of coronary artery disease: recent acute myocardial infarction, coronary artery bypass surgery, or percutaneous transluminal coronary angioplasty. Patients with angina pectoris

who are not functioning optimally are also well served by the program. Other patients who may benefit from participation, but who are, at this time, less frequently enrolled, are those who have had cardiac valve surgery or replacement, patients following correction of a congenital cardiac defect, and those with occlusive peripheral vascular disease.

Elderly cardiac patients should be recruited and enrolled as vigorously as younger patients. For seniors, some aspects of the program such as vocational and nutritional issues will be less emphasized, but others, such as the maintenance of functional capacity through exercise conditioning to promote independent living will be very relevant.[7]

Finally, some patients who are felt to be at high risk for the development of overt clinical coronary disease may benefit from the program. The principles of primary prevention of coronary artery disease, the staff, and the program activities are the same as for the secondary prevention aspects of the rehabilitation program.

Program Staff

The size of the cardiac rehabilitation team may vary considerably in terms of the number of persons and disciplines taking part. Generally speaking, any person who might have a positive impact on the outcome for a particular patient is an appropriate member of the team.

Physician. Each program must have a medical director to assume overall leadership of the program. Treatment protocols must be written and approved, emergency procedures determined, staff training and patient review conferences conducted, and regular reports to referring physicians written. The medical director must stay current with developments in cardiac rehabilitation so that new program activities are included as their value is made clear.

Clinical Coordinator. Most cardiac rehabilitation programs employ a registered nurse, usually one with coronary care unit or other dysrhythmia monitoring experience, as clinical coordinator of the program. Exercise physiologists, physical therapists, and occupational therapists can also function as the clinical coordinator. The coordinator must have strong leadership, organizational, teaching, and personal relations skills in order to make the program succeed. In addition, the coordinator must be firmly grounded in knowledge and understanding of cardiac rehabilitation, the clinical course, and complications associated with the participants' diagnoses. If at all possible, prior experience in a cardiac rehabilitation setting is desirable before assuming the clinical coordinator's role.

Physical Therapist. The physical therapist can assume responsibility for the progressive activity program during phase I and assist with exercise leadership in phase II. If motivated and trained, the therapist can participate in the patient and family education program. A graduate degree in exercise physiology is a superb background for involvement in cardiac rehabilitation.

Occupational Therapist. The skills of the occupational therapist are too often not utilized in the cardiac rehabilitation program. Many patients, especially those with significant physical limitations, and those with heavy physical demands at work, could be well served by a comprehensive job site and task analysis and suggestions for changes that will simplify the tasks and make the work- or homesite more efficient. When properly trained, the occupational therapist can also help with the progressive ambulation program and patient education.

Nutritionist. Nutritional assessment and counseling is required if the cardiac patient is to realize optimal benefits from the program: weight loss, correction of lipid abnormalities, and control of glucose intolerance or other conditions which require nutritional guidelines for effective management. Access to nutritional consultation services should be arranged early in the development of the program.

Psychologist/Psychiatrist. Many patients with cardiac disease will have problems with anxiety, depression, anger, hostility, or stress that may prevent a complete recovery if not modified or corrected. The clinical psychologist or psychiatrist, especially one who is behaviorally oriented, can help program participants by identifying specific emotional problems, providing stress management training, and, occasionally, referring them for more intensive counseling or psychotherapy that is not in the province of the cardiac rehabilitation program.

Vocational Rehabilitation Counselor. When it becomes apparent that a patient will have to change employment because of the cardiovascular condition and its sequelae, a vocational rehabilitation counselor should be contacted. Each state has a federally supported Division of Vocational Rehabilitation with counselors who serve specific communities. The counseling services are provided at no cost to the patient and may include a review of prior work experience, aptitude testing, assessment of employability, brokering of needed services from other professionals or agencies, and retraining for a new vocation. Some communities have private rehabilitation counselors who perform much of the same tasks as counselors in the state-federal program, but are not limited by the regulatory restrictions of government agencies. They can often complete the evaluation, training, and placement more quickly.

Other Personnel. Additional staff who might join the program include a medical social worker and clergyman.

It should be recognized that a cardiac rehabilitation program can be satisfactorily conducted with a small staff; a large number of professionals from many disciplines, although desirable, is not crucial. Many programs have succeeded with a medical director and a nurse as the only regularly involved staff. In this situation, the nurse must function as coordinator, educator, and exercise leader, and must broker nutritional, psychological, and vocational rehabilitation services.

THE CARDIAC REHABILITATION PROGRAM

This segment of the chapter provides the practical guidelines for establishing and conducting a cardiac rehabilitation program. Acute myocardial infarction serves as the model for this discussion. The principles and techniques presented apply to patients with other conditions, and the clinician must be able and willing to make modifications to adapt to special circumstances or patient needs. The discussion of the program proceeds according to the outline of phases and components already presented.

Phase I

Cardiac rehabilitation should begin on admission to the hospital with the first contact between the patient and a member of the health care team. The patient and family members should realize very soon during the course of hospitalization that the entire hospital team has been trained to think in terms of long-term rehabilitative care and that all will strive to achieve an optimal outcome for the patient.

Physiological Component

The main effort of the primary physician, nursing staff, technicians, therapists, and other staff is to deliver the highest quality medical and surgical care. The prime function of activity counseling during phase I is to institute a program of progressive activity, which can be tailored to the needs of each patient, and which is designed to make the patient fully independent in self-care and activities of daily living by the time of discharge. Low-level calisthenics can be added, if desired.

Not only will the progressive activity program promote functional independence, it will also help to prevent the deconditioning effects of bed rest.[4, 15, 74, 82, 97, 98] The major effects of bed rest, discussed in greater detail in Chapter 23, include reduced vital capacity, lower maximal breathing capacity, a decreased physical work capacity with higher heart rates at submaximal work loads, and reduced maximal cardiac output and maximal oxygen consumption capability. In addition, deconditioned patients may have varying degrees of orthostatic intolerance characterized by tachycardia, hypotension, and vasodepressor reactions occurring with a change in body position, usually from recumbent or seated to standing. These reactions might include lightheadedness, weakness, visual blurring, or syncope.

For some time, a controversy waged about how soon mobilization should begin following myocardial infarction.[1, 50, 56, 68, 121] There is now general consensus that early, appropriately aggressive ambulation is safe, is not associated with an increase in complications (re-infarction, congestive failure, myocardial rupture, extension of infarction, dysrhythmias, venous thrombosis and pulmonary embolism, or ventricular aneurysm formation), may prevent psychosocial disability, and reduces the duration and cost of the hospital stay.[5] Patients who are free of complications or who have minor complications such as first-degree heart block, sinus bradycardia, transient hypotension, intraventricular conduction disturbance (*e.g.,* left bundle branch block), premature ventricular contractions fewer than 6 per minute, sinus tachycardia on admission, or a third heart sound generally do well and can be ambulated relatively quickly and discharged in 7 to 10 days.[14, 72] Patients with serious complications (ventricular tachycardia, ventricular fibrillation, pulmonary edema, cardiogenic shock, persistent sinus tachycardia, atrial fibrillation or flutter, hypotension, extension of the infarct, second- or third-degree heart block) must be approached individually. Ambulation may be delayed and prolonged, while mortality is greater and hospitalization longer in this group.

The progressive activity program is often administered by the cardiac rehabilitation nurse, the physical therapist, and the occupational therapist under the supervision of the program director and attending physician. In some hospitals, this function is carried out by the staff nurses. This can be successful, but on a busy, understaffed service, ambulation duties may have a lower priority than the bedside care of those more acutely ill.

During and after each exercise session the nurse or therapist must look for indicators of a poor response to activity: ischemic chest pain (angina pectoris), symptoms of pump failure including those of pulmonary vascular congestion (especially dyspnea and cough), and low cardiac output (easy fatigability, weakness, apathy, inattention, poor memory). Significant dysrhythmias and repolarization changes should be noted by those watching the telemetry monitors. If telemetry is not available, staff members working with the patient should be taught to recognize rhythm changes by taking an apical pulse. Not only will dysrhythmias be noted, but changes in heart rate will be more reliably detected than by palpating a peripheral pulse. Generally, an increase in heart rate of more than 20 beats over the resting pulse suggests that the activity may be requiring an effort that is excessive. A resting pulse greater than 100 beats per minute should be reported, since this may reflect early pump failure.

Almost all activities of daily living can be performed at an energy cost of 4 METS or less (one MET equals the energy cost of seated rest, or 3.5 cc/kg/min oxygen consumption). Activities of 4 METS or less correlate with a class III or IV functional classification of the New York Heart Association (Table 34-1). One activity of daily living above 4 METS is climbing stairs, which exerts 5 METS. It is better for the patient to attempt climbing stairs under supervision in-hospital than to negotiate the steps at home in an unsupervised situation. In this way, the inability to climb stairs will be identified before going home and the activity can be avoided. However, if steps are successfully managed in-hospital, then both the patient and physician are reassured about this aspect of returning to normal life.

Because sitting in a chair imposes less of a cardiovascular burden than lying down, it is acceptable for the patient to sit at the bedside in the coronary care unit once pain has remitted and major complications are ruled out. The patient may sit up several times during the day and should be seated while the bedclothes are being changed.

The patient must participate in self-care from the beginning, thus avoiding a sense of dependency.

To leave the ward to go to the rehabilitation medicine department for exercise or therapy may be encouraging to the patient. He or she may see patients with severe physical disabilities, which often helps the cardiac patient to put things into a more realistic perspective.

Any progressive activity program should be constructed for easy administration. A single order such as "Begin cardiac rehabilitation, step 3" or "Begin postinfarction rehabilitation program" should be all that is necessary to carry the program through to completion.

Absolute or relative contraindications to an increase in activity include shock or symptomatic hypotension, pump failure, ominous ventricular dysrhythmias, and angina pectoris.

A low-level treadmill exercise evaluation is often performed prior to discharge from the hospital. This procedure is quite useful in selecting those patients who are at high risk for a repeat acute event, such as new infarction or sudden cardiac death, and for assessing the pre-discharge clinical and functional status.

Table 34-1
New York Heart Association Functional Classification System

Class	Limits of Activity	METS	Oxygen Consumption (cc/kg/min)
I	No limitations, no symptoms with ordinary activity	≥7	≥24.5
II	Slight limitation; comfortable at rest; symptoms with ordinary activity	5–6	17.5–21
III	Marked limitation; comfortable at rest; symptoms with less than ordinary activity	3–4	10.5–14
IV	Discomfort with any activity; may have symptoms at rest	1–2	3.5–7

Table 34-2
Treadmill Evaluation Protocols

Protocol	Stage	Time (min)	Speed (MPH)	Grade (%)	MET
Naughton	1	2	2	0	2.5
	2	2	2	3.5	3.4
	3	2	2	7.0	4.4
	4	2	2	10.5	5.3
	5	2	2	14	6.3
	6	2	2	17.5	7.3
Balke	1	2	3	0	3.3
	2	2	3	2.5	4.3
	3	2	3	5.0	5.4
	4	2	3	7.5	6.3
	5	2	3	10	7.4
	6	2	3	12.5	8.4
	7	2	3	15	9.5
	8	2	3	17.5	10.5
Modified Bruce	0	3	1.7	0	2.3
	½	3	1.7	5	3.5
	1	3	1.7	10	4.6
	2	3	2.5	12	7

Exercise-induced ischemic ST-segment depression is the most useful prognostic indicator observed at the early postinfarction evaluation. The 30% to 40% of patients who have 1 mm or more of ST-segment depression with exercise have a risk of subsequent events 3 to 20 times greater than patients with a normal repolarization response, and a 1-year risk of death or reinfarction of 5% to 15%.[19, 112, 120] Patients with angina pectoris at the time of the pre-discharge treadmill exercise evaluation have a high probability of developing angina later in convalescence and should therefore be carefully monitored during their participation in the rehabilitation program.[19] The presence of frequent and complex ventricular dysrhythmias suggests severe underlying myocardial ischemia, regional left ventricular wall motion abnormalities, and left ventricular dysfunction.[10, 11]

The pre-discharge, or early postinfarction (10–21 days) exercise evaluation is usually terminated upon completion of a 5-MET stage in the absence of earlier end points such as angina pectoris, ominous dysrhythmias, falling systolic blood pressure, dyspnea, or fatigue. The protocol selected should begin at a low work load (2–3 MET) and increase in 1-MET increments each stage. The Naughton or modified Bruce protocols are acceptable for this purpose (Table 34-2).

In addition to identifying patients who are at increased risk, the early postinfarction exercise evaluation can select patients who are at significantly reduced risk. For example, those patients who do not have exercise-induced ischemic ST segments have a 1-year risk of death or reinfarction as low as 2%.[19, 112, 120]

In a significant number of patients, important clinical information will be uncovered at the time of the low-level exercise evaluation, which will cause an adjustment of medication, addition of another medication, or a recommendation for further evaluation.

The pre-discharge treadmill evaluation is also an opportunity to provide counseling regarding a return to sexual activity. It has been shown that the energy cost of conjugal sex is approximately 5 METS in middle-aged men.[49] If this work load is completed without evidence of myocardial ischemia, the patient should be told that sexual activity may be resumed as soon as both patient and partner feel comfortable doing so. Because there is often a great deal of anxiety about returning to normal sexual activity, it may be important to discuss the issue with the spouse as well as the patient. Angina pectoris that occurs with intercourse can be treated with prophylactic nitrates.[53] The energy cost of intercourse is the same for any of the conventional sexual positions, making them safe for most couples.[39] The likelihood of death during intercourse is greater in extramarital sex, which suggests that emotional factors may be important precipitators.[115]

Finally, the early post-myocardial infarction exercise test has been shown to have a positive influence on the patient's feelings of self-confidence and subsequent physical activity at home, especially for activities that are similar to treadmill exercise (walking, running, climbing stairs).[29]

For those patients who have no abnormalities on the predischarge treadmill evaluation, and who will be enrolled in the phase II, early post-hospitalization program, the data obtained from the exercise should be used to write an initial activity prescription for exercise training, appropriate activities of daily living, and recreation. If the phase II program is located in the hospital, it is often helpful to have the patient attend at least one phase II session prior to discharge so that the patient becomes familiar with the procedures, facilities, and staff. In addition, the patient's expectation of participation in the phase II program is created, thereby increasing the probability that this will occur. (The writing of the activity prescription based on the treadmill evaluation is described in a later section.)

Nutritional concerns should be identified and a program of modification should be started during phase I. Unfortunately, many hospitals do not promote a low-fat, low-cholesterol diet, and patients are given traditional meals such as bacon and eggs for breakfast during their hospitalization. It seems prudent to provide a diet that meets certain minimal criteria: reduced fat (no more than 30% total calories), low cholesterol (300 mg or less daily), reduced calories if the patient is obese, and other modifications as indicated by attendant conditions such as diabetes, hypertension, and certain medications. This diet should be continued until 6 to 8 weeks following the infarct when blood lipids can once again be reliably assessed and a definitive nutritional prescription written.[96]

Psychosocial Component

The successful recognition and management of psychosocial issues are extremely important in cardiac rehabilitation, and are necessary if an optimal outcome is to be achieved. As indicated previously, the most common responses to the acute event are anxiety and depression.[13, 41] Many, if not most patients, will resolve these feelings during hospitalization and will adopt a constructive, realistic attitude toward their situation. Others, especially those who tend to be hypochondriacal or chronically depressed or dissatisfied, may have extended emotional disability following hospitalization.[13] This emotional disability may be characterized by a greater sense of personal disability, and reduced likelihood of returning to normal vocational and recreational activities. Good coping skills tend to prevent these responses.

Denial has been found to be a mechanism used by some patients as a way of coping with the anxiety following a heart attack. Patients who use denial have less anxiety, a lower hospital mortality, and an improved vocational outcome following infarction.[107, 108] In contrast, the patient who denies his or her disease may be more susceptible to a return to stressful and unhealthful behaviors when the acute illness is over, and a poor outcome may result.[100] The practitioner should probably not try to break down a patient's denial of the obvious clinical realities—to do so would not only remove a useful defense, but also might remove the only viable defense the patient has, leaving the patient anxious and depressed.

During phase I, the psychosocial assessment is often informal and consists of questions to the patient and spouse regarding mood state, financial concerns, past history of emotional upset, home care resources, and the family support systems. If available, the in-hospital psychosocial assessment can be performed by a medical social worker or clinical psychologist who works with the rehabilitation team. The advantage of doing so for the patient and family is that they can meet with a professional trained in the evaluation and management of psychosocial problems and the procedures for appropriate referrals to other professionals or agencies. Although there has been little systematic research on the efficacy of in-hospital psychosocial interventions, there is some evidence that providing informational or emotional support can help patients handle the crisis of coronary care following heart attack and can reduce the time in the hospital.[77]

The social issues usually encountered during phase I are largely financial: dealing with the immediate loss of income and the inability to meet financial obligations. The patient or the spouse or both should be questioned about these matters and an appropriate referral to social services arranged.

Vocational Component

Most persons who have an acute myocardial infarction can, and will, return to work. The usual expectation is that 70% to 80% will do so, but percentages approaching 30% have been noted.[37, 75] Members of the rehabilitation team should be optimistic about the patient's likelihood of returning to work, and usually to the job held prior to the infarction.

In some cases, a return to the previous job will be impossible. When this situation occurs, immediate steps to provide intense vocational assessment and counseling should be instituted. A visit by a vocational rehabilitation counselor during hospitalization may create a sense of hope and expectation that a productive working life will be sustained.

Most phase I programs do not have a vocational rehabilitation counselor as a regular member of the team. This is unfortunate, since the counselor can reinforce the importance of returning to work in the rehabilitation process, identify potential sources of vocational disability which can be addressed early in the program, and help identify specific job tasks which may require special exercise training during phase II. The reasons for this lack of participation are not entirely clear, but there are several possible explanations. A heavy case load may preclude assuming additional clients. Most cardiac patients return to work without intervention by a vocational rehabilitation counselor. Program directors may fail to ask the counselor to participate, or fail to understand the contributions which can be made by the vocational rehabilitation counselor. The role of the vocational rehabilitation counselor in minimizing the number of cardiac patients who fail to return to work has not been systematically studied.

Educational Component

The goal of the educational program is to provide the information and techniques that will help the patient to assume responsibility for future health outcomes. The patient and family education program is started during hospitalization. Each member of the rehabilitation team is responsible for participating in the education effort, although certain persons may be identified as assuming major roles in the organization and provision of the teaching program.

Information that is given to the patient or a family member must be clearly understood, reinforced, and consistent from one team member to another. Often, a patient will ask the same question of several persons. Unclear or inconsistent responses create anxiety and perhaps distrust toward the rehabilitation staff. The education program should include comprehensive topics that are regularly reinforced. During phase I, time is often so short in the hospital that only highlights can be provided; detailed instruction often must wait until phase II.

The approach to patient education may be either formal or informal. In a formal program, teaching is done classroom-style with a group of patients who are at different postinfarction or postoperative stages. This approach has the advantages of ensuring that topics are covered completely, of making efficient use of the educator's time, and of permitting an interaction and sharing of thoughts and problems among the patients and with the educator. In the informal approach to patient education, the topics are covered by the therapist or educator on an individual basis, often at the same time as the supervised daily activity sessions. Advantages of this approach include the ability to individualize instruction to the level of understanding of the patient being taught, the opportunity to change the plan of learning to respond to specific patient needs, and the opportunity to re-educate and reinforce areas of deficient knowledge or understanding multiple times during the course of hospitalization. However, with the informal approach there is greater risk of omitting or not adequately covering a topic. Individual instruction tends to be more time-consuming and may be less stimulating to the educator because each topic must be repeated as each new patient is served. Each rehabilitation team and institution must decide which approach to use. Generally, hospitals which have a large in-patient service will find the formal approach more efficient, whereas hospitals with few acute myocardial infarction patients will often find the informal method more satisfactory.

There are several important generalizations to recall when initiating an in-patient education program. Each member of the rehabilitation team must have the same basic information regarding coronary artery disease and the philosophy and practices of the rehabilitation program. Information given to the patient must be consistent. All members of the rehabilitation team have a patient education responsibility and must be prepared to answer questions as they arise. Individuals do not retain what is taught during a time of personal anxiety,[89] and health care providers need to recognize that many of the questions asked by patients are a reflection of their anxiety. Understanding, compassionate, and consistent responses to any inquiry may have a substantial impact on allaying patient fears and concerns. Because retention of information given during hospitalization may be inadequate, the patient education program must continue after hospitalization, in phase II.

Phase II

Phase II is the most rigorous of the cardiac rehabilitation program phases. It is designed especially for early post-hospitalization patients, but may also serve those who are at high risk for developing coronary disease or those persons with heart disease who require a structured program to ensure compliance. For patients who graduate from a phase I program, phase II typically begins within 2 weeks of discharge from hospital. Early phase II entry seems to help recently hospitalized patients avoid feelings of frustration, depression, worry, anxiety, and doubt.[125] The phase II program is usually held in a hospital or clinic, lasts 8 to 12 weeks, is often telemetry monitored during exercise sessions, and requires close physician supervision. The primary goal of the phase II effort is to provide the information and experience that will permit the patient to pursue an independent cardiac rehabilitation/wellness program after graduating from the structured program.

Physiological Component

While the medical leadership of the cardiac rehabilitation program does not usually provide primary care for patients in the program, the program staff can often help to optimize care through the recognition of new or previously unreported symptoms or complications. For example, the cause of brief episodes of light-headedness may be seen to be due to short bursts of ventricular tachycardia, or the recent onset of exertional dyspnea may be found to be due to early left ventricular failure. Program staff must be continually alert for changes in a patient's clinical status and any significant change should be reported immediately to the treating physician. The concept here is that an optimal rehabilitation outcome cannot be realized without the highest quality traditional medical care. The staff of the cardiac rehabilitation program must participate in that care through diligent observation for any change in the clinical status of program participants.

EXERCISE: EVALUATION. Exercise conditioning is the cornerstone of the phase II program. Exercise sessions are usually held three times each week and are 1 hour long. For persons with heart disease, exercise must be carefully prescribed after observing the patient's response to a graded exercise test. This test may be conducted on a bicycle ergometer or on a treadmill. The latter device is most often used in the United States. The following comments regarding exercise testing in the cardiac rehabilitation setting are not meant to substitute for comprehensive training in exercise testing, but represent some important points for the practitioner. Several recent texts give a more detailed discussion of the subject.[28, 33]

Exercise testing in the rehabilitation setting is done to assess functional capacity, evaluate the efficacy of certain treatments, (*e.g.,* the effect of antiarrhythmic therapy on exercise-induced dysrhythmias), and obtain information necessary for writing the exercise and activity prescriptions. Additional reasons for doing the exercise test are to assess the severity of coronary disease and to estimate prognosis. In rehabilitation, the exercise test is not performed to establish a diagnosis unless there has been a change in symptoms that requires clarification, since the nature of the underlying cardiac problem is already known.

There are many treadmill exercise protocols which have been well established in clinical practice and which provide reasonably accurate estimations of the energy cost of each stage. For patients entering phase II soon after hospitalization and those with significant symptoms or a history of functional limitations, a protocol that starts at a low work load and that increases in 1-MET increments is preferred. The Naughton, Balke, and modified Bruce protocols are satisfactory (see Table 34-2).

During the exercise test, the electrocardiogram (ECG)—usually a full 12-lead scalar tracing—and blood pressure should be monitored and recorded each minute. Since functional capacity assessment is a major goal of the procedure, the patient should not hold on to the treadmill railing during the test. Holding on invalidates the estimate of oxygen consumption (METS) because most patients who hold on assist themselves, thereby reducing the energy cost of a given work load.[88, 127] If the patient is at least 3 weeks from the onset of the acute cardiac event, and if no untoward responses to the exercise are noted, exercise should continue to a symptom-limited maximal effort. For most patients who have recently left the hospital, the limiting symptom will be generalized fatigue, leg fatigue, or shortness of breath. The deconditioning associated with bed rest and extended relative inactivity almost always precludes exhaustion as the limiting symptom. In some patients who have had uncomplicated myocardial infarctions, a symptom-limited maximal test may be performed safely less than 3 weeks post-event. However, for most communities, the 3-week guideline establishes a safe and prudent practice.[40]

It is important to constantly look for evidence of intolerance to exercise during the exercise evaluation and to stop the test if it becomes unsafe. Ventricular tachycardia, multifocal premature ventricular beats, second- or third-degree heart block, angina pectoris, symptomatic supraventricular dysrhythmias, or a reproducible fall in systolic blood pressure of 10 mm Hg or more is a clear indication to stop the procedure.[40, 114]

Abnormal repolarization in the absence of symptoms poses a special problem: is it due to silent ischemia or does it represent a false-positive repolarization response? The clinician must look for possible causes of a false-positive response such as hyperventilation, a recent meal, digitalis, hypokalemia, anemia, intraventricular conduction defect, left ventricular hypertrophy, hypoxemia, mitral valve prolapse, or female gender.[40] A thallium myocardial perfusion study may help to resolve the issue in appropriate cases.[81] From a practical standpoint, when a patient with known ischemic heart disease who is not taking digitalis has abnormal repolarization in the absence of symptoms, especially if the ST depression is 2 mm or more, the clinician should assume that the ST-segment change represents silent ischemia and should terminate the procedure. The decision to stop exercise is reinforced if there is an associated drop in systolic blood pressure.

The classical abnormal repolarization response is 1 mm or more of ST-segment depression with straightening or downsloping. In the past 10 to 15 years is has been recognized that a J-point (the point where the QRS segment ends and the ST segment begins) depression with an upsloping ST segment that remains at least 1.5 mm below the PQ segment 0.08 seconds after the J point also represents an abnormal repolarization response.[110]

EXERCISE: PRESCRIPTION. Once the exercise test has been completed, information obtained from the study is used to write the exercise prescription and to provide guidelines for work and recreational activities. Most exercise training following myocardial infarction is undertaken in a medically supervised setting. However, it has been shown that low-risk patients can be trained at home as safely and as effectively as in a group setting.[73]

The exercise prescription has four components: the type of exercise, intensity, frequency, and duration of exercise sessions.

Type of Exercise. The majority of exercise training in cardiac rehabilitation is aerobic. Aerobic exercises are dynamic and use large muscle masses in continuous motion. Common examples of aerobic activities include walking, jogging, running, cycling, swimming, cross-country skiing, and floor exercise such as jazzercise. With aerobic activity, ventilation, oxygen consumption, heart rate, and systolic blood pressure, all rise.[94] In the patient with normal blood pressure, diastolic blood pressure will remain at the resting value or will fall slightly. Systolic pressure will rise to a plateau, which is usually between 170 and 230 mm Hg at maximal effort, although higher values are often seen and are not necessarily abnormal.

The response to isometric, or static, exercise is characterized by little or no increase in heart rate, ventilation, or oxygen consumption, and a marked increase in both systolic and diastolic blood pressure.[69, 76] Isometric exercise can be recognized by activities in which there is muscle contraction but no joint motion. Common examples of isometric exercise include carrying a suitcase or briefcase (forearm isometrics) and overhead arm work (shoulder girdle isometrics). Many practitioners counsel against having patients perform isometric activities because of the marked pressor response and the associated increase in myocardial oxygen consumption. This conservative approach is appropriate for patients who have poor response to dynamic treadmill exercise (New York Heart Association class II or III), since a sustained isometric effort may produce myocardial ischemia, ventricular dysrhythmias, or left ventricular failure.[46] Patients with good dynamic exercise capacity—that is, greater than 6 METS—tolerate static exercise well. Most patients will be able to tolerate the brief isometric tasks required for normal living without incident.

Most cardiac rehabilitation programs use a variety of stationary exercise devices for exercise training such as a bicycle ergometer, rowing machine, treadmill, mini-trampoline, steps, a cross-country skiing machine, arm ergometer, or pulley weights. Free weights or other weight training equipment (e.g., universal gym, isokinetic devices) may be added to the conditioning prescription. Recent data suggest that the hemodynamic and symptom responses of cardiac patients to weight lifting are acceptable, and that weight lifting can be performed, at least in selected patients, without ECG or rhythm abnormalities.[30, 47] These exercises are especially beneficial to patients who have physically active jobs that require considerable muscle strength. When prescribing strength training in cardiac rehabilitation, it is probably best to use relatively low weight and frequent repetitions, thereby avoiding the marked pressor response of isometric, high resistance, isokinetic, or high weight–low repetition isotonic exercise. The role of weight training in cardiac rehabilitation has not been adequately investigated.

Intensity. The intensity of exercise, or how hard the patient exercises, is calculated from the patient's heart rate response to the treadmill exercise evaluation. The procedure is quite simple. The first step is to identify the clearance heart rate. This is the highest heart rate, determined from the exercise test, that is safe for exercise. For most, this will be the highest heart rate obtained during the procedure; for others, it will be the highest heart rate that occurred in the absence of angina pectoris, ominous dysrhythmias, abnormal blood pressure responses, or abnormal repolarization. The target heart rate range, which determines the exercise intensity, is calculated by multiplying the clearance heart rate by 0.7 and 0.85. This heart rate range permits the patient to vary the exercise intensity while avoiding a maximal or potentially unsafe effort, thus minimizing the possibility of cardiovascular complications during exercise conditioning.

Frequency. The frequency of supervised exercise conditioning should be three times per week in most programs. Additional exercise sessions at home may be prescribed once the patient has demonstrated the ability to self-monitor exercise intensity appropriately and to perform prescribed exercise safely. The risk of orthopedic injury increases with more than four exercise sessions a week,[22] although this risk can be minimized if the additional exercise is relatively atraumatic, such as walking, cycling, or swimming.

Duration. The duration of each exercise session is usually 1 hour. On arrival at the exercise site, patients weigh themselves, check their heart rate, apply electrodes, connect a telemetry unit, and report to the program supervisor. The exercise session begins with 5 to 10 minutes of warm-up exercises (e.g., stretching, light calesthenics, walking) that bring each person's heart rate into the lower end of the target heart rate range. Thirty or more minutes of aerobic exercise within the target heart rate range follow, and the session is concluded with another 5 to 10 minutes of cool-down exercises similar to those performed during warm-up. Each participant's heart rate and blood pressure are taken and recorded prior to leaving the facility. If values are inappropriate (too high or too low), or if the patient is symptomatic, the program medical director should be contacted, the patient detained, and a decision regarding evaluation and management made. Fortunately, these events are uncommon. Cardiac rehabilitation exercise is generally very safe. An early review of cardiovascular complications during exercise training of 13,570 cardiac patients in 103 programs documented one nonfatal event every 34,673 hours of patient participation and one fatal complication every 116,402 hours.[45] A recent report of data from 167 cardiac rehabilitation programs, involving 51,303 outpatients who exercised for a total of over 2,350,000 patient-hours documented 21 cardiac arrests (1 per 111,996 patient-hours of exercise), and 8 nonfatal myocardial infarctions (1 per 293,990 patient-hours of exercise). Of the 21 arrests, only 3 were fatal, resulting in a fatality rate of 1 per 783,972 patient-hours of exercise. There were no fatal myocardial infarctions.[116] The safety of exercise training following myocardial infarction is at least partly due to the careful screening and exclusion of patients with symptomatic heart failure, unstable angina pectoris, uncontrolled dysrhythmias, high degrees of atrioventricular block, recent thromboembolic disease, or uncontrolled metabolic disease such as diabetes.

Work and Recreational Activities. The same principles that were used to write the exercise prescription for conditioning can be applied to the prescription for work or recreational activities. First, find the clearance heart rate from the most recent exercise evaluation. Eighty-five percent of the clearance rate is the highest heart rate that is permissible for work or play. The MET level at which 85% of the clearance rate occurred can be determined from the exercise protocol. Tables, such as Table 34-3, which give the approximate energy cost of vocational and recreational activities, can be used to help make the decision regarding the appropriateness of returning to a specific task or activity. Generally, if there are no indicators of myocardial ischemia on the symptom-limited treadmill exercise, there will be none during the performance of job tasks. The treadmill exercise evaluation can also provide clearance for performing tasks following a meal,[52] in a cold environment,[66] and for activities which combine static and dynamic exercise.[21] Actually, the patient can perform any task that does not generate a heart rate that exceeds that at which ischemia occurs.

The patient's heart rate is the key to monitoring all activities. This is the one simple physiological parameter that the patient can assess with reasonable accuracy and which tracks myocardial oxygen demand.[52] The patient is taught to take the pulse immediately upon completing a task or exercise, using either the radial or carotid artery, counting for no more than 15 seconds. Multiplying by the appropriate factor (4 for a 15-second count; 6 for a 10-second count) will give a close approximation of the last minute exercise heart rate.

Cardiac patients should maintain their exercise conditioning program throughout the year. Extremes of temperature should not be a deterrent for most patients. Many larger communities with shopping malls have developed a "Walk the Mall" program, which permits regular exercise in any weather. Typically, brochures which outline a walking route and give distances between specific points in the mall are provided free of charge at mall entrances.

Table 34-3
Energy Cost of Common Vocational and Recreational Activities

MET Range	Vocational	Recreational
2–4	Desk work, typing	Card games
	Driving	Archery
	Light welding	Horseshoes
	Interior carpentry	Flying
	Scrubbing, waxing	Bowling
	Using hand tools	Fishing from boat
	Machine assembly	Golf with cart
	Crane operation	Shuffleboard
	Gas station work	Gardening
		Horseback riding, horse walking
		Cycling at 6 mph
		Walking at 2–3 mph
		Playing music
5–6	Bricklaying	Skating, roller, and ice
	Housepainting	Tennis, doubles
	Mowing lawn	Dancing
	Paperhanging	Fishing, wading
	Power sanding	Volleyball
	Pneumatic tool operation	Sledding
	Lifting and carrying up to 65 lbs	Cycling at 8 mph
		Walk-jog at 4 mph
7–8	Digging, shoveling	Badminton
	Plumbing	Tennis
	Moving van work	Skiing, downhill and water
	Using hand axe, saw	Swimming
	Snow shoveling	Hunting
	Lifting and carrying up to 65–85 lb	Cycling 11–12 mph
		Walk-jog at 5 mph
		Canoeing, kayaking
		Hiking cross country

For patients who do not have access to a shopping mall, or who prefer to exercise outdoors, simple guidelines to activity in inclement weather will permit safe exercise throughout the year. When it is hot, exercise should be done in the cooler times of the day, early morning or late evening. Fluid should be taken before starting the exercise and frequently during the exercise session, especially if sweating is significant. Waiting to take fluid until thirsty is not appropriate; some dehydration will already have occurred. Water is the best replacement fluid. Expensive ergogenic liquid mixtures are not necessary for the exercising cardiac rehabilitation patient, nor are salt tablets either indicated or needed. The conditions in which the greatest potential heat stress will be realized are high temperature, high humidity, and low wind. Unless the patient is highly fit and well acclimatized to a hot environment, exercise outdoors should be avoided when these conditions exist.

During the cold months, outdoor exercise can be both comfortable and enjoyable for most cardiac patients. They should dress in layers, so that clothing can be removed or put on as conditions dictate. The first layer should be a material such as polypropylene that wicks moisture away from the skin. Cotton is not a good material for the first layer. Wool makes an excellent second layer. It is warm and also has the important wicking property. The outer layer should protect against wind and wetness; Gore-tex is a fabric that works well for this purpose. None of the layers should be bulky. Since a significant amount of heat is lost from the scalp, a cap of some kind is important when exercising in the cold. Mittens provide more warmth and protection for the hands than gloves. Patients who develop angina pectoris with cold exposure should wear a mask when active in the cold. Breathing warm air will often reduce or prevent the anginal attacks. If the day is windy, the first segment of the exercise session should be taken into the wind; that way, the wind will be at the back on the return trip and excessive fatigue and chilling that might occur at the end of the exercise session due to walking or running into the wind can be avoided.

Altitude exposure places a significant burden on the visitor to high places. Heart rate, blood pressure, and ventilation increase, and maximal oxygen consumption capability is reduced about 3% for every 1000 feet of elevation above 6000 feet.[42, 99] For the cardiac patient, going to altitude can pose some problems and will raise questions about how to monitor oneself and gauge appropriate levels of activity. It has been shown with cardiac patients taken to altitude that exercise capacity is reduced, heart rates and blood pressure at submaximal activity levels are higher, and the rate–pressure product at which angina pectoris occurs is the same as at low altitude.[8] Therefore, the heart rate guidelines given in the exercise prescription at low altitude apply when the patient visits a high altitude community. Less work will be possible, and some tasks that could be performed at low altitude may not be possible at high altitude, but if the clearance heart rate is not exceeded, the stay at altitude should be both safe and comfortable.

EXERCISE: RESULTS. Exercise conditioning is clearly the cornerstone of the cardiac rehabilitation program. The benefits of exercise in the cardiac rehabilitation setting are incompletely defined, but are sufficiently substantial to warrant further study and continued inclusion of exercise training in the rehabilitation program.

The cardiac patient responds to an exercise conditioning program in much the same way as the person without heart disease: maximal oxygen consumption increases, rest and submaximal heart rate and systolic blood pressure are lower, and maximal ventilatory capacity and oxygen pulse (oxygen consumption/heart rate) increase.[16] Although no direct observations have been made in patients with coronary artery disease, peripheral training adaptations are believed to occur as in normal persons who are trained: oxidative enzymes and the capillary-fiber ratio should increase, resulting in improved oxygen extraction and a widened arteriovenous oxygen content difference.[51, 118] Although there is some controversy regarding the ability of normal persons to obtain full training benefits while taking a beta-adrenergic blocking agent,[126] all published studies of exercise training of cardiac patients on beta blockade have shown that conditioning does occur.[64, 80, 86, 117] Many cardiac patients will not show an improvement in ejection fraction or myocardial perfusion with exercise training, suggesting that the major site of training benefits is peripheral, not central.[20, 103] This probably explains why cardiac patients improve while training on beta blockade, since it has been shown in normal volunteers that beta blockade does not affect peripheral adaptations.[126] However, some studies have suggested that central training adaptations do occur in some patients with coronary disease, especially if the patient is able to exercise at high intensity and if the training program has been undertaken for a year or more.[27, 34, 55, 123]

The reduction in both systolic blood pressure and heart rate at rest and with submaximal exercise following conditioning are especially important for the patient with angina pectoris. The rate-pressure product (systolic pressure × heart rate) is directly and linearly related to myocardial oxygen demand.[61] Furthermore, in patients with stable, predictable angina pectoris, the rate-pressure product at which angina occurs is relatively constant and reproducible.[91] Because of the decrease in submaximal heart rate and systolic pressure following training, the rate-pressure product is also reduced. As a result, the critical rate-pressure product at which angina occurs will not be reached until a higher work load is achieved following training than was observed before exercise training began. The benefit for the patient is the ability to perform more difficult tasks at higher work loads without experiencing angina.

The effect of exercise conditioning on the progression of existing coronary artery disease has not been adequately studied. One study which attempted to evaluate the effect of exercise training intensity on the rate of progression of coronary disease in 120 patients who had serial coronary angiograms an average of 20 months apart suggested that an inverse relationship between amount of exercise and progression exists: that higher levels of fitness are associated with a reduced rate of progression of coronary disease.[111] However, the study was not controlled for other factors that might affect the progression of coronary disease.

Exercise conditioning may have a significant effect on several of the modifiable risk factors for coronary artery disease. Blood pressure may be lower at rest and at submaximal exercise, blood lipids may be improved (especially triglycerides and high-density lipoprotein cholesterol [HDLC]; body fat and weight usually decrease, and glucose tolerance improves.[44, 79] In addition, persons who become fit often find it easier to manage the stresses of daily living, have an improved self-image, and less depression.[17, 101, 106] In addition, a major psychological effect of exercise training in coronary disease patients is a feeling of increased confidence.[87] The effect of these changes on the natural history of coronary disease is not yet clear.

Does exercise-based cardiac rehabilitation affect mortality of persons with coronary artery disease? This question is often asked and the answer is not entirely clear. In nine randomized clinical trials of cardiac rehabilitation, only one showed a significant reduction in cardiac mortality.[12, 57, 60, 83, 90, 92, 102, 119, 122] However, when the data from the nine trials were pooled, cardiovascular mortality over an average 45½ month follow-up was 14.2% in 1,675 control patients, and 9.6% in 1,671 intervention patients (p < 0.001). Nonfatal recurrent myocardial infarction was the same in both groups, 10.5% and 10.1%, respectively.[70]

NUTRITION. Nutritional assessment and counseling are important aspects of the physiological component of the cardiac rehabilitation program. The evaluation that must be performed in order to write a comprehensive nutritional prescription includes documentation of the composition of the patient's diet through dietary recall, checklist, or diary; assessment of body weight, body composition, ideal body weight, blood lipid profile, activity level, and medications (e.g., potassium wasting diuretics); and assessment of any associated medical conditions in which nutrition plays an important therapeutic role, such as diabetes or hypertension.

The evaluation and nutritional prescription should be completed in the first week of the rehabilitation program. Specific nutritional goals should be negotiated with the patient for weight loss or gain, changes in body composition, or blood lipids. As with all goal setting in the rehabilitation environment, the goals should be short-term, realistic, and attainable. Nothing fosters success like having succeeded. For example, a grossly overweight patient may need to lose 100 pounds. To agree on a goal of 100 pounds is inappropriate; it is too big a task, will take too long, and is unlikely to be accomplished. A goal of 6 pounds lost in a 6-week period is far more realistic, is clearly attainable, and will give the patient a significant feeling of success when the goal is met.

The nutritional intervention includes specific nutritional prescription, nutritional counseling, and nutritional education. The patient's spouse is strongly encouraged to participate in all aspects of the nutritional program. This is particularly important if the spouse is the person in the household who prepares the food. The nutritional education program should include information about good nutrition, the role of fat and cholesterol and heart disease, the importance of fiber, the potential harm in fad diets, how to read food labels, how to order "heart-healthy" food from a menu, and how to shop for healthy foods. If facilities and staffing permit, cooking classes can provide a firsthand experience in the preparation and serving of heart-healthy food.

Whether a cholesterol-lowering diet affects the natural history of coronary artery disease is not entirely clear. The data to date suggest that the value of nutritional intervention may be significant. In three randomized, controlled trials of rehabilitation after myocardial infarction, the rehabilitation group showed reduced mortality and a significant lowering of cholesterol.[12, 57, 119] In the Oslo Diet-Heart Study, post-myocardial infarction patients on a cholesterol-lowering diet had a 17.6% reduction in serum cholesterol compared to a 3.7% reduction in the control group.[67] After an 11-year follow-up, there was a statistically significant reduction in the rate of fatal recurrent myocardial infarction in the experimental group as compared to the control. More recently, data from the uncontrolled Leiden Intervention Trial, a study of the effect of a cholesterol-lowering diet in patients with angiographically proven coronary artery disease, have shown a greater rate of stabilization or regression of coronary lesions in those subjects who had the lowest ratios of total to HDLC.[63] The data seem to support the value of a vigorous nutritional program in the cardiac rehabilitation setting.

Psychosocial Component

Psychosocial issues may be a significant source of disability for the patient with cardiac disease. The most common and potentially debilitating emotional responses are anxiety and depression.[9, 13, 41, 125] For many patients, these responses are transient and do not impede a return to normal living patterns, and therefore do not affect participation in the phase II program. In contrast, 15% to 30% of depressed patients will remain depressed and anxious 6 to 12 months following the infarct.[108] Patients who have a pre-event history of depressive tendencies, hypochondriasis, or chronic dissatisfaction are apt to have an extended untoward emotional response to an acute myocardial infarction.[13] In addition, these people consider themselves to be more disabled and are less likely to return to full normal vocational and avocational life following their heart attack than patients who have demonstrated good coping skills prior to the acute event.

Inability to cope with stress, financial problems, marital and job discord, or unhealthful behaviors (*e.g.,* cigarette smoking, poor eating habits) may delay or prevent a successful rehabilitation outcome. Social isolation and job stress have recently been found to be associated with an increased risk of death in men who survived a myocardial infarction.[95] The higher levels of both stress and isolation were found in men with the least education.

The practitioner may underestimate the degree of psychosocial morbidity following infarction, and a significant number of patients—up to one-third—may become unnecessarily disabled.[71] While most cardiac rehabilitation programs do not include traditional psychotherapy and counseling in the psychoso-

cial component, an evaluation for emotional characteristics that may affect the patient's outcome of the program should be undertaken early in the course of the program. Important potential impediments to the success of the program can thus be identified and referral to appropriate services arranged.

Stress management is the major psychosocial intervention provided by most cardiac rehabilitation programs. The course is conducted by someone with an interest in behavioral medicine and experience in group stress management leadership. A typical course is 8 weekly sessions of 1 to 1½ hours' duration.

Early reports regarding psychological interventions in the different phases of cardiac rehabilitation are encouraging. The recent work of Freidman and associates on the benefit of modifying the type A, coronary-prone, behavior pattern following myocardial infarction is promising.[31, 32, 85] They have shown that the type A behavior pattern can be altered by counseling, which is, in turn, associated with a significant reduction in the subsequent rate of nonfatal myocardial infarction.

Stress management and relaxation training may improve certain psychological characteristics such as assertiveness and social anxiety, factors which should help to keep the patient from adopting a "sickness role" during late convalescence.[66] These and other behavior therapy approaches form the basis of psychological interventions in cardiac rehabilitation. Important behavioral issues commonly encountered include diet and weight control, smoking, maintenance of regular exercise, type A behavior patterns, stress responses, and compliance. The status of behavioral strategies has been reviewed by Blumenthal and colleagues.[6]

Controlled studies of the effect of exercise-based rehabilitation programs on the psychological functioning of cardiac patients have yielded variable results. Two pertinent studies have been reported from the National Exercise and Heart Disease Project (NEHDP). In the first, low-level exercise (72% of age-corrected maximal heart rate) was associated with positive psychosocial changes.[104] This exercise was undertaken by all of the 651 subjects recruited for the NEHDP to evaluate compliance prior to randomization to either the exercise group or the control group. Whether the psychological improvement—primarily a reduction of depression—was due to exercise or to the "group effect" of volunteering and enrolling in a supportive rehabilitation study, is not clear. Late follow-up of the control and exercise groups at 6 months, 1 and 2 years showed almost no group differences of psychosocial variables.[105]

A second, more recent study measured the effect of a 3-month exercise and education cardiac rehabilitation program on 28 participants and 20 control subjects.[93] Patients who underwent treatment showed significant improvements in cardiovascular functioning, compliance with treatment, understanding of heart disease, psychosocial functioning (less job-related stress, more physical and sexual activity, more active use of leisure time), and positive self-perceptions (self-concept, health, body concept, progress toward goals) in comparison to control subjects. These changes persisted in a repeat evaluation 4 months after completion of the program.

In many cardiac rehabilitation programs, the psychosocial assessment of the patient is performed in a perfunctory, unsystematic fashion. Very often, an impression of the patient's emotional status is obtained from staff conversations with the patient; no documentation of specific sources of psychosocial disability is sought; and no effort is made to direct the patient to sources of support and care. At this time, there is no "best" approach to psychosocial evaluation of the cardiac patient, and there is no instrument or group of testing instruments which can be recommended for this purpose.

In the cardiac rehabilitation program of which I am director, three pencil-and-paper psychometric instruments are administered during the first week of participation in the program. These evaluations are completed in a quiet area in the rehabilitation facility. Except in unusual circumstances, the patient is not permitted to complete the instruments at home. The time requirement for completing the instruments is approximately 30 minutes. The psychometric tests are:

1. The SCL-90, a 90-item checklist of symptoms that relate to nine different domains: psychoticism, paranoid ideation, phobic anxiety, somatization, interpersonal sensitivity, anxiety, depression, hostility, and obsessive-compulsiveness.[24] The SCL-90 is a screening instrument which alerts the psychologist to the need for additional assessment or intervention.
2. The Lazarus Hassles Scale lists 134 potential sources of stress in the patient's life.[58] The patient identifies the items that represent current hassles and indicates, on a scale of 1 to 4, the intensity of the hassle.
3. The Bortner Scale is a simple scale of type A – type B behavior pattern. (The Jenkins Activity Scale is a more validated instrument than the Bortner Scale and may also be used to assess coronary prone behavior.[54])

The psychometric instruments are scored and given to the consulting psychologist for interpretation. The results of the tests are reviewed with the patient by the medical social worker at a psychosocial intake interview. In addition, a social work data base is obtained at the intake interview, the need for agency or specialist referral is discussed, and specific psychosocial goals are set. Because an acute cardiac illness such as heart attack can be very disruptive to the psychodynamic balance of a family, family members should be included in the rehabilitation program during all phases of rehabilitation.[18] Arrangements for the spouse to enter a support group may be made, although these groups are not always as successful as those comprising patients.[3, 43] Family counseling may be scheduled, and other services brokered as needs are identified.

Vocational Component

For many patients, especially those who are younger, returning to work constitutes a successful rehabilitation outcome. The majority of patients who are employed at the time of the infarction and who desire to return to work will do so, usually without any special intervention on the part of the rehabilitation program staff. Those patients with significant complications from their illness, those who are older, and those with physically taxing jobs may require a special vocational effort on their behalf.

Predictors of vocational outcome in coronary artery disease have been studied and reviewed.[26, 35, 109] Factors associated with a decreased likelihood of returning to work include low education level and advanced age,[38] blue collar work status,[84] the degree of emotional disability,[36, 62, 124] an unstable and unsatisfying work history,[2] lower social class, and a negative perception of health.[35] Data regarding the severity of heart disease as a predictor of vocational outcomes have not been consistent. In some studies, the severity of disease has been associated with a less positive outcome.[2, 25, 35, 78] In others, the severity of the disease and its complications have been less of a factor than the level of emotional stress.[2, 35] From a programmatic point of view, the presence of significant disease or complications should not cause a patient to retire, unless those symptoms occur with work and limit job performance.

The purpose of the vocational component is to minimize vocational disability through job evaluation, work hardening, work simplification, and return to work planning. Although not all of these activities will be required for all, or even most patients, it is desirable to have each aspect of the vocational program available in case it is needed.

All patients who enroll in the cardiac rehabilitation program should have a job evaluation performed by one of the staff during the first week of participation. A simple job assessment form, suitable for both the screening and initial return to work planning stages is shown in Figure 34-1. For patients with physically taxing jobs, it is important to identify the specific muscle groups required to perform job tasks. Low-resistance, high-repetition isotonic or isokinetic strengthening exercises involving those muscles should be added to the exercise prescription.

When the patient has anxiety or concern about his or her ability to perform job tasks, if the job requires heavy or frequent physical effort, or if symptoms are noted or anticipated with job tasks (chest pain, dyspnea, palpitations, easy fatigability), referral to an occupational therapist for further evaluation, work hardening, or work simplification activities should be considered.

Any patient who has significant limitation to activity from chest pain, heart failure, or dysrhythmias should be seen by an occupational therapist for work simplification instruction in activities of daily living. In selected instances, a home visit by the therapist may yield as much benefit for the disabled cardiac patient as it does for the patient with a severe neuromuscular disorder.

Educational Component

For most patients, cardiac rehabilitation requires a modification of life-style. Exercise is promoted as an important aspect of living. Smoking must be given up, stressors must be recognized and stress responses managed, and a new nutritional pattern adopted. Making, and adhering to, major changes in life-style requires much information: what changes are necessary, why the changes are important, how to make and sustain these changes. The purpose of the educational component of the phase II program is to provide the information necessary for the patient to assume responsibility for his or her own health outcomes. Program staff can indicate what changes need to be made and how they can be made, but staff cannot ensure that the patient will make the necessary changes. Acceptance of self-responsibility by the patient is the key to life-style change and long-term rehabilitation success.

The typical cardiac rehabilitation program will have a weekly class for all current program participants. The format of the sessions may vary: lecture, discussion, demonstration, film, and so on. Hand-outs which reinforce the material presented are helpful. Topics will also vary. The same general themes that were presented in phase I are expanded and typically include an overview of cardiac rehabilitation/wellness, stress and stress management, nutrition, risk factors for coronary artery disease, the benefits of exercise, effects of temperature and altitude on exercise, recognizing symptoms and warning signals of heart disease, access to the health care system if the need should arise, drugs used in cardiovascular disease, and smart medical consumer practices. As with all program components, an evaluation of the educational offerings will assure the maintenance of a quality program that addresses the needs of the patients it serves.

Phase III

Phase III is the maintenance program. All components of the phase II program are addressed, with emphasis on exercise conditioning. Exercise is not usually monitored, either by staff or telemetry, because the patient should be quite competent in self-

(*Text continues on p. 685*)

Healthsouth Rehabilitation Center of Denver
1000 South Colorado Boulevard
Glendale, Colorado 80222

Job Analysis

Job Analysis for ______________________________ Date ______________

Job Title ______________________ Company ______________________

Responsibilities ____

____

_________________________________ Emp. Since ___________________

I. Physical Tasks	Requirements (how much, how often)	Objects Involved (equipment, tools)	N/A*
1. Walking			
2. Standing			
3. Stooping/bending			
4. Carrying	lbs.; how far?		
5. Kneeling/squatting			
6. Lifting	lbs.; how high?		
7. Climbing steps/ladders			
8. Pushing/pulling	lbs.		
9. Driving			
10. Other:			

Comments: ____

____

____

II. Work Environment	Exposure (how much, how often)	Effects	N/A*
1. Poor air quality			
2. Crowded/dense conditions			
3. Accessibility barriers			
4. Temp. extremes/changes			
5. Chemicals			
6. Noise			
7. Wet or humid			
8. Scaffolding/ladders			
9. Equipment operation			
10. Other:			

Comments: ____

____

____

Figure 34-1. Vocational assessment form. *(Continued)*

III. Stress Factors	Frequency/Intensity (how much, how often)	Effects	N/A*
1. Irregular hours			
2. Time pressures			
3. Work overload/fatigue			
4. Job like/dislike			
5. Relationships with others			
6. Employer/supervisor attitudes			
7. Unclear responsibilities			
8. Preoccupation with symptoms			
9. Side effects of medication			
10. Workaholic tendencies			
11. Other:			

Comments: _____

_____

_____

Assessment:

Job is physically safe/appropriate without modifications: _____

Job is physically OK with following modifications: _____

_____

_____

Job is not physically safe/appropriate.   Temporarily _____ Permanently _____

Job is environmentally OK _____ Not OK _____

Work environment needs following modifications: _____

_____

_____

Job stress is _____ is not _____ a critical issue.

Job is too stressful to continue _____

Job stress can be modified as follows: _____

_____

_____

Vocational Recommendations:

Referral _____

Return to work; no changes _____ Retirement: _____ full _____ partial

Continue disability/sick leave until _____ (return to work date)

Return to work with following changes: _____

_____

Change jobs _____

Retraining _____

Other _____

_____

Analysis performed by: _____

1/87

*N/A = Non-applicable or None

monitoring by the completion of phase II and must assume this responsibility in phase III.

Often the program is held in a community facility rather than a clinic, hospital, or rehabilitation center. The patient's nutritional, psychosocial, vocational, and educational status is monitored, and reinforcing educational activities are planned. Some activities which may help the patient maintain life-style changes include a program newsletter, periodic meetings of program graduates, and booster sessions for stress management techniques.

REFERENCES

1. Acker JE: Are we mobilizing early enough? Bibl Cardiol 36:50, 1977
2. Acker JE: Factors affecting the employment of patients located in coronary care units for myocardial infarction. J Tenn State Med Assoc 61:1200, 1968
3. Adsett CA, Bruhn JG: Short-term group psychotherapy for post-myocardial infarction patients and their wives. Can Med Assoc J 99:577, 1968
4. Bassey EJ, Fentern PH: Extent of deterioration in physical condition during postoperative bed rest and its reversal by rehabilitation. Brit Med J 4:194, 1974
5. Bloch A et al: Early mobilization after myocardial infarction. A controlled study. Am J Cardiol 34:152, 1974
6. Blumenthal JA, Califf R, Williams RS et al: Continuing medical education. Cardiac rehabilitation. A new frontier for behavioral medicine. J Cardiac Rehabil 3:637, 1983
7. Brammell HL: Rehabilitation of the elderly cardiac patient. In Brody SJ, Ruff GE (eds): Aging and Rehabilitation, pp 241–255. New York, Springer Publishing, 1986
8. Brammell HL, Morgan BJ, Niccoli SA et al: Exercise tolerance is reduced at altitude in patients with coronary artery disease. Circulation (Suppl II) 66:371, 1982
9. Brown MA, Munford A: Rehabilitation of post MI depression and psychological invalidism: A pilot study. Intl J Psychiatry Med 13:291, 1984
10. Califf RM, McKinnis RA, McNeer JF et al: Prognostic value of ventricular arrhythmias associated with treadmill exercise testing in patients studied with cardiac catheterization for suspected ischemic heart disease. J Am Coll Cardiol 2:1060, 1983
11. Calvert A, Lown B, Gorlin R: Ventricular premature beats and anatomically defined coronary heart disease. Am J Cardiol 39:627, 1977
12. Carson P, Philips R, Lloyd M et al: Exercise after a myocardial infarction: A controlled trial. J R Coll Physicians Lond 16:147, 1982
13. Cay EL, Vetter NJ, Philips AE: Practical aspects of cardiac rehabilitation: Psychosocial factors. Ital Cardiol 3:646, 1973
14. Chaturvedi NE et al: Selection of patients for early discharge after acute myocardial infarction. Brit Heart J 36:533, 1974
15. Chobanian AV et al: The metabolic and hemodynamic effects of prolonged bed rest in normal subjects. Circulation 49:551, 1974
16. Clausen JP: Circulatory adjustments to dynamic exercises and effect of physical training in normal subjects and in patients with coronary artery disease. Prog Cardiovasc Dis 18:459, 1976
17. Council on Scientific Affairs: Physician-supervised exercise programs in rehabilitation of patients with coronary disease. JAMA 245:1463, 1981
18. Davidson DM: The family and cardiac rehabilitation. J Fam Practice 8:253, 1979
19. Davidson DM, DeBusk RF: Prognostic value of a single exercise test 3 weeks after uncomplicated myocardial infarction. Circulation 61:236, 1980
20. DeBusk RF, Hung J: Exercise conditioning soon after myocardial infarction: Effects on myocardial perfusion and ventricular function. Ann NY Acad Sci 382:343, 1982
21. DeBusk RF, Pitts W, Haskell WL et al: A comparison of cardiovascular responses to combined static-dynamic and dynamic effort alone in patients with chronic ischemic heart disease. Circulation 59:977, 1979
22. Dehn MM, Mullins CB: Physiologic effects and importance of exercise in patients with coronary artery disease. Cardiovasc Med 2:365, 1977
23. Dehn MM, Mullins CB: Design and implementation of training regimens. In Wenger NK, Hellerstein HK (eds): Rehabilitation of the Coronary Patient, pp 321–376. New York, John Wiley & Sons, 1984
24. Derogatis LR: SCL-90: Administration, scoring, and procedures manual for the revised version. Baltimore, Clinical Psychometric Research, 1977
25. Directory of Cardiac Rehabilitation Units—1981. Dallas, American Heart Association, 1981
26. Doehrman SR: Psycho-social aspects of recovery from coronary heart disease: A review. Soc Sci Med 11:199, 1977
27. Ehsani AA, Heath GW, Hagberg JM et al: Effects of intense exercise training on ischemic ST segment depression in patients with coronary artery disease. Circulation 64:1116, 1981
28. Ellestad MH: Stress Testing: Principles and Practice, 3rd ed. Philadelphia, FA Davis, 1986
29. Ewart CK, Taylor CB, Reese LB et al: Effects of early postmyocardial infarction exercise testing on self-perception and subsequent physical activity. Am J Cardiol 51:1076, 1983
30. Featherston JF, Holly RG, Amsterdam EA: Physiological responses to weight lifting in cardiac patients. Med Sci Sports Exerc (Suppl 1) 19:593, 1982
31. Freidman M, Thoresen CE, Gill JJ et al: Feasibility of altering type A behavior pattern after myocardial infarction. Circulation 66:83, 1982
32. Freidman M, Thoresen CE, Gill JJ et al: Alteration of type A behavior and reduction in cardiac recurrences in postmyocardial infarction patients. Am Heart J 108:237, 1984
33. Froelicher F: Exercise Testing and Training. New York, LeJacq Publishing, 1983
34. Froelicher V, Jensen D, Genter F et al: A randomized trial of exercise training in patients with coronary heart disease. JAMA 252:1291, 1984
35. Garrity T: Vocational adjustment after first myocardial infarction: Comparative assessment of several variables suggested in the literature. Soc Sci Med 3:705, 1973
36. Gelfand D, Hage J: Factors relating to unsuccessful vocational adjustment of cardiac patients. J Occup Med 2:62, 1960
37. Gelfand R, Flanders B, Haywood LJ: Return to work after myocardial

infarction in a lower socioeconomic population. J Natl Med Assoc 73:855, 1981

38. Goesset JD: Prediction of job success following heart attack. Rehab Counselor Bull, 1969
39. Griffith GC: Sexuality and the cardiac patient. Heart Lung 2:70, 1973
40. Guidelines for exercise testing. A report of the Joint American College of Cardiology/American Heart Association Task Force on assessment of cardiovascular procedures (subcommittee on exercise testing). Circulation 74:653A, 1986
41. Hackett TD, Cassem NH: Psychological adaptation to convalescence in myocardial infarction patients. In Naughton J, Hellerstein HK, Mohler IC (eds): Exercise Testing and Exercise Training in Coronary Heart Disease, p 253. New York, Academic Press, 1973
42. Hansen JE, Vogel JA, Stelter GP et al: Oxygen uptake in man during exhaustive work at sea level and high altitude. J Appl Physiol 41:832, 1976
43. Harding AL, Morefield MA: Group intervention for wives of myocardial infarction patients. Nurs Clin North Am 11:339, 1976
44. Hartung GH, Squires WG, Gotto AM: Effect of exercise training on plasma high-density lipoprotein cholesterol in coronary disease patients. Am Heart J 101:181, 1981
45. Haskell WL: Cardiovascular complications during exercise training of cardiac patients. Circulation 57:920, 1978
46. Haskell WL: Coronary heart disease. In Skinner JS (ed): Exercise Testing and Exercise Prescription for Special Cases, p 209. Philadelphia, Lea & Febiger, 1987
47. Haslam D, McCartney N, McKelvie R et al: Hemodynamics during weight lifting in cardiac patients. Med Sci Sports Exerc (Suppl 2) 19:S94, 1987
48. Heart Facts. Dallas, American Heart Association, 1987
49. Hellerstein HK, Friedman EH: Sexual activity in the post-coronary patient. Arch Intern Med 125:987, 1970
50. Herrick JB: Clinical features of sudden death. JAMA 59:2015, 1912
51. Holloszy JO: Adaptations of muscular tissue to training. Prog Cardiovasc Dis 18:445, 1976
52. Hung J, McKillop J, Savin W et al: Comparison of cardiovascular response to combined static-dynamic effort, to postprandial dynamic effort and to dynamic effort alone in patients with chronic ischemic heart disease. Circulation 65:1043, 1982
53. Jackson G: Sexual intercourse and angina pectoris. Br Med J 2:16, 1978
54. Jenkins CD, Rosenman RH, Friedman M: Development of an objective psychological test for the determination of the coronary-prone behavior pattern in employed men. J Chronic Dis 20:371, 1967
55. Jensen D, Atwood JE, Froelicher V et al: Improvement in ventricular function during exercise studied with radionuclide ventriculography after cardiac rehabilitation. Am J Cardiol 46:770, 1980
56. Jetter WW, White PD: Rupture of the heart in patients in mental institutions. Ann Int Med 21:783, 1944
57. Kallio V, Hamalainen H, Hakkila J et al: Reduction of sudden deaths by a multifactorial intervention programme after acute myocardial infarction. Lancet 2:1091, 1979
58. Kanner AD, Coyne JC, Schaefer C et al: Comparison of two modes of stress measurement: Daily hassles and uplifts versus major life events. J Behav Med 4:1, 1981
59. Kaplan NM: Clinical Hypertension, 4th ed. Baltimore, Williams & Wilkins, 1986
60. Kentala E: Physical fitness and feasibility of physical rehabilitation after myocardial infarction in men of working age. Ann Clin Res (Suppl 9) 4:1, 1972
61. Kitamura K, Jorgenson CR, Gobel FL et al: Hemodynamic correlates of myocardial oxygen consumption during upright exercise. J Appl Physiol 32:516, 1972
62. Klein R, Dean A: The physician and post-myocardial infarction invalidism. JAMA 2:145, 1966
63. Kromhout D, Arntzenius AC, van der Velde EA: Diet, total/HDL-cholesterol, and coronary lesion growth. The Leiden intervention trial. Circulation (Suppl II) 70:II-1, 1984
64. Langosch W, Seer P, Brodner G et al: Behavior therapy with coronary heart disease patients: Results of a comparative study. J Psychosom Res 26:475, 1982
65. Laslett JL, Paumer L, Scott-Baier P et al: Efficacy of exercise training in patients with coronary artery disease who are taking propranolol. Circulation 68:1029, 1983
66. Lassvik C, Areskog NJ: Angina pectoris during inhalation of cold air—Reactions to exercise. Br Heart J 43:661, 1980
67. Leren P: The Oslo Diet—Heart Study: Eleven year report. Circulation 42:935, 1970
68. Levine SA, Lown B: Armchair treatment of acute coronary thrombosis. JAMA 148:1365, 1952
69. Lind AR, McNicol GW: Cardiovascular responses to static and dynamic exercise. Ergonomics 8:379, 1965
70. May GS, Everlein KA, Furberg CD et al: Secondary prevention after MI: A review of long-term trials. Prog Cardiovasc Dis 24:331, 1982
71. Mayou R, Foster A, Williamson B: Medical care after myocardial infarction. J Psychosom Res 23:23, 1979
72. McNeer JF et al: The course of acute myocardial infarction. Feasibility of early discharge of uncomplicated patient. Circulation 51:410, 1975
73. Miller NH, Haskell WL, Berra K et al: Home versus group exercise training for increasing functional capacity after myocardial infarction. Circulation 70:645, 1984
74. Miller PB, Johnson RL, Lamb LE: Effects of four weeks of absolute bed rest on circulatory function in man. Aerospace Med 35:1194, 1964
75. Mitchell DK: Principles of vocational rehabilitation: A contemporary view. In Long C (ed): Prevention and Rehabilitation in Ischemic Heart Disease, p 316. Baltimore, Williams & Wilkins, 1980
76. Mitchell JH, Wildenthal K: Static (isometric) exercise and the heart: Physiological and clinical considerations. Ann Rev Med 25:369, 1974
77. Mumford E, Schlesinger HJ, Glass GV: The effects of psychological intervention on recovery from surgery and heart attacks: An analysis of the literature. Am J Pub Health 72:141, 1982
78. Nagle R, Gargola R: Factors influencing return to work after myocardial infarction. Lancet 2:7722, 1971
79. Oberman A, Cleary P, Larosa JC et al: Changes in risk factors among participants in a long-term exercise rehabilitation program. Adv Cardiol 31:168, 1982
80. Obma RT, Wilson PK, Goebel ME et al: Effect of a conditioning program in patients taking propranolol for angina pectoris. Cardiology 64:365, 1979
81. Okada RD, Boucher CA, Strauss HW et al: Exercise radionuclide imaging approaches to coronary artery disease. Am J Cardiol 46:1188, 1980
82. Pace N: Weightlessness: A matter of gravity. N Engl J Med 297:32, 1977
83. Palatsi I: Feasibility of physical training after myocardial infarction and its effect on return to work, morbidity and mortality. Acta Med Scand (Suppl) 559:1, 1976
84. Pell A, D'Alonzo CA: Myocardial infarction in a one-year industrial study. JAMA 166:322, 1958
85. Powell LH, Friedman M, Thoresen CE et al: Can the type A behavior pattern be altered after myocardial infarction? A second year report from the Recurrent Coronary Prevention Project. Psychosom Med 46:293, 1984
86. Pratt CM, Welton DE, Squires WG Jr et al: Demonstration of training effect during chronic β-adrenergic blockade in patients with coronary artery disease. Circulation 64:1125, 1981
87. Prosser G, Carson P, Phillips R et al: Morale in coronary patients following an exercise programme. J Psychosom Res 25:587, 1981
88. Ragg KE, Murray TF, Karbonit LM et al: Errors in predicting functional capacity from treadmill exercise stress test. Am Heart J 100:581, 1980
89. Reader GG: The physician as teacher. Health Education Monographs 2:34, 1974
90. Rechnitzer PA, Cunningham DA, Gull A et al: Relation of exercise to recurrence rate of myocardial infarction in men: Ontario exercise-heart collaborative study. Am J Cardiol 51:65, 1983
91. Robinson BF: Relationship of heart rate and systolic pressure to the onset of pain in angina pectoris. Circulation 35:1073, 1967
92. Roman I, Gutierrez M, Luksic I et al: Cardiac rehabilitation after acute myocardial infarction: 9-year controlled follow-up study. Cardiology 70:223, 1983

93. Roviaro S, Holmes DS, Holmsten RD: Influence of cardiac rehabilitation program on the cardiovascular, psychological, and social functioning of cardiac patients. J Behav Med 7:61, 1984

94. Rowell LB: Human cordiovascular adjustments to exercise and thermal stress. Physiol Rev 54:75, 1974

95. Ruberman W, Weinblatt E, Goldberg JD et al: Psychosocial influences on mortality after myocardial infarction. N Engl J Med 311:552, 1984

96. Rubies-Pratt J, Joven J: How soon after myocardial infarction should plasma lipid values be assessed? Br Med J 290:470, 1985

97. Ryback RS, Lewis OF, Lessard CS: Psychobiologic effects of prolonged bed rest in young, healthy volunteers (study II). Aerospace Med 42:529, 1971

98. Saltin B et al: Response to exercise after bed rest and after training. Circulation (Suppl VII) 38:1, 1968

99. Saltin B, Grover RF, Blomqvist CG et al: Maximal oxygen uptake and cardiac output after 2 weeks at 4300m. J Apply Physiol 25:400, 1968

100. Sanne H: Readaptation after myocardial infarction. Washington, DC, International Exchange of Information in Rehabilitation, 1979

101. Schomer HH, Noakes TD: The psychological effect of exercise training on patients after a myocardial infarction. A pilot study. S Afr Med J 64:473, 1983

102. Shaw LW: Effects of a prescribed supervised exercise program on mortality and cardiovascular morbidity in patients after myocardial infarction. Am J Cardiol 48:39, 1981

103. Sklar J, Niccoli SA, Leitner M et al: Changes in ventricular function after cardiac rehabilitation are not related to changes in myocardial perfusion. Circulation (Suppl II) 66:371, 1982

104. Stern MJ, Cleary P: The national exercise and heart disease project. Psychosocial changes observed during a low-level exercise program. Arch Intern Med 141:1463, 1981

105. Stern MJ, Cleary P: The national exercise and heart disease project. Long-term psychosocial outcome. Arch Intern Med 142:1093, 1982

106. Stern MJ, Gorman PA, Kaslow L: The group counseling v. exercise therapy study. A controlled intervention with subjects following myocardial infarction. Arch Intern Med 143:1719, 1983

107. Stern MJ, Pascale L, Ackerman A: Life adjustment post-myocardial infarction: Determining predictive values. Arch Intern Med 137:1680, 1977

108. Stern MJ, Pascale L, McLoone J: Psychosocial adaptation following an acute myocardial infarction. J Chronic Dis 29:513, 1976

109. Steward MJ, Gregor FM: Early discharge and return to work following myocardial infarction. Soc Sci Med 18:1027, 1984

110. Stuart RJ, Ellestad MH: Upsloping S-T segments in exercise stress testing. Six year follow-up study of 438 patients and correlation with 248 angiograms. Am J Cardiol 37:19, 1976

111. Sylvester R, Camp J, SanMarco N: Effects of exercise training on progression of coronary arteriosclerosis in men. In Milvy P (ed): The marathon: physiological, medical, epidemiological and psychological studies. Ann NY Acad Sci 301:495, 1977

112. Theroux P, Waters DD, Halphen C et al: Prognostic value of exercise testing soon after myocardial infarction. N Engl J Med 301:341, 1979

113. Thom TJ, Kannel WB, Feinleib M: Factors in the decline of coronary heart disease mortality. In Connor WE, Bristow JD (eds): Coronary Heart Disease. Prevention, Complications, and Treatment, p 5. Philadelphia, JB Lippincott. 1985

114. Thomson PD, Kelemen MH: Hypotension accompanying the onset of exertional angina: A sign of severe compromise of left ventricular blood supply. Circulation 52:28, 1975

115. Ueno M: The So-called coition death. Jpn J Legal Med 17:330, 1963

116. VanCamp SP, Peterson RA: JAMA 256:1160, 1986

117. Vanhees L, Fagard R, Amery Al: Influence of beta adrenergic blockade on effects of physical training in patients with ischemic heart disease. Br Heart J 48:33, 1982

118. Varnauskas E, Bjorntorp M, Fahlen I et al: Effects of physical training on exercise blood flow and enzymatic activity in skeletal muscle. Cardiovasc Res 4:418, 1970

119. Vermuenlen A, Lie KI, Durrer D: Effects of cardiac rehabilitation after myocardial infarction: Changes in coronary risk factors and long-term prognosis. Am Heart J 105:798, 1983

120. Weld FF, Chu K-L, Bigger JT Jr et al: Risk stratification with low-level exercise testing 2 weeks after acute myocardial infarction. Circulation 64:306, 1981

121. Wenger NK: Introduction to the pros and cons of early mobilization and of the convalescent phase in rehabilitation. Bibl Cardiol 36:45, 1977

122. Wilhemsen L, Sanne H, Elmfeldt D et al: A controlled trial of physical training after myocardial infarction: Effects on risk factors, nonfatal reinfarction and death. Prev Med 4:491, 1975

123. Williams RS, McKinnis RA, Cobb FR et al: Effects of physical conditioning on left ventricular ejection fraction in patients with coronary artery disease. Circulation 70:69, 1984

124. Williamson TB: The value of industrial rehabilitation following cardiac infarction. Proc R Soc Med 70:656, 1977

125. Wishnie H, Hackett T, Cassem N: Psychological hazards of convalescence following myocardial infarction. JAMA 215:1291, 1971

126. Wolfel EE, Hiatt WR, Brammell HL et al: Effects of selective and non-selective β-adrenergic blockade on mechanisms of exercise conditioning. Circulation 74:664, 1986

127. Zeimetz GA, Moss RF, Butts N et al: Support versus non-support treadmill walking (abstr). Med Sci Sports Exerc 11:112, 1979

35

Rehabilitation of the Patient With Pulmonary Disease

Robert D. Rondinelli

Nicholas S. Hill

Pulmonary rehabilitation has been defined as

> an art of medical practice wherein an individually tailored, multidisciplinary program is formulated which, through accurate diagnosis, therapy, emotional support and education, stabilizes or reverses both the physio- and psychopathology of pulmonary diseases and attempts to return the patient to the highest possible functional capacity allowed by his pulmonary handicap and overall life situation.[32]

The official position stated by the American Thoracic Society includes two principal objectives of any pulmonary rehabilitation program: "To control and alleviate as much as possible the symptoms and pathologic complications of respiratory impairment" and "to teach the patient how to achieve optimal capability for carrying out his/her activities of daily living."[58]

A number of excellent reviews outlining comprehensive pulmonary rehabilitation programs have been published.[33, 41, 54, 57] These programs involve the coordination of inpatient and outpatient resources of a regional medical facility with local home-care efforts. Such programs provide select patients with thorough diagnostic evaluations, medication adjustments, evaluation, and treatment by physical, occupational, and respiratory therapists and educational, psychological, and emotional support as needed. Integrated and intensive multidisciplinary pulmonary rehabilitation has been shown to improve exercise tolerance, decrease symptomatology, and improve psychological well-being for patients who successfully participate.[4, 30]

The major thrust of pulmonary rehabilitation has been toward patients with chronic obstructive pulmonary disease (COPD), which includes emphysema, chronic bronchitis, and asthma. Although this chapter will focus on rehabilitation of the COPD patient, the scope will be broadened as appropriate to include other chronic pulmonary disorders, including motor unit and spinal cord diseases, and the ventilator-assisted or dependent patient.

Epidemiology

Chronic pulmonary disease has become a leading health problem nationwide. In 1977 more than 34,000 deaths (more than 2.5% of total U.S. deaths) were attributable to COPD. The age-adjusted death rate showed a 22% increase since 1968. By contrast, the overall age-adjusted rate for all causes of death decreased by 18%, and deaths primarily related to heart disease declined by 22% over the same period. COPD now ranks as the fifth leading cause of death in the United States. By recent estimates, COPD accounts for 4.7 million hospital days/year and $6.5 billion in direct and indirect medical costs.[23] By 1980, according to the Department of Health and Human Services, respiratory-related illnesses had become the leading cause of lost work days, and chronic respiratory diseases were the fourth largest cause of major activity limitation and the sixth leading cause of premature retirement due to disability.[76]

PATHOPHYSIOLOGY

Respiratory impairment and pulmonary disability can result from a wide range of conditions.

The human respiratory system consists of conductive tubes and pumps that bring air and blood into intimate contact, a membrane barrier across which gas transfer takes place, and a control system that monitors gas tensions and adjusts flow rates to allow narrow ranges of arterial oxygen and carbon dioxide tensions to be monitored.

Inhaled air first passes through the upper airway (nasal and oral pharynx, larynx, and trachea) where it is humidified, warmed, and screened for particles. The lower airway (below the carina) consists of major bronchi, bronchial divisions, bronchioles, and alveolar ducts of increasing number and cross-sectional area and decreasing resistance to air flow. A ciliated columnar epithelial lining, rich with mucous glands, extends from the trachea to the respiratory bronchioles. A thin "mucous blanket" is secreted atop the beating cilia and continually moves toward the glottis. Foreign particles are adsorbed by this sticky coating and thereby removed. Additional airway protection is provided by macrophages, IgA, and occasional lymphocytes.

Pulmonary arteries carry deoxygenated blood to gas-exchanging areas of the lung. They divide and follow airways and comprise a compliant, low-pressure system requiring minimal work from the right ventricle.

The respiratory muscles comprise two functional groups. The *inspiratory* muscles include the diaphragm (the most important muscle of breathing), the external intercostals, and the accessory muscles (scalenes, trapezius). The *expiratory* muscles include the internal intercostals and abdominal muscles. At rest and during sleep, diaphragmatic contraction forces the abdominal contents away from the thorax and elevates the ribs in bucket-handle fashion. As ventilatory demand increases with exercise, intercostal and accessory muscles actively contribute to respiratory effort. Expiratory muscles come into play during exercise and also help expel secretions or foreign materials from the airway during coughing and sneezing. Normal respiratory muscle function depends on proper structure and compliance of the chest wall.

Medullary respiratory control centers, by mechanisms not entirely understood, integrate input from central and peripheral chemoreceptors and regulate ventilation to maintain normal blood gas levels in the face of changing metabolic demands. Central chemoreceptors are most sensitive to changes in arterial carbon dioxide partial pressure ($PaCO_2$) or pH; whereas, the peripheral chemoreceptors, located in the carotid bodies, contribute mainly to hypoxic ventilatory response and hypoxic potentiation of the carbon dioxide response.

Respiratory Insufficiency

Respiratory insufficiency occurs when any one or combination of the components of the respiratory system functions inadequately, disrupting gas exchange and causing symptoms. An increased airway resistance in COPD may be secondary to bronchospasm or edema of airways due to chronic inflammation and increased secretions with mucous gland hyperplasia. In emphysema, increased airway resistance results from destruction of supporting structures leading to early collapse of the airway during expiration.

Cigarette smoking is without doubt the single most-important cause of COPD in the United States today. Cigarette smoke predisposes to chronic bronchitis by irritating airways and paralyzing ciliary motion, thereby preventing removal of particulates. Evidence suggests that cigarette smoke enhances the development of emphysema by inhibiting alpha₁-antiprotease and by increasing the number of alveolar polymorphonuclear cells which, in turn, release a proteolytic enzyme (elastase) that destroys lung parenchyma.[38]

Interstitial lung disease results from inflammatory cell infiltration and fibrosis of interstitial spaces and alveolar walls. Replacement of normal lung architecture by these elements renders the lungs noncompliant and increases work of breathing. In addition, the thickening of alveolar walls and damage to alveolar capillaries interferes with gas exchange to produce hypoxemia. Interstitial lung diseases may commonly arise from unknown causes, such as idiopathic pulmonary fibrosis, or in association with sarcoidosis or heavy occupational exposure to asbestos or silica.

Pulmonary vascular disorders, which cause increased resistance in pulmonary vessels, may lead to pulmonary hypertension and secondary hypertrophy and dysfunction of the right ventricle (cor pulmonale).[29] Cor pulmonale most often occurs in hypoxemic patients with COPD, but can also occur in association with other hypoventilatory disorders, with recurrent emboli and primary pulmonary hypertension.

Severe kyphoscoliosis reduces lung volumes and compromises respiratory muscle efficiency. Symptoms of dyspnea predictably occur when the angle of curvature exceeds 90°, and hypoventilation with cor pulmonale will occur when the angle exceeds 120°.[9] Weakness of the respiratory muscles (less than 25% normal) impairs the bellows activity of the chest wall, limiting ventilatory capacity and causing hypoventilation. Progressive neuromuscular weakness, due to Guillain-Barré syndrome or myasthenia gravis (acutely) and muscular dystrophy or amyotrophic lateral sclerosis (chronically), often causes hypoventilatory failure.

Severe weakness of the expiratory muscles impairs cough and sneeze mechanisms, but does not cause hypoventilation because passive elastic forces achieve expiration at rest. In patients with C5-C6 cervical fractures, diaphragmatic function remains intact (the phrenic nerve arises from the third through fifth cervical segments); whereas, expiratory muscles (innervated from thoracic and lumbar segments) are paralyzed. Consequently, such patients retain approximately 60% of their inspiratory capacity and ventilate well, but have a severely weakened cough and great difficulty clearing secretions during respiratory infections.[44]

Disorders of ventilatory control often occur in combination with post-poliomyelitis or prior strokes. Central alveolar hypoventilation is quite unusual. The sleep apnea syndrome is more common and most likely caused by a relative central insensitivity to ventilatory stimuli in combination with peripheral abnormalities, such as decreased oropharyngeal or nasopharyngeal dimensions. Sleep apnea usually is seen in obese males with a long history of snoring and arises when intermittent upper airway obstructions occur during sleep. As oxygen saturation falls, the sleep pattern is disrupted and such patients become severely sleep-deprived and develop marked hypersomnolence.[72]

Respiratory Failure

Respiratory failure indicates an inability of the respiratory system to maintain arterial blood gas (ABG) tensions within an acceptable range. Although precise limits are somewhat arbitrary, respiratory failure is said to occur when the $PaCO_2$ exceeds 50 mm Hg (ventilatory failure), when the arterial oxygen partial pressure (PaO_2) is below 50 mm Hg (oxygenation failure), or when both ventilatory and oxygenation failure are present. Respiratory failure is considered to be chronic when the blood gas abnormality persists for more than 30 days.

Ventilatory Failure

Failure to maintain adequate levels of alveolar ventilation is caused by dysfunction of the same components of the respiratory system previously discussed with regard to respiratory insufficiency. Ventilatory failure, particularly chronic, most frequently arises from lower airway obstruction and increased air flow resistance.

Whether a patient experiences respiratory insufficiency or respiratory failure following traumatic spinal cord injury depends on the level of trauma. The diaphragm is innervated by the phrenic nerve (at C3–C5). Spinal cord trauma below C3, sparing the phrenic nerve, leaves diaphragm function intact and adequate ventilation can be sustained. Lesions above C3 eliminate all but the accessory muscles of breathing and ventilatory failure ensues. Although lower cervical and high thoracic cord lesions leave diaphragm function intact, they eliminate intercostal and abdominal muscle function, severely impairing the cough mechanism. Such patients have difficulty clearing secretions and may develop ventilatory failure during bronchitic or pneumonic episodes. Ventilatory failure arising from dysfunction of the respiratory center can result from suppression of ventilatory drive by drugs or trauma. Many of these conditions can be stabilized by either continuous or intermittent ventilatory assistance, with rehabilitation to optimize the patient's living situation.

Hypoxemia inevitably accompanies the hypercapnia of ventilatory failure unless oxygen supplementation is given. Severe hypoxemia may also occur without hypercapnia, a condition referred to as *oxygenation failure*. For practical purposes, oxygenation failure is caused by shunt or ventilation-perfusion mismatch, or both. Deoxygenated blood that bypasses gas exchange entirely (shunt) or perfuses regions of lung with low ventilation-perfusion ratios mixes with fully oxygenated systemic arterial blood from better ventilated areas and lowers PaO_2. Diffusion abnormalities rarely contribute to hypoxemia unless transit time across the pulmonary capillaries is shortened, as with exercise or high cardiac output states.[83]

Acute oxygenation failure most commonly results from severe respiratory infections, such as bacterial or viral pneumonias; diffuse parenchymal injury or widespread pulmonary edema, such as the adult respiratory distress syndrome (ARDS); or acute pulmonary circulatory failure, caused by acute pulmonary embolism. Chronic hypoxemia is most often seen in combination with ventilatory failure, but may also occur alone in patients with interstitial fibrosis or congenital shunts, such as arteriovenous malformations.

When ventilatory or oxygenation failure occurs, the respiratory system is stressed beyond tolerable limits and available energy substrates are quickly used. As the demand for work from the muscle exceeds the ability to supply energy, contractile force declines and muscle fatigue occurs.[64] As fatigue progresses, the muscle becomes increasingly inefficient, performing less work at a given energy expenditure. If energy supply is limited, as with cardiogenic shock, the respiratory muscles are particularly prone to fatigue. Malnutrition, chronically weakened respiratory muscles, and chronic increases in the work of breathing also predispose to acute respiratory muscle fatigue.

Fatigue of the diaphragm is manifest by increased respiratory rate and paradoxical motion of the abdomen. Rather than pushing the abdomen outward with inspiration, the weakened diaphragm is drawn into the chest and the abdomen moves inward.

Studies on experimental animals have shown that respiratory muscle fatigue contributes to acute respiratory failure and leads inevitably to hypercapnia and death unless the respiratory system is rested. With prompt intubation of the airway and assisted ventilation, weakened respiratory muscles can be adequately rested and the energy supply restored.[3] Aminophylline and certain beta-agonist agents may enhance the function of fatigued respiratory muscles.[79]

The role of respiratory muscle fatigue in chronic respiratory failure is not clearly understood. Patients with chronic respiratory failure may maintain steady levels of hypercapnia for months or years, such that a severe energy imbalance contributing to their respiratory insufficiency seems unlikely. However, a small increase in the demand for respiratory work, such as walking at a normal pace, may precipitate acute respiratory muscle fatigue in a patient with chronic respiratory insufficiency. Repeated acute bouts of fatigue may conceivably lead to a state of "chronic fatigue." In such patients, intermittent ventilatory assistance may provide sufficient rest periods to allow muscle recovery from fatigue and improve overall respiratory muscle performance. It is also possible that reversal of nutritional imbalances or resetting of the respiratory center to a lower level of hypercapnia contributes to improved ventilation in patients with chronic respiratory failure who benefit from intermittent ventilatory assistance.[31]

Prognosis for Pulmonary Patients

Once respiratory insufficiency has developed, the prognosis depends largely upon the pathophysiological basis for the insufficiency, the degree of impairment of gas exchange, and other individual factors. The prognosis of severe COPD is closely related to the degree of airway obstruction. Mortality of patients with a forced expiratory volume in 1 second (FEV_1) of less than 0.75 liters approaches 30% at the end of 1 year and 50% at the end of 3 years.[14] Hypercarbia and cor pulmonale also portend a worse prognosis. Death is most often related to a superimposed acute problem such as bronchitis, pneumonia, pulmonary embolism, or pneumothorax. Smoking cessation improves prognosis in these patients, even when the underlying lung disease is severe.[63]

Prognosis in patients with restrictive disease depends upon whether the restriction is related to parenchymal lung disease, chest wall stiffness, or muscle weakness. The course of interstitial lung disease is quite variable; occasional patients actually remit, others rapidly progress to terminal stages, and most follow an intermediate course. When a terminal stage is reached, patients generally do poorly with little response to therapy. Patients with severe kyphoscoliosis, in contrast, can survive for long periods of time with severe dysfunction. When the angle of curvature exceeds 120°, patients with kyphoscoliosis usually develop respiratory insufficiency and hypercarbia, but they respond well to intermittent ventilatory assistance. A wide array of neuromuscular diseases also causes restrictive lung disease. Some, such as Guillain-Barré syndrome, cause a rapid, usually reversible, onset of respiratory failure; whereas, others, such as Duchenne muscular dystrophy, cause a slowly progressive and largely predictable decline of respiratory function and eventual onset of respiratory failure.[37] Knowledge of the natural history of these various disorders allows timely intervention with ventilatory support and avoidance of more serious complications.

Goals for a Pulmonary Rehabilitation Program

Ensuing disabilities of pulmonary impairment are likely to be permanent and progressive, so that realistic goals of rehabilitation should be well understood by patient and physician. With the normal ageing process, FEV_1 declines at a rate of approximately 30 cc/year,[39] and this rate of decline is accelerated to 45 to 55 cc/year in patients with COPD.[14] The rate of spirometric decline does not appear to alter appreciably in spite of comprehensive ongoing rehabilitation programs. Likewise, survival estimates are not significantly enhanced by multidisciplinary treatment as opposed to more "casual" follow-up provided by individualized physician management.[14]

Documented beneficial effects from multidisciplinary pulmonary treatment include reduction in average number of hospital days per year[68] as well as subjective improvement in dyspnea severity as it relates to patient functional mobility and self-care. Broader goals for any such rehabilitation program should include development of a cost-effective management system to coordinate inpatient and outpatient resources so as to lessen the medical, psychological, social, vocational, and economic burdens on the individual, family, and community.

PATIENT EVALUATION

A comprehensive patient evaluation should be done at the outset in all cases in order to ensure that prospective patients are medically appropriate and in need of multidisciplinary rehabilitation treatment, that reasonable and realistic goals can be identified, and that a comprehensive problem-oriented treatment plan can be articulated which addresses medical, therapeutic, and educational aspects of patient care.

Functional History

Patients who may benefit from pulmonary rehabilitation should initially be evaluated by a physiatrist or pulmonologist with expertise in pulmonary rehabilitation. The patient's current pulmonary medical status, history of pulmonary and associated diseases, and rate of progression of symptoms are assessed, with particular attention to previous clinic visits and hospitalizations, relative success of previous medical and therapeutic interventions, and the home or community-support services used thus far to minimize symptoms and maintain functioning outside a hospital setting.

The history must include specifics on functional mobility, performance of basic and advanced self-care activities, and vocational and avocational pursuits to determine the degree of disability and handicap. The degree to which dyspnea and fatigue limit performance of such activities should be noted. The degree of dyspnea should also be graded in terms of distance walked (feet, the number of blocks), number of stairs or flights of stairs climbed, and routine performance of dressing, feeding, other routine daily activities, household chores, and community activities. Details of life-style change, socialization processes, and involvement in recreational pursuits, hobbies, and employment activities should be recorded along with an estimation of the rate of progressive loss of function.

A number of dyspnea indices exist,[47, 69] which allow the quantification of symptoms according to functional impairment in conversation and self-care performance. Moser and colleagues[49] proposed a dyspnea classification system for functional pulmonary disability (Table 35-1). This classification has practical applications for initial goal planning and establishing expectations of outcome, since class 1 patients are already maximally functional and might benefit most from education in preventive care. Patients in classes 2 to 4 might benefit from a comprehensive program emphasizing physical restoration, whereas class 5 patients might benefit most from a program of narrowed scope with emphasis upon education and counseling to improve energy conservation and emotional and psychological well-being.

Objective Assessment

Physical Examination

A complete physical examination should be performed initially, including attention to the upper airway structures, neck and chest, extremities, heart, abdomen, and lungs. The examiner should first observe the patient's breathing pattern and respiratory rate, also noting any evidence of respiratory distress, pallor, cyanosis, or other discoloration. The patient should be inspected for scoliosis or chest wall deformities and coordination of breathing muscles. During quiet breathing, inspiration should consist of slow outward motion of the chest and abdomen and accessory muscles should not be in use. Inward (paradoxical) motion of the abdomen or chest wall (Hoover's sign) during inspiration suggests diaphragmatic dysfunction. Palpation is a more sensitive way than inspection alone to detect contraction of the accessory muscles. The expiratory muscles are relaxed during quiet breathing in normal subjects. Strength of abdominal muscles should be tested by having the patient tense his or her abdomen.

Nasal flaring and degree of mucosal congestion or inflammation should be noted. Lymph nodes should be palpated and the larynx auscultated for inspiratory stridor.

The lungs should be percussed and auscultated posteriorly and anteriorly to best assess upper lobes. The ratio of inspiratory time to expiratory time can be ascertained by auscultating over the larynx while the patient performs a forced expiratory maneuver. Prolongation of audible expiratory sounds beyond 3 seconds suggests airway obstruction.

The cardiac examination should pay special attention to evidence of cor pulmonale or pulmonary hypertension. Increased intensity of pulmonic second sound (P_2) and the presence of a right-sided gallop, murmur of tricuspid regurgitation, distention of neck veins, or a right ventricular heave are helpful signs. Extremities should be examined for clubbing of fingernails, cyanosis, and edema.

Laboratory Examination

Routine bloods should be screened for abnormalities of hematocrit or electrolytes. An electrocardiogram should be obtained to seek evidence of cor pulmonale. Pulmonary functions should be performed by trained, qualified personnel. They should consist of spirometry to measure the forced vital capacity (FVC), or the amount of air exhaled during a complete, forceful expiration; FEV_1, the amount expelled in the first second of the FVC; and the maximal mid-expiratory flow rate (MMEF), the average flow rate between 25% and 50% of vital capacity. The maximum voluntary ventilation (MVV), the maximum volume of air exhaled in a 12-second period in liters per minute is also usually obtained. The FEV_1 and MVV correlate with functional capacity, and the FEV_1/FVC ratio serves as a good index of the degree of obstruction. Predicted normal rates for pulmonary function studies are based on age, height, and sex. In general, an FEV_1 of 1 liter indicates severe ventilatory impairment, and an FEV_1/FVC ratio of less than 75% indicates airway obstruction.

Arterial blood gases should also be obtained routinely on room air. Normal PaO_2 at sea level is between 80 and 90 mm Hg. Alveolar hypoventilation ($PaCO_2$ of more than 43) is increasingly likely with greater degrees of respiratory insufficiency; pH helps determine whether alterations in $PaCO_2$ are acute or chronic.

Table 35-1
A Classification of Functional Pulmonary Disability

Class	Functional Ability
1	No substantial restriction of normal activity, but noted dyspnea on strenous exertion May be employable
2	No dyspnea with essential activities of daily living (ADLs) or on level walking, but noted dyspnea on climbing stairs and inclines Employment usually limited to sedentary occupations
3	Dyspnea with certain ADLs (*e.g.*, showering or dressing) Able to walk at own pace for a city block, but unable to keep up with individuals of comparable age Generally employable at only highly sedentary occupations
4	Dependent on others for some ADLs Not dyspneic at rest, but becomes dyspneic with minimal exertion
5	Housebound and often limited to bed or chair Dyspneic at rest and dependent upon assistance from others for most ADLs

(From Moser K, Bokinsky G, Savage R et al: Results of a comprehensive rehabilitation program. Physiologic and functional effects on patients with chronic obstructive pulmonary disease. Arch Intern Med 140:1596–1601, 1980)

Other laboratory tests may be of occasional value, including microscopic sputum examination in patients with chronic bronchitis. The presence of many leukocytes may indicate infection. Alpha$_1$-antitrypsin deficiency is an unusual hereditary cause of emphysema, which can be detected through serum protein electrophoresis. Detection should be sought in younger individuals with severe emphysema, since documentation of the condition is of use mainly in genetic counseling.

Exercise Assessment

Exercise assessment is useful to quantify functional limitations objectively and to obtain a baseline for future comparison. (The rationale, benefits, and limitations of exercise assessment are discussed in a later section, "Therapeutic Exercise.")

Skin Testing

Skin testing is particularly important in evaluating patients with chronic cough, suspicious chest x-ray abnormalities, or constitutional symptoms, and is used mainly to screen for infection by tuberculosis. Following injection of 0.1 ml, 5 units purified protein derivative (PPD) intradermally, an area of induration (not just erythema) more than 10 mm in diameter indicates infection with mycobacterial strains. Multiple prong tests, such as the Tine test, have less sensitivity than the PPD and their use should be discouraged.

A positive PPD test, regardless of size, cannot determine activity of infection. This can only be assessed by using other clinical indicators, such as sputum analysis and chest x-ray. Control skin tests with common antigens, such as mumps or *Candida,* are helpful in interpreting negative reactions that could be due to anergy. Conversion of the PPD reaction from negative to positive over a brief period of time can be related to the "booster phenomenon,"[75] which is that the size of the PPD reaction increases an average of 4 mm when the test is repeated within months of the first test.

Evaluation for Rehabilitation

The following criteria are intended to serve as selection guidelines for patients entering into a comprehensive pulmonary rehabilitation program. Patients meeting each of these criteria can be expected to participate actively and derive significant benefit from such a program.

SELECTION CRITERIA FOR ENTRY INTO A PULMONARY REHABILITATION PROGRAM

1. Symptomatic chronic pulmonary disease, which necessitates frequent and repeated inpatient hospital treatments over time (four or more per year), or more frequent combinations of inpatient and outpatient management for acute exacerbations relating to the disease
2. Functional pulmonary disability (Moser's classes 2–5) and interest in a program designed to restore maximum physical and functional activity levels
3. Willingness to participate actively in the program and comply with recommendations
4. No concomitant medical condition that would otherwise imminently contribute to deterioration of pulmonary status (*e.g.,* congestive heart failure, myocardial infarction, dysrhythmia, malignancy) or undermine the expected benefits of the program
5. No psychological or social impairments that would otherwise impair compliance or interfere with the rehabilitation program (*e.g,* alcoholism, organic brain syndrome)
6. Recent (6 months or less) change in pulmonary functional disability, increasing the likelihood of reversals. In cases of long-standing functional impairment, prior opportunity for adequate trial of pulmonary rehabilitation has not been provided.
7. Adequate financial and social support, and feasibility to ensure timely participation and compliance with all aspects of the program

MANAGEMENT ISSUES

In directing a comprehensive multidisciplinary pulmonary rehabilitation program, the clinician must address a variety of management issues, including education in preventive care, optimization of medications, applications of respiratory care, therapeutic exercise, and education in energy conservation and work simplification. Attention must be paid to nutritional aspects of patient management, as well as psychological and social issues. Special equipment is required in some cases. The following section is intended to provide a practical overview of the major options and strategies available and an appropriate rationale for their specific use.

Preventive Care

Preventive care has an important role in minimizing complications and stabilizing the progression of chronic lung disorders. Important preventive measures include avoidance of environmental toxins and irritants, good bronchial hygiene, and timely vaccinations.

By far the most important pulmonary irritant is tobacco smoke. Cigarette smoking is responsible for an estimated 350,000 deaths per year in the United States, including 120,000 from lung cancer, 170,000 from coronary artery disease, and 60,000 from COPD. It is the major cause of COPD.[28]

Smoking cessation reduces mortality from coronary artery disease and lung cancer to rates approaching those in nonsmokers after 10 to 15 years. In addition, progression of disease and symptoms of chronic cough and dyspnea are usually ameliorated in patients with COPD within months of smoking cessation.[63]

Smoking cessation is one of the most important aspects of a pulmonary rehabilitation program. Unfortunately, cigarette smoking is potently addictive and patients are sometimes unable to give up smoking even in the face of severe respiratory failure. Formal smoking cessation programs have high failure rates approaching 70% to 80% after 1 year.[22] However, many smokers do eventually quit and intensive efforts at helping them appear worthwhile.

Simple physician advice alone may be helpful[65] and should routinely be provided in a firm and factual manner to smoking patients. The physician should emphasize the risks of continued smoking and the benefits of quitting.

Smoking cessation programs may also be effective and may employ self-help materials obtained from the American Lung Association, American Cancer Society, or American Heart Association. Through a multifaceted behavioral approach, patients are taught to identify and avoid cues that trigger their smoking behavior. Hypnosis, relaxation imagery, and acupuncture techniques are directed toward the psychological aspects of cigarette addiction.

Nicotine is almost certainly the physiologically addicting

substance in cigarette smoke, and the nicotine withdrawal syndrome can be alleviated if nicotine is administered by some other means.[34] Nicotine chewing gum has been approved for use by the Federal Drug Administration as an adjunct to smoking cessation programs. It is less effective if given without concomitant psychological support.[35]

Patients with an allergic component to their disease should minimize potential irritants in the home environment by eliminating pets, rugs, drapes, feather pillows and cushions, and removing as much dust as possible. Hyposensitization programs consisting of a series of injections containing known allergens may be helpful in selected individuals when environmental controls fail to alleviate symptoms effectively.

Industrial pollutants and exposure to occupational irritants at the worksite are of additional concern.[48] Exposure to asbestos or silica particles is particularly hazardous, but chemical fumes and excessive dust can also pose problems. Employers should be notified of a patient's illness in order to arrange protection from such irritants. In some cases, air purifiers, conditioners, humidifiers, and dehumidifiers can help modify the environment and alleviate symptoms. If satisfactory arrangements are not provided, patients should be advised to seek alternative occupations or obtain necessary disability dispensation.

In patients with chronic bronchitis, measures aimed at controlling secretions can bring about substantial symptomatic improvement. (Methods for postural drainage and chest physiotherapy are discussed later, under Chest Physical Therapy.) Such patients are subject to frequent exacerbations of symptoms, often due to infection. Broad spectrum antibiotics, such as ampicillin, tetracycline, or trimethoprim-sulfamethoxazole, are often administered to these patients at the first sign of an exacerbation in the hope that infection can be curtailed. Scientific evidence is lacking to support this approach and some exacerbations appear to be viral rather than bacterial in origin.[66] Nevertheless, many physicians have the clinical impression that symptoms can be alleviated by administration of antibiotics, particularly when purulent secretions are present. Antibiotics are occasionally administered by intermittent or continuous regimens in patients prone to frequent exacerbations of bronchitis.

Influenza and pneumococcal vaccines have proven effective in decreasing the likelihood of infectious respiratory illness in populations at risk.[16] The influenza vaccine is usually polyvalent, affording protection against influenza B, as well as several strains of influenza A. Administered as a single 0.5 ml intramuscular injection, the vaccine should be given to all high-risk individuals, including the elderly and those with respiratory disease, but not to patients with egg allergy.

Amantadine should be administered to high-risk individuals who have not been vaccinated or have received vaccine within the previous two weeks of a new influenza outbreak.[16] Amantadine also affords protection against influenza A, but not influenza B. Amantadine is also effective in reducing intensity and duration of illness if begun within 24 to 48 hours after the onset of symptoms. The dosage of amantadine is 100 mg, twice daily, for the duration of the outbreak unless renal dysfunction necessitates a reduction in dosage.

Pneumococcal vaccine contains capsular polysaccharide antigens from 23 subtypes of *Streptococcus* pneumonia.[15] Like the influenza vaccine, the pneumococcal vaccine should be administered to high-risk individuals, including those with splenic dysfunction or chronic lung disease. Because of frequent allergic reactions to repeated doses of the vaccine, it is recommended that the vaccine be administered only *once*.[15] The vaccine is judged to be 70% effective among individuals who are over age 55, although it fails to protect those with severe immunodeficiencies. The vaccine is well tolerated, can be administered simul-taneously with the influenza vaccine, and only rarely causes febrile symptoms or severe local reaction.

Medications

Optimization of bronchodilators and other respiratory medications is an integral part of comprehensive pulmonary rehabilitation. Medications must be tailored to individual patient needs and based upon the severity of disease, evidence of response to medication, and the nature and severity of side-effects.

The sympathomimetics consist of a number of adrenergic drugs that stimulate beta$_2$-adrenergic receptors, causing bronchodilatation. They are used as first-line agents in the treatment of bronchospasm.[62] None of the sympathomimetics are entirely beta$_2$-specific; they also stimulate beta$_1$ receptors, causing side-effects such as tachycardia and muscle tremulousness.

Nonspecific adrenergic stimulants (Table 35-2) are generally not used in the therapy of asthma except for certain special circumstances. Subcutaneous epinephrine has a highly potent and rapid onset of action and is still used in emergency situations for treatment of acute, severe bronchospasm. It should be avoided in elderly patients or in those with coronary artery disease. Ephedrine is a common component of over-the-counter asthma preparations, but its lack of beta$_2$ selectivity or potency renders it similarly unattractive.

Isoproterenol, like epinephrine, is a short-acting, potent bronchodilator lacking beta$_2$ selectivity which has been supplanted by the more selective beta$_2$ agonists that are popular today. The beta$_2$ agonists differ mainly in terms of potency and duration of action. Because of conflicting reports, it is difficult to rank them in order of beta$_2$ selectivity, and physician or patient preference often determines choice. The beta$_2$ selective agents have very similar efficacies and side-effects when used at equipotent doses.

In general, administration of beta$_2$ selective sympathomimetics by metered dose inhalers (MDI) is preferred for treatment of bronchospasm as the first line of therapy.[74] This route allows delivery of medication directly to the target organ at the lowest possible dose and minimizes systemic side-effects. The major limitation of MDI is that their proper use requires coordination of hand and breathing motions and many patients practice poor technique. Ideally, the MDI should first be shaken and held a few centimeters in front of the open mouth. The patient exhales to residual volume and slowly inhales to total lung capacity, activating the MDI shortly after inhalation starts. The patient then holds his breath for 10 seconds and waits a few minutes before repeated inhalation. Various spacers and reservoirs have been developed to improve delivery of medication in patients who are unable to learn proper technique. Obviously, MDI cannot be effectively used by small children or patients with severe neuromuscular or cognitive defects.

Beta$_2$ selective bronchodilators can also be administered in inhaled solutions with a nebulizer, but proof that it provides a more effective means of administration of bronchodilators is lacking. Nevertheless, patients with copious airway secretions sometimes report greater subjective improvement after administration of bronchodilators with a nebulizer as opposed to an MDI. Orally ingested beta agonists should be reserved for patients who fail to use MDI properly or who achieve inadequate control of bronchospasm, despite optimal use of MDI and theophyllines.

The methylxanthines (see Table 35-2) are a group of chemical compounds, including caffeine, that consist of methyl substitutions on xanthine, a product of purine catabolism.[46] Theophylline is the methylxanthine with the greatest bronchodilator

Table 35-2
Nonspecific Adrenergic Stimulants

Drug	Mechanism of Action	Routes of Administration	Dose	Duration of Action	Side-Effects
Sympathomimetic: Nonspecific agonists Epinephrine	Stimulation of airway beta$_2$-adrenergic receptors causes bronchodilation	Subcutaneous	.3–.5 ml 1 : 1000	20–30 min	Tachycardia Tremulousness
Ephedrine		Oral MDI*	15–50 mg 750 μg	3–4 hr	
Beta agonist Isoproterenol		MDI*	340 μg	1–2 hr	
Beta$_2$ agonists Isoetharine		MDI* Inhaled solution	340 μg 5 mg	1–4 hr	
Metaproterenol		MDI* Oral Inhaled solution	650 μg 10–20 mg 15 mg	1–5 hr 3–4 hr 2–6 hr	
Terbutaline		MDI* Oral Subcutaneous	250 μg .5–5 mg .25 mg	3–4 hr 4–6 hr 2–4 hr	
Albuterol		MDI* Oral	90 μg 2–4 mg	3–6 hr 4–6 hr	
Bitolterol		MDI*	370 μg	5–8 hr	
Methylxanthines: Aminophylline	Bronchodilatation may be due to phosphodiesterase inhibition and increased intracellular CAMP†	IV	Loading dose 4–6 mg/kg over 20–30 min Continuous infusion 0.2–0.9 mg/kg Obtain levels after 3–4 half-lives (T½ = 3–4 hr up to 12–16 hr)		Nausea, vomiting, diarrhea, tremulousness, palpitation, headaches, third heart sound at high serum levels (40 mg/ml)
Theophylline		Oral	100–300 mg		
Anticholinergics:	Suppress vagal-mediated cholinergic stimuli				Dry mouth, blurred vision
Atropine		Nebulizer	0.025–0.05 mg/kg	4–6 hr	Tachycardia (rare) Urinary retention (rare)
Ipratropium		MDI* Nebulizer	18 g	4–6 hr	
Cromolyn:	Stabilizes mast-cell membrane	MDI* Nebulizer	800 g		
Corticosteroids:	Enhance bronchodilatation by potentiating beta receptor responsiveness. Decrease inflammation and mucus production contributing to airway resistance by inhibiting arachidonic acid conversion pathways and suppressing leukocyte migration and release of lymphokines from lymphocytes				*Short-term:* Fluid retention, hypokalemia, insomnia, psychosis (rare) *Long-term:* Adrenal suppression, cushingoid features, osteoporosis, systemic hyperkalemia, hyperglycemia, cataracts, immune suppression
Hydrocortisone		IV	100 mg every 6 hr		
Methylprednisolone (Medrol)		IV Oral	40 mg every 6 hr 30–50 mg/day × 7 days and taper		
Prednisone		Oral	40–60 mg/day × 7 days and taper		
Beclomethasone		MDI*	84 μg	6–8 hr	
Flunisolide		MDI*	50 μg	12 hr	

*MDI, metered dose inhalers. Doses for inhalers in μg/puff; usually by 2–3 inhalations
†CAMP, cyclic adenosine monophosphate

activity. The bronchodilating mechanism of action of theophylline was long thought to be related to phosphodiesterase inhibition, resulting in elevation of intracellular cyclic adenosine monophosphate (CAMP). However, recent studies have shown that intracellular theophylline concentrations are too low to substantially inhibit phosphodiesterase and that some other unknown mechanism is likely.

Using theophylline preparations requires close attention to serum levels because of the narrow therapeutic index, and it is desirable to keep the serum level within the therapeutic range—between 10 to 20 mg/ml. The major factors that effect the serum level of theophylline are route of administration, dose, patient lean mass, and rate of metabolism. Liver failure, decreased liver perfusion (heart failure), advanced age, and a number of drugs, including cimetidine, erythromycin, allopurinol, and oral contraceptives, all decrease theophylline metabolism. Cigarette smoke and phenytoin both increase theophylline metabolism. Acute febrile illnesses can also affect theophylline metabolism in unpredictable ways, and these conditions must be borne in mind when administering theophylline. Serum levels must be monitored when initiating the drug, when adding a drug that might alter theophylline metabolism, or if symptoms or persisting bronchospasm occur that raise the question of non-therapeutic theophylline levels.

Intravenous aminophylline requires an initial loading dose of 4 to 6 mg/kg lean body mass, infused over 20 to 30 minutes and should be halved in patients already taking theophylline. The continuous infusion rate is selected, based upon the conditions discussed above, but usually ranges from 0.2 to 0.3 mg/kg lean body mass. Theophylline levels should be obtained after 3 to 4 half-lives and used to adjust the infusion rate.

Oral theophylline is now available in slow-release preparations and can usually be administered twice or even once daily. In order to minimize side-effects, it is generally preferable to begin theophylline at lower doses (100–300 mg, twice daily) and increase gradually unless urgent bronchodilatation is needed.

In addition to its bronchodilator action, theophylline also prevents respiratory muscle fatigue,[79] increases cardiac output and right ventricular ejection fraction, inhibits mast-cell degranulation, and enhances mucociliary clearance. Thus, there are a number of possible advantages in using theophylline to treat patients with COPD.

Anticholinergic agents (see Table 35-2) have recently gained importance with improved understanding of the role of the cholinergic nervous system in bronchospasm.[86] Asthmatic patients characteristically have airway hyperactivity to cholinergic substances. The vagus nerve may potentiate bronchospasm in response to emotional and exertional stimuli, which can be reversed by anticholinergic agents.

Although many anticholinergic agents are available in Europe, fewer are available in the United States, where substantial clinical experience has accumulated for only one agent—atropine. Although atropine can be administered by a variety of routes, bronchospasm is best treated by use of a nebulized solution, which delivers medications directly to the airways and minimizes systemic side-effects. The appropriate dose ranges from 0.025 to 0.05 mg/kg and is adjusted based on airway response and side-effects. Usually, 2 to 4 mg of atropine are diluted in 2.5 ml of saline and administered over 5 minutes, every 4 to 6 hours.

An atropine derivative, ipratropium, is now approved for use in Europe in both MDI and nebulizer preparations.[73] It appears to have equal efficacy to atropine in bringing about bronchodilatation, but because it is poorly absorbed, it causes fewer systemic side-effects.

The anticholinergics appear most effective for treatment of psychogenic and exercise- or cold-induced bronchospasm and in older patients with chronic bronchitis and emphysema. They should be added to sympathomimetics and methylxanthines when symptomatic control is inadequate and can also be used in combination with corticosteroids and cromolyn.

Cromolyn sodium (see Table 35-2) has no direct bronchodilator activity, but it reduces bronchospastic responses to exercise and acute inhalation of allergens and is an effective prophylactic agent in the treatment of asthma, primarily in children with allergic asthma.[26] Evidence of its benefit in adults with COPD is not so clear, although it may help lower the steroid requirement in patients with severe, persisting bronchospasm. It presumably acts to stabilize mast-cell membranes and prevent release of bronchoconstrictor substances. It produces essentially no systemic side-effects and should be tried in patients with allergic asthma who are not adequately controlled with inhaled sympathomimetics alone. A trial is also warranted in patients with COPD who are steroid-dependent or who have poorly controlled bronchospasm, despite optimal use of other bronchodilators. Because of its expense, it should be considered a second-line agent in the therapy of bronchospasm.

Corticosteroids are primarily of value in the control of severe, acute episodes of bronchospasm that cannot be adequately controlled by other medications.[85] Corticosteroids are also used chronically for control of persisting, poorly responsive bronchospasm in asthmatics and in selected patients with COPD.

The mechanism of action of corticosteroids in control of bronchospasm is not completely understood and is most likely multifactorial. Corticosteroids would be ideal agents for the treatment of hyperreactive airway disease were it not for their severe side-effects. During short-term administration, they are well tolerated, even inducing euphoria in many patients. However, long-term corticosteroid administration, particularly at moderate to high doses, causes a number of undesirable side-effects and should be avoided unless absolutely necessary in patients with obstructive lung disease. Minimal dosing schedules, including alternate-day dosing, can minimize long-term side-effects and are preferable to daily administration whenever possible.

Corticosteroid medications differ with regard to potency, amount of mineralocorticoid activity, and duration of action. Most often, during acute, severe exacerbations of asthma or COPD, patients are treated with intravenous corticosteroids. Short-acting hydrocortisone, 100 mg every 6 hours, or longer-acting methylprednisolone, 40 mg every 6 hours, is commonly prescribed. Once the patient manifests improvement on the intravenous medication, oral preparations (usually prednisone or methylprednisolone) can be started and the dose gradually tapered over 7 to 10 days. Slower tapering may be necessary in some patients to avoid relapse, and occasional patients may not tolerate tapering at all.

Roughly one-fourth of patients with stable COPD will experience significant improvement in air flow during a trial of prednisone, 40 to 60 mg/day, administered over a 2- to 4-week period, and some physicians recommend a routine steroid trial in most patients with severe COPD.[67] However, the benefits of this approach have never been shown to exceed the risks of long-term adverse side-effects, and chronic steroid therapy for COPD should probably be reserved for special situations, such as the patient with highly reactive airways who is unresponsive to optimal bronchodilator therapy.

Inhaled corticosteroids offer an alternative to systemic administration,[85] but they are ineffective in controlling acute exacerbations. They should be introduced in patients having frequent asthmatic exacerbations after the acute illness has been stabilized and oral steroids are being tapered. Inhalations should be performed in the same manner as inhaled bronchodilators, except that the inhalations should follow beta-agonist administration and the patient should rinse his or her mouth with water afterward to reduce chances of developing oral moniliasis. When used properly, inhaled corticosteroids reduce the frequency of exacerbations, lower the requirement for daily steroids, and virtually eliminate systemic side-effects.[85]

Therapy

Chest Physical Therapy

An important aspect of chest physical therapy involves the re-education of the patient in proper breathing techniques in order to maximize the efficiency of ventilation and to increase exercise tolerance. Training should involve hands-on demonstration of several specific techniques, which are then performed actively and repeatedly with the patient at rest and eventually incorporated into the patient's repertoire of activities.

Proper breathing techniques assume particular importance for the COPD patient who experiences a state of physiological obstruction to outflow of air from the lungs during expiration. This phenomenon causes air trapping and impairment to gas exchange in the alveoli and small airways and is perceived as increased difficulty in breathing. Impaired gas exchange contributes to muscle fatigue and further difficulty with the breathing mechanism. As the obstructed patient experiences increasing difficulty in breathing, the accessory muscles are called upon increasingly to assist the diaphragm and thereby set up an inefficient compensating mechanism.

Diaphragmatic breathing involves retraining the patient to use his or her diaphragm while relaxing accessory muscles, thereby restoring breathing efficiency. Diaphragmatic breathing is most likely to help the dyspneic patient with normal diaphragmatic excursions. Its benefit in patients with severe diaphragmatic flattening may be less apparent. Among the benefits expected with this technique are increased tidal volume, decreased functional residual capacity, and increased maximum oxygen uptake.[71]

To perform diaphragmatic breathing, the patient is instructed to lie supine or semi-reclined and relax, with one hand placed flat below the xiphoid process on the abdomen and the other on the chest wall (Fig. 35-1). The patient attempts to move the diaphragm as much as possible on inspiration and relax the abdomen while simultaneously inhibiting movement of the chest wall as much as possible. While inhaling slowly, the patient can feel the abdomen rise, while the chest wall remains stationary. This technique can be practiced with the use of small (3-lb)

weights on the abdomen to enhance focus on the diaphragm and should be practiced until it is learned effectively. It can gradually be incorporated into the patient's ADLs.[71]

A second technique—*pursed-lip breathing*—helps the patient prevent air trapping due to small airway collapse during exhalation and, consequently, promotes greater gas exchange in the alveoli.[51] The patient is instructed to sit comfortably erect, with feet placed flat on the floor, in a position which promotes maximum diaphragmatic excursion on inspiration. The patient inhales slowly through the nose and counts to 2, then purses the lips (as if to whistle) and exhales softly while counting from 2 to 6. The expiration phase should last two to three times as long as inspiration, with the patient avoiding forceful exhalation. Pursed-lip breathing is effectively combined with diaphragmatic breathing, and these techniques can be generalized and performed anywhere during routine ADLs.

During physical exertion, the COPD patient is likely to experience an increased rate and shallowness of breathing. Controlled respiratory rate and deep-breathing techniques improve tidal volume and increase PaO_2.[50] In order to maintain effective gas exchange, the rate and depth of breathing should be controlled in a rhythmic cadence. Patients should be instructed to set their cadence prior to initiating an activity and to continue the cadence during the activity. For example, a patient might approach stair climbing by setting a breathing cadence, using diaphragmatic or pursed-lip techniques. The patient then climbs two or three steps and pauses to rest while continuing the use of controlled breathing; then advances to climb two or three more steps, maintaining the same cadence until the activity is completed.

In patients with paralysis or severe paresis of the respiratory muscles, *glossopharyngeal breathing* provides a mechanism to maintain normal alveolar ventilation as a viable alternative to mechanically assisted ventilation. The technique involves using the tongue, jaws, cheeks, and pharynx to act as a pharyngeal pressure pump, forcing air into the lungs. The larynx provides the valve mechanism to retain the incremental volume and expiration is accomplished passively. When properly executed, this technique may increase vital capacity from .25 liters to 1.34 liters and allows measurable increase in independent breathing tolerance in otherwise ventilator-assisted individuals.[20] It also provides a mechanism for sighing or augmenting cough in patients with motor unit disease, phrenic nerve injury, or spinal cord injury.

The technique of *segmental breathing* deserves mention and is frequently administered or taught by respiratory therapists to patients postoperatively as a means of preventing focal atelectasis. The therapist applies manual pressure to the thoracic

Figure 35-1. Diaphragmatic breathing technique.

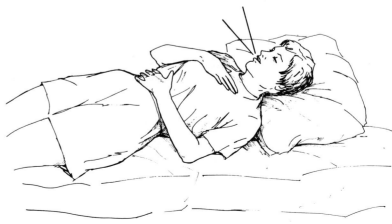

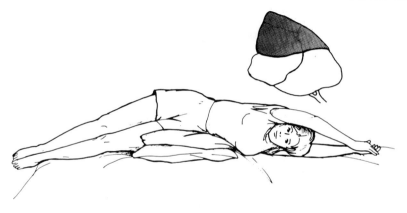

Figure 35-2. Postural drainage of right lower lung from left lateral decubitus position.

cage to resist respiratory excursions in a particular region where pressure is being directly applied. This facilitates expansion of adjacent regions of the thoracic cavity and presumably facilitates ventilation of those alveolar segments subserved. To date, there is no objective evidence that such techniques are effective in the COPD patient.[71]

A number of chest therapy techniques are available to assist in bronchial drainage of excessive mucus. The most important of these is *postural drainage*, the use of gravity-assisted positioning to improve the flow of mucus out of airways. Drainage of a particular segment is facilitated by tilting the lung at a 45° angle with respect to the segmental outflow. Individual patients may not be able to tolerate severe inclinations for the length of time necessary to achieve this effect and may need to adjust their positions according to individual comfort. In general, the patient should be placed in a Trendelenburg-type position, using a bed and pillows (Fig. 35-2) or other inclined support. The hips should be maintained above head level. A variety of positions are applicable and each designed to maximally drain a particular segment. Initially, the patient should remain in a particular position for 2 to 5 minutes and gradually increase to 15 minutes as tolerated. Therapy may be recommended on a four-times-a-day or every-four-hour basis in severe cases. It appears best to do postural drainage immediately prior to breakfast and again in the evening prior to bed (never on a full stomach as this may predispose to aspiration). Postural drainage may be facilitated by inhalation and nebulizer therapy immediately before treatments and after using oral or inhalant bronchodilators if indicated.[71]

Specific indications for postural drainage include sputum production exceeding 30 ml/day or moderate sputum production in patients too debilitated to raise their secretions effectively by alternative means. In patients with pulmonary edema or pleural effusion, this technique is contraindicated and should also be avoided in cases of patients sustaining acute chest trauma, myocardial infarction, hemorrhagic conditions, or pulmonary embolism.[71]

Manual percussion of the chest wall may serve to loosen mucous plugs and assist in moving mucus to the larger airways. Percussion is done by cupping the hands and alternatively clapping against the lower rib cage. This technique is most effective when applied during postural drainage with the assistance of a helper, although it can be done independently to the anterior and lateral aspects of the chest with the patient lying supine or in the lateral decubitus position.

Vibration is a second manual technique performed by a helper placing one hand over the other on the patient's rib cage. A steady, even vibration is produced across the rib cage and should be done only while the patient exhales through pursed lips.

Finally, controlled coughing is important to avoid airway

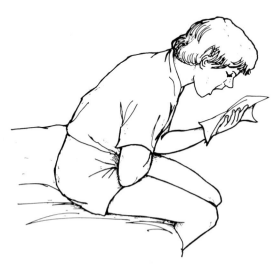

Figure 35-3. Controlled coughing technique.

collapse. The patient is taught to avoid forceful (explosive) coughing and to initiate a timed, deliberate cough of sufficient force to tear loose mucus without causing airways to collapse. The patient is instructed to sit comfortably and lean the body slightly forward over the hips (Fig. 35-3). Using diaphragmatic breathing, the patient should inhale and hold briefly, then cough two or three times in succession while exhaling slowly through pursed lips. After a short pause, the patient should inhale again and repeat the sequence. This strategy is designed to avoid uncontrollable or ineffective triggering of the cough reflex.

Therapeutic Exercise

Physical training leads to measurable improvement in work capacity that can be related to changes in hemodynamic and ventilatory functions, as well as rates of metabolic substrate use and energy production. The general principles of exercise training to improve endurance are presented elsewhere in Chapter 18 and need only be briefly summarized here before developing a rationale for exercise prescription in the pulmonary patient.

Physical training involves repeated exposure of an individual to a given workload or stress in order that physiological adaptation to that workload takes place. A "training effect" will occur in predictable fashion provided that the intensity of training stimulus exceeds that load to which the individual is regularly exposed and that the workload increases as individual performance improves during the course of training. In addition, the duration and frequency of training stimulus will vary to some degree in reciprocal fashion with intensity of workload and are both important additional determinants of training effect.[8]

In general, in order to evoke a cardiovascular training effect, the exercise must effectively engage a large proportion of the body muscle mass. Mode-specificity of training is important such that the maximum benefit through training toward performance of a particular activity will occur when the mode of training employs that particular activity. The specific effects of endurance training in physically unimpaired individuals include lowering the resting and submaximal exercise heart rate, increasing stroke volume to maintain cardiac output, increasing maximal oxygen uptake ($\dot{V}O_2$), and increasing oxidative metabolic capacity of endurance-trained muscles.[2, 8]

In order for an observable training effect to occur, exercise intensity must exceed a threshold, which is generally estimated to be 60% to 70% of predicted maximal heart rate or at least 50% of $\dot{V}O_2$ max for a sustained period of 30 minutes per session and four sessions per week over a 4-week period.[8]

Determinants of fitness derived from endurance training in the physically unimpaired individual may not be directly applicable to the COPD patient. Such patients are faced with symptomatic limitations, largely due to mechanical (ventilatory) as opposed to cardiovascular factors. The minute ventilation requirement for a given work rate is greater because the relative fraction of physiological dead space to lung volume is higher and because inadequate oxygen delivery leads to an earlier shift to anaerobic metabolism. The patient experiences dyspnea and is forced to discontinue exercise before the normal anaerobic threshhold is reached. Consequently, the COPD patient is unlikely to endure exercise of sufficient intensity to induce training effects.[80]

There is no widespread acceptance of objective criteria to guide and develop exercise protocols in COPD patients similar to those existing for healthy or cardiac-impaired individuals. The exercise performance of the COPD patient is limited by the subjective end point of dyspnea. Consequently, it is difficult, if not impossible, to objectively define maximum exercise tolerance according to measurable physiological parameters. Target heart rate may not be a reliable indicator of physiological work loads because the stroke volume response to maintain cardiac output is reduced and the target heart rate is likely to be reached at lesser work loads.[8]

A number of workers have found exercise testing with treadmill[18, 55, 60, 70] or cycle ergometry[5, 13] to be a useful prelude to exercise training, both for baseline assessment of fitness and determination of appropriate intensity for the subsequent exercise program. Conventional pulmonary function testing parameters have been shown to be poor predictors of exercise tolerance among COPD patients afflicted to similar degrees and, consequently, are less accurate than the alternative treadmill exercise testing.[61]

The 12-minute walk test originally described by Cooper for healthy individuals is recommended as a practical measure to estimate exercise tolerance in COPD patients.[43] The test measures the distance a patient can cover in 12 minutes, ambulating on a level surface. The standard time allows for uniformity in assessment of endurance among patients with varying degrees of severity. The test uses a modality that is familiar to all and requires no elaborate apparatus. It has been shown to be practical with the results applicable to everyday activities. It is an appropriate test of oxygen uptake and endurance.

A variety of exercise training programs have been applied to patients with COPD. All studies seem to show improvement in endurance and exercise performance whether treadmill, cycle ergometer, or non-treadmill-type walking was employed. Table 35-3 summarizes these studies and the effects of endurance

---

Table 35-3
Exercise Training Programs for the COPD Patient

	VC	Tidal Volume	MVV	FVC	FEV$_1$	MMEF	V$_E$	PaO$_2$	PaCO$_2$	$\dot{V}O_2$	AVDO$_2$	Resting Heart Rate	Resp. Rate	Dyspnea	Exercise Tolerance
Paez et al[55] (treadmill)	No Δ				No Δ			No Δ	No Δ	↑		No Δ			↑
Petty et al[59] (treadmill evaluation, progressive ambulation, and stair climbing)			No Δ	No Δ	No Δ			↑						↓	↑
Brundin[13] (cycle ergometer)	↑		↑		No Δ							No Δ	↓	↓	↑
Chester et al[18] (treadmill evaluation, cycle ergometer)			No Δ	No Δ		↓				↓	No Δ	No Δ			↑
McGavin, Gupta, McHardy[43] (12-minute walk test, stair climbing)			No Δ	No Δ			No Δ			No Δ		No Δ		↓	↑
Unger, Moser, Hanson[77] (treadmill evaluation)	No Δ			No Δ		No Δ	↓			↓				↓	↑
Belman, Wasserman[8] (cycle ergometer)	No Δ	No Δ	No Δ	No Δ	No Δ		No Δ			No Δ					↑
Pineda, Haas, Axen[60] (treadmill)	No Δ		No Δ	No Δ	No Δ	No Δ	No Δ	No Δ	No Δ	No Δ					

VC, vital capacity; MVV, maximum voluntary ventilation; FVC, forced vital capacity; MMEF, maximal mid-expiratory flow; V$_E$, volume of expired gas; $\dot{V}O_2$, oxygen consumption; AVDO$_2$, arteriovenous oxygen content difference; ↑, increase; ↓, decrease; No Δ, no change

training on conventional pulmonary functions and physiological parameters. In general, no significant or consistent trends in improvement in spirometry or ABGs were seen. One study showed an improvement in arteriovenous oxygen difference ($AVDO_2$), suggesting a more efficient peripheral extraction of oxygen with treadmill training, but also noted that improved work performance was probably due to learning effects (adjustment of stride length) which decreased the total aerobic cost of the activity.[55]

It appears that the cardiovascular training effects seen in the physiologically unimpaired individual are not determinants of improved fitness in pulmonary patients. Perhaps alternative factors such as increased motivation[8] and improvement in neuro-muscular coordination[2, 55] or psychological adaptation and desensitization to dyspnea explain the improvement. Whatever the mechanisms, physiological or psychological, the response to exercise training in pulmonary patients can be dramatic, and the direct benefits include improved performance in ADLs, psychological well-being, enhancement of appetite, and improved sleep patterns.

COPD patients participating in protracted endurance training programs on an outpatient basis improve work performance as much as inpatients participating in shorter, more intense programs.[13, 59] Simple walking, when prescribed in a progressive exercise program, can reduce dyspnea and remarkably improve distance walking and stairclimbing.[59] Such gains can be safely made by starting with an initial structured outpatient program on a daily basis for one week, tapering to three times a week for the second week, and then tapering the third week to an exclusive home exercise program.

The goal of exercise training in COPD patients is to challenge the patients physiologically without bringing about undue dyspnea or fatigue.[5] Recommendations include monitoring the heart rate to maintain a range of 80% to 85% of the maximum achieved heart rate determined by progressive exercise testing with a treadmill or cycle ergometer. The maximum achieved heart rate is invariably less than the age-predicted maximum due to dyspnea or muscle fatigue. Because of age and severity of deconditioning, many COPD patients will reach a target heart rate of 110 to 120 beats/minute with mild exercise levels. They may initially tolerate only short periods of less than 5 minutes/session, and an early goal would be to increase the number of sessions per day and consolidate the exercise to achieve a 20-minute session that can be sustained on a daily basis.

The patient should exercise to tolerance levels (avoiding undue fatigue or dyspnea) while monitoring the heart rate and stop when the pulse exceeds 120 or there are more than 6 premature beats per minute.[59] Training sessions, incorporating use of the 12-minute walk test to monitor improvement and performance, can be modified and continued on an outpatient basis.

Supplemental oxygen appears to be a beneficial adjunct to exercise programs for COPD patients in two ways.[11, 40] Portable oxygen supplementation facilitates exercise for strengthening in those patients capable of endurance training and also permits endurance training in patients who might otherwise not tolerate even minimal exercise levels. Consequently, assessment of oxygen saturation at rest and during exercise on room air is recommended. In patients with significant desaturation during physical training (below 85%–95%), supplemental oxygen should be provided in the form of low-flow nasal oxygen (1–3 liters/min) to enhance exercise performance, relieve dyspnea, and protect patients with coronary artery disease from possible dysrhythmias.

Ventilatory muscle endurance training using isocapnic hyperpnea, requires a rebreathing apparatus that is not readily available or practical for most pulmonary rehabilitation programs. However, a variety of hand-held muscle trainers, using a variable orifice to control inspiratory or expiratory resistance, are available. These are readily applicable to home use and may provide a useful adjunct to improving exercise capacity through ventilatory muscle strengthening. It has been shown that respiratory muscle training may improve exercise capacity in COPD patients.[7] However, there are no studies contrasting the benefits of respiratory muscle training to other forms of endurance training in these patients. Whether significant additional benefit is to be gained by using ventilatory muscle training techniques remains to be demonstrated.[5]

The breathing techniques described above appear to promote work tolerance during endurance exercise training or ADL performance in the COPD patient. Significant improvement in gas exchange parameters of emphysematous patients practicing controlled deep breathing at 8 to 12 breaths/minute have been demonstrated, including a significant decrease in respiratory rate, increase in tidal volume, minute ventilation, and oxygen saturation at rest.[50] Thus, improved exercise performance may be achieved by decreasing respiratory rate and relaxing the accessory muscles, thereby improving breathing efficiency.

Occupational Therapy

Improvements in performance of basic and advanced self-care activities of the COPD patient can be achieved through a combined effort by physical and occupational therapists to provide education and training in upper body exercises with coordinated breathing to promote flexibility and endurance; training in relaxation exercises; proper body mechanics, pacing techniques, and principles of energy conservation; and application of principles of work simplification to routine ADLs and leisure pursuits.

Patients should be instructed to exercise from a seated position with feet firmly on the floor and to maintain proper posture during bending and sitting activities. Flexibility exercises may incorporate trunk and arm flexion and extension with cross-body reaching or employ the use of a towel or dowel held with both hands while performing "wand" maneuvers overhead and behind the neck. Alternate arm and leg straight-raising exercises should be performed by inhaling during raising, and exhaling during lowering of each limb. Pursed-lip breathing during exhalation is recommended.

Patients can be taught to distinguish between states of tension and relaxation and enhance control of the latter through relaxation exercises. Such exercises are performed while sitting comfortably or lying supine with head and knees supported. The patients are instructed to clench the arm, forearm, and fist to a count of two, then relax to a count of four. They should alternate arms, then alternately contract and relax each leg in similar fashion; they may repeat the entire sequence several times in succession while using diaphragmatic and pursed-lip breathing techniques. In some cases, relaxation training is facilitated through the use of visual imagery and pre-recorded tapes.

Patients should be instructed in proper body mechanics for lifting and bending and in coordinating breathing with activity (inhale during reaching and extending, exhale during pushing or lifting). They should avoid holding their breath during physical exertion.

Patients can be taught to pace themselves by planning ahead when performing an activity, resting between activities, avoiding work to the point of fatigue, and quitting when tired. Fear of dyspnea may inhibit a patient from performing activities and they may not know how active they can or should be. Strategies to promote energy conservation should be reviewed in detail and should include the following principles.

1. Store items or materials needed for the performance of a chore or activity in a single area.
2. Place objects necessary for a particular project close to where they are needed before commencing an activity.
3. Remain seated whenever possible and make workspace accessible to avoid unnecessary reaching, bending, or stooping.
4. Use both hands while moving objects and use a wheeled cart to move heavy or bulky items.
5. Work consistently from right-to-left (or left-to-right) to avoid unnecessary movement back-and-forth.
6. Perform activities slowly and consistently.
7. Rest frequently (at least 10 minutes per hour working) and alternate light and heavy chores.
8. Use pursed-lip breathing with prolonged expiration during performance of tasks that are physically demanding.

Principles of work simplification should be discussed as they apply to basic and advanced ADLs. For example, bathing can be facilitated with equipment such as a bath stool and hand-held shower. Grooming can be simplified by keeping hair cut short and avoiding an elaborate hair style. Aerosol sprays should be avoided whenever possible. Dressing can be made easier through the use of extended reachers and long-handled shoe horns, and patients should be encouraged to wear loose, comfortable clothing and to avoid restrictive undergarments. A home environmental assessment should be completed with recommendations made for structural modifications and adaptive equipment as needed.

A sample outpatient therapeutic prescription for a COPD patient is summarized in Table 35-4.

Rehabilitation Equipment

Rehabilitation of the patient with chronic pulmonary disease often requires optimal use of respiratory therapy equipment to assist in removal of secretions and in delivery of medication, to provide ventilatory support, and to maintain airway access. A number of items of respiratory therapy equipment are likely to be prescribed as part of a pulmonary rehabilitation program and are listed in Table 35-5.

Humidifiers, Nebulizers, Suctioning, IPPB

Humidifiers increase the water vapor content of a gas by enhancing evaporation.[45] The simplest humidifier (bubble humidifier) is most often used for increasing the humidity of oxygen administered through nasal prongs or a face mask, thereby improving patient comfort. The patient's upper airway still provides the bulk of gas humidification as air enters the lungs. When the patient's upper airway is bypassed by endotracheal or tracheostomy tubes, delivery of heated, fully saturated gas is mandatory or airway desiccation and damage will occur. Heated humidifiers with special bubble systems of moistened paper to increase the surface area of contact between gas and water provide sufficient heat and humidity to fulfill this need.[45]

Nebulizers generate aerosols consisting of liquid particles suspended in a gas.[45] Unlike humidifiers, nebulizers can also trap solubilized medication in the suspended liquid particles and deliver it to the lower airways and are frequently used to administer bronchodilators. Nebulizers can also deliver larger volumes of liquid to lower airways than can humidifiers alone and, thus, are effective in loosening copious dry secretions.

The hand-held jet nebulizer can easily be installed with a simple air compressor for use in the patient's home. Ultrasonic

Table 35-4
A Sample Therapeutic Prescription for a COPD Patient

Diagnosis: COPD

Prognosis: Favorable, patient on stable self-medication program

Goals:
- Improve endurance and efficiency.
- Optimize oxygen needs and control of secretions.
- Increase independence in ambulation and self-care activities.
- Reduce anxiety and improve self-esteem through enhanced body awareness.

Precautions:
- Supplemental oxygen needed during exercise.
- Discontinue and notify physician if patient becomes severely dyspneic with exercise or develops ventricular premature beats of more than 6/min.
- Patient to self-monitor heart rate and maintain less than 120 beats/min.

Respiratory Therapy:
- Conduct ear oximetry at rest and during exercise to determine portable oxygen flow rate needed to maintain oxygen saturation of at least 90% at all times.
- Instruct patient in diaphragmatic and pursed-lip breathing techniques.
- Instruct patient and family in postural drainage techniques.
- Instruct patient and family on home portable oxygen use.
- Instruct in use of metered-dose inhaler prior to exercise.

Physical Therapy:
- Assess baseline endurance, using 12-minute walk test.
- Begin incremental exercise program to improve endurance through ambulation and stair climbing. Begin with 5-minute sessions, followed by rest periods between sessions. When patient tolerates 20 minutes total exercise per day, begin consolidating sessions. Initial treatments on daily basis during weeks 1 and 2, taper to 3 times per week over weeks 3 and 4, and then taper to home program with self-monitoring over weeks 5 and 6.
- Review proper body mechanics and coordinate with breathing patterns, using diaphragmatic and pursed-lip breathing when appropriate.

Occupational Therapy:
- Assess upper extremity mobility, strength, and endurance. Develop exercise program to improve same for home applications with self-monitoring.
- Evaluate basic and advanced self-care activities and provide adaptive aids to improve independence with dressing, hygiene, bathing, cooking, and other chores.
- Train patient in energy conservation and work simplification techniques.
- Evaluate home environment and make recommendations for workspace modifications and equipment to improve safety, efficiency, and independence.
- Provide relaxation exercise training with visual imagery techniques.

nebulizers produce high frequency sound waves that aerosolize water upon striking the surface. Variations in the ultrasonic frequency and amplitude alter the particle size and volume output, respectively, and allow greater particle size selectivity than with standard jet nebulizers.[45]

Hazards in the use of nebulizers include aerosolization of bacteria from a contaminated water source, requiring close attention to recommended cleaning regimens. High-volume nebulizers can deliver substantial quantities of fluid that are absorbed in the airways and can cause fluid overload. Overheated nebulizers can also cause airway burns and temperatures should be monitored.

Table 35-5
Equipment

Item	Function/Indications	Type	Advantages	Disadvantages
Humidifier	Increases water content of air administered via face mask or nasal prong; increases patient comfort with supplemental oxygen system	Bubble humidifier	Inexpensive Disposable	Inefficient
		Heated humidifier	Prevents desiccation of upper airway when endotracheal or tracheostomy tube used	Needs temperature monitoring to avoid burns
Nebulizer	Generates aerosol of liquid particles suspended in gas; can serve as humidifier and deliver medication suspended in liquid particles to lower airways; can serve to loosen thick secretions and induce sputum production	Jet nebulizer	Hand-held, easily used at home; operates with simple air compressor	
		Ultrasonic nebulizer	Greater selectivity of particle size	
Suctioning	Indicated in chronic airway intubation or severely impaired cough; assists with clearing secretions	Hand-held		
IPPB	Used with nebulizer to deliver medication or saline; provides positive airway pressure to assist with inspiration			Additional expense over nebulizer may not be justified
Supplemental Oxygen	Maintains oxygen tension between 65–95 mm Hg; delivers oxygen at set rate to nasopharynx	Nasal cannula	Doesn't interfere with speech or eating; allows fairly reliable control of F_IO_2 concentration	Uncomfortable
		Venturi mask	More accurate F_IO_2 concentration than nasal cannula	Confining; interferes with speech and eating
		Standard face mask	Delivers F_IO_2 more than 40%; utilizes high oxygen flow	Confining; interferes with speech and eating
		Trans-tracheal oxygen cannula	Provides more efficient chronic delivery of oxygen concentration; avoids discomfort of nasal oxygen and prongs	
Negative Pressure Ventilator	Creates intermittent subatmospheric pressure around thorax and abdomen to assist inspiration. Tidal volume determined by surface area over which negative pressure is applied and compliance of patient's chest wall and lungs	Iron lung	Most efficient and reliable	Heavy and bulky; restricts motion
		Portalung	Lightweight (50 kg); fits on standard bed; efficient and reliable	
		Poncho wrap		Negative pressure to anterior chest and upper abdomen only. Less efficient and requires greater negative pressure
		Chest cuirass	Portable; easy to apply	Difficult fitting patients with chest wall deformities

(Continued)

Table 35-5—Continued
Equipment

Item	Function/Indications	Type	Advantages	Disadvantages
Rocking Bed	Displacement of abdominal contents with gravity assistance to effect diaphragmatic motion. "Head down" position effects exhalation; head-up position effects inhalation		Assists disphragmatic motion in bilateral diaphragmatic paralysis	Inefficient
Pneumobelt	Abdominal bladder inflates and deflates to provide intermittent positive pressure to abdomen, thereby displacing diaphragm upward and assisting exhalation. Gravity assists inhalation by returning diaphragm to original position when bladder deflates			Must use in seated position; not conducive to nocturnal use
Positive Pressure Ventilators	Provide ventilatory assistance to patients with acute and chronic respiratory insufficiency, requiring round-the-clock support. Usually administered by artificial airway		Volume-limited	Delivers preset tidal volume to maintain reliable alveolar ventilation
Tracheostomy	Provides prolonged airway intubation	Cuffed Portex Soft-Seal	Minimizes airway trauma. Short-term application. Patient unable to speak. Excellent suctioning capability	
		Fome-Cuff	Maintains low cuff pressures in patients with prior airway trauma	
		Fenestrated cuff	Allows patients to speak who require only intermittent ventilatory assistance	

Suctioning of the airway is indicated in patients with chronic airway intubation or severely impaired cough.[42] Tracheobronchial suctioning is necessary in those patients with endotracheal tubes or chronic tracheostomies because the artificial airway impairs cough and damages tracheal mucosa, disrupting the flow of mucus from lower airways.

Tracheobronchial suctioning through an artificial airway requires practice, skill, and adherence to prescribed technique[27] to minimize the likelihood of respiratory infection, airway trauma, or bleeding and aggravation of hypoxemia.

Intermittent positive pressure breathing (IPPB) devices are generally used with a nebulizer and provide positive airway pressure to the patient to assist with inspiration. They previously achieved great popularity in the treatment of patients with exacerbations of COPD or pneumonia, but have recently fallen into disfavor because several large, randomized, controlled trials have failed to show any benefit of IPPB over standard nebulizers despite the added expense.[17] IPPB may still be useful to augment tidal volumes in patients with neuromuscular disease and weakened respiratory muscles.

Oxygen Supplementation

Supplemental oxygen is used to maintain arterial oxygen tension in an acceptable range, generally between 65 and 95 mm Hg. In patients with acute myocardial infarction, exacerbations of asthma, or carbon monoxide poisoning, supplemental oxygen is justified even if no hypoxemia is initially present. Chronic supplemental oxygen is indicated for patients with chronic arterial hypoxemia (PaO_2 less than 55 mm Hg). The Nocturnal Oxygen Therapy Trial, a multicenter randomized trial in hypoxemic COPD patients, demonstrated improved survival in patients treated with continuous as opposed to nocturnal oxygen supplementation (12 hours daily). Based upon results of this and other trials, it is recommended that not only patients with severe COPD and PaO_2 of less than 55 mm Hg, but also those with PaO_2 levels of less than 60 mm Hg and polycythemia or evidence of cor pulmonale on electrocardiogram, echocardiogram, or x-ray should use continuous oxygen supplementation.[52]

The most convenient means of oxygen administration is by nasal cannula, which delivers humidified oxygen to the nasopharynx at a set rate. The final inspired oxygen concentration is determined not only by the rate of oxygen delivery, but also by the patient's ventilatory rate and other factors such as structure of the nasal passages and extent to which the patient breathes through his or her nose as opposed to the mouth. Fortunately, because nasal cannulae deliver oxygen even if only a single prong is in the nose or the patient is a mouth breather, adjustments of the oxygen flow rate allow fairly reliable control of the inspired oxygen concentration. Particularly in COPD patients with hypercapnia, in whom $PaCO_2$ may rise further with oxygen supplementation, oxygen flow rates should be started at low levels (less than 1 liter/min) and carefully titrated upward in 0.5 to 1 liter/min increments until the desired PaO_2 is reached.

Other means of delivering supplemental oxygen use face masks. The Venturi mask delivers a more accurate inspired oxygen concentration than nasal cannulae.

In order to deliver inspired oxygen concentrations exceeding 40%, a standard face mask using high oxygen flows can be used.[45] Inspired oxygen concentrations exceeding 60% can be achieved by using a non-rebreathing reservoir mask. Unfortunately, face masks are not a reliable way of delivering oxygen supplementation in severely hypoxemic patients. Dyspneic patients often find face masks confining and uncomfortable and masks frequently fall off unattended patients. Because room air is usually entrained around even a well-positioned mask during inspiration, it is difficult to achieve inspired oxygen concentrations exceeding 60%. The mask also interferes with talking and eating, necessitating removal during these activities. When PaO_2 cannot be maintained above 50 mm Hg in an acutely ill patient despite optimal oxygen supplementation, airway intubation is usually necessary with possible institution of positive end-expiratory pressure (PEEP).

For chronic oxygen delivery in outpatients, nasal prongs offer the most convenient means of low-flow oxygen delivery. Low-oxygen delivery through a chronically implanted trans-tracheal catheter is currently undergoing evaluation[19] and may be advantageous in patients requiring high oxygen flows or in individuals who are uncomfortable with nasal prongs. Oxygen systems for home delivery consist of three basic types: oxygen concentrators, tank delivery systems, and liquid oxygen systems.[58] Each has advantages and disadvantages. The concentrator, which extracts oxygen from room air by means of a molecular sieve, is the least expensive for patients receiving less than 2 liters/min. For patients who wish easy portability, the liquid system generally works best.

Ventilatory Assist Systems

Body ventilators function by applying pressure to the thorax or abdomen to assist ventilation. They are less reliable than positive pressure systems in assisting ventilation and do not allow direct access to the airway; hence, they are disadvantageous in managing patients with acute respiratory failure. However, for selected patients with chronic respiratory failure, body ventilators may be preferable because they cost less, are easier to operate, and spare the airway.[31]

NEGATIVE PRESSURE VENTILATORS. Negative pressure ventilators function by intermittently creating a subatmospheric pressure around the thorax and abdomen, allowing air at atmo-spheric pressure to enter through the mouth and expand the chest. The efficiency of negative pressure ventilators (measured as the tidal volume achieved for a given negative pressure) is determined by the surface area over which the negative pressure is applied and the compliance characteristics of the patient's chest wall and lungs. The most effective negative pressure ventilator, the iron lung, can be synchronized to the patient's respiration rate and negative pressure can then be adjusted to achieve the desired minute ventilation. Despite its efficiency and reliability, the weight and bulkiness of the iron lung limit its acceptability to patients. A modified version, the Portalung (Portalung, Inc., Boulder, CO) has recently been introduced (Fig. 35-4) and weighs approximately 50 kg and will fit on a standard bed. Powered by a Thompson Maxi-vent negative pressure ventilator (Puritan-Bennet Corp., Boulder, CO), it matches the iron lung in efficiency and reliability.

The "poncho wrap," "nylon jacket," or "rain coat" ventilator consists of a nylon outer garment that fits over a rigid chest piece and is tightened around the neck, arms, and legs. When a negative pressure pump generates subatmospheric pressure within, the chest piece prevents collapse of the nylon jacket and chest expansion occurs. Because the negative pressure is applied to the anterior chest and upper abdomen only, slightly greater negative pressures are necessary to generate effective tidal volumes.

The "chest piece," "tortoise shell," or cuirass ventilator consists of a fitted rigid shell that fits over the anterior chest and upper abdomen (Fig. 35-5). It is the least efficient and should be used in patients with relatively stable chronic respiratory failure who require intermittent ventilatory assistance.

All negative pressure ventilators restrict patient motion. Patient discomfort (primarily back pain) is a frequent problem, particularly in patients with kyphoscoliosis. Careful placement of pillows, occasional repositioning, and nonsteroidal anti-inflammatory drugs can alleviate the discomfort, but for some patients who are unable to tolerate these ventilators other alternatives must be sought.

The rocking bed and the exsufflation belt, or "pneumobelt" (Fig. 35-6), function by displacing abdominal contents and affecting diaphragmatic motion. Both are relatively inefficient ventilators and should be reserved for patients with mild chronic respiratory failure. Both also function poorly in excessively thin or obese patients or in those who have severe kyphoscoliosis. The rocking bed and pneumobelt can be helpful in patients with bilateral diaphragmatic paralysis.

Most patients with respiratory failure, particularly acute respiratory failure, receive positive pressure ventilation by an artificial airway. Positive pressure ventilation allows direct control over ventilation and access to the airway and is generally prefer-

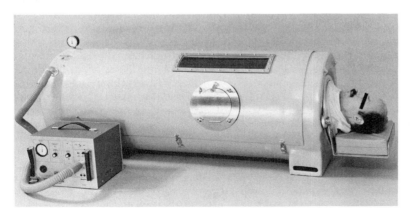

Figure 35-4. The Portalung (Puritan-Bennet Corporation, Boulder, CO) shown is a modified version of the tank ventilator. Porthole allows limited access to patient and neck seal is identical to that of an iron lung.

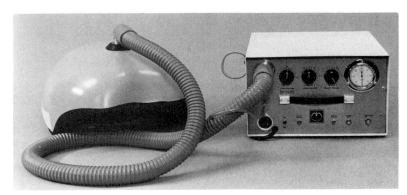

Figure 35-5. Molded part of the chest cuirass ventilator (Lifecare, Inc., Woburn, MA) is fitted over anterior chest to allow generation of intermittent negative pressure. The negative pressure ventilator is a Monaghan 170C.

Figure 35-6. Pneumobelt (Puritan-Bennet Corporation, Boulder, CO) is powered by a Bantam positive pressure ventilator. Inflation of the rubber bladder contained within the corset displaces abdominal contents inward, forcing diaphragm upward and assisting exhalation.

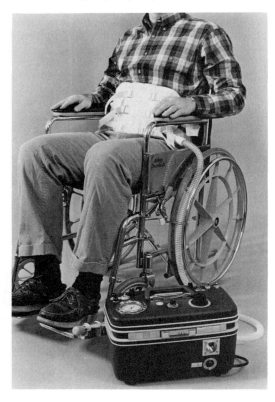

able in managing patients with acute respiratory problems or those with severe respiratory insufficiency requiring round-the-clock ventilatory assistance.

POSITIVE PRESSURE VENTILATORS. Positive pressure ventilators refer to devices that deliver supra-atmospheric pressure to the upper airway, forcing air into the lungs. Modern positive pressure ventilators are usually volume-limited; that is, they deliver a pre-set tidal volume and thereby maintain reliable alveolar ventilation.[27]

To initiate ventilation with a positive pressure ventilator, selections of respiratory rate, tidal volume, inspiratory flow rate, forced inspiratory oxygen rate (FiO_2), high pressure limit, and ventilator mode must be made. The variety of ventilator modes available depends on the specific ventilator, but most ventilators offer a control mode in which the ventilator delivers the selected volume at the selected rate, regardless of the patient's breathing pattern; an assist mode in which the ventilator delivers the selected tidal volume when it senses patient inspiratory effort as indicated by a negative pressure deflection; and an intermittent mandatory ventilation (IMV) mode in which the ventilator delivers controlled ventilation while the patient breathes spontaneously from a separate breathing circuit. IMV is the ventilatory mode commonly selected for patients receiving chronic ventilatory assistance. Other settings must be individualized, taking into consideration the patient's weight, metabolic needs, and desired blood gas levels.

Although positive pressure ventilation is usually administered through an artificial airway, certain patients with chronic respiratory insufficiency can adapt to receiving ventilatory assistance through a mouthpiece, face mask, or nose piece. The positive pressure system can be attached to a wheelchair and used for daytime supplemental ventilatory assistance, and a negative pressure ventilator used at night. Alternatively, some patients learn to sleep with a face or nasal mask strapped on and the positive pressure system can be used for nocturnal ventilatory assistance. Difficulties with aerophagia and swallowing secretions can arise with the nocturnal use of the face mask, and many patients find the arrangement intolerable.

Chronic Tracheostomies

Indications for tracheostomy include prolonged endotracheal intubation (3–4 weeks), bypass of an upper airway obstruction (*i.e.,* tumor, foreign body, or trauma), and prevention of chronic aspiration and control of excessive secretions in patients with marginal respiratory status. Tracheostomies have a number of advantages over chronic oro- and nasotracheal intubation, including freedom of the mouth for speech and eating, improved airway stability, easier replacement should the tube fall out, and decreased airway trauma. Thus, when prolonged airway intubation is anticipated, early tracheostomy should be performed. Caution must be used in changing tracheostomy tubes until the wound is well healed, because false lumens can result from improper tube placement. Once the tube has been in place for at least a week, replacement is usually quite simple.

The choice of tracheostomy tube depends upon the patient and likely duration of use. Speech is facilitated by so-called "talking traches" that contain a separate lumen for compressed air channeled toward the vocal cords. Patients can also learn to speak, using the leak around the deflated cuff of a standard tracheostomy tube. Ventilator tidal volumes are increased to compensate for air loss through the leak.

For chronic ventilation in patients able to speak and requiring only intermittent ventilatory assistance, fenestrated tracheostomy tubes have advantages. They consist of a fenestrated outer and a continuous inner cannula. The inner cannula can be removed and replaced with a small plug that allows the patient to breathe through the fenestration and upper airway, or can be left in place for attachment to a positive pressure ventilator.

Complications of tracheostomy include wound infection, hemorrhage, subcutaneous emphysema, acute tracheitis, accidental extubation, and swallowing difficulties. Chronic complications include tracheitis, ulceration, hemorrhage, tracheomalacia, granuloma formation, and stricture. Some complications, such as infection or accidental decannulation, can be avoided by meticulous care procedures. Tracheitis and hemorrhage can be ameliorated by gentle suctioning. It is particularly important to avoid over-distention of the tracheostomy cuff to prevent tracheal damage that could lead to granuloma formation and stenosis. A small air leak around the cuff is desirable and cuff pressure should be kept below 10 to 12 mm Hg. The minimal amount of air necessary to inflate the cuff adequately should be recorded and monitored.[27]

Nutrition and the Pulmonary Patient

Nutritional assessment and management in chronically disabled patients is discussed fully in Chapter 28. However, patients suffering from chronic pulmonary disease may be at particular risk of malnutrition, such that the subject deserves particular additional emphasis.

Clinically detectable malnutrition is prevalent among hospitalized patients,[10] and the risk of clinically detectable malnutrition increases with increased length of hospital stay.[81] Hospitalized patients with COPD may be at particular risk.[36] Malnutrition may play a particular role in acute respiratory failure in patients suffering from COPD[25] and survivability among patients with end-stage COPD may be significantly shortened in those patients experiencing precipitous weight loss.[78] Percent of change of ideal body weight and creatinine-height index have been correlated with such spirometric parameters as FEV_1 diffusing lung capacity for carbon monoxide (DLCO), and maximum inspiratory pressure among emphysematous patients.[53]

The chronic pulmonary patient may experience appetite suppression or disincentive to eat for a variety of reasons. The sensation of dyspnea in itself may be a significant deterrent toward swallowing or feeding, and arterial oxygen desaturation can occur in such patients during meals.[12] The possibility of hyperinflation associated with COPD and concomitant diaphragmatic flattening may cause impingement upon the stomach, decreasing the volume of food that can be eaten and causing a feeling of distention or other discomfort during digestion of a normal-sized meal. Polymedications are a frequent additional problem. Commonly used medications in the pulmonary patient group may contribute to gastric irritation, may cause nausea and vomiting, alter taste or suppress appetite, or may interfere with bio-availability of vitamins and other nutrients. In patients requiring chronic oxygen by nasal cannula or tracheostomy, oxygen delivery may have negative effects upon the senses of smell and taste.[56]

Nutritional status and metabolic substrate utilization have been linked to respiratory mechanisms of ventilatory control and gas exchange. The respiratory quotient (RQ) is determined to be the ratio of carbon dioxide production to oxygen uptake and varies with metabolic substrate. When carbohydrate is the primary metabolic substrate, the RQ is 1. It is somewhat lower at .7 for fat and .8 for protein substrates. Among patients receiving total parenteral nutrition (TPN), glucose loading can have a profound effect upon VCO_2,[1] whereas VO_2 increases to a lesser degree. As TPN patients experience glucose loading, the RQ shifts toward 1, reflecting the greater rate of carbon dioxide production, and there is a concomitant increase in minute ventilation. The clinical significance of these observations toward chronic pulmonary patients remains questionable; however, an increase in RQ, associated with hyperalimentation in ventilator-assisted patients with fixed ventilatory responses, can result in hypercapnia and respiratory failure.[21]

The hypoxic ventilatory response seen in normal subjects can be suppressed by clinical semi-starvation within 10 days by caloric restriction to 500 calories/day, a level frequently seen among hospitalized patients whose only source of nutrition is 2 to 3 liters of intravenous D_5 with electrolytes.[24] Suppression of the hypoxic ventilatory response is associated with significant decrease in basal energy expenditure and is reversible with refeeding. The respiratory effects of amino acid infusions in normal persons subjected to semi-starvation for 1 week have also been examined and shown to alter respiratory chemosensitivity and minute ventilation in the semi-starved state.[82]

Clinical malnutrition may have profound effects upon host-defense in the pulmonary-comprised patient, including cell-mediated and humoral mechanisms in general.[84]

A parallel may exist between the normal response to starvation, including weight loss, decreased oxygen consumption, and decreased lean body mass, and the weight loss seen in COPD patients. However, COPD patients have been shown to have increased basal energy expenditure over that predicted for height, weight, and age and appear to have increased oxygen consumption, which may be related to loss of diaphragmatic excursion and decrease in muscle efficiency. It is postulated that the greater energy requirements necessitated by loss of respiratory muscle efficiency in emphysematous patients may predispose to relatively greater weight loss with caloric restriction.[84]

A careful nutritional assessment of the chronic pulmonary patient should identify patients of moderate to high nutritional risk, and, hopefully, identify those factors contributing to their nutritional impairment. Recommendations include an initial dietary prescription, based upon determination of energy needs and adjusted upward or downward according to whether the patient needs to gain, maintain, or lose weight. A diet composed of 60% carbohydrates, 12% to 15% protein, and the remainder fats has been recommended.[56]

In patients experiencing undue fatigue or dyspnea during meals, it may be useful to perform ear oximetry to titrate oxygen needs during eating and provide supplemental oxygen by nasal cannula if indicated. Activity schedules should be coordinated to allow rest periods before and after meals, and breathing treatments (including postural drainage) should be performed 1 hour prior to meals. If postprandial loading or distention is a problem, multiple small feedings may be preferable to three large meals and patients should be encouraged to review their menus to avoid gas-producing foods altogether or limit their intake to tolerable levels. In some cases, sodium restriction may be desirable and patients should be counseled on foods high in sodium. In addition, any suggestions of ways to allow sodium restriction, yet enhance palatability of foods, may be helpful and encouraging to the patient. Patients on chronic steroids may be susceptible to osteoporosis and will benefit from calcium supplementation or high-calcium foods containing milk or milk products. Information concerning excellent sources of calcium can readily be provided by a dietary consultant.

Psychosocial Issues

Space limitations preclude an adequate discussion of the variety of functions and services provided by psychology and social service health professionals that are a necessary part of any pulmonary rehabilitation team approach. Formal neuropsychological testing may elucidate cognitive and emotional dysfunctions contributing to impairment or disability (an association between chronic hypoxemia of COPD and organic brain dysfunction has been made).[52] Psychological and social counseling are invaluable adjuncts, which need to be provided to patients and families confronted with a chronic and progressive disability and should cover issues of dependency, changing social roles, coping with physical distress, sexuality, and perspectives on death and dying. Furthermore, as increasing emphasis continues to be placed on cost containment at all levels of health care delivery, social service planning and coordination of activities are essential to ensure that patients have access to equitable resources in terms of home equipment, support services, and follow-up as needed. Several excellent texts have addressed these topics in considerable detail.[33, 54, 57]

REFERENCES

1. Askanazi J, Rosenbaum S, Human A et al: Respiratory changes induced by the large glucose loads of total parenteral nutrition. JAMA 243:1444–1447, 1980
2. Astrand P, Rodahl K: Textbook of Work Physiology: Physiological Bases of Exercise, 2nd ed. New York, McGraw-Hill, 1977
3. Aubier M, Trippenbach T, Roussos C: Respiratory muscle fatigue during cardiogenic shock. J Appl Physiol 51:499–508, 1981
4. Barach A, Petty T: Is chronic obstructive lung disease improved by physical exercise? JAMA 234:854–855, 1975
5. Bell C, Kass I, Hodgkin J: Exercise conditioning. In Hodgkin E, Zorn E, Connors G (eds): Pulmonary Rehabilitation Guidelines to Success. Boston, Butterworth & Co, 1984
6. Belman M, Kendregan B: Exercise training fails to increase skeletal muscle enzymes in patients with chronic obstructive pulmonary disease. Am Rev Resp Dis 123:256–261, 1981
7. Belman M, Mittman C: Ventilatory muscle training improves exercise capacity in chronic obstructive pulmonary disease patients. Am Rev Resp Dis 121:273–280, 1980
8. Belman M, Wasserman K: Exercise training and testing in patients with chronic obstructive pulmonary disease. Basics of RD. Am Thoracic Soc 10:1–6, 1981
9. Bergofsky E: Respiratory failure in disorders of the thoracic cage. Am Rev Resp Dis 119:643–668, 1979
10. Bistrian B, Blackburn G: Prevalence of malnutrition in general medical patients. JAMA 235:1567–1570, 1976
11. Bradley B, Garner A, Belleu D et al: Oxygen-assisted exercise in chronic obstructive lung disease. Am Rev Resp Dis 118:239–245, 1978
12. Brown S, Casciarri R, Light R: Arterial oxygen desaturation during meals in patients with severe chronic obstructive pulmonary disease. South Med J 76:194–198, 1983
13. Brundin A: Physical training in severe chronic obstructive lung disease. Scand J Resp Dis 55:25–36, 1974
14. Burrows B: Course and prognosis in advanced disease. In Petty T (ed): Chronic Obstructive Pulmonary Disease, 2nd ed. New York, Marion Dekker, 1985
15. Centers for Disease Control: Update: Pneumococcal polysaccharide vaccine usage—United States. Ann Intern Med 101:348–350, 1984
16. Centers for Disease Control: Recommendations for the prevention and control of influenza. Ann Intern Med 105:399–404, 1986
17. Cherniak R, Svanhill E: Long-term use of intermittent positive pressure breathing (IPPB) in chronic obstructive pulmonary disease. Am Rev Resp Dis 113:721–728, 1976
18. Chester E, Belman M, Bahler R et al: Multidisciplinary treatment of chronic pulmonary insufficiency. 3. The effect of physical training on cardiopulmonary performance in patients with chronic obstructive pulmonary disease. Chest 72:695–702, 1977
19. Christopher K, Spofford B, Branmin P et al: Transtracheal oxygen therapy for refractory hypoxemia. JAMA 256:494–497, 1986
20. Collier C, Dail C, Affeldt J: Mechanics of glossopharyngeal breathing. J Appl Physiol 8:580–584, 1956
21. Covelli M, Waylon-Black J, Osen M et al: Respiratory failure precipitated by high carbohydrate loads. Ann Int Med 95:579-581, 1981
22. Cummings S: Kicking the habit: Benefits and methods of quitting cigarette smoking. West J Med 137:443–447, 1982
23. Deaths due to chronic obstructive pulmonary disease and allied conditions: MMWR 35:507–510, 1986
24. Doekel R, Zwillich C, Scoggin C et al: Clinical semi-starvation. Depression of hypoxic ventilatory response. N Engl J Med 295:358–361, 1976
25. Driver A, McAlevy M, Smith V: Nutritional assessment of patients with chronic obstructive pulmonary disease and acute respiratory failure. Chest 82:568–571, 1982
26. Falliers C, Tinkelman D: Alternative drug therapy for asthma. Clin Chest Med 7:383–392, 1986
27. Feldman S, Crawley B: Tracheostomy and Artificial Ventilation in the Treatment of Respiratory Failure, 3rd ed. Baltimore, Williams & Wilkins, 1977
28. Fielding J: Smoking: Health effects and control. N Engl J Med 313:491–498, 555–561, 1985
29. Fishman A: Chronic cor pulmonale. Am Rev Resp Dis 114:775–794, 1976
30. Fishman D, Petty T: Physical, symptomatic and psychological improvement in patients receiving comprehensive care for chronic airway obstruction. J Chron Dis 24:775–785, 1971
31. Hill N: Clinical applications of body ventilators. Chest 90:897–905, 1986
32. Hodgkin J, Farrell M, Gibson S et al: Pulmonary rehabilitation. Official ATS statement. Am Rev Resp Dis 124:663–666, 1981
33. Hodgkin J, Zorn E, Connors G: Pulmonary Rehabilitation. Guidelines to Success. Boston, Butterworth & Co, 1984
34. Hughes J, Hatsukami D, Pickens R et al: Effect of nicotine on the tobacco withdrawal syndrome. Psychopharm 83:82–87, 1984
35. Hughes J, Miller S: Nicotine gum to help stop smoking. JAMA 252:2855–2858, 1984
36. Hunter A, Carre M, Larsh N: The nutritional status of patients with chronic obstructive pulmonary disease. Am Rev Resp Dis 124:376–381, 1986
37. Inkley S, Oldenburg F, Vignos P: Pulmonary function in Duchenne muscular dystrophy related to stage of disease. Am J Med 56:297–306, 1974
38. Janoff A: Biochemical links between cigarette smoking and pulmonary emphysema. J Appl Physiol 55:285–293, 1983
39. Kory R, Callandar R, Baron N et al: The Veterans Administration–Army Cooperative Study of pulmonary function. I. Clinical spirometry in normal men. Am J Med 30:243–258, 1961
40. Leggett R, Flenley D: Portable oxygen and exercises tolerance in patients with chronic hypoxic cor pulmonale. Br Med J 2:84–86, 1977
41. Lertzman M, Cherniack R: Rehabilitation of patients with chronic obstructive pulmonary disease. Am Rev Resp Dis 113:1145–1168, 1976
42. Mathewson H: Respiratory Therapy in Critical Care. St Louis, CV Mosby, 1976
43. McGavin C, Gupta S, McHardy G: Twelve-minute walking tests for assessing disability in chronic bronchitis. Br Med J 1:822–823, 1976
44. McMichan J, Michel L, Westbrook P: Pulmonary dysfunction following traumatic quadriplegia. JAMA 243:528–531, 1980
45. McPherson S: Respiratory Therapy Equipment. St Louis, CV Mosby, 1981
46. Miech R, Stein M: Methylxanthines. Clin Chest Med 7:331–340, 1986
47. Morgan W: Pulmonary disability and impairment: Can't work? Won't work? Basics of RD, Am Thoracic Soc 10:1–5, 1982
48. Morgan W, Seaton A: Occupational Lung Disease, 2nd ed. Philadelphia, WB Saunders, 1984
49. Moser K, Bokinsky G, Savage R et al: Results of a comprehensive rehabilitation program. Physiologic and functional effects on pa-

tients with chronic obstructive pulmonary disease. Arch Intern Med 140:1596–1601, 1980

50. Motley M: The effects of slow deep breathing on the blood gas exchange in emphysema. Am Rev Resp Dis 88:484–492, 1963

51. Mueller R, Petty T, Filley G: Ventilation and arterial blood gas changes induced by pursed lips breathing. J Resp Dis 124:376–381, 1970

52. Nocturnal Oxygen Therapy Trial Group: Continuous or nocturnal oxygen therapy in hypoxemic chronic obstructive lung disease. Ann Intern Med 93:391–398, 1980

53. Oppenbrief D, Irwin M, Rogers R et al: Nutritional status and lung function in patients with emphysema and chronic bronchitis. Chest 83:17–22, 1983

54. O'Ryan J, Burns D: Pulmonary Rehabilitation. From Hospital to Home. Chicago, Year Book Medical Publishers, 1984

55. Paez P, Phillipson E, Masangkay M et al: The physiologic basis of training patients with emphysema. Am Rev Resp Dis 95:944–953, 1967

56. Peters J, Burke K, White D: Nutrition and the pulmonary patient. In Hodgkin J, Zorn E, Connors G (eds): Pulmonary Rehabilitation Guidelines to Success. Boston, Butterworth & Co, 1984

57. Petty T; Pulmonary rehabilitation. In Petty T (ed): Chronic Obstructive Pulmonary Disease, 2nd ed. New York, Marion Dekker, 1985

58. Petty T, Neff T, Creagh C et al: Outpatient oxygen therapy in chronic obstructive pulmonary disease. Arch Intern Med 139:23–32, 1979

59. Petty T, Nett L, Finigan N et al: A comprehensive care program for chronic airway obstruction (methods and preliminary evaluation of symptomatic and functional improvement). Ann Intern Med 70:1109–1120, 1969

60. Pineda H, Haas F, Axen K: Treadmill exercise training in chronic obstructive pulmonary disease. Arch Phys Med Rehab 67:155–158, 1986

61. Pineda H, Haas F, Axen K et al: Accuracy of pulmonary function tests in predicting exercise tolerance in chronic obstructive pulmonary disease. Chest 86:564–567, 1984

62. Popa V: Beta-adrenergic drugs. Clin Chest Med 7:313–329, 1986

63. Report of the Surgeon General: Smoking and Health. DHEW Publ (PHS) #79-50066, 1949

64. Roussos C, Grassino A, Macklem P: Inspiratory muscle fatigue and acute respiratory failure. Canad Med Assoc J 122:1375–1377, 1980

65. Russell M, Wilson C, Taylor C et al: Effect of general practitioners' advice against smoking. Br Med J 2:231–235, 1979

66. Sacks F: Chronic bronchitis. Clin Chest Med 2:79–89, 1981

67. Sahin S: Corticosteroids in chronic bronchitis and pulmonary emphysema. Chest 73:389–396, 1978

68. Sahn S, Petty T: Results of a comprehensive rehabilitation program for severe COPD. In Petty T (ed): Chronic Obstructive Pulmonary Disease. New York, Marion Dekker, 1978

69. Shanfield K, Hammond M: Activities of daily living. In Hodgkin J, Zorn E, Connors G (eds): Pulmonary Rehabilitation Guidelines to Success. Boston, Butterworth & Co, 1984

70. Snider G: Clinical Pulmonary Medicine. Boston, Little, Brown & Co, 1981

71. Soria C, Waltman W, Price M: Breathing and pulmonary hygiene techniques. In Hodgkin J, Zorn E, Conners G (eds): Pulmonary Rehabilitation Guidelines to Success. Boston, Butterworth & Co, 1984

72. Stohl K, Cherniack N, Gothe B: Physiologic basis of therapy for sleep apnea. Am Rev Resp Dis 134:791–802, 1986

73. Storms W: Ipratropium bromide (Atrovent): A new anticholinergic bronchodilator for the treatment of asthma. Immunol Allergy Prac 8:32–38, 1986

74. Theodore A, Beer D: Pharmachotherapy of chronic obstructive pullmonary disease. Clin Chest Med 7:657–671, 1986

75. Thompson N, Glassroth J, Snider D et al: The booster phenomenon in serial tuberculin testing. Am Rev Resp Dis 119:587–597, 1979

76. Tockman M, Khoury M, Cohen B: The epidemiology of COPD. In Petty T (ed): Chronic Obstructive Pulmonary Disease, 2nd ed. New York, Marion Dekker, 1985

77. Unger K, Moser K, Hanson P: Selection of an exercise program for patients with chronic obstructive pulmonary disease. Heart Lung 9:68–76, 1980

78. Vanderburg E, Van de Woestigne K, Gyselen A: Weight changes in the terminal stages of chronic obstructive lung disease. Am Rev Resp Dis 96:556–565, 1967

79. Viires N, Aubier M, Musciano D et al: Effects of aminophylline on diaphragmatic fatigue during acute respiratory failure. Am Rev Resp Dis 129:396–402, 1984

80. Wasserman K, Whipp B: Exercise physiology in health and disease. Am Rev Resp Dis 112:219–249, 1975

81. Weinsier R, Hunker E et al: Hospital malnutrition: A prospective evaluation of general medical patients during the course of hospitalization. Am J Clin Nutr 32:418–426, 1979

82. Weissman C, Askanazi J, Rosenbaum S et al: Amino acids and respiration. Ann Intern Med 98:41–44, 1983

83. West J: Respiratory Physiology—The Essentials. Baltimore, Williams & Wilkins, 1974

84. Wilson D, Rogers R, Hoffman R: Nutrition and chronic lung disease. Ann Rev Resp Dis 132:1347–1365, 1985

85. Zement I: Steroids. Clin Chest Med 7:341–354, 1986

86. Zement I, Au J: Anticholinergic agents. Clin Chest Med 7:355–366, 1986

36

Treatment of the Patient With Chronic Pain

Nicolas E. Walsh

Daniel Dumitru

Somayaji Ramamurthy

Lawrence S. Schoenfeld

GENERAL OVERVIEW

Pain is purely subjective, difficult to define, and often difficult to describe or interpret. It is currently defined as an unpleasant sensory and emotional response to a stimulus associated with actual or potential tissue damage.[31, 98] However, pain has never been shown to be a simple function of the amount of physical injury; it is extensively influenced by anxiety, depression, expectation, and other psychological variables. It is a multifaceted experience, an interweaving of the physical characteristics of the stimulus with the motivational, affective, and cognitive functions of the individual. The result is behavior based upon an interpretation of the event, influenced by present and past experiences.

Acute pain is a biological symptom of an apparent nociceptive stimulus, such as tissue damage due to disease or trauma. The pain may be highly localized and may radiate. It is generally sharp and persists only as long as the tissue pathology itself persists. Acute pain is generally self-limiting, and as the nociceptive stimulus lessens, the pain decreases. Acute pain usually lasts less than 3 months.[98] If it is not effectively treated, it may progress to a chronic form.

Chronic pain is a disease process. Differing significantly from acute pain, it is defined as pain lasting longer than the usual course of an acute disease or injury. The pain may be associated with chronic pathology or may persist after recovery from a disease or injury. As with acute pain, treatable chronic pain due to organic disease is managed by effectively treating the underlying disorder. Chronic pain is often poorly localized and tends to be dull, aching, and constant. The associated signs of autonomic nervous system response may be absent, and the patient may appear exhausted, listless, depressed, and withdrawn.

Proper management of pain requires an understanding of its complexity and a knowledge of the non-neurological factors which determine its individual expression. The treatment of pain with physical modalities is as ancient as the history of man, but the use of interdisciplinary rehabilitation techniques has gained acceptance only within the last few decades.

Epidemiology

Nearly everyone experiences acute pain. Its incidence approximates the cumulative total of all acute diseases, trauma, and surgical procedures.

Chronic pain is less frequently experienced, but is reaching epidemic proportions in the United States. There are more than 36 million individuals with arthritis, 70 million with back pain, 20 million with migraine headaches, and additional millions with pain due to gout, myofascial pain syndromes, phantom limb pain, and reflex sympathetic dystrophies.[18] The pain resulting from cancer afflicts approximately 1 million Americans and 20 million individuals worldwide. Moderate to severe pain occurs in about 40% of patients with intermediate stage cancer and in 60% to 80% of patients with advanced cancer.[17, 44, 147] Back pain, as a general condition, episodically affects nearly 75% of the population in most industrial nations. It is estimated that at least 10% to 15% of the working population of industrial nations are affected by back pain each year.[138]

In studies of the general population, patients have identified the head and lower extremities as the most common sites of acute pain and have identified the back as the most common site of chronic pain (Fig. 36-1).[30]

Etiology

Chronic pain is not merely a physical sensation. In the affective component of chronic pain, most patients show a degree of depression resulting from anger, jealousy, and anxiety. For many individuals depression is the primary factor in the perception or experience of pain. Fifty percent to 70% of chronic pain patients have either a primary depression or a depression secondary to their pain syndrome. Chronic pain, with accompanying depression, often leads to extensive periods of down time and prolonged inactivity.[22] Prolonged immobility and inactivity alter cardiovascular function, impair musculoskeletal flexibility, and cause abnormal joint function.[21, 53, 111] Prevention involves the encouragement of patient activity as soon as it is reasonable.

The motivational component is concerned with the vocational, economic, and interpersonal reinforcement contingencies that contribute to the learning of pain behavior and the maintenance of chronic pain. Over 75% of chronic pain patients display behavioral characteristics, which include difficulties with job or housework, leisure activities, sexual function, and vocational endeavors.[133] The patient may also have significant functional limitations due to multiple previous surgeries with little success and prolonged convalescence, disuse/physical deconditioning syndrome, or narcotic medication.[56]

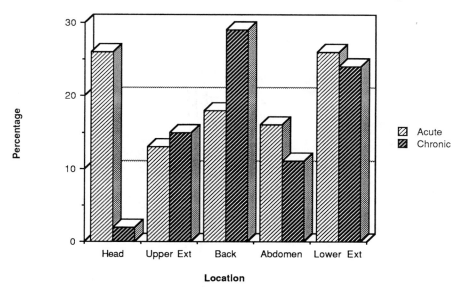

Figure 36-1. The back is the most common site of chronic pain; acute pain is most often located in the head or lower extremities.

The cognitive component is involved with how patients think and the part that pain plays in their belief systems and views of self. The more the patient views pain as a signal, which mandates a reduction of activity and protection of the affected part, the more difficult it is for the physician to achieve compliance with exercise, stretching, and other elements of the treatment program. Viewing pain as a result of sensory input, affective state, cognition, and motivation requires a multidimensional evaluation process with treatment interventions directed at those components most responsible for the pain experience.

Pain Pathways

Pain is a central perception of multiple primary sensory modalities. This interpretive function is complex, involving psychological, neuroanatomical, neurochemical, and neurophysiological factors of both the pain stimulus and the memory of past pain experiences. The peripheral mechanisms for sensing and modulating pain have been extensively studied during the past 20 years. The pathways for pain sensation from the initial stimulus of the nociceptors to the central nervous system is summarized in Figure 36-2.[12, 35, 122] There appear to be several descending systems which play a role in control of the modification of the ascending pain pathways, which are summarized in Figure 36-3.[7, 78, 84, 134]

Polynodal nociceptors respond to stimuli that damage tissue. This stimulation results in impulses ascending in the A-delta or C fibers to the marginal layers of the dorsal horn of the spinal cord. The A-delta fibers primarily synapse in laminae I and V, whereas C fibers synapse primarily in laminae II. Deeper regions of the dorsal horn may be polysynaptically involved in the processing of noxious stimuli.

The major ascending nociceptive pathways are the spinothalamic and spinoreticular tracts. The ascending pain pathways involve both oligosynaptic and polysynaptic neurons. The oligosynaptic pathways are fast conducting with discrete somatotopic organization resulting in rapid transmission of nociceptive information regarding site, intensity, and duration of stimulus. The oligosynaptic tracts provide somatic information by way of the posterior ventral nuclei of the thalamus to the post central cortex. The sensory discriminatory characteristics are delineated from the neospinothalamic portion of the lateral spinothalamic tract and the nonproprioceptive portion of the dorsal columns.

Polysynaptic pathways are slow conducting with a lack of somatotopic organization resulting in poor localization, dull aching, and burning sensations. The nociceptive impulses transmitted through this system result in suprasegmental reflex responses related to ventilation, circulation, and endocrine function. Pathways contributing to this slow conducting system are the paleospinothalamic tract, spinoreticular tract, spinocollicular tract, and the dorsal intercornual tract, as well as the spinomesencephalic tract. The polysynaptic tracts form the brain stem reticular activating system with projections to the medial and interlaminar nuclei of the thalamus. From these nuclei diffuse radiation occurs to the cerebral cortex, limbic system, and basal ganglia.

There are multiple levels of processing and convergence of nociceptive information in its ascending transmission to the cerebral cortex. In addition, there appear to be several descending pain control systems which play a role in the control and modification of the ascending pain pathways. The most complete studies have been of the periaqueductal gray region of the midbrain (PAG). Stimulation of the PAG neurons and the subsequent descending impulses result in release of endogenous opioids at the nucleus raphe magnus (NRM) and nucleus locus ceruleus (NLC). Endogenous opioids activate the serotoinergic cells in the NRM and norepinergic neurons in the NLC. The axons of both of these monoaminergic neurons descend in the dorsolateral tract to interneurons, predominately in laminae I, II, and V. These monoamines activate opioid-secreting interneurons. The morphine-like transmitter released may vary, depending on what type of receptor in the periphery has been activated. Both A-delta and C afferent fibers are inhibited by descending influences in the dorsal horn. These opioid inhibitory interneurons may be influenced by innersegmental and descending pathways, but the innersegmental and segmental mechanisms have not been established. These interneurons may function either by presynaptic inhibition on the terminals with the primary nociceptive afferents preventing the release of substance P, or by postsynaptic inhibition on second order neurons. Cells in the raphe magnus are activated by ascending sensory pathways transmitted to the reticular formation as well as by descending input from cells in the periaqueductal gray region.

Other descending monoamine systems include locus ceruleus to the dorsal horn; interneurons, nucleus reticularis, magnicellularis to the dorsal horn interneurons; and the mesencephalic lateral reticular formation to the dorsal horn inter-

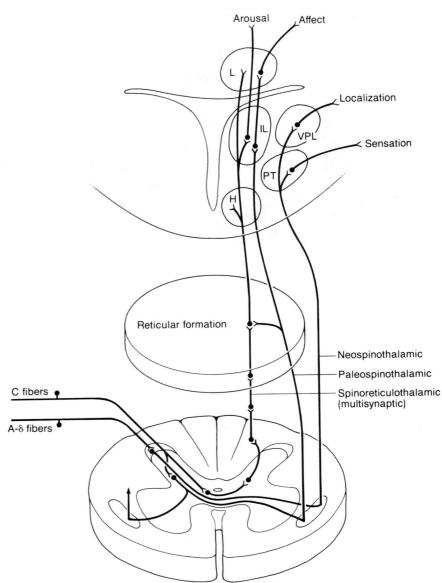

Figure 36-2. Ascending pathways for pain sensation, from nociceptors to central nervous system (L, Limbic System; IL, Intralaminar Thalamic Nuclei; VPL, Ventral Posterolateral Thalamic Nuclei; PT, Posterior Thalamic Nuclei; H, Hypothalamus).

neurons. It has been suggested that monoamines are involved with supraspinal and spinal nociceptive mechanisms. Hormonally based descending pathways have been described but are poorly understood.

Resolution of Pain

Acute pain is frequently the result of tissue damage in which the initial pain leads to an increase in anxiety, which magnifies the pain experience. The amount of anxiety generated (and pain) seems to be more influenced by the setting in which the pain develops than by personality variables. With the healing process comes a reduction or termination of the anxiety and acute pain perception. When acute pain, which functions as a warning signal, fails to respond to treatment with conventional medical therapies, illness behavior and chronic pain develops. The anxiety characteristic of acute pain is replaced by hopelessness, helplessness, and despair. When pain relief fails, physical activities decrease and suffering and depression increase.

Acute pain usually resolves when the source of nociperception is removed or cured. Acute pain, by definition, resolves

quickly and is often readily treated by a single modality. The cause of acute pain can be documented by the findings on physical examination and diagnostic procedures. When indicated, appropriate operative intervention can be carried out on the basis of these findings. A short course of analgesic medication usually controls postoperative pain and a return to full painless function can be anticipated in a matter of weeks. Acute pain control requires the administration of an efficacious analgesic dosage. Too little analgesia promotes suffering and anxiety, thus defeating the purpose of prescribing medication, but fear of drug addiction contributes to the under-utilization of analgesic medication, and physicians tend to under-medicate in terms of frequency and dosage of pain medications.[64, 124] By prescribing low oral doses of narcotics at infrequent intervals, physicians inadvertently force patients to adopt pain behavior in order to obtain adequate narcotic analgesia. Pain behavior is characterized by high verbalization of pain, decreased activities of daily living, high demand for medication, dependency, and the inability to work. Addiction in the acute pain situation is extraordinarily rare, probably less than 0.1%.[3, 143]

Unfortunately a significant minority of acute pain patients

set a reasonable time frame for the resolution of the acute pain process. Patients should be advised when the pain medication will no longer be needed. The patient's attention should be directed to a gradual return of full activity on a prescribed schedule. Follow-up appointments should be planned at specified intervals so the patient does not need to justify a visit.

Pain Reinforcing Factors

Chronic pain syndrome is a learned behavior pattern reinforced by multiple factors. These behaviors are frequently found in individuals who are depressed and inactive, and who lack the skills or opportunity to compete in the community. It is these environmental factors which promote pain behavior, regardless of the etiology of the pain that distinguishes the chronic pain patient from the population at large. Patients often develop a new self-image and see themselves as disabled by their pain. This self-perceived disability justifies their inactivity, their manipulation of others, and their attempts to collect compensation from society. The typical patient has often been unemployed or on sick leave for long periods of time. Our data indicate that individuals who have been removed from the labor market due to pain for less than 6 months have a 90% chance of returning to full employment; those removed from the labor force due to pain for more than 1 year have less than a 10% chance of returning.

Individuals with chronic pain syndrome receive gains from their pain behavior, hence they foster it to maintain those positive reinforcers. Physicians reinforce the pain behaviors by lacking knowledge of this chronic disease process, failing to identify the chronic pain behavior, and prolonging prescription of inappropriate medications. The physician's failure to acknowledge and direct the patient toward recovery tends to validate the chronic pain syndrome by providing an undiagnosable and untreatable problem. Family members also tend to reinforce the chronic pain behavior. They allow the individual to become inactive and cater to the patient's requests and needs over prolonged periods of time. In some instances, chronic pain patients provide role models for pain or disability behavior for other family members.[46, 47]

WORKERS COMPENSATION. In 1911, Workers Compensation laws were enacted in the United States, which required employers to assume the cost of occupational disability without regard to fault. These laws have dramatically influenced the recovery from injury. In many instances they have become counterproductive; financial compensation may discourage return to work, the appeal process may increase disability, an open claim may inhibit return to work, and recovering patients may be unable to return to work. Often the accident and the resulting symptoms represent the patient's solution to life's problems.[10]

LITIGATION. Disability, along with pain and suffering, greatly determines the amount of compensation awarded in workers compensation cases. The patient/client's pain behavior may be reinforced, maximized, and groomed with the hope of a large cash settlement. As a result of this reinforcement, the pain behavior develops into a learned response. The pain also becomes the disability for which the patient/client is seeking compensation. Therefore, a learned behavior becomes a determining factor in the amount of compensation awarded.[9]

Alteration of the disability laws could decrease the number of acute pain patients who develop the behavioral disease of chronic pain syndrome. Changes that might discourage the development of chronic pain include allowing an injured worker to continue working at a job he or she is physically able to accomplish during the recuperation period, rapid adjudication of dis-

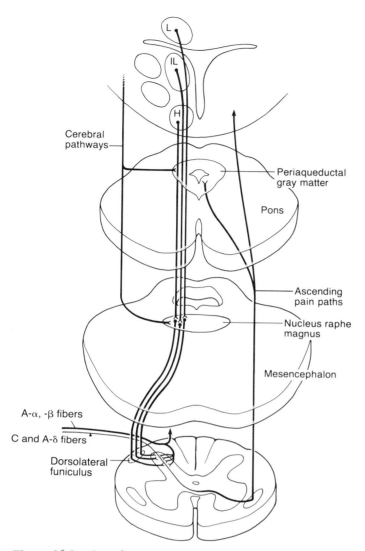

Figure 36-3. Central nervous system structures that modify ascending pain pathways (L, Limbic System; IL, Intralaminar Thalamic Nuclei; H, Hypothalamus).

continue to experience pain, which may progress into a more complex disease entity. Pain, a symptom of physiological malfunction, now becomes the disease itself. Chronic pain represents a complex interaction of physical, psychological, and social factors in which the pain complaint is a socially acceptable manifestation of the disease. The etiology of chronic pain may be persistent nociceptive input, such as arthritis or terminal cancer; psychological disorders, such as anxiety, depression, and learned behavior; or social factors, such as job loss, divorce, and secondary gain.

The optimal treatment for chronic pain is prevention. Once the disease state of chronic pain commences, reinforcers such as monetary compensation, absence of job-related problems, manipulation of the environment to satisfy unmet needs, and retirement from the competitive world obstruct resolution of the disease. Therapies designed for acute pain are often contraindicated for chronic pain.

Prevention of chronic pain requires identifying contributing factors and resolving them early in the acute stage. Aspects worthy of attention include psychological stress, drug or alcohol abuse, and poor posture or muscle tone, as well as significant psychological and operant pain mechanisms. Physicians should

ability and compensation claims, and physicians restricting the patient's use of addicting and depressant medication to less than 1 month. The extensive use of conservative intervention to include physical therapy and stress management early in treatment could also prevent the emergence of chronic pain syndrome.[123, 140]

Complications of Chronic Pain

Chronic pain is an elusive disease complicated by iatrogenic, idiopathic, and psychosocial factors. These complications encompass physical, psychological, and environmental issues.

PHYSICAL. The chronic pain patient often develops secondary pain loci due to inactivity. Decreased range of motion, myofascial pain, and weakness due to disuse may also develop.[137]

Medically induced drug addiction and dependence are particularly serious problems for both chronic pain patients and their physicians.[110, 139] It has been estimated that 30% to 50% of chronic non-malignant pain patients have a significant drug dependency problem.[59, 68] Substance abuse, dependence, and addiction are negative prognostic factors in outcome studies.[89] Treatment of the drug impairment is essential and results in a greater overall improvement in functioning.[41]

PSYCHOLOGICAL. Depression is a common complication noted with chronic pain.[45] These patients often manipulate family, friends, and co-workers to achieve secondary gain. Chronic pain causes considerable distress to spouses and family members;[119] sexual dysfunctions[67] are common. Twenty-five percent of spouses report clinical depression, and over 35% rate their marriage as maladjusted.[1]

ENVIRONMENTAL. Nearly one-third of the American population has persistent or recurrent chronic pain. One-half to two-thirds of these individuals are partly or totally disabled for varying lengths of time. Bonica estimates $70 billion a year is spent on medical needs, lost working days, and compensation.[148] Data compiled in 1982 suggest that lost wages and social support systems cost the taxpayer between $15,000 and $24,000 per chronic pain patient per year.[20]

Current Theories of Pain

Gate Control Theory

The gate control theory of pain was developed by Melzack and Wall to account for mechanisms by which other cutaneous stimuli and emotional states alter the level of pain.[94] They suggested that within the substantia gelatinosa of the dorsal horn there are interneurons that presynaptically inhibit transmission of nociceptive information to the ascending tracts. These interneurons are activated by large-diameter afferents and inhibited by small-diameter afferents. In addition, they suggested that the brain exerted descending control on this system, relying on the fact that cognitive factors are known to influence pain behavior.

Several studies have failed to provide support for the gate control theory. It remains significant, although incorrect in detail. The gate control theory of pain has altered the concept of pain as solely an afferent sensory experience, broadening the concept to include the affective and motivational factors involved in the human pain experience.[71] The gate control theory has been modified extensively during the past 20 years. It still represents the first attempt to describe a pain modulating system that responds to input by noxious stimuli, innocuous afferent impulses, and descending control.

Biochemical Theory

The biochemical theory of pain has evolved since the discovery of the endorphins. The endogenous opioid system consists of three families of opioid peptides: beta endorphin, enkephalin, and dynorphin/neoendorphin. The beta endorphins are primarily concentrated in the pituitary and the basal hypothalamus. The other endogenous opioids are distributed extensively in the central nervous system. The dynorphins/neoendorphins, and enkephalins are found in the caudate nucleus, amygdala, periaqueductal gray, locus ceruleus, and dorsal horn of the spinal cord. In addition, the enkephalins are found in the nucleus raphe magnus and the thalamic periventricular nuclei. The dynorphins/neoendorphins are found in the hypothalamus and substantia nigra.[7]

The endogenous opioids are involved in analgesia, as well as multiple other clinical events. There are at least seven different opiate receptors, of which the mu, delta, and kappa appear to be involved in analgesia.[130] The others are associated with such functions as respiration, appetite, hallucinations, dysphoria, immune function, temperature regulation, memory, and blood pressure control. The beta endorphins may function in the modulation of local blood flow and immune function.[102] The discovery of multiple opiate receptors and multiple endogenous opioid compounds provides an explanation for the multiple effects of the endogenous opioids. Within the peripheral and central nervous system the enkephalins act as neurotransmitters and the beta endorphin acts predominately as a hormone. Endogenous opioids are only one part of a complex modulatory system involved in the collating, processing, and filtering of information concerning tissue damage.[150] Other possible neural peptides having analgesia or antinociceptive properties are calcitonin, cholecystokinin, somatostatin, and neurotensin.[102, 131]

Chronic Pain Theory

The chronic pain theory encompasses many of the physical, motivational, cognitive, and affective components of pain. The anatomical pain pathways are relatively clear and represent a mechanism for nociceptive pain in the animal model. Multiple pain mechanisms exist in the human model due to the complex integration of nociceptive stimuli, conceptual and judgmental factors, sociocultural influences, and the motivational and emotional states of the individual. Pain mechanisms include nociceptive pain, central pain, psychogenic, and operant pain. The human perception and reaction to pain are a blending of these mechanisms. The nociceptive pain mechanism is detailed in the pain pathways, as previously described, and represents pain originating from tissue damage such as pain from cancer, degenerative joint disease, myofascial pain, and trauma. Central pain originates from denervation occurring after a cerebral vascular accident, spinal cord injury, or amputation. This pain may be due to a loss of the peripheral modulating influences on the central nervous system resulting in an unmodulated activity of afferent A-delta and C fibers.

Psychosis is the interpretation of emotional distress as aversive and unpleasant sensation and its description in terms of pain language and behavior. The psychological states that are interpreted in this manner include anxiety, neurosis, hysteria, and depression. This mechanism of pain is often overlooked in chronic pain patients. Operant or learned pain behavior is often a major factor in chronic pain. Although the initial precipitating event causing the pain may be quite minor, the pain behavior is often long-lasting, owing to reinforcement by environmental influences. Pain behavior may be directly reinforced by family and physician attention, or the delivery of medication. Indirect reinforcement (physical or psychological demands) occurs with avoidance of aversive consequences, which would have to be met if there were no pain. Operant pain behavior is also reinforced through a punishment cycle, when an injured party is over-protected and "punished" if he or she begins to function more independently.

Diagnostic and Clinical Evaluation

Physical Examination

In establishing the etiology of pain it is essential to consider its characteristics, its chronology, the limitations it imposes on the patient, and the results of previous therapy. This is accomplished by a thorough pain evaluation including a detailed history, a comprehensive physical examination, and appropriate tests. Most pain patients present a complex array of physical, motivational, cognitive, and affective manifestations and therefore require detailed psychological and social evaluations.

A detailed history of the pain complaint identifies the pain in terms of its location of origin, radiation, quality, severity, and time intensity attributes, mode of onset, duration, time of occurrence, and factors that aggravate and relieve it. Previous treatments for pain should be noted, including comments regarding usefulness in the reduction of pain. Medications currently being taken, as well as those used in the past, should be recorded, along with the patient's perceptions as to the results achieved by each. The details of physical therapy, including types of modalities, exercise, and effective regimes, should be recorded. An inquiry as to the patient's attempts at biofeedback, relaxation, and hypnopsis are also helpful. Information regarding associated findings including sensory deficits, muscle weakness, and altered body function should be obtained. It should be determined if compensation is involved, if the patient is working, and if not, the employment history. The physical examination and related diagnostic studies should be directed toward evaluating the site of pain and related regions. This process is useful in acquiring objective data to substantiate the clinical history.

Physical examination begins when the patient is first seen and continues through every contact made with the patient. This provides the opportunity for the physician to evaluate how the pain affects motion and activities. Physical examination always includes examination of related components of the spine, musculoskeletal system, and neurological evaluations. Painful regions need to be compared with normal areas on the contralateral side of the patient for sensation, temperature, and sensitivity to palpation.

Functional evaluation measures the appropriateness of the patient's functional capabilities for the level of impairment. Objective, quantitative measurements give a baseline with which to evaluate progress and long-term outcome.

Diagnostic Procedures

LABORATORY TESTS. Laboratory findings in acute and chronic pain usually have no features distinct from those found with a primary disease. Drug screening tests of the blood and urine may provide valuable information as to the variety and type of pain medications being ingested. Serum drug level testing provides data to determine the bioavailability of medications being taken by the patient.

RADIOGRAPHY. Radiographic procedures are extensively used in the evaluation of pain. Spinal radiography has minimal value in the evaluation of most low back pain conditions because of the equal prevalence of abnormalities in symptomatic and asymptomatic populations, that is, low specificity and predictive value.[49, 63] In a specific diagnosis of low back pain in sciatica due to herniated nucleus pulposus, plain radiography has been shown to have no value.[121, 136]

The x-ray and computed tomography (CT) scan demonstrate anatomical or structural disorders, which account for a low percentage of functional abnormalities. However, CT scanning and myelography are well established in the diagnosis of disk herniation, with 24% to 50% of asymptomatic individuals showing abnormalities on myelography,[61] discography[62] and CT scan.[153] The clinical usage of diagnostic tests requires a careful correlation between clinical signs, symptoms, and test results.

PSYCHOLOGICAL EVALUATION. The assessment of psychological issues in the overall evaluation and treatment of chronic pain patients is an important component of any pain management program.[33] Psychological evaluation often involves the use of questionnaires, inventories, and the clinical interview. Psychophysical methods of pain assessment[91] (tourniquet test, cold pressor test, and visual analogue scales) often augments the psychological evaluation.

The *McGill Pain Questionnaire*[25] is an often-used instrument designed to measure three dimensions of the pain experience: sensory, affective, and evaluative. The *Minnesota Multiphasic Personality Inventory (MMPI)* has been used in the United States perhaps more than any other psychological instrument in the assessment of personality factors contributing to the experience of chronic pain.[45] The typical *MMPI* profile for a chronic pain patient denotes increased levels of hypochondriasis, depression, and hysteria. The clinical interview helps to identify the affective, motivational, cognitive, and personality components of the chronic pain patient. The emphasis of this evaluation is on the patient's behavioral response to pain, adjustments to impairment/disability, primary/secondary gain, and motivation.

ELECTRODIAGNOSIS. Electrodiagnosis is an objective neurophysiological extension of the physical examination. It typically includes the determination of nerve conduction velocities (NCV) and needle electromyographic studies (EMG) of individual muscles. In addition, a relatively new technique known as somatosensory evoked potentials (SSEP) has expanded the armamentarium of the electromyographer.[2, 73, 118]

Electromyography and evoked potential studies demonstrate the pathophysiological changes associated with or due to structural abnormalities. The documentation of existing pathology is vitally important to the comprehensive management of complex painful conditions.[105] Careful clinical correlation is essential when interpreting all tests related to chronic pain.

ANESTHETIC PROCEDURES. The subsequent response of the body and mind to pain results in sympathetic nervous system and psychogenic responses. Although clinical examination and appropriate investigations can help in delineating the contribution of the various mechanisms in an individual patient, many patients do not exhibit clearcut mechanisms of pain. In these patients differential diagnostic blocks may be valuable. Clinicians employing the differential blocks are frequently impressed by their usefulness in pointing to mechanisms not suspected when considering the results of previous clinical examinations and laboratory workup.[16, 113, 115]

Thiobarbiturates such as Pentothal and thiamylal are useful in differentiating the patients who have somatic pain from those who have psychogenic or malingering pain.[115, 129]

THERMOGRAPHY. Thermography is a new and controversial method of evaluating pain. This procedure uses measurements of infrared radiation from the body for diagnostic purposes. The infrared energy emissions from one area of the skin, representing skin temperature, are recorded for comparison with patterns from adjacent skin areas. Thermal patterns that are bilaterally symmetrical are considered normal.

Thermography is based on the hypothesis that localized irritation of sympathetic nerves results in sympathetic nervous system stimulation. The increased output of the autonomic nervous system constricts the small arterioles in the skin, producing diminished temperature in the area that the sympathetic nerves innervate. The nerve topography of the vessels in the sympathetic chain are different from those of the somatasensory nervous system.[55] Thermography is reported to provide objective evidence of physiological dysfunction in pain patients.[24] However, it has not yet been shown to be a valid assessment of pain other than of that due to neurovascular compression syndromes and autonomic nervous system etiology.

The diagnostic reliability of thermography is still unknown. The studies to date have failed to use a carefully selected control population, or the observers were not blinded and, therefore, were subject to observer bias. In the absence of carefully controlled experiments with a large sample size, the accuracy of thermography in the diagnosis of the evaluation of back pain, spinal lesions, and similar pain syndromes is still speculative.[5, 34, 86, 100]

CLINICAL MANAGEMENT

The primary goals of treating a patient with pain are alleviating the pain and enhancing the patient's quality of life and functional capabilities. The management of acute pain is based on pharmacological, psychological, medical, and surgical innovations or advancements within the past century. And yet, the management of chronic pain has been recognized as a major health care problem only in the last 25 years. It remains unclear why some people become chronic pain patients and others resolve their acute pain without significant difficulty.

Multidisciplinary Approach

The chronic pain problem is multifaceted. No single physician has the resources to care comprehensively for the complex psychological, social, legal, medical, and physical problems involved in chronic pain. Therefore, the multidisciplinary team approach is necessary. Using an interdisciplinary approach does not mean the patient is referred from one specialist to another, as this tends to result in conflicting and overlapping treatment and a loss of hope of treatment in the patient. Ideally, the team should work together to provide a unified explanation of the illness and a comprehensive treatment program. The multidisciplinary pain service has the advantage of offering a variety of coherent treatment approaches to the patient. This type of program recognizes that a multifaceted problem requires a multifaceted approach, as well as continuity of care in which the patient is an active participant.[15]

The core group for the multidisciplinary treatment service includes a physiatrist, an anesthesiologist, and a clinical psychologist or psychiatrist. This group may vary considerably according to local needs, resources, and available expertise. However, the team must have the knowledge to manage the psychological and social problems with optimal medical and anesthetic treatments. They must also have a thorough understanding of physical treatments and the rehabilitation process.

The multidisciplinary pain approach begins with a complete clinical evaluation. Comprehensive medical and psychosocial evaluations with particular emphasis on functional capabilities and behavioral responses to pain are essential. All previous medical records are needed to avoid repeating appropriately performed studies and unsuccessful treatment approaches. This comprehensive clinical evaluation also includes functional capabilities to determine impairment level. The psychosocial evaluation focuses upon the behavioral response to pain, adjustments to the physical impairment, and the degree of motivation. The *MMPI* and other written tests are used for generalized screening.

The multidisciplinary team functions at several levels within the treatment process. They attempt to identify and resolve documentable organic problems when present, and to improve the patient's ability to cope with the pain through medication, psychological intervention, and patient education. In addition, considerable effort is devoted to improving the patient's functional outcome as measured by increased activity time, improved activities of daily living, increased distance walked, and increased tolerance for specific homemaking or vocational activities. To accomplish these objectives the multidisciplinary team must use many skills. In many cases, the chronic pain patient is so entrenched in pain behavior that a behavior modification approach is essential. These patients are often characterized by low levels of activities of daily living, high demand for medication accompanied by physical and psychological dependency, high verbalization of pain, and the inability to work.

Pain Treatment Centers

The organization and operation of the multidisciplinary pain clinic have been discussed by Grabois.[52] Many behavior modification programs use the Fordyce Model.[45, 77] This approach uses the general principles of interruption of the pain behavior reinforcement cycle, reward of healthy behavior, appropriate goals which the patient must achieve, measurement of improvement by functional assessment as well as pain level, and psychosocial adjustment. Particular emphasis is placed on detoxification and medication reduction, pain reduction, increased activity, and modification of pain behavior.

If the patient is on pain medications and determined to be physically or psychologically dependent, he or she must be detoxified. This is routinely done by establishing the equivalent dosage of each medication type (*e.g.,* narcotics, benzodiazepines, barbiturates, alcohol). Narcotic medications are replaced with methadone, and long-acting barbiturates are replaced with phenobarbital or pentobarbital. Medication equivalents are placed in orange juice or in capsulated form and decreased at a rate of 5% to 10% per day. The medication is then given on an around-the-clock basis at fixed intervals. Gradual reduction of the pain ingredients occurs without significant side-effects of withdrawal. The patient is not aware of the timing of the decrease, but has been informed of the concept before starting the program. Nonsteroid anti-inflammatory drugs (NSAIDs) and tricyclic antidepressants are routinely integrated as long-term medications. The pain management program is designed to *reduce* and not eliminate pain, while increasing the patient's functional capabilities.

The patient with chronic pain usually exhibits a decreased activity level, which results in a disuse syndrome. The exercise programs are based on the initial specific and general exercise that the individual can perform. The exercise regimen is progressive, with the goals rising along with the patient's ability. Rewards for accomplishing tasks are a mainstay of this program with no reinforcement given for pain behavior. The achievable goals provide success and confidence and allow for frequent reinforcement when they are met. Cooperation by all staff members is essential; they must consistently ignore pain complaints and encourage improved function. Psychological intervention is used as indicated. The chronic pain behavior modification programs report short-term success rates in medication reduction, increased activity, and more productive behavior patterns. Statistics suggest 60% to 80% improvement in patients with chronic pain without major psychosocial components, 30% to 50% in patients with significant psychosocial components, and approximately 20% in patients with major psychiatric components or secondary gains.[27, 52]

Multidisciplinary chronic pain treatment is a focused unified approach to the chronic pain syndrome. In this country, pain treatment centers differ widely in organization and emphasis. They are generally multidisciplinary centers that use some combination of anesthesiologists, clinical psychologists, dentists, neurologists, orthopedists, pharmacists, physiatrists, and psychiatrists. The goals of these centers are to diminish, if not eliminate, chronic pain; increase the patient's functional capabilities to allow for a more active life; and decrease the patient's dependence on drugs for pain control.

Physical Treatment Modalities

Physical modalities are valuable adjuncts to the successful management of acute and chronic pain. Therapeutic heat and cryotherapy are time-honored interventions in treating musculoskeletal pain. More recent acceptance of transcutaneous electrical nerve stimulation (TENS), acupuncture, and cold laser have increased the methods available to the physician in controlling pain.

Pain arising from the musculoskeletal system is often caused by muscle spasm,[82] and heat and cold applications are primarily directed at reducing spasmodic muscle shortening. The shortened muscle may be a result of direct muscular trauma, or underlying primary neurological or skeletal disease. Investigators have studied the muscle spindle and its firing rate in relation to thermal changes.[97] They found direct and indirect effects on the muscle spindle from both heat and cold applications in alleviating pain associated with the shortened muscle.[37, 42, 106] The return of the muscle to its normal resting length is also believed to promote the reduction and resolution of pain,[72] but precisely how muscle spasm is relieved is not completely understood.

Cryotherapy

Cold has four distinct applications in medicine: to stop or slow bleeding; to induce hypothermia; to decrease spasticity; and to relieve pain.[96] It may be applied in three forms: solid, liquid, and gaseous. Ice is a common form of direct cold therapy. It is usually rubbed in a circular fashion over the localized painful area. Immersing a body part in water combined with ice chips may provide pain relief. Cold applied directly to an injured area in acute musculoskeletal trauma serves to reduce hemorrhage and vasodilation, blunts the local inflammatory response, decreases edema production, and reduces pain perception. The so-called RICE (rest, ice, compression, and elevation) method is commonly prescribed for acute sports-related injuries.[103]

In addition to acute musculoskeletal injuries, cryotherapy has been shown to benefit chronic painful conditions. Pain may be alleviated by direct or indirect mechanisms.[81] The direct effect is the decrease in temperature of the affected area. Reduced pain sensation is presumed to result through an indirect effect on the nerve fibers and sensory end organs. Additionally, the decreased

temparature reduces the firing rate of the muscle spindle and decreases the painful muscle tone.[81, 106]

The direct application of ice massage has been shown therapeutically efficacious in several clinical trials. Grant demonstrated the beneficial effects of direct ice application on a large population of young individuals sustaining acute and chronic musculoskeletal trauma.[54] Pegg provided evidence suggesting that chronic inflammatory joint disease improved clinically with cold in regard to pain, stiffness, and range of motion.[108] Patients with low back pain also responded well to controlled clinical trials employing cryotherapy.[80]

The application of cold as a vapocoolant spray was popularized by Travell in treating myofascial pain syndromes.[144, 145] A counterirritant effect is presumed to provide the mechanism of muscle spasm relief and pain alleviation. The combination of vapocoolant spray, stretching, and trigger point injection has been reported to provide significant pain relief in the myofascial pain syndromes.[146]

Adverse effects have also been reported with the use of cold.[81] The major reaction is hypersensitivity. Patients with Raynaud's and peripheral vascular disease should not have their limbs exposed to cold temperatures, as this produces vasoconstriction. In addition, patients who display a marked cold pressor response are poor candidates for cryotherapy.

Heat Therapy

Heat is commonly used to treat pain. It is generally accepted that therapeutic heat is best tolerated in the subacute and chronic phases of a disease process. The physiological responses produced by heat are increased collagen extensibility, increased blood flow and metabolic rate, and inflammatory resolution. Decreased joint stiffness, muscle spasm, and pain are also recognized effects of heat.

Therapeutic heat is believed to have direct and indirect effects on the muscle spindle. Local elevated temperatures have been shown to directly decrease the spindle sensitivity,[97] and superficial heating of the skin has been shown to indirectly quiet spindle excitability.[42] This mechanism is similar to that proposed for reduced muscle spindle activity with the application of cold. It is also believed that the pain threshold may be raised by the direct and indirect actions of heat.

Pain associated with numerous conditions has been successfully treated with therapeutic heat application. Musculoskeletal contractures respond well to deep heat used in association with prolonged stretch.[74] Joint stiffness, associated with chronic inflammatory diseases, particularly affecting the limbs, respond to superficial heating with decreased pain and increased range of motion and function. Bursitis, tenosynovitis, and epicondylitis also may respond to heat with decreased pain and symptom resolution.

TENS Therapy

The use of electrical currents dates back to the Greeks who applied torpedo fish to individuals suffering from pain.[142] Electricity eventually fell into disrepute until Melzak and Wall proposed their gate control theory of pain.[94] This gate control model provided the theoretical basis for the utilization of electrical current in pain control. They found that the preferential activation of large afferent fibers (using TENS) would inhibit the transmission of painful impulses. The exact physiological basis by which TENS produces pain control is unknown.

Available equipment can produce a variety of specific wave forms, and the most effective one has not yet been determined.[156]

Therefore, it is clinically efficacious to try different wave forms when a particular one fails to achieve optimal pain suppression.

Electrode placement for a TENS unit must be based on a knowledge of anatomical and physiological principles. The painful area is often initially chosen as the site for an electrode placement. The actual landmarks for the electrode may be a dermatome, peripheral nerve, motor point, or acupuncture point. Electrode arrangement over the painful area may be linear, triangular, or criss-cross. Occasionally electrodes may also be placed on nonpainful areas.[87]

The conventional short-duration, high-frequency TENS has recently been applied with a current of low frequency and long duration (acupuncture-like TENS). It appears TENS may achieve pain relief by stimulating large sensory afferent fibers and inhibiting pain perception, or by enhancing the production of endogenous opioids.

TENS has also been used extensively to manage chronic pain. The results have been less promising and more variable than those in acute pain trials. Generally, patients who have fewer surgical interventions, less analgesic treatments, and limited use of narcotics respond more favorably to TENS.[23] Patients with radiculopathy, peripheral neuropathy, reflex sympathetic dystrophy, phantom limb pain, and peripheral nerve injury have all demonstrated good pain control with TENS.[23, 99, 154]

There are relatively few side-effects related to TENS. The major problem is one of skin irritation related to the conducting paste or tape that secures the electrodes. Currently, the use of TENS in patients with demand cardiac pacemakers is inadvisable.[154]

Acupuncture

Acupuncture (originating from the Latin *acus* or "sharp point" and *punctura,* "to puncture") is an ancient Chinese therapy practiced for more than 2,500 years to cure disease or relieve pain. Thin metal needles are inserted into specific body sites and slowly twisted manually or stimulated electrically. Various sensations may be produced, ranging from a dull ache or warmth, to that of a pinprick. The Chinese believe acupuncture achieves its beneficial results by restoring the balance between *yang* (spirit) and *yin* (blood), which flow in 14 channels or "meridians" containing 361 acupuncture sites.

Researchers have considered acupuncture to be a form of neuromodulation. Two theories have been proposed for its use in pain control. First, acupuncture may stimulate large sensory afferent fibers and suppress pain perception through the gate control theory of pain. Second, the needle insertion may act as a noxious stimulus and induce endogenous production of opiate-like substances to effect pain control.[92]

It has been demonstrated that there is a significant overlap between traditional acupuncture sites, myofascial trigger points, and muscular motor points.[93] The sensation induced by the application of an acupuncture needle is very similar to the dull ache often experienced by the patient when a trigger point is injected. The insertion of a needle, regardless of the substance injected, appears to produce the beneficial pain relief and is termed the *needle effect.* The injection of trigger points may share not only similar areas of needle insertion, but also associated mechanisms of pain control.

Acupuncture has been used in a wide variety of painful conditions. The insertion of a needle is considered an invasive procedure, and many states require a physician to perform or supervise the treatment. Uniform agreement does not yet exist as to the preferred time necessary for an adequate trial of acupuncture. Failure of an acupuncture trial is not a contraindication to a repeat trial. Localized hyperemia has been reported to occur frequently following needle insertion. Infrequently, syncopal episodes, hematoma formation, and pneumothorax have also been reported. Caution is suggested in the use of electrical acupuncture with patients who have cardiac pacemakers.[85]

Laser Treatment

Light amplification by stimulated emission of radiation (LASER), which can result in tissue destruction (hot laser), is an accepted treatment in many surgical procedures.[29] A relatively new infrared (cold laser) therapy is reportedly incapable of tissue destruction and has been used empirically on a variety of painful conditions.[19] The effectiveness of this technique has not been scientifically demonstrated and its mode of action, if any, remains totally speculative.

The effectiveness of a gallium arsenide cold laser was compared with a sham laser in a double-blind cross-over study of patients with carpal tunnel syndrome. Subjective pain relief and serial electrodiagnostic studies with both true and sham lasers were investigated. No statistically significant objective or subjective therapeutic effects were demonstrated.[158] Therefore, it is advisable to use cold laser therapy cautiously. More controlled studies are needed to determine its scientific credibility, mode of action, and efficacy.

Therapeutic Exercise

During acute injuries to the musculoskeletal system, a muscle may shorten as a protective reaction to pain. Treatment typically consists of immobilization combined with compression and cryotherapy. As the pain subsides, mobility is restored gradually. If normal range of motion is not achieved, the muscle may become chronically shortened and result in additional pain.

Prolonged muscle shortening will add to the painful condition by producing contracted soft tissue structures. In the chronic phase of pain, the optimal treatment methodology combines stretching movements, strengthening exercises, heat or cold, and massage. The patient is also educated regarding proper body mechanics and the need to continue the prescribed therapeutic exercise regimen outside of formal therapy sessions.

Therapeutic exercise, prescribed to correct a specific abnormal condition, is often used to treat chronic painful conditions. The primary goal is to aid the patient in achieving pain control. This may be accomplished through the restoration of normal muscle tone, length, strength, and optimal joint range of motion. Finally, the patient is urged to continue a home program after formal therapy sessions have ceased.

Therapeutic exercise consists of passive movements, active-assistive exercises, active exercises, stretching, and relaxing exercises. Each may be used alone or in combination to achieve the desired effect.[8, 75, 146, 151]

Behavioral Treatment Modalities

Among the treatment goals of pain management are the decrease in illness behavior (reduced drug use and visits to physicians) and the increase in well behavior (increased physical activities, mobility, and return to gainful employment). This may be accomplished by blocking noxious sensory input, decreasing tension and depression, rearranging reinforcement contingencies, or by assisting in the learning of new behaviors.[50] Biofeedback, cognitive behavior, operant pain hypnosis, and relaxation training can assist in the treatment of chronic pain behavior.

Biofeedback[6] has found some use in the treatment of chronic pain.[26, 43] Typically biofeedback teaches muscle relaxation (through EMG) or temperature control. The instrumentation is reported to be somewhat useful, although clinical experience suggests that relaxation without instrumentation is of equal value. Through biofeedback training the patient learns self-regulation of pain.

Cognitive behavior modification helps the patient learn self-coping statements and problem-solving cognitions[40] in order to alter the cognitive structures (schemata, beliefs) and cognitive process (automatic thoughts, images, and internal dialogue) associated with the pain experience. Cognitive strategies of imaginative inattention, imaginative transformation of pain, focused attention, and somatization in a dissociative manner have been found helpful.

The operant approach involves the identification of behaviors to be produced, increased, maintained, or eliminated. Reinforcement is then regulated to achieve the desired outcome. Activity and walking programs are followed to the prescribed level, not discomfort. All medication is prescribed by schedule. Family and friends are instructed to avoid reinforcing all pain behavior.

Relaxation methods[36, 132] to reduce tension may include deep muscle relaxation, deep diaphragmatic breathing, meditation, yoga, and autogenic training. Patients may also be taught self-hypnosis.[6] Hypnosis has the advantage of providing relief without unpleasant side-effects, with no reduction of normal functioning, and no development of tolerance. Hypnotic strategies can suggest analgesia or anesthesia, can substitute another feeling for pain, can move the pain perception to a smaller or less vulnerable area, can alter the meaning of pain, can increase tolerance to pain, or, in some individuals, dissociate the perception of body from the patient's awareness.

Pharmacological Intervention

Two groups of patients are encountered in the clinical management of chronic pain. The first group includes individuals with acute and recurrent pain due to chronic medical illness such as rheumatoid arthritis, cancer, and burn injuries. Primary therapy is usually directed at the underlying cause of pain. When the therapy is successful, the pain treatment is successful. Treatment commonly includes NSAIDs. Narcotic analgesics are used sparingly, on a limited basis, using time duration regimens to limit the development of psychological dependence.

The second group of patients consists of individuals who have chronic pain without organic etiology. Pharmacological intervention is the most common means of treatment for chronic pain. Substances may be divided into three categories: NSAIDs, narcotics, and adjuvant drugs.

Nonsteroidal anti-inflammatory analgesics include aspirin, acetaminophen, and the newer NSAIDs. These drugs are peripherally active analgesics that do not inhibit nociception or alter the perception of the pain input. They are best considered remittent agents that alter the pathological processes which generate pain. Aspirin and other NSAIDs reduce pain by interfering with prostaglandin (PG) sensitization of nociceptors and inhibiting the synthesis of prostaglandins. Additional NSAID actions include inhibition of tissue reaction to bradykinin, suppressed release of histamine, and decreased vascular permeability. This improves the environment of the nociceptor, increasing pain control by decreasing sensitivity. With the exception of acetaminophen, the NSAIDs also possess anti-inflammatory effects which reduce local heat, swelling, and stiffness. These drugs are used to treat acute and chronic pain patients with pain of low to moderate severity.

NSAIDs are often chosen over narcotics because they have fewer side-effects, including, no constipation, very little sedation, no psychological or physical dependence, and no development of tolerance. The mainstays of non-narcotic analgesic therapy are aspirin and acetaminophen. Acetaminophen is an excellent alternative to aspirin in patients who are unable to tolerate other NSAID medication. All NSAIDs have ceiling effects, but the ceilings for some of these drugs are higher than that of aspirin.[65]

Although aspirin, acetaminophen, and other NSAID compounds are available over the counter, they all have potential side-effects. The most common complication, involving the gastrointestinal tract, is seen in between 5% and 10% of patients. These drugs produce in varying degrees gastrointestinal, hematological, renal, and hepatic toxicities. The side-effects from prolonged use of all NSAIDs are similar to those occurring with aspirin, but there are significant differences in the potential for side-effects. Aspirin, in the nonsalicylated salsalate form (Disalcid), remains the preferred drug for the chronic pain patient. The newer NSAIDs have not been proven to offer any major advantage over aspirin, although their cost is much greater. Notable exceptions are patients unable to tolerate acetylsalicylic acid or who demonstrate difficulty with compliance.

Narcotic medication is useful and appropriate in the treatment of acute, recurrent, or cancer pain. Acute and recurrent pain are usually best managed by diagnosis and treatment of the underlying cause of the pain. The narcotic medication is used as an adjunct to provide relief during a period of temporary, excruciating pain. Narcotic analgesics are also preferred for relief of intractible pain due to cancer. The greatest obstacle to treating postoperative pain, pain related to cancer, acute pain, and recurrent pain due to chronic disease is the excessive concern of the physician regarding addiction. Repeated studies report that a high percentage of house officers tend to overestimate their patient's potential for addiction and, consequently, undermedicate them.[88] Ironically, undermedication may increase the potential for addiction due to the operant conditioning, anxiety, and dependent behavior created by inadequate pain relief. Psychological dependence has not been a major problem in acute pain or cancer pain patients who receive appropriately dosed narcotic analgesics for moderate to severe pain.[70]

Narcotic medications should be avoided in the treatment of chronic pain patients. There is almost no justification for the use of narcotic drugs in the patient with chronic pain having no organic etiology. The long-term use of narcotic drugs with these patients often produces behavioral complications that are more difficult to manage than the initial pain problem. The hazards of tolerance, physical dependence, and psychological dependence present major problems in the long-term management of this patient group. Deficits of cognition and motor function, as well as the masking of psychological disorders, are common. The indiscriminate use of narcotic medications in an attempt to control chronic pain only enhances chronic pain behavior.

Morphine is the prototype of the narcotic drugs and is commonly prescribed by many clinicians.[17] Pain relief is often obtained by titrating the dose to the patient's needs. At equianalgesic doses there is no significant pharmacological evidence to suggest the choice of one narcotic over another,[66] but there are significant differences in their action times, equianalgesic dose, and parenteral/oral ratio (Table 36-1). Inappropriate drug dosing often occurs because of a lack of knowledge or attention to equianalgesic doses, resulting in inadequate pain relief.

All clinically useful narcotics produce similar side-effects in equianalgesic doses. The undesirable side-effects of narcotics on the central nervous system include unwanted sedation, mental clouding, inability to concentrate, lethargy, impairment of mental and physical performance, constipation, nausea and vomiting, tolerance, physical dependence, psychological dependence, and

Table 36-1
Narcotic Medications

| Drug | Equianalgesic Dosage (mgs)* | | | | Action Times | | | |
	IM	PO	IV	Rectal	Half-Life (hrs)	Duration (hrs)	Onset (min)	Peak (min)
Alphaprodine (Nisentil)	50		0.4–0.6		2.6	0.5–1.5	5–10	30–60
Butorphanol (Stadol)	2		1			3–4	10	30–60
Codeine	130	200			3	4–6	15–30	60–120
Fentanyl (Innovar)	0.1					1–2	5–15	30
Hydromorphone (Dilaudid)	1.5	7.5	1			2–4	15–30	30–90
Levorphanol (Levo-Dromoran)	2	4	1			4–5	60	60–90
Meperidine (Demerol)	75	300	50		3–4	2–4	10–15	30–60
Methadone (Dolphine)	10	20†	5			6–8	10–15	60–120
Morphine	10	30†	5			2–4	20	30–90
Nalbuphine (Nubain)	10		5			3–6	10–15	30–60
Oxycodone hydrochloride	15	30				4–5	10–15	60–90
Oxymorphone hydrochloride (Numorphan)	1		0.5	10		4–5	5–10	30–90
Pentazocine (Talwin)	60	180			2–3	2–3	10–15	30–60
Anileridine (Leritine)	30	50				2–3		
Propoxyphene (Darvon)		300				4–6	15–60	120–180

* Equal in analgesia to 10 mg of morphine administered subcutaneously or intramuscularly
† For chronic dosing only; for single dosing use 60 mg

impaired respiration. These side-effects inhibit the chronic pain patient whose goal is to maintain a normal life-style.

Oral administration of medication is preferred in the treatment of all pain. A time-contingent round-the-clock schedule for pain medications is superior to an as-needed schedule. This form of administration minimizes alterations in plasma levels and provides optimal pain control. The schedule should be based on such variables as potency, duration of the analgesic effect, and efficacy of the analgesic medication. A regularly scheduled dosage optimizes the reduction of pain by minimizing the peaks and valleys of pain intensity. Generally it is better to begin the initial dose of medication too high rather than too low. Starting suboptimally and titrating upward results in the patient's experiencing anxiety due to a lack of adequate analgesic.

The as-needed, or PRN, schedule does not have a place in the control of chronic pain. Such a schedule results in operant conditioning, craving, a sense of dependence, and anxiety about the drug wearing off. In chronic pain management, the drugs with longer duration of action are usually preferred. There is considerable patient-to-patient variation with respect to effective analgesic dosage.[101, 152]

The adjuvant analgesic drugs produce or potentiate analgesia by mechanisms not directly mediated through the opiate receptor system. This group includes a wide variety of compounds with no proven specific analgesic properties: tricyclic antidepressants, anticonvulsants, and antispasmodics. The use of these drugs is often based on anecdotal data, clinical surveys, or limited drug trials.

Tricyclic antidepressants, such as amitriptyline (Elavil), doxepin (Sinequan), and imipramine (Tofranil), have been used in the treatment of chronic pain syndromes. One of the primary mechanisms of tricyclic compounds is to block the re-uptake of the neurotransmitter serotonin in the central nervous system. This enhances pain inhibition by way of the dorsolateral pathway.[7, 149] In addition, amitriptyline is a potent sedative drug, which may be used as a sleeping medication in chronic pain patients. The combination of antidepressant effect, enhanced cortical serotonergic mechanism, and improved sleep contrib-

utes to these medications being the most useful group of psychotropic agents presently used in pain management.[4]

Anticonvulsants such as phenytoin (Dilantin) and carbamazepine (Tegretol) have been used in the management of pain syndromes affecting the central nervous system. Their applications include trigeminal neuralgia, post-herpetic neuralgia, causalgia, and phantom pain syndromes. While the mechanism is unclear, they appear to have a stabilizing effect on excitable cell membranes, which decreases afferent and deafferent second-order neuron activity. Carbamazepine may have a central serotonin action similar to that of amitriptyline.[114]

Other anticonvulsants suggested for pain usage are valproic acid (Depakene) and clonazepam (Clonopin). They increase the effectiveness of gamma amino butyric acid (GABA) induced inhibition in the pre- and postsynaptic systems. These drugs appear to be most effective in the treatment of neuralgias and neuropathies.

Antispasmodics such as baclofen (Lioresal) are presumed to act by inhibiting gamma transaminases and their re-uptake at gamma receptor sites. Valproic acid and clonazepam act in a similar fashion.[112, 141]

In addition to these medications, a number of other adjuvant medications have been used. These include methotrimeprazine, chlorpromazine, and fluphenazine. Butyrophenones are anecdotal in the management of pain disorders, with haloperidol being the most often reported. Antihistamines, amphetamines, steroids, and cannabinoids are also reported anecdotally. Steroids such as prednisone and dexamethasone are thought to interfere with prostaglandin sensitization of nociceptors. Serotonin antagonists such as ergot alkaloids, the beta blocking agents such as propranolol, and the antihistamines such as hydroxyzine, all function by antagonizing transmitters that directly activate nociceptors. These medications have been used extensively in the treatment of migraine and cluster headaches. Lithium and calcium blocking agents have been proposed as drugs to interfere with the release of transmitters involved in the pain process.[102]

Benzodiazepines and barbiturates are two groups that have

little or no place as adjuvant drugs in chronic pain management. Long-term use of these medications may result in psychological and physical dependence as well as interference with cognition and motor function. Benzodiazepines, because of their claimed muscle relaxant properties, are often prescribed to patients with pain. However, their role as muscle relaxants is questionable in clinical studies. In addition to the adverse effects of dependency, it has been suggested that these medications adversely affect the serotonin system. These medications are depressants which, with long-term use, lower pain tolerance and tend to induce clinical depression as well as psychological and physical dependence. Due to their sedative effects, depressants often act as potent reinforcers of pain in drug-seeking behaviors. Chronic use of these medications may result in physical and mental incapacitation, emotional instability, and the inability to deal with initial physiological or psychological problems. Benzodiazepines deplete serotonin, alter sleep patterns, and increase pain perception. It is recommended that these two groups of medications should not be part of the long-term management of chronic pain. The only possible indication for these sedatives or for anti-anxiety agents is for the short-term (less than 1 month) treatment of a self-limited crisis unrelated to the particular pain problem, or as an adjunct when detoxifying a patient from narcotic medication.

Anesthetic Procedures

Blocking the nerve with a local anesthetic agent is one of the most common procedures in the management of chronic pain. Nerve block by itself, however, is not effective in relieving pain completely for a long period in the majority of patients. Therefore, nerve blocks should be considered as only one of the therapeutic modalities used in a multidisciplinary pain clinic. Other factors, such as psychological problems and associated muscle tightness and weakness, should be treated by using other appropriate modalities. Nerve blocks are helpful in many patients by interrupting the pain process. It is the experience of many clinicians that when pain is temporarily interrupted by a local anesthetic block, the patient's pain is permanently relieved. Nerve blocks are also useful in delineating the pain mechanisms and in blocking the pain when the patients are required to take part in physical therapy to mobilize the muscles and joints. Patients who have a nerve block followed by appropriate physical therapy display excellent results. The best results have been shown in patients requiring manipulation and mobilization of the knee and other joints. There are various nerve block techniques used in pain clinics; the most common and useful include epidural, use of a local anesthetic or narcotic, and peripheral nerve block.[16, 120]

An epidural with a local anesthetic or narcotic can provide prolonged relief by placement of a catheter in the epidural space, which can be left in place for several days to a few weeks. A local anesthetic or narcotic can be administered intermittently or by continuous infusion, providing somatic and sympathetic block and analgesia for physical therapy. This is the most commonly applied technique in patients who have low back and lower extremity pain while they undergo physical therapy and mobilization.[116]

Peripheral nerve block, such as suprascapular nerve block, is very useful in patients who have shoulder discomfort, frozen shoulder, or shoulder pain of other etiology. Patients can tolerate stretching and physical therapy after a suprascapular block with local anesthetic. In the upper extremities, brachial plexus blocks, especially continuous blocks performed by axillary or supraclavicular route, are of great value in patients requiring physical therapy. Other peripheral blocks, such as the lateral femoral

cutaneous nerve block for patients with meralgia parasthetica, the femoral nerve block for patients with thigh and knee pain, and sciatic nerve and intercostal blocks, have been extremely useful in managing chronic pain patients. Depot-types of steroids, injected into the epidural space, have been extremely useful in relieving nerve root irritation and inflammation in patients who have a herniated disk. They have also been effective in patients who have nerve root irritation secondary to radiation or a malignancy. The steroid preparations employed are Depo-Medrol and Aristospan Intralesional. Although steroid preparations may be used to produce anti-inflammatory action, the steroid preparations contain various preservatives such as benzyl alcohol, which may produce serious side-effects including paralysis. Only Depro-Medrol and Aristospan have been extensively used without producing significant neurological damage.

The steroids are injected into the epidural space close to the involved root. These injections can be performed at any level including cervical, thoracic, or lumbar. The steroid preparations stay in the epidural space for 2 to 3 weeks. Repeat injections, if necessary, are given a minimum of 2 to 4 weeks apart. Many clinicians give a series of three injections regardless of successful response following the first injection. The preferred procedure is to administer one injection and wait 2 weeks in order to assess the patient's response. If the patient is significantly pain-free, no further injections are administered. If the patient does not respond to two or three injections of epidural steroid, steroid treatment is discontinued. If three injections have failed to offer relief, it is unlikely any pain relief will be provided through further steroid treatment. If the patient receives only short-term pain relief, steroid injections are discontinued. Frequent injections of epidural steroid can produce problems related to chronic steroid administration as well as a remote possibility of infection.

Many clinicians combine the steroid injections with the administration of a local anesthetic agent. When this is done, the patient needs to be observed because the sympathetic block may produce postural hypotension and the patient may become unable to ambulate. No single technique has been proven to be more successful than another. Many clinicians use the caudal approach, using large volumes of local anesthetic agent or saline mixed with the steroid. This gives a 60% success rate as opposed to an 80% or higher success rate with a lumbar epidural technique, since caudally administered agents may not reach the site of pathology at L4-L5 or L5-S1 levels in significant concentration, owing to the leak through the sacral foraminae. Epidural steroid injection is also a useful technique in patients who have neural irritation. In addition, steroids may be injected into the subarachnoid space, especially in patients who have had multiple surgeries and in whom the epidural space has been obliterated. These patients, especially those with arachnoiditis, show significant pain relief. Epidural steroids can produce an initial increase in pain for 8 to 24 hours.[116]

COMMON PAIN SYNDROMES — DETECTION AND TREATMENT

Myofascial Pain

Myofascial pain syndromes are commonly seen when evaluating and treating patients for chronic pain. They are characterized by pain originating from small circumscribed areas of local hyperirritability and myofascial structures resulting in local and referred pain.[144] The pain is aggravated by stretching the affected area, cooling, and compression, often giving rise to a characteristic pattern of referred pain.[146] Although the exact pathophysiology of the trigger point phenomenon has not been identified, myofascial pain syndromes appear to be initiated by trauma, tension, inflammation, and other factors. The trigger point acts as a source of chronic nociception. The resultant muscle dysfunction and altered mechanics lead to the referred pain and associated phenomenon.

Trigger points may occur in any muscle or muscle group of the body. They are commonly found in muscle groups that are routinely overstressed or those that do not undergo full contraction and relaxation cycles. In the upper body, the group of muscles involved commonly include the trapezius, levator scapulae, and infraspinatus. In the lower body they include the gluteus group, tensor fasciae latae, quadratus lumborum, and gastrocnemius muscles.

Trigger points are best located by deep palpation of the affected muscle, which reproduces the patient's pain complaint both locally and in a referred zone. Trigger points are usually a sharply circumscribed spot of exquisite tenderness. When they are present, passive or active stretching of the affected muscle routinely increases the pain. The muscle in the immediate vicinity of the trigger point is often described as ropy, tense, or having a palpable band. Compared with equivalent pressure in palpation to normal muscle, the trigger point region displays isolated bands, increased tenderness, and referred pain.

The most reliable method of treating trigger points consists of routine, regular stretching to restore the normal resting length of the muscle. Methods to interrupt the pain cycle include injection or needle stimulation of the hypersensitive trigger points,[14, 57, 76, 117, 135] coolant sprays,[146] relaxation therapy, and pressure techniques.[117] After interrupting the pain cycle, the treatment is directed at restoring the normal resting muscle length with a regular routine stretching program of the involved muscle groups. This may be accomplished with physical modalities including heat, cold, and correction of poor body mechanics. Psychological intervention may be necessary if long-standing stress and tension are the underlying cause of the problem.

A long-term home modality and stretching program is essential in the management of patients with myofascial pain. Attention to body mechanics, stress, and daily routines may significantly alter their functional capabilities.

Peripheral Neuropathy

Pain is a common feature of peripheral neuropathy due to diabetes, amyloidosis, alcoholism, polyarteritis, Guillain-Barré syndrome, brachial neuritis, porphyria, and riboflavin deficiency. This pain may be of either a constant or intermittent nature and is often described as burning, aching, or lancinating. It may occur with or without signs of sensory loss, muscle weakness, atrophy, or reflex loss.

There are few placebo-controlled, double-blind, cross-over studies concerning the effectiveness of medications in alleviating the pain of peripheral neuropathy. The pilot studies suggest that placebos are effective therapy for painful neuropathy. Amitriptyline, fluphenazine, imipramine, and placebos, all demonstrated the same benefit for patients with painful diabetic neuropathy.[95] Because of the significant placebo response in studies of patients with peripheral neuropathy, early treatment with low doses of tricyclic antidepressants may be helpful. Pain due to alcoholic neuropathy is resolved after the correction of nutritional deficiencies. Pain due to polyarteritis may resolve after corticosteroid treatment, whereas pain due to cryoglobulinemia may resolve with plasmapheresis, and pain due to brachial neuritis and other self-limiting conditions resolves spontaneously in weeks to months. Pain secondary to diabetic neuropathies rarely resolves completely. Drugs that induce painful peripheral neu-

ropathies include isoniazid (Laniazid) and hydralazine (Hydralyn), which cause a decrease in tissue levels of pyridoxal phosphate; and nitrofurantoin (Furadantin), which has neurotoxic effects.

The patient with chronic painful peripheral neuropathy has many of the associated problems of chronic pain, including depression, inactivity, disuse syndrome, and significant alteration of life-style. Psychological intervention and physical therapy are important aspects of treatment in these patients. Conventional physical therapy modalities, TENS, and general conditioning programs are often helpful, as are psychological programs and other nonpharmacological methods of pain control.

Reflex Sympathetic Dystrophy and Causalgia

A contributing factor in many chronic pain syndromes is over-activity of the sympathetic nervous system. This is often reported as continuous burning pain in an extremity after trauma. *Causalgia* refers to partial injury to a major nerve followed by the symptoms of sympathetic system over-activity. *Reflex sympathetic dystrophy* refers to cases of minor injury or no injury, with resulting over-activity of the sympathetic nervous system. Examples include shoulder-hand syndrome, post-traumatic edema, Sudeck's atrophy, and various other syndromes in which sympathetic over-activity seems to be the primary etiological factor.

The etiology of the sympathalgia is not distinct. The most common aspect of a sympathalgia is burning pain. Associated with hyperpathia are hypersensitivity to touch and relief of pain with an appropriate sympathetic nerve block. The patient may also show evidence of over-activity of the sympathetic nervous system, including hyperhydrosis and vasoconstriction. These symptoms result in cooling the extremity. When accompanied by disuse, this may produce trophic changes including shiny thin skin, loss of hair, and demineralization of bone.

Diagnosis of sympathetic dystrophies is difficult. The patient's pain is usually diffuse and does not correspond to dermatomal or peripheral nerve patterns. Thus, these patients are often diagnosed as having psychogenic pain. Anatomic or pharmacologic nerve blocks may establish the diagnosis. Psychogalvanic reflex tests and thermography are also useful in documenting sympathetic nervous system hyperactivity.

The most effective treatment of a sympathetic dystrophy consists of an appropriate sympathetic nerve block using a local anesthetic agent.[120] Phenoxybenzamine has been reported effective in the treatment of causalgia.[51] If the problem originates in the head, neck, upper extremity, or upper thorax, a stellate ganglion or a cervical sympathetic block at the C6 level may be employed.[83] If the pain is in the upper abdominal area, sympathetic denervation can be achieved using the celiac plexus block. Pain originating in the lower extremities requires a lumbar paravertebral sympathetic block at the L2 level.[116] Patients with a history of long-standing pain may receive only temporary pain relief from the local anesthetic blocks. These patients may require intravenous regional guanethidine or reserpine when the nerve block ceases to provide pain relief. This technique can be applied to extremities, and is useful when local anesthetic blocks are contraindicated.[11, 60]

If the patient does not receive pain relief from sympathetic blocks or the intravenous regional technique, then permanent interruption of the sympathetic pathways should be considered. This can be accomplished by a neurolytic injection of the sympathetic trunk or surgical sympathectomy.

In conjunction with sympathetic blocks or guanethidine injection, physical therapy should be instituted. Often the patient receives spontaneous pain relief with the sympathetic block, but when the extremity is moved during physical therapy the patient experiences significant pain. This pain is secondary to tight muscles or stiffness of the joint, where the noxious input is carried through somatic fibers. These patients may be aided in the performance of physical therapy by somatic blocks, such as brachial plexus block or an epidural block.

When treating a patient with long-standing pain due to sympathetic dystrophy, it is important to consider the psychological aspects. Patients who develop reflex sympathetic dystrophy are usually overly tense. Their enhanced sympathetic pain, secondary to psychological tension, may be a contributing factor to this condition. Appropriate psychological and psychiatric consultation for relaxation training and biofeedback, in addition to other treatment modalities, may be beneficial.

Phantom Limb Pain

Phantom limb pain involves an amputated portion of the body. The etiology of phantom pain appears to be related to deafferentation of neurons and their spontaneous and evoked hyperexcitability. Pain may be continuous, in character with intermittent exacerbations. It is often reported by patients as cramping, aching, or burning, with occasional superimposed electriclike components. Recent studies have suggested that between 50% to 85% of amputees have phantom limb pain.[69, 125] The current data do not suggest a predisposition for phantom pain among traumatic amputees, elderly amputees, those with pain in the amputated limb before amputation, or poor preamputation interpersonal relationships.[125] Phantom limb pain does not appear to be correlated with amount of time following amputation or use of a prosthesis.

Multiple modalities, adjuvant medications, and anesthetic and surgical procedures have been used in the treatment of phantom limb pain with varying long-term success. Although at least 68 methods of treating phantom limb syndromes have been identified, successful treatment of persistent types is not commonly reported.[69, 126, 127] Transcutaneous nerve stimulation, tricyclic antidepressants, anticonvulsants, or chlorpromazine have been used with varying success. Chemical sympathectomy or neurosurgical procedures have also had variable success. Treatments yielding a temporary decrease in pain include analgesics, anesthetic procedures, stump desensitization, physical modalities, and sedative/hypnotic medication. One survey reported treatments reducing stump problems also resulted in decreased phantom pain.[125, 128] Therapeutic regimens have had less than a 30% long-term efficacy in the treatment of phantom limb pain.

Phantom limb pain is reported to be more frequent in patients with stump pain. In the early evaluation of phantom limb pain, it is important that stump pain due to a neuroma is ruled out as the etiology of the pain complaints. *Stump pain* is pain at the site of the extremity amputation. This sharp, often jabbing, pain in the stump is usually aggravated by pressure or by infection in the stump. Pain is often elicited by tapping over a neuroma in a transected nerve. The increased sensitivity of sprouts from cut peripheral nerves to noradrenaline and adrenaline may partially explain why adrenergic-influenced emotional states (*i.e.,* stress or anxiety) occasionally provoke attacks of phantom limb pain.

Neuroma and Scar Pain

Injury to the nerve with a resulting neuroma or entrapment of the branches of the nerve in scar tissue can produce disabling pain. Neuromas are suspected when numbness appears in the distribution of a particular nerve and when pain is produced by palpation of the neuroma. It has been shown that the nerve fibers in the neuroma develop alpha receptors, which respond to catecholamines with spontaneous firing and pain production. Painful neuromas are difficult to treat; many patients continue to have pain despite multiple attempts at surgical excision of the neuroma. Suspected scar pain can be evaluated by picking up the scar from the deeper tissues with two fingers and palpating. If this does not reproduce the patient's pain, the pain is probably not originating in the scar tissue. Pain due to neuroma or scar tissue can be associated with reflex sympathetic dystrophy. Diagnosis can be established by infiltration of the scar or the neuroma with a local anesthetic agent, resulting in complete pain relief.[115]

Repeated injection of a local anesthetic agent has proven to be an extremely useful technique. This should be followed by appropriate physical therapy to the scar, usually ultrasound followed by stretching or deep massage of the scar. This type of treatment has provided permanent or prolonged pain relief for longer than 6 months in many patients. When the local anesthetics, with or without steroids, do not provide prolonged relief, other methods should be considered. Cryoanalgesia using a cryoprobe and freezing the neuroma for 1 minute at $-20\,°C$ has been used with good success. The advantage of using a cryoprobe lies in the fact that it is a physical method of blocking the nerve without producing further neuroma or neuritis. Neurolytic agents such as phenol or alcohol have been used to relieve neuroma and scar pain. Incomplete block with these agents can result in neuritis producing severe pain. These neurolytic techniques should be employed only after repeated injections of local anesthetics produce consistent pain relief proportional to the duration of action of the local anesthetic agent. Although surgical revision of the scar is often considered, it is not very successful when the scar cannot be stretched out and there is significant nerve entrapment.

Cancer Pain

Pain is one of the greatest fears and a major source of morbidity for patients with cancer.[28, 90, 109] Clinical experience suggests that patients with cancer pain are treated most effectively with a multidisciplinary approach, including multiple modalities, appropriate analgesic drugs, neurosurgical and anesthetic procedures, psychological intervention, and supportive care.[17, 44, 147] The goals of pain therapy for cancer patients are a significant relief of pain to maintain the functional status they choose, a reasonable quality of life, and a death relatively free of pain.

Noninvasive treatment measures are often used singularly for mild to moderate pain and in combination with drug therapy for moderate or severe pain. Commonly used noninvasive measures include cutaneous stimulation, thermal modalities, and behavioral intervention. Their advantages include low risk of complications, low cost, and few serious side-effects.

Non-narcotic, narcotic, and adjuvant analgesic drugs are the primary therapy for patients with cancer pain. Anesthetic, psychiatric, behavioral, and occasionally neurosurgical approaches are commonly used with pharmacological intervention. This combination of treatment is estimated to provide adequate pain relief in at least 90% of the patients with cancer pain.

Narcotic analgesics are the drugs of choice for relief of intractable pain due to cancer.[17] Methadone is an extremely useful analgesic in the treatment of cancer pain due to its long duration of action once steady-state plasma levels are attained. The object is to titrate the level of analgesic to the optimal dose that prevents the recurrence of pain. Oral medications should be used whenever possible because they facilitate ambulatory care, encourage greater independence, and do not represent heroic intervention to the patient. It is important to remember that the maximum recommended dosages of narcotic medications were derived mainly from postoperative parenteral single-dose studies and are not applicable to administration by mouth in the long-term treatment of pain in advanced cancer. Dependency and respiratory depression should not be feared because they are seldom a problem. The most serious side-effects of drug therapy, which should be prevented or treated, include constipation and nausea.

Supportive care is designed to maintain the cancer patient in an outpatient setting, with pain a common cause for readmission to the hospital. Nerve blocks and neurolytic procedures are most often employed to provide pain relief in the thoracic and abdominal regions.[16, 120] These procedures are often done in the outpatient setting and often provide pain relief for up to 6 months. Supportive care may involve a hospice, hospital-based care teams, visiting nurses, and social services. The primary goal of the physician is to maintain the quality of life for the cancer patient to the end, allowing the patient a death with dignity.

It is essential that, during a cancer patient's hospitalization, outpatient treatment, and everyday activities, they maintain their functional skills, strength, and mobility. Progressive immobilization is an insidious aspect of this disease and is often iatrogenic. Although radiation and chemotherapy may transiently render a patient unable to perform activities, the patient needs to be consistently evaluated and involved in active physical, occupational, corrective, and recreational therapy programs. The physiatrist may offer multiple methods of combating immobility and its morbidity.

There are multiple invasive measures to control cancer pain. The most common is the surgical removal of all or part of the tumor in the hope of relieving pain and effecting a cure. Radiation therapy or chemotherapy may also relieve pain by shrinking the tumor. Common invasive anesthetic procedures include trigger point injections and nerve blocks. Myofascial pain syndromes are often the result of inactivity and disuse, and are commonly found in the cancer patient. Multiple neurosurgical procedures have been used for the control of cancer pain.[13, 48]

Herpetic Neuralgia

Herpes zoster (shingles) is a reactivation of the varicella (chicken pox) virus, which has remained latent. The viral inflammation of the dorsal nerve root and ganglion causes vesicle formation and severe burning, aching, and lancinating pain in a radicular distribution. During the acute stage, NSAIDs and sympathetic blocks provide excellent pain relief. The majority of patients recover from the acute episode in approximately 2 weeks without sequelae. However, some patients develop post-herpetic neuralgia. It is uncommon in patients under age 40, but occurs in over 50% of patients over 60.

Multiple reports indicate that postherpetic neuralgia may be prevented if the patient is treated with a sympathetic block within 1 month after the onset of herpes zoster.[113] Post-herpetic neuralgia is, thus, a preventable syndrome, but it is a difficult problem once established. A significant number of patients will experience pain relief with sympathetic blocks. If the syndrome is allowed to progress untreated for 3 months to a year, it becomes more difficult to treat.[116]

The most effective treatment for the management of established post-herpetic neuralgia is the use of a tricyclic antidepressant such as amitriptyline (Elavil) in small doses.[112] Most patients obtain pain relief with 25 mg to 75 mg administered at bedtime. If the patient does not get complete pain relief with administration of tricyclics alone, fluphenazine (Prolixin) may be added, beginning with 1 mg at bedtime and progressing as needed to a maximum dosage of 1 mg three times a day. Anticonvulsants, such as Dilantin, have been also administered with variable results.[141] Success in achieving pain relief using subcutaneous infiltration of local anesthetic and triamcinolone with two injections per week for 2 weeks has been reported.[38] TENS is beneficial in some patients, particularly when other techniques have given partial relief. Peripheral nerve blocks and destructive neurosurgical procedures have not proved useful in treating established post-herpetic neuralgia.

Pain in Spinal Cord Injury

The precise etiology underlying pain in spinal cord injuries is not known, but recent evidence suggests that trauma-induced alterations of the pain pathways are primarily involved.[107, 157] Hypersensitivity of the structures in the ascending pathway may play a role. Studies indicate that 50% of all spinal cord–injured patients have pain which is mild to moderate in severity; approximately 20% experience severe pain.[79, 155] Patients describe their pain as having one or more of the following components: burning in body parts below the injury, deep aching sensation over and around the site of injury, and radicular with lancinating characteristics. Burning pain in spinal cord–injured patients may be a variation of deafferentated pain occurring as a result of loss of inhibitory or augmentation of excitatory influences. The most effective treatments of this type of pain include tricyclic antidepressants and neuroaugmentive techniques.[32]

Spinal fracture site pain results from an alteration of body mechanics causing pain sensitive structures to be stretched or compressed. This mechanical pain may be the result of vertebral end-plate fractures, annulus fibrosus tears, or internal disk herniation following a spinal fracture.[104] Fracture site pain or mechanical pain is often exacerbated by activity. NSAIDs, trigger point injections, TENS, cognitive/behavioral techniques, and adjuvant medication may be used. Orthotics may also be used to decrease the mechanical stress and alleviate the underlying etiology.[39]

Radicular pain in these patients may be secondary to compression of nerve roots by a herniated nucleus pulposus, fracture fragment, dislocated vertebra, or the results of traumatic arachnoiditis. This type of pain is most effectively treated with anticonvulsants, with TENS used as a useful adjuvant.[58]

REFERENCES

1. Ahern D, Adams AE, Follick MJ: Emotional and marital disturbances in spouses of chronic low back pain patients. Clin J Pain 1:69–74, 1985
2. American Association of Electromyography and Electrodiagnosis: Guidelines in Electrodiagnostic Medicine. Rochester, 1984
3. Andrews IC: Management of postoperative pain. Int Anesth Clin 21:31–42, 1983
4. Aronof GM, Evans WO: Doxipam as an adjuvant in the treatment of chronic pain. J Clin Psychol 43:42–47, 1982
5. Ash CJ, Shealy CN, Young PA, Van Beaumont W: Thermography and the sensory dermatome. Skeletal Radiol 15:40–46, 1986
6. Barber J, Adrian C (eds): Psychological approaches to the management of pain. New York, Brunner/Mazel, 1982
7. Basbaum AI, Fields HL: Endogenous pain control mechanisms—Brainstem spinal pathways and endorphin circuitry. Ann Rev Neurosci 7:309–38, 1984
8. Bassmajian JV: Therapeutic Exercise, 4th ed. Baltimore, Williams & Wilkins, 1984
9. Beals RK: Compensation and recovery from injury. West J Med 140:233–237, 1984

10. Behan RC, Hirschfeld AH: The accident process—Toward more rational treatment of industrial injuries. JAMA 186:300–306, 1963
11. Benzon HT, Chomka CM, Brunner EA: Treatment of reflex sympathetic dystrophy with regional intravenous reserpine. Anesth Anal 59:500–502, 1980
12. Bishop B: Pain: Its physiology and rationale for management. Part I. Neuroanatomical substrate for pain. Phys Ther 60:13–37, 1980
13. Black P: Management of cancer pain—An overview. Neurosurgery 5:507–518, 1979
14. Bonica JJ: Management of myofascial pain syndromes in general practice. JAMA 164:732–738, 1957
15. Bonica JJ: Pain Research and Therapy: Past and Current Status and Future Needs. In Ng LKY, Bonica JJ (eds): Pain, Discomfort, and Humanitarian Care, pp 1–46. New York, Elsevier/North Holland, 1980
16. Bonica JJ: Local anesthesia and regional blocks. In Wall PD, Melzack R (eds): Textbook of pain, pp 541–557. Edinburgh, Churchill Livingstone, 1984
17. Bonica JJ: Management of Cancer Pain. In Zimmermann M, Drings P, Wagner G (eds): Pain and the Cancer Patient, pp 13–27. Berlin, Springer-Verlag, 1984
18. Bonica JJ: History of pain concepts and pain therapy. Semin Anesth 4:189–208, 1985
19. Brasford JR: Low energy laser treatment of pain and wounds: Hype, hope, or hokum? Mayo Clin Proc 61:671–678, 1986
20. Brena SF, Chapman SL, Decker R: Chronic pain as a learned experience. In Ng LKY (ed): New Approaches to Treatment of Chronic Pain, pp 76–83. Washington, DC, U.S. Department of Health and Human Services, 1981
21. Browse NL: The physiology and pathology of bed rest, pp 1–221. Springfield, IL, Charles C Thomas, 1965
22. Cailliet R: Disuse syndrome—Fibrocytic and degenerative changes. In Brena SF, Chapman SL (eds): Management of Patients with Chronic Pain, pp 63–71. New York, Sectrum Publications, 1983
23. Canthen JC, Renner EJ: Transcutaneous and peripheral nerve for chronic pain states. Surg Neurol 11:102–104, 1975
24. Chafetz N, Wexler CE, Kaiser JA: Thermography of the lumbar spine with CT correlation—A blinded study. Radiology 157(P):178, 1985
25. Chapman CR, Casey KL, Dubner R et al: Pain measurement: An overview. Pain 22:1–31, 1985
26. Chapman S: A review and clinical perspective on the use of EMG and thermal biofeedback for chronic headaches. Pain 27:1–43, 1986
27. Chapman SL, Brena SF, Bradford LA: Treatment outcome in a chronic pain rehabilitation program. Pain 11:255–268, 1981
28. Cleeland C: The impact of pain on the patient with cancer. Cancer 54:2635–2641, 1984
29. Council on Scientific Affairs: Lasers in medicine and surgery. JAMA 256:900–907, 1986
30. Crook J: The prevalence of pain complaints in a general population. Pain 18:299–314, 1984
31. DeJong RH: Defining pain terms. JAMA 244:143, 1980
32. Donovan WH, Dimitrijevic MR, Dahm L: Neurophysiological approaches to chronic pain following spinal cord injury. Paraplegia 20:135–146, 1982
33. Duckno PW, Margolis R, Tait RC: Psychological assessment in chronic pain. J Clin Psychol 41:499–504, 1985
34. Edeiken J, Shaber G: Thermography: A reevaluation. Skeletal Radiol 15:545–548, 1986
35. Edmeads J: The physiology of pain: A review. Prog Neuropsychopharmacol Biol Psychiatry 7:413–419, 1983
36. Edmonston W Jr: Hypnosis and Relaxation. New York, John Wiley & Sons, 1981
37. Eldred E, Lindsley DF, Buchwald JS: The effect of cooling on mammalian muscle spindles. Exp Neurol 2:144–157, 1960
38. Epstein E: Intralesional triamcinolone therapy in herpes zoster and post herpetic neuralgia. Ear Nose Throat Mon 52:416, 1973
39. Farkash AE, Portenoy RK: The pharmacological management of chronic pain in the paraplegic patient. J Am Paraplegia Soc 9:41–50, 1986
40. Fernandez E: A classification system of cognitive coping strategies for pain. Pain 26:141–151, 1986
41. Finlayson RE, Maruta T, Morse RM: Substance dependence and chronic pain: Experience with treatment and follow-up results. Pain 26:175–180, 1986
42. Fischer E, Solomon S: Physiological responses to heat and cold. In Licht S (ed): Therapeutic Heat and Cold, 2nd ed, pp 126–169. Baltimore, Waverly Press, 1965
43. Flor H, Haag G, Turk D: Long-term efficacy of EMG biofeedback for chronic rheumatic back pain. Pain 27:195–202, 1986
44. Foley KM: The treatment of cancer pain. New Engl J Med 313:84–95, 1985
45. Fordyce WE: Behavioral Methods for Chronic Pain and Illness, pp 41–221. St Louis, CV Mosby, 1976
46. Fordyce WE: Environmental factors in the genesis of low back pain. In Bonica J, Liebeskaind J, Albe-Fessard B (eds): Advances in Pain Research and Therapy, pp 659–666. New York, Raven Press, 1979
47. Fordyce W, McMahon R, Rainwater G: Pain complaint—Exercise performance, relationship and chronic pain. Pain 10:311–321, 1981
48. Freidberg SR: Neurosurgical treatment of pain caused by cancer. Med Clin North Am 59:481–485, 1975
49. Frymoyer JW, Newberg A, Pope MH: Spine radiographs in patient with low back pain. J Bone Joint Surg 66A:1048–1055, 1984
50. Fulton WM: Psychological strategies and techniques in pain management. Semin Anesth 4:247–254, 1985
51. Ghostine SY, Comair YG, Turner DM et al: Phenoxybenzamine in the treatment of causalgia—Report of 40 cases. J Neurosurg 60:1263–1268, 1984
52. Grabois M: Pain clinics—Role in the rehabilitation of patients with chronic pain. Ann Acad Med 12:428–433, 1983
53. Granger C (ed): Functional Assessment in Rehabilitation. Baltimore, Williams & Wilkins, 1984
54. Grant AE: Massage with ice in the treatment of painful conditions of the musculoskeletal system. Arch Phys Med Rehabil 45:233–238, 1964
55. Gross D: Pain and autonomic nervous system. Adv Neurol 4:93–104, 1974
56. Guck TP, Meilman PW, Skultety FM, Dowd ET: Prediction of long-term outcome of multidisciplinary pain treatment. Arch Phys Med Rehabil 67:293–296, 1986
57. Gunn CC, Milbrandt WE, Little AS, Mason KE: Dry needling of muscle motor points for chronic low back pain. Spine 5:279–290, 1980
58. Hachen HA: Psychological, neuropsychological, and therapeutic aspects of chronic pain — Preliminary results with transcutaneous electrical stimulation. Paraplegia 15:357–367, 1977
59. Halpern L: Substitution-detoxification and its role in the management of chronic benign pain. J Clin Psychiatry 43:10–14, 1982
60. Hannington-Kiff JG: Intravenous regional sympathetic block with guanethidine. Lancet 1:1019–1020, 1974
61. Hitselberger WE, Witten RM: Abnormal myelograms in asymptomatic patients. J Neurosurg 28:204–206, 1968
62. Holt EP: The question of lumbar discography. J Bone Joint Surg 50A:720–726, 1968
63. Horal J: The clinical appearance of low back disorders in the city of Gothenburg, Sweden. Acta Orthop Scand (Suppl) 118:8–73, 1969
64. Houde RW: The use and misuse of narcotics in the treatment of chronic pain. Adv Neurol 4:527–536, 1974
65. Houde RW, Wallenstein SL, Beaver WT: Evaluation of analgesics in patients with cancer pain. In Lasagna L (ed): International Encyclopedia of Pharmacology and Therapeutics. New York, Pergamon Press, 1966
66. Huber SL, Hill CS: Pharmacologic management of cancer pain. Cancer Bull 32:183–185, 1980
67. Infante M: Sexual dysfunction in the patient with chronic back pain. Sex Disabil 4:173–178, 1981
68. Jaffe J: Drug addiction and drug abuse. In Goodman LS, Gillman A: The pharmacological basis of therapeutics, pp 284–324. New York, Macmillan, 1985
69. Jensen TS, Krebs B, Nielsen J, Rasmussen P: Immediate and long term phantom limb pain in amputees—Incidence, clinical characteristics, and relationship to preamputation limb pain. Pain 21:267–278, 1985
70. Kanner RM, Foley KM: Patterns of narcotic drug use in cancer pain clinic. NY Acad Sci 362:161–172, 1981
71. Kelly DD: Central representations of pain and analgesia. In Kandel

ER, Schwartz JH: Principles of Neural Science, pp 331–343. New York, Elsevier/North Holland, 1985

72. Kendall HO, Kendall FP, Boynton DA: Posture and pain. New York, Robert E Krieger, 1952

73. Kimura J: Electrodiagnosis in Diseases of Nerve and Muscle: Principles and Practice. Philadelphia, FA Davis, 1983

74. Kottke FJ, Pauley DL, Rudolph PA: The rational for prolonged stretching for correction of shortening of connective tissue. Arch Phys Med Rehabil 47:345–352, 1966

75. Kraus H: Therapeutic exercise, 2nd ed. Springfield, IL, Charles C Thomas, 1963

76. Kraus H: Triggerpoints. NY State J Med 73:1310–1314, June 1, 1973

77. Kroening RJ: Pain clinics structure and function. Semin Anesth 4:231–236, 1985

78. Kruger L, Mantyh P: Changing concepts in the anatomy of pain. Semin Anesth 4:209–217, 1985

79. Lamid S, Chia JK, Kohli A, Cid E: Chronic pain in spinal cord injury: Comparison between inpatients and outpatients. Arch Phys Med Rehabil 66:777–778, 1985

80. Landen BR: Heat or cold for the relief of low back pain? Phys Ther 47:1126–1128, 1967

81. Lehmann JF, DeLateur RJ: Therapeutic Heat and Cold, 3rd ed. Baltimore, Williams & Wilkins, 1982

82. Lehmann JF, DeLateur BJ: Ultrasound, shortwave, superficial heat and cold in the treatment of pain. In Wall PD, Melzack R (eds): Textbook of Pain, pp 717–723. New York, Churchill Livingstone, 1984

83. Lewis R Jr, Racz G, Fabian G: Therapeutic approaches to reflex sympathetic dystrophy of the upper extremity. Clin Iss Reg Anesth 1:1–6, 1985

84. Liebeskind J, Sherman J, Cannon JT, Terman G: Neural and neurochemical mechanisms of pain inhibition. Semin Anesth 4:218–222, 1985

85. Lorenz KY: Acupuncture: A neuromodulation technique for pain control. In Aronoff GM (ed): Evaluation and Treatment in Chronic Pain, pp 539–547. Baltimore, Urban & Schwarttenberg, 1985

86. Mahoney L, McCullough J, Csima A: Thermography as a diagnostic aid in sciatica. Orthop Trans 7:104, 1983

87. Mannheimer JS, Lampe GN: Clinical Transcutaneous Electrical Nerve Stimulation. Philadelphia, FA Davis, 1984

88. Marks RW, Sacher EJ: Undertreatment of medical patients with narcotic analgesia. Ann Int Med 78:173–181, 1973

89. Maruta T, Swanson DW, Finlayson RE: Drug abuse and dependency in patients with chronic pain. Mayo Clin Proc 54:241–244, 1979

90. McGivney WT, Crooks GM: The case of patients with severe chronic pain in terminal illness. JAMA 251:1182–1188, 1984

91. Melzack R (ed): Pain Management and Assessment. New York, Raven Press, 1983

92. Melzack R: Acupuncture and related forms of folk medicine. In Wall PD, Melzack R (eds): Textbook of Pain, pp 691–700. New York, Churchill Livingstone, 1984

93. Melzack R, Stillwell DM, Fox EJ: Trigger points and acupuncture points for pain: Correlations and implications. Pain 3:3–23, 1977

94. Melzack R, Wall PD: Pain mechanisms: A new theory. Science 150:971–977, 1965

95. Mendel CM, Klein RF, Chappell DA: A trial of amitriptyline and fluphenazine in the treatment of painful diabetic neuropathy. JAMA 255:637–639, 1986

96. Mennell JM: The therapeutic use of cold. JAMA 74:1146–1157, 1975

97. Mense S: Effects of temperature on the discharge of muscle spindles and tendon organs. Pflugers Arch 375:159–166, 1978

98. Merskey H (ed): Classification of chronic pain—Descriptions of chronic pain syndromes and definitions of pain terms. Pain (Suppl)3:S1–S225, 1986

99. Meyer GA, Fields HL: Causalgia treated by selective large fiber stimulation of peripheral nerve. Brain 95:163–168, 1972

100. Mills GH, Davies GH, Getty CJM, Conway J: The evaluation of liquid crystal thermography in the investigation of nerve root compression due to lumbosacral lateral spinal stenosis. Spine 11:427–432, 1986

101. Moertel CG: Relief of pain with oral medications. Aust NZ J Med 6:1–8, 1976

102. Morely GK, Erickson DL, Morley JE: The neurology of pain. In Baker AB, Joynt RJ (eds): Clinical Neurology, chap 18, pp 1–81. Philadelphia, Harper & Row, 1986

103. Nicholos JA, Hershman EB: The lower extremity and spine in sports medicine. St Louis, CV Mosby, 1986

104. O'Brien JP: Mechanisms of spinal pain. In Wall PD, Melzack R (eds): Textbook of Pain, pp 240–251. New York, Churchill Livingstone, 1984

105. Oh, SH: Clinical Electromyography. Baltimore, University Park Press, 1984

106. Ottoson D: The effects of temperature on the isolated muscle spindle. J Physiol 180:636–648, 1965

107. Pagni CA: Central pain due to spinal cord and brain stem damage. In Wall PD, Melzack R (eds): Textbook of Pain, pp 481–495. London, Churchill Livingstone, 1984

108. Pegg SMG, Littler TR, Littler EN: A trial of ice therapy and exercise in chronic arthritis. Physiotherapy 55:51–56, 1969

109. Peteet J, Tay V, Cohen G, MacIntyre J: Pain characteristics and treatment in an outpatient cancer population. Cancer 57:1259–1265, 1986

110. Portnow JM, Strassman HD: Medically induced drug addiction. Int J Addiction 20:605–611, 1985

111. Powers JH: The abuse of rest as a therapeutic measure in surgery. JAMA 125:1079, 1944

112. Raferty A: The management of postherpetic pain using sodium valproate and amitriptyline. Irish Med J 72:399–401, 1979

113. Raj PP, Ramamurthy S: Differential nerve block studies. In Raj PP (ed): Practical Management of Pain, pp 173–177. Chicago, Year Book Medical Publishers, 1986

114. Rall TW, Schleifer LF: Drugs effective in the therapy of epilepsies. In Goodman L, Gillman A: The Pharmacological Basis of Therapeutics, pp 201–226. New York, Macmillan, 1986

115. Ramamurthy S, Winnie AP: Diagnostic maneuvers in painful syndromes. In Stein JM, Warfield CA (eds): International Anesthesiology Clinics, Pain Management, pp 47–50. Boston, Little, Brown, 1983

116. Ramamurthy S, Winnie AP: Regional anesthetic techniques for pain relief. Semin Anesth 4:237–246, 1985

117. Ready LB, Kozody R, Barsa JE, Murphy TM: Trigger point injections versus jet injection in the treatment of myofascial pain. Pain 15:201–206, 1983

118. Reiner S, Rogoff JB: Instrumentation. In Johnson EW (ed): Practical electromyography, pp 338–393. Baltimore, Williams & Wilkins, 1980

119. Rowat KM, Knafl KA: Living with chronic pain: The spouse's perspective. Pain 23:259–271, 1985

120. Rowlingson JC, Chalkley J: Common pain syndromes—Diagnosis and management. Semin Anesth 4:223–230, 1985

121. Scavone JG, Latshaw RF, Rohrer GV: The use of lumbar spine films—Statistical Evaluation at a university teaching hospital. JAMA 246:1105–1108, 1981

122. Schmidt RF: Somatovisceral sensibility: Cutaneous senses, proprioception, pain. In Schmidt RF, Thews G (eds): Human Physiology, pp 224–233. New York, Springer-Verlag, 1983

123. Seres JS, Newman RI: Negative influence of the disability compensation system—Perspectives for the clinician. Semin Neurol 3:360–369, 1983

124. Sharap AD: The knowledge, attitudes, and experience of medical personnel treating pain in the terminally ill. Mt Sinai J Med 45:561–580, 1978

125. Sherman RA, Sherman CJ: Prevalence and characteristics of chronic phantom limb pain among American veterans. Am J Phys Med 62:227–238, 1983

127. Sherman R, Sherman C, Gall N: A survey of current phantom limb treatment in the United States. Pain 8:85–99, 1980

126. Sherman RA, Sherman CJ: A comparison of phantom sensations among amputees whose amputations were of civilian and military origins. Pain 21:91–97, 1985

128. Sherman RA, Sherman CJ, Parker L: Chronic phantom and stump pain among American veterans—Result of a survey. Pain 18:83–95, 1984

129. Shoichet RP: Sodium amytal in the diagnosis of chronic pain. Can Psychiatr Assoc J 23:219–228, 1978

130. Sjolund BH, Eriksson MBE: Endorphins and analgesia produced by peripheral conditioning stimulation. In Bonica JJ, Abe-Fessard D, Liebeskind JC (eds): Advances in Pain Research and Therapy, 3rd ed, pp 587–599. New York, Raven Press, 1979
131. Smith G, Covino BG: Acute Pain. London, Butterworth, 1985
132. Smith J: Relaxation Dynamics. IL, Research Press, 1985
133. Snow BR, Pinter I, Gusmorino P et al: Incidence of physical and psychosocial disabilities in chronic pain patients: Initial report. Bull Hosp Jt Dis Orthop Inst 46:22–30, 1986
134. Snyder SH: Opiate receptors and internal opiates. Sci Am 236:44–56, 1977
135. Sola AE: The treatment of myofascial pain syndromes. In Benedetti C, Chapman CR, Moricca G (eds): Advances in Pain Research and Therapy, pp 467–485. New York, Raven Press, 1984
136. Spangfort E: The lumbar disk herniation—A computer aided analysis of 2,504 operations. Acta Orthop Scand 142:1–95, 1972
137. Steinberg FU: The Immobilized Patient—Functional Pathology and Management. New York, Plenum Medical Book, 1980
138. Steinberg GG: Epidemiology of low back pain. In Stanton-Hicks M, Boas R (eds): Chronic Low Back Pain, pp 1–13. New York, Raven Press, 1982
139. Stimmel B: Pain, analgesia, and addiction: An approach to the pharmacologic management of pain. Clin J Pain 1:14–22, 1985
140. Strang JP: Chronic disability syndrome. In Aronoff GM (ed): Evaluation and Treatment of Chronic Pain, pp 603–624. Baltimore, Urban & Schwarzenberg, 1985
141. Swerdlow M: Anticonvulsant drugs in chronic pain. Clin Neuropharmacol 7:51–82, 1984
142. Taub A, Kane K: A history of local analgesia. Pain 1:125–138, 1975
143. Torda TA: Management of acute and post-operative pain. Int Anesth Clin 21:27–47, 1983
144. Travell J: Ethyl chloride spray for painful muscle spasm. Arch Phys Med Rehabil 33:291–298, 1952
145. Travell JG, Ringer SH: The myofascial genesis of pain. Postgrad Med 11:425–434, 1952
146. Travell JG, Simons DG: Myofascial pain and dysfunction—The trigger point manual. Baltimore, Williams & Wilkins, 1983
147. Twycross RG, Lack SA: Symptom control and far advanced cancer: Pain relief. London, Pitman, 1984
148. Wallis C: Unlocking pain's secrets. Time 123(24):58–66, 1984
149. Walsh PD: Antidepressants in chronic pain. Clin Neuropharmacol 6:271–295, 1983
150. Watkins LR, Mayer DJ: Organization of endogenous opiate and non-opiate pain control systems. Science 216:11–85, 1982
151. Wells P: Movement education and limitation of movement. In Wall PD, Melzack R (eds): Textbook of Pain, pp 741–750. New York, Churchill Livingstone, 1984
152. White PF: Patient-controlled analgesia: A new approach to the management of postoperative pain. Semin Anesth 4:255–266, 1985
153. Wiesel SW, Tsourmas N, Feffer H: A study of computer assisted thermography—The incidence of positive CAT scans in an asymptomatic group of patients. Spine 9:549–551, 1984
154. Woolf C: Transcutaneous and implanted nerve stimulation. In Wall PD, Melzack R (eds): Textbook of Pain, pp 679–680. New York, Churchill Livingstone, 1984
155. Woolsey RM: Chronic pain following spinal cord injury. J Am Paraplegia Soc 9:51–53, 1986
156. Yel C, Gonyea M, Lemke J, Volpe M: Physical therpy: Evaluation and treatments of chronic pain. In Aronoff GM (ed): Evaluation and treatment of Chronic Pain, pp 251–261. Baltimore, Urban & Schwarzenberg, 1985
157. Young PA: The anatomy of the spinal cord pain paths—A review. J Am Paraplegia Soc 9:28–38, 1986
158. Ysla R, McAvley R: Effects of low power infra-red laser stimulation on carpal tunnel syndrome: A double blind study. Arch Phys Med Rehabil 66:577, 1985

37

Rehabilitation of the Patient With Lower Back Pain

Toni Jo Hanson

John L. Merritt

Lower back pain is among the most common clinical problems. Eighty percent of Americans will experience, at some time during their lives, lower back pain sufficient to disrupt their job or normal daily activities. Approximately 2½ million Americans have an impairment related to chronic back pain. It is the leading cause of worker's compensation expenditure and ranks second as a cause of lost work time. However, only a very small percentage of patients with back pain account for the major portion of these compensation costs.[18, 34, 61, 66, 68, 112, 134, 135]

Establishing an appropriate and effective management strategy for back pain is therefore essential for proper patient care, both by the primary care physician as well as the specialist who manages musculoskeletal disorders, such as the physiatrist, neurologist, rheumatologist, or orthopedic surgeon.[81, 87, 98, 100] This chapter will provide a practical guide for the evaluation, diagnosis and rehabilitation of the patient with lower back pain.

PATIENT EVALUATION

The examination of the back can be an intimidating, expensive, and time-consuming process. A large array of historical, physical, and special diagnostic tests are available and have been described in voluminous articles and books on back pain.[32, 49, 68, 82, 84, 113, 119, 134, 138] Most back pain syndromes can, however, be readily defined by developing a systematic history and physical examination and by plain radiographs; complex, expensive, and invasive procedures can be avoided in most cases. The keys to such a practical and efficient evaluation are a systematic approach and careful interpretation of symptoms and signs.

HISTORY

Obtaining a history from the lower back pain patient can be especially tedious, unproductive, and time-consuming if the examiner does not proceed in a systematic fashion. Key questions must be asked and responses recorded and interpreted.

After a review of the significant past medical history, specific inquiries are made regarding the back pain. The onset and duration of symptoms, frequency of painful episodes, factors that increase and decrease the pain, and previous interventions and treatments and their effects are essential components of the history. Mode and manner of onset and rapidity of symptom development and evolution are requisites to understanding the pathomechanics of the back pain.[113] Previous back pain episodes and their outcome should be recorded.

Inquiries should include these questions:

- Does lying down, sitting, standing, walking, bending, lifting, or changing positions increase or decrease your pain?
- Is your pain worse or better during sleep?
- Does the pain waken you?
- What do you do when you have pain to get relief?
- What medications are you currently taking?
- What medications have you tried?

Information about analgesics, including narcotics, steroids, nonsteroidal anti-inflammatory drugs, and muscle relaxants may need specific inquiry. The history should include past diagnostic tests and results as well as previous treatments, including physical therapies and chiropractic or surgical interventions and their responses. Past physical therapy needs additional specific delineation and should include questions about heat, diathermy, ultrasound, electrical stimulation, cryotherapy, massage, exercises, orthoses, education, manipulation, and traction and the results of these treatments. The impact on the patient's ability to perform activities of daily living, including vocational and avocational activities, must be recorded. Information on the type of work, days of missed work, and current status of employment can provide a basis for the patient's comprehensive rehabilitation. Worker's compensation or litigation issues should be defined.[22, 115, 134] These issues may surface in the initial interview, but not always as a conscious omission by the patient. Demographic data on the patient will include age, sex, type of work, specific tasks involved in work, and recreational activities.

Localization of pain is important. It is best defined by asking the patient to point to the affected sites. This area of pain is then recorded by the examiner on a diagram (Fig. 37-1A). We find it useful to record these sites with a red pen or pencil. Later, during the examination, areas of tenderness can be added to the same diagram with red "X" marks. This diagram is useful in developing an overall gestalt of the pain as well as providing a quick visual reference for subsequent evaluations.

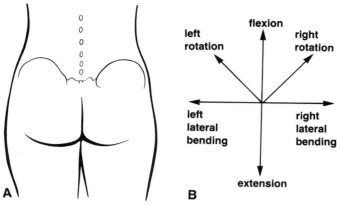

Figure 37-1. Localization of pain diagrams. (*A*) Regions of pain are marked, as indicated by patient. (*B*) Record of degree and direction of painful arcs of spinal motion: 0 = normal arc of motion, −1 = 25% reduction, −2 = 50% reduction, −3 = 75% reduction, −4 = total lack of motion in the corresponding arc; short intersecting lines indicate pain in the respective arc of motion.

In addition, some investigators find a patient-completed pain drawing can be helpful in describing characteristics of the pain, such as pain quality (sharp, dull) and presence of radiation. These pain drawings can also provide insight into nonorganic components and somatization of symptoms.[109]

Data on the presence of gait difficulties, numbness and tingling, weakness, muscle atrophy, and bowel, bladder, and sexual dysfunctions are essential in ruling out a neurological component. Increased pain or radiation of pain with coughing, sneezing, or the Valsalva maneuver may point to nerve root irritation, but may also occur in nonradicular, acute back pain syndromes.

Specific questioning about constipation should be included, since pain, inactivity, and many medications and, less frequently, neurological impairments may predispose to constipation. In the presence of straining associated with constipation, the pain may increase.

EXAMINATION

Just as a systematic history is important, so too is a methodical back examination. The first and often most important clue to the back examination is the simple, overall observation of the patient: posture, carriage, movement, and expressions. These general, usually subliminal, observations can, however, be biased by the physician's own recent experiences as well as his or her changing moods. Therefore, a number of conscious, specific observations need to supplement the overall impression. These specific observations should be recorded as objectively as is practical.

A useful objective clinical scoring system for nonorganic findings has been developed by Waddell.[130] This system can be incorporated into the physical examination. One point each is given for nonorganic (1) tenderness, (2) regionalization, (3) simulation, (4) overreaction, and (5) distraction. A score of "3" or more has been shown to represent significant manifestations of chronic pain behavior and indicates a need for further psychological assessment as part of the rehabilitation plan.

Gait

Observation of gait should include notation of velocity, cadence, and patterns of motion of the lower extremities, pelvis, and trunk. Gait velocity is usually decreased in the presence of back pain.

Nonorganic and hysterical components are usually obvious to the trained observer and can be differentiated from true antalgic patterns. An antalgic gait is one distinguished by the avoidance of pain. Weight-bearing on a painful extremity (foot, ankle, knee, hip) is characterized by a short stance phase on the affected side; hip disease can be identified by a concomitant lateral lurch (lateral shift of the center of gravity) during stance phase. In contrast, antalgic gaits of spinal origin are characterized by short steps with equal stance phase and a reduced cadence. The hips, knees, and trunk are usually slightly flexed, and the trunk is held rigidly in an effort to avoid the usual trunk and pelvic rotations.

Weakness, trunk lurches, foot drop, and lack of push-off will offer tips to neurological involvement before the formal neurological portion of the examination. Heel and toe walking can augment these findings and may provide insight into lesser degrees of weakness not detectable on manual muscle testing.

Posture

Clinical observations of posture have been described[32, 113] and can be supplemented with objective measurements using a large array of complex devices and gadgets that have appeared over the years. Quantification of posture, however, is also possible with a number of simple and reliable tests.[80, 85]

On the assumption that the curvature of the spinal segment can be determined by the angle formed by the tangent of one point on the curve with the tangent of another point on the curve, Loebl described a method of measuring four spinal segments using a commercially available gravity inclinometer (Fig. 37-2). We have found these simple measures to be quite reproducible and useful in documenting changes in posture. The gravity inclinometer measurement of lumbar lordosis, when combined with a simple measurement of lumbar depth and an overall visual observation, can provide quick and useful documentation of posture. Pelvic obliquity, muscular atrophy, listing, scoliosis, and kyphosis can similarly be measured when they are observed.

Spinal Motion

Spinal and trunk mobility can similarly be quantified by a number of simple and repeatable tests. The most popular measure of spinal mobility, the fingertip-to-floor test, is not, however, reliable. We studied its repeatability in 50 normal subjects and found the coefficient of variation to be over 80%.[85] The test is greatly affected by factors such as hip and lower extremity flexibility.

The modified Schober test is a quick, simple, and repeatable method of quantifying lumbar spine flexion (Fig. 37-3). It can be readily incorporated into the general back examination. A number of other skin distraction methods described by Moll and associates measure spine extension and lateral flexion.

Because limitation of spinal motion has been shown to correlate with the presence of lower back disability, accurate measurement of spinal motion is becoming increasingly important.[83, 107, 126] Some disability guidelines include the measurement of spinal motion in the calculation of disability and impairment.

Although it is not an accurate method of quantifying motion of the lumbar spine, a diagram of spinal motion can provide a quick visual reference of degree and direction of restricted arcs of spinal motion (Fig. 37-1B). Painful arcs can be added to the motion diagrams to provide the examiner with an overall visual impression, which is useful in the differential diagnosis of a number of common lower back syndromes.

Palpation

Palpation is an essential, but often overlooked, component of the lower back examination.[84, 113, 114] Foci of tenderness and the presence of spasm and abnormal contour require a careful hands-on evaluation. This is often best performed by a comparison of findings in standing and prone relaxed positions. After gentle palpation of the spine and of the paraspinal muscles, areas of tenderness to percussion should be noted.

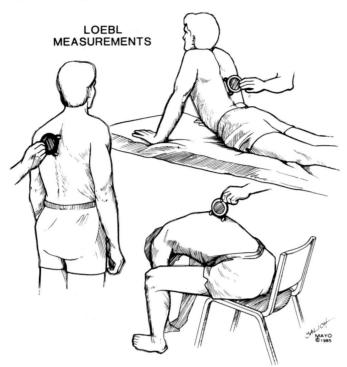

Figure 37-2. Loebl measurements. Spinal tangents are measured with an engineer's inclinometer. From these measurements, curvature of spinal segments is calculated. (Merritt JL, McLean TJ, Erickson RP, et al.: Measurement of trunk flexibility in normal subjects: Reproducibility of three clinical methods. Mayo Clinic Proceedings 61:192–197, 1986. By permission of the Mayo Foundation.)

Figure 37-3. Modified Schöber flexion test. (*A*) With subject standing erect but relaxed, top of sacrum (0) is identified by the spinal intersection of a horizontal line joining the dimples of Venus, and points 10 cm above and 5 cm below are marked. (*B*) Subject bends forward maximally, and distance between the upper and lower marks is measured in centimeters. This value minus 15 represents lumbar flexion. (Merritt JL, McLean TJ, Erickson RP, et al.: Measurement of trunk flexibility in normal subjects: Reproducibility of three clinical methods. Mayo Clinic Proceedings 61:192–197, 1986. By permission of the Mayo Foundation.)

Segmental instability, common in degenerative disease of the lower lumbar disks, can be suspected by the presence of a positive Larson test, performed with the patient in a prone position. Tenderness elicited with pressure over the spinous processes of the involved segment is reduced or eliminated with active splinting of the segment. (This only occurs with an unstable spine segment.) Tenderness from soft tissue injuries will persist despite active splinting.

Muscle spasm is best defined by the presence of a persistent, palpable increase in muscle tone accompanied by localized tenderness. In the presence of chronic lower back pain, the examiner may detect tenderness in muscle attachment sites of the pelvis and hip, including the regions of the trochanteric and ischial bursae. Lowered pain threshold, altered gait and spinal mechanics, secondary muscle and soft tissue contractures, prolonged sitting, and sleeping in a fetal position may all contribute to such localized soft tissue tenderness. These must be carefully defined, however, because they may be important secondary sources of pain. Frequently, they become a major contributor to the pain. In addition, they are generally amenable to physiatric interventions.

A digital rectal evaluation should not be dismissed, since it can detect pelvic floor myalgia or other pelvic pathology.[45, 118] In addition to the traditional rectal examination, gentle and systematic palpation of the coccyx, sacrum, levator ani, coccygeus, and pyriformis muscles and their associated ligaments and attachments should be performed.

Neurological Assessments

A quick systematic neurological examination is mandatory. This includes manual muscle testing of the trunk and lower extremities, testing of the deep tendon reflexes and Babinski reflex and a sensory survey. Straight leg raising tests (SLR) are performed to detect nerve root irritation.[65] The classic positive SLR is a reproduction of radicular pain at 30°. Radicular pain reproduced at greater angles probably represents less significant nerve root irritation. Back and leg pain can be produced in the absence of nerve root irritation.[52, 59, 60] Nonradicular pain may be caused by soft tissue tightness or spasms in the back, glutei, or hamstrings. The location and angle of occurrence of pain should be recorded in an effort to distinguish true radicular pain from soft tissue pain.

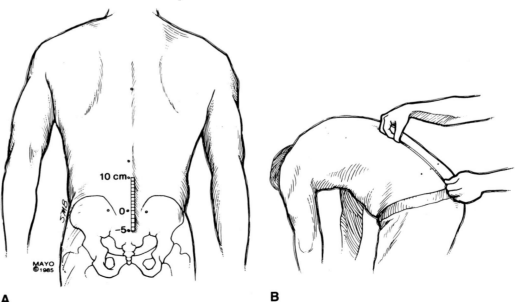

A

B

Even with a soft tissue pain source, the SLR can still be used as an index of improvement during treatment. The crossed SLR test, the "three-stage SLR," the "bowstring" test, Kernig test, and a number of other variations of the standard SLR test can be used as further confirmation of dural or root irritation. Of all the maneuvers performed during the physical examination, the positive crossed SLR test has the highest correlation with myelographic findings of a herniated disk (greater than 90%).[68] Significant inconsistency observed during sitting and supine SLRs may provide insight into psychogenic processes.[130] Electromyography is a valuable adjunct in delineation and confirmation of neurological findings.[125, 136]

Special Tests

Examination of the sacroiliac, hip, and other lower extremity joints may require special examination techniques, including the Fabere (Patrick), Gaenslen, and pelvic rock tests. The Hoover test is a technique of special interest and facilitates the detection of malingering because it allows the recognition of submaximal effort. The jolt test is a provocative method used to document pain enhancement or radiation due to sudden mechanical load-

ing of the erect spine. While standing on tiptoes, the patient is asked to suddenly drop to a foot-flat position. A positive jolt test is characterized by an exacerbation or radiation of pain.

Leg length can be measured from the anterior superior iliac spine to the prominence of the medial malleoli (true leg length) or from the umbilicus to the medial malleoli (apparent leg length).[113]

Trunk Strength

The lower back examination is not complete without an evaluation of the strength of the supporting musculature of the trunk. Abdominal muscles, back extensors, and lateral trunk muscles can be evaluated with the patient in a recumbent position. Abdominal strength can be assessed by asking the patient to attempt to sit up from a supine position; abdominal muscle strength can be graded as illustrated (Fig. 37-4):

Abdominal oblique muscles can be graded with the trunk rotated, as when the sit-up was performed.
A similar method can be used to grade back extensors. Lying prone with a pillow under the abdomen and hips, the

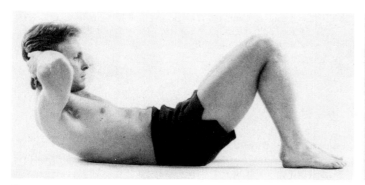

A

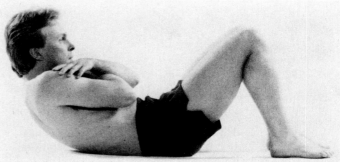

B

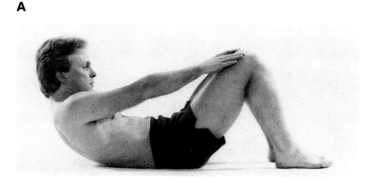

C

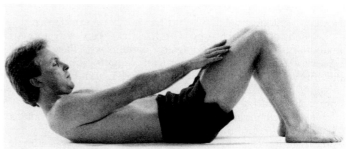

D

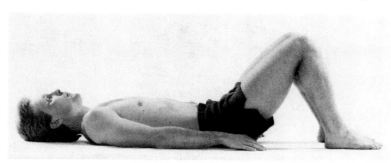

E

Figure 37-4. Grades of abdominal strength: (*A*) normal (ability to perform sit-up with hands and arms above the head); (*B*) good (ability to sit up with hands and arms folded across the chest); (*C*) fair (ability to sit up with arms extended parallel to the trunk); (*D*) poor (unable to perform sit-up with arms extended); (*E*) trace (palpable contractions only) or absent (no voluntary muscle contractions).

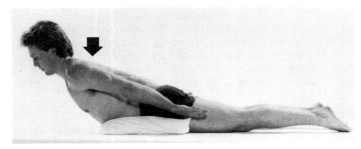

A

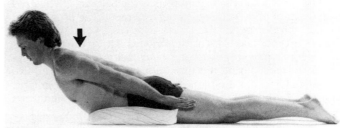

B

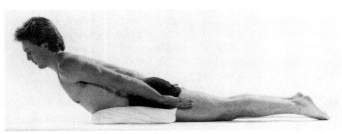

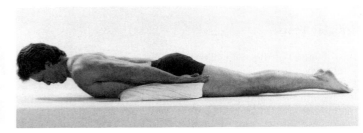

C

D

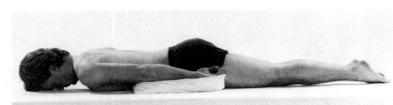

E

Figure 37-5. Grades of back extensor strength: (*A*) normal (full extension against maximal resistance); (*B*) good (full extension against some resistance); (*C*) fair (full extension but without resistance); (*D*) poor (unable to extend fully); (*E*) trace (palpable muscle contractions only) or absent (no detectable extensor muscle function).

patient is asked to extend his or her trunk and hold against resistance applied by the examiner (Fig. 37-5).

Lateral trunk muscles can be tested with the patient lying on his or her side; the patient is asked to flex the trunk laterally against gravity.

However, grading is difficult and has not been standardized.

Results of clinical testing of trunk muscles are only approximations and may be biased against patients who have a heavy upper torso or those with longer trunk lengths. The majority of patients will have good, fair, or poor grades, and these approximations are not sensitive enough to be useful in monitoring a comprehensive back rehabilitation program.

Recent technological developments, trunk dynamometers, are able to measure trunk strength with good repeatability in a clinical setting (Fig. 37-6).[56] Isometric, isotonic, and isokinetic trunk dynamometers are now available.[9, 102, 108, 123] One type of trunk dynamometer can measure trunk flexors, extensors, rotators, and lateral flexors simultaneously. Digital and graphic recordings during these evaluations can provide specific impulse, torque, power, movement, and velocity data. Graphic display of these data can be helpful in detecting patterns of effort and overall performance. This new technology may enable more precise prescription and monitoring of back rehabilitation programs.

Figure 37-6. Three-dimensional trunk dynamometer.

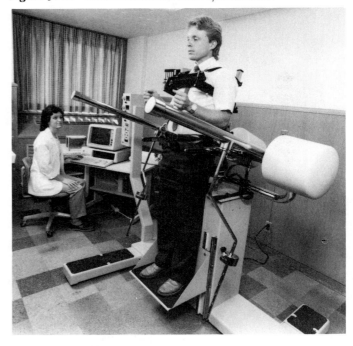

Radiological Tests

Modern technology has provided the clinician with increasingly sophisticated evaluation tools. The plain radiograph, however, remains the cornerstone of radiological tests. Standard antero-

posterior (AP) and lateral spine films can provide much useful information.[52, 140] These films allow visualization of degenerative disk disease (Fig. 37-7), spondylitis (Fig. 37-8), compression fractures, metabolic bone disorders, bone tumors, congenital anomalies, transitional vertebrae, Schmorl's nodes (Fig. 37-9A), and scoliosis. Focused views and oblique views of the lumbosacral level (Fig. 37-10 & 37-11), which allow visualization of the facet and sacroiliac joints, can be added. Flexion-extension views are frequently added whenever spinal instability is suspected. Computed tomography (CT) is helpful in further defini-

tion of a localized process (Fig. 37-12). However, care must be taken in ascribing specific symptomatology to these radiological findings.

Computed tomography (CT), myelography (with or without CT) (Fig. 37-13), isotopic bone scans, and magnetic resonance imaging (MRI) are now allowing increasingly refined definition of soft tissues, including intervertebral disks, nerve roots, intraspinal contents, and surrounding muscle, fascia, and ligaments.[11, 13, 47, 75, 124] Interpretation of these newer techniques also requires special skills and experience to properly correlate findings with clinical pictures.[2, 12, 14, 40, 89, 127] One illustration of too much reliance on radiological techniques for diagnosis is diskography. Diskography, a visualization technique of specific lumbar disks, seemed promising a few years ago. Now, however, it is infrequently performed because it fails to differentiate between symptomatic and asymptomatic disk disease.

The majority of back pain patients will not require sophisticated radiological evaluation beyond the basic AP, lateral, and oblique x-rays. The careful clinical examination is still, and is likely to long remain, the basis of diagnosis and management of the patient with lower back pain.

DIFFERENTIAL DIAGNOSIS

Clues to diagnosis in the patient with lower back pain are assembled in an ongoing fashion by the clinician during the complete history and physical evaluation process. Differential diagnosis of lower back pain includes an especially large array of regional and referred etiologies (Table 37-1). Although the list is long, the vast majority of cases will fit within a few diagnostic categories (Table 37-2).[41, 76, 113, 119, 128, 129]

Eight common syndromes presented next as case studies illustrate principles that should be helpful in differentiating among lower back pain syndromes and in constructing effective, specific rehabilitation programs.

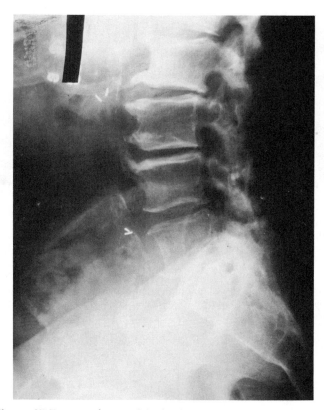

Figure 37-7. Lateral view of the lumbar spine demonstrating multi-level disk space narrowing, a vacuum sign at the L3 interspace, osteophytosis, and low-grade spondylolisthesis of L2 on L3.

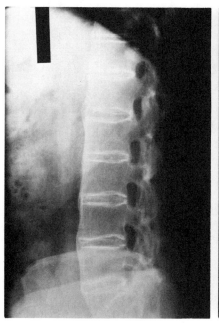

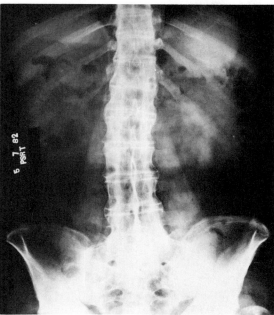

A **B**

Figure 37-8. (*A*) A lateral x-ray film demonstrating classical bony changes of far-advanced ankylosing spondylitis including calcification of the anterior longitudinal ligament, squaring of the vertebral bodies, and fusion of the facet joints with progressive loss of spinal motion (bamboo spine). (*B*) AP view of the same patient. Note obliteration of sacroiliac joints and syndesmophyte formation laterally along the vertebral bodies.

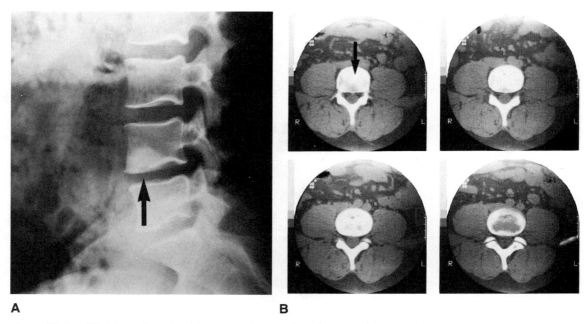

A   **B**

Figure 37-9. (*A*) Schmorl's node with surrounding reactive sclerosis and associated narrowing of fourth lumbar interspace. Schmorl's nodes are usually an incidental finding and not generally considered a cause of back pain. (*B*) CT scans demonstrate reactive sclerosis surrounding Schmorl's node.

Figure 37-10.   Three-quarter view of lumbar spine demonstrates unilateral spondylolysis of the right L5 pars interarticularis. Note the normal pars interarticularis at the L3 and L4 levels.

Figure 37-11.   Left oblique radiograph demonstrating degenerative joint disease of the facets at the L3 , L4, and L5 levels; the L2 facet appears normal.

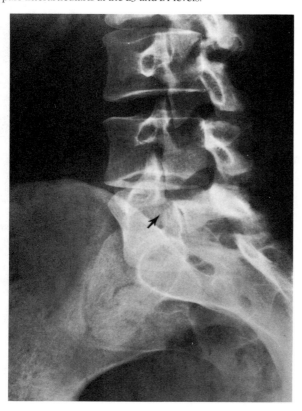

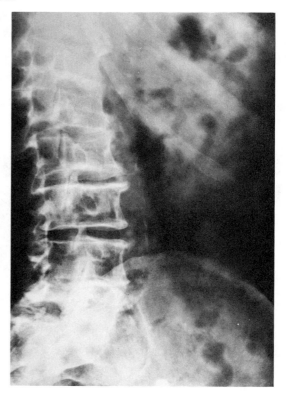

REHABILITATION OF COMMON BACK SYNDROMES

CASE 1

A 64-year-old computer executive and hobby farmer presents with a 5-year history of pain in the lower back and buttocks. He reports no acute precipitating event and describes an insidious onset and a gradually increasing intensity over this period. The pain is increased with prolonged standing or sitting, and especially when he is on his tractor. It decreases when he gets up or moves about, or if he lies down with his knees and hips flexed (in a fetal position). He has had 5 weeks of chiropractic adjustments and 6 sessions of ultrasound without benefit. There are no leg or foot radiating symptoms and no cough/sneeze effect is present.

On his examination, he identifies the pain as located in the lumbosacral triangle and upper buttocks. It is symmetrical. He has a mild reduction in lumbar flexion as well as right and left trunk rotation and a moderate reduction in lumbar extension

(*Text continues on page 736*)

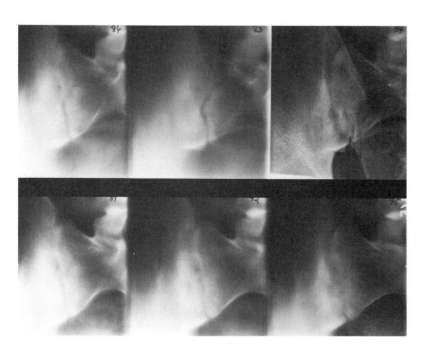

Figure 37-12. Tomograms of the right sacroiliac joint identify destructive arthritis.

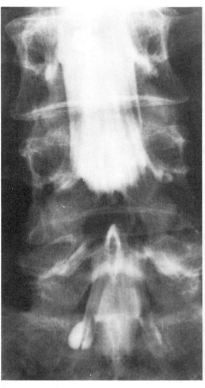

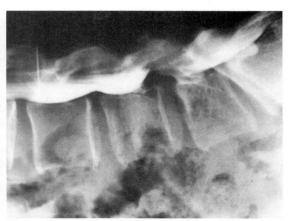

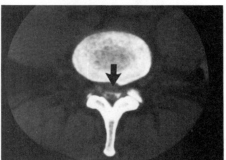

Figure 37-13. Large anterior extradural defect at L4 interspace on AP view (*A*) and lateral view (*B*) myelogram. (*C*) CT scan shows anterior epidermal soft tissue mass from a large central disk herniation.

B

A   C

Table 37–1
101 Causes of Lower Back Pain

Back strain syndromes
  Iliolumbar ligament
  Multifidus muscle
  Interspinous ligament
  Acute facet strain
  Sacroiliac strain
  Postural strain
  Annulus tear (?)
  Nonspecific strain
Chronic post-traumatic strain
Tension myalgia
  General
  Lumbar
Pelvic floor myalgia
Bursitis
  Trochanteric
  Ischial
  Multifidus
  Gluteal
  Interspinous
Compression fracture
  Osteoporosis
  Trauma
Ankylosing spondylitis
Other B-27 spondylitis variants
  Reiter's syndrome
  Psoriatic
  Juvenile rheumatoid
  Inflammatory bowel disease
Paget's disease
Infectious
  Tuberculous spondylitis
  Brucellar spondylitis
  Osteomyelitis
  Fungal
    Coccidioidomycosis
    Cryptococcosis
  Parasitic
    Echinococcosis
Disk space infection
Coccyx fracture/trauma
Osteitis condensans ilii
Sacroiliac instability
Referred
  Internal organ
    Thoracic, abdominal
    Retroperitoneal
    Cardiac
    Aortic (aneurysm)
    Renal
    Pancreatic
    Gastric
    Abscess, retroperitoneal
Protruded/herniated disk
Degenerative disk disease (DDD)
Facet degenerative joint disease (Facet DJD)
Segmental instability
Spondylolisthesis
Degenerative spondylolisthesis
Diffuse idiopathic skeletal hyperostosis (DISH,
  Forestier's)

Postoperative, chronic nonspecific
Leg length difference (>2 cm)
Psychogenic
  Somatization
  Learned pain behavior
Malingering
Spinal stenosis
  Lateral recess stenosis
Arachnoiditis
  Primary
  Secondary
  Postoperative
  Post-myelographic
Congenital
  Asymmetrical vertebrae
  Asymmetrical facets
  Other
Scoliosis
  Congenital and infantile
  Juvenile idiopathic
  Neuromuscular
  Degenerative
Scheuermann's juvenile kyphosis
Charcot's arthropathy (neuropathic arthropathy)
Metabolic
  Gout
  Chondrocalcinosis (pseudogout)
  Hemochromatosis
  Ochronosis
  Osteomalacia
    Primary (rickets)
    Secondary (renal)
Urologic
  Urolithiasis
  Infection
  Obstruction
Gynecologic
  Endometriosis
  Infection (PID)
  Tumor
  Ovarian
  Mittelschmerz
  Tubal
Tumor
  Lymphoma
  Myeloma
  Metastatic
    Breast
    Prostate
    Lung
    Thyroid
    Kidney
  Spinal, primary
    Benign
      Osteoid osteoma
    Malignant
      Sarcoma
      Chordoma
      Other
Calvé-Perthes disease, vertebra plana (aseptic
  necrosis)
Radiation necrosis
Neurofibromatosis (von Recklinghausen's
  disease)
Dysplasia

Table 37-2
15 Common Back Pain Syndromes

Cause	Pain (:⋰⋱:), Tenderness (x) Pattern	Painful Arc, ROM Diagram	Special Signs	Radiological Findings	Treatment
Disk herniation			List to contralateral side Loss of lordosis +/− Neuro signs + SLR Corkscrewing Antalgic gait	X-rays often normal +CT, MRI scans +Myelogram	Bed rest Traction (?) Extension exercises (?) Surgery Superficial heat
Degenerative disk disease			+ Larson test Incomplete reversal of lumbar lordosis	+ X-rays: narrow disk spaces hypertrophic changes facet sclerosis	Exercises: flexion isometrics Back school Reduction of spine stress Shoe inserts
Spondylolysthesis			Palpable "step-off" + Larson test	+ X-rays: lateral and oblique views	Exercises: flexion isometrics Back school Traction (?) Shoe inserts
Spinal stenosis			Pain (LB, legs) with walking Relief with rest & flexion Neg or subtle neuro signs: Babinski, increased reflexes	X-rays: Degenerative changes + CT scan + Myelogram	Surgery or trial of: Flexion exercises Shoe inserts, cane, corset, TENS
Tumors and other visceral sources			Constant or organ-specific pain Nocturnal pain Normal back examination	+/− X-rays +/− Bone scan CT or MRI scan may be indicated	Surgical or medical management
Strain syndrome: Multifidus muscle			List to ipsilateral side Antalgic gait Lordosis normal or increased Tenderness in multifidus muscle	Normal	Exercise: isometrics Short rest breaks Heat, massage Cryotherapy Injections Back school
Strain syndrome: Ilio-lumbar ligament			No list Tender in regions of origin & insertion of ligament Neg Larson test	Normal	Exercise: isometrics Short rest breaks Heat, massage Cryotherapy Injections Back school
Strain syndrome: Interspinous ligament			No list Localized tenderness in interspinous space Neg Larson test	Normal	Exercise: isometrics Short rest breaks Ultrasound Cryotherapy Injections Back school

(Continued)

Table 37-2—Continued

Cause	Pain (::::), Tenderness (x) Pattern	Painful Arc, ROM Diagram	Special Signs	Radiological Findings	Treatment
Strain syndrome: Acute facet		-2, -1, -2, -3, -1, -3	Sudden, non-traumatic onset; List to contralateral side; Characteristic painful arc pattern	Normal	Manipulation; Mobilization; Exercises: flexion, rotation, isometrics; Back school
Strain syndrome: Postural		0, 0, 0, 0, 0, 0	Pain on history only; Normal back examination; Poor posture & body mechanics	Normal	Posture principles; Back school; Lumbar roll; Special chair
Ankylosing spondylitis		-3, -2, -2, -3, -3, -3, -3	Morning stiffness; "Jelling"; Limited motion entire spine; + SI stress test; Loss of lordosis; Flexed posture	+ X-rays; + SI tomograms; Vertebral body "squaring"; "Bamboo" spine; Costovertebral & facet fusion	NSAIDs; Heat; Exercise: extensor strengthening; ROM; Flexor stretches; Posture training
Compression fracture, osteoporosis		-3, -1, -1, -2, -2, -2	Localized tenderness & paraspinal muscle spasms that correlate with X-ray findings	+ X-rays; + Bone scan; Decreased bone density (densitometry)	Limited bed rest; Limited corset use; Exercises: isometric extensor pectoral stretches; Posture training; Shoe inserts
Tension myalgia (fibrositis)		0, 0, 0, 0, 0, 0	Increased tenderness in multiple trigger points; Increased muscle "tone"; Sleep disorder	Normal	Reassurance; Relaxation training; Posture training; Heat & massage; Injections; Sleep Rx (Tricyclic Rx); Exercise (stretching/fitness)
Pelvic floor myalgia		0, 0, 0, 0, 0	Normal back examination; Tender pelvic floor muscles & attachments on rectal exam; + Pyriformis stretch test	Normal	Pelvic floor relaxation training; Short wave diathermy; Thiele's massage; Hydrotherapy
Chronic postoperative LBP		-3, -2, -2, -3, -3, -3	Multiple tender trigger points; Skin hyperesthesia; "Old" neuro findings	Postoperative & degenerative changes; Arachnoiditis on myelogram, CT, MRI	Exercises: strengthening isometrics; Fitness program; Back school; Pain management program

and lateral flexion bilaterally. The only arc of motion that causes increased pain is extension (Fig. 37-14). The Schober flexion test is 4.5 cm (normal is greater than 5 cm). Lumbar lordosis is normal but fails to reverse on full voluntary flexion. Gait, heel, and toe walking are normal; there is no list. Muscle testing and deep tendon reflexes are normal. Straight leg raising (80° bilateral) is limited by hamstring tightness. The jolt test is negative. The Larson test is positive at L5. Waddell score[130] is zero.

Radiological examination reveals narrowed disk spaces at L4–L5 and L5–S1, sclerosis of the facet joints, and "hypertrophic changes" (Fig. 37-15).

Diagnosis: Degenerative disk disease with associated degenerative joint disease of the lumbar facet joints.

Management/Discussion: Two primary functions of the intervertebral disk are to impart flexibility to the spine and to function as a shock absorber.[10, 17, 19] The latter role is thought to reduce mechanical stress on pain-sensitive structures that may be vulnerable to impact or torsion loading during daily activities. Pain-sensitive structures include the nerve root and its dural sheath, facet joints, vascular structures, periosteum, muscles, and

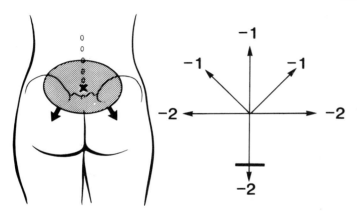

Figure 37-14. Patient exhibits tenderness localized at L5 and S1 spinous processes and increased pain on extension; Larson's test is positive. Diagnosis: degenerative disk disease with degenerative joint disease.

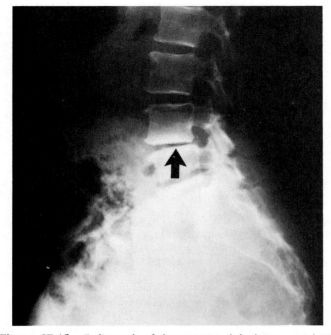

Figure 37-15. Radiograph of degenerative disk disease at L4–L5. Note vacuum sign, reactive sclerosis, and spondylolisthesis at the L4–L5 interspace (secondary to degenerative disease).

many ligaments.[30, 50] When disk material degenerates, there is a slow replacement of the soft semi-liquid, gel-like hydrophilic nucleus pulposus with a more dense, less hydrophilic, less compressible, and more granular fibrous tissue.[46, 58] The resultant decreased efficiency of the shock absorbing function of the disk may cause increased mechanical stresses on one or more pain-sensitive structures during daily activities that were previously well-tolerated. The increased density and reduced water content of these degenerated disks also result in narrowing of the intervertebral spaces. There is consequently a functional lengthening and, therefore, a laxity of ligaments and muscles that span those segments. This may further increase stresses on the same pain- or pressure-sensitive structures. Tolerance of vibration-related stresses is particularly reduced when degenerative disk disease is present. Degenerative disk disease is a consequence of the aging process and is therefore among the most common causes of mechanical back pain in middle-age or older patients.

The most popular of lower back exercises are Williams' exercises.[138] Although a variety of back exercises are known by that eponym, the original Williams' back exercises include only spinal flexion exercises. The rationale behind Williams' exercises is that flexing the spine and reducing lumbar lordosis will reduce axial loading on pain- and pressure-sensitive posterior spinal structures (such as the facet joints); this should in turn reduce pain due to mechanical loading of these structures.[25, 27, 93, 143] Back flexion exercises therefore continue to play a prominent role in the management of lower back pain secondary to degenerative disk disease.

Trunk strengthening exercises, in contrast, are designed to reduce mechanical stresses on pain-sensitive structures by improving the mechanical efficiency of the spinal-muscular support. Although the magnitude of such a muscular contribution is debated and to date has not been well-quantified, a role for trunk muscles in providing supplementary support of the spine has long been recognized and anatomically described.[121] Unless that role is shown to be insignificant, trunk strengthening exercises remain a rational addendum to a flexion exercise program. Particular attention should be given to strengthening the abdominal oblique muscles, if strengthening is prescribed, since they are the major contributor to increased intra-abdominal pressure generated by trunk muscles during heavy lifting.[91] Strengthening spinal extensors may also improve the efficiency of shock absorption by concentric and eccentric activity of the intersegmental spinal extensor muscles.[111] Trunk strengthening, when prescribed, should be predominantly isometric to reduce stresses during active flexion in isotonic activities such as sit-ups.

Lumbar supports can provide some reduction in mechanical stresses on the lumbar spine by providing a substitute for inactive or weak trunk musculature. Their judicious use may be reasonable, especially during heavy chores or during exposure to vibration, but it must be monitored and limited to short periods of time to prevent possible loss of strength and flexibility and possible psychological dependence. Lumbar rolls and pads are frequently used. These, when placed in a chair or seat, or when they are a part of the seat, can reduce axial loading on the spine and increase sitting tolerance.[3, 4, 5] Soft shock-absorbing shoe inserts have also been reported to reduce impact stresses on the feet and spine from walking and standing, thus reducing back pain associated with degenerative disk disease.[142]

Lumbar traction by simple bar hanging or pelvic gravity suspension, or other gravity or low-friction controlled methods, may reduce lumbar facet loading and segmental muscle spasm, widen the intervertebral space, and therefore temporarily reduce pain.[55, 78, 105] Traction may be empirically prescribed. If it is helpful and can be easily accomplished at home, it can be added to the patient's home treatment program. Nonsteroidal anti-inflammatory agents, heat, cold, and other nonspecific analgesic measures can also be added.

Essential interventions must include alterations in posture and improvements in body mechanics in order to best minimize mechanical stresses during daily activities. Efforts to teach body skills to the patient can be well provided through organized programs such as back schools.[31, 43, 44, 79, 110] Improvement in posture, body mechanics, and back skills are currently among the most readily demonstrated methods of reducing lumbar mechanical stresses.[33, 35, 48, 70]

A rational prescription for a patient with degenerative disk disease may therefore include the following:

- Flexion exercises
- Isometric strengthening of trunk muscles
- Bar-hanging traction
- Lumbar roll for sitting

- Lumbar support for repeated or heavier chores
- Shock-absorbing shoe inserts
- Heat, cryotherapy, and analgesics for acute flares
- Patient education in posture and body mechanics, including attendance in a back school or back skills program

CASE 2

A 23-year-old intensive care nurse with lower back and left buttock pain of 3-days' duration presents explaining that her pain began as she was bending over a bed transferring a patient. She felt a "pull" in her back and left buttock immediately after transfer, but developed a constant pain of increasing intensity over the remainder of the day. She finished the workday and went to bed early with a heating pad, but slept poorly. The next morning she was "stiff," called in sick, and stayed in bed for 2 days, with minimal improvement.

On examination, she localizes her pain in the lumbosacral triangle, left more than right, with extension into the left buttock and upper left posterior thigh. There is tenderness in the region of the left multifidus muscle. All lumbar motions are restricted 25 to 50% with painful arcs on flexion, extension, right lateral flexion, and right rotation (Fig. 37-16). There is a slight list to the left, slight antalgic gait, and a normal lordosis with incomplete reversal of lordosis on active trunk flexion. Schober flexion test is 4.6 cm; jolt and Larson's tests are negative. Manual muscle testing and deep tendon reflexes are normal. Straight leg raising tests are limited to 80° right and 70° left with back pain only on the left. The Waddell score is zero. Lumbar radiographs are normal (Fig. 37-17).

Diagnosis: Lumbosacral strain syndrome; multifidus strain.

Management/Discussion: Back strain syndromes are among the most common causes of back pain, clearly making up the majority of acute syndromes. Most are probably due to muscle and ligament strains or facet joint sprains. Most resolve spontaneously without sequelae and with a few days of rest or with curtailed activities. Bed rest has historically been prescribed for acute back strain syndromes. Bed rest is not, however, always necessary. In fact, the traditional full-week bed rest trial for acute

diskogenic disorders may be inappropriate for acute muscle, ligament, or facet strains. Recent studies have shown no advantage of a prolonged bed rest period.[21] Restricted activity with a prescription for a soft lumbosacral support, adherence to good posture, and care to observe proper body mechanics may be more beneficial. Local heat, cryotherapy, analgesics, and deep sedative massage may provide adjunctive, temporary relief.

These simple management methods are adequate for most,[53, 63, 71] but it has been argued that no medical intervention may have equally good results.[94, 95] This is logical, since muscle, ligament, and facet strains will heal as long as reinjury is avoided while healing is occurring. Some lumbosacral strain syndromes persist, however, and a few become chronic, possibly because of larger tears of muscles, ligaments, or the facet capsules or a reinjury before healing is complete.[92] Scarring and soft tissue contractures may further contribute to persistent pain. Prolonged or habitual muscle spasm may cause additional pain. An aggressive therapeutic program of deep heat, soft tissue mobilization, and muscle relaxation techniques, together with gentle but

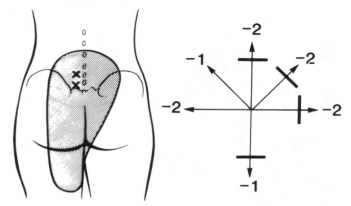

Figure 37-16.   Patient has tenderness in insertion and body of the multifidus muscle; lumbar antalgic gait; list to the left; negative Larson's test; pain on spinal flexion, extension, right lateral flexion, and right rotation. Diagnosis: left multifidus strain syndrome.

Figure 37-17. (A) Normal lumbar spine, lateral radiograph. (B) Normal lumbar spine, three-quarter view.

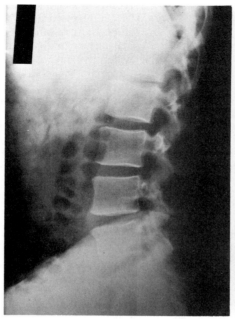

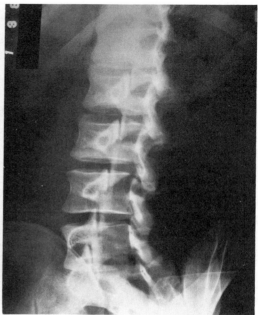

A   B

progressive lumbar stretching and isometric strengthening, may abort many of these more ominous chronic back strain syndromes. General strengthening with emphasis on knee extensor and leg strengthening, endurance training, and training in proper body mechanics and back skills are essential adjuvants in resolving and preventing more chronic pain states.

Early recognition and treatment of potentially chronic strains are skills obtained only by experience. Early referral for physiatric evaluation and intervention is warranted. Once such pain has become established, drug dependence, deconditioning, fear, and chronic pain behavior often become dominant features, and an inpatient pain management program may be required as part of a comprehensive rehabilitation program. Early, aggressive physiatric treatment in conjunction with maintenance of modified, appropriate work and activity levels is a requisite to the prevention of the evolution of simple back strain syndromes into chronic disabling pain.

CASE 3

A 32-year-old assembly-line worker in a tractor factory comes in for an evaluation of back and leg pain of 12 days' duration. While standing and bending over the assembly line, he noted a deep nagging pain in his left lower back and left posterior thigh. He finished his work day but was "stiff and sore" all evening and awoke frequently that night. On awakening the next morning, he was unable to straighten up and had pain in his left lower back, buttock, posterior thigh, calf, and heel. He saw his local physician who noted no weakness and prescribed 7 days of bed rest at home. He reported some improvement, but admitted that he had not actually been at absolute bed rest during most of the time, spending most of the day in a soft comfortable chair. He returned to work but could not complete the morning's work because of a full recurrence of his pain.

On examination, the patient localized his pain to the lumbosacral triangle (left greater than right), the left buttock, posterior thigh, and calf to the heel and lateral foot. There is a list toward the right, a loss of lumbar lordosis, and an antalgic gait. There is a marked restriction in trunk flexion and left lateral flexion due to pain and moderate reductions in all other arcs of motion (Fig. 37-18). The Schober flexion test is 1.5 cm, and the Larson's test is negative. The jolt test is positive with radiation. Manual muscle testing and knee reflexes are normal. The ankle jerk is diminished on the left, but is normal on the right. Left straight leg raising causes lower back, left leg, and foot pain at 30°. Right straight leg raising at 60° causes back pain only. The Waddell score is zero. Radiographs of the lumbar spine are normal.

Diagnosis: Acute lumbar disk protrusion suspected; acute left L5 or S1 radiculopathy.

Management/Discussion: Lumbar disk protrusions are due to degenerative or traumatic weakening and subsequent tearing of the annulus fibrosus.[38, 106] This usually occurs before degenerative fibrosis has occurred in the nucleus pulposus. Nucleus pulposus fragments then protrude posteriorly or posterolaterally and often impinge on pain-sensitive structures such as the nerve roots or dural sheaths.[24, 137] Pain, weakness, or numbness can result, with classic root signs as illustrated in this case.[7, 29, 62, 122]

The basic management principle is to reduce intradiskal pressure, thus allowing the nucleus material to retract and the associated edema of the nerve root to resolve.[16, 20, 101] Strict bed rest is the most effective way to reduce disk pressures for a prolonged time. Hospitalization may be warranted to enforce bed rest if it cannot be accomplished at home. Oral analgesics are appropriate. Muscle relaxants, such as benzodiazepines,

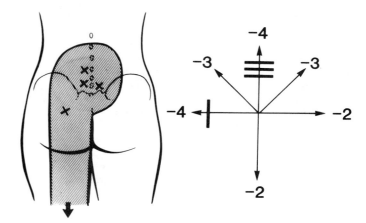

Figure 37-18. Patient complains of pain in the back, leg, calf, and feet. He lists to the right and has loss of lordosis, antalgic gait, marked loss of spinal motions in all planes, and decrease of pain with flexion or left lateral flexion. Straight leg raising causes pain 30° on the left. There is decreased ankle jerk reflex on left. Diagnosis: disk herniation suspected, left L5 on S1 radiculopathy.

have not been shown to be superior to aspirin, but their sedative side-effects may improve psychological tolerance to enforced bed rest. Generally, they should not be prescribed for more than 2 weeks. Local heat may be more effective and less addictive in reducing associated muscle spasms.

A bedside commode with armrests is preferable to bed pans for bowel and bladder care. Attention to proper body mechanics, as well as a soft lumbar orthosis applied in bed before getting on the commode, may provide support during toileting. Stool softeners and high-fiber foods or supplements reduce constipation, an adverse effect of bed rest, and straining with its untoward effects on intraspinal pressure. Bed positioning should be arranged so that excessive lumbar flexion is avoided. Slight flexion may reduce small protrusions by tightening annulus fibers. Larger protrusions, however, may not reduce with flexion, and some may instead protrude more if the annulus tear is large. Flexion of the hips and knees is allowed in order to reduce stretching of the nerve root over protruded disk material. The upper trunk should not be higher than the pelvis, except during meals, in order to avoid axial loading of the spine, which is associated with higher intradiskal pressures. Sitting is to be avoided, except during bowel movements. Sitting is associated with high intradiskal pressures, which are more than double those of lying supine and 40% higher than those of standing. The lowest intradiskal pressure is in a supine position with 90° hip and knee flexion.[97, 99, 104]

Attempts at reduction of a disk protrusion by a progressive passive spinal extension program can be made in selected cases, but careful identification of these cases requires special training and experience. The rationale for passive extension disk reduction techniques is based on the premise that intradiskal vectors are dependent on the position of adjacent vertebrae.[82] As a flexed position shifts vectors posteriorly, extension may shift vectors anteriorly, thus reducing forces favorable to posterior or posterolateral protrusion. Similarly, appropriate lateral shifting may centralize lateral vectors. In general, these procedures may be tried under trained and experienced direction when small protrusions are suspected and when initial attempts do not increase radicular symptoms. A small lumbar roll or pad may help maintain extension when supine. According to the same rationale, periods of prone lying may help to reduce small disk protrusions.

Lumbar traction is a long and deeply ingrained treatment of lumbar disk protrusion. It is based on the premise that one can reduce intradiskal pressure or even create a negative intradiskal pressure with application of external distracting forces. However, since the classic work of Judovich, it has been known that external forces must exceed 50% of body weight in order to overcome body surface friction.[55] Low-force traction (less than 20 kg) simply serves to keep the patient in bed. This, however, may be an appropriate goal for many individuals. A large number of low friction traction devices and tables have been developed and marketed. Popular systems use split tables or gravity to reduce friction and improve efficacy of traction forces.

Although these heavy lumbar traction systems can, in fact, reduce intradiskal pressures, they cannot be tolerated for long periods of time. The benefit of further periodic reduction in, or even negative, intradiskal pressure, instead of simple enforced bed rest, remains to be demonstrated in controlled trials. The contribution of traction after 3,000 years still remains controversial, although dramatic results are certainly seen in some individual cases.[78, 131]

A reasonable treatment prescription for an acute disk protrusion could include:

- 7 days of enforced bed rest
- Careful bed positioning
- Analgesics, muscle relaxants
- Stool softeners, bedside commode
- A progressive, passive extension program
- Possibly, periodic heavy lumbar traction

Surgical intervention is reserved for those patients who fail such a rest trial or those with progressive neurological deficits, bowel or bladder involvement, or intractable pain.[64, 73, 88, 103, 117, 133] Radiological demonstration of a protruded or extruded disk is necessary before surgical intervention. In the case presented, as in most cases of acute disk protrusions, the patient's symptoms and signs resolved with an enforced rest program. In this case, invasive studies such as myelography were not indicated, but the disk can be delineated with an MRI scan (Fig. 37-19).

The next, often neglected, steps in conservative management involve a post-rest management strategy. Mobilization of the patient from a bed rest period should not be precipitous, but should include early, but gradual and progressive, ambulation. Because intradiskal pressures are higher during sitting than during standing or walking, once total bed rest is over, the patient should be assisted directly in standing and walking. Ambulation with an assistant, walker, cane, or in parallel bars can transfer axial loading from the spine to the upper extremities. A soft lumbar support can further reduce intradiskal pressure while mobilizing the patient. There is no need to interpose bedside sitting, and, in fact, prolonged sitting should be delayed. Flexion and isometric exercises, as well as bending, twisting, or lifting, should be delayed until the annulus tear has had adequate opportunity to form a good scar—at least 6 weeks. Prolonged sitting without lumbar pads, back rests, armrests, or opportunity to frequently change positions should be minimized during this period. These restrictions may preclude a return to employment at this time. Observance of good posture and body mechanics is essential in order to avoid recurrence during this period. At a follow-up visit in 6 to 8 weeks, if there are no signs of disk protrusion, root irritation, or muscle spasms, a very gentle isometric exercise program should commence.[8] Instruction in a weaning program from the corset or other assistive devices is also reviewed, if not already completed. Instructions in back

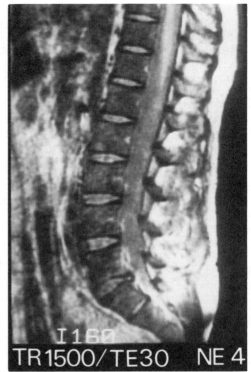

A

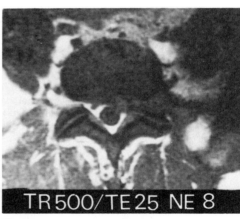

B

Figure 37-19. (*A*) Sagittal view MRI scan depicting L5 disk protrusion. (*B*) Obliteration of fat with effacement of left S1, nerve root.

skills and back care principles, including attendance in a back school, are especially appropriate at this time.[6]

A protruded disk, even if managed successfully (medically or surgically) inevitably will develop into a degenerative disk.[132] The principles previously discussed for the management of degenerative disk disease then apply.

CASE 4

A 62-year-old man, a night watchman, presents with buttock and calf pain, left greater than right, of 2-years' duration. The pain has been more intense over the last few months and is now severely interfering with his work. The pain is worse with standing and especially worse with walking. It is often associated with a sensation of weakness and numbness in his legs. He can now walk only 50 to 60 meters before the pain prevents further walking. He can, however, get prompt relief by sitting down and bending forward or by squatting. Bending, lifting, and coughing are not particularly bothersome, except for bending backward, which also causes leg numbness and weakness.

On examination, he has no current pain or tenderness. Peripheral pulses, gait, and the jolt and Larson's tests are all normal. Lumbar lordosis is decreased. Lumbar motions are only mildly reduced in all planes with no painful arcs (Fig. 37-20). Manual muscle testing and knee jerk reflexes are normal. Ankle jerks are absent on the left and barely detectable on the right. Straight leg raising is limited to 70° bilaterally only by tight hamstrings. The Schober flexion test is 4.4 cm. The Waddell score is zero.

Radiographs of the lumbar spine show multiple degenerative disks and facets and diffuse hypertrophic changes. An electromyogram shows mild bilateral L5 and S1 radiculopathies. Myelography with CT shows spinal stenosis (Fig. 37-21).

Diagnosis: Spinal stenosis (pseudoclaudication).

Management/Discussion: Spinal stenosis is a consequence of advanced degenerative hypertrophic changes in a setting of a narrow spinal canal.[24, 57, 68, 69] The characteristic feature is a claudication-like leg pain or weakness when walking that is relieved by rest and especially spinal flexion. If symptoms are sufficiently limiting and the patient is medically able, surgical decompression is indicated, since no physiatric measures are definitive.[15, 36, 120] If, however, the patient is not able or willing to undergo surgery, a program of flexion exercises and a lumbar corset, flexion jacket, or Williams' brace and a cane may reduce somewhat the neural element irritation.[138] Shock-absorbing shoe inserts may also be a reasonable prescription.[142] A transcutaneous electrical nerve stimulator (TENS) used during ambulation may further reduce pain associated with spinal stenosis but cannot affect weakness or numbness.

CASE 5

A 17-year-old high school girl who is an aggressive athlete, specializing in the broadjump and volleyball, reports with back pain of 6-months' duration. The pain was worse after broadjumping and volleyball games and persisted for a day or two afterward. Rest in bed for 2 to 3 hours usually relieved the pain. Over the last 2 months, however, the pain has been constant and she has stopped sports participation. No medical intervention has been employed.

On examination, she localizes the pain to the midline lower back region. It extends into the right and left upper thighs. All spinal motions are full and she reports increased pain only on extension (Fig 37-22). There is no lateral list, and there is a complete reversal of lumbar lordosis on active spinal flexion. Schober flexion test is 7.2 cm. Gait, manual muscle testing, and

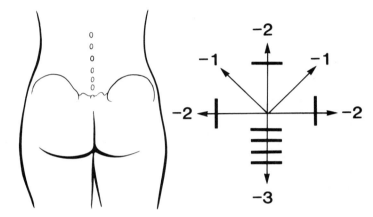

Figure 37-20. Patient has no resting pain and no tenderness. There is loss of lumbar motion in all planes. Local pain occurs on active lumbar extension. There are decreased ankle jerk reflexes. Diagnosis (primarily by history): spinal stenosis.

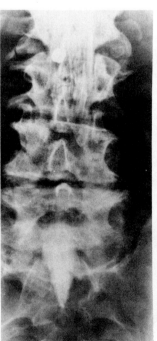

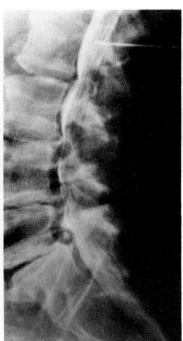

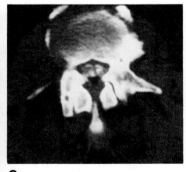

Figure 37-21. AP (*A*) and lateral (*B*) films from water-soluble contrast myelogram and (*C*) follow-up CT show lumbar spondylosis with bulging annuli and thickening of the ligamenta flava, which produces marked spinal canal stenosis at the L3–L4 and L4–L5 interspaces.

A **B** **C**

deep tendon reflexes are normal. Straight leg raising is negative at 90° bilaterally. There is localized tenderness at the L5-S1 interspace. A slight palpable step-off is detected at the same level. Larson's test is positive at the L5-S1 interspace and the jolt test is positive. The Waddell score is zero.

Lumbar radiographs show bilateral L5 spondylolysis and a grade 1 spondylolisthesis at the L5-S1 level.

Diagnosis: Bilateral spondylolysis with low-grade spondylolisthesis.

Management/Discussion: Although spondylolysis itself does not usually cause symptoms, its consequence, spondylolisthesis, is frequently symptomatic, either from its associated mechanical instability or from traction on or compression of neural elements.[54] Spondylolisthesis is graded according to

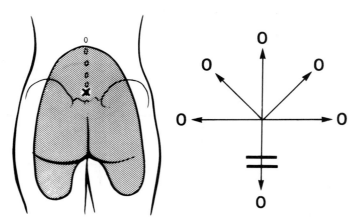

Figure 37-22.   Patient exhibits normal lumbar motions, but increased pain on active extension. She tests positive to Larson's test at L5. Her neurological exam is normal. Diagnosis: low-grade spondylolisthesis.

Meyerding by the percentage of displacement of one vertebral body upon the adjacent vertebral segment, as follows: grade 1, to 25% (Fig. 37-23); grade 2, 26 to 50%; grade 3, 51 to 75%; grade 4, 76 to 100% (Fig. 37-24).[139]

Although surgical fusion often may be indicated, it is not always successful. Effective nonsurgical treatment is available for low-grade spondylolisthesis. The basic principle in a conservative program is to reduce the lumbosacral angle and thereby reduce the anteriorly directed shear forces on supporting soft tissues. A spine flexion program seems most appropriate and has been shown to be effective in reducing symptomatology and maintaining function. It may include flexion exercises, posture training with emphasis on minimizing lumbar lordosis, isometric abdominal strengthening, and a lumbar support. Extension exercises are contraindicated.[39] Bar-hanging and gravity traction systems in a flexed spine position may provide additional symptomatic relief. Soft shock-absorbing shoe inserts can be helpful. However, activities that increase lordosis or are associated with sudden jolts should be avoided.[86]

A cause of spondylolisthesis without spondylolysis is marked degenerative disk disease, resulting in degenerative spondylolisthesis (Fig. 37-23).[1, 26] This occurs most frequently at the L4-L5 intradiskal space. Reverse spondylolisthesis (retrolisthesis) may also be seen in the mid and upper lumbar spine in the presence of significant degenerative disk disease. Management of degenerative spondylolisthesis is most similar to that of degenerative disk disease, already discussed in Case 1, with emphasis on isometric strengthening of trunk musculature and use of a lumbar orthosis. Surgical intervention (fusion) is not frequently indicated. Spondylolisthesis, as a result of multiple-level laminectomies, may also be seen.[116]

CASE 6

A 34-year-old janitor has a history of recurrent episodes of acute back pain. Most episodes have occurred as a "sharp catch" when bending and twisting at the same time and then attempt-

Figure 37-23.   Degenerative spondylolisthesis most frequently occurs at L4–L5, the least stable lumbar segment, and has a high correlation with pseudoclaudication. Lateral radiograph (*A*) demonstrates grade 1 spondylolisthesis at L4–L5 and to a lesser degree at L5–S1. Note sclerosis of facet joints on the AP view (*B*).

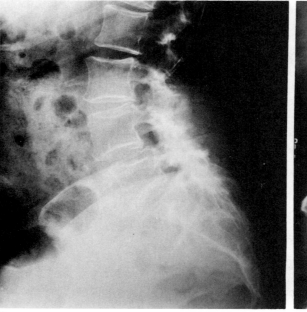

A

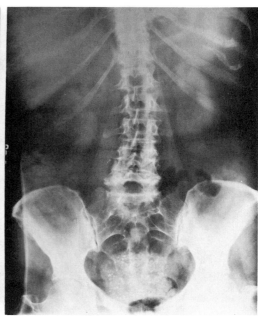

B

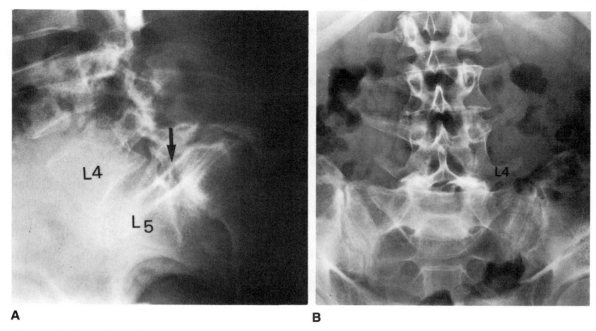

Figure 37-24. (*A*) Lateral view of grade 4 spondylolisthesis at L5 on S1 with associated spondylolysis. Note complete anterior displacement of L5 on the sacrum. (*B*) AP radiograph of the same patient.

ing to straighten up. He sometimes feels a "click," but not always. He would not be able to straighten up for 2 or 3 days, if he did not visit his local chiropractor for a session of spinal manipulation, which usually quickly afforded relief of pain and stiffness. Most often, heavy lifting was not involved. The present episode occurred the day before when bending over and repositioning a chair. No radicular symptoms were reported. He saw his local physician and was told to go to bed. There was no change in his symptoms overnight, so he has come to see if anything else can be done or if these episodes can be prevented.

On examination, he localizes his pain to the lumbosacral triangle with extension into the left buttock and upper thigh. His gait is antalgic on the left, with a list to the right side. Lordosis is reduced and reversal is incomplete on attempted trunk flexion. Schober flexion test is 3.2 cm. Manual muscle testing, deep tendon reflexes, and Larson's test are normal. The jolt test is positive. The straight leg raising test is limited to 60° on the left only by localized lower back pain, and to 80° on the right by tight hamstrings. There are two areas of localized tenderness—at the L5 spinous process and in the adjacent left paravertebral muscle belly. Spinal extension, left lateral flexion, and right rotation are markedly restricted by increased pain (painful arcs) (Fig. 37-25). The Waddell score is zero. Lumbar radiographs are normal.

Diagnosis: Acute facet syndrome.

Management/Discussion: The patient was placed on his left side on the examination table. Gentle lumbar manipulation was performed, after which his pain was immediately relieved except for a mild residual "soreness." He was able to straighten up and move his trunk in all planes without pain. He returned to work. Three weeks later, he returned with similar symptoms and signs and was again relieved. A slightly different lumbar mobilization method was employed, which did not use an "end-arc thrust." He was also given a flexion exercise program to do at home twice daily. He returned with the same problem two additional times

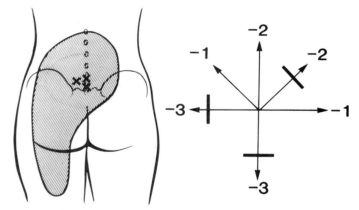

Figure 37-25. Patient presents with tender L5 and left lower lumbar paraspinals, loss of lordosis, and a list to the right. The neurological exam is negative. Pain is increased with active extension, left lateral flexion, and right rotation. Diagnosis: acute facet strain.

over the next 3 months and was treated similarly. Finally, he was instructed in a self-administered "lumbar rotation" mobilization technique and has been able to resolve all further episodes of pain himself. He was instructed in body mechanics and lifting techniques but does not always observe them.

This common but dramatic back syndrome has been dubbed "acute facet syndrome," based on the supposed anatomical and functional correlations of the facet joints with the pattern of painful arcs characteristic of this syndrome.[67, 90, 141] However, little direct evidence of a facet etiology is currently available other than the observation of equally dramatic results with image intensifier-controlled facet joint injections.[28, 72, 74] Because of the benign nature of the syndrome, which is characterized by prompt resolution of symptoms with simple, readily available measures, specific pathological confirmation is not available.[77]

Other proposed etiologies include deep segmental muscle strain and spasm. These segmental muscle spasms are supposedly relieved by quick or prolonged muscle stretching during manipulation or mobilization techniques.[37] This theory does not, however, account for the occasional sudden "click" associated with the onset or resolution of the symptoms. Another, but also less likely, theory is the displacement of small "hard" disk (meniscal) fragments.[114] The younger age and the absence of demonstrable disk disease in many patients with this syndrome, its infrequency in older patients with known degenerative disk disease, and the general lack of dramatic response to spinal manipulation in patients with known degenerative disk disease cast doubt on a disk fragment etiology.

Despite a lack of unanimous agreement on the functional pathology of this syndrome, it has unique clinical features that distinguish it and its management from other common back strain syndromes.

The acute facet syndrome is characterized by a sudden onset, usually when the patient has attempted to straighten up from a flexed and twisted position. This is in contrast with the onset of disk protrusion pain, which is usually a slow crescendo over several hours. Pain from acute muscle and ligamentous strain is also less intense on onset and builds over the next few minutes or hours. Both acute disk herniations and acute facet syndromes produce a list to the side opposite the pain. The pattern of painful arcs for a disk protrusion is pain on flexion (Fig. 37-19). The pattern for muscle or ligamentous strain is pain with flexion, lateral flexion, and rotation to the opposite side (those motions that stretch the involved ligaments or muscles) (Fig. 37-16). The painful arc pattern for an acute facet strain is increased pain on extension, on lateral bending to the same (painful) side, and on rotation to the opposite side (Fig. 37-25). These motions are those that would increase loading on an ipsilateral (painful) facet joint. The facet syndrome is most common on the left side, probably because most people are right-handed and would pick up a small object by left rotation.[67]

One feature of this syndrome is the consistent and prompt response to lumbar mobilization and manipulation techniques. In contrast, manipulation techniques rarely afford more than a transient relief for acute or chronic muscle or ligamentous strains, and they are useless or even contraindicated in cases of disk protrusion.[23, 42]

In addition to manipulation, treatment may include a flexion exercise program, although such a program has not always been routinely helpful in relieving acute symptoms, nor is it necessarily useful in preventing recurrences. Lumbar traction also has its proponents, but relief is not as dramatic or prompt as it is with manipulation. A program of regular flexion exercises and regular home traction may keep the facet capsule stretched and reduce facet joint sprains, but the mechanism by which this would be beneficial remains to be delineated.

A rational treatment approach may thus include:

- Prompt reduction by lumbar mobilization (preventing loss of work and prolonged immobility)
- Instruction in body mechanics, including lifting and bending techniques to prevent recurrences
- Regular daily lower-back flexion exercise program

CASE 7

A 35-year-old elementary school teacher presented with a 3-year history of neck, back, and shoulder pain. She reported generalized morning stiffness and pain that improved after getting up and moving about, but which worsened as the day progressed. She reported that she usually obtained 7 hours of sleep at night. She generally slept lightly and often felt tired and unrefreshed in the morning upon awakening. She found heat and rest to provide temporary relief. There were no radicular features.

On examination, she is noted to have protracted cervical spine and scapulae and a mildly increased lumbar lordosis. There is no list. Manual muscle testing, deep tendon reflexes, gait, and jolt and Larson's tests are normal. All spinal motions are normal without painful arcs. Schober flexion is 5.7 cm. Straight leg raising is negative and limited to 70° bilaterally only by tight hamstrings. No true muscle spasms are present, but there are multiple areas of increased tenderness in the classical parascapular, paracervical, paralumbar, and gluteal trigger point sites (Fig. 37-26). The Waddell score is 2, due to observed "overreaction" and "regionalization." All distraction and simulation tests are negative and her increased tenderness is limited to classical trigger point sites. Radiographs of the cervical, thoracic, and lumbar spine are normal (Fig. 37-17).

Diagnosis: Tension myalgia (fibrositis).

Management/Discussion: Fibrositis is an old name for an often vaguely described syndrome whose etiology has eluded clinicians for centuries. Attempts at identifying a "lesion" by laboratory, electromyography, radiography, direct biopsy, and, more recently, by electroencephalography have failed to identify any specific lesion. The diagnosis still remains one of exclusion with a high index of suspicion. Criteria for diagnosis have been described based on historical and physical findings, but no general consensus has been widely accepted.[144] Even harmonious agreement on the very existence of this syndrome, and, if it does exist, its name, has not been reached. Other names have included fibromyositis, fibromyalgia, tension myositis and muscle attachment syndrome.[118] We prefer to use the term "tension myalgia," as it is the most descriptive name for this syndrome, and it does not imply an etiological assumption.

Although a specific rheumatological, neurological, or biochemical abnormality could still be uncovered, it seems most likely that this syndrome may be a result of the notorious pain-spasm cycle. Considering it as such can lead to an appropriate and effective therapeutic program. The well-known pain-spasm cycle can be initiated by continuing muscle contraction, even if no true spasms are present. The cycle may thus begin as psychological stresses or anxiety, which result in increased muscle tension. Persistently increased muscle tension may cause diffuse muscle pain in the involved muscles, their attachments, or their

Figure 37-26. Patient shows normal spinal motions. She has increased tenderness in multiple "trigger points" and a normal neurological exam. Diagnosis: tension myalgia.

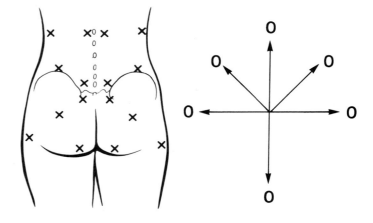

associated tendons or bursae. Increased tenderness in many of the classical trigger points may be explained by such a scenario. However, many trigger points represent naturally tender sites that are not associated with muscles, attachments, tendons, or known bursae. Increased tenderness and pain in these sites may be a result of a generally lowered pain threshold associated with psychological tension. Myalgia can be derived from muscle or psychological tension, hence the name "tension myalgia."

Poor posture is another cause of muscular strain and fatigue. It can result in pain in the muscle and its associated ligaments and attachments. This pain, if persistent, may trigger the pain-spasm cycle of tension myalgia. Studies by Smythe and Moldofsky have indicated a stage IV sleep abnormality associated with this syndrome. Such a sleep disorder may also contribute to a lowered pain threshold and increased pain in the classical trigger points. Evaluation of sleep quality, including morning fatigue and tiredness, may lead to adjunctive therapy with amitriptyline or other tricyclic agents.

Remote sources of pain (from degenerative disk disease, injuries to muscles, ligaments, other soft tissues, or from more ominous sources such as tumor or infection) could also trigger a pain-spasm cycle. Accordingly, tension myalgia can be secondary to other painful syndromes, complicating diagnosis and management.

The management strategy should be directed toward breaking the pain-spasm cycle. Reassurance should be provided, directed at answering questions and reducing anxiety. Describing what has been found, and not found, on examinations and a full discussion of the syndrome are the cornerstones of management. Statements such as, "We didn't find anything," or, "It must all be in your head," are likely to increase anxiety, as patients may then assume something is wrong but has been overlooked. Rather, after a thorough general and musculoskeletal examination, a detailed review of normal and abnormal findings followed by a discussion of tension myalgia can be quite reassuring. Reassurance alone may be a significant factor in reducing muscle and psychological tension and in raising the pain threshold.

In addition, cryotherapy, local heat, and massage can temporarily relieve pain and reduce muscle tension. Trigger point massage, trigger point injections, and spray and stretch techniques can also provide temporary, but often significant, relief. Any of these physical pain relief measures can prove helpful, as temporary symptomatic relief may be essential for the more lasting results from learned relaxation techniques.

Relaxation techniques are designed to reduce, by conscious effort, "resting" muscle tension. They can be of a general nature (general relaxation) or directed at specific muscles or groups (trapezius relaxation techniques). Myoelectric biofeedback can be used to assist with the learning of relaxation techniques. These techniques can become essential to self-management and the prevention of a recurrence of tension myalgia. Improving the general level of fitness, body mechanics, and the quality of sleep are all important in the treatment and prevention of tension myalgia.

CASE 8

A 48-year-old construction worker with no previous history of back pain fell 12 feet onto a hard wooden surface when his ladder slipped. He experienced immediate pain in his entire back. Pain was later restricted to his lower back, buttocks, and upper legs. Initial examination indicated only muscle spasms, and x-rays showed no fractures. He was treated in a local hospital for 5 days with bed rest, hot packs, massage, and a lumbar corset. After discharge, outpatient physical therapy was continued 3 times a week for the next 9 weeks. This provided only temporary relief of pain. Two attempts to return to work

were unsuccessful. Over the next 12 months consultations with several other physicians yielded no specific diagnosis. Further treatments included epidural and trigger point injections and a trial of TENS; all provided only temporary and partial relief of his symptoms. He eventually obtained an attorney after his worker's compensation benefits were discontinued by the insurance carrier. Now, 18 months after his injury, he seeks an opinion concerning his diagnosis, if more can be done, and if he has an impairment rating.

On examination, he localizes his pain diffusely over the entire lower back, both buttocks, and both entire lower extremities. He has diffuse tenderness over the entire back, sacrum, and both buttocks. There is superficial tenderness of the sacral skin when it is gently rolled. No true muscle spasm, however, can be found by palpation when he is examined lying relaxed and prone. He moves his back slowly and reluctantly and reports pain in all directions. The Schober test is 3.3 cm and spinal flexion measured by gravity goniometers is 30°. Manual muscle testing reveals "giving way" in all lower extremity groups in both lower extremities. No muscle atrophy is apparent on examination or on measurement of lower extremity circumferences. Deep tendon reflexes are normal. His gait is normal, but he exhibits partial falling motions and trunk lurches associated with incomplete knee buckling on attempted tandem walking. He reports back and leg pain bilaterally on straight leg raising at 70°. He has tight hamstrings. He is able to do a sit-up but reports back and leg pain during the sit-up. The Larson and jolt tests are negative. Simulated passive trunk rotation does not produce pain, and seated straight leg raising is full without pain.

X-rays of his lumbar spine reveal only mild degenerative disk disease at the L4, L5 and L5, S1 levels. An MRI scan is normal. His trunk muscle strength and trunk flexibility are evaluated with a computer-controlled isotonic dynamometer. This shows limitation of all trunk motions and deconditioning in all trunk muscle groups, especially in the trunk rotator (abdominal oblique) groups. A work capacity evaluation reveals regular and frequent reports of back and leg pain when bending, twisting, and sitting more than 30 minutes. He declines to lift more than 15 pounds or to lift above his shoulders during the testing.

Diagnosis:

Traumatic back strain syndrome; resolved.
Degenerative disk disease, lumbar spine, mild; unrelated.
Superimposed generalized deconditioning.
Superimposed pain amplification syndrome.

Management/Discussion: This case represents a chronic post-traumatic, soft tissue back injury. No bony or neurological lesion is demonstrable, but early descriptions may include evidence of muscle or ligament strains or contusions. As time passes, there may be less evidence of soft tissue injury, and nonorganic signs become more prominent.[130] In this case, there are four nonorganic signs. Nonorganic *regionalization,* both in pain localization and on muscle testing, is present. There is nonorganic *tenderness,* both over the sacrum and on gentle superficial skin rolling. Note that this increased superficial tenderness is in sites other than classic trigger point sites. The SLR sitting *distraction* test is positive. There is *overreaction* on tandem walking evaluation. Only the passive trunk rotation *simulation* maneuver is negative. The Waddell score is 4.

The Waddell score is a reliable and objective method of assessing nonorganic signs on physical examination. A score of 3 or greater is associated with significant nonorganic behavior and is an indication for further psychological investigations and treatment. This is not to say that such physical demonstrations are conscious, nor that the patient is malingering or faking the pain.

This pain amplification may be the result of repetitive, learned behaviors. Such a patient is, however, not likely to respond to more passive therapeutic modalities and interventions.

The term *pain amplification syndrome,* or Matheson's term *symptom magnification syndrome,* may be preferable to older terms like *functional pain* or *chronic pain behavior,* which have a history of overuse and imprecision. Terms such as *pain amplification syndrome* should, however, be used only upon evidence of significant nonorganic physical findings or documented significant inconsistencies on objective testing by dynamometers.

It is important to state clearly and early one's conclusion that incidental radiographic findings are unrelated. One must also recognize the historical likelihood of early soft tissue injuries, but to record if there is no evidence of current ongoing signs.

Finally, a diagnosis of deconditioning is appropriate if it is documented by objective dynamometric testing or is supported by a functional capacity or work capacity evaluation. This deconditioning may play as large a role in limiting rehabilitation as do nonorganic and psychological factors.

Family and employer support, psychological and vocational counseling, relaxation, training in good body mechanics, physical reconditioning, a work-hardening program, and early settlement of litigation are all essential for a return to a high-quality and productive life. Direction of the rehabilitation of such an injury-related, chronic back pain syndrome requires the full resources available to the physiatrist.

REFERENCES

1. Alexander E Jr, Kelly D, Davis CH Jr et al: Intact arch spondylolisthesis. J Neurosurg, 63:840–844, 1985
2. Anand AK, Lee BCP: Plain and metrizamide CT of lumbar disk disease: Comparison with myelography. AJNR 3(5):567–571, 1982
3. Andersson BJG, Ortengren R, Nachemson A, Elfstrom G: Lumbar disc pressure and myoelectric back muscle activity during sitting. I. Studies on an experimental chair. Scand J Rehab Med 6:104–114, 1974
4. Andersson BJG, Ortengren R: Lumbar disc pressure and myoelectric back muscle activity during sitting. II. Studies on an office chair. Scand J Rehab Med 6:115–121, 1974
5. Andersson BJG, Ortengren R, Nachemson A, Elfstrom G: Lumbar disc pressure and myoelectric back muscle activity during sitting. IV. Studies on a car driver's seat. Scand J Rehab Med 6:128–133, 1974
6. Andersson BJG, Ortengren R, Nachemson A: Quantitative studies of back loads in lifting. Spine 1(3):178–185, 1976
7. Andersson H, Carlsson C: Prognosis of operatively treated lumbar disc herniations causing foot extensor paralysis. Acta Chir Scand 132:501, 1966
8. Bartelink DL: The role of abdominal pressure in relieving the pressure on the lumbar intervertebral discs. J Bone Joint Surg (Br) 39:718, 1957
9. Biering-Sorensen F: Physical measurements as risk indicators for low back trouble over a one-year period. Spine 9(2):106–119, 1984
10. Brown T, Hansen RJ, Yorra AJ: Some mechanical tests on the lumbosacral spine with particular reference to the intervertebral discs. J Bone Joint Surg (Am) 39:1135, 1957
11. Burton CV: Lumbosacral arachnoiditis. Spine 3(1):24–30, 1978
12. Cacayorin ED, Kieffer SA: Application and limitations of computed tomography of the spine. Radiol Clin North Am 20(1):185–206, 1982
13. Carrera GF, Haughton VM, Syvertsen A et al: Computed tomography of the lumbar facet joints. Radiology 134:145, 1980
14. Carrera GF, Williams AL, Haughton VM: Computed tomography in sciatica. Radiology 137:433, 1980
15. Ciric I, Mikhael MA, Tarkington JA et al: The lateral recess syndrome. J Neurosurg 53:433, 1980
16. Colonna PC, Friedenberg ZB: The disc syndrome: Results of the conservative care of patients with positive myelograms. J Bone Joint Surg (Am) 31:614, 1949
17. Coventry MB: Anatomy of the intervertebral disk. Clin Orthop 67:9, 1969
18. Damkot DK, Pope MH, Lord J, Frymoyer JW: The relationship between work history, work environment and low-back pain in men. Spine 9(4):395–399, 1984
19. Dandy WE: Loose cartilage from intervertebral disk simulating tumor of the spinal cord. Arch Surg 19:660, 1929
20. Deyo RA, Diehl A, Rosenthal M: How many days of bed rest for acute low back pain? N Engl J Med 315:1064–1070, 1986
21. Davis PR: The use of intra-abdominal pressure in evaluating stresses on the lumbar spine. Spine 6(1):90–92, 1981
22. Deyo RA (ed): Occupational back pain. State of the Art Reviews. Spine 2(1):7–30, 1987
23. Doran DM, Newell DJ: Manipulation in treatment of low back pain: A multicentre study. Br Med J 2:161–164, 1975
24. Ehni G: Effects of certain degenerative diseases of the spine, especially spondylosis and disc protrusion, on the neural contents, particularly in the lumbar region. Mayo Clin Proc 50:327, 1975
25. Eisenstein S, Parry C: The lumbar facet arthrosis syndrome—clinical presentation and articular surface changes. J Bone Joint Surg (Br) 69(1):3–7, 1987
26. Epstein NE, Epstein JA, Carras R et al: Degenerative spondylolisthesis with intact neural arch: A review of 60 cases with an analysis of clinical findings and the development of surgical management. Neurosurgery 13:555, 1983
27. Fahrni WH: Conservative treatment of lumbar disc degeneration: Our primary responsibility. Orthop Clin North Am, 6:93, 1975
28. Fairbank JCT, Park WM, McCall IW, O'Brien JP: Apophyseal injection of local anesthetic as a diagnostic aid in primary low-back pain syndromes. Spine 6:598–605, 1981
29. Falconer MA, McGeorge M, Begg AC: Observations on the cause and mechanism of symptom-production in sciatica and low-back pain. J Neurol Neurosurg Psychiatry 11:13, 1948
30. Farfan HF, Sullivan JD: The relation of facet orientation to intervertebral disc failure. Can J Surg 10:179, 1967
31. Fisk JR, DiMonte P, Courington SM: Back schools. Past, present, and future. Clin Orthop 179:18–23, 1983
32. Fish JW (ed): A Practical Guide to Management of the Painful Neck and Back: Diagnosis, Manipulation, Exercises, Prevention. Springfield, IL, Charles C Thomas Publisher, 1977
33. Forscell MZ: The Swedish Back School. Physiotherapy 66(4):112–114, 1980
34. Frymoyer JW, Pope MH, Costanza MD et al: Epidemiologic studies of low-back pain. Spine 5:419, 1980
35. Garfin SR, Pye SA: Bed design and its effect on chronic low back pain—a limited controlled trial. Pain 10(1):87–91, 1981
36. Getty CJM: Lumbar spinal stenosis: The clinical spectrum and the results of operation. J Bone Joint Surg (Br) 62:481, 1981
37. Glover JR, Morris JG, Khosla T: Back pain: A randomized clinical trial of rotational manipulation of the trunk. Br J Ind Med 31:59, 1974
38. Goldthwait JE: The lumbo-sacral articulation: An explanation of many cases of "lumbago," "sciatica" and paraplegia. Boston Med Surg J 164:165, 1911
39. Gramse RR, Sinaki M, Ilstrup D: Lumbar spondylolisthesis, a rational approach to conservative treatment. Mayo Clin Proc 55:681, 1980
40. Grubb SA, Pipscomb HJ, Guilford WB: The relative value of lumbar roentgenograms, metrizamide myelography, and discography in the assessment of patients with chronic low back syndrome. Spine 12(3):282–285, 1987
41. Hadler N: Regional back pain. N Engl J Med 315(17):1090–1092, 1986
42. Haldeman S: Spinal manipulative therapy. Clin Orthop 179:62, 1983
43. Hall H: The Canadian Back Education Units. Physiotherapy 66(4):115–117, 1980
44. Hall H, Iceton JA: Back school. An overview with specific reference to the Canadian back education units. Clin Orthop 179:10–17, 1983
45. Hallin RP: Sciatic pain and the piriformis muscle. Postgrad Med 74:69, 1983
46. Harris RI, Macnab I: Structural changes in the lumbar interver-

tebral discs: Their relationship to low back pain and sciatica. J Bone Joint Surg (Br) 36:304, 1954

47. Haughton VM, Syvertsen A, Williams AL: Soft-tissue anatomy within the spinal canal as seen in computed tomography. Radiology 134:649, 1980

48. Hayne CR: Back schools and total back-care programmes—a review. Physiotherapy 70(1):14–17, 1984

49. Helfet AJ, Gruebel Lee (eds): Disorders of the Lumbar Spine, Philadelphia, JB Lippincott, 1978

50. Hirsch C, Ingelmark B, Miller M: The anatomic basis for low back pain. Acta Orthop Scand 33:1, 1963

51. Inman VT, Saunders JB: The clinico-anatomical aspects of the lumbosacral region. Radiology 38:669, 1942

52. Inman VT, Saunders JB: Referred pain from skeletal structures. J Nerv Ment Dis 99:660, 1944

53. Jackson CP, Brown MD: Is there a role for exercise in the treatment of patients with low back pain? Clin Orthop 179:39–45, 1983

54. Jackson DW, Wiltse LL, Dingeman RD, Hayes M: Stress reactions involving the pars interarticularis in young athletes. Am J Sports Med 9(5):304–312, 1981

55. Judovich BD: Lumbar traction therapy and dissipated force factors. Lancet 74:411–414, 1954

56. Kahanovitz N, Nordin M, Verderame R et al: Normal trunk muscle strength and endurance in women and the effect of exercise and electrical stimulation. Part 2: Comparative analysis of electrical stimulation and exercises to increase trunk muscle strength and endurance. Spine 12(2):112–118, 1987

57. Kavanaugh GT, Svien HJ, Holman CB et al: "Pseudoclaudication" syndrome produced by compression of the cauda equina. JAMA 206:2477, 1968

58. Kellgren JH, Lawrence JS: Osteo-arthrosis and disk degeneration in an urban population. Ann Rheum Dis 17:388, 1958

59. Kellgren JH: Observations on referred pain arising from muscle. Clin Sci 3:175, 1938

60. Kellgren JH: The anatomical source of back pain. Rheumatol Rehabil 16:3, 1977

61. Kelsey JL, White AA III: Epidemiology and impact of low-back pain. Spine 5:133, 1980

62. Kelsey JL: Epidemiology of radiculopathies. In Schoenberg B (ed): Advances in Neurology, vol 19, pp 385–398. New York, Raven Press, 1978

63. Kendall PH, Jenkins JM: Exercises for backache: A double-blind controlled trial. Physiotherapy 54:154, 1968

64. Konings JG, Williams FJB, Deutman R: The effects of chemonucleolysis as demonstrated by computerised tomography. J Bone Joint Surg (Br) 66:417, 1984

65. Kortelainen P, Puranen J, Koivisto E, Lahde S: Symptoms and signs of sciatica and their relation to the localization of the lumbar disc herniation. Spine 10(1):88–92, 1985

66. Kosiak M, Aurelius JR, Hartfiel WF: The low back problem—an evaluation. J Occup Med 10:588, 1968

67. Kraft G, Levinthal D: Facet synovial impingement: A new concept in the etiology of lumbar vertebral derangement. Surg Gynecol Obstet 93:439–443, 1951

68. Krueger BR: Low back pain and sciatica. In Spittell JA (ed): Clinical Medicine. Vol 4, Chap 50, pp 1–27. Philadelphia, Harper & Row, 1985

69. Lancourt JE, Glenn WV Jr, Wiltse LL: Multiplanar computerized tomography in the normal spine and in the diagnosis of spinal stenosis: A gross anatomic-computerized tomographic correlation. Spine 4:379, 1979

70. Lankhorst GJ, Van-de-Stadt RJ, Vogelaar TW, Van der korst JK, Prevo AJ: The effect of the Swedish Back School in chronic idiopathic low back pain. A prospective controlled study. Scand J Rehab Med 15(3):141–145, 1983

71. Lidstrom A, Zachrisson M: Physical therapy on low back pain and sciatica—an attempt at evaluation. Scand J Rehab Med 2:37–42, 1970

72. Lippitt A: The facet joint and its role in spine pain: Management with facet joint injections. Spine 9(7):746–750, 1984

73. Love JG, Walsh MN: Protruded intervertebral disks: Report of one hundred cases in which operation was performed. JAMA 111:396, 1938

74. Lynch M, Taylor J: Facet joint injection for low back pain—a clinical study. J Bone Joint Surg (Br) 68(1):138–141, 1986

75. Maravilla KR, Lesh P, Weinreb JC, Selby DK, Mooney V: Magnetic resonance imaging of the lumbar spine with CT correlation. AJNR 6:237–245, 1985

76. Maruta T, Swanson DW, Swenson WM: Low back pain patients in a psychiatric population. Mayo Clin Proc 51:57, 1976

77. Maslow GS, Rothman R: The facet joints: Another look. Bull, NY Acad Med 51:1294–1311, 1975

78. Mathews JA, Hickling J: Lumbar traction: A double-blind controlled study for sciatica. Rheumatol Rehabil 14:222–225, 1975

79. Mattmiller AW: The California Back School. Physiotherapy 66(4):118–121, 1980

80. Mayer TG, Tencer AF, Kristoferson S, Mooney V: Use of noninvasive techniques for quantification of spinal range-of-motion in normal subjects and chronic low-back dysfunction patients. Spine 9(6):588–595, 1984

81. McGill CM: Industrial back problems, a control program. J Occup Med 10:174, 1968

82. McKenzie RA (ed): The Lumbar Spine: Mechanical Diagnosis and Therapy. Waikanae, NZ, Wright & Carman Ltd, 1981

83. Mellin G: Correlations of spinal mobility with degree of chronic low back pain after correction for age and anthropometric factors. Spine 12(5):464–468, 1987

84. Mennell JM: *Back Pain.* Boston, Little, Brown & Co, 1960

85. Merritt J, McLean T, Erickson R, Offord K: Measurement of trunk flexibility in normal subjects: Reproducibility of three clinical methods. Mayo Clin Proc 61:192–197, 1986

86. Micheli LJ: Back injuries in gymnastics. Clin Sports Med 4(1):85–93, 1985

87. Million R, Hall W, Nilsen KH, Baker RD et al: Assessment of the progress of the back pain patient. 1981 Volvo award in clinical science. Spine 7(3):204–212, 1982

88. Mixter WJ, Barr JS: Rupture of the intervertebral disc with involvement of the spinal canal. N Engl J Med 211:210–215, 1934

89. Modic M, Masaryk T, Boumphrey F et al: Lumbar herniated disk disease and canal stenosis: Prospective evaluation by surface coil MR, CT, and myelography. AJNR 7:709–717, 1986

90. Mooney V, Robertson J: The facet syndrome. Clin Orthop 115:149, 1976

91. Morris JM, Lucas DB, Bresler B: Role of the trunk in stability of the spine. J Bone Joint Surg (Am) 43-A:327–351, 1961

92. Murphy KA, Cornish RD: Prediction of chronicity in acute low back pain. Arch Phys Med Rehabil 65(6):334–337, 1984

93. Murphy RW: Nerve roots and spinal nerves in degenerative disk disease. Clin Orthop 129:46, 1977

94. Nachemson A: A critical look at the treatment for low back pain. Scand J Rehab Med 11:143–147, 1979

95. Nachemson A: Physiotherapy for low back pain patients—a critical look. Scand J Rehab Med 1:85–90, 1969

96. Nachemson A: Recent advances in the treatment of low back pain. Int Orthop 9(1):1–10, 1985

97. Nachemson A: The influence of spinal movements on the lumbar intradiscal pressure and on the tensile stresses in the annulus fibrosus. Acta Orthop Scand, 33:183–207, 1963

98. Nachemson AL: The lumbar spine–An orthopaedic challenge. Spine 1:59, 1976

99. Nachemson A: Towards a better understanding of low-back pain: A review of the mechanics of the lumbar disc. Rheumatol Rehabil 14(3):129–143, 1975

100. Nachemson A: Work for all. For those with low back pain as well. Clin Orthop 179:77–85, 1983

101. Nachemson A, Elfstrom G: Intravital dynamic pressure measurements in lumbar discs—a study of common movements, maneuvers and exercises. Scand J Rehab Med 1:1–40, 1970

102. Nordin M, Kahanovitz N, Verderame R et al: Normal trunk muscle strength and endurance in women and the effect of exercise and electrical stimulation. Part 1: Normal endurance and trunk muscle strength in 101 women. Spine 12(2):105–111, 1987

103. Onofrio BM: Injection of chymopapain into intervertebral discs. J Neurosurg 42:384, 1975

104. Ortengren R, Andersson BJG, Nachemson AL: Studies of relationships between lumbar disc pressure, myoelectric back muscle

activity, and intraabdominal (intragastric) pressure. Spine 6(1):98–103, 1981

105. Oudenhoven RC: Gravitational lumbar traction. Arch Phys Med Rehabil 59:510–512, 1978

106. Pearce J, Moll JMH: Conservative treatment and natural history of acute lumbar disc lesions. J Neurol Neurosurg Psychiatry 30:13–17, 1967

107. Pearcy M, Portek I, Shepherd J: Three-dimensional x-ray analysis of normal movement in the lumbar spine. Spine 9:294, 1984

108. Porterfield JA, Mostardi RA, King S et al: Simulated lift testing using computerized isokinetics. Spine 12(7):683–687, 1987

109. Ransford AO, Cairns D, Mooney V: The pain drawing as an aid to the psychological evaluation of patients with low-back pain. Spine 1:127–134, 1976

110. Robinson GE: A combined approach to a medical problem. The Canadian Back Education Unit. Can J Psychiatry 25(2):138–142, 1980

111. Rose DL: The decompensated back. Arch Phys Med Rehabil 56(2):51–58, 1975

112. Rowe ML: Low back pain in industry. J Occup Med 11:161, 1969

113. Saunders HD: Evaluation, Treatment and Prevention of Musculoskeletal Disorders, Minneapolis, MN, Viking Press, 1985

114. Schiotz EH, Cyriax J (eds): Manipulation, Past and Present. London, William Heinemann Medical Books, 1975

115. Seres JL, Newman RI: Negative influences of the disability compensation system: Perspectives for the clinician. Semin Neurol 3:360, 1983

116. Shenkin HA, Hash CJ: Spondylolisthesis after multiple bilateral laminectomies and facetectomies for lumbar spondylosis. J Neurosurg 50:45, 1979

117. Simmons JW, Stavinoha WB, Knodel LC: Update and review of chemonucleolysis. Clin Orthop 183:51, 1984

118. Sinaki M, Merritt JL, Stillwell GK: Tension myalgia of the pelvic floor. Mayo Clin Proc 52:717, 1977

119. Spengler DM: Low Back Pain. New York, NY, Grune & Stratton, 1982

120. Spengler DM: Current concepts review—Degenerative stenosis of the lumbar spine. J Bone Joint Surg 69(2):305–308, 1987

121. Stillwell GK: The law of Laplace: Some clinical applications. Mayo Clin Proc 48:863, 1973

122. Storino HE, Siekert RG, MacCarty CS: Protrusion of lumbar discs causing marked bilateral weakness of the legs. Minn Med 41:687, 1958

123. Suzuki N, Endo S: A quantitative study of trunk muscle strength and fatigability in the low-back-pain syndrome. Spine 8(1):69–74, 1983

124. Teplick JG, Haskin ME: CT and lumbar disc herniation. Radiol Clin North Am 21:(2):259–288, 1983

125. Tonzola RF, Ackil AA, Shahani BT et al: Usefulness of electrophysiological studies in the diagnosis of lumbosacral root disease. Ann Neurol 9:305, 1981

126. Triano JJ, Schultz AB: Correlation of objective measure of trunk motion and muscle function with low-back disability ratings. Spine 12(6):561–565, 1987

127. Van Damme W, Hessels G, Verhelst M et al: Relative efficacy of clinical examination, electromyography, plain film radiography, myelography and lumbar phlebography in the diagnosis of low back pain and sciatica. Neuroradiology 18:109–118, 1979

128. Waddell G, Bircher M, Finlayson D, Main CJ: Symptoms and signs: Physical disease or illness behaviour? Br Med J 289(6447):739–741, 1984

129. Waddell G, Main CJ: Assessment of severity in low-back disorders. Spine 9(2):204–208, 1984

130. Waddell G, McCulloch JA, Kummel E et al: Nonorganic physical signs in low back pain. Spine 5:117–125, 1980

131. Weber H, Ljunggren AE, Walker L: Traction therapy in patients with herniated lumbar intervertebral discs. J Oslo City Hosp 34:61–70, 1984

132. Weber H: Lumbar disc herniation: A controlled, prospective study with ten years of observation. Spine 8:131, 1983

133. Weber H: The effect of delayed disc surgery on muscular paresis. Acta Orthop Scand 46:631, 1975

134. Wiesel SW, Feffer HL, Rothman RH (eds): Industrial Low Back Pain: A Comprehensive Approach. Charlottesville, VA, The Michie Company Law Publishers, 1985

135. Wiesel SW, Feffer HL, Rothman RH: Industrial low-back pain. A prospective evaluation of a standardized diagnostic and treatment protocol. Spine 9(2):199–203, 1984

136. Wilbourn AJ: The value and limitations of electromyographic examination in the diagnosis of lumbosacral radiculopathy. In Hardy RW (ed): Lumbar Disc Disease, pp 65–109. New York, Raven Press, 1982

137. Willberger JE Jr, Pang D: Syndrome of the incidental herniated lumbar disc. J Neurosurg 59:137, 1983

138. Williams PC: Low Back and Neck Pain: Causes and Conservative Treatment. Springfield, IL, Charles C Thomas Publisher, 1974

139. Wiltse LL, Newman PH, Macnab I: Classification of spondylolysis and spondylolisthesis. Clin Orthop 117:23, 1976

140. Witt I, Vestergaard A, Rosenklint A: A comparative analysis of x-ray findings of the lumbar spine in patients with and without lumbar pain. Spine 9:298, 1984

141. Wood L: Acute locked facet syndrome and its treatment by manipulation under local periarticular anesthesia—Part 1: Clinical perspective and pilot study proposal. J Manipulative Physiol Ther 7(4):211–217, 1984

142. Wosk J, Voloshin AS: Low back pain: Conservative treatment with artificial shock absorbers. Arch Phys Med Rehabil 66(3):145–148, 1985

143. Yang KH, King AI: Mechanism of facet load transmission as a hypothesis for low-back pain. Spine 9(6):557–565, 1984

144. Zohn DA, Mennell JM: Musculoskeletal Pain: Diagnosis and Physical Treatment. Boston, Little, Brown & Company, 1976

38

Management of Cervical Pain

Parminder S. Phull

In chronic pain clinics, cervical pain is second in frequency to low back pain.[10] Overall, 45% of working men have had at least one attack of stiff neck, 23% at least one attack of brachial neuralgia, and 51% both of these symptoms. The frequency of cervical pain symptoms almost doubles from age 25 to 45.[28] Pain-sensitive structures in the neck include the vertebral bones, ligaments (anterior and posterior longitudinal ligaments), the nerve roots, the articular facets and capsules, muscles, and the dura. Neck pain can originate from any of these structures or other structures in the neck region, or can be referred from other visceral and somatic structures (Table 38-1).

CERVICAL ANATOMY

A knowledge of cervical anatomy is essential to the understanding of cervical disorders, related pain syndromes, and their treatment.

The cervical spine is composed of seven cervical vertebrae (Figs. 38-1, 38-2, 38-3), which support the head (which weighs 8 to 12 lbs) and are connected to a less mobile thoracic spine. The cervical vertebrae are held together by five intervertebral disks, (there is no disk between C1 and C2), 14 facet (apophyseal) joints, 12 joints of Luschka, and a system of short and long ligaments and muscles. The cervical bodies are larger the more distal they are from C1. In adults, the cervical spine is normally held in a lordotic position, with a slight scoliosis to the left at the cervicothoracic junction in 80% of the people and to the right in 20%.[40] The cervical spine is the most mobile segment of the vertebral column.

A typical cervical vertebra (Fig. 38-4) is made up of a transversely elongated body, a pedicle on each side that runs posterolaterally, laminae, and a spinous process that runs posteriorly and can be palpated behind the neck in the midline. The upper and lower surfaces form the articulating surfaces for the facet joints. The facet joints are angled at 45° both posteriorly and laterally, thereby allowing movements not only in flexion and extension, but also in lateral bending and rotation. The cranial surfaces of the cervical vertebral bodies are concave transversely with upturned sides, which bear the facet joints and are rounded off anteroposteriorly. The inferior surfaces are concave from side to side. All seven cervical vertebral bodies have foramina (foramen transversum) in the transverse processes, which distinguish

them from the thoracic or lumbar vertebrae. The vertebral artery, vertebral vein, and sympathetic nerves pass through these foramina in the upper six cervical vertebrae. The vertebral artery occasionally passes the foramen transversum of the seventh cervical vertebra on the left, but the vertebral veins may pass

---

Table 38-1
Common Conditions Causing Pain

Musculoskeletal Causes
Osteoarthritis
Diffuse idiopathic skeletal hyperstosis (DISH)
Cervical spondylosis
Disk disease
Rheumatoid arthritis
Fracture
Neoplasm
Thoracic outlet syndrome (cervical rib, first rib, and clavicular compression syndromes)
Osteomyelitis

Neurological Causes
Nerve root syndromes
Cervical myelopathy
Neuritis (brachial, occipital)
Torticollis
Meningitis
Cord tumors

Soft Tissue and Muscular Pain
Acute cervical strain
Cumulative trauma, overstrain syndromes
Tendinitis, bursitis
Postural disorders
Fibrositis, fibromyalgia, and myofascial syndrome
Pharyngeal infection

Referred Pain
Heart and coronary artery disease
Apex of lung: Pancoast's tumor
Migraine
Muscle tension and myofascial pain
TMJ syndrome
Diaphragm, gallbladder, pancreas, hiatus hernia

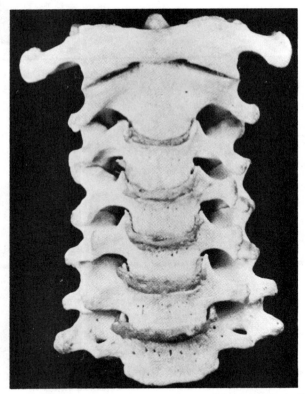

Figure 38-1. Anterior view of cervical spine. (Sherk HH, Parke WW: Normal Adult Anatomy. Philadelphia, JB Lippincott, 1983)

Figure 38-2. Posterior lateral view of cervical spine in normal configuration. (Sherk HH, Parke WW: Normal Adult Anatomy. Philadelphia, JB Lippincott, 1983)

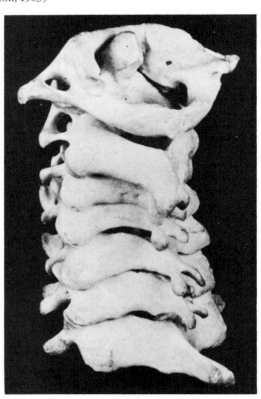

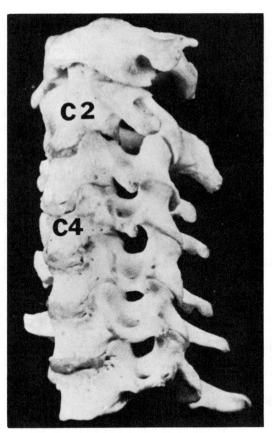

Figure 38-3. Lateral oblique view of cervical spine showing articulated pillars formed by articular processes. (Sherk HH, Parke WW: Normal Adult Anatomy. Philadelphia, JB Lippincott, 1983)

through on both sides. The third, fourth, fifth, and sixth cervical vertebrae are fairly similar. All have relatively short, split spinous processes. The cervical spinous processes are the shortest of any of the vertebrae, becoming longer in the fifth and especially the sixth vertebrae.

The first and second cervical vertebrae are unique. The first cervical vertebra (Fig. 38-5)—the *atlas*—supports the head. It is composed of a solid ring of bone with two lateral pillars, the superior and inferior surfaces of which form articular facets on each side. The atlas lacks a body and pivots about a bony process called the *dens* or odontoid process, which in essence is the fused bodies of C1 and C2. The short anterior arch of C1 articulates in the vertical plane with the ondontoid process of C2—the *axis* (Fig. 38-6)—thus forming a true pivot joint between C1 and C2 with rotation limited only by attachment of muscles and ligaments. The spinous process of C1 is a very small tubercle and is usually very difficult to palpate clinically. The spinal process of C7 is the most prominent cervical spinous process and is easily palpated posteriorly in the midline.

A strong ligament called the *ligamentum nuchae* extends as a fibrous band between the occipital crest, the bifid spines of the cervical vertebrae, and the investing layer of deep cervical fascia, which encloses the trapezius muscles.

The uncovertebral joints (joints of Luschka), first described by von Luschka in 1858, lie between the body of one cervical vertebra and the pedicular base of the subsequent vertebra (Fig. 38-7). They are absent at birth but appear between the first and second decades of life. They appear as clefts in the posterolateral part of the normal fibrocartilage of the intervertebral disk. Ulti-

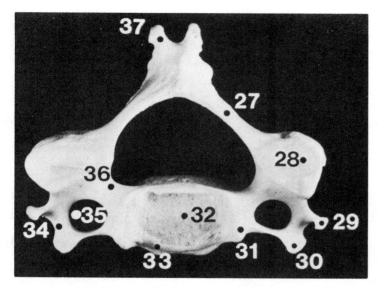

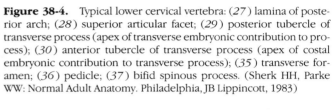

Figure 38-4. Typical lower cervical vertebra: (*27*) lamina of posterior arch; (*28*) superior articular facet; (*29*) posterior tubercle of transverse process (apex of transverse embryonic contribution to process); (*30*) anterior tubercle of transverse process (apex of costal embryonic contribution to transverse process); (*35*) transverse foramen; (*36*) pedicle; (*37*) bifid spinous process. (Sherk HH, Parke WW: Normal Adult Anatomy. Philadelphia, JB Lippincott, 1983)

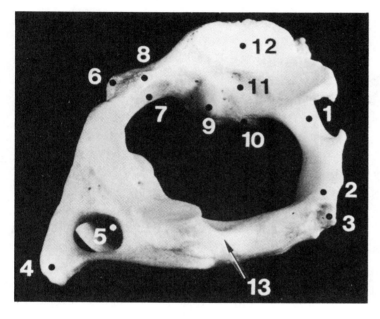

Figure 38-5. The first cervical vertebra, or atlas: (*1*) groove for vertebral artery; (*2*) posterior arch of atlas; (*3*) posterior tubercle; (*4*) transverse process; (*5*) transverse foramen; (*6*) transverse tubercle; (*7*) facet for dens; (*8*) anterior arch of atlas; (*9*) process for transverse ligament; (*10*) interior articular process; (*11*) lateral mass; (*12*) superior articular fovea; (*13*) strut of bone converting arterial groove into a foramen (occurs in 37% of cases). (Sherk HH, Parke WW: Normal Adult Anatomy. Philadelphia, JB Lippincott, 1983)

mately they develop a synovial lining, hyaline cartilage, meniscus folds, and a joint capsule. With age they may spread through the whole of the disk. Hence, Luschka joints are secondary fissures in originally normal disks and are not true joints. Produced by the shearing stresses during movements of the cervical vertebral bodies, they facilitate gliding and rotation of adjacent cervical vertebral bodies. They do undergo arthritic changes, including pannus formation, erosions, and osteophyte formation, as do other synovial joints, and are at times the source of pain in arthritic disease.[31]

The intervertebral disks make up about one-fourth of the height of the spinal column. They undergo dehydration or shrinkage from weight-bearing during the day and rehydrate at rest during the night. The disks are relatively thicker in the cervical region, which is a major factor in the flexibility of the cervical spine. The ratio of disk length to vertebral body height is 1 : 3 to 1 : 2. Cervical disks are also thicker anteriorly; their total height is 8 mm more anteriorly than posteriorly. Disks are composed of a fibrocartilaginous annulus and a viscoelastic nucleus pulposus. The annulus is made of crisscrossing concentric lamellae of fibrocartilage between adjacent vertebrae, which provide strength and stability but restrict excessive mobility. The nucleus pulposus absorbs stresses and distributes forces uniformly in all directions.

The cervical spine moves in flexion, extension, lateral flexion, and rotation. Nodding occurs at the atlanto-occipital joints. The occipital-atlantoaxial complex allows sizable quantities of motion in flexion, extension, lateral bending, and especially rotation. In order to protect the vital medullary structures, more free space is available for the spinal cord here than anywhere else in the spine. In addition, the axis of rotation is placed as close to the spinal cord as possible to permit a large magnitude (47%) of spinal rotation without bony impingement. A large amount of axial rotation is allowed at C1–C2, but virtually none between the occiput and C1, where the vertebral arteries enter the calvaria. The axial rotation is much less at C2–C3, largely because of the yellow ligament which begins here.[48]

Flexion, extension, lateral bending, and rotation are possible at C2 to C7. The orientation of the facet joints at about 45° to vertical in the sagittal plane allows both lateral bending and

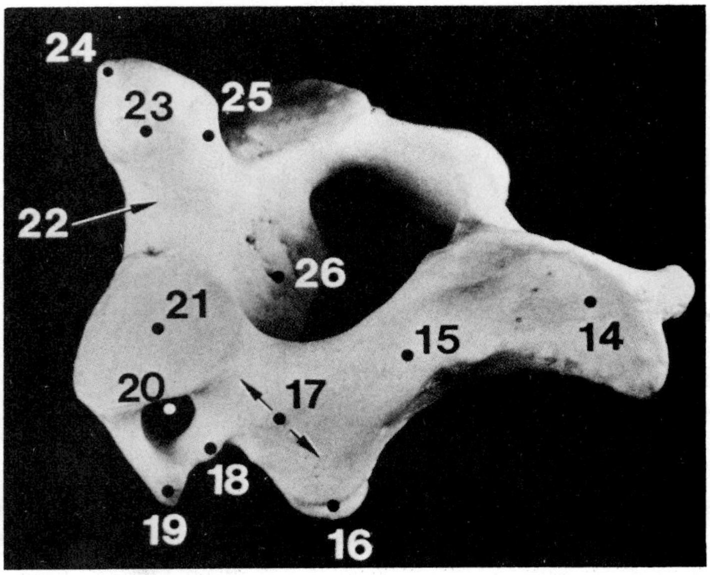

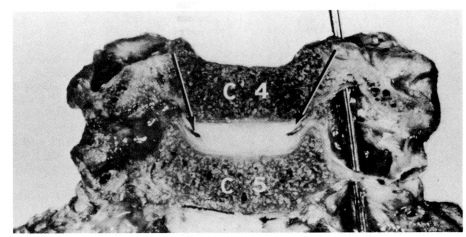

Figure 38-6. The second cervical vertebra, or axis: (*15*) lamina of neural arch; (*16*) inferior articular process; (*17*) pars interarticularis of neural arch; (*18*) posterior tubercle of transverse process; (*19*) anterior tubercle of transverse process; (*20*) transverse foramen; (*21*) articular facet of superior articular process; (*22*) dens (neck area); (*23*) attachment of alar ligament; (*24*) apex attachment of apical ligament; (*25*) posterior articular surface of dens; (*26*) vertebral body of axis. (Sherk HH, Parke WW: Normal Adult Anatomy. Philadelphia, JB Lippincott, 1983)

Figure 38-7. Frontal section of C4 disk with arrows indicating the uncovertebral joints. These do not appear until the latter part of the first decade and are not uniform with regard to the level or side of their occurrence. (Sherk HH, Parke WW: Normal Adult Anatomy. Philadelphia, JB Lippincott, 1983)

rotation. In the lower cervical vertebrae, the greatest amounts of flexion and extension movement occur between C5–C6 and the least at C2–C3 and C7–T1. The total range of available flexion and extension in the cervical region is 90°. About three-quarters of this movement is due to extension.[34] About 10° of flexion and 25° of extension occur at the atlanto-occipital joints.[39] The remainder of the movement occurs at the lower part of the cervical spine. In full flexion the anterior longitudinal ligament is lax, while the posterior longitudinal ligament is taut; extension reverses them. The size of the intervertebral foramina increases in flexion and decreases in extension by about one-third. Hence, in cervical radiculopathies the force of cervical traction should be in flexion.

The length of the cervical canal increases in flexion. The posterior longitudinal ligament and the ligamentum flavum are lax in extension, becoming thicker and reducing the dural diameter by 2 mm to 3 mm.

The intervertebral foramina are short tunnels bounded ventromedially by the disk and the uncovertebral joint (joint of Luschka) and dorsolaterally by the facet joint and the superior articular process of the subjacent vertebra. The intervertebral foramina are largest at the C2–C3 level, becoming smaller at lower cervical levels. The intervertebral foramina transmit the lateral terminations of the anterior and posterior nerve roots, spinal radicular arteries, intervertebral veins and plexuses, and

an extension of the epidural space containing areolar and fatty tissue with small arteries, veins, and lymphatics. The roots occupy one-fourth to one-third of the foraminal space. The anterior root lies anterior and inferior to the posterior root and in close proximity to the apophyseal joint.[20]

The cervical enlargement of the spinal cord extends from C3 to T2 and is greatest in diameter at the C6 level. Because of the difference in the growth of the vertebral components and the neural components, the spinous process overlies the cord segment numerically by one segment, that is, the C6 spinous process overlies the C7 cord segment. With increasing age, the vertebrae and disks lose height, resulting in the relative lengthening of the cord. In cervical spondylosis a cord segment and its emerging roots may be at the same level as the corresponding disk.

DIAGNOSIS

Clinical Examination

A good clinical examination consists of a thorough history and a systematic physical examination of the head, neck, upper thorax, shoulder, and arms. During the examination, the physician should observe the patient's gait, general posture, and head position and how naturally and rhythmically the head and neck move with the body.

After observing for normal contour of the cervical region and the major anatomic landmarks, the clinician looks for normal cervical lordosis, the position of the scapula on either side, sagging of the scapula or winging of the scapula, which may identify weakness of the trapezius, serratus anterior, or rhomboid major and minor. Palpation of bony structures should be done with the patient in a relaxed position. The neck is supported with one hand while the other is used to palpate. The hyoid bone lies at the level of the C3 vertebra. The superior border of the hyoid cartilage has a notch and lies at the C4 level, while the lower border is at the C5 level.

Below this is the trachea and cricoid rings. Lateral to the first cricoid ring lies the carotid tubercle, which is the anterior tubercle of the transverse process of C6. The carotid artery lies anterior to the carotid tubercle, which is a useful landmark for stellate sympathetic ganglion blocks.

The palpable posterior cervical landmarks include the occiput, the inion in the middle of the superior nuchal line, and the round mastoid process on either side of the superior nuchal line. The spinous process of C2 can be palpated just below the occiput. The spinous process of C7 is the most easily palpable cervical spinal process. The apophyseal joints can be felt as small rounded nubbles deeper to the posterior cervical muscles, about 1 inch lateral to the midline in a relaxed patient.

Examination of the soft tissues should be done keeping in mind the location of the various muscles in the neck. The posterior triangle usually needs careful palpation; it includes the whole group of muscles posterior to the sternocleidomastoid. The sternocleidomastoid is examined by asking the patient to turn the head to the opposite side, which causes the muscle to stand out for easy palpation. The trapezius is palpated from its origin at the inion to the spinous process of T2, the spine of the scapula, and the clavicle. The rhomboids and the supraspinatus muscles lie deep to the trapezius.

A sudden electric shock–like sensation traveling down the spine and spreading into one or more extremities on flexion of the neck was first described by Jean Lhermitte in 1932[24] and has since been referred to as Lhermitte's phenomenon or sign. It has been reported in patients with cervical cord tumors, cervical spondylosis, radicular myelopathy, and multiple sclerosis. It has also been reported in patients with high velocity missile injuries of the brain.[23] Self-limiting delayed onset Lhermitte's sign has been described following mild head and neck injuries without neurological loss or signs of cord compression.[6]

Specialized Tests

Head Compression Test

Axial compression of the head onto the cervical spine, leading to pressure and shearing forces on the apophyseal joint surfaces, intervertebral disks, or pressure on stiff ligaments and muscle structures, may lead to either local pain in the soft tissues or radicular pain. Radicular pain or paresthesias that are referred to the upper limbs is strongly suggestive of nerve root irritation. However, if the pain remains in the neck, soft tissues, or joints, it is suggestive of soft tissue pathology.

The head compression test should be performed with the patient sitting. The examiner places one hand across the other on the top of the patient's head and gradually exerts increasing downward pressure. The head may be tilted to either side, backward or forward.[28]

Spurling's Test

Spurling's test (Fig. 38-8) is another compression test. The head is turned in axial rotation to one side and bent laterally to that side. With the head in this position, a vertical blow is delivered to the uppermost portion of the cranium. A positive test is the development of pain in the neck, shoulder, or arm that is felt on delivery of the blow and results from compression of the nerve root or irritation of other pain-sensitive structures. The opposite side can be tested in a similar fashion by positioning the head to the opposite side.

Figure 38-8. Spurling's test is based on several biomechanical factors. If there is some pathological compromise or irritation of the nerve root, the irritation is aggravated when the root passes through the invertebral foramen. In order to demonstrate this, the head is positioned as shown, with the coupled motion of axial rotation and lateral bending further compromising the space available in the foramen. When the test is positive, a vertically directed blow of moderate impact produces an additional lateral bending movement that reduces this space, irritates the nerve root, and causes some combination of neck, shoulder, or arm pain. (Punjabi MM, White AA: Clinical Biomechanics of the Spine. Philadelphia, JB Lippincott, 1978)

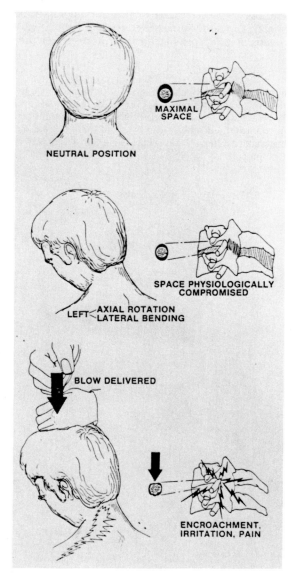

Head Distraction Test

The head distraction test is done with the patient seated and the head in a neutral position. The examiner places an open hand under the patient's chin with the other hand under the patient's occiput and gradually applies distracting force on the head, thereby distracting the foramina, disks, and joints. Nerve root compression may be relieved by the opening of the intervertebral foramina. This also relieves pressure on the apophyseal joints.[28]

Valsalva's Maneuver

Forced expiration against a closed glottis, or Valsalva's maneuver, increases venous and cerebral spinal fluid pressure. In the presence of an intraspinal tumor or a herniated disk, the action produces pain, which radiates in a dermatomal distribution. Vigorous coughing or sneezing, likewise, will elicit this pain.

Costoclavicular Maneuver, Hyperabduction Maneuver, and Adson's Test

There are several maneuvers to test for compression of the subclavian artery at the thoracic outlet, either from cervical rib, ligamentous structures, scalene muscles, or other thoracic outlet abnormalities. In performing the costoclavicular maneuver (Fig. 38-9), the patient sits upright with the arms resting on the thighs.

Figure 38-9. Costoclavicular syndrome can be produced by asking the patient to adduct his other scapula, forcing the clavicle against the first rib. Symptoms should be reproduced with a diminished radial pulse to confirm the diagnosis. (Ambrosia RD: Musculoskeletal Disorders, Regional Examination and Differential Diagnosis, 1st ed. Philadelphia, JB Lippincott, 1977)

While the radial pulse is felt, the patient is asked to thrust the shoulders backward, thus narrowing the space between the clavicle and the first rib. Obliteration or reduction in the intensity of the radial pulse suggests vascular compromise between the clavicle and the first rib.

In performing the hyperabduction maneuver (Fig. 38-10), the arm is abducted from 90° to 180° and externally rotated with the patient sitting upright. Obliteration or reduction of the radial pulse during the maneuver suggests vascular compromise beneath the pectoralis minor muscle.

Adson's test (Fig. 38-11) is performed with the patient sitting upright with the hands on the thighs. The radial pulse is felt while the patient is asked to extend his neck and turn the head to the affected side, take a deep breath, and hold it. This maneuver narrows the space between the anterior and middle scalene muscles, so that the obliteration or reduction in the volume of the radial pulse suggests vascular compromise at this level.

Dysphagia Test

Soft tissue swelling, hematoma, vertebral subluxation, or cervical osteophytic projections may produce pain or restriction of swallowing, which can be clinically observed and verified by swallowing studies.

Figure 38-10. Hyperabduction maneuver. The patient abducts his arm above his head. Where the neurovascular bundle is compressed under the coracoid process and pectoralis minor muscle, symptoms should be reproduced along with a diminished radial pulse. (Ambrosia RD: Musculoskeletal Disorders, Regional Examination and Differential Diagnosis. Philadelphia, JB Lippincott, 1977)

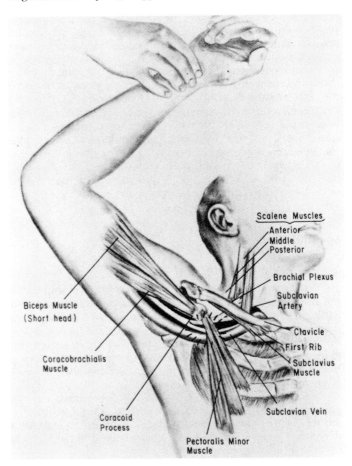

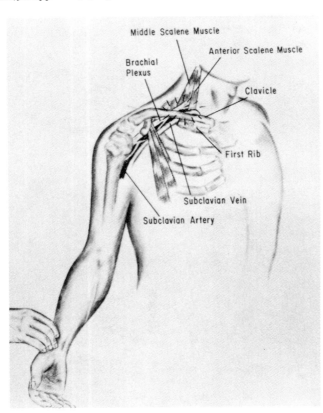

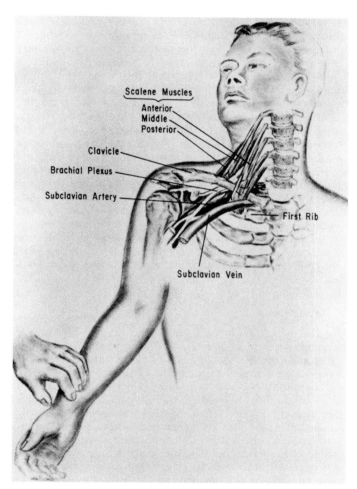

Figure 38-11. Adson's test reproduces compression of the neurovascular structures in the neck. The patient is asked to inhale deeply and turn the head to the affected side. A diminution of the radial pulse and reproduction of the patient's symptoms indicate constriction of the neurovascular bundle in the scalene muscles. (Ambrosia RD: Musculoskeletal Disorders, Regional Examination and Differential Diagnosis. Philadelphia, JB Lippincott, 1977)

Ophthalmological Tests

Sympathetic system involvement in cervical disorders may present as pupillary signs that may vary from time to time and on the two sides. Horner's syndrome follows complete interruption or paralysis of the sympathetic fibers, resulting in miosis, vasomotor and sweating changes, and ptosis on the affected side. The presence of such signs and symptoms indicates the need for ophthalmological evaluation.

Shoulder Depression Test

To perform the shoulder depression test, the examiner stands behind the patient who tilts his head to one side. With one hand supporting the head and the other hand on the patient's shoulder, the examiner exerts downward pressure on the shoulder and distracting pressure on the head in the opposite direction. This force creates a tug on the nerve roots, root sleeves, and adhesions, resulting in radicular pain or paresthesias.[28]

COMMON CONDITIONS CAUSING NECK PAIN

A number of diseases involve the cervical spine, including congenital abnormalities, trauma, infections, neoplasm, degenerative disk disease, and a number of systemic diseases. The cervical spine is involved in cases of rheumatoid arthritis (86%), diffuse idiopathic skeletal hyperostosis (DISH),[35] ankylosing spondylitis, and juvenile polyarthritis. Other diseases that present as cervical problems and pain include fibrositis, fibromyalgia, myofascial pain syndrome, torticollis, and thoracic outlet syndromes.

MYOFACIAL PAIN SYNDROMES AND FIBROSITIS FIBROMYALGIA

Symptoms

Myofascial pain syndromes and fibrositis fibromyalgia are a heterogeneous group of painful conditions which present with pain in muscles, their attachment site, and fascia. They represent probably the most frequent cause of pain in human beings.[1] A variety of terms have been used to describe these syndromes, including myofibrositis, rheumatoid myositis, and acute and chronic muscle strains and spasms. All these conditions are characterized by tenderness and pain located in skeletal muscles and fascial sheaths.

The myofascial syndrome is either primary or secondary. A primary myofascial syndrome is one in which the disorder is primarily confined to the skeletal muscles, fascia, or both, with physical findings confined to the muscles or fascia without the presence of neurological, orthopedic, or other disease processes. It is often related to soft tissue strain or injury and presents either as an acute condition or as a chronic condition such as chronic cervical strain syndrome after a whiplash injury. Secondary myofascial syndrome involves an underlying neurological, orthopedic, or rheumatological disease, but the manifestations of pain are primarily in the skeletal muscles, fascial sheaths, or both. Examples of this would include an old laminectomy scar with persistent pain, chronic adhesive arachnoiditis, carcinomatosis, reflex sympathetic dystrophy, and musculoskeletal pain in osteoarthritis.[16]

The diagnosis of myofascial syndrome is made by the process of elimination and by demonstration of exquisite tender areas (*trigger points*) in the appropriate areas of skeletal muscles. Trigger points are areas in the skeletal muscles or fascial sheaths, which on local pressure produce exquisite pain that radiates as paresthesias to other, usually distal, areas of the body. The trigger points in the cervical region are usually in the periscapular and trapezius areas. The common trigger points are at the superior portion of the trapezius muscle in the suboccipital region, palpation of which produces pain radiation to the occipital region and at times to the ear, scalene muscle, midtrapezious region, and superior medial angle and border of the scapula.[46]

Fibrositis fibromyalgia is a syndrome of generalized chronic and predominantly axial musculoskeletal aches and pain, characteristically modulated by weather, cold and heat, overexertion, anxiety, emotional stress, and nonrestoring sleep pattern with morning stiffness and daytime fatigue. It has characteristic localized areas of tender points on palpation that do not generally refer pain distally in a recognizable pattern. Patients are often unaware of the existence of these tender areas. These patients usually lack stage-4 non-REM sleep and commonly have headaches and irritable bowel syndrome.[50] The common tender areas in fibrositis are: in the suboccipital region, 2 cm below the occipital crest and 1 cm lateral to the midline; midpoint of upper border of trapezius; 3 cm lateral to midline at midscapular level; second costochondral junction; lateral epicondyle; interspinous ligaments of L4–S1; and upper half of gluteus medius and pes anserinus.[42]

Treatment

The treatment of myofascial pain syndrome is multifaceted and includes injection of the trigger points with either local anesthetics (0.25% bupivacaine or 0.5% procaine) or local anesthetics and corticosteroids.[46] Often trigger points need to be injected bilaterally and at multiple sites. Trigger point injections in the lower cervical and periscapular region have the potential risk of pneumothorax. In injecting trigger points around the shoulders, the risk of pneumothorax is greatly reduced if the needle is directed tangential to the chest wall and perpendicular to the ribs, so that the tip of the needle stays out of the thoracic cavity. Fortunately these trigger points are usually quite superficial, and it is not necessary to go very deep. The usual result is significant relief of symptoms for several weeks, but the duration varies from person to person. The frequency of injections is determined by duration of relief of symptoms. The trigger point injections are followed by gradual stretching of the muscles, which is facilitated with the use of heat or fluoromethane or ethylchloride spray. The muscles are sprayed medial to lateral in a fairly brisk sweeping motion in the direction of radiation of pain from the trigger point. Patients may be given fluoromethane for use at home.

Muscle strengthening exercises to tolerance level are very helpful in reducing the extent and frequency of pain and in musculoskeletal reconditioning. Ultrasound diathermy combined with sinusoidal electrical stimulation also helps resolve the trigger points. At times trigger points can be resolved with local massage and pressure over the trigger points (myotherapy). There is a remarkably high degree (71%) of correspondence between the trigger points and acupuncture points,[27] and therefore body acupuncture treatments may also be beneficial in relieving pain. Acupressure treatments probably also accomplish the same.

Narcotics should be avoided with myofascial syndromes, since this is a chronic condition and the potential for narcotic dependence is high. Often the symptoms can be controlled with the use of nonsteroidal anti-inflammatory drugs, such as naproxen and ibuprofen. Tricyclic antidepressants like amitriptyline are also helpful in managing symptoms. To treat the host of economic, social, and personal problems that beset these patients, autorelaxation, biofeedback, hypnosis, and individual and group therapy may be of help.

Soft Tissue Injuries of the Neck

Soft tissue injuries of the neck are also referred to as whiplash, cervical strain, cervical sprain, hyperextension, or acceleration injuries. The resulting syndrome is due to damage to cervical muscles, ligaments, disks, blood vessels, and nerves. The degree of damage to these structures varies from patient to patient.

A variety of mechanisms produce soft tissue neck injuries. Automobile accidents account for most of them. Sudden acceleration of the head and the neck, if of sufficient magnitude, may produce soft tissue injuries. Severy and co-workers[41] used anthropomorphic dummies and human volunteers to document extreme hyperextension as the main mechanism of whiplash injuries in rear-end collisions. Organic and electroencephalographic (EEG) brain lesions, as well as injuries to the esophagus, anterior cervical muscles and ligaments, and the intervertebral disks, have been documented in animal studies.[25, 29, 49] Reported clinical cases support the experimental findings. A partial solution to the problem of rear-end collision is the use of head restraints in all seats of every automobile.[30]

Rear-end collisions result in more severe and disabling injuries than front-end or side collisions. There is a built-in restraint to hyperflexion as the chin hits the sternum, a restraint that is lacking in hyperextension force injuries and in injuries of lateral momentum when the head momentum force is checked by the head striking the shoulder. There is no structural restriction to hyperextension until the occiput strikes against the dorsal spine, which is far beyond the normal limits of hyperextension.

In a front-end collision, an unrestrained passenger may strike the windshield, suffering a head injury and at the same time injuring the posterior cervical structures (tearing or straining the muscles and at times suffering partial or complete ligament tears). Correct use of head rests or seat extensions reduces or prevents hyperextension momentum, and internal padding of safety belts and use of air bags restrict the hyperflexion force and head impact during hyperflexion momentum.

Symptoms

The symptom complex varies vastly among patients, depending on the extent and nature of damage at impact. Cerebral symptoms may be present in two-thirds of patients.[17] Brief unconsciousness occurs in about 10% of patients. Some present with symptoms of confusion, mental dullness, or mild amnesia immediately after the injury. EEG changes have been identified after rear-end collisions.[45] Headache may begin within a few minutes after the collision and may last intermittently for several months. Neck ache is the most common early symptom, which may develop into soreness and stiffness over the neck and shoulder areas. Swallowing difficulty may last for a couple of days. Swelling and soreness in the anterior neck muscles usually disappear in about a week to 10 days, but may last longer. This is usually superseded by soreness of the posterior neck muscles. Periodic exacerbations during the recovery period are not uncommon.

Radiating pain is frequently associated with soft tissue neck injuries. Occipital headaches with radiation to occiput and eyes are not uncommon. Radiation to upper scapular and interscapular areas occurs in one-third of patients. Pain and numbness radiating into hands or arms is infrequent and carries a poor prognosis for recovery.[17] Actual nerve deficit is rare. Non-neurogenic radiation of pains, aches, paresthesias, and numbness resulting from chronic irritation of musculoligamentous, joint, and intervertebral disk structures does not follow a root or peripheral nerve distribution pattern. Non-neurogenic referred pain patterns have been experimentally produced in volunteers by injections of hypertonic saline solution into locations in cervical muscles and ligaments.[13, 19] Stimulation of the annulus during diskography similarly produces distant radiating pain.[8] Neurogenic pain, in contrast, is characterized by its clearly defined pattern of sensory, motor, reflex and electromyographic (EMG) impairment matching the distribution of nerve root pain.

Visceral symptoms like dizziness, and ringing and buzzing in the ears may accompany neck injuries. At times they are due to injury to the visceral nervous system in the neck or are side-effects of central nervous sytem injury or vascular impairment.

Patients examined soon after a whiplash injury may show few clinical findings. They may lack local soreness or muscle tightness and have pain-free normal range of motion. A few hours or a couple of days later, however, tenderness, tightness, spasm, and limited range of motion may develop. These symptoms worsen over the next few days. Patients with mild sprain may improve in about 1 week, but the symptoms may last for several weeks or months in moderate and severe injuries. Deconditioning that develops during this period may further prolong the duration of symptoms and disability.

A forward-held head position is often seen after soft tissue neck injuries. This position is probably analgesic, since it does not depend upon muscle contraction, but it unfortunately produces cumulative overstrain on the supporting posterior structures, the muscles and ligaments. If it is not counteracted by correction of posture with a gentle stretching and an active strengthening exercise program, it will cause prolongation of symptoms. Physical findings after soft tissue injuries may resolve weeks and months before symptoms abate.

Roentgenographic Findings

Absence of bony damage must not be assumed. Adequate radiographic examination must be done to study both bony and soft tissue structures. A minimal radiographic examination should include anteroposterior, lateral, and ondontoid views. Additional views may be needed depending on circumstance and might include pillar and oblique views.

A flexion and extension study may be indicated to rule out spinal instability.

An increase in the prevertebral space would suggest evidence of bleeding from anterior tissues or bones. An increase in the interspinous space suggests the possibility of a posterior ligamentous tear. Another indication is a posterior deviation in spinal curvature. Abrupt reversal of smooth cervical lordosis at one level often suggests a serious cervical injury. Smooth curves would suggest muscle spasms and compensatory muscle spasm or comfortable postures in an attempt to reduce pain. Failure to improve in a few weeks or progression of symptoms or physical signs necessitates further radiographic examination.

Treatment

Because of the large variation in the severity of injury, subjective symptoms, and clinical findings, treatment must be individualized. During the acute stage, rest to the injured parts and use of cervical supports are indicated. A soft contoured collar is usually sufficient to provide adequate support and is better tolerated by the patients. The cervical collar should hold the neck in a comfortable neutral position. As symptoms improve during the first few days, gradual mobilization should be started in the form of collar-free periods, which can gradually be lengthened. Active mobilization exercises should be started and, later, isometric strengthening exercises can be added. During the acute stages of the injury, ice is better in controlling the swelling, but later during the mobilization phase, heat is more advantageous to control the pain and facilitate movement. Moist heat or heating pads and warm showers are adequate in most cases, but if the symptoms do not resolve in a short time period, formal physical therapy and deep heat may be needed. Cervical traction is helpful in subacute and chronic cases. Analgesic medications and muscle relaxants may be needed for short periods of time. The use of narcotics may be required in some cases for short periods of time; however, nonsteroidal anti-inflammatory medications are preferred. Transcutaneous nerve stimulation (TENS) is sometimes helpful in controlling pain in selected cases. An early return to activity and work should be encouraged whenever possible. Undue delay in resumption of activity has a deleterious effect on the emotional adjustment of the patient.

Consultation with another physician should be sought when recovery does not occur as anticipated to assure the patient as well as the treating physician that no other problem is being overlooked. A further work-up at this time is usually indicated, which may include an EMG and nerve conduction studies, somatosensory evoked responses, repeat x-ray examination, cineradiography, and flexion and extension studies. If the signs and symptoms point to one intervertebral pathology, then further studies including computed tomography (CT) scan, myelography, diskography, and magnetic resonance imaging (MRI) may be indicated.

Patients with chronic pain may learn to live with their symptoms with the use of home traction units, TENS, heat, and trigger point injections (see Chapter 36 for methods of chronic pain management.)

Prognosis

Short-term follow-up studies indicate that factors extrinsic to the injury itself such as litigation and secondary gains may play an important role in the prognosis. Greenfield and Ilfeld studied short-term prognostic factors in 179 consecutive soft-tissue injury patients and noted that presence of shoulder, arm, and hand pain indicated slower prognosis. Upper back and interscapular pain needed a more intense treatment program.[50] Long-term studies reveal that a significant number of patients continue to have neck symptoms related to injury.[17] A significant number of patients without roentgenographic signs of pre-existing intervertebral disk degenerative disease at the time of injury develop disk narrowing and spur formation. There is no statistical correlation between the development of degenerative changes and continuation of symptoms.[41]

Poor prognostic factors include symptoms or findings of arm numbness or pain, a sharp reversal of the cervical curve, limitation of motion at one intervertebral level, wearing a collar for more than 12 weeks, needing home traction, or restarting physical therapy more than once.[17]

Cervical Spondylosis, Myelopathy, and Radiculopathy

Cervical spondylosis—the most common disorder of the cervical spine—is osteoarthritis involving the vertebral bodies, intervertebral disks (amphidiarthrodial joint), uncovertebral joints of Luschka, and apophyseal joints. Each of these joints may be involved to a varying degree. The presenting symptoms depend on the degree of involvement of these joints and their secondary effects on the cervical spinal nerve roots, spinal cord, and vertebral arteries. Most patients with cervical spondylosis have osteoarthritis elsewhere in the body, which frequently is asymptomatic. Cervical spondylosis increases after age 50 and is almost universal after age 70.[12,18] Pallis, Jones, and Spillane[32] studied 50 patients over age 50 who entered the hospital for reasons unrelated to the spine or nervous system and found that 75% had significant radiological evidence of cervical spondylosis; 75% had narrowing of intervertebral foramina; 50% had objective signs of cord involvement; and 40% had signs of root involvement. The positive signs were impaired vibration sense at the ankle, brisk knee and ankle jerks, and extensor Babinski responses. Few patients had any complaints.

Common symptoms of cervical spondylosis include stiffness, limitation of movement, crepitus on active or passive movements, muscle spasms, and local pain and tenderness. Lateral flexion, rotation, and extension are more limited than flexion. Pain is usually in the upper middle cervical region and may be referred to the occipital, scapular, or shoulder regions. Upper disk pain is perceived in the head and upper neck region, and lower disk pain in the neck, shoulder, and proximal and distal arm and hands. Pain is made worse with movement.

On radiographic examination the most obvious findings are reversal of normal cervical lordosis, narrowing of the intervertebral disk spaces, anterior and posterior osteophytes, osteophytes on the uncovertebral joints, and osteophytes laterally situated on the vertebral bodies. These various osteophytes encroach on the spinal canal and the intervertebral foramen. The anteroposterior diameter of the spinal cord is important for development of myelopathy, though that alone may not account for all cases. Edwards and LaRocca[11] reported the possibility of cervical myelopathy in patients with a static diameter of less than 13 mm. (A *static* anteroposterior diameter of the cervical canal is the shortest distance from the middle of the posterior surface of the vertebral body to the spinolaminar line, which is drawn through the anterior surface of the lamina on neutral lateral cervical x-rays). Penning[33] pointed out a dynamic diameter of less than 11 mm as being important in cervical myelopathy. (A *dynamic* anteroposterior canal diameter is the distance from the margin of the vertebral body to the anterosuperior margin of the inferior lamina on extension lateral cervical x-rays). Hayashi and colleagues[15] radiographically evaluated the aging changes in the cervical spine in 100 subjects. They documented a greater narrowing of the dynamic diameter of the cervical canal than of the static diameter, though both decreased with age, except at the C2–C3 level. Posterior osteophytes at C5–C6 or C6–C7 and retrolisthesis at C3–C4 or C4–C5 were the major levels of stenosis associated with changes in dynamic canal stenosis. Some subjects had critical static and dynamic canal stenosis without evidence of myelopathy, while others with signs of myelopathy were without critical static and dynamic stenosis. Hence, other factors besides spinal stenosis play a part in the development of myelopathy. These factors may include changes in the cord, repeated trauma or soft tissue entrapment from disk protrusion, and infolding of the ligamentum flavum.

Cervical spondylotic myelopathy is the most common disease of the spinal cord after middle age. Its onset is insidious and diagnosis is made only several years after onset. The neurological signs and symptoms are variable and depend on the site, extent, severity, and rate of evolution of the lesions. Gait disturbance and lower extremity weakness are the most common symptoms. Radicular symptoms may also be present, which reflects the degree of associated nerve root compression. The most common clinical signs are the presence of spasticity and weakness in the lower extremities. However, spasticity and weakness in the proximal and distal muscles of the upper extremities are also frequently seen. Patients can be divided into categories according to the predominant cord syndromes.[5] In the transverse myelopathy group there is corticospinal tract involvement combined with posterior column or spinothalamic tract involvement. A predominantly motor system syndrome is seen in some patients who have evidence of severe corticospinal tract involvement with or without anterior horn cell involvement and with an often present but relatively insignificant sensory deficit. Brown-Séquard syndrome, with ipsilateral corticospinal deficit and contralateral analgesia, is relatively uncommon. Occasionally patients may present with central cord syndrome with upper extremity weakness and sensory loss, but with lower extremities spared. The usual indications for surgery in cervical myelopathy are progressive decline in spinal cord function and sagittal narrowing of the spinal canal to less than 13 mm.

In cervical radiculopathy, root involvement may be single or multiple, unilateral or bilateral, symmetric or asymmetric. Both the motor and sensory roots may be involved with both motor and sensory symptoms (Table 38-2). Sensory symptoms are more common and disabling than motor symptoms. The sensory symptoms include pain, paresthesias, hyperesthesias, and hypoesthesia. Pain may be referred to the neck, head, periscapular, pectoral, and shoulder regions with radiation of symptoms into different parts of the upper extremities. Radicular pain is present in more than half of these patients. The onset of pain is slow and progressive in most cases. Some patients present with atrophy in the intrinsic muscles of the hands with radiographic evidence of osteophytes corresponding to levels of atrophy, but without disabling sensory symptoms. The neuralgic pain is often shooting, stabbing, and intermittent with dermatomal or sclerotomal distribution. Roots pains are usually proximal and rarely extend beyond the elbows, whereas paresthetic symptoms such as "pins and needles," cold or hot sensations, or numbness are often distal.

Table 38-2
Cervical Radiculopathies

Disk Space Involved	Root Involved	Clinical Presentation	Reflex Changes	Muscles With EMG Changes
C4–C5	C5	Hypoesthesia, lateral aspect of shoulder Weak deltoid & biceps	Decreased biceps reflex	Rhomboid Deltoid Supraspinatus Biceps Serratus anterior
C5–C6	C6	Hypoesthesia, lateral aspect of forearm & thumb Weak deltoid & biceps	Decreased biceps & brachio-radialis reflexes	Same as for C4–C5 plus pronator teres, extensor carpi radialis longus
C6–C7	C7	Hypoesthesia, index & middle fingers Weak pronators & hand grip	Decreased triceps reflex	Triceps Pronator teres Flexor carpi radialis Extensor digitorum communis anconeus
C7–C8	C8	Hypoesthesia, ulnar finger Weak intrinsic hand muscles		Intrinsic hand, triceps, & forearm

Treatment

Aims of treatment are to relieve pain, relax muscle spasm, enable the patient to rest, and protect the injured part to allow healing, rebuild muscle strength and endurance, restore functional and normal range of motion, and restore normal function.

ANALGESICS. Narcotic analgesic medications should be avoided if possible, since most often shoulder and neck pains are chronic with recurrent acute episodes. Aspirin and other nonsteroidal anti-inflammatory drugs are a better choice for controlling pain and for their anti-inflammatory effects. Phenylbutazone and indomethacin are often effective in reducing acute inflammatory reaction in radiculitis or bursitis. Local injection of steroids into a bursa or around the bicipital tendon at times can dramatically improve the acute inflammatory process in a localized shoulder problem.

Muscle relaxants are often used to relieve muscle spasm, but their effectiveness is variable and controversial. Cyclobenzaprine and diazepam are more effective than other agents, but both of them are quite sedating.

HEAT AND COLD. Heat is helpful in symptomatic treatment of painful muscle spasms (see Chapter 3). Pain, muscle spasms, and guarding are common symptoms seen in intervertebral disk disease with or without nerve root irritation. Relaxation of painful muscle spasms is a result of excitation of exteroceptors of the skin and its subsequent direct effect on the spindle mechanism. Short-wave diathermy, which heats skin, subcutaneous fat, and superficial layers of muscles, is quite effective in relieving muscle spasm when used for 20 to 30 minutes. Superficial heat, like hot packs, hydrocollator packs, or radiant lamps or heat cradles, also achieves muscle spasm relaxation owing to the skin's reaction to the heat. Use of heat is followed by active and passive exercises and deep and friction massage.

Heat is also used to stretch contractures. It is essential to selectively heat the fibrous tissue that limits the motion. Stretching exercises should be carried out during and after the use of heat. Microwave heat at 915 MHz for 30 minutes with direct contact applicators is most effective in working on diffuse fibrosis of muscles. Short-wave diathermy with induction coil is only effective in heating superficial muscle layers. Ultrasound is most effective in heating the deepest layers of muscles and in working on joint contractures (See Chapter 13).

Application of cold with the use of ice packs or ice massage reduces muscle spindle sensitivity and thus reduces muscle spasm. Heat or cold and low-dose ultrasound treatments can be used to disperse trigger points in myofascial syndrome or fibrositis.

MASSAGE. Massage is useful in relaxing muscle spasm, in improving circulation, and in dispersing tender areas in spasmotic muscles. It is often used after heat or cold treatments and in conjunction with stretching postures and stretching exercises (see Chapter 14).

EXERCISE. Complete rest to the cervical region is sometimes necessary for a few days after the acute onset of cervical pain or cervical strain. Cervical mobilization and exercises should be started as soon as the acute symptoms allow. The exercises should include cervical mobilization exercises, shoulder mobilization exercises, and muscle strengthening exercises for the cervical, periscapular, and upper extremity muscles. Exercises should be done within the limits of pain production. Local muscle spasm, such as in the trapezius and rhomboid muscles, often responds to maximum contraction against resistance followed by relaxation. Isometric exercise with resistance applied

by the hands to flexion, extension, lateral flexion, and rotation to either side is usually well tolerated initially.

Stretching exercises to the cervical muscles (especially to the trapezius and sternocleidomastoid) must also be included. This is easily accomplished by pulling the arm down with the opposite arm while stretching the neck muscles by laterally bending the neck to the opposite side and flexing and extending the neck slowly in the laterally flexed position and slowly rotating the neck first to one side and then to the other side. Slowly executing all movements of the cervical spine, usually brings about marked relief of muscle spasm, tension, and pain and restores cervical motion. (See Chapter 18 for more discussion on the effects of exercise.)

CERVICAL TRACTION. Cervical traction is very helpful in relieving cervical muscle spasm, stretching cervical muscles, and in relieving pain in early cervical radiculopathies with degenerative arthritis. Traction may be applied in a consistent or intermittent form and either in a vertical or horizontal position. Correctly applied, it stretches the cervical spine and enlarges the intervertebral foramina and thereby relieves compressive forces on the nerve roots.

Intermittent traction is applied manually, either as cervical manipulation or with the use of a motorized cervical traction unit (Fig. 38-12). It can be adjusted to the desired weight, period of traction, and period of relaxation desired. Traction and relaxation timing is measured in seconds and usually arbitrarily selected based upon the physician's clinical experience and patient tolerance. During the traction phase, the paracervical muscles tend to resist the forces of pull by contracting, while during the nontraction phase they relax as the forces are reduced to zero. Traction has a massagelike effect of reducing muscle spasm and thus allowing more effective subsequent traction.[44]

There is no agreement as to the amount of weight required to produce vertebral distraction.[14, 21] Often a 5- to 10-pound weight is used, which is inadequate even to support the head weight. Jackson[20] advocates beginning with a 15- to 20-pound weight and gradually increasing to 35 to 50 pounds in more muscular individuals. The traction is applied for 15 to 30 minutes on a daily basis, or at least three times a week. The force of traction should be with the head in 15° to 20° of flexion, with the force applied over the occiput and not over the mandible. Occipital force is not only better tolerated during traction but is also more effective in distracting the posterior cervical structures and

Figure 38-12. Motorized intermittent verticle cervical traction.

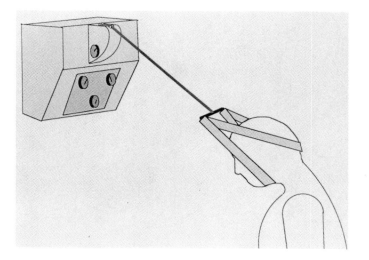

increasing the intervertebral foramina size. During traction the patient sits facing the traction unit at a distance of about 1 to 2 feet so that the traction of pull is approximately 60° to the horizontal (Fig. 38-13). The position of the halter should be adjusted to reduce pressure on the mandible.

Horizontal traction (Fig. 38-13) is most often used in hospitalized patients with acute pain. It allows prolonged traction with the patient in a more relaxed position. Since the traction time is longer, weight tolerance is less.[40] Starting weight is usually 5 pounds for 1 to 2 hours, three times a day. Gradually the weight is increased to tolerance as the patient is able to tolerate a greater amount of weight (8 to 10 pounds) for most of the day and night, with rest periods for meals. The angle of pull should be maintained in flexion at about 45° to the horizontal.

If the traction is found to be helpful under a supervised setting, then the patient should be educated in the use of a home unit (Fig. 38-14) and supplied with it. Use of a home unit follows principles similar to those for intermittent traction units. At times a home unit alone suffices to relieve the symptoms. The home unit attaches to a door, with the patient sitting about 2 feet away facing it; a water bag or weights are used for resistance.

CERVICAL ORTHOSES. Cervical collars are used to immobilize and rest the cervical region; to reduce mechanical stresses on the joints, ligaments, and muscles; and to relax and relieve painful muscle spasm and let the tissues heal. The type of collar used depends largely on the degree and extent of immobilization needed. The cervical collars can be broadly divided into four groups. The *tubular* collars are those that extend from the upper cervical or submandibular region to the lower cervical region. These collars are made either of soft materials like foam, felt wraps, or cervical ruffs[44] made out of 1-inch stockinette padded with surgical cotton and tied in front, or of more firm materials like Plastizote, plastic, or molded leather. These collars primarily work as a reminder to the patient to not move the neck to the extremes of ranges of motion.

The second group of cervical collars are the *mandibular and occipital extension* collars, including those made of firm Plastizote (Philadelphia) or polyethylene. They limit anteroposterior cervical motion to approximately 30% of normal, allowing 43% of normal rotation and 67% of lateral bending.[14, 21]

The next group of cervical orthoses have *sterno-manubrial and upper thoracic extensions,* and also mandibular and occipital extensions as well. Although they are more effective in restricting cervical movements than other collars, the degree of effectiveness depends on the rigidity and fit of the proximal and distal extensions. The most effective of these orthoses is the four-poster adjustable orthosis. The four-poster cervical orthosis consists of a chin piece and an occipital piece connected with four adjustable uprights to sternal and posterior thoracic plates. The four posts are easily adjustable. The SOMI (sternal occipitalmandibular immobilizer) has three uprights that attach to the mandibular and occipital pieces anchored to a firm suprascapular and sternal piece, and soft posterior straps. These orthoses are not often needed in managing cervical pain. The fourth group of orthoses include the *Halo-type cervical orthosis,* which is attached to a sub-biparietal diameter with metal pins that penetrate the outer table of the skull and are attached with a mechanism of metal rods to a polyethylene jacket.

For most situations a soft tubular cervical orthosis is adequate to rest the cervical region. It is desirable to support the neck in a neutral, comfortable position with the head tilted slightly forward so that the anterior cervical muscles are relaxed and the cervical foramina open. Motions to be limited are flexion and extension and rotation beyond the limits of comfort. The addition of an occipital extension is often helpful to limit extension.

In a well-fitted collar the edges should be padded sufficiently to prevent pressure discomfort. Posteriorly, its superior edge should fit under the occiput below the superior nuchal line; the inferior border should rest on the trapezii without pressing on the lower cervical or upper thoracic spinous processes. Anteriorly, the superior edge should be shaped to prevent pressure on the mandibular angles and, if a chin piece is used, pressure should be widely distributed and not focused just on the mental protuberance. Inferiorly, the collar should be cut out over the clavicles to permit pressure to be borne on the manubrium.[44]

Active cervical mobilization should be started as soon as the

Figure 38-14. Home door traction unit.

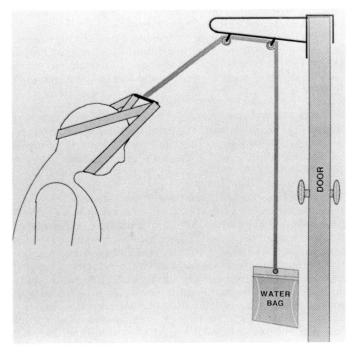

Figure 38-13. Horizontal cervical traction.

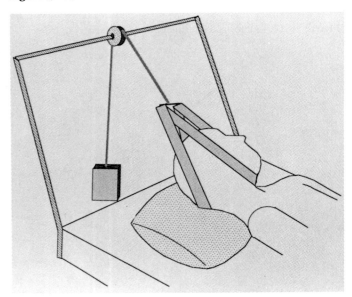

acute symptoms settle. This should be in the form of active range-of-motion exercises within the limits of discomfort and gentle cervical isometric muscle strengthening exercises.

Vertebral Artery Insufficiency Syndrome

Large osteophytes projecting laterally from the vertebral bodies may compress the vertebral artery causing intermittent symptoms of circulatory ischemia of the brain. A variety of symptoms have been described including cervical pain, headache, lightheadedness, dizziness and vertigo, syncopal attacks, ataxia, cerebral incoordination with staggering gait, diplopia, nystagmus, facial numbness, dysesthesias and atypical facial neuralgia, dysphagia, speech disturbance, Horner's syndrome, tinnitus, and precordial pain. Presenting symptoms are almost always triggered by increases in neck movements either by extension or turning of the head toward the side of the lesion. The symptoms result from direct compression of the vertebral artery by the osteophytes or irritation of the nerves that supply the vertebral artery, thus causing reflex vascular spasm. Development of ischemic symptoms depends on the adequacy of the carotid circulation. Many factors negatively influence blood flow in the vertebral and carotid circulation, including atheromatosis; cholesterol emboli from plaques; congenital anomalies; disorders of bone, joint, and muscles in the cervical region; cervical collars; carotid sinus compression, trauma; and usual and unusual neck movements.

Bilateral vertebral angiography demonstrates the size of the arteries and the location of the lesion, but angiography is not without risk. The definitive treatment is surgical decompression of the artery and excision of the offending osteophytes.

Thoracic Outlet Syndrome

The term *thoracic outlet syndrome* (TOS), first suggested by Rob and Standoven in 1958,[36] helped to unify a number of syndromes involving neurovascular compression problems at the thoracic outlet. It includes scalenus anticus syndrome, costocervical syndrome, brachial plexus compression syndrome, subcoracoid pectoralis minor syndrome, and the first thoracic rib syndrome. The symptoms in these syndromes result from the compression of the neurovascular bundle (brachial plexus, subclavian artery, and subclavian vein as it passes from the neck to the arm.[4, 26]

The thoracic outlet consists of the space between the inferior border of the clavicle and the upper border of the first rib (Fig. 38-15). This space is compartmentalized by the scalene muscles which arise from the transverse processes of the cervical vertebrae and insert on the first or the second rib. The scalenus anterior arises from the anterior tubercles of the transverse processes of the third to the sixth cervical vertebrae and inserts on the scalene tubercle on the inner border of the first rib. The scalenus medius originates from the posterior tubercles of the transverse processes of all the cervical vertebrae and inserts on the first rib behind the groove for the subclavian artery. Scalenus posterior arises from the transverse processes of the fifth and sixth cervical vertebrae and inserts on the second rib. The subclavian vein exists through the space formed by the clavicle, first rib, and anterior scalene muscle. The brachial plexus and subclavian artery exit between the anterior and middle scalene muscles, the clavicle, and the first rib. The next potential site of compression is the point at which the neurovascular bundle passes beneath the tendinous portion of the pectoralis minor where the pectoralis minor inserts on the coracoid process of the scapula. Hence, the various components of the neurovascular bundle can be compressed at several sites. The subclavian vein can be compressed between the scalenus anterior, the clavicle, and the first rib; the brachial plexus (with or without compression of the subclavian artery) between the scalenus anterior, scalenus medius, and first rib; compression of the neurovascular bundle by the scissor action between the clavicle and the first rib; and the compression of the neurovascular bundle as it passes underneath the tendinous insertion of pectoralis minor[3] (Fig. 38-16).

In addition to the anatomic relationships of these structures, several other factors may contribute to narrowing of the thoracic outlet. Hyperabduction of the arm above the head results in the axillary nerve being moved through 180° thus pulling the nerves and vessels across the coracoid process and the head of the humerus. Clavicular rotation in abduction further narrows the retroclavicular space. These dynamic factors may play a role in some patients. The static factors that are important in some patients include increased muscular bulk in those involved in vigorous occupations. The increased muscular bulk reduces the space for the neurovascular structures. Lack of adequate muscle tone and bulk in inactive middle-aged adults leads to sagging shoulders and thus compression of the neurovascular structures at the thoracic outlet. Drooping shoulder syndrome has been described as a separate entity.[7, 42] This syndrome is primarily

Figure 38-15. Relationship of the neurovascular bundle to the clavicle scalenus muscles and first rib. (Kelly TR: Thoracic outlet syndrome: Current concepts and treatment. Ann Surg 190:657, 1979)

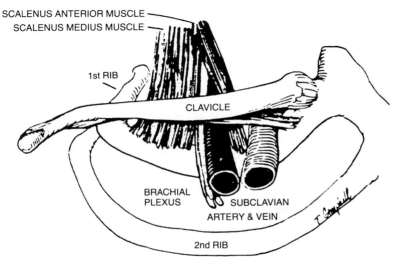

SCALENUS ANTERIOR MUSCLE
SCALENUS MEDIUS MUSCLE
1st RIB
CLAVICLE
BRACHIAL PLEXUS
SUBCLAVIAN ARTERY & VEIN
2nd RIB

limited to women and presents as pain and paresthesias involving the shoulder and arms in patients with excessively long necks and low-set shoulders. Brachial plexus stretch produced by low-hanging shoulders, rather than compression, has been suggested as the cause for the symptom.[43] There is absence of vascular, motor, or sensory involvement. Reflexes are usually normal, as are the conduction studies. There is immediate relief of symptoms by passive shoulder elevation and exacerbation of symptoms on palpation of the brachial plexus or passive downward traction of the arm.[43] On radiographic examination of the

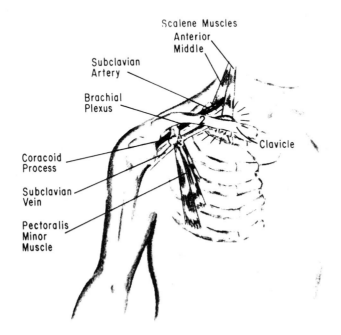

Figure 38-16.   Costoclavicular space and its relationship to the neurovascular bundle. (1) Brachial plexus and subclavian artery can be compressed between the scalene muscles. Compression by a cervical rib can also occur at this level (see Fig. 38-18). (2) Compression of the neurovascular bundle can occur between the first rib and clavicle. (3) Elevation of the arm may compress the neurovascular bundle against the coracoid process by the pectoralis minor. (Ambrosia RD: Musculoskeletal Disorders, Regional Examination and Differential Diagnosis. Philadelphia, JB Lippincott, 1977)

Figure 38-17.   Schematic diagram showing anatomical strictures that may compress the neurovascular bundle against the first rib, resulting in venous signs and symptoms. (Kelly TR: Thoracic outlet syndrome: Current concepts and treatment. Ann Surg 190:657, 1979)

neck, the second or lower thoracic vertebrae are visible above the shoulders on a lateral view of the cervical spine.

Several congenital factors may encroach the space between the first rib and the clavicle and play a part in the pathogenesis.[37] A cervical rib, whether complete or incomplete or represented by a fibrous extension, may encroach on the interscalene interval and on the retroclavicular space. The cervical rib originates from the transverse process of C7 and attaches directly or by a ligament to the first rib. It is the most common bony abnormality, but only less than 10% of these patients have symptoms. Abnormalities of the first rib such as bifid rib, which at times may be represented as a bony protuberance or anomalous reduction of the anterior curvature of the clavicle, may also encroach the space between the first rib and the clavicle. Scalene muscles vary considerably in their insertion to the first rib and the arrangement of their fibers.[3, 4] The subclavian artery or portions of the brachial plexus may pass through instead of between the scalene muscles. Abnormalities related to both the origin and insertion of scalenus anterior are either secondary to direct compression or due to significant space reduction.

Fracture of the clavicle with malunion or nonunion and excessive callus formation may impinge on the subjacent neurovascular structures. A single or repeated subacromial dislocation of the humerus may be the inciting cause in some patients. Severe injuries to the thorax may stretch the brachial plexus or thrombose the artery or the vein and thus initiate the symptoms.

At times in an arteriosclerotic extremity, an unusually vigorous activity may cause thrombosis or further narrowing and compression of the vessels. Ischemic symptoms will develop in an extremity where previous minimal compression was not sufficient to cause symptoms.

Any condition that affects the normally narrow rigid thoracic outlet space will impinge on the neurovascular complex and cause symptoms. These conditions include tumors of the upper lobe of the lung and displacement of the first rib by cervicothoracic scoliosis (Fig. 38-17).

Signs and Symptoms

Signs and symptoms vary greatly depending on whether the brachial plexus, subclavian artery, or subclavian vein is being compressed.[22, 35] There may be both vascular and neural symptoms (see Fig. 38-17). Compression of the brachial plexus is associated with pain, numbness, and paresthesias, and motor symptoms may be associated with weakness and atrophy of

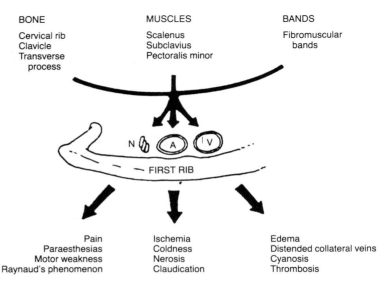

muscles. Pain is usually localized to the neck and shoulder regions with radiation to the suprascapular region, and paresthesias, numbness, and hypoesthesia in the ulnar nerve (C8 and T1) distribution involving the arm, forearm, and hand. Activities involving abduction of the shoulders such as combing the hair, painting walls, and hanging pictures cause worsening of the symptoms.

Arterial symptoms include pain, weakness, coldness, and easy fatigability of the arm. Radial pulse may be dampened or absent on different arm maneuvers. Raynaud's phenomenon, ulceration, and gangrene in advanced cases may be present. Abduction or elevation of the arm may exacerbate the symptoms. In presence of venous obstruction, the arm may be aching with swelling, cyanosis, and edema. Distended collateral veins around the shoulder and anterior chest may be seen. Thrombosis of the subclavian vein (Paget-Schoetter or "effort thrombosis") is frequently noted.[22]

Three clinical maneuvers are usually employed to assess the arterial involvement, as already noted: the costoclavicular maneuver (see Fig. 38-9), hyperabduction maneuver (see Fig. 38-10), and Adson's test (see Fig. 38-11). During these maneuvers the examiner monitors the radial pulse and auscultates the supra- and infraclavicular areas. A positive test is associated with decreased or absent radial pulse. A bruit may also be heard. Each of these maneuvers, if positive, has also been described as independent syndromes.

Diagnosis

The diagnosis of thoracic outlet syndrome is often a diagnosis of exclusion. Bony abnormalities are present in about 20% of cases, as cervical rib, long transverse ligament, clavicular abnormalities, bifid first rib, or fusion of the first and the second ribs.[22]

Roentgenographic examination of the cervical region is essential not only to document these abnormalities but also to see arthritic changes and neural encroachment with nerve root compression (Fig. 38-18). A radiographic examination of the chest should also be done to rule out an apical lesion of the lung.[26] A subclavian arteriogram may document subclavian artery compression, at the medial border of the first rib in 90% of the patients with radial pulse abnormalities.[22] Venography may document venous thrombosis in patients with venous symptoms.[22] EMG and nerve conduction studies are helpful in ruling out brachial plexus involvement and in ruling out such other causes as radiculopathies or compressive neuropathies, including carpal tunnel syndrome.[9, 22] EMG and nerve conduction abnormalities are not seen in patients free of neurological deficits even when vascular signs exist on clinical tests. In patients with clear neurological deficits, F-wave latency may be increased on the affected side. Reduced or absent ulnar sensory action potential and evidence of "denervation" in the ulnar innervated muscles may also exist.

Treatment

The treatment depends on the cause of the neurovascular compression. The basis of conservative treatment is the premise that an elevation and slight abduction of the shoulder girdle decreases the compressive forces on the neurovascular bundle at the thoracic outlet. Emphasis is also placed on strengthening the shoulder girdle muscles and on correction of posture. Heat or ice is often used in combination with stretching exercises. The muscles that usually need to be stretched are pectoralis minor and scalene muscles. In simple shoulder-shrugging exercises the shoulder girdle is elevated to the ears, contraction is held in the

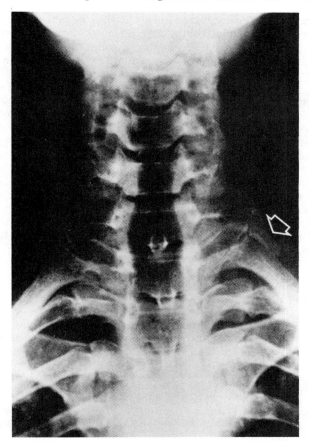

Figure 38-18. Roentgenogram of the neck verifies cervical rib (*arrow*) as source of a neurovascular disturbance in the upper extremity. (Ambrosia RD: Musculoskeletal Disorders, Regional Examination and Differential Diagnosis. Philadelphia, JB Lippincott, 1977)

elevated position for 3 to 5 seconds, followed by lowering of the shoulder to the relaxed position. The exercises should be done seven to ten times at a sitting, and five to ten times a day.[26] The goal of this exercise is to reduce muscular tension through muscle contraction and relaxation.

Resistance exercises are done to increase strength, endurance, and postural tone of the shoulder girdle elevator muscles. With hypertrophy of the shoulder girdle elevator muscles, the shoulder girdle obtains an overall elevation and widening of the thoracic outlet. The primary shoulder strengthening exercise is done with a prescribed amount of weight held in the hands, with the arms by the side of the trunk; elevation of the weight is done using the shoulder girdle muscles. Too heavy weights that would depress the shoulders should be avoided. The weight is increased as the muscles get stronger.

Sleeping posture can be adjusted with the use of pillows to maintain the shoulders in an abducted and slightly elevated posture. Usually three pillows are needed. With the patient in the supine position, one pillow is placed to support the head and neck in slight flexion and two pillows are placed lengthwise just under the scapulae on either side to force the scapulae into abduction and slight elevation.[26] The pillows may be pinned to each other and to the mattress to prevent wandering during the night. When sitting, the use of an arm chair to support the weight of the arms also helps. When standing, the arms can be rested by placing the hands on the waist or on the belt to help reduce downward pull of the shoulder girdle. The patient should also be advised to avoid repetitive overhead activity and carrying weights that might depress the shoulder girdle. Women with large breasts may be helped by the use of an underwire support bra so that the weight of the breasts can be supported on the thorax rather than be carried by the shoulders. Cervical traction may be helpful if there is associated cervical disease.

If symptoms fail to respond to conservative treatment, surgery should be considered, especially if sensory symptoms of coldness, paresthesias, and intolerable pain, and motor involvement with progressive weakness, fatigue, and in coordination of the hand persist.[38] Severe venous symptoms of venous congestion, cyanosis, and persistent edema of the arm and arterial symptoms of ischemic coldness, fatigue, and pain in the arm and hand from subclavian artery plaque formation, aneurysmal dilatation, and emboli rarely improve with conservative management.[38] The basic operation most commonly effective is transaxillary intraperiosteal resection of the first rib and all anomalous structures at the thoracic outlet.[44, 47] The results of surgery have been reported to be good in 85% of properly selected cases.[47]

REFERENCES

1. Bennett RM: The fibrositis/fibromyalgia syndrome, current issue and perspective. Proceedings of a symposium, introduction, Am J Med (Suppl 3A) 8:1, 1986
2. Bland JH, O'Brien R, Bouchard RE: Palmar erythema and spider angiomata in rheumatoid arthritis. Ann Intern Med 48:1026, 1953
3. Brown C: Compressive, invasive referred pain to the shoulder. Clin Orthop 173:55–62, 1983
4. Caldwell JW, Crane CR, Krusen EM: Nerve conduction studies: An aid in the diagnosis of the thoracic outlet syndrome. South Med J 64(2):210–212, 1971
5. Candall PH, Batzdorf U: Cervical spondylotic myelopathy. J Neurosurg 25:57–66, 1966
6. Chan RC, Steinbok P: Delayed onset of Lhermitte's sign following head and or neck injuries. J Neurosurg 60:609–612, 1984
7. Clein LJ: The drooping shoulder syndrome. Can Med Assoc J 114:343–344, 1976
8. Cloward RB: Cervical discography— a contribution to the etiology and mechanism of neck, shoulder, and arm pain. Ann Surg 150:1052, 1959
9. Daube JR: Nerve conduction studies in thoracic outlet syndrome. Neurology 25:347, 1975
10. Dolibar M: Role of the physical therapist at pain treatment centers. Phys Ther 64(6):905, 1984
11. Edwards WC, LaRocca H: The developmental segmental sagittal diameter of the cervical canal in patients with cervical spondylosis. Spine 8:20, 1983
12. Elias F: Roentgen findings in the asymptomatic cervical spine. NY State J Med 58:3300, 1958
13. Feinstein B, Langton JNK, Jameson RM, Schiller F: Experiments on pain, referred from deep somatic tissue. J Bone Joint Surg 36A:981, 1954
14. Fisher SV, Bowar JF, Awad EA, Gullickson G: Cervical orthoses' effect on cervical spine motion: Roentgenographic and goniometric method of study. Arch Phys Med Rehabil 58:109–115, 1977
15. Hayashi H, Okada, K, Hamada M et al: Etiologic factors of myelopathy. Clin Orthop 214: 200–209, 1987
16. Hench P: Secondary fibrositis. Am J Med (Suppl 3A) 8:60–62, 1986
17. Hohl M: Soft-tissue injuries of the neck in automobile accidents— Factors influencing prognosis. J Bone Joint Surg 56A:1675, 1974
18. Hult L: The Munkfors investigation: A study of the frequency and course of the stiff neck, brachialgia and lumbo sciatica syndromes as well as observations on certain signs and symptoms from the dorsal spine and the joints of the extremities in industrial and forest workers. Acta Orthop Scand 23 (Suppl 16):1–76, 1954

19. Inman VT, Saunders JB de CM: Referred pain from skeletal structures. J Nerv Ment Dis 99:660, 1944
20. Jackson R: The Cervical Syndrome. Springfield, IL, Charles C Thomas, 1956
21. Johnson RM, Hart D, Simmons EF et al: Cervical orthoses. J Bone Joint Surg 59A:332–339, 1977
22. Kelley TR: Thoracic outlet syndrome: Current concepts of treatment. Ann Surg 190(5):657–662, 1979
23. Leaver RC, Loeser JD: Lhermitte's phenomenon after high velocity missile injuries of the brain. J Neurosurg 34:159–163, 1971
24. Lhermitte J: Etude de la commation de la moele. Rev Neurol 1:210–239, 1932
25. Macnab I: Acceleration injuries of the cervical spine. J Bone Joint Surg 46A:1797, 1964
26. McGough EC, Pearce MB, Byrne JP: Management of thoracic outlet syndrome. J Thorac Cardiovasc Surg 77(2):169–174, 1979
27. Melzack R, Stillwell DM, Fox EJ: Trigger points and acupuncture points for pain: Correlation and implications. Pain 3:3–23, 1977
28. Nakano KK: Neck pain. In Kelley WN, Harris ED, Ruddy S, Sledge CB (eds): Text Book of Rheumatology, 2nd ed, pp 416–435. Philadelphia, WB Sanders, 1985
29. Ommaya AK, Faas F, Yarnell P: Whiplash and brain damage. JAMA 204(4):285, 1968
30. O'Neill B, Haddon W Jr, Kelley AB, Sorenson WW: Automobile head restraints. Am J Public Health 62:399, 1972
31. Orofino C, Sherman MS, Schechter D: Luskcha's joint—a degenerative phenomenon. JBJS 42A:853–858, 1960
32. Pallis C, Jones AM, Spillane JD: Cervical spondylosis: Incidence and implications. Brain 77:274, 1954
33. Penning L: Some aspects of plain radiography of the cervical spine in chronic myelopathy. Neurology 12:513, 1962
34. Penning L: Functional Pathology of the Cervical Spine. Amsterdam, Exceptra Medica, 1968
35. Resnick D, Shaul SR, Robin JM: Diffuse idiopathic skeletal hyperostosis (DISH): Forestier's disease with extraspinal manifestations. Radiology 115:513, 1975
36. Rob CG, Standoven A: Arterial occlusion complicating—Thoracic outlet compression syndrome. Br Med J 2:709–712, 1958
37. Roos DB: Congenital anomalies associated with thoracic outlet syndrome of anatomy, symptoms, diagnosis and treatment. Am J Surg 123:771–778, 1976.
38. Roos DB: Essentials and safeguards of surgery for thoracic outlet syndrome. Angiology 32(1):187–193, 1981.
39. Schmorl G, Junghans H: The Human Spine in Health and Disease. New York, Grune Stratton, 1959
40. Schutt CH, Dohan FC: Neck injury to women in auto accidents. JAMA 206:2689, 1968.
41. Severy DM, Mathewson JH, Bechtol CD: Controlled automobile medical phenomena. Can Serv Med J 11:727, 1955
42. Smythe HA: Nonarticular rheumatism and the fibrositis syndrome. In Hollander JL, McCarty DJ (eds): Arthritis and Allied Conditions, pp 874–884. Philadelphia, Lea & Febiger, 1972
43. Swift TR, Nichols FT: The drooping shoulder syndrome. Neurology 34:212–215, 1984
44. Thistle HG: Neck and shoulder pain: Evaluation and conservative management. Med Clin North Am 53(3):511–524, 1969
45. Torrs F, Shapiro S: Electroencephalogram in whiplash injury. Arch Neurol 5:28, 1961
46. Travel J, Simons DG: Myofascial Pain and Dysfunction—The Trigger Point Manual. Baltimore, Williams & Wilkins, 1983.
47. Urschel HD Jr, Rosyuk MA: Management of thoracic outlet syndrome—Current concepts. N Engl J Med 286:1140, 1972
48. White AA, Panjabi MM: Clinical Biomechanics of the Spine. Philadelphia, JB Lippincott, 1978
49. Wickstrom JK, Martinex JL, Rodriguez RP Jr, Hains DM: Hyperextension and hyperflexion injuries to the head and neck of primates. Paper presented at Wayne State University, May 1969
50. Wolfe F: The clinical syndrome of fibrositis. Am J Med (Suppl 3A) 81(7) 1986

39

Rehabilitation of the Patient With Arthritis and Connective Tissue Disease

Jeanne E. Hicks

Lynn H. Gerber

During the past decade, there has been increased interest in what rehabilitation can offer patients with rheumatic disease and increased awareness of significant improvements that have resulted from rehabilitation interventions. Both have helped to place the specialty on a more rational basis.[210] Whereas rheumatology is dedicated to the understanding and control of disease activity, rehabilitation medicine aims to maintain or restore function or prevent dysfunction by the use of physical modalities and techniques, exercise, orthotics, assistive and adaptive devices, energy conservation and joint protection techniques, and vocational planning.[90]

Rheumatic disease bridges a broad spectrum, including both articular and nonarticular disorders. This chapter is confined mainly to articular disorders.

Arthritis involves a joint or joints in an inflammatory and destructive or a noninflammatory mechanical degenerative process. It may affect one or many joints, be an acute process which completely resolves (septic joint), or be a chronic event (rheumatoid arthritis). Arthritis may involve all the joint structures: synovium, cartilage, tendons, capsule, bone, and surrounding muscle. It is often part of a systemic rheumatic disease (connective tissue disease): rheumatoid arthritis (RA), juvenile rheumatoid arthritis (JRA), systemic lupus erythematosus (SLE), polymyositis (PM), scleroderma (PSS). These diseases are usually chronic, remitting, and relapsing; they are variable in their course and affect multiple organ systems in addition to joints. They require long-term treatments with drugs, which may have a significant impact on appearance, sleep, psychological function, and reproductive ability. The physiatrist directing the rehabilitation team must bear all these issues in mind when evaluating and devising a treatment plan.

This chapter emphasizes the importance of a good initial evaluation and periodic reevaluation of the arthritis patient and the rational and stage-specific manner in which rehabilitative treatments are applied to the problems of patients with rheumatic diseases.

ARTHRITIC DISEASES AND THEIR CHARACTERISTICS

Classification

The important determinants in classifying arthritis are whether the disorder is inflammatory or noninflammatory, symmetrical or asymmetrical, or accompanied by systemic and extra-articular manifestations (Fig. 39-1).

A good history and physical examination and appropriate laboratory and x-ray studies will often allow a specific diagnosis to be made. Clinical features that suggest inflammatory rather than noninflammatory disease include acute painful onset, fever, erythema of the skin over the joint or joints involved, warmth of the joint or joints, and tenderness that usually parallels the degree of inflammation.[186]

Laboratory and x-ray findings that suggest an inflammatory process include an increased peripheral white blood cell count with left shift, an elevated erythrocyte sedimentation rate, a group II joint fluid (Table 39-1), and x-ray demonstration of soft tissue swelling, evidence of periostitis, bony erosions, or uniform cartilage loss (Table 39-2).

Inflammatory arthritis falls into four different groups. *Inflammatory connective tissue disease* includes RA, JRA, SLE, dermatomyositis-polymyositis (DM-PM), and mixed connective tissue disease (MCTD). *Inflammatory, crystal-induced disease* includes gout and pseudogout. *Inflammation induced by infectious agents* includes bacterial, viral, tuberculous, and fungal arthritis. Finally, *seronegative spondyloarthropathies* include ankylosing spondylitis (AS), psoriatic arthritis, Reiter's disease, and inflammatory bowel disease (IBD).

Noninflammatory arthritis may be classified as degenerative: osteoarthritis (OA) and aseptic necrosis (AN); or metabolic: lipid storage disease, hemochromatosis, ochronosis, hypogammaglobulinemia, and hemoglobinopathies.[10, 216]

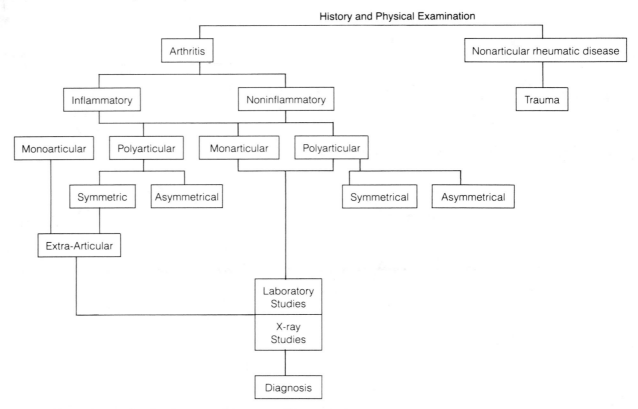

Figure 39-1. Steps in the classification and diagnosis of rheumatic disease.

Table 39-1
Synovial Fluid Analysis

Fluid Group	*Color*	*Clarity*	*Viscosity*	*Mucin Clot*	*Cells/mm³*	*White Blood Cells % Polymorphonuclear Leukocytes*
Normal	Pale yellow	Transparent	High	Good	< 200	< 25%
Group I (noninflammatory)	Yellow or straw	Transparent	High	Good	< 2000	< 25%
Group II (moderately inflammatory)	Yellow or straw	Transparent to opaque, slightly cloudy	Variably decreased	Fair to poor	3,000–50,000	> 70%
Group III (highly inflammatory, septic)	Variable: yellow-greyish, purulent	Opaque, cloudy	Low	Poor	50,000–100,000 (usually 100,000 or more)	> 75% of blood usually close to 100%
Group IV (hemorrhagic)	Red	Opaque	High	Good	Up to normal count in blood	May be same as normal blood

---

A number of diseases have systemic manifestations (Table 39-3), many of which need the attention of the rehabilitation physician in addition to treatment of the arthritis itself. In some diseases (RA, SLE, JRA, gout, AS) a number of set criteria delineated by the American Rheumatism Association (ARA) must be fulfilled before making a definite or probable diagnosis.[15] Preliminary criteria have been developed for PSS and Reiter's syndrome.

Demographic Information

Many types of arthritis tend to have specific distribution in terms of age, sex, race, and geographical appearance. Severity of disease may vary with age and sex. Genetics and occupation may also be influencing factors. It is helpful to be familiar with those proportions of the population that are more susceptible to certain diseases[101] (Table 39-4).

Table 39-2
Radiographic Findings in Rheumatic Diseases

Disease	Anatomical Distribution	Types of Changes Seen
Rheumatoid arthritis	Symmetrical: Most frequent: MCP, MTP, wrist, PIP Often: Knee, hip, ankle, shoulder, C-spine	Juxtarticular osteoporosis, soft tissue swelling Marginal erosion Subluxation Late: bony eburnation
Osteoarthritis	Asymmetrical: Most frequent: Hip, knee, DIP, 1st CMC, C-spine Less frequent: Ankle, shoulder	Joint space narrowing Marginal osteophyte Cortical sclerosis and cyst
Spondyloarthropathies	Asymmetrical: Most frequent: Sacroiliac joint, heel	Soft tissue swelling, sausage fingers (Reiter's, PsA) New bone formation, fluffy periosteal bone, and syndesmophytes
AS	Vertebral column, hip, shoulder	Enthesopathic ossification and/or erosion, especially heel
Reiter's	Knee, ankle	Bony ankylosis
PSA	CMP, PIP, DIP, MPT	
Septic	Asymmetrical: Knee, ankle, wrist, hip, small joints	Soft tissue swelling Joint space enlargement Periosteal elevation Late: bony destruction
Gout	Asymmetrical: 1st MTP, small joint, knee	Soft tissue swelling Soft tissue speckled calcification, gouty tophi Erosion of bone with marginal overhangs
Pseudogout	Symmetrical: knee, wrist, hip	Chondrocalcinosis Subchondral cysts
SLE	Symmetrical: Small joints of hands, feet, wrists Articular osteonecrosis: Hip, knee, shoulder, ankle	Suchondral lucency (crescent sign) Sunchondral sclerosis Subchondral collapse and remodeling of bone Late: joint space loss
PSS	Symmetrical: Small joints of hands and feet	Acro-osteolysis (bone resorption) Soft tissue calcification Sausage digits

Osteoarthritis

OA is the most common form of arthritis. Its prevalence increases with age. In radiological studies of the hands, 7% of males and 2% females age 18 to 24 show evidence of OA; by age 75 to 79, virtually all had evidence of OA. Below age 45 males are affected more often than females. Above age 45 females are affected more often and tend to have more severe disease than males.[2, 148, 184] Females more commonly have OA of the distal interphalangeal (DIP), proximal interphalangeal (PIP), first carpometacarpal (CMC), and first metatarsophalangeal (MTP) joints; males more often have hip involvement. Knee involvement is seen equally in the two sexes, age 55 to 64.[139] Severe OA of the knee is seen more commonly in females age 65 to 74 (6.9% *vs.* 2% in males). Age 55 to 64 hip involvement is twice as common in females (1.6% *vs.* 0.79% in males). Hip involvement in males increases at age 65 to 74 (2.3% *vs.* 1.2% in females).[177]

Rheumatoid Arthritis

RA is universal and found in all populations, but some populations and ethnic groups have a lower incidence rate. There is a low prevalence among African blacks (0.1% definite RA, and 0.8% probable),[225] a medium-high prevalence in Israeli males (0.5%–1.3%) and females (1.2%–3.1%),[1] and a high prevalence in rural Germany (males 5.7% and females 3.0%).[24] Prevalence rates are influenced depending on which set of criteria are used to diagnose RA and whether the RA is definite or probable.

There is a limited concordance of the disease in twins and a twofold increase among first-degree relatives of patients with RA, but no specific pattern of inheritance.[221]

Systemic Lupus Erythematosus

SLE is one of the most frequent serious disorders of young women. It is more common in black females,[77] North American Indians,[179] and Chinese populations.[219] SLE occurs in relatives of patients with the disease, with a frequency between 0.4% and 5% (several hundred–fold increase over that of the general population).[154, 155] Monozygotic twins have a 50% chance of being concordant for SLE.

Scleroderma

PSS occurs rarely and is more common in black females. There is no geographical preference or genetic inheritance.[227]

Table 39-3
Systemic Manifestations of Rheumatic Diseases

System	Disease
Skin	Juvenile chronic arthritis (Still's variety)
	Psoriatic arthritis
	Reiter's syndrome
	Colitic arthritis
	Sarcoid arthritis
	Septic arthritis (especially *Neisseria gonorrhoeae* and meningitides)
	Hyperlipoproteinemia
	Systemic lupus erythematosus
	Amyloidosis
Nasopharynx and ear	Reiter's syndrome
	Rheumatoid arthritis
Eye	Juvenile rheumatoid arthritis
	Reiter's syndrome
	Rheumatoid arthritis
	Sarcoid arthritis
Gastrointestinal tract	Colitic arthritis
	Scleroderma
	Whipple's disease
Heart and circulation	Amyloidosis
	Polymyositis
	Juvenile rheumatoid arthritis
	Reiter's syndrome
	Ankylosing spondylitis
Respiratory tract	Sarcoidosis
	Polymyositis
	Rheumatoid arthritis
Nervous system	Systemic lupus erythematosus
	Rheumatoid arthritis
Renal system	Amyloidosis
	Gout
	Systemic lupus erythematosus
	Rheumatoid arthritis
Hematological system	Rheumatoid arthritis
	Systemic lupus erythematosus

Juvenile Rheumatoid Arthritis

JRA is the commonest arthritis found in childhood. It has a prevalence rate of 0.16 to 1.1 per 1000 population. Systemic onset JRA begins at any age during childhood and affects boys and girls equally. Occasionally it may have an adult onset. Rheumatoid factor (RF)–negative polyarthritis begins at any age during childhood with a female preponderance. RF-positive polyarthritis begins after age 8. Pauciarticular arthritis usually begins before age 5 and occurs mainly in females. Studies have indicated a hereditary predisposition to JRA among first-degree relatives and a 40% concordance among monozygotic twins.[122]

Polymyositis

PM has a worldwide distribution. It is basically a rare disease with five to ten new cases per million population per year.[166] It has a 2 : 1 ratio in favor of females with a higher incidence in black females. Two peaks occur; one in childhood (ages 5–15) and one in adulthood (ages 45–64).[169]

Spondyloarthropathies

Spondyloarthropathies include a spectrum of diseases (AS, Reiter's, psoriasis, and IBD), all of which are relatively rare; the incidence is one case per 1000 population for each type. The conditions present between the ages of 15 and 45. The incidence of Reiter's is high in males, 60 : 1, and AS 3 : 1. Psoriasis and IBD have an equal incidence in males and females.[35]

Etiology and Pathophysiology of Arthritis

Because the designation *rheumatic disease* includes such a broad spectrum of processes and syndromes, a classification system (see Fig. 39-1) may be useful that groups arthritides to some extent by etiology.

Rheumatoid Arthritis

The etiology of RA remains unclear, although much has been learned in the past two decades about the inflammatory process, its relationship to the immune system, and molecular genetic regulation. Of the two hypotheses currently in vogue, one suggests that RA is an autoimmune disorder; the other proposes that specific external agents initiate the response, which then is perpetuated or amplified by the immune host response. Data in support of the first hypothesis are derived from the fact that antibodies against autologous immunoglobulin G are present in many patients with RA, which may represent a primary abnormality in the regulation of cells that control immunoglobulin synthesis.[223] This primary defect may alter the control mechanisms, so that stimulation and control of these events are unbalanced and the response to endogenous immune products goes awry.[98]

A more likely explanation for the etiology of RA is that specific external agents initiate an inflammation response, and in the susceptible host, the inflammation leads to continual disease activity. Infectious agents can cause synovitis. Some replicate in the joint space (mycobacterial, staphylococcus, smallpox); some enter the joint space and cause synovitis through initiating a local immune response (rubella, spirochete). Another type of arthritis follows gastrointestinal disease (*e.g., Shigella, Salmonella,* and *Yersinia*). No organism is recovered from the joint, though a reactive arthritis occurs, and the inflammatory process is initiated by a remote infection.

Putting the pieces of the puzzle together in a coherent picture that conforms to Koch's postulates is not yet possible. Several components need to be acknowledged in the understanding of this process: an inciting agent, most likely exogenous and possibly a wide range of antigens; a genetic susceptibility; and an abnormality in the host immune response.[25]

The mechanism of tissue injury in RA has been demonstrated to include the following components of the immune system and its associated mediators of inflammation.[109] In the affected host, a stimulus initiates an inflammatory response directed against self or nonself, which sets into motion complement, leukocyte phagocytosis, lysosomal enzyme release, and several small mediators that initiate clotting and fibrolysis. In the joint, the local reactions are helper T-cell mediators which are attracted to macrophages and dendritic cells. Antibody synthesis is initiated, thus perpetuating the immunological activities already begun. Some of the joint mononuclear cells are capable of producing proteinases, prostaglandins, and other small mediators of inflammation.

As the high intensity inflammation subsides, repair takes place, often with the proliferation of fibroblasts and scar tissue. While we are unsure of what triggers all this, once the process is

Table 39-4
Demographic Data on Rheumatic Diseases

	Prevalence Rate	Peak Age (years)	Sex	Race	Geographical Preference
Osteoarthritis (primary)	4% (age 20–30) 80% (> age 60)	Males before 45; females after 45	Equal	None	
Rheumatoid arthritis	1%–2%	25–55	2–3 times higher in females	Higher in whites; lower in Japanese	
Systemic lupus erythematosus	1 : 1000; 1 : 700 in white females; 1 : 245 in black females	15–25	90% female	3 times higher in blacks 40*	New Zealand; Rochester, MN; San Francisco; Oahu, Hawaii
Scleroderma	Rare (5-million)	30–40	3 times higher in females	3 times higher in blacks	None
Juvenile rheumatoid arthritis	0.16–1.1 : 1000	1–3 8–12	(F/M 2 : 1)		None
Spondyloarthropathies					
Ankylosing spondylitis	1 : 1000	15–45	3 : 1		None
Reiter's syndrome	1 : 1000	15–45	60 : 1 males	None	
Psoriasis	1 : 1000	15–45			
Inflammatory bowel disease	1 : 1000	15–45			
Polymyositis	Uncommon (5–10 : million)	(Bimodal)† 5–15 45–65	2 times higher in females; 10.8–4.6 black females to black males; 2.7–3.7 white females to white males	3 times higher in blacks	None

* Kelley W, Harris E, Ruddy S, Sledge CB: Textbook of Rheumatology. Philadelphia, WB Saunders, 1985
† Shulman LR: Epidemiology of the rheumatic diseases, pp 1–293. New York, Gower Medical Publishing, 1984

in place it often continues for a longer period than would be expected to successfully clear antigen. Hence, the host immunoregulatory system, which is genetically controlled, must be abnormal.

Osteoarthritis

In marked contrast to RA, OA seems to be a local phenomenon. The etiology of OA remains obscure, but the pathological processes have been well described. Cartilage degeneration is the hallmark of the disease. The cause of the degeneration is unknown, but the possibilities include collagen framework damage secondary to fatigue or abrasion; changes in synthesis of proteoglycan or its degradation; and defects in synovial fluid and chondrocyte function.[168]

Other factors play an important role in the progression of OA. The location of the osteoarthritic lesion determines progression. A cartilage lesion at the apex of the femoral head will undergo significant osteoarthritic changes, but lesions inferior to the fovea will not. Medial lesions of the patella are less likely to develop OA than lateral or central lesions, suggesting that local topographical variations exist. The amount of cartilage loading as well as bony resilience may be factors in developing OA.[204]

In some patients, OA is secondary to a pre-existing joint abnormality: rheumatoid arthritis, congenital hip dislocation, Legg-Calvé-Perthes disease, and avascular necrosis of bone. Some possible risk factors include age, weight, sports that may result in repetitive microfractures,[147, 200] and repetitive occupational activities.

Regardless of cause, or the initial event, OA is associated with a progressive destruction of articular cartilage, which leads to fibrillation, abrasion, and shearing. The underlying exposed bone is damaged and attempts repair by formation of a new bone.

Spondyloarthropathies

Spondyloarthropathies are polyarticular disorders that involve the vertebral column. These arthritides share a number of additional features, including mucocutaneous lesions, sacroiliitis, heel pain, and the B27 antigen. Antecedent gastrointestinal infection, caused by *Salmonella, Shigella,* and *Yersinia,* has stimulated interest that these diseases may be caused by a gramnegative organism. The most convincing data in support of this came from the well-documented *Shigella* epidemics, in which Reiter's syndrome occurred in 344 of 150,000 infected persons[201] and 9 of 602.[186] No case occurred in anyone who was not infected. Arthritis with some additional features of Reiter's syndrome has followed *Salmonella*[248] and *Yersinia* infections.[5] In psoriatic arthritis and ankylosing spondylitis the data are less convincing, but evidence has linked the development of guttate psoriasis and streptococcal infection. The presence of B27 antigen appears to be the crucial link in expression of the disease.

The pathology found in the axial skeleton occurs at the sites of insertion of ligaments and capsules into bone. The peripheral joint pathology is essentially indistinguishable from that of RA and shows synovial proliferation and fibrosis.

The etiology of spondyloarthropathies is most likely to be an infective agent, possibly gram-negative bacteria, which interacts with a susceptible gene host: B27 in AS and Reiter's, and perhaps B27, B38, and C6 in psoriatic arthritis.

Systemic Lupus Erythematosus

SLE is a multisystemic disease that is associated with abnormalities of immune regulation and immune complex–mediated tissue injury. It has been called a classic autoimmune disease, due to an abundance of auto-antibodies generated against cytoplasmic and nuclear cellular components. The etiology of SLE is obscure, but viral inclusion bodies have been implicated because of electron microscopic observations made in lymphocytes and vessel walls.[83] Virus has never been isolated in patients with SLE; even those diseases with documented infectious etiologies are often multifactorial. Family members with SLE are more likely to have immunological abnormalities than are controls.[27, 251] Hormonal influences are important in the expression of SLE, and women in the childbearing years appear to be at greater risk,[160] and those taking progestational oral contraceptives are at higher risk than those taking estrogen-based oral contraceptives.[134]

The pathogenesis of SLE depends upon abnormalities in humoral and cellular immunity. Lymphopenia is common and is inversely related to disease activity. B-lymphocytes are normal in number, but are hyperactive. T-lymphocytes are often decreased most markedly in the T-suppressor lymphocyte subpopulation. Natural killer cell activity is diminished, but there is an increased number of lymphocytotoxic antibodies.[255]

Systemic Sclerosis

PSS is a progressive disorder in which microvascular obliterative lesions in multiple organs terminate in fibrosis and atrophy. Patients with scleroderma have capillary abnormalities and small artery lesions, which appear late with organ involvement. The pathogenesis of organ involvement is most likely due to injury to the endothelial cell lining of vessels. Disturbing the lining activates the clotting system with the release of vasoactive peptides. These factors stimulate smooth muscle cells to migrate in, proliferate, and deposit connective tissue, which results in the proliferative vascular lesion of scleroderma. The etiological agent is obscure and no strong hypotheses exist as to its nature.

Dermatomyositis-Polymyositis

DM-PM is an inflammatory disease of muscle and skin often associated with profound weakness of all skeletal muscle, including the heart. There are five subtypes, each of which may have a different etiology.[30] They are group 1, primary idiopathic polymyositis; group 2, primary idiopathic dermatomyositis; group 3, DM-PM associated with neoplasia; group 4, DM-PM associated with vasculitis; and group 5, DM-PM associated with collagen vascular disease.

Two leading hypotheses may explain the etiology of DM-PM: (1) abnormal recognition of self, and (2) viral infection. Immunoglobulins have been demonstrated in vessel walls, especially in intramuscular blood vessels, suggesting these deposits are immune complexes to muscle. These deposits are seen in a variety of muscle-wasting conditions and may be nonspecific. Cellular immunity is abnormal with DM-PM, as demonstrated by myotoxic activity of the lymphocytes in patients with DM-PM. Skeletal muscle antigens cause lymphocytes of patients with DM-PM to proliferate, suggesting that the lymphocytes are inappropriately responding to these antigens.

Crystal-induced Synovitis

Crystal-induced synovitis can be caused by uric acid, calcium pyrophosphate, hydroxyapatite, and cholesterol crystals. Best understood is gout, which is a familial disorder, in which there is a deficiency of hypoxanthine-guanine phosphotransferase, resulting in an over-production of uric acid. Hyperuricemia results and, as the concentration of urate in the blood rises, monosodium urate crystals precipitate in the tissue. It has been shown that injecting urate crystals subcutaneously will cause tophus formation, and when injected into joints will cause gouty attacks. Other factors involved in the pathogenesis of the gouty attack include elevated temperature, which increases joint urate concentration; lowered pH, which may precipitate an attack; and trauma and aging, which are thought to increase the likelihood of an attack.

Pseudogout, or calcium pyrophosphate dehydrate deposition (CPPD), can be hereditary or sporadic. The etiological agent is the calcium pyrophosphate crystal, which is formed secondary to a disorder of local pyrophosphate metabolism. The crystals adhere to leukocytes and often immunoglobulin is adsorbed, which stimulates phagocytosis and the perpetuation of inflammatory arthritis.

Infectious Arthritis

A wide variety of infectious agents can cause arthritis secondary to the infection itself or as a consequence of the host's immunological response. The organisms can be viral (hepatitis, rubella, mumps, herpes); bacterial (gram-positive: *Staphylococcus*, *Streptococcus*, *Pneumococcus*; and gram-negative: *Neisseria*, *Hemophilus influenza*; *Pseudomonas*) or fungal (tubercle bacillus).

PATIENT EVALUATION

The physical examination and laboratory and x-ray findings are essential to the proper diagnosis and treatment of rheumatic diseases. Many schemes have been developed in an attempt to construct an organized approach to the classification of rheumatic diseases, including algorithms that sort signs and symptoms around the presence or absence of inflammation, symmetry, and number of involved joints. However, these categories are not very helpful in sorting out the underlying pathophysiological processes that need therapeutic intervention.

A practical approach is suggested by James Fries[85] in which eight specific types of musculoskeletal pathology are distinguished. Patients can have more than one type of pathology; for example, enthesopathy and synovitis present in patients with psoriatic arthritis (Table 39-5).

Laboratory Tests

The laboratory evaluation of blood, urine, and synovial fluid, coupled with radiographic evaluations, can usually establish a proper diagnosis. The following determinations are made: CBC, sedimentation rate, SMA-12, RF, and antinuclear antibody (ANA). An HLA-B27 determination is done if spondylitis is suspected.

Joint fluid is easy to obtain in the presence of effusion. Analysis of fluid is essential in the diagnosis of crystal-induced arthritis and joint infection, and it is helpful in differentiating traumatic and inflammatory arthritis. However, rarely will the diagnosis of RA, OA, psoriatic arthritis (PSA), or AS be made on the basis of joint fluid alone; rather the fluid is confirmatory of these diagnoses. Joint taps must be done when a question of

Table 39-5
Evaluation of Rheumatic Diseases

Pathology	Examples	Laboratory Tests	Other Organs Involved
Synovitis	Rheumatoid arthritis	Latex, x-rays	Lung, heart, skin nodules
	Psoriatic arthritis/ Reiter's syndrome	X-rays	Skin
Enthesopathy	Ankylosing spondylitis	HLA-B27, sacroiliac joint x-rays	Heart
	Psoriatic arthritis/ Reiter's syndrome		Skin, mucous membranes
Cartilage Degeneration	Osteoarthritis	X-rays	
Crystal Arthritis	Gout	Serum uric acid, joint fluid	Skin, kidney
	Pseudogout	Joint fluid	
Joint Infection	Bacterial	Joint culture	Vaginal infection
	Viral		Bacteremia
	Fungal		Hepatitis
Joint Effusion	Trauma	Joint fluid	
	Reactive arthritis		
	Metabolic/endocrine disorders		Thyroid, liver
Vasculitis	Scleroderma	Muscle biopsy, EMG	Any organ
	DM-PM	Antinuclear antibody	Heart
	SLE	Erythrocyte sedimentation rate	Any organ
	Polymyalgia rheumatica		
Tissue Conditions			
Local	Tendinitis		
	Muscle spasm		
Generalized	Fibrositis		

infection is raised and should be made prior to injecting steroid or other material into the joint. Classification of joint fluid into categories will help differentiate inflammatory, noninflammatory, septic, and hemorrhagic arthritis (see Table 39-1).

Radiographic Assessment

Radiography is often the most valuable technique for differentiating among arthritides.[209] Marginal erosion of bone with juxta-articular osteoporosis is the hallmark of RA. Nonuniform joint space loss in association with bony sclerosis and marginal osteophytes are the characteristic changes in OA. Spondyloarthropathies classically have involvement of the sacroiliac joints, either symmetrical as in AS, or asymmetrical as in Reiter's and psoriatic arthritis. Bony changes include periosteal new bone formation and ankylosis. Gout and pseudogout often involve only a few joints. In gout, there are soft tissue tophaceous deposits and marginal erosion with large bony overhangs, and in pseudogout, calcinosis in fibrocartilage. Early in joint infection, the x-ray films may be negative, or there may be some joint space widening. If the process continues and osteomyelitis develops, periosteal reaction can occur, indicating bony destruction. Typical radiographic findings in patients with rheumatic diseases are presented in Table 39-2.

Functional Assessment

Rehabilitation assessment for patients with rheumatic diseases includes both process and outcome measures. *Goniometry,* the measurement of joint range of motion (ROM), is standardized and widely used, as is manual muscle testing. Quantifiable mea-

sures of spine motion are particularly useful for patients with rheumatic diseases.[174] They can help chart progressive loss of spinal mobility, which prompts interventions designed to preserve posture and chest expansion programs, as in the management of patients with spondyloarthropathy.

Patients with arthritis often have stiffness rather than pain that limits function. Both symptoms are difficult to measure. However, duration of morning stiffness may be quantified. Pain can be measured in terms of severity in a descriptive way (mild, moderate, severe), or by using a visual analog scale,[127] which is quite reliable.

Fatigue is a frequent problem for patients with rheumatic disease. Its cause is multifactorial: medication, chronic inflammation, abnormal posture and gait which are energy inefficient, abnormalities of the sleep cycle, and atrophy of muscle secondary to disease or chronic pain. Fatigue is difficult to quantify because it can mean a decrease in stamina, true muscle weakness, and lack of motivation, all resulting in an inability to complete tasks. A visual analog of fatigue has been used with some success, but it has an imprecise reference. Tests of stamina and endurance have not been perfected for clinical use in this patient population.

Despite reliable, sensitive indices of strength, ROM, and grip strength, other measures are needed for evaluation of patients with rheumatic disease. The American Rheumatism Association in 1949 devised a functional scale for patients with RA.[229] This scale was a simple, global assessment that rated patients' functional status as independent (class I), able to perform with pain (class II), able to do some activities (class III), and unable (class IV). Subsequent efforts were made to improve upon that effort by increasing the sensitivity of the measure.

Two generations of functional assessments have been used in evaluating patients with rheumatic disease. The first set looked primarily at performance of patients in ambulation, self-care, and other activities of daily living.[46, 66, 136] Most had some testing of reliability and validity, and were relatively easy to use. The problem with them was that they defined function very narrowly and excluded psychological, social, and vocational functions. The newer functional indices are more comprehensive and offer a broader view of patients' functioning. They also have demonstrated validity and reliability.[86, 132, 170]

When rheumatologists were asked what functional measures were important to use in evaluation of patients with rheumatic diseases, the consensus was mobility, pain, self-care, and role-activity.[32] The evaluations needed may vary, since some rheumatic diseases involve only joints (OA), others primarily kidneys, skin, and central nervous system (SLE), others still different organ systems. Table 39-6 identifies standard and functional assessments likely to be needed for each of the rheumatic diseases.

Compliance

Sackett and Hayes indicate six key elements that influence compliance: demographic features, nature of the disease, therapeutic regimens, settings in which treatment is given, patient–doctor relationship, and sociobehavioral features of the patient.

Good patient–physician communication leads to better compliance,[99] and those diseases that require long-term treatment and multiple or frequent dosing are likely to result in lower levels of compliance. These studies indicate that patients with rheumatic disease who have chronic illness and require long-term, multi-modality interventions have a lower level of compliance than those with acute, short-term needs. Other studies have suggested that compliance is dependent in large measure upon individual patient's health beliefs, including the importance of the treatment goal, how likely the treatment is to achieve the goal or to reduce the disability, and the physical, psychological, and financial barriers to treatment.[213]

Specifically, rehabilitation programs have been associated with improved function.[61, 137] Compliance with the use of splints[78] was 40% to 78%, and was lower[187, 196, 242] in those patients with arthritis whose families did not expect them to use the devices. Compliance with exercise programs was 55% in one study[37] and 40% in another, but 90% in a study with visual feedback.

In view of this information, in order to improve patient compliance it is generally believed that good doctor–patient communication is important and that the treatment regimen must be clearly spelled out and agreed upon.[118] Educating the patient is also recommended. The treatment should be as simple as possible with one type of intervention planned and additional ones added after goal achievement is met or nearly met.

TREATMENT OF ARTHRITIC CONDITIONS

Pharmacological Management

Pharmacological management of rheumatic diseases often requires the use of a variety of drugs, the pharmacology and pharmacokinetics of which may influence physical and psychological functioning.

Aspirin

Aspirin, or ASA, is the foundation of management of rheumatic conditions and the symptoms of pain, fever, and inflammation. It has been shown to block the synthesis of prostaglandins (PG) in the anterior hypothalamus,[17] which is responsible for the antipyretic effect. The analgesic effect of ASA is not entirely understood. Musculoskeletal pain may be mediated by bradykinin, a synthesizer of prostaglandins, which sensitize nerves to painful stimuli. ASA blocks PG synthesis. At higher doses than those used for analgesia (e.g., 5.3 g/day), ASA reduces joint inflammation and swelling.[29] The mechanisms for this action are multi-factorial. Aspirin affects leukocyte migration and vascular permeability, both of which may be influenced by PG synthesis.[135] The toxicities of ASA include allergy, tinnitus and hearing loss, gastrointestinal blood loss, ulcer, chemical hepatitis, and reduced glomerular filtration rate. For patients who have clinically significant gastrointestinal symptoms, enteric-coated preparations (Easprin, Ecotrin, Measurin) are usually well tolerated.

NSAIDs

Newer agents in use form the group of drugs called non-steroidal anti-inflammatory drugs (NSAIDs). These drugs also suppress inflammation through the inhibition of synthesis of prostaglandins. They inhibit the cyclo-oxygenase effect on platelets and effects on leukocyte migration. Toxicities include gastro-

Table 39-6
Functional Scales for Rheumatic Diseases

	MMT	Range of Motion	Pain	Fatigue	Activities of Daily Living	Ambulation	Cognition	Role/Social Interaction
OA		++	++		+	++		
RA	+	++	++	+++	++	++		++++
Spondyloarthropathies		++	++		+	+		+
DM-PM	++			+++	++	++		++++
PSS		++	++	+	++			++
SLE	+			+++	+	+	++	++++
Gout (crystals)			+++			++		
Fibrositis			+++	+++				++

+, possibly useful evaluation; ++, recommended evaluation; +++, strongly recommended evaluation; ++++, must evaluate

intestinal bleeding, pancreatitis, hepatotoxicity, decreased renal blood flow, and allergic interstitial nephritis. Some have more gastrointestinal toxicity than others and cause more sodium retention. A review of the comparative NSAID toxicities is available.[21]

NSAIDs are widely used as first-line drugs in the treatment of RA, JRA (only Tolectin and Naprosyn have been approved for use in children by the Federal Drug Administration), OA, and spondyloarthritis. A list of those NSAIDs currently used in the USA is provided in Table 39-7.

Aspirin and NSAIDs are likely to provide significant clinical relief for patients with OA, RA, JRA, and spondyloarthritis. These drugs are not usually effective by themselves in controlling RA and vasculitic syndromes.

Antimalarials

Antimalarials are effective in discoid[49] and SLE[60] with improvement in skin involvement, and in RA.[19, 82] The arthritis and arthralgias associated with SLE also improved. One study showed improvement in the course of glomerulonephritis.[45] Patients with RA improved in joint count, grip strength, walk time, and sedimentation rate. The antimalarials are slow-acting, taking 4 to 6 weeks before a therapeutic effect is observed. They are as effective as other slow-acting antirheumatic drugs (SAARDs).[65]

The mechanism of action of these drugs is varied. They have been shown to impair enzymatic reactions, including phospholipase, cholinesterase-hyaluronidase, and proliferation of lymphocytes. They seem to block depolymerization by DNA'ase and interfere with DNA replication. The incidence of side-effects and toxicities varies widely. Gastrointestinal disturbance is quite common, and retinopathy is infrequent but of greatest concern; it rarely occurs before a cumulative dose of 300 grams is reached, specifically in chloroquin, but routine ophthalmologic examinations should be performed.

Gold

Parenteral gold, more recently oral gold, has been used in the treatment of synovitis in patients with RA. Gold is thought to work by inhibiting lysosomal enzymes or by inhibiting phagocytic activity in macrophages and polymorphonuclear leukocytes. It also inhibits aggregation of human gamma globulin *in vitro,* a phenomenon that is thought to be an inflammatory antigenic stimulus in RA. These events have been observed when parenteral gold is used. The oral preparation alters all mediated immunity, inhibits DNA synthesis *in vitro,* and suppresses humoral immunity.[157]

Adverse effects of gold compounds include rash, stomatitis proteinuria, and hematological disorders (leukopenia, thrombocytopenia). This drug is not used in patients with SLE, partly because it may flare the skin involvement. Recent literature suggests it may be useful in treating patients with peripheral arthritis associated with psoriasis.[58] Gold is not contraindicated in treating patients with Felty's syndrome.

D-Penicillamine

D-penicillamine has been effective in the treatment of seronegative or seropositive RA.[121] The patterns of response to penicillamine are similar to those observed with gold. Toxicities include leukopenia, thrombocytopenia, proteinuria, skin rash, stomatitis, gastrointestinal upset, and a variety of autoimmune syndromes including Goodpasture's, PM, and SLE. The mechanism of action is unknown, but it is neither cytotoxic nor anti-inflammatory.

Steroids

Glucocorticoids and therapeutics for rheumatic diseases are inseparable, and probably have been tried in every rheumatic disease either systemically or locally. Exogenous glucocorticoids influence leukocyte movement, leukocyte function, and humoral factors; inhibit recruitment of neutrophils and monocytes into inflammatory sites;[76] cause lymphocytopenia by inducing margination or redistribution of lymphocytes out of the circulation; modify the increased capillary and membrane permeability that occurs at an inflammatory site, reducing edema and antagonizing histamine-induced vasodilation; and inhibit prostaglandin synthesis.

Daily steroid use stimulates Cushing's syndrome in which hypertension, hirsutism, acne, striae, obesity, psychiatric symptoms, and wound healing problems occur. With exogenous steroid use, there is an increased incidence of glaucoma, cataracts, avascular necrosis, osteoporosis, and pancreatitis.[18] The side-effects are in part dependent upon the particular glucocorticoid employed and the dose. Alternate-day steroids are associated with fewer untoward effects. The oral route is usually selected for ease of administration, but glucocorticoids can safely be given intramuscularly or intravenously. They can be used intra-articularly and are best delivered in a suspension that is not water-soluble.

Low-dose glucocorticoids are traditionally used in treating patients with RA (less than 15 mg po qd). Higher doses are used in treating patients with SLE, vasculitis, and DM-PM (up to 100 mg qd prednisone). Benefit of steroid therapy to patients with AS, PSS, and PSA has not been shown.

Anti-hyperuricemic Agents

Pain and inflammation of crystal-induced arthritis are frequently adequately controlled using NSAIDs. While these drugs are effective in controlling symptoms, they do not alter the metabolism of the substances forming crystals, nor do they influence their excretion. Probenecid competes with the tubular transport mechanism for uric acid, reduces the reabsorption of uric acid, and hence increases its excretion.[237] Many other drugs have a uricosuric effect in man. Their use is widespread and their toxicities are well known, including nephrolithiasis, which is

---

Table 39-7
NSAIDs in Use

Indole Derivatives
  Indomethacin (Indocin)
  Sulindac (Clinoril)
  Tolectin (Tolmetin)
  Zomepirac (Zomax)

Pyrazolones
  Phenylbutazone (Butazolidin)

Phenylpropionic Acids
  Ibuprofen (Motrin)
  Naproxen (Naprosyn)
  Fenoprofen (Nalfon)

Fenamates
  Mefenamic acid (Ponstel)
  Meclofenamate (Meclomen)

Oxicam
  Piroxicam (Feldene)

preventable if the urine is alkalinized and fluids increased. Acute gout can be precipitated as the uric acid levels are lowered; gastrointestinal symptoms are not infrequently seen. A second approach toward controlling serum urate levels is that of regulating production of uric acid by inhibiting xanthine oxidase. This is done by using allopurinol as an analog of hypoxanthine. It, too, can precipitate an acute attack of gout and can cause xanthine renal stones. Side-effects include rash and rarely blood dyscrasia. Allopurinol should not be used with azathioprine.[140]

Cytotoxic Drugs

Immunoregulatory drugs have been used in the management of rheumatic diseases in an attempt to restore a balanced immune response by eliminating certain cell subsets. None of these drugs has cured patients with rheumatic diseases, but they have produced control and long-term remissions.[97] There are three general classes of cytotoxic agents currently used: (1) alkylating agents (cyclophosphamide, chlorambucil) which crosslink DNA, preventing replication; (2) purine analogs (azathioprine), which incorporate into cellular DNA leading to inhibition of nucleic acid syntheses; and (3) folate antagonists (methotrexate), which cause intracellular deficiency of folate. These drugs all cause marrow suppression and gastrointestinal intolerance. Cytoxan causes alopecia, hemorrhagic cystitis, and gonadal suppression. Methotrexate causes cirrhosis and is highly teratogenic and can cause severe mucosal ulceration. Aza-

thioprine is associated with increased incidence of infection, and oncogenesis is usually of the lymphoid variety. A review of the therapeutic application of these drugs is presented in Table 39-8. Other types of immunoregulatory drugs are called immune enhancers, such as levamisole, which augments the effector phase of the inflammatory response.

Experimental Treatment

Experimental techniques including total nodal lymphoid irradiation, therapeutic apheresis, and antilymphocyte serum have all been used with some success in patients with rheumatic diseases, primarily RA and SLE.

Cyclosporin A, an antifungal agent has been shown to have suppressive effects on T-helper lymphocytes. Because of this mechanism it has been used in treatment of RA and PSA.

Surgery: Soft Tissue and Reconstructive Procedures

The surgical procedures relevant for arthritis include synovectomy, arthrodesis, tendon repair and realignment, osteotomy, and joint replacement. Each of these procedures has specific indications.[187] Much has been written about the degree of success of these procedures and the attendant complication rates.

Table 39-8
Therapeutic Application of Drugs in Rheumatic Diseases

Diseases	Recommended Medications	Probable Mechanisms	Precautions
OA	ASA	Inhibition of PG synthetase	Allergy bleeding
	NSAID		Bleeding diathesis
	Intra-articular steroids		Renal failure
RA	ASA, NSAID	As above	As above
	Anti-malarials	Block lysosomal enzymes	Retinal toxicity, psoriasis
	Gold	Inhibits phagocytic activity of macrophages	Nephritis, rash, marrow suppression
	D penicillamine	Unknown	
	Steroids	Interferes in lymphocyte migration; decreases membrane permeability	Nephritis, cytopenia, SLE, PM
	Azathioprine	Inhibits DNA synthesis	Lymphoid tumors Not used with allopurinol
	Methotrexate	Causes intracellular folate deficiency	Cirrhosis, leukopenia
	Cyclophosphamide	Prevents DNA replication	Ovarian cystitis
Spondyloarthritis	ASA, NSAID	As above	As above
	Gold	As above	As above
	Methotrexate	As above	As above
Gout	NSAID		
	Uricosurics	Increases excretion of uric acid	Often need to alkalinze urine
	Allopurinol	Inhibits xanthine oxidase	Do not use with azathioprine
	Colchicine	Inhibits microtubular assembly and inhibits lysosomal-enzyme release	
SLE	NSAID	As above	As above
	Steroids	As aboe	As above
	Anti-malarials	As above	As above
	Azathioprine	As above	As above
PSS	D penicillamine	Unknown	As above
	Colchicine	As above	As above
DM-PM	Steroids	As above	As above
	Azathioprine	As above	As above
	Methotrexate	As above	As above

Synovectomies

Synovectomies were first performed by Volkmann in 1877 for tuberculosis of the knee. Today they are sometimes performed on RA patients, most commonly to relieve pain and inflammation associated with chronic swelling uncontrolled by medication, to retard the progression of joint destruction (a controversial issue), and to prevent and retard tendon rupture. Other indications include the alleviation of decreased range of motion caused by very hypertrophied synovial tissue, and denervation effect.

Synovectomies can be performed on the knee, hip, ankle, wrist, metacarpophalangeal joint, shoulder, and elbow. Regrowth of synovium commonly occurs postoperatively so the procedure is not a curative one.

The major contraindications for synovectomy are very active polyarticular disease (controversial), poor general medical condition, poor motivation of the patient, and stage IV joint destruction.[104]

Arthrodesis

Arthrodesis is performed less often today than in the past because of the popularity and success of joint replacement. It may still be the best procedure to eradicate resistant infection that has destroyed significant bone. The stability provided by an arthrodesis should be permanent. Adolescents and young adults with many more years of activity might well be considered for an arthrodesis in selected instances rather than a joint replacement, which often does not stand the stress placed on it by a young, vigorous patient. An arthrodesis of an ankle is preferred to a joint replacement at this time. Hip replacement is preferred to arthrodesis of the hip, since such replacements have proved quite durable.

Common indications for arthrodesis of a joint are to relieve persistent pain, to provide stability where there is mechanical destruction of a joint, and to halt progress of the disease (infection or RA).

Contraindications for arthrodesis include significant bilateral joint disease (joint replacement is indicated more in this instance) and arthrodesis of the same joint on the contralateral side.

The most common joints for arthrodesis are the ankle, first metacarpophalangeal, proximal interphalangeal, wrist, and knee. Other joints that can be fused are the hip, sacroiliac (rare), shoulder, and elbow. Joints should be fused in optimal positions of function.[67]

Tendon Surgery

Tendon surgery is common in RA for the following:

Ruptured extensor tendons in the fingers
Ruptured central slip tendon of the extensor expansion of the extensor digitorum communis in the fourth and fifth digits (correction of boutonnière deformity)
Long extensor tendon of the thumb
Flexor tendon rupture in digits (less common)
Extensor tendon realignment when tendons have slipped in an ulnar direction over the metacarpophalangeal joints in the hand; commonly combined with synovectomy
Ruptured Achilles and patellar tendons in SLE.[183]

Osteotomies

Osteotomy is most commonly performed on the knee in unicompartmental OA to help correct varus and valgus deformities, and valgus deformity in JRA.[129]

Joint Replacements

Patients with RA, JRA, OA, and AN in SLE may require joint replacement. Common indications for replacement are persistent pain despite adequate medical and rehabilitative management, loss of critical motion in the involved joint, and loss of functional status.

Main contraindications for joint replacement are inadequate bone stock and periarticular support, serious medical risk factors, and the presence of significant infection in any body system. Other contraindications include lack of patient motivation to cooperate in a postoperative rehabilitation program, advanced age, and inability of the procedure to increase the patient's total functional level.[75, 185, 207, 218, 240]

The three most frequently replaced joints are the hip, the knee, and the metacarpophalangeal joints. Other joints for which replacements are done are the wrist, the shoulder, the elbow, the MTP joints, and the ankle. The latter has not been very successful.

Common complications of joint replacement include loosening, early or late infection, dislocation, fracture of bone adjacent to component, and wearing out of component parts. Other complications are nerve injury, heterotopic ossification, and pulmonary embolus.

Infections are more common in patients with RA or SLE and in those taking steroids or immunosuppressive medication.[75, 185, 207, 218, 240]

Postoperative Rehabilitation Management

The rehabilitation management goals of a total joint replacement program are to relieve pain, to redevelop comfortable musculoskeletal function, and to develop joint protection techniques in order to avoid overstressing the prosthetic joint.

The postoperative management of hip replacement includes

1. Referral of the patient for rehabilitation on the third to fifth postoperative day
2. Active-assisted ROM exercises of the hip in all directions (guard against excessive flexion or internal rotation and adduction)
3. Use of a tilt table
4. Progression to parallel bars as hypotension is overcome
5. Practice in swing and stance in place, then taking consecutive steps (stop if fatigued)
6. Progression outside of parallel bars with crutches (three-point gait for unilateral replacement, four-point gait for bilateral replacement)
7. Quadriceps exercises (bilaterally)
8. Restriction of hip flexion to 90° for 3 months
9. Written home instruction and adaptive devices to compensate for limited flexion of hip (elevated toilet seat)
10. When the patient becomes pain-free, use of isometric exercises to increase hip muscle strength.

The postoperative management of knee replacement includes

1. Referral of the patient to rehabilitation on the third and fifth postoperative day
2. Active-assisted ROM exercises of the knee. If the knee was immobilized in flexion, the goal is to regain full extension to facilitate maximal quadriceps muscle function
3. Use of gentle prolonged stretching without eliciting cocontraction, in the third postoperative week if necessary to achieve knee extension
4. Gait training as outlined for hip arthroplasty.

Total metacarpophalangeal joint replacement includes

1. Referral of the patient for rehabilitation on the third to fifth postoperative day
2. Construction of static and dynamic splints
3. Instructions to the patient on monitoring anti-edema measures
4. An initial exercise program of active-assisted ROM exercises with control of the arc of motion.

Rehabilitation Interventions

Rehabilitation treatment plans must be individualized for the patient's needs; they should be practical, economical, and valued by the patient to enhance compliance. Treatment is best begun early in the disease process so that the patient identifies this as part of the overall management plan.

There is scientific and clinical rationale for the use of many specific rehabilitation treatments; others are based on clinical judgment.

Rehabilitative rheumatology treatments and techniques must be monitored carefully and periodic reevaluation of the patient with adjustments in treatment made.

Rest

Rest is an accepted treatment for inflammatory rheumatic disease. It can be provided by bed rest, local rest with splints (orthotics), or rest periods during the day. Both beneficial and adverse effects of local and systemic rest exist.[255a]

As early as 1875 local rest was prescribed for joint disease by James Sayre. After splint removal, joints were found to be stiff and passive ROM was introduced to restore motion to the stiff joint. Hugh Thomas[239] developed the Thomas splint to immobilize joints fearing ROM could increase inflammation.

More recently investigators have studied animals with induced arthritis. Rats with polyarthritis from Freund's adjuvant who run freely develop more arthritis than those restricted in cages.[206] Brandt found that, days after transection of the anterior cruciate ligament, dogs could be prevented from developing OA if the knee were pinned in flexion and rested.[199] Clinical studies describe Heberden's nodes occurring on the sound hand of patients with hemiplegia,[167] and likewise Bywater and Thompson found subcutaneous nodules and erosions of RA only on the non-hemiplegic side of patients with strokes. Thus, there is evidence more severe arthritis occurs with a limb in use.

ADVERSE EFFECTS IN THE ABSENCE OF ARTHRITIS. Local Rest. Investigations[6, 74, 241, 252] have found that local rest in animals causes both an increase in connective tissue and joint stiffness and that cartilage integrity decreases. These changes may become permanent after 1 to 2 months.

Systemic Rest. The adverse effects of systemic rest include deconditioning, osteoporosis, hypercalcemia/hypercalciuria, muscle atrophy and weakness, orthostatic intolerance, ataxia, diminution in heart and stroke volume, and an increase in pulse rate. Investigations[102] have documented the loss of lean body mass with rest of 2 to 3 weeks' duration, which is due to muscle atrophy. Incorporation of isotonic exercise preserves lean body mass and allows loss of fat. Total body water, intracellular fluid volume, red cell mass, and plasma volume are decreased with rest.[214]

BENEFICIAL EFFECTS ON ARTHRITIS. Local Rest. A number of studies[88, 111, 139, 189] demonstrate that patients with inflammatory arthritis achieve a decrease in inflammation when individual inflamed joints are rested for a week or more in casts or splints.

For patients, the awkwardness and visual non-appeal of splints limit their use.

Systemic Rest. Studies[7, 149, 177, 202] report overall improvement in patients with rheumatoid arthritis who have been hospitalized from 1 to 10 weeks. The most severely inflamed joints improved the most, while endurance, strength, and ROM did not significantly deteriorate after 3 weeks of rest. Therefore, it is rational to hospitalize patients with severely inflamed joints if medical and rehabilitative outpatient and home management have proved inadequate. The worst joints improve following 1 to 2 weeks of hospitalization.

Exercise

It is common clinically to see atrophy and weakness of muscles around painful and inflamed arthritic joints. In addition, inactivity and improper positioning of the joints lead to ROM deficits and decreased endurance.[255a]

Arthritis patients may lose muscle strength and bulk due to inactivity. A muscle can lose 30% of its bulk in a week and up to 5% of its strength a day when maintained at strict bed rest.[143, 180] Other factors contributing to loss of strength are myositis, myopathy secondary to steroids, inhibition of muscle contraction due to joint effusion, and direct effects of the disease itself on muscle. For example, in RA some destruction of muscle fibers occurs as well as intermuscular and perimuscular adhesions, which may impair blood flow. Muscle fascicles adhere to one another and the entire muscle may adhere to the intermuscular septum and perimuscular fascia causing inhibition of muscle contraction and normal movement. Myositis of muscle can occur with RA, PM, SLE, and PSS causing weak, painful, and easily fatigable muscle.

The biomechanical advantage of joints is compromised by the weak muscles. Normally, muscles function to provide postural stability and distribute forces of impact and stress across joints during activity. Normal joint function requires that muscles contract and relax synchronously. Atrophic muscles around joints do not coordinate well and are deficient in both static endurance and strength. If the quadriceps is atrophied the hamstring may exert an overpull causing excess flexion at the knee. A muscle with normal tone is in slight contraction all the time and there is no slack in the muscle tendon apparatus allowing it to be optimally ready for function. There is decreased tone and increased spasm in muscle surrounding arthritic joints resulting in less coordinated motion of the joint.[22]

Exercise programs for patients with arthritis are known to increase and maintain ROM, re-educate and strengthen muscles, increase static and dynamic endurance,[107, 159, 193, 192, 194] enable joints to function better biomechanically, increase bone density,[8] and increase the patient's overall function and well-being.[71]

Exercise prescriptions must take into account the degree of joint inflammation, mechanical derangement, and presence of joint effusion in each of the joints to be treated; the condition of surrounding muscles; the patient's overall level of endurance; and condition of the cardiorespiratory system. Programs need to be periodically reevaluated and adjusted according to the disease activity and stage of the joints at any given time.

When prescribing therapeutic exercise for arthritic patients, the physician should specify which muscles are weak and need to be strengthened, the degree of weakness, and the type and the duration of the exercise to be used. Specific directions for exercise should be written out by the therapist, reviewed, and given to the patient. If the patient and the family are instructed in the purpose and necessity of the exercises, then compliance improves.

An exercise program should be progressive and start with relieving pain of the involved joints with appropriate modalities; increasing ROM if needed by stretching and an active or active-assisted ROM program; increasing muscle tone by muscle re-education (increasing the ability of the patient to relax and contract the muscle completely in a synchronous manner); increasing the static strength and endurance of the muscle by isometric exercise; introduction of an isotonic exercise program for endurance and for strengthening (if joints permit); and finally recreational exercise.

PASSIVE EXERCISE. Passive exercise is beneficial for patients with severe muscle weakness due to polymyositis or neuropathic disease associated with stroke, peripheral neuropathy, and vasculitis.[90] However, it should be avoided as much as possible in an acutely inflamed joint, since both Merritt and Hunder[173] and Agudelo et al[4] found it caused increased inflammation in dogs with urate-induced arthropathy. Passive exercise also increases intra-articular pressure in the presence of joint effusion and has been associated with rupture of the joint capsule.[130]

ACTIVE EXERCISE. Active exercise uses three types of muscle contraction[50]: static or isometric contraction, highly suited for arthritis patients; isotonic or dynamic contraction, most suited for patients without acutely inflamed or biomechanically deranged joints, since it stresses the joint throughout its range; and isokinetic contraction, which is not recommended for arthritis patients but is used after the acute phase of sports injuries of the knee to rebuild an atrophied quadriceps muscle.

STRENGTHENING EXERCISE. Strengthening of a muscle may be achieved by isometric, isotonic, or isokinetic exercise, but not all of these forms of exercise are appropriate for the arthritic.

Isometric (static) exercise is ideally suited for restoring and maintaining strength in patients with muscle atrophy from rheumatic diseases, and for the recovery phase of DM-PM.[119] Hettinger, Muller and Rhomert,[180, 181] and Liberson[158] have demonstrated as little as two-thirds maximal contraction held for 1 to 6 seconds daily can increase strength. Repetitive contractions of 6 seconds each increase static endurance of muscle.[158] Machover and Sapecky demonstrated a significant increase (27%) in quadriceps strength in patients with RA on an isometric strengthening program.[159] This program consisted of three maximal contractions held for 6 seconds with 20 seconds rest between each daily. The knee was in 90° of flexion. The opposite quadriceps had a crossover effect with a 17% increase in strength.

An advantage of isometrics is that maximal muscle tension can be generated with minimal work, muscle fatigue, and joint stress. Forceful, repetitive resistive exercise through full joint range is associated with increased joint inflammation, intra-articular pressures, and juxta-articular bone destruction.[131] Merritt and Hunder demonstrated that in white rats with uric acid synovitis, isometric exercise of the knee did not increase the joint temperature or joint fluid white count.[173] Relaxation of tight muscle around joints is also facilitated by isometrics.

Since DeLateur[52] has shown that strength obtained by isometric training is not fully transferable to isotonic tasks, the addition of isotonic exercise into the arthritic program is warranted where appropriate.

DeLorme progressive resistive exercises (PRE) of isotonic high intensity, high resistive (high weight) and low repetition, build strength but are time-consuming and put much stress across joints. DeLateur[51] has shown that low weight, low intensity, prolonged exercise can build strength as well as static endurance of muscle if carried to the point of fatigue. The DeLateur method with low weights is suited to patients with noninflamed joints, few ligamentous problems, and minimal x-ray changes.

Dynamic high resistive exercise often causes exacerbation of inflammation in general, increases muscle fatigue and joint pain, and secondarily decreases joint ROM.[40] PRE and isokinetic exercise is not recommended for persons with arthritis. In addition, DeLateur[53] has found that the strength gains with isokinetic exercise do not exceed those obtained with a low weight, isotonic strengthening program.

ENDURANCE. Patients with systemic rheumatic disease have overall limited endurance and their ability to continue static or dynamic tasks is impaired. Isotonic endurance exercise can lead to an increased functional level in RA patients.[70, 71, 234, 255a]

Dynamic, low-repetition, low-resistance isotonic exercises to build strength and endurance are appropriate after articular inflammation and pain have been controlled and when sufficient isometric static strength and endurance have been achieved. Lifting light weights through a short arc of motion is appropriate, and swimming, bicycling, gardening, and weaving improve endurance. Dynamic endurance exercise for arthritis has proven usefulness. Ekblom and co-workers in 1975 reported a study of stage II and III RA patients who were trained for 6 weeks with bicycle ergometer and quadriceps strengthening exercises.[71] They showed improved mobility and cardiovascular function occurred, in comparison to the control group, without joint flares. This was also seen at 6-month follow-up.[70]

Further studies revealed increased size in type I and II quadriceps muscle fibers without joint flares with both short-term training[194] and with longer 7-month training on ergometer cycles.[193] Nordemar in 1981[192] described RA patients who were trained 4 to 8 years on a bicycle ergometer at home and a self-suited exercise program consisting of jogging, skiing, swimming, and cycling. He found improved activities of daily living (ADL) performance in the exercised group as well as less progression of x-ray changes in arthritis, more improvement in hamstring strength, and less sick leave. Harkcom and colleagues[108] also reported benefit from aerobic exercise in RA patients.

Bone mineralization is thought to be partially dependent on muscle contraction. Exercise has been shown to have a positive effect on bone mineralization in postmenopausal women.[9] Exercise may increase bone mass and may be useful in the management of senile osteopenia.[8] Patients with rheumatic disease develop osteopenia from disuse, medication, and calcium and collagen metabolism abnormalities.[106] Most studies that support the positive effects of exercise in these areas cite the use of isotonic and some resistive exercises.[8]

STRETCHING EXERCISES. Stretching may be used to prevent contractures and maintain or restore ROM by breaking capsular adhesions. These exercises must be graded according to the degree of inflammation, pain present, and pain tolerance of the patient. Heat (to increase collagen extensibility) and cold (to decrease pain) may be used prior to stretching exercises.

Passive stretching to preserve or increase ROM should not be done if there is acute inflammation, since it may increase it. It may be used for mechanically deranged joints in which active stretching should be avoided.

Active-assisted stretching can be used for maintaining or increasing ROM when the problem is subacute and pain is decreased. The patient initiates muscle contraction and the therapist or an assistive device serves as an aid.

Active stretching is done in the absence of pain and inflammation to maintain ROM. It may be facilitated by the use of pulleys. Active stretching exercises in a pool are excellent. Devices may be needed to facilitate stretching for hip flexion contractures in JRA, and knee flexion contractures in RA,[84] and hemophiliac arthropathy.[228] In adhesive capsulitis, traction with overhead pulleys combined with transcutaneous electrical nerve stimulation (TENS) can be used.[238]

RECREATIONAL EXERCISE. Patients with rheumatic diseases often want to participate in recreational exercise programs. Care must be taken to advise the patient which activities or programs would be beneficial for him or her and to relate use of recreational exercise with the condition of the joints (*i.e.*, inflamed, subacute, chronic, mechanical derangement problems). The use of preset rate-limited devices (Cybex) or of muscle contraction against high resistive forces on Nautilus machines should be avoided. Light weights and minimal repetitions on the Nautilus are permitted patients with OA and RA with no inflammation, minimal x-ray changes, and no ligamentous laxity. If isotonic weight lifting is done it should be with light weights, minimal repetitions, and a short arc of motion. Swimming is an excellent form of isotonic exercise for arthritis patients because gravity is eliminated and ROM of the joints is less painful. ROM and stretching exercises and pool jogging or walking are good. Local chapters of the Arthritis Foundation have aquatic courses for arthritics and often make heated pools available. The YMCA also has special pool exercise programs.

Adaptive devices and special hand grips are available to help patients in specific sports (table tennis, golf, gardening, bowling).

Dry land jogging, which involves repetitive joint motion and offers little chance for increase in strength, is not recommended if arthritis of the knee or hip is present. If osteophytes appear on knee films with no joint narrowing and no pain, jogging can be permitted.

It is a good rule that a patient should be made as strong as possible by isometrics and strength and endurance increased by light isotonic exercises before recreational exercise is begun.

Indications of both excess therapeutic and recreational exercise include post-exercise pain at 2 or more hours, undue fatigue, increased weakness, decreased ROM, and joint swelling. If these occur, the program should be adjusted.

Treatment With Heat and Cold Modalities

Therapeutic heat can be applied using a number of devices and techniques.[90, 113] The effect on the tissue, location, surface area, depth of the tissue, and acuteness or chronicity of the arthritis must be considered in selection of modalities.

Investigations on the use of superficial and deep heat and cold modalities have produced conflicting data. We do have some knowledge of the effects of these various modalities on skin, muscle and joint temperature, pain threshold, elasticity of tendon, relaxation of spasticity in muscle, and influence on synovial fluid enzyme activity, cell count, and volume. Using these data, plus clinical observation, recommendations can be made as to the appropriate use of heat and cold for acute or chronic arthritis.

HEAT. The use of superficial heat for pain relief in patients with arthritis is well known. Patients report that warm baths, heated pools, hot packs, and warm mineral springs provide relief of pain and decrease the stiffness in their joints. Normal intra-articular temperature is reported to be lower than body temperature.[124] Skin and joint temperature is increased to 34° to 37.5 °C in patients with active arthritis.[126] Superficial moist heat

applied for 3 minutes causes elevation of the soft tissue temperature 3 °C to a depth of 1 cm.[152] In inflamed knee joints the joint temperature is decreased 2.2 °F with application of superficial heat.[123] On the other hand, microwave application of deep heat to the knee increases the temperature by 8.4 °F; shortwave diathermy by 9.8 °F. Lehman demonstrated that ultrasound elevated the temperature in the pig hip joint 4 °C more than did the application of microwave or shortwave diathermy.[151] Painful stimuli, apprehension, alarm, or smoking lowers skin temperature and elevates knee joint temperature, as do active and passive exercise.

When joint temperature is increased from 30.5 °C to 36 °C as it is in active RA the collagenase enzyme from a rheumatoid synovium is four times as active with lysis of cartilage.[112] Increasing joint temperatures could contribute to perpetuating inflammation and joint destruction. Ultrasound as a deep heating modality has the capability of increasing joint temperature to this level in superficial and deep joints.

Dorwart, Hansell, and Schumacher[59] showed that prolonged superficial heat (4 hours) elevates the volume and white count of joint fluid in acute crystalline-induced arthritis. A temperature increase of 5 °C increases the enzymes in urate-induced synovitis. There are no studies to indicate if superficial heat applied for 20 minutes (a clinically acceptable time) causes the same phenomena or if the same effect is seen in RA as in crystalline disease. Mainardi and associates[162] found no increase in joint destruction in the hand in RA with the use of superficial heat.

Warren, Lehman, and Koblanski[247] noted that rat tail tendon distended more when heated to 45 °C than to 39 °C and prolonged stretching could produce longer lasting and greater deformation of rat tail collagen when heated.[246] Deep heat affects the viscoelastic properties of collagen. As tension is applied, stretch is effected, and an increase of "creep" (the plastic stretch of ligamentous structures placed under tension) occurs.[133] Heat may enhance the efficacy of stretching if applied to appropriately chosen joints.

Both superficial and deep heat can raise the threshold for pain after application.[150] They produce sedation and analgesia by acting on free nerve endings (both peripheral nerves and gamma fibers of muscle spindles).[79]

COLD. Cold modalities decrease skin and muscle temperature.[142] However, Hollander found cold packs elevated knee joint temperature.[123] The application of cold to rheumatoid joints may inhibit collagenase activity in the synovium.

Some clinical studies have shown more relief of pain with ice in patients with RA than with deep heat by diathermy. The pain threshold of the shoulder as measured with an algesimeter was higher immediately and 30 minutes after treatment with ice than it was with shortwave diathermy.[26]

Other investigations[141] found the increase of joint ROM to be the same with either ice or superficial heat applied daily for 5 days with 9-day interval between the two treatments.

Cold decreases muscle spasticity[175] and muscle spindle activity and raises the pain threshold. Cold should not be used in patients with Raynaud's phenomenon, cold hypersensitivity, cryoglobulinemia, or paroxysmal cold hemoglobinuria.[198] The abrupt application of cold causes discomfort and produces a stressful response.[198]

At the current time we lack controlled clinical trials in the use of modalities. At best, information can be gleaned from noncontrolled studies and clinical observation in order to choose the appropriate modalities in treating patients with arthritis.

In treating the acutely inflamed or early subacute joint, the goal is pain relief. One is careful not to use interventions which may perpetuate inflammation. The use of cold seems most logical as it can decrease the pain threshold, relax surrounding spastic muscles, and is associated with decreased collagenase and cell count in the joint fluid. Hollander's report in 1949 of increased joint temperature after use of cold needs to be further investigated.[123]

Later in the subacute period, when inflammatory pain is subsiding and stiffness is present, and the patient may have lost some ROM, either cold or superficial heat with TENS is appropriate before starting active-assistive ROM and isometric exercise. When inflammation has fully subsided, superficial heat for pain is appropriate. If tight periarticular structures remain, ultrasound or cold and TENS followed by stretching to increase joint ROM is suitable. TENS has been reported to relieve joint pain in RA[164, 165] and pain in RA neuropathy.[66]

Orthotics

Splints and orthotics are used to unweight joints, stabilize joints, decrease joint motion, or preserve joints in a position of maximal function. Splints may be prefabricated but are best when molded to fit the individual patient. (See also Chapter 16.)

UPPER EXTREMITY. Orthotics for the upper extremities are mainly confined to the wrist and hand and include resting splints, functional wrist splints, thumb post splints, ring splints, and dynamic splints. Resting splints immobilize the hand and wrist and are used at night for patients with active RA, carpal tunnel, or extensor tendinitis. The role of splints in preventing deformity in RA has not yet been scientifically proven. The clinical recommendation is to use both resting and functional splints in early RA and that they probably help in delaying ulnar deviation and in reducing pain, synovitis, and edema. Functional wrist splints extend to the mid-palmar crease, permit finger function, block wrist flexion, and are used for activities during periods of inflammation. They provide wrist and ligament support. A functional thumb post splint may be used to relieve pain in CMC and interphalangeal (IP) pain associated with OA. The same type of splint with a longer wrist extension is useful for De Quervain's extensor tendinitis of the thumb. A functional wrist cock-up splint can help relieve pain in carpal tunnel syndrome.

Small ring splints (Bunnell and boutonnière orthoses can reduce swan neck or boutonière deformity (Fig. 39-2).

For patients who have had MCP replacements or who have a radial nerve neuropraxia, a dynamic outrigger splint allows some exercise of the fingers in extension and flexion and enhances muscle re-education. They provide gentle stretch through limited range while supporting the wrist and MTPs. Splints to help reduce ulnar deviation are also available (Fig. 39-3).

Elbow orthotics are rarely used. However, braces with dial locks are used to reduce flexion contracture at the elbow.

Compliance with splints has been assessed in a number of studies.[78, 188] Compliance is best when family members expect the patient to be compliant and when the patient uses splints to relieve pain. Cosmesis is a major factor for non-use, as well as fear of discrimination in the work place.

LOWER EXTREMITIES. The most useful orthotics in arthritis are for the foot and ankle. Those for the knee have been less successful, and there are none generally used for the hip.

Foot-Ankle. Excess pronation at the subtalar joint, loss of the medial arch, and subtalar movement commonly seen in RA[95] can cause pain, contribute to tarsal tunnel syndrome, and cause strain on the knee and hip. Control of pronation by bringing the calcaneus perpendicular to the floor often relieves pain and

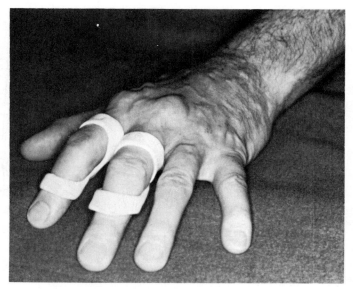

Figure 39-2. Swan neck ring splint.

Figure 39-3. Dynamic ulnar deviation splint with metacarpophalangeal hinge.

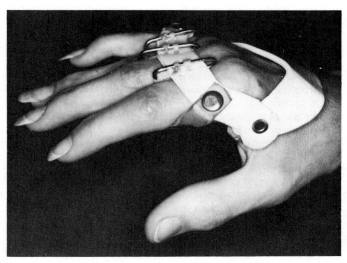

helps to balance the weight-bearing column. The first step toward control is to fit the patient with a shoe with a good heel counter and a soft or rigid orthotic insert lined with Spenco. The sole should not be too soft. This will minimize the flotation effect on heel strike and stance during gait and decrease stress, hypermobility, or instability at the ankle or a higher joint level. If pronation is not controlled by a shoe, a newly devised hindfoot orthotic, which can be fabricated in the office has been proven in a gait study to decrease hindfoot pronation and attendant pain[94] (see Fig. 39-4). A beveled heel that makes a 20° angle with the floor can decrease ankle motion and pain.[250] For the very painful or arthritically involved ankle from traumatic OA post-fracture or RA, a short-leg patellar tendon–bearing orthosis which shifts weight away from the ankle to the patellar tendon is useful.[153, 233]

Fascitis of the heel may be relieved with a cup insert or an insert with a depression in the area of the tender fascia.

Appropriate wide-toe-box shoes should be used to accommodate a wide forefoot, cocked toes, and hallux valgus seen in RA or JRA and the hallux valgus deformity seen in OA. A soft insert is added, as well as metatarsal reliefs (cookie inside the shoe or

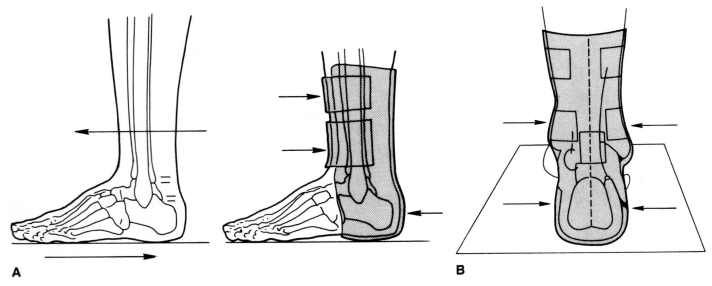

Figure 39-4. (*A*) A hindfoot orthotic. (*B*) Rear view.

external bar on the sole of the shoe—we prefer the former as being safer). A rocker bottom shoe can facilitate roll-over in the presence of a painful ankle.[55]

Knee. Bracing for the knee may be for pain, instability caused by ligamentous laxity, significant quadriceps weakness, or excess recurvatum.[39, 212, 224]

A useful brace for quadriceps weakness is a double upright Klenzak set at 5° plantar flexion at the ankle to put the knee in slight recurvatum during heel strike and stance.[232] The Klenzak can be used for a unilateral problem or for the weaker side when the problem is bilateral (as in PM). A Lenox Hill orthosis may be used to control medial-lateral or rotational instability.

A knee-ankle-foot orthosis (KAFO) with ischial weight-bearing and dial lock at the knee can be employed to reduce knee pressure and may be adjusted to relieve medial or lateral compartmental stresses in OA or RA. This orthosis is difficult to fit with severe valgus deformities and in the obese patient. Compliance in the use of KAFOs is poor.

A knee joint replacement is most often the best recommended procedure for severe knee pain refractory to medical and rehabilitative management. However, when there are serious medical problems which prohibit joint replacement, knee orthoses may be tried.

Smaller knee orthoses, such as hinged orthoses, Swedish knee cage, or Lerhman orthoses, may be used to help control recurvatum and give some medial-lateral support. A knee orthosis to help prevent dislocation of the patella is available and often effective. A shoe with a beveled heel at 20° also decreases knee flexion and promotes a more stable extended knee.[250] Orthoses with a dial lock turned 1° or 2° daily can be used to reduce knee flexion contracture.

SPINAL ORTHOSES. Spinal orthoses are used primarily to relieve pain or to support an unstable spine. A lumbar spinal orthosis or thoracic orthosis with mold and form insert will often offer support for painful back musculature, compression fracture, or disk disease and relieve pain. This type of orthosis may reduce lordosis, reinforce abdominal muscles, and unload the spine.[34, 195] For thoracic compression fractures prone to gibbous deformity or an unstable spine, lumbar or thoracic, a Jewitt orthosis or a molded polypropylene body jacket is needed.

A lumbosacral corset does not limit motion but provides some abdominal support and relieves painful lower lumbar musculature.

The cervical spine is involved in RA, OA, JRA, and spondyloarthropathies. A variety of collars provide different levels of support.[114] A soft cervical collar only minimally limits motion, but provides some pain relief. A Philadelphia collar offers slightly more support and some limitation of extension. A four-poster collar substantially limits flexion and extension, particularly at the C4-5, C-5, and C-6 levels.[44] A halo is needed to completely control C1-2 instability.

Assistive Devices and Adaptive Aids

These aids and devices compensate for limited ROM and pain and help promote independence for arthritics. To help ensure patient acceptance, the appliance should be affordable, easy to use, and improve patient function.

Ambulation and transfer skills are extremely important for persons with arthritis and gait aids and devices may be needed.

GAIT AIDS. If joint pain is a problem, secondary to loss of cartilage, effusion, or active synovitis, the painful joint needs to be unloaded. Weight reduction is encouraged, since a 1-kg weight loss results in a 3- to 4-kg decrease in load across the hip joint.[28] A straight cane or quad cane is good for balance but is not very efficient in unloading the limb, but a forearm crutch is. The elbow should be in 30° flexion when such a device is in use.

Custom hand-grip pieces can be made by making a mold of the patient's hand in a functional position of weight-bearing, or commercially made hand pieces on canes are available. Platform crutches distribute weight on the forearm reducing the need for wrist extension. Forearm attachments for walkers and wheelchairs are available.

For significant loss of strength or endurance, a small lightweight wheelchair is recommended. There are also small motorized scooters, such as the sporty Amigo chair.

ADAPTIVE DEVICES FOR TRANSFER. Chronic hip or knee pain, limited motion, or proximal muscle weakness make transfers from low-level chairs, toilets, and beds difficult. Upper extremities may be needed for push-off, but when these are inca-

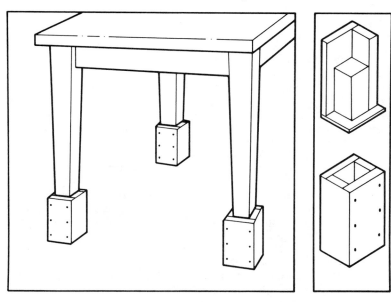

Figure 39-5. Blocks for elevating chair or table legs.

pacitated by RA, such simple motion becomes impossible. Independence in making transfers can be restored by elevating the seat with a cushion or placing 3-inch or 4-inch blocks under each leg of chairs, tables, and beds (Fig. 39-5). Chairs with motorized seats, elevated toilet seats, or clamp-on tub seats are helpful.

Transfers in and out of the car are facilitated by the use of an extra-thick seat cushion and a mounted grab bar to increase leverage. In the car the use of the side, rear-view, and wide-angle mirrors for patients with limited cervical ROM due to OA and spondyloarthropathies becomes essential. A spinner bar for the steering wheel and a large handled door opener and ignition piece are adaptations for the patient with significant hand problems. Patients with back pain benefit from a firm seat and back cushion, such as a Sacro-Ease; those with neck pain need adjustable neck supports or pillows.

Self-Care

Dressing, undressing, and other daily self-care activities can be time- and energy-consuming tasks for persons with RA, SLE, and PM. Adaptive and self-care aids such as long-handled reachers, shoe horns, elastic shoelaces, long-handled sponges, brushes and toothbrushes, Stirex scissors, button hook, zipper hook, toilet paper holder (when grip strength is weak), and large handled items are all helpful devices which also conserve energy. Clothing made with elastic and Velcro is easier to don than that with buttons and hooks. Wrinkle-resistant fabrics that do not require ironing and lightweight fabrics and wools (mohair, alpaca) are useful. Large buttons and partial zippering before putting on the garment may facilitate dressing, as will stretch straps and waists, garments with large raglan sleeves, and those with smooth linings. Capes, ponchos, and down jackets are easy to put on, warm, and lightweight.

DEVICES IN THE KITCHEN. Useful kitchen devices include food processors, long-handled reachers, built-up handles on utensils, electric knives, mounted wedge-shaped jar openers and lightweight aluminum pans. Lining pans with aluminum foil saves scrubbing. Bringing together items involved in a work area (*e.g.,* kitchen stove, work area, sink, and refrigerator) is helpful. A microwave oven cuts down on food preparation time. A kitchen cart loaded with needed utensils cuts down on walking.

ENVIRONMENTAL DESIGN. Slopes, stairs with deep steps, high curbs, and buses or cars may be difficult to negotiate for someone with disease of the hips and knees. Appropriate placement of steps, lowered curbs, suitably graded inclines, and ramps are helpful. Buses that kneel to accept passengers are available in many communities. Indoors, thick carpets increase friction and are difficult to walk on or negotiate in a wheelchair. In the bathroom, guard rails are best for safety. The bathtub should have non-skid strips or an entire non-skid surface. Door openings should be wide enough to accept a wheelchair. Chest-high storage cabinets and work surfaces are best; special door handles are available. For those patients in wheelchairs, proper positioning of door knobs, light switches, and kitchen equipment is necessary. Large-handled pencils and eating utensils are helpful. Devices to help with spray cans are available. The ARA provides a catalog of available assistive devices.[16]

Education

Patient education should include a discussion about the natural history of the disease and the likely impact that it will have on life-style, job, and leisure activities. Many systemic rheumatic diseases are chronic and have periods of remission and exacerbation which affect function.

A good rapport between physician and patient must exist in discussing these problems. The physician must take a comprehensive approach to the patient in order to assist him or her in habilitation or adjustment to the chronic disease process. In addition, educational groups consisting of arthritis patients who gather to hear experts in the field and talk about aspects of medical and rehabilitative management are very informational and supportive. These groups are sponsored by hospitals, the YMCA, and the Arthritis Foundation.

Some studies relate that education increases patient compliance, while others report that it provides increased knowledge about the disease process, enhanced communication with physician and family, and improved coping ability.[215, 231, 244] Other studies reveal no knowledge differences.[125, 178]

JOINT PROTECTION. In 1965, Cordery[47] observed that arthritic patients change their life-style and habits to protect their joints and use devices that make work easier rather than persist with activity that causes pain. Melvin also has described practical suggestions about joint preservation.[171]

Elements in a program of joint protection for arthritic patients include avoiding prolonged periods in the same position; minimizing stress on particular joints by promoting good posture; maintaining ROM, strength, and good joint alignment; reducing pain; unloading the joint when very painful; avoiding over-use during acute periods of pain; using appropriate adaptive equipment and splints when necessary; and modifying tasks to decrease joint stress. Joint protection and its companion, energy conservation, are based on data which suggest that use enhances joint inflammation, and rest diminishes inflammation.

ENERGY CONSERVATION. In systemic rheumatic disease accompanied by fatigue, conserving energy to maximize function is an important part of the arthritic's life-style.

Mechanisms for conserving energy include:

Maximizing biomechanical function of joints (by use of proper orthotics and assistive devices) to effect energy-efficient ambulation and hand function
Use of appropriate adaptive aids and clothing
Proper environmental design
Rest periods throughout the day
Maintaining ROM and strength
Maintaining proper posture.

Good body posture, sitting or standing, balances the weight of the head and limbs on the body framework so that gravity helps to maintain joint position with minimal muscle activity. Significant changes in posture cause muscles to exert more energy to pull against the force of gravity. For example, standing takes 25% more energy than sitting to perform activities. Ideal posture cannot be maintained unless care is taken to preserve ROM and strength of muscles around the joints.[87]

PSYCHOSOCIAL INTERVENTIONS. Rheumatic disease has major impact on the patient's mobility, activities of daily living, general life-style, self-image, family life, sexuality, and work. Major patient reactions ranging from denial and repression to depression occur, as well as other components of chronic illness, such as anger, bargaining, and acceptance. Belief that there is a particular personality type prone to developing RA has been dropped. However, premorbid personality is an important determinant of the patient's reaction to illness. Patients with arthritis, in addition to coping with pain, may have to deal with both losses in function and in physical attractiveness, due to the disease and medication side-effects, and the reactions of friends, spouse, and family. The unpredictability of systemic disease complicates the coping process.[23, 42, 191, 226, 230]

Some families adjust well, maintaining good communication, support, and flexibility in family routines. Other families are not able to reorganize and adjust to the needs of a person with arthritis. Psychiatric support for both patients and family is often needed. Group therapy including discussion about body image, job status, family relationships, and coping mechanisms is effective and has been used for a variety of arthritic groups.[172]

SEXUAL ADJUSTMENT. About 50% of normal, well-educated, financially successful, and maritally stable U.S. adults admit to sexual dysfunction or difficulties.[18] According to Ehrlich,[69] "sexual orientation of the person who has a musculoskeletal disorder is not necessarily very different from that of someone who does not. However, arthritis may impose certain limitations or alterations that influence the sexual life as they do other activities of daily living."

Particular sexual problems in the arthritic arise as a result of mechanical problems associated with decreased range of mo-

tion, pain, and stiffness; depression, with decreased self-image and interest; drug therapy resulting in decreased libido; psychosocial problems in the family unit related to the patient's arthritis; and fatigue.[236]

Mechanical Problems. Arthritic involvement of the hips, knees, lumbar spine, hands, and shoulders commonly cause mechanical or painful problems that interfere with sexual performance. Sixty-seven percent to 75% of all patients with arthritic hips have some mechanical sexual disability.[48] Analgesics and warm baths prior to intercourse may help. In women with more advanced disease a posterior approach by the man for intercourse may be successful. With severe limitation of motion, either unilateral or bilateral hip replacements may be requisite to achieve intercourse. After hip surgery, intercourse should not be resumed at all for 6 weeks, and hip flexion over 90° should be avoided.[20] Neither pain, stiffness, nor limitation of motion of the knees should mechanically limit intercourse, but a change in position may be required for more comfort. For those patients with back pain (OA, spondyloarthropathies, disk disease) a lateral position for both the man and the woman is preferable.

Significant problems in the joints of the hands and arms (as in RA) are more restrictive for the man than the woman, and a side-lying position may alleviate this. In both men and women, arthritis of these joints may interfere with the early stages of love-making involving caressing and manual stimulation.[254]

Self-image. Often arthritic patients experience a decrease in self-image, a feeling of helplessness, and ultimately depression, which in turn is associated with decreased libido. Chronic pain may reduce a woman's efforts to make herself more attractive for her partner, and it is difficult to reassure the woman who has significant joint deformities that she is still physically attractive. A man may abstain from sexual relations rather than cause his arthritic spouse pain and the spontaneity is reduced. Appropriate counseling may help alleviate these problems.

Medications. Certain medications are associated with decreased libido (Aldomet, steroids). High-dose steroids used in SLE and DM-PM may affect physical appearance and contribute to decreased self-image or acceptance by one's spouse. Immunosuppressive medications may interfere with conception.

Psychosocial Problems. Psychosocial problems in the family unit may lead to decreased sexual relationships between husband and wife. Such problems include inability to work, inadequate finances, limited acceptance by friends, and limited participation in social or recreational events. Misunderstanding and anxieties of the children about the chronic disease of the parents also contribute to tension and adversely influence sexual relationships.

Fatigue. Fatigue associated with systemic diseases can be a major factor in limiting sexual activities. Energy conservation is essential.

Successful treatment of musculoskeletal disease does not necessarily serve as a sexual restorative, but rather understanding, counseling, alterations in sexual positions, or appropriate joint replacements are needed.

VOCATIONAL ASPECTS. A vocational assessment should be part of the work-up for rheumatic disease patients and should cover educational level, work history and achievements, physical functional level, and social and psychological adjustment. Musculoskeletal conditions rank second to disease of the circulatory system in restricting activities, make up 41% of persons referred to vocational rehabilitation, and are the second most frequent cause of work disability.[243]

The arthritic patient's ability to remain in the work setting depends upon the stage of arthritis and the concomitant functional limitations imposed by it; the duration of the disease; the use of the proper medical and rehabilitation treatment to ensure a maximal functional level; the type of job the person has; and the willingness of the employer to allow for modifications in the job or to make environmental changes.[117]

Rehabilitation using a team approach has been associated with improved functional level in terms of ADL, mobility, and economic independence.[61, 137]

The more flexibility or control over work conditions that a person has, the more likely he or she is able to maintain a job.[117, 245] This is called *locus of control*.

The first step in vocational counseling is to see if adjustments can be made in the job setting so that the patient can continue working. If changes cannot be made, then the patient may have to receive training for another vocation. Remaining in the work force or being a homemaker is an important goal for the person with arthritis, and rehabilitative care and the support of the family help ensure success.

Specific Diseases

Osteoarthritis

OA, the most common type of arthritis, is an asymmetrical noninflammatory disease which has no systemic component. Most frequently it becomes clinically significant after retirement. There are three types of osteoarthritis: primary, secondary, and erosive inflammatory.

In primary OA the joints that develop OA in order of decreasing frequency are the knees, first MTP joints, DIP joints, CMC, joints, hips, cervical spine, and lumbar spine. It spares the elbows and shoulders, except if it is secondary osteoarthritis caused by an injury, fracture, or occupational-related task. In a population of mill workers in North Carolina, Hadler[117] relates specific tasks to development of secondary osteoarthritis as measured by x-ray films.

In OA the main impact on function results from involvement of large weight-bearing joints, which can cause pain and limit mobility. Back involvement ranks next. OA of the hands (CMC, PIP, DIP joints) is generally not associated with significant impairment of function in daily activities except significant CMC arthritis, which can cause difficulty at work with repetitive or manual labor tasks. Middle-age females who have a clinical syndrome, inflammatory erosive osteoarthritis described by Ehrlich,[68] have painful swelling and redness of the PIPs and DIPs resembling RA in appearance and interfering with ADL. It often burns out in 5 years, with no long-term disability.

A 1983 study by Krammer, Yelin, and Epstein[144] indicated 26% of patients with significant OA still work full time, even though 44% indicated they were always symptomatic. The mean number of bed days for a person with OA was 12.2 per year.

The course of OA is slow and variable. In one study, the mean time from onset of hip pain to severe loss of motion was 8 years (ranging from 18 months to 23 years).[203] In some people, the disease stabilizes[205] and does not progress. OA of the knee has a worse prognosis than the hip,[116] and varus deformity and early development of pain appear to be unfavorable prognostic factors.

ASSESSMENT. Rehabilitative assessment includes evaluating the biomechanical joint deficits as they relate to joint function

as well as studying the impact of the joint defect on contiguous joints and the patient's comfort and independence.

Since OA is basically a degenerative process, pain is usually local and results from altered biomechanics of the involved joint, and stress and strain on periarticular structures (tendons, muscles, nerves), which may result in radiating pain to other sites. Specifically, pain can be caused by periosteal elevation by spurs, trabecular microfractures, and capsular distension with fluid accumulation and associated crystal deposition disease (pseudogout).

Many people with OA by radiography are clinically asymptomatic, most studies show 25% to 30% having no symptoms.[43] However, the severity of symptoms when they occur seems to correlate with the extent of x-ray findings.[148] Joint stiffness in the morning and after periods of inactivity is common. Limited joint motion occurs as the OA progresses and may be compounded by poor positioning of joints, particularly at night.

Treatment plans should include methods to decrease pain, preserve and restore ROM and strength, reduce joint loads, prevent or reduce contractures, and preserve joint alignment.

PROBLEMS OF SPECIFIC JOINTS. Hip. Osteophytes on x-ray are often an indication of the presence of OA; subchondral cysts, sclerosis, and joint space narrowing usually follow. Hip pain, usually located around the greater trochanter, can be confused with trochanteric bursitis; it may radiate to the groin, the anterior thigh, the knee, and sacroiliac joints. Unilateral hip disease has a high association with increased leg length on the affected side.[100] A lift for the opposite shoe is indicated if there is more than ¼-inch discrepancy.

An important goal is to maintain at least 20° to 30° of hip flexion to assume normal gait. OA of the hip is associated with loss of motion in all planes and weakness of the abductors and extensors of the hip. Hip effusion may cause inhibition of contraction of the gluteus medius. Lurching to the same side or a Trendelenburg gait may be seen.

The patient should maintain hip extension by lying in the prone position for 30 to 40 minutes twice daily. For tight hip flexors unresponsive to active stretching exercise, prolonged stretching of the hip flexors may be effected in the supine position with a pillow under the affected buttocks and a 10- to 20-lb weight supported by a sling from the knee. Isometric exercise should emphasize both the abductors and extensors.

Knee. In contradistinction to the hip, osteophytes on a knee joint x-ray without any other changes (joint space narrowing, cysts, *etc.*) are not usually an indication of OA, since they are seen with the aging process after age 40. Knee problems may be uni-, bi-, or tri-compartmental. Pain in the knee with OA may be due to loss of cartilage, mechanical compression of the medial knee compartment with varus deformity or the lateral compartment with valgus deformity, stretch on the medial and lateral collateral ligament, microfractures and subchondral fractures, capsular distension by effusion, associated syndromes such as anserine bursitis or prepatellar bursitis, chondromalacia patella, or PPD (seen in 28% of OA patients by age 80[71]). Pain can be referred medially from the hip. As much as possible identification of the mechanism of the pain should be determined before treatment. Moderate or large effusions should be tapped and the fluid should be checked for CPPD crystals. Steroid and lidocaine should be instilled if no indication of infection is present. Effusion can inhibit voluntary contraction of the quadriceps[190] and contribute to atrophy and is associated with instability and valgus or varus deformity. ROM of the knee in the presence of joint effusion increases intra-articular pressure.

Pain and swelling of the knee lead to restricted ROM and

contractures of the joint capsule and hamstrings. If the knee cannot fully extend, it depends on the weakened quadriceps for stability, causing increased mechanical stresses and further joint dysfunction. Deep knee bends may increase intra-articular pressure and thus should be avoided.[92]

The amount of valgus or varus deformity of the knee can be reduced using a medial or lateral wedge and a flare of the sole of the shoe.

The patient should avoid the use of a pillow under the knee at night, since this encourages knee and hip flexion contracture, plantar flexion at the ankle, and venous obstruction in the popliteal area. A functionally important goal is to maintain extension. More than 10° of flexion contracture results in less than optimal knee biomechanics and increased stress with weight-bearing.

For strengthening, non-weight-bearing quadriceps isometric exercises should be done twice daily by patients with OA of the knee. With patella-femoral disorders isometrics with the knee extended are best to avoid patella-femoral compression.

Foot. Fifty percent of patients with OA have significant foot problems.[92] The most commonly encountered problems are hallux valgus (with or without bunions), hallux rigidus and cocked toes, metatarsal head callouses, and abrasions on the dorsum of the toes.

Ensuring properly fitting shoes is essential. (See section on foot-ankle orthotics.) If hallux rigidus or painful first MTP are present, mobility at the toe-off portion of the gait cycle will be decreased; a rocker sole will help facilitate toe-off. The physician must be sure that the problem is a foot problem and not compensation for a more proximal problem (*e.g.,* rotation of the tibia or hip).

Carpometacarpal Joint (CMC). The CMC is frequently affected by OA. The use of a thumb post splint to immobilize the thumb in a functional abducted position will relieve pain and allow for performance of functional activities. In severe OA, fusion in a functional position may be necessary.

Rheumatoid Arthritis

RA is a systemic rheumatic disease which primarily affects the synovial lining of diarthrodial joints. It can affect almost any and all of the peripheral joints with relative sparing of the axial spine except for the upper cervical (atlantoaxial joints). The end result of the process is joint pain, swelling, and malfunction. The muscles that surround the painful and inflamed joints or biomechanically compromised joints are painful and often atrophied or myositic. Ankylosis may occur with total restriction of joint motion. If it occurs with the joint in a nonfunctional position, then there are increased problems with ADL, mobility, and energy expenditure. OA often coexists with RA. Pain and deformity may cause problems with self-image and sexuality.[93]

The systemic nature of the disease is associated with fatigue and overall decreased endurance. Involvement of the cardiorespiratory system leads to further compromise of endurance. Involvement of the skin can lead to poorly healing ulcers of the lower extremity. Neuritis and vasculitis can impair mobility and function. Side-effects from chronic use of anti-inflammatory medications can cause additional problems.

PROGNOSIS AND MANAGEMENT. Clinically 80% of those initially diagnosed as having possible or probable RA are misdiagnosed or experience complete remission. Definite or classical RA may take three courses: intermittent mild disease with partial or complete periods of remission lasting 1 month to 1 year or more

(about 30% of patients); long clinical remission of 12 to 30 years; and progressive disease with rapid or slow, but relentless, deterioration. There are two subgroups: those who respond to medical therapy and those who do not (less than 3% of those with definite or classical RA). It is these two subgroups that experience the greatest adverse impact on function that the disease may impose.[110]

When we speak of prognosis in RA we tend to refer to the morbidity of the disease. The morbidity is increased in patients in whom the disease has an insidious onset, is seropositive, has radiographic evidence of erosive disease, and has persistent synovitis. The disease is hard to control in this group and they need more medical services.

Radiographic evaluation adds information about mechanical function. For example, if a patient is a Steinbrocker functional class III and has only grade-2 x-ray changes, it is likely that aggressive rehabilitation with attention to joint and systemic problems will improve function to that of a class II.

In terms of work performance, Yellin found that patients in class I or II had a 0.44 probability of disability from work, whereas in class III or IV the probability rose to 0.72. In those with class I or II disease of less than 5 years, the probability of disability was 0.33 compared to 0.7 in those with disease of greater than 5 years' duration.[253]

Although anti-rheumatic drugs have not been shown to definitely reverse the radiological abnormalities of RA, it is our clinical impression that patients being treated today have a much better functional outcome than they did 20 years ago. This is probably due to prompt specialty care, improved anti-inflammatory medications with restricted use of steroids, exercise to improve joint ROM, strength and endurance, and appropriate and timely joint replacements.

Rehabilitation of patients with RA requires a team of health care professionals and a significant time commitment and effort on the part of the patient and family. The disease may result in changes in life roles—homemakers need assistance and those working may need to make significant adaptations in the work setting or change their vocational status. Techniques of energy conservation and joint protection are essential. Flexibility in the work place is more likely to result in a person remaining on the job. The self-employed patient who exhibits locus of control does better than those who work for others.

Comprehensive management of the RA patient has been said to be associated with better control of the activity of the disease. Thus, since 1965, emphasis has been placed on prevention of disability by early diagnosis and aggressive medical and rehabilitative management. Some studies indicate that outpatients with class II and III RA who had comprehensive rehabilitation suffered 50% less deterioration in their ADL and in the clinical manifestation of their disease and enjoyed 25% improvement in economic status than a control group receiving conventional treatment.[137]

Particular attention needs to be given to the physical effects of the disease; the degree of inflammatory involvement in the joints; the degree of integrity of the joints radiologically and clinically; the state of the capsule, ligaments, and tendinous structures surrounding the joints; the condition and function of the key muscles surrounding the joints and skin; and state of the cardiopulmonary system. Similarly the psychosocial, sexual, and work impact of the disease needs assessment.

The specific main goals in the management of RA center around pain control; improvement of altered biomechanics; improvement and maintenance of strength, endurance, and ROM of joints; and improvement of self-image and adjustment to disability.

JOINT-SPECIFIC PROBLEMS. Shoulder. Glenohumeral arthritis is associated with pain in the shoulder girdle, which is referred to the neck, back, and upper arm. Decreased motion of the joint and soft tissue contracture and muscle atrophy follow.

Limitation of internal rotation (IR) is seen early. Proximal subluxation of the humeral head occurs late in the disease. Weakness of the rotator cuff may cause superior subluxation in about 33% of RA patients; about 21% of patients develop rotator cuff tears; an additional 24% have fraying of the tendons.[73] The insertion of the rotator cuff tendon into the greater tuberosity makes it vulnerable to erosion by synovitis.[249] Adhesive capsulitis, subcromial and subdeltoid bursitis, and dilation of the biceps tendon sheath are not uncommon associated problems.

In addition to pain control with modalities, local steroid injection into the specific affected area is often useful. A ROM program to increase and prevent loss of mobility is crucial. For functional activities the shoulder must have 30° to 45° flexion and 10° of IR. Care must be taken to assess the degree of radiographic involvement and joint stability when prescribing mobilization so as not to injure a compromised joint. When pain and inflammation subside, Codman exercises and the use of a cane (wand) can increase flexion and IR and external rotation (ER). "Wall walking" is good for chronic capsulitis. In the presence of adhesive capsulitis a technique of abduction-ER-flexion traction for 1 hour a day in conjunction with TENS has been successful in decreasing pain and increasing ROM.[238] Isometric strengthening should first focus on the deltoid with the shoulder adducted, then wrist-restricted isometrics in IR and ER and finally triceps and biceps isometrics are added.

Instruction in joint protection is essential to avoid overusing the shoulder.

Arthroplasty should be considered before end-stage erosion and soft tissue contraction occur.

Elbow. Elbow involvement is common in RA (20%–65%),[146] with loss of full extension an early problem. Preservation of flexion is needed for ADL. In severe disease, lateral stability may be lost and cause significant pain and disability in ADL function. Olecranon bursitis and accumulation of RA nodules which may breakdown easily are annoying to the patient.

Bursitis may be caused by staphylococcus infection and care must be taken not to inject the bursae of the elbow with steroid before a culture is done. Wearing a padded Heel-bo is useful to relieve pressure.

Lateral and medial epicondylitis is common. Acute epicondylitis is managed with modalities. Steroid injection may be necessary. Stretching exercise should not be forceful, since articular damage may occur easily in the arthritic elbow.

Hand and Wrist. Hand and wrist function as a unit. With weakness of the extensor carpi ulnaris the carpal bones rotate (the proximal row in an ulnar direction and the distal ones radially), resulting in ulnar deviation of the MCPs.[220] A power grasp[128] and weakened intrinsics[235] accentuate these problems.

Synovial proliferation increases pressures in the wrist joint, so that ligaments, tendons, and cartilage may begin to be destroyed. When the ulnar collateral ligament is stretched or ruptures, the ulnar head springs up. Synovium can cause median nerve compression. In advanced disease the carpus becomes significantly compacted.

In the hand, muscle weakness and contraction occur and grip strength decreases. Swan neck deformity—flexion of the DIP and MP with hyperextension of the PIP—occurs. Boutonnière deformity results when the extensor hood of the PIP is stretched, causing the PIP to pop up in flexion and the IP joint to hyperextend. With incomplete profundus contraction, limitation of full flexion occurs at the DIP joints. Similarly tight intrinsics prevent full flexion of the PIP joints with the MPs in extension.

Three types of deformity occur at the thumb[182]: A boutonnière-type at the IP joint (Nalebuff, type I), volar subluxation at the CMC joint during adduction (type II), and, in severe disease, exaggerated adduction of the first metacarpus, flexion at the MCP, and hyperextension at the DIP joint. Flexor tenosynovitis and De Quervain's thumb extensor synovitis are common.

Rehabilitative hand care involves appropriate resting and functional splints, joint protection techniques, and postoperative care. These may help decrease synovitis, relieve pain and edema, correct deformity, and, although not proven, help retard deformity.

Hip. About 50% of patients with RA have radiographic hip involvement.[64] Synovitis of the hip can cause pain radiating to the groin, whereas trochanteric bursitis causes pain radiating over the lateral thigh. Collapse of the femoral head and remodeling of the acetabulum which is pushed medially (petrusio) occur in 5% of RA patients. Reduction in internal rotation is an early finding with hip involvement. Synovial cysts can develop around the hip joint and communicate with the trochanteric bursae. Hip effusion can inhibit contraction of the gluteus medius muscle.

ROM exercises are important first to maintain at least the crucial 30° of hip flexion. A tight tensor fascia lata should be stretched. Stretching in abduction helps to relieve pain. Stretching of the internal and external rotators, extensors, and adductors should be followed by isometric strengthening exercise for the hip abductors and extensors.

Ultrasound may be best avoided in RA of the hip as it is somewhat difficult to assess the state of the inflammatory process in this deep joint, and ultrasound may aggravate an acute or subacute process.

Knee. The knees are commonly involved in RA and synovial inflammation and proliferation and effusion are easily seen. Quadriceps atrophy occurs within weeks of the onset of the disease and leads to increased forces through the patella to the femoral surface. Loss of full knee extension also occurs early and fixed contractions may ensue.[105]

Knee flexion is associated with increased articular pressure, and caution must be observed in performing ROM exercises on a knee with significant fluid. Outpouching of the posterior joint space may occur, creating a popliteal or Baker's cyst. Fluid from this popliteal portion does not readily return to the anterior joint space, but rather adds increased pressure to the popliteal space. There may be uncomfortable fullness or pain in the popliteal space and rupture into the calf may simulate thrombophlebitis. If rupture occurs, a hematoma may be seen below the malleoli.[145] Observe the patient from the rear while he is standing to check for a popliteal cyst.

Meniscal cartilage and cruciate ligaments can be easily destroyed by proliferative synovitis. Collateral ligaments become stretched. Tests for knee stability are always indicated in an examination. X-rays should be taken in the standing position to assess the cartilage and joint space.

Treatment is directed to the particular focal intra- or periarticular problem.

The patient should be instructed in early ROM exercise to preserve knee extension and flexion. Ninety degrees of knee flexion is needed to kneel and 100° to climb stairs. A pillow under the knee at night is to be avoided, because this will encourage a knee flexion contracture. Stretching of the hamstrings is important. Initially, strengthening of the quadriceps mechanism by isometrics in 30° flexion, if done early in the disease process, helps to maintain the biomechanical advantage of the knee. Isotonic exercise should follow for the non-inflamed joint.

Moderate to large effusions that inhibit contraction of the quadriceps and contribute to knee pain are best removed. Deweighting the knee is indicated with acute flares. Bracing the knee for instability is possible (see earlier in orthotics section).

Inflamed peri-articular or articular structures respond favorably to ice massage. When the joint is subacute or chronic, moist hot packs and TENS can be used.

Ankle and Foot. Ankles are less frequently involved than knees. Ankle involvement is usually present in severe RA. Synovial involvement can be prominent and is seen anterior and posterior to the malleoli. In acute disease, stretching and erosion of collateral ligaments around the ankle occur, resulting in incongruity and usually pronation of the hindfoot. Subtalar joint involvement is common and patients experience more pain walking on uneven ground.[57] About 50% of patients with RA have forefoot problems: widening at the metatarsal area, prominent MTP joints (due to subluxed metatarsal heads), hammer toe deformities, and hallux valgus of the great toe. Areas of skin breakdown are common on the dorsum of the toes (hammer toes), and callous is seen under the MTP heads. Plantar fasciitis and sub-Achilles bursitis may occur. Rupture of the Achilles tendon due to diffuse granulomatous inflammation may be seen. Gait is typically flat-footed with little heel strike or toe-off; pronation of the hindfoot can be prominent. Appropriate footware is extremely important.

Polymyositis

PM is a systemic rheumatic disease which affects skeletal muscle. The clinical picture is predominantly one of profound weakness of the shoulder and hip girdle muscle, as well as of the neck and pharynx. In severe cases the diaphragm, intercostals, and abdominal muscles are involved. Ten percent of patients also have distal muscle weakness, and some have weakness of the respiratory muscles. The muscle weakness is often compounded by steroid myopathy and atrophy of disease; a fair amount of muscle pain may be experienced when the inflammation is active. There may be complete remission of the disease or episodic periods of remission and exacerbation, which are often unpredictable and pose problems with functional activities and maintaining work status.

PROGNOSIS. The heterogenicity of the disease makes predicting prognosis and responses to medical and rehabilitative management difficult.[93, 119]

Before the introduction of steroid treatment in 1940 there was a 50% mortality[197] rate. Currently good nursing and medical and rehabilitation care have improved the prognosis of the disease. Several factors in general tend to influence prognosis:

Adults fare better than children
Those with associated carcinoma have a higher mortality rate
Those most severely affected at the onset of the disease have a poor prognosis
Late treatment results in a poor outcome.

The prognosis and particular functional problems seen with this disease depend on the type of PM-DM. There are five types.[30] Type I disease has an onset which is insidious, beginning in the pelvic girdle and later progressing to the shoulder girdle and neck muscles. Weakened posterior pharyngeal and laryngeal muscles result in dysphagia and dysphonia. Remission and exacerbations are quite common. Moderate to severe arthritis may be present as well as Raynaud's phenomenon. The skin over the knuckles and elbows is often atrophic. In contradistinction to type I, type II has an acute onset. Proximal muscle weakness and an erythematous heliotropic rash is seen on the skin of the eyelids and dorsum of the hands. Muscle tenderness is encountered in 25% of cases; subacute joint findings are common, as are systemic manifestations of malaise, fever, and weight loss.

Type III PM is associated with malignancy and is most common in males over age 40. Often muscle weakness precedes the diagnosis of malignancy by 1 to 2 years. The muscle weakness is usually progressive and does not respond well to steroids. Dysphagia and respiratory muscle weakness are common events. The mortality rate is high, and death is often the result of respiratory failure and pneumonia.

Type IV PM-DM involves children. The muscle weakness is rapidly progressive and problems with dysphagia, dysphonia, and respiratory weakness are quite common. It is important to remember that late exacerbations occur after 7 years of remission. The propensity for the development of severe joint contractures and muscle atrophy is frequent. Skin problems in the form of calcinosis universalis (cutaneous and muscle calcification), particularly over bony prominences, contribute to skin breakdown and draining lesions and joint contracture.

Type V disease is associated with other collagen vascular diseases, namely RA, SLE, and PSS. The functional problems associated with the individual collagen disease often dominate the clinical picture.

Rehabilitation intervention must be tailored to suit the needs of each patient depending on the disease type.

Patients with PM and associated collagen vascular disease (PSS, RA, SLE) have muscle weakness plus the added problems of the additional disease, which needs to be addressed from a rehabilitation standpoint.

Adults with type I and II disease can recover completely or be left with residual muscle weakness and fatigue, which can respond to rehabilitation management. But patients with PM and associated malignancy are not expected to recover from the disease. The rehabilitation goals are short-term. Ambulation mobility and self-care functions will progressively decline. Preserving ROM and strength will aid in keeping the person functional as long as possible. To not be able to continue in the work force for long is difficult for a middle-aged person to accept. Disability support payments and community support efforts need to be mobilized early on. Psychological support in coping with a chronic illness is needed. Good medical backup to contend with the problems of respiratory compromise and infection will be needed.

Children with type IV disease need to be watched carefully for contractures.

PROBLEMS AND INTERVENTIONS. Musculoskeletal System. The functional problems that arise depend on the muscle groups involved and the extent of the weakness.[119] For example, weakness of the pelvic girdle muscles is associated with difficulty in rising from a chair or a prone position, difficulty going up stairs, difficulty getting in and out of a bath tub, frequent falls with difficulty returning to the standing position, waddling gait, and toe walking caused by heel cord tightness (common in children). Shoulder girdle weakness causes functional problems with dressing (difficulty pulling on shirt, hooking a bra), grooming (combing hair, showering, shaving, brushing teeth), difficulty picking up heavy objects on a shelf, and difficulty eating. Neck weakness causes difficulty lifting and holding the head off a pillow and holding the head up while in a sitting position.

Respiratory muscle weakness (intercostals, diaphragm) results in difficulty with respiration, causing shallow and sometimes inefficient respiration. Distal muscle weakness (seen in 5%–10%) may cause foot drop and problems with hand activities.

Rehabilitation goals in the acute phase consist of maintaining ROM of the joints and preventing joint contractures. In the recovery phase the goals are to increase and regain muscle strength, maintain ROM, return to functional ADL and ambulatory activities, and to restore previous life-style activities as much as possible.

Joint contractures are prevented by active and passive ROM exercise and proper positioning and splint use when the patient is on bed rest. If contractures are already present other techniques are necessary to restore joint ROM. Contractures of the ankle, hip, and knee are common in childhood dermatomyositis and make ambulation difficult. Likewise, they may occur in the upper extremity (shoulder, elbow, wrist) and make ADL difficult. Static or isometric exercises are recommended initially when enzymes have decreased because they cause the least amount of fatigue. Isotonic resistive exercises are to be avoided because they easily fatigue muscle, cause general fatigue, and may contribute to muscle inflammation. Appropriate assistive and adaptive devices and ambulatory aids are needed.

If pharyngeal and laryngeal weakness are present, referral to a speech pathologist to teach the patient techniques to avoid aspiration of food and prevent respiratory infection is needed. If respiratory muscle weakness is present, chest physical therapy breathing techniques, proper positioning, suctioning, postural drainage, breathing exercises (if not in acute stage) are indicated. Tidal volume should be checked daily with a bedside spirometer. A collar may be provided to support the neck when neck flexor or extensor weakness is present.

For muscle pain, gentle muscle massage may produce a sedative relaxing effect on the muscle. The use of heat therapy is poorly described in the literature. Microwave therapy which heats superficial and deep muscle is described as being useful.

Joint pain and arthritis (usually wrists, fingers, knees) usually respond to steroids and are limited and non-deforming. DM-PM with associated rheumatic disease (RA, SLE, PSS) is frequently associated with arthritis, which can be deforming; therefore, the use of modalities, splints, and joint conservation techniques are needed.

Iatrogenic steroid problems cause vertebral compression fractures in the thoracic and lumbar spine resulting in back pain and muscle spasm. Interventions include a corset to decrease spinal mobility, heat modalities to relieve pain, and a long-handled reacher and shoehorn. If aseptic necrosis of the femoral head causes pain in the hip and groin on weight-bearing, unweighting the hip is indicated. Deep heat (ultrasound) to the hip may relieve pain.

Steroid myopathy presents with atrophy of muscle and increased muscle weakness. Repeated enzyme tests, electromyography (EMG), and muscle biopsy should be done. If the enzymes have remained normal, and if the EMG reveals no increased acute activity and the biopsy reveals no increased active inflammation, the steroid should be reduced and the exercise program continued.

A number of problems can occur with the respiratory system. In addition to respiratory insufficiency, aspiration pneumonia may result due to weak pharyngeal and laryngeal muscles. Primary interstitial fibrosis[63] of the lung has been reported. Patients with PM associated with SLE, RA, and PSS may have lung disease associated with these diseases. Pulmonary rehabilitation may be indicated.

Cardiovascular complications with DM-PM include[31] con-gestive heart failure (3.3%), cardiomyopathy (1.3%), cor pulmonale (0.7%), and electrocardiogram abnormalities (50%).[31] They are most common in type I and type V disease. Rehabilitation includes cardiac precautions, energy conservation techniques, and an endurance program.

Dermatological problems include pressure sores over bony prominences (sacrum, elbows, heels). Extensive calcinosis seen in childhood DM-PM causes breakdown of the skin over bony prominences of joints with drainage of calcium oxalate. Vasculitis with ulcerations of the finger tips and toes may occur in the overlap syndromes. Preventive measures include proper positioning, good nutrition with adequate protein intake, use of an egg-crate mattress pad or waterbed, and padded support over elbows, knees, and heels. Restoration measures include appropriate treatment if deep pressure sores are present.

Raynaud's syndrome precipitated by cold and stress is usually mild when it occurs, unless associated with collagen vascular disease. Symptoms include painful cold fingers and color changes from white to blue. Wearing gloves and using biofeedback have been useful.

Systemic Lupus Erythematosus

SLE is a chronic inflammatory disease that can affect any organ in the body. The most frequently involved sites are skin, joints, pleuropericardium, kidneys, and central nervous system. Its course is quite varied in severity and duration.

The rehabilitation team is often consulted with respect to a number of functional problems. Fatigue is a common problem, partly due to the chronic inflammatory process, but it also can be secondary to a disturbed sleep/wake process or myositis. Treatment may include an energy conservation training program during which physical activity is interrupted by rest. Naps are taken during the day and sleep can be promoted by the use of relaxation tapes.

Pain is quite common in the small joints of the hands and feet due to arthralgias and arthritis. Joint pain can also result from avascular necrosis of bone. Joint deformity is also seen. Control of joint pain has been successful using acupuncture and acupressure techniques, heat, cold, and TENS.[163, 165] These techniques are more effective in treating arthralgias than in treating avascular necrosis, which requires unweighting of the lower extremity, which, when unsuccessful, requires joint replacement to control symptoms.

The rashes of lupus are usually not responsive to nonpharmacological treatments, but the skin ulceration that can occur as a result of active Raynaud's syndrome responds to hand-warming techniques.[96] Temperature biofeedback is often effective in controlling vasospastic disease.

Patients with renal disease often have diminished stamina and fatigue. Improvement will occur with good blood pressure control and management of edema. In patients with nephrotic syndrome and significant edema, care must be taken to position the limb in the most functional position to minimize contracture; compression pumps and garments can be used to help with and maintain the reduction of limb edema. Precautions must be taken for patients with cardiac failure. They must be compressed slowly or not at all, since they may not tolerate any additional fluid load resulting from compression.

One of the major challenges to the rehabilitation team is the request to evaluate and treat patients with central nervous system involvement. Stroke, psychosis, depression, and memory deficits, all have a significant impact on function.[157] Treatment is aimed at the underlying problem. Spasticity may be controlled with baclofen (Lioresal) or diazepam (Valium) or local motor point blocks. Treatment of flaccidity using braces or adaptive equipment should be offered. Speech therapy can provide strategies to enhance memory using lists and cues.

The patient with SLE has to overcome major obstacles to successfully cope with this multifaceted illness. Support groups and family have been shown to be helpful in increasing compliance and are an essential component in the rehabilitation process.

Systemic Sclerosis

PSS (scleroderma, progressive systemic sclerosis) gets its name from the fibrosis-like changes that occur in skin and epithelial tissues of the affected organ. In addition, heart, lung, kidney, gastrointestinal tract, and small vessels also can be involved. While there are no cures, treatment is thought to prolong life.[211] The rehabilitation management depends on the extent and severity of the involvement.

Skin involvement occurs in 90% of patients and is often accompanied by Raynaud's syndrome, a condition in which there is vasospasm of the digital arteries often leading to ulceration of the finger tips. The skin involvement often evolves through three phases. There is an early painless edematous phase, during which range of motion may be limited but pain and weakness are not a problem. In a subsequent phase, the skin becomes tight and bound to deeper structures, the dermis becomes thin, and there is hair loss and decreased sweating. This period is associated with significant morbidity with loss of joint motion, itching of the skin, and an overall decrease in functional level. The third stage is usually associated with increased elasticity of the skin.

Rehabilitation interventions are directed at maintaining ROM, increasing skin elasticity, and preserving or increasing function. The techniques for accomplishing this include heat, paraffin, or ultrasound.[246] The management of Raynaud's syndrome may require nothing more than education about hand protection in the cold and the use of warm mittens. For those who are significantly affected there is evidence that temperature biofeedback is helpful in controlling vasospasm, although it has proven most effectivee in laboratory settings, and less so in daily situations. However, the treatment may be of some use in that patients report feeling that they are more in control of their environment.

Exercise to maintain ROM is essential and should be done daily or twice daily. Strengthening exercise should be prescribed with caution and only after inflammatory myositis with abnormal levels of muscle enzymes has been ruled out. A variant of PSS, eosinophilic fasciitis, a syndrome that has tight skin as one of its features, may be precipitated by unusually strenuous exercise, reinforcing the concern that strengthening exercise should be used with caution.

Pulmonary involvement takes the form of pleuritis, interstitial fibrosis, and pulmonary hypertension. Symptoms include chest wall pain, pleurisy, and dyspnea. Educating the patient about breathing mechanics and practicing chest wall expansion may help improve ventilation. TENS may relieve chest wall pain. Energy conservation training and use of adaptive equipment may increase functional independence.

Weight loss, constipation, and dysphagia are gastrointestinal symptoms that accompany PSS. The speech pathologist or occupational therapist may be helpful in demonstrating techniques that can improve mastication and swallowing.

The course of PSS is variable. All rehabilitation intervention must be on an individual basis and frequently reviewed to evaluate goal achievement. Supportive measures to preserve mobility and independence should be included as rehabilitation goals.

Spondyloarthropathies

The spondyloarthropathies encompass a number of diseases: AS, psoriatic arthritis, Reiter's syndrome, and arthritis of inflammatory bowel disease. AS has a propensity for axial skeletal involvement, but also affects such large joints as the hip and shoulders. Psoriatic arthritis and Reiter's syndrome are predominantly peripheral arthropathies with less frequent sacroilliitis and spondylitis (20%). Peripheral joint involvement is seen in 20% of IBD patients and axial involvement is seen in 10%.

With axial involvement a number of rehabilitation problems occur, including limitation of motion of the cervical and lumbar spines, paravertebral muscle spasm, and decreased chest expansion due to thoracic and costovertebral involvement. Loss of both cervical extension and lumbar lordosis are frequent. Visual impairment is associated with the former.[14]

Reiter's syndrome is associated with fusion of the tarsal and metatarsal joints and Achilles tendon shortening.[80]

Key elements in a rehabilitation program include maintaining critical ROM, posture, and strength; relieving pain; and providing appropriate orthotics.

A ROM program to maintain critical joint motion is prescribed[91] (e.g., maintaining at least 75° of shoulder abduction, 110° elbow flexion, 90° wrist supination, 15° hip flexion, 30° knee flexion, and the ability to obtain neutral position at the ankle and functional grasp at the hand). In addition, encouraging good posture is extremely important, and a firm mattress or bed board should be recommended. The patient should rest in the prone position to encourage extension of the spine. Lying on the side is to be avoided as this encourages cervical and thoracic kyphosis. Use of good postural habits in walking and sitting is requisite.

Appropriate exercise should be prescribed to promote spinal extension and ROM of the neck, shoulders, and hips. Swimming is excellent for isotonic and ROM exercise.

Mirror devices for the car or prism glasses for reading are helpful for patients with limited neck motion, as are long-handled reachers and shoehorns. All preventive and restorative rehabilitation strategies help ensure maximal function and psychological and vocational adjustment.[36, 103]

PEDIATRICS AND GERIATRICS

Pediatrics

The two rheumatic diseases primarily affecting the pediatric age group are JRA and type-IV DM-PM. Others include SLE, PSS, and vasculitis.[38]

Juvenile Rheumatoid Arthritis[33a]

JRA is a systemic disease. It is manifested by three disease types and the outcome depends on the type. In general there is some similarity to RA in terms of joint and systemic evolvement. However, there are also specific differences in the areas of both functional problems and the psychosocial impact of the disease on the child.

Recently early identification of the disease, advances in drug therapy, appropriate and well-timed surgical intervention, and active ongoing rehabilitation programs have contributed to better functional outcome. Many patients who in the past were wheelchair-bound are now functionally ambulatory.

MANIFESTING DISEASE TYPES. There are three main ways for JRA to present, the most frequent of which is a pauci-articular arthritis involving five or fewer joints, often including the knee and ankle. Pauci-articular arthritis is usually subdivided further into that which has an early age of onset (6 and under) and particularly affects girls and has a high risk of chronic iridocyclitis, and that affecting boys at age 9 and over, who tend to belong to the spondylitis group with positive HLA B27. In this latter group, ankles and feet tend to stiffen quickly.

The second type of JRA is polyarticular in which more than five joints are involved during the first few months of the disease. This group is further divided into those patients who have a positive immunoglobulin-M RF and are usually older, with an adultlike seropositive disease, and those patients who are seronegative.

The final and rarest type of JRA is systemic. In this type the child is acutely ill with fever, rash, lymphadenopathy, and at times pericarditis, myocarditis, and liver dysfunction. Initially, symptoms may only include arthralgia, but ultimately arthritis develops in varying severity, from a mild form affecting wrists, knees, and ankles, to an extremely severe form affecting all the joints. With persistently active arthritis, hip involvement is common.[13] This is asymptomatic initially and manifested merely by loss of movement.

Special problem areas exist which deserve the attention of the rehabilitation specialist. Growth retardation, in general, may limit full stature. Abnormalities in growth related to specific joints result in a number of problems: short toes and fingers, leg-length discrepancies, and micrognathia (small mandible). These abnormalities are due to premature closure of epiphyseal plates caused by intra-articular inflammation disturbing the development of the growth plate. Iritis and blindness are other major problems with which to contend.

It is important to remember that joint contractures and loss of ROM occur rapidly in JRA and must be managed quickly and efficiently.

SPECIFIC PROBLEMS. Much information is available about specific management of JRA-related problems.[11, 12, 208]

Upper Limbs. The wrist is often involved in JRA, and wrist flexion contracture can occur rapidly. A cock-up resting splint should be used at night. If the wrist is inflamed or forearm muscles are weak, contributing to wrist flexion, a functional splint should be used for activities. If a wrist flexion contracture is present, serial casting may be needed.

If there is proximal interphalangeal involvement, the resting splint should include the hand as well as the wrist. During the day with IP joint contractures, a dynamic outrigger splint should be employed.

If the elbow is acute, a hinge splint can be used. ROM exercises to maintain extension, pronation, and supination is important. If a contracture exists serial casting can be done.

Neck. Every effort should be made to avoid flexion contracture at the neck. Proper positioning at night with the use of a single thin pillow, like a pediatric Wall pillow, is recommended. When there is acute pain a soft cervical collar is worn. Sometimes torticollis becomes a problem, and a firmer plastazote collar may help. A collar is recommended for desk work.

Lower Limbs. Knee involvement should be managed promptly. If the joint is acute, a posterior resting splint should be used at night to prevent flexion contracture. If contracture already exists, a posterior splint may increase the danger of tibial subluxation and should not be used. Rather, the contracture

should be reduced with a skin traction device or by serial casting. Occasionally soft tissue release is necessary.

Valgus deformity frequently occurs and a supracondylar osteotomy may be needed to achieve realignment if conservative measures fail.

A hip flexion deformity contributes to knee flexion problems and care must be taken to maintain hip extension.

An acute hip joint is most often associated with acute muscle spasm and rapid formation of a flexion contracture. Often skin traction is used during acute hip pain to prevent contracture, with the patient lying supine in bed; 1 kg of weight for each 10 kg of body weight is used. In the child with a tendency for knee flexion contracture, use of light hip traction during the night reduces the chances of the formation of hip and knee contractures. There should be periods of lying prone during the day to encourage maintenance of hip extension. If hip contracture is not responsive to conservative treatment, a soft tissue release may be needed. Joint replacement may be needed in severe disease.[222]

Ankle-foot. Particular attention should be paid to management of the foot, and the use of proper shoe type and orthoses as well as ROM exercise is important.[56]

Spine. Significant loss of motion, particularly in extension, can occur. The use of a small Wall pillow while the child is supine at night gives support without causing unwanted flexion.

Compliance. Both the parents and the child should understand treatment regimens to ensure compliance. Many treatments are done at home with parents supervising.

Psychosocial. The disease has an impact on the child's self-image, socialization, sexuality, and integration into school activities.[115]

Efforts should be made to keep acute admissions to hospitals at a minimum so the child can participate as fully as possible in school, family, and social activities. He or she should be allowed to participate as much as desired but given clear guidelines about limitations. Particular advice should be given in regard to sports activities.

Guidance and support are needed during adolescence to deal with issues of vocation and sexuality.

Geriatrics

The elderly are often subject to multiple pathology. It is most unusual for the aged to have no other limitations on health or function than arthritis. Anyone treating the elderly arthritic must take this into consideration. Additionally, age is not always the best predictor of response to therapeutic intervention, and the physician does the patient a disservice to assume that patients have no rehabilitation potential simply because they are elderly.

Several considerations should be added to the traditional rehabilitation evaluation of the elderly with arthritis.

Does the patient look older-younger than the stated age? This may be a predictor of less or greater rehabilitation potential.

Does the patient have other illnesses or take medications that might affect cardiopulmonary performance, or neurological or mental status?

Is there strong family support for rehabilitation and for carrying out rehabilitation goals post-hospitalization?

As the body ages, muscle power declines but is still quite functional. The ability to sustain a maximal contraction as well as to change direction of motion quickly diminishes. Proprioception and spatial orientation decrease and difficulty is experienced in balancing and righting oneself. Falls are more common. Any exercise program must take this into account.

Those elderly who age normally and are active in the community are quite functional.[120] The late-stage arthropathic problems seen in some elderly are usually the end-stage, fixed deformity type of OA or RA associated with minimal pain at rest and more pain during physical activity. Attempts to stretch out contractures in the elderly are usually unsuccessful, and straightening joints using passive stretch is often painful. Surgical interventions and occasionally serial casting may help. Relief of pain may be achieved using analgesia, heat, and TENS. Most of the rehabilitation interventions should be done early in the course of the disease, and attempts to prevent contracture and preserve strength are the desired approaches.[3, 33, 41, 89, 217] Patients should be taught proper posture and adaptation of furniture and toilet.

If the therapeutic goals are realistic and the patient is committed, they are likely to succeed. Self-care activity is often the first goal and needs to be approached using adaptive aids and a maintenance program to support the required levels of strength and motion. Pain relief is critical if the patient is to carry out a series of movements. The physician should select a modality not likely to be hazardous. Hydrotherapy or pool use is very effective in enhancing total body movement and in providing a relaxing environment. The elderly must be well supervised in this setting both to ensure that the temperature is not unduly stressful to the cardiac status and that no anxiety or panic reactions occur while in the water.

Foot problems are very common in the arthritic and even more common in the elderly. Proper footwear should provide adequate depth to clear tops of toes and cushioning of the heels and metatarsals. Foot hygiene and prompt care of skin breakdown are essential to prevent infection in a patient with possible vascular compromise of the lower extremity.

REFERENCES

1. Abramson JH, Adler E, Ben Hader S et al: Studying the epidemiology of rheumatoid arthritis in Israel methodological considerations. Arthritis Rheum 7:135, 1964
2. Acheson RM, Collart AB: New Haven survey of joint disease XVII. Relationship between some systemic characteristics and osteoarthritis in a general population. Ann Rheum Dis 34:379–387, 1975
3. Agate J: Physiotherapy problems and practice in the elderly: A critical evaluation. In Wright V (ed): Bone and Joint Disease in the Elderly, pp 237–255. London, Churchill Livingston, 1983
4. Agudelo CA, Schumacher HR, Phelps P: Effect of exercise on urate crystal-induced inflammation in canine joints. Arthritis Rheum 15:609–616, 1972
5. Aho K, Ahroneu P, Lassus A et al: HLA-27 in reactive arthritis. A study of Yersinia arthritis and Reiter's disease. Arthritis Rheum 17:521,1974
6. Akeson WH, Amiel D, LaViolette D, Secrist D: The connective tissue response to immobility: An accelerated aging response? Exp Gerontol 3:289–301, 1968
7. Alexander GJM, Hortas C, Bacon PA: Bed rest, activity and the inflammation of rheumatoid arthritis. Br J Rheumatol 22:134–140, 1983
8. Aloia JF, Cohn SH, Babu T et al: Skeletal mass and body composition in marathon runners. Metabolism 27:1793, 1976
9. Aloia JF, Cohn SH, Ostuni JA et al: Prevention of involutional bone loss by exercise. Ann Intern Med 89:356, 1978
10. Anderson R: Polyarticular arthritis. In Kelly W, Harris ED, Ruddy S, Sledge CB (eds): Textbook of Rheumatology, 2nd ed, pp 401–415. Philadelphia, WB Saunders, 1985
11. Ansel BM: Joint manifestation in children with juvenile chronic polyarthritis. Arthritis Rheum 20:204, 1977
12. Ansel BM: Rehabilitation in juvenile chronic arthritis. Arthritis Rheumatol Rehab Suppl:74–76, 1979
13. Ansell BM, Unlu M: Hip involvement in juvenile chronic polyarthritis. Ann Rheum Dis 29:687, 1970
14. Arnett F: Spondyloarthropathies. In Gall E, Riggs G (eds): Rheumatic Diseases, Rehabilitation and Management, pp 429–437. City, Butterworth & Co, 1984
15. Arthritis Foundation Primer on Rheumatic Diseases, 8th ed, Arthritis Foundation Appendix I, pp 207–212. New York, Contact Associates, 1983
16. Arthritis Health Profession Section of the Arthritis Foundation: Self-Help Manual for Patients with Arthritis. Arthritis Foundation, 1980
17. Avery DD, Penn PE: Blockade of Pinogen induced fever by intra hypothalamic injections of salicylate in the rat. Neuropharmacology 13:1179, 1974
18. Axelrod L: Adverse reactions to glucocorticoids. In Miller RR, Greenblatt DJ (eds): Handbook of Drug Therapy, p 809. New York, Elsevier, 1979
19. Bagnall AW: The value of chloroquine in rheumatoid arthritis—A four year study of continuous therapy. Can Med Assoc J 77:182, 1957
20. Baldursson H, Brattstrom H: Sexual difficulties and total hip replacement in rheumatoid arthritis. Scand J Rheumatol 8:214–216, 1979
21. Ballet AJ: Non-steroidal anti-inflammatory drugs. In Kelly WN, Harris ED, Ruddy S, Sledge CB (eds): Textbook of Rheumatology, pp 752–769. Philadelphia, Saunders, 1985
22. Banwell BF: Exercise and mobility in arthritis. Nurs Clin North America 19(4):605–616, 1984
23. Barem J: A review of the psychological aspects of rheumatic diseases. Semin Arthritis Rheum 11:352–361, 1981
24. Behrend T, Lawrence JS: Prevalence of rheumatoid arthritis in rural Germany. Int J Epidemial 1:153, 1972
25. Bennett JD: The infections etiology of rheumatoid arthritis: New considerations. Arth Rheum 21:531, 1978
26. Benson TB, Copp EP: The effects of therapeutic forms of heat and ice on the pain threshold of the normal shoulder. Rheumatol Rehabil 13:101–105, 1974
27. Block SR, Winfield JB, Lockshin et al: Studies of twins with SLE. A review of the literature presentation of 12 additional sets. Am J Med 59:533, 1975
28. Blount WP: Don't throw away the cane. J Bone Joint Surg [Am] 2:695–698, 1956
29. Boardman PL, Hart FD: Clinical measurements of the anti-inflammatory effects of salicilates in RA. Br Med J 2:264, 1967
30. Bohan A, Peter JB: Polymyositis and Dermatomyositis (first of 2 parts). N Eng J Med 292:344, 1975
31. Bohan A, Peter JB, Bowman RL, Pearson CM: A computerized analysis of 153 patients with polymyositis and dermatomyositis. Medicine 56:255, 1977
32. Bombardier C, Tugwell P, Sinclair A et al: Conferences on outcome measures in rheumatological trials. J Rheumatol 9:798, 1982
33. Boum J: Rehabilitation aspects of aging in the elderly. In William TF (ed): Rehabilitation in the Aging, pp 177–197. New York, Raven Press, 1984
33a. Brewer EJ, Giannini EH, Person DA: Juvenile Rheumatoid Arthritis, 2nd Ed. Philadelphia, WB Saunders, 1982
34. Bunch WH, Keagy RD: The spine. In Bunch WH, Keagy RD (eds): Principles of Orthotic Treatment, pp 84–90. St Louis, CV Mosby, 1976
35. Calin A: The epidemiology of ankylosing spondylitis: A clinician's point of view. In Lawrence R, Shulman L (eds): Epidemiology of the Rheumatic Diseases, pp 51–60. New York, Gower, 1984
36. Calin A: Spondyloarthropathies. Orlando, Grune & Stratton, 1984
37. Carpenter JO: Medical recommendations followed or ignored? Factors influencing compliance in arthritis. Arch Phys Med Rehabil 57:241–246, 1976
38. Cassidy JE: Juvenile rheumatoid arthritis. In Kelly W, Harris ED, Ruddy S, Sledge CB (eds): Textbook of Rheumatology, 2nd ed, pp 1247–1275. Philadelphia, WB Saunders, 1985

39. Cassuan A, Wunder KE, Fultonberg DM: Orthotic management of the unstable knee. Arch Phys Med Rehabil 58:487–491, 1977

40. Castello BA, El Sallab RA, Scott JT: Physical activity, cystic erosion and osteoporosis in rheumatoid arthritis. Ann Rheum Dis 24:522, 1965

41. Chamberlain A: Mobility in the elderly arthritic. In Wright V (ed): Bone and Joint Disease in the Elderly, pp 222–236. London, Churchill Livingstone, 1983

42. Cobb S: Contained hostility in rheumatoid arthritis. Arthritis Rheum 2:419–425, 1959

43. Cobb S, Merchant WR, Rubin T: The relation of symptoms to osteoarthritis. J Chronic Dis 5:197–204, 1957

44. Colachis SC Jr, Strohm BA, Ganter EL: Cervical spine motion in normal women: Radiographic study of the effect of cervical collars. Arch Phys Med Rehab 54:161–169, 1973

45. Conti JJ, Mignon-Conte MA, Fournie JJ: Lupus nephrite: Treatment with indomethaum-hydroxycloraquine combination and comparison with cortico steroid treatment. Press Med 4:91, 1975

46. Convery RF, Minteer MA, Amiel D et al: Polyarticular disability: A functional assessment. Arch Phys Med Rehabil 58:494, 1977

47. Cordery JC: Joint protection: A responsibility of the occupational therapist. Am J Occup Ther 19:285, 1965

48. Currey HLF: Osteoarthrosis of the hip joint and sexual activity. Ann Rheum Dis 29:488–493, 1970

49. Davidson AM, Birk AR: Quinine bisulfate as a desensitizing agent in the treatment of lupus erythematosus. Arch Dermatol 37:247, 1938

50. DeLateur BJ: Exercise for strength and endurance. In Basmajcain JV (ed): Therapeutic Exercise, 4th ed, pp 90–92. Baltimore, Williams & Wilkins, 1984

51. DeLateur BJ, Lehman JF, Fordyce WE: A test of the DeLorme axion. Arch Phys Med Rehabil 49:245–248, 1968

52. DeLateur B, Lehman J, Stonebridge J, Warren JC: Isotonic versus isometric exercise: A double-shift transfer-of-training study. Arch Phys Med Rehabil 53:212–226, 1972

53. DeLateur BJ, Lehmann JF, Warren CG et al: Comparison of effectiveness of isokinetic and isotonic exercise in quadriceps strengthening. Arch Phys Med Rehabil 53:60–64, 1972

54. DeLorme TL: Restoration of muscle power by heavy resistive exercise. J Bone Joint Surg 27:645–667, 1945

55. Demopoulous JT: Orthotic and prosthetic management of foot disorders. In Jahss MH (ed): Disorders of the Foot, p 1785. Philadelphia, WB Saunders, 1982

56. Dhanedraw M, Hutton WC, Klenerman L et al: Foot function in juvenile chronic arthritis. Rheum Rehabil 19:20–24, 1980

57. Dixon L: The rheumatoid foot. In Hill AGS (ed): Modern Trends in Rheumatology, vol 2, pp 158–173. London, Butterworth & Co, 1971

58. Dorwart BB, Gall EP, Schumacher et al: Chrysotherapy in psoriatic arthritis. Arthritis Rheum 21:513, 1978

59. Dorwart BB, Hansell JR, Schumacher HR Jr: Effects of cold and heat on urate crystal-induced synovitis in the dog. Arthritis Rheum 17:563–571, 1974

60. Dubois EL: Quinacrine (atobine) in treatment of systemic and discoid lupus erythematosus. Arch Int Med 94:131, 1954

61. Duff I, Carpenter J, Neukom J: Comprehensive management in patients with rheumatoid arthritis. Arthritis Rheum 5:635–645, 1974

62. Duncan ME: Transcutaneous nerve stimulation in rheumatoid neuropathy. Rheum Rehabil 21:187, 1982

63. Duncan PE, Griffin JP, Garcia A, Kaplan SB: Fibrosing alveolitis in polymyositis. Am J Med 57:621, 1974

64. Duthie R, Harris C: A radiographic and clinical survey of the hip joints in sero-positive rheumatoid arthritis. Arth Orthop Scand 40:346, 1969

65. Dwosh IL, Stein HB, Urowitz MB et al: Azothiaprine in early rheumatoid arthritis. Comparison with gold and chloraquine. Arthritis Rheum 20:685, 1977

66. Ebert OR, Fasching V, Rohlfs V et al: Repeatability and objectivity of various measurements in RA. Arthritis Rheum 19:1278, 1976

67. Edmondson AS, Crenshaw AA (eds): Campbell's Operative Orthopedics, 6th ed. St Louis, CV Mosby, 1980

68. Ehrlich GE: Inflammatory osteoarthritis. The clinical syndrome. J Chron Dis 25:317–328, 1972

69. Ehrlich G: Rehabilitation Management in Rheumatic Diseases. Baltimore, William & Wilkins, 1986

70. Ekblom B: Effect of short-term physical training on patients with rheumatoid arthritis. A six month follow-up study. Scand J Rheumatol 4:87–91, 1975

71. Ekblom B, Lovgren O, Alderin M et al: Effect of short-term physical training on patients with rheumatoid arthritis I. Scand J Rheumatol 4:80–86, 1975

72. Ellman MH, Leven B: Chondrocalcinosis in elderly persons. Arthritis Rheum 18:43–47, 1975

73. Ennevaara K: Painful shoulder joint in rheumatoid arthritis. Acta Rheumatol Scand (Suppl) 11:1–116, 1967

74. Evans EB, Eggers GWN, Butler JK, Blumel J: Experimental immobilization and remobilization of rat knee joints. J Bone Joint Surg [Am] 47:737–758, 1960

75. Ewald F: Reconstructive surgery and rehabilitation of the elbow. In Kelly W, Harris Ed, Ruddy S, Sledge CB (eds): Textbook on Rheumatology, 2nd ed, pp 1838–1855. Philadelphia, WB Saunders, 1985

76. Fauci AS, Dale DC, Bolow JE: Glucocosteroid therapy. Mechanisms of action and clinical considerations. Ann Intern Med 84:304, 1976

77. Fessel WN: Systemic lupus erythematosus in the community. Arch Int Med 134:1027, 1974

78. Fienberg J, Brandt K: Use of resting splints by patients with rheumatoid arthritis. J Occup Ther 35:173–178, 1978

79. Fischer E, Solomon S: Physiological responses to heat and cold. In Licht S, Kamenetz HL (eds): Therapeutic Heat and Cold, pp 126–169. New Haven, E Licht, 1965

80. Fox R, Colin A, Gerber RC, Gibson D: The chronicity of symptoms in Reiters syndrome. Ann Intern Med 91:190–193, 1979

81. Frank E, Anderson C, Rubinstein D: Frequency of sexual dysfunction in "normal" couples. N Engl J Med 229:111–115, 1978

82. Freedman A, Bach F: Mepacrine and rheumatoid arthritis. Lancet 2:231, 1952

83. Fresco R: Virus-like particles in SLE. N Engl J Med 283:1231, 1970

84. Fried DM: Splints for arthritis. In Licht S (ed): Arthritis and Physical Medicine, pp 185–314. New Haven, E Licht, 1969

85. Fries JF: General approach to the rheumatic disease patient. In Kelly W, Harris ED, Ruddy S, Sledge CB (eds): Textbook of Rheumatology, 2nd ed, pp 361–365. Philadelphia, WB Saunders, 1985

86. Fries JF, Spitz P, Kraines RG et al: Measurement of patient outcome in arthritis. Arthritis Rheum 23:137, 1980

87. Furst G, Gerber L, Smith C: Rehabilitation through learning: Energy conservation and joint protection. A work book for persons with rheumatoid arthritis. US Dept Health and Hanover Services. Baltimore, Natl Institutes of Health, 1982

88. Gault SJ, Spyker JM: Beneficial effect of immobilization of joints in rheumatoid arthritides: A splint study using sequential analysis. Arthritis Rheum 12:34–44, 1969

89. Gerber L: Aids and appliances. In Wright V (ed): Bone and Joint Disease in the Elderly, pp 256–274. London, Churchill Livingstone, 1983

90. Gerber L: Rehabilitation of patients with rheumatic diseases. In Kelly W, Harris ED, Ruddy S, Sledge CB (eds): Textbook of Rheumatology, 2nd ed, pp 1769–1785. Philadelphia, WB Saunders, 1984

91. Gerber L: Psoriatic arthritis: Pharmacologic, surgical and rehabilitative management. In Gerber L, Espinoza L (eds): Psoriatic Arthritis, pp 147–165. Orlando, Gwen & Stratton, 1985

92. Gerber L, Hicks J: Rehabilitation in the management of patients with osteoarthritis. In Moskowitz R, Howell DS, Goldberg VR, Manalan H (eds): Osteoarthritis, pp 287–315. Philadelphia, WB Saunders, 1984

93. Gerber L, Hicks JE: The scope of rehabilitative interventions in the treatment of patients with systemic rheumatic diseases. In Hadler N (ed): Arthritis in Society, pp 230–251. London, Butterworth & Co, 1985

94. Gerber L, Hunt G: Ankle orthosis for rheumatoid disease. Arthritis Rheum, 28(4):547, 1985

95. Gerber L, Hunt G: Evaluation and treatment of the rheumatoid foot. Bull NY Acad Med 61(5):359–368, 1985

96. Gerber LH, Smith C, Novick A et al: Autogenic training in the treatment of Raynaud's phenomenon. Arch Phys Med Rehabil 59:522, 1978

97. Gerber NL, Steinberg AD: Clinical use of immuno-suppressive drugs. Part I, II. Drugs 11:36, 90, 1976
98. Gershon RK, Eardley DD, Durum S et al: Contrasuppression. A novel immunoregulatory activity. J Exp Med 153;1533, 1981
99. Gerstein HR: Patient non-compliance within the context of seeking medical care for arthritis. J Chronic Dis 26:689–698, 1973
100. Gofton JP: Studies in osteoarthritis of the hip. Part IV. Biomechanisms and clinical considerations. Can Med Assoc J 104:1007–1011, 1971
101. Gordis L: Keynote address. The role of epidemiology in the study of rheumatic disease. In Lawrence R, Shulman L (eds): Epidemiology of the Rheumatic Diseases, pp 6–15. New York, Gower Medical Publishing, 1984
102. Greenleaf JE, Bernauer EM, Juhos JT et al: Effects of exercise on fluid exchange and body composition in man during 14-day bed rest. J Appl Physiol 43:126–132, 1977
103. Gross M, Brandt KD: Educational support groups for patients with ankylosing spondylitis: A preliminary report. Patient Counseling Health Ed 3:6–12, 1981
104. Gschwend N: Synovectomy. In Kelly W, Harris ED, Ruddy S, Sledge CB (eds): Textbook of Rheumatology, 2nd ed, pp 1793–1818. Philadelphia, WB Saunders, 1985
105. Gupta PT: Physical examination of the arthritis patient. Bull Rheum Dis 20:596, 1970
106. Hahn TJ, Hahn BH: Osteopenia in patients with rheumatic diseases: Principles and diagnosis of therapy. Semin Arthritis Rheum 6:165, 1975
107. Halstead LS: Team care in chronic illness. A critical review of the literature of the past 25 years. Arch Phys Med Rehabil 57:507, 1976
108. Harkcom TM, Lampman RM, Banwell BF, Castor WC: Therapeutic value of graded aerobic exercise training in rheumatoid arthritis. Arthritis Rheum 28(1):32–39, 1985
109. Harris ED: Pathogenesis of RA. In Kelly W, Harris ED, Ruddy S, Sledge CB (eds): Textbook of Rheumatology, 2nd ed, p 887. Philadelphia, WB Saunders, 1985
110. Harris ED: Rheumatoid arthritis: The clinical spectrum. In Kelly W, Harris ED, Ruddy S, Sledge CB (eds): Textbook of Rheumatology, 2nd ed, pp 915–950. Philadelphia, WB Saunders, 1985
111. Harris R, Copp EP: Immobilization of the knee joint in rheumatoid arthritis. Ann Rheum Dis 21:353–359, 1962
112. Harris ED Jr, McCroskery PA: The influence of temperature and fibril stability on degradation of cartilage collagen by rheumatoid synovial collagenase. N Engl J Med 290:1–6, 1974
113. Harris R, Millard JB: Paraffin wax baths in the treatment of rheumatoid arthritis. Ann Rheum Dis 14:278, 1955
114. Hartman JT, Palumbo F, Hill BJ: Cineradiography of braced normal cervical spine: Comparative study of five commonly used cervical orthoses. Clin Orthop 109:97–102, 1975
115. Henoch MJ, Batson JW, Baum J: Psychosocial factors in juvenile rheumatoid arthritis. Arthritis Rheum 21:229–233, 1978
116. Hernborg JS, Nilsson BE: The natural course of untreated osteoarthritis of the knee. Clin Orthop 123:130–137, 1977
117. Hicks JE: Arthritis: Impact of function in the work setting and comprehensive rehabilitation management. Special report of the President's Committee on the Handicapped: Impact of musculoskeletal problems on employment, May 4, 1984
118. Hicks JE: Compliance: A major factor in the successful treatment of patients with rheumatic disease. Compr Ther 11(4):31–37, 1985
119. Hicks JE: Comprehensive rehabilitative management of patients with polymyositis. In Dalakas M (ed): Polymyositis. London, Butterworth & Co (in press)
120. Hicks J, Steneman MG: Rehabilitation can restore elders' independent lives. J West Gerontol Soc 5(2):10–12, 1980
121. Hill HFH: Treatment of rheumatoid arthritis with penicillamine. Semin Arthritis Rheum 6:361, 1977
122. Hochberg MC: The epidemiology of juvenile rheumatoid arthritis: Review of current status and approaches for future research. In Lawrence R, Shulman L (eds): Epidemiology of the Rheumatic Diseases, pp 220–233. New York, Gower, 1984
123. Hollander JL, Horvath SM: Changes in joint temperature produced by diseases and by physical therapy. Arch Phys Med Rehabil 30:437–440, 1949
124. Hollander JL, Stoner EK, Brown EM et al: Joint temperature measurement in evaluation of anti-arthritic agents. J Clin Invest 30:701, 1951
125. Holsten DJ, Morris AD, Moeschberger M: Effects of an organized educational program on patient understanding of rheumatoid arthritis and compliance with medical treatment. Presented at the 12th Scientific Meeting of the Allied Health Professions Section of the Athritis Foundation, Miami Beach, FL, December 1976
126. Horvath SM, Hollander SL: Intra-articular temperature as a measure of joint reaction. J Clin Invest 28:469–473, 1949
127. Huskisson EC, Jones J, Scott PJ: Application of visual analog scales to the measurement of functional capacity. Rheumatol Rehabil 15:185–187, 1976
128. Inglis AE: Rheumatoid arthritis in the hand. Am J Surg 109:368, 1965
129. Insall JN: Reconstructive surgery and rehabilitation of the knee. In Kelly W, Harris ED, Ruddy S, Sledge CB (eds): Textbook of Rheumatology, 2nd ed, pp 1870–1896. Philadelphia, WB Saunders, 1985
130. Jayson MIV, Dixon ASJ: Intra-articular pressure in rheumatoid arthritis of the knee III: Pressure changes during joint use. Ann Rheum Dis 29:401, 1970
131. Jayson MIX, Rubenstein D, Dixon AS: Intra-articular pressure in rheumatoid geodes. Ann Rheum Dis 29:496, 1970
132. Jette AM: Functional capacity evaluation: An empirical approach. Arch Phys Med Rehab 61:85, 1980
133. Jordon EE, Kowalski K, Fritts M: Changes in rat muscle fiber with forceful exercise. Arch Phys Med Rehabil 48:296–303, 1967
134. Jungers P, Dongodos M, Pelissier C et al: Influence of oral contraceptive therapy on activity of SLE. Arthritis Rheum 25:618, 1982
135. Kaley G, Weiner R: Prostaglandin E, a potential mediator of the inflammatory response. Ann NY Acad Sci 180:338, 1971
136. Katz S, Downs TD, Cash HR et al: Progress in development of an index of ADL. Gerontologist 10:20–30, 1970
137. Katz S, Vignos PJ, Moskavitz RN et al: Comprehensive outpatient care in rheumatoid arthritis. JAMA 206:1249–1254, 1968
138. Kellgren JH, Lawrence JS: Osteoarthritis and disk degeneration in an urban population. Ann Rheum Dis 17:388–397, 1958
139. Kelly M: Rheumatoid arthritis: The active immobilization of acutely inflamed joints. New Zealand Med J 60:311–315, 1961
140. Kelly WN, Holmes EW: Antihyperuricemia drugs. In Kelly W, Harris ED, Ruddy S, Sledge CB (eds): Textbook of Rheumatology, 2nd ed, pp 495–497. Philadelphia, WB Saunders, 1985
141. Kirk JA, Kersley GD: Heat and cold in the physical treatment of rheumatoid arthritis of the knee—A controlled clinical trial. Ann Phys Med 9:270–274, 1968
142. Knutsson E, Martensson E: Effects of local cooling on monosynaptic reflexes in man. Scand J Rehab Med 1:126, 1969
143. Kohke F: The effects of limitation of activity upon the human body. JAMA 196:825–830, 1966
144. Krammer JS, Yelin E, Epstein W: Social and economic impacts of four musculoskeletal conditions. Arthritis Rheum 26(7):901–907, 1983
145. Kroog G, Thevathason EM, Gordon DA, Walker IH: The hemorrhage crescent sign of acute synovial rupture. Ann Intern Med 85:477, 1976
146. Laine V, Vainio K: The elbow in rheumatoid arthritis. In Hymans W, Paul WD, Herschel H (eds): Early Synovectomy in Rheumatoid Arthritis, p 112. Amsterdam, Excerpta Medica, 1969
147. Lane NE, Bloch DA, Jones HH et al: Long distance running bone density and osteoarthritis. JAMA 225:1147–1152, 1986
148. Lawrence JS, Bremmer JM, Beer F: Osteoarthritis. Prevalence in the population and relationship between symptoms and x-ray changes. Ann Rheum Dis 25:1–24, 1966
149. Lee P, Kennedy AC, Anderson J, Buchanan WW: Benefits of hospitalization in rheumatoid arthritis. Q J Med (New Series) 43:205–214, 1974
150. Lehmann JF, Brunner GD, Stow RW: Pain threshold measurement after therapeutic application of ultrasound, microwaves, and infrared. Arch Phys Med Rehabil 39:560, 1958
151. Lehmann JF, McMillan JA, Brunner GD, Blumberg JB: Comparative study of the efficiency of short-wave microwave and ultrasound diathermy in heating the hip joint. Arch Phys Med Rehabil 40:510–512, 1959

152. Lehmann JF, Silverman DR, Baum BA et al: Temperature distribution in the human thigh, produced by infrared, hot pack and microwave application. Arch Phys Med Rehabil 47:291–299, 1966

153. Lehmann JF, Warren GC, Pemberton DR et al: Load bearing function of patellar tendon bearing braces of various designs. Arch Phys Med Rehabil 52:128, 1971

154. Lehman TJA, Hamson V, Singson BH et al: Serum complement abnormalities in the antinuclear antibody positive relatives of children with systemic lupus erythematosus. Arthritis Rheum 22:954, 1979

155. Leonhardt T: Family studies in systemic lupus erythematosus. Acta Med Scand 416:51, 1964

156. Lewis AJ, Watz DT: Immunopharmacology of gold. In Ellis JP, West GB (eds): Progress in Medicinal Chemistry, vol 19, pp 1–58. New York, Elsevier Biochemical Press, 1982

157. Liang MH, Roger M, Larson M et al: The psychosocial impact of systemic lupus erythematosus and rheumatoid arthritis. Arthritis Rheum 27:13, 1984

158. Liberson WT: Brief isometric exercises. In Basmajian JV (ed): Therapeutic Exercise, 4th ed, pp 236–256. Baltimore, Williams & Wilkins, 1984

159. Machover S, Sapecky AJ: Effect of isometric exercise on the quadriceps muscle in patients with rheumatoid arthritis. Arch Phys Med Rehabil 47:737–741, 1966

160. Maddock RK: Incidence of SLE by age and sex. JAMA 191:137, 1965

161. Magora F, Aladjemoff L, Tannenbaum J, Magora A: Treatment of pain by transcutaneous electrical stimulation. Acta Anasthesiol Scand 22:589–592, 1978

162. Mainardi CL, Walter CM et al: Rheumatoid arthritis failure of daily heat to affect its progression. Arch Phys Med Rehabil 60:390–393, 1979

163. Mann SC, Buragar FD: Preliminary study of acupuncture in rheumatoid arthritis. J Rheum 1:126, 1974

165. Mannheimer C, Lard S, Carlsson CA: The effect of transcutaneous electrical nerve stimulation (TENS) on joint pain in patients with rheumatic arthritis. Scand J Rheum 7:13, 1978

164. Mannheimer C, Carlsson CA: The analgesic effect on TENS in patients with rheumatoid arthritis: A comparative study of different pulse patterns. Pain 6:329, 1979

165. Masi AT, Medger TA Jr: Epidemiology of the rheumatic diseases. In McCarty DJ (ed): Arthritis and Allied Conditions, 9th ed, pp 11–30. Philadelphia, Lea & Febiger, 1979

167. McEwen C: Herberden's nodes: Heredity in hypertrophic arthritis of the finger joints. JAMA 115:2024, 1940

168. Meachim G, Brooke G: Pathology of OA in Osteoarthritis: Diagnosis and Management, pp 29–34. Moscowitz R et al (eds): Philadelphia, Saunders, 1984

169. Medsger TA, Dawson WN, Masi AT: The epidemiology of polymyositis. Am J Med 48:715–723, 1970

170. Meenan RF, Gertman PM, Mason JH: Measuring health status in arthritis: The arthritis impact measurement scales. Arthritis Rheum 23:146, 1980

171. Melvin JL: Rheumatic Disease Occupational Therapy and Rehabilitation. Philadelphia, FA Davis, 1982

172. Menuchin S: Families and Family Therapy. Cambridge, MA, Harvard University Press, 1974

173. Merritt JL, Hunder GG: Passive range of motion, not isometric exercise, amplifies acute urate synovitis. Arch Phys Med Rehabil 64:130–131, 1983

174. Merritt JL, McLean TJ, Erickson RP et al: Measurement of trunk flexibility in normal subjects: Reproducibility of three clinical methods. Mayo Clin Proc 61:19–97, 1986

175. Miglietta O: Action of cold on spasticity. Am J Phys Med 52:198–202, 1973

176. Mikkelson WM, Duff IF, Dodge HJ: Age-sex specific prevalence of radiographic abnormalities of the joints of the hands, wrists, and cervical spine of adult residents of the Tecumseh, Michigan, community health study area. J Chron Dis 23:151–159, 1970

177. Mills JA, Pinals RS, Ropes MW et al: Value of bed rest in patients with rheumatoid arthritis. N Engl J Med 284:453–458, 1971

178. Moll JMH, Wright V, Jeffrey MR et al: The cartoon in doctor-patient communication. Ann Rheum Dis 36:225–231, 1977

179. Morton RO, Steinberg AD, Gershwin ME, Brady C: The incidence of systemic lupus erythematosus in North American Indians. J Rheumatol 3:16, 1976

180. Muller EA: Influence of training and activity on muscle strength. Arch Phys Med 51:449–462, 1970

181. Muller EA, Rohmert W: Die Geschwindigkeit der Muskelkraft-Zunahme bei isometrischem Training. Int 2 Angew Physical 19:403–419, 1963

182. Nalebuff EA: Diagnosis, classification and management of rheumatoid thumb deformities. Bull Hosp Joint Dis 24:119, 1968

183. Nalebuff EA, Millender LH: Reconstructive surgery and rehabilitation of the hand. In Kelly W, Harris ED, Ruddy S, Sledge CB (eds): Textbook of Rheumatology, 2nd ed, pp 1818–1833. Philadelphia, WB Saunders, 1985

184. National Center for Health Statistics: Osteoarthritis in adults by selected demographic characteristics W.S. 1960–1972. Series 11, No 20, 1966

185. Neer CS: Reconstructive surgery and rehabilitation of the shoulder. In Kelly W, Harris ED, Ruddy S, Sledge CB (eds): Textbook of Rheumatology, 2nd ed, pp 1855–1870. Philadelphia, WB Saunders, 1985

186. Neer HR: An experimental epidemic of Reiter's syndromes. JAMA 198:693, 1966

187. Nicholas J, Hicks J, Gerber L, Magness J: Rehabilitation in joint and connective tissue disease. In Syllabus of the American Academy of Physical Medicine and Rehabilitatiaon, pp 10–15. Chicago, 1983

188. Nicholas JJ, Gwen H: Splinting in rheumatoid arthritis. I. Factors affecting patient compliance. Arch Phys Med Rehabil 63:92–94, 1982

189. Nicholas JJ, Ziegler G: Cylinder splints: Their use in the treatment of arthritis of the knee. Arch Phys Med Rehabil 58:264–267, 1977

190. Nichols PIR: Osteoarthrosis. In Rehabilitation Medicine, Chap 7. London, Butterworth, 1980

191. Noldofsky H, Chester WJ: Pain and mood patterns in patients with rheumatoid arthritis: A prospective study. Psychosom Med 32:309–318, 1970

192. Nordemar R: Physical training in rheumatoid arthritis: A controlled long term study II. Functional capacity and general attitudes. Scand J Rheumatol 10:25–30, 1981

193. Nordemar R, Berg U, Ekblom B, Edstrom L: Changes in muscle fibre size after physical performance in patients with rheumatoid arthritis after 7 months' physical training. Scand J Rheumatol 5:233–238, 1979

194. Nordemar R, Edstrom L, Ekblom B: Changes in muscle fibre size and physical performance in patients with rheumatoid arthritis after short-term physical training. Scand J Rheumatol 5:70–76, 1976

195. Norton PL, Brown T: The immobilizing efficiency of back braces. J Bone Joint Surg [Am] 39:111, 1957

196. Oakes TW, Ward JR, Gray RM et al: Family expectations and arthritis patient compliance to a hand resting splint regimen. J Chron Dis 22:757–764, 1970

197. O'Leary PA, Waisman M: Dermatomyositis. Arch Dermatol 41:1001, 1940

198. Olson JE, Stravino VP: A review of cryotherapy. Phys Ther 52:840, 1972

199. Palmoski MJ, Brandt KD: Immobilization of the knee prevents osteoarthritis after anterior cruciate ligament transection. Arthritis Rheum 25:1201–1208, 1982

200. Panush RS, Schmidt C, Caldwell JR et al: Is running associated with degenerative joint disease. JAMA 225:1152–1154, 1986

201. Paronen I: Reiter's Disease; A study of 344 cases observed in Finland. Acta Med Scand (Suppl 212) 131:1, 1948

202. Partridge REH, Duthie JJR: Controlled trial of the effect of complete immobilization of the joints in rheumatoid arthritis. Ann Rheum Dis 22:91–99, 1963

203. Pearson JR, Riddel DM: Idiopathic osteoarthritis of the hip. Ann Rheum Dis 21:31–39, 1962

204. Pedley RB, Meachim G: Topographical variation in patellar subarticular calcified tissue density. J Anat 128:737–745, 1979

205. Perry GH, Smith MJ: Spontaneous recovery of the joint space in degenerative hip disease. Ann Rheum Dis 31:440–448, 1972

206. Phelps JM, Kaklamahis P, Glynn LE: In Glynn LE: 1967 Heberden

Oration: The chronicity of inflammation and its significance in rheumatoid arthritis. Ann Rheum Dis 27:105–121, 1968

207. Poss R, Sledge C: Surgery of the hip in rheumatoid arthritis and ankylosing spondylitis. In Kelly W, Harris ED, Ruddy S, Sledge CB (eds): Textbook of Rheumatology, 2nd ed, pp 1916–1929. Philadelphia, WB Saunders, 1985

208. Rennebohm R, Correll JK: Comprehensive management of juvenile rheumatoid arthritis. Nurs Clin North Am 19(4):647–662, 1984

209. Resnick D, Niwayama G (eds): Diagnosis of Bone and Joint Disorders. Philadelphia, WB Saunders, 1981

210. Robinson HS, Halderman J, Imrie J et al: Evaluation of a province wide physiotherapy monitoring service in an arthritis control program. J Rheum 7:387, 1980

211. Rodman GP: Progressive systemic sclerosis and penicillamine. J Rheumatol 8(7):116–120, 1981

212. Rubin G, Dixon M, Danisi M: Prescription of procedures for knee orthosis and knee ankle foot orthosis. Orthotics Prosthetics 31:3–15, 1977

213. Sackett OH, Hayes RB (eds): Compliance with Therapeutic Regimens. Baltimore, John Hopkins University Press, 1976

214. Saltin B, Blomqvist G, Mitchell JH et al: Response to exercise after bed rest and after training. Circulation (Suppl VII), American Heart Association Monograph Number (23) 37, 38:VII-1-VII 78, 1968

215. Schmitt A, McBriar W: Assessing the quality of education provided to rheumatoid arthritis patients in a suburban-rural setting: Presented at the 14th Scientific Meeting of Allied Health Professions Section of the Arthritis Foundation, Denver, June 1979

216. Schmidt F: Approach to monoarticular arthritis. In Kelly W, Harris ED, Ruddy S, Sledge CB (eds): Textbook of Rheumatology, 2nd ed, pp 391–400. Philadelphia, WB Saunders, 1985

217. Schutt AH: Physical medicine and rehabilitation in the elderly arthritic patient. J Am Geriatrics Soc 25(2):76–82, 1977

218. Scott R, Sledge C: The surgery of juvenile rheumatoid arthritis. In Kelly W, Harris ED, Ruddy S, Sledge CB (eds): Textbook of Rheumatology, 2nd ed, pp 1910–1916. Philadelphia, WB Saunders, 1985

219. Serdula MK, Rhoads GG: Frequency of systemic lupus erythematosus in different ethnic groups in Hawaii. Arthritis Rheum 22:328, 1979

220. Shapiro JS: A new factor in the etiology of ulnar drift. Clin Orthop 68:32, 1970

221. Shulman L, Lawrence R: Current topics in rheumatology. In: Epidemiology of Rheumatic Diseases. New York, Gower Publishing, 1984

222. Singsen BH, Isaacson AS, Bernstein BH et al: Total hip replacement in children with arthritis. Arthritis Rheum 21:401–406, 1978

223. Sites DP, Stabo JD, Fudenberg HH et al: Basic and Clinical Immunology, 4th ed. Los Altos, Lange Med Publications, 1982

224. Smith EM, Juvinoll RC, Corell EB et al: Bracing the unstable arthritic knee. Arch Phys Med Rehabil 51:22, 1970

225. Solomon L, Beighton P, Valkenburg HA: Rheumatic disorders in the South African Negro: Part I. Rheumatoid arthritis and ankylosing spondylitis. Afr Med J 49:1292, 1975

226. Spergel P, Ehrlich G, Glass D: The rheumatoid arthritic personality. Psychosomatics 19:79–86, 1978

227. Stallone R: The epidemiology of systemic sclerosis. In Lawrence R, Shulman L (eds): Epidemiology of the Rheumatic Diseases, pp 169–174. New York, Gower, 1984

228. Stein H, Kickson RA: Reversed dynamic slings for knee flexion contractures in the hemophiliac. Bone Joint Surg [Am] 51:282, 1975

229. Steinbrocker O, Tiraeger CH, Batterman RC: Therapeutic criteria in rheumatoid arthritis. JAMA 140(8):659–662, 1949

230. Stitt FN, Frane M: Mood changes in rheumatoid arthritis. J Chronic Dis 30:135–145, 1977

231. Stross J, Mikkelsen WM: Educating patients with osteoarthritis. J Rheum 4:313–316, 1977

232. Sugarbaker PH, Lampert MH: Excision of quadriceps muscle group. Surgery 93(3):462–466, 1983

233. Swezey RL: Below-knee weight-bearing brace for the arthritic foot. Arch Phys Med Rehabil 56:176–179, 1978

234. Swezey R: In Athritis Rational Therapy and Rehabilitation. Philadelphia, WB Saunders, 1978

235. Swezey RL, Fiegenberg DS: Inappropriate intrinsic muscle action in the rheumatoid hand. Ann Rheum Dis 30:619, 1972

236. Swinburne WR (ed): Clinics in rheumatic disease: Sexual counseling for the arthritic. 23:639–651, 1976

237. Talbott JH, Bishop C, Norcross et al: The clinical and metabolic effects of Benemid in patients with gout. Trans Assoc Am Physicians 64:372, 1957

238. Tewfik IE, Christopher RP, Pinals RS et al: Adhesive capsulitis (frozen shoulder): A new approach to its management. Arch Phys Med Rehabil 64:29, 1983

239. Thomas HO: Diseases of the Hip, Knee, and Ankle Joints with Their Deformities, Treated by a New and Efficient Method, 3rd ed. London, Lewis, 1978

240. Thomas WH: Reconstructive surgery and rehabilitation of the ankle and foot. In Kelly W, Harris ED, Ruddy S, Sledge CB (eds): Textbook of Rheumatology, 2nd ed, pp 1896–1910. Philadelphia, WB Saunders, 1985

241. Thompson M, Bywaters EGL: Unilateral rheumatoid arthritis following hemiplegia. Ann Rheum Dis 21:370–377, 1962

242. Treuish FV, Krusen F: Physical therapy applied at home for arthritis. Arch Int Med 72:231–238, 1943

243. US Dept of Health, Education, and Welfare: Acute conditions: Incidence and associated disability, US, 1974–75. Vital Health Statistics, USDHEW Publication No. HRA 10(114):77-1541, 1977

244. Vignos P, Parker W, Thompson H: Evaluation of a clinic education program for patients with rheumatoid arthritis. J Rheum 3:155–165, 1976

245. Walliston KA, Kaplan GD, Maides SA: Development and validation of the health focus of control (HLC) scale. J Consult Clin Psychol 4:530–535, 1976

246. Warren CG, Lehman JF, Koblanski JN: Heat and stretch procedures: Evaluation using rat tail tendon. Arch Phys Med Rehabil 57:122, 1976

247. Warren CG, Lehman JF, Koblanski JN: Elongation of rat tail tendon: Effect of load and temperature. Arch Phys Med Rehabil 52:465–474, 1977

248. Warren CPW: Arthritis associated with samonella infection. Ann Rheum Dis 29:483, 1970

249. Weiss JJ, Thompson GR, Doust V, Burgener F: Rotator cuff tears in rheumatoid arthritis. Arch Intern Med 135:521, 1975

250. Weist DR, Waters RL, Bontrager EL et al: The influence of heel design on a rigid ankle foot orthosis. Orthotics Prosthetics 33:3, 1979

251. Winchester RJ, Nunez-Roldon A: Some genetic aspects of systemic lupus erythematosus. Arthritis Rheum 25:833, 1982

252. Woo SLY, Matthews JV, Akeson WM et al: Connective tissue response to immobility. Arthritis Rheum 18:257–264, 1975

253. Yellin E, Meenan R, Nevitt M, Epstein W: Work disability in rheumatoid arthritis: Effects of disease, social and work factors. Ann Int Med 93:551–556, 1980

254. Yoshino S: Sexual problems of women with rheumatoid arthritis. Arch Phys Med Rehabil 62:122–123, 1981

255. Zuaifler NJ, Woods VL: Etiology and Pathogenesis of SLE. In Kelly W, Harris ED, Ruddy S, Sledge CB (eds): Textbook of Rheumatology, 2nd ed, pp 1042–1053. Philadelphia, WB Saunders, 1985

255a. Hicks, JE, Nicholas, JJ: Treatments Utilized in Rehabilitative Rheumatology. In Hicks, JE, Nicholas, JJ, Swezey, RL (eds): Handbook of Rehabilitative Rheumatology, pp 31–79. Atlanta, American Rheumatism Association, 1988

40

Rehabilitation of the Patient With Peripheral Vascular Disease of the Lower Extremity

Margaret C. Hammond

Geno Merli

R. Eugene Zierler

A major tenet of rehabilitation medicine is the prevention and early diagnosis of complications of chronic disease and disability. Each of the vascular diseases in this chapter, arteriosclerosis obliterans, vasospastic disorders, lymphedema, and venous disease, results in significant acute or chronic functional impairment. Promotion of understanding and reduction in risk factors, combined with proper medical management, can do much to improve disease prognosis.

ARTERIOSCLEROSIS OBLITERANS

Pathophysiology

Arteriosclerosis obliterans is a disease of the large and medium-size arteries, particularly of the lower extremities, characterized by occlusive lesions. The earliest lesion or fatty intimal streak is of unclear etiology. It is commonly found in children and consists of a flat, lipid-rich collection of macrophages and smooth muscle cells.[59] As smooth muscle cell proliferation occurs, the atheroma progresses to a fibrous plaque. Advanced lesions may develop ulceration, thrombosis, hemorrhage, and calcification. Resultant complications include progressive narrowing or occlusion of the lumen producing ischemia, rupture, atheromatous emboli, and aneurysm formation from weakening of the vessel media.

Atherosclerosis affects most segments of the arterial system with a local distribution of lesions. Lesions tend to develop at major arterial bifurcations and sites of acute vessel angulation, presumably owing to disrupted laminar flow and the formation of eddy currents, which cause local intimal damage. The disease does not affect all arteries to the same extent, but shows a predilection for the coronary arteries, carotid bifurcation, aortoiliac, and lower extremity vessels. The lower extremity site most commonly affected is the arterial segment between the superficial femoral and popliteal arteries in Hunter's canal. In nondiabetics, aortoiliac disease is the second most likely location, whereas in diabetics, popliteal disease and tibial disease are more likely to follow femoral disease.

The initial symptom of lower extremity atherosclerosis is intermittent claudication. In this condition, blood flow is adequate to meet the metabolic demands of the resting extremity but cannot meet increased muscular demands in response to exercise. A consistent amount of exercise will produce pain in the calf, thigh, or buttock muscles with the severity and location of pain depending on the level of the occlusive lesions. Generally, hip girdle pain signifies aortic or common iliac disease, thigh claudication represents aortoiliac or common femoral disease, and calf pain represents superficial femoral or popliteal artery disease. However, the more distal muscle groups are usually the most ischemic with exercise, so calf claudication may be due to any proximal level of disease.[73] Other symptoms of intermittent claudication include weakness, fatigue, numbness, paresthesia, and muscular cramping. The discomfort subsides shortly after rest and does not require a positional change for relief.

The differential diagnosis of intermittent claudication (Table 40-1) includes such neuromuscular problems as spinal stenosis with pseudoclaudication, arthritis of the hip or knee, herniated intervertebral disk, peripheral neuropathy, popliteal artery entrapment,[80] tarsal tunnel syndrome, plantar neuroma, and McArdle's disease (absent muscle phosphorylase).

Progression of the disease is usually slow, resulting in gradual arterial occlusion and compromised lower extremity perfusion. Pre-existing, high-resistance intramuscular collateral vessels may dilate and convey arterial flow when a stenosis or an occlusion develops in a main artery. When an increased pressure gradient develops across a potential collateral bed as a result of arterial occlusion, flow in the distal re-entry vessels (which is normally directed away from the main artery) is reversed, increasing flow velocity and causing collateral vessel dilatation.[42] Tissue hypoxia and acidosis produce decreased peripheral resistance, enhancing the pressure gradient and contributing to collateral vessel dilatation.[4] Provided there are no sudden occlusions or emboli, collateral flow is usually adequate to meet the metabolic demands of resting muscle.

The prognosis of intermittent claudication is not necessarily grim. Seventy-five percent of nondiabtic patients with intermittent claudication will remain symptomatically stable for up to 5 years, and 50% may actually show improvement during the first few years after diagnosis.[48] However, disease progression and symptoms can be variable: while disease progressed over a 3-year period in 52% of patients in one study, 20% were not symptomatically worse.[74] Conversely, significant progression of both disease and symptoms may also occur within the first year.[48] Associated morbidity in the form of amputation is actually low,

Table 40-1
Differential Diagnosis of Intermittent Claudication

Neurospinal Disorders
  Spinal stenosis
  Herniated lumbar disk
  Spinal claudication or pseudoclaudication

Neuropathic Disorders
  Diabetic
  Ischemic
  Other peripheral
  Entrapment (tarsal tunnel syndrome)
  Plantar neuroma

Musculoskeletal Disorders
  Arthritis (hip, knee)
  Poplitial cyst
  Osteoporosis

Miscellaneous
  McArdle's disease

being between 3% and 7% in 5 years for nondiabetic patients,[38, 48] and 34% in 5 to 10 years for diabetic patients.[66]

Limb ischemia does represent a continuum of disease severity. Intermittent claudication may progress to ischemic rest pain, tissue necrosis, and gangrene. Rest pain occurs when blood flow is not adequate to meet the resting metabolic needs of the distal extremity. There is a persistent dull pain, numbness or dysesthesias in the foot, especially of the toes and metatarsal heads. Such dysesthesia may be described as coldness, deadness, tingling, burning, or a sensation of walking on gravel. These symptoms are typically worse at night and are better when the feet are in a dependent position, as this increases arterial flow. The diabetic patient with peripheral neuropathy may not feel pain and may present with a chief complaint of ulceration or gangrene.[27]

A number of factors may compromise the already limited blood flow. As the patient attempts to relieve discomfort by dangling the legs, the resultant dependent edema may limit arterial flow, particularly to the skin. Edema may also be due to congestive heart failure or hypoproteinemia. Other extrinsic factors that affect arterial flow by promoting edema include a weak calf muscle pump due to stroke or neuropathy, inactivity, and arthritis. In addition, injury, trauma, or infection may increase tissue metabolic requirements and exacerbate ischemia.

Epidemiology

Arteriosclerosis obliterans presents as a symptomatic disease predominantly in men between age 50 and 70. In an English study, the overall incidence of intermittent claudication was 2.2% in men and 1.2% in women.[29] Emphasizing the diffuse nature of this disease, there was a 36% incidence of coronary artery disease in patients with intermittent claudication.[30] The overall survival rate for patients with intermittent claudication is 73% at 5 years, in contrast to 93% at 5 years for normal age-matched controls.[38] Patients are at greater risk for mortality from other vascular diseases than for morbidity associated with limb loss.[83] In addition, most patients with arteriosclerosis obliterans can be expected to die from arterial disease, of either cerebral or cardiac etiology.[6]

Risk Factors and Associated Diseases

A number of factors predispose to the development or acceleration of arteriosclerosis obliterans. The ankle-arm systolic pressure gradient, an indirect measure of the degree of atherosclerosis between the heart and ankle, increases depending on the presence of risk factors such as hyperlipidemia, hypertension, and smoking.[35] The lipid theory of atherosclerosis cites the role of cholesterol in the initiation and maturation of arterial lesions. Serum cholesterol is derived from hepatic synthesis, dietary absorption, or mobilization from tissue pools. In patients with significant arteriosclerosis obliterans, the mean plasma cholesterol was found to be more than 50 mg/dl higher than in controls.[38, 39]

Hypertension exacerbates atherosclerosis with each incremental increase in pressure, directly increasing the risk of coronary artery disease.[25] Hypertension was found in 25% of patients with symptomatic disease of the aortoiliac and femoropopliteal arteries, but was found in only 9% of age-matched controls.[38] The mechanism appears to be related to endothelial injury from hypertensive pressure or hemodynamic shearing. Ironically, in advanced stages of disease, elevated pressures may be needed to allow flow through stenotic vessels.

A strong association exists between cigarette smoking and arteriosclerosis obliterans.[29, 38, 76] Not only does smoking potentiate platelet aggregation,[44] but it also produces vasospasm. In a prospective study of subjects with mild intermittent claudication, those who smoked at least 40 pack years had a 3.3 times greater vascular reconstruction rate than those who smoked less.[16]

Diabetes mellitus is associated with an earlier onset of atherosclerosis and a more rapid disease progression.[27] Distal vessels are more involved than are aortoiliac vessels; however, the disease is qualitatively similar to that seen in nondiabetics. Anatomically there may be extensive involvement with multiple stenotic areas, but no distinct lesions can be identified in the small vessels to distinguish the disease from atherosclerosis.[42] The concomitant finding of calcific medial sclerosis renders vessels incompressible, and may result in artifactually high values when Doppler ultrasound is used to noninvasively measure the arterial pressure. Long-term prognosis for limb viability is worse in diabetics due to rapid disease progression, extensive distal disease, peripheral neuropathy, and decreased ability to contain infection.

Other risk factors for generalized atherosclerosis include obesity, hyperuricemia, a sedentary life-style, and a positive family history.

Diagnosis

Physical Examination

Findings on physical examination that are related to ischemia include trophic skin changes (thin, shiny, hairless appearance), dependent rubor (an erythematous or dusky color), and decreased temperature. Arterial pulses are decreased or absent to palpation and may be associated with bruits. Delayed capillary filling and dependent rubor with pallor upon leg elevation may be found.

Diagnostic Tests

Supplementing a careful history and physical examination, diagnostic tests serve to establish the diagnosis, document the location and severity of stenosis or occlusion, evaluate the relative importance of multilevel disease, and assess the presence of collateral vessels or vasospasm. They also provide a baseline from which to assess disease progression, therapeutic results, or the degree of functional impairment.

Diagnostic tests can assess blood flow or pressure. Noninvasive flow studies include a regional flow assessment with plethysmography, Doppler evaluation of single vessel flow, and indirect testing through calorimetry and thermography. In mild to moderate atherosclerosis, total limb blood flow is usually normal at rest due to compensatory distal vasodilation. Therefore, it must be evaluated under conditions of increased flow to assess the physiological severity of the disease. Stress and maximal vasodilation may be induced by using a treadmill or bicycle ergometer. In the normal extremity, the resistance of the main conduit arteries is low and only a small pressure gradient is present across the vascular system. With isotonic exercise, peripheral vasodilation and a decrease in resistance occur in response to the metabolic demands of exercising muscle. Whereas exercise results in a markedly increased flow rate in a normal extremity, the corresponding increase in a limb with atherosclerosis is much less. This failure to increase flow during exercise is one physiological basis of intermittent claudication. Creating temporary limb ischemia with a pneumatic cuff, and resultant reactive hyperemia, is another method of inducing maximal vasodilation. In the presence of atherosclerotic lesions there is decreased maximal flow, an increased time to peak flow values, and increased time for return to baseline flow. If blood flow is limited by arterial disease, pulses may disappear with exercise or hyperemia-induced vasodilation.

The clinical use of pressure measurements relies on a drop in pressure across sites of stenosis where arterial resistance is increased. A ratio of ankle-to-arm systolic pressures measured with a pneumatic cuff and Doppler flow detector provides a useful indication of the severity of disease. An index of .9 or greater is considered normal, while an index of .7 to .9 indicates mild disease, .4 to .6 moderate to severe claudication, and less than .4 severe claudication. With an index greater than .5, occlusion of a single vessel is likely.[73] This test has less validity in a diabetic who may have incompressible vessels. As with flow studies, test sensitivity can be increased by stressing the circulation with exercise or reactive hyperemia. A patient with true intermittent claudication will show a definite decrease in ankle systolic pressure compared to resting values when exercised to the point of pain.

Whereas the previously described tests measure regional blood flow, other techniques assess local tissue perfusion. Transcutaneous measurements of oxygen tension assess skin oxygen content, which has been shown to correlate with the extent of occlusive disease, the potential for cutaneous wound healing, the determination of optimum amputation level, and the possible effectiveness of bypass procedures.[15, 23, 82]

Arteriography defines the anatomical lesion by severity and site of stenosis or obstruction. This test is generally performed prior to reconstructive arterial surgery. Magnetic resonance imaging (MRI) may be used for evaluation of aortoiliac disease and for follow-up after revascularization; however, it currently has too many limitations to replace preoperative arteriography.[81]

Management

Medical Management

Candidates for medical management include those with mild to moderate arterial disease and only symptoms of intermittent claudication. Other candidates include those with recent onset of disease who do not yet have fully developed collaterals, and patients who have failed vascular reconstruction, have distal lesions not amenable to reconstruction, or who are high surgical risks for other reasons.

As a first approach, the patient must be educated about his or her disease in order to reduce his or her fear of pain and to provide reassurance that amputation is not imminent. The physician can then focus on risk factors, associated diseases, and the manifestations of atherosclerosis itself. A new set of patient behaviors may be required, highlighting the need to provide the patient with patience, understanding, and positive reinforcement until such behaviors can be incorporated into the patient's daily activities. Patient management should follow these steps:

1. Educate the patient.
2. Reduce risk factors.
3. Treat associated disease.
4. Perform daily foot care.
5. Prescribe shoes and protective foot devices.
6. Institute measures to decrease edema.
7. Use medications: analgesics, others.
8. Provide local wound care.
9. Prescribe therapeutic exercise.
10. Prescribe orthotics.

Since smoking is a major contributing factor, both in terms of operative risk and promotion of disease progression, patients must stop tobacco use. Hypertension should be controlled, although diastolic pressures of 90 to 95 mm Hg may be allowed in order to maintain perfusion through stenotic vessels. The onset of intermittent claudication or its exacerbation can occur if antihypertensive treatment is too aggressive. Although the role of dietary cholesterol intake is still unclear, an overall reduction in calories to control body weight, restriction of high-sucrose-content foods which may reduce serum very-low-density lipoproteins, and a daily limitation of cholesterol intake to less than 300 mg seem prudent.

Associated or commonly found diseases which exacerbate atherosclerosis require attention. Treatment of congestive heart failure will maximize cardiac function and lessen peripheral edema. Arterial oxygenation can be improved with treatment of chronic obstructive pulmonary disease or anemia. Diabetes must be controlled because of its association with arterial disease progression and neuropathy.

The lower extremities require special attention from the patient. Overall tissue oxygen demand should be decreased by avoiding trauma, inflammation, and heat, with 92°F the maximal allowed temperature of water. Meticulous foot care is essential. The patient should inspect and wash the feet daily, and avoid prolonged soaking. Professional nail care, treatment of fungal infections and ingrown toenails, and daily lanolin applications to maintain skin pliability are recommended. Patients may wear oxfords with a wide toe-box in early disease, but may require a custom-molded insole with medial support in later stages. In the diabetic, autonomic denervation and peripheral neuropathy resulting in altered weight-bearing forces increase the vulnerability to foot lesions and necessitate custom footwear. As mentioned previously, edema can decrease arterial perfusion. Patients may find that elevating the head of the bed 6 to 8 inches will allow pain-free sleep with minimal edema formation.[45] At night, protective heel devices (*e.g.,* boots, pads) are critical for protection from the weight of the foot compressing against the bed. Lastly, mechanical injury from narrow shoes, restrictive clothing, bed siderails, and wheelchair footrests must be avoided.

Medical management also includes use of analgesic medication (aspirin or acetaminophen) and drugs acting directly on the vascular system. Vasodilators such as alpha-adrenergic blocking agents, beta-adrenergic stimulating agents, and smooth muscle relaxants do not significantly increase blood flow to ischemic tissues or exercising muscle. Pentoxifylline, a methylxanthine derivative, affects red blood cell flexibility and has been associated with significant increases in walking distances in a double-blind study of patients with intermittent claudication.[57]

Should an ischemic ulcer develop, the patient should avoid weight-bearing and protect the involved foot with lamb's wool separation of the toes. Hydrotherapy, routine wound dressing, and antibiotics may be indicated. Some physicians will allow ambulation as long as gangrene is dry and edema absent. Patients on bed rest will require daily physical therapy to prevent tissue atrophy and joint contractures, especially since patients tend to keep the leg in a flexed position of comfort.

Surgical Management

Indications for surgical intervention, such as endarterectomy or bypass grafting, include intractable ischemic pain, severe ischemia with nonhealing ulcers or gangrene, and increasing disability. The physiatrist and physical therapist may assist in postoperative mobilization. Knee flexion is generally prohibited after across-knee procedures until graft patency is ensured, at approximately 3 days; extreme knee flexion should be avoided indefinitely. Progressive weight-bearing and ambulation is usually initiated on the first postoperative day.

Therapeutic Exercise

The goals of therapeutic exercise are to increase arterial blood flow, decrease the oxygen demand of the tissue, improve the efficiency of oxygen extraction, and increase the patency of collateral vessels. Patients with infrequent rest pain (1–3 times per week) may participate in a trial of training.[37] Exercise therapy is contraindicated in the presence of ischemic ulcers.

A number of studies support the use of exercise in the presence of intermittent claudication. The physician should first consider obtaining a baseline treadmill study to evaluate cardiac work tolerance and the presence of angina, hypertension, or ST segment depression with exercise. Treadmill testing is also useful for assessing the musculoskeletal and pulmonary factors that can affect walking ability. Training may consist of walking, jogging, bicycling, or swimming; the upright exercise posture is preferable to the horizontal, as it improves lower extremity perfusion.[69] In a program of group therapy three times per week with each session including walking, jogging, leg stretching, and leg relaxation, patients doubled their walking distance after 3 months. Additional but less significant improvement was noted for another 6 months.[17] Interestingly, patients with aortoiliac disease responded as well as those with femoropopliteal disease.[21] If exercise is limited to walking, patients should walk three to five times per day to or just beyond the onset of claudication. In patients with superficial femoral artery occlusion, symptomatic improvement can be expected in those with an ankle-arm ratio greater than 0.6.[83] Low-level pain-free endurance training is also effective in increasing walking distance, exercise time, and energy expenditure. Its theoretical advantages include a decrease in anaerobic metabolism, which may trigger claudication pain.[7]

Multiple factors affect the exercise capacity of patients with intermittent claudication. Sorlie found a two- to tenfold increase in lower leg blood flow in subjects with atherosclerosis at maximum exercise, compared to a 20-fold increase in normals.[69] In addition, a greater oxygen extraction in claudicants persists into the postexercise period.[70] This may be due to an increased red blood cell passage time as a consequence of decreased flow, or it may be due to an increased tissue oxidative capacity.[17] Vasodilation after exercise is due to regional hypoxia, hypercapnia, and low pH. Release of metabolites from the catabolism of adenosine nucleotides may play a role in the local regulation of muscle blood flow.[71] A provocative study by Matsen and colleagues evaluated transcutaneous oxygen pressures and ankle blood pressure during treadmill exercise. The pressure of oxygen in the skin decreased after exercise and then returned to preexercise values.[47] Exercise produces a decrease in muscular resistance causing limited arterial flow to be shunted from skin to muscle. Of clinical concern is the hypothesis that exercise may reduce cutaneous oxygen delivery to levels associated with impaired local cutaneous wound healing.

Exercise training can produce several effects on exercise capacity. Zetterquist showed a greater arteriovenous oxygen difference without a change in arterial inflow as a training effect of walking.[84] Although no change in total calf blood flow was found by Dahllof, training may cause a redistribution of flow.[18] Patients may also learn to vary their ambulation pattern, walking more slowly and with more pain tolerance.[16] A more efficient use of muscles and a change in gait have also been suggested as mechanisms for increasing walking distances. Other general effects of training may include improved muscular coordination, joint mobility, general fitness, and balance.

Orthotics

Although infrequently used, orthotics may play a role in treating the patient with arteriosclerosis obliterans. An ankle-foot orthosis may decrease plantar flexion activity and work during the push-off phase of the gait cycle, contributing to subjective improvement and longer walking time.[28] Occasionally, a patient who refuses amputation for ischemic or neuropathic ulcers may ambulate safely with a patellar tendon–bearing orthosis.[24]

VASOSPASTIC DISORDERS

Raynaud's syndrome is a condition of unknown etiology which manifests as episodic digital arterial vasospasm in response to cold exposure or emotional stress. Specific theories for the etiology include abnormal sympathetic (nerve) activity, abnormal digital vessels, or an immunological process. Women constitute 70% to 90% of patients with Raynaud's syndrome, although 30% of a general population may report similar symptoms.[56] Raynaud's disease is the primary or idiopathic form of cold sensitivity, while Raynaud's phenomenon refers to cold sensitivity associated with some underlying disease process. Such diseases include connective tissue disorders, atherosclerotic arterial disease, thromboangiitis obliterans, occupational diseases involving vibration injury, and drug-induced states (beta-blocking drugs or oral contraceptives).

The minimal clinical criterion for Raynaud's syndrome includes a skin color change in response to cold or stress. The classic triad presents as digital or occasionally proximal hand pallor with numbness, which persists for the duration of the cold stimulus. Cyanosis then develops after 10 to 30 minutes of warmth as the small amount of flowing blood desaturates. Lastly, a reactive hyperemia and rubor of the skin develops. Severe pain is rarely associated with the process.

Diagnosis can be readily confirmed with an ice water immersion test and serial digital pulp temperature measurements.

A general history and physical examination are necessary to diagnose associated diseases. Treatment is directed primarily at symptom relief. Avoidance of cold, nicotine, and exacerbating drugs is essential. Sympatholytic or direct vasodilators are of limited benefit. Calcium channel blockers (nifedipine) may be helpful. Biofeedback has benefited some individuals by teaching them to warm their hand or dilate the blood vessels. Additional measures include relaxation training and stress management if stress is the inciting factor.

LYMPHEDEMA

The term *lymphedema* should be confined to patients with swelling of an extremity or other body part secondary to a malformation or obstruction of lymphatic channels. Lymphedema can be classified into the following primary and secondary categories.[61]

CLASSIFICATION OF LYMPHEDEMA

Primary lymphedema
    Hereditary (Milroy's disease)
    Congenital
    Praecox
    Tarda
Secondary lymphedema
    Obstructive/obliterative
    Inflammatory

It is the purpose of this section to review the pathophysiology, diagnosis, and management of lymphedema of the lower extremity.

Pathophysiology

The primary function of the lymphatics is to clear the interstitial space of excess proteinaceous fluid and return it to the blood circulation. When this protein-rich fluid (1–5 g/dl) is not adequately removed, lymphedema develops. Four factors regulate this fluid production: the capillary blood pressure (hydrostatic), the osmotic pressure of plasma proteins in the blood, the interstitial pressure (hydrostatic), and the osmotic pressure of protein in the interstitial fluid (Fig. 40-1).

The lymphatic system is composed of three major components: the terminal lymphatic capillaries, which absorb lymph from the interstitial space; the major lymphatic vessels, which transport lymph to the thoracic duct; and the lymph nodes, which are mechanical filters and serve an immunological function. The terminal lymphatics begin in the superficial dermis as valveless vessels which follow the vascular pathways. In the lower extremities, the major lymph vessels are arranged as superficial and deep systems with tricuspid valves every 2 mm to 3 mm (Fig. 40-2). The superficial system is divided into a medial and lateral group. The medial lymphatics begin on the dorsum of the foot and course along the greater saphenous vein, ending in the inguinal lymph nodes (Fig. 40-3). The lateral lymphatics begin on the lateral aspect of the foot, cross in front of the leg below the knee, and follow the medial lymphatics into the inguinal nodes. There are a few posterior channels that arise from the lateral aspect of the foot and Achilles tendon and course along the lesser saphenous vein to the popliteal area. The posterior lymphatics then pierce the deep fascia to join the popliteal node. Efferent channels from this node follow the deep lymphatics and drain into the inguinal nodes (see Fig. 40-3D). The deep lymphatics are not visualized on lymphangiography because there is no

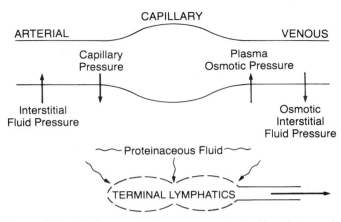

Figure 40-1. Under normal circumstances, terminal lymphatic capillaries remove excess proteinaceous fluid from interstitial space and return it to the blood.

Figure 40-2. Enlarged lower limb lymphatic vessel. The "beaded" appearance is produced by the dilatation of the lymphatic, which is immediately upstream from a valve cusp. (Kinmonth JB: The Lymphatics: Surgery, Lymphology and Disease of the Chyle and Lymph Systems. London, E Arnold, 1982)

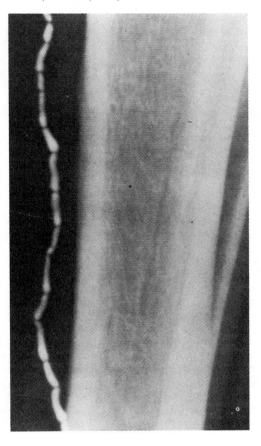

communication between the superficial and deep systems. The deep lymph vessels follow the course of the deep arteries and veins. These also drain into the inguinal nodes. From the inguinal nodes, efferent lymphatics accompany the major vascular structures through the retroperitoneal area[6] (Fig. 40-4). In the thorax they form the thoracic duct which joins the venous system

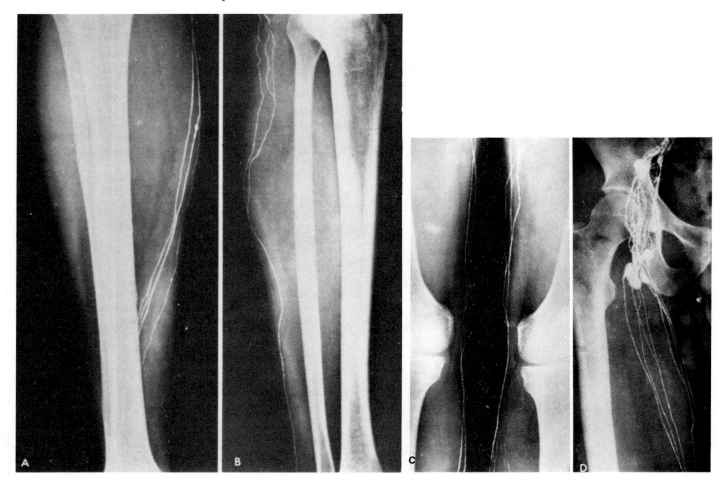

Figure 40-3. Examples of the medial lymph trunks. Below the knee: (*A*) anteroposterior projection; (*B*) postero-oblique view. Lower limb: (*C*) medial trunks grouped closely together as they pass the knee joint; (*D*) vessels in the thigh are filled and spread out over the anteromedial aspect. (Kinmonth JB: The Lymphatics: Surgery, Lymphology and Disease of the Chyle and Lymph Systems. London, E Arnold, 1982)

at the junction of the internal jugular and subclavian veins[58] (Fig. 40-5).

The lymphatic channels are unique because their endothelial cells have a microfibril attachment.[12, 13] These allow the endothelial junctions to remain open when pressure rises in the interstitial space.[12, 13] Large plasma proteins (albumin predominantly) are filtered through the pores and are returned to the venous system. The movement of lymph through these channels depends upon external forces such as pulsation of the arteries, muscular pump action, peristaltic activity of the intestines, respiratory movement, and blood pressure. Recently, Olszewski and Engeset have measured the frequency and amplitude of rhythmic contractions in the subcutaneous lymphatics of the human leg at rest.[54] These results suggest that the intrinsic contractility of the lymphatic wall is also a force in the propulsion of lymph in the resting leg.

The lymph nodes are variable in size, with major groupings located in the inguinal and retroperitoneal areas. The nodes, which have their own blood and nerve supplies, act as filtering areas for the afferent lymph channels. A dynamic cell population is present in the nodes consisting predominately of lymphocytes. The filtration process results in a greater resistance to lymph flow, but a greater opportunity for lymphocytes to act.

Diagnosis

The two major categories of lymphedema are labeled primary and secondary. The patient history is probably the most important factor in differentiating these two groups. The physical examination, although often not very specific, is important in distinguishing lymphedema from other causes of edema.

Primary Lymphedema

One classification system proposes three major clinical groups of primary lymphedema distinguished by the age of onset. The first group includes congenital and hereditary forms. The congenital form often presents in an individual without a past family history of lymphedema. The hereditary form (Milroy's disease) is transmitted as an autosomal dominant trait. The clinical characteristics are predominantly an enlargement of an extremity at birth with firm, non-pitting edema (Fig. 40-6). The child's development and activities are not impaired.

The second group is lymphedema praecox, a term first used by E. V. Allen.[2] This group is composed primarily of females in the second and third decades of life. It presents spontaneously without an apparent etiology. The edema is initially soft and pitting, but becomes firm and non-pitting over time (Fig. 40-7).

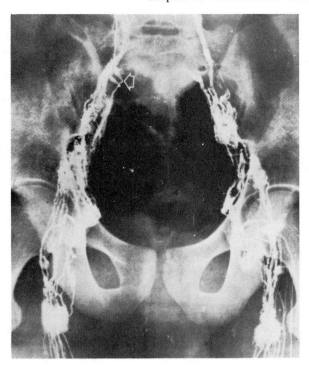

Figure 40-4. Efferent lymphatic vessels appear on a normal iliac lymphangiogram. Their valve ampullae may be quite large (see *arrow*) without being abnormal. (Kinmonth JB: The Lymphatics: Surgery, Lymphology and Disease of the Chyle and Lymph Systems. London, E Arnold, 1982)

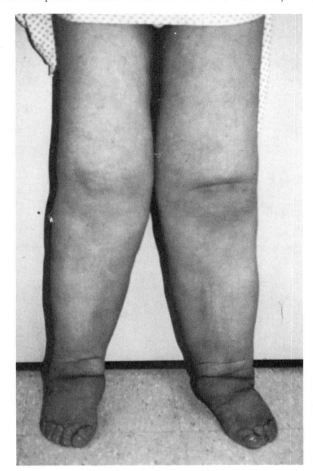

Figure 40-6. Congenital lymphedema.

Figure 40-5. Efferent lymphatic vessels in normal upper portion of the thoracic duct, with segmentation of the contrast material and fish-tail appearance near valves. (Kinmonth JB: The Lymphatics: Surgery, Lymphology and Disease of the Chyle and Lymph Systems. London, E Arnold, 1982)

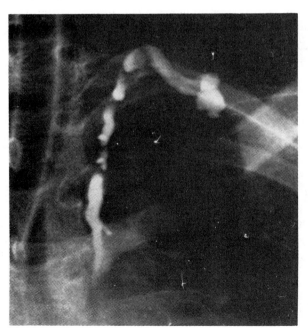

There is no pain or ulceration, but recurrent infection can occur in this group.

The lymphedema tarda group was added by Kinmonth and co-workers for those patients who develop lymphedema after the age of 35 years[43] (Fig. 40-8). This also occurs without an obvious etiology. The edema is non-pitting and firm. Pain and ulceration do not occur, but recurrent infections are common. Both the praecox and tarda forms of lymphedema may represent congenital lymphatic disease with delayed onset of symptoms.

A second classification proposed by Kinmonth and colleagues used lymphangiographic anatomy as the criteria for separation of lymphedema[43] into two major types, hyperplasia with large numerous dilated lymphatics, and hypoplasia with abnormally few and small lymphatics. Such a classification requires lymphangiography to be performed distally as well as proximally. We do not advocate lymphangiography because of its risk and the lack of any benefit in long-term management and prognosis.

Other conditions that have been associated with primary lymphedema (congenital type) include Turner's syndrome,[3] Noonan syndrome,[50] Fabry's disease,[26] congenital absence of nails,[46] distichiasis,[22, 58] and pleural effusions (yellow nail syndrome).[65]

Secondary Lymphedema

On a worldwide basis, secondary lymphedema is the most frequent type. Infection is the predominant etiology in third-world countries, whereas malignancy is the major cause in the

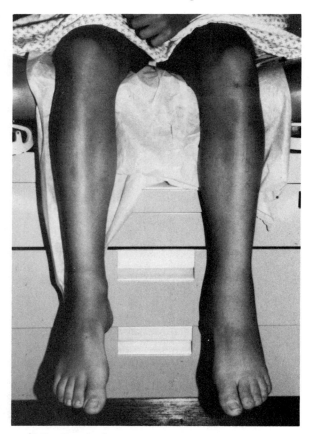

Figure 40-7.   Lymphedema praecox.

Figure 40-8.   Lymphedema tarda.

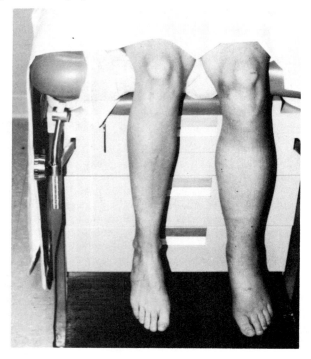

western world. The pathophysiology of secondary lymphedema is the obstruction or removal of lymphatic channels, either by extranodal or intranodal malignant disease, radiation, surgical excision, trauma, or infection. Therefore, two groups exist under the heading of secondary lymphedema: obstructive/obliterative and inflammatory.

The obstructive/obliterative type is caused predominantly by malignancy. This results from tumor invasion or compression, surgical removal, or radiation. Smith, Spittell, and Schirger reported 80 cases of secondary lymphedema with the most common underlying lesion being prostate cancer in men and lymphoma in women.[78] Lymphedema may precede the diagnosis of malignancy. The edema is predominantly unilateral, pitting or non-pitting, and regresses slightly with elevation.

The inflammatory type may result from frequent infections with residual limb edema, which becomes firm and non-pitting over time. Filariasis, tuberculosis, typhoid fever, and influenza have all been reported as causes for this process. Lastly, Nathan and co-workers and Silver, Tsongaris, and Eaton reported sarcoidosis as an etiology of lymphatic obstruction.[51, 67] In one patient, the edema was present for 10 years before the other manifestations of sarcoidosis appeared.

The workup of these patients requires a thorough history and physical, supplemented by laboratory tests as indicated. Computed tomography and MRI of the abdomen and pelvis add additional information. Venography and arteriography are reserved for those cases in which additional anatomical information is required for diagnosis and prognosis.

Management

The approach to managing lymphedema is based on mobilization of fluid and prevention of long-term complications (Table 40-2).

Every effort must be made to define the etiology of lymphedema prior to beginning a regimen of therapy. In the past, bed rest and leg elevation were the predominant treatment. With the need for appropriate use of hospital time, an outpatient course of therapy may be established which allows indepen-

---

Table 40-2
Guidelines for Lymphedema Care

A. *Define Etiology*
1. History and physical examination
2. Laboratory
3. Venography*
4. Arteriography*
5. CT scan or MRI*

B. *Treatment in Hospital*
1. Pneumatic compression
2. Gradient elastic compression stocking
3. Education of patient and family on use of compression device at home and care of the involved extremity
4. Antibiotics
5. Diuretics

C. *Discharge*
1. Extremity compression prescribed for 2 to 4 hours/day
2. Use of gradient elastic stocking
3. Skin care
4. Observation for signs and symptoms of infection

---

* If clinically indicated

dence in activities of daily living, but still achieves the mobilization and control of lymphatic fluid.

When new patients are evaluated, the extremities are measured (length and circumference) and photographed for future assessment of therapy. Lymph is mobilized by extremity compression with a commercially available device (Jobst, Venodyne, Flotron). A 3- to 5-day hospitalization is required for an intensive course of extremity compression. This will define the efficacy, tolerability, and safety of pneumatic compression. During the hospitalization, an educational program for family and patient is provided. Following discharge, daily compression for 2 to 4 hours per day with either a rented or purchased device is recommended, with further adjustment of the treatment as dictated by the patient's life-style. Graded compression stockings must always be worn during daily activities; they are removed in the evening for skin care and laundering. The patients are re-evaluated initially in 1 month and subsequently every 4 to 6 months for 2 years. After this course, a once-per-year and as-needed regimen for care is followed.

The above regimen of care is used as the standard approach. Modifications are made for the patient with individual problems. The most frequently encountered problem is the previous use and failure of a pneumatic compression device. These patients are admitted in order to assess the safety and efficacy of the more sophisticated sequential compression devices (Wright Linear Pump, Lymphapress). These patients must be monitored during the initial use of these devices because of the rapid mobilization of fluid. Training in the use of the machine is necessary, and because these devices are expensive, efficacy must be established.

Another problem is presented by the patient with cellulitis and swelling, which occur frequently in the secondary lymphedema group, but can also occur in the praecox and tarda primary lymphedema group. In our experience, the use of oral antibiotics on an outpatient basis has not been efficacious. These patients are admitted and treated with intravenous antibiotics (cephlosporin, second generation, or erythromycin if patient is penicillin-allergic) for 7 to 10 days and compression beginning once the inflammation has subsided. The portal of infection is commonly the skin. Emphasis must be made on early and aggressive treatment of cellulitis of the extremity, since delay will result in a longer recovery time. Recurrent episodes of cellulitis can be prevented by small daily doses of oral penicillin. Leg swelling may be exacerbated by urinary tract infections.

Diuretics are rarely used to mobilize fluid because the risks outweigh the benefits. Diuretics are used in selected cases of excessive edema when the cardiopulmonary system would be compromised by the excessive mobilization of fluid during pneumatic compression. In these cases diuretics are used in conjunction with pneumatic compression.

Skin care is performed twice daily with moisturizing cream. Foot care with topical antifungal creams or powders is also necessary to reduce the possibility of secondary infection of the affected extremity.

Lymphangiosarcoma is a malignant tumor that can occur in patients with chronic lymphedema. It appears as a nonhealing bruise with satellite lesions. This lesion should be biopsied and referral to an oncologist made upon confirmation of the diagnosis.

Only 15% of patients with primary lymphedema will eventually require operation. Surgical intervention is indicated in this group when medical management has failed and severe disfigurement is present or function is impaired. The operations can be divided into debulking procedures (Charles, Thompson, Homans) and drainage procedures (lymphaticovenous shunt, small bowel pedical graft). Despite some favorable results, the surgical treatment of lymphedema has been generally disappointing. The drainage procedures cannot be recommended, and the debulking operations should only be considered in extremely severe cases as an alternative to amputation.

VENOUS DISORDERS

Venous disease is a common medical problem in the United States. There is a wide spectrum of disease which is served by many disciplines, both surgical and medical. In the following sections, the anatomy, pathophysiology, assessment, and management of acute and chronic venous disease will be presented.

Anatomy

Veins are thin-walled tubes containing bicuspid valves, which can alter their cross-sectional shape from a flat to circular configuration (Fig. 40-9).[77] This physiological ability allows the veins to serve as capacitance vessels and to maintain unidirectional flow. The presence of a sinus adjacent to the valve leaflets prevents them from coming in contact with the vein wall and facilitates rapid closure when pressure is reversed (Fig. 40-10).[78] This creates an area of stasis behind the valve leaflets, which is believed to be a nidus for thrombosis in low-flow states (Fig. 40-11).[63] There are more valves in the distal deep venous system than in the superficial system.

The superficial venous system is composed of the greater saphenous vein, the lesser saphenous vein, and their tributaries (Fig. 40-12).[14] The greater saphenous vein originates at the me-

Figure 40-9. Cross-sections of venous lumen at various transmural pressures. (Sumner DS: Hemodynamics and pathophysiology of venous disease. In Rutherford RB [ed]: Vascular Surgery, 2nd ed, pp 148–166. Philadelphia, WB Saunders, 1984)

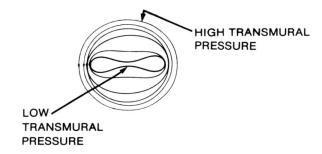

HIGH TRANSMURAL PRESSURE

LOW TRANSMURAL PRESSURE

Figure 40-10. Longitudinal section through a venous valve shows open and closed positions.

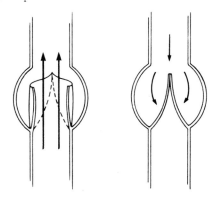

dial end of the dorsal venous arch of the foot and ascends anterior to the medial malleolus. The lesser saphenous vein has its origin at the lateral end of the superficial venous arch of the foot and courses posterior to the lateral malleolus. Both of these veins receive tributaries and perforating veins. More than 100 perforating veins have been identified in the lower extremity.

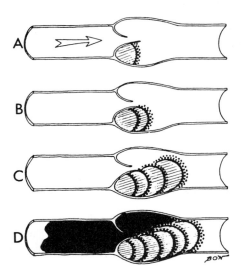

Figure 40-11. (*A*) Propagation of a deep vein thrombus behind a valve leaflet. (*B, C*) Deposition of successive layers of fibrin, platelets, and so on. (*D*) Retrograde extension occurs once the vein is completely blocked. (Bergan JJ, Yao JS [eds]: Venous Problems. Chicago, Year Book, 1978)

The perforating veins join the superficial and deep veins by penetrating the crural fascia, and they contain valves which normally direct flow from superficial to deep. The deep veins accompany the named arteries in the muscular compartments of the leg. Varying anatomical patterns of the deep veins exist.[14]

Pathophysiology

The pathophysiology of acute venous disease is related to Virchow's triad of stasis, intimal injury, and hypercoagulability. Stasis is the primary factor that results from surgery, paralysis, or immobilization.[14, 52, 62] The reduction in blood flow velocity establishes a nidus for deep vein thrombosis, as noted in Figure 40-11.[63] Recently, Steward, Schaub, and colleagues have shown by electron microscopy intimal damage secondary to the vasodilatation accompanying general anesthesia.[60, 72] (Fig. 40-13). These intimal tears are believed to be an initiating event in the development of deep vein thrombosis. Hypercoagulability, the third factor, is primarily the result of an imbalance between thrombosis and hemorrhage. Stasis and surgery are conditions conducive to clot formation. Seyfer and associates demonstrated a decreased antithrombin III level in trauma and surgical patients who developed deep vein thrombosis.[64] Owen and colleagues showed that plasmin activity was impaired in neurosurgical patient days prior to the onset of thrombosis.[55] All the above mechanisms may contribute in various degrees to the formation of acute deep vein thrombosis.

The primary mechanism for chronic venous disease is related to increased pressure in the deep venous system secondary to incompetent valves. Perivalvular laxity of tissue and postthrombotic damage are etiologies for valvular incompetence.

Figure 40-12. Radiographic anatomy of major vessels of the lower limbs.

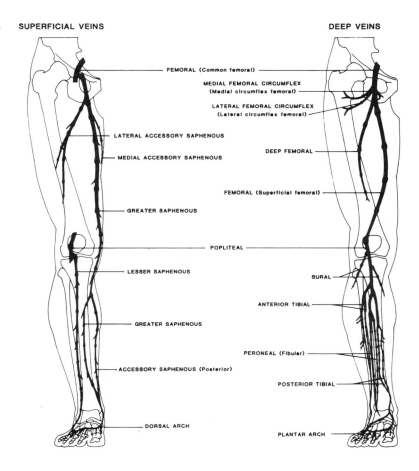

SUPERFICIAL VEINS

DEEP VEINS

FEMORAL (Common femoral)

MEDIAL FEMORAL CIRCUMFLEX
(Medial circumflex femoral)

LATERAL FEMORAL CIRCUMFLEX
(Lateral circumflex femoral)

LATERAL ACCESSORY SAPHENOUS

MEDIAL ACCESSORY SAPHENOUS

DEEP FEMORAL

FEMORAL (Superficial femoral)

GREATER SAPHENOUS

POPLITEAL

LESSER SAPHENOUS

SURAL

ANTERIOR TIBIAL

GREATER SAPHENOUS

PERONEAL (Fibular)

ACCESSORY SAPHENOUS (Posterior)

POSTERIOR TIBIAL

DORSAL ARCH

PLANTAR ARCH

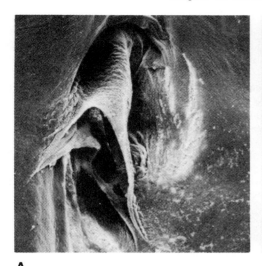
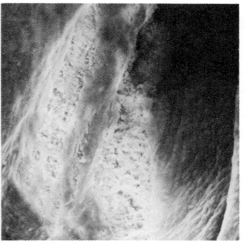

A   **B**

Figure 40-13. (*A*) Scanning electron microscopy photomicrograph of the venous confluence of an operated dog. Endothelial and basement membrane damage is visible. (*B*) Damaged vein wall under higher magnification.

The resulting reflux flow causes ambulatory venous hypertension and the various symptoms and signs of chronic venous insufficiency.

Valvular incompetence of the primary type is seen in the superficial venous system and is associated with varicose veins. This condition does not result from damage to the valve cusps, but to dilatation of the valvular ring with failure of the valve leaflets to coapt. This laxity is secondary to a decreased collagen content in the walls of varicose veins and is inherited by a polygenic mechanism.[79] This alteration in physiology causes retrograde flow during exercise (Fig. 40-14) with venous dilatation, elongation, and tortuosity.[20]

Valvular damage from the post-thrombotic process is due to inflammatory changes in the valve leaflets. This damage results in abnormal pressure gradients, reflux flow, and the typical clinical sequelae.[20] The main difference between primary varicose veins and deep venous insufficiency is the pressure of valvular incompetence and obstruction in the deep venous system with abnormally high venous pressures during leg exercise.

The venous hypertension of deep venous insufficiency results in histological tissue changes. Browse and Burnard demonstrated increased growth of new capillaries in the epidermis and dermis.[8] These capillaries have been shown to be abnormally permeable to hemoglobin and fibrinogen.[8] Interstitial hemoglobin is degraded, leaving a brown hemosiderin pigment which results in a bronze skin color. Interstitial fibrinogen is converted to fibrin, which polymerizes and forms a barrier to the diffusion of oxygen and other nutrients into the tissue. This barrier explains the high oxygen content of venous blood and the increased risk of tissue necrosis and ulceration.[19] Thus, ambulatory venous hypertension is responsible for the pigmentation, edema, subcutaneous fibrosis, and ulceration that characterize chronic venous disease.

Diagnosis

The accuracy of clinical evaluation for acute deep vein thrombosis is highly nonspecific.[1, 5, 49] This limitation of signs and symptoms is related to the fact that various nonthrombotic disorders can cause similar manifestations. Contrast venography is the standard objective method for the assessment of acute deep vein thrombosis. Although venography has been available for at least three decades, it has not been routinely used due to concern

Figure 40-14. Pressure changes in the veins of the foot produced by various degrees of valve dysfunction. (DeWeese, JA: Venous and lymphatic disease. In Schwartz SI, Lillehei RC, Shires GT et al [eds]: Principles of Surgery, 2nd ed. New York, McGraw-Hill, 1974)

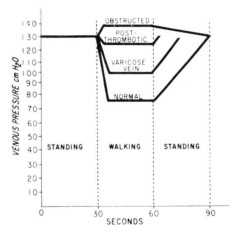

over the rare contrast-related problems of allergic reactions, local venous or skin injury, and secondary thrombophlebitis.[33, 75] Noninvasive testing has provided another method of assessing deep vein thrombosis. Venous Doppler, impedance plethysmography (IPG), phleborrheography, and iodine-125 fibrinogen scanning are a few of the methods available in the United States. IPG is the most frequently used study. Hull and colleagues demonstrated the sensitivity and specificity of this method to be 95% and 98%, respectively.[33] The venous Doppler examination is easy to perform, but requires an experienced technician because the interpretation is entirely subjective.[40] The above tests are most accurate for thrombosis in the deep veins proximal to the knee.

Radioiodine-labeled fibrinogen scanning depends on the incorporation of this isotope into the clot and increased uptake measured by a surface radioisotope detector. The test is accurate for calf vein thrombosis but requires 48 hours for assessment.[32] Hull and co-workers combined IPG and I-125 scanning for the assessment of deep vein thrombosis and reported a 97% sensitivity and 94% specificity.[9] One approach to assessment of acute deep vein thrombosis is venography, but if circumstances advise against this, then IPG is used. Another approach is the use of a venous Doppler examination, resorting to venography when the Doppler is not diagnostic.

Chronic venous disease is ten times more prevalent than arterial disease of the lower extremities in the United States. Lower extremity venous disease can be divided into varicose veins and postphlebitic (or post-thrombotic) syndrome.

Varicose veins can be primary or secondary (Table 40-3). Patients with primary varicose veins often have a family history and are predominantly female (Fig. 40-15). Connective tissue laxity is believed to be the underlying mechanism, and terminal valve incompetence of the greater and lesser saphenous veins is the major abnormality. Secondary varicose veins are usually associated with chronic abnormalities of the deep venous system and are the result of ambulatory venous hypertension. Rare causes of varicosities include arteriovenous fistula with resultant valvular incompetence.

Postphlebitic syndrome (PPS) occurs in approximately 20% of patients following deep vein thrombosis.[53] It has been estimated that PPS affects 0.5% of the population of Great Britain and the United States and causes an estimated loss of 500,000 working days each year in England and Wales and 2 million in the United States.[31] As already mentioned, the underlying mecha-

nism for this syndrome is the destruction of venous valves by thrombosis resulting in abnormal lower extremity venous pressures.

The symptoms most frequently experienced with chronic venous disease are pain and heaviness (Table 40-4). The pain is described as an aching throughout the leg. Frequently this symptom is interpreted as degenerative joint disease, except that no specific joints are involved. The heaviness increases as the day progresses with relief by rest overnight. This symptom is attributed to increased venous volume of the extremity that occurs with normal activities of daily living. The signs of chronic venous disease are edema, distended superficial veins (varicosities), skin pigmentation, subcutaneous fibrosis, dermatitis, and ulceration (Figs. 40-16—40-19). The signs of chronic venous disease can be grouped into three stages (see Table 40-4). This classification directs the degree and intensity of care. Stage I is characterized by edema and pigmentation; in stage II varicosities, edema, skin pigmentation, and dermatitis appear; and in stage III varicosities, edema, skin pigmentation, dermatitis, and ulceration are seen.

Management

After diagnostic studies have confirmed the presence of deep vein thrombosis, therapy is initiated with heparin or thrombolytic agents. Constant intravenous heparin infusion is the preferred initial treatment. Heparin is begun with a bolus of approximately 5000 units followed by an infusion of 1000 units per hour. The activated partial thromboplastin time (aPTT) is assessed in 6 hours, and the dose is adjusted up or down to maintain a value of $1^1/2$ to $2^1/2$ times the control. A platelet count is done every other day. Warfarin is begun on the evening of the third day of heparin therapy at 10 mg daily. Heparin therapy is discontinued when the prothrombin time has been in the therapeutic range (ratio 1.3 to

Table 40-3
Varicose Veins

Primary
1. Hereditary
2. More common in women

Secondary
1. Pregnancy-related
2. Occupational
3. Rare (arteriovenous fistulae)
   a. Klippel-Trenauny
   b. Congenital arteriovenous fistulae
   c. Traumatic arteriovenous fistulae

Figure 40-15.   Varicose veins.

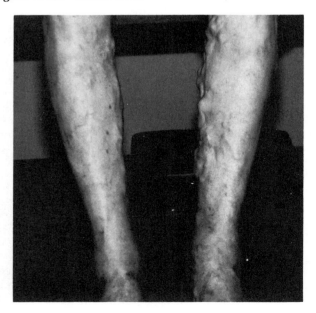

Table 40-4
Chronic Venous Disease

Symptoms
1. Pain
2. Heaviness

Signs
1. Edema
2. Varicosities
3. Subcutaneous fibrosis
4. Skin pigmentation
5. Dermatitis
6. Ulceration

Stages
1. Stage I
   a. Edema
   b. Skin pigmentation
2. Stage II
   a. Edema
   b. Skin pigmentation
   c. Dermatitis
   d. Varicosities
3. Stage III
   a. Edema
   b. Skin pigmentation
   c. Dermatitis
   d. Varicosities
   e. Ulceration

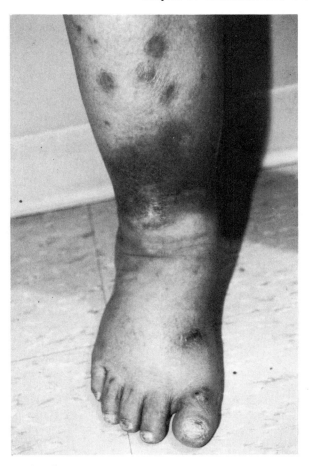

Figure 40-16. PPS.

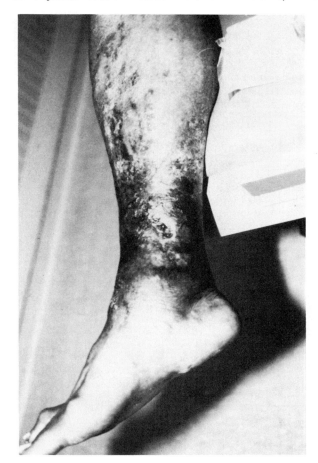

Figure 40-17. PPS.

1.7) for at least 48 hours. Warfarin or adjusted-dose heparin are then used to prevent early recurrence of the deep vein thrombosis. The latter method has been documented by Hull and associates.[31] Treatment for the prevention of recurrence is maintained for 3 to 6 months.

Thrombolytic therapy with streptokinase or urokinase is reserved for extensive deep vein thrombosis or pulmonary embolism with compromised cardiopulmonary status or threatened limb viability. Kakkar and Lawrence demonstrated that successful thrombolysis of deep vein thrombosis does not prevent venous hemodynamic deterioration or the postphlebitic syndrome.[41]

Patients with calf vein thrombosis are placed on bed rest for 72 hours, followed by gradual mobilization. Proximal vein thrombosis requires 7 days of bed rest with gradual mobilization and bathroom privileges with assistance if pain and swelling have subsided. All patients wear gradient elastic stockings when they are mobilized.

Patients with chronic venous disease are managed according to the staged classification (Table 40-5). Stage I patients wear calf-length gradient elastic stockings during the day to improve lower extremity external support and to reduce the abnormal pressure gradient on the superficial veins. This support will reduce edema and prevent hemoglobin leakage into the interstitial tissues resulting in hemosiderin skin pigmentation. Gradient elastic stockings can be custom-made by such companies as Jobst or Sigvaris. Off-the-shelf 20 to 30 mm Hg Jobst or Sigvaris graded stockings are also available. They have an 8- to 10-month longevity and are economical. Topical skin moisturizing lotions are recommended twice per day. Exercise such as walking, bicycling, and swimming are encouraged.

Stage II patients have edema, skin pigmentation, dermatitis, and varicosities. The retrograde pressure from incompetent valves is more significant in this stage resulting in varicosities and their sequelae. Gradient elastic stockings are the principal treatment. Skin care is essential with moisturizing lotions and judicious use of topical steroid cream for short periods. Surgical consultation is requested to assess the need for removal of varices. Patient education to observe for infection, avoidance of trauma, and skin care are very important.

Ulceration is the disabling complication of stage III disease. The approach to management of stage III is to reduce venous pressure and edema, and provide ulcer care. Gradient compression stockings are important, as in the other stages, to decrease transmural venous pressure. Improvement in edema has been achieved by use of an external pneumatic compression boot (Fig. 40-20). The device is portable and easily applied. It is worn 2 to 4 hours per day. It will improve circulation, increase fibrinolysis, and reduce edema. Ulcers are cleaned with either peroxide, Dakin's solution or potassium permanganate once per day. Bio-occlusive dressings (Table 40-6) can be applied and changed every 2 to 7 days. These dressings promote formation of good granulation tissue and rapid healing compared to traditional methods.

Mechanical treatment with hydrotherapy at 100°F can be used instead of the above agents with ulcers greater than 3 cm to promote debridement. If the ulcer is larger than 3 cm and has not responded to the previous medical regimen, surgical assess-

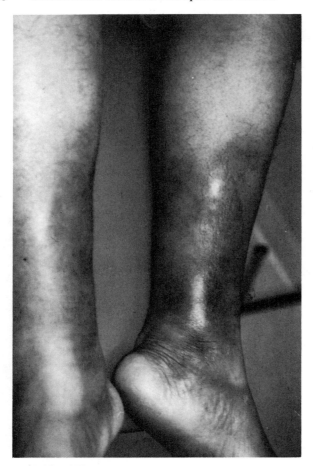

Figure 40-18.   PPS.

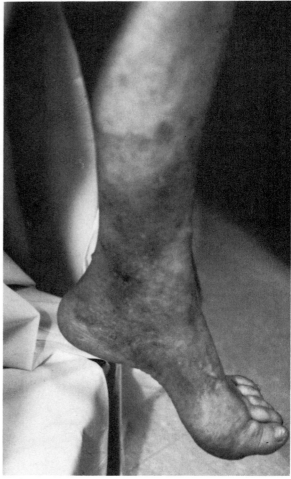

Figure 40-19.   PPS.

Figure 40-20.   External pneumatic compression boot.

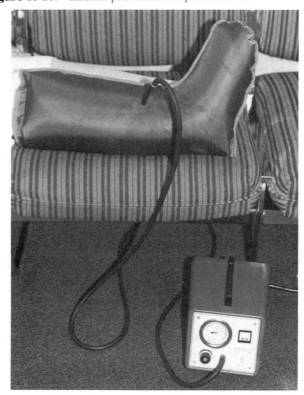

Table 40-5
Staged Treatment of Chronic Venous Disease

Stage I
1. Gradient elastic stockings
2. Skin care

Stage II
1. Gradient elastic stockings
2. Skin care
3. Topical steroids for dermatitis
4. Surgical consultation

Stage III
1. Gradient elastic stockings
2. Ulcer care
   a. Antiseptic solution
   b. Bio-occlusive dressings
3. External compression boots

Table 40-6
Bio-Occlusive Dressings

Polyurethane Films
Opsite
Tegaderm
Bio-occlusive

Polyethylene Oxide Hydrogel With Polyethylene Film Backing
Vigilon

Hydrocoloid Particles of Gelatin and Pectin in Hydrophobic Polymer
Duoderm

Unna Boot
Semi-rigid dressing containing calamine, zinc oxide, and gelatin

ment is recommended. Split-thickness skin grafting is used to close the ulcerated areas. Frequently, concomitant skin grafting and ligation of incompetent perforating veins is performed in an attempt to correct the pathophysiological problem of abnormal venous pressure.

REFERENCES

1. Albrechtsson V, Olsson CB: Thrombotic side effects of lower limb phlebography. Lancet 1:723, 1976
2. Allen EV: Lymphedema of the extremities: Classification, etiology, and differential diagnosis: A study of three hundred cases. Arch Intern Med 54:606–624, 1934
3. Alvin A, Diehl J, Lindsten J et al: Lymph vessels hypoplasia and chromosomal aberrations in 518 patients with Turner's syndrome. Acta Derm Venereol (Stockh) 47:25–33, 1967
4. Barner HB, Kaiser GC, William VL, Hanlon CR: Intermittent claudication with pedal pulses. JAMA 204:958–962, 1968
5. Bettman MA, Paulin S: Leg phlebography: The incidence, nature and modification of undesirable side effects. Radiology 122:101–104, 1977
6. Bloor K: Natural history of arteriosclerosis of the lower extremities. Ann R Coll Surg Engl 28:36–52, 1961
7. Boyd CE, Bird PJ, Teates CD et al: Pain free physical training in intermittent claudication. J Sports Med 24:112–122, 1984
8. Browse ML, Burnard KG: The Postphlebitic Syndrome: A New Look at Venous Problems. Chicago, Yearbook Medical Publishers, 1976
9. Browse NL, Clemenson G, Thomas ML: Is the postphlebitic leg always postphlebitic? Relation between phlebographic appearances of deep-vein thrombosis and late sequelae. Br Med J 281:1167–1170, 1980
10. Browse NL: Normal lymphographic appearances: Chest and thoracic duct. In Kinmonth JB (ed): The Lymphatics, p 59. London, Edward Arnold, 1982
11. Browse NL, Normal lymphographic appearances: Lower limb and pelvis. In Kinmonth JB (ed): The Lymphatics, p 19. London, Edward Arnold, 1982
12. Casley-Smith JR: The fine structure, properties and permeabilities of the lymphatic endothelium: How these determine the function of the lymphatic system. In Collete JM, Jantet G, Schoffeniels E (eds): New Trends in Basic Lymphology. Proceedings of the symposium of the Council of International Organic Medicine Sciences, p 19. Basel, Switzerland, Birdhaiiser Verlag, 1967
13. Casley-Smith JR: The functioning of the lymphatic system under normal and pathological conditions: Its dependence on the fine structure and permeabilities of the vessels. In Ruttimann A (ed): Progress in Lymphology. Proceedings of the International Symposium on Lymphology, pp 348–359. West Germany, Georg Thieme Verlag, 1967
14. Clark C, Cotton L: Blood flow in deep veins of the leg: Recording technique and evaluation of methods to increase flow during operations. Br J Surg 55:211–214, 1968
15. Clyne CAC, Ryan J, Webster JHH, Chant ADE: Oxygen tension on the skin of ischemic legs. Am J Surg 143:315–317, 1982
16. Cronenwett JL, Warner KG, Zelenock GB et al: Intermittent claudication. Current results of nonoperative management. Arch Surg 119:430–436, 1984
17. Dahllof AG, Holm J, Schersten T: Exercise training of patients with intermittent claudication. Scand J Rehabil Med (Suppl) 9:20–26, 1983
18. Dahllof AG, Holm J, Schersten T et al: Peripheral arterial insufficiency: Effect of physical training on walking tolerance, calf blood flow and blood flow resistance. Scand J Rehabil Med 8(1): 1976
19. DeWeese JA: Problems of acute deep venous thrombosis: The interpretation of signs and symptoms. Angiology 20:219–223, 1969
20. DeWeese JA: Venous and lymphatic disease. In Schwartz SI, Shires GT, Spenser FL, Storer EH (eds): Principles of Surgery, 3rd ed, pp 985–1010. New York, McGraw-Hill, 1979
21. Ekroth R, Dahllof AG, Gundevall B et al: Physical training of patients with intermittent claudication: Indications, methods and results. Surgery 84:640–643, 1978
22. Falls HF, Kertesz DE: A new syndrome combining pterygivim colli with developmental anomalies of the eyelids and lymphatics of the lower extremities. Trans Am Ophthalmol Soc 62:248–272, 1964
23. Franzeck UK, Talke P, Bernstein EF et al: Transcutaneous PO$_2$ measurements in health and peripheral arterial occlusive disease. Surgery 91:156–163, 1982
24. Friedmann LW: Selecting the therapeutic alternative for rehabilitating patients with occlusive arterial disease. Vasc Surg 11(5):321–332, 1977
25. Fuchs JA: Medical management of atherosclerosis. In Rutherford RB (ed): Vascular Surgery, 2nd ed, pp 313–327. Philadelphia, WB Saunders, 1984
26. Gemignani F, Pietrini V, Tagliavini T et al: Fabry's disease with familial lymphedema of the lower limbs: Case report and family study. Eur Neurol 18:84–90, 1979
27. Guggenheim W, Koch G, Adams AP et al: Femoral and popliteal occlusive vascular disease. A report on 143 diabetic patients. Diabetes 18:428–433, 1969
28. Honet JC, Strandness DE, Stolov WC, Simons BC: Short-leg bracing for intermittent claudication of the calf. Arch Phys Med Rehabil 49:578–585, 1968
29. Hughson WG, Mann JI, Garrod A: Intermittent claudication: Prevalence and risk factors. Br Med J 1:1379–1381, 1978
30. Hughson WG, Mann JI, Tibbs DJ et al: Intermittent claudication: Factors determining outcome. Br Med J 1:1377–1379, 1978
31. Hull R, Delmore T, Carter C et al: Adjusted subcutaneous heparin versus warfarin sodium in the long-term treatment of venous thrombosis. N Engl J Med 305:189–194, 1982
32. Hull R, Hirsh J, Sackett DL et al: Combined use of leg scanning and impedance plethysmography in suspected venous thrombosis: An alternative to venography. N Engl J Med 296:1497–1500, 1977
33. Hull R, Hirsh J, Sackett DL et al: Replacement of venography in suspected venous thrombosis by impedance plethysmography and I^{125} fibrinogen leg scanning. Ann Intern Med 94:12–15, 1981
34. Hutchison K, Oberle K, Crockford P et al: Effects of dietary manipulation on the vascular status of patients with peripheral vascular disease. JAMA 249:3326–3330, 1983
35. Janzon L, Bergentz SE, Ericsson BF, Lindell SE: The arm-ankle pressure gradient in relation to cardiovascular risk factors in intermittent claudication. Circulation 63:1339–1341, 1981
36. Johnson HD, Pflung J: The anatomy of the veins and lymphatics. In: The Swollen Leg: Causes and Treatment, p 29. Philadelphia, JB Lippincott, 1975
37. Jonason T, Jonzon B, Ringquist I, Oman-Rydberg A: Effect of physical training on different categories of patients with intermittent claudication. Acta Med Scand 206:253–258, 1979
38. Juergens JL, Barker NW, Hines EA Jr: Arteriosclerosis obliterans: Review of 520 cases with special reference to pathogenic and prognostic factors. Circulation 21:188–195, 1960
39. Jeurgens JL, Bernatz PE: Atherosclerosis of the extremities. In Juergens JL, Spittell; JA Jr, Fairbairn JF II (eds): Peripheral Vascular Diseases, 5th ed, pp 253–273. Philadelphia, WB Saunders, 1980
40. Kakkar VV: The diagnosis of deep vein thrombosis using I^{125} fibrinogen test. Arch Surg 1034:152–159, 1972

41. Kakkar VV, Lawrence D: Hemodynamic and clinical assessment after therapy for acute deep vein thrombosis. Am J Surg 150:54–63, 1985

42. Kempczinski RF, Bernhard VM: Management of chronic ischemia of the lower extremities. In Rutherford RB (ed): Vascular Surgery, 2nd ed, pp 547–557. Philadelphia, WB Saunders, 1984

43. Kinmonth JB, Taylor G, Tracy C, Marsh J: Primary lymphedema. Clinical and lymphographic studies of a series of 107 patients in which the lower limbs were affected. Br J Surg 45:1, 1957

44. Levine PH: An acute effect of cigarette smoking on platelet function: A possible link between smoking and arterial thrombosis. Circulation 48:619–623, 1973

45. Lippmann HI: Medical management of "trophic" ulcers in chronic arterial occlusive disease. Angiology 29:683–690, 1979

46. Maisels DO: Anonychia in association with lymphedema. Br J Plast Surg 19:37–42, 1966

47. Matsen FA, Wyss CR, Pedegana CR et al: Transcutaneous oxygen tension measurement in peripheral vascular disease. Surg Gynecol Obstet 150:525–528, 1980

48. McAllister FF: The fate of patients with intermittent claudication managed nonoperatively. Am J Surg 132:593–595, 1976

49. McLachlin J, Richards T, Paterson JC: An evaluation of clinical signs in the diagnosis of venous thrombosis. Arch Surg 85:738–744, 1962

50. Miller M, Matulsky AC: Noonan syndrome in an adult family presenting with chronic lymphedema. Am J Med 65:379–383, 1978

51. Nathan MPR, Pinsker R, Chase PH et al: Sarcoidosis presenting as lymphedema. Arch Dermatol 109:543–544, 1974

52. Nicolaides AN, Kakkar VV, Rennery JTG: Soleal sinuses and stasis. Br J Surg 57:307, 1970

53. O'Donnell TJ, Browse NL, Burnand DG et al: The socio-economic effects of iliofemoral venous thrombosis. J Surg Res 22:483–488, 1977

54. Olszewski WL, Engeset A: Intrinsic contractility of leg lymphatics in man. Lymphology 12:81, 1979

55. Owen J, Kvam D, Nossel HL et al: Thrombin and plasmin activity and platelet activation in the development of venous thrombosis. Blood 61:482–482, 1983

56. Porter JM: Ragnaud's syndrome and associated vasospastic conditions of the extremities. In Rutherford RB (ed): Vascular Surgery, 2nd ed, pp 697–707. Philadelphia, WB Saunders, 1984

57. Porter JM, Cutler BS, Lee BY et al: Pentoxyfylline efficacy in the treatment of intermittent claudication: Multicenter controlled double blind trial with objective assessment of chronic occlusive arterial disease patients. Am Heart J 104:66–72, 1982

58. Rabinow M, Johnson GF, Verhagen AD: Distichiasis-lymphedema: A hereditary syndrome of multiple congenital defects. Am J Dis Child 119:343–347, 1970

59. Ross, R: The pathogenesis of atherosclerosis—An update. N Engl J Med 314:488–500, 1986

60. Schaub R, Lynch P, Steward G: The response of canine veins to three types of abdominal surgery: A scanning and transmission electron microscopic study. Surgery 411–426, 1980

61. Schirger A, Peterson LF: Lymphedema. In Juergens JL, Spittell JA, Failbain JF (eds): Peripheral Vascular Diseases, 5th ed, p 524. Philadelphia, WB Saunders, 1980

62. Seifert J, Lob D, Staephasius E et al: Blood flow in muscles of paraplegic patients under various conditions measured by a double isotope technique. Paraplegia 10:185–191, 1972

63. Sevitt S: Pathology and pathogenesis of deep vein thrombi. In Bergan JJ, Yao JST (eds): Venous Problems, pp 257–269. Chicago, Year Book Medical Publishers, 1976

64. Seyfer A, Seaber A, Dombrose F et al: Coagulation changes in elective surgery and trauma. Ann Surg 193:210–213, 1981

65. Sidgelman SS, Heckman BH, Hasson J: Lymphedema, pleural effusions, and yellow nails: Associated immunologic deficiency. Dis Chest 56:114–117, 1969

66. Silbert S, Zazecla H: Prognosis in arteriosclerotic peripheral vascular disease. JAMA 166:1816, 1958

67. Silver HM, Tsongaris NT, Eaton OM: Lymphedema and lymphography in sarcoidosis. Arch Intern Med 117:712–714, 1966

68. Smith RD, Spittell JA, Schirger A: Secondary lymphedema of the leg: Its characteristics and diagnostic implications. JAMA 185:80–82, 1963

69. Sorlie D, Myhre K: Lower leg blood flow in intermittent claudication. Scand J Clin Lab Invest 38:171–179, 1978

70. Sorlie D, Myhre K, Mjos OD: Exercise and post-exercise metabolism of the lower leg in patients with peripheral arterial insufficiency. Scand J Clin Lab Invest 38:635–642, 1978

71. Sorlie D, Myhre K, Saugstad OD, Giercksky KE: Release of hypoxanthine and phosphate from exercising human legs with and without arterial insufficiency. Acta Med Scand 211:281–286, 1982

72. Steward G, Schaub R, Niewiarowski S: Products of tissue injury: Their induction of venous exothelial damage and blood cell adhesion in the dog. Arch Pathol Lab Med 104:409–413, 1980

73. Strandness DE: Diagnostic considerations in occlusive arterial disease. Vascular Surgery 11:271–277, 1977

74. Strandness DE, Stahler C: Arteriosclerosis obliterans: Manner and rate of progression. JAMA 196:1–4, 1966

75. Strandness DE, Sumner DS: Ultrasonic velocity detector in the diagnosis of thrombophlebitis. Arch Surg 104:180–183, 1972

76. Strong JP, Richards ML: Cigarette smoking and atherosclerosis in autopsied men. Atherosclerosis 23:451–476, 1973

77. Sumner DS: Hemodynamics and pathophysiology of venous disease. In Rutherford RB (ed): Vascular Surgery, 2nd ed, pp 148–166. Philadelphia, WB Saunders, 1984

78. Sumner DS: Applied physiology in venous problems. In Bergan JJ, Yao JST (eds): Surgery of the Veins, pp 3–23. New York, Harcourt Brace Jovanovich, 1985

79. Svejcar J, Prerovsky I, Linhart J, Kruml J: Biochemical differences in the composition of primary varicose veins. Am Heart J 67:572–574, 1964

80. Turner GR, Gosney WG, Ellingson W, Gaspar M: Popliteal artery entrapment syndrome. JAMA 208:692–693, 1969

81. Wesbey GE, Higgins CB, Amparo EG et al: Peripheral vascular disease: Correlation of MR imaging and angiography. Radiology 156:733–739, 1985

82. White RA, Nolan L, Harley D et al: Noninvasive evaluation of peripheral vascular disease using transcutaneous oxygen tension. Am J Surg 144:68–74, 1982

83. Wilson SE, Schwartz I, Williams RA, Owens ML: Occlusion of the superficial femoral artery. What happens without operation. Am J Surg 140:112–116, 1980

84. Zetterquist S: The effect of active training on the nutritive blood flow in exercising ischemic legs. Scand J Clin Lab Invest 25:101–111, 1970

41

Rehabilitation of the Patient With Diseases Affecting the Motor Unit

Robert G. Taylor

James S. Lieberman

The initial phase in the management of any disorder is a complete evaluation to establish the best diagnosis and permit prognosis for progression or improvement of the existing disorder. This statement is never more true than for the disorders of the motor unit, in which the course of the disease can vary from static and nonprogressive to rapidly progressive toward disability, or even to death. In addition, many of these disorders are hereditary, so proper management may also require genetic counseling.

There are many excellent books reviewing the subject of neuromuscular disorders, ranging from the clinically oriented by Brooke[7] to the encyclopedic review of muscle function and disorders edited by Engel and Banker.[16] In addition, there are books reviewing the techniques for muscle biopsy, processing of the tissue, and interpretation of the results[14, 51] and books on the treatment of these disorders.[16, 30] As a result we will not attempt to cover all details of each disorder but merely highlight generalities that we feel can be of assistance to the clinician who must evaluate, diagnose, or treat a patient suspected to have one of these disorders.

Motor unit disorders may involve the anterior horn cell, its axons, the neuromuscular junction, or innervated muscle fibers. In the absence of a positive family history, which would prompt early evaluation, the presenting symptom is almost always weakness or abnormal fatigue[18] or, in the case of the metabolic disorders, exercise intolerance (fatigue) and muscle cramps or pain.[7] There is no sensory abnormality in patients with disorders of the motor unit, and their central nervous system function remains normal.

PLAN OF TREATMENT

Our emphasis will be directed toward the treatment, rather than diagnosis, of patients with various neuromuscular disorders. Since the treatment plan should be based on prevention or minimization of complications, we will discuss the disorders in groups. The hereditary disorders are easily grouped because the prognosis for many of these disorders is somewhat predictable. The acquired disorders, amyotrophic lateral sclerosis (ALS) and the inflammatory myopathies, must be discussed separately because of their more variable course and the probability for therapeutic intervention in the very near future.[7] Even though they are hereditary, it is necessary to also discuss the metabolic disorders of muscle function as a separate group, because the presenting symptoms and prognosis are quite different from the other neuromuscular disorders. We will not attempt to discuss the neuromuscular disorders acquired secondary to trauma to nerves, muscles, or their vascular supply, because the etiology for these is usually relatively obvious and treatment is relatively specific and frequently of an emergency nature.

The motor unit diseases, regardless of their etiology, are usually managed by similar rehabilitation techniques. However, the treatment plan will vary significantly depending on the particular features and prognosis of the condition being treated. The initial phase of rehabilitation management is a complete evaluation of the patient, adequate to permit a specific diagnosis and classification of the disorder. This is essential, since the appropriate rehabilitation program must include a prognosis for the patient's disorder as a part of the basic consideration. The treatment program chosen for a patient must be based upon the current residual function, plus the anticipated disease course, which is based on the natural history of progression for the patient's particular disease. A useful classification system for planning treatment places these disorders into groups based on the expected rate of progression (Table 41-1).

Generalizations are also possible for the management of patients with these disorders. All patients must receive general primary medical care appropriate for their age and associated medical conditions (e.g., dental care, vaccinations, routine pediatric evaluation).[18, 28] The general goals for treatment of patients with these disorders are

- Early diagnosis and establishment of a rehabilitation plan, which must consider the anticipated rate of progression of the disorder
- Maintenance of independence in activities of daily living (ADL) and ambulation for as long as possible
- Anticipation and prevention of complications
- Counseling of patient and family regarding the anticipated progress of their disorder, including genetic counseling in the case of the hereditary disorders
- Assistance to the patient in leading as normal a life as possible, within the limits of functional abilities

Table 41-1
Motor Unit Disorders Classification According to Usual Rate of Progression

Rapidly Progressive Disorders
   Duchenne muscular dystrophy
   Werdnig-Hoffmann disease
   Amyotrophic lateral sclerosis

Slowly Progressive Disorders
   Limb girdle muscular dystrophy
   Facioscapulohumeral muscular dystrophy
   Myotonic muscular dystrophy
   Familial proximal spinal muscular atrophy
   Becker muscular dystrophy
   Charcot-Marie-Tooth disease

Static Disorders
   Congenital myopathies
   Poliomyelitis (late loss of function may occur)

Table 41-2
Motor Unit Disorders Classification According to Functional Ability

Stage	Function
Early	Patient still ambulatory
Middle	Wheelchair ambulation
Late	Patient is dependent for almost all activities

It should be rather obvious that the specific modes of management used will vary because of the rate of progression of the patient's particular disorder, and the management methods will also vary with the stage of the disorder for that patient[28]:

Early, still ambulatory
Middle, wheelchair ambulatory
Late, fully dependent

The goals will be discussed in more detail in the section on management. It must be remembered that these disorders add severe personal, emotional, and economic impact on the patients and their families, in addition to physical impairment.

PATIENT EVALUATION

The major findings contributing to disability in any patient with a motor unit disease are weakness and contracture. The pattern of weakness is quite variable; however, neuropathic disorders usually show distal more than proximal involvement. The opposite is true for myopathic disorders. The exceptions are patients with myotonic muscular dystrophy, in whom the weakness is greater distally than proximally, and patients with proximal spinal muscular atrophy, in whom proximal weakness predominates. Contractures are more common in the myopathic than in the neuropathic disorders, and the most severe contractures are seen in the patients with Duchenne muscular dystrophy (DMD). Significant contractures are more common in the muscles that cross two joints. In evaluating the patient it is most important to determine the stage of the disease that the patient appears to be in at that time. A very convenient classification of the stages of these diseases is based on the patient's functional ability at the time of evaluation (Table 41-2).[28]

Complicated protocols for patient evaluation are necessary in order to compare progression of a disorder between different patients or between clinics,[8, 9] and to determine if a therapeutic intervention is capable of significantly altering the natural progression of a disorder. However, detailed evaluations of this type are not required in order to develop a treatment plan for a particular patient.[33] Patients must be evaluated, based on symptoms, to rule out other diseases that can worsen the natural progression of their neuromuscular disorder.

Patient History

The history is the most important element in the evaluation of a patient suspected of having a neuromuscular disorder. The significant elements are the age of onset and rate of progression of the disorder. An acute onset with rapid and major loss of function would suggest postinfectious polyneuropathy or a toxic problem rather than one of the herditary disorders. The distribution of the weakness is also a very significant clue. The patient with distal weakness will have difficulty grasping or holding an object, while the patient with proximal weakness will experience difficulty lifting an object as if to place it on a shelf. The patient with myotonic muscular dystrophy will have difficulty releasing an object once it has been grasped, but the patient may not be aware that this is abnormal, since it has been present since the patient's earliest recollection. If the patient requires assistance from the upper extremities to rise from a chair or to ascend stairs, this suggests weakness of the hip and knee extensor muscle groups. Muscle pain and tenderness are uncommon complaints for patients with the hereditary neuromuscular disorders; however, these are relatively common complaints for patients with the acquired disorders of muscle function, particularly Guillain-Barré syndrome and the inflammatory myopathies.

The history must also include an assessment of the patient's social environment, including availability of support or assistance from family or friends, which is perhaps the most important factor in determining whether or not the patient will be able to remain at home or will require an institutional living environment to provide for his or her needs. Assessing the patient's living environment is also important in helping to determine the assistive devices he or she will need. It is important to determine the activities the patient enjoys and is accustomed to, since assistive devices may be needed or modified to allow the patient to successfully continue the desired activities.

Physical Examination

The physical observation of the patient will allow estimation of areas of significant atrophy, or abnormal hypertrophy of individual muscles or of muscle groups. It also allows an estimate of whether the involvement is greater in the proximal or distal muscle groups. The physical examination permits evaluation of the residual muscle strength, from which an estimate can be made as to the activities the patient may be capable of continuing and the assistive devices that may be necessary. The extremities are inspected for evidence of edema or abnormal tenderness that could suggest an inflammatory response in the underlying muscles.

The major joints must be examined for passive range of motion in order to identify contractures that may be present. Contractures are soft tissue ankylosis occurring at a joint limiting the range of motion for that joint. In patients with contractures, it is important that passive motion be used, because their weakness limits a full range of active motion. Mild flexion contractures at the elbows may not present a handicap, but flexion contractures at the hips and knees can preclude ambulation in the patient with weak hip and knee extensor muscles.[27, 50] Toe-walking in a boy with DMD can occur as a mechanism to compensate for the weak knee extensor muscles long before actual contracture occurs. The back must be examined for evidence of scoliosis.

Laboratory Studies

The laboratory test most useful in monitoring the progress or level of activity for the muscle diseases is the serum creatine kinase (CK). In the rapidly progressive disorders the CK will be markedly elevated. However, these elevations will decrease as the patient's level of physical activity decreases and as the total muscle mass is decreased by the disease.[8, 26] The CK levels can also be of assistance in attempting to identify whether the mother and sisters of patients with Duchenne muscular dystrophy are carriers for that disorder.[16, 26]

Electrodiagnostic testing is a very important part of the evaluation of a patient suspected to have a neuromuscular disorder. The nerve conduction studies can confirm the presence or absence of a peripheral neuropathy. The electromyogram (EMG) can confirm whether the disorder is neuropathic or myopathic. An additional very important role for the EMG is to help identify the muscle most appropriate for muscle biopsy. Since trauma to the muscle from the EMG needle can produce histological changes in the muscle that make interpretation difficult, we recommend that the EMG be limited to one side of the body. Since these disorders are usually symmetrical, an appropriate muscle from the other side of the body can then be recommended for the biopsy.

The best muscle for biopsy will depend on the experience of your team. For diagnostic biopsy we do not feel the "needle" biopsy is adequate. In our experience the muscles most available for open biopsy are the quadriceps (we usually try to use the vastus lateralis) or in the upper extremity we prefer the deltoid or biceps. The EMG will help to identify a muscle that is definitely involved, but not so severely involved that it represents only end-stage disease and would not be of assistance for diagnosis. The muscle biopsy, like the EMG, can help to confirm whether the muscle is normal or abnormal. If the muscle biopsy is abnormal it can usually be classified as myopathic or neuropathic in origin. Perhaps the most significant finding available from the muscle biopsy is whether or not it is an inflammatory myopathy, as those disorders are treatable.

Laboratory evaluation may assume a much more important role in the future when the gene responsible for these disorders has been identified.[32] Gene probes can be developed that will permit identification of those persons who are carriers of these disorders, in particular, the carriers of the sex-linked disorders in which the carrier female is asymptomatic.[49]

The new genetic techniques also have the potential to assist in identification of suspected carriers of other disorders, such as Charcot-Marie-Tooth disease, myotonic muscular dystrophy (MMD), spinal muscular atrophy, and the other sex-linked muscle diseases including Becker muscular dystrophy.[49]

PATIENT MANAGEMENT

Role of the Physician

It is very common for the physician faced with care of a patient with a diagnosis of one of the known neuromuscular disorders to assume that the prognosis for the patient is one of progressive loss of function, which can be rapid or slow, leading to an early death for the patient. This is a very negative approach and should not be tolerated, as the ability of most of these patients to function within their family or social environment can usually be improved to a significant degree after evaluation by a concerned and knowledgeable rehabilitation team. The rehabilitation team must include the patient and his or her caretakers, or others involved in the patient's social support system, as well as the usual team of physicians, nurses, and therapists. A major determinant as to what can be done to improve the patient's quality of life-style will be determined by what economic and personal support is available to the patient. A skilled medical social worker is an invaluable part of the team at this point to evaluate this aspect of the patient's support system. The support system will frequently be the major factor determining whether it is possible for the patient to continue to live independently, remain in the family home with parents or spouse or significant other providing the care required, or will require institutional care. All efforts should be made to permit the patient to remain at the most independent level possible.

A physician who assumes that the only role in care of these patients is anticipation and prevention, or minimization, of complications that are common for these disorders has ignored the major responsibility, which is to help assist them in maintaining the maximum independence possible for as long as possible. For patients with a rapidly progressive disorder, independence is lost early. However, attention and direction toward activities at which they can be productive or successful can significantly improve their quality of life. Obviously, the efforts required to assist in development of this type of plan requires innovation and are rarely covered in the usual medical school curriculum.

Koch, Arego, and Bowser[29] have reviewed the appropriateness and cost effectiveness of out-patient care for the patients with the various neuromuscular disorders covered by the Muscular Dystrophy Association, and concluded that it is best to attempt to try to keep these patients in the out-patient setting. The out-patient setting permits these patients to try to maintain the maximal control over their environmental situation, and allows them to continue to explore areas of interest within their capabilities.

Duchenne Muscular Dystrophy

The patient with DMD, an X-linked hereditary disorder, has weakness which is rapidly progressive. He will develop contractures and will display all three stages of progression. This disorder is the most severe of the muscular dystrophies and the patient is vulnerable to all of the expected complications. As a result we will use the patient with DMD as our example to discuss management for these disorders.

Early Stage (Patient still ambulatory)

The major efforts for this patient in the early stage is to confirm that his muscle weakness and inability to keep up with his peers is due to DMD. This requires a detailed history and physical examination.

A careful family history must be made to identify involved male siblings and male children of any of the mother's female relatives to suggest or confirm genetic transmission by the X-linked recessive pattern. The patient's mother and all sisters must be evaluated for possible carrier status. Failure to warn a woman of the fact that she is a definite or probable carrier can lead to medicolegal action. At the present time it is not possible to prove that a woman is not at risk to be a carrier, so caution must be exercised. However, now that the gene responsible for DMD has been identified,[32] and a deficient protein has been identified,[52] there is optimism that definite identification of carrier and noncarrier status for women could be available within a few years. Genetic counseling is usually not necessary for patients, since they are not usually capable of reproduction. However, sexual counseling for these boys in early adolescence can frequently help avoid, or at least reduce, emotional problems they might develop regarding the subject of sex and their limited social exposure.

The boy with DMD is still in the pediatric age group during this stage and must receive routine prospective care, including the medical care given to all individuals: routine immunizations, dental care, and so on.[28] This patient probably requires slightly more than routine medical care because extra effort is needed to prevent or minimize the effects of routine childhood illnesses, which can be more severe because of his weakened state. An attempt must be made to maximize his self-care capabilities and independence in his ADL for as long as possible, because it will help to delay the burden for others to provide care when he loses those abilities. Prevention of contractures is primarily a role of supervision until the later portion of this stage when the patient's strength further declines, and the effort required to maintain his independence begins to exceed his capability.

At this stage the patient's muscles are becoming so weak that they are no longer able to develop the force necessary to prevent the contractures from developing. The usual progression of the loss of strength for boys with DMD is for the proximal muscles, about the hips and shoulders, to become weaker at a much more rapid rate than the more distal muscles. In the upper extremities, flexion contractures are much more common than contractures in extension, except following injury. Contractures in extension at the elbow and wrist, even though rare, must be avoided at all cost as they can prevent the hand from being brought toward the midline to assist in ADL. Indeed mild flexion contractures may functionally benefit active elbow flexion by improving the mechanical advantage through the lever mechanism, which can reduce the effort required to initiate flexion.

In this early stage weakness and inability to run, jump, and keep up with one's peers are the main complaints given by the patient or his parents. Assistive devices to enable the patient to run or jump are not available. The question, then, is what can be done to improve the patient's strength? The usual approach for weak muscles is strengthening exercises. However, there are the questions of how much exercise is appropriate and whether exercise above a certain level will do harm to the patient's muscles.[19, 21, 24, 26, 50] For the present it is recommended that exercise training programs for patients with motor unit diseases should be started early in the course of the disease when muscle fiber degeneration and weakness are minimal, and should emphasize submaximal exercise levels.[12, 19] An active exercise program should be properly supervised in order to reduce the possibility of overwork injury to the muscles with resultant reduction in muscle function.[50] If at all possible, an exercise program should be developed to include activities that the patient enjoys, since this will maintain his interest and willingness to participate. The program should include activities that have potential for him to master, since this will facilitate his ability to continue these activities in his later and more dependent years. Any exercise program, to be considered, must not make excessive demands on the patient's family, either in terms of transportation time or participation, because this will reduce time available for the patient at school, care of the patient at home, and for family interaction. Gardner-Medwin[20] has stated that therapy efforts aimed solely at ambulation as the only goal even if achieved will soon be lost.

In the later portion of this stage the patient will show a progressive reduction in most activities. Most of this is a result of his reduced physical capacity; however, fear of falling also becomes a major factor in reducing the patient's mobility. Early evidence of this is the patient's decision to walk around the periphery of the room, using the walls or furniture for support, in preference to taking the shorter route across the room.

Major, and functionally limiting, joint contractures do not start to develop until the later part of the early stage of DMD. It is important to maintain ambulation as long as is reasonably practical, since contractures develop rapidly once ambulation ceases. There is no question that the most effective mechanism for prevention of contractures in the lower extremities is ambulation, or maintenance of the standing position, in which the patient's body weight exerts a significant stretching force on the flexor muscles at the hips, knees, and the plantar flexor muscle group at the ankles. When contractures do start to occur, local heat can assist in stretching them; it will not, however, improve the contractile ability of the muscles.[18, 24] Fowler[18] pointed out that crutch assistance for ambulation for these patients is rarely of benefit because of the significant weakness of their shoulder stabilizing muscles. Toe-walking while these patients are still ambulatory will occur long before ankle plantar flexion contractures occur. Most of these boys will toe-walk in the late period of their ambulatory phase in order to maintain stability in extension at the knee. Toe-walking is a compensatory maneuver that permits the patient to continue ambulation. Surgical release of the heel cords at this point will usually result in the patient becoming unable to ambulate.[20, 21]

Minor loss of function, such as loss of active or passive supination of the forearm, is frequently missed or ignored during this stage. Only careful attention by the patient's family to passive range of motion of the significant joints can retard the onset or progression of contractures that will limit the patient's ability to assist in self-care. The major element for prevention of these contractures is activity plus passive range of motion by the family. The frequency of exercises required exceeds what can be provided by a therapist, since the exercises must be performed at least daily.

The question of orthoses for these patients has received almost as much discussion as exercise.[20, 27, 41, 42, 45, 46, 50] Static orthoses for prevention of contractures have a place, but they are poorly tolerated and rarely effective for prevention of ankle plantar flexion contractures. The main question regarding orthoses for these boys is whether knee-ankle-foot orthoses for the lower extremities in combination with surgical release of the ankle plantar flexion contractures and the iliotibial band produces functional ambulation that is better than wheelchair mobility. Gardner-Medwin[20, 21] states that "the boys seem to take to wheelchairs with relief, and indeed with enthusiasm" in preference to the time and effort involved in attempts at continued ambulation.

Most physicians will feel significant pressure, more from the patient's parents than from the patient, to "do something" to help the poor child. The compulsion to do something rather than be objective frequently can result in a "doing something, even if it is wrong" approach by the physician. Swash[46] states that the benefits of intervention frequently do not outweigh the disability and discomfort caused by the intervention. He concluded that many programs have been advocated for patients with muscular dystrophy and eventually all have been found to be ineffective after careful evaluation.

Scoliosis is usually not a significant problem while the patient is still ambulatory. However, if it starts in this early phase, it will probably progress at a fairly rapid rate as further mobility is lost.

Middle Stage (Wheelchair mobility)

Selection of a wheelchair appropriate for the patient's abilities is a very important element at this stage. It is tempting to prescribe a motorized wheelchair as the patient's initial chair, knowing that the patient will soon require one for mobility. However, a significant amount of maturity (judgment and responsibility) on the patient's part must be demonstrated to avoid the use of this device as a hazard or weapon. Although motorized wheelchairs have provided a significant degree of independence for the nonambulatory patient, there has been a report of death due to hypothermia when a patient was forced to remain out of doors overnight in cold weather because of failure of his motorized wheelchair.[23] The objective to be remembered in selecting the proper wheelchair is that it should be his passport to mobility, not a prison to which he is confined.[21]

It is very important to maintain the patient's maximum ability for self-care for as long as possible throughout this stage in order to try to minimize his feeling of total dependence. Efforts should include continuation of activities introduced in the early stage that the patient continues to be proficient at, such as hobbies and particularly vocational skills that can be a later source of income. The patient needs to believe that he can be a productive member of society.

Contractures can develop at a very rapid rate after the patient becomes wheelchair-bound, and scoliosis may also become a major problem. At present, the most effective method to prevent the development or retard the rate of progression of scoliosis is the use of the custom-made plastic body jacket.[21] In order to be effective, the body jacket must be started while the spinal curvature is still minimal. These jackets are only capable of stopping, or retarding, progression of the scoliosis, and they are *not* capable of reversing a curve that is already present. For some patients the combination of maximum lordosis and an increased pelvic tilt is capable of producing the respiratory compromise and discomfort similar to that commonly seen with scoliosis. For either problem it may become necessary to consider surgical stabilization of the spine, in hope of improving pulmonary function and reducing discomfort. Rideau and colleagues[37] suggest that monitoring the vital capacity can be an important indicator for the need and timing of surgical intervention for scoliosis.

Respiratory therapy for instruction in exercises to facilitate ventilation and clearing of secretions (progressive problems as dependency increases in this stage) can be very important. Humidifiers can help decrease viscosity of secretions. There are devices and training techniques that can help the patient to learn the deep voluntary inspiration that is of major assistance in reducing the incidence of atelectasis, which can progress to a much more serious complication, pneumonia. In the later portion of this stage postural drainage and chest percussion techniques should be learned by all caretakers, in addition to techniques for use of suction devices to assist in clearing secretions from the oropharynx.

Additional assistive devices and equipment are available: (1) special mattresses or pads to reduce pressure on bony prominences and assist in prevention of pressure sores; (2) a hospital bed, which can significantly assist in positioning the patient for comfort, as well as in preparation for transfer to or from a wheelchair; (3) raised toilet seats are a necessity now if not already obtained during the earlier stage; (4) grab bars for the toilet (a necessity); (5) a hand-held shower head and bathtub seat and grab bars; (6) a hydraulic or similar lift to assist the caretakers in getting the patient from the wheelchair to the tub seat and back; and (7) clothing adaptations to assist in patient dressing and undressing.

Late Stage (Totally dependent patient)

In this stage the major efforts are not toward traditional rehabilitation, as the patient's function will not improve, but maintenance of any activities that the patient is still capable of doing, in addition to general nursing care and prevention or minimization of the medical (nonmusculoskeletal) problems that can or will occur. The major problems are usually respiratory or later cardiac problems. Urinary tract problems are much less common for the patient with neuromuscular disorders than for the spinal cord injured patient.

Joint range of motion for gentle stretching to reduce the rate of progression of contractures is still indicated, since maintenance of passive range of motion at the hips can significantly facilitate nursing care. Again these exercises or routines, must be performed by the caretakers because the frequency required is greater than a physical therapist can provide.

Other than the extreme work load for nursing care placed on the patient's family or other caretakers, the major problems relate to pulmonary and cardiac complications. The major cause of death for DMD patients is respiratory failure, and an important factor in maintaining adequate respiratory function is preventing or minimizing the progression of scoliosis. Labored respirations, nightmares, and altered sleep patterns can be early evidence of impending respiratory failure. Sleep disturbances are considered by most physicians to result from hypoventilation in the DMD patient. Redding and co-workers[36] reported that sleep disturbances can occur in these boys in the absence of objective evidence of hypoventilation.

Advocates of mechanical ventilation for DMD patients when they become minimally able to maintain adequate function on their own claim that ventilation significantly extends meaningful life: Alexander and group, 2 to 7.5 years, average 3.4[1]; Bach, O'Brien, Krotenberg, and Alba, 10 months to 22 years, average 8.4 years.[3] Despite these claims, the use of mechanical ventilation in these patients is not uniformly accepted. Colbert and Schock[10] surveyed Muscular Dystrophy Association clinics regarding their use of respirators. Only 44% of the responding clinics indicated that respirators were used routinely and that was for patients with DMD and ALS. As more patients and their families become aware that mechanically assisted ventilation can assist in prolonging life, they also should be made aware that such an option exists long before an emergency situation arises. We are aware of two patients who experienced no obvious respiratory problems at their accustomed altitudes of 100 to 200 feet above sea level, but who died of acute respiratory decompensation when taken to altitudes of about 6000 feet on weekend outings with their families.

Often the patient and his family are afraid of the tracheostomy usually required for assisted ventilation. An alternative method is mouth intermittent positive pressure ventilation as described by Bach, O'Brien, Krotenberg, and Alba.[3] They suggest that the patients will accept this method for assisted ventilation more readily than tracheostomies, and they report significant prolongation of "useful life." However, the question of appropriateness of mechanically assisted ventilation for the patient with a progressive disorder is controversial in terms of ethics as well as cost. We recommend that the physician and, if possible, the patient and his or her family consult the local ethics committee for assistance in making a decision on whether or not to institute assisted ventilation. It is imperative that all parties be aware of the responsibilities and effort required and be willing to accept them.

Periodic electrocardiograms (ECG) should be performed on patients with DMD. It is not possible to rely on clinical symptoms alone, because the patients' very low levels of physical activity prevent them from displaying the usual symptoms of shortness of breath or angina customarily used in classifying the severity or progression of heart disease. In clinical practice these patients can abruptly progress from class I to class IV heart disease and do not demonstrate the warning signs provided in classes II and III. Any evidence of congestive heart failure should prompt treatment by traditional measures.

We have omitted discussion of the question of mental *versus* social retardation in these boys, since this is a question that is still under active evaluation. It must be remembered that many of the older articles on this subject have stated that at least one-third of the patients with DMD are mentally retarded.

Other Disorders

Treatment plans for patients with the more slowly progressive disorders or the static disorders are the same as those described for DMD patients at similar levels of functional loss. However, these other disorders may permit more plan modifications to allow for significantly greater social and vocational involvement.

Werdnig-Hoffmann Disease

Even though it is a rapidly progressive disorder, infantile spinal muscular atrophy (Werdnig-Hoffmann disease) is not treated in a manner similar to DMD for two reasons: the onset is usually at or shortly after birth, and this disorder is usually rapidly progressive to death by age 2. Because of this rapid progression in an infant it is rare that the child with this form of the disorder will require traditional rehabilitation measures. In the more slowly progressive form of this disease, the child may reach adolescence or even adulthood. For these older patients the rehabilitation measures are similar to those described for DMD at a similar functional level.

Myotonic Muscular Dystrophy

MMD differs from the other muscular dystrophies because the weakness is distal more than proximal. It is a multisystem disorder characterized by frontal balding, cataracts, and testicular atrophy, in addition to the muscle disorder. The frontal balding and wasting of the facial muscles give these patients a very characteristic appearance, sometimes described as "hatchet faced." MMD is one of the most common of the neuromuscular disorders with an estimated incidence of 13 per 100,000 live births and a prevalence estimated at between 3 and 5 per 100,000 population.[7] This disorder is transmitted as an autosomal dominant trait, and since most patients are capable of reproduction, it will eventually become the most common of these disorders. The most characteristic feature of DMD is myotonia, with stiffness and difficulty releasing objects that have been grasped. However, since this has been present since the patient's first memory it is rare for the myotonia to be the presenting complaint. The presenting complaint is usually weakness in the hands. The impaired relaxation of the muscles can be improved significantly with membrane-stabilizing drugs such as phenytoin, carbamazepine, or procainamide. However, the decision whether or not to use one of these compounds must follow a careful evaluation and discussion with the patient to determine whether the major problem is the impaired relaxation or the weakness. If the weakness is the major problem, the patient's symptoms can be made worse by use of these drugs, since the myotonia can actually increase the patients' ability to grasp and hold an object.

MMD patients commonly have myocardial conduction defects, and frequent ECG studies are indicated to monitor the degree of the heart block and to watch for dysrhythmias. The clinical laboratory is of little assistance in monitoring these patients as the CK is usually normal. The EMG is very helpful in identifying these patients because the motor unit action potentials will be the low-amplitude, brief-duration potentials seen in most muscle diseases, but with distal involvement greater than proximal. The very characteristic waxing and waning myotonic high frequency discharges are also present.

These patients can have problems during general anesthesia. When the neuromuscular junction–depolarizing muscle relaxants are used they can cause increased and sustained muscle contraction rather than the expected muscle relaxation.

The MMD patient has little need for the usual rehabilitation therapies, since contractures are rare. Exercises are usually not indicated because the problem is one of muscle overactivity, but most patients will require orthoses for their foot drop, and some will require orthoses for wrist weakness. Most patients will sooner or later require a properly fitting wheelchair.

THE ACQUIRED DISORDERS

Amyotrophic Lateral Sclerosis

The motor neuron disease ALS results from degeneration of motor nerves throughout the nervous system and involves the upper as well as the lower motor neurons. When involvement of the lower motor neurons predominates, flaccid weakness of the involved muscles occurs and the muscles will atrophy rather rapidly. When upper motor neuron involvement predominates, spasticity will occur. Fasciculations are a common feature of this disorder, although they are not unique to ALS.

ALS affects males considerably more frequently than females and the onset is commonly during their most productive years (over age 40). The etiology is unknown and, in spite of many claims for treatment, there are no cures or effective treatments or procedures available to arrest the progression of this disorder.[7] As a result, for the present, treatment must be aimed at rehabilitation measures to maximize the patient's independence in self-care and techniques to reduce or minimize the burden of their care on others.[13]

The clinical laboratory is of little or no assistance in confirming the diagnosis of ALS, since the serum enzyme levels are usually normal and there are no specific diagnostic tests. Histological examination of muscle biopsy specimens can confirm that partial denervation and perhaps some reinnervation has occurred, but cannot provide any evidence of the upper motor neuron problems that are a major factor in this disorder. The EMG will show evidence of denervation and partial reinnervation in a very widespread pattern that could not be a result of peripheral nerve involvement or a segmental lesion.

Sensation is usually not impaired and the intellect does not deteriorate the way the muscles do, so the psychological impact of this disorder on the patient is severe. Because of this the patient is forced to observe his or her own progressive deterioration and increasing dependence while still able to understand that the situation can only become worse. Brooke[7] comments that these patients will usually become wheelchair-dependent within 12 to 18 months, and progress from this level to bedbound and unable to move over a relatively short period of time. Death is usually due to respiratory failure. Bowel and bladder functions are rarely involved, but bulbar involvement of speech or swallowing present major problems.

Since cure is not possible, the traditional rehabilitation approaches of maximizing the patient's residual capacity for self-care, or methods to reduce dependency on others for care, are the main efforts.[13] In the early stage exercises to improve muscle function can help, but the question of possible overwork injury to the muscles is always present. When weakness becomes prominent, instruction in energy conservation and work simplification are appropriate. Occupational therapists can be of considerable assistance in this area. Assistive devices to aid ambulation are necessary, but as the weakness progresses a prescription for an appropriate wheelchair is necessary. The decision as to whether the wheelchair should be manual or powered will depend on the activities the patient must do, and the rate of progression of his or her disease.

The major problems in the later stage are the bulbar involvement with associated loss of speech, difficulty swallowing, and respiratory failure. Loss of speech requires the skills of a speech pathologist to assist in developing a mechanism for communication. Problems with swallowing will commonly require feeding measures such as nasogastric feeding tubes or even a gastrostomy. It must be remembered that patients with feeding problems of this type must be in the near-erect position during feeding to help minimize gastroesophageal reflux and aspiration. Aspiration can become such a significant problem that tracheostomy and even laryngeal closure may be necessary to prevent or at least minimize the resulting respiratory complications.[7] Respiratory problems should be anticipated and the patient should be started fairly early on programs to assist in maintenance of self-ventilation, such as incentive spirometers.[13] Most patients will require assisted ventilation prior to their demise because of respiratory failure. In regard to the decision of when assisted respiration should be started, the physician is urged to inform the patient and caretakers long before the problem arises. When in doubt, a local bioethics group should be consulted.

The Inflammatory Myopathies

The inflammatory myopathies are probably one of the most important of the muscle disorders to accurately diagnose because they are treatable. The etiology of these disorders is unknown, but they are assumed to be autoimmune in origin.[6, 7] Even though they are quite rare, the outcome can be devastating, or even fatal, if untreated. This group of diseases is usually classified into five groups:

1. Primary idiopathic polymyositis
2. Primary idiopathic dermatomyositis
3. Dermatomyositis or polymyositis associated with neoplasia
4. Childhood dermatomyositis or polymyositis associated with vasculitis
5. Polymyositis or dermatomyositis associated with other collagen vascular diseases.[6]

The clinical symptoms are symmetrical weakness, involvement of proximal more than distal, slowly progressive disease with or without dysphagia. The CK will be very elevated when the disease is progressing, but can be normal at other times. The EMG can be helpful in assisting with the diagnosis for this disorder; the EMG pattern of low-amplitude, brief-duration motor unit action potentials plus fibrillation potentials, positive sharp wave potentials, and high frequency discharges is very characteristic.

The treatment for these disorders is medical, using the various medications for immunosuppression, with little role for rehabilitation except for prevention of contractures and prescription of assistive devices. In the recovery phase many of these patients will benefit from rehabilitation to facilitate their recovery or improve their ability to perform ADL.

STATIC DISORDERS

The Congenital Myopathies

As a group the congenital myopathies are usually considered to be relatively nonprogressive, and most patients will show improvement in neuromuscular function with growth. As a result, patients with these disorders deserve aggressive efforts at correction or prevention of contractures so that activity can be maximized as ability for function improves with age.[7]

Post-Poliomyelitis

Conventional teaching suggests that, after the acute phase of poliomyelitis, no further loss of neuromuscular function is to be expected and the patient's muscle strength and ability to function will continue to improve with use. More recent experience has shown that many of these patients will demonstrate significant reduction in function, occurring relatively acutely 20 to 40 years after their acute episode.[22] This is no longer thought to be a reactivation of the previous polio virus or early signs of ALS. The major question that remains to be resolved is whether the increased loss of function is a result of a wearing-out of surviving anterior horn cells (or axons), or a result of overwork insult to the muscle fibers of the surviving motor units. In addition to the symposia results in the book by Halstead and Wiechers,[22] an entire issue of the journal *Orthopedics* (volume 8, July 1985) was devoted to this subject.

Another question yet to be resolved is whether therapeutic exercise for these patients will improve their functional ability or only accelerate their loss of functional capacity. It has been observed that their neuromuscular function will continue to deteriorate if they continue their usual active life-style. These patients will benefit more from a significant modification of their life-style than from assistive devices, which also are necessary.

PERIPHERAL NEUROPATHIES

Charcot-Marie-Tooth Disease

A hereditary disorder, Charcot-Marie-Tooth disease is transmitted as an autosomal dominant disorder. Thus, it is rare to find a patient with this diagnosis in the absence of other family members with similar, but perhaps milder or even more severe, evidence of this disorder. As with all peripheral neuropathies there is greater distal than proximal involvement of musculature.[15, 40]

Early signs are relatively symmetrical atrophy of the muscles of the leg distal to the knees and pes cavus. These patients undergo slowly progressive weakness, and most remain fully functional throughout most of their adult life. Often the weakness of the leg muscles will result in foot drop and ankle instability, which will benefit from orthotic devices. Contractures are not usually a problem, and strengthening exercise programs usually will not signifiantly improve the patient's functional ability to any significant degree. Occupational therapy can help many of these patients with assistive devices and techniques to increase their efficiency in performing ADL. The neuropathy in these patients is a demyelinating process and electrodiagnostic studies can confirm the very marked slowing of the nerve conduction velocities.

Acute Inflammatory Demyelinating Polyneuropathy

Also known as Guillain-Barré syndrome (GBS), acute inflammatory demyelinating polyneuropathy is an acute onset of weakness, which can involve any or all muscle groups including the muscles of respiration. Symptoms will reach the maximal functional loss usually in less than 4 weeks. The acute phase is usually followed by a plateau phase of variable duration before there is evidence of improvement. It is reported that most patients with GBS recover with little or no residual; however, 10% to 23% will require assisted ventilation and 7% to 22% are left with significant residual disability.[2]

The neuropathy in these patients is a demyelinating disorder and electrodiagnostic studies are indicated to assist in confirming the diagnosis and are also frequently of value to assist in monitoring the patient's progress.

Activities such as exercise should be limited, even during the early portion of the recovery period, to avoid potential further damage to the motor units.[4, 24] The mainstay of treatment for the GBS patient in the early and plateau phases is good and intensive nursing care and attention to prevention of complications. Since many of these patients are bed-bound for long periods, special attention is required for proper bowel and bladder care and prevention of pressure ulcers. Even though this is primarily a motor neuropathy, pain can be a significant problem and narcotic analgesics may be required. Since the report by Hughes and others,[25, 35] corticosteroids are no longer considered appropriate treatment for this disorder. As already mentioned, a significant number of these patients will require mechanical ventilation and, if that must be continued for more than a very few days, a tracheostomy will be necessary to permit adequate pulmonary toilet.

Passive devices to help prevent contractures plus passive range-of-motion exercises are essential to help maintain joint range of motion.[24, 35] These patients frequently will need considerable supervision of their activities by physical and occupational therapists to facilitate their progress in the recovery phase. The use of plasmapheresis is probably no longer a controversial subject, since the report by the Guillain-Barré Syndrome Study Group[48] confirms that it "appears to be of benefit in patients with GBS of recent onset."

METABOLIC DISORDERS OF MUSCLE FUNCTION

Metabolic disorders are probably the rarest of the disorders of muscle function. They are unique for representing functional abnormalities resulting from the absence, or the abnormality of function, of a specific enzyme system. As a result, these disorders receive considerable interest from the muscle physiologists as isolated abnormalities of muscle function that cannot be duplicated in the laboratory.

The presenting symptoms for these patients are fatigue and muscle cramps—not muscular weakness, as that usually does not occur until the later stages. Contractures of the joints are rare. Fatigue is a major presenting complaint because of the inability of the muscles to produce the adenosine triphosphate required for muscle function, or in extreme cases, for survival of the muscle fibers. In addition to fatigue the presenting complaint for many will be muscle cramps or contracture of the muscles during or following activity. Fatigue and muscle cramps are problems that are commonly experienced by almost all normal individuals,[38] so that when the patient's symptoms persist and all conventional studies are normal, the patient is commonly considered to have a psychosomatic problem and they are referred for psychiatric consultation. Few psychiatrists have a sound background in muscle physiology and they are not likely to make the correct diagnosis for the patient. However, the relaxation techniques they occasionally recommend may be very appropriate for the patient.

There is very little role for rehabilitation in the care of these patients, other than making them aware of the limits of their endurance and cautioning them against overactivity that can cause pain and destruction of muscle fibers. At the present time our best laboratory monitor for evidence of injury to the muscle fibers is the CK levels. CK levels significantly above the normal range confirm that muscle fibers are being injured and possibly destroyed.[26]

Using the example of the best known of these disorders, McArdle's disease (absence of muscle phosphorylase), the patients do not have access to the glycogenolytic pathway for energy production for short bursts of high energy output or effort. Some physicians and other professionals have recommended aerobic exercise programs to improve endurance. However, since these patients do not have access to the glycogenolytic pathway, they have been totally dependent on their aerobic pathway for energy supply for their muscles since childhood, except for the facilitated transport of glucose that may have occurred as a compensatory mechanism.[5] Therefore, exercises of any type have potential to accelerate damage to their muscles and little probability for improving their functional ability. Our advice for these patients is to exercise as much as possible, or tolerable, within the limits of pain or muscle discomfort. In our opinion pain that persists for more than a few minutes, or at most a few hours, is a warning from the body that a tissue is in jeopardy of being injured. If the CK levels remain elevated for more than 24 hours, this is probably objective evidence that muscle fibers have been or are on the verge of being destroyed, and that the level of exercise that caused these changes is excessive for this patient. This autosomal recessive disorder is quite rare, and the presenting symptoms are exercise intolerance and muscle cramps. The patient may also describe episodes of pigmenturia (myoglobinuria) following strenuous effort. The CK is usually not elevated except following effort. However, the patient may have chronic elevation of the CK even with normal or minimal ADL in later years. The patient's muscles produce little or no elevation of lactate on the forearm ischemic exercise test,[31] but greater than normal elevation of ammonia.[11, 17, 43, 44, 47] The EMG is usually normal, but when abnormal will show myopathic changes. The definitive test to confirm the diagnosis is biochemical analysis for the enzyme on muscle tissue removed at biopsy.

By now the list of the metabolic disorders of muscle is quite long and their clinical presentations are quite variable. A few of the better known of these disorders are listed in Table 41-3. Most patients present with exercise intolerance, muscle pains, or cramps, and many will experience myoglobinuria following strenuous effort. Many of these disorders, such as acid maltase deficiency, cause major abnormalities in organ systems other than muscle. As a group, the metabolic disorders are genetically transmitted in an autosomal recessive pattern. At present there is no method or procedure to substitute for the enzyme deficiency in these patients. However, one of the metabolic disorders does have potential for treatment by substitution. Patients with carnitine deficiency commonly have presenting symptoms of muscle weakness, as opposed to exercise intolerance. A few reports describe marked improvement in some of the patients with this disorder but not in others when given oral L-carnitine.[7] A recent article describes an episode of acute rhabdomyolysis in a patient who had a partial deficiency of muscle carnitine palmityl transferase that may have been precipitated by therapy with ibuprofen.[39]

Table 41-3
Metabolic Disorders of Muscle

Phosphorylase deficiency (McArdle's disease)
Phosphorylase kinase deficiency
Phosphofructokinase deficiency
Phosphoglyceromutase deficiency
Lactate dehydrogenase deficiency
Acid maltase deficiency
Carnitine palmityl transferase deficiency
Myoadenylate (AMP) deaminase deficiency

Alcoholic myopathy, the acute form that will occasionally follow episodes of binge drinking, can have symptoms of muscle pains, tenderness, and swelling with muscle cramps, and laboratory findings that can be confused with McArdle's disease; however, symptoms and findings clear with abstinence.[7,34]

REFERENCES

1. Alexander MA, Johnson EW, Petty J, Stauch D: Mechanical ventilation of patients with late stage Duchenne muscular dystrophy: Management in the home. Arch Phys Med Rehabil 60:289–292, 1979
2. Arnanson BGW: Acute inflammatory demyelinating polyradiculoneuropathies. In Dyke PJ, Thomas PK, Lambert EH, Bunge R (eds): Peripheral Neuropathy, 2nd ed. Phialdelphia, WB Saunders, 1984
3. Bach JR, O'Brien J, Krotenberg R, Alba AS: Management of end stage respiratory failure in Duchenne muscular dystrophy. Muscle Nerve 10:177–182, 1987
4. Bensman A: Strenuous exercise may impair muscle function in Guillain-Barré patients. JAMA 214:468–469, 1970
5. Bogusky RT, Taylor RG, Anderson LJ et al: McArdle's disease heterozygotes—Metabolic adaptation assessed using ^{31}P-nuclear magnetic resonance. J Clin Invest 77:1881–1887, 1986
6. Bohan A, Peter JB: Polymyositis and dermatomyositis. N Engl J Med 292:343–347, 403–407, 1975
7. Brooke MH: A Clinician's View of Neuromuscular Diseases, 2nd ed. Baltimore, Williams & Wilkins, 1986
8. Brooke MH, Fenichel GM, Griggs RC et al: Clinical investigation in Duchenne dystrophy: 2. Determination of the "power" of therapeutic trials based on the natural history. Muscle Nerve 6:91–103, 1983
9. Brooke MH, Mendell JR, Fenichel GM et al:; Clinical trial in Duchenne dystrophy. I. The design of the protocol. Muscle Nerve 4:186–197, 1981
10. Colbert AP, Schock NC: Respirator use in progressive neuromuscular diseases. Arch Phys Med Rehabil 66:760–762, 1985
11. Coleman RA, Stajich JM, Pact VW, Pericak-Vance MA: The ischemic exercise test in normal adults and in patients with weakness and cramps. Muscle Nerve 9:216–221, 1986
12. De Lateur BJ, Giaconi RM: Effect on maximal strength of submaximal exercise in Duchenne muscular dystrophy. Am J Phys Med 58:26–36, 1979
13. DeLisa J, Mikulic MA, Miller RM, Melnick RR: Amyotrophic lateral sclerosis: Comprehensive management. Am Fam Physician 19:137–142, 1979
14. Dubowitz V: Muscle Biopsy a Practical Approach, 2nd ed. London, Bailliere Tindall, 1985
15. Dyck PJ: Inherited neuronal degeneration and atrophy affecting peripheral motor, sensory, and autonomic neurons. In Dyke PJ, Thomas PK, Lambert EH, Bunge R (eds): Peripheral Neuropathy, 2nd ed. Philadelphia, WB Saunders, 1984
16. Engel AG: Duchenne dystrophy. In Engel AG, Banker BQ (eds): Myology—Basic and Clinical. New York, McGraw-Hill, 1986
17. Fishbein WN, Armbrustmacher VW, Griffin JL: Myoadenylate deaminase deficiency: A new disease of muscle. Science 200:545–548, 1978
18. Fowler WM: Rehabilitation management of muscular dystrophy and related disorders: II. Comprehensive care. Arch Phys Med Rehabil 63:322–328, 1982
19. Fowler WM, Taylor MN: Rehabilitation management of muscular dystrophy and related disorders: I. The role of exercise. Arch Phys Med Rehabil 63:319–321, 1982
20. Gardner-Medwin D: Controversies about Duchenne muscular dystrophy. (2) Bracing for ambulation. Dev Med Child Neurol 21:659–662, 1979
21. Gardner-Medwin D: Rehabilitation in muscular dystrophy. Int Rehabil Med 2:104–110, 1980
22. Halstead LS, Wiechers DO: Late Effects of Poliomyelitis. Miami, Symposia Foundation, 1984
23. Hayes RM, Jaffe KM, Ingman E: Accidental death associated with motorized wheelchair use: A case report. Arch Phys Med Rehabil 66:707–710, 1985
24. Herbison GJ, Jaweed MM, Ditunno JF: Exercise therapies in peripheral neuropathies. Arch Phys Med Rehabil 64:201–205, 1983
25. Hughes RAC, Newsom-Davis J, Perkins GD, Pierce JM: Controlled trial of prednisolone in acute polyneuropathy. Lancet 22:750–753, 1978
26. Jackson MJ, Round JM, Newham DJ, Edwards RHT: An examination of some of the factors influencing creatine kinase in the blood pf patients with muscular dystrophy. Muscle Nerve 10:15–21, 1987
27. Johnson EW: Pathokinesiology of Duchenne muscular dystrophy: Implications for management: Arch Phys Med Rehabil 58:4–7, 1977
28. Johnson EW, Kennedy JH: Comprehensive management of Duchenne muscular dystrophy. Arch Phys Med Rehabil 52:110–114, 1971
29. Koch SJ, Arego DE, Bowser B: Outpatient rehabilitation for chronic neuromuscular diseases. Am J Phys Med 65:245–257, 1986
30. Maloney FP, Burks JS, Ringel SP: Interdisciplinary Rehabilitation of Multiple Sclerosis and Neuromuscular Disorders. Philadelphia, JB Lippincott, 1985
31. McArdle B: Myopathy due to a defect in glycogen breakdown. Clin Sci 10:13–35, 1951
32. Monaco AP, Neve RL, Colletti-Feener C et al: Isolation of candidate cDNAs for portions of the Duchenne muscular dystrophy gene. Nature 323:646–650, 1986
33. Moxley RT, Brooke MH, Fenichel GM et al: Clinical investigation in Duchenne dystrophy. VI. Double-blind controlled trial of nifedipine. Muscle Nerve 10:22–33, 1987
34. Perkoff GT, Hardy P, Velez-Garcia E: Reversible acute muscular syndrome in chronic alcoholism. N Engl J Med 274:1277–1285, 1966
35. Pollard JD: A critical review of therapies in acute and chronic inflammatory demyelinating polyneuropathies. Muscle Nerve 10:214–221, 1987
36. Redding GJ, Okamoto GA, Guthrie RD et al: Sleep patterns in nonambulatory boys with Duchenne muscular dystrophy. Arch Phys Med Rehabil 66:818–821, 1985
37. Rideau Y, Glorion B, Delaubier A et al: The treatment of scoliosis in Duchenne muscular dystrophy. Muscle Nerve 7:281–286, 1984
38. Rowland LP: Cramps, spasms and muscle stiffness. Rev Neurol (Paris) 141:261–273, 1985
39. Ross NS, Hoppel CL: Partial muscle carnitine palmitoyltransferase—A deficiency. Rhabdomyolysis associated with transiently decreased muscle carnitine content after ibuprofen therapy. JAMA 257:62–65, 1987
40. Sabin TD: Classification of peripheral neuropathies: The long and the short of it. Muscle Nerve 9:711–719, 1986
41. Shapiro F, Bresnan MJ: Current concepts review—Orthopaedic management of childhood neuromuscular disease. Part III: Diseases of muscle: J Bone Joint Surg 64-A:1102–1107, 1982
42. Siegel IM: The management of muscular dystrophy: A clinical review. Muscle Nerve 1:453–460, 1978
43. Sinkeler SPT, Daanen HAM, Wevers RA et al: The relation between lactate and ammonia in ischemic handgrip exercise. Muscle Nerve 8:523–527, 1985
44. Sinkeler SP, Wevers RA, Joosten EM et al: Improvement of screening in exertional myalgia with a standardized ischemic forearm test. Muscle Nerve 9:731–737, 1986
45. Sutherland DH, Olshen R, Cooper L et al: Pathomechanics of gait in Duchenne muscular dystrophy. Dev Med Child Neurol 23:3–22, 1981

46. Swash M: Corrective procedures and orthotics in progressive neuromuscular diseases. A neurologist's view. In Dimitrijevic MR, Kakulas BA, Vrbova G (eds): Recent Advances in Restorative Neurology: 2. Progressive Neuromuscular Diseases, pp 2–10. New York, Karger, 1986

47. Taylor RG, Lieberman JS, Portwood MM: Ischemic exercise test: Failure to detect partial expression of McArdle's disease. Muscle Nerve 10:546–551, 1987

48. The Guillain-Barré Syndrome Study Group: Plasmapheresis and acute Guillain-Barré syndrome. Neurology 35:1096–1104, 1985

49. Thompson MW: The genetic transmission of muscle diseases. In Engel AG, Banker BQ (eds): Myology—Basic and Clinical, pp 1151–1179. New York, McGraw-Hill, 1986

50. Vignos PJ: Physical models of rehabilitation in neuromuscular disease. Muscle Nerve 6:323–338, 1983

51. Walton J: Disorders of Voluntary Muscle. London, Churchill Livingston, 1981

52. Wood DS, Zeviani M, Prelle A et al: Is nebulin the defective gene product in Duchenne muscular dystrophy? N Engl J Med 316:107–108, 1987

42

Rehabilitation of the Patient With Burns

Phala A. Helm

Steven V. Fisher

Rehabilitation of the burn patient can be exciting, challenging, and thoroughly rewarding. These patients have extremely complex problems requiring expertise of many specialties. Often, needed disciplines shy away from burn care, which is unfortunate because they have much to offer.

Classification of the burn injury is important for planning the treatment regimen for the patient. Burns may be classified by causative agent, depth, and percent of total body surface area burned (Table 42-1 and Fig. 42-1). Other factors considered are body part burned, age of patient, pre-existing illnesses, and other associated injuries such as smoke inhalation, and fractures.[38]

PATHOPHYSIOLOGY

Normal Skin

The epidermis and dermis comprise the two identifiable layers of skin. Epidermal cells begin in the basal layer and gradually move to the surface. As the cells approach the surface, they undergo keratinization and flatten, leaving a thin layer of keratin fiber on the surface that provides a protective barrier to bacterial invasion and fluid loss. The epidermal cells line not only the basal layer of the epidermis, but also the hair follicles and sweat glands which are deep in the dermis.

The dermis consists of vascular connective tissue which supports and provides nutrition to the epidermis and skin appendages, the sweat glands, hair follicles, and sebaceous glands. The dermis gives the skin strength and elasticity by an interlacing of collagen and elastic fibers. The skin thickness varies with age and body location, with thicker skin over the back and posterior neck, and thinner skin over the medial aspect of the arms and legs.

Local Effects of Heat Injury

Thermal destruction of the skin causes a chain of events which may be classified as local and systemic. The amount of tissue destroyed depends on local and systemic reactions to heat damage, the duration and intensity of thermal exposure, and the characteristics of the area burned. In children the rete pegs are not well developed in most body areas, and in the elderly they have become thin and atrophic, thus increasing the damage with burn injury because of fewer protective layers of epithelium.[38]

It is very difficult, even for the most experienced, to determine with certainty the depth of burn for 3 to 5 days post-burn. Shortly following the burn injury, histamine is released into the local area which causes intense vasoconstriction, and within a few hours there is vasodilatation and increased capillary permeability, which permits plasma to escape into the wound. Damaged cells swell, and platelets and leukocytes aggregate and stick to vessel walls, causing thrombosis and ischemia and further damage.

Second- and third-degree burns impair the body's defenses against infection and cause loss of massive amounts of body fluids through open wounds. The evaporative loss results in a heat loss and a large caloric drain on the patient. Bacterial contamination of the burn wound may occur immediately and local burn wound sepsis results.

Systemic Effects of Heat Injury

Some of the major systemic effects of burns include acute hypovolemia with loss of fluid into the extravascular compartment and subsequent burn shock, pulmonary changes with hyperventilation, and marked increase in oxygen consumption. The high incidence of upper airway obstruction is probably related to direct damage by inhalation of noxious gases and because of this, the patients are subject to pneumonia. Blood viscosity increases and platelets increase their adhesiveness. Acute gastric dilatation and gastrointestinal ileus commonly occur in the first three days post burn. Immunologic competence is depressed for many reasons including depression of immunoglobulins.[10]

Skin Regeneration and Scarring

Healing and regeneration of skin in partial-thickness burns arise from the epithelial linings including the hair follicles and sweat glands. Depending upon the depth, healing is completed within 14 to 21 days. The new skin again becomes active as a temperature regulator and as a barrier for bacteria. After epithelialization there is continued healing with regeneration of the peripheral nerves, sometimes associated with symptoms of pain and itch-

Table 42-1
Burn Classification

Causative Agent
1. Thermal
   a. Heat
   b. Cold
2. Electrical
3. Chemical
4. Radiation

Depth of Burn
1. Older Terminology
   a. 1st degree: Epidermis injured
   b. 2nd degree: Dermis partially damaged
   c. 3rd degree: All dermis destroyed
   d. 4th degree: Muscle, nerve and bone damaged
2. Newer Terminology
   a. Superfiical partial thickness: Epidermis and upper part of dermis injured
   b. Deep partial thickness: Epidermis and large upper portion of dermis injured
   c. Full thickness: All skin destroyed

Size of Burn: Rule of Nines
1. Head = 9% body surface area (BSA)
2. Each upper extremity = 9% BSA
3. Each lower extremity = 18% BSA
4. Anterior trunk = 18% BSA
5. Posterior trunk = 18% BSA
6. Perineum = 1% BSA

American Burn Association Classification
1. Minor
   a. <15% BSA partial thickness (10% in child)
   b. <2% BSA full thickness (not involving eyes, ears, face or perineum)
2. Moderate*
   a. All 15%–25% BSA (10%–20% in child)
   b. 2%–10% BSA full thickness (not involving eyes, ears, face or perineum)
3. Major*
   a. All >25% BSA partial thickness (20% in child); ≥10% BSA full thickness
   b. All burns to face, eyes, ears, feet, perineum
   c. All electrical
   d. All inhalation
   e. All burns with fracture or major tissue trauma
   f. All with poor risk secondary to age or illness

* Most moderate and all major burns should be hospitalized.

ing. It should be noted that split-thickness autografts have no dermal appendages.

Although epithelium covers the wound, dermal scarring occurs in the burn wound on a continuous basis for several months after injury. The healing process is ongoing from 6 months to 2 years until the skin is mature. By that point the vascularity of the wound has returned to near normal and there is no further collagen deposition in the wound.

PATIENT MANAGEMENT

Acute Phase

Resuscitation

An immediate estimate of the total percent of surface area burned is a priority in management to determine if intravenous fluid therapy is needed to prevent or treat burn shock. A shift of body fluids to involved areas can cause intravascular hypovolemia and massive edema of both injured and uninjured tis-

sues. If treatment is inadequate acute renal failure and death can occur. Several formulas are available for calibrating fluid requirements (Brooke, Evans and Baxter formulas); however, the formulas serve only as guidelines, since individual adjustments must be made, based on the patient's response. It is important that the fluids contain sodium and that fluid replacement be completed within 48 hours.

Escharotomy

An *escharotomy* is an incision through the burned tissue to relieve increased tissue pressure (Fig. 42-2). Massive edema of the extremities can cause neurovascular compromise, which could result in amputation. Early assessment of blood flow is essential. This can be evaluated by physical examination, Doppler studies, and by measuring tissue pressures with a wick catheter. If using tissue pressure as a guide, escharotomy is indicated when tissue pressure exceeds 40 mm Hg. Escharotomies are done on other parts of the body, such as the chest when chest expansion is limited and interferes with breath-

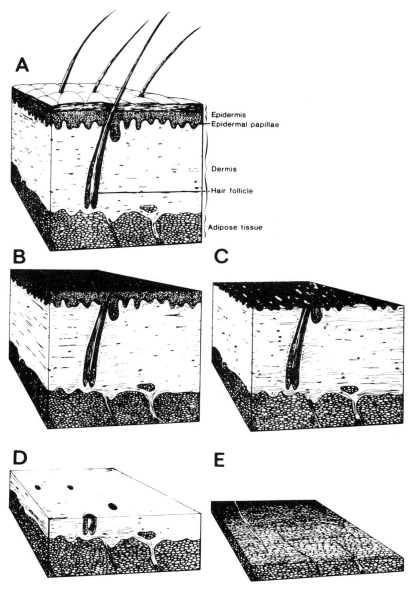

Figure 42-1. Depth of burns: (*A*) normal skin; (*B*) superficial partial thickness (first degree); (*C*) superficial partial thickness (second degree); (*D*) deep partial thickness (second degree); and (*E*) full thickness (third degree).

Figure 42-2. Escharotomies on the dorsum of the hand.

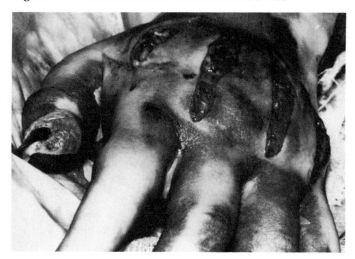

ing. To prevent compartment syndromes fasciotomies are recommended.

Wound Coverage

TOPICAL ANTIBACTERIAL AGENTS.   Following resuscitation the burn wound is cleansed, devitalized tissue is removed, and a topical antibacterial agent is applied. There are a number of effective topical agents used for the prevention of burn wound sepsis. Among the various agents available are mafenide, silver nitrate, gentamicin, povidone-iodine, and silver sulfadiazine (currently in widest use because of comfort and fewer side-effects). There is no single agent universally effective and no one agent superior over another in terms of patient survival.

BIOLOGICAL DRESSINGS.   A *biological dressing* is a skin substitute used for temporary coverage of the burn wound. These skin substitutes are skin grafts from cadavers, human fetal membranes (homografts or allografts), and skin grafts from pigs (heterografts or xenografts). The recommended uses for the dressing are immediate coverage of a superficial partial thickness burn; wound debridement; a "test" dressing (if it adheres, the wound bed is ready for autografting); and wound coverage following excision of burn eschar. In addition, closing a wound with a biological dressing prevents fluid loss, decreases pain, inhibits bacterial growth on clean wounds, and encourages growth of granulation tissue. The biological dressing should be changed every several days until the wound is healed or ready for autografting. If left in place too long it becomes incorporated into the burn wound, making removal extremely difficult. It can also become dry and adherent to the wound, restricting range of motion.

SYNTHETIC DRESSINGS. Synthetic skin substitutes were developed to cover open wounds until the wound healed or until it could be autografted. They are used in place of xenografts or homografts. For the synthetic skin to be an effective replacement for certain biological dressings it had to meet certain criteria. A product was needed that was readily available, non-allergenic, relatively inexpensive, easily removable, and which had a permeable membrane. One additional criteria was that it come in large sheets that would conform to various tissue planes. A product that met this criteria, and which is widely used, is Biobrane. It has a bilaminar structure with silicone on the outside, and nylon bonded to the bottom which is covered with collagen.[37] Opsite is another synthetic skin composed of a thin transparent elastic adhesive coated polyurethane film, permeable to water vapor.

Surgical Management

Debridement

Debridement is the removal of devitalized tissue (eschar) down to a viable tissue level to prepare the wound bed for definitive coverage. Removal of eschar aids in healing by preventing bacterial proliferation. Types of debridement are mechanical with scissors and forceps (Fig. 42-3) and wet-to-dry dressings; enzymatic; and surgical (tangential, fascial, and full-thickness excisions).

MECHANICAL DEBRIDEMENT. Mechanical debridement is best accomplished either during hydrotherapy or immediately following. Removal of dressings when they are dry is effective in debridement of dead tissue as it adheres to the dressing. All areas should be cleansed gently to remove topical agents so that the wound is completely visible before sharp debridement begins. Hydrotherapy, without wound care, is poor patient management.

Wet-to-dry dressings can also be very effective in removal of eschar or exudate. Coarse mesh gauze, soaked in warmed antibacterial solution or normal saline, is applied to the wound and left to dry. With this technique the eschar softens, sticks to the dressing, and then is debrided as the dressing is removed.

ENZYMATIC DEBRIDEMENT. An enzymatic debriding agent such as Travase (sutilains) will selectively digest necrotic tissue without harming viable tissue. Since there is increased fluid drainage through the wound with enzymatic debridement, no more than 20% of the body surface area should be treated at one time. Other side-effects include bleeding, body temperature elevation, and pain. The enzyme should not be used in conjunction with hexachlorophene or iodine preparations, since enzyme activity will be impaired.[9]

SURGICAL DEBRIDEMENT. The two primary surgical techniques used for wound debridement are fascial and tangential (or sequential) excision (Figs. 42-4 and 42-5). Fascial excision removes nonviable burn tissue and a variable amount of viable tissue and is reserved for patients with very deep burns. It is believed that skin grafts have a much better "take" on fascia than on fat. The problem with fascial excision is that fat does not regenerate and thus can cause severe cosmetic deformities.

The most widely employed technique in surgical debridement is eschar removal by tangential excision, usually performed at 1 to 10 days post-burn. The principle of tangential excision is to shave thin layers of burn eschar sequentially until viable tissue is apparent. There can be a significant amount of blood loss and different methods are used to control this. Tourniquets are used for the extremities by the more experienced surgeon, since there is the danger of sacrificing normal tissue by excising too deep. Some surgeons control bleeding with microcrystalline collagen, thrombin, epinephrine, and electrocautery.

Heimbeck reports that early excision and grafting in comparison to the standard nonoperative treatment has shown decrease in hospital stay, slight fall in overall patient mortality, decrease in systemic sepsis, decrease in deaths due to burn wound sepsis, and a decline in nursing turnover.[18]

Figure 42-3. Mechanical debridement.

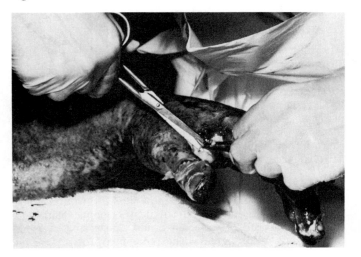

Figure 42-4. Surgical debridement by excision.

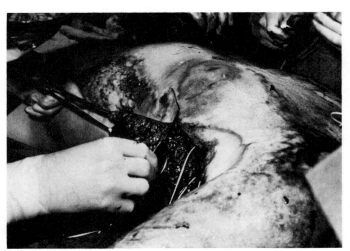

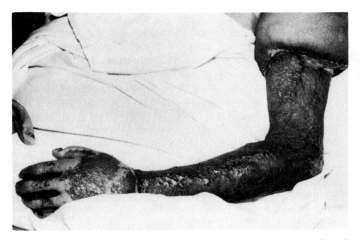

Figure 42-5. Patient's arm after surgical debridement by fascial excision.

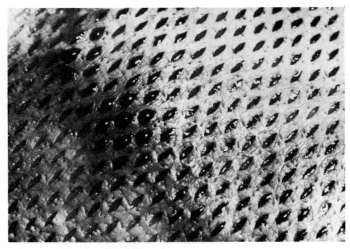

Figure 42-6. Tanner mesh split-thickness skin graft.

Skin Grafting

With the exception of small wounds, all full-thickness wounds require skin grafting. Deep partial-thickness wounds that are slow in healing may also require skin grafting. Some investigators believe that grafting of deep partial-thickness wounds prevents the development of thick scar tissue. *Autografting* is the removal of skin from one part of the body and transferring it to another part. Split-thickness skin grafts are primarily used, whereas full-thickness grafts are used more for reconstructive procedures.

There are a variety of split-thickness skin grafts, each with different indications for use. The Tanner mesh graft is expandible skin that can be used to cover large wounds (Fig. 42-6). Expansion of the skin can be varied, with better cosmetic results with a 1.5:1 expansion rather than, for example, with a 6:1. Postage stamp grafting is the application of squares or rectangles of various dimensions spread evenly over the wound. This type of grafting often leaves a poor cosmetic result because of hypertrophic scarring of the uncovered areas. Sheet grafting is another method used and involves using a piece of split-thickness skin without meshing or cutting it into small squares. This method is used on smaller burn wounds and on the face, neck, and hands for better cosmetic results. The part grafted should be immobilized for at least 4 or 5 days.

Rehabilitation

Wound Care

Wound care, debridement, and subsequent skin care are extremely important considerations for functional and cosmetic outcome and therefore have direct bearing on rehabilitation. Aggressive wound care is important to delineate wounds prior to early surgical intervention, to protect and promote good granulation tissue until grafting, or to promote rapid healing in moderate to deep partial-thickness wounds which tend to have prolonged healing times and subsequently increased scarring.[16] The goals of wound care are:

1. To prevent or control infection
2. To preserve as much tissue as possible
3. To prepare the wound for earliest possible closure by primary healing or grafting.

Cleaning techniques include local care, spray or nonsubmersion hydrotherapy, and submersion with or without agitation of the water. The choice depends on the depth of injury, extent and location of the wound and the overall condition of the patient. All areas should be scrubbed gently, but thoroughly. When manual debridement is indicated, it should be done following the cleansing process. Daily wound care, which must be aggressive and vigorous, should always be done with as little trauma as possible to the wound and granulation tissue.

Positioning

In the acute care period, contracture prevention by proper positioning is fundamental to the overall program. The burn patient is obviously extremely uncomfortable and seeks relief by moving the extremities and trunk into a relaxed position to remove the stretch from the burned tissue. To do so he primarily flexes and adducts the extremities into a position of comfort (Fig. 42-7). Since contractures develop rapidly in these patients, antideformity positioning should begin immediately. It is only logical to stress abduction and extension (Fig. 42-8). What is often forgotten is the alternating of positions so that opposing deformities or pain problems are not created by trying to prevent these flexion-adduction contractures. To aid in positioning, the addition of orthopedic frames and shoulder boards to the bed allow for innovative techniques.

Another salient issue in positioning is the type of bed used. Often the air-fluidized beds are used on burn units for relief of pressure in decubiti prevention and for more even distribution of pressure over wounds and grafts. Although the pressure is better distributed, contractures can be encouraged because the patient sinks into the bed or often assumes a fetal position. The Roho mattress can be as effective as the air-fluidized beds for pressure distribution, and superior in preventing contractures.

Splinting

If voluntary positioning becomes a problem, as with the elderly, the noncompliant, and children, splinting becomes an important adjunct to care. If normal range of motion is maintained, there is no need to apply splints with two major exceptions. Exposed tendons should be splinted in a slack position in an attempt to prevent rupture, whereas exposed joints should be splinted for protection.

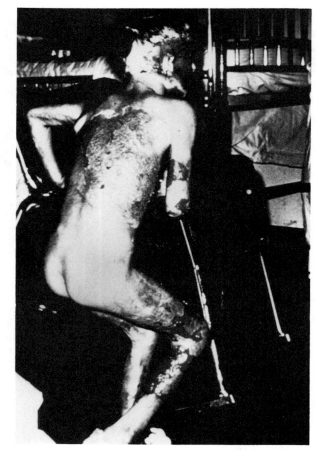

Figure 42-7. Deformities will develop if the patient is allowed to remain in the position of comfort.

Figure 42-8. Therapeutic positioning. (Helm PA, et al: Burn injury: Rehabilitation management in 1982. Arch Phys Mod Rehabil 63:6–16, 1982)

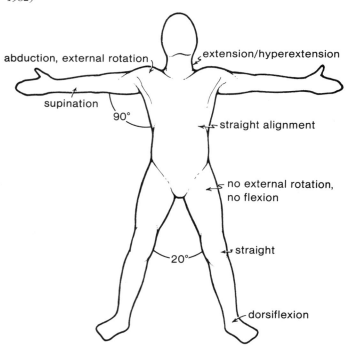

The major splints used in the acute phase are resting hand splints, dorsiflexion splints to the ankles for tight heelcords and peroneal nerve palsies, knee-extension dorsiflexion splints to prevent "frog leg" position (particularly in children) and elbow extension splints for limited elbow extension with the precaution that the patient should have close to full elbow flexion.

Opposite deformities can be created by prolonged immobilization with splinting; therefore frequent assessments of joint range of motion is necessary. The transparent face mask is frequently applied early in the acute phase. The plastic mask is made from a plaster model of the face and is applied over new grafts and over newly healed skin. Its advantages include conforming well to the contours of the face, transparency to allow viewing of the skin to verify appropriate pressure distribution, and when worn properly, preventing severe cosmetic deformities. Many centers are also using the silicone face masks immediately post-grafting and prior to application of the transparent face mask (Fig. 42-9).

Exercise and Ambulation

Throughout convalescence gentle sustained stretch is more effective than multiple repetitive movements in stretching burned tissue. Before the therapist begins an exercise program, the area to receive treatment must be viewed after cleansing; otherwise, an unrecognized injury to vital structures could be compounded by the exercise program. Exercise programs may be indicated three to four times daily to more involved areas, and without exception the patient should exercise between therapy sessions. Active exercises to the lower extremities, whether burned or not, assist in the prevention of thrombophlebitis. Escharotomies, heterografts, synthetic dressings, and tangential excisions are not contraindications for exercise; however, exercises should be discontinued for 4 or 5 days to joints proximal and distal to those autografted and, sometimes, homografted areas.

In the acute period trunk mobilization is needed to prevent the robot-type posture that frequently occurs. Burns to the anterior trunk can cause rounding of the shoulders with a sunken chest, and shoulder elevation, as well as limited trunk rotary movements. To counteract these problems, vigorous trunk flex-

Figure 42-9. Silicone face mask.

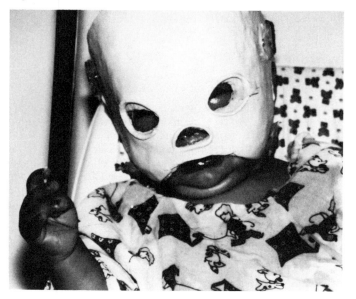

ion-extension and rotation exercises and bilateral shoulder horizontal abduction exercises are necessary (Fig. 42-10). Every part of the body that has received a burn should be exercised in some manner.

Assistive devices, if needed to get the patient ambulatory or to keep him ambulatory, should be used (Fig. 42-11). A wheeled walker with an adjustable overhead attached bar can be used for patients with upper extremity burns to help stretch and increase range of motion of shoulders and elbows, as well as reduce edema in the arms. Ambulatory patients have fewer problems with lower extremity contractures and endurance. Patients with burns to the feet requiring deep excision or partial foot amputations should be fitted early with extra-depth shoes, molded insoles, or inserts. Early application of proper footwear prevents later secondary complications of knee, hip, and back pain.

HAND BURNS

Burn injuries to the hands have a profound effect on the patient's return to normal function; therefore, hand therapy is stressed during both acute and post-acute phases.

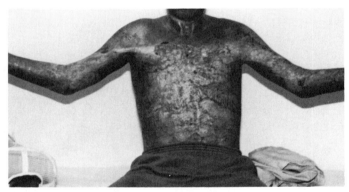

Figure 42-10. Position for bilateral shoulder horizontal abduction exercise.

Figure 42-11. Ambulation assistive devices.

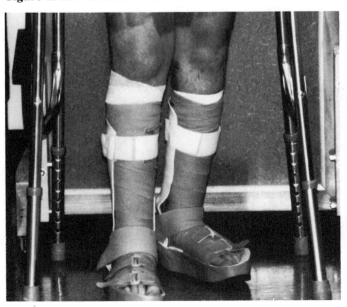

Edema

Edema is a major cause of the typical "clawed" burned hand with hyperextension of the metacarpophalangeal (MCP) joints, flexion of the proximal and distal interphalangeal (IP) joints, and the thumb in adduction and external rotation (Fig. 42-12). Anti-deformity positioning is best treated with a resting hand splint, positioning the wrist in slight extension (see Fig. 42-23A and B), the MCP joints in 60° to 90° flexion, the proximal and distal IP joints in full extension, and the thumb in palmar abduction. It may be necessary to wear the splints continuously until edema resolves and the patient is actively using his hands. Edema is also treated through elevation and active exercise. Immediately post-injury, the arms may be elevated with Robert Jones skeletal traction, with bedside troughs or night-time stands.

A complication of the pneumatic tourniquet with prolonged application as reported by Bruner is the adverse effects upon tissues of the hand, called the *post-ischemic hand syndrome.*[7] His findings of puffiness of the hand and fingers, stiffness of the hand and finger joints, color changes in the hand (congested in the dependent position), subjective sensations of numbness, and objective evidence of weakness without real paralysis, are frequently encountered in the post-operative burn patient.

Exposed Tendons and Joints

Exposed tendons in the hand can be a serious problem, since they have a tendency to rapidly dehydrate, denature, and subsequently, rupture. Exposed tendons should therefore be covered with a moist gauze or biological dressing to prevent drying. Continuous splinting should be used to maintain the tendon in a slack position until permanent wound closure is obtained. Tendons that appear denatured or charred may ultimately revascularize and should not be debrided prematurely. If the dorsal hood mechanism is exposed, the interphalangeal joints should be splinted in extension until wound closure. Only then can gentle active range of motion begin. If the dorsal hood ruptures, the typical boutonniere deformity develops (Fig. 42-13). Immediately after rupture, immobilization of the finger for 6 weeks in extension may allow scar tissue to form across the extensor surface and provide a substitute for the destroyed extensor mechanism (Fig. 42-14). Active motion can then be started.[21]

If joint capsules are exposed but not open, they may be

Figure 42-12. Edematous "clawed" hand.

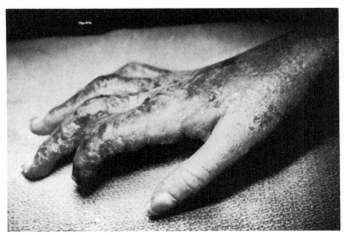

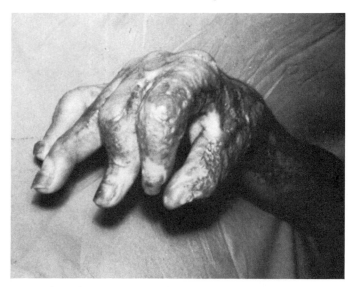

Figure 42-13.   Boutonniere deformity.

gently actively exercised and protectively splinted. If the joint is open and/or draining, it will probably undergo spontaneous ankylosis; therefore functional positioning should be encouraged.

Exercise

Primary considerations in exercising the burn hand include intrinsic muscle stretching by mobilizing the metacarpals and stretching the intrinsic muscles by hyperextension of the MCP joint in combination with flexion of the proximal IP joint. Traction applied to the joints with passive movement allows for additional ligamentous stretch.

Splinting

It is not unusual for the burned hand to require customized splinting. Dynamic, as well as static, splinting is used. Custom-conforming splints are used primarily on the flexor surfaces of

Figure 42-14.   (*A*) Rupture of extensor hood. (*B*) Finger splinted in full extension. (*C*) Active extension of finger after 6 weeks. (*D*) Active flexion of finger after 6 weeks.

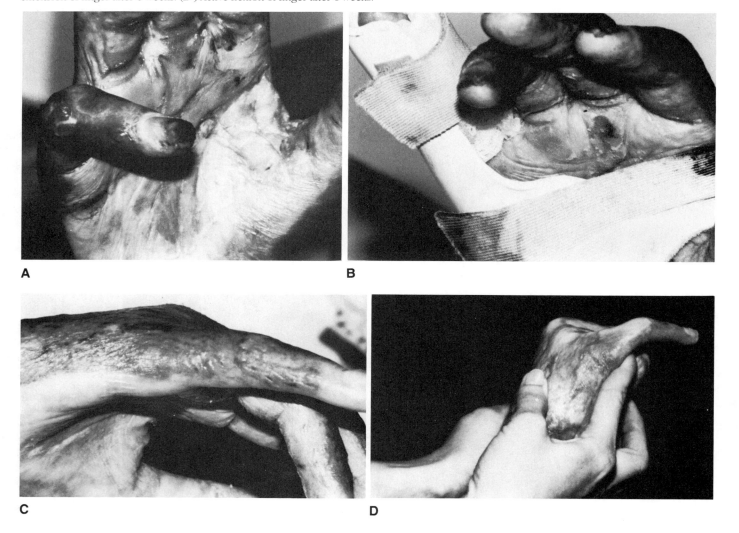

A

B

C

D

the hand in patients who have developed contractures or banding over the palmar aspect. The pressure of the splint produces softening, flattening, and lengthening of the scar band. Splints may be used for *serial splinting,* with the splint being applied at maximum tension and constant pressure; and as the contracture improves, the splint is remodeled.

Dynamic splinting can be effective in correcting contractures. Nail hooks, leather loops over the phalanges, flexion wrap, or flexion glove may be used for dynamic stretch in extension contractures (see Fig. 42-23F and G). A custom-made elastomer foam insert placed at the first web space is helpful in maintaining the space and in decreasing an adduction contracture of the thumb.

The successful splinting of the hand requires therapist innovation as well as significant patient cooperation. Rehabilitation of a child's hand is different from that of the adult's and bears special mention. The child's hand is small, making it difficult to fabricate properly fitting hand orthoses, and children have a tendency to flex the hand causing splint movement and thus producing pressure ulcers. Unfortunately the young child cannot express pain complaints appropriately. For dorsal hand burns, it may be necessary to position the MCP as well as the IP joints in extension. In the uncooperative child, serial casting is very beneficial and passive range-of-motion exercises are critical. Play activities become a much more important feature of the exercise program.[34]

ELECTRICAL INJURIES

Mechanism of Injury

Electrical injuries constitute only a small number of most burn unit admissions; however, they probably represent the most devastating type of thermal injury. These injuries are arbitrarily divided into low voltage (no greater than 500 to 1000 volts) and high voltage, those greater than 1000 volts. Home injuries usually involve 110 to 220 volts with 60-cycle current and cause little cutaneous and very rare deep muscle damage. These low voltage accidents, however, can be associated with cardiac standstill or rhythm irregularities. The most common low-voltage burn injury

is in the child who bites an electrical cord and sustains a burn of the commissure of the lips.

Generally, the greater the voltage the greater the amperage and, consequently, the more severe the injury. As current flows through the body, electrical energy is converted to heat expressed as Joule's law:

$$\text{Power or heat} = \text{Amperage}^2 \times \text{Resistance}$$

It is therefore apparent that amperage is of greater importance in causing tissue destruction than voltage. Damage is primarily related to tissue resistance and sensitivity to heat. The most resistant or nonconductive tissue is bone, followed by cartilage, tendon, skin, muscle, blood, and nerve. Although blood vessels and nerves offer little resistance and relatively little heat is produced, these structures seem to be particularly sensitive to heat damage and sustain injury despite their low resistance.[4, 25, 26]

Soft Tissue and Bone Damage

Tissue destruction is always greatest in areas of the body with small volume such as fingers, toes, wrists, or ankles. One must therefore be knowledgeable of this "iceberg-type" injury in which the cutaneous injury may give no indication of the possible underlying muscle, bone, and nerve damage.

The acute surgical treatment is early diagnosis and debridement of necrotic tissue. In all burn patients, the greatest number of amputations occur from electrical injuries.[32] Bone that is exposed, must be covered with moist dressings to prevent desiccation of the periosteum. Some surgeons drill bur holes in exposed bone to stimulate granulation tissue formation for eventual bone coverage (Fig. 42-15).

Localized Nerve and Central Nervous System Injury

Local neuropathies may occur both in tissues that are directly burned and in tissue through which electrical energy passes. Patients who have had current pass through their legs often complain of weakness manifested by inability to stand on the feet

Figure 42-15. (A) Burr holes with protruding granulation tissue. (B) Wound coverage 4 weeks later.

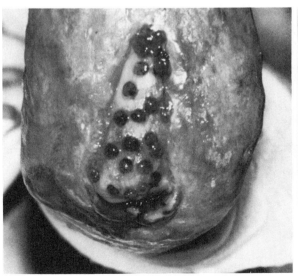
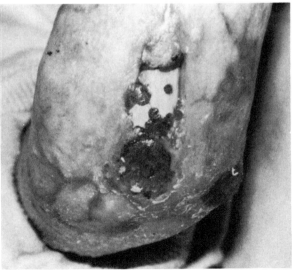

A

B

for long periods of time and general lack of stamina. Electrodiagnostic tests are worthwhile to diagnose subtle peripheral neuropathies.

Central nervous system damage may result in memory loss, personality changes, and spinal cord pathology. Symptoms of central nervous system injury may not be evident up to 2 years post-injury; therefore long-term patient follow-up is needed.

Cataracts

Electrical contact on the head or shoulders may predispose a patient to cataract formation. Cataracts may form within 1 month or as late as 3 years post-injury. Therefore, serial eye examinations should be performed for at least 3 years post-injury.

NEUROLOGICAL INJURIES

Localized Neuropathies

Peripheral neurological complications in the burn patient are not uncommon; however, they are frequently undiagnosed, since neurological assessments are difficult in patients with multiple concurrent problems. To a great extent the majority of nerve injuries are preventable and therefore a clear understanding of their etiology is essential. Certain patients are predisposed to peripheral nerve compromise because their nerves are diseased, as seen in diabetics and alcoholics. Elderly patients develop neuropathies because their peripheral nerves do not tolerate pressure well and because they are less mobile; therefore, they maintain prolonged positions that place their nerves at risk.[20, 22]

Brachial Plexus

There are several bed positions the burn patient may assume, and intraoperative positions in which he is placed, that put the brachial plexus at risk. In conjunction with these at-risk positions, loss of muscle tone in the anesthetized patient and immobility of the patient in bed add to the problem of positioning risks. Possible mechanisms of injury to the plexus during anesthesia have been reported by several authors. Jackson and Keats reported that plexus stretch injury could occur in patients positioned supine with shoulders abducted 90° or more, and externally rotated. In addition, if the upper arm is posteriorly displaced (hung below table level), added tension is placed on the plexus. The mechanism creating the injury is compression of the plexus between the clavicle and first rib, causing tension and stretch with these particular shoulder and arm movements.[28] Ewing wrote that when the humerus is abducted in external rotation, its head forms a prominence in the axilla where the nerve trunks pass; the nerves may become angulated with resultant stretching. The nerve trunks to the upper extremity are anchored at the vertebral column and by fascial attachments in the axilla; they pass under a tendenous arch formed by the insertion of the pectoralis minor. Even though nerves are extensible, there is a limit to their stretch.[14]

It has been recommended that, to prevent compression-stretch injury to the brachial plexus, the patient be positioned in 15 cm of arm horizontal adduction, lifting the clavicle off of the first rib. Dhuner reported that 40 minutes was the shortest time in the operating room within which injury to the brachial plexus occurred.[8] Other at-risk positions are prone and side-lying. In the prone position the patient usually lies with arms abducted 90° or greater and externally rotated.[8] One or two pillows under the chest will adduct the extremities and lift the clavicle off of the

first rib. Patients positioned on their side, with the opposite arm abducted, elbow extended, and then suspended from an IV pole or overhead frame, can develop a traction injury to the brachial plexus. This position may be used in the surgical suite for grafting of the axilla or lateral chest wall, for bed positioning to decrease edema of the extremity, or to prevent axillary contractures.

One additional problem that can occur is a stretch injury of the plexus following an axillary contracture release, particularly if the contracture has been long-standing. All structures can become tight with prolonged limited mobility; therefore, the surgeon often chooses to do staged releases to try to prevent a stretch injury from occurring. In a stretch injury, the upper trunk (C5 and C6) of the brachial plexus is primarily involved; generally the patient completely recovers, but it may take several months.

Suprascapular Nerve

Injury to the suprascapular nerve is often overlooked, since function is not markedly impaired and the burn usually involves the posterior shoulder girdle on the side of injury (Fig. 42-16A). The suprascapular nerve passes through a fibro-osseous tunnel of the suprascapular notch to innervate the supraspinatus and infraspinatus. As reported by Rask, hyper-protraction of the shoulder overstretches the nerve with resultant swelling and unrelenting pain in the shoulder region. A hyper-protracted position can occur when the patient tries to stretch the skin in the posterior shoulder girdle by forward flexion and horizontal adduction of the arm. Injury can be prevented by stabilizing the scapula.[35]

Ulnar Nerve

The primary area of involvement of the ulnar nerve in the burn patient is at the elbow in the cubital tunnel. The roof of the tunnel is the arcuate ligament, which extends from a fixed point on the medial epicondyle to a movable attachment on the olecranon. The floor of the tunnel is formed by the medial ligament of the elbow. Wadsworth reports that the capacity of the tunnel is maximal with elbow extension when the arcuate ligament is slack.[43] When the elbow is flexed to 90°, the arcuate ligament becomes taut and the medial ligament bulges, decreasing the capacity of the tunnel and putting the nerve at risk (Fig. 42-16B). He also noted that pronation of the forearm could cause surface contact with the cubital tunnel, whereas supination of the forearm lifts the tunnel containing the ulnar nerve away from the surface. Unfortunately many burn patients assume the position of elbow flexion and forearm pronation in the supine and prone positions, causing elbow flexion pronation contractures; this probably accounts for the majority of ulnar neuropathies. In the operating suite the patient is frequently positioned in the same manner. An injury at this level usually spares the flexor carpi ulnaris and ulnar half of the flexor digitorum profundus because the fibers to these muscles are located deep in the central part of the nerve.[43]

Another circumstance predisposing a patient for an ulnar neuropathy is subluxation of the ulnar nerve onto the medial epicondyle, thereby essentially leaving it unprotected from pressure. In cases of heterotopic bone at the elbow, entrapment of the ulnar nerve in an osseous tunnel has been reported.

Radial Nerve

The radial nerve is most frequently involved in the burn patient by compression in the spiral groove where the nerve winds around the humerus and virtually lies on bone. Compression injuries at this level may be secondary to the arm resting on

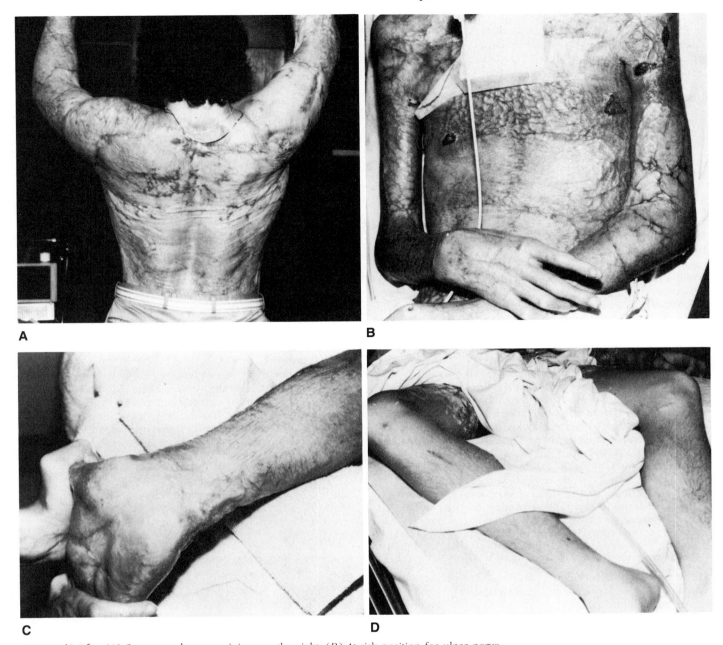

Figure 42-16. (*A*) Suprascapular nerve injury on the right. (*B*) At-risk position for ulnar nerve injury. (*C*) At-risk position for median nerve injury. (*D*) At-risk position for peroneal nerve injury.

the side rails of the bed, hanging over the edge of the operating table, or slipping off the edge of an arm board. In these cases, the triceps muscle is usually spared, since it is innervated at a higher level.

Restraints at the distal forearm-wrist level can injure the superficial cutaneous branch of the radial nerve, causing paresthesias of the dorsum of the hand and thumb.

Median Nerve

Most injuries to the median nerve occur at the wrist level and are usually due to extremes of positioning used to gain range of motion (Fig. 42-16*C*). Prolonged or repeated hyperextension of the wrist irritates the nerve at the carpal tunnel, which can cause paresthesias in the thumb, index, middle, and ring fingers, and weakness of the thenar muscles. Sustained stretch to the wrist in

a hyperextended position, either with splints or exercise programs, should be performed with caution.

Femoral Nerve

Femoral nerve dysfunction in the burn patient is uncommon; however, it has been known to be injured in the femoral triangle after hematoma formation, secondary to obtaining femoral blood samples. Femoral blood withdrawal is often necessary in the extensively burned individual.

The nerve is also susceptible to injury in patients on anticoagulant therapy who have had a retroperitoneal hemorrhage. Mant and associates studied 76 patients receiving heparin anticoagulation for venous thromboembolism and found a 7% incidence of retroperitoneal hemorrhage.[31] Reinstein and coworkers studied femoral nerve dysfunction after retroperitoneal hemorrhage with computed tomography and were able to localize the hematoma. They found that localization of the hematoma within the tight iliacus muscle compartment could produce femoral nerve injury by compressing the nerve against the taut psoas tendon. It is reported that 75% of the patients experience complete recovery of nerve function with conservative management.[36]

Peroneal Nerve

The peroneal nerve has several peculiarities that make it vulnerable to injury. Studies of the nerve by Berry and Richardson showed that the nerve is applied to the periosteum of the fibula for a total of 10 cm, is exposed over the bony prominence for about 4 cm covered only by skin and fascia, and has limited longitudinal mobility of about 0.5 cm.[6] Although compression injuries of the peroneal nerve are notoriously associated with the lateral decubitus position, metal stirrups, and leg straps, less attention is given to positions of the leg that cause stretch injuries. When a patient maintains a position of externally rotated hips, flexion of the knees, and inverted feet (frog leg) (either because the bed is too short, because a urinal is placed between the thighs in the male patient, or when there are tender medial thigh/perineum burns), the peroneal nerve is placed on a stretch and can be injured in a matter of hours, due to its limited longitudinal mobility (Fig. 42-16D). This type of injury usually involves the common peroneal nerve and moderate-to-good recovery is reported at about 3 months.[6]

Another source of injury that cannot be ignored is pressure at the fibular head from heavy bulky dressings. Windowing of the dressings over the fibular head helps relieve pressure.

Occasionally patients with deep burns on the dorsum of the feet and ankles complain of numbness between the great and second toes. On examination, extensor digitorum brevis atrophy may be noted; otherwise, there is no weakness in the common peroneal distribution. The distal deep peroneal nerve at the anterior tarsal tunnel may be destroyed or may be compressed, causing these signs and symptoms.

Tourniquet Paralysis

Most articles on tourniquet paralysis usually begin with the statement "since the pneumatic tourniquet has been employed it has virtually eliminated the danger of nerve palsy." However, the pneumatic tourniquet used to establish a bloodless field has not prevented this complication to the extent reported. Aho and colleagues report that faulty gauges on pneumatic tourniquets can sometimes be the cause of the problem.[1] Tourniquet inflation to 500 mm Hg instead of the intended 250 mm Hg can cause direct pressure injury of the nerve at the cuff edge. The radial nerve is most vulnerable, but ulnar and median nerves can also be damaged. It is reported by Sunderland that the nerve lesions heal in 3 to 6 months and are only exceptionally permanently damaged.[39] In cases of paralysis, the tourniquet time has varied from 28 minutes to 2 hours and 40 minutes.[1, 7]

Peripheral Neuropathy

Generalized peripheral neuropathy is the most common peripheral neurological disorder seen in the burn patient. It usually occurs in patients with burns greater than 20% of the total body surface area with the exception of electrical injuries, in which the total body surface burn may be less. The incidence ranges from 15% as determined by Henderson, Koepke, and Feller, to 29% as reported by Helm and associates.[19, 20, 24] The etiology of peripheral neuropathies is uncertain; however, metabolic complications and neurotoxic drugs have been implicated. The patient may have symptoms of paresthesias and signs of mild to moderate weakness in the muscles of the distal extremities. On manual muscle testing, most patients eventually appear to recover their strength, although they complain of lack of endurance and easy fatigability for years post-burn.[19, 20, 24]

BONE AND JOINT CHANGES

Bone Growth

Growth disturbances in burns may be due to premature fusion of the entire epiphyseal plate or only a portion of the plate, and subsequent growth arrest.[27, 28] Premature fusion of the epiphyseal plate can cause bone shortening and should be a consideration in children who have scar tissue crossing joints, or especially who have persistent joint contractures. Partial epiphyseal plate fusion may cause bone deviation and deformity.[27, 28] Pressure treatment of scar tissue as reported by Leung and colleagues can cause regressed skeletal growth in the chin and thoracic cage from wearing a face mask and body suit. The face was noted to be "birdlike" due to the slow growing mandible and the thoracic cage developing a roundish appearance.[30] Shortened legs, hands, and feet have occurred (Fig. 42-17).

Growth stimulation has also been found by some investigators and is described as growth spurts in children and increased shoe size in adults. It is postulated that skeletal growth is stimulated through stasis or passive hyperemia or a chronic inflammatory process.

Figure 42-17.   Growth disturbance in a 56-year-old burned at age 6.

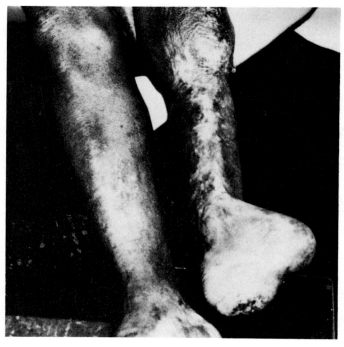

Osteophytes

Evans and Smith report that osteophytes are the most frequently observed skeletal alteration in adult burn patients. They are most often seen at the elbow and occur along the articular margins of the olecranon or coronoid process.[11, 13]

New Bone Formation

Heterotopic Ossification

New bone formation begins as heterotopic calcification and is seen on x-ray as a fluffy shadow. In at least 50% of patients this calcification will be absorbed; in the remainder it can ossify. Calcification and ossification have been reported to occur as early as 5 to 6 weeks post-burn, but usually develop in 3 to 4 months. Teperman and group reported that bone scans assist in making early diagnosis; in one patient the positive bone scan preceded positive radiological findings by 3 weeks. Rarely are there any detectable chemical changes by laboratory tests. One of the earliest signs of heterotopic ossification is loss of joint range of motion and this change can precede x-ray findings by 5 days.[40] The most common site involved is the elbow, followed by the hip in children and the shoulder in adults.

Patients who are predisposed for the development of heterotopic ossification are those with full-thickness burns to the upper extremities of greater than 20% total body surface area. Other commonalities for development are immobility, repeated minor trauma, and pressure (particularly over the medial epicondyle).

Once the diagnosis of heterotopic ossification has been made, forceful passive movements of the extremity are contraindicated because this type of exercise can make the condition worse. Only gentle movement within the patient's active range should be performed. Operative treatment is indicated if there is no spontaneous resolution of the heterotopic calcification. Most surgeons will not operate until the bone is mature, which can take 12 to 18 months. Incidence of true heterotopic ossification probably ranges between 0.1% and 3.1%.

Bony Changes in Electrical Burns

New bone formation at amputation sites in the electrical burn has been reported to involve long bones, or more specifically, above-elbow, below-elbow, above-knee and below-knee stumps (Fig. 42-18). Helm and colleagues reported 23 out of 28 long-bone amputations (82%) developed new bone at the amputation site.[21] Of the 61 amputations studied, 78% of upper extremity and 90% of lower extremity long-bone amputations had new bone formation. The average time from amputation to diagnosis of new bone was 38 weeks. Five patients (11.6%) required surgical revision of the stump and an additional 3 patients (7%) required replacement of their prosthesis secondary to new bone formation. It has not been determined what causes this high rate of new bone formation in the electrical amputee; however, it has been postulated that perhaps the effect of high voltage on bone is similar to long-term low voltage/amperage stimulation for promoting callous formation at fracture sites.[23]

Vrabec and Kolar studied bone changes in the electrical burn and described bony changes directly related to the action of the passage of electric current as osteochisis (bone split), "bone pearls" from the melting of bone minerals, bony necrosis, and periosteal new bone caused by inflammatory reaction as a result of avulsion of the periosteum. Other authors have reported lucent "holes" in the bone and bone swelling.[42]

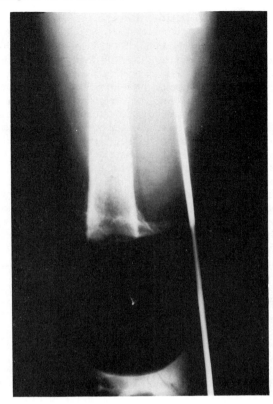

Figure 42-18.   Bone spur in an electrical burn, above-knee amputee.

Scoliosis and Kyphosis

Asymmetrical burns of the trunk, hips, and shoulder girdle can cause the patient to favor the side of the body burned and shift weight to the same side. A functional scoliosis can develop because of the pain in maintaining correct posture. A functional scoliosis can change to a structural scoliosis with vertebral wedging if a child has a growth spurt before this is corrected.[12] Burns on the anterior neck, shoulders, and chest wall may produce a rounding of the shoulders and sunken chest. This is caused by burn scar shortening and by the patient assuming a protective posture. The result can be a kyphotic thoracic spine if not corrected with proper exercise and positioning programs. Surgical excision of adherent scar tissue to the anterior chest wall is not usually successful for correcting this abnormality.

Septic Arthritis

Septic arthritis can easily be overlooked in the severe burn patient. Inability to make the diagnosis is due to lack of the usual clinical signs and symptoms. Some septic joints are pain-free and some are covered with burn wounds that mask the usual fusiform swelling and local tenderness.

The two primary causes of a septic joint in burns are penetrating burns into joints and bacteremia. Septic arthritis may cause gross dislocation because of capsular laxity, or cartilage and bone destruction,[11] or it may result in severe restriction of movement or ankylosis. It occurs most frequently in the hips, knees, wrists, and joints of the hands.

Subluxations and Dislocations

Joint subluxation in the hands and feet is commonly seen in burn patients. Generally the burn is over the dorsal aspect of the part, and as the burn wound contracts, it pulls the joint into hyperextension. If allowed to persist the joint will sublux. This is more commonly seen in the MCP and metatarsophalangeal (MTP) joints. An ulnar neuropathy can accentuate the problem in the fourth and fifth digits (Fig. 42-19). A hyperextended thumb at the MCP joint can also easily subluxate. Prevention in the hand begins in the acute phase of treatment by splinting the MCP joints in flexion to approximately 60° to 90°, thereby keeping the collateral ligament on a stretch. This is done in conjunction with an exercise program stressing joint flexion. The MTP joints of the toes become more of a problem post-healing as the burn scar contracts. Simple application of surgical high shoes with a metatarsal bar worn 24 hours a day keeps the toes in an anti-deformity position.

Hip dislocation can be a problem in children if the hip is allowed to remain in an adducted and flexed position. Shoulder dislocations are reported to occur in extreme positions of abduction and extension.

LONG-TERM REHABILITATION

The post-acute rehabilitative phase of treatment can be five to ten times longer than the acute phase of treatment, and it is during this period that the patient undergoes a multitude of physical and emotional changes. It is usually during this time that the patient and family realize how devastating this insult has been to the body. They frequently react in adverse ways that can affect outcome if proper support is not available. The physicians and therapists assume a new role when rehabilitation, rather than survival, is the primary issue.

Skin and Wound Care

Rarely does the patient leave the hospital with completely healed wounds and donor sites; therefore, continuation of the wound care program with hydrotherapy, debridement, and dressing changes is necessary. Once the wounds are healed, or there are only spotty areas open, hydrotherapy should be discontinued because of the ultimate drying effect on the skin. This will, in turn, cause the skin to crack and make it more susceptible to bacteria invasion.

Additional problems can occur post-healing such as skin breakdown, blistering, ulceration, and allergic reactions. Newly formed skin is especially fragile and even the slightest trauma, as from stretching exercises, pressure from splints and garments, or from minor bumps, can cause abrasions and blisters (Fig. 42-20). Blisters can be drained with a sterile needle and flattened with a dressing. If denuded areas are created by large blisters, mercurochrome is excellent for treatment. These areas will usually dry, crust, and heal. All open wounds, however, should be gently cleansed with a mild soap. Ulcerations or chronic open wounds have a tendency to develop in tight bands of scar tissue in the axilla and cubital and popliteal fossae. These wounds are generally deep and repeated splitting of the wounds with exercise prolongs healing and causes increased scarring. If the wound is clean, application of a biological dressing and placing the part at rest will speed the healing process.

Allergic reactions post-healing that produce moist, weeping wounds can be frustrating, since finding the irritating agent is sometimes difficult. The most common agents that cause these

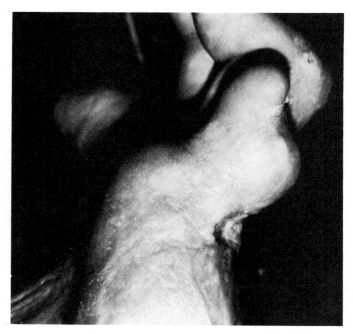

Figure 42-19.   Severe subluxation of fifth metacarpal joint.

Figure 42-20.   Fragile skin with multiple open wounds.

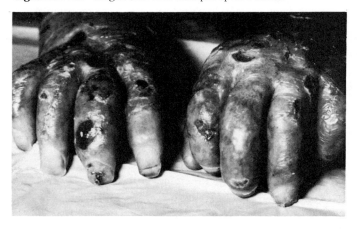

reactions have been skin lubricants (particularly those products with mineral oil), pressure garments, and various soaps used to cleanse the skin. All of these agents should be discontinued for 2 to 4 days before beginning substitution with different products, one at a time.

In the healed burn skin there is often lack of normal lubrication and suppleness. Dryness and decreased elasticity contribute to skin problems such as cracking, pruritis, and skin breakdown. Patients who are treated in settings where there is no hands-on technique suffer from hypersensitive skin and scar pain. Skin lubrication helps alleviate some of these problems and should be considered an essential part of the overall treatment program performed by the therapists. Massage of healed burn wounds can accomplish skin lubrication, decrease skin hypersensitivity, and increase skin pliability. A variety of lotions have been found to be nonirritating, as Aloe Vera moisturizers, vitamin E ointment, cocoa butter, and Corrective Concepts moisturizers. Pruritic symptoms frequently require oral antihistamine medication as well as pressure garments to make the patient more comfortable.[16]

Exercise

Techniques

Maintaining range of motion of a joint post-healing or post-grafting is more difficult than in the acute phase. Burn scars contract, form bands, and thicken, and joint range of motion is affected. Remolding of the burn scar is possible while the scar is actively undergoing internal changes, such as collagen degradation and deposition and myofibroblastic activity. Once the burn scar matures, stretching of skin contracture is of no benefit.

By far the most effective stretching technique for skin contractures is slow sustained stretch. The part being stretched should be visible and should be palpated along the line of pull to ensure that the skin does not rupture. Stretching can be done manually with weights, traction, and serial casting. The technique of applying paraffin to the part being mobilized and allowing 30 minutes of sustained stretch has been very rewarding in gaining range of motion; at the same time it decreases joint discomfort and lubricates the skin (Fig. 42-21). The paraffin temperature must be lowered to 116° to 118° Fahrenheit to prevent burning of hypesthetic skin.[17]

Another important principle in the exercise program is to put the entire length of a burn scar on a total stretch (Fig. 42-22). In other words, if a scar crosses multiple joints, all involved joints are stretched simultaneously. A joint does not have full range of motion unless full range is obtained in combined movements.

Finally, all patients should be on a generalized strengthening program for reconditioning after prolonged inactivity. Resistive exercises of opposing muscle groups are also beneficial in contracture prevention and treatment. Exercises for endurance and coordination are frequently overlooked in burn rehabilitation, but are an essential aspect of the total program.

Specialized Splinting

Without the benefit of custom-made splints, exercise programs would be in vain. A joint contracture may be stretched to full range, but maintaining that range is in part dependent on static and dynamic positioning accomplished with splinting. So often the mistake is made to splint joints in full extension for prolonged periods because the patient looks anatomically cor-

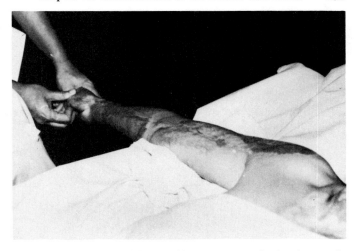

Figure 42-22. The total length of burn scar is involved in the stretch.

rect; however, function is sacrificed. This unfortunately is true especially for elbows, which are often placed in extension.

Experienced therapists are able to make splints that control more than one joint and, at the same time, apply pressure over thick bands of scar tissue. Major areas of concern in the convalescent period are hands. Difficult areas requiring specialized splints are

Palmar contractures (Fig. 42-23C and D)
Cupping of the palm (Fig. 42-23E)
Fifth-digit flexion contracture (Fig. 42-23H)
Tight thumb–index web space (Fig. 42-23I)
Ruptured extensor hood mechanism
Neck flexion contracture
Hip flexion-abduction external rotation in children
Ankle-dorsiflexion contractures

There is another area of major concern, yet no effective splint has yet been devised, and that is for pronation contractures of the forearm. As mentioned earlier, serial casting or serial splinting can be extremely effective in reducing contractures. The more common splints need not be addressed since their indications are obvious.

Modalities

There are certain modalities commonly used in rehabilitation medicine clinics that have been found useful in treating specific burn complications.

Electrical stimulation, using an alternating current, is helpful in treating tendon adherence to underlying scar tissue. Bipolar, pulsed, or surged alternating current helps reduce edema and increases joint range of motion. The transcutaneous electrical stimulator is useful for treatment of various pain problems, particularly those involving the shoulder from prolonged or faulty positioning.

Ultrasound for treatment of painful joints of the hands makes the patient much more comfortable and thus makes it easier to tolerate exercises. In our experience, ultrasound to the elbow has not been beneficial for heterotopic calcification. Ice massage, combined with ultrasound, decreases hypertrophic scar pain. Painful scar tissue is generally located over the lateral chest wall, medial arm, and volar wrist.

Figure 42-21. Sustained stretch to gain range of motion.

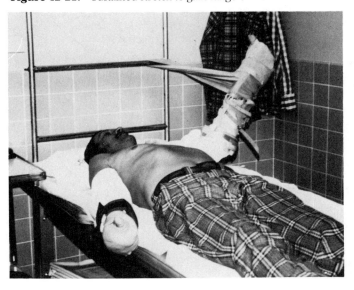

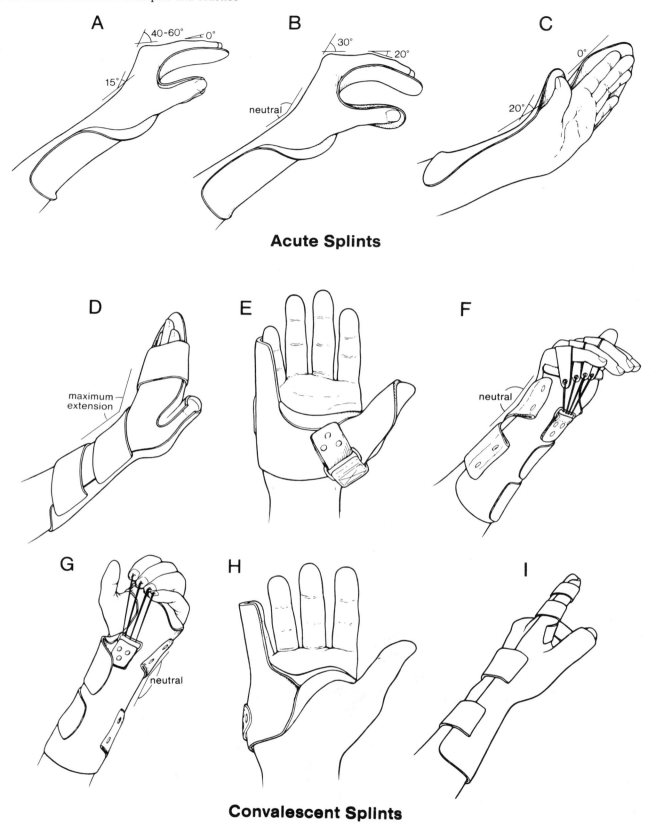

Acute Splints

Convalescent Splints

Figure 42-23.   Common hand splints. (Helm PA, et al: Burn injury: Rehabilitation management in 1982. Arch Phys Med Rehabil 63:6–16, 1982)

Intermittent compression units or similar devices are valuable in reducing edema in extremities, primarily the edematous hand. Post-healing hand edema, secondary to circumferential burns of the forearm, hands with reflex sympathetic dystrophy, and hands with post-ischemic hand syndrome, usually respond well with elevation and compression. Persistent edema can be devastating, if allowed to persist, since it can result in a "frozen hand."

Continuous passive motion (CPM) machines can never take the place of the hands-on exercises by the therapists. Occasionally CPM is indicated when the patient is resistant to the exercise program from fear of pain, in children who seem to relax better with CPM, and in those who need additional range-of-motion treatments for exceptionally tight areas.

Biofeedback has been used with success for relaxation purposes in those patients with sleep disorders, which is often the case for burn patients. Amputees with phantom pain have also responded to this type of treatment. It continues to be useful in burns, as in other types of patients, for muscle re-education following a neurological insult.

Burn Sequelae

Hypertrophic Scarring

It is well known that hypertrophic scar and scar contracture can result from deep partial- and full-thickness burns. An excellent review on hypertrophic scarring and the effects of pressure was done by Jensen and Parshley.[29] They reported on areas of the skin affected by the scar, noting that the epidermis was not thickened and did not contribute to the depth of the hypertrophic scar. They also reported

> the regenerated epidermis lacks rete pegs and interconnections that attach it to the dermis; hence it is cosmetically abnormal with respect to color, texture, and friability and is prone to abrasion with minor trauma.[29]

They noted that changes in the dermis involving fibroblasts, myofibroblasts, mast cells, collagen, mucopolysaccharides, and vasculature cause a metabolically active abnormal mass of thick tissue. In hypertrophic scars collagen forms large nodules rather than loose wavy bundles as seen in normal dermis. In granulation tissue and hypertrophic scars, capillaries proliferate and are thought to have a mediating effect on hypertrophic scar formation. The mechanism for contraction of hypertrophic scar is thought to be the myofibroblast.[29]

It has been known for years that external pressure in the form of special garments that provide at least 25 mm Hg or more of pressure (above capillary pressure) can flatten scar tissue if worn continuously until the scars lose redness and soften. It is postulated that pressure inhibits blood flow with occlusion of vessels in the scar affecting fibroblastic activity and reduces tissue water content, thereby reducing the amount of ground substance. Prolonged pressure may also have detrimental effects; therefore, one should be certain there are indications for its use. Burn scars that lose their redness within 8 to 10 weeks may not become hypertrophic.

Other Residual Defects

After the surgeon has completed all of the reconstructive procedures and the patient is, from a medical standpoint, totally rehabilitated, there are certain residual defects that affect the remainder of the burn patient's life (Table 42-2). These range

Table 42-2
Burn Sequelae

Defect	Cause
Hypopigmentation, hyperpigmentation	Melanin abnormality and donor site choice
Sensory impairment	Sensory nerve fibers fail to penetrate thick scar tissue
	Damaged in full-thickness burns
Abormal skin lubrication	Loss of sebaceous glands due to depth of burn
	Unable to penetrate heavy scar
Abnormal hair growth	Hair follicle damage
	Cannot penetrate thick scar
Abormal sweating, heat intolerance	Loss of sweat glands due to depth of burn
Cold intolerance	Abnormal vasomotor response
Pruritis	Dry skin from lack of lubrication
Fragile Skin	Loss of normal elasticity; thin
Ingrown hairs, pustules	Hair cannot penetrate thick scar and becomes infected
Permanent tanning	If exposed to direct sunlight before 12–18 months post-born
Marjolin's ulcer	Chronic recurring ulcers
	Poorly nourished scar tissue
Calloused feet (Fig. 42-24)	Deep excision of feet
	Skin adherence to bone
	Bony abnormality
Cosmesis	Permanent scarring
	Flattened facies
	Body part amputated
Joint pain	Repeated minor trauma to hands and knees
	Joint pinning
Psychological, social	All of the above
Fatigability	
Lack of endurance	

from sensory impairment, cold intolerance, and calloused feet (Fig. 42-24) to social and psychological problems.

Disability Determination

The rating of permanent impairment is a physician's function and is an appraisal of the nature and extent of the patient's illness or injury as it affects performance. Permanent disability is not a purely medical condition, but is based on a person's impairment and multiple psychosocial and economic factors. The evaluation of disability is much more complex and factors such as age, sex, education, economics, and social relationships are involved.

The evaluation of the burn victim requires the physician to consider such unique factors as heat and cold intolerance, sensitivity to sunlight, pain, chemical sensitivity, changes in apocrine function, and objective findings of decreased coordination, sensation, strength, and contractures. If scars affect sweat glands, hair growth, nail growth, or range of motion, they may affect performance and cause impairment. Every state as well as private and governmental agencies have different criteria on which to base impairment ratings. However, utilizing the generally accepted methods of evaluating impairment as well as considering

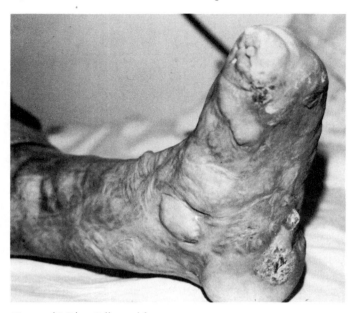

Figure 42-24. Calloused foot.

the unique factors of the burn patient, the physician may, with relative objectivity, establish an impairment rating.[2]

The physician has the ultimate responsibility in deciding when the burn patient is medically capable of returning to work and some unique factors must be considered. Open wounds in employees involved in food handling should not be allowed. In other management areas, open wounds can be aggravated by irritants and dirt or constant friction or pressure on the skin, and the employee should refrain from any duties which inhibit wound closure. New immature skin is delicate and fragile, and laborers, especially those with hand burns, can easily reinjure freshly burned skin. Cold intolerance is a very common problem after thermal injury and employees working in cold climates or refrigerated areas may be unable to tolerate the discomfort and be unable to perform job responsibilities.[15]

Psychological Aspects of Burn Care

A major burn represents both a physical and psychological trauma to the individual. Alterations in appearance and function after the injury are apparent, both in terms of incidence and their implications. Less apparent, however, is the emotional impact of severe, sudden stress followed by an often long and extremely painful recovery process. Well over half of the burn patients develop severe emotional consequences after a major burn.[5]

Post-traumatic stress disorder is quite common among burn patients. Some characteristics of stress disorder are re-experiencing the trauma through vivid intrusive recollections or dreams, exaggerated startle response, numbing of responsiveness to the outside world, problems with memory and concentration, avoidance of cues associated with the burn, and intensified distress when reminded of the burn.[3] If the individual with stress disorder was injured in a work setting, returning to the same work situation may be difficult or impossible because of the emotional reaction from cues associated with the burn. Psychological treatment processes designed to help the individual to define the experience in a way such that he or she would experience the least trauma and consequently the most control over the outcome are critical in the rehabilitation process. Stress and pain

reduction mechanisms such as relaxation or hypnosis can help the individual experience less pain, and subsequently less trauma, with reduced long-term psychological effects. Behavior management strategies are employed to maximize patient control over his or her own treatment, improve therapy compliance, and reduce psychological trauma. Goal-directed individual and group psychotherapy are also beneficial.

Attention must be devoted to the milieu in which treatment is administered. The patient uses cues in the burn care setting to determine how he or she defines the experience. These cues are associated both with staff and other patients' behavior. Other patients screaming in pain or a staff nurse who shows signs of tension while approaching a dressing change can serve to sensitize the patient to the upcoming procedure. Both staff and patients benefit from increased control of the situation.

Provision of adequate levels and appropriate types of medication as well as the use of behavioral management strategies on the part of the burn staff can assist greatly to diminish the amount of distress and pain. Giving patients choices among acceptable alternatives with regard to medication is also helpful. Use of additional pre-procedure medications on a routine basis helps to further diminish the pain and trauma sensitization, while allowing the patient periods of greater alertness during other times of the day. The patient will have more self-control and greater participation in the rehabilitation process, and involving the patient in as many decisions as possible serves to minimize any sense of passivity or helplessness. It also sets the stage for assumption of more and more control and active participation in the rehabilitation process. A growing body of research shows that active psychological intervention on the part of the psychologist as well as the burn unit personnel and rehabilitation staff is critical in the patient's recovery.[41] Patients who receive instructions on how to cope with pain and stress of a burn do substantially better in terms of a sense of psychological well-being and sense of control over the outcome of their injuries.

REFERENCES

1. Aho K, Sainio K, Kianta M, Varpanen F: Pneumatic tourniquet paralysis: Case report. J Bone Joint Surg 65B:441–443, 1983
2. American Medical Association's Council on Scientific Affairs: Guide to the Evaluation of Permanent Impairment. Chicago, American Medical Association, 1984
3. American Psychiatric Association: Diagnostic and Statistical Manual of Mental Disorders, 3rd ed. Washington, DC, 1980
4. Artz CP: Electrical injury. In Artz CP, Moncrief J, Pruitt BA Jr (eds): Burns: A Team Approach, pp 351–362. Philadelphia, WB Saunders, 1979
5. Avni J: Severe burns. Adv Psychosom Med 1:57–77, 1980
6. Berry H, Richardson PM: Common peroneal nerve palsy: A clinical and electrophysiological review. J Neurosurg Psychiatry 39:1162–1171, 1976
7. Bruner JM: Safety factors in the use of the pneumatic tourniquet for hemostasis in surgery of the hand. J Bone Joint Surg 33A:221–224, 1951
8. Dhuner KG: Nerve injuries following operations: A survey of cases occurring during a six-year period. Anesthesiology 11:289–293, 1950
9. Dimick AR: Debridement: Surgical, mechanical, and biochemical. In Dimick AR (ed): Practical Approaches to Burn Management, pp 21–26. Deerfield, Flint Laboratories, Division of Travenol Laboratories, 1977
10. Dimick AR: Pathophysiology. In Fisher SV, Helm PA (eds): Comprehensive Rehabilitation of Burns, pp 9–15. Baltimore, Williams & Wilkins, 1984
11. Evans EB: Bone and joint changes secondary to burns. In Lewis SR (ed): Symposium on the Treatment of Burns, pp 76–78. St Louis, CV Mosby, 1973

12. Evans EB: Scoliosis and kyphosis. In Feller I, Crabb WC: Reconstruction and Rehabilitation of the Burned Patient, p 264. Ann Arbor, National Institute for Burn Medicine, 1979

13. Evans EB, Smith JR: Bone and joint changes following burns: A roentgenographic study—preliminary report. J Bone Joint Surg 41A:785–799, 1959

14. Ewing MR: Postoperative paralysis in the upper extremity: Report of five cases. Lancet 1:99–103, 1950

15. Fisher SV: Disability determination. In Fisher SV, Helm PA (eds): Comprehensive Rehabilitation of Burns, pp 401–411. Baltimore, Williams & Wilkins, 1984

16. Head MD: Wound and skin care. In Fisher SV, Helm PA (eds): Comprehensive Rehabilitation of Burns, pp 148–176. Baltimore, Williams & Wilkins, 1984

17. Head M, Helm P: Paraffin and sustained stretching in the treatment of burn contracture. Burns 4:136–139, 1977

18. Heimbach DM, Engrav LH: Surgical Management of the Burn Wound. New York, Raven Press, 1984

19. Helm PA: Neuromuscular considerations. In Fisher SV, Helm PA (eds): Comprehensive Rehabilitation of Burns, pp 235–241. Baltimore, Williams & Wilkins, 1984

20. Helm PA, Johnson ER, Carlton AM: Peripheral neurological problems in the acute burn patient. Burns 3:123–125, 1977

21. Helm PA, Kevorkian GC, Lushbaugh MS et al: Burn injury: Rehabilitation management in 1982. Arch Phys Med Rehabil 63:6–16, 1982

22. Helm PA, Pandian G, Heck E: Neuromuscular problems in the burn patient: Cause and prevention. Arch Phys Med Rehabil 66:451–453, 1985

23. Helm PA, Walker SC: New bone formation at amputation sites in electrically burn-injured patients. Arch Phys Med Rehabil 68:284–286, 1987

24. Henderson B, Koepke GH, Feller I: Peripheral polyneuropathy among patients with burns. Arch Phys Med Rehabil 52:149–151, 1971

25. Hunt JL: Electrical injuries. In Fisher SV, Helm PA (eds): Comprehensive Rehabilitation of Burns, pp 249–266. Baltimore, Williams & Wilkins, 1984

26. Hunt JL et al: The pathophysiology of acute electrical injuries. J Trauma 16:335–340, 1976

27. Jackson DM: Destructive burns: Some orthopaedic complications. Burns 7:105–122, 1980

28. Jackson L, Keats AS: Mechanism of brachial plexus palsy following anesthesia. Anesthesiology 26:190–194, 1965

29. Jensen LL, Parshley PF: Postburn scar contractures: Histology and effects of pressure treatment. J Burn Care Rehabil 5:119–123, 1984

30. Leung KS, Cheng JCY, Ma GFY et al: Complications of pressure therapy for post-burn hypertrophic scars: Biochemical analysis based on 5 patients. Burns 10:434–438, 1984

31. Mant MJ, O'Brien BD, Thong KL et al: Haemorrhagic complications of heparin therapy. Lancet 1:1133–1135, 1977

32. Meier RH III: Amputation and prosthetic fitting. In Fisher SV, Helm PA (eds): Comprehensive Rehabilitation of Burns, pp 267–310. Baltimore, Williams & Wilkins, 1984

33. Nothdurft D, Smith PS, LeMaster JE: Exercise and Treatment Modalities. In Fisher SV, Helm PA (eds): Comprehensive Rehabilitation of Burns, pp 96–147. Baltimore, Williams & Wilkins, 1984

34. Pullium GF: Splinting and positioning. In Fisher SV, Helm PA (eds): Comprehensive Rehabilitation of Burns, pp 64–95. Baltimore, Williams & Wilkins, 1984

35. Rask MR: Suprascapular nerve entrapment: A report of two cases treated with suprascapular notch resection. Clin Orthop 123:73–75, 1977

36. Reinstein L, Alevizatos AC, Twardzik FG, DeMarco SJ: Femoral nerve dysfunction after retroperitoneal hemorrhage: Pathophysiology revealed by computed tomography. Arch Phys Med Rehabil 65:37–40, 1984

37. Robson M: Synthetic burn dressings: Round table discussion. J Burn Care Rehabil 6:66–73, 1985

38. Solem LD: Classification. In Fisher SV, Helm PA (eds): Comprehensive Rehabilitation of Burns, pp 9–15. Baltimore, Williams & Wilkins, 1984

39. Sunderland S: Nerves and Nerve Injuries. Edinburgh and London, F & S Livingstone, 1968

40. Teperman PS, Hilbert L, Peters WJ, Pritzker KPH: Heterotopic ossification in burns. J Burn Care Rehabil 5:283–287, 1984

41. Tobiasen JM, Hiebert JM: Burns and adjustment to injury: Do psychological coping strategies help? J Trauma 25:1151–1155, 1985

42. Vrabec R, Kolar J: Bone changes caused by electric current. In Transactions of the Fourth International Congress of Plastic and Reconstructive Surgery, Rome, 1967, pp 215–217. Amsterdam, Excerpta Medica, 1969

43. Wadsworth TG: The external compression syndrome of the ulnar nerve at the cubital tunnel. Clin Orthop 124:189–204, 1977

43

Rehabilitation of the Injured Athlete

Jeffrey A. Saal

The field of sports medicine is new terrain for the modern physiatrist. Historically, the orthopedic contribution to sports medicine came almost exclusively from surgical practitioners, and only recently have physiatrists shown a growing involvement and interest in the area of rehabilitative care of injured athletes. By virtue of the physiatrist's background and training, he or she becomes an ideal practitioner of sports medicine. The physiatrist must apply his background and knowledge in anatomy and pathophysiology of musculoskeletal injury and combine this with an understanding of modern rehabilitative procedures.

Experience is the other extremely important ingredient. To successfully treat and rehabilitate the injured athlete, the physiatrist needs to be familiar with treating a variety of athletes at varying levels of competition. For instance, it is extremely difficult to treat the injured tennis player if one is not well versed in the biomechanics of the tennis serve and the mechanical characteristics of the equipment in use. It is, therefore, imperative for the physiatrist with an interest in sports medicine to develop a knowledge base of the biomechanics of running, throwing, swimming, and jumping.[150] This, in combination with the knowledge of musculoskeletal biomechanics, will establish minimum requirements for beginning to treat the injured athlete. Practical experience can be gained by working with local teams and participating in sports injury clinics.

The responsibility of the sports medicine practitioner also includes education and dissemination of pertinent information to the community. This involves community-level education in injury prevention, proper equipment selection, and the counseling of young athletes with respect to proper training methods and the use and abuse of ergogenic aids. The diagnosis, treatment, and rehabilitation of the injured athlete has widespread implications to all segments of society. It should not be looked on as a trivial matter, nor as a matter which only affects elite athletes.

REHABILITATION GOALS

Goal setting is an important aspect of rehabilitative care. In the field of athletic medicine, goals can be defined based upon the type of injury and the competition level of the injured athlete. The first competition level is recreational athletics. Those who engage in recreational athletics can be subdivided into the occasional recreational athlete, such as the individual who runs two

or three times a week or plays tennis two or three times a week but does not compete in formal events. The second category of recreational athlete is the competitive recreational athlete. This is an individual who is a serious athlete involved in continual training to improve performance while competing in races or matches and whose needs and desires to return to competition are extremely high.

The third level of competition is the institutional level. This is subcategorized into the high school athlete and the university level athlete. These athletes have commitments to their institution and to their team. They are extremely motivated to improve and are on tight training schedules due to their athletic and academic calendars. Decisions regarding care must consider these scheduling needs and must also consider the school seniority status of the competitor. The college senior who is participating in his last year of a sport with no intention of continuing in the professional ranks would obviously have a different goal than an individual who is a junior in high school fighting very hard for a collegiate scholarship.

The professional athlete is involved at a unique level of competition. In this arena, the athlete has many pressures to perform and continue to participate at a high level of efficiency. Team sports such as baseball, basketball, and football have organized sports medicine programs for the team members. The nonaligned athlete such as track and field participants, tennis players, and motorcycle racers do not have organized health care and usually pursue their care on an individual basis.

The last category of competition level is the Olympic athlete. This is a special individual who has chosen to put aside other goals and endeavors to participate in the Olympic competition. These individuals do not always have financial support and often do not even have medical insurance. The donation of time and effort can be a rewarding experience both for the athlete and the sports medicine physician. Olympic athletes have only one opportunity to perform. This performance must be at the ultimate level attainable by that individual. The rehabilitation goals for these individuals, therefore, are geared toward the one moment of truth.

Age and sex categories of the athletic participants also are worthy of consideration in planning treatment goals and strategies. The pediatric athlete has specific physiological as well as emotional needs which must be dealt with in the rehabilitative care plan.[75, 86] The geriatric population continues to participate in many athletic endeavors, most frequently tennis, golf, and walking. Their rehabilitation should also be goal oriented, to allow them the opportunity to maintain health and fitness through these exercise programs. The woman athlete has special problems, specifically bone mineralization and endocrinological disorders.[16, 66] The former may predispose the woman athlete to stress fractures and overuse injuries. Both factors must be taken into consideration in her rehabilitative care. Specific questions regarding exercise during pregnancy and the postnatal periods must also be considered.[127]

PATHOPHYSIOLOGY OF INJURY AND HEALING

The Inflammatory Process

An adequate understanding of how injuries affect living tissue and how healing occurs is extremely important. During the first 7 days following an injury the acute inflammatory process is in full swing. Hemorrhage and infiltration of cellular elements occur at a rapid pace. This period should be looked upon as a productive phase and should not be unduly interrupted.

The chemical mediators of the inflammatory response set the stage for the development of pain, effusion, and edema. The chemical mediators of the inflammatory response can be divided into three categories. The first category is vasoactive substances, which cause vasodilation and increased vascular permeability. These substances affect the contractile elements in the endothelial and periendothelial cells, leading to dilation of the vessels and opening of the junctions between cells in the post-capillary venules, causing edema. Examples of vasoactive substances are histamine, anaphylatoxins, kinins, and prostaglandins. Histamine, stored in basophils and tissue mast cells, is released by the interaction of antigen and IgE with these cells during immediate hypersensitivity reactions.

Anaphylatoxins are polypeptide fragments derived from the complement components of C3 and C4. These components are potent mediators of vascular permeability and, therefore, enhance edema formation. Kinins are best represented by bradykinin, which has the ability to stimulate histamine release from mast cells and to stimulate prostaglandin synthesis in a variety of tissues. Kallikreins cleave bradykinin to form precursor kininogens in plasma while also activating plasminogen to form plasmin.

Prostaglandins are a group of compounds derived from polyunsaturated fatty acids. The most important prostaglandins are of the II series which are derived from arachidonic acid, a component of the phospholipid present in all cell membranes. The prostaglandins cause vasodilation and potentiate edema induced by other agents and sensitize tissue to painful stimuli. They also act synergistically with other mediators such as bradykinin and histamine. The synthesis of prostaglandins is inhibited by anti-inflammatory drugs. Corticosteroids of the glucocorticoid variety are the most potent inhibitors of prostaglandin synthesis. The potency of prostaglandin synthesis inhibition by glucocorticoids parallels the relative inflammatory potency of these drugs. Dexamethasone has greater capability than prednisolone, which in turn has a greater capability than hydrocortisone. The potent anti-inflammatory effect of glucocorticoids appears to be based not only upon inhibition of prostaglandin synthesis, but on several other mechanisms as well.[63]

The second category of chemical mediators of the inflammatory process are chemotactic factors, which cause increased cell motility and direct cell movement to the inflammatory focus.

The third category are degradative enzymes that are released in inflammatory exudates. They catalyze the hydrolysis of tissue components, including proteins, carbohydrates, and lipids.[63]

The initial phases of the inflammatory response are reparative and necessary. However, continuation of the initial inflammatory response past the initial healing phases can be destructive and, therefore, deleterious to the ultimate outcome. The goal of initial rehabilitative procedures is to help limit and curtail the inflammatory response and work on the sequelae of pain, effusion, and immobility.

The next 2 weeks following injury, days 7 through 21, are marked by collagen proliferation produced by the newly infiltrated fibroblasts and cellular fibrin matrix. The collagen fibers are initially laid down in a random pattern. Unless specific stresses are placed upon the healing tissue to force the tissue to comply with Wolff's law, the newly produced collagen will become useless scar tissue.[1, 2] Stretching of the collagen tissue will force the collagen fibrils to become aligned in an organized pattern and, therefore, enhance range of motion and limit exuberant and unnecessary scar formation.[3] Elastin fibers, which are the most prominent component of ligaments (70% to 80% of the dry weight of the ligamentum nuchae), serve an important role in the maintenance of the tensile strength of tissue.[205] Stretching of ligamentous tissue has been demonstrated to cause proliferation of elastin fibrils, whereas ligamentous tissue that has been immobilized has an absence of elastin fibrils and therefore poor tensile strength.[3, 28, 152]

Loss of strength secondary to immobility and injury is a well-recognized phenomenon.[17, 18, 147] It should be noted that inflammation and joint effusion are also important inhibitors of muscle strength and can cause rapid atrophy of juxta-articular musculature.[44, 55] This loss of strength will lead to delays in the rehabilitation process and ultimately to delays in returning the athlete to participation.

Several key points can be garnered from an understanding of the inflammatory process and its sequelae. First, the initial phase of healing following the injury is an extremely important restorative process. If this initial phase of biochemical restoration is inappropriately shortened by the early injudicious use of corticosteroids, normal tissue healing will not occur.[113, 192] This can secondarily lead to weakened support structures and prolonged disability. However, if the initial phase is prolonged, it will lead to excessive edema and scar formation as well as pain, loss of motion, and weakness. Nonsteroidal anti-inflammatory agents introduced within 24 hours of an ankle inversion injury have been demonstrated to speed the rehabilitation process and not adversely affect the mechanical integrity of tissue.[205]

The second key point concerns the proliferative phase of the inflammatory process. Early mobilization during this phase will enhance normal collagen and elastin fiber deposition. This early mobilization will also lead to strengthening of tendons and ligaments.[195, 196] If the patient is immobilized throughout this phase, soft tissue contracture will occur as well as poor nutrition to intra-articular tissues.[1] Therefore, shortening of the proliferative phase sets the stage for beginning functional rehabilitation.

Potential Sites of Injury

Mechanism of Injury

To formulate the care plan, the physiatrist must understand the types of specific injuries and their effect upon performance. The nuances of the rehabilitation plan as it relates to these particular injuries must be appreciated as well.

The mechanism of sports-related injury can be divided into three categories. The first category is *overuse*. The common factor in overuse injuries is repetitive microtrauma to a particular anatomic structure.[11] Frictional forces, tractional forces, and cyclical loading forces can cause secondary inflammation of involved structures resulting in pain and disability. An example of frictional forces would be bursal inflammation over a bony prominence. An example of tractional forces would be the development of plantar fasciitis in a runner.[42] An example of cyclical loading of impact forces would be a lower extremity stress fracture.[136]

The second mechanism of sports-related injury is *direct contact*. An obvious example of this would be an acromioclavicular joint separation in a football player secondary to direct impact to the shoulder girdle.

A third category is *soft tissue failure*. A single violent muscular contraction or effort can injure a structure without specific overuse and without any contact; examples of this would be a pulled hamstring and an Achilles tendon rupture.

Specific Structures

LIGAMENTS. Ligaments are designed to prevent the occurrence of excessive or abnormal movements at joints and bony articulations. Ligament tissue is tough and unyielding but, at the same time, flexible enough to offer no resistance to normal movement. The collagen fibers in ligament tissue are arranged in semi-regular bundles (in contrast to tendons which are regular). Ligaments may contain variable amounts of elastin fibers for flexibility. Each synovial joint possesses a fibrous capsule, which consists of parallel interlacing bundles of ligament tissue. The fibrous capsules often possess two or more localized thickenings in which the fiber bundles are parallel to one another, forming collateral ligamentous structures. Additionally, some joints have accessory ligaments to act as collaterals to restrain excessive and unwanted motion.[28]

An overload placed on a ligament can cause tearing of the structure. Depending on the degree of abnormal movement and the force and time period by which it is applied, varying amounts of tearing can occur.[156] Ligament injuries are graded from I to III.[5, 32] The grade I injury is basically a stretch injury with no significant consequent instability. The grade II injury causes greater disruption of the ligament architecture and will cause a low degree of instability. The grade III injury constitutes a total tear of the structure and, as a consequence, joint instability of a greater degree. Degrees of instability can be appreciated on physical examination, and there exists a specific test for instability at the knee, ankle, elbow, wrist, and shoulder.[49, 94, 95, 168] Occasionally, stress x-ray views or examination under anesthesia is necessary to establish a precise diagnosis of instability.[106]

Ligament injuries are extremely common; 42% of sports-related knee injuries are ligamentous in nature[60] (Table 43-1). Ligamentous injuries of the ankle are the most common type of sports injury.[49]

An inversion ankle sprain causing stretch of the anterior talofibular ligament is an example of a common grade I ligamentous injury. If the inversion sprain is severe, this can manifest itself as a grade II or even a grade III lesion. A valgus injury to the knee causing a medial collateral ligament injury, with a physical examination finding of 5° to 15° of laxity noted on valgus stress testing with the knee at 30° of flexion, would constitute a grade II injury. A noncontact torsional injury to the knee causing an isolated total tear of the anterior cruciate ligament with the consequent finding of a positive Lachman's test on physical examination is an example of a grade III ligamentous lesion.[120] Grade I lesions will cause pain and usually only low levels of soft tissue swelling and joint effusion. The grade II and III lesions will cause greater degrees of swelling of soft tissues and greater joint

Table 43-1
Common Sports-Related Ligament Injuries

Upper Extremity
  Ulnar collateral, elbow
  Carpal ligaments
  Shoulder capsule

Lower Extremity
  Ankle
  Lateral ligaments
  Medial ligaments
  Knee
  Medial collateral ligament
  Lateral collateral ligament
  Anterior cruciate ligament
  Posterior cruciate ligament

effusion. Instability is not a characteristic of grade I lesions due to the remaining integrity of the ligamentous and capsular structures.

Grade II lesions will cause a slight degree of instability, which the patient will often note and find uncomfortable. Grade II lesions, therefore, will often need some external support during the rehabilitation phase. An example of a grade II ligamentous injury that necessitates external support during the rehabilitation process is injury of the medial collateral ligament of the knee. During the rehabilitation process, a hinged cast brace can be used to facilitate stability and allow ligament healing while permitting the patient to participate in a graded exercise program. Grade II lesions may also necessitate some external support after the rehabilitation process when resuming sport competition.[190]

A joint that sustains a grade III ligamentous injury will be frankly unstable.[94, 95] This structure will need constant support until the ligamentous structure can be reconstructed, reconstituted, or substituted for by external support mechanisms.[155] The individual who suffers an anterior cruciate ligament injury who elects not to undergo a primary or secondary reconstruction of the anterior cruciate ligament and associated capsular injuries will need an external support to limit rotational instability.[69, 131]

The same forces that disrupt ligaments can also damage the internal articular structures. Therefore, it is imperative to look for associated joint injuries and internal derangements which may have occurred at the same time as the ligamentous injury.[45] For example, ignoring an osteochondral fracture of the talar dome in an individual who has sustained an ankle inversion injury will delay the institution of the proper care plan.

When planning the rehabilitation of ligamentous injuries, one should take into consideration the degree of ligamentous injury as well as the level of competition of the injured athlete.[133] Stability and maintenance of range of motion as well as strengthening of juxta-articular musculature and improvement of proprioceptive responses are necessary components of the treatment program. The specific aspects of the treatment program will be discussed later in this chapter.

TENDONS. The intrinsic properties of the tendon unit facilitate movement. Based upon their tensile strength (which is one-half that of steel) and their ability to absorb contractile energy from the working muscle unit, tendons form an integral part of the locomotive network. Collagen fibers of the tendon unit are arranged in regular bundles. Areolar tissue (loose connective tissue) permeates the tendon fascicles and allows the ingrowth of vasculature and nerve supply. The condensing of this connective tissue on the surface of the tendon forms the epitendineum or so-called tendon sheath. Tendons are rather flexible and can be angulated around bony surfaces and under retinaculae to affect the final direction of pull on the musculotendinous unit. Tendon synovial sheaths occur when tendons must pass underneath ligamentous bands and retinacular fibro-osseous tunnels.[56] The synovial sheaths are double-walled with a thin film of synovial fluid in the cavity. Some tendons, such as the Achilles tendon, only contain a mesotendineum, which is the coalescence of the two sheath layers into a single unit.[121] The vascular supply of the tendon unit is precarious and is often implicated as a major causative factor in injuries of the supraspinatus tendon and Achilles tendon.[188] Tendon calcification appears to occur at these zones, theoretically due to tissue hypoxia.[200]

Most tendon injuries are secondary to overuse. Repetitive frictional and tractional forces placed upon the tendon unit contribute to the insult. Fatigue of the muscle unit with secondary alteration in biomechanical efficiency as well as loss of muscle shock absorption also contribute to injury development. These injuries will promote tendon swelling and, secondarily, abnormal gliding of these previously flexible structures.[11, 86] Adhesions can develop within the synovial sheath causing crepitation, which can often be heard by both the examiner and the patient (termed *tenosynovitis*). De Quervain's stenosing tenosynovitis commonly occurs in rowers. Limitation of articular motion will often occur as a consequence both of pain and of shortening of the tendon unit.

Poor flexibility and poor absolute and endurance strength of the muscles attached to the tendon unit have been implicated as causative factors in the development of tendon injuries.[56, 151, 167] Primary tendon degeneration can also occur and present as tendinitis. Degenerative tendinopathy appears to be a distinct pathological entity, with poor correlation to overuse and the development of this condition.[109] Crystal-induced inflammation has also been implicated as a potential cause of this condition. Tendon rupture occurs most frequently at sites of degenerative changes within the tendon substance. These degenerative changes may be related to primary degenerative tendinopathy or degenerative alteration of the microstructure due to previous

injury or of the peripheral zones surrounding primary calcifying tendinopathy.[200]

Tendon injuries can occur as a secondary mechanism as the tendon unit tries to protect an injured joint. Successful treatment will, therefore, necessitate accurately diagnosing and treating the primary joint pathology. The biomechanical derangement of other joints in the kinetic chain will often be causative factors in injury. For example, a baseball pitcher may change his delivery motion due to a rotator cuff injury and secondarily injure his elbow.[169]

Pain and low-grade swelling of the soft tissues without joint effusions, along with the loss of normal flexibility with the preservation of stability, are the manifestations of tendon injuries. Tendon injuries are extremely common in the athletic population. The most common locations for tendon injuries are the Achilles tendon and the wrist extensor tendons originating at the elbow[31, 151] (Table 43-2).

When planning the treatment and rehabilitation of tendon injuries, the primary goals are reduction of pain, swelling, and inflammation. Surgical consultation should be sought in cases of tendon rupture. The judicious use of flexibility and strengthening programs are paramount. Careful instruction of the injured athlete regarding proper equipment selection, maintenance exercises, as well as pre- and post-activity flexibility programs are important treatment principles.[188]

BURSAE. Bursae occur in the same anatomical circumstances as tendon sheaths. The bursa is simply a flattened sac of synovial membrane supported by dense irregular connective tissue. Its function is to create an environment of discontinuity between opposing structures in order to facilitate low-friction, free movement.

The same type of injury pattern that can cause damage to the tendon structures will also cause injury to the bursae. The inflamed bursa will increase the friction in the movement plane with resultant pain and motion loss. If the bursa is situated close to the body surface, then actual swelling can be appreciated on physical examination. Bursal inflammation is a component of the so-called shoulder impingement syndrome, either as a primary or secondary effect.[87, 114, 168] Excessive friction and traction upon the rotator cuff and its associated subacromial bursa can lead to

Table 43-2
Tendon Injury in Sport

Site	Sport	Motion Type
Rotator cuff	Baseball, tennis	Throwing
Elbow extensor tendon	Tennis	Gripping
Elbow flexor tendon	Baseball, tennis	Throwing
Triceps tendon	Weight lifting	Pushing
Anconeus tendon	Baseball	Throwing
Distal biceps tendon	Weight lifting	Pulling
Abductor pollicis tendon	Rowing	Pulling, gripping
Ilio-tibial band	Running	Running
Popliteus tendon	Running	Running
Patellar tendon	Basketball, bicycle	Jumping, pushoff
Pes anserinus	Running	Running (hills)
Plantar fascia	Running	Running
Achilles tendon	Running	Running
Flexor hallicus tendon	Dancing	Planatarflexion
Posterior tibial tendon	Running	Running
Hamstring tendon origin	Running	Running
Flexor digitorum longus	Running, dancing	Running, dancing

secondary inflammatory change in both the cuff and bursal structures. As the inflammatory process becomes chronic, scar tissue will form, leading to loss of motion and increased friction with joint movement.

Instability is not a primary component of bursal injury, but bursal inflammation can develop as a consequence of joint instability with the development of secondary frictional forces. An example is pes anserine bursitis secondary to rotational instability of the knee joint.

Specific modalities to reduce the inflammatory response affecting the bursa and vigorous attempts at improving and maintaining joint motion are key components of treatment. This is a specific circumstance in which intrabursal corticosteroid infiltration can have a dramatic positive effect. Infection must be considered and ruled out prior to corticoid infiltration. It is imperative that the primary cause of the bursal inflammation be sought. The development of bursitis can be a primary event, such as with olecranon and prepatellar bursitis. In the sporting population, biomechanical aberration plays an important role in the development of secondary bursal pathology, such as in subtrochanteric bursitis secondary to poor flexibility of the iliotibial band and gluteus medius tendon structures in runners.[22, 23] Biomechanical malalignment of the lower extremity secondary to excessive foot pronation can lead to frictional forces applied to the inflexible tendons with the secondary development of bursitis.[42]

FASCIA. Mesodermal cells are differentiated during development into specialized functional units. The fascia is a form of less-specialized connective tissue permeating all areas of the body. Its primary function is to compartmentalize structures and to facilitate movement by establishing low-friction tissue planes. Superficial fascia facilitates freedom of movement and deep fascia, with its more dense connective tissue make-up, forms the intermuscular septa and compartments of the upper and lower extremities. The most important sports-related injury involving fascially contained structures are compartment syndromes.

A compartment syndrome develops as the result of increased pressure within a tissue compartment. Normally, during exercise, compartment pressures rise to tolerable limits (less than 30 mm Hg) and fall rapidly after the exercise is discontinued. Muscle mass will increase by 20% of resting state during exercise. In the abnormal state, the intercompartment pressure rises to levels greater than 30 mm Hg and can remain elevated for prolonged periods of time, even following the cessation of exercise, causing damage to the soft tissue components of the compartment. This can lead to muscle necrosis as well as myelin degeneration of the nervous tissue that courses through the involved compartment.[145, 146] The diagnosis can be established by measuring compartment pressures before, during, and after exercise. Equipment for this purpose is commercially available.

Exertional compartment syndromes of the lower extremities are most commonly found in the running athlete. Runners with exertional compartment syndromes will present with pain and occasionally small muscle hernias. They may also experience loss of sensation in the distribution of the sensory nerves that course through the involved compartment and weakness of the compartment musculature. Early in the clinical course, the symptoms and signs may only be present during exercise or immediately following exertion. However, in chronic situations, the clinical signs will often occur with minimal exertion and even at rest.[22] Upper extremity compartment syndromes in motorcycle racers and weight lifters have also been reported.[118]

Flexibility treatment programs may reduce the repetitive forces on the compartment by both stretching out the fascia and the musculotendinous unit which courses through the compart-

ment. Careful attention should be given to any biomechanical abnormalities of the lower extremity that could be corrected by equipment changes and orthoses.[40] A surgical approach with fasciotomy may be necessary in refractory cases, producing best results in the lower extremity with anterior and lateral calf compartment syndromes and poor results with deep calf compartment syndrome. Excellent results have been obtained in upper extremity cases.[118] It should be kept in mind that a 20% decline of muscle strength in the affected compartment can occur following fasciotomy.[145]

MUSCLE. Muscles are the prime movers of the locomotion system. Muscles are expected to contract, elongate, and stretch in an appropriate phasic pattern dependent upon circumstance. The key in the prevention of all types of muscle injury is the synchronized action of agonist units as prime movers (with secondary and tertiary movers) with phasic relaxation of antagonist units.

Muscles can themselves fall victim to injury not only by direct contusion, but also by overzealous stretching,[65] causing muscle tearing. The degree of tearing is graded from I to III depending upon the amount of structural disruption. A grade I injury would be considered a common pulled muscle. With a grade II injury, there is a greater disruption but the muscle unit remains intact. A grade III lesion involves total tearing of the muscle unit. The hamstring muscles are by far the most common group of muscles that suffer from this type of injury. Tearing injuries of the biceps and pectoralis major are also not uncommon in weight-lifting enthusiasts. In addition, the use of anabolic steroids may increase the frequency of musculotendinous rupture. The mechanism can be explained by the decreased elasticity of the tendon due to fibrous tissue deposition combined with rapid muscle bulk and strength gain that overpowers the relatively inelastic attachment.

Hamstring pulls are an extremely frequent sports-related injury and are the most frequent reason for loss of practice time in all sports. The diagnosis is not difficult, but the treatment and specifically the prevention can often be difficult and frustrating. Muscles that span two joints may be more likely to rupture than those over a single joint. Special attention to stretching these muscles is, therefore, quite important.

Myositis ossificans can develop as a consequence of muscle injury. The most frequent location is the quadriceps. This type of heterotopic ossification may be precipitated by early injudicious stretching of an injured muscle that has suffered significant hemorrhage.[198] Cryotherapy and electrical muscle stimulation to pump out hemorrhage, along with guarded movement for the first 24 to 48 hours, can be important. Evacuation of encapsulated hematoma, whenever possible, can be valuable. The use of oral corticosteroids at the first signs of heterotopic bone formation may be helpful to reduce the degree of ossification.[*]

In acute muscle injuries, the early use of ice can reduce hemorrhage. Beginning ultrasound to enhance soft tissue extensibility and to facilitate stretching should be reserved until hemorrhage has ceased. Anti-inflammatory medication may be useful at this stage. Education of the injured athlete in proper flexibility routines can be the most important portion of this rehabilitation program.

Predisposition to muscle strains occurs when the muscles are cold and have impaired muscular circulation, and the athlete suffers from local and general overfatigue and insufficient training.[50] An insufficient pre-exercise flexibility program appears to be the major determinant in the development of muscle

---

*Personal communication

strains.[20, 35, 51, 98] The absolute strength of the muscle does not appear to be an important factor in the prevention of muscle strain injuries.[187]

CARTILAGE. The articular surface of most bones is formed of a special variety of hyaline cartilage that facilitates movement, absorbs shock, and protects the subchondral bone. Articular cartilage is typically from 1 mm to 2 mm thick, but may be as thick as 5 mm to 7 mm in the larger joints. Young cartilage is typically white, smooth, and glistening to the naked eye. Aging cartilage is thinner, less cellular, more brittle, and has a yellow opacity and irregular surface. Articular cartilage is porous, which enhances this tissue's shock-absorbing capability. Microscopically, chondrocytes (mature cartilage cells) are imbedded in a matrix of water, proteoglycans, lipid, collagen, noncollagenous protein, and electrolytes. The meniscus of the knee joint is composed of white fibrocartilage: dense, white, fibrous tissue arranged in bundles.[177] The knee meniscus transmits one-half of the contact force of the medial compartment[202] and even a higher percentage of the load in the lateral compartment. This force transference capability of the menisci protects the articular cartilage from repetitive trauma and secondary development of degenerative changes. Degenerative changes appear rapidly after meniscectomy, for instance, in the anterior cruciate-deficient knee. The menisci also play a significant role in stability of the knee, especially with the knee at 90° of flexion.[161]

Meniscal injuries of the knee are frequent in the sporting population. Fifty-two percent of sports-related knee injuries involve meniscal tears.[32] The injury mechanism is a combination of torsion and impact stress placed upon the joint with secondary tearing of the cartilage substance. Capsular disruption with meniscal cartilage separation can also occur. Joint effusion, pain, loss of motion, clicking, and occasionally locking are the hallmark manifestations of meniscal injury. Joint line tenderness is the typical finding on physical examination. Symptoms may be reproduced by loading of the involved joint compartment with the appropriate valgus or varus maneuver and rotational forces applied (*i.e.,* McMurray's test or lateral grind test).[106]

Meniscal injuries can often be confused with fat pad lesions, loose bodies, osteochondritis dissecans, degenerative joint disease, patellofemoral osteoarthritis, ganglion cyst, and plica syndrome.[106]

Injury and damage to articular cartilage (*e.g.,* in the patellofemoral joint) is an extremely common disorder.[100, 128] It is the most common running-related knee complaint.[105] The subsequent development of degenerative disease in a previously injured joint is an important sequela of articular cartilage damage. Until recently, articular cartilage was considered metabolically inert. However, research conducted over the last 25 years has shown this tissue has surprisingly active metabolism. The process involved in replacement or repair of cartilage takes place under avascular conditions and is extremely complex. Anaerobic glycolysis is the major metabolic pathway used by articular cartilage.[177]

The diagnosis of articular cartilage injuries can be difficult. An accurate history must be taken that includes any acute injury, overuse, or previous injury of that particular joint which has led to pain, joint effusion, crepitation, and loss of motion. Radiographic and radionuclide diagnostic procedures as well as arthroscopic evaluation of the affected joint is often necessary to both localize and grade the severity of the articular cartilage damage.[54, 106] Degenerative changes noted on examination do not necessarily ensure that the pain generator is indeed the cartilage. Correlation with the history and physical examination is imperative.

Planning the treatment program for patients with suspected meniscal injuries and articular cartilage injuries will necessitate a precise and accurate diagnosis of the painful lesion. This should be followed by a program to progressively restore motion, and strengthen the juxta-articular musculature.[46] Muscle strengthening in a protected range of motion and modalities and drugs to reduce inflammation are the cornerstones of the restorative protocol. The key goal is to reduce shear stress, absorb shock, and limit torsion to the involved joint in order to minimize repetitive insult and thereby control synovitis. Appropriate and timely surgical intervention must be carefully planned.

Preserving as much of the meniscus as possible is important in order to delay the subsequent development of degenerative arthritis.[45] Arthroscopic partial meniscectomy has been a mainstay in the surgical treatment of meniscal injuries.[54] Newer techniques of meniscal repair are currently being used in an attempt to maintain meniscal function, such as meniscorrhesis. Meniscal repair should be considered in all cases whenever possible. Early arthroscopic debridement of acute osteochondral injuries may be appropriate and should be considered at the time of diagnosis.[106]

BONE. Bone is essentially a highly vascular, live, constantly changing, mineralized connective tissue. Its collagen framework varies from an almost random network of coarse bundles to a highly organized system of parallel fibered sheets of helical bundles. There are two basic categories of mature bone: one is dense in texture and termed *cortical bone;* the other consists of a meshwork of trabeculae called cancellous or trabecular bone.

Of major interest to sports medicine physicians is the high incidence of stress fractures in the sporting population.[135, 136] Three types of stress are transferred to bone, presumably producing these stress fractures: compression impaction, distraction with pulling of periosteum (postulated as a cause in some shin splint syndromes),[101] and direct muscle concentration. Clinical stress fractures stem from training errors roughly 75% of the time.[136] Anatomical discrepancies such as leg length discrepancies and biomechanical aberrations such as hyperpronation of the feet have been implicated in the development of lower extremity stress fractures in runners. Poor shoe selection or changes in running shoes at the same time other portions of the training regimen are changed have also been implicated.[53] The tibia is involved in 34% of stress fractures in runners, the fibula 24%, and the metatarsals 20%[136] (Table 43-3). A history of acute pain onset after a change in the training regimen should raise a

Table 43-3
Incidence of Lower Extremity Stress Fractures in Runners

Bone	Incidence
Femoral neck	7%
Femoral upper shaft	5%
Distal femoral shaft	2%
Fibula	24%
Tibia metaphysics	7%
Tibia upper shaft	12%
Tibia midshaft	4%
Tibia distal shaft	11%
Metatarsals	20%
Second	11%
Third	7%
Other	2%
Sesamoid	
Os calcis, talus, navicular	2%

high index of suspicion with the examiner; point tenderness is a hallmark physical examination sign. Radiographic confirmation is necessary, but is often nonconfirmatory, especially early in the course. Radionuclide bone scanning is, therefore, often necessary to ensure a proper diagnosis.[21, 184]

A discussion of all fracture types that occur in athletes is beyond the scope of this chapter. Clavicular fractures, rib fractures, and carpal navicular fractures are some of the more common fractures encountered in a sports medicine population. Upper extremity stress fractures can also occur in a variety of sporting circumstances.[149] Stress fractures of the pars interarticularis are an important part of the differential diagnosis of low back pain in athletes.[104]

One basic step in treatment is to determine what degree of immobilization is needed to ensure fracture healing. It is also imperative to determine the causes of fracture for preventive purposes. Stress fractures of the tarsal navicular will necessitate nonweight-bearing and cast immobilization for 8 to 12 weeks, and occasionally surgery.[197] Femoral stress fractures may require nonweight-bearing for 4 to 6 weeks. If the fracture is distracted, surgery may be necessary. Stress fracture of the pars interarticularis may need immobilization.[140] Abstinence from athletic activity for a period of at least 12 weeks is necessary after acute pars interarticularis fracture.[140] The majority of the other stress fractures can be successfully treated with rest followed by reconditioning and a progressive return to activity, guided by the degree of pain remaining.

NERVOUS TISSUE. The most frequent nerve injuries encountered in sports are usually secondary to compression or traction. Elongation of a nerve to greater than 15% of resting length has been demonstrated to cause cessation of vascular supply.[175] The resultant ischemia appears to be a major causative mechanism in the development of these types of injuries. Some of the other more frequent types of nerve injuries to athletes occur secondary to repetitive trauma from overuse. The overuse phenomenon usually combines frictional forces placed upon the nerve along with compression forces, resulting in ischemia and mechanical deformation upon exertion.

Upper extremity nerve injuries in athletes are common. Brachial plexus traction injuries are common in football, hockey, and wrestling[29, 134, 170] (Table 43-4). These injuries are commonly referred to as "stingers" or "burners." The brachial plexus lesions are secondary to contralateral lateral bending of the cervical spine coupled with ipsilateral shoulder depression. A C6 radiculopathy secondary to cervical flexion and axial loading, as can occur in a football tackle, with nerve root compression and traction may be a more frequent cause of the stinger.[164] Electrodiagnostic evaluation can differentiate these two conditions.

Median nerve injuries in the forearm are also common upper extremity problems[176] (see Table 43-4). These are most frequently noted in baseball pitchers, tennis players, musicians, motorcycle racers, and weight lifters. The most frequent symptoms are deep aching in the forearm compartment and paresthesias in the second and third digits.[186] The pain and par-

Table 43-4
Sports-Related Peripheral Nerve Injuries

Nerve Injury	*Related Sporting Activity*
Median nerve	
Forearm	Pitching, tennis, motorcross
Wrist	Music playing, weight lifting
Posterior interosseous nerve	Tennis
Ulnar nerve	
Elbow	Pitching, weight lifting, tennis
Forearm	Pitching
Wrist	Bicycling, gymnastics
Palm	Bicycling
Axillary nerve	Football
Suprascapular nerve	Skiing, football, rugby, hockey, tennis
Accessory nerve	Wrestling, tennis
Long thoracic nerve	Backpacking, wrestling, tennis
Musculocutaneous nerve	Tennis, weight lifting
Digital nerve	Bowling
Tibial nerve	
Popliteal space	Any
Tarsal tunnel	Running
Peroneal nerve	
Popliteal space	Football, soccer
Compartmental	Running
Sensory	Skiing, ice skating following ankle injuries
Sural nerve	Skiing, ice skating
Sciatic nerve (pyriformis)	Sprinting, jumping
Femoral nerve	Hurdling, dancing
Obturator nerve	Dancing
Ilioinguinal nerve	Running
Lateral femoral cutaneous nerve	Weight lifting
Thoracic outlet syndrome	Swimming, pitching
Brachial plexus stretch injuries	Football, hockey, rugby
Cervical nerve root	Tennis, football, rugby
Lumbar nerve root	All sports

esthesias are most often experienced only at times of exertion, with the athlete often asymptomatic at rest. Carpal tunnel entrapment of the median nerve is common in musicians, who comprise an interesting subset of the athletic population. Ulnar nerve lesions at the cubital tunnel are frequently seen in the throwing athlete.[72] A chief complaint of medial elbow pain along with paresthesias in the fourth and fifth digits is often noted. Later, symptoms of forearm aching and hand fatigue may be noted by the athlete. The symptoms are exertionally related and the athlete is often asymptomatic at rest.[43] No changes are usually noted on gross neurological examination, especially early in the clinical course. Posterior interosseous nerve entrapment at the supinator channel may occur in tennis players. The symptoms are lateral elbow pain, deep aching dorsal forearm pain, and occasionally deep aching into the carpus itself.[186] Quadrilateral space entrapment of the axillary nerve[115] and thoracic outlet symptomatology are also encountered in the sporting population.[73] Direct contusion of the axillary nerve is not uncommon in football. Axillary nerve injuries following glenohumeral dislocation are also encountered. Thoracic outlet syndromes occur most frequently in swimmers and baseball pitchers.[64]

Suprascapular nerve injuries can occur as an isolated incident after shoulder trauma, either from a direct blow or following a brachial plexus stretch injury.[29] Backpacking injuries of the long thoracic nerve can also occur.[108] Repetitive tennis serving and throwing may be associated with some cases of suprascapular nerve injury. A direct blow to the shoulder girdle can also potentially injure this nerve.

Lower extremity nerve injuries include sural nerve and superficial sensory peroneal nerve injuries secondary to boot-top compression, such as in skiers and ice skaters.[123] These sensory nerves can also be injured at the time of ankle inversion injury. Common peroneal nerve injury at the fibular head and above is also frequently seen as a sequela of ankle inversion injuries.[139] Common peroneal nerve injury is also frequently encountered in patients who have experienced a rotational knee injury resulting in anterior cruciate ligament tearing. The peroneal nerve can also be injured in the anterior tarsal region, as a boot-top injury or secondary to ankle trauma.[19] Tibial nerve entrapment in a fibrotic popliteal space secondary to prolonged immobilization after knee injury has been encountered. Tibial nerve injury secondary to rotational instability has also been recognized.[161] Saphenous nerve injuries can mimic the knee pain of internal derangement. These injuries have been noted following meniscal repair surgery and following a variety of knee injuries.

Tarsal tunnel entrapment of the tibial nerves is important in the differential diagnosis of arch pain, heel pain, and foot paresthesias in runners and dancers.[89, 110, 111] Interdigital nerve injury of the foot (*i.e.,* Morton's neuroma) is also a common malady in the same population.

Other interesting nerve injuries to be aware of are obturator nerve injuries in dancers[8] and deep palmar ulnar nerve injuries and pudendal nerve injuries in bicyclists.[174] Piriformis entrapment of the sciatic nerve has also been described in jumpers and sprinters.[158, 183] Femoral nerve stretch injuries can be an unusual cause of anterior thigh and hip pain in hurdlers and dancers. Obviously, the most frequent type of nerve injury affecting the lower extremity is lumbar nerve root injury, which can often be a masquerader for all types of lower extremity pain problems.[175] Cervical nerve root injuries likewise can mimic a peripheral nerve entrapment in the upper extremity.[10] Double crush lesions should also be considered.[176]

Planning the basic treatment program for sports-related nerve injuries necessitates an accurate diagnosis. This is followed by the identification of precipitating stresses and secondary risk factors in the injury development. Appropriately planned surgical decompression should be considered if conservative measures fail.

Brachial plexus stretch injuries will usually resolve with a careful period of observation. The athlete should not return to full athletic activities until strength is normal. In severe injuries, this can take as long as 4 months.

Careful electrophysiological grading of all nerve injuries is extremely important in treatment planning. Post-exertional electrodiagnostic studies are sometimes necessary to establish the diagnosis of a sports-related peripheral nerve injury.[176]

Forearm entrapments of the median nerve often respond to local steroid infiltration and stretching programs. A careful analysis of the pitcher's form and the equipment used by the tennis player is also a key element in treatment. Surgical decompression in refractory cases may be required. Ulnar nerve injuries are usually best treated by rest. Ulnar nerve transposition with or without flexor arcade decompression is sometimes necessary to treat refractory cases of ulnar neuritis. Valgus instability of the elbow should also be noted and an appropriate strengthening program designed. Surgical stabilization procedures should be planned if instability does not respond to conservative means. Posterior interosseous nerve entrapments often respond to stretching programs, steroid injection, and rest. These should be followed by tennis equipment changes, such as lowering string tension and increasing racquet grip size. Strengthening of forearm extensor musculature should be done following the cessation of the inflammatory process.

Tarsal tunnel syndrome in runners often responds to rest and orthotic balancing of a pronated foot. Occasionally, surgical decompression is necessary. Morton's neuroma in the early stages can respond to orthotic devices that place the foot in a neutral position and allow even weight distribution across the metatarsal joints. Pads to spread the metatarsal heads may need to be added for additional comfort. A change in running shoes and local steroid injection can also be helpful. In the later stages, surgery will often be necessary.

Peroneal nerve and tibial nerve injuries about the knee may require an external neurolysis followed by treatment of the primary knee pathology. Peroneal nerve traction injuries secondary to ankle inversion sprains usually resolve spontaneously.

MANAGEMENT AND REHABILITATION OF SPORTS-RELATED INJURIES

General Principles

The goal of rehabilitation is to restore an optimal state of health and function to its utmost potential. This process of functional restoration must take into consideration the type of athlete, the age of the athlete, the level of performance of the athlete, the structure involved, the level of conditioning of the athlete prior to the injury, as well as the level of conditioning the athlete must return to. The rehabilitation process can be divided into phases, each of which is part of the overall plan to restore function:

Phase I   Control of the inflammatory process
Phase II   Control of pain
Phase III   Restore joint range of motion and soft tissue extensibility
Phase IV   Improve muscular strength
Phase V   Improve muscle endurance
Phase VI   Develop specific sport-related biomechanical skill patterns (*i.e.,* coordination retraining)
Phase VII   Improve general cardiovascular endurance
Phase VIII   Maintenance programs

These principles have long been applied in other rehabilitation situations and are well known to the practicing physiatrist. As in other forms of rehabilitation, the maintenance of motivation in the sports-injured individual appears to be the key ingredient to success.

Surgical Planning

The appropriate timing of surgical referral is an integral part of the rehabilitation continuum. The constant status reevaluation of the injured athlete allows the physician to develop reasonable therapeutic goals and guidelines.[52] Decisions regarding surgery must start with an accurate diagnosis. Careful workups, which include thoughtful radiographic radionuclide bone scans, electromyograms, and arthrograms, may be indicated according to the specific site and severity of the injury. The diagnostic algorithm for each injury is beyond the scope of this chapter, but it should become familiar to all sports medicine physicians.

The social profiling of the injured athlete to determine his or her goals and needs is imperative before planning any surgical intervention. Problems that are obviously surgical in nature such as grade III ligament injuries should be referred to the surgeon member of the sports medicine team immediately. Injuries that, in due time, are obviously not responding to nonoperative rehabilitation should also be referred to the surgeon for consultation and surgical consideration.

The SAID Principle

The SAID (Specific Adaptation to Imposed Demands) principle is an important concept in sports rehabilitation. It states that the body responds to a given demand with a specific predictable adaptation.[4] If one can define the specific goals of the rehabilitation process, then the program designed can be tailored to meet that need. For instance, identifying a weak supraspinatus muscle in a throwing athlete with rotator cuff tendinitis and impingement syndrome will necessitate isolated strength training to that particular muscle group as part of the rehabilitation process.[6]

The Team Approach

Careful communication between the sports medicine physician and the trainer or physical therapist is imperative to ensure a good outcome. The team approach to sports medicine improves care. The thoughtful sports-minded surgeon, working with the physiatric team member, is an invaluable combination.

Timing

It is quite obvious that the rehabilitation process should begin immediately after injury and should be terminated only at the point when the injured athlete can successfully return to his or her previous level of competition. A careful outlining of the rehabilitation goals prior to embarking upon the functional restoration program will eliminate the athlete's frustration and discouragement. Early diagnostic intervention with the establishment of a precise diagnosis is the key to unlock the rehabilitation plan. An improper or imprecise diagnosis can lead to major pitfalls in the treatment regimen. Early intervention will lead to control of the inflammatory processes and speed the recovery of normal articular and soft tissue range of motion. Early exercise will also enhance the early development of muscular strength, which has been shown to correlate with the development of stronger ligaments and tendons.[90, 152, 195, 196]

Phases of Treatment

Phase I: Control of Inflammation

The control of inflammation that occurs secondary to an injury can be best accomplished by the early application of ice and elevation of the appropriate structure. Cryotherapy serves as a cornerstone of rehabilitation of the injured athlete, effectively controlling edema and reducing pain. Ice can be applied in the form of crushed ice in a plastic bag, iced immersion tub, or as ice massage. The use of crushed ice in a bag is specifically applicable to an acutely injured knee. In this situation, the extremity is elevated and ice is applied directly to the knee and held on with an Ace wrap. Limiting the initial development of joint effusion will speed the recovery process.[1] The ice is applied for 12 to 15 minutes, followed by a rest period, and then reapplication. Immersion tubs are applicable to subacute lower extremity muscle injuries of the calf or hamstring. The use of ice massage finds its greatest use in the treatment of tendinitis and is especially useful prior to and after exercise.[188]

The prescription of rest is also an important component of the treatment process during the inflammatory phase. The amount of rest should be specifically prescribed to the injured athlete and guidelines for progressive activity established. Nonweight-bearing of the involved lower extremity during this early phase will help curtail the inflammation; the use of a sling or splint in the upper extremity serves the same purpose.

Compression wrapping is also an important procedure early after injury. The use of a horseshoe-shaped compression wrap on an ankle that has sustained an inversion sprain can significantly help to reduce edema.[49] When compression is combined with the other early components of treatment which may include ice, elevation, rest, immobilization, and nonweight-bearing, early control of the inflammatory process can be gained.

Nonsteroidal anti-inflammatory medications are extremely useful during this initial phase. The early use of anti-inflammatory medication appears to speed recovery by both curtailing the inflammatory response and controlling pain. The use of glucocorticoids during the acute phase of injury must be done cautiously. The powerful anti-inflammatory effect of these drugs can reduce the potential of the normal healing process and thereby actually prolong the phases of rehabilitation.[84, 113, 192] For instance, an acutely torn ligamentous structure during the first 7 days would be harmed by the systemic or local application of corticosteroids. During the proliferative phase of the inflammatory process, especially after the 14- to 21-day mark, the use of glucocorticoids can help reduce an unchecked inflammatory response and control unwanted edema. The injection of glucocorticoids into tendon sheaths, bursae, and joints can rapidly reduce an inflammatory response. Once again, the careful timing of the use of these procedures is imperative. The infiltration of a tendon itself with glucocorticoids should be avoided. Achilles tendon rupture and patellar tendon rupture have been reported after corticosteroid injection into these structures.[113] However, tendon sheath injection, such as into an inflamed abductor pollicis longus tendon, can markedly reduce the inflammatory response in the structure and speed the rehabilitation process. Direct intratendinous injection of corticosteroids into the rotator cuff should be avoided as well. The use of an intrabursal injection into the subacromial bursa, combined with a careful injection into the biceps tendon sheath as it rests in the intertubercular groove, can reduce the unwanted inflammatory response in the peritendinous structures and enable the later phases of rehabilitation to proceed. Injecting muscle pulls with corticosteroids, either during the acute or subacute stages, is not usually useful. But if one can identify a specific area of restricting fibrosis in the musculotendinous unit in the subacute to chronic phase, careful corticosteroid injection followed by friction massage can be useful. The intra-articular injection of corticosteroids into a joint with synovitis in an individual who has had a previous osteochondral injury can be a useful treatment modality.

Continuing the use of nonsteroidal anti-inflammatory agents throughout all the phases of rehabilitation is often necessary. Therefore, it is strongly advised to carefully monitor for the development of possible side-effects of these drugs.[73]

Electrical stimulation is useful in the reduction of edema. Pulsed electrical current, coupled with ice therapy, is an effective means of controlling early edema.[14] Higher pulse rates of greater than 75 Hz and above will produce a tetanic muscle contraction and can be useful for control of acute pain. Lower frequencies of 1 to 5 Hz are useful in chronic pain control.[119] Iontophoresis can be a useful means for delivering corticosteroids to superficially placed inflamed soft tissue structures.[68, 70] This technique can be useful in cases of patellar tendinitis, Achilles tendinitis, wrist extensor tendinitis with lateral elbow pain, and occasionally rotator cuff injuries.

During the later phases of the inflammatory process, ultrasound can be useful to enhance local circulation to remove the byproducts of the inflammatory process. The key role of ultrasound in this phase, however, appears to be enhancement of soft tissue extensibility, which facilitates early motion. Phonophoresis can also be a successful way of delivering corticosteroids to superficial structures.[77, 78] Patients tend to find phonophoresis more comfortable than iontophoresis.

Contrast baths are an ideal way to help reduce resistant edema in later phases of the inflammatory process. This is especially useful in soft tissue injuries about the ankle.

The duration of phase I is determined by edema and effusion control. Once joint effusion can be eliminated or minimized and interstitial edema controlled, the later phases of the rehabilitation process can proceed. Occasionally, arthrocentesis to remove an excessive or stubborn knee joint effusion is necessary. It should be noted that the presence of hemarthrosis of the knee following an acute injury is a strong indicator of anterior cruciate ligament tear.[45]

Phase II:
Controlling Pain

Controlling of pain after sports-related injury is accomplished while controlling the inflammatory process. The use of ice, rest, immobilization, and nonweight-bearing are once again important components. All throughout the rehabilitation process, pain will need to be controlled. The use of ice is often the most successful method. Icing prior to and after strengthening workouts is also beneficial.

The use of nonsteroidal anti-inflammatory medications, as mentioned earlier, can be useful for the control of pain as well as inflammation. The use of acetylsalicylate should be avoided during the early phases of injury because of its antiplatelet activity, which persists for the life of the platelet (other nonsteroidal anti-inflammatory agents have an antiplatelet effect that is entirely dose-related).[73] The use of opiate and nonopiate analgesic medications can be necessary during the very early phase of the post-injury treatment but should be used judiciously.

The use of transcutaneous electrical nerve stimulation (TENS) is a useful modality for treatment of acute pain following injury. TENS can allow the injured athlete to participate in the range of motion and strengthening programs. Acupuncture can

be a useful way to control both acute post-injury pain as well as pain that limits function during the rehabilitation process. Acupuncture can also be used in lieu of anesthesia for examination of a joint to aid in the diagnosis of suspected acute knee and ankle ligament injuries. Acupuncture can be an extremely useful and reliable tool. Both TENS and acupuncture raise central nervous system levels of endorphins.[182]

Protection of the injured structure can be accomplished by taping, padding, or bracing. In the case of an unstable knee, the use of a cast brace or knee immobilizer is useful. In the case of an injured ankle, rigid taping combined with a compressive wrap serves a protective function. The use of slings to limit arm motion in the case of acute acromioclavicular joint injuries can help control post-injury pain. Cervical spine injuries that result in segmental instability will necessitate immobilization until bone and soft tissue healing is sufficient to limit the instability. The use of a cervical collar for pain control after cervical facet or ligamentous injury can be useful. The period of immobilization or protection of the particular body part will need to be adjusted for each injury. Careful reevaluation during the early phases of the program will help in deciding on the continuance or discontinuance of any taping, bracing, or protective equipment.

Phase III:
Restore Joint Range of Motion and
Soft Tissue Extensibility

Prior to the inception of any strengthening program, joint range of motion and soft tissue flexibility must be improved. Limited range of motion can be attributable to muscular spasm, soft tissue contracture, intra-articular blockade, and pain. Ascertaining the causative factor or factors for the loss of motion will determine the treatment regimen necessary.

The use of ice and TENS is helpful in the presence of muscle spasm. The use of ultrasound, followed by a stretching program and friction massage, may be prescribed for soft tissue contracture. Intra-articular blockade, if due to a locked meniscus, will need operative intervention; but not if it could be secondary to the development of intra-articular fibrosis. Pain inhibiting joint motion can mimic intra-articular pathology. Pain abolition with TENS, acupuncture, or local anesthetic infiltration can aid in diagnosis and can be useful to break the pain cycle and enhance motion.

Range-of-motion programs can be divided into passive, active assistive, and active programs. An additional phase should be added, which can be termed a full flexibility program, beginning after joint range of motion is attained. During the initial phases of range-of-motion restoration, careful passive techniques are used. These require both a skilled therapist and a cooperative patient. The use of static stretch and proprioceptive neuromuscular facilitation techniques, such as contraction-relaxation, the contraction of the contralateral extremity, and the contraction of antagonistic muscle can all be effective.[144, 193] The use of the stationary bicycle to enhance knee range of motion by continually adjusting the seat height is valuable.

Active-assistive range of motion should begin as early as the patient can tolerate and is especially useful at times when the patient is not actually in the therapy gymnasium. Active-assistive programs can be used, for instance, in shoulder injuries with the use of pulleys to help enhance motion.

Active range-of-motion exercise can begin as the individual reaches the limits of normal range. The athlete should be taught specific exercises to be certain that full range of motion can be obtained. The full flexibility program geared to attain maximal soft tissue flexibility can be begun at the end of this phase.

The presence of instability must be noted and taken into consideration. Obviously, in a situation of an unstable joint, vigorous range-of-motion exercises in certain planes are not advisable. For instance, in an individual who has suffered an anterior glenohumeral dislocation, the avoidance of the extremes of abduction and external rotation during the first 6 weeks of the rehabilitation process is important. Subsequently, the gradual stretching of the anterior capsule can be accomplished, but, theoretically, the maintenance of some level of anterior capsule contracture may be of benefit to prevent further recurrences.[7] As previously mentioned, a hinged cast brace can be extremely beneficial with grade II medial collateral ligament injury.

Phase IV:
Improve Muscular Strength

After the injured athlete has regained his range of motion, the program is progressed from phase III to phase IV. There are times when phase III and phase IV treatment principles are used concurrently; for example, the early use of isometric strengthening after ankle injury even prior to normalizing joint range of motion. In most cases, it is advised to gain at least 75% of the range of motion before beginning strengthening programs. There are four basic types of strengthening programs: manual resistance, isometric, isotonic, and isokinetic. The exercises can be further subdivided into concentric contractions and eccentric contractions. Special programs for isolated muscle groups and hydrotherapy programs will be discussed later in this section.

The major principle to keep in mind is one of progressive resistance exercise.[48] This type of exercise must be performed on a regular basis at a minimum of three times per week. The initial programs involve progressive resistance exercise to the muscle groups designated as the prime movers of that particular injured area. Subsequently, the program should involve the contralateral uninvolved extremity as well as strengthening and conditioning for the total body. Programs using frequently adjustable progressive resistive exercise techniques appear to achieve maximum benefit.[4, 52] One such program is the daily adjustable progressive resistance exercise technique (DAPRE). The DAPRE technique is based on the principle that strength can be redeveloped more quickly after injury than it was developed initially.[52] The key component of the program consists of performing maximal repetitions during the third and fourth sets, with the number of repetitions performed used as a basis for adjusting the resistance used during the fourth set and on the next day.[14, 24]

Maintenance strength programs are begun once the injured extremity has reached 90% to 95% of strength compared to the uninjured side. But because the uninjured extremity has been strengthened as well, the use of absolute comparative percentage strength figures must be looked upon critically. Evaluation techniques for quantifying strength will be discussed later in Evaluation Procedures. The limits of performance must be persistently extended to improve muscle strength. The rate of improvement appears to depend upon the willingness of the subject to overload.[37, 47]

To achieve maximum intensity of muscle contraction, the highest possible percentage of muscle mass should be involved in any given moment.[15, 24] In order to achieve this end, good form is of utmost importance. The components of proper form include proper speed in raising and lowering the weight, full range of motion, and a movement pattern that begins from a pre-stretched or supra-range-of-motion position. The resistance should be accelerated in a smooth fashion and briefly halted at the position of full muscle contraction. The speed used in raising and lowering the weight will also train the muscle to develop the appropriate speed of contraction for the type of sporting activity designated.[38, 141]

Different sports require a greater degree of strength in certain muscle groups; other sports require greater endurance of muscle groups. For instance, the absolute muscle strength of a single contraction is an important component of shotput and discus throwing. The muscles of the trunk are used to rotate and accelerate the body, while powerful quadriceps muscles accelerate the trunk forward. The football lineman also needs the ability to maximally contract the muscles quickly to burst forward (quadriceps) as well as push forward (pectoralis musculature). Greater muscular endurance is necessary in alpine ski racing, and the greatest muscular endurance is necessary in cross-country skiing. Further discussion of improving muscular endurance and the development of specific sport-related skill patterns will be discussed during the phase V and phase VI sections of the rehabilitation program.

Concentric exercise programs are the most frequently used. Recently, eccentric training programs have been developed for the treatment of tendinitis.[188] Eccentric programs are felt to be beneficial in increasing the length of the musculotendinous unit while applying an increasing load. The speed of the contraction is modified during this specialized eccentric program to gradually increase the speed of movement while increasing the load on the tendon. This type of eccentric loading program parallels normal musculotendinous unit function in movement patterns. It has been suggested that concentric programs may place greater stress on the musculotendinous unit and are unable to increase the length of the soft tissues. Some authors have reported that patients will often report increased symptoms with concentric contraction and decreased symptomatology with eccentric programs. Eccentric programs are specifically applicable to wrist extensor tendinitis, patellar tendinitis, Achilles tendinitis, and rotator cuff tendinitis.[188]

Pre-stretching of the musculotendinous unit is important prior to beginning strengthening programs.[144, 187] Following the strengthening session, stretching should once again be done followed by the icing of the injured part to reduce post-exercise inflammatory flare-ups.

The use of overload to attain muscle fatigue appears to be the most important factor in strengthening programs. Initial gains in muscle strength are related to improved levels of motor unit activity. After the first two weeks of training, additional force gains are made through muscle hypertrophy.[36, 47, 67]

The ability to synchronize the firing ratios of the motor units is a consequence of weight training programs. Improvement in strength correlates with increased synchronization patterns. Therefore, the use of carefully concentrated exercise performed at the proper skill level and proper speed will allow synchronization of the motor units and improve the ability of the muscle to gain strength more rapidly.[9, 24, 27, 47] Overzealousness during the initial phases of the strengthening program can result in reactive inflammatory changes or joint synovitis. Carefully progressing the strength program is, therefore, imperative.

Numerous techniques of progressive resistive exercise have been described since the initial descriptions of DeLorme.[48] No particular program appears to have significant advantage over any other. An adjustable progressive resistance exercise routine using four sets of exercise is one example. The first set is carried out at a weight at which 12 to 15 repetitions can be accomplished. For the second set, the amount of resistance is adjusted so that only 10 repetitions can be carried out. For the third set, the weight is further adjusted so that a maximum of 6 repetitions can be carried out. During the fourth set, the weight is adjusted so that a maximum of 2 or 3 repetitions can be carried out. Often, assistance needs to be added to perform the last movement. This type of strengthening program provides exercise of the aerobic as well as the anaerobic pathways and, when speed adjustments are made during the later sets, both fast-twitch and slow-twitch fiber development can be attained.[137]

Isometric exercises are the initial phase of the strengthening program. The isometric phase can be carried out early on while still protecting joint motion. Manual resistance exercises can begin once the joint can be moved. In this situation, the therapist uses a carefully graded manual resistance to act as the progressive resistor. As the patient is able to accomplish this with comfort, the therapist can note the range that will be appropriate to work within. It is important that the contractions be carried out in the pain-free range.[124] In the patient with a patellofemoral compression syndrome, the pain-free range will often be between 0° and 30° and also between 90° and 45° of flexion. Exercises which are carried out in the midrange arc of 30° to 45° of flexion will increase the contact forces of the patellofemoral articular cartilage surfaces, thereby causing secondary pain.[97, 162] Rotator cuff strengthening programs should also be carried out in the pain-free ranges of abduction and rotation.[6] Neutral trunk stabilization programs should be used to strengthen patients with lumbar injuries.

Once the patient is carefully progressed through the manual resistance program and isometric program, pain-free ranges can be carefully adjusted. Isometric contractions are optimally held for 5 to 6 seconds with a rest period of between 10 and 20 seconds. This ensures a proper muscle blood flow and removes the substrate of muscular contraction. The isometric contraction should be carried out frequently during the day, in sets of 10 to 12 repetitions.[4] The goal is to transfer this isometric strength development to the isotonic and/or isokinetic programs. Individuals who carry out isometric exercises of a greater frequency develop greater endurance, which transfers better to progressive resistive exercises.

The concept of specificity of exercise should constantly be kept in mind. Since most athletic endeavors rely on dynamic muscle contraction, merely training the muscle with static contractions, that is, isometric contractions, may not transfer to the playing field,[4, 83, 116, 117] even though this method can increase absolute static strength.[165]

After the patient can successfully perform isometric and manual resistance exercises, progression to either an isotonic or isokinetic program begins. An isokinetic program is often preferable during this phase of the strengthening program because of its ability to control speed while maintaining force.[122, 142] Studies have demonstrated that isokinetic training and isotonic training both eventually reach the same degree of absolute strength, but the isokinetic program participants reach that goal sooner with less post-workout soreness.[163]

Isokinetic equipment also allows the therapist to train the individual first at slow speed and later at high speed. This training at high speed is specifically transferable to the type of high speed contraction most often encountered in the majority of sporting activity.[141] Some conditions such as patellofemoral compression syndromes should ideally be trained at high speed, especially in terminal extension (0° to 30°).[75, 162] The isokinetic equipment also acts as a dynamometer, which permits quantification of force velocity curve and torque measurements.[58, 74] These evaluation procedures serve not only as baselines and benchmarks in treatment, but also as a motivating force for the patient. Using isokinetic dynamometry, the physiatrist can determine when the patient has reached his or her strength goals as a sign of readiness to return to athletic participation.[180, 181] Training at high speeds appears to have carry-over benefits to torque developed at lower velocities, while training only at lower velocities primarily benefits only the lower part of the velocity

curve.[38, 52] Newer forms of isokinetic dynamometry allow for smooth transference of torque with only minimal stress applied to the joint surfaces.[180]

Isotonic programs can use free weights, elastic bands, universal-type exercise machines, or cammed equipment such as Nautilus. Free weights are useful in isolation patterns, such as using dumbbells for the upper extremity after rotator cuff injury. Specifically training the supraspinatus muscle has been demonstrated to be particularly useful in the shoulder impingement syndrome.[6] Isolation patterns can also be carried out for the anterior, middle, and posterior fibers of the deltoid. With higher weight, free weights should be used only in a buddy system and by patients who are skilled lifters. For the novice, the use of weight machines such as the Universal machine and Hydragym are especially useful. Isolation patterns are difficult to obtain, but the ease of use of the machine and the multiple stations make this type of equipment extremely practical. The use of cammed equipment such as Nautilus has many distinct advantages. This type of equipment is designed with a cam, which varies the resistance offered by a given load to try to match the average torque curves for each of a large number of muscle groups. This theoretically eliminates the "dead areas" which are noted in certain portions of the range of motion when an individual trains with free weights. Another advantage to cammed equipment is the individualized stations, which allow adjustment of foot rests and seat height. This can be specifically advantageous for the reconditioning of lumbar spine patients. Careful instruction of the patient using Nautilus equipment is imperative to avoid injury. Both eccentric and concentric contractions can be accomplished using cammed equipment.

The use of elastic bands is extremely practical, especially for home strengthening programs. The elastic bands can be used not only to supply resistance, but also for flexibility programs. The elastic band technique can be applied to ankle programs, shoulder programs, and knee programs. Isolation patterns can be accomplished with the use of elastic bands. This type of exercise is also extremely practical because the patient is able to travel with the exercise equipment. Maintenance programs using elastic bands can be helpful.

The specific way a joint is loaded by weight must also be taken into consideration. For example, the most efficient way to load the patellofemoral joint for quadriceps strengthening during knee rehabilitation for patellofemoral compression syndrome would be to load the joint from above.[97] In this particular situation squats are done from full knee extension to 20° of flexion. This particular program places minimum stress on the articular cartilage and applies maximal strengthening to the quadriceps musculature.[9] The patellar tendon can be lengthened through this program and can be incorporated into the specialized eccentric programs. Angled leg press in the restricted ranges of 0° to 30° of flexion and 45° to 90° of flexion can also be useful for the rehabilitation of patellofemoral problems.

Electrical muscle stimulation (EMS) is particularly useful during periods of immobilization. Cutting portals in cast braces following surgery and applying EMS pads is a useful part of the early phase of treatment.[61, 82] The type of contraction developed with the EMS is a concentric isometric contraction that, by itself, may not be transferable to dynamic activity. Total reliance on EMS strengthening not only is uncomfortable and impractical, but also does not meet the principle of specificity of exercise. There is good transference of the strength gained through EMS to isokinetic programs.[61, 82] A specialized type of electrical stimulator, the "Russian" type of electrical stimulator, is becoming popular in the United States. This type of stimulator uses an alternating current of high pulse rate and high intensity to produce strong involuntary muscle contractions with associated stimulation of local blood flow. Strength gains reported in the Russian literature using this type of electrical stimulator are much greater than what is noted with standard EMS units.[52] Carefully controlled studies need to be carried out to determine true efficacy of these units.

Occasionally, the buoyancy produced by water is useful during the initial phase of strengthening programs. An individual can be placed in the pool and, with the use of a life vest, can begin to use the water and his or her body weight as resistance for strengthening. This is particularly effective with victims of running injuries to the lower extremity. These hydro programs allow the individual to maintain lower extremity strength and range of motion and aerobic endurance as well. This satisfies not only physiological goals, but also the psychological goals of the injured athlete. The use of a stationary bicycle with varying seat heights to improve knee and ankle range of motion as well as progressive resistance can be beneficial during this phase. This type of combined program is particularly useful for a patient with patellofemoral compression syndrome as well as for the injured runner.

The establishment of programs to develop strength in an isolated muscle group is necessary in a variety of clinical situations.

A strength maintenance program should follow the structured and supervised rehabilitation program. Teaching baseball pitchers and tennis players to maintain a level of strength in their supraspinatus muscle coupled with rotator cuff stretching has been found to be extremely effective in the prevention of recurrent rotator cuff injuries.[6, 87, 168] The maintenance of trunk strength with the use of the oblique abdominals, latissimus dorsi, and spinal extensor musculature should be a priority for the athlete recovering from any one of the varieties of spinal pain conditions.

The post-surgical patient must have a carefully planned program. Careful attention to the type of surgery carried out and the time of healing that is necessary postoperatively must be carefully noted. Specific programs for rehabilitation of the individual who has undergone an anterior cruciate repair or reconstruction have been developed by several authors.[143, 160, 180, 189, 191] These particular programs take into consideration the type of surgery carried out and whether an intra-articular graft was made. The basic postoperative rehabilitation phases are rest, flexibility, strengthening, and coordination.

A balance of quadriceps and hamstring forces is necessary for proper function. Specific emphasis on hamstring muscle strengthening is appropriate. Pushing weight resistance from 30° of flexion to full extension will add an element of protection to the patellofemoral joint, but will create large forces to the anterior cruciate ligament. Resistance applied from 90° of flexion to 30° of flexion protects the anterior cruciate ligament but loads the patellofemoral joint. Some authors have recommended a compromise to push low weight through a full range of motion rather than larger weights through lesser ranges of motion.[160, 180, 191] During the later phases of postoperative rehabilitation, progressively less protection and progressively greater resistance at increased motion are employed. The later phases of rehabilitation include running and subsequently cutting and jumping as well.[40] Before beginning the rehabilitation of the postoperative anterior cruciate ligament patient, careful attention to the postoperative protocol of the operating surgeon is necessary.

Postoperative rehabilitation for the individual who has undergone an arthroscopic meniscectomy is obviously more rapid and much less controlled than for the patient who has undergone a ligament reconstruction procedure.[26] Full return to function after an anterior cruciate ligament repair is assumed to be a

minimum of 12 months but can be as early as 6 to 8 months. The return to play after an arthroscopic partial meniscectomy can be as short as 2 to 3 weeks with a maximum of 10 to 12 weeks dependent upon the degree of internal derangement.[33]

Phase V:
Improve Muscular Endurance

Costill has demonstrated the necessity for combining strength and endurance programs into the muscle rehabilitation portions of the program. Since there is a specific response to the type of exercise performed, an exercise program must be tailored to meet the needs of the individual.[83] Steadman has employed a group of exercises that challenge the muscles in three different ways.[191] High-repetition, moderate-weight sets are performed initially, followed by a rapid, low-resistance repetition until fatigue. The last step is to hold an isometric contraction for approximately 1 minute. This type of program improves not only absolute strength but also endurance, as well as stresses the anaerobic pathway necessary for burst-type activities.[36] Gaining muscle endurance necessitates stressing the aerobic pathways and improving the oxidative enzyme capacity of slow-twitch muscle fibers[47], and this will necessitate higher repetition work at lower weight levels.[15, 24] These types of muscle endurance sets are useful as maintenance programs also. Isolating the specific muscle contractions necessary for endurance training is based upon the activity the athlete is engaged in.

The threshold of change in the development of muscular endurance is unclear. Therefore, the degree of intensity placed upon the muscle cannot be clearly defined. In one study, strength scores improved significantly when preceded by a program using high-repetition work. Therefore, it would seem appropriate to start the athlete on a high-repetition, low-weight program before embarking on a higher resistance program.[52] This would appear to allow time for cellular adaptation to occur and to enhance the eventual strength gains of the program participant.

The use of the stationary bike with variable resistance is extremely beneficial in lower extremity muscle endurance programs. Swimming and other hydro exercises are useful in upper extremity muscular endurance programs. The maintenance of muscle endurance has been demonstrated to be a significant factor in the prevention of injury. It is not uncommon to see injuries occurring late in competition or on the last ski run of the day. This appears to be related to depletion of oxidative enzymes in slow-twitch fibers leading to fatigue of the musculature and inability of the musculature to protect the joint.[59]

Phase VI:
Develop Specific Sport-Related
Biomechanical Skill Patterns

Before starting this recoordination phase of the program, the athlete must have gained joint range of motion and soft tissue flexibility. The patient has increased muscular strength and has improved muscular endurance. Work has also been undertaken to improve the speed of contraction through the use of high-speed lifting techniques. The athlete is now ready to begin specific training and specific retraining in the development of biomechanical and neurophysiological skill patterns necessary for the specific sport.

The concept of specificity of exercise states there is poor carry-over from one type of exercise to another. In other words, to train an athlete who needs power, strength, and skill in running with only pool training would be inappropriate, due to the poor carry-over from the pool exercises. As was alluded to previously, the use of isometric strengthening solely as a strength development technique only trains that particular muscle to obtain a static concentric contraction at that particular joint angle.[124, 165] Therefore, strengthening activities must be carried out through the full arc of motion and specifically through the full arc of motion used in the particular sporting endeavor. Training the particular enzyme systems that are physiologically necessary for the neuromuscular skeletal system to carry out its function should precede this phase.

The neurophysiological learning process to develop coordinated skill patterns is based upon constant repetition with careful attention to perfecting the movement.[62, 85] Substitution patterns must be avoided to reduce the possibility of a substitution engram pattern programming. Substitution patterns arise when certain muscle groups are either weak or inflexible or there is not full joint and soft tissue range of motion available to carry out the perfect movement. The most efficient engram patterning occurs with slow methodical repetition with minimal forced application. As the movement can be carried out with greater degrees of precision, the speed and force can be increased. While the speed and force are being increased, it is imperative to watch for the development of substitution patterns. If substitution patterns develop, the speed and force must be reduced. Due to the neurophysiological principle of central nervous system irradiation, force should be minimized and replaced by coordinated movements of associated articulations to perform the movement.[85] An example of this would be the throwing motion. The acceleration of the throwing arm is most efficiently accomplished by trunk rotation. The rotator cuff muscles function as stabilizers of the glenohumeral joint in order to maintain instantaneous center of rotation of the humerus and glenoid.[107] If excessive force is applied by the shoulder girdle musculature during the throwing motion, overuse injuries will occur, with poor accuracy and early fatigue.[6, 168, 169]

The retraining of a baseball player's throwing motion after upper extremity injury should follow the principle described above. After a careful warm-up and capsular stretching program, the athlete can begin throwing using a long toss technique with very little velocity applied. Careful attention should be given to hip rotation and trunk acceleration. Once the athlete can comfortably carry out this short toss regime, a greater distance can be placed between the thrower and the catcher. This is then progressed to increasing the velocity of the toss by limiting the arc of the thrown ball. After the athlete can successfully throw from the outfield on a line drive to second base, the line drive distance is increased so that the ball will reach home plate in one or two bounces. After this can be successfully accomplished, the patient can be placed in a particular position, either as outfielder, infielder, or pitcher, and specific throwing can be undertaken. Velocity of the toss should be the last element worked on. Careful coordinated action with trunk rotation and follow-through are imperative. Each throwing session should be preceded by a careful warm-up and closed with a careful cool-down stretch and icing routine.

The redevelopment of running and cutting skills after lower extremity injury is carried out in a similar fashion. The use of rolling slant boards to retrain proprioception of the ankle joint has been found to be useful in the rehabilitation of the ankle after repeat inversion sprains.[49] Careful progressive running should be carried out initially with fast walking and careful attention to gait style, eliminating possible substitution patterns and asymmetry. After the individual can carry out a normal gait pattern, then slow running is begun. The slow running is limited to only the speed which can be accomplished pain-free without causing recurrent joint effusion, and without substitution patterns. The individual is then progressed from slow running to faster running. The fast running is done initially on soft surfaces such as grass or a track. The track appears to be best due to its constancy of terrain, which may not always be obtainable on grass surfaces. The use of protective equipment such as ankle taping or knee braces during this phase is continued. The athlete should gradually increase the stride length.

After the patient can successfully run at 75% of maximum speed without pain or recurrent swelling, slowly running in lazy S's and figure-eights is begun. The figure-eights are made closer and run tighter and tighter as the athlete begins to actually start cutting. After this can be successfully achieved, specific agility drills can be carried out using jumping in and out of obstacles and jumping on top and over obstacles such as automobile tires and wooden boxes. The amount of jumping is dependent upon the sport that the athlete is involved in. The use of plyometric exercises appears to be valuable in this phase but can cause injury due to joint and soft tissue overload.[62] Ski racers have obviously a greater need for this type of training technique than long-distance runners.

High-speed sprinting is also begun during this phase, followed by high-speed cutting. The progression through these running phases should be carried out slowly, methodically, and best accomplished under the direction of a skilled physical therapist, athletic trainer, or coach. The principles outlined above should be carefully adhered to to avoid the development of unnecessary substitution patterns. The recurrence of pain or swelling during this phase may necessitate medical reevaluation.

Similar programs have been devised for swimmers using kickboards and progressively lengthening stroke patterns. Careful technique is stressed and speed is the last element to be refined.

If the athlete is a part of an organized athletic program during this phase, he or she should work with the coaching staff if possible. The coach should look for specific flaws in technique that can be retrained during this phase to establish the necessary coordination engrams. The coaches and therapists must stress the repetitive training of only precise movements. The repetition of imprecise movements will be deleterious to both the performance and health of the athlete. Psychological support from the coaching staff, treating physician, and treating therapist/trainer is exceedingly important during this phase in order for the athlete to regain his or her confidence.

Phase VII: Improve General Cardiovascular Endurance

During the entire functional restoration program the injured athlete is not allowed to remain sedentary. At the earliest possible moment he or she is begun on either stationary bike or pool exercises. The aerobic capacity of the athlete should not be allowed to drop during the early phases of the program. This particular phase, therefore, is more of a "topping off" of the aerobic needs of the athlete.

The aerobic needs of a soccer player are different from the aerobic needs of a football lineman. The football lineman is mostly operating in the anaerobic category, whereas the soccer player is placing great demands on the aerobic enzymatic system. The cardiovascular reconditioning program should also be tuned to the particular sport. Long distance swimmers and sprint swimmers should be trained in the pool doing their particular stroke, whereas running athletes should be trained using running programs. Consistency is the key to the development of aerobic capacity. Rapid drop-offs in aerobic capacity occur with cessation of this type of training. A five times per week aerobic program of at least 30 minutes per session with the athlete exercising at greater than 75% of his or her heart rate is recommended. Obviously, considerations must be made for the middle-aged athlete who may have pre-existing cardiac disease. Early recognition of possible cardiovascular abnormalities or disease is important.[132, 166, 194, 201]

Substitution of one aerobic program for another during the rehabilitation program will often be necessary. Early in a program, swimming may be the aerobic program of choice. Later, this may be progressed to running in the pool, and later on will be progressed to a running program as already described. Some athletes may not be able to resume their previous levels of activity and will be forced to switch from running activities to either bicycling or swimming training on a permanent basis. Bicyclists are able to use stationary turbo trainers to train indoors, or they can use standard stationary bike equipment. The Schwinn Air Dyne bicycle couples both arm and leg motion and is a beneficial form of aerobic training. This bicycle enables the athlete to use large muscle groups in the upper and lower extremities in varying patterns. Rowing machines, seated pedal cycles, and cross-country ski machines are other ways to improve aerobic function.

Phase VIII: Establish Maintenance Programs

Programs for flexibility, strength, and aerobic maintenance should be designed and instructed to enable the patient to maintain fitness upon completing the last phase of rehabilitation.

Evaluation Procedures

Setting guidelines and goals during the rehabilitation program facilitates the transition between phases. Ultimately, the decision of returning the athlete to participation should be aided by some objective classification.[92] Isokinetic testing using the Cybex II, Lido, or similar isokinetic device is extremely helpful in this regard.[58, 74, 181] Isokinetic testing can yield information regarding strength deficiencies that need attention during the rehabilitation process and can help to establish guidelines in regard to the appropriate timing of return to play. There may be a side-to-side difference in strength of around 20% of which the athlete is unaware. This has been noted in studies following knee injuries and after Achilles tendon injuries, in which a side-to-side difference of 30% or more was noted without subjective sensation. These observations demonstrate the necessity for objective measurements in muscle strength in the rehabilitation procedure.[79, 80]

These testing devices, by accommodating resistance against a lever moving at a set angular velocity (e.g., 100°/sec), can measure dynamic strength at every point in the range of motion. Muscles are made to contract at the speed of the machine, and no matter how hard the person may push, the testing lever will not move faster than the predetermined angular velocity. Conversely, if the person applies less torque force to the lever than that which is set, no resistance will be encountered. In this way, injury is avoided because no weight is left to fall on the tested limb. The Cybex machine incorporates a dual channel recorder, dynamometer, and electrogoniometer, which provide a continuous printout curve of the joint angles and peak torque across the entire range of motion of the limb being tested. Different speeds can be evaluated, which is important considering the velocity-specific training effects that have been demonstrated in numerous studies.[83, 141, 157]

In general, return to athletic activity is not recommended if there is a significant (10% to 20%) side-to-side difference in strength. In general, when the injured extremity has reached 80% of the unaffected side strength, the more vigorous aspects of the training program can begin. For example, in lower extremity programs, the 60% to 80% mark would generally allow the beginning of jogging and running programs. After knee ligament injuries, attaining an 80% mark with normal coordination could qualify an individual to return to action.

Isokinetic strength evaluations have been found to be beneficial in pre-participation evaluations also.[25] They can pinpoint deficiencies in strength and deficiencies in specific speeds of contraction and thereby help in designing preseason rehabilitation programs.[39] Isokinetic evaluation protocols have been established for strength (defined as maximum slow-speed torque capability) and power (defined as fast-speed torque capability for which muscle tension must be developed in brief time limits at functional limb velocities); exercise protocols for power endurance (defined as the number of repetitions to 50% fatigue during maximum effort) have also been designed. Isometric time rates of tension development at peak torque and fatigue are also available.

During testing, optimal positioning and stabilization minimize the effect of possible body movements. Avoidance of substitution patterns are important also in the testing procedure. Locating the true or best possible axis of rotation to allow maximum functional range of motion and smooth comfortable movement for the patient is imperative. The appropriate selection of test speeds should take into account the functional speed demands and capability of the joint and muscle group being tested.[71, 91, 181] Isokinetic evaluation procedures can be performed for upper extremity, lower extremity, and trunk musculature.

A range-of-motion assessment is another important evaluation procedure to help establish guidelines during the rehabilitation process. Careful and accurate recording of the joint range of motion will assist in decision-making when used in combination with strength evaluation procedures.

Flexibility Programs

For many years, flexibility training was an ignored aspect of injury rehabilitation and injury prevention. Now, however, the literature supporting flexibility training continues to grow, as it is repeatedly demonstrated to reduce sports injury in many environments.[11, 20, 35] Flexibility programs with a sound scientific foundation should be incorporated into sports training programs.[50, 51] One such program, the proprioceptive neuromuscular facilitation (PNF) procedure, is a proven, effective means of passive stretching.[193] A PNF procedure involves an initial passive static flexibility maneuver of the agonist, followed by a 3-second maximum voluntary contraction of the agonist, followed by a concentric contraction of the antagonist, and then static stretching of the agonist once again. This type of flexibility program has been found to be more effective than use of passive static flexibility methods alone.[193]

Flexibility programs can enhance concentric contraction velocities of the musculature as well as reduce the subjective symptoms of muscle soreness after vigorous exercise.[93] Flexibility programs are especially useful in the prevention of overuse injuries.[86, 167] As discussed by Beck and Day, a careful assessment of pre-participation flexibility will allow the designing of better pre-participation rehabilitation programs.[11]

Taping and Bracing

Taping and bracing are useful for both the prevention of injury and the protection of injured structures. The goal of the appliance or taping procedure should be determined before the brace or taping procedure is selected. Taping ankles and knees can help support previously injured ligamentous structures during athletic competition. Knee taping can be useful to help stabilize the knee after a collateral ligament injury during the return to play phase. There are a variety of knee braces used to support the anterior cruciate-deficient knee, but there is inadequate scientific information to determine which of these braces are effective. Initial brace designs used dynamic rotation control, whereas new designs use extension control.

Recurrent shoulder dislocation can sometimes be managed, specifically in a football player, with the use of a harness to limit the extremes of external rotation and abduction. Depending on the position that the athlete plays, this type of device is useful in returning an athlete to the playing field after the shoulder dislocation has been successfully rehabilitated. Cast braces limit the extremes of extension in a previously dislocated elbow and enable an athlete to return to competition with the hinges locked at the degree of motion desired. Hinged cast braces are also an extremely important component during the postoperative knee ligament rehabilitation process.

There are a variety of knee supports which may be useful in the treatment of soft tissue afflictions. Patellar tendinitis can often be controlled with the use of a knee brace which exerts pressure on the patellar tendon.[159] Recurrent patellar subluxation can often be controlled with the use of a brace that has a buttress to limit patellar motion. Occasionally Neoprene knee sleeves are employed to warm the knee of a person with degenerative arthritis and provide comfort. Elbow counter force braces can provide symptomatic relief for the athlete suffering from elbow extensor tendinitis, but its mechanism of action is poorly understood.[151, 188] Controlling cervical extension is one way to protect a previously injured cervical nerve root in football players.

Knee braces prescribed to prevent collateral ligament injuries of the knee in football players have gained recent popularity. This type of brace uses a single metal upright; some possess a biaxial or polycentric hinge. At present, however, there is inadequate scientific evidence to support their routine use.[173]

Molded orthotic devices to control subtalar joint alignment have become popular for the treatment of running injuries. A careful evaluation for the presence of a correctable malalignment coupled with evidence that the malalignment contributed to the injury is necessary before prescribing these devices.[41]

Pre-Participation Examinations

The preseason physical examination serves several important functions, including pinpointing previously injured areas and designing injury prevention programs.[76] It can also better identify potentially injurable areas, such as in an individual with poor muscle strength and poor flexibility,[39] and possible life-threatening cardiovascular abnormalities such as idiopathic hypertrophic subaortic stenosis and other varieties of aortic outflow problems.[138, 194]

An adequate understanding of the nutritional aspects of sporting activity is important for all sports medicine practitioners.[88] Proper counseling and sound advice based upon scientific information rather than food faddism serve an integral function in the care of athletes.

REHABILITATION ALGORITHMS FOR SPECIFIC INJURY TYPES

The information presented in earlier sections of this chapter combined with the algorithms shown here will assist the sports medicine physician in planning appropriate treatment programs.

A treatment program must, by necessity, be flexible enough to handle mid-program changes determined by changes in clinical status and differing responses to a variety of treatments. Therefore, rigid interpretation of these algorithms is inappropriate.

Tendinitis Rehabilitation Algorithm

Figure 43-1 shows an algorithm for tendinitis rehabilitation. Major goals include the following:

1. Reduce tendon, tendon sheath, and related soft tissue inflammation
2. Enhance muscle tendon unit flexibility
3. Enhance muscle tendon unit strength
4. Identify and correct athletic form, equipment, and biomechanical problems that predispose to repeat injury.

Comments

Phonophoresis and iontophoresis are controversial, but have been found to be useful by many sports medicine specialists in the treatment of tendinitis.

Acupuncture may be useful as an adjunctive treatment to reduce pain early in the treatment, but probably should not be used as stand-alone treatment.

Corticosteroid injection into the tendon substance is contraindicated. Corticosteroid injection into a tendon sheath or into a contiguous bursa that is inflamed is beneficial.

Individualize the sports-specific retraining to meet the clinical circumstance.

Surgical treatment may be necessary in refractory cases.

Rotator Cuff Tendinitis

Figure 43-2 presents an algorithm for the rehabilitation of shoulder impingement. Major goals include the following:

1. Reduce rotator cuff tendon and overlying bursa inflammation
2. Enhance rotator cuff tendon flexibility
3. Enhance strength of rotator cuff musculature with specific attention to the supraspinatus
4. Retrain athletic form to avoid substitution patterns
5. Identify and rehabilitate cervical pathology that may contribute to the syndrome
6. Strengthen scapular stabilizers.

Comments

The use of phonophoresis and iontophoresis is controversial, but have been found to be useful by many sports medicine specialists in the treatment of this condition.

Acupuncture may be useful as an adjunctive treatment to reduce pain, but should probably not be a stand-alone treatment.

The decision to perform surgery may come earlier than the

(Text continues on page 861)

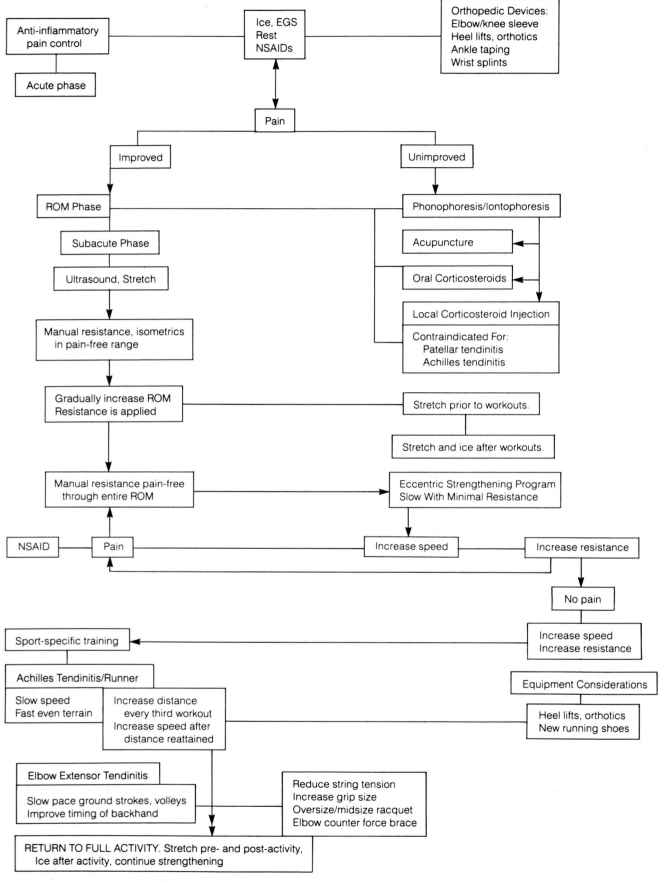

Figure 43-1.   Tendinitis rehabilitation algorithm.

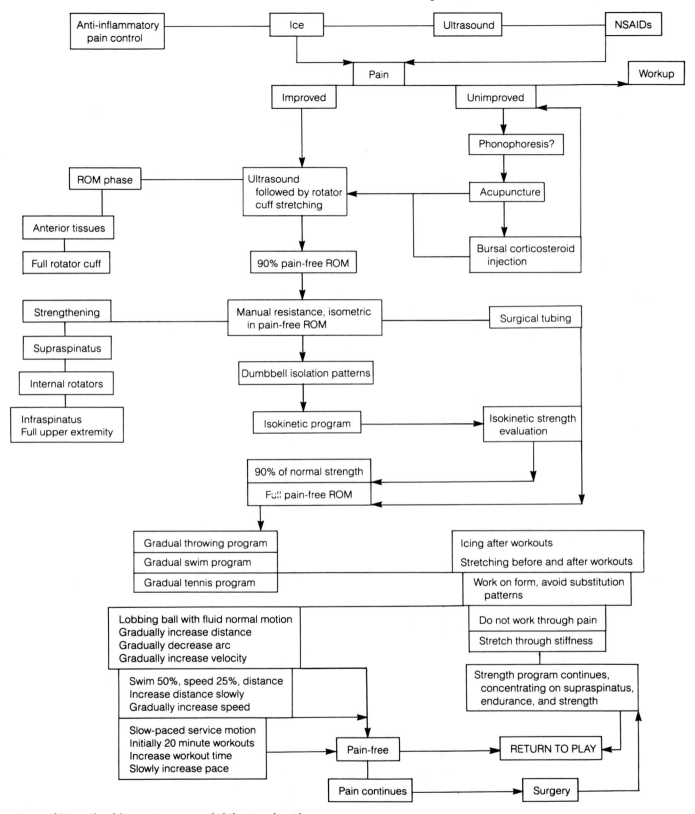

Figure 43-2.   Shoulder impingement rehabilitation algorithm.

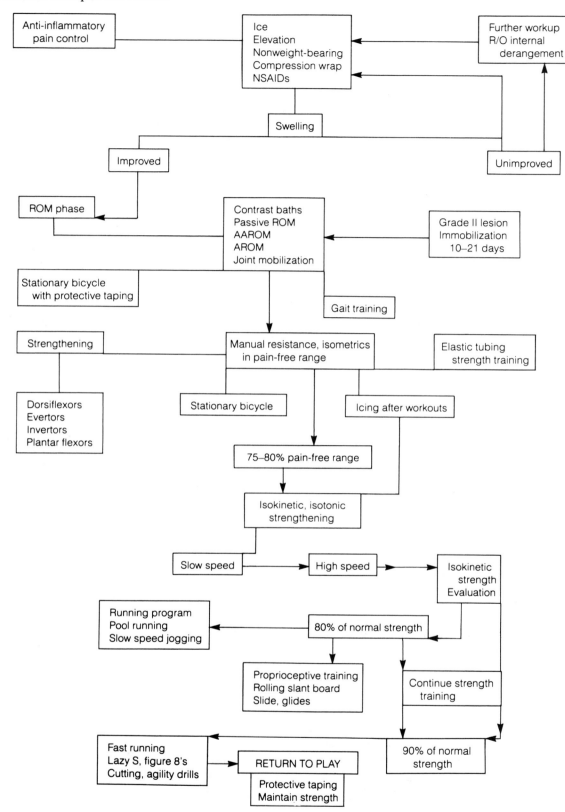

Figure 43-3. Ankle ligament injury rehabilitation algorithm.

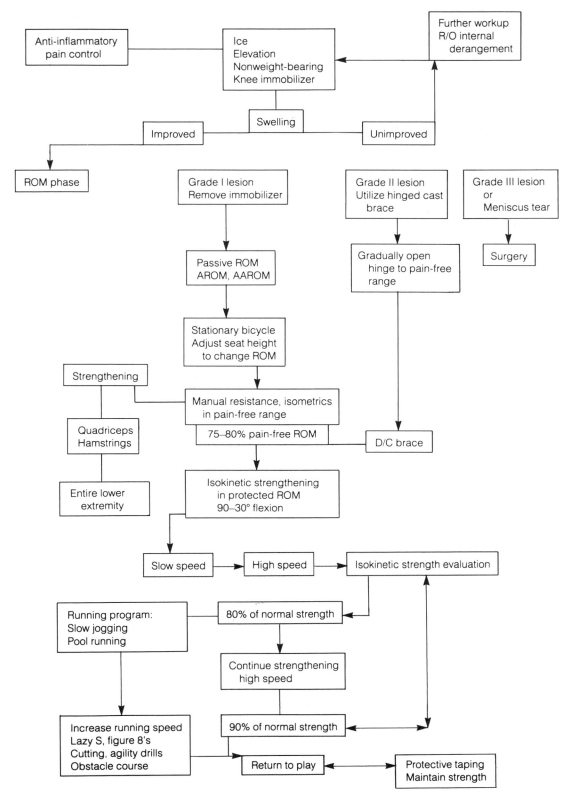

Figure 43-4. Knee collateral ligament injury rehabilitation algorithm.

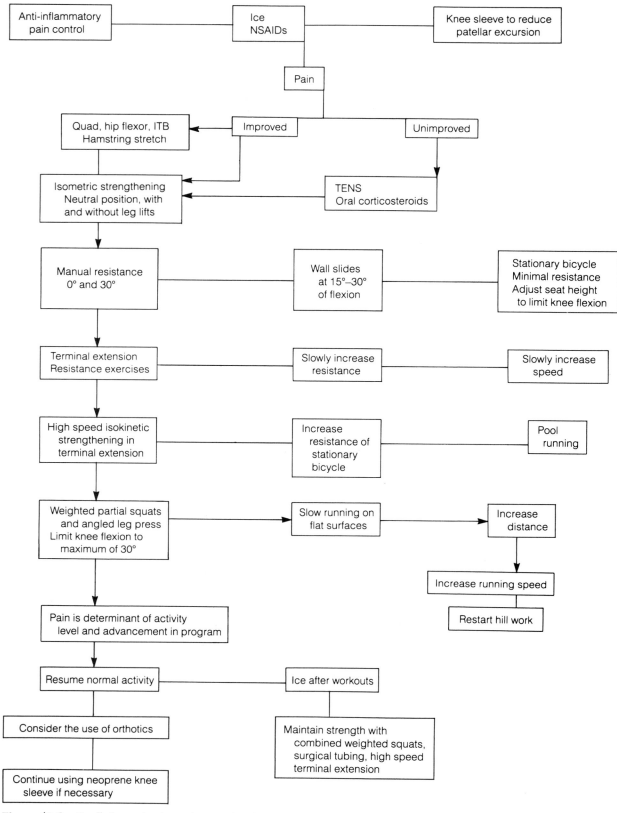

Figure 43-5.   Patellofemoral pain syndrome rehabilitation algorithm.

last phase of the algorithm, depending on the degree of disability, the results of diagnostic tests, and social decisions concerning season of play and school eligibility.

Identify shoulder instability syndromes that may contribute to the injury process.

Ankle Ligament Injury Rehabilitation

Figure 43-3 presents an algorithm for the rehabilitation of ankle ligament injury. Major goals include the following:

1. Reduce and control post-injury inflammation
2. Enhance strength and endurance of ankle stabilizing musculature
3. Regain full articular range of motion of the ankle and midfoot structures.

Comments

Nonweight-bearing for grade I ligament injuries may be limited to the first 24 to 72 hours. Nonweight-bearing for the grade II ligament injuries may be necessary for the first week but can be discontinued when the athlete can walk comfortably without recurrence of swelling.

The use of cast immobilization should be reserved for those individuals who demonstrate significant ligament laxity or poor clinical response to anti-inflammatory control in the first 72 hours. Ankle taping can be useful in the initial phase to limit motion and reduce pain.

Be sure to identify midfoot sprain and tibiofibular ligament (*i.e.,* interosseous membrane) sprain.

Recurrent ankle injuries should be treated more aggressively in the strengthening phases and maintenance phases.

Continued pain with recurrent swelling should be a signal to look for a possible osteochondral injury or the development of capsular fibrosis or associated tendinitis.

Knee Collateral Ligament Injury Rehabilitation

Figure 43-4 presents an algorithm for the rehabilitation of knee collateral ligament injury. Major goals include the following:

1. Allow ligament healing to occur
2. Strengthen quadriceps and hamstring musculature
3. Regain full range of motion after ligament healing
4. Do not rely upon strength parameters as sole criteria for return to action. Retraining is imperative before competition resumption.

Comments

A grade II lesion may necessitate a minimum of 4 to 6 weeks of protective range bracing to ensure proper ligament healing.

Strict criteria regarding return to play are not available. Therefore, these decisions must be based upon the combined criteria of strength parameters, coordination skills, and social factors.

Attention to total lower extremity strength is important.

Patellofemoral Pain Syndrome Rehabilitation

Figure 43-5 presents an algorithm for the rehabilitation of patellofemoral pain. Major goals include the following:

1. Enhance strength of quadriceps muscle and be certain the vastus medialis is functioning well
2. Enhance flexibility of lateral patellar supporting soft tissue and hamstrings
4. Regain full patellar mobility
5. Strengthen within arcs of motion that minimize shear and compression stress to patellofemoral articular surfaces
6. Find the pain-free ranges within which to strengthen by careful physical therapy assessment.

Comments

The use of knee sleeves to guard patellar motion may be useful but there is no scientific evidence of their effectiveness.

Orthotic devices to control subtalar joint motion may be useful to correct some varieties of patellofemoral malalignment and thereby reduce pain.

Acupuncture and TENS used together may be beneficial to reduce pain and enhance the strength restoration process. Surgical options may need to be explored in refractory cases. Arthroscopic evaluation, debridements, and patellar realignment procedures may be appropriate. A plica masquerading as patellofemoral pain must also be considered.

Counseling in regard to long-term activity modification may be necessary in certain cases.

REFERENCES

1. Akeson WH: An experimental study of joint stiffness. J Bone Joint Surg 43A(7):1022–1034, 1961
2. Akeson WH, Amiel D, LaViolette D: The connective tissue response to immobility: A study of chrondroitin-4 and 6-sulfate and dermatan sulfate changes in periarticular connective tissue of control and immobilized knees of dogs. Clin Orthop 51:183–197, 1967
3. Akeson WH, Woo SLY, Amiel D et al: Connective tissue response to immobility. Clin Orthop 93:356–362, 1973
4. Allman FL: Exercise in sports medicine. In Basmajian JV (ed): Therapeutic Exercise, pp 485–509. Baltimore, Williams and Wilkins, 1984
5. Andrews R, Axe MJ: The classification of knee ligament instability. Orthop Clin North Am 16(1):69–82, 1985
6. Aronen JG: Shoulder rehabilitation. Clin Sports Med 4(3):477–483, 1985
7. Aronen JG, Regan K: Decreasing the incidence of recurrence of first time anterior shoulder dislocations with rehabilitations. Am J Sports Med 12:283–291, 1984
8. Balaji M, DeWeese J: Adductor canal outlet syndrome. JAMA 245(2):167–170, 1981
9. Basmajian JV, Harden TP, Regenos EM: Integrated actions of the four heads of quadriceps femoris: An EMG study. Anat Rec 172:15–20, 1972
10. Bateman J: Nerve injuries about the shoulder in sports. J Bone and Joint Surg 49:785–792, 1967
11. Beck JL, Day RW: Overuse injuries. Clin Sports Med 4(3):553, 1985
12. Bergfeld J: Functional rehabilitation of isolated medial collateral sprains. First, second, and third degree sprains. Am J Sports Med 7:207–209, 1979
13. Bird CB, McCoy JW: Weight-lifting as a cause of compartment syndrome in the forearm. J Bone Joint Surg 64A(3):406, 1983
14. Blackburn TA, Rehabilitation of anterior cruciate ligament injuries Orthop Clin North Am 16(2):241–269, 1985
15. Bonde-Petersen F, Grandal H, Hansen JW, Hvid N: The effect of varying the number of muscle contractions on dynamic muscle training. Eur J Applied Physiol 18:468–473, 1966
16. Bonen A, Keitzer HA: Athletic menstrual cycle irregularity: Endocrine response to exercise and training. Phys Sports Med 7:83–95, 1984
17. Booth, FW: Time course of muscular atrophy during immobilization of hind limbs in rats. J Applied Physiol 43:656–661, 1977

18. Booth FW, Seider MJ: Effects of disuse by limb immobilization on different muscle fiber types. In Pette D (ed): Plasticity of Muscle. New York, de Gruyter, 1980

19. Borges JF, Hallet M, Selkoe JD et al: The anterior tarsal tunnel syndrome. J Neurosurg 54:89–92, 1981

20. Borms J: Importance of flexibility in overall physical fitness. Int J Phys Ed 21:15–26, 1984

21. Brill DR: Bone imaging for lower extremity pain in athletes. Clin Nucl Med 8:101–106, 1983

22. Brody D: Techniques in the evaluation and treatment of the injured runner. Orthop Clin North Am 13:541–558, 1982

23. Brody DM: Running injuries. Clin Symp 32:1–36, 1980

24. Burger RA: Optimal repetitions for the development of strength. Res Q 33:334–338, 1962

25. Cahill BR, Griffith EH: Effect of preseason conditioning on the incidence and severity of high school football knee injuries. Am J Sports Med 6:180–184, 1978

26. Campbell D, Glenn W: Rehabilitation of knee flexor and knee extensor muscle strength in patients with meniscectomies, ligamentous repairs, and chondromalacia. Phys Ther 62(1):10–15, 1982

27. Chu DA: Comparisons of selected electromyographic data under isokinetic and isotonic stress load. Menlo Park, Stanford University, 1974

28. Chvapil M: Physiology of Connective Tissue. London, Butterworth, 1967

29. Clancy WG, Brand RL, Bergfeld JA: Upper trunk brachial plexus injuries in contact sports. Am J Sports Med 5:209–216, 1977

30. Clein LJ: Suprascapular entrapment neuropathy. J Neurosurg 43:337–342, 1975

31. Clement DB: Taunton JE, Smart GW: Achilles tendinitis and peritendinitis: Etiology and treatment. Am J Sports Med 12(3):179–184, 1984

32. Collins HR: Screening of athletic knee injuries. Clin Sports Med 4(2):217, 1985

33. Colville JM, Jackson DW: Reasonable expectations following arthroscopic surgery. Clin Sports Med 4(2):279–293, 1985

34. Cooper RR, Miso S: Tendon and ligament insertion. J Bone Joint Surg 52A(1):1–19, 1970

35. Cornelius WL: A flexibility method designed to establish suitable internal environment for strength. Int Gymnast Techn (Suppl) 2:33–34, 1981

36. Costill DL, Coyle EF, Fink WF et al: Adaptations in skeletal muscle following strength training. J Applied Physiol 46:149, 1976

37. Costill DL, Fink WJ, Habansky AJ: Muscle rehabilitation after knee surgery. Phys Sports Med 5:71–74, 1977

38. Coyle EF, Feiring DC, Rotkis TC et al: Specificity of power improvements through slow and fast isokinetic training. J Applied Physiol 51(6):1437–1442, 1981

39. Crouch L: Neck injuries: Prevention to avoid rehabilitation. Nat Strength Conditioning Assoc 1:29–31, 1979

40. Curl WW, Markey KL, Mitchell WA: Agility training following anterior cruciate ligament reconstruction. Clin Orthop 172:133–136, 1983

41. D'Ambrosia RD: Orthotic devices in running injuries. Clin Sports Med 4(4):611–618, 1985

42. D'Ambrosia RD, Drez D: Orthotics. In D'Ambrosia RD, Drez D (eds): Prevention and Treatment of Running Injuries. Thorofare, NJ, Slack, 1982

43. Dangles C, Bilos Z: Ulnar nerve neuritis in a world champion weightlifter. Am J Sports Med 8(6):443–445, 1980

44. DeAndrade JR, Grant C, Dixon AS: Joint distention and reflex muscle inhibition in the knee. J Bone Joint Surg 47:313–322, 1965

45. DeHaven KE: Diagnosis of acute knee injuries with hemarthrosis. Am J Sports Med 8:9–14, 1980

46. Dehne K, Kriz FK Jr: Rationale of immediate immobilization and the restoration of joint function. J Bone Joint Surg 49A:1235, 1967

47. DeLateur BJ: Exercise for strength and endurance. In Basmajian JV (ed): Therapeutic Exercise, Baltimore, Williams & Wilkins, 1984

48. DeLorme TL: Restoration of muscle power by heavy-resistance exercises. J Bone Joint Surg 27A:645–667, 1945

49. Derscheid GL, Brown WC: Rehabilitation of the ankle. Clin Sports Med 4(3):527–544, 1985

50. de Vries HA: Electromyographic observations of the effect of static stretching upon muscle distress. Res Q 32:468–480, 1961

51. de Vries HA: Evaluation of static stretching procedures for improvement flexibility. Res Q 33:222–230, 1962

52. Dickinson AD, Bennett KN: Therapeutic exercise. Clin Sports Med 4(3):417–429, 1985

53. Drez D: Running footware, examination of the training shoe, the foot and functional orthotic devices. Am J Sports Med 8:140–141, 1980

54. Drez D: Arthroscopic evaluation of the injured athlete's knee. Clin Sports Med 4(2):275–278, 1985

55. Edstrom L: Selective atrophy of red muscle fibre in the quadriceps in long-standing knee-joint dysfunction. J Neurol Sci 11:551–559, 1960

56. Elliott DH: Structure and function of mammalian tendon. Biol Rev 40:392–421, 1965

57. Elliott DH: The biomechanical properties of tendon in relation to muscular strength. Ann Phys Med 9:1–7, 1967

58. Elsner RC, Pedegana L, Lang J: Protocol for strength testing and rehabilitation of the upper extremity. J Orthop Sports Phys Ther 4(4):229–235, 1983

59. Ericksson E: Anatomical, histological and physiological factors in experienced downhill skiers. Orthop Clin North Am 7:159–165, 1976

60. Ericksson E: Sports injuries of knee ligaments. Their diagnosis, treatment, rehabilitation, and prevention. Med Sci Sports 8:133–144, 1976

61. Eriksson E, Haggmark T: Comparison of isometric muscle training and electrical stimulation supplementing isometric muscle training in the recovery after major knee ligament surgery. Am J Sports Med 7(3):169–171, 1979

62. Fahey TD: Physiological adaptation to conditioning. In Fahey TD (ed): Athletic Training: Principles and Practice. pp 57–78. Palo Alto, CA, Mayfield Publishing, 1986

63. Fearon DT, Austen FK: Acute inflammatory response. In McCarty DJ Jr (ed): Arthritis and Allied Conditions, 9th ed, pp 214–228. Philadelphia, Lea & Febiger, 1979

64. Frankel S, Hirata I: The scalenus anticus syndrome and competitive swimming. JAMA 215(11):1796–1798, 1971

65. Friden J, Sjostrom M, Ekblom B: Myofibrillar damage following intense eccentric exercise in man. Int J Sports Med 2:1–6, 1981

66. Frisch RE, Wyshak G, Vincent L: Delayed menarche and amenorrhea in ballet dancers. N.Engl J Med 303:17–19, 1980

67. Fuglsang-Fredriksen A, Sheel U: Transient decrease in number of motor units after immobilization in man. J Neurol Neurosurg Psychiatry 41:924–929, 1978

68. Gangarosa LP, Park N, Wiggins CA, Hill JM: Increased penetration of nonelectrolytes into mouse skin during iontophoretic water transport (iontohydrokinesis). J Pharmacol Exp Ther 212(3):377–381, 1980

69. Giove T, Sayers J, Kent G et al: Non-operative treatment of the torn anterior cruciate ligament. J Bone Joint Surg 65A:184–192, 1983

70. Glass JM, Stephen RL, Jacobson SC: The quality and distribution of radiolabeled dexamethasone delivered to tissue by iontophoresis. Int Soc Tropical Dermatol 19:519–525, 1980

71. Gleim G, Nicholas J, Webb J: Isokinetic evaluation following leg injuries. Physician Sports Med 6:74–82, 1978

72. Godshall R, Hansen C: Traumatic ulnar neuropathy in adolescent baseball pitchers. J Bone Joint Surg 53A:359–361, 1971

73. Goodman AG, Gilman LS, Gilman A: The Pharmacological Basis of Therapeutics, 6th ed. New York, Macmillan, 1980

74. Goslin BR, Charteris J: Isokinetic dynamometry: Normative date for clinical use of lower extremity (knee) cases. Scand J Rehabil Med 11:105–109, 1979

75. Grana WA, Kriegshauser LA: Scientific basis of extensor mechanism disorders. Clin Sports Med 4(2):247–251, 1985

76. Grant T, Puffer J: Cervical stenosis: A developmental anomaly with quadriparesis during football. Am J Sports Med 4:291–321, 1976

77. Griffin JE, Touchstone JC: Ultrasonic movement of cortisol into pig tissue. I. Movement into skeletal muscle. Am J Phys Med 42(1):77–84, 1963

78. Griffin JE, Touchstone JC, Liu AC: Ultrasonic movement of cortisol

into pig tissue. II. Movement into paravertebral nerve. Am J Phys Med 44(1):20–25, 1965

79. Grimby G: Isokinetic training. Int J Sports Med 3:61–64, 1982

80. Grimby G: Progressive resistance exercise for injury rehabilitation: Special emphasis on isokinetic training. Sports Med 2:309–315, 1985

81. Gudas, CJ: Patterns of lower extremity injury in 224 runners. Compr Ther 6(9):50–59, 1980

82. Haggmark T, Eriksson E: Cylinder or mobile cast brace after knee ligament surgery. Am J Sports Med 7:48, 1979

83. Halling A, Dooley J: The importance of isokinetic power and its specificity to athletic conditions. Athletic Training 14:83–86, 1979

84. Halpern AA, Horowitz BG, Nagel DA: Tendon ruptures associated with corticosteroid therapy. West J Med 127:378–382, 1977

85. Harris FA: Facilitation techniques and technological adjuncts in therapeutic exercise. In Basmajian JV (ed): Therapeutic Exercise, 9th ed., pp 110–178. Baltimore, Williams & Wilkins, 1984

86. Harvey JS Jr: Overuse syndromes in young athletes. Clin Sports Med 2(3):595–607, 1983

87. Hawkins RJ, Hobeika PE: Impingement syndrome in the athletic shoulder. Clin Sports Med 2(2):391–405, 1983

88. Hecker AL (ed): Nutritional aspects of exercise. Clin Sports Med 3(3). Philadelphia, WB Saunders, 1984

89. Henricson AS, Westlin ND: Chronic calcaneal pain in athletes: Entrapment of the calcaneal nerve? Am J Sports Med 12:152–154, 1984

90. Hirsch G: Tensile properties during tendon healing. ACTA Orthop Scand (Suppl) 153:1–145, 1974

91. Hislop HJ, Perrine JJ: The isokinetic concept of exercise. Phys Ther 47:114–117, 1967

92. Holland DP: Exercise prescription and therapeutic rehabilitation in sports medicine. Athletic Training 17:283–286, 1982

93. Hortobagyi T, Faludi J, Tihanyi J, Merkely B: Effects of intense "stretching" flexibility training on the mechanical profile of the knee extensors and on the range of motion of the hip joint. Int J Sports Med 6:317–321, 1985

94. Hughston JC, Andrews JR, Cross MJ et al: Classification of knee ligament instabilities. I. J Bone Joint Surg 58A:159, 1976

95. Hughston, JC, Andrews JR, Cross MJ et al: Classification of knee ligament instabilities. II. J Bone Joint Surg 58A:173, 1976

96. Hughston JC, Andrews JR, Waddell DD et al: The suprapatellar plica: Its role in internal derangement of the knee. Presented at the American Academy of Orthopaedic Surgeons, Dallas, February 1978

97. Hungerford DS, Barry M: Biomechanics of the patellofemoral joint. Clin Orthop 144:9–15, 1979

98. Hupprich FL, Sigerseth PO: The specificity of flexibility in girls. Res Q 19:25–33, 1950

99. Imbriglia JE, Bolland DM: An exercise-induced compartment syndrome of the dorsal forearm—A case report. J Hand Surg 9A(1):142–143, 1984

100. Insall J: Current concepts review: Patellar pain. J Bone Joint Surg 64A:147, 1982

101. Jackson DW: Shin splints: An update. Phys Sports Med 6:49–61, 1978

102. Jackson DW: Low back pain in young athletes: Evaluation of stress reaction and discogenic problems. Am J Sports Med 7:364–366, 1979

103. Jackson DW, James CM, McBryde AM: Injuries in runners and joggers. In Schneider RC et al (eds): Sports Injuries, Mechanism, Prevention and Treatment. Baltimore, Williams & Wilkins, 1985

104. Jackson DW, Wiltse LL, Cirincione RJ: Spondylolysis in the female gymnast. Clin Orthop 117:68–73, 1976

105. James SL, Bates BT, Osternig LR: Injuries to runners. Am J Sports Med 6:40–50, 1978

106. Jensen JE, Conn RR, Hazelrigg G, Hewett JE: Systematic evaluation of acute knee injuries. Clin Sports Med 4(2):295–312, 1985

107. Jobe FW, Tibone JE, Perry J, Moynes D: An EMG analysis of the shoulder in throwing and pitching. Am J Sports Med 11(1):3–5, 1983

108. Johnson J, Kendall H: Isolated paralysis of the serratus anterior muscle. J Bone Joint Surg 3:567–574, 1955

109. Jozsa L, Balint BJ, Reffy A, Demel Z: Hypoxic alterations of tenocytes in degenerative tendinopathy. Arch Orthop Traumat Surg 99:243–246, 1982

110. Kaplan PE, Kernaham WT: Tarsal tunnel syndrome. J Bone Joint Surg 63A:96–99, 1981

111. Keck C: The tarsal-tunnel syndrome. J Bone Joint Surg 44A:180–182, 1962

112. Kelemen MH, Stewart KJ: Circuit weight training: A new direction for cardiac rehabilitation. Sports Med 2:385–388, 1985

113. Kennedy JC, Baxter-Willis R: The effects of local steroid injections on tendons: A biochemical and microscopic correlative study. Am J Sports Med 4:11–18, 1976

114. Kennedy JC, Hawkins R, Krissoff WB: Orthopaedic manifestations of swimming. Am J Sports Med 6:309–322, 1978

115. Kirby JF, Kraft GH: Entrapment neuropathy of the anterior branch of axillary nerve. Report of case. Arch Phys Med Rehabil 53:338–340, 1972

116. Knapik JJ, Wright JE, Mawdsley RH, Braun JM: Isokinetic, isometric and isotonic strength relationships. Arch Phys Med Rehabil 64:77–80, 1983

117. Knapik JJ, Wright JE, Mawdsley RH, Braun J: Isometric, isotonic, and isokinetic torque variations in four muscle groups through a range of joint motion. Phys Ther 63:939–947, 1983

118. Kutz JE, Singer R, Lindsay M: Chronic exertional compartment syndrome of the forearm: A case report. J Hand Surg: 10A(2):302–304, 1985

119. Lampe GN, Mannheimer JS: Clinical Transcutaneous Electrical Nerve Stimulation. Philadelphia, FA Davis, 1984

120. Larson RL: Physical examination in the diagnosis of rotatory instability. Clin Orthop 172:38–44, 1983

121. Leach RE, James W, Wasilewski S: Achilles tendinitis. Am J Sports Med 9(2):93–98, 1981

122. Lesmes GR, Costill DL, Coyle EF, Fink WJ: Muscle strength and power changes during maximal isokinetic training. Med Sci Sports 10:266–269, 1978

123. Lindenbaum B: Ski boot compression syndrome. Clin Orthop Rel Res 140:109–110, 1979

124. Lindh M: Increase of muscle strength from isometric quadriceps exercise at different knee angles. Scand J Rehabil 11:33–36, 1979

125. Logan JG, Rorabeck CH, Castle GSP: The measurement of dynamic compartment pressure during exercise. Am J Sports Med 11(4):220–223, 1983

126. Lothm M, Fried A, Leavy M et al: Radial palsy following muscular effort. J Bone Joint Surg 53B:500–506, 1971

127. Lutter JM: Health concerns for women runners. Clin Sports Med 4(4):615, 1985

128. Lutter LD: The knee and running. Clin Sports Med 4(4):655, 1985

129. Mann RA et al: Running symposium. Foot Ankle 1:199, 1981

130. Marinacci AA: Neurological syndromes of the tarsal tunnels. Bull Los Angeles Neurol Soc 33:90–100, 1968

131. Markey KL: Rehabilitation of the anterior cruciate deficient knee. Clin Sports Med 4(3):513–526, 1985

132. Maron BJ, Roberts WC, McAllister HA et al: Sudden death in young athletes. Circulation 62:218–229, 1980

133. Marshall JL, Rubin RM: Knee ligament injuries—A diagnostic and therapeutic approach. Orthop Clin North Am 8:641–668, 1977

134. Marshall T: Nerve pinch injuries in football. J Ky Med Assoc 68(10):648–649, 1970

135. McBryde AM: Stress fractures in runners. In D'Ambrosia R, Drez D (eds): Prevention and Treatment of Running Injuries. In American Academy of Orthopaedic Surgeons: Instructional Course Lectures, vol 33. St Louis, CV Mosby, 1984

136. McBryde AM: Stress fractures in runners. Clin Sports Med 4(4):635, 1985

137. McDonagh MJN, Davies CTM: Adaptive responses of mammalian skeletal muscle to exercise with high loads. Eur J Applied Physiol 52:139–155, 1984

138. McKeag DB: Preseason physical examination for the prevention of sports injuries. Sports Med 2:413–431, 1985

139. Meals R: Peroneal nerve palsy complicating ankle strain. J Bone Joint Surg 59A(7):966–968, 1977

140. Micheli LJ: Back injuries to dancers. Clin Sports Med 2(3):473–484, 1983

141. Moffroid M, Whipple R: Specificity of speed of exercise. Phys Ther 50(12):1692–1700, 1970

142. Moffroid M, Whipple R, Hofkoch J, Lowman E, Thistle H: A study of isokinetic exercise. J Am Phys Ther Assoc 49(7):735–747, 1969

143. Montgomery JB, Steadman JR: Rehabilitation of the injured knee. Clin Sports Med 4(2):333–343, 1985

144. Moore MA, Hutton RS: Electromyographic investigation of muscle stretching techniques. Med Sci Sports 12:322–329, 1980

145. Mubarak SJ, Gould RN, Lee YF et al: The medial tibial stress syndrome: A cause of shinsplints. Am J Sports Med 10:202–205, 1982

146. Mubarak SJ, Hargens AR: Compartment Syndromes and Volkmann's Contracture. Philadelphia, WB Saunders, 1981

147. Muller EA: Influence of training and of inactivity on muscle strength. Arch Phys Med Rehabil 51:449–462, 1970

148. Murray MP, Baldwin J, Gardner G et al: Maximum isometric knee flexor and extensor muscle contractions—Normal patterns of torque versus time. Phys Ther 57(6):637–643, 1977

149. Mutch Y, Mori T, Suzukiy, Sugiura: Stress fractures of the ulna in athletes. Am J Sports Med 10:365–367, 1982

150. Nicholas JA, Grossman RB, Hershman EB: The importance of a simplified classification of motion in sports in relation to performance. Orthop Clin North Am 8(3):499, 1977

151. Nirschl RP: The etiology and treatment of tennis elbow. J Sports Med 2:30B, 1974

152. Noyes FR: Functional properties of knee ligaments and alterations induced by immobilization: A correlative biomechanical and histological study in primates. Clin Orthop 123:210–242, 1977

153. Noyes FR, Matthews DS, Mooar PA et al: The symptomatic anterior cruciate deficient knee. J Bone Joint Surg 65A:163–174, 1983

154. Noyes FR, McGinniss GH, Grood ES: The variable functional disability of the anterior cruciate ligament-deficient knee. Orthop Clin North Am 16(1):47–67, 1985

155. Noyes FR, Pekka AM, Matthews DS et al: The symptomatic anterior cruciate deficient knee. J Bone Joint Surg 64A:154–162, 1983

156. Noyes FR, Torvik PJ, Hyde WB, DeLucas JL: Biomechanics of ligament failure. J Bone Joint Surg 56A(7):1406–1418, 1974

157. Osternig LR, Hammil J, Sawhill J, Bates BT: Influence of torque and limb speed on power production in isokinetic exercise. Am J Phys Med 62(4):163–171, 1983

158. Pace JB, Nagle D: Piriform syndrome. West J Med 124:435–439, 1976

159. Palumbo PM: Dynamic patellar brace: A new orthosis in the management of patellofemoral disorders. Am J Sports Med 9(1):45–49, 1981

160. Paulos L, Noyes FR, Grood E, Butler DL: Knee rehabilitation after anterior cruciate ligament reconstruction and repair. Am J Sports Med 9(3):140–149, 1981

161. Perry J, Antomelli D, Ford W: Analysis of knee joint forces during flexed knee stance. J Bone Joint Surg 57A:961, 1975

162. Pevsner DN, Johnson JRG, Palzina ME: The patellofemoral joint and its implications at the rehabilitation of the knee. Phys Ther 59:869–874, 1979

163. Pipes TU, Wilmore J: Isokinetic vs. isotonic strength training in adult men. Med Sci Sports 7:262–274, 1975

164. Poindexter DP, Johnson EW: Football shoulder and neck injury: A study of the "stinger." Arch Phys Med Rehabil 65:601–602, 1984

165. Rasch PJ, Morehouse LE: Effect of static and dynamic exercises on muscular strength and hypertrophy. J Applied Physiol 11:29, 1957

166. Raskoff WJ, Goldman S, Cohn K: The "athletic heart." JAMA 236:158–162, 1976

167. Renstrom P, Johnson RJ: Overuse injuries in sports: A review. Sports Med 2:316–333, 1985

168. Richardson AB: Overuse syndromes in baseball, tennis, gymnastics and swimming. Clin Sports Med 2(2):379–390, 1983

169. Richardson AR: The biomechanics of swimming: The shoulder and knee. Clin Sports Med 5(1):103–113, 1986

170. Robertson W, Eichman P, Clancy W: Upper trunk brachial plexopathy in football players. JAMA 24(14):1480–1482, 1979

171. Roles NC, Maundsley RH: Radial tunnel syndrome: Resistant tennis elbow as a nerve entrapment. J Bone Joint Surg 54B:499, 1972

172. Rosentsweig J, Hinson M, Ridgway M: An electromyographic comparison of an isokinetic bench press performed at three speeds. Res Q 46(4):471–475, 1975

173. Rovere GD, Haupt HA, Yates CS: Prophylactic knee bracing in college football. Am J Sports Med 15(2):111–116, 1987

174. Russell W, Shitty C: Traumatic neuritis of the deep palmar branch of the ulnar nerve. Lancet 1:828–829, 1947

175. Saal JA: Electrophysiologic evaluation of lumbar pain: Establishing the rationale for therapeutic management. SPINE: State of the Art Rev 1(1):21–46, 1986

176. Saal JA: The multiple crush lesion of the median nerve in the presence of clinical root compression. Instructors' Course, Academy of Physical Medicine and Rehabilitation, Los Angeles, 1983

177. Saal JA: Synovial joints and range of motion. In Fahey TD (ed): Athletic Training: Principles and Practice. Mayfield Publishing, 1986

178. Saal JA: The pseudoradicular syndrome. Spine (in press)

179. St Pierre RK, Andrews L, Allman F, Fleming LL: The Cybex II evaluation of lateral ankle ligamentous reconstructions. Am J Sports Med 12(1):52–56, 1984

180. Sherman WM, Pearson DR, Plyley MJ et al: Isokinetic rehabilitation following surgery: A review of factors which are important to developing physiotherapeutic techniques following knee surgery. Am J Sports Med 10(3):155–161, 1981

181. Simmons W, Rath D, Merta R: Calculation of disability using the Cybex II system. Orthopedics 5(2):181–185, 1982

182. Sjolund BH, Terenius L, Eriksson M: Increased cerebrospinal fluid levels of endorphins after electroacupuncture. Acta Physiol Scand 100:383, 1977

183. Solheim LF, Siewers P, Paus B: The piriformis muscle syndrome. Acta Orthop Scand 52:73–75, 1981

184. Spencer RP, Levinson ED, Baldwin RD et al: Diverse bone scan abnormalities in "shin splints." Clin Sci 12:1271–1272, 1979

185. Spinner M: The anterior interosseous-nerve syndromes with special attention to its variations. J Bone Joint Surg 52A:84–94, 1970

186. Spinner M: Injuries to the Major Branches of Peripheral Nerves of the Forearm. Philadelphia, WB Saunders, 1972

187. Stanish WD: Neurophysiology of stretching. In D'Ambrosia R, Drez D (eds): Prevention and Treatment of Running Injuries. Thorofare, NJ, Slack, 1982

188. Stanish WD et al: Tendinitis analysis and treatment. Clin Sports Med 4:593–608, 1986

189. Stanitski CL: Rehabilitation following knee injury. Clin Sports Med 4(3):495–511, 1985

190. Steadman JR: Rehabilitation of first and second degree sprains of the medial collateral ligament. Am J Sports Med 7:300–302, 1979

191. Steadman JR: Rehabilitation after knee ligament surgery. Am J Sports Med 8(4):294–296, 1980

192. Sweetham R: Corticosteroid arthropathy and tendon rupture. J Bone Joint Surg 51B:397–398, 1969

193. Tanigawa MC: Comparison of the hold-relax procedure and passive mobilization on increasing muscle length. Phys Ther 52:725–735, 1972

194. Thompson PD, Stern MP, Williams P et al: Death during jogging or running. JAMA 242:1265–1267, 1979

195. Tipton CM, James SI, Mergner W: Influence of exercise in strength of medial collateral ligaments of dogs. Am J Physiol 218:894–902, 1970

196. Tipton CM, Schild RJ, Tomanek RJ: Influence of physical activity on the strength of knee ligaments in rats. Am J Physiol 212:783–787, 1967

197. Torg JD, Pavlov H, Cooley LR et al: Stress fractures of the tarsal navicular. J Bone Joint Surg 5:700–712, 1982

198. Urist MR et al: Transmembrane bone morphogenesis across multiple-walled diffusion chambers. Arch Surg 112:612, 1977

199. Uthoff HK: Calcifying tendinitis, an active cell-mediated calcification. Virchows Arch 366:51–58, 1975

200. Uthoff HK, Sarkar K, Maynard JA: Calcifying tendinitis. Clin Orthop 118:164–168, 1976

201. Virmani R: Jogging, marathon running, and death. Hosp Phys 18:A28–A39, 1982

202. Walker PS, Erkmann MJ: The role of the meniscus in force transmission across the knee. Clin Orthop 109:184–191, 1975

203. Wancura I, Konigg R: On the neurophysiological explanation of acupuncture analgesia. Am J Chin Med 2:193, 1974

204. Williams JGP, Sperryn PM: Sports Medicine, 2nd ed. Baltimore, Williams & Wilkins, 1976

205. Woo SLY, Matthews JV, Akeson WH et al: Connective tissue response to immobility: A correlative study of biochemical and biomechanical measurements of normal and immobilized rabbit knees. Arthritis Rheum 18:257–264, 1975

44

Osteoporosis

Charles H. Chesnut III

Osteoporosis, the most common of the metabolic bone diseases, may occur as a primary or secondary medical condition. Primary osteoporosis, occurring without apparent association with other medical diseases, is usually classified as postmenopausal osteoporosis in the elderly woman and as senile osteoporosis in the elderly man. Secondary osteoporosis occurs in association with other diseases (*e.g.*, Cushing's disease), medication (*e.g.*, heparin), or physiological aberration (*e.g.*, disuse). A classification of osteoporosis is provided in Table 44-1.[11]

DEFINITION

Common to all osteoporotic conditions is a reduction in bone mass, both absolutely[2] and per unit volume, to a level leading to fracture (especially of the spine, hip, and wrist) after minimal trauma. Bone mass reduction may be termed *skeletal osteopenia,* with the term *osteoporosis* usually referring to such reduction to the point of fracture, although it should be noted that the two conditions may be differentiated only by findings after a fall or other trauma. Although bone mass is reduced in osteoporosis, current data (with some exceptions[3]) suggest that the bone that is present is normal.

EPIDEMIOLOGY

Osteoporosis has become a public health problem of epidemic proportions, responsible for 1.2 million or more fractures per year in the United States.[41] Seventy percent of fractures in people aged 45 and older are attributable to osteoporosis;[27] 1.7% of people 45 to 64 years of age and 2% of those aged 65 years and older have an osteoporosis-related fracture yearly.[28] One-third of women over age 65 will have vertebral fracture;[41] by age 80, one of every three women and one of every six men will have had a hip fracture.[32] Hip fractures are found in 12% to 20% of cases[16] and result in long-term nursing home care for one-half of the survivors.[32]

In addition, in the future there will understandably be an increase in the incidence and prevalence of osteoporosis. The average live expectancy at birth in the year 2050 for women in the United States will be 81 years,[24] and the current figure of 23 million white women 55 years of age and older will increase.

The morbidity of the osteoporotic fracture (particularly of the hip) is considerable for society and for the patient, since the deterioration in the quality of life following fracture may be catastrophic. Economically, the expense of osteoporotic fracture is overwhelming; in the United States direct and indirect costs of osteoporosis are estimated to be at least $6.1 billion annually.[26]

PATHOGENESIS

Osteoporosis is a heterogeneous disease with multiple causes. Although the pathogenesis of bone mass loss, and fractures, in secondary osteoporosis may be readily apparent (*e.g.*, corticosteroid excess in Cushing's disease or the lack of muscle effect on bone with subsequent negative bone remodeling sequences in paraplegia and disuse osteoporosis), the exact pathogenesis of primary osteoporosis may be more difficult to define. However, the pathogenesis of primary osteoporosis may be approached from the standpoint of osteopenia (bone mass loss) and osteoporosis (bone mass loss to a point of fracture). Osteopenia may be due to multiple causes, including inadequate bone mass at skeletal maturity (age 13 to 25 for women) and/or subsequent age-related and postmenopausal bone loss.[31, 48] Regardless of the pathogenesis of the osteopenia, osteoporosis with fracture is principally due to low bone mass; it should, however, be noted (Fig. 44-1) that other determinants of fracture include bone quality (the trabecular architecture[38] and the ability to heal trabecular microfractures[20] may contribute to bone quality or lack thereof) and the propensity to fall. The latter determinant consists of the decreased neuromuscular coordination of the elderly (resulting in their inability to break a fall's impact) and such environmental factors as confusion and dizziness due to medications, the use of "throw rugs" with subsequent increased slips and falls, and so on. The propensity to fall in the elderly population may be of equal importance to bone quantity, owing to the increased number and traumatic severity of falls in this age group.[1, 33]

The pathogenetic basis of inadequate bone mass, particularly in the elderly, may also be considered from the standpoint of cellular, hormonal, and tissue abnormalities.

Table 44-1
Classification of Osteoporosis

A. Primary osteoporosis: basic etiology unknown, no associated disease
    1. Postmenopausal osteoporosis: elderly women
    2. Senile osteoporosis: elderly men
B. Secondary osteoporosis: secondary to inherited or acquired abnormalities/diseases or to physiological aberrations
    1. Hyperparathyroidism
    2. Cushing's disease
    3. Multiple myeloma
    4. Hyperthyroidism (endogenous and iatrogenic)
    5. Idiopathic hypercalciuria
        a. Due to renal calcium leak
        b. Due to renal phosphate leak
    6. Malabsorption (including partial gastrectomy)
    7. 25-OH vitamin D deficiency
        a. Due to chronic liver disease
        b. Due to chronic anticonvulsant therapy (phenytoin, barbiturates)
    8. 1,25 (OH)$_2$ vitamin D deficiency due to lack of renal synthesis
        a. Due to chronic renal failure
    9. Adult hypophosphatasia
    10. Osteogenesis imperfecta tarda
    11. Male hypogonadism (Klinefelter's syndrome)
    12. Female hypogonadism (Turner's syndrome)
    13. Conditions consistent with hypoestrogenism secondary to anorexia and/or exercise
        a. Anorexia nervosa
        b. Exercise-induced amenorrhea
    14. Conditions associated with disuse
        a. Paraplegia/hemiplegia
        b. Immobilization
        c. Prolonged bed rest (?)
    15. Alcoholism
    16. Diabetes mellitus (?)
    17. Rheumatoid arthritis
    18. Chronic obstructive pulmonary disease
    19. Systemic mastocytosis
    20. Conditions associated with the use of medications
        a. Corticosteroids
        b. Heparin
        c. Anticonvulsants
        d. Excess thyroid hormone
    21. Malignancy

Cellular Abnormalities

Conclusive evidence of cellular abnormalities contributing to the pathogenesis of osteoporosis is lacking, principally owing to an inability to define abnormalities of bone cells (osteoblast, osteoclast, or osteocyte) specific for osteoporosis and separate from abnormalities of bone cells occurring with aging alone. For instance, it may be that failure of the osteoblast (the cell responsible for bone formation), due to either decreased cell number or decreased cell activity, may accompany advancing age but is not specific for osteoporosis.

Hormonal Abnormalities

Many hormonal agents may affect bone cell function and bone mass; however, although there are numerous age- and menopause-related alterations in the physiology of these hormones, a

DETERMINANTS OF OSTEOPOROTIC FRACTURE

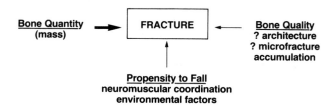

Figure 44-1.   Determinants of osteoporotic fracture, including bone quality, bone quantity, and propensity to fall (see text).

specific pathogenetic hormonal abnormality in osteoporosis (excluding the osteopenia associated with hypercorticism and hyperparathyroidism) has not been conclusively defined. Estrogen deficiency is, however, most frequently incriminated in the pathogenesis of postmenopausal osteoporosis; indeed, estrogen deficiency of whatever etiology (including early oophorectomy[39] and a functional hypogonadism associated with strenuous exercise[17]) may be considered a prime risk factor for bone mass loss. The specific mechanism of estrogen's effect on bone is unclear; no estrogen receptors exist in bone.[5] A reasonable hypothesis for estrogen's effect is its apparent ability to decrease bone resorption via a decrease in the responsiveness of the osteoclast (the bone cell primarily responsible for bone resorption) to endogenous circulating parathyroid hormone.[25] Estrogen deficiency from any cause would therefore result in increased skeletal responsiveness to parathyroid hormone and increased bone resorption, a transient increase in the serum calcium level, and a resultant decrease in parathyroid hormone secretion; with such a decrease a reduced production of the active form of vitamin D, 1,25(OH)$_2$ cholecalciferol, would be expected, with a consequent decrease in calcium absorption.[21] A number of these hormonal perturbations are demonstrated in osteoporotic populations; however, estrogen deficiency alone is an incomplete pathogenetic explanation for osteoporosis, since all postmenopausal females are relatively estrogen deficient but not all develop osteoporosis. The serum level of immunoreactive parathyroid hormone increases with aging,[29] and it is also increased in about 10% of postmenopausal osteoporotic women; in the latter group this increase in parathyroid hormone may be related causally to bone loss. However, in the majority of postmenopausal osteoporotic women parathyroid hormone is normal or low compared with that of normal elderly women via the mechanisms noted previously, and in these patients the pathogenetic contribution to osteoporosis is unclear.

A number of vitamin D abnormalities occur with aging, although an abnormality specific for osteoporosis (rather than simply aging) has not been defined. Decreased levels of 1,25(OH)$_2$ vitamin D are noted with increasing age; a postulated defect in the osteoporotic elderly person of the renal 25(OH)D 1α-hydroxylase enzyme in response to parathyroid hormone has not been conclusively proven.[40, 47] Nevertheless, calcium absorption does decrease with advancing age and is even lower in postmenopausal osteoporotic women.

A deficiency of the hormone calcitonin could also contribute to ongoing bone loss; calcitonin inhibits the production and activity of osteoclasts and thus decreases osteoclastic bone resorption. Serum levels of immunoreactive calcitonin are indeed lower in women than in men and also decrease with age; in addition, a decreased calcitonin secretion in response to calcium stimulation has been noted in some,[49] but not all,[50] osteoporotic populations.

Tissue Abnormalities

Although cellular and hormonal abnormalities undoubtedly contribute to osteopenia and osteoporosis, the basic abnormality in all types of osteoporosis is a disturbance of the normal bone remodeling sequence at the tissue level. Therefore, to fully understand the pathogenesis of osteoporosis, knowledge of bone remodeling is necessary.

Bone is constantly turning over (remodeling); the skeleton is a reservoir for calcium, and remodeling provides calcium to the organism without sacrificing the skeleton. In addition, remodeling allows bone mass to respond to increased and decreased muscle activity (as an example, bone mass increases in a tennis player's dominant arm). As noted in Figure 44-2B, the initial event in bone remodeling with normal bone turnover is an increase in bone resorption, as mediated by the osteoclast. This event is typically followed within 40 to 60 days with an increase in bone formation, as mediated by the osteoblast. Bone resorption and formation are normally, presumably homeostatically, "coupled": an increase or decrease in resorption produces a corresponding increase or decrease in formation, so that the net change in bone mass is zero. In postmenopausal osteoporosis, and possibly in senile osteoporosis as well (Fig. 44-2C), bone resorption is thought to be increased over normal resorption levels, without a corresponding increase in bone formation, leading to a net loss in bone mass. In this case, bone remodeling is described as "negatively uncoupled." In other forms of osteoporosis, particularly that associated with corticosteroid-induced osteoporosis, a primary decrease in bone formation may occur (Fig. 44-2D); the end result is the same in either situation, that is, a net loss of bone mass and presumably an increased risk for fracture. Abnormalities of bone remodeling at the tissue level will therefore contribute to the pathogenesis of the disease.

ETIOLOGY AND RISK FACTORS

In secondary osteoporosis, specific etiologies are easily defined; in postmenopausal osteoporosis, however, multiple etiological factors (Table 44-2) may act independently or in combination in an individual patient to produce diminished bone mass. Presumably, the presence of one or more of these factors in the elderly woman increases the risk of accelerated bone loss and subsequent fracture; the "weighting" of each of these risk factors in terms of relative importance as an etiological factor is undefined, although presumably estrogen depletion, calcium deficiency, diminished peak bone mass, and diminished physical activity are the most important of the risk factors in Table 44-2.

In senile osteoporosis, alcoholism and testosterone depletion must be considered as significant risk factors; unfortunately, however, the specific etiology of osteopenia and osteoporosis in men may be difficult to delineate.[36, 44]

Table 44-2
Etiological Factors Contributing to the Risk of Osteopenia/Osteoporosis

1. Estrogen depletion
   a. Postmenopausal state (natural or artificial)
   b. Exercise-induced amenorrhea, anorexia nervosa
2. Calcium deficiency
   a. Inadequate calcium intake
   b. Malabsorption
   c. Lactose intolerance
3. Diminished peak bone mass at skeletal maturity; varies with sex (men > women), race (blacks > whites), and heredity
4. Diminished physical activity
5. Testosterone depletion
6. Aging (over age 65 in men)
7. Leanness (adipose tissue is the major source of extragonadal estrogen production postmenopausally)
8. Alcoholism, smoking
9. Excessive coffee intake (>4–6 cups daily) and excessive dietary protein intake: increased calcium loss in the urine
10. Medications: corticosteroids, thyroid hormone, heparin

CLINICAL PRESENTATION

The first clinical indication of osteoporosis, either primary or secondary, will usually be a fracture. Fractures of the proximal femur and the distal forearm will usually follow a fall or other significant trauma; patients will present with pain and subsequent roentgenographic studies will confirm a fracture at these sites. Fractures of the vertebrae, however, may be associated with minimal trauma, and although usually associated with significant pain, they may occasionally be asymptomatic.

The natural history of the vertebral fracture usually begins with acute pain at the site of the fractured vertebra; the fracture may follow lifting, coughing, or, on occasion, simply turning the torso. There may be radiation of pain laterally from the vertebral column, paravertebral muscle spasm, and percussion tenderness over the affected vertebra. The pain is typically sharp, increased with movement, and usually reduced somewhat with bed rest. Such severe and frequently disabling pain may persist for 2 to 3 weeks and then continue with lesser severity for 6 to 8 weeks, usually subsiding at this time until the next fracture occurs. The persistence of pain beyond 6 months at the site of a previous vertebral fracture should suggest causes other than osteoporotic fracture for the pain complex, including psychiatric, pathological (metastatic), or medicolegal etiologies. In some younger (50 to 65 years of age) patients, clusters of fractures may occur, with the disease relentlessly progressing to four to six spinal fractures. The cause of this most aggressive form of osteoporosis is unclear but may be associated with an accelerated trabecular bone loss soon after the menopause.

It is unlikely that osteoporosis produces acute, severe pain in the absence of fracture (although paraspinous muscle spasm may produce a more chronic pain, typically of lesser severity). It is possible that painful vertebral microfractures of individual

Figure 44-2. Pathogenesis of osteoporosis at the tissue level: disruption of normal bone-remodeling sequences. (*A* and *B*) Bone trabecula at zero time and normal bone turnover. (*C* and *D*) Two possible mechanisms of abnormal bone remodeling. (Chestnut CH, Kribbs PJ: Osteoporosis: Some aspects of pathophysiology and therapy. J Prosthet Dent 48:407–412, 1982)

OSTEOPOROSIS DUE TO DISRUPTION OF NORMAL
BONE REMODELING SEQUENCES

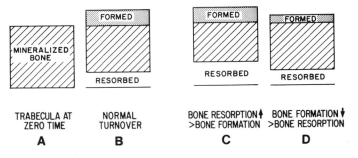

trabeculae may develop; such microfractures may not be visible on a roentgenogram but may be noted on a radionuclide bone scan.

Following a number of fracture events in the spine, the collapsed and/or anteriorly wedged vertebrae may lead to deformity of the back, with subsequent kyphosis (the typical "dowager's hump" deformity), loss of height, and a chronic back pain in either the mid-thoracic or the lumbosacral area, which is undoubtedly secondary to mechanical deformity and paraspinous muscle spasm. This chronic back pain is typically of lesser intensity than the pain associated with the acute fracture event; it radiates laterally, is associated with exertion, and is relieved to a certain extent with rest. In addition, with the progressive spinal deformity and height loss, an abdominal protuberance and resultant gastrointestinal discomfort (bloating and constipation) may occur, as well as some degree of pulmonary insufficiency secondary to thoracic cage deformity. Also, in some severely affected patients, the spinal kyphosis may be sufficient to produce a painful rubbing of the lower ribs on the iliac crest.

DIAGNOSIS

An absolute diagnosis of osteoporosis will be made only if an atraumatic fracture exists (of the spine, femur, and/or distal ulna or radius). However, it is obviously of value from the standpoint of patient management to evaluate the patient at risk for fracture prior to a fracture occurring, as well as to determine the cause of the fracture in patients in whom a fracture has occurred. The diagnosis of osteoporosis may therefore be approached from the standpoint of evaluating the patient at potential risk, as well as evaluating the patient who already has fractures and, by definition, the disease. Diagnostic procedures, most frequently the radionuclide bone scan, may also be used in evaluating the pain complex of osteoporosis.

Prior to describing such diagnostic evaluations a brief outline of the noninvasive quantitation of bone mass is indicated, since the noninvasive techniques are currently an integral part of the diagnostic workup. Since the amount of bone mass present is the principal determinant of fracture, a noninvasive technique for quantitating bone mass would consequently be of value in the diagnosis of osteoporosis and in following a response to therapy.

Noninvasive Techniques for Quantitating Bone Mass

A number of noninvasive procedures have been developed over the past 20 years to quantitate bone mass, including single- and dual-photon absorptiometry (SPA and DPA, respectively), computed tomography (CT), and total body calcium by neutron activation analysis (TBC-NAA).[8, 10] Such techniques quantitate bone mass at the spine, wrist, and hip, the principal areas usually involved in osteoporosis; in addition, a number of the techniques provide assessment of bone mass throughout the entire skeleton. The axial and appendicular sites noted above exhibit varying proportions of cortical (compact) and trabecular (cancellous) bone; it should be remembered that trabecular bone is metabolically more active than cortical bone, appears to be preferentially altered in osteoporosis, and is the type of bone most affected by medications used in treatment of osteoporosis. It should also be kept in mind that roentgenograms of the spine are relatively insensitive in quantitating bone mass, since 30% to 35% of bone mass must be lost before roentgenographic demineralization is detected.

Attenuation or absorption of ionizing radiation by bone is the basic principle used in the majority of the noninvasive techniques; in SPA and DPA the source of such radiation is radionuclides, and in CT it is x-rays. Figure 44-3 shows a generally linear relationship between bone mass and radiation attenuation: the greater the amount of bone present, the greater the attenuation of ionizing radiation, and subsequently the less radiation quantitated in a detector. TBC-NAA quantitates total body calcium by quantitating the gamma emission of calcium-49 after conversion by NAA of stable calcium-48 to radioactive calcium-49. Since 99% of total body calcium is in the skeleton, TBC essentially measures total skeletal mass.

The ideal noninvasive technique quantitates primarily trabecular bone at the spine and possibly at the hip with an acceptable precision and accuracy; such procedures should be of reasonable cost and be associated with low radiation exposure. In addition, ideally such techniques should also significantly discriminate between normal and osteoporotic populations, should predict which patients are at risk for subsequent fracture, and should be readily applicable to assessing therapeutic response. As noted in Table 44-3, currently available techniques satisfy these ideal criteria to varying degrees. For instance, SPA exhibits a reasonable cost, low radiation exposure, logistical simplicity, and quite acceptable precision. However, with the exception of the SPA ultradistal and os calcis measurements, this parameter quantitates primarily cortical bone mass at the wrist, which is neither the site nor the type of bone usually involved in osteoporosis. No definitive evidence exists that measurement of wrist bone mass significantly predicts spine or hip bone mass or bone mass change. Also, this technique cannot discriminate between osteoporotic and age-matched normal populations, cannot predict the future risk for fracture, and cannot assess response to therapy with most medications used in the treatment of osteoporosis (with the exception of estrogens, which do have some effect on cortical bone mass). Although the SPA ultradistal site and the os calcis measurements do assess primarily trabecular

Figure 44-3. Principles of SPA, DPA, and CT. In practice, a scan is performed across the radius or ulna (SPA) or a lumbar (DPA and CT) or thoracic (CT) vertebra. Below is noted the absorption profile, demonstrating a generally linear relationship between bone mass and radiation attenuation. Computer integration of the hatched area below baseline is performed, and compared with calibration standards, providing units of bone mass and/or density (g, g/cm, g/cm^2: SPA and DPA; mg/cc: CT). (*D*, detector; *S*, source of ionizing radiation [SPA: iodine-125, DPA: gadolinium-153, CT: x-ray]; ---, direction of scan; *B*, baseline count rate) (Chestnut CH: Bone imaging techniques. In Becker KL [ed]: Principles and Practice of Endocrinology. Phildelphia, JB Lippincott, 1987)

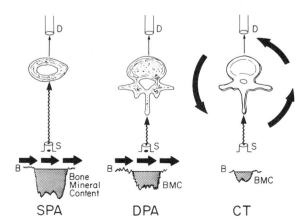

Table 44-3
Noninvasive Techniques for Quantitating Bone Mass

Technique	Site Measured	Cortical/Trabecular (%)	Precision/Accuracy (%)	Discrimination	Response to Therapy	Radiation	Cost
Single-photon absorptiometry	Radius/ulna						
	Distal	80–95/20–25	±2–4/±3–4	−	±*	10 mrem	$75–125
	Ultradistal	25/75	±2–4/?	?	?		
	Os calcis	20/80	±2–4/?	?	?		
Dual-photon absorptiometry	Spine: L1–L4†	35/65	±2–5/±2–4	±	+	10 mrem	$150–200
	Femur: neck:	75/25	±3–5/?	−	?	10 mrem	$50–75
	trochanter	50/50	±3–5/?	−	?	10 mrem	
Computed tomography	Single energy spine: T12–L4‡	5/95	±3–5/±6–30§	±	+	500–750 mrem	$125–175
	Dual energy spine: T12–L4‡	5/95	±5–10/±5	?	?	750 mrem	?
Total bone calcium by neutron activation analysis	Total skeleton	80/20	±2/±5	±	+	2000 mrem	$750

* Estrogens
† Total vertebral body including spinous process
‡ Area of interest within vertebral body
§ ? due to marrow fat
(Chesnut CH: Bone imaging techniques. In Becker KL [ed]: Principles and Practice of Endocrinology. Philadelphia, JB Lippincott, 1987)

bone, the sites measured (extreme distal radius and ulna and the heel) are subject to mechanical stresses and loading forces, as well as local hormonal interactions, which are quite different from those encountered at the spine and hip sites. Consequently, cortical SPA, the ultradistal SPA, and the os calcis measurement are of limited value as primary bone mass quantitating techniques in osteoporosis.

The DPA and CT techniques are currently the most promising of available methodologies, since they quantitate bone mass at the two principal target sites of osteoporosis, the spine and the hip. Measurement of the total skeleton with DPA is available but is used primarily in research studies. The cost of these techniques is higher than with SPA; radiation dosage is high with CT, although quite acceptable with DPA; and quality control and patient logistics may be more acceptable with DPA than with CT (see Table 44-3). Precision and accuracy are quite reasonable with DPA, although in the elderly accuracy may be compromised by the presence of extraskeletal calcification, such as in osteophytes and the aorta. Marrow fat provides a significant error in accuracy for single-energy CT; dual-energy CT may correct such an error, but precision may consequently decrease and, most importantly, radiation dosage may increase. Dual-energy CT is rarely used outside research laboratories. With both DPA and CT, difficulties may arise in accuracy owing to previously compressed vertebral bodies, kyphosis, and vertebral sclerosis. DPA quantitates both trabecular and cortical bone mass of the entire vertebral body, including the spinous and transverse processes, the posterior elements, and calcification within the surrounding tissues. CT, as performed in most practitioners' laboratories, measures almost exclusively trabecular bone within the vertebral body; in terms of fracture risk such a measurement may provide a biologically more important quantitation of bone mass than a measurement of the entire vertebral body.

Femoral bone mass may be measured at multiple sites with DPA; such a measurement is technically difficult but can be accomplished with acceptable precision and radiation exposure.

The contribution of bone mass quantity to the risk of subsequent hip fracture however is unknown; previous studies have shown virtually no discrimination in terms of femoral bone mass between populations with and without hip fracture.[14]

Although SPA, DPA, and CT lack the ability to discriminate between normal populations and populations with osteoporotic fractures,[15, 37] DPA and CT can be used in following the response of bone mass to therapy.

TBC-NAA has been used in the past as a noninvasive research technique for monitoring the response to osteoporosis therapy; it is a precise and accurate procedure, but its high radiation dosage, cost, limited availability, predominantly cortical bone mass measurement, and lack of definitive discriminatory ability make it less acceptable for widespread use in quantitating bone mass.

When used appropriately, the noninvasive techniques (particularly CT and DPA) are of definite value in the clinical evaluation of the osteopenic or osteoporotic patient. The clinical situations in which they may be used are as follows:

1. In selected perimenopausal and postmenopausal patients in defining their risk for subsequent fracture, when combined with the assessment and presence of historical risk factors (see Table 44-2)
2. In defining the need for prophylactic estrogen therapy
3. In screening for significant bone loss in conditions in which osteopenia is an accompanying manifestation, such as steroid-induced osteopenia and exercise-induced amenorrhea
4. In following response to treatment
5. In research endeavors such as epidemiological studies

There appears to be little justification for the use of noninvasive bone mass quantitating techniques in mass screening of all perimenopausal women[14, 23] or in quantitating the severity and progression (exclusive of therapy) of disease in the osteoporotic patient

Diagnostic Evaluation of the Patient at Risk for Osteoporosis

The patient at risk (most typically the immediately post-menopausal woman concerned about her future risk for osteoporosis) requires a relatively brief evaluation, consisting of the following:

1. A brief history is taken to determine the presence of the risk factors noted in Table 44-2 and to exclude medical conditions resulting in the secondary osteoporoses noted in Table 44-1.
2. A brief physical examination is performed to exclude the secondary osteoporoses.
3. A *minimal* laboratory evaluation in this group (Table 44-4) might include determination of calcium, phosphorus, and alkaline phosphatase levels plus a 24-hour urinary calcium-creatinine value; the overall cost–benefit ratio of even these minimal procedures is however unproven. In primary osteoporosis, results of laboratory tests typically are normal; the role of blood and urine tests (with the exception of the urinary calcium value) is to exclude other diseases, and this can frequently be accomplished by the history and physical examination.
4. A measurement, noninvasively, of bone mass, usually at the spine (either DPA or CT), will be of value in the individual patient with positive risk factors. If such a bone mass measurement is low, more aggressive prophylactic therapy (*i.e.,* estrogen) may be indicated; if a bone mass measurement at the spine is normal, activity and increased calcium intake may be sufficient.

Diagnostic Evaluation of the Patient With Osteoporosis (Fractures)

The patient with osteoporosis, who is most frequently female and in her late 50s or 60s, may present with one to five or six vertebral fractures and requires a more thorough evaluation, consisting of the following:

1. A complete history is obtained, again to determine the presence of risk factors and specifically to exclude medical condi-

tions resulting in the secondary osteoporoses. This latter evaluation is most important since multiple myeloma, hyperparathyroidism, and hyperthyroidism are not uncommon in this elderly age group.
2. A more thorough physical examination is performed, but again primarily to exclude the secondary osteoporoses. Signs of hyperthyroidism or hyperparathyroidism, alveolar ridge resorption resulting in dental osteopenia and missing teeth and dentures, proximal muscle weakness and discomfort in osteomalacia, and steroid excess should be kept in mind.
3. As noted in Table 44-4, a *maximal* laboratory evaluation in this group may be indicated; again, laboratory test results are frequently normal in primary osteoporosis and the main function of the laboratory evaluations noted are to exclude other diseases, such as primary hyperparathyroidism with determination of ionized and total calcium, parathyroid hormone, and phosphorus values; multiple myeloma with protein electrophoresis and complete blood cell count; and possible vitamin D abnormalities with the vitamin D congeners noted. The 24-hour urine collection for calcium, normalized for creatinine, remains a mainstay of the evaluation of the patient with osteoporosis; a general assessment of dietary calcium adequacy and dietary calcium gut absorption and the exclusion of idiopathic hypercalciuria can be accomplished with this parameter; if the urinary calcium value is low, either inadequate calcium intake or absorption or a vitamin D abnormality must be considered; if the value is high, either dietary calcium excess or idiopathic hypercalciuria is a possibility. The urinary hydroxyproline and GLA (γ-carboxyglutamic acid or osteocalcin, a noncollagenous bone protein measurable in serum) protein levels can monitor possible states of high bone remodeling, which may respond more to antiresorptive therapeutic agents; low remodeling as measured by a low GLA protein and urinary hydroxyproline would indicate an inactive and senescent bone, and such a condition may respond more favorably to bone forming agents. Lastly, the iliac crest bone biopsy is used primarily to exclude osteomalacia or other metabolic bone diseases, although such biopsies can also be used to define high and low bone turnover.
4. A noninvasive measurement of spinal bone mass will be of value as a baseline measurement to monitor response to therapy over time. Quite obviously such a measurement will also quantitate the severity of the disease, but this should not be the primary indication for such procedures.

Table 44-4
Laboratory Evaluations in the Diagnosis of Osteoporosis

Minimal	Maximal
Serum calcium	The above tests plus the following:
Phosphorus	Ionized calcium
Alkaline phosphatase	iPTH
Urinary calcium/creatinine	25-OH vitamin D
(24-hour collection)	1,25(OH)$_2$ vitamin D
	GLA protein
	Protein electrophoresis
	Thyroid function tests
	SMA-12 studies (renal and liver functions)
	Complete blood cell count
	Urinary hydroxyproline (24-hour collection)
	Iliac crest bone biopsy with tetracycline labeling

Diagnostic Evaluation of the Osteoporotic Patient With Back Pain

The osteoporotic patient may have acute or chronic back pain related to recent compression fractures, to mechanical derangement of the spine such as kyphosis, and/or to paraspinous muscle spasm. The radionuclide bone scan can be used in the diagnostic evaluation of back pain, as well as in determining the current metabolic activity of the disease. Increased radionuclide accretion at the site of a recent fracture (usually a vertebral body, but also the hip) indicates ongoing bone formation and bone healing; normal radionuclide accretion indicates that healing is complete and that the metabolic activity of the disease at that site is normal. A positive scan correlates well with the presence of acute pain, indicating the need for continued aggressive therapy such as a back brace, potent analgesia, and so on; a normal scan on the other hand reflects reasonable healing and a subsequent lesser need for aggressive therapy. A bone scan typically returns to normal within 4 to 6 months after fracture.

Continued back or hip pain in the presence of a normal bone scan suggests a nonskeletal origin of the pain, such as paraspinous muscle spasm, psychogenic factors, or medicolegal problems. The combination of a positive bone scan and a negative roentgenogram of the same site, in the absence of metastatic disease, may indicate a microfracture (stress fracture) of a vertebral body or proximal femur; such a microfracture may progress in time to a radiographically demonstrable macrofracture. Aggressive therapy, including short-term immobilization, may prevent completion of such an incipient fracture.

The currently available diagnostic procedures are expensive; whether the performance of these procedures is cost-effective in every patient with fracture, in only patients with back pain, and/or in patients at high risk for osteoporosis is unproven; their use is to be decided on by the individual practitioner.

THERAPY

Treatment of osteoporosis may be divided into treatment of symptoms and treatment of the underlying disease (skeletal osteopenia).

Symptomatic Therapy

Symptoms, and their associated therapies, of hip and wrist fractures are covered in standard orthopedic texts. Spinal compression fractures may result in acute and severe pain, may be due to either primary or secondary osteoporosis, and may necessitate significant limitation of activity, analgesia, and a back support (which reduces spinal movement and resultant pain). Rarely intercostal nerve blocks may be necessary to alleviate the severe pain associated with recent fractures.

Limitation of activity may involve short-term bed rest; it is important, however, that extensive and prolonged bed rest, with its consequent spinal immobilization (a situation at the tissue level in which bone resorption may exceed bone formation), be avoided. Increased bone wasting may otherwise occur. In addition, a flexible back brace is indicated should a back support be used; a rigid back brace with near-total spine immobilization may increase bone loss if it is used over an extensive period of time (months).

The acute pain phase may last for 2 to 8 weeks; the patient may be reassured that eventually the fractured vertebral body will heal and pain will lessen with time. Unfortunately, in a number of patients, the acute pain phase may be replaced within 2 to 4 months following fracture by chronic and frequently severe lumbosacral discomfort.[19] This discomfort may be secondary to lumbosacral muscle spasm, in turn secondary to the accentuated lumbar lordosis compensating for the thoracic kyphosis. This chronic pain phase may last for 6 to 10 months and may be managed with mild analgesia, muscle relaxants, rest periods reclining to alleviate muscle spasm, a flexible lumbar back support, and time.

During this difficult period of acute and/or chronic back pain the patient may also be using specific pharmacological therapies; it should be noted that these therapies (with the possible exception of calcitonin) are not expected to alleviate pain symptomatology but rather to treat the underlying skeletal osteopenia of osteoporosis. On the other hand, if such therapy can increase bone mass, or slow down bone mass loss, further fractures may not occur; in the absence of fractures, the pain complex will then obviously improve.

Therapy for Skeletal Osteopenia

General Measures

Treatment of the secondary osteoporoses may be accomplished by treatment of the underlying disease (for instance, in the thyrotoxic patient, alleviation of the hyperthyroid state).[12] The ideal goal of treatment, however, in any form of osteoporosis and osteopenia should be either prophylactic or restorative, depending on the patient's bone mass and fracture history. Since an inadequate skeletal mass is the primary determinant of increased fracture risk in the osteoporotic patient, in an aging person with a relatively normal bone mass and no previous fractures, the therapeutic goal would involve a slowing of age-related bone loss. On the other hand, in patients with a low bone mass and a history of previous fracture, treatment should involve not only slowing of age-related bone loss but also restoration of bone previously lost.

In terms of the previously described sequences of bone remodeling (see Fig. 44-2), prophylaxis and/or restoration may be accomplished by decreasing bone resorption,[11] and/or increasing bone formation.[41] In preventing osteopenia, a decrease in bone resorption may suffice if bone formation is maintained at its normal level or if bone formation decreases to the same degree as bone resorption. Restoration of bone mass, however, ideally would require both an increase in formation as well as a decrease in resorption. An increase in resorption with a greater increase in formation, or a decrease in resorption with a lesser decrease in formation, will also result in the desired net positive bone mass change. In other words, these manipulations of bone remodeling will result in a "positive uncoupling" of the normal coupling mechanisms previously described.

As noted in Table 44-5, several therapeutic agents can slow the loss of bone mass by decreasing bone resorption ("anti-bone resorbers"). The primary efficacy of these therapeutic modalities may be prophylactic, that is, they may prevent significant bone loss. Such anti-bone resorbing agents would be used in patients in whom bone mass has not decreased below a hypothetical fracture threshold, most typically immediately after menopause (Fig. 44-4). In this clinical situation, bone mass remains above the fracture threshold and presumably will be sufficient to prevent fractures. On the other hand, the use of the anti-bone resorbing agent as a single therapy in patients with osteoporotic fractures

---

Table 44-5
Mode of Action of Osteoporosis Therapies

Decreased bone resorption ("Anti-bone resorbers")
  Calcium
  Estrogen
  Calcitonin
  Diphosphonates*
  25(OH) Vitamin D, 1,25(OH)₂, Vitamin D*

Increased bone formation ("Positive bone formers")
  Sodium fluoride*
  Testosterone*
  Anabolic steroids*
  ? 1,25(OH)₂, Vitamin D*
  ? Exercise

Other
  Thiazides (urinary calcium)*

*Experimental

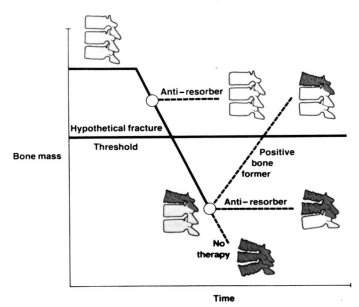

Figure 44-4. Therapy for osteoporosis based on bone mass; darker vertebrae represent compression fractures. (Chestnut CH: Treatment of postmenopausal osteoporosis. Comp Ther 10:41–47, 1984)

(and most frequently a low bone mass) is of questionable value; bone mass (inadequate) would indeed be maintained, but since there would be no restoration of previously lost bone mass, the patient would remain at risk for further fractures because of deficient bone mass.

As again noted in Table 44-5, a number of therapeutic agents are capable of increased bone formation ("positive bone formers"); such agents appear capable of restoring previously lost bone mass and, at least theoretically, preventing further fractures. These positive bone formers increase bone mass and may elevate the skeletal mass above the hypothetical fracture threshold, thus decreasing the occurrence of further fractures.

The combination of a positive bone forming agent with an anti-bone resorbing agent would, according to this therapeutic rationale, be of particular value in the patient with osteoporotic fractures and low bone mass, both preventing further loss and replacing bone previously lost.

Specific Measures

CALCIUM. Hypothetically, calcium administration should be of value in osteoporosis as an anti-bone resorber since it is a major component of hydroxyapatite crystal and presumably can decrease parathyroid hormone–mediated bone resorption by a slight and transient elevation in the serum calcium level. In addition, calcium absorption is lower in osteoporotic women compared with age-matched normal women; also, calcium intake is deficient in teenage, perimenopausal, and postmenopausal women in the United States. Whether calcium is of value in preventing bone loss over an extended period of time is, however, unproven; current data indicate a decrease in hip fractures in patients receiving high calcium intake[30] and in those who were previously calcium deficient.[4] Other evidence, however, suggests that up to 2000 mg of calcium daily is not beneficial in preventing either cortical or trabecular bone loss.[34, 43]

It appears that a significant proportion (perhaps 40%) of the population, perhaps those with chronically low calcium intake, may respond to increasing calcium intakes with a stabilization of bone mass for a significant period of time; at the present time,

however, it is impossible to identify these patients. It therefore appears reasonable to increase calcium intake to a minimum of 1000 mg/day in these populations since calcium is generally safe (in the absence of previous nephrolithiasis), comparatively inexpensive, and logistically simple to ingest. The source of calcium may be either milk and dairy products or calcium supplements; in terms of the latter, calcium carbonate is perhaps the most efficacious, since 40% of this calcium preparation is elemental calcium.

As shown in Table 44-6, excessive calcium intake may result in elevated urinary calcium levels, and rarely a predisposition to kidney stones; urinary calcium excretion of up to 250 mg/24 hr is acceptable in a person without a history of nephrolithiasis.

It appears unlikely that oral calcium alone can restore previously lost bone mass; adequate calcium intake should, however, be mandatory in therapeutic programs attempting to prevent bone loss or to treat the osteoporotic patient who has already experienced significant bone loss.

VITAMIN D. A multivitamin with 400 IU of vitamin D should be included in the therapy of postmenopausal osteoporosis; this is primarily to treat a mild vitamin D deficiency that may exist in the elderly. Use of vitamin D greater than 1000 IU/day is contraindicated if only postmenopausal osteoporosis is being treated; stimulation of parathyroid hormone–mediated bone resorption may occur. Whether the active forms of vitamin D are effective in osteoporosis in increasing calcium absorption and bone formation is unproven.

ESTROGENS. The estrogen compounds are anti-bone resorbers, which slow, and possibly prevent, bone mass loss by decreasing the responsiveness of bone to parathyroid hormone. As such, estrogens only maintain bone mass with no restoration of bone previously lost; therefore, their use as sole therapeutic modalities in women with low bone mass and spinal compression fractures is questionable (see Fig. 44-4). The status quo of an already compromised bone mass is maintained, but presumably the patient would remain at risk for fracture. Therefore, it would appear that the primary value of estrogens in osteoporosis would be prophylactic or in combination with agents that stimulate bone formation.[7]

A daily dosage (cycled) or 0.625 mg of conjugated equine estrogen (Premarin) or equivalent, or 0.3 mg of Premarin daily plus 1500 mg of calcium,[18] is indicated to prevent bone loss; transdermal estrogen (Estraderm) remains an experimental estrogen preparation in the treatment of osteoporosis, but initial studies indicate potential efficacy.[6]

Side-effects to estrogen administration include endometrial carcinoma, thromboembolic disease, and a questionable association with gallbladder disease and breast carcinoma. Endometrial cancer can be prevented by cycling estrogen with a progestational agent but at the expense of recurrent menstrual periods after the menopause. In the woman receiving "unopposed" estrogen (without progesterone) who has not undergone a hysterectomy, a pelvic examination and possibly endometrial biopsy are indicated at yearly intervals.

For maximum benefit, estrogen should be given as soon as possible after the menopause and continued (if there are no contraindications) through perhaps age 60 to 65. Osteoporosis therapy with estrogens alone after the age of 65 would appear to be of limited value, if an effect on bone mass is the primary reason for estrogen administration.

CALCITONIN. Calcitonin is an anti-bone resorbing agent (see Table 44-5) that decreases bone resorption by inhibiting osteoclast activity.[9] Studies indicate short-term efficacy of syn-

Table 44-6
Available Therapies for Osteoporosis

Medication	Usual Dosage*	Side-Effects
Calcium	1000–2000 mg/day	Urinary calcium
Multivitamin with D_2 or D_3	400 IU/day	
Estrogen	0.625 mg/day (Premarin or equivalent) cycled 21/30 days with/without progesterone	Endometrial carcinoma, thromboembolic disease
Calcitonin (salmon)	50–100 MRC units/day or every other day IM/SQ (Calcimar or equivalent)	Flushing, local irritation
Diphosphonates (EHDP)[†]	Not yet defined	
Sodium fluoride[†]	44–88 mg/day	Gastric upset, tendonitis, arthritis, plantar fasciitis
Anabolic steroids (stanozolol)[†]	2 mg tid cycled (Winstrol or equivalent) 21/30 days	↓ High density lipoproteins, liver toxicity, masculinization
Thiazides (?)[†]	50 mg/day (Hydrodiuril or equivalent)	↑ Cholesterol, blood sugar, ↓ serum K^+

* Oral unless otherwise specified
[†] Experimental therapy, not approved for use by the FDA

thetic salmon calcitonin (Calcimar or equivalent) in slowing bone loss and transiently increasing bone mass by a transient uncoupling of coupling mechanisms.[22] Proof of long-term efficacy is lacking, probably owing to an apparent "resistance" (possibly due to a down-regulation of receptor sites) to drug action after 16 months of therapy. Although alteration of the amount and duration of therapy may alleviate this apparent loss of drug effect (50 MRC units of Calcimar every other day may be superior to 100 MRC units every day), the expense and route of administration (intramuscularly or subcutaneously) of calcitonin prevents its extensive use in the osteoporotic patient. The drug is, however, quite safe, and would be an alternative to estrogen therapy in prophylaxis if a more suitable route of administration can be found; the use of calcitonin in a nasal spray is under evaluation and may prove to be a most reasonable prophylactic agent.

In addition, calcitonin may have an analgesic effect by a stimulation of endorphins; it may be of value in the management of the pain of acute fracture at a dosage of 50 to 100 MRC units every day or every other day for 1 to 2 weeks after fracture. Calcitonin would be indicated in patients unable to take estrogen and in combination with positive bone formers for patients with osteoporosis.

DIPHOSPHONATES. Diphosphonates are currently experimental, potentially beneficial anti-bone resorbers since they chemisorb to bone crystal, thus decreasing bone resorption and overall bone remodeling.[9] Currently under evaluation in the treatment of osteoporosis, EHDP (ethane-1 hydroxy-1, 2-diphosphonic acid [Didrone]) has proven effectiveness in the treatment of Paget's disease of bone and, to a lesser extent, in heterotopic ossification. The medication is quite safe; the exact dosage to be used has yet to be defined.

SODIUM FLUORIDE. Sodium fluoride is an experimental agent proven to increase bone formation, presumably by stimulating the osteoblast. When fluoride is administered, a new bone crystal is produced, fluorapatite. Concern has arisen regarding the structural integrity and possibly greater fracture potential of such bone. Data, however, suggest satisfactory skeletal strength in

patients treated with sodium fluoride.[42] The drug would consequently be of value in increasing bone mass and conceivably in preventing fractures; as shown in Figure 44-4, sodium fluoride, alone or in combination with an anti-bone resorbing agent, would be of value in patients with compromised bone mass and previous fractures, since presumably this medication could elevate bone mass above a hypothetical fracture threshold.

The therapeutic dosage for sodium fluoride is 44 to 88 mg/day in divided doses; because of its poor gastric absorption, fluoride is best taken on an empty stomach. Should the patient by unable, because of gastric irritation, to tolerate fluoride on an empty stomach it may be given with meals with a subsequent increase of 1 tablet per day (*i.e.,* four 22-mg tablets could be taken daily if the patient takes the medication with meals, rather than the three 22-mg tablets taken daily on an empty stomach).

Side-effects of sodium fluoride include gastric upset, tendonitis/fasciitis, and possibly exacerbation of arthritic symptoms. Perhaps 35% of patients will be unable to tolerate sodium fluoride; in addition, about 25% of osteoporotic patients show only a limited response to such therapy.

ANABOLIC STEROIDS. A primary increase in bone formation, possibly due to osteoblastic stimulation, without a corresponding increase in bone resorption, is noted following treatment of postmenopausal osteoporotic patients with the anabolic steroid stanozolol.[13] With persistent use a bone mass increase over 2 years is observed following anabolic steroid therapy; it would therefore appear that this group of agents would be of value in both slowing bone loss and in restoring bone mass previously lost, in a fashion similar to sodium fluoride.[9] Whether testosterone preparations would have similar effects on bone mass is unproven.

The side-effects of anabolic steroids, however, prevent their widespread use in osteoporosis; indeed, these agents are not approved for such therapy by the Food and Drug Administration. Side-effects include elevation of hepatic enzymes, fluid retention, androgenic effects, and a significant reduction in high density lipoproteins. Although these effects appear to be dose related and are generally transient, the physician using these agents should be aware of their potential side-effects and should balance the need for an effective treatment against possibly less desirous drug actions. The usual dosage of stanozolol is 2 to 6 mg/day for 21 of 30 days.

EXERCISE. A reasonable exercise program should be an integral part of any osteoporosis treatment program; exercise may decrease bone mass loss, and increase bone mass, by increasing bone formation to a greater extent than bone resorption.

Weight-bearing exercise is usually recommended, such as walking and aerobics. It has also been shown that swimming may be of benefit to spinal bone mass.[35] In general, exercise should be performed up to, and slightly beyond, the point of bone pain, although it may frequently be important to reduce exercise in the patient after an acute fracture. A flexion exercise program may be contraindicated; extension or isometric exercises seem to be more appropriate for patients with postmenopausal osteoporosis.[46]

General Recommendations for Osteoporosis Treatment

In patients with essentially normal bone mass and without fractures, but at high risk for development of significant osteopenia, increased calcium intake, vitamin D in a multivitamin form, an exercise program, and avoidance of "environmental" risk factors such as alcoholism and cigarette smoking should be prescribed. Estrogens may also be used in the absence of contraindications to these medications.

On the other hand, for patients with low bone mass and fractures, calcium and vitamin D supplements, exercise, and a positive bone former such as sodium fluoride should be prescribed. Estrogens or calcitonin could be added for combination therapy, particularly if a therapeutic response is lacking from initial therapy.

The rationale of the first therapeutic regimen is the prevention of significant bone loss, and that of the second regimen is the restoration of bone mass previously lost and the prevention of further loss.

Therapy for Secondary Osteoporosis

In secondary osteoporosis the primary aim in many situations may be discontinuation of the osteopenia-producing agents (*e.g.*, corticosteroids, heparin, thyroid medication) or treatment of the underlying pathological process (*e.g.*, hyperthyroidism); unfortunately, few studies are currently available that assess the value of the osteoporosis therapies in preventing and treating the osteopenia and osteoporosis associated with other disease processes. Presumably such treatment programs would be of value; in corticosteroid-induced osteopenia there are data suggesting a decrease in bone mass loss that with a regimen of calcium, vitamin D replacement (50,000 IU of vitamin D orally weekly for 12 weeks), sodium fluoride 22 to 44 mg orally daily,[2] and possibly thiazides may be of value, although definitive data establishing efficacy of this therapeutic regimen in steroid-induced osteopenia are lacking. It should be noted that on this regimen, 24-hour urinary calcium should be monitored at 1- to 2-month intervals for significant hypercalciuria.

Monitoring Response to Therapy

The ultimate determinant of therapeutic success is the absence of new fractures; the occurrence of new fractures after 8 to 12 months indicates therapeutic failure and necessitates reevaluation of therapy. Monitoring bone mass at different skeletal sites (particularly the spine) by currently available techniques may be advantageous in defining trends in bone mass change; presumably stabilization of bone mass, or an increase in bone mass over time indicates a beneficial therapeutic response. However, with certain therapies (*e.g.*, sodium fluoride and possibly diphosphonates) an increase or stabilization of bone mass may occur, but without a positive effect on bone quality; in these situations, roentgenography must be the primary method for following response to treatment.

REHABILITATION MEDICINE AND OSTEOPOROSIS

To date, physical therapy and rehabilitation medicine have been underused as therapeutic disciplines by the specialties usually providing care to the osteoporotic patient. Undoubtedly, however, physical therapy and rehabilitation principles can be of value in the management of the osteoporotic patient.[45]

Therapeutic measures would include management of acute and chronic pain and the complications of a severe kyphosis, as well as preventative measures aimed at modifying environmental factors contributing to fracture. In terms of pain management, the measures previously noted would be enforced by physical medicine and rehabilitation specialists; an area in which their expertise is of particular value is in the designing of a properly fitted back support. In terms of chronic pain, the physical medicine and rehabilitation specialist can be of particular assistance in instructing the patient in an exercise program, particularly incorporating extension exercises.[46] Prevention of increasing kyphosis would also be related to exercise, improved posture, use of sheepskin for sleeping to decrease the possibility of pressure sores over the kyphotic spine,[45] and so on. Preventative measures that would be reinforced would be prevention of falls due to environmental modification (*e.g.*, use of a cane for better balance, use of rubber-heeled shoes, absence of "throw-rugs," presence of a night light).

An area of specific concern is that of disuse osteoporosis, particularly in terms of paraplegia and quadriplegia. Disuse and immobilization appear to increase bone mass loss, ostensibly owing to decreased muscle action on bones, with an acute increase in bone remodeling (bone resorption greater than bone formation), followed by a more chronic decrease in bone remodeling with a greater decrease in bone formation than in bone resorption. In addition, in the paraplegic or quadriplegic patient there may be a component of abnormal piezoelectric effects on bone cells, owing to the disruption of neuronal transmission, which may result in decreased osteoblast function. In any case, significant bone loss occurs with disuse.

Therapy for disuse osteoporosis may be directed primarily at restoring the normal use of the affected skeletal part; studies with bed-rest volunteers and studies of spaceflight–related osteopenia have shown that restoration of normal activity may result in reversal of the osteopenia associated with these clinical situations. There is, however, little evidence that bone mass restoration can be accomplished in cases of paraplegia or hemiplegia; use of such medications as calcitonin and diphosphonates in this clinical situation may be of value, although definitive therapeutic studies denoting their efficacy have not been performed.

REFERENCES

1. Baker SP, Harvey AH: Fall injuries in the elderly: Symposium on falls in the elderly: Biological aspects and behavioral aspects. Clin Geriatr Med 1:501–508, 1985

2. Baylink DJ: Glucocorticoid-induced osteoporosis. N Engl J Med 309:306–308, 1983

3. Burnell JM, Baylink DJ, Chesnut CH III et al: Bone matrix and mineral abnormalities in postmenopausal osteoporosis. Metabolism 31:1113–1120, 1982

4. Burnell JM, Baylink DJ, Chesnut CH, Teubner EJ: The role of calcium deficiency in postmenopausal osteoporosis. Calcif Tiss Int 38:187–192, 1986

5. Chen TL, Feldman D: Distinction between 2-fetoprotein and intracellular estrogen-receptors: Evidence against presence of estradiol receptors in rat bone. Endocrinology 102:236–240, 1978

6. Cherkowski RJ, Meldrum DR, Steingold KB et al: Biological effects of transdermal estrogen. N Engl J Med 314:1615–1620, 1986

7. Chesnut CH: An appraisal of the role of estrogens in the treatment of postmenopausal osteoporosis. J Am Geriatr Soc 32:604–608, 1984

8. Chesnut CH: Bone imaging techniques. In Becker JL (ed): Principles and Practice of Endocrinology. Philadelphia, JB Lippincott, 1988

9. Chesnut CH: Drug therapy: Calcitonin, bisphosphonates, anabolic steroids, and hPTH (I-34). In Riggs, Melton (eds): Osteoporosis: Pathogenesis, Diagnosis, and Treatment. New York, Raven Press, 1988

10. Chesnut CH: Noninvasive methods of measuring bone mass. In Avioli LV (ed): The Osteoporotic Syndrome: Detection, Prevention and Treatment, 2nd ed. New York, Grune & Stratton, 1987

11. Chesnut CH III: Osteoporosis. In Andres R, Bierman EL, Hazzard WR (eds): Principles of Geriatric Medicine, pp 801–812. New York, McGraw-Hill, 1985

12. Chesnut CH: Treatment of postmenopausal osteoporosis. Comp Ther 10:41–47, 1984

13. Chesnut CH, Ivey JL, Gruber HE et al: Stanozolol in postmenopausal osteoporosis: Therapeutic efficacy and possible mechanisms of action. Metabolism 32:571–580, 1983

14. Cummings SR: Are patients with hip fractures more osteoporotic? Am J Med 78:487–494, 1985

15. Cummings SR, Black D: Should perimenopausal women be screened for osteoporosis? Ann Intern Med 104:817–823, 1986

16. Cummings SR, Kelsey JL, Nevitt MC, O'Dowd KJ: Epidemiology of osteoporosis and osteoporotic fractures. Epidemiol Rev 7:178–208, 1985

17. Drinkwater BL, Nilson K, Chesnut CH et al: Bone mineral content of amenorrheic and eumenorrheic athletes. N Engl J Med 311:277–281, 1984

18. Ettinger B, Genant HK, Cann CE: Postmenopausal bone loss is prevented by treatment with low-dosage estrogen with calcium. Ann Intern Med 106:40–45, 1987

19. Frost HM: Managing the skeletal pain and disability of osteoporosis. Orthop Clin North Am 3:561–570, 1972

20. Frost HM: The pathomechanics of osteoporosis. Clin Orthop 200:198–225, 1985

21. Gallagher JC, Riggs BL, DeLuca HF: Effect of estrogen on calcium absorption and serum Vitamin D metabolites in postmenopausal osteoporosis. J Clin Endocrinol Metab 51:1359–1365, 1980

22. Gruber HE, Ivey JL, Baylink DJ et al: Long-term calcitonin therapy in postmenopausal osteoporosis. Metabolism 33:295–303, 1984

23. Hall FM, Davis MA, Baron DT: Bone mineral screening for osteoporosis. N Engl J Med 316:212–214, 1987

24. Hazzard WR: Aging and cardiovascular disease: Coping with success. In Kietz AD (ed): Aging—Its Chemistry, pp 162–173. Washington, DC, American Association for Clinical Chemistry, 1980

25. Heaney RF: A unified concept of osteoporosis. Am J Med 39:877–880, 1965

26. Holbrook TL, Grazier K, Kelsey JL, Stauffer RN: The frequency of occurrence, impact and cost of selected musculoskeletal conditions in the United States. Chicago, American Academy of Orthopedic Surgeons, 1984

27. Iskrant AP, Smith RW: Osteoporosis in women 45 years and older related to subsequent fractures. Publ HHN Rep 84:33–38, 1969

28. Kelsey JF: Osteoporosis: Prevalence and incidence. In Proceedings of the NIH Consensus Development Conference, April 2–4, 1984

29. Marcus R, Madvig P, Young G: Age-related changes in parathyroid hormone and parathyroid hormone action in normal humans. J Clin Endocrinol Metab 58:223–230, 1984

30. Matkovic V, Kostial K, Simonovic I et al: Bone status and fracture rates in two regions of Yugoslavia. Am J Clin Nutr 32:540–549, 1979

31. Mazess RB: On aging bone loss. Clin Orthop 165:239–252, 1982

32. Melton LJ III, Riggs BL: Epidemiology of age-related fractures. In Avioli LV (ed): The Osteoporotic Syndrome, pp 45–72. New York, Grune & Stratton, 1983

33. Melton LJ, Riggs BL: Risk factors for injury after a fall: Symposium on falls in the elderly: Biological aspects and behavioral aspects. Clin Geriatr Med 1:1–15, 1985

34. Nilas L, Christiansen C, Rodbro P: Calcium supplementation and postmenopausal bone loss. Br Med J 289:1103–1106, 1984

35. Orwoll ES, Ferar JL, Oriatt SK, Huntington K: The effect of swimming exercise on bone mineral content (abstr). Clin Res 35:194A, 1987

36. Orwoll ES, Meier DE: Alterations in calcium, vitamin D, and parathyroid hormone physiology in normal men with aging: Relationship to the development of senile osteopenia. J Clin Endocrionol Metab 63:1262–1269, 1986

37. Ott SM: Should women get screening bone mass measurements? Ann Intern Med 104:874–876, 1986

38. Parfitt AM, Matthews CHE, Villaneuva AR et al: Relationships between surface, volume, and thickness of iliac trabecular bone in aging and in osteoporosis. J Clin Invest 72:1396–1409, 1983

39. Richelson LS, Wahner HW, Melton LJ, Riggs BL: Relative contributions of aging and estrogen deficiency to postmenopausal bone loss. N Engl J Med 311:1273–1275, 1984

40. Riggs BL, Hamstra A, DeLuca HF: Assessment of 25-hydroxy vitamin D 1α-hydroxylase reserve in postmenopausal osteoporosis by administration of parathyroid extract. J Clin Endocrinol Metab 53:833–835, 1981

41. Riggs BL, Melton LJ: Involutional osteoporosis. N Engl J Med 314:1676–1686, 1986

42. Riggs BL, Seeman E, Hodgson SF et al: Effect of the fluoride/calcium regimen on vertebral fracture occurrence in postmenopausal osteoporosis: Comparison with conventional therapy. N Engl J Med 306:446–450, 1982

43. Riis B, Thomson K, Christiansen C: Does calcium supplementation prevent postmenopausal bone loss? N Engl J Med 316:173–177, 1987

44. Seeman E, Melton LJ, O'Fallon WM, Riggs BL: Risk factors for spinal osteoporosis in men. Am J Med 75:977–983, 1983

45. Sinaki M: Postmenopausal spinal osteoporosis. Physical therapy and rehabilitation principles. Mayo Clin Proc 57:699–703, 1982

46. Sinaki M, Mikkelsen BA: Postmenopausal spinal osteoporosis: Flexion versus extension exercises. Arch Phys Med Rehabil 65:593–596, 1984

47. Slovik DM, Adams JS, Neer RM et al: Deficient production of 1, 25-dihydroxyvitamin D in elderly osteoporotic patients. N Engl J Med 305:372–374, 1981

48. Smith DM, Khairi MRA, Johnston CC: The loss of bone mineral with aging and its relationship to risk of fracture. J Clin Invest 56:311–318, 1975

49. Taggart HM, Chesnut CH, Ivey JL et al: Deficient calcitonin response to calcium stimulation in post-menopausal osteoporosis? Lancet 2:475–477, 1982

50. Tiegs RD, Body JJ, Wahner HW et al: Calcitonin secretion in postmenopausal osteoporosis. N Engl J Med 12:1097–1100, 1985

Index

Page numbers followed by the letter f refer to figures; those followed by the letter t refer to tabular material.

Verbalization. *See* Speech